P9-AOU-105

THE HANDBOOK OF NURSING

Editors

JEANNE HOWE, R.N., Ph.D.
Formerly Associate Professor
School of Nursing and Health Sciences
Western Carolina University
Cullowhee, North Carolina

ELIZABETH J. DICKASON, R.N., M.A., Ed.M.
Professor
Department of Nursing
Queensborough Community College
Bayside, New York

DOROTHY A. JONES, R.N., C., M.S.N., F.A.A.N.
Associate Professor
School of Nursing
Boston College
Chestnut Hill, Massachusetts

MARTHA J. SNIDER, R.N., Ed.D.
Associate Professor
College of Nursing
University of Florida
Gainesville, Florida

Consulting Editor

MARGARET E. ARMSTRONG, R.N., M.S.
Research Associate Professor
College of Nursing
University of Utah
Salt Lake City, Utah

THE HANDBOOK OF NURSING

A WILEY MEDICAL PUBLICATION
JOHN WILEY & SONS
NEW YORK • CHICHESTER • BRISBANE • TORONTO • SINGAPORE

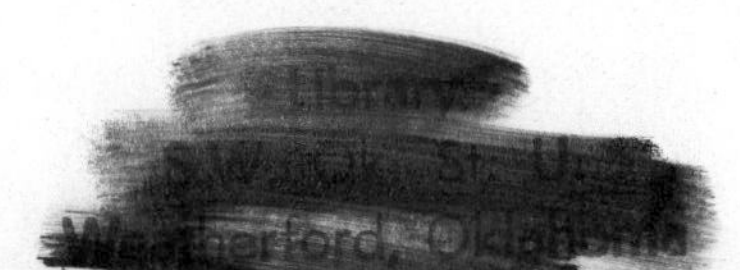

The authors and publishers have made a conscientious effort to ensure that the drug information and recommended dosages in this book are accurate, and in accord with accepted standards at the time of publication. However, pharmacology is a rapidly changing science, so readers are advised, before administering any drug, to check the pacakage insert provided by the manufacturer for the recommended dose, for contraindications for administration, and for added warnings and precautions. This recommendation is especially important for new, infrequently used, or highly toxic drugs.

Cover and interior design: Wanda Lubelska
Production supervision: Rosalind Straley, Pam Lloyd, and Audrey Pavey
Copyediting: Irene Curran and Anita Wayne

Library of Congress Cataloging in Publication Data:

Main entry under title:
The Handbook of nursing.

(A Wiley medical publication)
Includes index.
1. Nursing. I. Howe, Jeanne. II. Armstrong, Margaret E. III. Series. [DNLM: 1. Nursing process. 2. Nursing care. WY 100 H235]

RT41.H224 1984 610.73 83-25942
ISBN 0-471-89524-5

Printed in the United States of America

10 9 8 7 6 5 4 3 2 1

Portions of this book were previously published by the same authors in 1979 in a book entitled *McGraw-Hill Handbook of Clinical Nursing*.

CONTRIBUTORS

Susan E. Anderson, R.N., M.S., Ed.D.
Associate Professor
Salem State College
Salem, Massachusetts

Barbara J. Boss, R.N., Ph.D.
Associate Professor
School of Nursing
University of Mississippi Medical Center
Jackson, Mississippi

Beverly A. Bowens, R.N., M.N.
Trauma Clinical Nurse Specialist
University of Alabama Hospitals
University of Alabama in Birmingham
Birmingham, Alabama

Ann Ottney Cain, R.N., Ph.D.
Professor
School of Nursing
University of Maryland
Baltimore, Maryland

Judy B. Campbell, R.N., Ed.D.
Professor
Department of Nursing
Palm Beach Junior College, Central Campus
West Palm Beach, Florida

Mable Searcy Carlyle, R.N., M.N.
Assistant Professor
School of Nursing and Health Sciences
Western Carolina University
Cullowhee, North Carolina

Virginia L. Cassmeyer, R.N., M.S.N.
Associate Professor
School of Nursing
University of Kansas

Meredith Censullo, R.N., M.S.
Assistant Professor
Massachusetts General Institute
Boston, Massachusetts

Sherrilyn DeJean Coffman, R.N., M.S.
Assistant Professor
Department of Nursing
Miami-Dade Community College
Miami, Florida

Jeanette Coleman, R.N., Ed.D.
Formerly Assistant Professor of Nursing
School of Nursing
Maternal-Child Nursing Division
Columbia University
New York, New York

Ann Faas Collard, R.N., C., M.S.
Formerly Instructor
School of Nursing
Boston College
Chestnut Hill, Massachusetts
Doctoral Student
Brandeis University
Waltham, Massachusetts

Phyllis L. Collier, R.N., M.S.P.H.
Assistant Professor
School of Nursing
University of Rochester
Rochester, New York

Marilyn de Give, R.N., M.S.
Formerly Instructor and Clinician II
School of Nursing
University of Rochester
Rochester, New York

Elizabeth J. Dickason, R.N., M.A., Ed.M.
Professor
Department of Nursing
Queensborough Community College
Bayside, New York

Beverley H. Durrett, R.N., M.N.
Instructor, Allied Health and Biological Sciences
Polk Community College
Winter Haven, Florida

Mary E. Eddy, R.N., Ph.D.
Consultant
College of the Elms
Chicopee, Massachusetts

Joanne Kelleher Farley, R.N., D.N.Sc.
Associate Professor and Director of Continuing Education
School of Nursing
St. Anselm's College
Manchester, New Hampshire

Helen L. Farrell, R.N., M.S.N.
Supervisor of Adult Health Services
Buncombe County Health Department
Asheville, North Carolina

Annette Crosby Frauman, R.N., M.S.N.
Assistant Professor
College of Nursing
Clinical Nurse Researcher
Shands Teaching Hospital
University of Florida
Gainesville, Florida

Rosellen M. Garrett, R.N., Ph.D.
Chairperson and Associate Professor
Department of Nursing
University of Scranton
Scranton, Pennsylvania

Cyrena M. Gilman, R.N., M.N.
Unit Director, Pediatric Dialysis
Riley Hospital for Children
Indianapolis, Indiana

Karolyn Lusson Godbey, R.N., M.S.N., C.S.
Assistant Professor
College of Nursing
University of Florida
Gainesville, Florida

Patricia E. Greene, R.N., M.S.N., F.A.A.N.
Director of Cancer Nursing
American Cancer Society, Inc.
New York, New York

Diana W. Guthrie, R.N., Ed.S., F.A.A.N., C.
Adjunct Professor
Department of Nursing
Wichita State University
Associate Professor
Kansas Regional Diabetes Center
University of Kansas School of Medicine
Wichita, Kansas

Faye Gary Harris, R.N., Ed.D., F.A.A.N.
Professor
College of Nursing
University of Florida
Gainesville, Florida

Patricia Harris, R.N., C., M.S.N., P.N.P.
Pediatric Clinical Specialist
Independent Consultant
St. Louis, Missouri

Mary Fran Hazinski, R.N., M.S.N.
Cardiovascular Clinical Specialist
Children's Memorial Hospital
Chicago, Illinois

Sherry W. Honea, R.N., M.N.
Director of Nursing
Highlands Hospital
Asheville, North Carolina

Betty L. Hopping, R.N., M.N.
Associate Professor
School of Nursing
University of Kansas
Kansas City, Kansas

Sue E. Huether, R.N., Ph.D.
Associate Professor
College of Nursing
University of Utah
Salt Lake City, Utah

Mary Bigelow Huntoon, R.N., M.S.
Formerly Assistant Professor
School of Nursing
Boston University
Boston, Massachusetts

Jo Annalee Irving, A.R.N.P., M.S.N.
Assistant Professor
College of Nursing
University of Florida
Gainesville, Florida

Mary Marmoll Jirovec, R.N., M.S.
Doctoral Student
University of Michigan
Ann Arbor, Michigan

Dorothy A. Jones, R.N., C., M.S.N., F.A.A.N.
Associate Professor
School of Nursing
Boston College
Chestnut Hill, Massachusetts

Catherine Kneut, R.N., M.S.
Pediatric Clinical Specialist
Rhode Island Hospital
Providence, Rhode Island

Ruth Dailey Knowles, Ph.D., A.R.N.P., C.S.
Nurse Psychotherapist, Private Practice
Director, Peers, Inc.
Miami, Florida

Hilda Koehler, M.S., C.N.M.
Parent Educator
St. Luke's–Roosevelt Hospital Center
New York, New York

Cynthia S. Luke, R.N., M.S.N.
Assistant Professor of Nursing
East Carolina University
Director of Special Nursing Projects
Wilmington Area Health Education Center
Wilmington, North Carolina

Lynne McInerney, R.N., M.S.
Cardiac Rehabilitation Coordinator
General Hospital of Everett
Everett, Washington

Carol Ann McKenzie, R.N., C.N.M., Ph.D.
Formerly Associate Professor
Graduate Maternal-Newborn Nursing
Medical University of South Carolina
Charleston, South Carolina

Jean R. Miller, R.N., Ph.D.
Professor and Associate Dean of Research and Development
College of Nursing
University of Utah
Salt Lake City, Utah

Elaine Muller Morris, R.N., M.A., M.Ed.
Associate Professor
Department of Nursing
Queensborough Community College
Bayside, New York

Rhoda L. Moyer, R.N., M.N.
Adjunct Faculty
Southeast Institute
Chapel Hill, North Carolina
Nursing Consultant
Mandala Center
Private Practice and Training
Bridge Enterprises
Winston-Salem, North Carolina

Margaret Allen Murphy, R.N., C., M.A.
Assistant Professor
School of Nursing
Boston College
Chestnut Hill, Massachusetts

Annalee Oakes, R.N., M.A., C.C.R.N.
Associate Professor
Department of Nursing
School of Health Sciences–Nursing
Seattle Pacific University
Seattle, Washington

Rose Pinneo, R.N., M.S.N.
Associate Professor and Clinician II
School of Nursing
University of Rochester
Rochester, New York

Noreen King Poole, R.N., Ed.D.
Associate Professor
Department of Nursing
Palm Beach Junior College, Central Campus
West Palm Beach, Florida

Imogene Stewart Rigdon, R.N., M.S.N., C.N.
Doctoral Student
College of Nursing
University of Utah
Salt Lake City, Utah

Dorothy L. Sexton, R.N., Ed.D.
Associate Professor and Chairperson
Medical-Surgical Nursing Program
Yale University School of Nursing
New Haven, Connecticut

Bonnie Silverman, R.N., B.S.N.
Neonatal Nurse Clinician
Booth Memorial Medical Center
Flushing, New York

C. Marie Hall Smith, R.N., M.S.N.
Assistant Professor
Vanderbilt University School of Nursing
Clinical Specialist
Department of Pediatrics, Hematology
Vanderbilt University Medical Center
Nashville, Tennessee

Martha J. Snider, R.N., Ed.D.
Associate Professor
College of Nursing
University of Florida
Gainesville, Florida

Janet L. Snow, R.N., M.S.N.
Assistant Director
Division of Administrative and Professional Practices
Chicago Hospital Council
Doctoral Candidate
Rush University College of Nursing
Chicago, Illinois

Mary Suzanne Tarmina, R.D., R.N., M.S.
Assistant Professor
College of Nursing
University of Utah
Salt Lake City, Utah

Nora Doherty Tully, R.N., M.Ed.
Assistant Professor
Department of Nursing
Queensborough Community College
Bayside, New York

Laurie Weintraub, R.N., B.S.N.
Neonatal Nurse Clinician
Booth Memorial Medical Center
Flushing, New York

Mary P. Wieland, R.N., M.S.
Associate Director of Emergency Nursing
Assistant Professor
School of Nursing
Oregon Health Sciences University
Portland, Oregon

Cynthia Sarno Yeager, R.N., C., M.S.
Clinical Instructor
Middlesex Community College
Bedford, Massachusetts

Preface

The rapid and ongoing development of the art and science of nursing has significantly influenced the educational requirements, clinical practice, and responsibilities of nurses who provide professional care. *The Handbook of Nursing* provides practitioners and students with a reference that will enable them to practice more effectively in a variety of health care settings.

New federal cost-containment efforts are also affecting nursing practice. With the advent of Medicare's new diagnosis-related payment system (DRGs), the reimbursement revolution is under way. It is predicted that within the year, 80 percent of the hospitals in the United States will have been phased into this new system. It is essential that DRGs accurately reflect the many degrees of nursing care needed in each category. Hopefully, this book will assist nurses in identifying the various types and degrees of tangible and intangible care provided to each client through the nursing process.

The *nursing process*, a systematic and logical method for planning, providing, and evaluating care, is the organizational structure used throughout the book. *The Handbook of Nursing* identifies the nursing actions and essential supplemental information at each sequential phase of the nursing process. Thus, it is a reliable and versatile tool for providing care that conforms to standards of excellence for clients with a comprehensive range of health situations.

Many of our best researchers and practitioners have been intensely involved in the development of the nursing process as a comprehensive tool for providing care, and it is now an exciting, usable, practical instrument for the profession. The last five years have seen an explosion in the number of nurses who have learned its value, and others are quickly realizing their need to understand this method of thinking about client care. It is for all these nurses who desire to be competent in nursing planning and care that this book was written.

The book is divided into eight parts. Part I lays the foundation for what is to follow. Chapters 1 and 2 explain the rationale and use of *The Handbook of Nursing* and assist the reader in applying the nursing process. Chapters 3, 4, and 5 cover additional areas that apply in all practice settings and specialties: client teaching, life-span growth and development, and family.

Although the general concepts of nursing discussed in the first five chapters apply to all nursing specialties, other more focused techniques and concepts differ among specialists and across age levels. *The Handbook of Nursing* begins its treatment of these differences with the nursing care of parents and infants (Part II) and progresses to care of children and adolescents, adults, and the elderly (Parts III, IV, and VI). Mental health nursing and the general medical and surgical emergencies that are not age-related are covered in Parts V and VII. Health problems that can occur in any of several developmental levels or specialty settings (e.g., diabetes mellitus) are discussed thoroughly where they are most likely to occur, and they are referred to more briefly in appropriate other chapters.

Within each chapter, wherever possible, a consistent, process-oriented format is followed in discussing a particular health problem. Since health promotion and maintenance are vital roles of nursing, *prevention* (health promotion, population at risk, and screening) opens the discussion of each health problem.

Assessment (including health history, physical assessment, and diagnostic tests) leads to the establishment of *actual or potential nursing diagnoses* for each health problem. *Expected outcomes* are then established, which are followed by specific *interventions,* including guidelines and suggestions for client teaching. The process is completed by an *evaluation.* Complications are then discussed, and guidelines for reevaluation and follow-up are presented. Every chapter concludes with an annotated bibliography of recent sources of additional information.

It is important to recognize that within the framework of a reference book, every unique response of an individual client cannot always be anticipated. Therefore, the material presented and discussed under each health problem reflects the probable outline of a plan of care that will be observed for most clients. It is the responsibility of the nurse to carefully assess and evaluate those problems that reflect a client's unique response to a health problem.

The Appendixes include practical reference information: conversion tables, normal laboratory values, nutritional information, nomograms, and growth charts. Also in the Appendix, and unique to *The Handbook of Nursing,* are the DSM-III Classification Axes I and II Categories and Codes, as well as the nursing diagnoses approved for clinical testing by the Fifth National Conference of the North American Nursing Diagnosis Association. Each accepted diagnosis includes the diagnostic and etiological labels, defining characteristics, and definitions.

Because of the need for current, accurate, and often specialized information, authors were selected who are actively practicing or teaching (or both) within their content areas. All are nurses, and many are recognized leaders in their fields. Their experience and knowledge have produced a reference book that we believe is unsurpassed in its authority and usefulness.

Jeanne Howe
Elizabeth J. Dickason
Dorothy A. Jones
Martha J. Snider

Acknowledgments

The editors of the Handbook gratefully acknowledge the unselfish assistance of many who have helped with the preparation of this book. For their careful review and numerous suggestions regarding content and organization, the editors thank: Ann E. Aswegan, Madison, Wisconsin; Claire Dunbar, University of New Hampshire; Kathleen Field, Emory University; Carole Mandel, Boston College; Joyce S. Martin, Indiana University; Margaret A. Murphy, Boston College; Terry McCormick, Terre Haute, Indiana; Jinnette A. Pepper, University of Colorado; and Rachel E. Spector, Boston College.

Additionally, we would like to thank those who have helped us in our work: Judith H. Budd, Marda Messick, Judy Norton, Janet Quinn, Laura Rossi, Delores Schumann, and Mary Wagner.

We are also grateful to the staff of John Wiley & Sons, Inc. for their assistance in the management and production of this book. We would especially like to thank the following people: Andrea Stingelin, Executive Editor, Nursing; David P. Carroll, Editor; Janet Foltin, Assistant Editor; Mercedes Bierman, Director of Marketing; Margery Carazzone, Production Manager; and Rosalind Straley, Senior Production Designer.

Contents

PART I
INTRODUCTION

Part I Contents 3

1. Organizational Structure, Design, and Function 5
Dorothy A. Jones

2. Nursing: Process and Practice 13
Dorothy A. Jones

3. Health Education 33
Lynne McInerney

4. Human Development Through the Life Span 53
Mable Searcy Carlyle

5. Family Assessment and Nursing Intervention 79
Jean R. Miller

PART II
THE NURSING CARE OF PARENTS AND INFANTS

Part II Contents 95

6. Family Planning 97
Phyllis L. Collier

7. Pregnancy: The First, Second, and Third Trimesters 115
Nora Doherty Tully

8. Labor and Delivery 149
Susan E. Anderson

9. Recovery: The Fourth Trimester 175
Jeanette Coleman and Hilda Koehler

10. The Full-Term Infant 197
Elaine Muller Morris

11. The High-Risk Infant 223
Bonnie Silverman and Laurie Weintraub

12. Birth Defects: The Grieving Family 253
Bonnie Silverman and Elizabeth J. Dickason

13. The Family Unready for Childbearing 269
Cynthia S. Luke

14. The Infertile Family 281
Elizabeth J. Dickason and Carol Ann McKenzie

PART III
THE NURSING CARE OF CHILDREN AND ADOLESCENTS

Part III Contents 307

15. The Nervous System 311
Beverly A. Bowens

16. The Musculoskeletal System 345
Sherrilyn DeJean Coffman

17. The Endocrine System 371
Diana W. Guthrie

18. The Hematologic System 405
C. Marie Hall Smith and Patricia E. Greene

19. The Cardiovascular System 459
Mary Fran Hazinski

20. The Respiratory System 505
Janet L. Snow

21. The Urinary System 537
Annette Crosby Frauman and Cyrena M. Gilman

22. The Gastrointestinal System 567
Catherine Kneut

23. The Integumentary System 597
Patricia Harris

24. Communicable Diseases 621
Helen L. Farrell

PART IV THE NURSING CARE OF ADULTS

Part IV Contents 663

25. The Nervous System 669
Barbara J. Boss

26. The Sensory System 789
Sue E. Huether

27. The Musculoskeletal System 823
Rosellen M. Garrett

28. The Endocrine System 865
Virginia L. Cassmeyer and Betty L. Hopping

29. The Hematologic System 921
Mary Bigelow Huntoon

30. The Cardiovascular System 967
Rose Pinneo

31. The Respiratory System 1045
Dorothy L. Sexton and Mary E. Eddy

32. The Urinary System 1117
Margaret Allen Murphy

33. The Gastrointestinal System 1177
Mary Marmoll Jirovec

34. The Reproductive System 1231
Mary Suzanne Tarmina

35. The Integumentary System 1259
Meredith Censullo

PART V THE NURSING CARE OF ADULTS AND CHILDREN WITH MENTAL HEALTH PROBLEMS

Part V Contents 1293

36. Anxiety and the Affective Disorders 1297
Ruth Dailey Knowles

37. Interpersonal Problems of Adults 1319
Rhoda L. Moyer and Martha J. Snider

38. **Threats to Survival 1339**
Imogene Stewart Rigdon and Karolyn Lusson Godbey

39. **Disruptions of Perceptual and Cognitive Functions 1351**
Martha J. Snider

40. **Mental Health Problems of Children 1357**
Faye Gary Harris

41. **Person Abuse 1369**
Judy B. Campbell and Noreen King Poole

42. **Group Work in Inpatient Settings 1391**
Ann Ottney Cain

43. **Family Work in Inpatient Settings 1405**
Ann Ottney Cain and Jo Annalee Irving

PART VI THE NURSING CARE OF THE ELDERLY

Part VI Contents 1421

44. **Physical Changes of Normal Aging 1423**
Ann Faas Collard

45. **Coping with Loss and Aging 1449**
Cynthia Sarno Yeager

46. **Common Health Problems That Affect the Elderly 1463**
Joanne Kelleher Farley

PART VII NURSING CARE DURING EMERGENCIES

Part VII Contents 1491

47. **General Principles of Emergency Care 1493**
Mary P. Wieland

48. **Traumatic Injuries 1511**
Marilyn de Give and Annalee Oakes

49. **Medical Emergencies 1585**
Marilyn de Give

50. **Psychiatric Emergencies 1631**
Sherry W. Honea and Beverley H. Durrett

APPENDIXES

Appendix Contents 1643

A. **Diagnostic Tables 1645**

B. **Conversion Tables 1684**

C. **Clinical Laboratory Values 1690**

D. **Nomograms and Growth Charts 1693**

E. **Communicable Disease Table 1703**

F. **Dietary Tables 1713**

G. **Vital Statistics 1733**

INDEX

Index 1737

THE HANDBOOK OF NURSING

PART I

INTRODUCTION

PART I CONTENTS

CHAPTER 1
ORGANIZATIONAL STRUCTURE, DESIGN, AND FUNCTION 5

A Reference Textbook 5

Organizational Framework 5

Structure and Design 5

Headings Used Throughout the Book 8

Acquisition of Information and Cross-Referencing 10

Application of the Text to Clinical Practice 10

Authorship 11

CHAPTER 2
NURSING: PROCESS AND PRACTICE 13

Defining Health 13
The consumer of health care 13
The focus on prevention 13

Nursing and Health 15
Nursing theorists and health promotion 15
Defining nursing 15
Standards of nursing practice 18
Implementation of nursing standards and the nursing process 19
Quality assurance 29
Recording clinical data 30

Summary 30

CHAPTER 3
HEALTH EDUCATION 33

Biologically Inherent Differences in Learning 35

Developmental Differences in Learning 36

Cultural Variations in Learning 39

Socioeconomic State 44

Stage of Acceptance of Illness 44

Selecting Appropriate Methods 51

Evaluation 51

Summary 51

CHAPTER 4
HUMAN DEVELOPMENT THROUGH THE LIFE SPAN 53

Neonate (Birth to 1 Month of Age) 53

Infant (1 to 12 Months) 55
Second month 55
Third month 55
Fourth month 56
Ffth month 56
Sixth month 56
Seventh, eighth, and ninth months 56
Tenth, eleventh, and twelfth months 57

Toddler (1 to 3 Years) 57

Preschool Child (3 to 6 Years) 58

Middle Childhood (6 to 12 Years) 59

Adolescence (12 to 20 Years) 60

Hospitalized Children and Adolescents and Their Families 63
Guidelines for assessment of children and adolescents 63
Psychological support of the hospitalized child and family: separation anxiety 65

Young Adult (20 to 40 Years) 71

Middle Age (40 to 60 Years) 72

Maturity (60 Years and Over) 74

CHAPTER 5
FAMILY ASSESSMENT AND NURSING INTERVENTION 79

Family Impact on Health and Illness 79
Alternative family structures 80

PART I CONTENTS *(continued)*

Nursing Role: Assisting the Family 80
Common family problems 80
Additional difficulties of nontraditional family structures 82

Nursing Interventions for Common Family Problems 82

Acute Illness in the Family 83
Antestress period 84
Stress period 85
Poststress period 86

Counseling the Family Confronting Rehabilitation or Chronic Illness 87

Coping with Death in the Family 89
Stage I: living with terminal illness 90
Stage II: restructuring in the living-dying interval 90
Stage III: bereavement 90
Stage IV: reestablishment 91

Summary 91

1

Organizational Structure, Design, and Function

Dorothy A. Jones

A REFERENCE TEXTBOOK

A reference textbook, by virtue of its design, provides the reader with quick and complete access to information. Such a book is written in a style that presents the reader with immediate facts within a format that is easily understood and consistently followed.

The Handbook of Nursing has been designed as a comprehensive reference text that offers the practicing nurse easy retrieval of information about a variety of medical problems and related nursing care. This format increases the utility and applicability of the text to any health setting. The pages that follow describe this format in greater depth.

ORGANIZATIONAL FRAMEWORK

The Handbook of Nursing is organized around the nursing specialties—maternity, pediatrics, medical-surgical, aging, psychiatric and behavioral problems, and emergency care—and focuses upon medical problems, nursing problems, and related care that is concurrent with changes in a client's health status. The nursing process is the framework used to organize nursing care. Related components of this process, including nursing assessment, diagnosis, planning, intervention, and evaluation, are consistently discussed throughout the text in relation to each health problem described.

STRUCTURE AND DESIGN

Throughout the text an outline format is the predominant style used to communicate information. Because of the volume of material covered in this reference text, it was decided that this format would best provide the reader with the most salient facts about a topic. As it is not the function of this reference text to provide a complete, in-depth discussion of a particular health problem, the reader is directed to additional resources by an annotated bibliography included at the end of each chapter.

BOOK PARTS

The Handbook of Nursing is subdivided into seven parts (see Figure 1-1). Part I includes introductory chapters that contain essential concepts re-

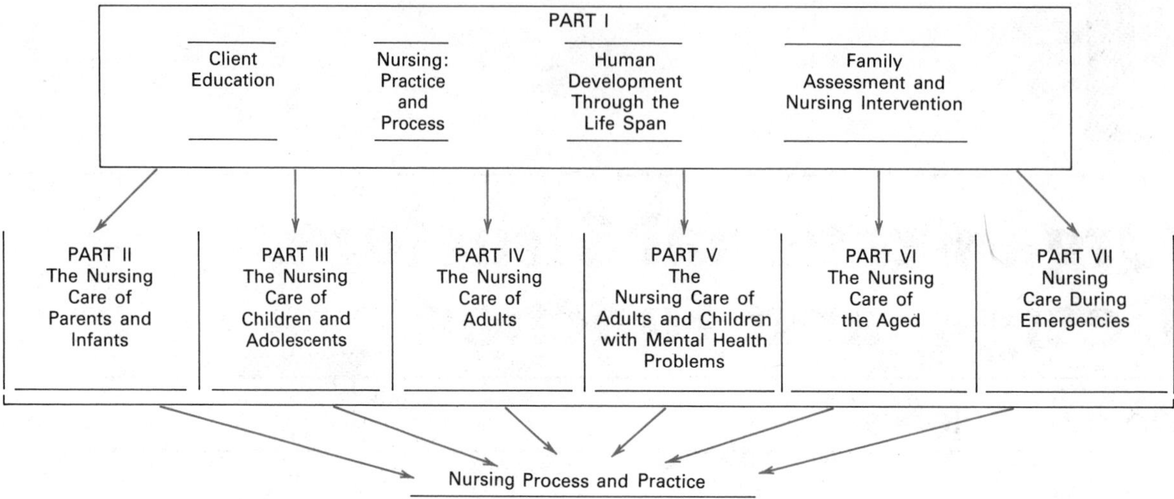

Figure 1-1 Organizational framework for *The Handbook of Nursing.*

lated to nursing practice regardless of clinical specialty (e.g., health education, nursing process, human development, and the family). Subsequent parts cover nursing care of parents and infants, nursing care of children and adolescents, nursing care of adults, nursing care of adults and children with mental health problems, nursing care of the aged, and nursing care during emergencies.

Part I: Introduction

Part I contains five chapters. Chapter 1 discusses the organization and design of the text. Chapter 2 presents the standards of nursing practice and their application to clinical practice. In addition, the chapter includes the American Nurses' Association Congress for Nursing Practice social policy statement along with an exploration of each of the components of the nursing process in a way that is introductory to its use throughout the book.

In Chapter 3, the teaching-learning process is addressed. Methods for assessing learning needs, along with teaching and learning strategies, are discussed.

Growth and development across the life span are presented in Chapter 4, followed by a discussion of family development and related components of assessment in Chapter 5. Because each of the chapters in Part I contains information that directly or indirectly affects all clients, cross references to these chapters are included in later discussions as necessary.

Part II: The Nursing Care of Parents and Infants

In Part II, the nursing process is applied to parents and families with reproductive concerns, women during pregnancy, delivery of the child, and care of term and preterm infants. Problems occurring during this period are discussed according to the format presented in Chapter 2. In addition, family problems of genetic defects, infertility, or psychological unreadiness for childbearing are elaborated upon in the last chapters of this part.

Part III: The Nursing Care of Children and Adolescents

The Nursing Care of Children and Adolescents details the nursing process as it applies to ill and high-risk infants and to children and adolescents. Health problems are arranged into chapters according to body systems. Respiratory, cardiovascular, and neurologic systems are examples of the topics covered. In addition, health problems within each body system (e.g., respiratory system) are further categorized under concepts that include abnormal cellular growth (e.g., structural birth defects), inflammation (e.g., pneumonia), obstruction (e.g., asthma), and other broad conceptual categories (see Table 1-1).

Part IV: The Nursing Care of Adults

Part IV addresses health concerns of young, middle, and older adults. Traditionally, this area

TABLE 1-1 MEDICAL-SURGICAL SUBCONCEPTS

Concepts	Definitions
Abnormal cellular growth	This category includes abnormal cellular growth and proliferation, structural birth defects, and neoplasms.
Hyperactivity and hypoactivity	This category includes those disorders whose underlying pathology is excessive or insufficient activity of cells (e.g., diabetes mellitus), organs (e.g., congestive heart failure), and so forth.
Metabolic disorders	Nutritional metabolic problems, toxicities, and other basically biochemical disorders fit into this classification.
Inflammations	Infectious processes as well as inflammatory disorders such as pancreatitis and dermatitis.
Obstructions	Refers to mechanical problems that interrupt normal function of organ, system, or related components (e.g., bowel obstruction).
Degenerative diseases	Degenerative disorders are problems that occur as a result of changes in or interruption in cell growth (e.g., Parkinson's disease).
Traumatic injuries	Most health problems that belong in this category are discussed in Part VII, Nursing Care during Emergencies.

of practice has been referred to as medical-surgical nursing. The content of these chapters is organized around body systems in a format similar to that of Part III, The Nursing Care of Children and Adolescents.

Obviously, many illnesses can be classified in more than one category. Aortic coarctation, for example, is both an abnormal cellular growth problem and an obstruction. The reader will find that decisions related to the placement of a problem have been made by the editors based upon where a particular problem is most likely to occur.

Part V: The Nursing Care of Adults and Children with Mental Health Problems

The Nursing Care of Adults and Children with Mental Health Problems focuses on changes in perception, affect, cognition, interpersonal relationships, societal norms, and activities of daily living and on situational crises. Family and group work are given special attention, and cross references are made to other chapters in the text as appropriate.

Part VI: The Nursing Care of the Aged

Part VI discusses nursing of the aged in relation to normal physiologic, psychologic, and sociocultural effects of aging; responses to losses; and health problems seen in atypical responses to aging. Because of the growing number of well elderly people, attention has been given to normal changes of aging as well as age-related health problems.

Part VII: Nursing Care during Emergencies

Nursing Care during Emergencies presents information on common medical and surgical emergencies as well as pediatric, obstetric, and psychiatric crises. Nursing care related to immediate needs of clients experiencing an emergency is presented. When appropriate, cross references are made to particular chapters throughout the text.

ARRANGEMENT OF CONTENT

To facilitate access to information, immediately following each part opening a list of the major headings in each chapter in that part is presented. This provides the reader with a quick overview of the content to be covered and will reduce the search time for finding a particular subject area.

Each medical disorder addressed is presented as a major or minor problem. A *major* (or commonly seen) problem is discussed completely, with all the components of the nursing process included. A *minor* problem is viewed as a rare problem, one less commonly seen. These problems are described briefly, and care is incorporated in the overall discussion of the problem.

HEADINGS USED THROUGHOUT THE BOOK

Each major problem is organized according to the following headings and related definitions.

DESCRIPTION

In narrative or outline format, the disease, or health problem, is described. Components such as etiology, incidence, pathophysiologic changes, and outcomes are considered as part of this discussion.

PREVENTION

Factors that need to be considered by the nurse to prevent the disorder are addressed (see Table 1-2).

Health Promotion

Health measures (including teaching) are listed that can be used by both the client and nurse to prevent illness. Immunization is often included in this discussion (see Table 1-3).

Population at Risk

Individuals at risk to develop the health problem are identified for purposes of directing health promotion activities.

Screening

Screening techniques or tools used to detect actual or potential risk factors, identification of carrier states, and subclinical problems are isolated when possible.

TABLE 1-2 HEALTH GOALS FOR THE NATION

Healthy infants
- Reducing low-birth-weight infants and birth defects

Healthy children
- Facilitating childhood growth and development; reduction of accidents

Healthy adolescents and young adults
- Reducing deaths and injuries from automobile accidents; decreasing substance abuse

Healthy adults
- Reducing heart attacks, strokes, cancer

Healthy older adults
- Increasing the proportion of functioning older adults; reducing death from pneumonia and influenza

SOURCE: Adapted from *Healthy People: The Surgeon General's Report on Health Promotion and Disease Prevention.* USDHEW, Public Health Service, Washington, D.C., PHS Publication No. 79-55071, 1979.

ASSESSMENT*

The data collection process contains three subparts: health history, physical assessment, and diagnostic tests.

Health History

Information that reflects the client's or significant others' report of signs, symptoms, or relevant factors contributing to a health problem is described. Data such as age, sex, race, and socioeconomic influences are identified as pertinent to the disorder being discussed. The rationale for collecting particular data is briefly stated wherever feasible, if it is not self-evident.

Physical Assessment

Information collected primarily through objective data is presented. Specific assessment pertaining to physical changes occurring in specific organs or body systems is included. Wherever feasible, a brief rationale for the physical assessment changes is included. For example,

* A complete discussion of the entire nursing process is presented in Chapter 2.

TABLE 1-3 HEALTH ACTIVITIES FOR HEALTH PROMOTION

Prevention
- Family planning
- Pregnancy, infant care
- Immunization
- Reduction of sexually transmitted diseases
- Reduction of hypertension

Protection
- Control of toxins
- Occupational safety
- Reduction of accidents
- Flouridation of water
- Control of infectious agents

Promotion
- Reduction of smoking, decrease in substance abuse (alcohol and drugs)
- Improvement in nutrition (balanced food consumption)
- Regular exercise and general fitness
- Stress management
- Promotion of optimal wellness

SOURCE: Adapted from *Healthy People: The Surgeon General's Report on Health Promotion and Disease Prevention,* USDHEW Public Health Service, Washington, D.C., PHS Publication No. 79-55071, 1979.

"hemorrhoids usually accompany cirrhosis because the fibrosed liver obstructs the flow of venous blood through the portal circulation."

Diagnostic Tests

Pertinent diagnostic tests and the findings usually associated with the health disorder are discussed. Tests that are not widely known receive a brief description.

NURSING DIAGNOSES: ACTUAL OR POTENTIAL

"Nursing diagnoses describe health problems in which the responsibility for therapeutic decisions can be assumed by a professional nurse . . . these problems encompass potential or actual disturbances in life processes, patterns, functions, or development, including those occurring secondary to disease" (Gordon, 1976). Use of the classification system (diagnostic nomenclature) approved by the Fifth National Conference on Nursing Diagnosis is incorporated. (Refer to Chapter 2 for a more complete discussion.) Nursing outcomes, care, and evaluation evolve from the diagnoses generated.

EXPECTED OUTCOMES

Expected outcomes are goals to be achieved by the client and facilitated by the nurse. Although each client's goals are individually planned, general outcomes are suggested.

Goals are stated in clear, realistic, measurable terms presented in the future tense, for example, "The client will lose 30 lb in the next 20 weeks" (long-term goal) or "The client will lose 1 to 2 lb by each weekly visit" (short-term goal). Goals are listed in order of priority and in response to a nursing diagnosis.

INTERVENTIONS

Nursing interventions clearly state the nursing actions to be used to attain the goals. Wherever advisable and feasible, a brief rationale is given. When physician interventions (surgery, drug prescription, etc.) are mentioned, they are identified and followed by the related nursing actions. Nursing interventions encompass prevention (health promotion), maintenance, and restoration.

EVALUATION

Standards for measuring achievement or lack of achievement of the goals of care are presented. This section contains two subparts: outcome criteria and complications.

Outcome Criteria

This section lists the criteria by which the nurse can measure the extent to which the interventions have been successful and the degree to which each of the goals has been attained. Outcome criteria are phrased as statements rather than as questions, for example, "The client has resumed normal activity without reports of fatigue."

Complications

Complications for which the nurse should be alert focus on (1) *assessment* of changes that indicate that the complication is occurring, (2) *revised outcomes,* and (3) *interventions* recommended for dealing with the complication.

Reevaluation and Follow-up

This section presents an outline of reevaluation data and follow-up care that are recommended to evaluate the client's long-term progress. Where feasible, time intervals at which reevaluation should be conducted are included.

ACQUISITION OF INFORMATION AND CROSS-REFERENCING

A reference book of such wide scope requires a system for coordinating related content areas so that the book's usability is maximized and repetition is minimized. Nursing care of diabetics, for example, is part of maternity, medical-surgical, pediatric, gerontologic, and emergency practice, but it is obviously undesirable to duplicate information in several different parts of the book. The discussions pertaining to diabetes have been arranged so that the main body of material is presented in the endocrinology chapter of Part IV, The Nursing Care of Adults, and information that pertains only to other specialty areas is found in those other parts of the book. Thus, information about gestational diabetes and nursing of diabetics during family planning, pregnancy, and delivery is included in the maternity section. The specific ways in which juvenile diabetes differs from adult diabetes are discussed in the pediatric section. The acute crises of insulin shock and diabetic coma are included under emergency nursing. Surgical management and the special aspects of nursing aged diabetics are contained in the medical-surgical and gerontologic sections of the book, respectively.

The main discussion of each health problem is included in the part of the book that best deals with the nursing care of clients who are most likely to encounter that particular problem. Thus, disorders that most commonly arise during childhood (e.g., acute leukemias and certain communicable diseases) receive their major discussion in the pediatric chapters.

The psychosocial aspects of care for persons with predominantly physical disorders is integrated into overall care. Fear of the possibility of recurring myocardial infarction is dealt with in the same section as the other problems related to the care of a client with myocardial damage. Body image distortions associated with amputation are included in the discussion of nursing care of amputees. Problems that result in behavioral disturbances are discussed in the psychiatric nursing section.

Cross-reference notations are inserted where appropriate to direct the reader to the specialty chapter and specific topic. In addition, the index can also be used by the reader to isolate content and identify where information is discussed throughout the text.

APPLICATION OF THE TEXT TO CLINICAL PRACTICE

This text was prepared with the needs of the acute care practitioner in mind, but it was also designed to be useful in other settings. Long-term chronic care in the home and community (nursing home) or ambulatory care facilities (hospital or other institution) is discussed as part of each care plan. The nurse working in any setting can use this resource to become better able to plan teaching, coordinate care, and provide direct services to clients with a variety of health needs.

Although a comprehensive list of care plans has been presented in this text, a basic and inevitable limitation accompanies them. The authors recognize the individuality of each client and by no means wish to imply that these plans can be generalized to accommodate all people. Rather, it is important for the reader to recognize that the care plans represent a typical approach to care. Any one care plan is by no means "all inclusive" and should be used as a guide and a resource for identifying actual or potential health problems and related care.

RELATION OF TEXT TO OTHER LITERATURE

This reference text is not intended to replace other books or eliminate the need for more comprehensive resources in one's professional library. Accordingly, each chapter includes a briefly annotated bibliography that supplements the information outlined by this book.

Readers will also note that two types of information have been omitted from this text. First, it is assumed that the knowledge and skills that constitute "fundamentals of nursing" have been mastered by practicing nurses and, therefore, need not be repeated. Second, because of the widespread availability of procedure manuals and the specificity and individualization among institutions as to how procedures are carried out, minimal book space has been given to instructions for nursing procedures.

In addition, it is important to note that pathophysiology is presented under the description section of each disease entity. Additional references to an extensive discussion of a particular problem are included in the bibliography in each chapter.

AUTHORSHIP

The expansion and deepening of knowledge in nursing and in the related sciences have brought about the end of the single-author broad-scope reference work. This handbook has been written by a large number of nursing authors, each selected for the ability to contribute up-to-date accuracy and clinical expertise. In conformity with the editorial board's conviction that the design and evaluation of nursing care are the prerogative and responsibility of professional nurses, each chapter focuses on the nursing management of care.

REFERENCES

Gordon, M.: "Nursing Diagnosis and the Diagnostic Process," *American Journal of Nursing,* **76**(8):1298, 1976.

BIBLIOGRAPHY

Healthy People: The Surgeon General's Report on Health Promotion and Disease Prevention, publication no. 79-55071, U.S. Department of Health, Education and Welfare, Public Health Service, 1979. Provides an updated analysis of our nation's critical health issues. Particular emphasis is placed upon risks to good health, health goals for each age group, and actions for health promotion.

Promoting Health/Preventing Disease: Objectives for the Nation. U.S. Department of Health and Human Services, Public Health Service, 1980. Presents an expansion of the Surgeon General's report by identifying objectives for 15 priority areas that need to be achieved in order to optimize health.

Standards of Nursing Practice, American Nurses' Association, Kansas City, Mo., 1973. Provides eight standards that organize and direct nursing care for individuals, families, and groups. It offers the nurse a guide for determining, implementing, and evaluating quality care.

2

Nursing: Process and Practice

Dorothy A. Jones

DEFINING HEALTH

Health is a familiar term to everyone. Although it is spoken of in positive terms, for example, "good health," it is defined differently by various health providers. Yet, most providers will agree that health is more than the mere absence of disease. For many, health encompasses the spiritual, emotional, social, and physical components of the total person as he or she interacts with the environment. This belief system is currently supported by proponents of the holistic health movement. A *holistic* definition of health encompasses the total interaction of the human being's body, mind, and spiritual components. The goals of the holistic movement entertain a view of an individual who is in control of and responsible for his or her state of health (Figure 2-1).

Dr. John Travis, developer of the Wellness Resource Center in Mill Valley, California, has expanded the holistic health beliefs in his work related to the promotion of wellness. Accordingly, he defines *wellness* as a dynamic state reflecting the growth and change within an individual physically, emotionally, and socially. He further suggests that "high level wellness is a means of giving good care to your physical self; using your mind constructively, expressing your emotions effectively, being creatively involved with those around you, being concerned about your physical and psychological environment and becoming aware of other levels of consciousness" (Travis, 1981). (See Figure 2-2.)

THE CONSUMER OF HEALTH CARE

It is important to note the reference to the consumer of health care as the *client*. This term has been used throughout this text in support of the idea that the client is a personal advocate of self-care. Further, it is felt that the term *patient* can connote a more passive role on the part of the individual in controlling care.

The goal is to have the client be an active participant in his or her own health care, freely making choices and being responsible for the outcomes. The use of the term *client* helps to broaden the scope of an individual's seeking, receiving, participating in, and evaluating health care and, more specifically, nursing care.

THE FOCUS ON PREVENTION

In the Surgeon General's report on health promotion (*Healthy People*, 1979), broad national goals were set forth to reduce death rates and disability. To accomplish this, 15 priority areas were identified (see Table 2-1) and specific, quantifiable objectives necessary for achieving these goals were set forth.

Because one major focus of the national health policy is on promoting health through preven-

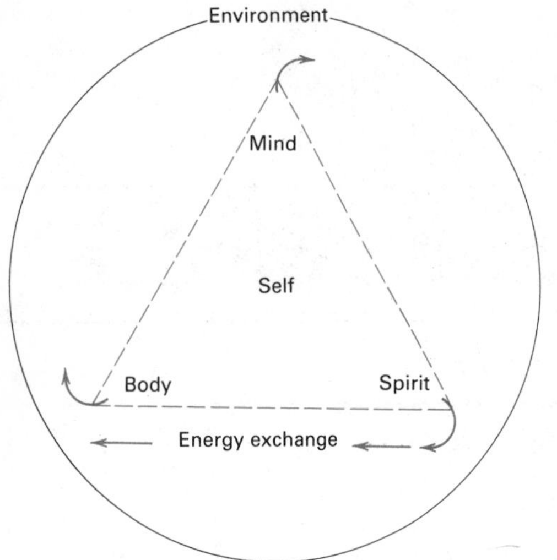

Figure 2-1 The interaction of mind, body, and spirit affecting the whole person.

tion of illness, attention is drawn to this aspect throughout this text under three headings: *Health Promotion*, *Population at Risk*, and *Screening*.

Health Promotion

Interventions that could prevent a particular health problem and promote optimal wellness are discussed.

TABLE 2-1 CATEGORIES OF DISEASE PREVENTION AND HEALTH PROMOTION

Preventive Focus
High blood pressure control
Family planning
Pregnancy and infant death
Immunization
Sexually transmitted diseases
Health Protection
Toxic agent control
Occupational safety
Accident prevention and injury control
Fluoridation and dental control
Control of infectious disease
Health Promotion
Smoking and health
Misuse of alcohol and drugs
Nutrition
Physical fitness and exercise
Control of stress and violent behavior

SOURCE: Adapted from the Surgeon General's report *Promoting Health/Preventing Disease*, U.S. Department of Health and Human Services, Washington, D.C., 1980.

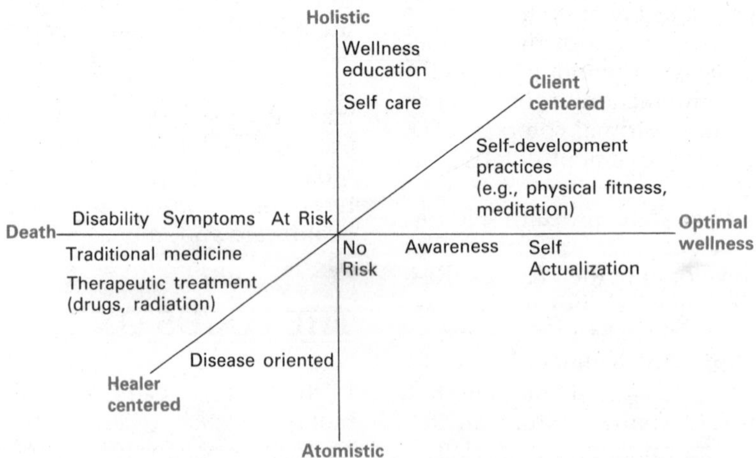

Figure 2-2 Interactive health model demonstrating optimal health and wellness. (From Jones, D. et al., *Health Assessment Across the Life Span*, McGraw-Hill, New York, 1984, p. 10. Used with permission. Adapted from *Wellness Workbook for Helping Professionals*, John W. Travis, M. D., Wellness Associates, 42 Miller Avenue, Mill Valley, CA 94941 (1981).)

Population at Risk

The population at risk for a particular health problem is identified so that appropriate preventive measures can be instituted through teaching and counseling.

Screening

Screening measures are isolated so that persons at risk for a particular health problem can be identified and measures enacted to prevent the onset of the problem and/or related complications.

NURSING AND HEALTH

Nursing over the years has consistently defined health in terms of the "whole person." It has had as its goal the prevention of illness, the promotion of health, and the optimization of an individual's state of wellness regardless of that person's actual level of health.

The evolution of nursing science has seen many nursing leaders express their views on health in various models of clinical practice. A *model* is "a symbolic depiction in logical terms of an idealized, relatively simple situation . . . a conceptual representation of reality" (Roy and Riehl, 1981). It is a broader term than *theory*. Theory represents the elements of a model. Models have evolved to guide and define nursing in several ways:

1. They provide an overall goal of practice.
2. They provide a framework for direct care by:
   a. Defining health.
   b. Offering a definition of the client.
   c. Providing direction for assessment and data collection.
   d. Directing nursing intervention.
   e. Allowing for nursing practice to direct the care of others by incorporating a chosen framework of practice as a guide for other role components, for example, consultation, change agent, researcher, or teacher.

NURSING THEORISTS AND HEALTH PROMOTION

Rogers offers a model that embraces a holistic view of human beings. She states, "the life process of unitary human beings is a phenomenon of wholeness, of continuity, of dynamic and creative change" (Rogers, 1970). When one's health is altered, repatterning of the life process is essential to regaining wholeness (see Table 2-2).

Orem, on the other hand, promotes a self-care model that supports the principle of holism and stresses the fact that the individual is responsible for his or her own health. Within this model, when illness occurs, self-care deficits develop that require nurses' assistance in a variety of levels until health is restored (see Table 2-2).

Johnson's view of the client is one of complexity and interrelatedness of systems. Accordingly, each system has a pattern that interacts to serve the whole. Nursing's role is to serve the client when his or her own resources fail (see Table 2-2).

Roy's nursing model is described in terms of an adaptation model. Nursing is concerned with the client's adjustments and adaptations to the stress of change. Disease is a manifestation of a client's inability to adapt to these stressors. Nursing serves the client by directing interventions toward helping the person develop coping mechanisms within the physiological, self-concept, role-function, and interdependence modes (see Table 2-2).

There are many other models of practice (see bibliography) that have been developed to guide the art and science of nursing. As models develop, nursing refines its conceptual base and identifies more clearly its scientific nature. For the present, nurses are encouraged to utilize a framework of practice that relies on the work of these and other theorists. In so doing nurses will be more articulate in describing their role in promoting health.

DEFINING NURSING

In 1980 the American Nurses' Association Congress for Nursing Practice developed a document entitled *Nursing: A Social Policy Statement*. In it, the congress defined the nature and scope of nursing practice and presented criteria for role specialization within nursing practice settings.

THE NATURE OF NURSING

According to the social policy statement, nursing is defined as "the diagnosis and treatment

TABLE 2-2 FOUR FRAMEWORKS FOR NURSING PRACTICE

Framework and Assessment Focus	Diagnostic Focus	Causality
Rogers: Life process model Behavioral manifestations of events in the human and environmental field. Holistic patterns of functioning (total pattern of events at a given point in space-time).	Pattern and organization of the life process that does not support maximum health potential and the creative-formative process. (No diagnostic classification.)	Multicausality found in human and environmental field interaction.
Roy: Adaptation model Adaptive responses to need deficits or excesses: Physiological mode: rest/exercise, nutrition, elimination, fluids and electrolytes, oxygen and circulation, regulation of temperature, regulation of senses, and regulation of endocrine system. Self-concept mode: physical self; personal self: moral-ethical, self-consistency, self-ideal, and self-esteem. Role-function mode: primary/secondary/tertiary roles; expressive/instrumental: role identity, role expectations, role interactions. Interdependence mode: cognitive/affective, parameters in relation to independency-dependency needs: affection achievement (love, support). Influencing factors: focal, contextual, and residual stimuli.	Potential problems in adaptation; actual maladaptation problems. (Diagnostic classification according to four adaptation modes: physiological, self-concept, role-function, and interdependence modes.)	Causality lies in need deficits or excesses produced by stressors (focal stimulus) or in coping mechanisms (cognator and regulator). Multicausality concept, but intervention focus is on primary cause.

Johnson (Grubbs): Behavioral system model Structural and functional level of behavioral system and the behavioral subsystem: Achievement Affiliative Aggressive/protective Dependency Eliminative Ingestive Restorative Sexual Coping effectiveness	Instability in the system; behavior at variance with the desired state; behavior that does not maintain equilibrium: Intrasubsystem insufficiency Intrasubsystem discrepancy Intersubsystem Incompatibility Intersubsystem dominance Inadequate coping/adaptation (Diagnostic classification according to eight subsystems, intrasubsystem or intersubsystem problem.)	Etiological classification according to source of stress/instability. *Etiology* used in singular sense.
Orem: Self-care agency model Eight universal self-care requisites, two developmental self-care requisites, and six health deviation self-care requisites (as well as interrelationships among these). Current repertoire of self-care practices (self and dependent): Degree of development Degree of operability Adequacy relative to demand	Presence of a deficit between existing powers of self-care agency and the demands on it. Actual or potential deficits in type and quality (therapeutic value) of self-care actions. (Diagnostic classification according to self-care needs in relation to (1) development, (2) health deviation, and (3) universal.)	Cause may be disease process; therapy used; or lack of knowledge, skills, resources, interest, or motivation.

SOURCES: Adapted from Rogers, M.: *An Introduction to the Theoretical Basis of Nursing*, Davis, Philadelphia, 1970; Roy, C.: *Introduction to Nursing: An Adaptation Model*, Prentice-Hall, Englewood Cliffs, N.J., 1981; Orem, D.: *Nursing: Concepts of Practice*, McGraw-Hill, New York, 1980; Grubbs, J.: *The Johnson Behavioral Model*, in J. P. Riehl and C. Roy (eds.), *Conceptual Models for Nursing Practice*, Appleton-Century-Crofts, New York, 1978; Gordon, M.: *Nursing Diagnosis: Process and Application*, McGraw-Hill, New York, 1982, pp. 75–76.

of human responses to actual or potential health problems" (American Nurses' Association, 1980). This definition is further divided into the following four defining characteristics:

1. Phenomena.
2. Theory application.
3. Nursing action.
4. Evaluation of effects (outcomes of one's actions).

Phenomena

Phenomena are those things with which nursing is concerned, i.e., those responses to actual or potential health problems.

Example:

1. Attending to a client's discomforts after surgery.
2. Teaching the client cholesterol reduction to decrease the risk of cardiac injury.

Theory

Theory provides a set of principles that guide and facilitate nursing practice. These principles reflect a model of nursing that provides a definition of the client and helps direct nursing action (e.g., assessment, goal setting, intervention, and evaluation).

Example:

1. Martha Rogers' life process model.
2. Sister Callista Roy's adaptation model.
3. Dorothea Orem's self-care model.

Actions

Actions are those activities (preventive, nurturative, and generative) in which a nurse engages in order to prevent an alteration in health or to promote wellness. Actions are determined by nursing diagnosis of an actual or potential problem and are the technical, interpersonal, and scientific interventions that result from the synthesis and evaluation of the client's health status.

Example:

1. Health teaching.
2. Washing the client.
3. Assisting the client with self-care activities.

Effects

The *effect* of a nursing action is often referred to as an *outcome*, that is, the result of nursing action, the thing to be evaluated. Achievement of the outcome through the establishment of standards or criteria helps to validate nursing practice and make nursing a valued resource.

STANDARDS OF NURSING PRACTICE

The standards of nursing practice were developed by the ANA's Congress for Nursing Practice in 1973. These standards "provide a means for determining the quality of nursing which a client/patient receives and provide a systematic approach to nursing practice" (American Nurses' Association, 1973). (See Table 2-3.)

The development of standards for nursing practice is essential to determining the quality of care provided by nurses in all settings. This means that nurses working within various agencies or clinical specialties must refine the standards to accurately reflect their applicability to a setting. To this end, various specialty groups have developed standards of care for practice. They are available from the American Nurses' Association.

WHY STANDARDS OF PRACTICE?

"'A professional association is an organization of practitioners who judge one another as professionally competent and who have banded together to perform social functions which they cannot perform in their separate capacity as individuals'" (Merton, 1958). A professional association, because of its nature, must provide measures to judge the competency of its membership and to evaluate the quality of its services. Studies show that the tendency for self-organization is characteristic of professions and the establishment and implementation of standards characteristic of the organization. . . .

"A profession's concern for the quality of its service constitutes the heart of its responsibility to the public. The more expertise required to perform the service, the greater is society's dependence upon those who carry it out. A profession must seek control of its practice in order to guarantee the quality of its service to the public. Behind that guarantee are the standards of the profession, which provide the assurance that service of a high quality will be provided. This is essential for the protection of both the public and the profession itself. A profession that does not maintain the confidence of the public will soon cease to be a social force.

TABLE 2-3 AMERICAN NURSES' ASSOCIATION STANDARDS OF NURSING PRACTICE

STANDARD I
The collection of data about the health status of the client is systematic and continuous. The data are accessible, communicated, and recorded.

STANDARD II
Nursing diagnoses are derived from health status data.

STANDARD III
The plan of nursing care includes goals derived from the nursing diagnoses.

STANDARD IV
The plan of nursing care includes priorities and the prescribed nursing approaches or measures to achieve the goals derived from the nursing diagnoses.

STANDARD V
Nursing actions provide for client participation in health promotion, maintenance, and evaluation.

STANDARD VI
Nursing actions assist the client to maximize his or her health capabilities.

STANDARD VII
The client's progress or lack of progress toward goal achievement is determined by the client and the nurse.

STANDARD VIII
The client's progress or lack of progress toward goal achievement directs reassessment of priorities, new goal setting, and revision of the plan of nursing care.

SOURCE: American Nurses' Association, 1973. Congress for Nursing Practice Standards of Nursing Practice. Reprinted with the permission of the American Nurses' Association.

"In recognition of the importance of standards of professional practice and the need to guarantee quality service, the various divisions on nursing practice of the American Nurses' Association have each formulated standards. The association recognizes that ongoing revisions of the standards of nursing practice will be necessary to reflect the enlarging scope of practice as well as the increasingly sharper delineation of the theoretical basis upon which the practice rests" (Congress for Nursing Practice Standards of Practice, 1974).

IMPLEMENTATION OF NURSING STANDARDS AND THE NURSING PROCESS

The standards of practice serve as a model of nursing care that reflects nursing action in delivery of direct care to clients. They further describe those activities for which nurses are responsible and accountable. Implementation of the standards of nursing practice can be accomplished through the enactment of a scientific problem-solving approach called the *nursing process*.

The nursing process focuses upon the client's health state and helps direct nursing intervention through several discrete steps that include:

1. Collecting data through assessment of client needs.
2. Generating nursing diagnoses based upon the data.
3. Establishing goals, or outcomes, of care.
4. Selecting appropriate interventions.
5. Evaluating care through the development of specific outcome criteria and reassessment of the client's need(s).

DEVELOPING A DATA BASE: ASSESSMENT

A data base, as developed within this text, is presented in terms of a health history, physical assessment, and diagnostic tests.

Health History

The health history focuses on facts (signs and symptoms) that reflect the client's responses to actual or potential health problems. In order to focus this data collection process on nursing problems, a system that looks at "human functional patterns" (Gordon, 1982) as a basis for assessment can be used. (See Tables 2-4 and 2-5.)

Physical Assessment

Specific physical and behavioral changes commonly assessed during a physical examination can be described by the nurse to add to an existing nursing data base. One-word lists should

TABLE 2-4 FUNCTIONAL HEALTH PATTERNS

Health perception–health management pattern. Describes client's perceived pattern of health and well-being and how health is managed

Nutritional-metabolic pattern. Describes pattern of food and fluid consumption relative to metabolic need and pattern indicators of local food supply

Elimination pattern. Describes patterns of excretory function (bowel, bladder, and skin)

Activity-exercise pattern. Describes patterns of exercise, activity, leisure, and recreation

Sleep-rest pattern. Describes patterns of sleep, rest, and relaxation

Cognitive-perceptual pattern. Describes sensory-perceptual and cognitive pattern (including memory)

Self-perception–self-concept pattern. Describes self-concept pattern and perceptions of self (i.e., body comfort, body image, feeling state)

Role-description pattern. Describes pattern of role-engagements and relationships

Sexuality-reproductive pattern. Describes client's patterns of satisfaction and dissatisfaction with sexuality pattern; describes reproductive patterns

Coping-stress-tolerance pattern. Describes general coping pattern and effectiveness of the pattern in terms of stress tolerance

Value-belief pattern. Describes patterns of values, beliefs (including spiritual), or goals that guide choices or decisions

SOURCE: Gordon, M.: *Nursing Diagnosis: Process and Application,* McGraw-Hill, New York, 1982.

be avoided and all changes should be described fully. Frequently, a head-to-toe approach is used for the purpose of collecting physical assessment data.

Diagnostic Tests

Within this text relevant diagnostic tests, unique to the health problem being described, are presented for information and to serve as a teaching resource.

NURSING DIAGNOSIS

The goal of assessment is to be able to state a nursing diagnosis clearly in order to determine care. Nursing diagnosis "describes health problems in which the responsibility for therapeutic decisions can be assumed by the licensed professional nurse" (Gordon, 1982). These problems encompass those actual or potential disturbances in human functional patterns.

Shoemaker further defines the process in the following way: "Nursing diagnosis is a clinical judgment about an individual family or community, which is derived through a deliberate systematic process of data collection and analysis. It provides a basis for prescriptions for definitive therapy for which the nurse is accountable. A nursing diagnosis is expressed concisely and includes the etiology of a condition when known" (Shoemaker, 1983).

Through a process of clinical reasoning (diagnosing), the nurse determines clusters of critical cues (Kim and Moritz, 1982) that lead to the formulation of a statement (diagnosis) with a clearly defined etiology (see Table 2-6). The selection of the etiology helps direct nursing interventions and results from the nurse's analysis of data collected during the assessment period. Lack of an etiology suggests there may be insufficient data to support the diagnosis at that time. With expansion of the data base, the diagnosis and related etiology may become clearer. Table 2-7 lists those nursing diagnoses accepted by the North American Nursing Diagnosis Association (NANDA) for clinical testing by the nursing community (Kim, et al., 1984).

ESTABLISHING OUTCOMES/SETTING GOALS

The development of clear, realistic goals helps the nurse to establish outcome criteria to measure the effectiveness of care. It is essential that the nurse realize that goals/outcomes will vary from client to client. In addition, goals should reflect mutual planning and be realistic and achievable within the time frame selected.

A *contract* is a negotiated statement between the nurse (provider) and the client that can help the individual achieve stated goals (see Figure 2-3). The use of a contract allows the client to participate not only in goal setting but in establishing outcomes. This is viewed by some as a way to increase the individual's compliance and personal control of life events.

SELECTING INTERVENTIONS

Nursing interventions should address the etiology of the problem stated as well as the goals developed. Although it is true that all nursing care should be individualized, this text provides standard or commonly accepted interventions used to promote care. In addition, if specific medical or surgical interventions are used, they are discussed under interventions along with related nursing care.

EVALUATING CARE

Evaluation of care is accomplished by the development of outcome criteria, followed by an assessment of the client's achievement of these outcomes. Outcome criteria should be stated in clearly measurable terms and should include a standard against which success or failure to achieve the goal can be determined. (Refer to Figures 2-4 and 2-5.)

CONTRACT

I, ______________________________ agree to participate in the following contract

with ______________ from ______________, 19____, to ______________, 19____,

for the purpose of achieving the goals listed below:

Goals: —to lose 30 pounds by ______________;
—to learn to control excessive weight gain through careful planning of well-balanced meals;
—to identify the times when my eating patterns change, recognize the precipitating behavioral changes and/or stress factors that accompany overeating, and learn to control the cause before it affects my eating habits.

I also agree to attend bimonthly meetings with ______________________________ at the Primary Health Clinic to evaluate intermediate achievements toward accomplishing my goals.

Within one month from the date of this contract, I will reevaluate my goals and make necessary changes. If I am not satisfied with my progress, I may cancel this contract and future meetings. Should I intend to terminate this contract, I will inform ______________ during our scheduled meeting time. I will also provide reasons for terminating the agreement.

At the completion of our scheduled meetings both ______________ and myself will decide if additional meetings are needed.

I further agree that this contract can become part of my health record, accessible to both the nurse and physician only.

Date ______________________________

Name of the Client ______________________________

Name of the Nurse ______________________________

A copy of this contract should be given to the client and reviewed as needed.

Figure 2-3 Sample teaching–learning contract between client and nurse. (From Jones D. et al., *Medical Surgical Nursing: A Conceptual Approach*, 2d ed., McGraw-Hill, New York, 1982, p. 59. Used with permission.)

TABLE 2-5 SAMPLE QUESTIONS USED TO ELICIT A FUNCTIONAL HEALTH PATTERN ASSESSMENT

Functional Assessment

Demographic Data	Tool
Name ______	Social security number ______
Address ______	Medicare/hospitalization ______
Occupation ______	Telephone ______
Employer ______	Emergency contact ______

Sample Questions to Include in Functional Assessment of Pattern Areas[a]

Health Perception/Health Management

What does "being healthy" mean to you?

What do you do to keep healthy? (describe)

How would you describe your present state of health?

To whom do you usually go to seek health care?

How does your health today compare to 1 year ago? 5 years ago?

What activities do you participate in on a regular basis to maintain your present state of health?

When did you have your last physical examination?

Did you receive your immunization? (type and date of immunization, reaction to immunization, comments)

Do you have allergies?

What is your blood type?

Describe for me the times when you've been ill.

Are you taking any medication now? (type of medication, frequency, amount, reaction)

Discuss your family and health.

Describe your usual day.

Describe your neighborhood, neighbors.

Do you own or rent your home? Describe the environment surrounding the home (e.g., near highway, factories, etc.).

Are there pollution hazards in your living, school, or working environment (e.g., water, air)?

What means of transportation are available to you (bus, train, car, etc.)?

Is your home fire-safe?

Do you socialize with friends, neighbors, relatives?

Have you made plans for your retirement?

If retired, are you enjoying it?

Nutritional and Metabolic Patterns

Describe a typical day's eating menu (include content of meals, snacking patterns; maintain log).

Are there particular foods you like or dislike? (Why?)

Are you on a special diet? (describe)

Are there particular foods that cause disturbances (e.g., indigestion)?

Are there times during the day when you feel hungry?

What is your present height/weight? How does it compare with 5 and 10 years ago?

Have there been any significant changes in your weight over the past year?

How do you feel about your present weight?

Who does your food shopping? Do you have a grocery list?

Do you have a food budget?

Do you eat out frequently?

What do you do to care for your teeth?

How often do you have your teeth checked?

Do you wear dentures?

TABLE 2-5 *(continued)*

Sample Questions to Include in Functional Assessment of Pattern Areas[a]

***Nutritional and Metabolic Patterns* (*continued*)**

How much fluid do you drink per day (e.g., how many glasses of water)?

Do you think alcohol is a problem for you? (describe)

Does stress affect your eating and drinking habits?

Does smoking affect your appetite?

Do you take vitamin supplements?

Have you noticed changes in your hair, nails, etc.?

Describe how you heal.

Do you have any difficulty tolerating hot or cold weather?

Elimination Patterns

What do you consider a normal bowel movement? (frequency, consistency)

Do you take any medication to maintain your regularity?

Do you ever experience constipation or diarrhea? Are these changes associated with stress? other associations?

What do you take when changes in bowel habits occur?

Describe your usual pattern of urination.

Do you wake up at night to urinate? (frequency)

Have you experienced any changes in your pattern of urination? (burning, frequency, leaking urine, dribbling)

Exercise and Activity Patterns

Describe the type, frequency, and amount of exercise you engage in on a regular basis.

Do you see daily exercise as important to your state of health?

Describe how you feel after exercising.

Are you satisfied with your present level of physical fitness? stamina?

Does your occupation involve physical activity?

Do you climb the stairs rather than take an elevator? How do you feel after climbing stairs?

What is your principal means of transportation?

Describe your leisure-time activities.

When you plan a vacation, is exercise an integral part of it?

Can you move about freely without discomfort (e.g., leg pain, chest pain)?

Sleep and Rest Patterns

How many hours of sleep do you get each night?

Do you feel rested when you wake up in the morning? Describe the first 10 min of your day.

Do you nap during the day? Is this a routine, or do you feel exhausted by a certain time?

Do you have difficulty falling asleep? Can you identify a reason or reasons why this is so?

Do you take anything to help you fall asleep?

Do you dream? Are you troubled by your dreams? Are there recurring themes in your dreams?

Do you relax during the day? evening?

Do you follow any routine to help you relax?

Do you use meditation?

TABLE 2-5 *(continued)*

Sample Questions to Include in Functional Assessment of Pattern Areas[a]

Congitive and Perceptual Patterns

Describe your hearing at this time.
Have you noticed any changes in your hearing in the past year? (describe)
Have you ever had wax removed from your ears? (describe)
Have you ever had a hearing test? When? Do you know the results?
Have you experienced changes in your balance?
Describe your present vision.
Is it as good as it was 1 year ago? 5 years ago?
Do you have routine eye examinations?
Do you wear glasses? contact lenses?
Do you have problems seeing at night?
Do you find that your activities are limited because of your vision?
Are you able to smell odors?
How does food taste? Have you noticed any changes in your taste perception?
Do you speak without interruption?
Are you able to express words and phrases the way you wish?
Can you perceive hot and cold without difficulty? Have you experienced any changes in your perception?
How would you describe your memory?
Has it changed over the past year? 5 years?
Can you concentrate without difficulty?
Describe your educational background.
When you experience pain, how do you handle it? What makes it better? Worse?
Do you think you are sensitive to pain?

Roles and Relationship Patterns

Describe your family unit. Who lives with you?
What are your primary responsibilities to the household?
Who makes decisions within your household? How are finances managed?
Are chores shared?
Who is the most significant person in your life?
Where is that person? Is he or she available to you?
Are there other individuals that you can turn to if necessary?
Have there been any major changes in your role(s) and/or responsibilities recently? (explain)
Do you foresee future changes in the coming years? Have you begun to make preparations for these changes?
Are there any family stressors? How are they being handled?
If individual is a parent:
- Describe your relationship with your children.
- Do you plan to expand your family?
- Are your parenting patterns different from those of your parents? (explain)

Describe your occupation (include work role and responsibilities).
How many hours do you work per week? Does this interfere with other aspects of your lifestyle?
Do you own your home?
Is your income adequate to maintain your lifestyle?
Do you take vacations? How frequently? What do you do on vacations?
Do you have many friends?
Do you have any plans for your retirement?

TABLE 2-5 *(continued)*

Sample Questions to Include in Functional Assessment of Pattern Areas[a]

Coping and Stress Management

How do you feel you handle stress?

Describe a stressful incident in your life and describe how you reacted.

What do you feel are major stressors in your life?

Do you feel that stress affects your health? (describe how)

Do you feel your life is more or less stressful than that of other people you know?

When you are under stress, do you cry, get angry, depressed, meditate, drink alcohol, take tranquilizers?

What makes you happy? sad?

Is it easy for you to express your emotions?

Has there been a significant loss in your life? How did you handle this loss?

Have you experienced many recent changes in your life? Do you expect any?

Would you like to make some life changes?

Do you feel you are coping well with your life at this point?

Self-perception and Self-conception

Do you feel good about yourself—the way you look? feel?

How would you describe yourself to another person? your physical appearance? your personality?

What would you describe as your strengths and weaknesses?

Are there things you would like to change about yourself? (describe)

Are you pleased with your life's accomplishments so far?

Do you have future goals you'd like to achieve? 5 years? 10 years?

Sexuality and Reproductive Patterns

What does being male/female mean to you?

Are you comfortable with your own sexuality?

Where did most of your sex education take place? school? home? friends? etc.

When did you begin having intercourse? Is it a satisfying experience for you?

Have you ever had venereal disease? (If so, what treatment did you have?)

Females

Describe your menstrual cycle (onset of menses, duration, dysmenorrhea, last menstrual period, etc.).

Have you ever been pregnant (abortions, miscarriages, etc.)?

Do you practice birth control?

Is this satisfying to you and your partner?

Have you experienced menopause? Describe the experience or expectations if it has not occurred.

Do you examine your breasts regularly?

Males

Do you ever experience problems with intercourse? impotence?

Do you have any feelings about male menopause?

Do you examine your testes?

TABLE 2-5 *(continued)*

Sample Questions to Include in Functional Assessment of Pattern Areas[a]	
Values and Belief Patterns	
Is religion important to your life? Do you participate regularly in church activities? Do you see religion as a support for you now? in the past? Do your religious beliefs influence the way you live your life?	Describe three things you value most in your life. Do you value health (if not mentioned above)? What changes would you make in your life to achieve optimal health?
Summary	
At the completion of this functional assessment, the nurse should make an overall determination of the client's life process and actual or potential problems that may exist.	These impressions should then be shared with the client and plans made with the individual to incorporate necessary changes to improve the client's overall pattern.

SOURCE: Jones, D. A., and Garrett, R. M.: "Application of a Conceptual Framework to the Practice of Nursing," in D. Jones, C. Dunbar, and M. Jirovec, (eds.): *Medical-Surgical Nursing: A Conceptual Approach,* 2d ed., McGraw-Hill, New York, 1982, pp. 30–32.

[a] The questions included in Table 2-5 are not all inclusive but are representative of the functional pattern areas being explored.

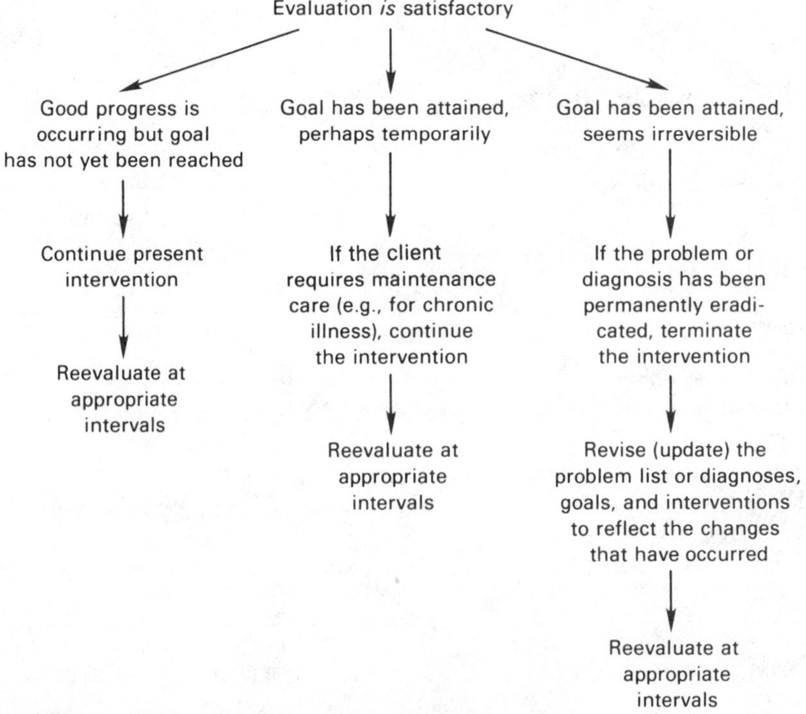

Figure 2-4 Flowchart of the decisions and actions that follow an evaluation of satisfactory progress or goal attainment.

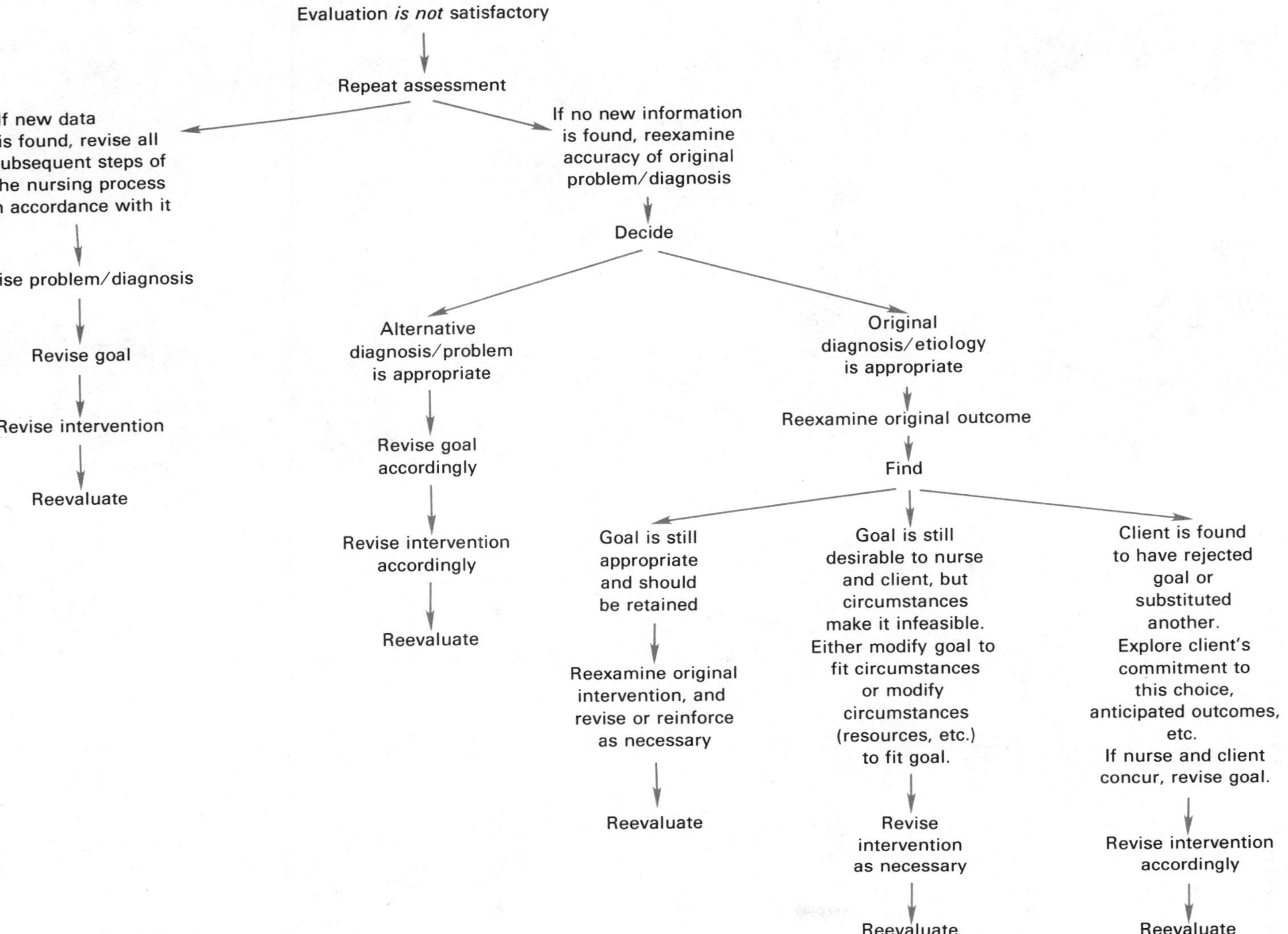

Figure 2-5 Flowchart of the decisions and actions that follow an evaluation of unsatisfactory progress toward goal attainment.

TABLE 2-6 COMPONENTS USED IN FORMULATING A NURSING DIAGNOSIS

Pattern
  Cognitive—perceptual pattern
Diagnosis
  Comfort, alteration in: pain
Definition
  Verbal report and presence of indicators of severe discomfort (pain)
Defining characteristics (signs/symptoms; cues)
  Communication (verbal or coded) of pain descriptors (Gordon)
  Guarding behavior—protective
  Self-focusing
  Narrowed focus (altered time perception, withdrawal from social contact, impaired thought process)
  Distraction behavior (moaning, crying, pacing, seeking out other people and/or activities, restless)
  Facial mask of pain (eyes lack luster, "beaten look," fixed or scattered movements, grimace)
  Alteration in muscle tone (may span from listless to rigid)
  Automatic responses not seen in chronic, stable pain (diaphoresis, blood pressure and pulse rate change, pupillary dilation, increased or decreased respiratory rate)
Etiology
  Knowledge deficit (pain management techniques) (Gordon)
  Injuring agents (biological, chemical, psychological)

SOURCE: Kim, M. J., and Moritz, D. A. (eds.): *Proceedings from the Third and Fourth National Conference on Nursing Diagnosis*, McGraw-Hill, New York, 1982.

In addition, when outcomes are not accomplished, a process of *reevaluation* occurs. At this time additional data collected may suggest a *complication* of the medical problem or referral for further evaluation. It may also mean that the outcomes set for the client were unrealistic or that the diagnosis may have been incorrect and a revised data base may have to be elicited.

Follow-up care refers to care given after an acute problem has been resolved and a time

TABLE 2-7 LIST OF NURSING DIAGNOSES ACCEPTED FOR CLINICAL TESTING BY THE NORTH AMERICAN NURSING DIAGNOSIS ASSOCIATION, APRIL 1982

Activity intolerance
Activity intolerance, potential
Airway clearance, ineffective
Anxiety
Bowel elimination, alteration in: constipation
Bowel elimination, alteration in: diarrhea
Bowel elimination, alteration in: incontinence
Breathing pattern, ineffective
Cardiac output, alteration in: decreased
Comfort, alteration in: pain
Communication, impaired: verbal
Coping, family: potential for growth
Coping, ineffective family: compromised
Coping, ineffective family: disabling
Coping, ineffective individual
Diversional activity, deficit
Family process, alteration in (formerly Family dynamics)
Fear
Fluid volume, alteration in: excess
Fluid volume deficit, actual
Fluid volume, deficit, potential
Gas exchange, impaired
Grieving, anticipatory
Grieving, dysfunctional
Health maintenance, alteration in
Home maintenance management, impaired
Injury, potential for: (poisoning, potential for; suffocation, potential for; trauma, potential for)
Knowledge deficit (specify)
Mobility, impaired physical
Noncompliance (specify)
Nutrition, alteration in: less than body requirements
Nutrition, alteration in: more than body requirements
Nutrition, alteration in: potential for more than body requirements

TABLE 2-7 (*continued*)

Oral mucous membranes, alteration in
Parenting, alteration in: actual
Parenting, alteration in: potential
Powerlessness
Rape-trauma syndrome
Self-care deficit: feeding, bathing/hygiene, dressing/grooming, toileting
Self-concept, disturbance in: body image, self-esteem, role performance, personal identity
Sensory-perceptual alteration: visual, auditory, kinesthetic, gustatory, tactile, olfactory
Sexual dysfunction
Skin integrity, impairment of: actual
Skin integrity, impairment of: potential
Sleep pattern disturbance
Social isolation
Spiritual distress (distress of the human spirit)
Thought processes, alteration in
Tissue perfusion, alteration in: cerebral, cardiopulmonary, renal, gastrointestinal, peripheral
Urinary elimination, alteration in patterns
Violence, potential for: self-directed or directed at others

SOURCE: Kim, M. J., McFarland, G. K., and McLane, A. M. (eds.): *Classification of Nursing Diagnoses: Proceedings of the Fifth National Conference*, Mosby, St. Louis, 1984.

period has elapsed. This care is usually guided by the outcome criteria set by the nurse at the previous meeting.

QUALITY ASSURANCE

Standards of practice do not undesirably constrain nursing practice or lessen its creativity and artistry. They are simply criteria by which the care of a nursing provider can be evaluated. *Quality assurance* is that process through which nursing standards for a particular group are developed. Furthermore, it is this same process that takes the necessary action to determine (evaluate) how well a standard has been achieved.

The Professional Standard Review Organization (PSRO) has enforced the development of quality assurance programs within various clinical facilities. These PSRO groups develop standards of care within specific agencies and set up various ways to evaluate individual care rendered by a nurse, physician, or other health care provider.

TABLE 2-8 CASE STUDY

R. J. was a 19-year-old college student who lived in a one-bedroom apartment with two other students. During midterm exams he felt tired frequently, ate very little, and developed headaches almost every day. He attributed his symptoms to the pressures of studying. The day of his last exam, however, friends began to comment that he "looked yellow," so he went to the student health service.

1. As the nurse in the student health service:
   a. What changes would you expect to find during your assessment, given R. J.'s preliminary history?
   b. What laboratory results would you expect to confirm a diagnosis of hepatitis?
   c. What questions would you ask during the health history to distinguish types A and B hepatitis. (See chart in Chapter 33.)
2. R. J. is confirmed to have type A viral hepatitis.
   a. What measures would you institute to prevent this problem from spreading to R. J.'s roommates?
3. As the nurse who admits R. J. to the hospital:
   a. What actual and potential nursing diagnoses would you expect to make?
   b. What expected outcomes would you set for R. J.'s care?
   c. How would you achieve those goals? (List interventions.)
   d. In evaluating your nursing care, what criteria would you set to determine R. J.'s recovery?

TABLE 2-9 SAMPLE SOAP FORMAT

S (subjective data)	What the client or family member says (e.g., "I have a backache").
O (objective data)	Information obtained from the client's records. Assessment of physical indicators. Observation of the client's facial expressions, etc. Changes in behavior, agitation.
A (assessment)	Overall impression or assessment of the problem (e.g., alteration in comfort due to the presence of a headache) with possible etiology of the discomfort included.
P (plan)	Plan of care includes interventions directed if possible toward etiology in diagnosis, e.g. medication as prescribed; the use of therapeutic touch to reduce muscle tension.
O (outcome)	Outcome indicates criteria against which improvement can be measured [e.g., client verbally reports decreased or absent pain, physical indicators (e.g., pulse rate) of pain are within normal limits, and behavior is reflective of the client's normal pattern of interaction].

SOURCE: Adapted from Jones, D., Dunbar, C., and Jirovec, M. (eds.), *Medical-Surgical Nursing: A Conceptual Approach*, 2d ed., McGraw-Hill, New York, 1982.

The *peer review process* is one evaluative mechanism whereby an individual's practice can be determined. Peer review is accomplished by evaluating the process and outcome of a client's health state based on the provider's achievement of standards of care. This can occur in the form of chart audit (or chart review) and/or through the direct observation of the care being delivered. Achievement of the desired standards is one measure that offers data regarding the quality of care offered in a particular agency or unit.

RECORDING CLINICAL DATA

It is critical in this day of cost containment that nursing care be clearly described in terms nurses identify and treat. This information should be identified on the client's record so that during a peer review audit process nursing's role will be clearly visible. Research related to the effects of nursing's performance on long-term client outcomes can be easily quantified. One method would be to evaluate the nurse's response to a data base, as described in Table 2-8.

A SOAP format (see Table 2-9) can be used to record information on specific problems. S, or subjective data, reflects client reporting; O, or objective data, reflects information obtained by the nurse; A refers to assessment of the problem; and P describes the plan. Outcomes of care (i.e., criteria) should also be identified.

SUMMARY

Throughout this presentation there is a continuous interaction between the nature of nursing (e.g., the definition of nursing), the standards of nursing practice, and the nursing process (see Figure 2-6). By clearly describing this interaction, the scope of a nurse's practice becomes easier to articulate to peers. The standards of practice serve to operationally guide nursing's implementation of the definition of nursing, while the steps of the nursing process serve as the vehicle to implement the definition of nursing.

The Handbook of Nursing utilizes the steps of the nursing process. Each description of a health problem is addressed in terms of those changes that accompany the disease process. This is followed by the development of the components of the nursing process as outlined in this chapter (see Figure 2-7).

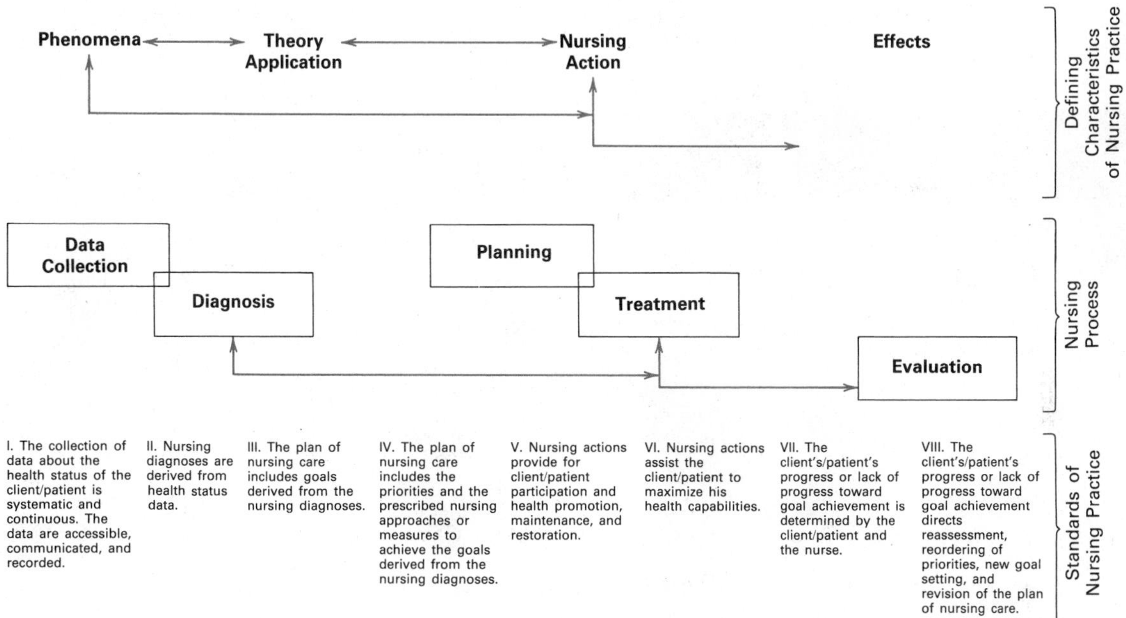

Figure 2-6 Defining characteristics of nursing practice: relationship to the nursing process and the standards of nursing practice. (From *Nursing: A Social Policy Statement*, American Nurses' Association, Congress on Nursing, Kansas City, Mo., 1980, pp. 14–15. Reprinted with the permission of the American Nurses' Association.)

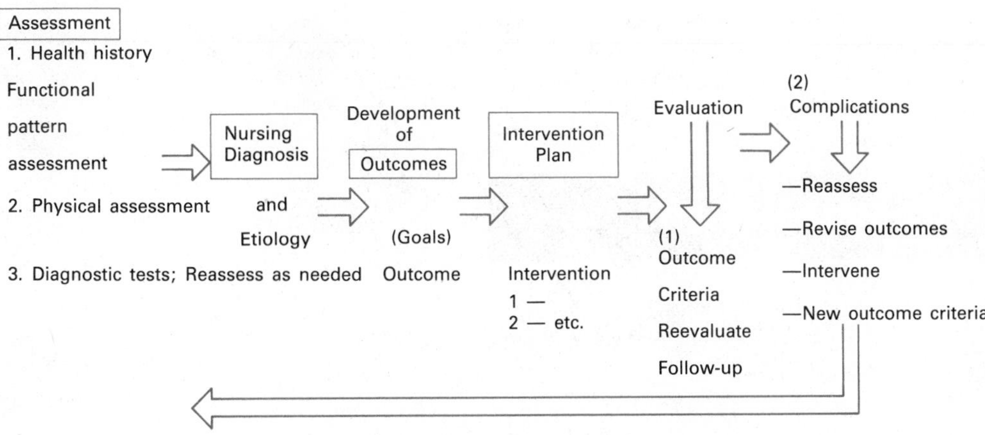

Figure 2-7 Interactive nursing process model.

Through presentation of this model, it is hoped that nurses engaged in clinical practice, regardless of the clinical setting, will adhere to a consistent form of practice and document their actions. By doing so, the role of nursing will be clearly visible and the scope of practice well defined.

REFERENCES

American Nurses' Association: *Nursing: A Social Policy Statement*, Kansas City, Mo., Congress on Nursing Practice, 1980, p. 9.

Gordon, M.: *Nursing Diagnosis: Theory and Process*, McGraw-Hill, New York, 1982, p. 2, 81.

Healthy People: The Surgeon General's Report on Health Promotion and Disease Prevention, publication no. 79-55071, U.S. Department of Health, Education and Welfare, Public Health Service, 1979.

Kim, M. J., and Moritz, D. A.: *Proceedings from the Third and Fourth National Conference on Nursing Diagnosis*, McGraw-Hill, New York, 1982, p. 255.

Kim, M. J., et al. (eds): *Classification of Nursing Diagnoses: Proceedings of the Fifth National Conference*, Mosby, St. Louis, 1984.

Merton, R.: "The Functions of the Professional Association," *American Journal of Nursing*, **58**:50, 1958.

Rogers, M.: *An Introduction to the Theoretical Basis of Nursing*, Davis, Philadelpia, 1970.

Roy, C., and Riehl, J., (eds.): *Conceptual Models for Nursing Practice*, 2d ed., Appleton-Century-Crofts, New York, 1981, p. 8.

Shoemaker, J.: "A Delphi Study on a Definition of Nursing Diagnosis," in Kim, M. J., et al. (eds.), *Proceedings from the Fifth National Conference of the North American Nursing Diagnosis Association*, Mosby, St. Louis, 1983.

Standards of Nursing Practice, American Nurses' Association, Congress for Nursing Practice, 1973, p. 2.

Travis, J.: *Wellness Workbook for Helping Professionals*, Wellness Associates, Mill Valley, Calif., 1981.

BIBLIOGRAPHY

Blattner, B.: *Holistic Nursing*, Prentice-Hall, Englewood Cliffs, N.J., 1981. Excellent text on holistic health principles as they apply to nursing.

Block, D.: "Criteria, Standards, Norms—Crucial Terms in Quality Assurance," *Journal of Nursing Administration*, **7**(9):20, 1977. Excellent resource on the development of standards of care.

Chaska, N.: *The Nursing Profession—A Time to Speak.* McGraw-Hill, New York, 1982. Excellent compilation of readings addressing a number of timely issues affecting nursing and the profession.

Chinn, P., and Jacobs, M.: *Theory and Nursing: A Systematic Approach*, Mosby, St. Louis, 1983.

Field, L.: "The Implementation of Nursing Diagnosis in Clinical Practice," *Nursing Clinics of North America*, **14–18**(3):479, 1979. Excellent article that discusses the use of nursing diagnosis in clinical practice.

Gebbie, C., and Lavin, C.: "Classifying Nursing Diagnosis," *American Journal of Nursing*, **74**(2):250, 1974. Classic article on the proceedings of the Initial Conference for Nursing Diagnosis Development.

Ginsberg, A. D.: *Clinical Reasoning and Patient Care*, Harper & Row, New York, 1980.

Gordon, M.: "Nursing Diagnosis and the Diagnostic Process," *American Journal of Nursing*, **76**(10):1298, 1976.

Gordon, M., and Sweeney, M. A.: "Methodological Problem and Issues in Identifying and Standardizing Nursing Diagnosis," *Advances in Nursing Science* **2**(1):1, 1979. Excellent article on problem research on the diagnostic process.

King, I.: *Toward a Theory for Nursing: General Concepts for Human Behavior*, John Wiley & Sons, New York, 1971.*

Neuman, B.: *The Neuman Systems Model Application to Nursing Education*, Appleton-Century-Crofts, New York, 1982.*

Parse, R. R.: *Man-Living-Health: A Theory of Nursing*, John Wiley & Sons, New York, 1981.*

Patterson, J. G., and Zderad, L.: *Humanistic Nursing*, John Wiley & Sons, New York, 1976.*

Roy, C.: *Introduction to Nursing: An Adaptation Model*, Prentice-Hall, Englewood Cliffs, N.J., 1976.*

Roy, C., and Roberts, S.: *Theory Construction in Nursing*, Prentice-Hall, Engelwood Cliffs, N.J., 1981.*

Soares, C. A.: "Nursing and Medical Diagnosis: Comparison of Variant and Essential Features," in N. L. Chaska (ed.), *The Nursing Profession: Views Through the Mist*, McGraw-Hill, New York, 1978. Presents a comprehensive discussion of the components of the diagnostic process.

Walker, L., and Avant, K.: *Strategies for Theory Construction in Nursing*, Appleton-Century-Crofts, New York, 1983.

* Excellent resources which describe in depth some of the current nursing theories being discussed today.

3

Health Education

Lynne McInerney

Over the past 20 years consumer awareness has developed in every conceivable realm of the marketplace. Sophisticated media have created a consumer who regards "informed choice" as an inalienable right, and the legal system has supported that contention. The health care delivery system is profoundly affected by this change; clients now want to know fully the progress and plan of treatment for their conditions. Professionals must meet this challenge by preparing educational programs that will allow the consumer to be able to maintain his or her health. Client education has always been regarded as something that ought to be done, but who should do it has not always been clear.

According to the American Nurses' Association, a professional nurse is responsible for the quality of nursing care that the client receives. Many licensure laws have specified teaching as a nursing responsibility. Such a responsibility includes teaching relevant facts about specific health care needs and encouraging appropriate modification of behavior. The health education process incorporates intellectual, psychological, and social dimensions, is based on scientific principles, and should result in behavior change. Often nurses have given facts or taught skills to clients, but they need to become more thoroughly involved in seeking behavior change and in evaluating the results of teaching:

> Much of the discrepancy over the role of the nurse as a teacher has been longstanding. Lack of knowledge on the part of the nurse, insufficient time to teach, poor preparation for teaching, and physician dominance have all contributed to the confusion. It is time to state unequivocably that patient teaching is a responsibility of the nurse in all settings. Nurses should be held accountable for delivery of this professional service. They must provide time for teaching and possess necessary knowledge to educate the public. To clearly establish the teaching role for the professional nurse, nurses must document and evaluate the effects of these teaching activities on the maintenance, retention, and attainment of maximum health (Jones, 1978).

Human beings are the most complex species in the phylogeneic order, requiring decades to develop fully into functioning, independent adults. Many factors determine and influence this growth and development. In order to recognize influential factors, one must organize the relevant information about learning. For the purposes of this chapter, four areas are highlighted: biological, developmental, cultural, and socioeconomic. Information gathered from these areas will constitute the background for the nurse's assessment of an individual's need for learning and will be essential in creating an appropriate learning environment and teaching strategy.

TABLE 3-1 BIOLOGICAL DIFFERENCES RELATED TO TEACHING STRATEGIES

Research Findings	Derived Stereotypes	Teaching Strategies
FEMALES		
Increased hearing acuity throughout life: Increased sensitivity to sound, especially mother's voice Increased startle response Increased ability to sing in tune	Generally more fearful than males, especially of the unknown.	Utilize audio equipment and verbal reinforcement for all visual input. Pace content and activities to individual's learning rate.
Earlier speaking and larger vocabularies than males: Increased facility for foreign languages Earlier reading Greater attention to social contexts (focus, speech patterns, subtle vocal cues) or metacommunications	More studious: better at languages, writing, social sentences; more intuitive; enjoy talking.	Allow adequate time for discussion, questions, and answers. Utilize group discussion sessions enhance scope of understanding and clarify social ramifications of newly acquired behaviors. Provide written instructions.
Better at fine motor skills.	Better at detailed, intricate work; poor at sports and activities requiring gross motor coordination.	When psychomotor skills are taught, allow more time for verbal explanation, demonstration, and return demonstration.
Use of both cerebral hemispheres for tasks involving spatial concepts. (This integration process increases reaction time.)	Poor at hard sciences, working with machines, and making decisions under pressure.	Allow more time for practice sessions and return demonstration when dealing with multiple learning tasks (e.g., administering specific doses of insulin based on Dextro-Stix test). Use three dimensional models and drawings as visual aids. Trouble shoot potential areas for complication by setting up problem situations the client must resolve.
MALES		
Earlier visual superiority.	Are better than females at jobs requiring supervision. Prefer to observe rather than interact.	Use visual aids to augment any verbal or written instructions. Provide time for the client to practice on his own before returning the demonstration.

TABLE 3-1 *(continued)*

Research Findings	Derived Stereotypes	Teaching Strategies
		Avoid group discussions in the early stages of learning; focus on visual input.
Different levels of responsiveness.	More curious about their environment. Poor attention spans. Poor students. Quick reaction time.	Make teaching sessions shorter and more frequent to avoid sensory overload. Remove superfluous stimuli from the immediate environment. Introduce each teaching aid individually as needed.
Better total body coordination or gross motor skills than females.	Better at sports than females. Hyperactive.	Allow for frequent stretch breaks. Allow more time for practice and return demonstration when teaching fine motor skills (i.e., insulin administration, dressing changes, etc.). Clearly define and demonstrate any required limitations in physical activity.
Use of right hemisphere in tasks involving spatial concepts; therefore, better manipulation of three-dimensional space and faster reaction time.	Better in hard sciences, working with machines, making decisions under pressure.	Discuss and/or demonstrate potential problems and appropriate interventions. Practice reviewing all alternatives to a problem before selecting appropriate response.

BIOLOGICALLY INHERENT DIFFERENCES IN LEARNING

There are biological differences between men and women, and in this age of role diffusion and confusion it is important to look at how these objective differences influence the way men and women learn (see Table 3-1).

Cultural understandings regarding biological abilities may vary widely and are often deeply felt and irrational, that is, unrelated to factual evidence. These cultural understandings form basic stereotypic roles and most learning environments have supported these roles. For instance, in the United States before the 1960s women were expected to be:

1. Gentle, warm, and sensitive.
2. Nonassertive, other-directed, supportive of others.
3. Passive, dependent.

Men were expected to be:

1. Aggressive, hard-driving, hard-playing.
2. Assertive, goal-oriented, blunt.
3. Active, independent.

Today, roles are in transition and are emerging into a more rational relationship which considers developmental and biological differences between individuals.

It is important to recognize the objective differences and separate these from subjective conclusions based on culturally ascribed roles. By doing so the nurse may maximize strengths and provide an optimal learning environment for either sex. Biological differences are noted from infancy and have implications for structuring the learning environment throughout life. When teaching strategies are based on objective research, the learner is able to achieve his or her goal and avoid the stigma of stereotypes and culturally ascribed roles. In essence, the bias in learning is removed. The key lies in structuring the learning environment to develop strengths and minimize limitations.

DEVELOPMENTAL DIFFERENCES IN LEARNING

Just as there are specific biological differences, there are changes in learning readiness and focus related to the developmental process. These changes require modifications in teaching strategies to promote learning (see Table 3-2). The learning environment should be aligned with the specific developmental level of the

TABLE 3-2 DEVELOPMENTAL DIFFERENCES IN LEARNING

Learning Style	Teaching Strategy
CHILDREN	
Egocentric: concerned only with how a specific event will affect "me." See themselves as the cause of all reactions in their environment.	Avoid all superfluous information and focus only on those aspects that will have direct impact. Answer questions specifically; avoid broad descriptions or additional information. Listen for "magical" thinking; use reinforcement to assure the child that a situation did not occur because of his or her misbehavior.
Concrete thought process: unable to deal with concepts or abstractions or focus attention for long periods.	Always use concrete terms and examples; avoid other people's experiences or stories with a moral; relate explanation to the child's own experience; use the child's language. Time is a concept; make it concrete by using a timer, the length of a TV program, when the sun rises or sets, etc. Explanations should be brief and restricted to events happening in the immediate time frame.
Learn best through play activities.	Utilize play activities to prepare for procedures; use drawing, clay, role play with dolls and toys; help child express anger with dolls. A child deals best with fear and pain through guided visualization: what color is it, what size box does it fit in, how does it taste and sound; repeat the process until the fear gradually dissipates. Make several play activities available at any given time.

TABLE 3-2 *(continued)*

Learning Style	Teaching Strategy
	If possible, allow for activities that require gross motor exercise. If possible, change the play environment (bed, chair, playroom, etc.).
Inseparable from significant others: not able to see themselves as individuals apart from their parents or siblings.	Encourage parents to remain with the child throughout a hospital stay. If possible, parents should be present during a traumatic procedure and always immediately following. Provide special toys or comforting blankets from home. Establish trust by keeping all promises that are made. Answer all questions honestly. Set aside the same time each day to review needs and progress with the child. Acknowledge the perception without contradicting it; deal with the fear that causes misperceptions. If you tell a child what he or she feels is not real, the child will cease to trust you.
ADOLESCENTS	
Egocentric: self-absorbed and self-conscious. Dealing with identity.	Explain procedures in relation to physical and social effect on adolescent. Set realistic goals for recovery period that include criteria for measuring expected outcomes. Structure time and interaction to allow for ventilation of feelings. Acknowledge fears and give reality feedback. Provide for and respect the adolescent's privacy.
Abstract thought process begins: now able to deal with concepts and transfer them to their own experience.	Address concepts such as pain, fear, loneliness, etc., when dealing with threatening procedures or lifestyle change. Structure time and interaction to allow for personal exploration of feelings. Encourage definition of values and decision-making skills by talking about priorities and alternative choices in behavior. Facilitate problem-solving behavior by including the adolescent in planning his or her care.
Strongly identified with a peer group.	Whenever possible, be flexible and allow choices but set firm limits.

TABLE 3-2 *(continued)*

Learning Style	Teaching Strategy
	Avoid criticizing maladaptive behaviors; place the emphasis on complimenting adaptive coping skills. Group teaching is very beneficial, but avoid singling out individuals as examples and use a democratic style of leadership.
ADULTS	
Reality-oriented and interested in control.	Determine the individual's priorities in the learning process (i.e., learn to administer an insulin injection *before* understanding diabetes as a disease). Develop teaching plan around the client's priorities. Always include client in the goal-setting and evaluation process. Set realistic goals that include criteria for measuring expected outcomes. Do periodic evaluations of progress. Build flexibility and choices into learning activity.
Problem-oriented.	Evaluate traditional methods of problem solving by asking how the individual has handled previous situations; listen for and identify coping mechanisms. Utilize or adapt teaching to the individual's traditional method of problem solving. Break learning tasks into subsets and define the goal of each subset clearly.
Concerned about preserving self-esteem. Dealing with intimacy.	Avoid all value judgments regarding the client's lifestyle or behavior; use objective research to point out causal relationships between behavior and disease. Develop a series of questions to determine baseline knowledge in a given area prior to planning teaching. Do not assume any previous level of knowledge.
ELDERLY	
Limited physically: strength decreases; speed, intensity, and endurance of neuromuscular reaction decrease.	Allow more time for the overall teaching plan to be accomplished. Set realistic goals based on the extended time necessary for healing to occur. Make teaching sessions short. Begin each session with a brief review of the previous lesson. Include a relative or close friend in the teaching process.

TABLE 3-2 *(continued)*

Learning Style	Teaching Strategy
	When dealing with psychomotor skills, begin teaching these as soon as physically possible, allowing for practice and return demonstration. Arrange for follow-up home teaching if psychomotor skills are not satisfactory by the time of discharge from the hospital setting.
Impaired perceptual ability: vision and hearing frequently affected.	Have any necessary equipment available (glasses, hearing aids, magnifying glass, etc.). Use a well-lighted area, preferably natural or indirect lighting. Use large, bold, clearly defined printing in any visual aid. Screen out all extraneous noise (phones, TV, radio, other conversations, air conditioners, machines, etc.). Speak slowly and clearly; maintain eye contact; do not elevate the pitch of your voice to speak louder. Use audiovisual programs very selectively and only as a review of material given on a one-to-one basis.
Egocentric: well-established patterns.	Focus only on those aspects of care that will directly affect the client; eliminate superfluous information. Speak directly when attempting to elicit information. Agree on a separate time for therapeutic interactions that are not directly related to the teaching plan.

learner. A frequent error made in client education is an attempt to teach in a didactic classroom approach similar to that used in school. This approach does not transfer well to a one-to-one relationship of bedside teaching or to instructing small groups of older clients in a clinic. Teaching strategies must be geared to the assessed level of ability and maturation.

CULTURAL VARIATIONS IN LEARNING

Belief systems are handed down through culture and are internalized over time. Belief systems contain the values by which people live their lives and provide moral yardsticks by which all behaviors and actions are judged in the cultural group. Belief systems underlie each person's perception of self in relation to God, family, other persons, and to the world as a whole. This perception is a vitally important component of how individuals choose to live their lives. People are motivated to learn those things perceived as being important. Clearly, in order to motivate individuals to change their behavior regarding health, the nurse must first understand what these values encompass. Knowing an individual's orientation to the various components that make up his or her value system will enable the nurse to appeal to those values that support change.

Because each culture has a unique orientation to these values, six areas present in every culture will serve as a useful evaluation tool in determining cross-cultural differences (Table 3-3). There are many degrees of adherence to these values, so that only the continuum or the direction may be recognized. In general, older persons tend to hold more strongly to "ways of the group" but when under stress many younger persons also search for structure and comfort in doing things the way the cultural group has done in generations past.

Cultures also vary in the degree of control individuals expect. A useful, brief tool to determine the emphasis held by a particular patient is found in Table 3-4. The continuum proceeds from no control (fate) to self-blame for becoming ill. Until the degree of inner control is evident for an individual, any teaching strategy may be ineffective.

SOCIOECONOMIC STATE

Just as adaptations in teaching strategy need to be made for sex, age, and culture, so must they be made to account for socioeconomic status, as that status might influence educational level, experience, and comprehension of abstract concepts. The nurse needs to recognize that stereotyping is possible and that teaching strategies should not be based on one's own style of learning but on the client's style.

The way a person comes to perceive and experience the world is directly related to the kinds of opportunities that are available for that person. The structure of the learning environment influences how one thinks and learns. It is reasonable to assume that children growing up in a disadvantaged environment may learn in different ways. Redman (1980) has taken some of these ways and applied them to teaching with an awareness of the person's background of life experiences (see Table 3-5). The table should be utilized with the understanding that these are generalizations. Individualizing education for the particular client will include gathering data to determine if indeed this person is thus affected by prior learning experiences.

STAGE OF ACCEPTANCE OF ILLNESS

Redman (1980) has also helped the nurse recognize that during illness there are stages of adaptation and that teaching is best done during the stage of reorganization of priorities when the client is looking for alternatives. Usually there is denial and anger before this stage and learning is inhibited. Similarly, a lack of readiness to learn is also seen following childbirth during the stage of "taking-in," according to Rubin (see Chapter 9). During the second phase of recovery, the "taking-hold" stage, the mother faces the implications of caring for the infant and is suddenly very eager for any assistance the nurse may provide.

Listed below are stages of adaptation to illness and typical phrases with which a client might express such feelings (Redman, 1972).

Stages of Adaptation	**Comments by Clients**
1. Disbelief, causing a flight to imaged health.	1. "I don't have TB. I feel perfectly happy."
2. Beginning awareness of condition: angry feelings emerge.	2. "Dammit! Why am I so tired all the time?"
3. Reorganization of priorities.	3. "I guess playing tennis isn't all *that* important."

TABLE 3-3 CONTINUUM OF VALUES

Six Common Areas Found in Each Culture	Teaching Strategies
HUMANKIND VS. NATURE (sense of destiny) This relates to how humans see themselves in relation to a high power (i.e., God, the universe). Some cultures place human beings in close proximity to God as His highest creation. It is a very personal and private relationship. There is no predominant belief in reincarnation, but rather one lifetime to resolve human weaknesses and perfect virtues. Humans are responsible and accountable for their actions. God is just: goodness is rewarded, evil punished.	Western civilization tends to see humans as the cause of their own fortune or misfortune and as highly likely to mobilize forces in their behalf. Appealing to these values can be beneficial in presenting alternative behaviors and outcomes. Preventing illness by promoting healthy habits has a real chance of success because the tendency is to try to control.
Other cultures and philosophies see human beings as part of the natural order of all living things and, as such, in no greater position of power. Humans are responsible for maintaining that order and for learning from life's lessons. All life events are regarded as opportunities to grow in perfection. Each reincarnated lifetime brings one closer to that goal, if nature's laws are not violated. Hardships may be regarded as part of the learning process or debts for transgressions of a previous life.	Some cultures tend to feel many factors influence an event and may be less likely to mobilize personal forces in their own behalf. There may be less urgency to resolve a situation and more thought put into the solution. Appealing to reestablishing the balance in one's life may be far more effective here. Living in harmony with mind, body, and spirit provides an excellent incentive for promoting healthy lifestyles. The tendency is to accept so the nurse should differentiate between the things one can change and those that one *cannot* change.
GOOD VS. BAD (in basic human nature) Each culture reflects about basic human nature through the socialization process. There are those cultures that believe that human beings need rigorous discipline and stringent rules and regulations in order to develop into responsible, law-abiding citizens. Left to their own means, humans would not have the integrity to make wise decisions. This has been the basis for many puritanical movements in history.	Cultures that overuse discipline and rigid structure frequently produce people who ignore their health in favor of adherence to group norms (i.e., success). They feel guilty about becoming ill and also feel they "deserve it" for failing in some area. The individual needs assistance in developing his/her own priorities within the system. Encouraging the group to incorporate positive health habits is essential. Making these habits a part of "the program" may succeed.
Other cultures subscribe to the belief that human beings are basically good and thus require little guidance to express themselves appropriately. There is a great emphasis on personal freedom and tolerance for individual expression.	Cultures that minimize discipline can create individuals who have little practice with schedules or goal setting. Exposing them to health habits that feel good and fit into a flexible lifestyle can work. Individualizing any plan is essential.
OPEN VS. CLOSED (sense of privacy) Every culture teaches its group certain norms regarding privacy. These laws govern everything from acceptable distance between people in social situations to how	It is important to respect the territorial bounds of an individual. Simple manners, such as knocking on doors before entering and asking permission to touch or sit close, can convey respect for a person's bounda-

TABLE 3-3 *(continued)*

Six Common Areas Found in Each Culture	Teaching Strategies
many people and whom one lives with. An individual's sense of privacy is developed to protect the ego boundaries of the personality. In some cultures the accepted distance between people in a social situation is approximately 3 ft, or arm's length. To come any closer, without being invited, is a breech of social conduct and is regarded as a threatening gesture. Touching someone without permission is a violation of his personal space and can be punishable by law. Family problems are considered confidential and are dealt with in the nuclear group.	ries. The way information is requested is just as crucial as the confidentiality clause. Interventions should be structured so that they meet the clients needs without violating privacy.
For other cultures, the acceptable distance between people in social situations may be a matter of inches. Touching is an integral part of communicating a complete thought. The basic unit of structure is the extended family, and this may include individuals who are not blood relatives. Living conditions frequently encompass housing several generations under one roof. Family problems may be shared with the entire extended family.	It is often difficult to adapt rules and environment to incorporate this orientation. Arrangements should be made for family members to stay with the client on a rotating basis to allow for as much contact as possible. The client should indicate which members will be involved in direct home care, and teaching sessions should be planned with these people present.
PRESENT VS. FUTURE (orientation to time) Every culture has a sense of its own life span and develops an orientation to time. Some cultures are *future* oriented. Specific life goals are defined at an early age, and there is a great sense of urgency about achieving them. People work, talk and act quickly in the pursuit of "getting ahead" of their own timetables and their neighbors. There are many rewards for being able to do more, better, quicker. Time is scarce.	Frequently, crisis events are the only times a person ever stops to evaluate life patterns. This presents a unique opportunity to help a person gain insight into behaviors that are maladaptive and consider alternatives. Helping the client understand the choices that are available and the associated benefits is important in facilitating adherence.
Other cultures are *present* oriented. There is no past, no future, only now. Although certain achievements are expected to occur someday, they are not planned for years in advance; they will evolve, in good time. There is no sense of urgency; time is not scarce. One can do nothing about the past and little about the future, until it arrives.	Compliance with prophylactic treatment tends to be a major problem. Teaching plans to create *daily* schedules for health care needs are necessary for clients with this frame of reference. Appointments should be made to coincide with the need for reinforcement. Frequent contact with health care professionals in satellite community clinics and home care visits will be effective in ensuring compliance.

TABLE 3-3 *(continued)*

Six Common Areas Found in Each Culture	Teaching Strategies
TIGHT VS. LOOSE (relation to other significant persons) Each culture determines the structural unit that will be vested with the responsibility for conveying group norms or values. How that unit is defined affects how its members will cope with life. The nuclear family (husband, wife, and children) is representative of a tight structure. This nuclear family, whether it be a large or small group, functions autonomously from other members of the extended family in its own dwelling. Frequently, family members are not even geographically close at hand, which further emphasizes the autonomy. Members of the group rely only on one another to meet their respective needs in life. Children are expected to leave home at a prescribed age and begin their own nuclear families.	Cultures that have families who are this tightly bound experience a great deal of stress. All the responsibilities for raising a family and dealing with life's events are vested in a very small unit that does not easily ask for assistance from the extended family and frequently ends up seeking support from agencies that have no vested interest in their personal survival. Developing the extended family as a support group would be the best choice. A viable alternative is to teach people to cultivate a broad circle of friends who will function as a support system during times of stress (see Chapter 5).
The extended family is a loose structure. This group usually consists of several generations living together or in close proximity and may also include aunts, uncles, cousins, and friends who are not blood relatives. Members of the extended family regard one another as vital contributors to their physical, emotional, spiritual, and financial well-being. It is expected that each member will be responsible for the life of the group as a whole.	The extended family offers a broad support system for any of its members who need assistance. Children growing up in this system can escape accountability for their actions by simply changing "parents" until the coast is clear. It is sometimes difficult to determine who is really in charge of anything, because everyone is! Compliance tends to diminish within such a system, so it is important to make a *contract* with one or two members who will ensure direct support in helping the client comply with treatment.
INTERNAL VS. EXTERNAL (locus of control) Each culture gives the individuals within it varying degrees of power. The degree to which people feel they can make changes in their lives and communities is a reflection of that power. The belief that one can or cannot effect change is called *locus of control.* No culture is predominantly internal or external regarding locus of control. Individuals within a culture who believe that life's events were or could be affected by their own behavior are said to have an *internal* locus of control. In other words, they feel they can make changes and control the destiny of their lives. Political leaders, executives, and entrepreneurs are ex-	These individuals respond very well to health promotion programs. In any plan of teaching they require an extra degree of control over their learning environment. Providing appropriate information, resources, and assistance may be all they will require in constructing their own plan of care.

TABLE 3-3 (continued)

Six Common Areas Found in Each Culture	Teaching Strategies
amples of individuals who are considered to be highly internal regarding locus of control.	
Individuals within a culture who believe that life's events were not or could not be contingent on their actions are said to have an *external* locus of control. They feel relatively helpless and powerless to control the destiny of their lives (see Table 3-4).	In approaching a teaching situation it is important that learning tasks be broken into simple subsets, with clear behavioral expectations for each task. Previous sessions should be reviewed before a new objective is begun. Having a significant person present during the teaching process to reinforce and encourage learning will help.

TABLE 3-4 STATEMENTS ABOUT YOUR HEALTH TO DETERMINE EMPHASIS ON INTERNAL OR EXTERNAL LOCUS OF CONTROL[a]

	Strongly Agree 1	Moderately Agree 2	Neutral 3	Moderately Disagree 4	Strongly Disagree 5
1. If I take care of myself, I can avoid illness.					
2. Good health is largely a matter of good fortune, so no matter what I do, if I am going to get sick, I will get sick.					
3. Getting help when I need it depends on my ability to talk with my doctor and other health resource people.					
4. When I feel ill, I believe it is because I have not been getting the proper exercise or eating right.					
5. If we are sad, we should try not to let anyone know.					
6. I will have better control of my life by increasing the knowledge I have of my disease.					
7. I can do only what my doctor tells me to do.					
8. I am directly responsible for my health and physical fitness.					
9. Stress can be associated with both pleasant and painful events.					
10. It is beneficial to communicate with my family, including children, about my disease.					

SOURCE: From "I Can Cope," a patient education program of the American Cancer Society, homework assignment 3, class 3, "Dealing with Daily Health."

[a] This questionnaire will be instrumental in determining how much control an individual feels he or she has over health issues. Each score should be looked at separately.

TABLE 3-5 EFFECTS OF SOCIOECONOMIC LEVEL ON THE LEARNING PROCESS

Lower Level	Teaching Strategies	Middle to Upper Level	Teaching Strategies
Uses inductive thought process. Events that are observed in the environment are grouped together in order to create theories.	Discuss details and observable events/symptoms first, then relate these to big picture.	*Uses deductive thought process.* Theories are postulated and tested by observing events in the environment.	Discuss the issues, the big picture, before going into details.
Usually problem-centered. Motivated to make change when there is a readily defined problem (i.e., "The problem with having diabetes is that I can't eat cake.").	Break broad issues into subsets and use the client's problem-solving mechanisms to define the problem and resolve it. Relate each problem and solution back to the broader issue.	May be *abstract-centered.* Able to think about cause and effect on a larger scale (i.e., "Having to change my whole lifestyle.").	Talk about cause-and-effect relationships on a broad level but get down to identifying the client's particular problem areas.
Learns more easily when content is related to actions.	Utilize modeling, demonstration, return demonstration teaching techniques.	Verbal-conceptual in approach to learning.	Provide written/verbal instructions.
Externally oriented. Behavior is motivated by tangible, observable events (i.e., "I am going to lose weight so I can wear that dress next week.").	Determine what is important to the client and base your strategies on rewarding those areas.	*Introspective.* Behavior is motivated by thinking of how the broad issue affects the individual (i.e., "I have to learn to handle anxiety in more productive ways than overeating.")	Guide client to look at health-related issues from a personal perspective by giving him or her information that raises awareness, followed by discussion of personal habits in those areas.
One-track focus. Deals best with single tasks in sequence.	Break broad issues into smaller subsets and limit information to topic at hand.	*Comprehensive focus.* May work on several aspects of task.	When discussing broad issues, enumerate the potential consequences and then deal with those that are relevant to the client.
Content-oriented. Wants to master the skill first.	Provide simple tasks and procedures first.	*Process-oriented.* Wants to know why and how before accepting task; remembers oral instructions. Aural skills are usually well developed.	Responds well to understanding global nature of problem or treatment first.
Uses visual, tactile senses as ways to reinforce learning.	Present pictures and three-dimensional objects as a way to reinforce learning. Audiovisual aids are more successful than only audio instruction.		Utilize audiovisual aids and listening as a way to reinforce learning.

Stages of Adaptation	Comments by Clients
4. Resolution and identity change.	4. "Lots of important people have been ill like this and still done work and been happy."
5. Recovery or rehabilitation.	5. "As long as I have to take life at a slower pace, I am glad I have my hobbies."

Behaviors related to health are learned (Figure 3-1). Smokers learn to smoke; eaters learn to overeat or undereat; worriers learn to worry. Understanding how people learn health habits is crucial to helping them change those behaviors that are maladaptive. Although the objective of health education has been to help people adopt healthier lifestyles or to comply with prescribed medical treatment, emphasis has been on dissemination of information, not on behavior change. Information and concepts are essential parts of learning but are only the first steps. An equal amount of effort must be placed on the values and attitudes regarding specific behaviors that are important to maintain health.

Because learning is defined as a change in behavior, it can occur in any one of the following *domains*:

1. *Cognitive:* Facts and concepts.
2. *Affective:* Attitudes and values.
3. *Psychomotor:* Physical and manipulative skills.

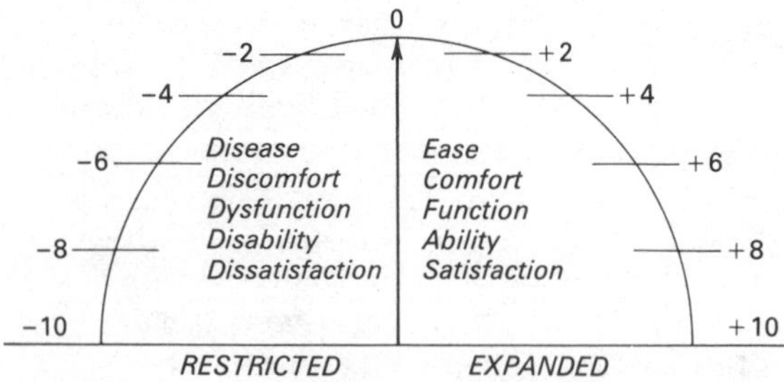

Figure 3-1 "Health is not just the absence of disease, it is a physical, psychological and spiritual sense of well being." (World Health Organization. Adapted from Pion, R., "Facilitated Learning in Health Care," *New Approaches to Counseling and Communication*, Medical Communications & Services Association, Seattle, Wash.)

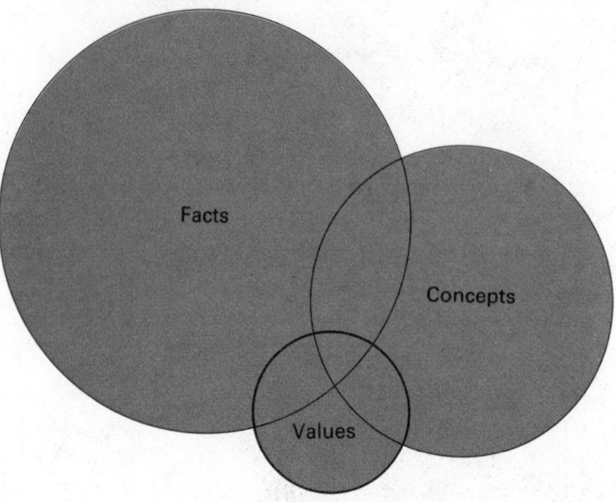

Figure 3-2 FACTS: Information that may be interpreted in a variety of ways, "other oriented" (e.g., heart disease is the number one killer in the United States). CONCEPTS: Truisms derived from grouping related facts that hold true with different combinations of facts and situations; "relationship centered" (e.g., smoking causes heart disease and cancer). VALUES: The criteria one uses for choosing among alternatives; a standard of preference that directs our performance; "me directed" (e.g., how am I handling smoking?). (From Fors, S., "Getting It Together," *Achieving High Level Wellness*, **1**(5): 200–206, Sept/Oct, 1977.)

The domains of learning are a useful way to regard how people learn. The phrase "simple to complex" may refer to levels in each domain. One generally acquires knowledge before being able to apply, analyze, or synthesize ideas. Usually, there is movement between domains; "nothing is purely cognitive, affective, or psychomotor. Rather, it should be noted that objectives overlap and when a psychomotor task is performed, cognitive and affective learning may also be present" (Jones, 1977). (See Figure 3-2.) In formulating a teaching-learning plan, the nurse should identify if the task or behavior is fairly complex and should be divided into smaller steps for easier learning (see Table 3-6).

With the baseline data of how learning takes place and how illness may affect learning, the nurse may then use the nursing process in planning for the *teaching-learning transaction* (TLT). This interaction is one in which specific objectives are met. The objectives must be those with which the client can agree and must promote

TABLE 3-6 DOMAINS OF LEARNING

COGNITIVE DOMAIN	
Knowledge	Recall of factual information.
Comprehension	Ability to translate or interpret information and summarize events.
Application	Translation of concepts learned in the classroom to the real situation.
Analysis	Investigation of the relationship of ideas, elements, principles; ability to distinguish fact from hypothesis; comparison between facts.
Synthesis	Combination of ideas to form a whole; formulation of hypotheses; design of an experiment.
Evaluation	Ability to problem solve, analyze, synthesize, make judgments based on the facts, and arrive at a solution.
AFFECTIVE DOMAIN	
Receiving (attending)	Awareness of color arrangement and design; willingness to receive information when others speak; tolerance for others; alertness to human values and judgment; some discrimination of music.
Responding	Willingness to respond by acquainting oneself with specific rules and regulations; assumption of responsibility for self and others; enjoyment of self-expression in art, music.
Valuing	Acceptance of others in speaking and writing effectively; identification with all human beings in their struggle for survival; commitment; willingness to hear all sides of an argument.
Organization	Conceptualization of values; adjustments regarding social issues; consideration of alternatives.
Characterization (value or value complex)	Willingness to change opinion in light of new data; tendency to be less rigid, making decisions after all the facts are in; development of a personal philosophy of life based on individual ideals and goals.
PSYCHOMOTOR LEVELS	
Imitation	Exposure to an observable action resulting in covert then overt repetition of the activity; performance often reflecting limited coordination of musculoskeletal system.
Manipulation	Development of skill in following directions, performing selected activities, then fixing the performance by practice; ability to carry out a specific activity according to a set of instructions and not merely by imitation.
Precision	Improved coordination, refined performance; ability to carry out an action without a model or set of directions.
Articulation	Coordination of multiple activities through establishment of an appropriate sequence, achieving harmony and consistency among different acts.
Naturalization	Proficiency at performing a single act skillfully in an almost routine, automatic, spontaneous way.

SOURCE: Adapted from *Taxonomy of Educational Objectives, Handbook I: Cognitive Domain*, by Benjamin S. Bloom, et al.

maintenance of self-care for the client. It is most useful to set the goals together with the client or with the family members.

Data may be collected from the client and family interview, review of medical records, review of current treatment and medical plan, and conferences with other health workers. Problems are identified and knowledge is built upon the baseline understanding demonstrated by patient and family. Learning outcomes or objectives should be chosen for the domains of learning. If the behavior sought after is one associated with facts or knowledge, the objective is classified as cognitive. (What does the client need to know?) If the person is to perform a physical task, the objective is psychomotor. (What motor skills should he or she possess?) If the desired behavior is a change of attitude, values or feelings, the objective is affective (review Table 3-6). Choose a behavioral outcome that is specific and time-related. Plan a definite sequence, usually going from simple to more complex ideas or skills. When the client chooses the sequence, a larger degree of control is perceived, but the sequence may vary from this "ideal." Client involvement in the plan is worth more, however, than a careful sequence.

Useful objectives or learning outcomes contain several major components:

1. A *doer*. This is the subject. When the learning has been achieved, *who* is to do the task?
2. A *behavior*, or product. *What* is the behavior that will demonstrate mastery, or *what* will be the results of the behavior? An action verb must be used that can be measured in order to determine the success of the learner (e.g., *list, demonstrate, walk*).
3. A *stimulus*, or condition. This is a *circumstance*: any experience or resource or special environmental influence that must be accounted for while learning or while doing the task.
4. A *standard of performance*, or criterion. This is the measure of how well the task will be performed. It may be something accomplished within a time limit, accurately recalled, something measured by testing, or appropriately demonstrated.

Guidelines for the teaching-learning plan are given in Table 3-7, and a model of the teaching-learning transaction is seen in Table 3-8. Table 3-9 contains a TLT for an individual client after learning problems have been identified. Note

TABLE 3-7 GUIDELINES FOR TEACHING-LEARNING PLAN

Teaching-learning transactions should be individualized to each client or group of clients.

Assessment of each learner, including limitations as well as strengths, before the learning experience facilitates the teaching-learning process.

Readiness to learn is critical to the teaching transaction and is often determined by the client.

Teaching plans should begin at the proper level for the client.

Mutual goals for the teaching-learning plan should be developed by the client and nurse, when possible.

Learning should be goal-directed with measurable outcomes established, when possible (cognitive, psychomotor, affective).

Intermittent evaluation is important to the teaching-learning process; therefore, a feedback mechanism should be established.

Teaching strategies should be varied and complement an individual's learning style and meet the client's readiness.

Client motivation to learn increases when information imparted will have a significant impact on an individual's life.

When possible, the client should be allowed a choice in acquiring new information.

Current lifestyle and cultural practice as well as family participation should all be incorporated into the teaching transaction.

The learning environment should be conducive to the learning process and, when possible, distractions should be eliminated.

The teaching plan should build in reinforcements, such as written directions for follow-up in the home and home visit, when possible.

The nurse should operate as a facilitator of the teaching-learning transaction, enhancing the learning experience whenever possible.

The nurse must be adept in the subject taught, be able to adjust to the level of the client, and establish rapport early.

SOURCE: Jones, D., et al. (eds.): *Medical-Surgical Nursing: A Conceptual Approach*, McGraw-Hill, New York, 1978.

TABLE 3-8 TEACHING-LEARNING TRANSACTION: SAMPLE

PROFILE OF THE LEARNER

Description of the population: factory blue collar workers, average intelligence, high school graduates (motivation to learn, strong support systems).

Learning environment: local school auditorium, limited resources.

Teaching-learning need: normal nutrition and a well-balanced diet.

GOALS OF THE TRANSACTION

Improve nutritional state through a well-balanced diet.

Change attitudes in eating habits and food selection.

CONSTRAINTS TO THE INTERACTION

Psychological: personal problems, attention span decreased, anxiety.

Physical: current health problem, pain.

Environment: uncomfortable seats, poor acoustics, poor equipment.

Sociocultural: limited income; content presented in conflict with cultural eating pattern.

Other: disinterest in attending the workshop.

STUDENT OBJECTIVES

After a workshop on the daily components of a balanced diet, the learner will do the following:

1. List in writing all the basic foods included in a balanced diet.
2. Pick out the basic foods from a menu given in class with 90% accuracy.
3. Plan a balanced diet according to guidelines presented in class.

CONTENT TO BE TAUGHT

Purpose of a balanced diet.

Health problems that can occur when an unbalanced diet is followed.

Basic components of normal nutrition.

Foods that should be used to achieve a balanced diet.

Nutritional value of each food discussed.

Discussion of a well-balanced menu and food selection.

ASSESSMENT OF ACHIEVEMENT

List of the basic foods with 100% accuracy.

Food selection with 90% accuracy.

Plan menu containing all the basic foods according to the class lecture.

An interview which reflects personal views.

STRATEGY FOR TEACHING/LEARNING

Film on a balanced diet.

Slide tape on food selection.

Lecture.

Small group discussions on menu planning, and health maintenance.

Food budgets.

Attending two nutritional laboratory sessions.

Lifestyle.

EVALUATION

Evaluation based on achievement of the objectives.

Follow-up test to evaluate compliance.

SOURCE: Jones, D., et al. (eds.): *Medical-Surgical Nursing: A Conceptual Approach*, McGraw-Hill, New York, 1978.

TABLE 3-9 TEACHING-LEARNING TRANSACTION FOR POST-DELIVERY LEARNING: EXAMPLE

PROFILE OF THE LEARNER

Biological, developmental status: age 22, female, first infant, first pregnancy.

Cultural, socioeconomic status: comes from group with shared privacy in extended family.

Teaching-learning need: caring for first infant, desires breastfeeding; has been told by relative that she will not make enough milk and must supplement with formula.

GOALS OF THE TRANSACTION

Select nutrients to support production of breast milk.

Learn skill of breastfeeding, including ways of solving minor discomforts.

Respond positively to infant, gaining satisfaction from process of providing nourishment.

CONSTRAINTS TO THE INTERACTION

Physical: recovering from normal birth and episiotomy discomfort.

Psychological: happy with child's sex, but feels inadequate during "taking hold" phase of emotional adjustment.

Sociocultural: no prior study of subject, read no literature; content may conflict with present eating pattern; does not drink milk; breastfeeding techniques conflict with mother-in-law's ideas.

Environment: time/space: to be discharged within 24 h; teaching environment has many interruptions.

STUDENT OBJECTIVES

Mother will write down list of foods she should increase or avoid during breastfeeding.

After viewing film on breastfeeding techniques, she will identify those that are comfortable for her to use.

Mother will demonstrate positive affective response to infant during feeding.

Mother will be able to verbalize signs of infant satisfaction after feeding.

With the aid of breastfeeding literature, mother will recall verbally the signs of breast engorgement, or mastitis, and will identify when to use home remedies and when to call physician.

CONTENT TO BE TAUGHT

Basic food groups and changes for lactation; need for milk and protein intake.

Need for extra fluid intake.

Weight control during lactation.

Correct positioning of infant, intervals of feeding, signs of satisfaction.

Minor difficulties that may arise during lactation.

ASSESSMENT OF ACHIEVEMENT

Infant has appropriate weight gain at first pediatrician examination.

Good tissue turgor and moist mucous membranes are noted; stooling is within normal range.

Mother's weight returns gradually to normal while she eats the recommended distribution of foods.

STRATEGY FOR TEACHING/LEARNING

Small group discussion on foods during breastfeeding.

Chart of illustrated weight loss.

Literature containing basic food groups for lactation.

Film on breast care and feeding techniques (if needed: demonstration for mother about use of breast pump, so that she may see the volume and appearance of her breast milk).

Illustrations of how baby will suck, grasp nipple.

Demonstrations of comfortable positions.

Small group sharing of feelings regarding interference by well-meaning relatives.

Literature on need to maintain breastfeeding alone, with no additional baby foods until after 3 months of age; literature on minor discomforts.

TABLE 3-9 *(continued)*

EVALUATION
Mother lists basic foods with 100% accuracy.
Mother identifies which foods should be omitted in own cultural diet.
Mother writes plan for adequate intake of dairy products.
Mother demonstrates to the nurse at least four comfortable positions she uses while feeding infant.
Baby appears able to grasp nipple well and is in a comfortable position.
Mother makes statements of satisfaction with own ability to feed.

the *constraints* of environment, time, learner involvement, feedback, measurement, and evaluation.

SELECTING APPROPRIATE METHODS

Once the direction of teaching has been determined, the techniques that will best facilitate learning in a particular domain must be selected. Facts and concepts belonging to the cognitive domain are best taught through written materials, audiovisual aids, lectures, and discussion. Motor skills in the psychomotor domain are best taught through activities: demonstration, practice, return demonstration. Attitudinal changes in the affective domain may be taught through role modeling, role playing, group discussion, and therapeutic interaction.

Learning may be reinforced through use of audiovisual programs; seeing someone else doing, responding, or sharing feelings allows a "second opinion" to back up the nurse's presentation.

Where possible, the TLT should occur in an environment free from extraneous distractions, one that is comfortable, well-lighted, and conducive to interactions. Unfortunately, most in-hospital client education does not have the benefit of such conditions, and the nurse must therefore adapt, fit into cramped spaces, or work with larger than ideal groups. One-to-one bedside TLTs should occur when the client is alert and expecting a lesson; the lesson should be limited to the client's ability to concentrate.

EVALUATION

Evaluation should be related to the progress the client makes as a result of the educational program. Progress is evaluated by the behavioral objectives written in the plan. The clearer and more measurable those objectives, the easier the ongoing evaluation becomes. Each session should be reviewed in regard to the appropriateness of the goal, materials, techniques, and learner responses. Client feedback and a changing medical regimen may often dictate a different order of priorities. Here are some basic questions that can aid the evaluation process. The answers to these questions influence the end results of the teaching-learning process and these answers need to influence further planning.

1. Was the client's knowledge adequately assessed?
2. Were the biological, developmental, cultural, and socioeconomic assessments taken into consideration in modifying the learning environment?
3. Were the educational needs adequately identified and defined?
4. Were the educational goals realistic and timely?
5. Was the priority of educational goals appropriate?
6. Did the behavioral objectives clearly measure the appropriate domains?
7. Did educational goals take into account the changing medical status of the client?
8. Were the family members involved? Should they have been?
9. Was the client's sense of control maintained?

10. Was positive praise and reinforcement given for achievement?

SUMMARY

This chapter has presented an overview of the client education process, an area of nursing that is assuming an important role in promoting self-care for the person who has health-related needs. Nurses may expand that role for a society that now asks to be educated about health maintenance.

REFERENCES

Jones, P., and Oertel, W.: "Developing Patient Teaching Objectives and Techniques: A Self Instructional Program," *Nurse Educator*, **2**(5):1–4, September–October 1977.

Redman, B. K.: *The Process of Patient Teaching in Nursing*, 2d ed., Mosby, St Louis, 1972.

Redman, B. K.: *The Process of Patient Teaching in Nursing*, 4th ed., Mosby, St. Louis, 1980.

BIBLIOGRAPHY

Barb, W. M., et al.: "The Relationship of Spatial Ability and Sex to Formal Reasoning Capabilities," *The Journal of Psychology*, 1980, pp. 104, 191–198. Good reference for biological differences in learning between the sexes.

Birren, J.: "Adult Capacities to Learn," in *Psychological Backgrounds of Adult Education*, R. Kuhler (ed.), Center for Study of Liberal Education for Adults, New York, 1963. Succinct chapter on adult learning by one of the foremost authorities in the field.

Gagne, R. M.: *Conditions of Learning*, 2d ed., Rhinehart and Winston, Chicago, 1970. Excellent overview of learning theories.

Jones, P., and Oertel, W.: "Developing Patient Teaching Objectives and Techniques: A Self Instructional Program," *Nurse Educator*, **2**:5, September–October 1977. Autotutorial approach to developing broad and behavioral objectives. Clearly differentiates between domains of learning and affords an opportunity to develop behavioral objectives using appropriate descriptive terms.

Kid, J.: *How Adults Learn*, Association Press, New York, 1963. Classic reference on adult learning by an expert in the field.

Mayer, R., and DeCecco, J.: *The Psychology of Learning and Instruction: Educational Psychology*, Prentice-Hall, Englewood Cliffs, N.J., 1968. Excellent resource book on writing behavioral objectives and constructing methods of evaluation.

Muhs, P. J., et al.: "Cross Sectional Analysis of Cognitive Functioning Across the Life Span," *International Journal of Aging and Human Development*, **10**(4), 1979–1980. A sound overview of learning readiness throughout the stages of development.

Pion, R. J.: "Facilitated Learning in Health Care," *New Approaches to Counseling and Communication*, Medical Communications & Services Association, Seattle, Wash., pp. 51–54. Defines the importance of educating for value change.

Redman, B. K.: *Issues and Concepts in Patient Education*, Appleton-Century-Crofts, New York, 1981. Excellent source of principles of learning for clients.

———: *The Process of Patient Teaching in Nursing*, 4th ed., Mosby, St. Louis, 1980. An overview of the teaching-learning process. Chapters on learning readiness and evaluation of health teaching are especially helpful.

Thorndike, E. L., et al.: *Adult Learning*, Macmillan, New York, 1928. A classic on the principles of adult learning.

Weller, C. V.: "Biological Aspects of the Aging Process," *Aging in Today's Society*, Tibbets and Donohue, 1960. Clearly defines the aging process and its effects on the learning ability curve.

Zanger, M. E., and Duffy, P.: "Contracting with Patients in Day to Day Practice," *American Journal of Nursing*, March 1980. Offers practical examples of when and how contracts can increase client compliance.

4

Human Development Through the Life Span

Mable Searcy Carlyle

Knowledge of human growth and development is basic to nursing practice. Obviously, the assessment phase of the nursing process draws heavily on the nurse's understanding of norms for physical and behavioral function. Nursing diagnosis requires that the practitioner be able (1) to recognize the range of effective, normal function, as well as deviations, and (2) to anticipate changes that can be expected to occur as time passes and the client's developmental characteristics undergo predictable modifications. The establishment of goals must take into consideration the person's developmental capacities and expected future development. Interventive efforts cannot succeed unless they are geared to the cognitive, affective, and physiologic status and potential of the client.

To assist the practitoner in understanding the client and his or her potential so that nursing care can be tailored to the individual, this chapter describes major growth and developmental characteristics and milestones for children and adults at various stages of the life span.

Inherent in every discussion of norms is the obvious limitation that a description of "the average person" is inadequate to reveal the richness of human variation. This chapter should in no way be interpreted as implying either what all people are like or what people should be like. Its purpose, rather, is to serve as a reference point to guide the nurse by identifying commonly occurring human characteristics and sequences of development.

NEONATE (BIRTH TO 1 MONTH OF AGE)

PHYSICAL DEVELOPMENT

Breathes immediately at birth. Can yawn, cough, sneeze, swallow, and regurgitate (all are protective reflexes). Moves extremities in random and uncoordinated fashion. Turns head from side to side. Has automatic grasp reflex strong enough for partial lifting of body. Blinks and closes eyes protectively. Sucking reflex is strong. Brushing of the baby's cheek elicits the rooting reflex, that is, turning of the head toward the stimulus and attempting to grasp with the mouth. Lifts head briefly when prone. Cries without tears; the character of the cry varies with circumstances.

1. *Temperature.* Temperature regulation is critically important for avoidance of metabolic imbalance and rapid deterioration, particularly in low-birth-weight neonates. Infant's body heat regulation mechanisms are immature, even at term. Sweat glands do not function until about 4 weeks.
2. *Size and proportions.* Weighs 6 to 8 lb at birth; gains about 6 oz per week. Head constitutes one-fourth of height. Legs and arms are relatively short.

PERCEPTUAL DEVELOPMENT

Looks at human face in preference to other visual stimuli. Hears at birth and better after the auditory canal is drained of amniotic fluid. Is startled by loud, sudden noises. May show preference for the high-pitched voice of mother and rhythmic sounds similar to the heartbeat (familiar prenatal sound). Responds to certain olfactory stimuli and is capable of scent discriminations; withdraws from strong odors like ammonia, and may recognize own mother's scent (pheromones) as separate from that of another lactating woman (Waletzky, 1976).

PSYCHOSOCIAL AND COGNITIVE DEVELOPMENT

Behavior is primarily at the reflex level. Shows evidence of very short memory; attention shifts as soon as an object is out of sight. Sleep-wake activities are organized into *behavioral states,* as follows:

In the initial hour or so after birth the infant experiences a period of pronounced alertness (coinciding with a similar state in the new mother, unless medication alters her behavior); during this period he actively participates in developing relationship (bond) to mother if they are together and in close contact. Newborns are able to elicit caretaking responses from others (e.g., by crying) and to respond to (and thereby reinforce) caretaking and comfort measures offered by others. Infant behavior consists of six different behavioral states:

1. Quiet sleep—Infant sleeps deeply without movements of the eyes, face, trunk, or extremities except for startles at rather regular intervals. Respirations are regular. Infant is not easily aroused by environmental stimuli, and startle response to them may be delayed.
2. Active sleep, also called light sleep—Eyes are closed but rapid eye movements are noticeable. Respirations are irregular, often more rapid than in quiet sleep. There is some limb movement in addition to startles. Mouthing and sucking occur at times. Baby startles in response to environmental stimuli and may awaken.

Drowsiness—Infant may open and close eyes but eyes appear unfocused. Lids may flutter. Response to stimuli may be delayed. Infant moves from this dozing state into sleep or greater alertness. Mild activity (wiggling, writhing) occurs.

4. Alert inactivity—Eyes are open and bright and infant seems intent upon the environment. There is little movement.
5. Alert activity—Characterized by a generally high level of motor activity including bursts of arm waving and kicking. Respirations are irregular. Skin may be quite flushed. Eyes are bright but not necessarily focused.
6. Crying—Infant cries intensely. The face flushes and grimaces. Crying is accompanied by vigorous motor activity.

Each baby has his or her own usual pattern of organizing the sequence and duration of these six behavioral states. One infant may may move rapidly from sleep to crying, for example, giving caretakers little time to prepare feedings and interact with the baby in a noncrying, awake state (Barnard et al., 1981).

NURSING CONSIDERATIONS

1. *Feeding and comforting.* Feeding time may be the most important part of the infant's day. Sucking is pleasurable and apparently a means of releasing tensions. The presence of the mother (or other primary caretaker) and ability to visualize the caretaker (e.g., bililight eyepatches should be removed for feedings) are important to support bonding. Talking with the baby sets the stage for the beginning of an active communication process. Mother and family members seem intuitively to raise the pitch of the voice when talking to an infant. Rhythmic sounds and movements are comforting. After feeding the infant should be turned on the right side to facilitate gastric emptying and help prevent aspiration.
2. *Parent education.* Parents, particularly if inexperienced, have many questions about care of the newborn. (See Chapters 10 and 11 for care of the full-term or preterm infant, respectively.) The behavioral states listed im-

mediately above are quite helpful in helping parents get acquainted with their baby's patterns of behavior. It is important that parents recognize the different kinds of cry that indicate hunger, anger, fear, pain, and so forth.

3. *Protection*. Care of the newborn is presented in detail in Chapters 10 and 11. Protection against chilling may require a heat source. Observation is needed for both drop and elevation of temperature. Dress and wraps should be just slightly more than would be comfortable to an adult. Because the head represents a significant portion of the body surface, the head should be bathed last to minimize cooling; a cap or head covering is important when going outside in cold weather.
4. *Stimulation*. During the alert states, soft music and bright colored mobiles may catch the infant's attention. Additional stimulation can be provided by moving the child to the area of family activity when he or she is awake.

INFANT (1 TO 12 MONTHS)

SECOND MONTH

PHYSICAL DEVELOPMENT

May roll over. Cries tears. Cannot open hand purposefully to grasp toy but will hold it when placed in hand.

COGNITIVE DEVELOPMENT

Learns by repetition. Is aware only of that which is in the perceptual field. Begins to develop patterned responses to certain stimuli, such as sucking when placed in feeding position. Begins to recognize familiar sounds such as mother's voice.

PSYCHOSOCIAL DEVELOPMENT

Smiles in response to stimulation; coos and squeals; responds to speaking voice. (Tactile stimulation is especially necessary for development during early life.)

NURSING CONSIDERATIONS

Teach parents to take precautions to prevent falls and rolling off surfaces as the child becomes more active. Holding during feeding, diapering, and other caregiving activities assists in meeting psychosocial needs. Child is learning to elicit a great amount of response from others. Repetitiveness in play is enjoyable and necessary for learning.

THIRD MONTH

PHYSICAL DEVELOPMENT

Motor development permits purposefully putting hand into mouth. Becomes able to swallow solid foods (extrusion reflex diminishes). Can hold head erect. Can focus eyes on bright objects and follow from side to side. Makes crawling movements when in prone position. Can arch back and hold up head in prone position. Strikes at toy but cannot grasp it.

COGNITIVE DEVELOPMENT

Behaves as if an object out of sight does not exist. Can wait for brief periods.

PSYCHOSOCIAL DEVELOPMENT

Laughs aloud, coos, blows bubbles, squeals, and seems to enjoy the noise. Smiles at mother's face. Cries less than when younger.

NURSING CONSIDERATIONS

In the interest of preventing allergies and obesity, pediatricians and nutritionists recommend delaying the introduction of solids until 4 to 6 months of age. There is no evidence that adding solids to the diet makes the baby sleep through the night. At whatever age solids are begun, only one new food should be introduced at a time, allowing a week or so before the next new food. Baby seems to respond more to change in texture than taste. Brightly colored mobiles are entertaining and provide visual stimulation. Prefers red, blue, green, and yellow. Music boxes provide auditory stimulation. Simple toys such as telephone-shaped rattle are enjoyable.

FOURTH MONTH

PHYSICAL DEVELOPMENT

Can seize an object and move it to mouth. Turns from back to side. Introduces thumb apposition in grasping. Supports part of weight with legs. Pushes feet against support. Reaches out with hands. Brings hands together, plays with them, and puts them into mouth. Drooling begins.

COGNITIVE DEVELOPMENT

Recognizes mother's face and some familiar objects. Is developing a vague idea that unseen objects exist.

PSYCHOSOCIAL DEVELOPMENT

Laughs aloud. Initiates social play. Sleep reaches a pattern of one or two naps and longer periods at night.

NURSING CONSIDERATIONS

Teach parents to take precautions to prevent ingestion or aspiration of objects in infant's environment and to prevent falls from rolling off surface. Gradual increase in sensory stimuli provides more opportunities to learn. Guard against fatigue from overstimulation, as the attention span remains short. Teething biscuits or teething rings are useful.

FIFTH MONTH

PHYSICAL DEVELOPMENT

No head lag when pulled to sitting position. Rolls from back to side. Can transfer toys from one hand to the other. Doubles birth weight.

COGNITIVE DEVELOPMENT

Recognizes mother from others. Attention span increases and child can play alone for an hour or so.

PSYCHOSOCIAL DEVELOPMENT

Turns head toward voice. Babbles vowels and "talks" to self. Splashes in bathwater. Lifts arms to be picked up.

NURSING CONSIDERATIONS

Increased opportunities for motor activity and play become important. Constant assessment of the environment for safety hazards is critical: child is at risk for falls, ingestions, burns, and suffocation or strangulation.

SIXTH MONTH

PHYSICAL DEVELOPMENT

Can sit alone briefly. Lifts head in anticipation of sitting and pulls into sitting position. Bears a large portion of weight on legs when held in standing position. Bangs objects on table. Holds bottle. Drops toy from hand to reach when another is offered. Lower incisors commonly erupt, although age at teething varies widely.

COGNITIVE DEVELOPMENT

Responds with attentiveness to new stimuli. May cry if play is interrupted. Begins to show food likes and dislikes. Begins to recognize the meaning of certain words and vocal tones.

PSYCHOSOCIAL DEVELOPMENT

May begin demonstrating separation anxiety and fear of strangers. Begins to act coy.

NURSING CONSIDERATIONS

This is a good time to introduce the cup. Cups designed not to spill are useful. Being placed so as to view older children playing is intriguing. Viewing one's reflection in a nonbreakable mirror is a pleasurable pastime.

SEVENTH, EIGHTH, AND NINTH MONTHS

PHYSICAL DEVELOPMENT

Sits alone by 8 months and pulls into standing position by ninth. Crawls forward and backward on abdomen, then creeps on hands and knees. Completes thumb-finger apposition and learns to pick up small objects with pincer grasp by 9 months. Hand-eye coordination is per-fected. Two upper incisors may erupt, making a total of four teeth.

COGNITIVE DEVELOPMENT

Becomes aware that objects exist although out of sight: "searches" for toy covered by blanket, for example. Can associate familiar happenings with unfamiliar ones. Attention span increases.

PSYCHOSOCIAL DEVELOPMENT

Says first words, usually *dada* and *mama*. Responds to *no, no* and cries when scolded. Is shy with strangers. Waves bye-bye and plays pat-a-cake. May feed self finger foods.

NURSING CONSIDERATIONS

Caution must be taken that objects small enough to be swallowed or aspirated are removed from play area. Some discomfort, drooling, and low fever may be expected with teething. Begin prevention of "nursing bottle" tooth decay: bedtime bottle (if not discontinued) should not contain any sugar-containing fluid, including milk. Counsel parents to minimize sweets in the baby's diet and not to add salt. The introduction of a variety of unseasoned foods helps develop an appreciation for natural flavors.

TENTH, ELEVENTH, AND TWELFTH MONTHS

PHYSICAL DEVELOPMENT

Learns to take a few steps alone, initially holding onto furniture or adult. May try to use spoon but seldom gets it to mouth with food still on it. Holds cup alone. Scribbles with crayon. Has tripled birth weight by 1 year. Bowel movements have decreased to one or two per day.

COGNITIVE DEVELOPMENT

Understands short commands. Responds rhythmically to music.

PSYCHOSOCIAL DEVELOPMENT

Negativism and self-assertion are the general attitude. Tantrums may begin. Resists going to bed. "Dances" to music. Enjoys simple games. May use two or three single words correctly.

NURSING CONSIDERATIONS

Setting of limits is necessary for the child in spite of tantrums. A regular bedtime needs to be established and enforced for the benefit of all. Great tolerance is needed by the parents as the child begins to participate in self-care activities such as feeding self. Soft, flexible shoes or bare feet are best for walking. Little weight gain is to be expected at this age because growth *rate* has decreased.

TODDLER (1 TO 3 YEARS)

PHYSICAL DEVELOPMENT

1. *Gross motor development skills.* Can walk, run, jump, step backward and sideways; can go down stairs alone, at first on buttocks, eventually learning to alternate feet. Learns to ride tricycle.
2. *Fine motor control.* Can build a tower of blocks, feed self, string beads, throw ball, help undress self, and put on simple garments. Can turn pages of a book.
3. *Toileting.* Voluntary control of sphincters is developing. Toilet training may reasonably begin around 18 months for most children. Manipulation of genitals for pleasure is common.
4. *Dentition.* At 15 months usually has first upper and lower molars. At 18 months has about 12 teeth. All 20 deciduous teeth are in by $2\frac{1}{2}$ years for most children.
5. *Sleep.* May sleep about 10 to 14 hours daily, usually including one or two naps.

COGNITIVE DEVELOPMENT

1. *General.* Demonstrates beginning memory. Experiments with environment and activity in order to expand knowledge. Is beginning to think of alternative ways to reach goals without having to act out each one.
2. *Language.* Verbal communication skills are developing. By 3 years can use a noun, verb, and object in a three-word sentence and has 300 or more words in vocabulary. Under-

stands more than is able to verbalize. Knows own name.

PSYCHOSOCIAL DEVELOPMENT

1. *Autonomy.* Is highly self-assertive, especially at 1 and 2 years, and insists on doing things without help or interference. Shows pride in independence.
2. *Separation.* Can now spend time away from mother without excessive anxiety if child has met caretaker in mother's presence and a period of adjustment has been provided.
3. *Play.* Plays imaginatively, imitating adult roles. Plays mostly alone even if in a group of children.
4. *Morality.* Conscience is developing. Tells self "No, no"; gradually incorporates beginnings of self-control in behavior.

NURSING CONSIDERATIONS

1. *Accident prevention.* Safety must be kept constantly in mind. The child should not be left unsupervised at any time. Lacks experience and cannot make good judgments about danger and cannot be relied upon to follow parents' instructions or warnings.
2. *Motor activity.* Mobility is a major means of learning and coping at this age and should not be restricted unnecessarily, especially when child is under stress, such as from hospitalization.
3. *Toileting.* Successful toilet training depends on three factors: child experiences discomfort when wet or soiled, there is motivation to alter the situation, and child recognizes pre-elimination sensations.
4. *Dental care.* Needs to be taught to brush teeth. Foods with concentrated sweets should be avoided. The first visit to the dentist should be made.
5. *Learning.* Repetition is necessary for understanding and for memory to develop; from this accumulation of experience, child can move to new learning. A wide variety of learning experiences can be had with safe objects in the home, such as pots and pans, boxes, colored egg cartons, and so forth. Bedtime stories are enjoyable and cognitively valuable. Simple explanations of events can be understood. Playing with genitalia is a part of the normal process of self-exploration.
6. *Baby-sitting.* Planning ahead of time for baby-sitting is wise; several short visits of mother and child with the sitter before the child is actually left make the transition smoother.
7. *Self-care.* Children need to be permitted to perform tasks they can accomplish, regardless of the fact that this can be time-consuming and messy for the parent.
8. *Psychosocial traits.* Toddlers should not be expected to share toys. Flare-ups of indignation are common. Guilt and shame are developmental hazards.

PRESCHOOL CHILD (3 TO 6 YEARS)

PHYSICAL DEVELOPMENT

1. *Growth.* Rate of growth slows. Birth length has doubled by age 4.
2. *Toileting.* Nighttime control of bowel and bladder is usually attained by age 3 or 4.
3. *Self-care.* Learns self-care skills. Washes and dries hands by age 3. Feeds self with some spillage at age 3. Brushes teeth by self at 3 or 4, but still needs supervision to ensure thoroughness. Undresses at 3; dresses self at 5.
4. *Motor activity.* Ability to judge distances and own strength is limited and accidents are common. Moves with speed and agility.
5. *Dentition.* Deciduous dentition is complete and the incisors may be lost.

COGNITIVE DEVELOPMENT

1. *Concept learning.* Learns basic concepts of the culture. Understands time concepts such as *morning, night, later,* and so on. Can count to 4 or 5. Knows at least the primary colors.
2. *Fantasy.* Fluctuates between reality and fantasy; may have some difficulty distinguishing between the two.
3. *Thought qualities.* Believes that whatever moves is alive (cars, vacuum cleaner, hospital equipment). Thinking is concrete. Is unable to analyze or synthesize. Perceives end results of change but does not understand the process. Focuses on certain details of object but usually not the object as a whole.

4. *Language.* Language skills rapidly increase. May have own private language and interpretations.

PSYCHOSOCIAL DEVELOPMENT

1. *Morality.* Learns to distinguish right and wrong and begins to demonstrate conscience.
2. *Sexuality.* Learns sex differences, sex roles, and sexual modesty.
3. *Body awareness.* Develops a body image and a body boundary. May masturbate as self-awareness develops.
4. *Family roles.* Enjoys doing simple chores. "Helps" family members.
5. *Social expansion.* Enlarges social interests to others outside the immediate family—playmates, neighbors, friends of parents, and so on.
6. *Concept of death.* Equates death and separation. Considers dying the result of a deliberate act: wants to know "Who killed him?"
7. *Magical thinking.* Believes that wishing makes things happen; for example, that anger can make a person disappear or die.
8. *Discipline.* Feels more secure when behavioral boundaries are set by adults. "Tests" to establish limits of acceptable behavior.

NURSING CONSIDERATIONS

1. *Growth.* Parents may worry because appetite decreases or is unpredictable as growth rate slows.
2. *Toileting.* May have accidents during periods of stress or illness.
3. *Family roles.* Planning the daily schedule to allow time for child to participate in the household activities promotes development of skills and builds self-esteem.
4. *Accident prevention.* Provide for safety needs: supply sturdy, safe toys; protect valuable household objects; and assign a safe play area. Watchful supervision is needed.
5. *Dental care.* Child should have already developed regular habit of brushing teeth and should be making twice-yearly visits to dentist.
6. *Stimulation.* Environmental opportunities influence learning to a great degree.
7. *Fantasy.* Dramatization of experiences by fabrication, exaggeration, or boastfulness is not intentional deceit. Equipment that moves or makes noise may produce fears.
8. *Teaching-learning.* Preoperative teaching probably has little meaning, but postoperative reteaching about what the child has experienced is now meaningful and helpful. The same is true of other experiences: learning and understanding require personal experience. Child is unable to comprehend the whole picture of an event; for example, when about to receive an injection, will focus only on the needle and the anticipated pain and not on the purpose of the injection.
9. *Morality.* The preschooler wants to "do right," and likes kind guidance. Condemns self (and others) when things to wrong.
10. *Sexual curiosity.* Plays "doctor." Peeking and asking to see others' bodies are natural.
11. *Body intactness.* Becomes greatly concerned about even the smallest injury. Bandage strips to small scratches and injection sites are reassuring. Intrusive procedures such as throat swabs and rectal temperatures are distressing.
12. *Death.* Although death is beyond understanding, the child should be permitted to experience death as it comes naturally within the family or circle of friends or to pets. Give explanations as they are asked for. Reassure the child that fantasies or wishes did not cause the death.
13. *General traits.* Difficulty in separating fantasy from reality and belief in magical thinking lead to feelings of insecurity. Is proud of accomplishments and enjoys praise. Is friendly, likes attention from others; appreciates jokes.

MIDDLE CHILDHOOD (6 TO 12 YEARS)

PHYSICAL DEVELOPMENT

1. *Body changes.* Growth is less dramatic than during babyhood or later during adolescence. General body configuration changes from childlike and begins to approximate adult proportions. The lower portion of the face enlarges as dentition becomes complete. The

nose enlarges. Hair becomes coarser and less manageable.

2. *Motor development.* Motor skills become refined with practice. Clumsiness (both gross-motor and fine-motor) and incoordination gradually diminish. Greater muscle strength is gained. The school-age child works and plays hard but tires easily.

COGNITIVE DEVELOPMENT

The child's thinking remains concrete. However, boundaries of knowledge and ability to process information expand at a tremendous rate. Develops ability to be reflective. Experience and memories accumulate from which to draw information and understanding. Increases use of language. Can consider alternative solutions to a problem.Can consider parts or the whole independently. Understands and uses classification systems (collections are a favorite activity). Understands the Piagetian principle of conservation; develops the concept of reversibility.

PSYCHOSOCIAL DEVELOPMENT

1. *Peer relations.* Learns to get along with agemates. Is loyal to friends. Chooses best friend, almost always of same sex.
2. *Sexuality.* Knows appropriate masculine and feminine social role. Is interested in sex differences. Plays games that involve male and female roles. Is interested in the opposite sex but won't admit it. Sexual exploration of own body and those of friends is common.
3. *Morality.* Is developing conscience, morality, and a set of values. Good sportsmanship becomes important. May take a strong stand for ideals.
4. *Self-awareness.* Develops an awareness of self as a growing, changing, and unique individual. Is curious about body functions and changes that are occurring.
5. *Family interactions.* Learns to be independent in self-care activities. Wants own room. Will accept responsibility for routine household tasks with occasional reminders. Likes to participate in family decision making.
6. *Social learning.* Develops attitudes about social groups and institutions. Likes to belong to clubs. Can permit own goals to be subordinate to the group goals. Puts on "good manners" in social settings. Family remains the primary agent of socialization, but peers are becoming more and more important.

NURSING CONSIDERATIONS

1. Behavior and level of understanding cannot be relied upon to be consistently as mature as adults often expect.
2. Participation in crafts and sports provides both boys and girls opportunity to refine motor skills. Hobbies, sports, crafts, arts, and other interests may supplement formal schooling in satisfying the need to learn.
3. Needs to have experiences by which to clarify values. Delegation of tasks supports this learning.
4. Some free time should be provided for introspection and learning about self.
5. Classroom groups, clubs, and sports groups become very influential in the socialization process.
6. The school-age period of curiosity is an ideal time for health teaching. Special effort should be made to eliminate anxiety and misinformation about body changes.

ADOLESCENCE (12 TO 20 YEARS)

PHYSICAL DEVELOPMENT

1. *Growth.* A growth spurt takes place between ages 10 and 16. For girls, this period of accelerated growth begins about 2 years earlier than for boys. Girls gain about 40 lb; boys gain about 55 lb (weight is attributed mostly to increase in bone and muscle tissue in both sexes). Girls retain more subcutaneous fat than boys.
2. *Function.* Muscle development is greater in males than in females and therefore males are usually stronger. Males develop larger hearts and lungs, have a higher systolic blood pressure, and maintain a slower heart rate at rest. Different body parts reach adult size at different times; extremities grow before the trunk does, resulting in awkwardness and a gangly appearance.

3. *Sequence of female sexual development.* The first visible sign of puberty in girls is usually the appearance of the breast bud, usually between the ages of 8 and 13. Growth of pubic hair follows the early breast development. Full growth of pubic hair takes about 3 years. Axillary hair begins about 1 year after the appearance of pubic hair. Menarche usually occurs just after the growth spurt; the average age for American girls is just under 13. Menstruation may be irregular for several months and accompanied by a certain amount of discomfort, such as backaches or cramps. Ovulation generally begins a year or so after menarche. The uterus reaches adult size about age 18 or 20. Skin changes resulting from increased androgen secretion may lead to acne vulgaris, which is of minor medical consequence but can be a major social or emotional consequence to the adolescent. (For additional information, see Chapter 34.)
4. *Sequence of male sexual development.* The first sexual change of puberty is increased growth of testes and the scrotum, which becomes redder, coarser, and wrinkled. The average age is about 13. About this time pubic hair begins to grow. About a year later, at the height of the growth spurt, the penis begins to grow in length and circumference. The prostate gland and seminal vesicles are maturing. The first ejaculation occurs about a year after the penis begins to grow. A temporary increase of the areola and elevation of the nipple occurs in about one-fourth of boys and is accompanied by breast tenderness. These breast changes disappear in a year or so. About 2 years after the beginning of the growth of pubic hair, facial, axillary, and body hair begin to grow. Body hair continues to spread until adulthood. The mustache comes first in sequence of facial hair. The larynx enlarges and the vocal cords double in length, causing the voice to deepen in pitch. As androgen secretion increases, it stimulates the growth of the sebaceous glands and the production of sebum. At the same time developmental changes of the skin, including enlargement of pores, may result in acne. (For additional information, see Chapter 34.)

COGNITIVE DEVELOPMENT

Begins to use formal thought process. Can deal conceptually and logically with abstractions, hypotheses, and hypothetical situations. Considers several solutions to a question. Can problem-solve in a systematic, adult manner, although people of course vary in their cognitive abilities, and young people do not consistently operate at a high level of formal cognitive process.

PSYCHOSOCIAL DEVELOPMENT

1. *Peer relationships.* Gradually achieves a new and more mature relationship with age-mates of both sexes. Enjoys participating in jokes and humorous activity but may have difficulty being the "victim" of jokes. May be highly competitive. Patterns behavior after role models (own age and older).
2. *Family relationships.* Embarrassed by family in public at age 13 or 14. Conflict with parents is much diminished after age 16 or 17.
3. *Independence.* Achieves increased emotional independence from parents and other adults. Becomes independent and self-directed in schedules and homework. May have employment outside the home.
4. *Career.* Is preparing for economic independence and meaningful work. Begins to explore career possibilities and interests. Ability or inability to set long-range goals influences choice. Aptitude and cultural and parental influence contribute to career choice.
5. *Morality.* Searches for new beliefs, resolves inconsistencies of old beliefs, and begins to crystalize a personal philosophy of life. The defense mechanisms of asceticism (attempt to deny entirely the instinctual drives toward pleasure) and intellectualization are widely used. Is acquiring a set of values and an ethical system as a guide to behavior. Is developing own ideology. Moral judgment continues to develop in terms of pleasing others and respect for authority. Most young people desire and achieve socially responsible behavior, although some define that in ways conservative adults do not. Becomes interested in social problems; may be active in service-oriented organizations or, later, in movements to promote social change.
6. *Egocentricity.* Because adolescents' thoughts are primarily about themselves, they assume that they are also the center of other people's thoughts. As a result of this egocentrism, negative or positive self-regard is magnified and the young person creates an "imaginary au-

dience" that is believed to share these same feelings about him or her.

7. *Body image.* The body image—the person's mental picture of his or her physical self—must change to incorporate rapid body changes. The body image is formed from a conglomerate of real and fantasied experiences. Self-esteem in adolescence is closely related to body image.
8. *Early and late puberty.* Variation in rate of maturation is of great concern to many adolescents. Early maturers may have the advantage of being admired by peers and becoming leaders of their age group; they also have the disadvantage of being expected to behave in a more mature way than others of their age. Late maturers may feel left out, unpopular with their peers, and worried that they are abnormal.
9. *Sexuality.* Their own and others' sexuality, including both sex role behavior in the broadest sense and sexual activity in the narrow meaning, are intensely interesting to adolescents. Sexual curiosity and fantasy are at a peak. Masturbation is nearly universal, particularly among males, and even in this "age of enlightenment" may be accompanied by fear of injury and feelings of guilt. Dating may be a major activity in middle and late adolescence. Most experiment with kissing and petting; many engage in intercourse.

NURSING CONSIDERATIONS

1. *Growth.* The gangly appearance and some of the awkwardness typical of adolescence are due to rapid growth and variation of growth rate of body parts. The sequential development of these characteristics may be somewhat variable between individuals but not nearly as variable as the age at which they appear. Puberty usually begins between the ages of 8 and 13 for females, and 12 and 16 for males. It can be very reassuring to know that different growth patterns are normal. Counsel adolescents that final adult height and age at which growth occurs are largely determined by heredity.
2. *Nutrition.* Nutrition education should include information about the hazards of food fads and unbalanced reducing diets. Adolescents may overeat as a means of coping with problems, such as loneliness. Obesity reduces pressures to participate socially or assume a sexual role. Adolescent may overeat in an attempt to become big in order to overcome feelings of being small and inadequate.
3. *Self-care.* Accident prevention and prevention of substance abuse are major health maintenance foci. Sessions for exploration of peer group values can be very effective in reducing dangerous activities and the need to use alcohol, tobacco, and other drugs. Adolescents can understand cause-and-effect relationships and can anticipate expected outcomes of behavior, but they are typically very present-oriented and do not take the long view of preventive health education. They are not as influenced by long-term hazards of poor health habits (unsound dieting, for example, or smoking) as they are by short-term advantages of good habits: expected outcomes such as good physical function, strength, athletic skill, and attractive appearance are more likely to induce good health habits than are threats of lung disease, cardiovascular disorders, or other negative results of poor habits.
4. *Sexuality and sex education.* Education of both sexes about the reproductive process, birth control methods, and prevention and treatment of venereal diseases should be begun at least by the onset of puberty and earlier if interest is shown. Cultural and religious guidelines for handling sexual behavior for both sexes should be discussed early within the family. Masturbation provides release of sexual tension and is not harmful. Menstruation should be fully explained well before the age of onset as a normal and natural occurrence. Reference to menstruation as an illness is unwarranted and should be avoided. Education well in advance of "wet dreams" will eliminate unnecessary concern in the young man. Learning that these spontaneous nighttime ejaculations are normal is reassuring to the adolescent.
5. *Self-concept.* The adolescent may feel that everyone on the street is gaping as he or she walks by. Wearing apparel, hair styles, and other fads are of extreme importance. The adolescent needs to understand that (1) body changes normally occur within a wide age range, (2) changes are not as conspicuous to others as the adolescent thinks, and (3) sexual identity is not dependent on the attainment of a certain size of body parts. The adolescent needs objective feedback from others in order

to form a realistic body image. Honest feedback is rare and must be handled delicately, as the adolescent is already highly sensitive about his or her appearance.

6. *Emotional control.* Adolescents must learn to deal with strong emotions not previously experienced. Phases of self-denial and overintellectualizing about self or others are common but may be brief. Role modeling by admired adults is highly influential.
7. *Morality.* Value system is based on the ideal, and the young person may become critical, impatient, and depressed when reality falls short of the ideal. Later comes to a resolution of conflicting standards and avoids self-condemnation and guilt feelings. May serve as junior scout leaders or athletic coaches for younger children, march for fund drives, and so forth. Later, "antiestablishment" efforts and experiences help in the formation of a personal value system.
8. *Independence.* Permission granted by adults for the adolescent to become more independent allows time to practice new behaviors while still in the family setting.
9. *Career planning.* Hobbies, after school jobs, career clubs, and role models help with career choice. Referral to career guidance counselor or other such persons may be useful.

HOSPITALIZED CHILDREN AND ADOLESCENTS AND THEIR FAMILIES*

This section provides an overview of general concepts important in the care of every child and family. It presents suggestions for adapting assessment techniques to children and adolescents; discusses young clients' and parents' responses to hospitalization, illness, and surgery; and carries the reader through the steps of the nursing process as they pertain to the care of children. The information contained here is intended for use in conjunction with the more specific information in later chapters about the nursing of children and adolescents.

* This section of the chapter was written by Mary Fran Hazinski, R.N., M.S.N.

GUIDELINES FOR ASSESSMENT OF CHILDREN AND ADOLESCENTS

SEQUENCE OF ASSESSMENT

1. Children must often be assessed in an informal way.
   a. Consider the child's physical and emotional tolerance levels.
   b. Obtain any resting vital signs or measurements (e.g., observation of color at rest, respiratory rate and effort during sleep, and monitored heart rate and blood pressure) *before* disturbing the child. The most uncomfortable or intrusive procedures should be performed last in the exam.
2. Adapt style of exam to the developmental level of the child.
   a. Infants are usually distracted by faces, gentle voices, brightly colored objects, rattles, and keys.
   b. Toddlers may feel extremely threatened by an exam (especially if forced into a reclining position). Try to perform the exam on the parent's lap.
   c. Preschool and school-age children often enjoy actively participating in their examination. Allow them some choices (e.g., the sequence of the exam), and provide appropriate explanations. You may wish to allow the child the opportunity to play with the exam equipment and the chance to examine you.
   d. Adolescents may become extremely self-conscious during a physical exam. Protect their privacy (as for any client) and drape the parts of their body not being examined.
3. Perform as much assessment as possible while the child is playing.
   a. Observe psychomotor, cognitive, and psychosocial skills.
   b. Note physical tolerance of activity (e.g., change in color or respiratory effort).
4. Include child *and* family in the assessment.
   a. Take cues from them to discover areas of concern.
   b. Parents may feel frustrated or guilty about child's illness—they may think that they have "failed" to keep child healthy.

c. Presence of a congenital lesion may cause parents to feel guilty for conceiving and giving birth to a less than perfect child.
   (1) Mourning process is often necessary (grief at loss of the awaited perfect child).
   (2) Parents may feel they are responsible for the child's condition. It is often very important for the nurse to differentiate between the term *congenital* (from birth, etiology not implicated) and the term *hereditary* (inherited), as parents often assume the two are synonymous.

d. Parents will need reassurance, support, and compassion.
e. Explore the emotional responses of the child and family to health and illness.
f. If parents do not usually provide child's care, health history must also be obtained from the child's primary caretaker.

5. The child's condition should determine priority of your assessment.
   a. Often specific diseases have very general manifestations (feeding or sleeping patterns may be affected first).
   b. Change in child's disposition (irritability or lethargy) is usually an important clinical sign.

HEALTH HISTORY

General Health

1. It is helpful to ask the parent and child to describe the child's health in a word or phrase and to assess the impact of the child's illness *on the child* (it is helpful to note days of school missed, for example, in school-age children).
2. Determine the child's exercise tolerance.
   a. Separate the physical limitations imposed by the parents from those self-imposed by the child.
   b. Note the child's daily sleep patterns (include duration and frequency of naps, rest periods).
   c. Determine whether the child interrupts play to rest (due to fatigue or dyspnea) and whether or not the child can "keep up" with peers in play and sports activities.
   d. Mother may compare one child's development and activity levels to those of other children in family; this may be a source of frustration if the children differ in play preference or athletic ability.
3. Emotional health and significance of illness to the child must be ascertained; preschool and school-age children often assume that illness and therapy are punishment.
4. Note current medications or diet the child is receiving.
   a. Purpose, dosage, schedule of medications, and the child's response to them must be noted.
   b. Note the child's favorite foods and any food allergies or foods restricted by special diet.
   c. Determine the child's comprehension of, physical and emotional response to, and compliance with therapeutic regimen.

Gestational and Neonatal Health History

1. It is important to determine the maternal and family response to the pregnancy and birth of the child.
   a. If the pregnancy was unplanned or undesired, and the child was born with congenital disease or serious illness, parental anger and guilt may be magnified.
   b. Assess any emotional, cultural, or financial problems the family may be experiencing as a result of the child's birth or illness.
2. Occasionally, maternal illness (e.g., first trimester rubella) or drug ingestion (e.g., thalidomide or stilbesterol) may be linked with illness or congenital abnormalities in offspring.
3. Prematurity and its treatment are associated with an increased incidence of some cardiovascular, respiratory, ophthalmological, neurological, and gastrointestinal disorders.

History of Growth and Development during Infancy and Childhood

1. Feeding difficulties may be a nonspecific sign of poor health; it is important to determine maternal response to such difficulties.
2. Note infant's attainment of developmental milestones; delayed achievement may result from frequent illness and hospitalization, as well as decreased stimulation.

Family Health History

1. Ascertain family history of congenital or hereditary diseases, cardiorespiratory disease, cancer, hematological disorders, neurological disease, renal disorders, endocrine disease, or gastrointestinal problems.

a. Family's previous experiences with health care personnel may affect their responses to the child's illness and to the present staff.
b. The occurrence of any unexplained infant deaths in the family may be the result of congenital defects or sudden infant death syndrome (SIDS).

2. Explore the impact of the child's illness on the child and family.
   a. Do parents have adequate health insurance and financial resources to support fees, tests, special medical equipment, diets, or medications required for the child's care?
   b. Explore importance of health to the family.
   c. Family coping strategies and support systems must be determined.

History of Present Illness

1. For any symptoms discussed, elicit the following information from the child and parents.
   a. Onset.
   b. Precipitating or alleviating factors.
   c. Severity (ask child to compare it to common childhood experiences or sensations).
   d. Distribution.
   e. Medications or therapies used to relieve symptoms and their efficacy.
2. To determine duration of symptoms, it may be helpful to refer to major holidays or the school-year cycle to help the child or parents place illness in a time frame.

PHYSICAL ASSESSMENT

Appropriate Measurement of Vital Signs

1. Heart rate and respiratory rate should always be counted for a full minute because there are often variations in rate during a 1-min period in children.
2. Infants are especially prone to heart rate slowing with vagal stimulation (during or following feeding, suctioning, and defecation), so child's activity at the time of vital sign measurement should be noted.
3. Refer to Tables 19-1 through 19-3 for normal vital sign ranges in children.
4. Note *trends* in the child's vital signs, as well as effect of any environmental stimuli (e.g., Does the child's respiratory rate remain rapid even when he or she is asleep, or is it elevated only when the child is active and playing? Is the child's heart rate much faster during the last several days, when child is also gaining weight and developing symptoms of congestive heart failure, or does heart rate only increase appropriately when child is febrile?)
5. The most frequent cause of high blood pressure measurements in hospitalized children is probably use of a cuff that is too small; cuff bladder should cover two-thirds of the child's upper arm (or thigh, if leg measurements are desired) and should not be wrapped more than $1\frac{1}{4}$ times around the extremity.

Daily Fluid Intake and Output

1. Caloric intake should be calculated for each hospitalized child (see Table 19-4 for maintenance requirements); discuss the child's nutritional status with physician or nutritionist if caloric intake is insufficient.
2. Monitor fluid intake and output as well as daily weight. Notify physician of the following weight changes within 24 h.
   a. More than 25 g in premature neonates.
   b. More than 50 g in infants.
   c. More than 200 g in toddlers or preschool children.
   d. More than 500 g in school-age children or adolescents.
3. Refer to Table 19-6 for calculation of daily pediatric fluid requirements.
4. If it is necessary to have an accurate measurement of the infant's urine output, it is usually easier (and more accurate) to weigh diapers before and after they are placed on the child than to attempt to collect and measure urine in a bag attached to the perineum. One mL of urine weighs approximately 1 g.

PSYCHOLOGICAL SUPPORT OF THE HOSPITALIZED CHILD AND FAMILY: SEPARATION ANXIETY

DESCRIPTION

Separation anxiety is most frequently seen in children 7 months through 4 years of age when they are abruptly or stressfully separated from their parents or primary caretakers. Theoretically, a child can demonstrate three distinct phases of response to the separation:

1. *Protest.* The child is frightened and cries frequently, actively pleading with departing parents to remain or calling for absent parents to return. When parents visit during this phase, the child usually acts pleased to see them but may cry during their visit, fearing their departure.
2. *Despair.* The child has been separated for a longer or more stressful period of time from the parents and is losing hope that they will return. The child is usually more withdrawn and may respond with anger or silence when parents visit.
3. *Denial.* This phase of separation is associated with the most significant negative psychological sequelae. The child appears to be resigned to abandonment and soon begins to participate more in activities of his or her environment. The child may not appear to be affected by the presence or the absence of the parents but, in fact, may be withdrawing as a defense mechanism. During this period, the child may readily form superficial relationships with members of the health care team, but this may represent evidence of emotional trauma rather than a "positive adjustment" to hospitalization.

PREVENTION

1. The child requires reassurance and support during separations from parents.
2. The child tolerates separation from parents best when:
   a. The child is physically and emotionally healthy.
   b. The duration of separation is short.
   c. The separation is not accompanied by other stresses (pain, illness, etc.).
   d. Home routines (feeding time and types of food, nap time, bedtime) are maintained during the separation.
   e. The child is cared for by a limited number of nurses (so that the child may become accustomed to the m and they can learn about the child and the child's routines, and so that the child is not constantly subjected to repeat separations).
   f. The child is returned to the home environment, and normal routines are resumed at home.
   g. Parents return at regular, predicted intervals.
   h. The child is frequently reminded that he or she is good and loved (so the child has less tendency to associate separation with punishment).

ASSESSMENT

Hospitalization can interrupt the child's normal sequence of development and thus introduce anxiety, pain, and separation from family and from the security of familiar surroundings. Although such a crisis can be devastating to the child, it can also help the child and parents grow

TABLE 4-1 DEVELOPMENTAL TASKS AND STRESSES OF HOSPITALIZATION: INFANT

Developmental Tasks	Potential Stresses of Hospitalization
Enormous amount of learning	Constant environmental stimuli
Maternal-infant bonding	Separation from mother (or primary caretaker)
Development of object permanence at approximately 7 months (stranger and separation anxiety)	Lack of consistency of schedule and personnel
Learning to respond to and signal environment	Decreased environmental (and caretaker) response to signals
Oral gratification	Feeding disruptions
Reflex: Organized responses to stimuli	Restricted movement
Erikson: Trust vs. mistrust	Possible parental guilt and/or anxiety
Piaget: Sensorimotor period	Pain

TABLE 4-2 DEVELOPMENTAL TASKS AND STRESSES OF HOSPITALIZATION: TODDLER

Developmental Tasks	Potential Stresses of Hospitalization
Beginning upright (pedal) locomotion	Movement restriction
Egocentricity/ability to choose	Loss of control
Learning toilet training	Inability to move to bathroom at will
Developing concept of body image	Fear of bodily harm
Ambivalence/rage	Pain/punishment relationship (may assume painful procedures are punishment)
Development of language	Lack of comprehension of child's speech by personnel
Erikson: Autonomy vs. shame and doubt	Possible need to regress in order to cope
Piaget: Sensorimotor period	Disruption in routines
Freud: Retentive vs. eliminative mode	Inconsistency of caretakers, rules

in their ability to deal with stress and to master new challenges. The support of a sensitive health care team can make hospitalization a positive experience for parent and child.

Tables 4-1 through 4-5 summarize major developmental tasks of children at the major age groups. They also include potential consequences of hospitalization at each age group. Please note that the tables list common coping strategies the child may employ for dealing with a stressful situation.

Assessment of Potential Sources of the Child's Anxiety

1. If the child must be hospitalized frequently, it becomes even more important that the experiences be as positive as possible.
2. Determine the sources of anxiety (nightmares, fantasies, medical treatments, hospital environment, family crisis, separation from family, etc.). Much assessment can be accomplished through play.

TABLE 4-3 DEVELOPMENTAL TASKS AND STRESSES OF HOSPITALIZATION: PRESCHOOLER

Developmental Tasks	Potential Stresses of Hospitalization
Verbal means of communication	Medical staff discussions perhaps partially heard and understood
Expanding imagination and curiosity	Fantasies produce anxiety
Easy body control with developing body image	Concern for bodily integrity and fear of mutilation
Developing conscience	Illness-punishment relationship (may feel hospitalization is punishment)
Family/sex role identification	Loss of routine and family support systems
Developing individual coping style	Possible criticism by health team personnel for regression or withdrawal
Erikson: Initiative vs. guilt	Heightened vulnerability
Piaget: Preoperational thought	Poor concept of time intervals even after advance preparation for tests and procedures
Importance of play and activities	Separation from toys, play area ("safe" surroundings)

TABLE 4-4 DEVELOPMENTAL TASKS AND STRESSES OF HOSPITALIZATION: SCHOOL-AGE CHILD

Developmental Tasks	Potential Stresses of Hospitalization
Importance of the school environment	Separation from school
Geared to meet expectations and "succeed"	Loss of control over body, schedule, illness
Critical self-appraisal	Discomfort arising from focus on body
Reality-oriented	Guilt associated with illness
Acquiring peer group and friends	Separation from friends, concern about being "different"
Enormous intellectual growth	Interference with ability to communicate fears and misunderstandings about illness and treatment as a result of strong ego defenses
Psychoanalytic theory: "Latency" years	Fears of bodily mutilation
Erikson: Industry vs. Inferiority	Boredom and frustration with inactivity
Piaget: Concrete operational thought	Incomplete explanations and exclusion from discussions of plan of care
Good concept of time	Lack of thorough preparation for treatments

a. Provide medical equipment and nonmedical toys and allow the client to play freely. Watch and listen for clues to the child's fears, concerns, opinions.
b. Request that the school-age client draw a self-portrait or a picture of his or her hospital unit, and then discuss it with the child.
c. It may be helpful to ask the child to "name one thing that is scary" as children often respond better to specific rather than vague or broad questions.

3. Determine the child's interpretation of the illness and severity of his or her condition (as noted earlier, school-age children often think illness or pain is a punishment). The child may need support in working through these ideas.

TABLE 4-5 DEVELOPMENTAL TASKS AND STRESSES OF HOSPITALIZATION: ADOLESCENT

Developmental Tasks	Potential Stresses of Hospitalization
Puberty and body changes	Threat to bodily integrity
Break from childhood	Restricted independence
Dependence vs. independence	Loss of control
Learning to resolve conflict between ideology and practicality	Disagreement with health care personnel about plan of care or hospital rules
Developing heterosexual interest	Separation from peer group and activities
Ability to deal with hypothetical	Severe anxiety or depression stemming from understanding of illness and prognosis
Erikson: Identity vs. role diffusion	Loss of individual clothes, comforts of room
Piaget: Formal operational thought	Insufficient answers from health care team to young adult's hypothetical or "what if" questions

4. Determine any concurrent psychosocial or developmental stresses the child may be experiencing.
5. Provide the child with sufficient opportunities to ask questions.
6. The child's comprehension, interpretation, and support of care regimen must be assessed; note any misconceptions the child may have about the illness or treatment.

Assessment of Potential Sources of Parent's Anxiety

1. Note family structure and support systems (see, also, *Family Health History,* above).
2. Determine the significance of the child's illness to the family.
   a. Note parents' (or primary caretaker's) description of child's health; note any misconceptions that may be increasing their anxiety.
   b. Assess family's interpretation of the severity of the child's illness.
   c. Note any concurrent stresses (financial or emotional) family members are encountering that may interfere with family support.
3. Allow family members to discuss fears and frustrations.
4. Identify economic, cultural, or social factors that may hinder parental compliance with the child's therapy (these must be addressed in teaching plan).

NURSING DIAGNOSES: ACTUAL OR POTENTIAL

1. Anxiety of child related to fear of the unknown, fear of bodily harm, lack of familiarity with or trust in health team members, separation from parents, pain, movement restriction, loss of independence, and misconceptions about cause and treatment of illness.
2. Anxiety of parents related to guilt, loss of control of child's care, inadequate or inaccurate understanding of treatment plan or of surgical or procedural risks or goals, inconsistent messages from health team members.
3. Delay in child's normal developmental sequence related to multiple caretakers, anxiety, loss of normal routines, pain, weakness, and separation from parents.
4. Anger of parents related to guilt or misconceptions regarding cause of child's illness, mistrust of health care personnel, inconsistent messages from health care team, loss of control over child's care, and anxiety.
5. Noncompliance with home care regimen due to inadequate knowledge and anxiety.

EXPECTED OUTCOMES

1. Child and parents will discuss accurately the child's disease and treatment plan.
2. Child and family members will discuss concerns and sources of stress in a constructive manner.
3. Child and family will demonstrate mutual support.
4. Child will demonstrate activities appropriate for age group, energy level, and prehospitalization developmental level.
5. Child (as appropriate) and parent(s) will demonstrate appropriate knowledge and skills to perform child's home health care, including:
   a. Indications for contacting physician or primary nurse.
   b. Appropriate timing and administration of medications (including what to do if medication dose has been forgotten).
   c. Potential side effects or cautions for medications.
   d. Appropriate diet.
   e. Appropriate activity (including any restrictions).
   f. Dressing changes or wound care.

INTERVENTIONS

1. Encourage child's and parent's discussion of fears or concerns, if such discussion appears to reduce their anxiety and clarify information (if discussion appears to be too threatening, use other, nonverbal modes of communication, such as art or therapeutic play).
2. Assist child in developing plan to eliminate sources of unwarranted fear:
   a. Some imagined sources of fear may be eliminated through discussion and carefully worded explanations.
   b. Other sources of anxiety may be conquered through use of therapeutic play and by participation in self-care whenever possible (offer child reasonable choices and some control over scheduling and treatment plan).
3. Provide the child with consistent health team members whenever possible and a consistent schedule to increase child's and

family's familiarity with environment and care regimen.

4. Assist parents with planning adequate rest periods for child.
5. Include parents or primary caretaker in child's plan of care; however, maintain integrity of the parental role, and do not make nurses out of parents. The child will need a "safe" person who does not give painful treatments or medications.
6. Familiarize the family with the child's care schedules and health team members and provide appropriate teaching regarding unit policies and rules.
7. Be sensitive to the learning needs of child and parents.
   a. Provide child and caretaker with sufficient opportunity to ask questions.
   b. Be aware that information *you* would like to give client and family is not always consistent with amount and type of information they actually need in order to care for the child. (Do not overwhelm them with excess information or speculation.)
8. Familiarize child and family with postoperative or postprocedure equipment and care routines.
   a. Be sensitive to what the child or parents *hear* (not always the same as what you may be saying).
   b. Consider the child's age and cognitive development when determining appropriate timing for preparatory teaching.
      (1) If the child does not yet understand the concept of time intervals, early preparation may only provide excessive time for fears to build up or may confuse child. In this case, it is usually best to prepare the child immediately before the event.
      (2) A child 4 years or older can usually comprehend discussion of future events and appreciate time intervals, so preparation should be planned to allow sufficient time for the child to mobilize emotional defenses before the procedure.
   c. Usually, younger clients are more concerned about what they will *feel;* older clients are often more curious about *why* and *how* things will be done.
   d. If child and family have sufficient energy and emotional strength, familiarize them with the postprocedure or postoperative care unit, unit personnel, routines, and visiting hours.
   e. Attempt to provide child and parents with a timetable of procedures that will include them (e.g., sequence of diagnostic tests, time parents should be present on unit to speak with physician, etc.).
   f. NOTE: Children often fear mutilation when they anticipate surgical procedures; nursing care should support children so that they feel comfortable enough to express these fears and work through them.
9. Provide teaching regarding parental assessment of child's condition at home, and home health care.
   a. Child and family should be taught when to seek medical care and how to reach members of the health care team.
   b. When parent or primary caretaker is sensitive and observant, determination of the child's health status becomes intuitive and accurate. Parent will bring the child to the physician with the complaint that "something's not right" when the child is ill; this is often the most sensitive indicator of child's health status. In this case, teaching should focus on reinforcement of the parent's observational skills and assistance in clarifying any associated symptoms the child may be demonstrating (e.g., when "something's not right," child is breathing very rapidly).
   c. When the child's caretaker is less observant or demonstrates more difficulty appreciating changes in the child's condition, teaching should include simple observational tasks and more frequent follow-up visits with health care personnel.
10. Teach child and parents appropriate level of physical activity for the child.
    a. Young children will often limit their activity appropriately if they experience dyspnea or other intolerance of exercise.
    b. Because of peer pressure adolescents and school-age children may frequently test limitations placed by physician, so the nurse must discuss the importance of such restrictions with the client as well as potential consequences of violations.

EVALUATION

Outcome criteria

These will be the same as the outcomes previously stated under *Expected Outcomes* above.

Complications

1. Child's and parents' anxiety accelerate, so they become unable to provide support for one another.
   a. Nursing care must focus on breaking the anxiety cycle by minimizing the variety of the child's and parents' sources of (potentially conflicting) information. Plans for the child's care should be presented thoroughly, with more time allowed for questions and preparation. Occasionally, it may be necessary to speak to the parents in a separate room (away from the child) so that they may discuss their questions or fears without inflicting them on the child.
   b. Reevaluation and follow-up: Child and parents should be able to repeat information regarding child's health care plan accurately. Child and parents should be able to interact without increasing one another's anxiety.
2. The child demonstrates withdrawn behavior or other evidence of anxiety (e.g., soiling, even though the child was previously "potty-trained," thumbsucking, etc.) that may be misinterpreted and criticized (by parents or staff) as immature behavior.
   a. Nursing care should support the child's coping and explore the sources of the child's anxiety (through play, discussion, etc.). The child may need help in verbalizing the sources of the anxiety; criticism to "act your age" may only increase the child's anxiety and guilt.
   b. Reevaluation and follow-up: The child's regressive behavior will not be criticized by health care staff, and sources of child's anxiety will be minimized so that the child will have to employ coping behaviors less frequently.
3. Child and parent are unable to discuss or demonstrate sufficient knowledge or skills to provide child's home care.
   a. Nursing care should determine the cause of the failure of the teaching plan (inconsistency of information, parent anxiety, etc.) and plan to resume teaching as soon as the impediments to learning have been removed.
   b. Reevaluation and follow-up: Child and parent will be able to discuss and demonstrate required home health care principles and techniques.
4. Child may demonstrate lack of preparation for procedure or surgery.
   a. The nurse should initially ascertain what preoperative or preprocedure teaching was performed and what the child's initial reaction to it was. If the teaching apparently was performed without interruption or distraction, and consistent information was given, the nurse must assess potential sources of the child's misinterpretation or denial of the information (e.g., overwhelming anxiety). The teaching should be resumed only after the source of the child's inability to prepare has been eliminated and if the child indicates willingness to hear the information.
   b. Reevaluation and follow-up: Child (or parents) will be able to discuss or demonstrate knowledge of child's plan of care and postoperative or postprocedure care.

YOUNG ADULT (20 TO 40 YEARS)

PHYSICAL DEVELOPMENT

Full physical maturity is achieved in the early twenties. The rate of physiological aging begins to overtake the rate of cellular growth.

COGNITIVE DEVELOPMENT

Intellectual ability continues to increase if stimulated. The person becomes more serious about schooling and may return to school after a few years or for additional education or skill development. Interest broadens into community and world affairs. May be active in civic projects.

PSYCHOSOCIAL DEVELOPMENT

Chooses, prepares for, and practices a vocation. Becomes independent of parents. Prepares for and adjusts to marriage or other intimate love relationship. Develops civic consciousness. Refines own value system. Develops a unique personal identity. Childbearing and child rearing are major concerns of those who have children and are strongly associated with both stress and satisfaction. Reworks patterns of responsibility and accountability. Adjusts to ongoing relationships, such as those with employer, spouse, parents, and children. Manipulates household activity patterns, including the spending of money, to accommodate changing family needs. The rapidity of change in all aspects of current-day life compounds the stresses with which people have traditionally had to cope.

NURSING CONSIDERATIONS

1. *Health maintenance.* Cumulative health history should be maintained. Baseline data (ECG, laboratory reports) should be collected for later reference. Periodic physical and dental examinations should be obtained to maintain health and check for silent diseases. Good health practices help maintain optimum health. Preventive practices should be taught, such as avoiding obesity and preventing stress-related illnesses.
2. *Mental health.* Prevention of and early intervention for mental health problems that arise with developmental crises (e.g., parenthood) or situational crises (e.g., divorce, death of a parent) of this age span can be critical to the well-being of the individual and the family. Crisis intervention, short-term marriage counseling, or participation in self-help groups (e.g., parents who have lost a baby to SIDS, Alanon) can be very effective. Person may need education about the need for counseling at times when stress is particularly great, with an effort to dispel the stigma attached to seeking counseling. May need to learn new coping mechanisms. Good mental hygiene should be as much a goal as absence of physical stress symptoms.
3. *Reproduction and child rearing.* With improved methods of birth control, the question is not only the number of children wanted and when to have them, but whether to have children at all. Knowledge about birth control should be available before the person becomes sexually active (see Chapter 6). Special health care needs of the pregnant woman and new mother need to be provided (see the chapters in Part II). Parents of both sexes may need education about child-rearing practices and stages of growth and development. Parents may also need guidance in providing health care for children as well as for the family as a whole.
4. *Work.* A multitude of vocational choices make it difficult for the young adult to make a selection. This task may be delayed because of the extended period of education required for some vocations. The young adult may still be a student and financially dependent on parents.
5. *Continuing education.* Because of rapidly changing technology and the growing philosophy toward lifelong learning, the adult may have continuing education either on the job or in preparation for a new job if the old one becomes obsolete. The availability of education and shorter work hours also permit expansion of interests and hobbies.
6. *Emotional and intellectual maturity.* Physical maturity has been achieved but emotional and intellectual maturity may not yet have been reached. The continuing examination of the values of parents and others and the lessening of peer influence permit the formation of an individualized value system. This is more difficult in the present society than previously because of the rapid changes in society and technology that cause issues to become complex or clouded. The current-day emphasis on "finding oneself" often produces frustration while the young adult resolves conflicts between self-development and concern for loved ones.

MIDDLE AGE (40 TO 60 YEARS)

PHYSICAL DEVELOPMENT

Progressive physiological changes occur throughout middle life.

1. *Musculoskeletal changes.* Decrease in bone density and mass permits the body to "shrink." Muscle tone decreases, and the body may ap-

pear flabbier. Some decrease in muscle strength occurs.

2. *Sensory changes.* Presbyopia (farsightedness) and decreases in acuity, night vision, and peripheral vision are frequently associated with aging. Presbycussis (impaired hearing acuity) is common; the ability to hear high-frequency sounds is often the first lost. Ability to taste decreases because of atrophy of taste buds. (For additional information, see Chapter 26.)
3. *Sleep pattern changes.* Especially for males, the amount of time in deep sleep diminishes and wakefulness increases, so that the client tends to feel less well rested upon awaking. Sleep needs usually decrease, although sleep patterns are highly varied from one person to the next (Burnside, 1979).

COGNITIVE DEVELOPMENT

Little change in cognitive ability occurs. Motivation for learning is influential and is related to the importance the individual places on the task. The person consciously draws upon past experience for problem solving.

PSYCHOSOCIAL DEVELOPMENT

1. *Family relations.* Assists teenage and young adult offspring to become responsible and happy adults. Works out money matters with teenagers. Establishes a division of labor for sharing the responsibilities of family living. Permits offspring to have affectional relationships and courtship experiences. Keeps communication systems open among family members. Maintains contact with extended family. Provides financing, if able, for offspring launching a career or continuing their education. Reallocates responsibilities with remaining members of household. Expands the family circle through release of young adults and recruitment of new members by marriage. Tries to reconcile conflicting loyalties and philosophies of life between the generations. Learns and adjusts to role as grandparent. Defines the role of grandparent (e.g., fun-seeker, parent surrogate, reservoir of family wisdom, or distant figure). Maintains a relationship with grandchildren. Redefines roles in marriage. Builds a new relationship with spouse, or may change marriage partners. Roles and tasks within the home may change. Adjusts to aging parents or loss of parents and reverses the caring and providing roles. Forgives parents for past hurts and real or imagined inadequacies.
2. *Social roles.* Achieves adult social and civic responsibility. Significance of friends increases, as does value placed on coworkers. Participation in civic matters increases.
3. *Occupation.* Reaches and maintains satisfactory performance in career. Develops heightened job productivity as a result of experience and accumulated knowledge. Redefines vocational aspirations and considers possible job change. The need for additional education may be identified. Adjusts to having reached "the peak." Women who choose earlier to work at home may now return to school or begin employment outside the home.
4. *Leisure activities.* Develops adult leisure-time activities. Development of interests and activities not only is enriching for the present but also is excellent preparation for the period when child rearing is completed and, later, when retirement comes.
5. *Acceptance of aging and preparation for future.* Readies self both financially and psychologically for retirement (see also item 4 immediately above). Continues integration of a philosophy of life. Is aware of the philosophical wisdom of the culture. Realizes death is inevitable.
6. *Sexuality.* Accepts changing body and body image. Adapts to changing sexual patterns. The female may experience increased interest in sexual activity as a result of freedom from fatiguing child care and decreased fear of pregnancy. The male may need increased time to produce erection and ejaculation; this change increases the time in sexual play and brings greater pleasure to both partners.

NURSING CONSIDERATIONS

1. *Health maintenance: physical examination.* The risk factors of aging, stress, and accumulation of environmental influences create a need for annual physical and dental examinations and periodic screening for the diseases most common to this age, such as cancer, hypertension, and diabetes.
2. *Health maintenance: sensory changes.* May need to use reading glasses for close work, limit driving to daytime, and learn to shift eyes to maintain wide visual field. Should have an

eye examination every 1 to 2 years during the period of greatest change, the forties. A suspected hearing loss indicates a need for evaluation and possible fitting for a hearing aid. Frequent examination of hearing may be indicated if working in noise-polluted area. (For additional information, see Chapter 26.)

3. *Health maintenance: nutrition education.* Nutrition teaching should be done to reduce caloric intake without producing nutritional shortages. Supplemental vitamins are not needed by the healthy adult with an adequate dietary intake. Adding spices to food to compensate for diminishing taste acuity may be contraindicated if there is evidence of other health problems, such as peptic ulcer or irritable colon. Salt use should be curtailed to help prevent hypertension.
4. *Health maintenance: exercise.* An exercise program should be planned and followed. Walking is an excellent form of exercise available to almost everyone. Physically taxing forms of recreation need not decrease if a pattern of exercise has been maintained. If new activities involving additional physical stresses are begun, a graduated plan of increased exercise is important.
5. *Sleep.* Decreased need for sleep may cause a great deal of worry about insomnia and result in habituation to drugs. The quality of sleep is more important than the quantity.
6. *Family relations.* With the shifting of family structure and increasing stresses, additional support systems, including counseling, may be needed. Marital therapy may be recommended if adjustments are difficult. If disabled parents require constant attention, family "vacations" or rest periods may be needed in order for the family to continue with its own developmental tasks.
7. *Sexuality.* Partners need to recognize the change in patterns of sexual functioning as normal. Impotence is more likely caused by fear of loss of sexual function than by any physical changes.
8. *Mental health.* Susceptibility to anxiety seems to increase with age. Depression is frequent in this age group. Diversity of pleasurable activities assists with coping. Hobbies or sports enjoyed as a child may be a beginning point for people with no interest at present. Vocational counseling may assist in developing a new career if that is desirable. A youth-oriented culture may make acceptance of the changes of aging difficult. (See also item 6, *Family relations,* immediately above.)
9. *Finances.* Financial obligations to adult children as well as to the primary family may interfere with saving for retirement. On the other hand, the opportunity to obtain long wished for luxuries may be available.

MATURITY (60 YEARS AND OVER)

See also Chapters 44 and 45.

PHYSICAL DEVELOPMENT

1. *General function.* Physiological changes include general diminution of function. There may be greater decline in the more complex functions than in simple ones. Aging takes place at different rates between individuals and also within each individual's various tissues and systems. Vulnerability to disease is increased. Ability to maintain homeostasis is decreased. The major change in cells is that cellular reproduction is at a slower rate.
2. *Body system changes.* Tissue changes occur. *Musculoskeletal* changes include decrease in bone mass, loss of elasticity in joints, degeneration of cartilage and connective tissue, and gradual decrease in muscle mass. There is decreased efficiency of the *nervous system,* manifested primarily in increased response time. Progressive loss of *sensory* functions compounds the effect of other declining functions. Alterations of the *integument* include wrinkling, sagging, growths and discolorations, loss of hair for men or growth of hair on women's faces, drying, and thinning. Alterations in the *pulmonary system* include decreases in breathing capacity, residual lung volume, and total lung capacity, with consequent decreases in basal oxygen and metabolic rate. Decreased bronchoelimination results from diminished cough reflex and decreasing efficiency of the ciliary mechanism. Changes in the *digestive system* include periodontal disease (preventable), decrease in digestive juices, slowed peristalsis, and interferences with absorption. Modifications in

the *cardiovascular system* include changes in vessel structure (narrowing and loss of elasticity), valvular disease, and arrhythmias. *Renal system* changes may include renal atrophy, which contributes to diminished renal function, and increased risk of lower urinary tract infections. Involutionary processes affect the renal system, both in decreased number of cells and the capacities of the remaining cells. Extrarenal disease increases with age. *Endocrine system* changes include both decreased hormone production and diminution of the effect of the hormones produced. *Immunologic* defenses are diminished. *Sexual* function is altered. Tissue changes may reduce the flexibility of the vagina and the firmness of the erect penis. Sexual response time is slowed but is compensated for by a lengthened arousal period.

COGNITIVE DEVELOPMENT

There is little if any change in IQ. Skills and abilities tend to become obsolete rather than lost through deterioration. Intellectual functioning may be somewhat slower but is compensated for by extra caution and fewer mistakes from inexperience. Memory losses affect the more recent events, whereas events of long ago are remembered. Meaningfulness affects what is remembered. Problem-solving ability is decreased because of the loss of recent memory, difficulty in making fine discriminations among stimuli, and fear of making mistakes. Learning performance may be altered by speed of response, level of motivation, and state of health. A decrease in learning ability has not been proven.

PSYCHOSOCIAL DEVELOPMENT

1. *Retirement.* Retirement introduces changed schedules, reduced income, and additional time for leisure and other uses. Readjustments in roles and relationships within the home may require considerable attention from both spouses. Readjusting social roles includes establishing affiliations with own age group and developing friendships that are no longer focused around the job.

   There may be a change in living facilities. The present dwelling may be too large, too expensive to maintain, or unsuitable for people with increasing disabilities. A location previously chosen for convenience to work, schools, and so on may no longer be desirable. A change in climate is often sought. Locating in an area with other retired people may be appealing to some; others may want to remain in their established setting. The retiree maintains ties with children, grandchildren, and possibly parents. Feelings of worth, pride, and usefulness need to be maintained. Volunteer work is often an aid in meeting these goals.
2. *Acceptance of inevitability of death.* Deaths of spouse, friends, and acquaintances are realities at this age. The increased awareness of the inevitability of one's own death facilitates setting of goals to be achieved before death. One goal may be one's preparation for death through strengthening religious beliefs or other vehicles of self-transcendance. The elderly ultimately teach others how to die through their own deaths.

NURSING CONSIDERATIONS

1. *Health maintenance: physical examinations.* Regular screening for degenerative disorders and chronic diseases (cancer, hypertension, and diabetes) is required at least yearly, as their likelihood increases with age and early recognition and treatment can greatly improve outcomes. Cumulative effects of past illnesses and previous poor health habits increase health risks. Many discomforts and functional limitations may result from the aging process, but changes should be evaluated for the presence of some underlying disease process and for appropriate supportive treatment for the symptoms of aging. Examination by an appropriately prepared person should be done before corrective items such as glasses and hearing aids are purchased.
2. *Health maintenance: nutrition.* Natural seasonings such as lemon or onion may increase flavor when taste and smell are declining. Teach to use caution with hot foods and liquids to avoid burns. Diminished intestinal absorption is a factor to consider, both in terms of nutrition and from a pharmacological standpoint. Maintaining adequate fluid intake (2000–3000 mL) is often forgotten by the aged, or they may limit their fluids to reduce urinary frequency. Acidic fluids will help maintain urine acidity and decrease

susceptibility to urinary tract infection. Teeth must function properly so that digestive juices can penetrate food and so that the person can ingest roughage to stimulate peristalsis. Twice-yearly dental examinations are necessary for denture wearers for preventive maintenance of fit as the tissues and structure of the mouth change.

3. *Health maintenance: exercise.* Slowing and increasing ease of fatigue may lead to sedentary behavior patterns. A regular exercise program helps promote good health and slows the aging process. Reasonable exercise, determined by past patterns, should be continued. Excessive fatigue is to be avoided. Body position should not be changed quickly (e.g., from sitting to standing) nor should the head be turned or tilted quickly, in order to avoid dizziness. Extremes in activity or environment may be less well tolerated than previously. Movement becomes slower and uneven. More time should be allowed for all activities.
4. *Health maintenance: sleep.* As sleep patterns change, 4 or 5 h at night and a short nap or two in the daytime are probably all that are required.
5. *Health maintenance: avoidance of infection.* Extra precautions should be taken to avoid respiratory infections or other infections, as immune response is diminished. Any illness that directly or indirectly decreases pulmonary function creates a high risk of pneumonia and demands immediate nursing intervention.
6. *Health maintenance: safety.* Teaching about preventive safety measures becomes especially important at this age. Evaluation of living quarters for hazards may decrease the risk of accidents. Falls, fires, and auto accidents (including pedestrian incidents) are major accident categories for the elderly. Diminishing agility, balance, and sensory perception (i.e., host factors rather than environmental factors) contribute to accident vulnerability; hence, *client* assessment is required in addition to evaluation of the environment. Interventions for host factors may include eyeglasses, teaching avoidance of abrupt position changes and drugs that can impair balance, and periodic reevaluation for safety in driving an automobile. Environmental interventions may include hand rails, adequate lighting, white strips on the edges of stairsteps, and the like.
7. *Sexuality.* The libido is generally not reduced until the eighties or so; therefore, an active sexual relationship can continue if one's mate is willing and able and if time and privacy are considered. Couples need to know that change in patterns of sexual behavior is a normal process. The possibility of alternative lifestyles is being considered by numerous aged people. Self-stimulation may be an alternative way of meeting sexual needs.
8. *Mental health.* Satisfactory use of time promotes good mental and physical health. Previous interests of adult life or childhood may be redeveloped at this time. Participation in service-oriented organizations may help fill this need. Participation in clubs and organizations is one method of developing a new set of friends. Retirement counseling is available at many places of employment. Anticipatory planning well ahead may reduce the impact of change. A spouse who previously spent most of the day at work may now be "underfoot" at home all day. Activities such as service organizations, volunteer work, consultation, or part-time work may be more rewarding than "play." Feelings of guilt and depression may result if these needs are unfulfilled.

   Loss of spouse and friends along with physical losses will result in depression and withdrawal of varying degrees. Counseling and other support services may be useful. Participation in religious groups of choice may provide comfort. An opportunity to express feelings and thoughts enhances acceptance of death. Observing others' dying is the only way the living can learn about dying.
9. *Living arrangements.* Caution should be recommended concerning changes in residence or location. Friends of long standing, the familiar climate, and the variety of people in the community may be more rewarding than recognized at first. A trial period at a new location before cutting the ties from the past may avoid a lot of regrets. Moving in with children may or may not be desirable for both parties. Independent living may be maintained longer with support from community agencies such as home health care,

housekeeping services, a regular visitor, and monitoring phone calls.

10. *Finances.* If previous financial preparation for retirement has not been adequate, additional sources of support may have to be solicited. Part-time jobs or hobbies may provide some financial gain.
11. *Social contributions.* Expertise developed through the years may be shared through a role as an "elder" consultant, and this role may serve to increase self-esteem and a feeling of usefulness.
12. *Lifelong learning.* The slowing or diminution of sensory and motor processes often causes others (and the aged person as well) to conclude that there has been a loss of intellectual ability. The person should be allowed to pace activities to enhance learning. The trend toward lifelong learning will tend in the future to prevent this obsolescence from occurring.

REFERENCES

Barnard, M. U., et al.: *Handbook of Comprehensive Pediatric Nursing,* McGraw-Hill, New York, 1981.

Burnside, I. M., Ebersole, P., and Monea, H. E. (eds.): *Psychosocial Caring Throughout the Life Span,* McGraw-Hill, New York, 1979.

Waletzky, L. R. (ed.): *Symposium on Human Lactation,* publication no. (HSA) 79-5107, U.S. Department of Health, Education and Welfare, Rockville, Md., 1976.

BIBLIOGRAPHY

Burnside, I. M. (ed.): *Nursing and the Aged,* 2d ed., McGraw-Hill, New York, 1981. A thorough and very helpful exploration of the middle-aged and old person's developmental tasks and vulnerabilities, including health problems, and the nursing process as it applies to maximize the well-being of older persons.

———, Ebersole, P., and Monea, H. E. (eds.): *Psychosocial Caring Throughout the Life Span,* McGraw-Hill, New York, 1979. This book is appropriate for a variety of professionals and paraprofessionals. It is useful as a reference for psychosocial development.

Butler, R. N., and Lewis, M. I.: *Aging and Mental Health: Positive Psychosocial Approaches,* 2d ed., Mosby, St. Louis, 1977. This fine book by the physician-director of the National Institute on Aging and a social worker-gerontologist realistically presents the problems and potentials of the elderly. Assessment and intervention for individuals and groups are presented in a manner that is very helpful to nurses. Government programs, in-service education materials, and social services for the aged and those who assist them are briefly reviewed in the appendixes.

Diekelmann, N.: *Primary Health Care of the Well Adult,* McGraw-Hill, New York, 1977. This book's focus is on the well adult and nursing interventions to meet well-care needs of young, middle-aged, and older adults. Activity, rest, safety, environmental health, and sexuality are among the topics presented.

Erikson, E. H.: *Childhood and Society,* 2d ed., Norton, New York, 1963. This book includes a chapter presenting the classic "eight ages of man," Erikson's *either-or* formulations of developmental tasks throughout the life span.

Howard, R. B., and Herbold, N. H. (eds.): *Nutrition in Clinical Care,* 2d ed., McGraw-Hill, New York, 1982. Excellent reference about food-related behavior and nutrition throughout the life span and in various states of health and illness.

Howe, J. (ed.): *Nursing Care of Adolescents,* McGraw-Hill, New York, 1980. This multiauthored book by and for nurses discusses the major substantive topics related to health and health deviations during adolescence (growth and development, response to illness and disability, nutrition, substance abuse, mental retardation, sexuality, health teaching and counseling, crisis, etc.) and describes settings and programs in which adolescents receive health care, including rehabilitation centers, street clinics, women's health clinics, juvenile detention institutions, and others.

Kastenbaum, R. J.: *Death, Society, and Human Experience,* Mosby, St. Louis, 1977. This excellent exploration of social and psychological aspects of death and dying includes discussions of "the death system" and the impact of death at various points in the life span.

Manaster, G. J.: *Adolescent Development and the Life Tasks,* Allyn and Bacon, Boston, 1977. This readable, psychology textbook summarizes current thinking about adolescents' physiological, cognitive, moral, sex-role, and personality development and the major developmental tasks—school, work, and interpersonal affiliations.

Murray, R., and Zentner, J.: *Nursing Assessment and Health Promotion through the Life Span,* 2d ed., Prentice-Hall, Englewood Cliffs, N.J., 1979. Developmental characteristics at each stage of life are described and nursing supports are presented.

Neugarten, B. L. (ed.): *Middle Age and Aging: A Reader in Social Psychology,* University of Chicago Press, Chicago, 1968. This valuable collection of readings deals with the psychology of the life cycle and theories of aging. Subtopics include family relationships, work, leisure, retirement, and death.

Ramsey, N. L.: "Effects of Hospitalization on the Child and Family," in M. J. Smith et al. (eds.), *Child and Family: Concepts of Nursing Practice,* McGraw-Hill, New York, 1982. Excellent and detailed description of how children and parents respond to illness, hospitalization, treatments, and related stressors; their fears and fantasies; and nursing techniques for assisting them in coping.

Schuster, C. S., and Ashburn, S. S.: *The Process of Human Development: A Holistic Approach,* Little, Brown, Boston, 1980. A comprehensive exploration of human development in western culture. The focus is on the healthy individual functioning at the highest potential. It is organized chronologically from conception through old age around the four domains. The idea of the uniqueness of the individual is not lost.

Scipien, G. M., et al. (eds.): *Comprehensive Pediatric Nursing,* 2d ed., McGraw-Hill, New York, 1979. This exceptionally useful textbook includes chapters about the nursing process as employed in the care of children and about growth and development and effects of illness at each age and stage of childhood.

Sheehy, G.: *Passages: Predictable Crises of Adult Life,* Dutton, New York, 1976. Primarily a journalistic rather than scientific or professional book, this best-seller examines the life tasks and crises of the postadolescent years.

Shneidman, E. S. (ed.): *Death: Current Perspectives,* 2d ed., Mayfield, Palo Alto, Calif., 1980. This is a collection of readings from the arts, sciences, and service professions. Intended as a textbook for college students in death and dying courses, it provides an excellent overview of social, demographic, and personal attitudes and practices related to dying.

Stevenson, J. S.: *Issues and Crises During Middlescence,* Appleton-Century-Crofts, New York, 1977. Provides insight into the middle years of adulthood and the crises that are likely to occur.

Tudor, M. (ed.): *Child Development,* McGraw-Hill, New York, 1981. Superb, in-depth, comprehensive treatment of the biological, social, behavioral, cognitive, language, perceptual, and motor development of children from conception to puberty. Multiauthored book by nurse specialists.

Woods, N. F.: *Human Sexuality in Health and Illness,* 2d ed., Mosby, St. Louis, 1979. This is an excellent nursing reference on the topic of normal human sexual behavior and related nursing care, including care and counseling of ill and handicapped persons.

Yaros, P., and Howe, J.: "Responses to Illness and Disability," in J. Howe (ed.), *Nursing Care of Adolescents,* McGraw-Hill, New York, 1980. Describes effects of illness and related phenomena on adolescents at varying stages of maturity and identifies nursing interventions for promoting favorable outcomes.

5

Family Assessment and Nursing Intervention

Jean R. Miller

The family is important in preventing physical and psychosocial problems throughout the family life cycle, restoring health during illness, promoting an optimal level of wellness during health and illness, and supporting its members during times of illness and when death occurs. In general, when caring for families the nurse must develop skill to (1) screen and assess individual and family problems, (2) teach clients and their families regarding prevention of illness and recovery from illness, (3) counsel families as they deal with adjustments related to illness, and (4) refer families to other health care providers when appropriate. In this chapter each of these responsibilities will be discussed as they relate to common family problems throughout the family life cycle, difficulties associated with acute and chronic illness, and death in the family.

FAMILY IMPACT ON HEALTH AND ILLNESS

The family's powerful impact on health is seen in assessment of each of its members. The foundation for health promotion activities is established in the home, as health habits related to eating, sleeping, and relaxing are initiated and reinforced in the home. The family also imparts a sense of self-identity, allowing for expression of emotions without fear of loss of love and affection.

When a family member experiences symptoms of altered health, other members are often the first to observe changes in health. Discussions about the symptoms can be the main stimulus for the ill member to seek professional health care.

The members of a family assist one another during acute illness, recovery, chronic illness, and death. They adjust their functions in the home when someone in the family is sick so that the ill member can assume an altered role function and recover more quickly. Because family members are the people in closest contact with an ill member, the family can be instrumental in encouraging its members to assume positive health behaviors. During the course of chronic illness, the family can be a source of aid by reinforcing appropriate behaviors that are conducive to prevention of other problems and maintenance of a healthy state. A family with a dying member also can be the main source of support to one another and the dying member, as supportive bonds of affection have been established over time.

The family needs to be viewed in the broadest sense. The traditional definition of a family is a group of two or more persons who are joined by marriage, blood, or adoption and who interact with one another but may not live together.

A broader and more useful definition is to view a family as a group of two or more persons who are joined by an agreement to share various aspects of life together. The latter definition allows the health professional to involve a greater range of persons in the care of the ill member.

ALTERNATIVE FAMILY STRUCTURES

Alternative family structures and the people who make up these family units are listed below.

1. *Single-parent families*: consist of either father or mother of one or more children.
2. *Three-generation families*: usually consist of elderly parents, their adult child, and the adult child's children.
3. *Blended families*: consist of a husband and wife who have been married previously and who bring one or more children into the new family.
4. *Unmarried single-parent families*: consist of unmarried single parents who are rearing their children or single parents who adopt children.
5. *Unmarried couples*: consist of couples of the same or opposite sex who are living together without having made a legally binding agreement.
6. *Commune families*: consist of married couples, unmarried couples, single persons, and children.

Each type of family tends to go throgh normal developmental crises that are typically experienced in traditional families. Alternative family types, however, often face additional difficulties that affect the emotional, social, and physical well-being of the family.

NURSING ROLE: ASSISTING THE FAMILY

Families offten experience similar difficulties as they pass through each stage of the family life cycle (Duvall, 1977). Most families manage these difficulties without professional assistance. Sometimes, however, the resistance of some families to disease is weakened by the strain associated with trying to cope with the various problems of everyday living. Often members from such families are seen in clinics and doctors' offices with complaints such as depression, headaches, and viral infections.

The goal of nursing is to assist families in mobilizing their resources to facilitate self-care. Knowledge of the types of stresses families normally experience when confronted with chronic health problems can be helpful to nurses in assessing and counseling clients and their families. Nurses also can assist families in anticipating stressful internal and external events. In this way families can be prepared to resist predictable problems and adapt to changes throughout the family life cycle.

The nurse needs to be sensitive to a family's readiness for anticipatory guidance. Some families welcome information and help concerning how they can best deal with upcoming events, whereas other families feel that the present is a large enough burden to bear. The nurse needs to be aware of differences in the desire for anticipatory guidance among families and must provide counseling measures accordingly.

The following section presents the major tasks for each stage of the family life cycle along with common crisis events and problems most often encountered in each stage. Some of the problems listed below will have a direct influence on family members' health. The nurse may use these potential problems listed under each major family task as a guide in determining if the problems normally encountered in family development are affecting the health of family members.

COMMON FAMILY PROBLEMS

1. Marital family: Early prechild couple (dyad).
   a. Communication problems.
      (1) Indirect messages.
      (2) Difficulty with open verbalization of differences and conflicts.
      (3) Lack of honesty and trust.

(4) Inconsistent or incongruent messages.
(5) Poor listening skills.

b. Roles and division of labor.
   (1) Lack of flexibility, i.e., rigidity about roles.
   (2) Lack of clarity as to who should perform which tasks.
   (3) Lack of skills to do tasks.
c. Sexual relations.
   (1) Insensitivity to partner's needs.
   (2) Tenseness and performance expectations.
d. Conflict management.
   (1) Unrealized expectations.
   (2) Misunderstandings.
   (3) Unestablished methods for dealing with conflict.
e. Extended family relations.
   (1) Relationships with extended family.
   (2) Autonomy and individuality of new family unit—establishing own traditions.
f. Decision making.
   (1) Who has the most power and influence and in what circumstances.
   (2) How income should be spent.
   (3) Whether or not to have children and when.
   (4) Purchase of a home and home furnishings.

2. Childbearing family.
   a. Psychological response to news of pregnancy.
      (1) Financial implications.
      (2) Fear of loss of freedom.
   b. Self-esteem of parents (parenting problems).
      (1) Physical and emotional implications for mother.
      (2) Father's value and importance in the process.
      (3) Fantasies about child.
   c. Sexual relations during pregnancy.
      (1) Feelings of unattractiveness by the woman.
      (2) Uncomfortable sexual positions.
      (3) Decreased sexual relations in the third trimester.
   d. Physical discomfort of pregnant mother.
   e. Fears concerning the well-being of the child.
   f. Increased tasks and responsibilities after the arrival of the child.
   g. Decreased time for interaction between the spouses after the birth of the child.
3. Preschool family.
   a. Parental differences in child-rearing styles due to upbringing.
   b. Lack of clarity regarding parental roles.
   c. Feelings of inadequacy regarding physical, psychological, social, and spiritual care of the children.
   d. Desires for adult interaction and activities by the parent staying at home with the children.
4. School-aged family.
   a. Overinvolvement between mother and children.
      (1) Satisfaction derived more from children than from spouse.
      (2) Frustration from feeling left out of main stream of adult activities.
   b. Overinvolvement between father and his work—satisfaction derived more from outside work than from spouse or children.
   c. Inadequate financial resources for child care.
5. Teenage family.
   a. Chaos from adolescent vacillating between adult and child behavior.
   b. Transition in adolescent development of self-identity through peer rather than family approval.
6. Launching family.
   a. Parental difficulty in allowing the adolescent to assume adult roles and responsibilities.
   b. Loss of children to homes of their own—impact of separation from child and loss of control (differentiation).
7. Middle-aged family.
   a. Feelings of inadequacy resulting from loss of active occupational life.
   b. Decrease in strength and vitality of younger years.
   c. Difficulties with communication between husband and wife.
      (1) Lack of common interests.
      (2) Misunderstanding of one another's feelings.
      (3) Lack of clarity and spontaneity in conversations.
      (4) Lack of expressions of positive and negative affect.
   d. Responsibilities of aging parents may lead to increased stress

8. Aging family.
   a. Increasing health and self-care problems.
   b. Difficulty with home maintenance.
   c. Difficulty with activities of daily living.
   d. Feelings of little worth and value in our culture.

ADDITIONAL DIFFICULTIES OF NONTRADITIONAL FAMILY STRUCTURES

1. Single-parent family.
   a. Finances, especially for female-headed households
   b. Extensive child care because of working parent.
   c. Discipline decisions.
   d. Need for male or female role models, i.e., surrogate fathering/mothering figure.
   e. Loneliness—need for support systems for parent.
2. Three-generation family.
   a. Lack of role clarity among the elderly and their adult children and grandchildren.
   b. Overdependence between elderly parent and adult children.
   c. Antagonism between elderly parent and adult children.
3. Blended family.
   a. Lack of acceptance between stepparents and stepchildren.
   b. Children pulled between parent and stepparent.
   c. Children manipulated by parent and stepparent.
   d. Discipline—who, when, how.
   e. Financial difficulties.
   f. Marital misunderstandings.
4. Unmarried single-mother family.
   a. Finances and employment.
   b. Child care.
   c. Schooling for adolescent.
   d. Loneliness and feelings of alienation.
5. Unmarried couple.
   a. Instability of the relationship and loss of other relationships.
   b. Legal difficulties with property and finances.
   c. Decisions about childbearing.
6. Commune family.
   a. Emotional and financial instability.
   b. Poor physical environment—lack of privacy, ownership, control.
   c. Conflict with the outside community.

NURSING INTERVENTIONS FOR COMMON FAMILY PROBLEMS

The nurse has numerous opportunities to assist a family through difficult times in the family life cycle. These opportunities are prevalent during well-child visits, but needs for counseling are also evident during the hospitalization of a family member. Sometimes the stresses of life cycle crises are such that normal resistance to disease is diminished and health breakdown results. It is important for the nurse to recognize that family conflict at certain stages of the family life cycle may contribute to illness in a family member.

Many families could benefit from anticipatory guidance so that they would know what to expect in the next stage of family development and how to handle the problems normally associated with that stage. For instance, information about how adolescents think, feel, and act and how this affects the family could be helpful to a family anticipating the movement of a child into adolescence. Teaching-learning activities for such instances are suggested in the next section. The ultimate aim is to help families help themselves through these life cycle changes.

ASSESSMENT

1. Determine in which stage the family is within the family life cycle.
2. Assess the extent to which normal difficulties are becoming problems.
3. Assess the family's readiness and motivation to deal with existing problems and/or prepare for the difficulties of the next stage.
4. Examples of normal life cycle difficulties.
   a. A mother exhibits impatience and anger toward her child during a well-baby visit. The nurse refocuses assessment questions toward the well-being of the mother and finds that she feels exhausted and de-

pressed. She seldom gets more than 4 h of sleep each night because the baby is awake much of the night and sleeps during the day.
b. An adolescent complains of frequent headaches. He admits to feeling anxious at home where he is manipulated by his parent and stepparent in a newly blended family.
c. An elderly person is hospitalized for high blood pressure, which continues to be elevated inspite of medication and diet. During hospitalization, the blood pressure drops considerably without additional treatment. On examination, continual tensions were found in the home where the elderly person lives with her adult child and husband. Frequent arguments occur between the elderly person and her son-in-law. The family has not adjusted to the addition of a new and dependent member in the household.

EXPECTED OUTCOMES

1. Clients will understand the nature of the problems as they are related to various stages in the family life cycle.
2. Clients will develop methods for coping with family life cycle problems.
3. Clients will prepare for the next stage of the family life cycle.

INTERVENTION

1. Determine which issues are of most concern to the family and which issues should be dealt with first.
2. Decide with the family what they consider desirable behavior for the next stage.
3. Discuss preferred methods of learning, that is, reading, watching, listening, discussing, practicing.
4. Implement teaching-learning strategies according to the nature of the content and the desires of the family.
   a. Attendance at large group lectures.
   b. Small group discussions and individual family discussions.
   c. Films and slide-tape programs (often available for client and family use at the bedside).
   d. Demonstrations and return demonstrations.
   e. Role playing.
   f. Reading material, that is, pamphlets, articles, books.
5. Counsel the family when the problems deal with interpersonal relationships that need discussion by the family members.
   a. Listen to the family's perception of the problem.
   b. Convey your feelings of warmth and acceptance.
   c. Assist the family in clarifying the issue(s).
   d. Encourage family members to discuss alternative ways of handling their problems.
   e. Provide information as needed.
   f. Reinforce appropriate behaviors.
6. Refer to other health professionals when the problems are too complex for the level of education and ability of the nurse.

EVALUATION

The family should be involved in the evaluation process from the beginning of the sessions so that there is a clear understanding of what the family wants to accomplish.

Outcome Criteria

1. The family is able to compare where they are in understanding a family-related problem to where they want to be before discharge from the hospital or completion of visits.
2. The family has new plans for additional learning if necessary.
3. The family feels satisfied with their ability to mobilize their resources.
4. Desired behavior changes have occurred.

ACUTE ILLNESS IN THE FAMILY

The hospitalization of a family member usually is a crisis event, although the family normally displays considerable resiliency during this time. In fact, Litman (1971) found that family relations were more close than disruptive in nature during hospitalization depending, of course, on the family's definition of the situation and its reaction to it. Naturally there are disruptions in home activities, inconveniences, emotional feelings of missing the client, and role reversals, especially when the wife/mother is hospitalized. In most situations, principles from crisis theory frameworks can be used to guide the nurse in problem solving and supporting the family.

There are two models for crisis intervention that are at polor extremes: the *screening/assessment model* and the *problem-solving model.* A third model, the *convergent model,* which is based on the work of Caplan (1961), optimizes the strengths and minimizes the weaknesses of the other two opposing models. In the hospital setting, the problem-solving approach is most frequently used by medical-surgical nurses, as there is time to deal only with present and future-oriented issues in a relatively structured manner. The community health nurse is more likely to use the convergent model because there is the possibility of relating to the family over time. More information on each of these models can be found in the book by Burgess and Baldwin (1981). Emphasis in the next section will be on the crises which are involved with hospitalization of a family member.

ANTESTRESS PERIOD

This is the time during which the family becomes aware of the possible seriousness of the situation, that is, diagnostic testing and evaluation take place.

ASSESSMENT

1. *Assess anticipatory fears.* When the client and family have a period of time to prepare for hospitalization, such as for elective surgery, necessary arrangements can be made and the client and family can organize resources for coping with the hospitalization. This is also a time when many people become anxious and worried about the consequences of the hospitalization. Assessments need to be made when the client arrives at the hospital to determine if the anxiety is within normal limits so that the anxiety will not interfere with optimal recovery.

   When the hospitalization is required for a sudden and serious illness, such as a heart attack, the client and family may arrive at the hospital in a very stressful state. Often there is considerable tension and conflict at home because the victim and his or her family often do not agree on whether or not the ill member should be taken to the hospital and by what method. Family members may be speaking very little to one another when they first arrive at the hospital or they may be verbalizing angry statements. Usually there is a sense of relief when the client is finally admitted to the hospital, although fears remain.
2. *Assess knowledge of hospital routine.* If the family has not been associated with the hospital setting, the members may exhibit random and meaningless behavior. They often do not know where to go while the client is being admitted and when they can be in the room with the client.
3. *Assess knowledge of the client's condition.* Because the laboratory tests have not been completed at this point, it is difficult to give the family an accurate assessment of the condition of their loved one. The family may have exaggerated ideas of the seriousness of the problem or they may not realize how serious the condition really is. Information such as "the blood pressure is within normal limits" is helpful.
4. *Assess the meaning of the crisis to the family.* The family may view the admission of the family member to the hospital as a threat to current adjustment, a temporary loss of their family member while he or she is in the hospital, or a permanent loss, such as by death. Knowledge of the family's perception is important so that misperceptions can be clarified.

EXPECTED OUTCOMES

1. The family will become acquainted with the hospital setting and assume ways of interacting with the client that are supportive.
2. The family will gain a beginning understanding of the implications and realities of the illness and hospitalization for the client and for family relationships.

INTERVENTIONS

1. Allow family members to ventilate their fears.
2. Convey understanding of the family's fears.
3. Discuss ways to handle stress if the family members appear as though they are unable to manage the tension, for example, take a walk, get some food, talk to one another.
4. Explain the hospital routine, that is, where to

wait for the doctor, when to be with the client, where to park, where to eat.
5. Explain how the family can help the client, for example, hold and/or stroke the client's hand, apply cold wash cloth to forehead if needed, give the client ice chips if allowed.
6. Explain the procedures and treatments that are being done to the client.
7. Give the family information that might be helpful and reassuring, for example, a general reading on the blood pressure, temperature, pulse.

EVALUATION

Outcome Criteria

1. The family is comfortable in the hospital environment.
2. The family knows the essential ways of helping the client feel comfortable.
3. The family has a beginning understanding of the client's condition.
4. The family has a beginning understanding of the meaning of the illness and of how the hospitalization will affect family relationships.

STRESS PERIOD

At the midway point of the hospitalization, stress increases as the diagnosis is clarified.

ASSESSMENT

1. Assess the individual coping behaviors of family members.
   a. Maladaptive coping behaviors that are normal for short periods.
      (1) Denial of the seriousness of the illness.
      (2) Inability to mobilize a plan of action for caring for the client and family.
      (3) Meaningless random activity.
      (4) Aggressive (verbal and nonverbal) behavior directed toward family members and/or others.
      (5) Withdrawal from family members and/or others.
   b. Later signs of adaptive coping responses.
      (1) Expression of feelings with one another.
      (2) Resumption of usual communication patterns.
      (3) Utilization of support from family members and friends.
      (4) Problem solving and decision making.
      (5) Rearrangement of household tasks and activities.
      (6) Reduction in unpleasant affect.
2. Assess the family's ability to communicate and plan with one another.
   a. Extent to which family members listen to one another.
   b. Expression of feelings to one another.
   c. Clarity of messages.
3. Assess the family's ability to manage everyday tasks during the crisis period, for example, cooking, cleaning, washing, chauffering, visiting client.
   a. Reallocation of tasks according to members' abilities and strengths.
   b. Teaching and learning new tasks while the ill member is unable to perform his or her role.
4. Assess outside support systems available to the family.
   a. Determine who knows that the family needs help.
   b. Assess the degree to which others may be able to provide assistance.

EXPECTED OUTCOMES

1. The family will manage the crisis with adaptive coping responses.
2. The family will maintain its communication system.
3. The family will maintain a reasonable degree of order in the home.
4. The family will receive needed assistance from their support system.

INTERVENTIONS

1. Provide information regarding client status.
2. Allow family to give emotional support to the client when possible, that is, hold client's hand, have caring visits, sit with the client.
3. Encourage family members to rest and eat in order to maintain their strength.
4. Accept maladaptive coping behavior when it is limited to high-stress periods.
5. Encourage adaptive coping behavior during less stressful times.
6. Refer to appropriate colleagues when coping strategies are maladative over long periods.
7. Plan how everyday tasks can be managed at home.

8. Encourage the use of outside support persons when available and needed.
9. Convey care and concern.

EVALUATION

Outcome Criteria

1. The family shows more adaptive coping responses than maladaptive responses.
2. The family maintains communication among its members.
3. The family maintains the necessary home tasks.
4. The family accepts assistance from outside sources.

POSTSTRESS PERIOD

This is the time when the main trauma is over.

ASSESSMENT

1. Assess readiness to accept reality.
2. Assess readiness to problem-solve regarding care of client and family.
3. Assess readiness to learn more about the client's condition and ways to assist the client at home.
4. Assess readiness to learn how to prevent future problems related to the illness.

EXPECTED OUTCOMES

1. The family will accept reality.
2. The family will learn how to manage the family and client at home.
3. The family will learn how to prevent problems associated with the disease in the future.

INTERVENTIONS

1. Encourage family to express their feelings with one another.
2. Confirm reality if unrealistic expectations are expressed. Assess readiness for acceptance of implications of illness.
3. Assist the family in clarifying the issues.
4. Assist the family in problem solving and making decisions.
5. Assist the family in seeking and accepting support from friends and extended-family members.
6. Prepare the client and family for discharge.
   a. Medications.
      (1) Value of the drug.
      (2) How the family can help the client remember to take the drug at the prescribed time.
      (3) Side effects.
   b. Diet.
      (1) Value of prescribed diet.
      (2) Ways to integrate prescribed diet into the total family eating patterns.
   c. Activities. Restrictions on activities, especially as it relates to using the shower or tub, climbing stairs, lifting, driving a vehicle, or resuming sexual activities
   d. Treatments. Prescribed treatments the family may help with, for example, oxygen therapy, dressings, hot packs, special exercises.
   e. Examples of special instructions.
      (1) How to give a bath and make a bed with the client in it.
      (2) How to use a wheelchair.
      (3) How to assist with crutch-walking.
      (4) How to suction the client.
      (5) How to change the home environment to make it safe, for example, modify the bathroom, remove rugs.
   f. Appointments. Clarify place, date, and time.
7. Teach the client and family how to prevent complications and further exacerbations of the disease.
   a. Provide information about the physiology and pathophysiology of the disease appropriate to the level of the learner.
   b. Show how adherence to the treatment plan will help prevent further problems.
   c. Involve the family in helping the client adhere to the treatment plan.
   d. Identify members of the family who might be at high risk for problems similar to those faced by the client.
   e. Teach high-risk family members how to prevent diseases in themselves.
8. Prepare the family for the normal mood swings the client may experience while recovering, for example, depression, overindependence or overdependence.
9. Prepare the family for their reactions to recovery of the client, that is, discouragement, tiredness, resistance to allowing the client to assume his or her former role in the family.

EVALUATION

Outcome Criteria

1. Family and client are making realistic plans to manage the recovery of the client and family at home.
2. Family and client understand the basic processes of the disease and how the treatment plan will affect these processes.
3. Family and client understand how to prevent future complications and occurrence of the disease.
4. Family and client know how to deal with anticipated problems associated with normal recovery.

COUNSELING THE FAMILY CONFRONTING REHABILITATION OR CHRONIC ILLNESS

Families with members who are recovering from illness or are chronically ill face special challenges. Many of these families, however, have healthy interpersonal relationships because the family is *cohesive* and *adaptable.* Community health nurses have used these two concepts for many years in assessing families, but they have needed a well-defined list of what dimensions to assess under the broader concepts, *cohesion* and *adaptability.* Olson, Sprenkle, and Russell (1979) found in their reviews of the family therapy literature that several dimensions clustered around cohesion and adaptability. These dimensions can be used by community health nurses and others in assessing the adequacy of functioning in families in cases where a member is recovering from illness or where chronic illness might be interfering with normal family functioning.

ASSESSMENT

Cohesion

Cohesion is defined as "The emotional bonding members have with one another and the degree of individual autonomy a person experiences in the family system" (Olson et al., 1979).

1. Independence. This is the degree to which persons meet their own needs.
   a. Healthy signs: moderate amount of independence or dependence of family members on one another.
   b. Unhealthy signs: high amount of independence or dependence of family members on one another.
2. Family boundaries. These are the unwritten rules that define who in the family participates with whom and to what degree.
   a. Function of boundaries is to protect the differentiation of the system/subsystem from interference by other systems/subsystems.
   b. Types of boundaries (Minuchin, 1974).
      (1) *Clear:* normal range of well-defined rules that enable the members to carry out their functions without undue interference.
      (2) *Diffuse:* blurred rules that contribute to constant communication and overconcern on the part of family members and consequent overload (*enmeshment*).
      (3) *Rigid:* rules that do not allow family members to communicate adequately and care for one another (*disengagement*).
   c. Healthy signs.
      (1) Semiopen external boundaries to outside systems.
      (2) Semiopen internal boundaries to subsystems within the family.
      (3) Clear generational boundaries.
   d. Unhealthy signs.
      (1) Completely open or closed external boundaries to outside systems.
      (2) Completely open or closed internal boundaries to subsystems within the family.
3. Coalitions. Coalitions are relationships in which two or more family members have a special bond that excludes other family members.
   a. Healthy sign: marital coalition clear and strong.
   b. Unhealthy signs.
      (1) Parent-child coalition in place of marital coalition.
      (2) Separation of one member as a scapegoat.
4. Time.
   a. Healthy signs.
      (1) Importance placed on time alone as well as the time together as a family.
      (2) Time alone permitted.

b. Unhealthy signs.
(1) Most of time spent apart from family (physically and/or emotionally).
(2) Most of time spent with family members; little time permitted to be alone.

5. Space at home (physical and emotional).
a. Healthy sign: maintenance of both private and family space.
b. Unhealthy signs.
(1) Maximum amount of separate space both physically and emotionally.
(2) Little or no private space.

6. Friends.
a. Healthy sign: some individual, couple, and family friends.
b. Unhealthy signs.
(1) Primarily individual friends and few family friends.
(2) Few family friends; couple and/or family friends usually seen together.

7. Decision making.
a. Healthy signs.
(1) Most decisions individually based but joint decisions on family issues.
(2) Individual decisions shared and made with the family in mind.
b. Unhealthy signs.
(1) Primarily individual decisions.
(2) Personal and family decisions made primarily by family.

8. Interests and recreation.
a. Healthy signs.
(1) Some spontaneous and some scheduled family activities.
(2) Individual activities supported with family being involved in some individual interests.
b. Unhealthy signs.
(1) Noninvolvement of family in any individual activities.
(2) Almost all activities and interests shared by family.

Adaptability

Adaptability is defined as "The ability of a marital/family system to change its power structure, role relationships, and relationship rules in response to situational and developmental stress" (Olsen et al., 1979).

1. Family power.
a. Healthy signs.
(1) Family members generally assertive.
(2) Control is equalitarian with fluid changes or democratic with stable leader.
b. Unhealthy signs.
(1) Passive and/or aggressive styles.
(2) No leadership or authoritarian leadership.

2. Negotiation styles.
a. Healthy signs.
(1) Democratic discipline with both predictable and unpredictable consequences.
(2) Good problem-solving and structured negotiations.
b. Unhealthy signs.
(1) Discipline is laissez-faire; very lenient or autocratic and overly strict.
(2) Endless or overly brief negotiations; poor problem solving.

3. Role relationships.
a. Healthy signs.
(1) Capable of making and sharing roles.
(2) Able to make changes in roles.
b. Unhealthy signs.
(1) Make drastic role changes.
(2) Have stereotyped roles; incapable of making decisions.

4. Relationship rules.
a. Healthy signs.
(1) Rules generally enforced.
(2) Few rule changes.
b. Unhealthy signs.
(1) Very fluid or rigid rules.
(2) Arbitrarily enforced or strictly enforced rules.

5. System feedback.
a. Healthy signs: constructive, system-enhancing behaviors that enable the family to grow and change.
b. Unhealthy signs: status quo maintained so that the family does not adapt to change.

EXPECTED OUTCOMES

1. The family will move toward a healthy degree of cohesion while supporting the ill family member.
2. The family will adapt in a healthy way to the changes in the condition of the ill family member.

INTERVENTIONS

The success of the interventions is mainly dependent on efforts of the family, although it would be very useful for nurses to be able to effectively apply the principles of counseling with the families.

1. Promote a healthy degree of cohesion in the family.
   a. Encourage family members to maintain a moderate amount of independence/dependence on one another.
   b. Assist the family in defining rules that enable the members to carry out their functions without undue interference.
   c. Promote the special bond between the husband and wife.
   d. Encourage the family to spend time together as well as separately.
   e. Encourage the maintenance of both private and family space.
   f. Promote individual, couple, and family friends.
   g. Encourage family members to make individual decisions as appropriate but to make joint decisions when the entire family is affected.
   h. Encourage both family and individual interests and recreation.
2. Promote a healthy degree of adaptability in the family.
   a. Assist the family members in being generally assertive with equalitarian or democratic leadership.
   b. Encourage negotiation styles that include democratic discipline with predictable consequences and structured problem solving.
   c. Establish role relationships that are flexible and shared when necessary.
   d. Reinforce agreed upon rules for healthy interaction; e.g., "When there is conflict between family members we will talk about it."
   e. Use therapeutic interaction to enhance appropriate behaviors (feedback) that will allow the family to grow and change; e.g., reinforce, promote independence in self-care by the client rather than continued dependence.

EVALUATION

Outcome Criteria

1. The family exhibits a healthy degree of emotional bonding with one another while allowing autonomy to individual members.
2. The family demonstrates an ability to change its power structure, role relationships, and relationship rules in response to situational and developmental stresses.

COPING WITH DEATH IN THE FAMILY

Death of a family member probably is the most difficult of all times for families regardless of whether the death is sudden or anticipated. Family members experience feelings of loss from an emotional standpoint as well as in a more practical sense, as the structure of a family is altered, affecting each member's roles and relationships. Additional strain occurs when family members do not go through the grieving process at the same time.

Preparing children for the death of a parent or sibling is a difficult but important responsibility of older family members. Children can be helped to realize that death is coming through ways adapted to their development and through the leads they provide. Younger children may need only to be reminded that their parent or sibling is very sick and may not always be with the family. Older children may need much more, including the medical facts and information about what is being done to keep their loved one alive. Children may derive satisfaction from helping and interacting with the dying family member, although it is wise not to overburden a child with too heavy a responsibility. Children can be a real source of comfort to the terminally ill and this may later be a source of comfort to them.

The stages of grief can be used to assess where the family and its individual members are in their adjustment to the loss. Knowledge of where the family is within each stage is helpful in determining intervention strategies. A four-stage model used with families of cancer patients (Giacquinta, 1977) is applied below and can be used with families experiencing any type of terminal illness.

STAGE I: LIVING WITH TERMINAL ILLNESS

ASSESSMENT

1. Assess the ability of the family and client to cope with terminal illness.
2. Assess the resources available to assist the family and client in coping with the terminal illness.

EXPECTED OUTCOMES

1. The family will deal with the shock of the diagnosis and the implications for the family.
2. The family will recover from initial disorganization.

INTERVENTIONS

1. Convey understanding of the family situation.
2. Develop a supportive relationship with the family.
3. Help the family solve everyday problems of life in an effort to reduce their feelings of helplessness.
4. Encourage use of outside supportive resources.

EVALUATION

Outcome Criteria

1. The family displays adaptive coping responses.
2. The family is able to solve everyday problems of life.
3. The family utilizes outside supportive resources.

STAGE II: RESTRUCTURING IN THE LIVING-DYING INTERVAL

ASSESSMENT

1. Assess the family members' abilities to reorganize their individual lives and their family life.
2. Assess the family's ability to confront reality.

EXPECTED OUTCOMES

1. The family will reorganize family life by adjusting roles and relationships.
2. The family members will recall or "frame memories" of the dying member from happier days so that the dying member remains part of the family rather than a symbol of death and sadness.

INTERVENTIONS

1. Gently assist the family in confronting reality.
2. Provide facts about the client's condition.
3. Encourage the family in the process of recollection and reminiscence.
4. Help the family prepare for the change in planning and mobilizing effective coping strategies.

EVALUATION

Outcome Criteria

1. The family demonstrates adaptability to the changing roles and relationships.
2. The family helps the dying member continue to feel like an important member of the family.
3. The family maintains a system of communication for supporting one another and planning for the future.

STAGE III: BEREAVEMENT

ASSESSMENT

1. Assess the family's ability to grieve appropriately.
2. Assess the family's provisions for their physical and emotional well-being.

EXPECTED OUTCOMES

1. The family members will actively mourn the loss of the loved one.
2. The family members will accept one another regardless of the reaction to the loss.
3. The family members will support one another and accept support from others.
4. The family members will maintain their physical health through rest, exercise, and proper nutrition.

INTERVENTIONS

1. Provide support, encouragement, and listening.
2. Assist the family to reduce some of the rou-

tine burdens and to do simple problem solving.
3. Accept initial feelings of disbelief, denial, anger, and depression, and then help the family move to the next stage.

EVALUATION

Outcome Criteria

1. The family is grieving the loss of their loved one.
2. The family is receiving support from others.
3. The family takes steps to maintain health of members.
4. The family demonstrates that it can do problem solving for daily living issues.

STAGE IV: REESTABLISHMENT

Assessment

1. Assess the reality of the family's perception of the loved one.
2. Assess the family's adjustment to new activities, roles, and relationships.

EXPECTED OUTCOMES

1. The family will move from the idealization of the loved one to a more realistic assessment.
2. Family members will return to everyday activities and routines.
3. The family will reenter the larger social system and interact with friends and acquaintances.
4. The family will adjust roles and relationships so that it can function adequately again.

INTERVENTIONS

1. Listen to statements of idealization about the loved one.
2. Encourage interaction between family members and with persons in the broader social environment.
3. Assist in decision making, if needed, as roles and relationships are readjusted.

EVALUATION

Outcome Criteria

1. The family is moving toward a realistic assessment of the loved one.
2. The family is adjusting roles and relationships.
3. The family is beginning to be involved in the larger social system.

SUMMARY

Nursing intervention cannot be truly successful without linking nursing actions to a client's family, regardless of who the client considers that family to be. This approach requires understanding, time, and energy on the part of the nurse, and yet the dividends are far greater than those of working with the client alone. The client and family benefit, but so does the nurse as she or he grows personally from the rewards of providing family as well as client care.

REFERENCES

Burgess, A. W., and Baldwin B. A.: *Crisis Intervention Theory and Practice*, Prentice-Hall, Englewood Cliffs, N.J., 1981.

Caplan, G.: *An Approach to Community Mental Health*, Grune & Stratton, New York, 1961.

Duvall, E. M.: *Marriage and Family Development*, 5th ed., Lippincott, Philadelphia, 1977.

Giacquinta, B.: "Helping Families Face the Crisis of Cancer." *American Journal of Nursing*, **77**(10):1585–1588, 1977.

Litman, T. J.: "Health Care and the Family: A Three Generational Analysis," *Medical Care*, **9**:67, 1971.

Minuchin, S.: *Families and Family Therapy*. Harvard University Press, Cambridge, Mass., 1974.

Olson, D. H., Sprenkle, D. H., and Russell, C. S.: "Circumplex Model of Marital and Family Systems: I Cohesion and Adaptability Dimensions, Family Types, and Clinical Applications," *Family Process*, **18**:3–28, April 1979.

Phipps, L. B.: "Theoretical Frameworks Applicable to Family Care," in J. R. Miller and E. H. Janosik (eds.), *Family-Focused Care*, McGraw-Hill, New York, 1980.

BIBLIOGRAPHY

Burgess, A. W., and Baldwin, B. A.: *Crisis Intervention Theory and Practice*, Prentice-Hill, Englewood Cliffs, N.J., 1981. This text answers the need for a comprehensive theory that includes a meaningful typology of crises, as well as implementation strategies for each type. Crisis intervention has proven to be of great practical value in application to such phenomena as a death in the family, rape, returning to work, divorce, war combat stress, child abuse, and natural disasters. Innovative theoretical concepts and practical clinical applications suggest new areas in which crisis theory can be successfully applied.

Haley, J.: *Problem-Solving Therapy*, Jossey-Bass, San Francisco, 1976. Jay Haley describes specific skills and techniques for solving problems that lead people to psychotherapeutic treatment. His approach is to cause a change in the client's behavior that will clearly eliminate the problem or alleviate the symptom. The principles of short-term counseling are applicable to the nonpsychiatric nurse.

Miller, J. R., and Janosik, E. H.: *Family-Focused Care*, McGraw-Hill, New York, 1980. The emphasis in this book is on working with normal families in community and hospital settings. Clinical examples are used to highlight the principles suggested for dealing with families in various stages of the family life cycle. Both teaching and counseling approaches are discussed.

Speedling, E. J.: *Heart Attack: The Family Response at Home and in the Hospital*, Tavistock, New York, 1982. This book recounts the experiences of members of eight families following a heart attack to the husband. It analyzes the impact of hospitalization on the family's ability to come to terms with the heart attack and to formulate plans for dealing with it both during the hospital stay and later at home. The book provides a framework for understanding families' experiences and also insights into how, if the clients' families had been incorporated in the therapeutic process, some problems would have been avoided, or at least alleviated.

Walsh, F. (ed.): *Normal Family Processes*, Guilford, New York, 1982. The investigation of family process has yielded a solid data base from which clinical understanding of the normal family has emerged. *Normal Family Processes* is the first volume to coherently synthesize and organize this knowledge. Walsh shows how Minuchin, Haley, Bowen, Framo, and other leading behavioral scientists have contributed to a workable definition of the normal family.

PART II

THE NURSING CARE OF PARENTS AND INFANTS

PART II CONTENTS

CHAPTER 6
FAMILY PLANNING 97

Description 99
Prevention 107
Assessment 107
Nursing diagnoses: actual or potential 109
Expected outcomes 109
Interventions 110
Evaluation 112

CHAPTER 7
PREGNANCY: THE FIRST, SECOND, AND THIRD TRIMESTERS 115

The First Trimester 115
Complications:
Spontaneous abortion 129
Missed abortion 130
Hydatidiform mole 130
Ectopic pregnancy 131
Hyperemesis gravidarum 131
Vaginal infection 131
Adolescent pregnancy 131
Elderly gravida 132

The Second Trimester 132
Complications:
Multiple pregnancy 134
Pregnancy-induced hypertension 137
Preexisting hypertension 138
Diabetes mellitus 138
Abnormal weight gain 140
Anemia 140
Bacteriuria 141
Varicose veins 141
Thrombophlebitis 141

The Third Trimester 141
Complications:
Placenta previa 143
Abruptio placentae 144
Cardiac dysfunction 147

CHAPTER 8
LABOR AND DELIVERY 149

First Stage of Labor 149
Complications:
Psychological stress 156
Physical stress 157
Ineffective early labor 157
Cervical dystocia 157
Uterine inertia 164
Vaginal bleeding 164
Elevated blood pressure 165
Elevated temperature 165
Postmaturity 165
Premature labor 166
Cardiac complications 166
Diabetes 166

Second Stage of Labor 167
Complications:
Lack of descent 169
Hypotension: vena cava syndrome 169

Third Stage of Labor 170
Complications:
Uterine atony 170
Laceration in the birth canal 171

Fourth Stage of Labor 172
Complications:
Hematoma 173
Urinary retention 173

CHAPTER 9
RECOVERY: THE FOURTH TRIMESTER 175

Vaginal Delivery 175

Cesarean Delivery 190
Complications:
Puerperal hemorrhage 192
Puerperal infection 193
Breast infection 194
Urinary tract infection 194
Thrombophlebitis 194
Psychologic disorders 195

PART II CONTENTS *(continued)*

CHAPTER 10
THE FULL-TERM INFANT 197

The Normal Full-Term Infant 197

Complications 213
Inhibited or disrupted bonding 213
Jaundice in the full-term infant 216
Infant of a substance-abusing mother 218

CHAPTER 11
THE HIGH-RISK INFANT 223

The Premature Infant 223

Complications 233
Respiratory distress syndrome 233
Apnea 238
Sepsis 239
Necrotizing enterocolitis 240
Hypoglycemia 241
Hypocalcemia 242
Hypothermia 243
Hyperbilirubinemia 244

The Postmature Infant 247
Meconium aspiration syndrome 248

Transport to a Regional Center 249

CHAPTER 12
BIRTH DEFECTS: THE GRIEVING FAMILY 253

Chromosomal Defects 253
Monosomy 253
Trisomy 253
Polyploidy 254
Mosaicism 254
Double fertilization 254
Abnormal structure 255

Single-Gene Defects 255
Autosomal dominant 255
Autosomal recessive 255
Sex-linked defects 256

Polygenic Defects: Multifactorial Disorders 257

Congenital Disorders: Environmental Factors 257
Teratogens 257
Viruses or bacteria 257

Birth Injuries 260
Drug effects 260
Anoxia 263
Trauma 263

Perinatal Grieving 263

CHAPTER 13
THE FAMILY UNREADY FOR CHILDBEARING 269

Adolescent and Adult Abortion 269
Complications:
Trauma to cervix 278
Infection (endometritis) 278
Future risk 278
Delayed grieving 278

CHAPTER 14
THE INFERTILE FAMILY 281

General Infertility Factors 281

Female Infertility Factors 285
Hypogonadotropic secretion 285
Occlusion of the oviducts 295

Male Infertility Factors 297

The Future in Infertility 300
Artificial insemination 300
In vitro fertilization and embryo transfer 301

Guide for Partners 301
Groups that can help 302
Books for couples who want to be parents 303

6

Family Planning

Phyllis L. Collier

In its broadest sense, *family planning* refers to the process of choosing and planning one's fertility options. For most people this means deciding whether to have children, how many to have, and when to have them.

In the past, children were an economic necessity, natural resources were plentiful, and information was lacking about control of bodily processes. Today, societal needs and attitudes have changed, technology has improved, and natural resources are diminishing. We are now more able to control fertility and have a greater need to do so. Fortunately, vital statistics for the past several years indicate a steadily declining birth rate in this country. In addition, behavioral and attitudinal studies have demonstrated that people from every demographic category—religious, ethnic, socioeconomic—prefer a smaller family.

A range of factors has been influential for this reduced birth rate.

1. In comparison with previous generations, there is improved technology to aid in effective family planning.
2. Abortion has been legalized in the United States and is associated with lower morbidity and mortality rates than childbirth.
3. Improved diagnostic procedures aid in early detection of pregnancy, in prediction of genetic conditions, and in finding the causes of infertility.
4. Less traumatic sterilization techniques have been developed for both males and females.
5. Legal and institutional restrictions for these services have been lessened, particularly those related to age, marital status, parity, and agreement of spouse. Laws and governmental regulations have attempted to ensure that these services are available and accessible to all persons.
6. The role of women is changing. Childbearing and rearing—"motherhood"—is only one of many alternatives now open to women.
7. Finally, it is natural that people who choose to have children wish to offer them the highest quality of life possible. Increases in the cost of living make it difficult for many families to provide the basic necessities of life, higher education, and other advantages to more than a few children.

One goal of health care is that every child should be planned for and wanted and that every individual or couple should be able to make fertility decisions that suit their personal desires and ensure their optimum well-being. This goal has been institutionalized into federal regulations and needs to be carefully incorporated into the approach of every family planning care provider.

The choices of whether or not to use a contraceptive method, which method to use, and how regularly to use it may be influenced by obvious outside factors as well as by complex internal feelings. The decision involves interrelationships, feelings about one's sexuality, and personal or family goals. The following factors frequently have a role in contraceptive decision making.

1. *Culture*: pregnancy and children seen as a symbol of masculinity or femininity; impor-

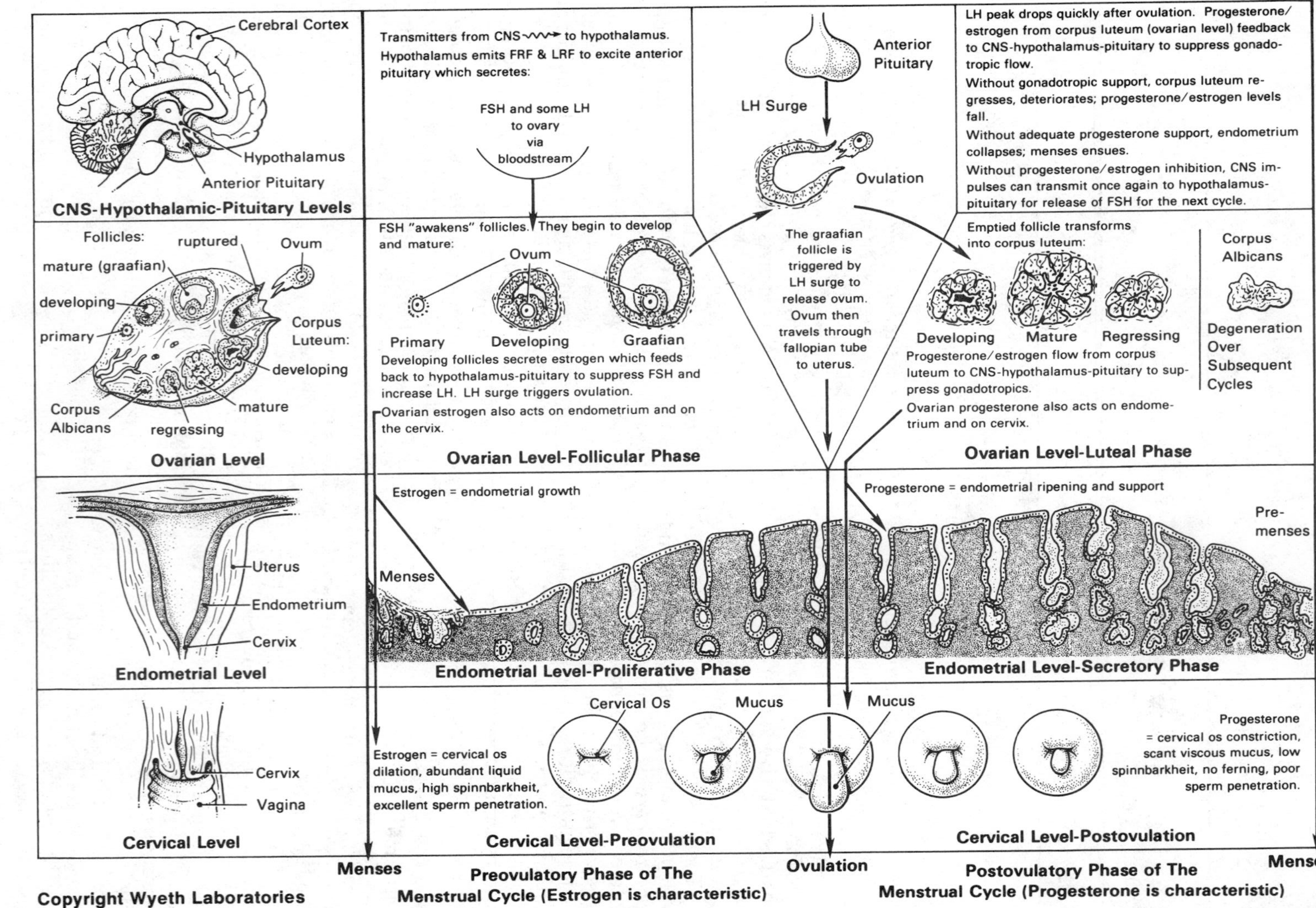

Figure 6-1 The normal menstrual cycle. (Courtesy of Wyeth Laboratories, Philadelphia, Pa.)

tance of sons or daughters; pressures from family or friends to have children.

2. *Religion*: may discourage use of some or all artificial methods of birth control; reproductive process viewed as a natural outcome.
3. *Daily activity pattern*: sedentary/mobile; regular/irregular hours.
4. *Personality*: habitual/forgetful; impulsive/methodical.
5. *Relationship with partner*: monogamous/more than one partner; agreement/disagreement or desirability of pregnancy and who is responsible for contraception; mutual satisfaction with method used; honesty/"gamesmanship."
6. *Feelings about body*: like/dislike touching self; sense of control/lack of control over body.
7. *Comfort with sexuality*: acceptance of self as a sexual being; freedom/guilt regarding sexual activity.
8. *Myths and misinformation*: all birth control interferes with sexual enjoyment, if you don't have an orgasm you won't get pregnant; birth control pills cause sterility.
9. *Psychological outlook*: pregnancy seen as a way of "getting even" with parents or partner or as punishment for sexual behavior.
10. *Balance of gratification and frustration with contraceptive method*: ease/difficulty of using method; severity of side effects; degree comforted by or indifferent to effectiveness rates.

Some of this information may be routinely solicited or volunteered during an assessment interview. Because of the nature of these factors, however, their true role in contraceptive decision making may never be fully understood, either by the client or the care provider.

DESCRIPTION

Contraception involves the use of a method, routine, or procedure to prevent, delay, or space pregnancy. Temporary methods prevent contraception from occuring during the time they are being used but provide no obstacle to fertility when they are discontinued. the *IUD, diaphragm, foams and jellies, condom, rhythm methods,* and *oral contraceptives* fall into this category.

Because the menstrual cycle is altered by oral contraceptives, which frequently cause a lighter menstrual period, and by IUDs, which may cause menstrual flow to be heavier and to last longer, the nurse's knowledge of the cycle physiology is essential when evaluating and counseling clients choosing birth control methods. Those teaching natural family planning methods will perhaps have to have the most detailed knowledge of the menstrual cycle (Figure 6-1).

Permanent methods of contraception are the surgical procedures of *tubal ligation* and *vasectomy,* which end the reproductive capacity. In women, sections of the fallopian tube are cut and tied or cauterized (tubal ligation), thus blocking the ovum from reaching the uterine cavity. In men, the vas deferens is cut and tied (vasectomy) so that sperm are no longer ejaculated. Sterilization does not affect physiologic processes such as ovulation, menstruation, production of sperm and semen or sexual responses. Although there has been some success at reversing these surgical procedures, all sterilization should be considered permanent contraceptive methods and should be performed only when no children or no more children are desired. The individual or couple considering sterilization should carefully evaluate their motivation for this alternative and seriously explore their feelings about terminating the ability to reproduce.

Tables 6-1 and 6-2 present a summary of contraceptive methods. Methods can also be classified by mode of action, ease of accessibility, or relationship to time of intercourse.

1. Mode of action.
   a. Chemical barriers—foam, cream, jelly, suppository.
   b. Mechanical barriers—diaphragm, condom, cervical cap.
   c. Hormonal—oral contraceptives, implants, injections.
   d. "Natural"—rhythm, basal body temperature (BBT), mucus method, symptothermal method, natural family planning, fertility awareness.
   e. Surgical blockage—tubal ligation, vasectomy.
2. Ease of accessibility.
   a. Over-the-counter purchase—foam, jelly, cream, suppository, condom.
   b. Prescribed by physician—IUD, diaphragm, oral contraceptives.
3. Relationship to time of intercourse.
   a. Used at time of intercourse—diaphragm, jelly, cream, foam, suppository, condom.
   b. Separated from intercourse—IUD, oral contraceptives, surgical sterilization.

TABLE 6-1 TEMPORARY METHODS OF CONTRACEPTION

ORAL CONTRACEPTIVES
0.5–2%[a,b]

Description of Action

Tablets contain varying doses of estrogens and progestogens. Primary action is suppression of ovulation by changing the gonadotropin feedback cycle. Cervical mucus may be altered, making it hostile to sperm, and an unfavorable endometrial environment may prevent normal implantation.

Instructions for Use

Take one pill daily for 21 days, at approx. the same time daily; stop for 7 days. Menses will begin 1–4 days after pill has been stopped. Restart new pack of pills on 29th day. Some packs contain seven placebo tablets that can be taken instead of stopping for a week.

Initially, begin pills on fifth day of menses or on the first Sunday following beginning of period or termination of pregnancy by abortion. If using the "Sunday method," use a second method of contraception for one to two cycles.

To establish regularity of use, take with an established daily activity. For early nausea, take at bedtime or with evening meal. For weight gain, reduce salt and caloric intake.

If one pill is skipped, take as soon as you remember and take next pill at regular time. There is a much higher risk of ovulation, if two or more pills are missed, therefore, follow instructions of care provider and use a second method of contraception for rest of cycle. Some spotting may occur. Pills should be completely stopped at end of pack and two to three normal cycles should occur before attempting pregnancy.

Side Effects

Minor: Mild nausea, breast tenderness, spotting, breakthrough bleeding, shorter and lighter periods, missed or "silent" periods, mood changes, chloasma, acne, increased vaginal itching or discharge, weight changes.
Other: Blood clots, heart attacks, strokes, hepatocellular tumors, gallbladder disease, hypertension, depression, decreased libido, prolonged amenorrhea after discontinuation.

Contraindications

Absolute: History or presence of thromboembolic phenomena, cerebrovascular accident, coronary artery disease, malignancy of the breast or reproductive system, hepatic adenoma, liver disease or dysfunction, pregnancy.
Probable: Migraine headaches, hypertension, gallbladder disease, diabetes or strong family history, sickle cell disease, acute mononucleosis, ovarian dysfunction, fibroceptic breast disease, undiagnosed vaginal bleeding, termination of a term pregnancy within the past 2 weeks, lactation, elective surgery planned within the next month, client age 40 or more.
Possible: Potential for infertility, i.e., late or irregular menstrual cycles; depression, asthma, epilepsy, varicose veins, heavy smoking.

TABLE 6-1 *(continued)*

	Care provider should be informed if any symptoms occur: chest, abdominal, or leg pain, shortness of breath, headache, blurred vision. **Advantages/Disadvantages** *Advantages:* Nearest to 100% effective; regular menstrual cycle, period predictable; decreased menstrual flow; decreased dysmenorrhea, mittelschmerz pain, premenstrual tension; decreased iron deficiency anemia; not related to time of intercourse. *Disadvantages:* Must be taken daily even if user is not sexually active; must be started at specific time to be effective.
MINIPILL (progestogen only) 1–2.5%	**Description of Action** Tablets contain only low doses of progestogens. Ovulation is inhibited only some of the time, but hostile cervical mucus and an unfavorable endometrial environment provide contraceptive effect. **Instructions for Use** Take one pill daily, without stopping. Start new pack of pills on day after completion of previous pack. If one pill is missed, take it as soon as you remember and take next pill at regular time. Also use a second birth control method until next menses begin. Menstrual bleeding may be regular or irregular with use. For increased protection against pregnancy, use a second birth control method at midcycle. **Side Effects** *Minor:* Irregularity in amount and duration of menses, spotting between periods, missed periods. *Other:* Edema, hirsuitism, alterations in liver function tests. **Contraindications** *Absolute:* Same as for combination pill (see *Oral Contraceptives*, above). *Probable:* Diabetes, acute mononucleosis, irregular menses, history of ectopic pregnancy, undiagnosed vaginal bleeding. Care provider should be notified immediately of abdominal pain, discomfort; minipill users are at higher risk for ectopic pregnancy. **Advantages/Disadvantages** *Advantages:* Fewer side effects than with estrogen-containing pills; can be used in presence of some medical problems; not related to time of intercourse. *Disadvantages:* Irregular periods, higher rate of ectopic pregnancy; must be taken daily even if user is not sexually active.
IUD 1.5–4%	**Description of Action** A plastic or polyethylene device in various shapes and sizes (Figure 6-4) is inserted into uterus by physician and usually re-

TABLE 6-1 *(continued)*

	mains there until user wishes it removed. Action of IUD is unknown, but it is thought to cause a local inflammatory reaction inside uterus that prevents implantation of fertilized ovum. Copper and progesterone have been added to some IUDs for extra antifertility effect. **Instructions for Use** Approximately 3–5 cm of IUD string will be in vagina. Insert finger to check for presence of string. (Can be checked by partner, also.) Notify care provider if no string is felt, string feels much longer than after insertion, or plastic tip of IUD is protruding. Use another method of birth control until reexamined. Insert during menses; remove at any time during the cycle. If pregnancy occurs with IUD in situ, IUD may need to be removed to decrease danger of infection. Replace every 3–5 years if IUD contains copper; every year if it contains progesterone. **Side Effects** *Minor:* Heavier and/or longer periods, cramps, spotting between periods. *Other:* Heavy bleeding, anemia (secondary to bleeding), pain, infections, pelvic inflammatory disease (PID), uterine perforation, spontaneous expulsion of device, embedding of IUD. **Contraindications** *Absolute:* Pregnancy, acute PID, gonorrhea. *Probable:* History of ectopic pregnancy, severe dysmenorrhea, recurrent PID, valvular heart disease, acute cervicitis, abnormal Pap smear results, allergy to copper (rare). *Possible:* Nullipara desiring children in the future (more likely to get uterine infection), history of gonorrhea or PID with desire for future children, cervical or uterine abnormalities, anemia, endometriosis, abnormal uterine bleeding, multiple sexual partners. Care provider should be informed if signs of infection occur: fever, pain, unusual vaginal bleeding, foul-smelling discharge. **Advantages/Disadvantages** *Advantages:* Little maintenance or attention needed after insertion; not related to time of intercourse. *Disadvantages:* Must be inserted and removed by care provider (no self-involvement); higher rate of ectopic pregnancy; IUDs containing copper or progesterone must be replaced more frequently.
DIAPHRAGM (with spermicide) 2–10%	**Description of Action** A dome-shaped rubber cap on a circular metal spring is inserted into the vagina. Used with spermacidal jelly or cream, it fits over cervix and blocks entry of sperm into uterus. Come in sizes 55–105 mm, in gradations of 5 mm, and must be individually fitted. Inserted and removed by the user.

TABLE 6-1 *(continued)*

	Instructions for Use Before insertion, put spermicidal jelly or cream in cup and on rim of diaphragm. In lying, standing, or squatting position ease diaphragm into vagina. Hook rim under symphysis pubis. Check to see that cervix is covered. (See Figure 6-3.) If intercourse is repeated, add an applicator of foam or jelly without removing diaphragm. Do *not* remove diaphragm or douche for 6–8 h after last intercourse. Special care after each use is necessary. Check for holes or tears periodically. Diaphragm fit should be rechecked if discomfort is felt, if there is a weight gain or loss of 20 or more pounds, and following pelvic surgery or end of pregnancy. **Side Effects** *Minor:* Mild irritation from spermicidal cream or jelly, cramps. *Other:* Allergy to rubber or spermicidal preparation, urinary retention, urinary tract infection (UTI) symptoms, pelvic pain. **Contraindications** *Probable:* Allergy to rubber or spermicide, prolapsed uterus, cystocele, rectocele, severe retroversion or anteversion of uterus, recurrent UTIs. Care provider should be notified of any difficulty voiding with diaphragm in place or symptoms of UTI. **Advantages/Disadvantages** *Advantages:* Few side effects; effective for infrequent intercourse; holds back menstrual flow during intercourse; offers some protection against sexually transmitted diseases. *Disadvantages:* Closely precedes sex act; may become dislodged during intercourse; can be messy.
FOAM, JELLY, CREAM, SUPPOSITORY 3–15%	**Description of Action** Spermicidal preparations inserted into the vagina slow down and kill sperm, thus preventing their entry into the uterus. Can be used alone or in conjunction with other methods. Inserted by the user just before intercourse. **Instructions for Use** Insert an applicator full of foam, jelly, or cream into vagina within 30 min of intercourse. Follow package instructions for insertion of suppositories; most require a waiting period before intercourse while suppository melts or effervesces. For all preparations, insert an additional application each time before intercourse is repeated. There is no need to douch after use; the preparations are absorbed into mucous membrane, but if douching is desired wait 6–8 h after last intercourse. Use with condom for increased effectiveness. **Side Effects** *Minor:* Mild irritation from spermicide. *Other:* Allergy to spermicide.

TABLE 6-1 ***(continued)***

	Contraindications *Probable:* Allergy to spermicide. **Advantages/Disadvantages** *Advantages:* Few side effects, easily available, no prescription needed; provides some protection against sexually transmitted diseases; aids in vaginal lubrication. *Disadvantages:* Closely precedes intercourse; most suppositories require waiting period; can be messy; taste may be unpleasant with oral sex.
CONDOM (with spermicide) 2–10%	**Description of Action** A thin rubber or skin sheath put over an erect penis creates a mechanical barrier that prevents sperm from getting into vagina. **Instructions for Use** Put condom on erect penis *before* any penetration. (Rolling on by partner may add to sexual pleasure.) If no tip on condom, allow $\frac{1}{2}$-in slack in front to catch semen. For increased ease of penetration, use prelubricated condoms or lubricate with a water-soluble jelly (such as K-Y), contraceptive foam, or saliva. Withdraw soon after ejaculation; semen is more likely to leak out when penis is flaccid. Hold onto condom when withdrawing to prevent slipping off. If condom breaks during intercourse, insert an applicator of foam or jelly immediately. Use with a spermicidal preparation for increased effectiveness. **Side Effects** *Minor:* Mild irritation from rubber. *Other:* Allergy to rubber. **Contraindications** *Probable:* Allergy to rubber, inability to maintain an erection. **Advantages/Disadvantages** *Advantages:* Male method, allows for shared contraception; easily available; few side effects; offers increased protection against sexually transmitted diseases; offers protection when female is allergic to male sperm. *Disadvantages:* Requires interruption of coitus to put on; can be messy; may reduce sensitivity of glans.
RHYTHM (alone) 14–20%	**Description of Action** A pattern of abstinence from intercourse around the time of ovulation or time of greatest fertility. Records must be kept of menstrual cycles and calculations made for "safe days." **Instructions for Use** BBT; charting the low preovulation temperature contrasted with the 0.8–1.0°F elevation on the day of ovulation gives indication of the "unsafe period."

TABLE 6-1 *(continued)*

	Side Effects None. **Contraindications** *Probable:* Irregular menstrual cycle, inability to understand and follow protocols. **Advantages/Disadvantages** *Advantages:* No side effects, no cost, acceptable for those with religious or other objections to artificial birth control methods; promotes learning about bodily systems. *Disadvantages:* Requires extensive education to learn and consistent follow through; irregular cycles or presence of cervicitis or vaginitis may make process more difficult to follow; problem if partner is not cooperative; abstinence may cause sexual frustration.
NATURAL FAMILY PLANNING (BBT plus cervical mucus) 2–20%	**Description of Action** This general term refers to such methods as fertility awareness, symptothermal, Billings, ovulation, and mucous methods. A variety of methods may be combined; "safe" and "fertile" days are calculated via evaluation of stretchability or pH of cervical mucus. BBT and/or traditional rhythm may also be included for a more reliable contraceptive result. **Instructions for Use** Each type of natural method requires detailed instructions. Until instruction completed by a trained counselor, a natural method should not be relied on. Preparation for use may include daily evaluation of changes in temperature and/or mucus over a period of several months. Client must develop familiarity with own menstrual cycle and learn normal ranges and factors that can alter symptoms. **Side Effects** None. **Contraindications** *Probable:* Same as *Rhythm*.
UNPROTECTED (chance) (sexually active) 90%	

[a] Number of pregnancies per 100 women-years of use.
[b] Range of theoretical to actual (Hatcher et al., 1982).

TABLE 6-2 PERMANENT METHODS OF CONTRACEPTION

Method	Procedure	Advantages/ Disadvantages	Postoperative Discomforts	Potential Adverse Effects
TUBAL LIGATION				
Laparotomy 0–2%[a]	Tubes cut and tied, ends buried in wall of uterus; Pomeroy, Irving, and Uchida techniques are variations of this procedure.	*Advantage:* May be done post partum. *Disadvantages:* Longer hospital stay, general anesthesia, greater cost.	General anesthesia recovery; postsurgical pain.	Hemorrhage, infection.
Laparoscopy 0.2–2%	Tubes cauterized and clamped, laparoscope plus CO_2 used to expand abdominal wall for visualization; termed "Band-Aid" surgery because of small incision.	*Advantages:* May be done under local anesthesia; short hospital stay (12–36 h); low morbidity rate. *Disadvantage:* Client not eligible if extremely overweight.	Abdominal fullness and tenderness; CO_2 may cause shoulder, rib, and abdominal soreness; constipation; fatigue; tender, itchy incision.	Hemorrhage, infection, muscle trauma, bowel injury. (If client is apprehensive about procedure, general anesthesia should be used.)
Minilaparotomy 0.2–0.6%	Performed under local or general anesthesia; $2\frac{1}{2}$–3 cm incision made near pubic hairline; each tube is grasped, tied, and cut (Pomeroy and similar techniques); cauterization used.	*Advantages:* Local or general anesthesia; short hospital stay; low morbidity; less damage to tube, raising chance of reanastomoses. *Disadvantage:* Somewhat more postop pain than from laparoscopy.	Postsurgical pain, abdominal fullness and tenderness.	Infection, bladder injury.
VASECTOMY 0.15%	Small incision on either side of scrotum; piece of vas deferens removed from each side and ends tied off.	*Advantages:* May be done under local anesthesia; inexpensive; low morbidity rate; no hospitalization. *Disadvantages:* Not immediately effective; 10–30 ejaculations needed to clear genitourinary track beyond incision.	Tenderness of scrotum, possible hematoma.	Infection, sperm granulomas, recanalization; one-half to two-thirds of clients develop sperm antibodies, but to date no adverse effect has been linked; possible pregnancy in partner unless contraceptives are used until two sperm-free specimens of semen have been obtained.

[a] All rates from Hatcher, R., et al., *Contraceptive Technology 1982–1983*.

PREVENTION

Health Promotion

1. Encourage acceptance of responsibility for sexuality and sexual behavior.
2. Promote knowledge about birth control methods and resources for care.
3. Encourage consistent use of chosen contraceptive method(s), unless pregnancy is desired.
4. Increase knowledge of family roles and functions.

Population at Risk

1. For unplanned pregnancy.
   a. Persons who are sexually active and not using a method.
   b. Persons using a contraceptive method incorrectly or irregularly.
   c. Persons ambivalent about pregnancy and/or contraception—may not use a method consistantly.
   d. Adolescents often deny that they may get pregnant and frequently have unprotected early sexual experience (see Chapter 13).
2. For complications with birth control methods.
   a. Persons who use a contraceptive method for which they have medical contraindications, for example, IUD used with chronic cervical infection.
   b. Women who smoke and use oral contraceptives are at higher risk for cardiovascular complications.
   c. Method users who are not aware of or who ignore danger signals related to a given method.
   d. Persons who do not get follow-up method checkups on schedule—asymptomatic problems may be occurring.

Screening

1. Intake interview and counseling session.
2. Identifying risk factors through health history.
3. Noting special risk factors in the family history, for example, strong history of breast cancer or diabetes.

ASSESSMENT

Initial assessment of the individual or family interested in conception control is done through history taking, physical examination, laboratory tests, and exploration of goals and motivations. The assessment should be conducted in a setting that ensures privacy and dignity for the client. The data gathered should be kept confidential. Assuring the client of this may provide more honest and complete information. An explanation of why the questions are being asked—particularly those questions that some clients may consider intrusive—is important. The assessment can be a learning experience for the individual or couple as well as a source of information for the care provider.

Health History

1. General health history with special attention to conditions that may contraindicate a specific birth control method (see column on contraindications in Table 6-1).
2. Family history for conditions that may place the client at higher risk of morbidity or mortality relative to a given contraception method. For example: With a strong family history of breast cancer or diabetes, oral contraceptive use may be questionable.
3. Age. Oral contraceptives are contraindicated for women over 35 to 40 years of age. Adolescents may need additional education and counseling related to method use.
4. Smoking habits. Smokers who also use oral contraceptives are at greater risk for cardiovascular complications.

Menstrual History

1. Age of menarche, plus interval and length of menses.
2. Amount of flow—heavy, moderate, light.
3. Regularity of menses. Irregular cycles may be a symptom of various conditions and should be evaluated, particularly before oral contraceptives are prescribed.
4. Symptoms of premenstrual tension—fatigue, fluid retention, breast tenderness, weight gain, mood changes.
5. Symptoms of midcycle ovulation—mittelschmerz, mucous viscosity, and higher pH. More distinct symptoms may enhance ability to use natural family planning.
6. Dysmenorrhea. Oral contraceptives may help to relieve dysmenorrhea, whereas an IUD may increase discomfort.
7. Spotting or bleeding between periods. This may be symptomatic of cancer, cervicitis or cervical erosion, vaginitis, traumatic intercourse, or side effects of IUDs and oral contraceptives.

8. Changes in menstrual cycle while using a given contraceptive method.
9. Date of onset of most recent menstrual period.
   a. May influence when a client can begin a chosen method. IUDs are usually inserted during a period and some oral contraceptives are begun on day 5 of the menses, whereas other methods can be initiated at any time.
   b. If menses are late, evaluate for pregnancy or other conditions before prescribing contraception.

Obstetric History

1. Number of pregnant.
2. Pregnancy outcomes—live births, stillbirths, spontaneous abortions, voluntary abortions. Problem patterns can be noted, such as habitual abortions. More than one voluntary interruption of pregnancy may indicate a need for special counseling regarding client attitudes and practices relating to conception control.
3. Types of delivery—vaginal, cesarean section.
4. Complications of pregnancy or delivery.
5. Birth weight of children. A pattern of high birth weights may indicate a diabetic or prediabetic condition in mother. Evaluate before prescribing oral contraceptives. Low birth weight may be associated with failure-to-thrive syndrome or delayed growth and development.
6. Number and general health status of living children. Provide opportunity for case finding and referral if problems are noted.
7. Problems with conception. Risks of amenorrhea after going off the pill may contraindicate oral contraceptives for a client who desires a future pregnancy but who has a history of problem conception.
8. Number of children desired in the future and at what intervals.
   a. Discussion may help clarify the wishes of a client who is vague or unsure about future conception.
   b. Desired timing for future pregnancies may influence method chosen. If pregnancy is desired within a short period of time, mechanical methods carry less risk of conception-delaying side effects. If no further children are desired, sterilization frees the individual or couple from both the need to use and the cost of temporary contraceptive methods.

Contraceptive History

1. Contraceptive method(s) presently and/or previously used—brand, type, size, or dose. If these are unknown, have client describe by color, shape, type of package or container.
2. Satisfaction with method(s)—partner satisfaction, if appropriate.
3. Length of time used.
4. Side effects experienced—minor, major.
5. Reasons for discontinuation—planned pregnancy, medical complications, partner dissatisfaction, fear of side effects, personal patterns and preferences.

Sexual History

1. Has client ever had intercourse? If not, client may wish to discuss feelings about becoming sexually active.
2. Frequency of intercourse.
   a. Clients who have infrequent intercourse may not wish to use a method that is active in the body at all times (e.g., pills, IUD).
   b. A highly sexually active client with multiple partners may wish to use a method that is not related to the time of intercourse.
3. Diversity of sexual contacts.
   a. If in a steady relationship, the client may wish to involve partner in decision making.
   b. If the client has no steady relationship, her decision will be more independent.
4. Presence of pain or bleeding with intercourse may indicate infections, trauma, or psychological factors.
5. Interference of contraceptive method(s) with sexual pleasure.
   a. Dislike of a method may cause a client to use it irregularly or discontinue it altogether.
   b. Partners may not agree about the same contraceptive methods.
6. Sexual problems.
   a. Lack of communication between partners about sexual satisfaction.
   b. Fear of being "unnatural" or perverted because of sexual experimentation and noncoital intercourse.
   c. Sexual dysfunction—lack of sexual desire, orgasmic impairment, vaginismus, premature ejaculation, impotence.

Exploration of Knowledge and Motivation about Contraception

1. Client's knowledge regarding anatomy and physiology of reproduction and contraceptive processes.
2. Stated reasons for desiring contraception.
3. Personal likes and dislikes and awareness of methods.
4. How serious are client and partner about preventing conception? Definite response, or ambivalence? (e.g., Did client seek health care for contraception?)
5. Feelings about touching own body or partner's body.
6. Cultural and family traditions of childbearing.
7. Fears about side effects of a particular contraceptive device, for example, impotence, cancer.
8. Feelings about ability to successfully use selected methods; e.g. for instance, have there been past failures?
9. Degrees of involvement or influence of partner in decision making.
10. Religious influences concerning use of any contraceptives.

Physical Assessment

The physical examination and diagnostic tests are geared to assessing and maintaining the general health state of the individual, ruling out contraindications to specific birth control methods. The initial visit and annual examinations should include but not be limited to:

1. Auscultation of heart and lungs; screen for cardiopulmonary problems.
2. Thyroid palpation; hypothyroid persons will have altered menses.
3. Inspection and palpation of breast and axillary glands for abnormal configurations: include teaching breast self-examination. Assess client's ability to perform self-examination.
4. Examination of extremities for edema, vascular changes.
5. Abdominal and pelvic, bimanual and rectovaginal exam.
6. Weight and blood pressure; any elevation while taking pill will cause reconsideration.

Diagnostic Tests

1. Hemoglobin/hematocrit. Anemic clients who use an IUD may be subject to additional blood loss. Supplementary iron medication may need to be prescribed.
2. Urinalysis for glucose and protein. Elevated glucose may indicate diabetes; evaluate before prescribing oral contraceptives.
3. Papanicolaou smear for detection of cervical carcinoma, other smears for vaginal infections, evaluation of estrogen levels.
4. Endocervical culture for *Neisseria gonorrhoeae* (rectum or throat, if indicated). IUDs should not be inserted if gonorrhea is present.
5. Serologic test for syphilis when any recent examination has not included serology.
6. Pregnancy test, if indicated. If client is pregnant, no new contraceptive method should be initiated. If pregnancy has occurred with the IUD in situ, removal of the device may be indicated if client wishes to continue pregnancy.

NURSING DIAGNOSES: ACTUAL OR POTENTIAL

1. Knowledge deficit due to lack of knowledge about personal anatomy/physiology and possible contraceptive choices.
2. Health management deficit. Poor health habits increase risk of harmful side effects related to given method.
3. Noncompliance with contraceptive regimen due to side effects, interference of method with lifestyle, or ambivalence about sexual behavior and contraceptive use.

EXPECTED OUTCOMES

1. Client will have increased knowledge and understanding of contraceptive methods as evidenced by an 85 percent accurate response to verbal questions following the initial educational session.
2. Client will be able to make an informed decision regarding first and second method preferences by end of initial education and counseling session.
3. Client will be able to reduce anxiety and tension during pelvic examination and method-initiation procedures, such as diaphragm fitting or IUD insertion, because of prior preparation.
4. Client will not get pregnant, unless by choice.
5. Client will follow her personal birth control plan, depending on method, by:

a. Using chosen method consistently and correctly with each intercourse.
b. Informing care provider immediately if any danger signals occur.
c. Adhering to follow-up visit routine established for each contraceptive method by a given care provider or family planning agency.
d. Gradually decreasing then eliminating smoking if using oral contraceptives.

6. Client will consult with care provider by phone or visit before discontinuing contraceptive method because of unforeseen problems (e.g., client or partner does not like method, client has difficulty using method, minor side effects are annoying, method and lifestyle are not compatible).

INTERVENTIONS

1. Orient client to methods of conception in easily understood language so that she can select a method.
   a. Clients should be given background information about anatomy and physiology in relation to contraceptive use (see Figure 6-1).
   b. Use of charts, drawings, and models to help make information more realistic and understandable. Actual birth control methods should be available for women to see and handle (see Figure 6-2).
   c. Basic content should include action, effectiveness, side effects and risks, contraindications, simple details on use, advantages and disadvantages.
   d. Initially, emphasize information that will be helpful in decision making but will not overwhelm the person with detail. For example: When presenting preliminary information on oral contraceptives, stress the need to take a pill regularly each day. Save information on when to start the pill, how to take it, what to do if pill is missed, and so on until the client has actually chosen to use the pill as a contraceptive.
   e. Group education allows a client to receive information and share experiences with persons in similar circumstances.
2. Discuss the influence of lifestyles, individual and partner preferences, and cultural and societal norms on fertility control and contraceptive use. This should aid women and their partners in decision making.

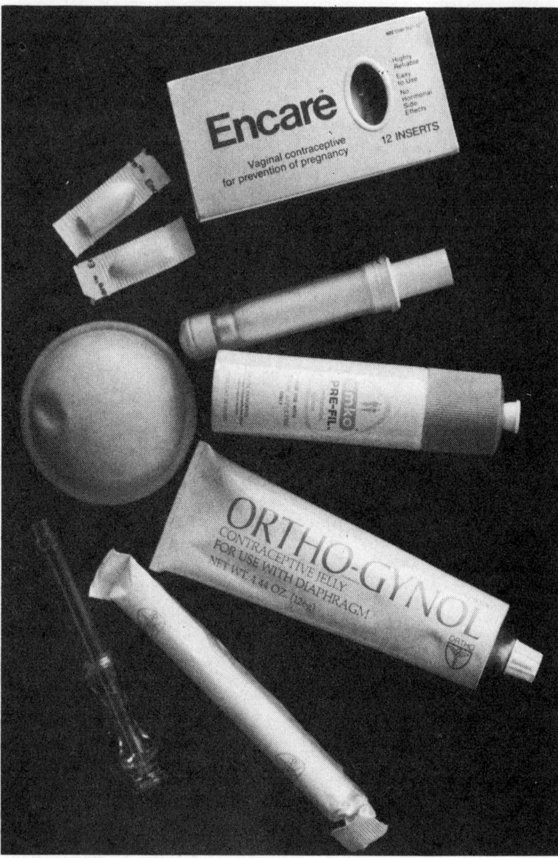

Figure 6-2 Types of foam, contraceptive jelly, and suppositories. (Photograph courtesy of Ronald Tringali, R.N., M.S.)

3. Prepare client for experience of obtaining a contraceptive method.
   a. Describe service routines—first interview, education and counseling services, laboratory work, fee payment (if appropriate).
   b. Explain which medical person will do each procedure and where in the facility each will be performed.
4. Provide support during gynecologic examination, support that includes the following nursing actions:
   a. Explain how a gynecologic examination is done and what procedures are included—speculum insertion, Pap smear, culture, breast and bimanual vaginal, abdominal examinations.

b. Allow the woman to meet the examiner while she is sitting in an upright position, not while she is flat on her back with her feet in the stirrups.
c. Explain each step of the examination as it is being done.
d. Suggest relaxation measures, such as deep breathing, if the client appears to be tense or anxious.
e. Incorporate client education into the routine; have the client participate when possible, such as during the breast examination.
f. Inform the client of her "normality" during the course of the examination; it is more reassuring to hear that "your uterus and ovaries seem to be perfectly normal" than to hear silence.
g. Encourage the client to ask any questions about the examination findings, contraceptive methods, and so on.
h. If the contraceptive method is initiated during the examination, provide additional care.
   (1) Diaphragm fitting. Show the client positions and techniques for insertion and removal of the diaphragm. Provide ample time for practice at her pace, without rushing (Figure 6-3).
   (2) IUD insertion. Note signs of tenseness, pain, or fainting during insertion. When there is no discomfort, instruct client on how to check IUD string. Provide for rest period on table if necessary (Figure 6-4).

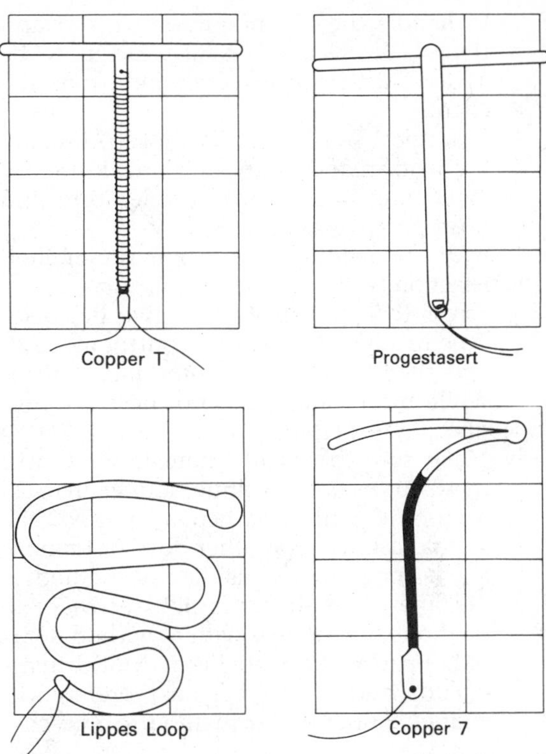

Figure 6-4 Types of approved IUDs.

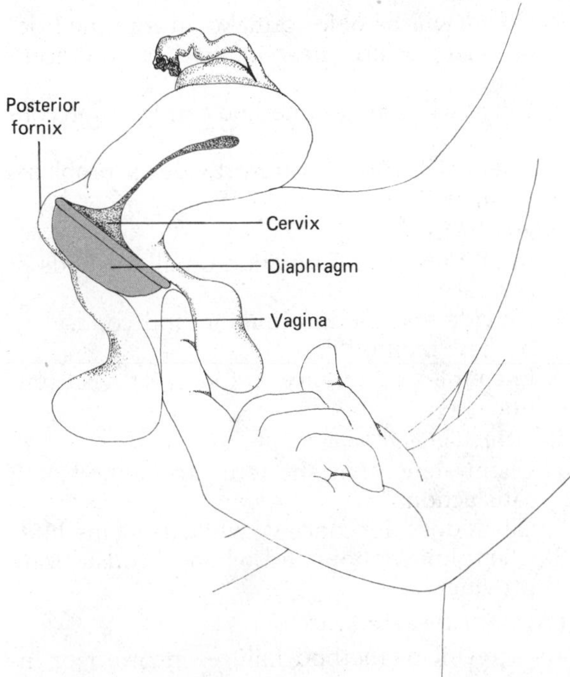

Figure 6-3 Insertion technique for the diaphragm. (Drawing by P. Rodriguez-Lovink.)

5. Ensure that the client understands the method's use and potential side effects or danger signals.
   a. Demonstrate method and have client repeat instructions and information.
   b. Provide literature along with the contraceptive information that the client can refer to at a later time.
   c. If the contraceptive method has been initiated during examination, review previous instructions and add additional details. For example: During the fitting of a diaphragm the emphasis was on learning

to handle the diaphragm and insert and remove it. Details on use can now be added, with greater attention from the client.

d. If surgical sterilization is chosen, prepare the woman and partner for procedures by explaining impact on lifestyle, pre- and postoperative care.

6. Provide homegoing instruction on method satisfaction. For example:
   a. Stress that the client must give her body time to adjust to the birth control method, and time to become comfortable with it, while incorporating it into the daily routine.
   b. Make sure the client understands that if minor problems continue (longer than 2–4 months) with a particular method, she should ask to try another dose or brand if she is committed to using that method.
   c. Tell the client that it is not necessary to continue indefinitely with a method if she or her partner does not like it. Motivations, circumstances, and personal preferences change, and another method can be chosen.
   d. Stress that client should not discontinue the method without consulting a care provider. Problems related to contraception can frequently be resolved without discontinuing the method.
   e. Provide a phone number where the care provider can be reached if questions or problems related to the method arise.
   f. Encourage adherance to follow-up visit routine as established by client and provider.

EVALUATION

Outcome Criteria

1. Client can recall verbally, with 85 percent accuracy, information taught regarding the contraceptive method prescribed.
2. Client is able to use method with ease, as evidenced by statements of comfort.
3. Client uses method with each intercourse and does not conceive.
4. Client who is smoking and using oral contraceptives has reduced smoking by at least half and is working toward abstinence.
5. Client knows any danger or other problems related to method in use.
6. Client has kept initial follow-up appointment.

Complications

CLIENT DISSATISFACTION

Client returns dissatisfied for a variety of reasons. It is understood that major side effects would cause a woman to return promptly for reevaluation and change of method. A number of other reasons for dissatisfaction may occur over time as a person's lifestyle, sexual partner, or motivation changes. Unplanned pregnancy can often occur at transition periods. Sometimes women unintentionally conceive around the anniversary of a significant life event, such as the death of a family member or previous abortion or perinatal death.

Assessment

1. Determine reasons for dissatisfaction (e.g., discomfort).
2. Reevaluate client's motivation for continuing to contracept.
3. Determine client's knowledge of and preference for new method.
4. Determine whether or not the new method will meet client needs.

Revised Outcomes

1. Client will be able to make an informed decision regarding new method of contraception.
2. Client will use new method correctly and consistently.
3. Client will consult care provider if problems occur with new method.

Interventions

1. Briefly review information on all methods of contraception.
2. Provide specific information and counseling on new method chosen.
3. Encourage adherence to follow-up visit routine.

Reevaluation and Follow-up

1. Client states that she is using method with satisfaction.
2. Client does not conceive while using method.
3. Client knows how and when to consult care provider.

UNPLANNED PREGNANCY

As a result of method failure, incorrect or inconsistent method use, or lack of motivation to use contraceptives, an unplanned pregnancy occurs.

Assessment

1. Method use/nonuse leading to pregnancy.
2. Client's feelings about pregnancy.
3. Decision making related to unplanned pregnancy.
4. Partner's response, if involved.
5. Knowledge of available options related to continuation or noncontinuation of pregnancy.

Revised Outcomes

1. Client will have increased knowledge related to options available.
2. Client will be able to make an informed, satisfactory decision regarding desired outcome of pregnancy, with minimal ambivalence.
3. Client will seek and follow through with care appropriate to decision.

Interventions

1. Discuss options available, that is, continuing the pregnancy and keeping the baby, adoption, abortion.
2. Discuss client's feelings, life situation, views of each alternative. Be especially alert to evidence of ambivalence of client or partner.
3. Provide support during decision-making process.
4. Assist with location of appropriate providers for prenatal care or abortion.

Reevaluation and Follow-up

1. Reevaluate client's goals when pregnancy terminates.
2. Assist with long-term fertility planning.
3. Encourage client to follow revisit routine as indicated.

BIBLIOGRAPHY

Boston Women's Health Book Collective: *Our Bodies, Ourselves*, 2d ed., Simon & Schuster, New York, 1976, Chap. 10. Includes detailed information on the menstrual cycle and methods of birth control. Written in lay language; good diagrams and pictures.

Britt, S. S.: "Fertility Awareness: Four Methods of Natural Family Planning," *Journal of Obstetric, Gynecologic, and Neonatal Nursing*, **14**:9–18, March/April 1977. Describes four types of "natural family planning"—the basal body temperature, calendar rhythm, ovulation, and "symptothermal" methods.

Deibel, P.: "Natural Family Planning: Different Methods," *MCN: The American Journal of Maternal Child Nursing*, **3**:171–178. May/June 1978. Describes in some detail the ovulation/mucus method. Includes color-coded graphs and charts for clients use. Also includes information on BBT.

Gorline, L.: "Teaching Successful Use of the Diaphragm," *American Journal of Nursing*, **79**:1732–1735, October 1979. Includes basic information about diaphragms, factors to assess regarding client readiness for this method, and approaches to teaching clients who elect diaphragm use.

Hatcher, R., et al.: *Contraceptive Technology 1982–1983*, 11th ed, Irvington Publishers, New York, 1982. Includes detailed information on philosophy and benefits of family planning, the menstrual cycle, contraceptive methods, abortion, sterilization, and sexually transmitted diseases and a special section on adolescent contraception. Incorporates suggestions for teaching and counseling. Updated edition published every 1 to 2 years. An excellent resource book.

Huxall, L.: "Update on IUD's," *MCN, The American Journal of Maternal Child Nursing*, **5**:186–190, May/June 1980. Presents current data on types of IUDs available, risks and benefits of each, contraindications to use, and management of problems.

Luker, K.: *Taking Chances: Abortion and the Decision not to Contracept*. University of California Press, Berkeley, 1975. Explores the process of contraceptive decision making, with emphasis on social and cultural factors that are influential. Includes implications for care providers. A classic study.

McCann, M., and Cole, L.: "Laparoscopy and Minilaparotomy: Two Major Advances in Female Sterilization," *Studies in Family Planning*, **11**:119–127, April 1980. A comparison of two surgical methods of sterilization, with emphasis on differences in procedural techniques, postoperative routines, surgical and postoperative complications, and failure rates.

Taylor, D.: "A New Way to Teach Teens about Contraceptives," *MCN: The American Journal of Maternal Child Nursing*, **1**:378–383, November/December 1976. Describes an interesting approach to helping adolescents make decisions about contraceptive use. The steps involved in purchasing a pair of jeans are compared to selection of a specific birth control method. Decision making in a common adolescent experience is applied to a new situation.

Tyrer, L.: "Advantages and Disadvantages of Nonprescription Contraceptives," *Medical Aspects of Human Sexuality*, **11**(7):55–56, July 1977. An excellent article for those who counsel clients using diaphragms, foams, jellies, and condoms, methods where high motivation and consistent use are important. Suggestions for history taking, education, and follow-up are given.

Williams, J: *Psychology of Women: Behavior in a Biosocial Context*, Norton, New York, 1977. Includes portions of female growth and development, the menstrual cycle, female sexuality, and birth control.

7

Pregnancy: The First, Second, and Third Trimesters

Nora Doherty Tully

THE FIRST TRIMESTER

DESCRIPTION

The period from the beginning of the last menstrual period (LMP) until the fourteenth week (or 1 to 12 weeks after conception) constitutes the first trimester of pregnancy. It is a period of multiple physical and psychological changes in the mother, a time for the mother to begin working through developmental tasks that will lead to effective parenting. For the fetus it is the crucial period of *organogenesis,* a time during which the maternal environment may be beneficial or hazardous for the infant. Fetal development is outlined in Table 7-1 and in Figure 7-1. For details of psychophysical changes in the expectant mother see Table 7-2.

Because it is estimated that 2 out of 100 babies born have some form of birth defect, it becomes important in prevention to reduce that number to the lowest possible figure. (Chapter 12 discusses in detail the possible problems affecting the developing fetus.) In addition, spontaneous and voluntary abortion are significant factors in the early months of pregnancy. (See Chapter 13 for care of the family unready for childbearing.) For those who determine to become parents, the highest quality of prenatal nursing care is mandated, for nurses are dealing with the future potential of quality of life for the woman and her child, a possible future potential of 120 years.

PREVENTION

Methods of preventing pregnancy until the couple is ready are discussed in Chapter 6.

Health Promotion

1. Teaching, beginning in early adolescence, about risk factors, need for maturity in parenting, and readiness for responsibility.
2. Use of media to communicate teratogenic dangers from chemicals, alcohol, drug use.
3. Promotion of good nutrition in childhood and during teenage and childbearing years.
4. Promotion of any programs that enhance the growth and development of children into responsible, well-adjusted adults.
5. Use of literature and media to promote prenatal care, early and continued throughout the pregnancy.

Population at Risk

1. Uninformed women, of all socioeconomic classes.
2. Immigrants, who speak English as a second language.
3. Young, single teenagers.

TABLE 7-1 FETAL DEVELOPMENT: APPLICATION TO PRENATAL CARE AND FETAL STUDIES

	Fetal Development	Application to Prenatal Care and Fetal Studies
	First Trimester	
Days:		
1–7	Cleavage—tubal transport and implantation.	Only affected by substances present or absent from tubal fluid.
8–14	Implantation completed. Primitive placental circulation begins and is functioning by 20 days.	As soon as substances can cross placenta, equilibrium usually occurs between mother and fetus with fetus getting maternal dose.
15	First missed menses.	
20–22	Neural fold develops and heart begins beating.	Brain growth can be inhibited. Heart defects may occur.
27–30	Arm and leg buds begin. Ear and eye development begins.	Phocomelia can occur. Cataracts can be caused. Immunoreactive pregnancy test begins to be positive.
32	Hand plates.	
34	Foot plates.	
36	Oral and nasal cavities contiguous.	Cleft lip and/or palate may result if teratogens are present in maternal system.
38	Upper lip joins	
30	Palate develops.	
48	Beginning of all internal and external organs are present.	
Week:		
8	Fetal period begins. External genitalia begin to differentiate. Heartbeat: 40–80 bpm; length: 40 mm; weight: 5g.	Exogenous hormones can affect differentiation of genitalia, gonads.
9	Eyelids close over eyes. Intestine still in proximal umbilical cord.	Ultrasonic B scan can distinguish amniotic sac, fetus.
10	Face looks more "human." Intestines into abdomen. Tooth buds begin. Weight: 14 g.	Calcium becomes more important in maternal diet.
11	Arms bend at elbow. Legs are slower to assume fetal proportions.	
12	Organogenesis almost complete. Sex clearly differentiated. Muscle movements still generalized, but can suck thumb. CR length: 87 mm; weight: 45 g.	Heartbeat can be heard with ultrasonic scan at about 120 bpm.
	Second Trimester	
Week:		
16	Ears stand out from head. Bones are storing calcium. Sucking, swallowing, respiratory movements are noted on ultrasonic scan (real time). CR length: 140 mm; weight: 200 g.	Diet contines to be very important. Liver is functioning and can metabolize some drugs. Drugs affect fetal systems in same way as in mother's now; i.e., intoxicated mother, drunk baby.

TABLE 7-1 *(continued)*

	Fetal Development	Application to Prenatal Care and Fetal Studies
	Second Trimester	
Week:		
20	Eyebrows, lanugo visible. Vernix because anabolic-catabolic exchange begins. Myelinization in brainstem. Respiratory movements stronger. Liver forming bile. Meconium present. CR length: 190 mm; weight: 464 g; biparietal diameter (BPD) of head: 4.8–5.0 cm.	Preterm infant: 1% viable but immature. Fetus metabolizes some drugs but not others. There is 400 mL amniotic fluid, and castoff fetal cells can be studied: chromosomes and Barr bodies can determine sex, genetic defects, etc.
24	Fingernails. Eyes begin to reopen. Reacts to light, pain, noise(?). Thick layer of vernix covers body. If born now, high incidence of respiratory failure due to lung immaturity. Now usually called premature infant; 15% rate of premature birth. CR length: 230 mm; weight 650–820 g; BPD: 5.8–6.2 cm.	Maternal emotions and habits are thought to have influence on fetus (studies are incomplete); smoking, excess alcohol, addicting drugs are all negative environmental agents.
	Third Trimester	
Week:		
29	Testes in inguinal canal. Skin translucent. Prominent clitoris; small, separated labia majora. Hypotonic, arms/legs not flexed, do not recoil. No resistance to scarf sign or heel to ear. Wrist shows square window when flexed. Weak suck, shallow. Moro reflexes. CR length: 270 mm; weight: 1000–1300 g; BPD: 7.3–7.8 cm.	<20% survive. Nitrogen, iron, and calcium being stored. Maternal diet very important. Period of most weight gain. All fetal structures develop ability to function.
32	Vernix all over. No lanugo on face. Hypotonic. Some hip flexion, ear flat, soft cartilage. Creases only over ball of foot. Hair fine, woolly, bunches out from head. Sucking, swallowing stronger. Nails to fingertips. CR length: 300 mm; weight: 1500–2100 g; BPD: 8.0–8.4 cm.	50% survive. Orange-stained fat cells begin to appear in amniotic fluid.
36	Vernix over whole body. Testes in upper scrotum. Rugae only over anterior portion. BPD: 8.9–9.3 cm.	Maternal antibodies stored. Fat developing.
37	Clitoris still exposed, but labia larger. Ear pinna two-thirds incurved. Sole creases two-thirds of foot. Weight of 2500 g usually attained; BPD: 9.0–9.4 cm.	97% survive. *Term period* begins as 38th week of gestation starts.

TABLE 7-1 *(continued)*

Week	Fetal Development	Application to Prenatal Care and Fetal Studies
	Third Trimester	
38 39 40 41 42 43	Testes in scrotum. Rugae cover scrotum. Weight: 2600–3600 g; BPD: 9.1–9.5 cm or more. Labia majora more prominent. Clitoris nearly covered. Lanugo on shoulders. Scant vernix. Ear cartilage firm in- creases: Sole crease over heel. No vernix or lanugo. Some weight loss. Skin wrinkled, often deeply creased. Desquamation over most of body. Nails extend well over fingertips. Pendulous scrotum. Deep creases over entire sole of foot.	98% survive. Amniotic fluid tests for fetal maturity: 1. Optical density, ΔOD_{450} = 0.00. Labor begins within 4 weeks and infant is mature (measures bilirubin in amniotic fluid). 2. Nile blue stains fetal fat cells orange. When 20% or more of cells in amniotic fluid are orange, baby is mature. 3. Creatinine >2 mg/100 mL (measures kidney maturity) indicates baby is mature. 4. L/S ratio of 2:1 indicates lung maturity. Correlates with CNS and liver maturity as well (tests may be changed by drugs).
	Postterm infant is one born after the beginning of the 42d week of gestation (288 days or longer); incidence, 4%. Small-for-gestational-age, large-for-gestational-age, and postmature infants vary in measurements from norm above.	Digitalis and aspirinlike drugs delay labor 1–2 weeks. Tests for deteriorating fetal condition: 1. Estriols, falling. 2. Oxytocin challenge test, positive. 3. Meconium in amniotic fluid. 4. Number of fetal movements on ultrasonic B scan less than normal.

NOTE: Average duration of pregnancy from LMP is 280 days, *or* 40 weeks, *or* 10 *lunar* months. Pregnancy really lasts 266 ± 8 days, *or* 38 weeks, *or* 9½ *lunar* months.

TABLE 7-2 NURSING INTERVENTION CORRELATED WITH MATERNAL DEVELOPMENT

Maternal Tasks, Concerns, and Problems	Signs and Symptoms	Nursing Interventions
	First Trimester	
	Weeks 1–4	
Tasks: To acknowledge pregnancy. To accept fetus.	*Subjective* Fatigue, thought to be due to ovarian hormone, relaxin.	Teach the importance of adequate sleep, rest periods, sitting while elevating legs, exercise, using good body mechanics.

TABLE 7-2 *(continued)*

Maternal Tasks, Concerns, and Problems	Signs and Symptoms	Nursing Interventions
To work through any conflicts with own mother in order to begin own mothering role.	Nausea, may be due to decreased maternal blood sugar, decreased gastric motility. Peak period from 60 to 100 days after conception.	Suggest intake of dry carbohydrate foods before arising; eating small, frequent carbohydrate foods and eliminating greasy, spicy foods. Teach about avoiding over-the-counter medications for nausea.
	Soreness, tingling of the breasts.	An early symptom of pregnancy.
	Objective:	
	Amenorrhea, but some women may have spotting at time of expected period.	Instruct on importance of seeking early prenatal care, avoiding any drugs during weeks 1–12 unless prescribed by physician.
	Elevated HCG levels.	Isoimmunologic test can be positive 26 days after conception.
	Elevated basal body temperature due to presence of corpus luteum.	Client using BBT can see sustained temperature elevation on graph.
		Pick up client's concerns and begin teaching at those points. Other instruction must wait until anxiety diminishes.
	Weeks 5–8	
Concerns:	*Subjective*	
Normality of symptoms, future changes in lifestyle.	Enlarging uterus causes pressure on blader, frequency of urination.	In the absence of pain, burning on urination, or hematuria, reassure client that these are due to pressure of the growing uterus. Omit fluids after 6 P.M. to prevent nocturia.
Changes in relationship with partner.		
Cost of care and how to manage.		
Normality of ambivalence to being pregnant.	Desire for sexual relations may decrease.	Explain that sexual desires vary during pregnancy due to both physical and psychological reasons.
	Objective:	
	Breasts enlarge, areolas darker. Enlarged Montgomery's tubercles.	Advocate use of a supporting bra, with adjustable cups, wide adjustable straps,

TABLE 7-2 *(continued)*

Maternal Tasks, Concerns, and Problems	Signs and Symptoms	Nursing Interventions
	These signs present by weeks 5–7: Ladin's—softening on anterior side of uterus above uterocervical junction. Goodell's—softening of cervix. Hegar's—softening of lower uterine segment. Positive pregnancy test for HCG using isoimmunologic methods. Chadwick's—a bluish discoloration of the vagina, present at 8 weeks.	and smooth interior to prevent irritation. Lab work at first visit includes type, Rh, CBC, hemoglobin, hematocrit, urinalysis, and often serology. High-risk population are screened for TB, sickle cell disease. Vaginal or cervical smears for gonorrhea, other infections, and a Pap smear may be done. Instruct client to obtain freshly voided specimen for isoimmunologic test.
	Weeks 9–12	
Problems: Exaggerated discomforts such as nausea, sleeplessness. Excessive need for reassurance that she is pregnant. Anger and rejection of idea of pregnancy. Depression, crying, extreme mood swings. Distance from sexual partner.	*Subjective:* Nausea subsides by 12 weeks. Frequency of urination subsides by 12 weeks.	Caution about self-medication with over-the-counter drugs.
	Objective: Gingivitis, hypertrophy of the gums.	Check on intake of vitamin C-rich foods. Advise dental checkup. Use lead apron if dental x-rays needed.
	Weight gain of 0–3 lb. Some may lose weight. Height of fundus is at the symphysis, rises about 1 cm per week thereafter. 12 weeks—fetal pulse detected by ultrasonic techniques.	Dietary teaching: weight gain should be about 1 lb/month in the first trimester, and at least 11 lb in each of the second and third trimesters (0.8 lb/week). Teach to report these warning signals of problems in first and second trimester: vaginal bleeding, fever, chills, pain, persistent vomiting, leaking of fluid from vagina.

TABLE 7-2 *(continued)*

Maternal Tasks, Concerns, and Problems	Signs and Symptoms	Nursing Interventions
	Second Trimester	
	Weeks 13–16	
Tasks:	*Objective*	
To accept fetus as a separate being.	Colostrum is present.	Advise the use of skin cream to soften crusts formed by colostrum. Remove crusts as part of bathing. Avoid soap on nipple. Suggest the external use of a solution of vinegar and water; use of loose, cotton undergarments; vulval pads, change frequently; tampons are contraindicated.
To manage shifts in dependency from the role of daughter to the role of mother.	Mucous plug formation in cervical canal.	
To continue working through of any conflicts with own parents.	Leukorrhea, profuse, thin, white vaginal discharge. Report if pruritis or foul odor develop: *Candida albicans*, trichomonal infections common.	
To use mimicry, role playing to help assume the role of mother.	Abdominal appearance of pregnancy.	Advise against tight, constricting clothing or wearing shoes with a heel higher than $1\frac{1}{2}$ in. Reinforce good body mechanics; introduce pelvic rock exercise, body toning exercise.
	Height of fundus is halfway between symphysis and umbilicus.	
	Weeks 17–20	
	Subjective:	
	Quickening—maternal perception of first fetal movements.	Instruct client to report any cessation of fetal movement lasting longer than 24 h.
	Often increased sexual desire.	Reinforce concept that variations in sexual interest do occur, that client's partner may not understand these variations. Good communication is essential.
Concerns:	*Objective:*	
Nutritional intake.	Increase in total blood volume that contributes to lightheadedness or fainting; occurs by 10–14 weeks; peaks at $8\frac{1}{2}$ months (34–36 weeks).	Advise client to get up slowly from a horizontal position.
Changing body image.		
Changing life-style and sexual needs.		
Profression of fetal growth.		
Warning signs of problems.	Hemodilution of pregnancy is result of increased plasma (40%) and small RBC increase. Hb of 11–12 g, and Hct may be 31–35%.	Include iron-rich foods in diet.

TABLE 7-2 *(continued)*

Maternal Tasks, Concerns, and Problems	Signs and Symptoms	Nursing Interventions
	The enlargement of varicosities of the saphenous system, vulva, and rectum, if preexisting or predisposed to varicosities, will be aggravated.	Avoid constricting bands around legs and long period of sitting and standing. Use of support hose and elevation of legs at a 90° angle at least twice a day may be indicated.
	Headaches.	Report severe headaches—do not take aspirin in large doses. Report visual disturbances; edema of the face, hands, or legs in the morning; scanty, concentrated urine.
	Fundus is slightly below the umbilicus.	Fetal heart tones are audible with stethoscope.
	Weeks 21–24	
Problems: Lack of acceptance of pregnancy. Depression, anger, anxiety continue. Numerous physical complaints, and focus on own concerns. Indications of no family support. Indication of inability to plan ahead.	*Objective:* Pelvic joints relaxing due to hormone relaxin.	Reinforce good body mechanics; use of squatting and tailor position.
	Possible pigment changes in skin—chloasma of face, linea nigra of abdomen, striae gravidarum.	Reassure patient that while these cannot be prevented, pigmentation will fade after delivery.
	Increased perspiration, oily secretions.	Teach hygiene if necessary.
	Dilation of right ureter due to pressure from dextrorotated uterus.	As urinary stasis and resultant pyelonephritis may result, reinforce need to report any signs of infection. Lying on side aids kidneys efficiency from now on.
	Weeks 25–28	
	Subjective: Leg cramps due to decreased calcium; when there is an increased phosphorus level, fatigue.	Advise exercise, particularly walking, and elevation of legs; as a substitute for milk, calcium tablets may be ordered to achieve Ca:P balance.
	Objective: Hemorrhoids and constipation due to slowed per-	Replace if external. Advise use of ice to the part, use of

TABLE 7-2 *(continued)*

Maternal Tasks, Concerns, and Problems	Signs and Symptoms	Nursing Interventions
	istalsis, pressure of uterus on lower colon and rectum.	the knee-chest position for up to 15 min. Avoidance of constipation by a regular elimination routine, liberal fluid and roughage intake, and exercise is best. Use of home remedies, over-the-counter preparations, and enemas are to be avoided.
Third Trimester		
	Weeks 29–32	
Tasks: To accept pregnancy. To continue to view fetus as a separate individual. To accept physical and psychological changes. To prepare for parenting. To prepare for labor and delivery.	*Subjective:* Fatigue recurs. Anxiety about future. Bad, fearful dreams.	Anticipatory guidance about classes in preparation for childbirth. Inform of the signs of labor; be aware of unrealistic attitudes toward labor. Employment may be terminated, usually by seventh month. Travel involving trips of over 2–3 h are unwise. If necessary, the woman should be instructed to change position frequently and to walk around.
	May feel faint in supine position, due to pressure on the inferior vena cava, which prevents the return of blood from lower extremities.	Advise a side-lying position such as a modified Sims position.
	Sexual desire again decreases due to physical discomfort.	Counseling about variations in desires, alternative sexual practices, and reassurance that this is normal.
Concerns: Baby's well-being and factors affecting this. Anxiety over possibility of deformed baby. Expenses. Process of labor and delivery. Acceptance of baby by other children.	*Objective:* Heartburn due to pressure of uterus on stomach, causes mild hiatus hernia, regurgitation of stomach acid into esophagus.	Antacids may be ordered by physician. Advise small meals and sitting up after eating. Advise against over-the-counter preparations.
	Blood pressure returns to prepregnancy level after a slight drop due to vasodilation.	Monitor blood pressure for changes. Blood pressure of 140/90 or an increase of 30 mmHg in the systolic read-

TABLE 7-2 *(continued)*

Maternal Tasks, Concerns, and Problems	Signs and Symptoms	Nursing Interventions
Present discomforts.	Pulse rate has risen to 15 bpm over normal due to increase in cardiac work.	ing or of 15 mmHg in the diastolic reading is considered a symptom of preeclampsia.
	Braxton Hicks contractions—painless, intermittent contractions.	Explain that these occur throughout pregnancy and are not labor contractions.
	Fundus is midway between the umbilicus and the xiphoid.	Prenatal visits will be every 2 weeks until the ninth month, when they will be weekly.
	Weeks 33–36	
Problems:	*Subjective:*	
High level of anxiety about self, process of labor.	Backache, change in gait.	Reinforce use of good body mechanics. Use of heat, analgesics, and rest as ordered by physician.
Continued nonacceptance of pregnancy.	Becomes impatient for ending of pregnancy.	
Behavior that neglects health practices.	Mood swings occur again as ambivalence about future is demonstrated.	
Lack of support from family or spouse.	*Objective:*	
Lack of preparation for or focus on needs of new baby.	Shortness of breath and other pressure symptoms increase (heartburn, feeling of fullness after eating, constipation, varicose veins, dependent edema in extremities, hemorrhoids).	Remind client to limit activities to avoid dyspnea; pillows may be needed at night. Symptoms will disappear when lightening occurs.
	Weeks 37–40	
	Subjective:	
	Lightening—descent of the presenting part into the true pelvis.	Relaxation and breathing techniques, support husband as coach.
	Aching in lower abdomen.	Teach signs of impending labor:
	Objective:	
	Fundus just below the diaphragm until lightening, then appears to tip forward.	1. Contractions increasing in intensity and frequency, which do not stop when walking. 2. Mucous plug, "bloody show," expelled. 3. Membranes may rupture anytime and should be reported to physician.

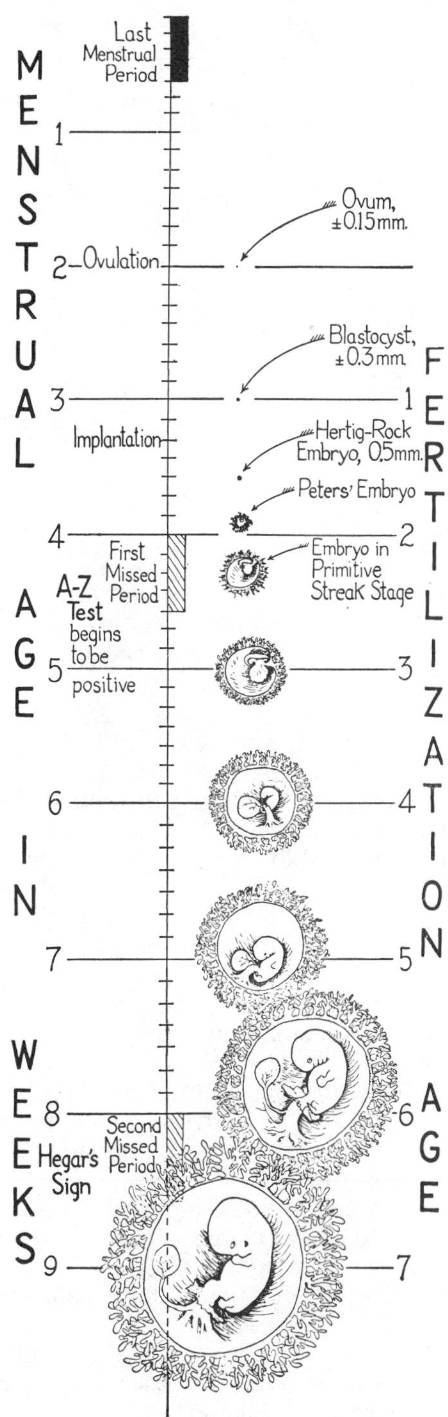

Figure 7-1 Menstrual age compared with fertilization age, showing the actual size of embryos in relation to mother's menstrual history (*left*) and fertilization age of embryo (*right*). Based on a 28-day cycle. (From Corliss, C. E., *Patton's Human Embryology*, McGraw-Hill, New York, 1976.)

4. Those with preexisting medical problems, or socioeconomic problems.
5. Any woman who is habituated to alcohol, smoking, or drugs.

Screening

1. Screening is best done during earliest clinic visits for those already pregnant.
2. In addition, screening for high-risk factors in genetic inheritance may be done in specific population groups. (See Chapter 12.)

ASSESSMENT

Health History

1. *Family history* should include information about cardiovascular diseases, diabetes mellitus, epilepsy, blood dyscrasias, hereditary diseases, congenital defects, tuberculosis, mental or emotional problems, and history of multiple pregnancies.
2. The father's present health status, blood type, significant health problems, and health history should be known, as well as his attitude toward this pregnancy.
3. For *family psychosocial* history see Chapter 5.
4. *Medical history* should include information about mother's own health in terms of conditions listed above, as well as any allergies, immunization record, recent viral disease, and exposure to drugs or pollutants. History of venereal disease exposure, gynecologic disorders, surgery of the pelvic area are important as well.
5. *Menstrual history* should include information about onset, character, interval, and duration and problems and attitudes toward menses.
6. *Obstetric history* should include information about gravidity and parity: *gravida* = number of times ever pregnant, *para* = number of deliveries after 20 weeks gestation; twins count as one para, as do stillbirths. Query client about number of pregnancies—full-term, preterm, abortions, stillbirths—and about the number of surviving children. For each pregnancy obtain information about date of delivery, gestation, length of labor, type of delivery, weight and condition of infant, and if there was a physical or mental problem in the infant. Also, any problems with infertility, plus experience with success or failure of contraceptive methods.

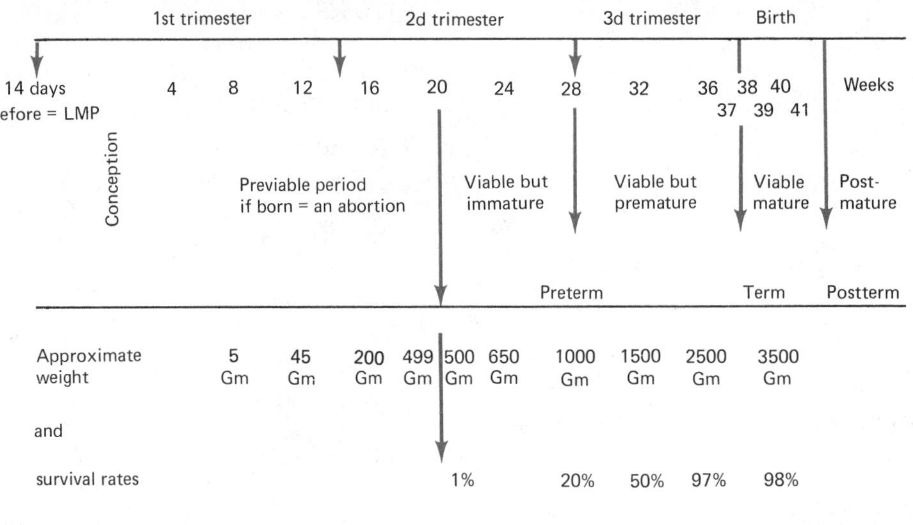

Figure 7-2 Dates, weights, and terminology related to fetal maturity. (From Dickason, E. J. and Schult, M. O., *Maternal and Infant Care*, 2d Ed., McGraw-Hill, New York, 1979.)

Physical Assessment

1. Medical examination.
   a. *Head.* Hair texture, eye, ear, nose, throat, thyroid, presence of chloasma, condition of teeth, tongue, gingiva.
   b. *Heart.* By 10 to 12 weeks rate increases up to 10 beats per minute (bpm), reflecting increased blood volume (+40 percent) and higher cardiac output (+50 percent). In first trimester, blood pressure decreases slightly but will increase later, thus baseline is important.
   c. *Lungs.* Volume expands as a result of relaxation of intracostal cartilage; during late pregnancy, dyspnea and orthopnea occur because of pressure of the uterus on the diaphragm.
   d. *Breasts.* Early changes are soreness, tingling, enlargement with areola darkening and enlargement of tubercles of Montgomery, colostrum begins by 14 weeks; blood supply markedly increases, with veins observable through skin.
   e. *Abdomen.* Enlargement occurs earlier in multigravida; striae, linea nigra are present; note amount of total body hair and hair distribution.
   f. *Extremities.* Note edema; varicose veins will become more marked due to increased blood volume and increased femoral venous pressure (up to 18 mmHg).
   g. *Baseline weight.* Weight gain pattern should be at least in range of 0–3 lb in first trimester, then 0.8 lb/week, totaling at least 27–30 lb; markedly overweight women should control calorie intake under physician's orders but should not attempt any weight loss.
2. Obstetric examination.
   a. *Pelvis.* Adequacy determined for vaginal delivery.
      (1) The diagonal conjugate, from lower margin of symphysis pubis to promontory of the sacrum, is normally 12.5 cm or larger.
      (2) The transverse diameter between both ischial tuberosities is normally 10.5 cm or larger;
      (3) The bispinous diameter is usually 10.5 cm.
      (4) X-ray pelvimetry is delayed until just before delivery in order to reduce exposure to radiaton.
   b. *Vagina.* Observe wall for weakness, anterior or posterior; palpate glands for enlargement, bluish discoloration (Chadwick's sign) should be present by 8 weeks.
   c. *Cervix.* Observe for erosion, type of mu-

cous discharge, color, consistency a softening occurs by seventh week (Goodell's sign); observe amount of dilatation, presence of scarring.

d. *External genitalia.* Observe for warts, infections, and signs of old scars, especially around meatus, perineal area, or anal sphincter.
e. *Fundus.* Estimate location, size, and consistency; note any displacement, signs of ectopic growth.
f. *Estimated date of delivery (EDD).*
   (1) Usually determined by *Nagele's rule*: date of LMP + 7 days − 3 months + 1 year.
   (2) Measurement of height of fundus: after 12 weeks, rises 1 cm/week above the symphysis pubis; or *MacDonald's rule*: height of fundus in centimeters × 8/7 = duration of pregnancy in weeks (Figure 7-3).
   (3) Date of quickening.
      (a) Primigravida = 20 weeks + 2 days after quickening = EDD.
      (b) Multigravida = 21 weeks + 4 days after date of quickening = EDD.

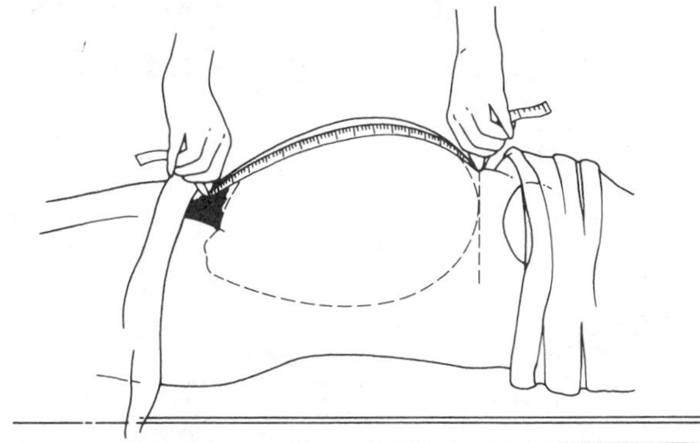

Figure 7-3 Measurement of fundal height.

Diagnostic Tests

1. *Blood work.* Complete blood count (CBC) will show evidence of hemodilution of pregnancy with

   RBC: 3.75^6–4.5^6 (million)
   Hemoglobin (Hgb): 11 ≥ 11 g/dL
   Hematocrit (Hct): 31 ≥ 31%
   WBC: 7,000–15,000

   a. Identification of mother's blood type and Rh factor and also, preferably, those of the father of the child.
   b. Serologic screening along with screening for rubella titer, sickle cell trait, glucose-6-phosphate dehydrogenase (G-6-PD).
   c. Blood glucose in high-risk population.
2. *Cervical mucus/cells.*
   a. Papanicolaou test (sometimes omitted because of confusing atypical cells found during pregnancy.
   b. Smears for infections—gonorrhea, trichomonas, candidiasis as indicated (see Table 7-3).
3. Chest x-ray: screening for tuberculosis and heart disease in high-risk populations.
4. Urinalysis: glucose, protein, cells; on subsequent visits, glucose and protein; culture if cells, casts, or RBC present; glucose tolerance test if glucose present.
5. Pregnancy diagnostic tests.
   a. Biologic tests: infrequently used tests that require a fasting morning specimen that is injected into a lab animal; changes in animal gonads caused by human chorionic gonadotropin (HCG) indicate presence of placental hormone in client.
   b. Isoimmunologic tests: tests based on antibody-antigen reaction with HCG-coated sheep red cells; HCG in client's urine does not allow agglutination in test tube or on 2-min slide test paper; a home test kit that uses a 2-h process is available.

NURSING DIAGNOSES: ACTUAL OR POTENTIAL

1. Alterations in physical status: potential: abnormal symptoms appearing in the first trimester.
2. Alterations in comfort: minor discomforts caused by physiologic changes of pregnancy.
3. Anxiety resulting from pregnancy: new prenatal procedures; potential: socioeconomic stresses.
4. Ineffective coping: potential: result of client's inability to meet developmental tasks.
5. Alterations in self-concept: potential: due to weight gain or loss; potential: due to changes in sexuality; potential: due to change in career status.
6. Lack of compliance: potential: due to knowledge deficit.

TABLE 7-3 VAGINAL INFECTIONS DURING PREGNANCY

Agent	Manifestation in Newborn if Untreated	Treatment during Pregnancy
Candidiasis: *Candida albicans*	Oral or GI thrush; diarrhea with grey, wet infected areas on buttocks	*Diagnosis:* Nickerson's medium or wet-mount slide. *Treatment:* Miconazole; AVC cream, nystatin. Treat partner. Maintain hand-washing technique in caring for infant.
Gonorrhea: *Neisseria gonorrhoeae*	Conjunctivitis, blindness; septicemia following maternal septicemia	*Diagnosis:* Gram stain of smear at first and thirty-sixth week clinic visits. *Treatment:* Probenecid plus penicillin or erythromycin. Treat all partners.
Herpes simplex type 2 (HSV): *Herpesvirus hominis*	During pregnancy increase in abortion and rate of stillbirth. Ascending infection after membrane rupture. Generalized neonatal infection appears in 4–7 days, skin vesicles, jaundice, bleeding, seizures, neonatal death.	*Diagnosis:* Check titer for rising levels of serum antibodies. Culture weekly during last 6–8 weeks of pregnancy. *Treatment:* No effective treatment. Often choose cesarean section if active lesions seen on genitalia or have been present during last 6 weeks. Mother must deliver within 4 h of rupture of membranes to prevent ascending infection. Vaginal delivery done if more than 4 h have elapsed since fetus considered already infected. Mother instructed on wound and skin precautions; baby isolated but not from mother.
Syphilis: *Treponema pallidum*	Primary and secondary maternal infection leads to stillbirth. Latent and tertiary leads to bone, tooth deformities and secondary symptoms in the newborn.	*Diagnosis:* Serologic tests, observation, wet mount of primary lesion. *Treatment:* Large dose of penicillin will reach fetus for intrauterine syphillis. Erythromycin not as effective but used in cases of penicillin sensitivity. Follow with serologic tests. Partner should be treated.
Trichomoniasis: *Trichomonas vaginalis*	No effects on fetus.	*Diagnosis:* Wet-mount saline slide. *Local treatment:* Careful acidic douche, AVC cream. *Systemic treatment:* Metronidazole (Flagyl) not used or only with caution during pregnancy. Partner must be treated.
Cor vaginale vaginitis: *Haemophilus vaginalis*	Chorioamnionitis; some cases of septicemia, neonatal death.	*Diagnosis:* Gram stain or culture for nonmotile rods. *Treatment:* AVC cream, suppositories.

EXPECTED OUTCOMES

1. Client will be aware of danger signs of pregnancy and will be able to return this information verbally.
2. Client will be aware of reasons for physical discomforts of pregnancy and will use comfort measures successfully.
3. Orientation to procedures and schedule will reduce anxiety.
4. Referrals will be made to social worker, nutritionist, dentist as needed, and client will be involved in plan.
5. Developmental tasks for both parents will progress smoothly.
6. Client will give evidence of compliance with care plan by keeping appointments and maintaining weight gain.
7. Client will understand and apply nutrition counseling to her own food habits and will be able to explain verbally the adjustments she will make in her diet.
8. Client will not use potentially adverse substances during the pregnancy.

INTERVENTIONS

1. Alert client to abnormal symptoms of the first trimester and what action to take:
   a. Bleeding or uterine cramping.
   b. Urinary infection, other infections.
   c. Severe mood swings, depression.
   d. Protracted vomiting, weight loss.
2. Elicit history of minor discomforts and answer any questions regarding care and future developments.
3. Explain prenatal procedures, interpret physician's instructions, determine client's level of understanding.
4. Provide appropriate literature and suggest ways of preparing for psychological growth tasks.
5. Provide support concerning variable psychological responses to pregnancy; explain variations in sexual responses that women and men may experience.
6. Teach about the following topics and include both parents in any planning.
   a. Nonpharmacologic relief of minor discomforts.
   b. Effects of use of drugs, alcohol, tobacco.
   c. Developmental changes of mother and fetus (Table 7-2).

EVALUATION

Outcome Criteria

1. Acceptance of the pregnancy is evidenced by compliance with plan of care and by verbal statements.
2. Client is maintaining weight gain pattern and diet, with understanding.
3. Fetal development is progressing normally.
4. Client participates regularly in clinic or physician follow-up.
5. Client refrains from ingesting and/or using drugs, alcohol, or tobacco.
6. Client accepts minor discomforts, uses learned comfort measures without undue anxiety.

Complications

SPONTANEOUS ABORTION

Spontaneous abortion is the unplanned loss of the conceptus before the end of the twentieth completed week of fetal development. When the fetus weighs less than 464 g or measures less than 16.5 cm crown to rump (CR) in length, it is thought to be nonviable. Incidence is 1 out of 15 pregnancies. Spontaneous abortion may be caused by a defective embryo or placenta (50 to 60%), unknown causes (20 to 30%), or maternal disease (15%) (Assali, 1975).

Abortions are also classified as *early*, occurring at 8 to 10 weeks, or *late*, occurring at 13 weeks or thereafter. A *habitual abortion*, the spontaneous loss of three or more successive pregnancies, usually occurs late and is most commonly due to an incompetent cervix. Treatment is by a cerclage procedure that sutures the cervix closed, accompanied by extensive bed rest.

Threatened abortion begins, without cervical dilatation, with early signs such as spotting and cramping. It may or may not progress to *inevitable abortion*, when cervical dilatation progresses in spite of bed rest and sedatives, so that products of conception are passed, *completely* or *incompletely*. In the case of incomplete passage, a dilatation and curettage (D&C) is necessary.

Assessment

1. Vaginal bleeding of varying degrees of severity.
2. Low hormonal levels of estrogen, HCG.
3. Lower abdominal aching, cramping that may progress in severity, and then cervical dilatation with rupture of membranes.

Revised Outcomes
1. Client will give evidence of compliance with plan of care by maintaining bed rest until bleeding ceases, refraining from sexual intercourse as directed, and collecting urines for hormonal assay.
2. Client's statements will indicate acceptance of loss of pregnancy, that process of grieving has begun.

Interventions
1. Bed rest, sedation, fluids, emotional support, analgesia as needed.
2. Instruct client to maintain abstinence from intercourse.
3. Collect 24-h urine for hormonal assay—assessment of HCG levels (1 IU/100 mL at time of first missed period up to 100 IU/100 mL in the 60–100 days after LMP; then it falls off sharply); estriol levels below 3 to 4 mg/100 mL in 24-h urine in the first trimester usually indicate fetal death.
4. Observe possible progression of signs and symptoms.
5. Observe amount of bleeding, cramping; do careful check for completeness of aborted fragments.
6. Provide explanations to father and mother.
7. Obtain consent for operative intervention; client will need a D&C if abortion is incomplete, usually under anesthesia with IV fluids and infusion of oxytocin.

Reevaluation and Follow-up
1. Cessation of bleeding; client returned for appointments.
2. Counseling given regarding future pregnancy spacing.
3. Client able to discuss feelings of loss.
4. Partner supportive in dealing with loss.

MISSED ABORTION

In the previable period, the retention of the conceptus for 4 or more weeks after intrauterine death is also called a *retained abortion*. The placenta may function for a time, confusing the pregnancy tests and signs. Retention of degenerating tissues can interfere with coagulation and platelet function and *disseminated intravascular coagulation* (DIC) can result. *Intrauterine fetal death* (IUFD) is death of the fetus after the age of viability; after the delivery of such an infant it is called a *stillbirth* and must be reported in vital statistics.

Assessment
1. Absence of fetal heart beat, cessation of movements.
2. Regression of signs of pregnancy—static uterine size.
3. In early weeks, mother may state that "something is not right."

Revised Outcomes
1. Pregnancy will be terminated with least possible trauma to mother.
2. No adverse effects of retention of dead fetus will occur.
3. Client's statements will indicate that grieving is in process.

Interventions
1. Obtain consent for required procedure, depending on week of gestation. Early—D&C; midtrimester—prostaglandin instillation into amniotic fluid; later pregnancy—oxytocin or prostaglandin induction.
2. Observe for symptoms of DIC.
3. Provide support during maternal anxiety about causes of intrauterine death and its effects.
4. Support client during grieving process.

Reevaluation and Follow-up
1. Fetus was delivered without trauma or complications.
2. Postpartum follow-up was sought.
3. Client participated in counseling regarding future pregnancy.
4. Client found support for grieving process.

HYDATIDIFORM MOLE

Hydatid, or molar, pregnancy is a developmental anomaly of the chorionic syncytium involving degeneration of the villi into fluid-filled grapelike vesicles. In the United States it is thought to occur in 1:2000 pregnancies. Studies indicate it may be more common in women with protein-deficient diets. Lack of, or destruction of, folic acid and amino acids in food preparation may interfere with the developing embryo. Molar pregnancy is associated with larger than usual uterine size for estimated gestational age, heavy vaginal bleeding, early hypertensive symptoms, i.e., before the twenty-fourth week, and hyperemesis. Urinary chorionic gonadotropin (UCG) levels are elevated to 35,000 IU/mL. Dilatation and curettage are indicated and follow-up is essential because of possibility of recurrent mole or development of choriocarcinoma, a highly malignant cancer. The client is followed with periodic evaluation for condition and continuing or recurring presence of HCG in urine.

ECTOPIC PREGNANCY

Ectopic pregnancy involves implantation of the fertilized ovum outside the uterus, usually in the fallopian tube. The average incidence is 1:200 pregnancies and varies widely with economic and social conditions and history of health care, as contributing to predisposing factors. Although the reason for tubal implantation (97 percent of ectopic pregnancies) is often unknown, delayed movement through the tube appears to be the major cause. Infection or salpingitis as a sequel to childbirth, surgery, abortion, or gonorrhea may result in adhesions and scar tissue. Health and function of the tube also may be affected by low fertility levels and by endometriosis.

Recurrence after one tubal pregnancy is possible as bilateral pathology may be present.

Assessment

1. Amenorrhea, followed by varying amounts of vaginal bleeding; uterine size enlarges to 8 weeks; all signs of early weeks of pregnancy are present.
2. Increasing lower abdominal pressure beginning about 3 to 5 weeks after LMP.
3. Syncope, "fainting in bathroom," rectal pressure from collection of unclotted blood in cul-de-sac.
4. Anemia, increased fatigue.
5. Possible abdominal pain, beginning about 10 to 12 weeks after LMP.

Revised Outcomes

1. Client's statements will indicate ability to cope with loss of pregnancy.
2. Client will demonstrate uneventful postoperative course, without fever or infection.
3. Client will be aware of implications for future pregnancies.

Interventions

1. Prepare for diagnostic tests—culdocentesis, ultrasound evaluation, blood tests, urinalysis.
2. Type and cross match for surgery if diagnosis confirmed.
3. If client is hypovolemic, treat symptoms, observe vital signs, provide fluid replacement, keep NPO.
4. Support client through grieving process.

Reevaluation and Follow-up

1. Postoperative care resulted in uneventful recovery.
2. Client abstained from sexual intercourse until fully recovered and now plans an interval before next pregnancy.
3. Beginning of acceptance of pregnancy loss was evidenced by verbal statements by couple.

HYPEREMESIS GRAVIDARUM

Hyperemesis gravidarum is a condition of constant and excessive vomiting continuing into the sixteenth week of pregnancy, resulting in loss of 5 percent or more of body weight. Without treatment, it may result in ketosis, liver or renal damage, neurologic disturbances, or death. Hospitalization to monitor fluid and electrolyte balance and treatment with antiemetics, IV fluids, tranquilizers, and vitamins are usual. Psychiatric assessment may be included as hyperemesis continues to have a mixed etiology. High levels of HCG are contributory as well as facets of rejection of the pregnancy.

VAGINAL INFECTION

During pregnancy, a higher pH than the norm, 4.0, and an increase in glucose levels in vaginal tissues can support the growth of commonly resident bacteria. The vaginal discharge may cause vulval irritation, itching, dysuria, and painful intercourse. The client should be screened for elevated glucose levels: persistent infections may indicate the presence of gestational diabetes. After identification of the causative organism, treatment is given only by means of a nonteratogenic drug; for example, Flagyl is not recommended during pregnancy for cases of *trichomonas*. Other interventions include frequent perineal hygiene with vinegar solution but no pressure-douching; use of vulval pads but no tampons; and ascertaining if infection is present in client's sexual partner (Table 7-3).

ADOLESCENT PREGNANCY

Adolescent pregnancy is complicated by immature physical development, interruption of education, and lack of achievement of developmental tasks. Often, the pregnancy is unplanned and unwanted. There is little, or late, prenatal care. Lack of family acceptance or of paternal support necessitates difficult decisions about abortion, adoption, or keeping the infant. The welfare of the infant is dependent upon decisions made under emotional stress.

The current incidence is 213,000 births and 135,000 abortions in girls 17 years old or less. Of these numbers, 11,000 births and 13,000 abortions occurred in girls younger than 14 years of age (*Morbidity and Mortality Report,* 1980). Although the numbers are lower than in previous periods, percentage of the total birth rate is higher.

Although prevention would be the ideal, at present, care to the pregnant adolescent is crisis-oriented rather than preventive. Sex education classes, availability of family planning services, and media campaigns have had little effect. The adolescent father has only recently been recognized as also needing help and as having rights and responsibilities. Whenever possible, he should be included in interventions and decision making. Comprehensive care is primary, for there are higher neonatal and infant mortality rates for the children of these girls as well as increased rates of prenatal and intrapartum maternal problems (see Chapter 13).

Assessment

1. Higher risk of anemia, poor nutrition, over- or underweight.
2. Increased incidence of preeclampsia, preterm delivery.
3. Psychosocial problems, poor adaptation, ambivalence, lack of family support resulting in increased anxiety about labor and parenting problems.
4. Difficulty in developmental tasks, both of adolescence and of pregnancy.

Revised Outcome

1. Client will receive explanations about each step of care that acknowledge her developmental level.
2. Adolescent will be cared for by a single reference person for personal support throughout the pregnancy and if possible the labor period.
3. Father of infant will be involved in decision making.
4. Client will recognize the importance of nutrition and maintain adequate diet.
5. Client will develop ability to solve problems in her own situation and plan for child care.
6. Young mother will show evidence of increased self-esteem.
7. Complications due to inadequate screening and/or care will be prevented.

Interventions

1. Provide continuity of care, with nutrition counseling and referral.
2. Encourage client to attend classes in pregnancy, labor, and child care that are geared to developmental level.
3. Refer client to social service and sometimes psychiatrist.
4. Attempt follow-through with same nurse, and one plan for pregnancy and labor, post delivery.
5. Teach family planning method of choice.

Reevaluation and Follow-up

1. Client participated in decision making about outcome of pregnancy.
2. Client participated in and displays knowledge learned at child care and prenatal classes.
3. Client made homegoing plans that will lead to positive results for mother and infant.
4. Client planned to use and learned how to use contraceptive method of choice.

ELDERLY GRAVIDA

This term is applied to those women having a first pregnancy after the age of 35 or subsequent pregnancies after the age of 40. There is two times the incidence of maternal mortality, a higher risk of complications from a preexisting chronic disease or obesity, and a higher risk of pregnancy-induced hypertension. In addition, Down's syndrome occurs in a 1:40 to 1:100 ratio, and there is increased risk of congenital defects. Delivery is often by cesarean section. There may be anxiety, ambivalence, and lack of support for the pregnancy. Diagnostic amniocentesis and genetic counseling will be recommended, but those families opposed to elective abortion may refuse counseling.

THE SECOND TRIMESTER

DESCRIPTION

The period between 15 and 28 weeks after the LMP (13 to 27 weeks after conception) constitutes the second trimester of pregnancy. The uterus enlarges to above the umbilicus, and the first fetal movements are felt. During this period of fetal growth, organogenesis is almost completed though cell growth in size and number continues. If delivery occurs, the chances of survival are slight (see Chapter 11). By the end of the second trimester, the expectant father usually will become more involved in the growth tasks of pregnancy, as well as attending to practical and financial concerns.

ASSESSMENT

Health History

In addition to the basic health history and physical examination as outlined in the beginning of this chapter, the obstetric course and reasons for delay in seeking care should be elicited.

Physical Assessment

1. *Abdominal palpation.*
   a. *Ballottement,* the rebound movement of the fetus when the uterus is tapped by the examiner, can be detected by the sixteenth week.
   b. By palpation the examiner can differentiate fetal movements by 20 weeks, and by 26 weeks infant parts can be felt through the abdominal wall.
2. *Fetal heart beat.* 100 to 180 beats per minute (120 to 160 average) can be heard with an ultrasound instrument at 13 to 16 weeks and by fetoscope by 20 weeks.

Diagnostic Tests

1. *Amniocentesis.* A sample of amniotic fluid is removed by tapping the amniotic sac with a needle inserted through the abdominal and uterine walls; fluid is studied for biochemical or cell chromosome structure (see Chapter 12).
2. *Ultrasonography.* Ultrahigh-frequency sound pulses are beamed into the body; pulse-echo responses outline the interface between types of soft tissue. (Because ultrasonography discriminates soft tissue types, it is a very accurate method of detecting any abnormal implantation, or the stage of fetal development, as well as major anomalies.)
3. *X-rays.* With progressive ossification the fetal skeleton is visible by 21 to 24 weeks; x-ray is rarely requested until the ratio between fetal size and maternal pelvic cavity must be measured at the time of labor.

NURSING DIAGNOSES: ACTUAL OR POTENTIAL

1. Alterations in client's physical status: potential development of abnormal symptoms during second trimester.
2. Alterations in physical status: potential: chronic preexisting disease may be intensified by advancing pregnancy.
3. Alterations in nutrition/iron needs as a result of increased fetal demands.
4. Difficulty in family coping: potential: stemming from a lack of support from family.
5. Alterations in self-concept: resulting from a changing body image.
6. Lack of knowledge about need for early and continued prenatal care.

EXPECTED OUTCOMES

1. Client will keep appointments and will be able to explain reasons for early and continued care.
2. Woman's statements indicate an understanding of physical changes during pregnancy as well as comfort measures.
3. Client will understand nutritional requirements and will maintain a hemoglobin of 11 g/dL or above.
4. Client will be able to describe signs of physical "warning signals," especially those of the second trimester.
5. Woman's statements indicate adequate support from family and significant other.
6. Client will give evidence of achieving first trimester developmental goals.

INTERVENTIONS

1. Explain normal changes of the second trimester and the nonpharmacologic measures for relief of minor discomforts. (See Table 7-2.)
2. Reinforce nutritional requirements and explain side effects if oral iron is prescribed. (See Table 7-4.)
3. Teach warning signals for this trimester and why and when to report to physician and/or clinic.
   a. Any bleeding.
   b. Signs of localized or regional infection.
   c. Any pain other than round ligament aching.
   d. Any signs of pregnancy-induced hypertension.

TABLE 7-4 DAILY DIET PLAN IN PREGNANCY

Food	Baseline Diet	Diet during Pregnancy
Milk	Adult: 2 cups Teenagers: 4 cups	4 cups 4 cups
Meat, fish, poultry, eggs, nuts, dried peas or beans	2 servings (2 oz each)	2 servings (3 oz each)
Vegetable/fruit	4 servings	4 servings
High-vitamin C fruit or vegetable	1 serving daily	1 serving daily
Dark green or deep yellow vegetable	1 serving every other day	1 serving every other day
Bread/cereal, enriched or whole grain	5 servings[a]	5 servings[a]

SOURCE: Lau Kee, B.: "Nutrition during Pregnancy," in E. J. Dickason and M. O. Schult (eds.), *Maternal and Infant Care*, 2d ed., McGraw-Hill, New York, 1979, p. 127.
[a] Four servings if one is a breakfast cereal.

(1) Generalized edema present on arising.
(2) Any change in color/concentration of urine.
(3) Unexplained rapid weight gain.
(4) Headaches, visual disturbances.
(5) Epigastric pain (often confused with heartburn).

4. Teach developmental changes in fetus.
5. Assess client's psychosocial responses to pregnancy stresses, ability to accept changing body image, and relationship with and support from family and significant others (Table 7-5).
6. Evaluate progress in developmental tasks of pregnancy; identify potential for positive and negative adjustments to parenting role.

EVALUATION

Outcome Criteria

1. Client keeps appointments and follows health care suggestions.
2. Weight gain is within normal pattern for trimester; hemoglobin remains above 11 g/dL.
3. Client can identify any warning signals and knows when to consult physician/clinic.
4. Client has begun preparing for the infant and plans to attend childbirth education classes.
5. Client is achieving second-trimester task of identifying the fetus as a growing baby, separate from herself.

Complications

MULTIPLE PREGNANCY

Without pharmacologic intervention, the incidence of multiple pregnancies has been highest in black women and lowest in Asian women. Ovulatory agents such as Clomid carry a 20 to 30 percent risk (see Chapter 14). With multiple gestation, there is a higher risk of perinatal morbidity and mortality because of the incidence of preterm and low-birth-weight infants.

The incidence of *monozygous*, or *identical*, twins differs from that of *dizygous*, or *fraternal*, twins. In about 1:200 pregnancies, there is splitting of a single fertilized egg within the first 2 weeks, resulting in monozygous twins. A double ovulation and fertilization resulting in dizygous twinning occurs in varying numbers depending upon heredity, race, maternal age, and ovulation-inducing drugs. Two-thirds of all twins in the United States are dizygous. In addition, placentation differs with zygosity:

1. *Monozygous twins* may be monochorionic (one chorion) and monoamnionic (one amnion), monochorionic and diamnionic (two amnions), or dichorionic (two chorions) and diamnionic (see Figure 7-4).
2. *Dizygous twins* can be only dichorionic and diamnionic.

TABLE 7-5 MAJOR CONCERNS EXPRESSED BY 100 PREGNANT WOMEN

Concern	Women, %
Baby	
Whether your baby will be healthy and normal	94
Whether your baby will be a boy or a girl	70
Self	
How you look	91
Your own health	80
Gaining too much weight	70
Change in your way of living	69
Being depressed	65
Doing all the housework	60
Being nervous	53
Medical care	
Medication you might receive during childbirth	77
What drugs are safe to take during pregnancy	70
Being able to follow the diet your doctor ordered	62
Whether the doctors will give you good care	58
Whether the nurses will give you good care	58
Whether the doctors are able to help you	57
Childbirth	
Baby's condition at birth	93
Unexpected things that might happen during childbirth	89
Pain of childbirth	83
Your condition during childbirth	81
Whether baby will be premature	70
Being cut when the baby is delivered	61
Being torn when the baby is born	58
Whether your baby will be overdue	56
Whether something might happen to baby during birth	69
Finances	
Managing the added cost of having a child	66
Being able to buy the things you need and want	55
Being able to buy the things your other children need and want	52
Subsequent pregnancies	
Type of birth control you will use after this baby is born	54

SOURCE: Glazer, G.: "Anxiety Levels and Concerns Among Pregnant Women," *Research in Nursing and Health,* **3**:110, 1980.

Intrauterine growth of twins proceeds as in a normal singleton pregnancy until 29 weeks gestation, when their weight gain is less than that of a singleton. The average birth weight of a twin is 2600 g. One complication of twin pregnancy is discordant intrauterine growth resulting in one SGA (small-for-gestational-age) or growth-retarded infant and one normal-sized infant. There may also be concordant transfusion syndrome in monochorionic gestation, which results in one twin's shunting blood from the other. The donor twin becomes anemic, growth-retarded, and hypotensive while the recipient twin is polycythemic, hypertensive, and much larger. Congenital anomalies are twice as frequent in twin pregnancies; conjoined twins are rare (1:38,000 to 1:165,000 live births). Risk of mortality is increased in twin gestation to 14 per-

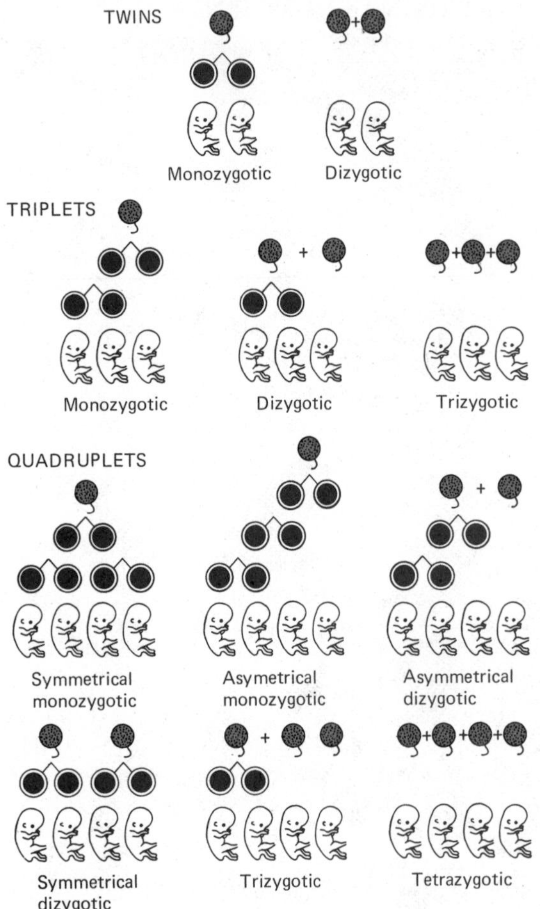

Figure 7-4 Diagrammatic illustration of possible embryological origins of multiple pregnancy. (From Hafez, E. S. E., "Physiology of Multiple Pregnancy," *Journal of Reproductive Medicine*, **12**:88, 1974, with permission.)

cent and is mostly due to premature delivery; however, there exists a difference between first and second twins. The second twin is frequently more hypoxic, as there may be placental separation before delivery. When more than 30 min have passed between the delivery of the first and second infants, the second twin is said to be "retained." As the interval increases, chances of survival for the second twin decrease. There is also an increased risk of intracranial hemorrhage, as there has been no chance for the second twin's head to mould, as well as an increased exposure to anesthesia. Cesarean section is becoming the delivery mode of choice for twin pregnancy to avoid these problems as well as that of interlocking twins (i.e., first twin presents as a breech and the second as a vertex with locking of the heads beneath the chins, thus preventing vaginal delivery of either).

Management of twin delivery should include special attention to the second twin, who is a higher risk for asphyxia. Careful observation for congenital anomalies, polycythemia, anemia, plus problems of prematurity, is necessary. It is important to offer support to the family, especially when the twins have not been diagnosed prenatally. Mothers of Twins clubs are available in most larger cities. If the infants require extended hospital care, an attempt should be made to discharge them together so as to avoid difficulties in family-infant attachment.

Assessment

1. Anemia, nutritional deficiency, and fatigue are potential.
2. Hyperemesis may occur early and last longer.
3. Pressure symptoms appear earlier—varicose veins, hemorrhoids, constipation, vena cava syndrome, backache, orthopnea.
4. Third-trimester bleeding may be due to large low-lying placenta.
5. Pregnancy induced hypertension occurs earlier than usual.
6. Preterm labor is common.
7. Fetal growth retardation or disproportional growth of one fetus can occur.

Revised Outcomes

1. Prenatal complications will be minimized with high-protein diet, bed rest in last 6 weeks, and more frequent evaluations.
2. Client will be aware of early hospitalization plan and will understand delivery alternatives.
3. Client's statements will indicate that she has accepted the idea of a multiple birth.
4. Client will understand the potential for differences in development and maturation of her infants.

Interventions

1. Teach the need for a high-protein diet with folic acid and iron supplements.
2. Provide extra care for pressure-induced discomforts.
3. Instruct client to maintain bed rest in side-lying position for last 6 weeks to promote renal function.
4. Observe for hemorrhage before and after delivery, plus delayed involution.

5. Prepare client for possibility of a complicated, preterm delivery.
6. Provide extra support for maternal bonding plus teaching to help client cope with more than one infant.

Reevaluation and Follow-up

1. Client maintained a hemoglobin of 11 g/dL or above throughout pregnancy.
2. Client maintained rest and comfort measures so that gestational age was optimum at birth.
3. Parents incorporated idea of multiple infants in family and planned appropriately.

PREGNANCY-INDUCED HYPERTENSION (PIH)

Pregnancy induced hypertension (preeclampsia) occurs in an incidence of 6 to 7:100 pregnancies. Preventive care has reduced the incidence of severe preeclampsia and eclampsia (convulsive state), but cases do occur and are accompanied by increased risk of stillbirths, abruptio placentae, chronic fetal distress, and intrauterine growth retardation. Rarely, there is a maternal death. The differential diagnosis from preexisting hypertensive states is the occurrence after the twentieth week of generalized vasospasm related to hypersensitivity to angiotensin II. This results in rapid weight gain due to sodium retention with generalized edema, elevation of at least 30/15 in systolic and diastolic blood pressures, and eventually proteinuria. Uncorrected, the condition will progress until there is severe preeclampsia and then eclampsia, a state of convulsions and coma.

Treatment has changed markedly over the last decade and early diagnosis is possible through use of the rollover test and/or infused angiotensin II to identify women sensitive to angiotensin II. When future potential hypertensives are identified, a program of modified bed rest, high fluid and protein intake, and more frequent evaluations is begun. A client with overt symptoms should be hospitalized for evaluation and management of hypertension. In severe cases, an emergency condition exists and delivery of the infant is planned as soon as the hypertension or convulsions are controlled. Symptoms of preeclampsia may occur at anytime after 20 weeks until 48 h after delivery; therefore, a woman is considered high risk with any of the following symptoms.

Assessment

1. Presence of abnormal weight gain and edema.
   a. Mild—more than 1 kg/week.
   b. Severe—5 kg/week plus orbital, pretibial edema.
   c. Eclampsia—over 30 kg total weight gain, severe facial edema, papilledema.
2. Presence of hypertension.
   a. Mild—elevation of 30/15 over baseline, fatigue.
   b. Severe—up to 160/110 at bed rest, headache, visual disturbances, tinnitus, amnesia, epigastric distress.
   c. Eclampsia—elevation of 60/30 over baseline, convulsion, coma.
3. Presence of proteinuria and oliguria.
   a. Mild—trace to 1+; may have state of hypervolemia.
   b. Severe—3–4+, or 5 g or more in 24 h.
   c. Eclampsia—loaded protein, oliguria, less than 600 mL/24 h; may be hypovolemic, shown by elevated hematocrit.
4. Visual disturbances caused by retinal vasospasm lead to retinal ischemia and papilledema; eye ground examinations done frequently to note progress of changes.
5. Vital signs. Compare all blood pressure readings with baseline. Do not allow diastolic to drop below 90 mmHg in severe states or placental perfusion will be compromised.
   a. Temperature—one-third of severely ill clients show temperature above 38°C.
   b. Respirations—observe for inhibition by magnesium sulfate, during coma may be rapid, stertorous.
   c. Pulse—reflects hypertension, will be strong, bounding in severe states.
6. Reflex responses from brachial, wrist, knee tendons; may be hyperactive in severe states before magnesium sulfate is effective.
7. Preconvulsion warning signs—amnesia, visual disturbances, epigastric pain due to edema of liver capsule.

Revised Outcomes

1. Client will be made aware of need for hospitalization and reasons for treatments.
2. Client will maintain rest, diet modifications, and fluid intake.
3. Within 24 to 48 h, blood pressure will be reduced to a safe level and fetal status will not be impaired.

Interventions

1. Place client in quiet room, reduce stress.
2. Begin frequent monitoring of vital signs, level of consciousness.

3. Encourage bed rest, in the side-lying position to promote renal function and prevent vena caval compression.
4. Increase protein in diet, low to moderate salt intake; severe hypertension will require clear fluids or only intravenous fluids at first.
5. Increase fluid intake for natural diuresis; evaluation of blood volume will guide fluid intake in severe cases, using CVP line.
6. Check hourly intake and output with Foley catheter in place for severe cases.
7. Test urine at every voiding for albumin, specific gravity; send urine for 24-h protein concentration, estriol levels.
8. Prepare client for various tests for fetal status: nonstress test (NST), OCT, ultrasound, amniocentesis.
9. Monitor drug infusion via electric infusion pump.
   a. Magnesium sulfate—loading dose of 4 g by IV push, then 1–2 g/h to maintain blood level of 4–8 mEq/L (at 10 mEq/L deep tendon reflexes disappear, at 15 mEq respirations are paralyzed).
   b. Hydralazine—initial dose of 5 mg if BP is over 110 diastolic, then by IV pump up to 20 mg/h titrated to maintain diastolic between 90 and 100 mmHg.
   c. Diazoxide—in crisis, 5 mg/kg by bolus IV may be attempted to promote decrease in blood pressure.
10. Check for adverse effects on deep tendon reflexes, respirations, and blood pressure. Monitor urine output to check that magnesium sulfate is being excreted. Urine output must be more than 100 mL/4 h to continue infusion; however, blood levels of $MgSO_4 \cdot 7H_2O$ are the best guide to therapy. Keep calcium gluconate ampules at bedside for antidote.
11. Expect delivery as soon as symptoms are controlled in severe cases. Trial induction of labor with pitocin, or cesarean will be planned.
12. Check infant carefully for transitional effects of maternal drugs.

Reevaluation and Follow-up

1. Client complied with plan of care.
2. Client maintained control of blood pressure by prescribed treatment.
3. Blood pressure was returned to normal levels as quickly as possible and infant delivered promptly.
4. Postpartum course uneventful.
5. Postpartum referral for follow-up of hypertension.

PREEXISTING HYPERTENSION

In pregnancy this presents as an elevated diastolic pressure before the twentieth week. Such an elevation may not have been previously diagnosed and may reflect underlying renal disease. A workup is essential before any antihypertensive therapy is instituted. Because severely elevated pressures may be discovered, cerebral hemorrhage is a risk as well as superimposed preeclampsia and abruptio placentae. When hypertension is severe, placental function is compromised and there is increased incidence of intrauterine growth retardation (IUGR) and chronic fetal distress. In addition, if antihypertensive medication is instituted, the infant must be observed closely during the recovery period after birth.

A woman who demonstrates an elevated diastolic pressure on admission to prenatal care, but demonstrates none of the other symptoms of preeclampsia, would be classified according to the following scale:

Elevated Diastolic	First or Second Trimester	Third Trimester
Mild	80	90
Moderate	90	100
Severe	120+	130+

Women with moderate to severe hypertension are treated by bed rest and controlled diet and are maintained on the prescribed antihypertensive drugs unless the particular drug affects placental blood flow (reserpinelike drugs). Hospitalization is always planned for evaluation and monitoring of fetal condition. Early delivery is planned if fetal condition deteriorates (Finnerty, 1977).

DIABETES MELLITUS

This inability to metabolize glucose properly is manifested in different degrees of severity (see classifications in Chapter 28). The incidence of diabetes mellitus is 1 : 100 to 1 : 200 pregnancies. It should be considered for a woman who: has a family history of diabetes, particularly in a parent or twin; has a history of spontaneous abortions or infections; has delivered an infant of 4000 g or larger; or has had a series of infants who had increasing birth weights, had unexplained congenital anomalies, or died in the perinatal period.

During pregnancy, a woman with diabetes is five times more likely to develop preeclampsia, and 20 percent of pregnant diabetics have hydramnios. Infections are more common as well. Infants of diabetic mothers (IDM) have a higher incidence of congenital anomalies and a higher perinatal mortality rate. Class A (gestational diabetes) infants are often large for gestational age (greater than 4000 g) and have a higher risk of respiratory distress syndrome (RDS), hypoglycemia, and hyperbilirubinemia. Infants of severely insulin-dependent women may have intrauterine growth retardation and early delivery may be planned to rescue a compromised fetus.

Maintenance of normal fasting glucose levels is the factor that distinguishes class A diabetics from more severe diabetics. Most clients with an abnormal FBS level will need insulin sometime in the pregnancy. The quality of metabolic control is most important. Investigators have found that mothers with acetonuria have had offspring with lower IQ levels than control infants. Thus dietary control and careful insulin prescription is essential. Oral hypoglycemic agents are not used as such agents cross the placental barrier, may contribute to anomalies, and cause prolonged neonatal hypoglycemia.

Each diabetic is followed closely in the clinic and may be admitted to the antepartum unit several times during the pregnancy for close observation and assessment. Most diabetics will be admitted soon after the thirty-fourth week of pregnancy for evaluation of possible early delivery. After 28 weeks, weekly estriols and NST evaluations are usually prescribed. The mother is taught to do fetal movement evaluation for $\frac{1}{2}$ to 1 h three times daily and record. Any change in fetal movement patterns, NST or CST (contraction stress test), or estriol levels will require admission for further evaluation. Timing of delivery is variable but no later than 38 weeks.

Class B-R diabetics, overt diabetics, require a carefully planned pregnancy. Those with prior onset of vascular complications should be encouraged not to conceive. Once pregnant, however, the control of acetonuria is essential. Clients are placed on a diet of 30 cal/kg, with carbohydrates giving 40 to 50 percent of the total calories and the remainder evenly divided between fats and proteins (Gabbe, 1978). Other researchers recommend a high-protein (125-g) daily intake.

Insulin therapy will change in response to metabolic demands of pregnancy as well as to the anti-insulin effects of increased estrogen levels. More frequent injections are usual as well as increases in dosage up to three times the nonpregnant dose.

Additional assessment will be required of a severely labile diabetic, and extended periods of hospitalization are not unusual. Timing of delivery may be early when parameters show that the infant is doing poorly.

The post delivery period is labile, and the client may be almost normoglycemic for 1 to 2 days, which reflects the sudden change in estrogen and other placental hormones. Careful monitoring of all parameters is essential as the return of insulin dependence is unpredictable. Control should be reestablished before discharge from the hospital.

Assessment

1. Glucose tolerance test demonstrates a prolonged glucose curve in latent, gestational diabetics.
2. Labile signs and symptoms of more severe diabetes appear in first trimester in formerly diet-controlled adult-onset clients.
3. Labile diabetic state ensues early for insulin-dependent clients. The first sign of pregnancy may be a hypoglycemic reaction as carbohydrate tolerance and insulin requirements change frequently.
4. Vaginal or urine infections occur that are difficult to resolve.
5. Preeclampsia is five times more common.
6. Fetal growth is under or over norms.

Revised Outcomes

1. Client will learn how diabetes and pregnancy interact and will return this information verbally.
2. Client will understand reasons for dietary control, changing insulin requirements, glucose regulation, hygienic skin care.
3. Client will understand the various procedures and lab tests to determine fetal status and will follow preparatory steps accurately.
4. Client will keep appointments every 2 weeks until the twenty-eighth week, and then weekly until delivery.

5. Client will be referred to visiting nurse, social worker, nutritionist as necessary.

Interventions

1. Clarify how diabetes and pregnancy interact.
2. Teach/reinforce understanding of dietary and insulin needs. Be sure client understands how to test urine or blood, measure and administer insulin and care for skin.
3. Evaluate compliance with frequent prenatal visits.
4. Instruct client about appropriate action for problems in control: hyperglycemia, hypoglycemia, infection, any other signs of illness or imbalance.
5. Prepare client for early admission midpregnancy for control studies and in ninth month for evaluation of fetal status: optimum delivery date.
6. Explain evaluations for diabetic status.
   a. FBS should be approximately 100 mg/dL.
   b. 2 h post prandial should be below 140 mg/dL.
   c. Fractional (double-voided) urines may show trace or 1+ in an attempt to prevent acetonuria.
   d. 24 h urine for total glucose; if carbohydrate loss is above 20 g/24 h, diet should be supplemented by that amount (Greene, 1975).
7. Explain evaluations for fetal condition.
   a. Hemoglobin A_{1c}, a fraction of adult hemoglobin, binds to glucose. Test may indicate degree of control in early weeks of pregnancy and should be done before 13 weeks gestation. In Joslin Clinic findings, if Hb A_{1c} was more than 8.5, anomalies occurred in 22 percent of the infants of diabetic mothers (Miller, 1981).
   b. Ultrasonic evaluation for fetal macrosomia, over 4000 g.
   c. Repeated nonstress tests in last weeks of pregnancy to follow fetal reactivity (see Chapter 8).
   d. 24 h urinary estriols, human placental lactogen levels.
8. Teach client reasons for potential changes in insulin requirements.
   a. Several injections daily, a mixture of regular and intermediate insulin, are to be given, with an additional dose of regular insulin in the evening.
   b. Insulin needs tend to increase early in pregnancy and may reach three times the nonpregnant dosage.
9. Teach client how to monitor her status at home with glucose oxidase–impregnated strips for testing capillary blood glucose.
10. Instruct mother to check level of fetal movements three times a day for $\frac{1}{2}$ to 1 h and record and to report any changes.

Reevaluation and Folow-up

1. Client complied with plan of care by maintaining control of diabetic diet and insulin requirements.
2. Client maintained a 1+ to normoglycosuria, without acetone.
3. Client reported abnormal symptoms appropriately.
4. Client accepted hospitalization as necessary.
5. Client remained free of postoperative and postpartum complications.
6. Client cooperated with postpartal follow-up for diabetic condition and parenting ability.

ABNORMAL WEIGHT GAIN

Optimum weight gain is 0.8 to 1.0 lb/week in the second and third trimesters. Obese clients approaching pregnancy may have diets high in carbohydrate, low in protein, accompanied by junk food snacking. All of the accompanying problems of obesity are aggravated by the normal weight gain of pregnancy: edema and hypertension may be noted early. Low-birth-weight infants have been born more frequently to these women after complicated deliveries. If delivery is by cesarean section, recovery is more difficult; suture lines may part, circulation to extremities may be impaired by immobility, and vascular changes already present may predispose to thrombophlebitis.

Diet control is recommended under guidance of nutritionist; weight loss is not advised, but weight gain can be kept within certain limits; and exercise during pregnancy promoted.

Inadequate weight gain may be the result of a preoccupation with maintaining a "slim" body image or of excessive nausea and vomiting. Nutritional counseling and extensive assistance may be necessary. Assessment of client's psychological state and acceptance of pregnancy may be indicated.

ANEMIA

Anemia during pregnancy is most often caused by inadequate supplies of iron or folic acid, as 2 mg additional iron daily must be absorbed from the diet to meet the requirements of the growing fetus, the expanded blood volume, and placental growth. Additional supplemental iron is often prescribed preventively, and a diet higher in protein and citrus foods is recommended. If hemoglobin is below 11 g/dL or hematocrit is below 31 percent, and oral iron fails to improve the anemia, parenteral iron is administered.

Blood loss as a cause of anemia may be treated with replacement transfusion in cases of placenta previa or abruptio or postpartum hemorrhage. For further discussion see Chapters 9 and 29.

BACTERIURIA

Infections can become established as urine forms pools in the bladder or looping ureter, particularly as a result of hormone-induced dilatation of smooth muscle of the ureter and bladder. Ascending infection can result. First signs are WBC and RBC in urine with culture counts of 100,000 organisms per millimeter. Later, symptoms of cystitis—frequency, burning, dysuria, or pyelonephritis—fever, chills, lumbar pain, may be evident. As bacteriuria has been implicated as a cause of premature labor and has also been a cause of some cases of intrauterine fetal growth retardation, even before cystitis develops, early treatment of signs is usually the optimal course.

VARICOSE VEINS

Dilated, tortuous superficial veins, usually in the lower extremities, occur most commonly in the saphenous system. In response to genetic predisposition, hormonal influences on vascular tone, and to marked increase in femoral venous pressure (up to 18 mmHg), varicose veins become distended early in the first trimester but worsen during the final months of pregnancy. The condition is aggravated by sitting or standing for long periods and by constipation. In addition, during later pregnancy, the enlarging uterus obstructs venous return and further aggravates constipation and related varicose veins of rectal and anal tissue. For discussion of treatment see Chapter 30.

THROMBOPHLEBITIS

Thrombophlebitis is caused by inflammation of the vein intima resulting in accumulation of fibrin and blood cells. The clot formation is usually attached firmly to the vein wall in the superficial venous system. Incidence is highest in women with preexisting varicose veins. Because of the normally elevated plasma fibrinogen state during pregnancy, mild problems may be aggravated.

In contrast, deep vein thrombophlebitis may occur during pregnancy, within 72 h of a traumatic birth, or after postpartum hemorrhage or infection. Deep vein thrombus can throw off emboli to the lungs and may do so as late as 3 weeks after delivery. Sites of thrombus may be deep femoral veins or the uterine or iliac veins after septic delivery. (For treatment, see Chapter 30.)

THE THIRD TRIMESTER

DESCRIPTION

The period between the end of the twenty-eighth completed week of gestation until the time of delivery is a period of rapid fetal growth in size and in ability to function. Every week of development in utero increases the chance of survival for an infant. The third trimester is also a period of completion of developmental tasks for the mother and father as they face taking up the parenting role.

The question of noncompliance arises when a woman first seeks care in the third trimester. The noncompliant person may not keep appointments or follow instructions. Psychosocial problems that may contribute to lack of self-care include poverty, distance from the health care center, care of other children, drug addiction, prostitution, or unfamiliarity with the health care system because of language barriers. Other factors contributing to lack of early prenatal care include continuing ambivalence or fears about the pregnancy, especially in single women or young teens.

ASSESSMENT

Health History

See first and second trimesters.

1. History of preparation for childbirth, client's prior feelings about childbirth.
2. Support system available to client.

Physical Assessment

1. Evaluation for underlying chronic disease is especially important when client is seen for the first time so near delivery.

2. Fundus should be between umbilicus and xiphoid.
3. Cervix will be firm, closed, and posterior until the last few weeks before delivery. Evaluation of effacement and dilatation should be done by vaginal exam as delivery approaches.
4. Estimated EDD should be compared with actual measurements of uterus, estimated size of fetus and cervical status.
5. Client's present complaints should be determined—fatigue recurs; pressure symptoms are common as delivery nears.

Diagnostic Tests

1. In addition to screening for genetic diseases, infections, chronic diseases, and blood constituents as in first and second trimesters, when the client is seen initially in the third trimester she should have a culture of the cervix for gonorrhea and a serologic test for syphilis.
2. Women following the prenatal care schedule will be retested for hematocrit, hemoglobin levels, and serology.
3. Tests for fetal maturity and condition are done when any question of early delivery is present, or when the pregnancy continues to post term.
   a. Amniocentesis.
      (1) Lecithin/sphingomyelin (L/S) ratio of less than 2:1 indicates fetal lung immaturity.
      (2) Creatinine increases with age after 32 weeks; a value of 2 mg/100 mL usually indicates a mature fetus.
      (3) Bilirubin disappears from the fluid by 36 to 37 weeks; unusual levels are present with fetal hyperbilirubinemia.
      (4) Fetal cell count is taken after staining with Nile blue; fat cells stained turn orange. If 20 percent or more cells stain orange, the fetus is usually more than 36 weeks.
   b. Antepartal fetal monitoring. Nonstress test is utilized with every high-risk pregnancy to determine fetal condition and ability to withstand stress of labor contractions. (See Chapter 8 for fetal distress.)
   c. Maternal hormone levels.
      (1) Estriols. Estriol levels indicate fetoplacental health. 24-h urine levels must be obtained in a series as falling levels or rising levels are indicative of diminishing function or adequate placental function. Blood levels can be determined, as well.
      (2) Human placental lactogen. Rising levels indicate placental function is adequate.
   d. Ultrasound evaluation for fetal size, biparietal diameter (Figure 7-5).

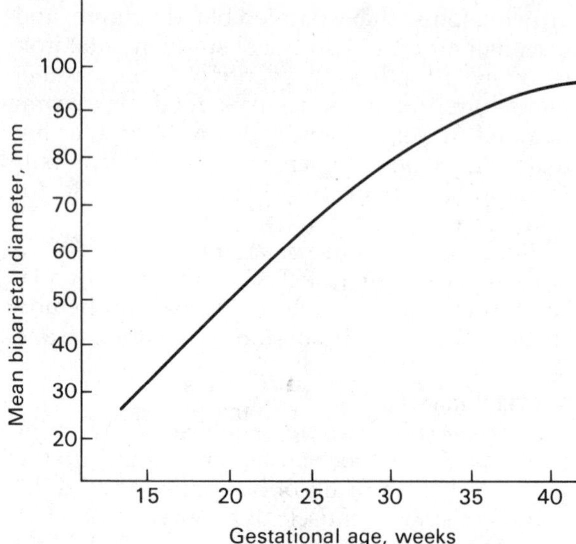

Figure 7-5 Composite curve of mean biparietal diameters as compared to gestational age. (From Weiner, S. N., et al., *Radiology,* **122**:781, 1977.)

NURSING DIAGNOSES: ACTUAL OR POTENTIAL

1. Alterations in physical status: potential: abnormal symptoms appear in the third trimester.
2. Alterations in physical comfort: due to pressure symptoms.
3. Anxiety about impending delivery due to physical, emotional, or economic reasons.
4. Ineffective coping: delay in seeking prenatal care because of inability to deal with pregnancy, economic hardship, knowledge deficits, inability to meet developmental tasks, inadequate support system.
5. Lack of compliance as a result of physical and/or psychosocial reasons.
6. Alterations in sexuality: due to advancing pregnancy.

EXPECTED OUTCOMES

1. Client will be aware of the danger signs of pregnancy in the third trimester and will be able to return the information verbally.
2. Client will be aware of potential physical discomforts and will utilize nonpharmacologic methods of alleviation.
3. Client will be referred to appropriate resource persons for any nonnursing problems.
4. Woman will make statements indicating acceptance of the pregnancy and will think of the fetus as separate from herself.
5. Woman's statements about sexual relations with partner will not indicate misinformation about sexuality during pregnancy.
6. Client will give evidence of compliance with care plan by keeping appointments, maintaining weight gain pattern, and attending available prenatal classes.
7. Client will learn about process of labor and delivery and will be able to state the signs of impending labor.

INTERVENTIONS

1. Alert client to abnormal symptoms of the third trimester and the appropriate action to be taken. In addition to the major warning signs of first and second trimester, emphasize the following signs.
   a. Cessation or change in character of fetal movements.
   b. Vaginal spotting progressing to painless bleeding.
   c. Rupture or leaking of membranes.
   d. Premature labor.
2. Teach nonpharmacologic measures to relieve discomforts.
3. Determine client's understanding of third-trimester developmental tasks and readiness to take up parenting.
4. Determine need for counseling about sexual misinformation.
5. Interpret physician's instructions for client and determine her level of understanding; explain reasons for more frequent visits—every 2 weeks in eighth month, every week in ninth month.
6. Interpret results of physical assessment, needs of the phase of pregnancy, lab tests.
7. Provide information about childbirth preparation.
8. Instruct on breast care and nipple rolling, if client will be breastfeeding.
9. Teach signs of impending labor, process of labor and delivery, and initial infant care.
10. Make arrangements for couple to see labor unit before admission.

EVALUATION

Outcome Criteria

1. See those of first and second trimester.
2. Client is achieving third-trimester tasks of preparing for parenting.
3. Client is keeping appointments.
4. Fetal development is progressing normally.
5. Client is maintaining diet and weight in the normal range.
6. Client plans to come to labor unit at the appropriate time.
7. Client is preparing for childbirth and for the infant.

Complications

PLACENTA PREVIA

Painless vaginal bleeding occurs after the twentieth week. Placental tissue has been formed by invasion of trophoblastic cells into uterine endometrium (decidua basalis), rupturing arterioles and venules to form lakes (lacuni) of maternal blood. Into these lakes fetal villi protrude. In placenta previa, the blastocyst implants in the lower uterine segment. The decidua here is less nourishing, the blood supply less adequate, and the placenta extends over a larger area, impinging on the internal os completely, partially, or marginally (see Figure 7-6). Any separation of the placenta from the slowly effacing cervix will open a direct line to maternal circulation. Bleeding can be any degree from spotting to massive

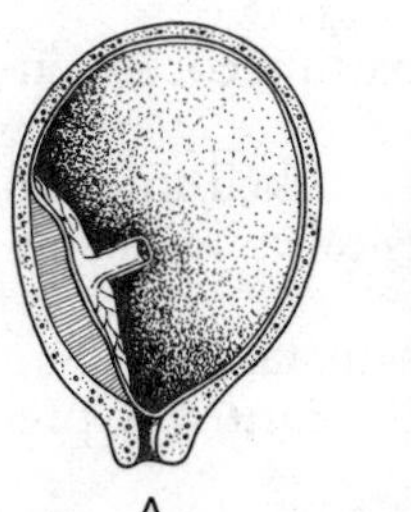

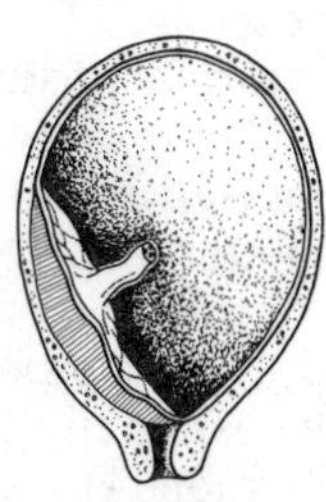

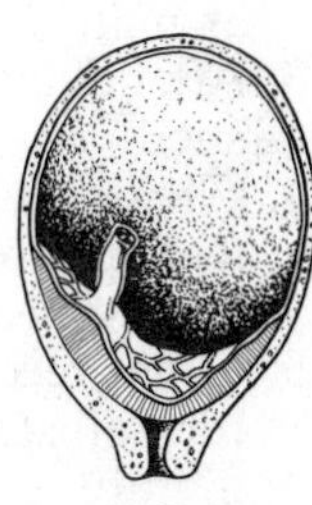

Figure 7-6 Types of placenta previa. (*a*) Total; (*b*) partial; (*c*) low-lying.

hemorrhage and is usually halted only by delivery of the fetus and placenta.

The incidence of placenta previa is thought to be 1:100 to 1:150 (Abdul-Karim, 1976). It is more common in older gravidas and in multiple pregnancy.

Assessment

1. Bleeding begins as painless spotting, increasing daily.
2. Hemoglobin and hematocrit fall; estriols decline.
3. Ultrasound indicates preterm infant.
4. In spite of bed rest, bleeding continues.
5. If bleeding occurs as labor approaches, may be confused with bloody show, but this bleeding is bright red and not mixed with mucus.

Revised Outcomes

1. Client will maintain complete bed rest.
2. Client will understand diagnostic testing, plan of care.
3. Client will express fears and receive support during anticipatory grieving.

Interventions

1. Admission for observation, assessment of fetal-placental function, condition (see Diagnostic Tests above).
2. Monitor bleeding, vital signs, pad count, serial hematocrits; type and cross-match blood.
3. Complete bed rest; sedation may be necessary.
4. Careful evaluation of cervical/placental condition without manipulation of cervix; ultrasound localization of placenta.
5. Usual intervention with cesarean section at last possible day to allow fetal maturity; preoperative preparation, explanations, consent.

Reevaluation and Follow-up

1. Lab tests indicated maintenance of adequate blood count.
2. Client maintained bed rest so that fetus was as mature as possible.
3. After delivery, normal postpartum course ensued.
4. Client felt supported as she worked through feelings about maternal physical condition affecting health of infant.
5. Client received intensive postnatal follow-up for adjustment, especially if infant was premature (see Chapter 11).

ABRUPTIO PLACENTAE

This is a condition of some degree of separation of the placenta before delivery. Maternal hypertension accompanies 40 to 50 percent of all premature separations. The incidence is complete 1:500 and partial 1:85 (Abdul-Karim). An increased incidence is seen in multiparity, folic acid deficiency, and in the woman with a previous premature separation. Maternal mortality is less than 1 percent when treatment is available, but fetal mortality from anoxia and immaturity is about 40 to 50 percent. Types of separation can be classified into grades:

Grade 0—no clinical symptoms; up to one-third separation.

Grade 1—external hemorrhage visible; up to two-thirds separation.

Grade 2—both internal and external hemorrhage; strong, erratic contractions; up to two-thirds separation.

Grade 3—internal hemorrhage only; almost total separation; severe, woodlike contraction; maternal shock; clotting defect; fetal death.

Assessment

1. Bleeding becomes evident by external, or related signs: hypovolemic signs, changes in contraction characteristics. (Fig. 7-7)
2. Fetal distress is always present, late decelerations, then bradycardia.
3. Maternal anxiety is always present.
4. Pain accompanies shock in cases of internal hemorrhage, placing great tension within uterus.

Revised Outcomes

1. Intensive monitoring of condition will follow prompt interpretation of signs and symptoms.
2. Client will be supported through all procedures and decisions as to method of delivery.

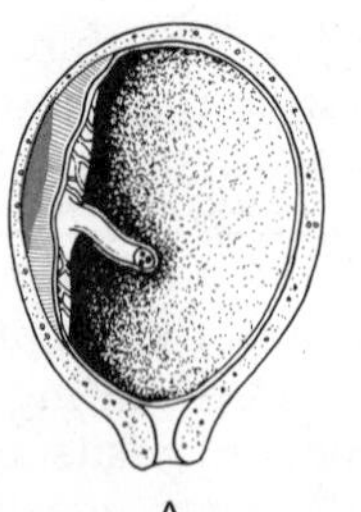

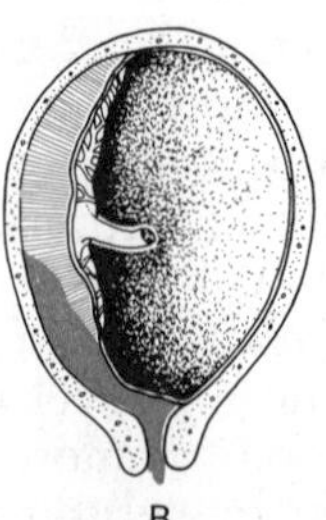

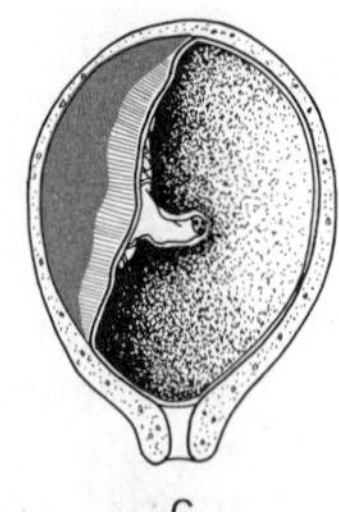

Figure 7-7 Types of placenta abruptio, premature separation of the placenta. (*a*) Partial separation (concealed bleeding); (*b*) complete separation (concealed bleeding); (*c*) partial separation (with hemorrhage apparent).

TABLE 7-6 ADDITIONAL HIGH-RISK CONDITIONS AFFECTING PREGNANCY OUTCOME

Problems	Diagnosis	Interventions
Rh-negative mother with rising antibody titer	No risk to mother Repeated amniocentesis required to measure bilirubin density, ΔOD_{450}, in amniotic fluid. Fetus may become either hyperbilirubinemic or extremely anemic. Infant may need exchange transfusion or, rarely, intrauterine transfusion.	Antibody titers must be done at regular intervals. Oxygen may be given during labor. Preterm induction may be done to deliver baby in order to do exchange transfusion. RhoGAM can be given mother after amniocentesis (see Chapter 10).
Polyhydramnios (hydramnios)	Aggravates all pressure symptoms, severe supine hypotension, pressure on renal vessels. Infant is usually small, often associated with GI or GU anomalies. Preterm labor is common.	Possibly repeated amniocentesis and removal of amniotic fluid. Fetal heart hard to auscultate, use ultrasound equipment, try to alleviate maternal anxiety. Expect and prepare for a compromised infant.
Systemic lupus erythematosus (SLE)	Chronic inflammatory disease of unknown cause: an autoimmune system disturbance that is four times more common in young women than in men. Early symptoms are confusing: arthritis is transient, weakness, weight loss, sun sensitivity in 40% with rash, itching and burning skin, fever. GI upset. Later renal and neurologic involvement are serious signs. Sometimes symptoms are precipitated by drugs. Lab tests show antinuclear antibodies (ANA) and LE cells (80%), plus anemia, low WBC.	Multiple discomforts are aggravated by pregnancy; advise conception during remission periods as perscriptions with corticosteroids, aspirin, are considered drug risks for fetus. Teach client to avoid stress; major problems are fatigue, depression. Observe for flareups. Follow during pregnancy very carefully.
Renal disease	Multiple underlying problems will affect pregnancy by changing renal excretory ability: chronic glomerulonephritis, nephrotic syndrome, solitary kidney, polycystic kidney, or severe diabetic renal changes. Proteinuria may be massive, hypertension, edema, vomiting, and accompanying discomforts of nausea, headache, palpitations, visual disturbances may allow the diagnosis to be confused with severe preeclampsia.	Risk is mainly to fetus unless mother goes into renal failure. Spontaneous abortion, preterm labor, and intrauterine death are possible. High protein, low-salt diet, antihypertensives added, and sometimes diuretics and cardiac glycosides. Bed rest in side-lying position is important. Urine infections are treated vigorously. See Chapter 32.

TABLE 7-6 *(continued)*

Problems	Diagnosis	Interventions
Hemoglobinopathies:[a] Folate deficiency anemia	Macrocytic anemia may occur. May underlie conditions such as abruptio placentae, spontaneous abortion, or preeclampsia.	Replacement with folate supplements, accompanying iron supplements. More frequent blood tests. Teach diet with adequate folic acid sources.
Thalassemia Major (Cooley's anemia Minor (heterozygous)	Autosomally transmitted disease. Hemoglobin has altered globin production because of defect in alpha or beta chain.	Screen populations from Mediterranean and Southeast Asian countries. See Chapter 18 for detailed account.
	Clients with *major* rarely become pregnant; those with *minor* have minimal anemia until under stress conditions such as pregnancy.	Supportive care if anemia worsens; blood transfusions.
Sickle cell Disease (SS)[b]	Autosomally transmitted disease. Hemoglobin has poor solubility for oxygen at low oxygen tensions, crystallizes into sickle shape, with sludging of cells, hemolysis, and hypoxia to vital organs. 25–50:100 pregnancies of sickle disease terminate in abortion, stillbirth, or neonatal death. Increased incidence of complications: preeclampsia, infection, premature labor, sickle crises.	Treatment of infections, prevention of stress conditions critical. High folic acid-bearing foods, iron supplements. Folic acid 1 to 2 mg qd often prescribed. Exchange transfusion in pregnancy when crises occur.
Trait (AS)[c]	Urinary infection, hematuria more common with sickle trait women.	Screen more frequently for bacteriuria.
Hemoglobin C Trait (CA)[d] Disease (SC)[e]	Homozygous state tolerated well with only mild anemia, but pregnancy may precipitate severe crises with maternal mortality 7:100, fetal death 35:100.	Best possible supportive care if homozygous client becomes pregnant. Genetic counseling; advise to avoid prenancy.
Disease (CC)	Very similar effects to sickle cell anemia.	
Erythrocyte enzyme deficiency: Glucose-6-phosphate dehydrogenase (G-6-PD) Pyruvate kinase (PK)	May cause chronic hemolytic process or trigger severe hemolytic crises from stress of certain drugs or metabolic stresses such as infection, pregnancy.	Screening of all clients with family history suggestingt enzyme deficiency. Over 40 oxidant drugs may precipitate crisis. Teach client to avoid stress conditions that may precipitate hemolytic crises.

[a] Incidence: 50:100 women show some signs of deficiency before pregnancy ends. [b] Incidence 1 to 3:1000 of U.S. blacks. [c] Incidence: 8 to 10:100 of U.S. blacks. Usually no overt symptoms. [d] Incidence: 2:100 of U.S. blacks. [e] Linked with sickle cell.

3. Blood loss will be replaced and shock prevented.
4. Fetal rescue will take priority.

Interventions

1. Monitor intensively both mother and fetus.
2. Provide oxygen by mask, IV replacement of fluids.
3. Monitor serial hemoglobin, hematocrit, and clotting time and fibrinogen levels.
4. Obtain consent for operative procedure and explain all procedures for preparation.
5. Keep expectant father informed.

Reevaluation and Follow-up

1. Blood pressure and adequate hemoglobin and hematocrit were maintained until delivery was possible.
2. Normal clotting time was maintained without complication of DIC.
3. Client began grieving process for loss of expected normal delivery, expected healthy infant, expected happy experience.
4. Intensive postnatal follow-up was provided for adjustment to parenting adaptation.

CARDIAC DYSFUNCTION

The incidence of cardiac disease has decreased as the major cause, rheumatic fever, has been brought under control. The overall incidence of cardiac disease was 0.5 to 1.5 percent in the last decade and is less today. Most of the persons demonstrating difficulty are those with treated congenital cardiac defects or advanced hypertensive cardiopathy. However, immigrants to this country may show changes due to rheumatic heart disease, as may a few older multiparas. Cardiac disease preexisting pregnancy will be complicated by the marked cardiovascular changes normally developing by the twelfth week: an average of 40 percent increase in circulating blood volume, physiologic hemodilution, and increased pulse rate and cardiac output. Functional classifications are useful to indicate heart function under the stress of pregnancy. Women in classes I and II may go through pregnancy with a minimum of difficulty if they follow prescribed precautions on rest, diet, and medication. Classes III and IV clients are at high risk for multiple problems and must be hospitalized during the last trimester. The periods of highest risk are during the greatest blood volume, peaking at 28 weeks, and then during labor and delivery. Pressure on the great vessels and dyspnea in the supine position must be carefully avoided. The influence of maternal posture on hemodynamics is critical and may require that the woman maintain bed rest in a side-lying position. Cardiac work may be elevated during labor and delivery, and special precautions must be taken to support respiratory and cardiac function and prevent bearing down during second stage. In the postdelivery period the radical readjustments in blood volume and intraabdominal pressure place the client at risk for hypotension and inadequate cardiac function. In addition, cardiac clients may be more prone to anemia, fluid retention, fatigue, and thrombophlebitis. Infants of mothers with mild to moderate Class I and II heart disease are smaller than normal infants and prematurity is a more frequent outcome for the pregnancy. (See Chapter 30)

Treatment in general follows these guidelines:

1. Extended rest in the side-lying or semi-Fowler's position.
2. Reduction of anxiety.
3. Prophylactic antibiotics.
4. Anticoagulants (depoheparin, not coumadins).
5. Moderate sodium restrictions with careful maintenance of protein levels in the diet.
6. Cardiac drugs are not deemed teratogenic, but diuretics and propranolol are used only with extreme caution because of adverse effects in the fetus.
7. Frequent assessment of fetal and maternal condition is done.

REFERENCES

Abdul-Karim, R. W.: "Antepartum Hemorrhage and Shock," *Clinics in Obstetrics and Gynecology*, **19**(3):533, 535, September 1976.

Assali, N. A. (ed.): *Pathophysiology of Gestation*, Vols. I and II, Academic Press, New York, 1975.

Finnerty, R.: "Hypertension in Pregnancy," *Angiology*, 10:545, 1977.

Grabbe, S. G.: "Diabetes in Pregnancy: Clinical Controversies," *Clinics in Obstetrics and Gynecology*, **21**(2):443, 1978.

Miller, E., Hare, J. W., Cloherty, J. P., et al.: "Elevated Maternal Hemoglobin A_{1c} in Early Pregnancy and Major Congenital Anomalies in Infants of Diabetic Mothers," *New England Journal of Medicine*, **304**:1331, 1981.

Morbidity & Mortality Report, National Center for Health Statistics, **29**(14):157, 159, April 1980.

BIBLIOGRAPHY

Abdul-Karim, R. W.: "Antepartum Hemorrhage and Shock," *Clinics in Obstetrics and Gynecology,* **19**(3):533, 545, September 1976. Medical management of crisis caused by hemorrhage.

Assali, N. A. (ed.): *Pathophysiology of Gestation,* Vols. I and II, Academic Press, New York, 1975. Entire two volume set covers in-depth pathophysiology of pregnancy. Especially pertinent for hormonal and anatomic changes during pregnancy.

Finnerty, R.: "Hypertension in Pregnancy," *Angiology,* **10:**545, 1977. Initial integration of hypertensive treatment for pregnancy-induced hypertension. Recognition of pathophysiology and early identification of need to avoid diuretics and severely restricted salt intake.

Glazer, G.: "Anxiety Levels and Concerns Among Pregnant Women," *Research in Nursing and Health,* **3:**107, 1980. Specific concerns identified in study of 100 women. Clinic clients were seen to have a significantly higher anxiety level than did private clients.

Grabbe, S. G.: "Diabetes in Pregnancy: Clinical Controversies," *Clinics in Obstetrics and Gynecology,* **21**(2):443, 1978. Entire volume on high-risk pregnancies, demonstrating the rapid changes in treatment taking place in the late seventies.

Jensen, M. D., and Bobak, I. M.: *Handbook of Maternity Care,* Mosby, St. Louis, 1980. Written for nurse practitioners; complete assessment of each part of perinatal care with nursing interventions.

Jovanovic, L., and Peterson, C. M.: "Management of the Pregnant Insulin Dependent Diabetic Woman," *Diabetes Care,* **3**(1)63, 1980. Intensive care program with client self-monitored glucose determination, diet, and titration of insulin.

Mercer, R. T.: "Teenage Motherhood: The First Year," *Journal of Obstetric, Gynecologic, and Neonatal Nursing,* **9**(1):16, 1980. Study of teenage mothers during the first year of parenting, focusing especially on infant progress.

Miller, E., Hare, J. W., Cloherty, J. P., et al.: "Elevated Maternal Hemoglobin A_{1c} in Early Pregnancy and Major Congenital Anomalies in Infants of Diabetic Mothers," *New England Journal of Medicine,* **304:**1331, 1981.

Morbidity & Mortality Report, National Center for Health Statistics, **29**(14):157, 159, April 1980.

Wheeler, L., and Jones, M. B.: "Pregnancy Induced Hypertension," *Journal of Obstetric, Gynecologic, and Neonatal Nursing,* **10**(3):212, 1981. Module on PIH, carrying CE credits. Presents problem of hypertension during pregnancy in a fairly complete and logical sequence.

8

Labor and Delivery

Susan E. Anderson

FIRST STAGE OF LABOR

DESCRIPTION

Labor is the physiologic process by which the uterus expels, or attempts to expel, the fetus and placenta at 20 weeks or more gestation. It is a complex process during which the nurse plays a major role in assessing, planning, and intervening to meet the physical and psychological needs of the mother, fetus, and family.

Labor is divided into three stages. The *first stage* is the period from the onset of labor through complete dilatation of the cervix. The *second stage* is the period from complete dilatation of the cervix through the birth of the fetus. The *third stage* is the period from the birth of the fetus through expulsion or extraction of the placenta and membranes. For the purposes of this chapter there is added a *fourth stage,* which is the first hour after the delivery of the placenta.

The first stage of labor is divided into three phases (Table 8-1):

Latent phase (Figure 8-1)—the period from the onset of labor to 2-cm dilatation.
Active phase (Figure 8-2)—the period from 3–7-cm dilatation.
Transition phase (Figure 8-3)—the period from 8–10-cm dilatation.

Friedman (1978) has classified phases of labor in a different way (Figure 8-5). His classifications are (1) the acceleration phase, (2) maximum slope, and (3) the deceleration phase. Friedman's *acceleration phase* is the "get going" phase, a period during which contractions begin to increase in frequency and intensity and dilatation increases from 2–4 cm. The *maximum slope* is the period during which the greatest dilation occurs in the shortest period of time, from 4–9 cm. The *deceleration phase* is the period from 9–10 cm during which contractions decrease in frequency but remain the same in intensity.

The onset of labor is a complex process attributed to a combination of multiple factors stemming from the maternal uterus, cervix, and pituitary and the fetal hypothalmus, pituitary, and adrenal cortex. Because the interaction of these physical and hormonal factors in initiating labor is still not clearly understood, there is no definitive theory as to the causes of labor. The onset of labor usually occurs after the thirty-seventh week of gestation. Preterm labor that occurs before week 37 is associated with high infant mortality and morbidity due to the prematurity of the infant.

ASSESSMENT

Health History

1. Preparation for childbirth.
   a. Clients may have attended prenatal classes of varying natures.
      (1) Psychoprophylactic techniques involve a conditioning of the response to pain that helps the client block pain by focusing on another stimulus. Exercises, breathing, and alternative focusing activities are included.
      (2) Relaxation techniques are based upon the alleviation of fear, apprehension, and tension through controlled breathing and relaxation exercises.

b. Clients may have had no prior preparation for childbirth.
   (1) Controlled breathing and relaxation techniques can be taught during the latent phase of labor.
   (2) Charts and pictures should be used to provide explanations of the physiology of labor to decrease fear and anxiety.

2. Support system(s) accompanying client.
   a. Husband or other close person.
   b. Trained labor coach or monatrice (LaMaze).
3. Date of LMP and EDC or expected date of delivery (EDD).
4. Parity.
   a. Abortions—less than 20 weeks gestation or below 500 g in weight.
   b. Premature births—20 weeks until the thirty-seventh week of gestation.
   c. Stillbirths—after 20 weeks gestation with no sign of life at birth.
   d. Full term—38 weeks gestation or more.
5. Last food intake to determine eligibility for certain types of anesthesia and to anticipate nutritional needs during labor.
   a. Time of last food intake.
   b. Amount and type of food ingested.
6. Medical conditions can be antagonized by labor and delivery, creating additional risks for the mother and fetus. Note the presence or history of:
   a. Diabetes.
   b. Epilepsy.
   c. Heart disease.
   d. Asthma.
   e. Urinary tract infection.
   f. Allergies.
   g. Varicosities.
   h. Hypertension.
   i. Accidents.
   j. Surgery, especially in pelvic region.
7. History of any drug intake; prescribed, over-the-counter, or drugs of abuse. Pay particular attention to any that may influence recovery of newborn or affect analgesics or anesthetics.

Physical Assessment

1. Vital signs should be within normal limits as established by the prenatal record.
2. Abdominal examination should reveal uterine fundus at the xiphoid process.
3. Leopold's maneuver should reveal:
   a. A longitudinal lie.
   b. Vertex as the presenting part.
   c. LOA (left occiput anterior) or ROA (right occiput anterior) position.
   d. Engagement of the presenting part.
4. External perineal examination may reveal:
   a. Vaginal discharge.
      (1) Bloody show indicates that cervical dilatation has begun.
      (2) Leukorrhea may indicate a vaginal infection and should be cultured.
   b. Vulvar or vaginal varicosities may cause excessive bleeding during the second stage of labor.
   c. Condyloma.
      (1) A pointed wartlike growth.
      (2) A flat, broad, moist growth indicative of secondary syphilis.
   d. Signs of lacerations or scars from prior deliveries.
   e. Ulcerations and lesions should be cultured for possible venereal disease: syphilis, gonorrhea, herpes (Lynch, 1982).
5. Internal examination is done to determine the status of:
   a. Membranes.
      (1) If there is a question as to whether or not the membranes have ruptured the fluid should be tested with nitrazine paper before any lubricants have been used for the vaginal exam. The alkalinity of the amniotic fluid will turn the paper dark blue.
      (2) If the membranes are ruptured the fluid should be clear with flecks of vernix, odorless, and not in excess of 1000–1500 mL.
      (3) If the membranes are intact note whether they are tense or bulging in front of the presenting part.
   b. Cervix.
      (1) The cervix should be soft and anterior (ripe), indicating that it is favorable for labor to progress.
      (2) A firm, posterior, unripe cervix may prolong labor or indicate false labor.
      (3) The cervix should be effaced 70 to 80 percent.
      (4) The cervix should be *at least* 1–2 cm dilated on admission, preferably 4–5 cm.
   c. Presenting part.
      (1) The presenting part is normally the vertex (Figure 8-1).
      (2) The position of the presenting part is determined by the location of the suture lines and fontanels in vertex pres-

entations and by the position of the sacrum in breech presentations. Normally the position is LOA. (See Figure 8-6.)

(3) Stations describe the descent of the presenting part into the pelvis relative to the ischial spines. (See Figure 8-9.) Normally at onset of effective labor the presenting part is at 0 station, at the spines, indicating engagement. Minus stations indicate centimeters above the spines, −1, −2, −3. Plus stations indicate centimeters below the spines, +1, +2, +3.

d. Contractions.

(1) Note the time of onset of regular contractions.

(2) The frequency of contractions is assessed by timing from the beginning of one contraction to the beginning of the next.

(a) Regular contractions, 3–5 min apart, increasing in frequency and intensity, usually indicate true active, effective labor (Figure 8-2).

(b) Irregular contractions indicate false labor, very early labor, or a posterior position.

(3) The duration of contractions is normally 30–60 s by palpation but may be recorded longer by monitor. With palpation one can only sense contractions over 25–30 mmHg pressure readings.

(4) Location and intensity of discomfort of contractions should be recorded.

(a) Discomfort in lower abdomen or groin indicates false labor.

(b) Fundal region discomfort radiating to the back usually indicates true labor.

(c) Sacral region discomfort is common with a posterior position.

(d) Intensity of discomfort usually increases as labor progresses.

Diagnostic Tests

These are done in the labor area when there is no prenatal record.

TABLE 8-1 CHANGES DURING THE FIRST STAGE OF LABOR

Stage	Physical Changes	Behavioral Changes
Latent phase: (see Fig. 8-1)	Contractions: mild Duration: 20–40 s Frequency: 5–10 min Dilatation: 0–2 cm, early effacement Primipara: 8–10 h or more Multipara: 3–5 h	Eager to be in labor but apprehensive and ambivalent. Receptive to teaching. Low pelvic cramps or backache.
Active phase: (see Fig. 8-2)	Contractions: moderate to strong pressure, 50–75 mmHg Duration: 40–60 s Frequency: 3–5 min Dilatation: 3–7 cm Primipara: 3–5 h Multipara: $1\frac{1}{2}$–2 h	Decreased response to environment. Begins breathing and relaxation techniques. Desires support, attention, and medication. Becomes increasingly tense, fearful, and restless with contractions. NOTE: Contractions require attention.
Transition phase: (see Fig. 8-3)	Contractions: strong pressure, 50–100 mmHg Duration: 60–90 s Frequency: 2–3 min Dilatation: 8–10 cm, effacement complete Primipara: 1.5 h Multipara: 0.5–1 h	Irritable, anxious, wants to go home. Withdraws from environment. May be nauseated, perspires, legs tremble.

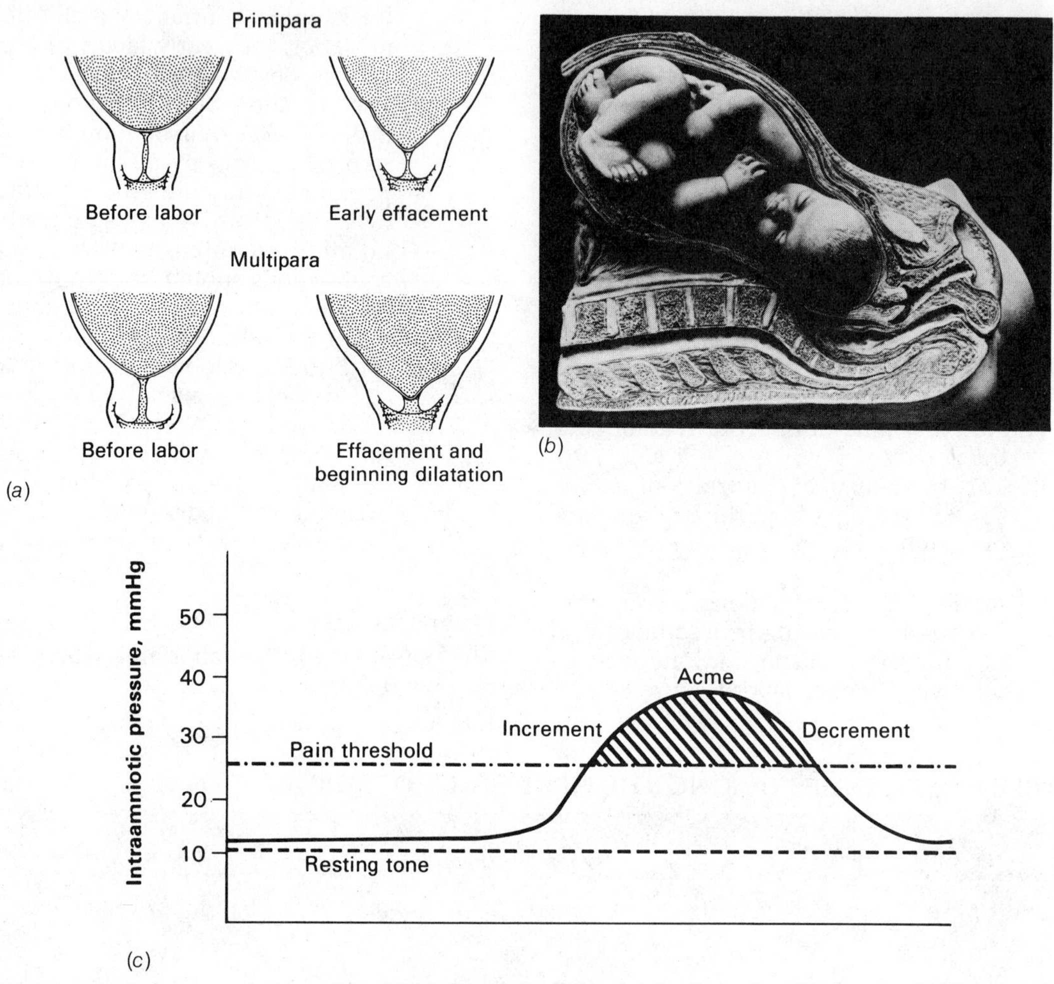

Figure 8-1 Prelabor and latent phase of labor. (*a*) Cervical status. (*b*) Fetal position: head in left occipitotransverse (LOT) position. (*c*) Contraction intensity. [(*a*) From Clinical Education Aid 13, Ross Laboratories, Columbus, Ohio 43216; (*b*) Reproduced with permission from the *Birth Atlas*, Maternity Center Association, New York.]

1. Urinalysis should indicate no bacteria, cells, sugar, or albumin, although trace or +1 albumin may be considered normal in a term pregnancy. Use clean voided midstream urine.
2. Hemoglobin and hematocrit should be within normal limits.
3. Blood type and Rh with a cross-match tube held in case of emergency.
4. Serology should be negative.
5. Rubella titer should be greater than 1:20 to ensure immunity.
6. Culture of any abnormally appearing vaginal discharge.

NURSING DIAGNOSES: ACTUAL OR POTENTIAL

1. Potential for excessive anxiety as a result of lack of knowledge, lack of support system.
2. Alteration in comfort secondary to physical changes of the labor process.
3. Potential threat to maternal/fetal well-being due to abnormal variations in labor process.
4. Potential ineffectiveness of support system.

EXPECTED OUTCOMES

1. Client will be free from excessive anxiety.
   a. Client will understand procedures and her current labor status.
   b. Client will receive support from the designated support system.
2. Client will be as free as possible of discomfort.
3. Client will be provided with an environment that will promote the well-being of mother and fetus.
4. Father or significant other will be informed and receive support by the nursing staff.

INTERVENTIONS

1. Provide explanations of:
   a. Physiological processes of labor.
   b. Changes in physical sensations as labor progresses.
   c. Approximate time parameters of labor progression.

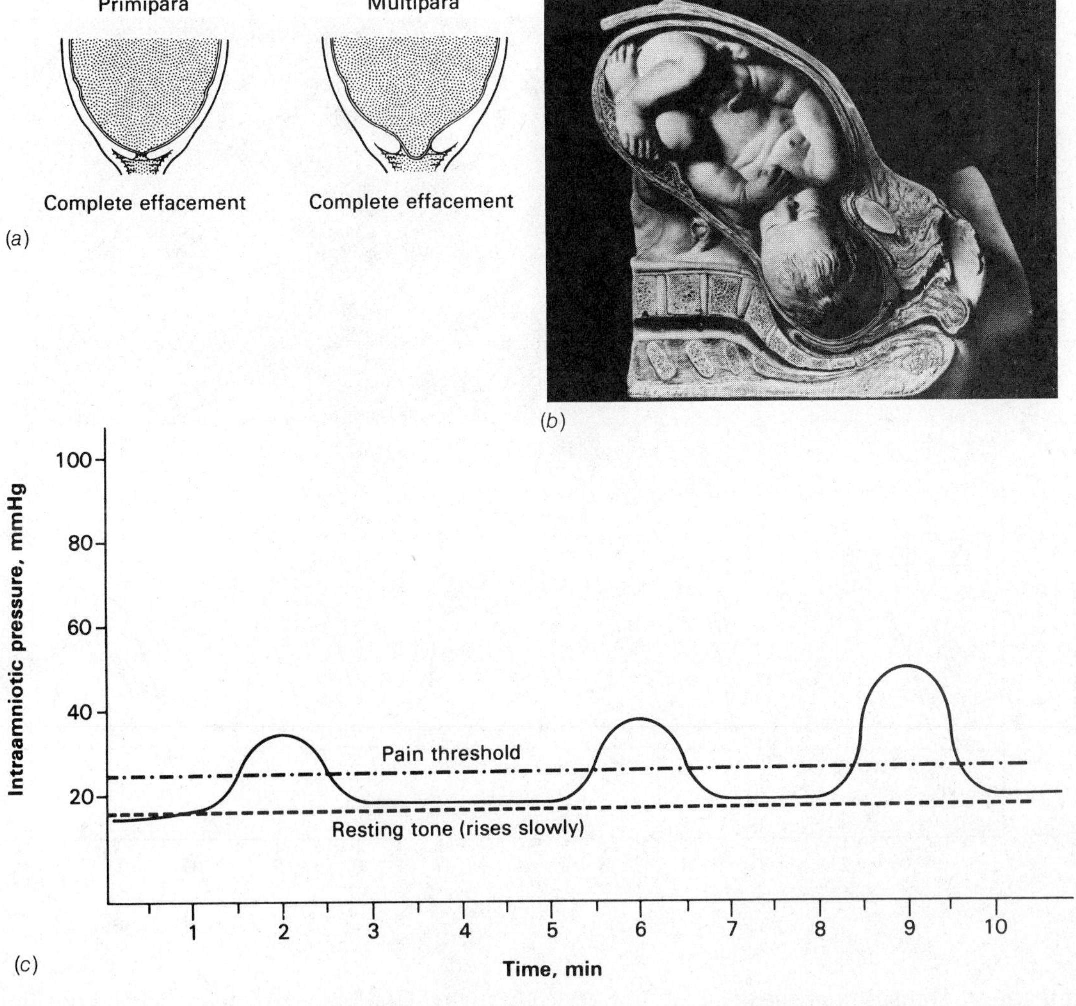

Figure 8-2 Active phase of labor. (*a*) Cervical status. (*b*) Fetal position: contraction and flexion completed. (*c*) Contraction intensity, acceleration phase: duration, 40 to 60 s; recurrence, every 3 to 5 min. [(*a*) From Clinical Education Aid 13, Ross Laboratories, Columbus, Ohio 43216; (*b*) Reproduced with permission from the *Birth Atlas*, Maternity Center Association, New York.]

d. Procedures such as enema, perineal prep, vaginal exams.
e. Breathing or relaxation techniques.

2. Provide comfort measures as needed by the client in the form of:
   a. Positioning.
      (1) Knee-chest to alleviate back discomfort.
      (2) Sim's position to promote relaxation.
      (3) Semi-Fowler's or side-lying position to prevent hypotension from caval compression.
   b. Back rub, especially for the sacral area.
   c. Effleurage, light stroking of skin over abdomen, thigh.
   d. Mouth care—hard candy, ice chips, or a wet gauze for dry mouth.
   e. Hygiene—keep client clean and dry and do perineal care.
3. Provide a safe environment for mother and fetus.
   a. Monitor maternal status.
      (1) Take blood pressure every 4 h unless not in normal range, then every $\frac{1}{2}$–1 h.
      (2) Take temperature, pulse, and respiration every 4 h unless membranes have

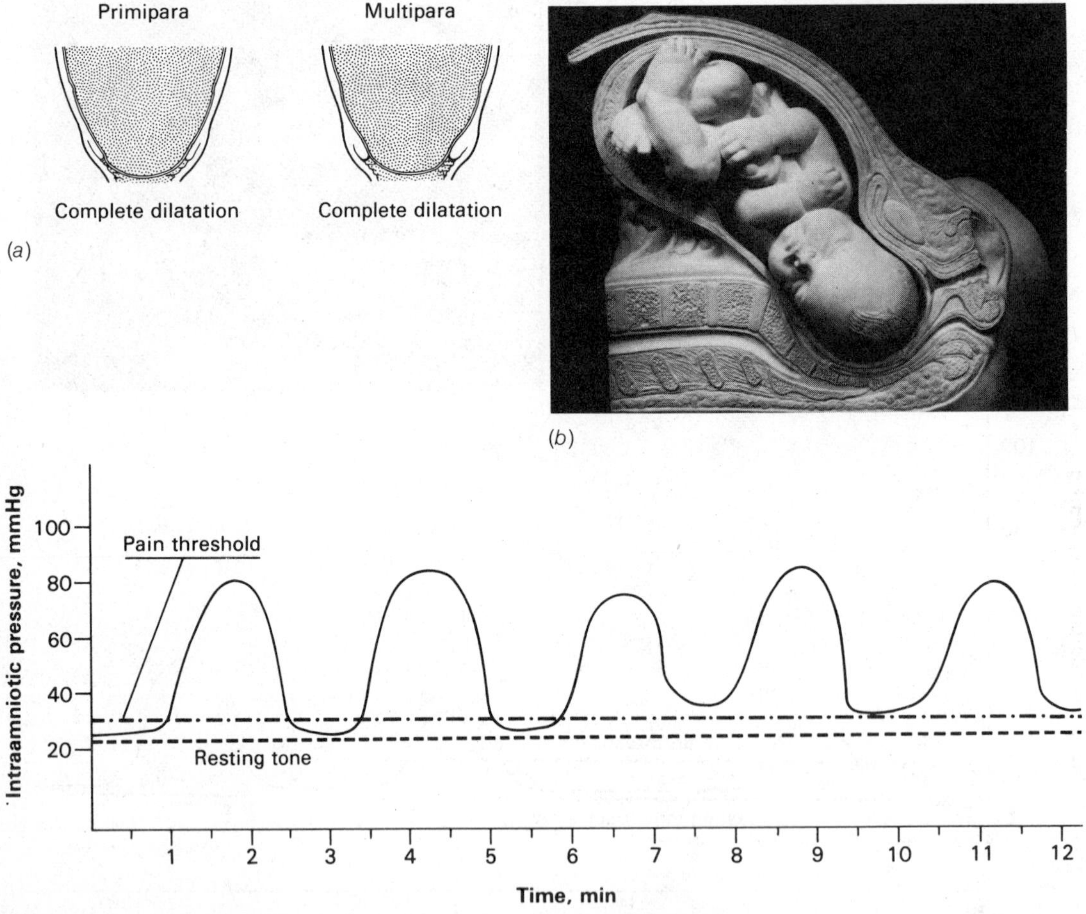

Figure 8-3 Transition phase of labor. (*a*) Cervical status: dilatation completed. (*b*) Fetal position: internal rotation in progress. (*c*) Contraction intensity: duration, 60 to 90 s; recurrence, every 2 to 3 min. [(*a*) From Clinical Education Aid 13, Ross Laboratories, Columbus, Ohio 43216; (*b*) Reproduced with permission from the *Birth Atlas*, Maternity Center Association, New York.]

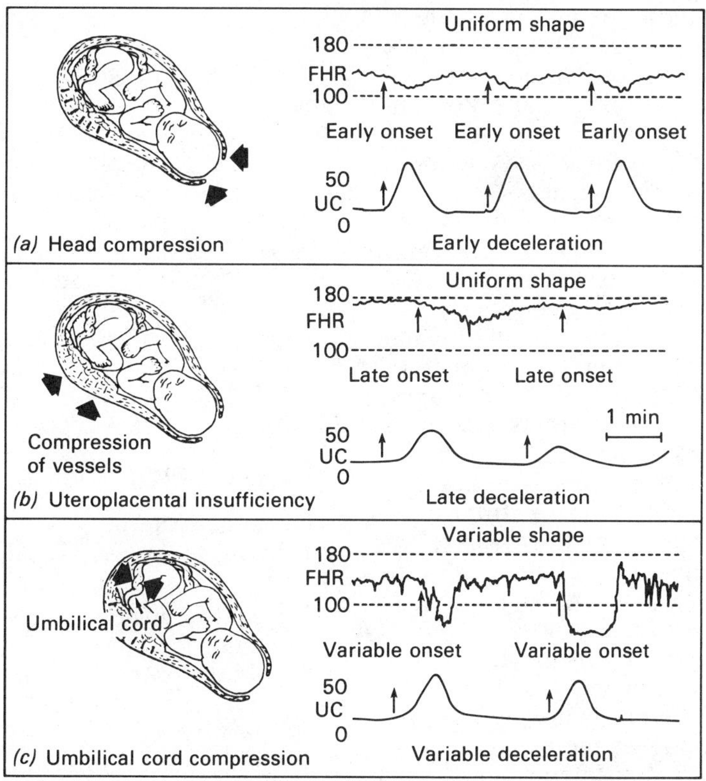

Figure 8-4 Types of decelerations seen on the monitor. (*a*) *Early decelerations,* due to reflex response to fetal head compression most often occur in the phase of accelerated labor. Uniform shape, beginning early in the contraction. (*b*) *Late decelerations* due to uteroplacental insufficiency result from decreased intervillous space as blood flow is restricted. Onset occurs late in relationship to the contraction. (*c*) Umbilical cord occlusion causes a *variable deceleration,* variable both in onset and in relationship to the contraction. (From Hon E., *An Introduction to Fetal Heart Monitoring*, Harty Press, New Haven, Conn., 1968.)

ruptured or temperature is elevated, then every hour.

(3) Note frequency, duration, and intensity of contractions every 15–30 min; in advanced labor every 15 min.

(4) Note progress in cervical dilatation every hour; however, once membranes have ruptured limit vaginal exams to prevent infection. (See Figure 8-3.)

(5) Note type and amount of vaginal discharge every 30 min.

(6) Note condition of bladder and encourage voiding.

b. Monitor physical status of the fetus.

(1) Use doptone or fetoscope to assess fetal heart rate and record every 15 min in active labor, then every 5 min in second stage.

(2) Apply the fetal monitor, either internally or externally, and observe for the following patterns:

(a) *Early decelerations* caused by head compression. These patterns have their onset at the time of beginning contraction and reflect the symmetrical curve of the contraction.

The patterns are innocuous and do not lead to fetal distress but may occur when contractions intensify, especially during transition and second stage.

(b) *Late decelerations* caused by uteroplacental insufficiency.
   (i) Drop in heart rate noted after the beginning of a contraction; these decelerations are symmetrical in shape.
   (ii) May be caused by placental separation or any condition reducing oxygen exchange at the placenta: abruptio placentae, placenta previa, oxytocin drip with hypertonic uterine contractions, and epidural anesthesia with hypotensive response in the client. May be present where there is prior placental insufficiency.
   (iii) Such patterns require immediate nursing action to allow optimum maternal/fetal exchange via the placenta.
   - Increase isotonic intravenous fluid to increase circulating blood volume.
   - Relieve vena caval compression that is causing maternal hypotension by positioning her on left side.
   - Administer oxygen at 6–8 L/min by nasal mask or cannulae.
   - Discontinue oxytocin drip until cause can be evaluated.

(c) *Variable decelerations* caused by cord compression.
   (i) These patterns are variable in shape and onset with regard to the contractions and may dip as low as 60 bpm. Fetal rate should return to baseline during interval.
   (ii) A change in maternal position is tried initially to relieve fetal pressure on the cord, oxygen by mask is begun.

(d) *Bradycardia* is a baseline fetal heart rate falling to 100 bpm or less.
   (i) May be caused by cord compression or separation of the placenta.
   (ii) Interventions are the same as for late decelerations.

(e) *Tachycardia* is a fetal heart rate rising above 160 bpm; often associated with amnionitis and/or severe hypoxia; indicative of fetal distress.

(f) *Decrease in variability* of the baseline can be induced by drugs such as scopolamine, atropine, magnesium sulfate, and diazepam. In the absence of such drugs it is indicative of severe fetal distress. (See Figure 8-4.)

EVALUATION

Outcome Criteria

1. Client is able to cope effectively with the psychological stress of the first stage of labor.
2. Client is able to deal with the physical discomforts of the first stage of labor.
3. Labor is progressing according to the normal curve. (See Figure 8-5.)
4. The physical status of the mother remains within normal limits.
5. The physical status of the fetus remains within normal limits.
6. The significant other is providing effective support.

Complications

PSYCHOLOGICAL STRESS

Assessment

1. Client does not cope effectively with psychological stress of labor.
2. Increased anxiety, restlessness, sweating.
3. History of unplanned pregnancy, separation from husband, complications with previous labor.
4. Ineffective support systems.

Revised Outcomes

1. Anxiety will be reduced to a manageable level.
2. Support system will become effective, augmented by intensive nursing care.

Interventions

1. Reinforce client teaching.
2. Provide support and encouragement to the significant person or take over role of supportive other by providing an alternative support system.

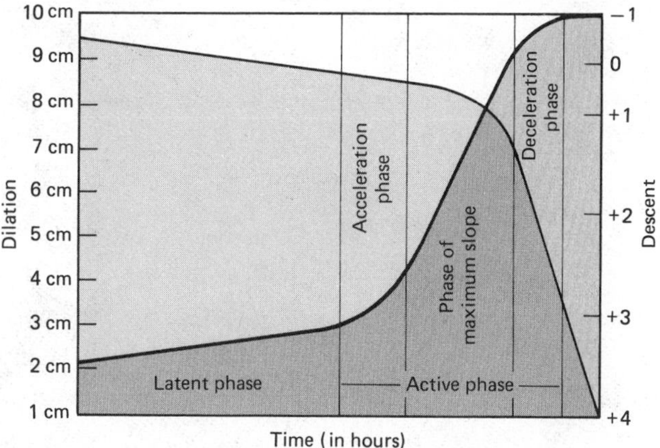

Figure 8-5 Dilatation and descent, normal curve. (From Friedman E. and Greenhill J. P., *Biological Principles and Modern Practice of Obstetrics*, Saunders, Philadelphia, 1974.)

3. Administer prescribed medication at correct interval.

Reevaluation and Follow-up

Continuous reassessment of client and support system.

PHYSICAL STRESS

Assessment

1. Client does not cope effectively with the physical discomforts of labor.
2. Client is restless and crying.
3. A posterior position may be causing excessive discomfort.
4. Client may be fatigued.

Revised Outcomes

Discomfort will be maintained at a manageable level for the client.

Interventions

1. Proceed to the next level of breathing.
2. Encourage supportive other or staff to use more direct commands when coaching.
3. Administer appropriate analgesics and observe for adverse reactions (Dickason, Schult, Morris, 1978). (See Table 8-2.)
4. Prepare for administration of anesthetic. (See Table 8-3.)

Reevaluation and Follow-up

1. Client's level of discomfort was reduced.
2. The degree of relief from analgesics or anesthetic allowed client to cope.
3. The effectiveness of support system's coaching increased.

INEFFECTIVE EARLY LABOR

Assessment

1. Mild irregular contractions do not effect cervical change.
2. Contractions do not increase in frequency or intensity.
3. Lack of progressive cervical effacement, dilatation.

Revised Outcomes

Cervical changes will be consistent with stage of labor. (Refer to Figure 8-5.)

Interventions

1. Prepare client for discharge or encourage to walk until effective labor begins.
2. Instruct client to return if membranes rupture or if contractions become regular, at 3–4 min apart.

Reevaluation and Follow-up

Remain informed as to client's labor status at home to determine appropriate entry time to hospital.

CERVICAL DYSTOCIA

Assessment

1. Strong regular contractions do not effect cervical changes.
2. Abnormal fetal position. (See Figure 8-6.)
3. Abnormal fetal presentation. (See Figure 8-7.)
4. Pelvic inadequacy.

Revised Outcomes

1. Change in woman's position will facilitate fetal progress.

TABLE 8-2 NARCOTICS, BARBITURATES, AND TRANQUILIZERS USED IN LABOR

Agent	Dosage	Onset	Duration	Maternal Effects	Infant Effects
			Narcotics		
Meperidine (Demerol, Pethidine)	30–100 mg IM 25 mg IV diluted in 5 mL normal saline[a]; SC not advised	10–20 min 3–5 min	2–3 h 1.5–2 h	70–90% relief of pain; sedation. Delays labor if dose excessive, but may enhance labor for some. Nausea and vomiting, hypotension, some respiratory depression, urine retention.	Rapid placental transmission. Possible CNS depression, respiratory depression. In newborn, large doses result in lowered oxygen saturation. Metabolites hinder adaptation to stimuli for more than 1 month.
Alphaprodine (Nisentil)	40–50 mg SC 15–20 mg IV	10 min 3–5 min	2–3 h 1.5–2 h	70–90% relief of pain; sedation. Delays labor if given too early or in excessive dose. Enhances labor for some. Similar to meperidine in effect, but *shorter* duration.	Rapid placental transmission. As there is shorter duration of action in mother, if dose/time interval observed, may not affect infant as much in newborn period. Studies incomplete.
Anileridine (Leritine)	30–40 mg SC 20–40 mg IM 15–20 mg IV	15–30 min 10–20 min 3–5 min	4–5 h 2.5–4 h 2–3 h	Similar to meperidine, but less sedation and sleep and short duration of side effects: respiratory depression, hypotension. Some antiemetic and antitussive effects.	Depressant effects on fetus may be more severe than for meperidine in equigesic doses. Must have Narcan available.
Morphine	8–10 mg SC 3–5 mg IV diluted in 5 mL normal saline[b]	15–30 min 3–5 min	4–5 h 1.5–2 h	Given in equigesic doses, morphine is no more depressing than other narcotics. Time/dose interval before birth is critical; therefore, not commonly used subcutaneously. Side effects: nausea and vomiting; slower respirations; hypotension; urinary retention, which may require intervention.	Rapid placental transmission. CNS depression in high doses. Respiratory depression counteracted by Narcan. Observe infant 2–3 h after delivery because of short action of Narcan.
Oxymorphone (Numorphan)	0.75–1.5 mg SC[c] 0.5–1.0 mg IM 0.5–0.75 mg IV	15–30 min 10–20 min 3–5 min	4–5 h 2.5–4 h 1.5–2 h	Pain relief and sedation. Similar effects as morphine. Maternal respiratory depressant.	Similar to morphine effects.

				May delay labor if given too early or in too large doses. Note that subcutaneous doses are not recommended during active labor as the duration is so long.	
Barbiturates[d]					
Secobarbital (Seconal)	50–200 mg PO	20–30 min	4–5 h	Sleep and sedation, but no analgesic or amnesia action. No effects on progress of labor, but must be given so that drug is completely metabolized before birth. Depressive effect on respiratory and circulatory systems with higher doses.	Attention depressed for 2–4 days after birth. Enhances microsomal liver metabolic rate. May affect action of other drugs.
Pentobarbital (Nembutal)	50–200 mg PO	20–30 min	4–5 h	Sleep and sedation, but no analgesic or amnesic action. No effects on progress of labor. Drug must be completely metabolized before birth.	Attention depressed for 2–4 days after birth. Enhances microsomal liver function, thus metabolizing other drugs faster.
Tranquilizers					
Promethazine (Phenergan)	25–50 mg IM 25 mg IV	15–20 min 3–5 min	3–4 h 2–3 h	Antihistaminic action adds extra sedation with narcotic. Potentiates narcotic; reduce dosage. Stimulates respirations, decreases nausea and vomiting. Some disorientation, hypotension, tachycardia may occur. No effect on labor progress.	CNS depression; equilibrates with maternal level within 15 min (intravenous route). Transitional effects depend on level/time of dose.
Promazine (Sparine)	25–50 mg IM 25 mg IV	15–20 min 3–5 min	3–4 h 2–3 h	Effective in combination with narcotic. Labile hypotension may occur. Other effects same as for promethazine.	CNS depression. Into fetal circulation within 4 min (intravenous route). Transitional effects depend on level/time of dose.

TABLE 8-2 *(continued)*

Agent	Dosage	Onset	Duration	Maternal Effects	Infant Effects
Tranquilizers					
Hydroxyzine hydrochloride (Vistaril)	50–100 mg IM only	15–20 min	3–4 h	Reduces nausea. Some sedation. Potentiates narcotic; reduce dose by 50%.	CNS depression. In high doses, observe for infant sedation.
Propiomazine (Largon)	20–40 mg IM 20–40 mg IV	15–20 min 3–5 min	2–4 h 2–3 h	Avoid combination in syringe with other drugs. May cause hypotension, some respiratory depression in adult.	Minimal CNS depression.
Diazepam (Valium)	5–10 mg IM 5–10 mg IV diluted in 5 mL normal saline[e]	10–15 min 2–3 min	5–7 h 5–6 h	*Not* used during labor. May be given intravenously during delivery only. Will potentiate any analgesic. Not recommended if mother is to breast-feed.	Into fetus in 4–6 min. Higher doses concentrate. Affects thermoregulation and responses, for up to 1 week after delivery. May affect pulse, respiration for 24 h.

[a] Dose reduced if given with tranquilizer.
[b] Give slowly over 2–3 min.
[c] For postoperative use only.
[d] Used only in very early labor to provide sleep.
[e] Give over 5-min period.

TABLE 8-3 REGIONAL ANESTHETICS USED DURING LABOR

Anesthetics	Period of Labor	Location of Injection	Comments	Precautions
Pudendal block	Second stage: expulsive phase	Pudendal nerves above and behind ischial spines. Anesthesia to second, third, and fourth sacral nerves.	Blocks sensation to entire perineum but not to uterus. Must allow 5–10 min for anesthetic to take full effect. Additional local to site of episiotomy. Does not cover pain of manual extraction of placenta or midforceps delivery. Recovery takes place within 1 h.	May have one-sided effect if placement is incorrect. Aspiration for blood is important as area is very vascular. Usually quite safe for mother and infant.
Peridural block: Lumbar epidural (continuous) for vaginal delivery	First stage: active labor, phase of maximum slope through second stage	Insertion at interspace between second, third, or fourth lumbar to block second, third, and fourth sacral nerves, higher block to tenth thoracic and fifth sacral. Blocks cervical and perineal pain, depending on dose and location of catheter.	Client may be in lateral decubitus or sitting on side of bed, neck must be flexed. Test dose always administered with 5-min wait for response. Plastic canula taped in place for future additional doses. When each dose is administered, check for bilateral anesthesia, vasodilation in legs, and toe temperature. Client will not have sensation to bear down. Must be coached. Recovery complete by 2–3 h, depending on dose and type of medication.	After dose is given, move client into supine position to distribute medication to both sides. Then semi-Fowler's position may be assumed. Check that catheter taping is secure. Watch for hypotension in first adjustment period; elevate legs to correct. Watch for vena cava compression. During recovery, no urge to void. Delayed recovery of sphincter control may persist after full recovery of leg movement. Watch for bladder distension.
Epidural for cesarean section		Anesthesia for cesarean section to sixth and seventh thoracic by insertion of catheter up toward first lumbar	Check effectiveness of anesthesia and signs for hypotension every 5 min for first 20 min.	Observe for vena cava compression and hypotension. Administer IV fluids and oxygen to prevent further hypotension and hypoxia in infant.

TABLE 8-3 *(continued)*

Anesthetics	Period of Labor	Location of Injection	Comments	Precautions
				Postural hypotension possible during recovery as well as voiding problems (see above).
Subarachnoid block:	Second stage or just prior to delivery	Insertion of needle at fourth lumbar through dura into spinal fluid.	Does not block contractions, but no urge to push. Must be coached.	Hypotension most common complication due to vena cava compression. Must position uterus with a lateral tilt.
Saddle block (low spinal)		Hyperbaric solution used to allow anesthetic to gravitate down toward sacral area. Anesthesia to tenth thoracic and to fifth sacral at level of umbilicus.	Administered in a sitting position; client remains upright 90–120 s for solution to descend, then lies supine with neck flexed on pillow. Must be well hydrated with IV fluids to alleviate hypotension. Postoperative: Usually quick recovery but keep flat 6–8 h as precaution against spinal headache. Watch for postural hypotension when first ambulatory.	Hypotension is most common complication. Other adverse effects (1) back pain from muscle trauma; (2) postpuncture headache from loss of spinal fluid and stretching of meninges (patient kept flat until hydration by IV fluids restores CSF); (3) postural hypotension when first ambulatory; (4) inability to void; (5) very rare, respiratory paralysis from medication rising in cord to affect nerves to thorax.
Spinal	Just prior to cesarean section or difficult delivery	Blocks to sixth, seventh, and eighth thoracic nerves.	Client in side-lying position with neck and knees flexed. Usually obliterates contractions, so forceps and fundal pressure may be necessary for vaginal delivery. Same as for "saddle block" above.	

SOURCE: Dickason, E. J., Schult, M. O., and Morris, E. M.: *Maternal and Infant Drugs and Nursing Intervention*, McGraw-Hill, New York, 1978.

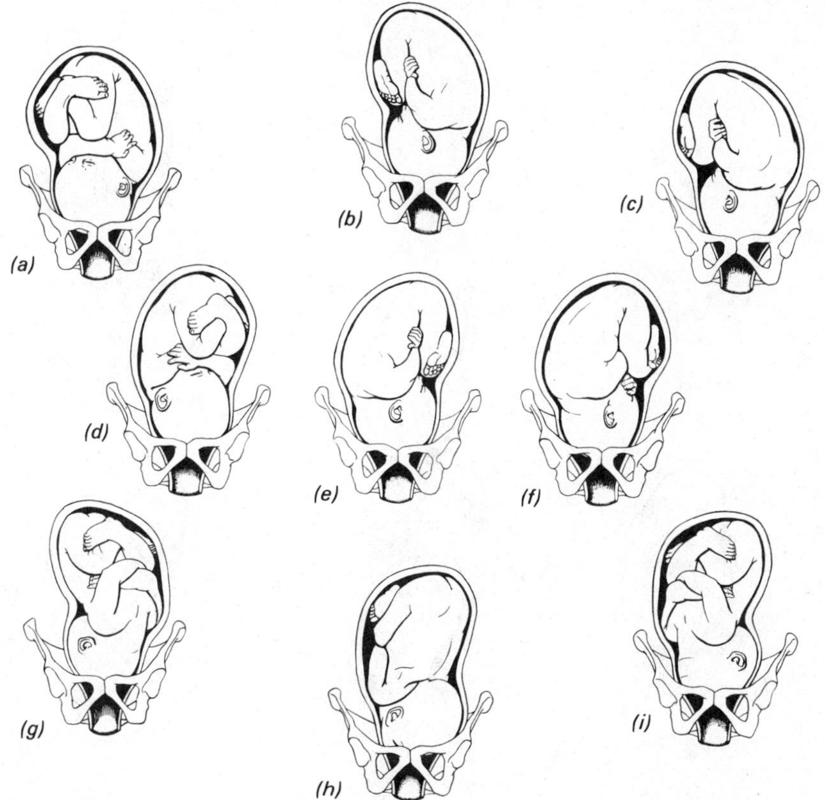

Figure 8-6 Positions of the fetus in cephalic presentation: (*a*) left occipitoposterior (LOP); (*b*) left occipitotransverse (LOT); (*c*) left occipitoanterior (LOA); (*d*) right occipitoposterior (ROP); (*e*) right occipitotransverse (ROT); (*f*) right occipitoanterior (ROA); (*g*) left mentoanterior (LMA); (*h*) right mentoposterior (RMP); (*i*) right mentoanterior (RMA). (From Ross Clinical Educational Aid No. 18. Courtesy of Ross Laboratories, Columbus, Ohio, 43216.)

2. Pelvic adequacy in relationship to presentation and position will be completely evaluated.

Interventions

1. Try a change in position to the right side; this may facilitate rotation of the fetus and promote more effective contractions.
2. Prepare the client for x-ray study of pelvic/fetal ratio.
   a. Explain the procedure.
   b. Transport client via wheelchair or stretcher, depending on the phase of labor.
   c. Allow a relative or close friend to accompany client.
   d. Carry an emergency delivery kit.
3. Prepare client for possible cesarean section.
   a. Obtain consent forms.
   b. Check laboratory work for CBC, Hgb, Hct, and type and cross match.
   c. Give abdominal prep, complete upper pubic shave.
   d. Insert a Foley catheter.
   e. Establish an intravenous infusion, with intra catheter.
   f. Reassure client and family with explanations of procedures.

Reevaluation and Follow-up

1. Any change of position of fetus evaluated by Leopold's maneuver and vaginal examination.

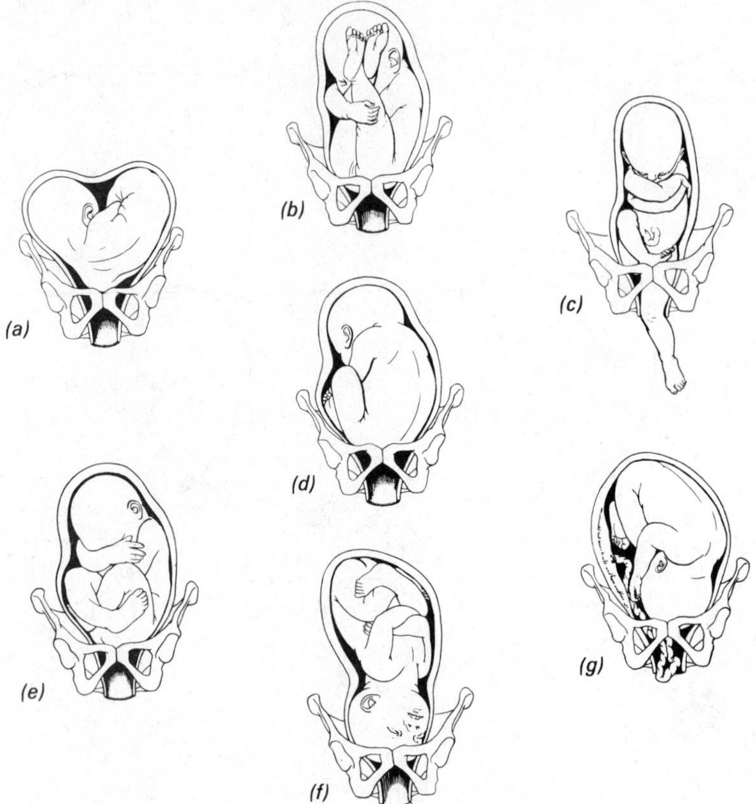

Figure 8-7 Less common types of presentation: (*a*) shoulder presentation; (*b*) frank breech; (*c*) incomplete breech; (*d*) left sacroanterior (LSA); (*e*) left sacroposterior (LSP); (*f*) brow presentation; (*g*) prolapse of cord. (From Ross Clinical Educational Aid No. 18. Courtesy of Ross Laboratories, Columbus, Ohio, 43216.)

2. Evaluation of cervical dilatation and effacement continued.
3. Client and family effectively prepared for surgery (see Chapter 9).

UTERINE INERTIA

Assessment

1. Pelvis is adequate.
2. Cervical dilatation is at least 2–3 cm.
3. Cervical effacement is more than 50 percent.
4. The presenting part is engaged.
5. Contractions are regular but mild and ineffective, requiring stimulation.

Revised Outcomes

The intensity and effectiveness of contractions will be increased.

Interventions

1. When ordered, establish a piggy back intravenous infusion for stimulation (usually 20 U Pitocin/500 mL D_5W).
2. Carefully monitor the flow rate; utilize IV infusion pump to control rate.
3. Observe for uterine hypertonicity and discontinue intravenous oxytocin if it occurs.
4. Monitor fetal heart rate, observing for late decelerations.

Reevaluation and Follow-up

Frequent reassessment of cervical dilatation to ensure that progress has been made without danger to mother or fetus.

VAGINAL BLEEDING

Assessment

1. The blood may be bright or dark red and amount may be a large gush or a slow trickle.
2. Vital signs may indicate shock.
3. The fetal heart may show late decelerations.
4. Pain accompanying the bleeding may indicate an abruptio placentae.

Revised Outcomes
1. Anxiety will be alleviated by close monitoring and explanations.
2. The source of bleeding will be identified and controlled.
3. The fetal/maternal unit will be free of complications related to bleeding.

Interventions
1. Pad count to determine the amount of vaginal bleeding.
2. Change body position to gain a tamponade effect by the presenting fetal part and thus decrease bleeding.
3. Monitor maternal vital signs noting signs of shock.
4. Do not perform vaginal exams, as there is risk of increasing bleeding.
5. Apply fetal monitor, observing for late decelerations.
6. Prepare client for ultrasound procedure to determine location of the placenta. Explain procedure and reassure client that it is not harmful to her or her fetus.
7. Arrange for lab work: Hgb, Hct, clotting factors, and type and cross match for several units.
8. Observe for development of clotting defect showing signs of bleeding without clotting, unusual bruisability, oozing at intravenous site, hematuria, bleeding from gums.
9. Reassure client and family, keeping them informed of status of mother and fetus.
10. Prepare for possible cesarean section.

ELEVATED BLOOD PRESSURE

Assessment
1. Blood pressure reading of 140/90, or 30 mm above normal systolic and 15 mm above normal diastolic. (See Chapter 7.)
2. Albuminuria, increased specific gravity, possible oliguira.
3. Edema, especially of hands and face.
4. Hyperreflexia.

5 Altered blood volume: elevated hematocrit.

Revised Outcomes
1. Blood pressure will be returned to normal limits.
2. Convulsions will be prevented.
3. Fetal health will be guarded.

Interventions
1. Monitor vital signs every 10–15 min and observe fetal monitor.
2. Restrict activity and sensory input.
3. Record intake and output; insert Foley catheter in severe preeclampsia, using hourly urines.
4. Employ seizure precautions.
5. Administer prescribed anticonvulsants and antihypertensives, usually by infusion pump.

Reevaluation and Follow-Up
1. Assess effectiveness of medications.
2. Evaluate output, minimum of 100 mL/4 h; evaluate vital signs. Do not allow diastolic to fall below 90 mmHg.
3. Continue to monitor fetal and maternal labor status.

ELEVATED TEMPERATURE

Assessment
1. Temperature above normal 98.6°F.
2. Fetal tachycardia and decreased variability in baseline fetal heart.
3. Membranes may be ruptured over 24 h and fluid may be cloudy with an odor.

Revised Outcomes
1. Temperature will be restored to within normal limits.
2. Fetal and maternal complications of infection will be minimized.

Interventions
1. Administer intravenous fluids with antibiotics as ordered.
2. Evaluate temperature every 1 h, fetal status every 15–30 min.
3. Prepare for induction of labor if membranes have been ruptured for over 24 h as ascending infection is hazardous to mother and fetus.

Reevaluation and Follow-up

Maternal/fetal status monitored and evaluated until temperature lowered or delivery accomplished.

POSTMATURITY

See Chapter 11.

Assessment
1. Fundal height may be below xiphoid due to fetal weight loss.
2. Biparietal head diameter indicates a term fetus, greater than 9.8 cm.
3. Blood estriol levels may be low, indicating decreasing placental function.
4. Amniotic fluid studies show mature L/S ratio; may show signs of chronic distress.
5. Gestation is 42 weeks or more, but labor does not begin.

Revised Outcomes

Fetus will be delivered in optimum state of well-being.

Interventions

1. Prepare client for nonstress test and, if positive, an oxytocin challenge test.
   a. Set up a piggyback intravenous infusion.
   b. Apply external fetal monitor.
   c. Titrate oxytocin drip until contractions occur at a rate of 3 in 10 min.
   d. Observe fetal heart rate for late decelerations.
2. Prepare client for induction if estriol levels are low and/or fetal heart shows late decelerations.

Reevaluation and Follow-up

Evaluation of fetal/maternal unit continued in order to minimize complications of postmaturity.

PREMATURE LABOR

Assessment

1. Gestation is 37 weeks or less and labor begins.
2. Height of fundus is below the xiphoid.
3. Ultrasound reveals biparietal diameter under 8.7 cm.
4. Amniocentesis reveals.
   a. L/S ratio below 2.0, indicating lung immaturity.
   b. Creatinine levels below 1.5 mg/100 mL, indicating renal immaturity.
   c. Lipid cells below 10 percent when stained with Nile blue (Tucker, 1978).
5. Membranes may or may not have ruptured, but signs of true labor are present.

Revised Outcomes

1. Optimum environment for fetal well-being will be provided.
2. Risk of fetal mortality due to prematurity will be decreased.

Interventions

1. Prepare client for ultrasound to determine biparietal diameters.
2. Prepare client for amniocentesis.
3. Remain with client for emotional support as well as monitoring of vital signs and fetal heart.
4. If labor has begun, but the cervix is less than 3 cm dilated or 50 percent effaced, membranes intact, take preventive measures:
   a. Place client on bed rest and decreased activity.
   b. Currently, ritodrine hydrochloride (Yutopar) is in use as a tocolytic agent to inhibit premature labor. Side effects are numerous and may be potent. Usually contraindicated for cardiac or diabetic conditions.
   c. *Dose:* 100 μg/min titrated to responses. Do not exceed 350 μg/min. Administer by infusion pump. Careful monitoring for maternal or fetal adverse reactions.
   d. *Side effects:* Tachycardia, premature ventricular contractions, decreased diastolic/increased systolic blood pressure, hyperglycemia. *Fetus:* tachycardia, neonatal hypoglycemia. (Foster, 1981)

Reevaluation and Follow-up

Monitor labor and fetal status to ensure against complications; bed rest maintained until labor ceased or delivery ensued.

CARDIAC COMPLICATIONS

Complications may occur as a result of the strain of labor and delivery, especially in a cardiac client of class 2 or 3 limitations.

Assessment

Signs of cardiac insufficiency—rales, edema, respiratory rate above 28 with dyspnea, pulse rate above 100 with palpitations.

Revised Outcomes

1. Mother will proceed through labor and delivery without developing congestive heart failure.
2. Adequate oxygenation of fetus will occur.

Interventions

1. Promote rest and decreased activity.
2. Position client in high Fowler's position.
3. Administer antibiotics as prescribed, monitor IV flow rate carefully.
4. Monitor heart rate and respirations every 15 min.
5. Ensure availability of oxygen, morphine, digitalis, and diuretics as prescribed; later observe for fetal/newborn effects.
6. Prepare client for epidural anesthesia. (See Table 8-3.)

DIABETES

Assessment

1. Woman may be hypoglycemic because of stress of labor and decreasing placental function.
2. Fetus is large for dates.

Revised Outcomes

1. Hyper- or hypoglycemia will not develop to threaten fetal/maternal well-being.
2. Delivery of a large fetus will not result in physical injury to mother or fetus.

Interventions

1. Prepare client for induction or cesarean section, depending upon fetal size.
2. Prepare for possible premature infant, as fetal size is not indicative of gestational age.
3. Test urine for sugar and acetone or do blood glucose readings every 4 h.
4. Administer insulin SC to cover the glucose in intravenous fluids (do not add to IV solution).

Reevaluation and Follow-up

Continued monitoring of sugar and acetone, fetal status, and labor progress to ensure against further complications to mother and fetus.

SECOND STAGE OF LABOR

DESCRIPTION

The second stage of labor is the period of labor from full dilatation of the cervix to complete delivery of the infant. It is the period of fetal descent through the vaginal canal. The mean duration is 20 min for multigravidas and 1–2 h for primigravidas (Figure 8-8).

ASSESSMENT

Health History

See first stage history.

Physical Assessment

Refer to Table 8-4.

1. Cervix is fully dilated.
2. There is an increase in bloody show.
3. There is pressure on the rectum with a desire to defecate.
4. Contractions occur every 3–5 min, lasting 90–110 s.
5. The presenting part is engaged and descending.
6. Client is totally preoccupied with contractions and may be irritable and exhausted; she may doze or experience amnesia between contractions.
7. Fetal monitor may reveal early decelerations associated with head compression.

NURSING DIAGNOSES: ACTUAL OR POTENTIAL

1. Potential for lack of descent of presenting part.
2. Potential for ineffective bearing down due to inappropriate positioning, excessive fear of physical harm, exhaustion, analgesia or anesthesia.
3. Potential threat to maternal/fetal well-being because of infection caused by fecal contamination, lacerations caused by uncontrolled pushing, or fetal hypoxia.
4. Potential for excessive anxiety as a result of loss of control associated with second stage.

EXPECTED OUTCOMES

1. Fetus will descend at an appropriate rate.
2. Client will be effective in her bearing-down efforts.
3. Client will be provided with an environment that will promote the safety and well-being of mother and fetus.
4. Client will be free of excessive anxiety and receive support from significant other.

TABLE 8-4 CHANGES DURING THE SECOND STAGE OF LABOR

Physical Changes	Behavioral Changes
Contractions: strong with several acmes Duration: 90–110 s Frequency: 3–5 min Dilatation: complete Primipara: 50 min Multipara: 20 min	May be nauseated and exhausted. If conditioned to push, may feel it as a relief. Fearful of losing control. Amnesia between contractions. Needs steady coaching.

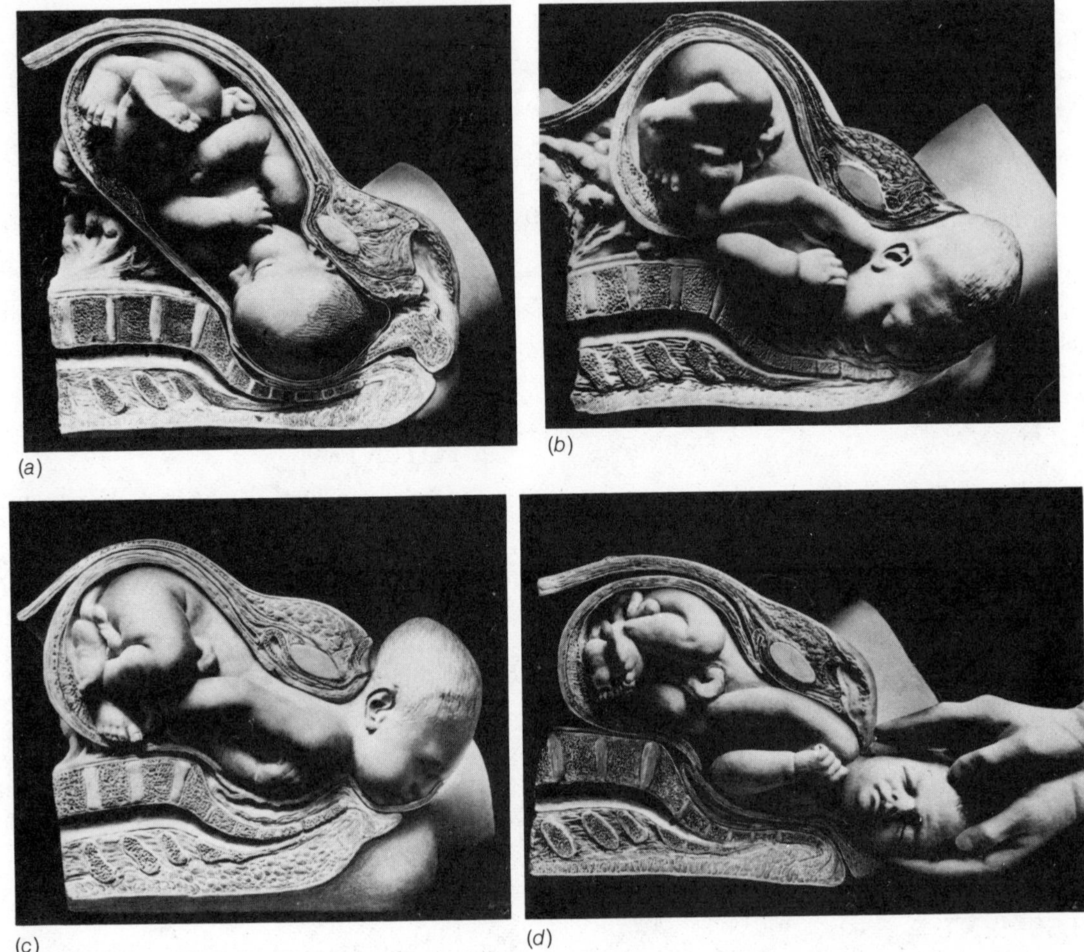

Figure 8-8 Second stage of labor. Fetal positions: (*a*) internal rotation completed; (*b*) extension and crowning; (*c*) extension completed; (*d*) delivery of head and external rotation. (Reproduced with permission from the *Birth Atlas*, Maternity Center Association, New York.)

INTERVENTIONS

1. Position client for effective pushing.
   a. Place in semi-Fowler's position with legs abducted, chin on chest, and hands grasping legs behind the knees.
   b. Client may push in Sim's position if fetus is in a posterior position.
   c. Client may push in kneeling or squatting position.
2. Encourage effective pushing with utilization of appropriate breathing techniques.
3. Coach client and provide emotional support.
4. Provide privacy by draping the client properly while she is pushing.
5. Minimize the chances of infection by keeping the bed linen clean and dry; cleanse perineum to prevent fecal contamination; maintain aseptic technique in the delivery room.
6. Minimize physical complications by observing for perineal bulging and crowning of presenting part and monitoring fetal heart every 5 min or after each contraction.
7. Decrease anxiety regarding the delivery process by explaining delivery room procedures, such as administration of anesthesia and use of stirrups and restraints if birthing room is not available.
8. Provide mirror in which parents can view the delivery.

EVALUATION

Outcome Criteria

1. Client will push effectively.
2. Fetus will descend and progress through delivery.
3. Maternal/fetal well-being will be maintained.

Complications

LACK OF DESCENT

Assessment

1. Presenting part does not descend despite strong contractions and effective pushing (Figure 8-9).
2. Vaginal exam reveals high station and increased molding of presenting part due to malpresentation, inadequate pelvic size.
3. Posterior position or malpresentation is slowing descent.
4. Time interval in second stage exceeds normal limits.

Revised Outcomes

Fetus will be delivered without harm to physical well-being.

Interventions

1. Monitor fetal heart rate.
2. Prepare for forceps delivery and possible Scanzoni's maneuver if position is posterior.
3. Prepare for possible cesarean section if pelvis is inadequate or there is a malpresentation.

Reevaluation and Follow-up

Continued monitoring of fetal/maternal unit until delivery accomplished.

HYPOTENSION: VENA CAVA SYNDROME

Assessment

1. Hypotension may result from use of anesthetics and the pressure of the gravid uterus on the inferior vena cava.
2. Blood pressure below client's baseline, pulse rising.
3. Client nauseated and light-headed.
4. Fetal heart shows late decelerations.

Revised Outcomes

Blood pressure will be restored to normal.

Interventions

1. Change position of mother to alleviate pressure of the gravid uterus, try left side first, then right in position to move uterus off vena cava.
2. If unable to change client's position, move the uterus to the left side of the body, place wedge under right flank.
3. Administer oxygen by mask.

Reevaluation and Follow-up

Blood pressure monitored until it returned to normal level.

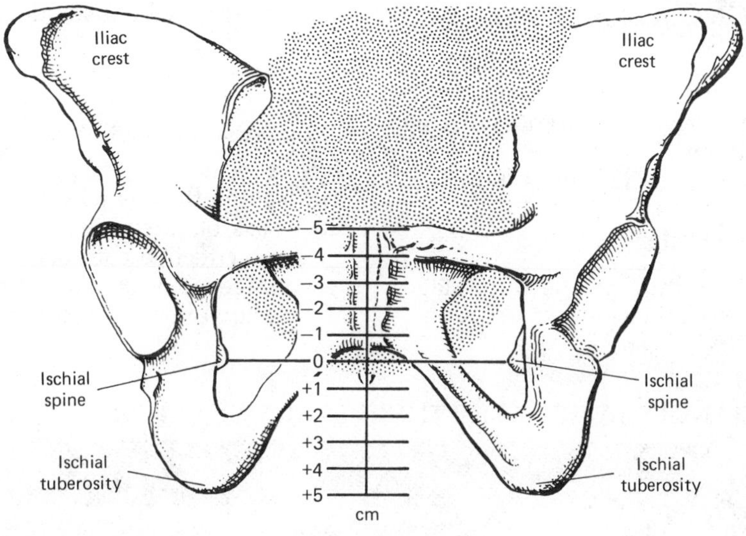

Figure 8-9 Stations of the presenting part. (From Ross Clinical Educational Aid, "The Phenomena of Labor." Courtesy of Ross Laboratories, Columbus, Ohio, 43216.

THIRD STAGE OF LABOR

DESCRIPTION

The third stage of labor includes the period of time from the delivery of the infant to the complete delivery of the placenta and membranes (Figure 8-10).

ASSESSMENT

Health History

See previous labor record.

Physical Assessment

Refer to Table 8-5.
1. A firmly contracting, rising uterus.
2. A gush of blood from the vaginal introitus.
3. Lengthening of the umbilical cord.

Diagnostic Tests

1. Cord blood for Rh and Coombs' test, serology.
2. Placenta may be sent to pathology if abnormal.
3. Maternal blood drawn if mother is Rh negative, for Fetaldex (presence of fetal blood constituents in maternal system).

NURSING DIAGNOSES: ACTUAL OR POTENTIAL

1. Potential for hemorrhage due to retained placenta, partial expulsion of placenta, uterine atony, or lacerations.
2. Potential for delayed interaction with infant.

EXPECTED OUTCOMES

1. Client will progress through the third stage of labor without complications.
2. Client and family will begin interaction with infant during the period of reactivity.

INTERVENTIONS

1. Monitor vital signs and contractility of fundus every 15 min.
2. Administer oxytocins as ordered, usually 20 U into remaining IV fluids.
3. Provide time for infant and parents to interact and for infant to breast-feed if desired. Maintain overhead warmer or skin-to-skin maternal infant contact to prevent heat loss in baby.

EVALUATION

Outcome Criteria

1. Client will have no physical problems regarding lacerations or expulsion of placenta and membranes.
2. Reactions of parents to newborn will be within normal limits.

Complications

UTERINE ATONY

Assessment
1. Fundus is boggy, above umbilicus, and out of midline.
2. Excessive vaginal bleeding; changes in vital signs may be delayed until a large amount of blood has been lost.
3. Bladder may be distended.

Revised Outcomes
1. Bleeding will be controlled and uterine tone returned.
2. Blood volume will be supported.

Interventions
1. Massage fundus with palm of hand.
2. Assess bladder status as a full bladder prevents effective contraction of the uterus; encourage voiding. Catheterize if client is unable to void and bleeding continues.

TABLE 8-5 CHANGES DURING THE THIRD STAGE OF LABOR

Physical Changes	Behavioral Changes
Contractions strong Duration: 120 s Frequency: 3–5 min Delivery of placenta completed	Must be asked to push, as relief of pressure diminishes sensation of contraction. Client may laugh or cry and ask about infant. May be excited or exhausted.

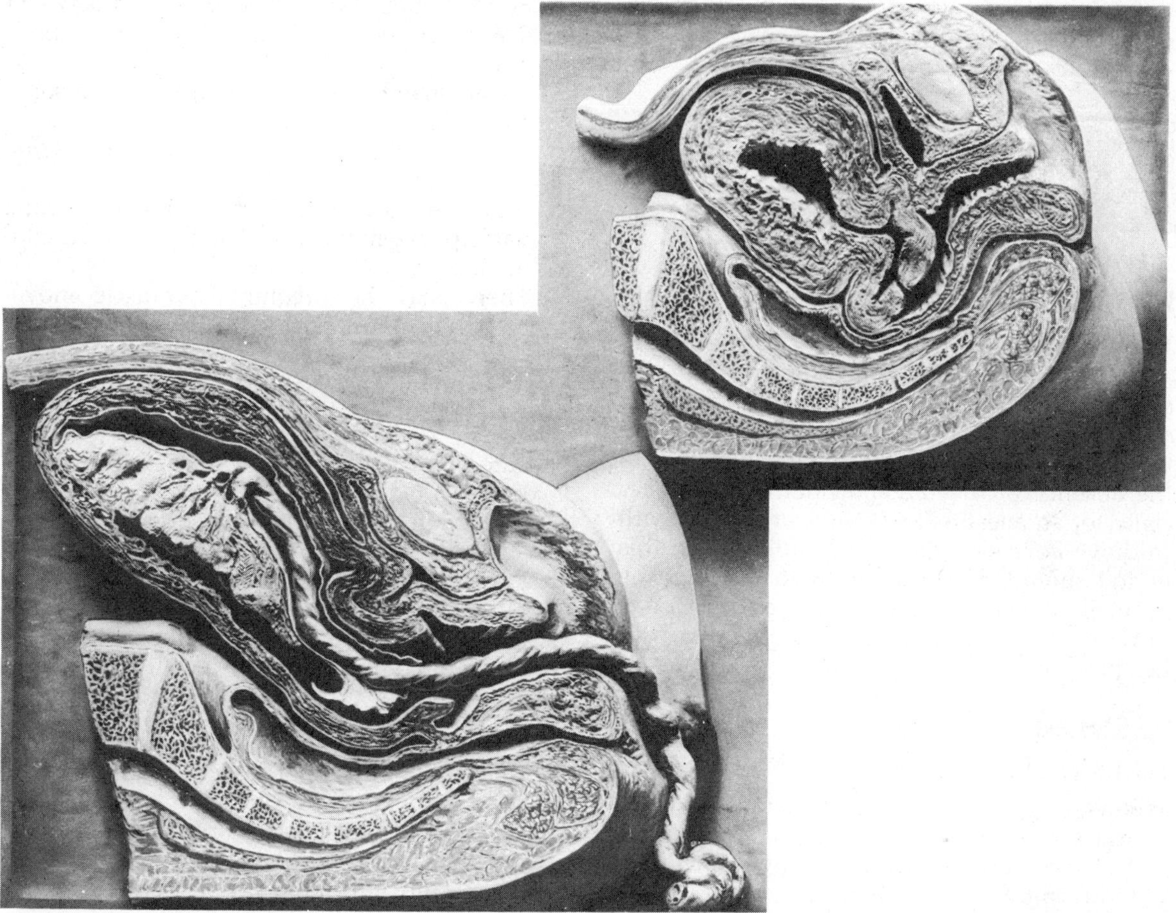

Figure 8-10 Third stage of labor: delivery of the placenta. Bottom left, separation of the placenta from the uterine wall; top right, contraction of the uterus after placental delivery. (Reproduced with permission from the *Birth Atlas*, Maternity Center Association, New York.)

3. Administer oxytocin as ordered. Methergine 0.2 mg IM may be ordered in addition to IV oxytocin if client normotensive.

Reevaluation and Follow-up

1. Bladder, fundus rechecked at frequent intervals, especially after oxytocin effect diminished.
2. Fundus began descent according to normal pattern and maintained firm tone.

LACERATION IN THE BIRTH CANAL

Assessment

1. Excessive vaginal bleeding, but uterus is firm.
2. Cervical or vaginal lacerations may be present: bleeding may not be clotted, may be bright or dark red; arterial or venous bleeding.
3. Clotting defect may be present; check prenatal history.

Revised Outcomes

Cause of bleeding will be discovered and treated.

Interventions

1. Notify physician as treatment is medical.
2. Prepare client to return to delivery room for suturing and cervical, vaginal exploration.
3. Prepare to obtain blood for transfusion or blood samples for analysis of clotting defect.

Reevaluation and Follow-up

1. Continued monitoring of lochia.
2. Bright and dark red bleeding ceased within the expected locial pattern.
3. Client received blood replacement when he-

moglobin, hematocrit fell. Vital signs remained within normal range.

FOURTH STAGE OF LABOR

DESCRIPTION

The fourth stage of labor is the period of 1 h after delivery of the placenta. For the client it is a period of immediate adjustment to the sudden change in abdominal pressure and blood volume and includes the immediate adjustment to the absence of the placental hormones. Especially for an anesthetized client, or a client with cardiovascular or endocrine complications, this period should be considered high risk. For the normally delivered mother, this period is a one of relief, rest, and time to get acquainted with her newborn. (See Chapter 9)

ASSESSMENT

Health History

1. Review labor record, noting length of labor and any complications of delivery.
2. Note type of anesthesia and any difficulty in induction.
3. Check for episiotomy type, lacerations, trauma.

Physical Assessment

Refer to Table 8-6.

1. Client may be sleeping after having seen and held infant.
2. Client may be excited and talkative regarding her labor and delivery experience.
3. Fundus should be firm and located between symphysis pubis and umbilicus and in midline.
4. Lochia may be heavy, darker red, with some small clots.
5. Perineum should be intact, although edema may be present.
6. Vital signs should reflect admission baseline data; pulse may be elevated due to excitement.
7. There may be involuntary muscle movements, such as spasmodic shivering.

NURSING DIAGNOSES: ACTUAL OR POTENTIAL

1. Alteration in comfort secondary to delivery process.
2. Alteration in fluid balance due to fluid restriction during labor and fluid loss.
3. Dysrhythm of sleep/rest activity as a result of fatigue, excitement.
4. Potential for threat to maternal well-being because of complications of fourth stage.

EXPECTED OUTCOMES

1. Client will be free of discomfort and able to rest.
2. Fluid balance will be restored and nutritional needs met.
3. Client and partner will begin adjustment to infant and new roles.
4. Recovery will occur without complications.

INTERVENTIONS

1. Provide quiet, nonstimulating environment.
2. Give client a partial bath and provide clean linen. A warm blanket may alleviate shivers and feeling of chilling.

TABLE 8-6 CHANGES DURING THE FOURTH STAGE OF LABOR

Physical Changes	Behavioral Changes
Uterus contracts Duration: 100 s Frequency: 5 min, unless receives oxytocins; then stays contracted until IV absorbed. Infant suckling will promote contraction. Mother may shiver and have chills.	Seeks reassurance of performance. Usually fatigued. Preoccupied with labor experience; needs to talk about it. Father of child or other family member should be with mother during this time, plus infant if possible.

3. Provide food and fluids as tolerated.
4. Encourage mother and father to talk about delivery. Provide reassurance about her performance. Encourage partner to support her.
5. Monitor fundus, lochia, bladder, and vital signs at regular intervals.
6. Apply ice to perineum to reduce edema and promote comfort.
7. Ensure that parents have time alone with infant for early acquaintance period.

EVALUATION

Outcome Criteria

Client will progress through fourth stage without complication.

Complications

HEMATOMA

Hematoma may occur anywhere within the birth canal as capillaries, arterioles or larger arteries, and veins tear or rupture because of pressure. It is usually found over the ischial spines on the midvaginal wall but also occasionally in the broad ligament rectal wall or higher up in the vaginal wall. Overt signs are quickly spotted when bleeding is into the labia. Pain out of proportion to usual postdelivery discomfort, perspiring, and changes in vital signs may be the only clues.

Assessment

1. Persistent perineal pain, rectal or low back pain.
2. Large swelling at labia or vaginal introitus or within vaginal wall.
3. Exquisite pain at site, client perspiring, trembling.

Revised Outcomes

Hematoma will be reduced and bleeding stopped.

Intervention

1. Prepare client for incision and evacuation of hematoma by physician.
2. Vaginal pack may be inserted.
3. Insert Foley catheter if hematoma is near urethra.
4. Place ice pack on perineum for short, frequent intervals; do not overchill.

Reevaluation and Follow-up

Continued monitoring of physical status of mother to ensure that intervention was effective.

URINARY RETENTION

Assessment

1. Fundus is displaced from midline.
2. A full bladder is palpated abdominally.
3. Client cannot void spontaneously.

Revised Outcomes

1. The bladder will be emptied at regular intervals.
2. Bladder distension will not occur to cause uterine atony or bleeding.

Interventions

1. Help client to bathroom unless physical status or anesthetic prevents ambulation.
2. Measure first voiding and assess for retention or overflow. Expect 500–1000 mL urine in first 12 h after delivery.
3. Catheterize only after trying several methods to promote voiding. Priority is to prevent uterine atony from bladder distension.
4. Observe for evidence of edema, trauma, infection.

Reevaluation and Follow-up

1. Client voided within 6 to 8 h after catheterization.
2. In event of trauma to urethral area: Foley catheter remained in place for 24–48 h to allow initial healing and reduction of edema.
3. No incontinence occurred subsequent to discharge.
4. No bladder infection present.

REFERENCES

Dickason, E. J., Schult M. O., and Morris, E. M.: *Maternal and Infant Drugs and Nursing Intervention*, McGraw-Hill, New York, 1978.

Foster, S. D.: "MCN Pharmacopoeia, Ritodrine," *MCN: American Journal of Maternal Child Nursing*, **6**:204, May/June 1981.

Friedman, E. A.: *Labor: Clinical Evaluation and Management*, Appleton-Century-Crofts, New York, 1978.

Lynch, J. M.: "Helping Patients through the Recurring Nightmare of Herpes," *Nursing 82*, **12**(10):52–57, October 1982.

Tucker, S.: *Fetal Monitoring and Fetal Assessment in the High Risk Pregnancy*, Mosby, St. Louis, 1978.

BIBLIOGRAPHY

Angelini, D. J.: "Nonverbal Communicaion in Labor," *American Journal of Nursing,* **78**(7):1220–1222, July 1978. Describes a variety of nonverbal expressions seen in laboring women and discusses nursing implications.

Crandon, A. J.: "Maternal Anxiety and Obstetrical Complications," *Journal of Psychosomatic Research,* **23**(2):109–111, 113–115, 1979. Two research studies supporting the need to decrease anxiety in clients in order to maximize maternal and fetal well-being.

El Sherif, C., McGrath, G., and Smyrski, J. T.: "Coaching the Coach," *Journal of Obstetric, Gynecologic, and Neonatal Nursing,* **8**(2):87–89, March/April 1979. Evaluates and discusses the role of the coach in labor. Provides guidelines for assessing coaching performance and how to support the coach.

Foster, S. D.: "MCN Pharmacopoeia, Ritodrine," *MCN: American Journal of Maternal Child Nursing,* **6**:204, May/June 1981. Pharmacologic effects and nursing implications for the administration of ritodrine for premature labor.

Gay, J.: "Theories Regarding Endocrine Contributions to the Onset of Labor," *Journal of Obstetric, Gynecologic, and Neonatal Nursing,* **7**(5):42–47, September/October 1978. An in-depth discussion of endocrine factors in influencing labor. Implications for nursing practice and theory are discussed.

Gray, J.: "Fetal and Maternal Monitoring: Nursing Care," *American Journal of Nursing,* **78**(12):2104–2105, December 1978. An entire series on fetal and maternal monitoring techniques. Explains procedures, normal values, and nursing care of monitored clients.

Kitzinger, S.: "Pain in Childbirth," *Journal of Medical Ethics,* **4**(3):119–121, September 1978. Describes pain and its control throughout the various stages of labor. Stresses the value of antepartal preparation as well as the need for a supportive environment.

Lynch, J. M.: "Helping Patients through the Recurring Nightmare of Herpes," *Nursing 82,* **12**(10)52–57, October 1982. Psychologic and physiologic effects of herpes, with a special segment on pregnancy and herpes effects.

McKay, S.: "Second Stage Labor—Has Tradition Replaced Safety?" *American Journal of Nursing,* **81**(5):1016, May 1981. Identifies complications of supine position and breath holding in second stage of labor. Proposes alternatives to Sim's position, squatting, kneeling positions, and exhaling during contractions.

Mozingo, J. N.: "Pain in Labor: A Conceptual Model Intervention," *Journal of Obstetric, Gynecologic, and Neonatal Nursing,* **7**(4):47–49, July/August 1978. Describes a model for intervening with the labor client in pain that uses education, purposeful activity, and supportive care.

9

Recovery: The Fourth Trimester

Jeanette Coleman and Hilda Koehler

VAGINAL DELIVERY

DESCRIPTION

The postpartum period is the stage in the maternity cycle that bridges the pregnant to nonpregnant state. It is part of a continuum: as the woman's health status before pregnancy significantly influences the events of gestation and birth, so too do those events determine her ability to cope with her altered physical self and the radical differences she will experience in adapting to the responsibilities and pleasures of motherhood.

During pregnancy, each body system undergoes profound change, but slowly. In the 6 weeks following birth, called the *postpartum period* (or puerperium, from the Latin *puer*, "child," and *parere*, "to bring forth") all these systems are rapidly restored: circulatory, respiratory, gastrointestinal, metabolic, renal, integumentary, musculoskeletal and, of course, reproductive. The uterus involutes, lochia is discharged, lactation is established or suppressed depending on the feeding choice of the mother, and the perineum and vaginal tissues heal. Total weight loss should be approximately 25 lb.

All the preparations the woman and her family made for the arrival of the new family member are now tested, as she, the father, other children, other residents of the household, and the baby adjust to each other. Parents learn their child is in reality a person with individual likes, dislikes, sensitivities, and sensory threshold. Parents must learn to provide physical care, love, security, and stimuli for their baby's cognitive growth and at the same time budget time and resources for themselves.

PREVENTION

Health Promotion

The postpartum phase, although one of profound change, is essentially a time of well-being. Conscientious monitoring of the total woman's adaptation to her new life experience can provide assurance to her and to those significant to her that she is recovering as expected. Additionally, vigilance provides clues to the earliest signs and symptoms of possible serious complications, so that early intervention can be implemented. Supporting wise health practices and recommending those not already followed will effect not just the health of the woman but potentially the health of her entire family.

ASSESSMENT

General Assessment

See Chapter 2.

Prenatal History

1. Did client receive prenatal care during this pregnancy? If so:
   a. Date of first visit, type of care.
   b. Health care provider(s).
   c. Number of kept or missed appointments.
2. Illnesses during this pregnancy.
   a. Kind of illness, date of occurrence.
   b. Treatment, resolution.
3. Exposure to infectious diseases during pregnancy.

a. Type and source of exposure.
b. Month of pregnancy, result of any titers to follow.

4. Immunization status
   a. Type of testing and results, that is, rubella titer, toxoplasmosis titer.
   b. Any immunizations received during pregnancy, reason.
5. X-ray procedures during pregnancy: dental, chest, other.
6. Prescription and nonprescription medications taken during pregnancy, reasons.
7. Laboratory tests/diagnostic procedures performed during pregnancy: date, type, results.
8. History of participation in childbirth education and parenting classes.

Labor and Delivery History

1. Date and time of:
   a. Admission to hospital.
   b. Onset of labor.
      (1) Spontaneous.
      (2) Induction (method).
   c. Rupture of membranes.
      (1) Spontaneous; description of characteristics of fluid.
      (2) Artificial; phase of labor.
2. Duration of labor.
   a. First stage: followed normal pattern?
   b. Second stage: completed cervical dilatation.
   c. Third stage: spontaneous placental expulsion or not.
3. Augmentation of labor.
   a. Method, dose and duration.
   b. Indication.
4. Medication received during labor and delivery with dose: time interval.
5. Intravenous fluids received during labor and delivery. Type and amount of solution.
6. Presence of maternal/fetal complications.
   a. Nonstress or oxytocin challenge test results.
   b. Intrapartum monitoring results.
7. Results of laboratory tests/diagnostic procedures.
   a. Maternal.
   b. Fetal/neonatal.
8. Summation of delivery events.
   a. Fetal presentation and position.
   b. Method of delivery.
      (1) Vertex: spontaneous, low or midforceps, vacuum extraction.
      (2) Breech: spontaneous, assisted.
      (3) Cesarean section: indication and type of incision.
   c. Type of anesthesia and duration, any problems.
   d. Condition of placenta and cord.
   e. Estimated blood loss.
   f. Episiotomy: description.
   g. Lacerations: perineal (degree), vaginal, cervical, other.
   h. Surgical procedures.
      (1) Tubal ligation.
      (2) Other.
9. Status of newborn.
   a. Sex.
   b. Birth weight, length.
   c. Apgar score at 1 and 5 min.
   d. Resuscitation.
      (1) Measures instituted.
      (2) Minutes until respiration sustained.
   e. Birth injuries: present, absent.
   f. Congenital defects: present, absent.
   g. Medications received in delivery room.
   h. Location of newborn.
      (1) With mother.
      (2) Transitional nursery.
      (3) Newborn nursery.
      (4) Intensive care nursery.
      (5) Transfer to tertiary center.
10. Support system during labor and delivery.
11. Parent-newborn interaction.
    a. Did mother and/or father have opportunity to interact with the baby immediately after birth? If so:
       (1) Type of contact.
       (2) Length of contact.
    b. Description of interactional response.
12. Summation of maternal status—fourth stage.
    a. Vital signs: TPR and BP
    b. Fundus: Location, height, consistency.
    c. Lochia, pads used in 1 h.
    d. Status of perineum, voiding.
    e. Medication.
       (1) Time narcotic was last administered.
       (2) Amount of oxytocin.
    f. Intravenous fluid volume.

Assessment of Current Health Practices and Habits

1. Nutrition.
   a. Height and prepregnant weight, total weight gain during pregnancy, current weight.

b. Sample of usual daily food and fluid intake.
c. Dietary restrictions or problems with nervous overeating, undereating, sporadic eating.

2. Elimination pattern.
3. Sleep pattern.
4. Exercise and recreation pattern.
5. Personal hygiene pattern.
6. Narcotic or other drug use: type, pattern of use.
7. Smoking pattern: type, amount per day.
8. Alcohol intake pattern: type, pattern of consumption.
9. Contraception history.
   a. Any difficulty conceiving?
   b. Contraceptive usage.
      (1) Method used before this pregnancy.
      (2) How long used.
      (3) Use effectiveness.
      (4) Other methods used, if any.
   c. Attitude toward family planning.
   d. Future plans for practice of family-planning behaviors.

Assessment of Health Education and Counseling Needs

Assess those needs related to the puerperium.

1. Self-care.
   a. Expected physiologic and emotional changes of the puerperium.
   b. Hygiene.
   c. Rest.
   d. Exercise.
   e. Nutrition.
   f. Resumption of sexual activity.
   g. Reportable signs and symptoms of illness.
   h. Measures to alleviate common discomforts.
   i. Available health care resources.
   j. Plan for continuity of care.
   k. Coping with conflicts related to changes in lifestyle.
      (1) Own self-image.
      (2) Adjustment of father, grandparents, significant others.
2. Client's other children: identify for each:
   a. Age.
   b. Present health status.
   c. Significant health problems.
      (1) Physiological.
      (2) Psychological.
      (3) Developmental.
   d. Preparation for new family member.

Physical Assessment

1. General appearance.
   a. May alternately appear extremely weary, then fully exhilarated.
   b. Note grooming, posture, facial expression, speech, mood.
2. Vital signs.
   a. Puerperal morbidity exists when the temperature is over 38°C (100.4°F) for any consecutive 48-h period, excluding the first 24 h after delivery.
   b. Transient bradycardia with pulse rates of 50 to 70 beats per minute is a common finding following delivery, lasting approximately 1 week to 10 days.
   c. Tachycardia is associated with excitement, anxiety, dehydration, increased bleeding, infection, pain, and cardiovascular and renal disease.
   d. A decrease in blood pressure may result from excessive blood loss during delivery.
3. Weight loss.
   a. Initial weight loss approximates 10–12 lb due to delivery of products of conception (including fetus, placenta, cord, membranes, amniotic fluid) and some blood loss.
   b. An additional 12-lb loss occurs by the end of the sixth week through diaphoresis and diuresis.
   c. With the exception of added weight of lactating breasts in mothers who are breastfeeding, failure to achieve prepregnant weight usually represents additional fat at the end of the postpartum period.
4. Integument.
   a. Pigmentary changes from pregnancy may be present, such as chloasma, linea nigra, striae gravidarum, spider nevi.
   b. Capillary breakage from the effort of giving birth gives rise to petechiae over face.
   c. Diaphoresis, reaching a peak on the third postpartum day and subsiding by the end of the first week, rids the body of accumulated fluid during pregnancy.
   d. Hair begins to fall out ("by handfulls") within a week after giving birth. (Due to increased peripheral circulation, hair loss during pregnancy is only between 70 and 150 hairs a day, whereas during postpartum it is between 500 and 600 hairs a day.)
5. Head, eyes, throat, and neck.

a. Headache, may occur as aftermath of spinal/epidural anesthesia; anxiety.
b. Eyes may be "blood shot" from capillary breakage at the effort of giving birth.
c. Throat may be sore from general anesthesia; there may be hoarseness or a voice change.
d. Thyroid enlargement may remain from pregnancy.
e. Dizziness secondary to blood loss, exertion, shift in center of gravity, postural hypotension.

6. Breasts and axillae.
   a. Inspect breasts for size, fullness, condition of skin, erectility of nipple; check use of brassiere for support, fit, comfort.
   b. Areola and nipples still heavily pigmented from pregnancy.
   c. Lactation begins approximately 48 h after a vaginal birth; 60 h after a cesarean. Breasts may be slightly full to seriously engorged: hard, nodular, dilated veins; hot-tender, painful-to-touch, shiny skin. Within 48 h after milk "comes in" veins should be less dilated and breasts softer, with or without treatment.
   d. Nipples may be flat or inverted, making it difficult or impossible for baby to nurse. With poor care and/or abuse nipples may be sore, tingling, red, cracked, bleeding.
   e. Milk glands under axillae may be distended.
7. Respiratory system.
   Findings are comparable to those of the nonpregnant state.
8. Gastrointestinal system.
   a. Appetite varies according to the individual.
   b. Bowel motility decreases following pregnancy, as the birth of the baby has resulted in a lessening of intraabdominal pressure. Gas accumulation may give cramps.
   c. Hemorrhoids may appear externally or increase in size following the birth event.
9. Reproductive system.
   a. Fundus should remain firm throughout the puerperium, with involution proceeding at rate of approximately one fingerbreadth per day (see Figure 9-1).
   b. Discomfort ("afterpains") associated with uterine involution is usually more pronounced in multiparas.

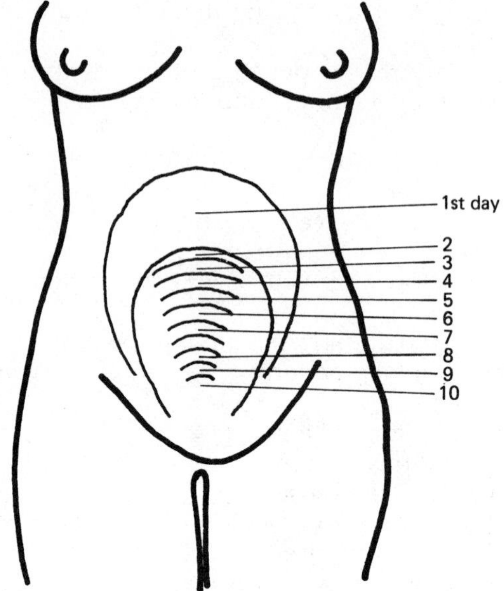

Figure 9-1 Descent of the uterus (involution). (Courtesy of the Carnation Company.)

   c. Inspect genital area with woman in both supine and side-lying positions. Perineum may be intact or have an episiotomy or repaired lacerations. Muscle tone is usually impaired. Check episiotomy site for redness, edema, ecchymosis, discharge, and approximation. Note any vulvar varicosities. Vaginal rugae return by 3 weeks post partum.
   d. Lochia (bloody vaginal discharge) should be bright red (lochia rubra) for about 4 days, then brownish pink (lochia serosa) for about 4 more days. A whitish yellow discharge (lochia alba) may continue until the woman resumes menses.
   e. External cervical os closes, slowly, admitting only a fingertip by the end of the first week post partum. The external os thereafter assumes the characteristic "fish mouth" shape of a woman who has borne a child.
10. Urinary system.
   a. Urethral edema subsequent to a traumatic or forceps delivery is common and may lead to difficulty voiding.

   b. Bladder tone may be relaxed; increased capacity and decreased sensitivity may lead to bladder fullness and distention or incomplete voiding.
   c. Diuresis should be expected, as the 2 or 3 L of extracellular fluid retained in pregnancy is excreted. If the client received prolonged administration of oxytocin, diuresis may be delayed.
11. Musculoskeletal system.
   a. Sore muscles in neck, back, arms, and/or legs are common from exertion of pushing.
   b. Abdominal muscles may be lax from distention due to pressure from the products of conception during pregnancy.
   c. Diastasis of the abdominal recti muscles (separation in midline of two abdominal muscles) is common. (See Fig. 9-7)
12. Cardiovascular system.
   a. Legs may have varicosities and/or edema as sequelae of pregnancy. Inspect and palpate for temperature, color, symmetry, and general condition.
   b. Positive Homan's sign may indicate thrombophlebitis.
   c. Increased progesterone during pregnancy predisposes women to blood-clotting problems.

Mental and Emotional Status

Usually assessment of a client's mental status can be readily obtained through the psychosocial history (see Chapter 5) and observations listed under general appearance. Additional information would be required when behaviors displayed indicate anxiety; depression; alterations in orientation, memory, perception, thought processes and content; inability to make judgments; inability to meet responsibilities of daily living; and difficulty in establishing and maintaining interpersonal relationships.

The birth experience drains physical and emotional energy. Mood swings are common, ranging from euphoria to tearfulness. Stress is increased by the many physiologic changes occurring in the body as it returns to a nonpregnant state and the mother begins to adjust to the increased responsibilities and role changes associated with the birth of a baby. All previous relationships experience at least a shift in emphasis. Jealousy may appear in response to the baby's presence, creating conflict within the family constellation, such as between husband/wife, parent/child, master/pet, spouse/in-laws. Excitement over the birth event as well as the mother's need to repeatedly recall experiences encountered during the process of labor and delivery often masks weariness.

Major emotional adjustments occurring during the early puerperium have been described by Rubin as the phases of "taking in" and "taking hold". The taking-in phase usually lasts 2 to 3 days. During this time the woman's behavior is characterized by dependency and passivity. The mother is trying to integrate her new experiences. She follows suggestions readily, is preoccupied with her own needs, especially with regard to food and sleep, and avoids decision making. As the mother starts to take hold, she begins to initiate caretaking responsibility for herself and her baby. She strives to gain control over her bodily functions and the change in her life situation. Although she may question her competence and seem overzealous in asking questions and seeking information, her concern is for excellence and being a "good" mother. Transitory depression, postpartum or maternal "blues", is frequently associated with the puerperium. It may be manifested by unexplained feelings of sadness, tearfulness, difficulty sleeping, or anorexia. Although the mother may experience this depression while in the hospital, it usually occurs when she has returned to her home (as so many new mothers are discharged from the hospital within 72 h of delivery). Transitory depression is thought to be precipitated by hormonal changes, role changes, environmental pressures, and interpersonal conflict. This depression is reactive in nature and is not to be confused with the more serious condition termed *postpartum psychosis* (Klaus and Kennell, 1982).

Parent-Infant Interaction

The parent-infant interactional processes have been an area of concentrated study by researchers representing various disciplines. Consequently, the literature contains multiple descriptions and definitions. The consensus is that optimum growth of both parents and infants increases as their commitment to each other is enhanced. However, as Campbell and Taylor (1980) insist:

Whether or not early and extended contact leads to other than experiential benefits, it should be offered to all mothers, fathers, and infants. The desirability of early contact stands quite independent of the idea that it is a facilitator of, much less a precondition for, subsequent optimal mother-infant interactions and relationships. Such a notion puts unnecessary constraints on human adaptability and resilience, and it fails to account for satisfactory attachments between most adults and their foster or adopted children, and satisfactory psychosocial development of most premature infants.

The process by which the infant becomes committed to the parent is termed *attachment*. Researchers have identified smiling, sucking, clinging, following, and crying as elements in the attachment process for the infant. The process by which the parent becomes committed to the infant is termed *bonding*. Klaus and Kennel's principles of bonding are presented in Table 9-1.

Diagnostic Tests

1. Hemoglobin should have dropped no more than 2 mg from admission. By the sixth week post partum value should be 12.0 g/dL or above.
2. Hematocrit should have dropped no more than 3 percent from admission. By the sixth week values should be 37 percent ±5.
3. Sedimentation rate may be elevated, clotting time faster.
4. Red blood cells are a normal finding in urine. Specific gravity is usually high, 1.020. There should be no glucose and no bacteria present.

NURSING DIAGNOSES: ACTUAL OR POTENTIAL

1. Fatigue in the immediate postpartum period related to increased expenditure of energy during the labor and delivery processes.
2. Potential: alteration in involutional progression related to decreased uterine muscle tone.
3. Alteration in comfort related to uterine cramps, perineal trauma, hemorrhoids, breast engorgement, nipple trauma.
4. Alteration in urinary elimination patterns related to paraurethral edema, decreased bladder tone and sensitivity, hesitancy associated with dysuria.

TABLE 9-1 PRINCIPLES OF BONDING

1. The phenomenon of mother-to-infant attachment is developed and structured so that a close attachment can optimally be formed to only one person at a time.
2. During the early process of the mother's attachment to her infant, it is necessary that the infant respond to the mother by some signal, such as body or eye movements.
3. People who witness the birth process often become strongly attached to the infant.
4. The processes of attachment and detachment cannot easily occur simultaneously.
5. Early events have long-lasting effects. Anxieties in the first day about the well-being of a baby with a temporary disorder may result in long-lasting concerns that may adversely shape the development of the child.

SOURCE: Klaus, M. H., and Kennell, J. H.: *Bonding: The Beginnings of Parent-Infant Attachment*, Mosby, St. Louis, 1983.

5. Alteration in bowel elimination related to sudden decrease in intraabdominal pressure, relaxed abdominal musculature, decreased fluid and food intake, perineal and rectal discomfort.
6. Potential: impairment of mobility related to weakness, dizziness, discomfort from perineal trauma.
7. Nutritional alteration related to excess weight gain in pregnancy and increased fluid and nutrient requirements for lactation.
8. Potential: delay in parent-infant bonding related to lack of readiness for parenthood.
9. Potential: difficulty in assimilating new roles related to ineffective coping with changes in lifestyle.
10. Potential: delay in performing activities for self and baby associated with insufficient knowledge and experiences.

EXPECTED OUTCOMES

1. The client will establish and maintain effective rest patterns.
2. The uterus will not be palpable above the symphysis pubis by the tenth postpartal day.
3. During hospitalization, the client will experience increased levels of comfort.
4. The client will void within 8 h after delivery and will not experience difficulty in emptying the bladder thereafter.
5. By the third postpartal day, the client will have a soft bowel movement and will maintain a pattern of regularity.
6. The client will be fully mobile by the time of hospital discharge.
7. After the immediate weight loss resulting from delivery, the client will loose an average of 2 lb/week until achieving optimum weight. The client will demonstrate understanding of proper nutrition by selecting and eating foods that meet the recommended daily requirements.
8. Parent(s) will give evidence of positive bonding throughout the puerperium by the type of verbal and nonverbal communication patterns used and behaviors demonstrated in meeting the needs of the infant, such as holding, feeding, cleansing, dressing, stimulation.
9. Parent(s) will give evidence of adapting to new roles by establishing effective communication and support systems, apportioning task assignments, providing for financial security, and readjusting relationships with significant others.
10. The client will satisfactorily demonstrate infant caretaking activities and will verbalize understanding of self-care necessary to establish her own healthful patterns of daily living.

INTERVENTIONS

1. Encourage rest periods based on assessment of individual client needs. Provide an environment conducive to rest. For example: subdue room lighting, provide privacy, turn off TV/radio, disconnect telephone, organize nursing activities for minimal disturbance, encourage mother to rest while baby sleeps, offer back rub and warm drink.
2. Monitor vital signs a minimum of each shift if findings are within normal parameters. (Follow agency protocols for variations.)
3. Monitor involutional progress every hour ×3 upon client's transfer to postpartum unit, then at least once per shift if findings remain within normal ranges. Note the following conditions:
   a. Fundal height, consistency, location.
   b. Lochial color, consistency, amount, and odor.
   c. Condition of perineum—signs of redness, edema, ecchymosis, discharge, and approximation.
4. Implement specific measures to promote comfort.
   a. Uterine cramps and afterpains.
      (1) Position woman as shown in Figure 9-2.
      (2) Encourage frequent voiding.
      (3) Administer analgesic.
      (4) Offer reassurance that cramps will lessen as involution is accomplished; explain relation to breastfeeding.
   b. Perineum.
      (1) Administer treatments such as sitz bath, application of hot/cold, witch hazel compresses, analgesic spray for episiotomy discomfort.

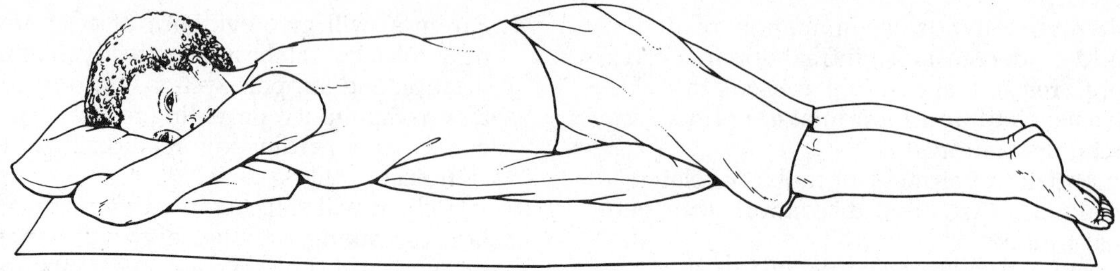

Figure 9-2 Prone position favors uterine descent.

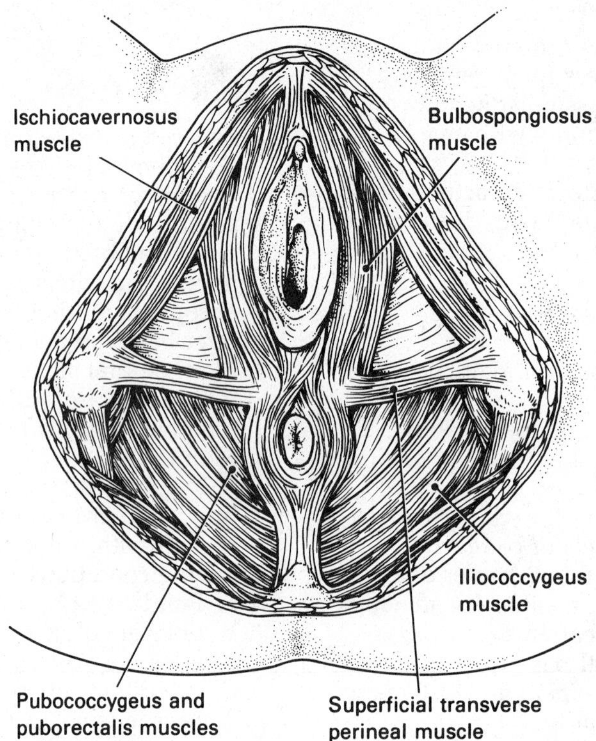

Figure 9-3 Perineal muscles will respond to Kegel exercises. Kegel exercise (also called pelvic floor or perineal tightening): (1) (Easiest to learn when passing urine)—start stream of urine, then voluntarily stop stream before voiding completely. (2) Start and stop stream until sure of the sensation of releasing and tightening muscles around urethra, vagina, rectum. (3) Remind mother to practice Kegel every time she visits bathroom, 5 contractions at least 3 times a day for the rest of her life. (4) Exercise of perineal muscles keeps swelling and therefore soreness at a minimum around sutures, increases blood supply for healing, ensures good pelvic floor support as prevention of incontinence problems as an older woman, and provides the basis for maximum pleasure during sexual stimulation and intercourse.

(2) Teach perineal care.
(3) Encourage Kegel exercise (see Figure 9-3).
(4) Administer treatments for hemorrhoids, such as sitz bath, witch hazel compresses.
(5) Instruct client to use a rubber ring when she is sitting on a hard chair.
(6) Offer medications—ointments, suppositories, stool softeners, analgesics.

c. Breast engorgement when not breastfeeding.

(1) Teach client to wear supportive bra and to avoid stimulating milk flow.
(2) Demonstrate exercises to reduce engorgement (see Figure 9-4).
(3) Reduce or moderate client's fluid intake.
(4) Apply ice packs to axilla for 15 min and on top of breasts for 15 min every 2–3 h.

d. Breast engorgement when breastfeeding.

(1) Teach client to wear supportive bra.
(2) Show exercises to reduce engorgement (Figure 9-4).

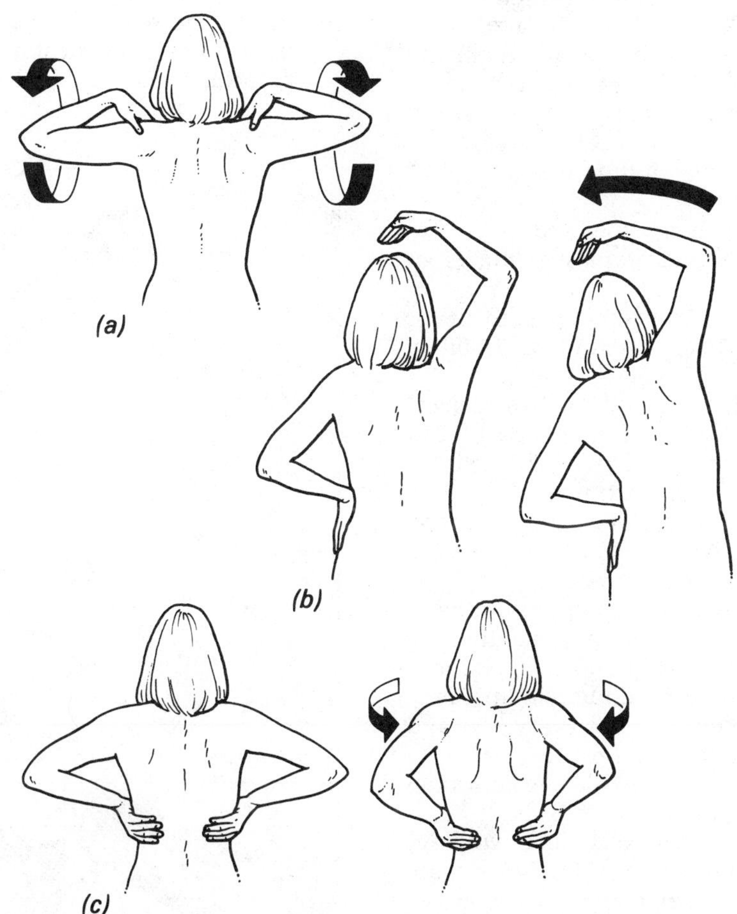

Figure 9-4 Exercises to relieve breast fullness. (*a*) With bra off, place hands on shoulders, raise elbows to shoulder height, and slowly rotate in wide circles. (*b*) Place left hand on hip, raise right arm over head, bend at the waist to left, and return. Repeat on other side. (*c*) Place both hands on rib cage, thumbs front; "wing" elbows as far as possible. Return elbows to sides and repeat.

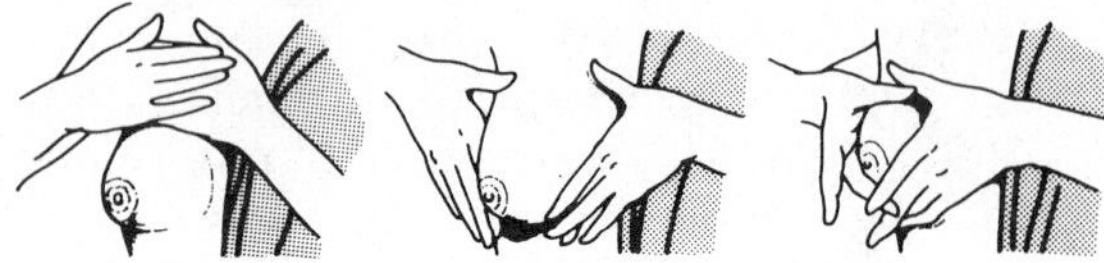

Figure 9-5 Breast massage. Apply lotion to hands so that they will move smoothly over the breasts. Start the hands well above the breast. Exert pressure evenly, thumbs across the top and fingers underneath. Do not touch the areola and nipple, but glide over them. Lift the breast from beneath and permit to drop lightly.

(3) Encourage client to massage breasts (Figure 9-5) after application of moist heat or during shower and manually express milk, or use breast pump.
(4) If additional relief is necessary, apply ice packs after the baby nurses.
(5) Continue liberal fluid intake.

e. Nipple trauma.
(1) Instruct client that support bra should not have plastic linings in cups.
(2) Have client expose nipples to air for 15 min after nursing, to facilitate drying.
(3) Have client expose nipples to light every 3–4 h, positioning breasts 12 in away from a 60–75-W light bulb for at least 15 min each time.
(4) Encourage client to position the baby in a variety of ways at each nursing period (see Figure 9-6).
(5) Show client how to apply ointment for cracked nipples after feeding.
(6) Use nipple shield only if necessary.

5. Monitor and promote bladder elimination.
   a. Encourage client to void every 6 h and measure first voiding.
   b. Encourage client to ambulate to bathroom as soon as condition permits.
   c. Institute measures to induce voiding, such as a comfortable, safe, and private environment; warm bedpan; warm water poured over perineum; warm sitz bath; sound of running water; flush toilet, open faucet.
   d. Provide adequate fluids.
   e. Check for bladder distention.
   f. Catheterize if necessary.
6. Monitor and promote bowel elimination.
   a. Encourage ambulation and exercise.
   b. Provide adequate fluids and roughage in diet. Warm drinks are often beneficial.
   c. Administer laxative or stool softener if indicated.
   d. Give enema or suppository if needed.
7. Facilitate mobility.
   a. Monitor state of equilibrium.
   b. Support as needed upon initial ambulation and during first shower.
   c. Suggest client tighten gluteal and perineal muscles and use a firm surface for sitting.
8. Weigh client at least once by time of discharge.
9. Encourage selection and intake of food and fluids to maintain health and meet the needs of lactation (see Table 9-2).

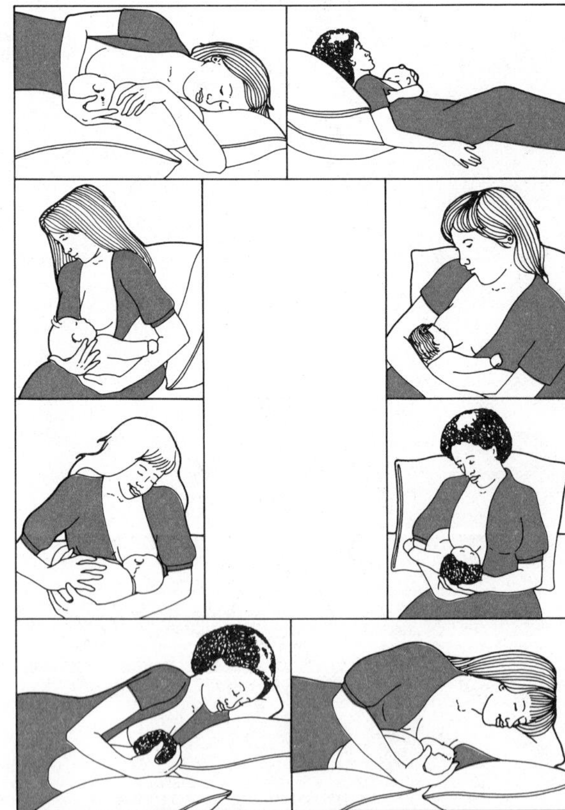

Figure 9-6 Examples of breastfeeding position changes. (Available from Vis-u-lac Breastfeeding Teaching Aids, 635 Bowen Street, Dayton, OH 45410.)

TABLE 9-2 DAILY FOOD GUIDE: THE BASIC FOUR FOOD GROUPS

Food Group	Main Nutrients	Amounts
Dairy Milk, yogurt, genuine cheese; products made with whole or skimmed milk	Calcium Protein Riboflavin	1 serving = 1 cup whole, skim, buttermilk; 8 oz yogurt; 1 oz genuine cheese Nonlactating: 2 or more cups per day Lactating: 4 or more cups per day
Meat Organ meats, beef, lamb, eggs, pork, poultry, veal, fish, dried beans/peas, nuts/seeds, peanut butter	Protein Iron Thiamine Niacin Riboflavin	1 serving = 2 to 3 oz lean boneless, cooked meat; 2 eggs; 1 cup cooked dried legumes; 4 tsp peanut butter 2 or more servings per day
Vegetables and Fruits	Vitamin A Iron Folic acid Vitamin C	1 serving = 1 fruit; 4 oz juice 4 or more servings, including 1 dark green or 1 dark yellow serving (vitamin A) per day and a citrus (vitamin C) food per day.
Grain Foods Bread, rolls, crackers Cereal Rice Pasta Potato Corn	Thiamin Niacin Riboflavin Iron Protein Plus roughage or fiber	1 serving = 1 slice bread; ½ cup pasta or rice; ½ cup cooked cereal; 1 medium potato; 2 graham crackers 4 or more servings per day (whole grain or enriched)

SOURCE: From Williams, S. R.: *Essentials of Nutrition and Diet Therapy*, 3rd ed., Mosby, St. Louis, 1982, p. 152.
NOTE: Add butter, margarine, oils, as desired or needed. Use additional amounts of foods as needed.

10. Provide milieu that fosters positive bonding.
    a. Provide privacy and time for parents to have physical, verbal, and nonverbal contact with their baby.
    b. Encourage parents to actively participate in the care of their baby.
    c. Counsel the mother and father to plan times when each can be alone with the baby.
    d. Avoid methods or language implying professional staff is "expert" and new parents are "inadequate."
11. Explore and discuss parents' expectations and needs related to role adaptation.
    a. Allow time and opportunity for parent(s) to express feelings and concerns about the birth experience and future expectations.
    b. Provide reassurance that condition of mother and infant are within acceptable range, as appropriate.
    c. Encourage parents to listen to each other and freely share joys, fears, frustrations, and hopes.
    d. Explore potential areas of conflict between parents and/or significant others and provide anticipatory guidance relevant to needs.
       (1) Discuss resources for securing help during the first weeks at home. Be financially realistic but urge parents to think of arrangements as an investment. Make referrals as indicated (housekeeping, financial assistance.)
       (2) Encourage father to take advantage of paternity leave plan if available.
       (3) Delineate clearly what can be expected from relatives or "baby nurse" so that potential conflict can be minimized.
       (4) Encourage parents to present a uni-

fied plan of child care to "well meaning" significant others and to support each other if resistance is met.

(5) Establish a plan with parents for receiving visitors at home.

(6) Inform parents of ways to assist newborn's siblings in adapting to the new family member. Encourage sibling visitation, telephone calls to children at home while mother is in the hospital. Provide anticipatory guidance regarding sibling responses to a new baby based upon principles of growth and development.

e. Give positive reinforcement for tasks completed.

f. Arrange for group interaction among parents on maternity unit and encourage attendance at parent workshops in the community.

12. Provide health education and counseling.

a. Self-care.

(1) Discuss the expected physiologic and emotional changes of the puerperium.

(2) Teach client to monitor her own involutional progression; instruct client to massage fundus to keep it well contracted and to observe characteristics of lochial discharge.

(3) Encourage healthful patterns of personal cleanliness, with emphasis upon a daily shower and techniques of breast and perineal care.

(4) Instruct client in measures of alleviating common discomforts, such as uterine cramps, perineal soreness, hemorrhoids, constipation, breast engorgement, nipple trauma.

(5) Teach signs and symptoms of reportable complications.

(a) Fever or chills.

(b) Lochia: foul-smelling, bright-red bleeding beyond the fourth postpartum day, presence of clots or tissue.

(c) Perineum/episiotomy: increased pain, edema, redness; sense of fulness, dragging sensation in the vagina.

(d) Bladder: dysuria, frequency, urgency.

(e) Breasts: marked engorgement, pain, redness.

(f) Any unusual sensation of pain—head, chest, abdomen, extremities.

(g) Prolonged lethargy, weepiness, feeling "blue".

(6) Explore dietary patterns and provide instruction based upon assessment of client's understanding of the basic four food groups: foods, portions, and nutrients provided (see Table 9-2). (See Appendix F)

(7) Teach abdominal toning; review perineal toning (see Figure 9-7).

(8) Discuss plans for meeting rest needs at home.

(9) Explore arrangements for simplifying lifestyle and obtaining maximum help with cooking, shopping, cleaning, laundry, and the like.

(10) Plan for progressive resumption of homemaking and/or employment activities.

(11) Discuss factors relating to resumption of sexual activity; include physiologic and psychologic reactions to sexual stimulation and measures that enhance pleasure and comfort.

(12) Assist in selection of family planning method and/or refer for follow-up care.

(13) Provide information regarding health care resources available to the postpartal family (community agency and/or individual health care providers).

(14) Establish a plan for continued health supervision and maintenance for self-care (Figure 9-8).

b. Infant care.

(1) Review or teach about normal newborn characteristics.

(2) Instruct parents in caretaking activities. Include:

(a) Techniques of breast and bottle feeding.

(b) Methods of formula preparation and storage.

(c) Intake requirements of infant, nutritional needs, weight pattern.

(d) Holding and positioning neonate.

(e) Skin care and bathing.

(f) Cord and circumcision care.

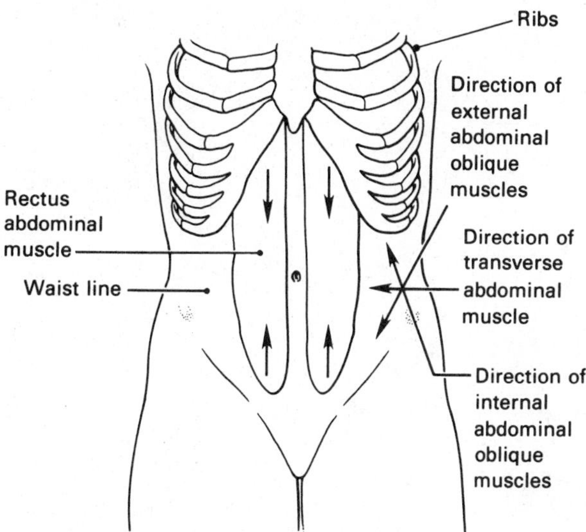

Figure 9-7 Abdominal musculature may need toning exercises. Remind mother of correct posture; contract abdominal muscles while in bed, at least 3 times a day, 5 times each, even if she has had a cesarean. Abdominal toning: (1) Lie flat on back on bed (on floor on carpet or blanket at home) with ankles crossed and hands palms down resting lightly across lower abdomen, elbows on bed but not using elbows for support. (2) Inhale deeply through nose. (3) In deliberate sequence, tighten abdominal, then buttocks, then perineal muscles; hold. (4) Very slowly (to slow count of 8) raise head (not shoulders) as though lifting head to look at toes; at same time very slowly blow air out as though making a candle flame flicker. (5) Very slowly lower head back to bed, continuing to blow out air unless supply depleted. (6) Release all muscles. (7) Repeat to total of 5, morning and evening first day, 6 twice a day the second day, 7 twice a day the third, working up to 10 bid.

(g) Diapering and clothing, stool patterns, voiding pattern, and rashes.
(h) Provision of stimulation and rest; sleep states.
(i) Factors to promote a safe environment, at home and when traveling.
(j) Techniques to determine body temperature and maintain environmental temperature.

(3) Provide information regarding reportable signs and symptoms of illness: what to report, when, and to whom.
(4) Establish a plan for continued health supervision and maintenance for infant.

EVALUATION

Outcome Criteria

1. The client will void spontaneously after delivery and will not show subsequent evidence of urinary dysfunction such as dysuria, urgency, frequency.
2. Lochial characteristics will progress from

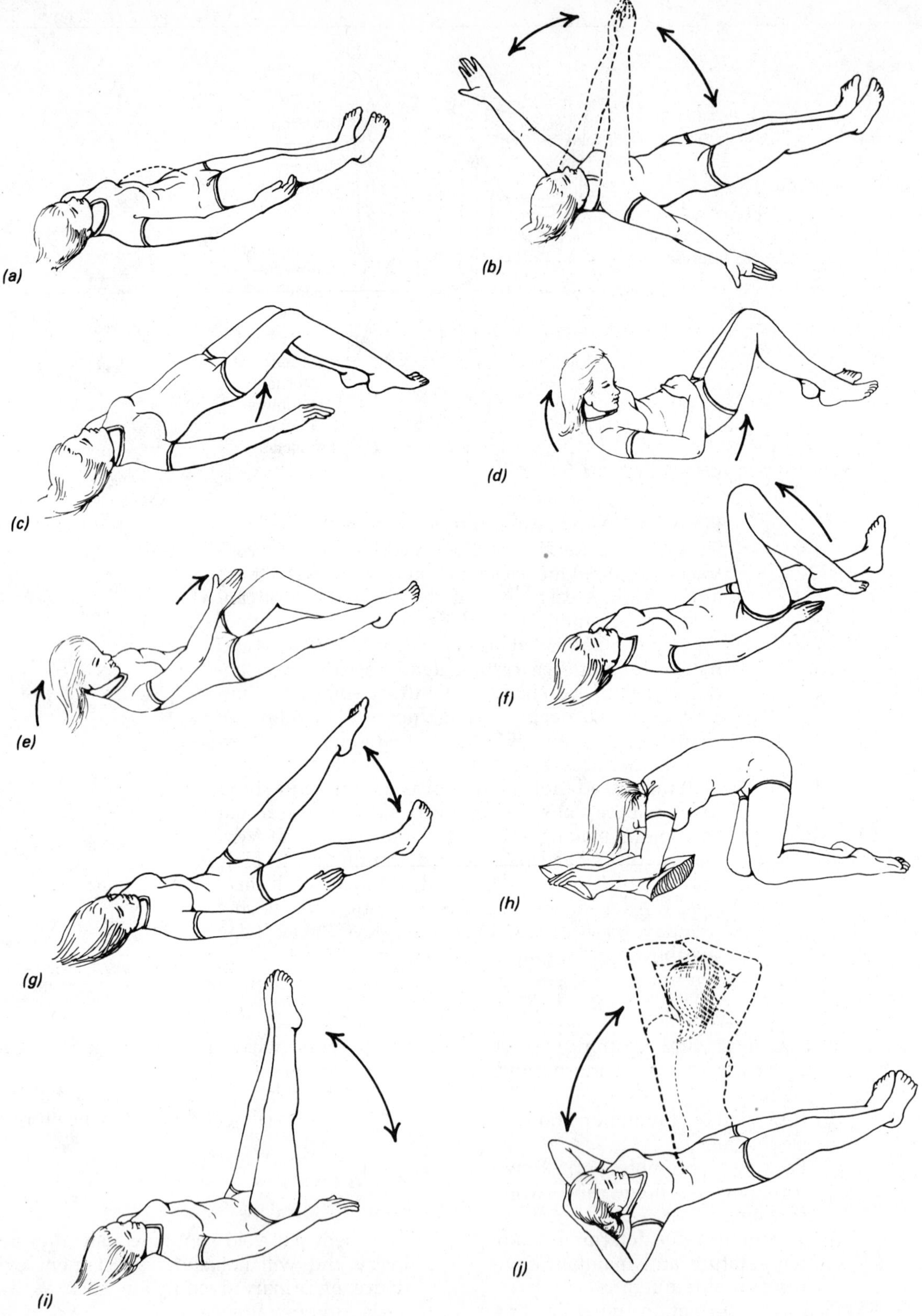

(a)
(b)
(c)
(d)
(e)
(f)
(g)
(h)
(i)
(j)

rubra to serosa to alba; amount of discharge will diminish and cease by the sixth week. Menstrual pattern will be reestablished. Foul odor will not be evident at any time and perineal area will show no signs or symptoms of infection throughout the puerperium.

3. By the sixth postpartum week, breast discomfort will have ceased. In non nursing mothers the breasts will be soft and will have returned to prepregnant size. Lactation will be well established in the nursing mother.
4. The uterus will involute at a rate of one-half fingerbreadth per day and will be only slightly larger than in the prepregnant state by the sixth week postpartum.
5. Bowel function will return to prepregnant pattern of regularity.
6. Abdominal muscle tone will improve; difficulty associated with walking and sitting will have become normal by the sixth week.
7. Immediately after delivery, weight loss will be at least 10 lb and prepregnant weight will be achieved in 6 weeks.
8. With the exception of anticipated variations in vital signs associated with the immediate postpartum period, mother's temperature, pulse, respiration, and blood pressure will be similar to prepregnant baseline levels at the first postpartum visit.
9. Hemoglobin will not be below 12/dL; hematocrit will not be below 37 percent.
10. At time of first postpartum visit, client will have implemented a plan of rest and sleep at home.
11. Parents will respond affirmatively to their baby by establishing eye contact, holding, touching, caressing, soothing, calling by name, and the like. Parent(s) will express reassurance that infant characteristics are "normal."
12. Parent(s) will demonstrate progressive confidence and competence in infant caretaking skills.
13. Parents will make positive statements about keeping their channels of communication open. Parents' verbal reports will reflect positive adaptation to changes in lifestyle, such as establishing new household routines, meeting necessary living expenses, making needed adjustments in relationships with significant others.
14. Sibling adjustment to new family member will progress in a positive manner.
15. Parents will resume sexual activity and will consistently use a family-planning method.
16. Client will implement a plan for continue health care supervision and maintenance for herself and infant.

←

Figure 9-8 Recommended postpartal exercises. (Note: Each exercise is to be repeated four times, twice daily, with a new exercise added each day.) (*a*) First day: Breathe in deeply; expand the abdomen. Exhale slowly, hissing; draw in abdominal muscles forcibly. (*b*) Second day: Lie flat on the back with the legs slightly apart. Hold arms at right angles to the body; slowly raise the arms, keeping the elbows stiff. Touch hands together and gradually return arms to their original position. (*c*) Third day: Lie flat on the back with the arms at the sides. Draw the knees up slightly. Arch the back. (*d*) Fourth day: Lie flat on the back with the knees and hips flexed. Tilt the pelvis inward and contract the buttocks tightly. Lift the head while contracting the abdominal muscles. (*e*) Fifth day: Lie flat on back with the legs straight. Raise the head and one knee slightly. Then reach for, but do not touch, the knee with the opposite hand. Alternate with the right and left hand. (*f*) Sixth day: Slowly flex the knee and then the thigh on the abdomen. Lower the foot to the buttock. Straighten and lower the leg to the floor. (*g*) Seventh day: Raise first the right and then the left leg as high as possible. Keep the toes pointed and the knee straight. Lower the leg gradually, using the abdominal muscles but not the hands. (*h*) Eighth day: Rest on the elbows and knees, keeping the upper arms and legs perpendicular with the body. Hump the back upward. Contract the buttocks and draw the abdomen in vigorously. Relax, breathe deeply. (*i*) Ninth day: Same as seventh day, but raise both legs at the same time, etc. (*j*) Tenth day: Lie flat on the back with the arms clasped behind the head. Then sit up slowly. (If necessary, hook feet under furniture.) Slowly lie back. (Reproduced with permission from Benson, R. C., *Handbook of Obstetrics and Gynecology*, Fifth edition, Lange Medical Publications, Los Altos, Calif., 1974.)

CESAREAN DELIVERY

DESCRIPTION

The birth of a fetus through an abdominal and uterine incision is an operative procedure commonly referred to as a *cesarean section*. Over the past few years the rate has steadily risen from 10 percent in the 1960s to 20 percent in 1980. All the following factors, alone and in combination, have been identified as contributing to deciding for a cesarean birth: placenta previa, preeclampsia, herpes virus type 2 infection, fetopelvic disproportion, fetal distress, abruptio placentae, maternal diabetes, Rh disease (erythroblastosis fetalis), and previous cesarian surgery. Additionally, some argue that the following factors have added to the increased rate of cesarean births: threat of malpractice ("defensive obstetrics"), emphasis in medical education on technologically oriented labor and birth, expansion of conditions for which a cesarean is the preferable birth method (e.g. breech presentation, atypical labor), economic/insurance coverage factors, and a change in the characteristics of the childbearing population (fewer women having many fewer babies at an older age; those with severe medical conditions now able to carry to term who were not previously able to do so).

Maternal and perinatal mortality and morbidity are higher for cesarean birth than for vaginal birth, both because of the conditions that led to the surgery and because of the increased risks associated with surgery and anesthesia. Common incision sites are the classical (vertical skin and vertical uterine incision) and the low cervical/Pfannenstiel "bikini" (horizontal incision through both skin and lower uterine segment). During the postpartal period the woman who has had a cesarean birth must receive both postsurgical and postdelivery care.

ASSESSMENT

Health History

1. Review prenatal record, noting any major health problem(s) occurring during pregnancy, history of previous cesarean delivery (see prenatal history).
2. Review labor, delivery and recovery room records noting indication for cesarean birth, status at time of transfer from recovery room to postpartal unit, status of neonate.

Physical Assessment

1. Client may be sleeping or drowsy from the effects of anesthesia/analgesia or may be experiencing pain and discomfort.
2. Vital signs stable with baseline data obtained from recovery room records.
3. Fundus firm, midline, at the level of the umbilicus or one fingerbreadth above ubilicus.
4. Lochia rubra, moderate amount, no foul odor.
5. Abdominal incision should not show signs of tissue separation, drainage, redness, unusual swelling or bruising. If dressing has been applied, it should be properly secured, no drainage noted.
6. IV fluids are usually administered 24–48 h postoperatively or
   a. Until client is retaining fluids taken by mouth, or
   b. Until bowel sounds are present.
7. Bowel sounds should be active by the third postoperative day.
8. Lung fields should be clear upon auscultation.
9. Indwelling catheter should be patent, draining at least 30 mL/h.
10. Client may show signs of grieving if cesarean birth was an emergency, baby is ill or defective, or baby did not survive.

Diagnostic Tests

Hemoglobin and hematocrit to follow, as unexpected drop in these parameters is not unusual.

NURSING DIAGNOSES: ACTUAL OR POTENTIAL

1. Alteration in comfort level secondary to tissue trauma, uterine cramps.
2. Potential: delay in involutional progression secondary to decreased uterine muscle tone.
3. Altered fluid and nutrition status related to nausea, vomiting, restricted fluid and food intake.
4. Impairment of urinary elimination related to decreased bladder tone, use of catheters.
5. Impaired bowel function related to decreased intestinal motility, decreased fluid and food intake, effects of immobility.

6. Altered respiratory function secondary to anesthesia, analgesics, immobility.
7. Potential: impairment of skin integrity related to poor wound healing.
8. Alteration in parenting related to separation of mother and infant.
9. Lowered self-esteem secondary to change in expected mode of delivery.

EXPECTED OUTCOMES

1. Vital signs will remain in a normal range.
2. Pain and discomfort will be minimized.
3. Effective rest pattern will be maintained.
4. Uterine involution will progress at the rate of approximately one-half fingerbreadth per day; lochial characteristics will remain in a normal range throughout the course of the puerperium.
5. If present, nausea and vomiting will cease and client will progress to unrestricted fluid and dietary intake.
6. Client will void within 8 h after removal of indwelling catheter and not experience difficulty in renal or bladder function.
7. Tissue healing will not be interrupted by adverse factors such as infectious organisms.
8. Abdominal distention will be minimized and bowel elimination will resume by the third postoperative/postpartal day.
9. Lung fields will sound clear throughout the puerperium.
10. Client will understand and comply with care regimens such as deep breathing, coughing, splinting abdomen, progressively ambulating, medications, and the like.
11. Client will verbalize positive feelings about cesarean birth and accept the neonate regardless of the baby's health status.

INTERVENTIONS

1. Institute measures to promote comfort and rest and minimize pain.
   a. Provide a quiet, nonstimulating environment.
   b. Reassure clients about her postoperative condition and status of neonate as appropriate to her situation.
   c. Administer pain medication as ordered.
   d. Implement comfort measures such as clean, wrinkle-free bed linens, positional changes, and backrub if desired by client.
2. Monitor vital signs according to client's responses. If stable, follow agency policy for postoperative/postpartal period. Report changes indicative of shock, infection immediately.
3. Monitor height, consistency, and location of fundus. To minimize discomfort in the immediate recovery period palpate fundus $\frac{1}{2}$ after administration of pain medication. Discomfort may also be alleviated if fundus is palpated from the side of the abdomen.
4. Monitor lochial characteristics.
5. Monitor incisional site, noting condition of wound and dressing, characteristics of drainage. If dressing has been removed, inspect incision for tissue separation, hematoma formation, drainage, redness, or other signs of infection.
6. Maintain intravenous infusion—check patency of tubing, rate of flow; observe for signs of infiltration.
7. Administer ice chips, surgical fluids; advance diet as ordered.
8. Indwelling catheter to drainage system. After catheter is removed, measure and record at least two voidings. Check for bladder distention, dysuria, frequency, urgency.
9. Maintain accurate intake and output record.
10. Administer antiemetics if nausea and vomiting are present. Provide mouth care.
11. Change position q2h. Teach and encourage progressive ambulation.
12. Monitor bowel function. Auscultate for return of bowel sounds, check for abdominal distention. Administer enema and/or suppositories as ordered.
13. Auscultate lung fields daily. Encourage deep breathing and coughing q2h for the first 24 h postoperative, then tid. Teach client to splint incision to reduce discomfort during such maneuvers. Instruct client in the use of incentive spirometer, IPPB (intermittent positive pressure breathing) if indicated.
14. Administer prophylactic antibiotics as ordered.
15. Offer positive reinforcement for all client's attempts to comply with care regimens or to engage in self-care activities.
16. Maintain regular care of postpartal woman as appropriate to the client's physical and psychosocial status. (See Vaginal Delivery earlier in this chapter.)
17. Arrange for mother to see baby as soon as possible according to status of both mother

and baby. Afford mother opportunity to touch and examine baby as desired. Breastfeeding can be started usually after 24 h. Use pillows and side-lying position to promote comfort. Instruct mother in use of analgesics and other drugs if breastfeeding is the chosen method. If baby is in the intensive care nursery, mother may be taken via wheelchair to the unit as her condition allows (usually after 24 h). Mother should be encouraged to participate in infant care activities appropriate to the situation.

18. Encourage client and family members to verbalize concerns regarding cesarean birth.
19. Assess knowledge and skills regarding self and infant care. Develop and implement a teaching plan based on client needs (see Vaginal Delivery).

EVALUATION

Outcome Criteria

1. Vital signs will remain within normal parameters.
2. Uterine involution will progress at the expected rate.
3. Skin integrity will be restored without complications.
4. Fluid and dietary intake will be adequate to maintain and promote well-being.
5. Bowel function will be restored before hospital discharge and difficulty in urinary elimination will not be experienced.
6. Client will be fully mobile by time of hospital discharge and independently engaged in self-care and infant care activities.
7. Client will comply with plan of continued health supervision for self and baby; she will understand the implications for subsequent pregnancies and will use family planning until fully recovered.

Complications

PUERPERAL HEMORRHAGE

A usually preventable cause of maternal death is hemorrhage, which may occur suddenly or result from a significant total blood loss from moderate but persistent bleeding. *Early* postpartum hemorrhage is defined as occurring within the first 24 h after birth; *late* postpartum hemorrhage occurs after the first 24 h to the twenty-eighth day. Average blood loss from birth is 200 mL; any amount greater than 500 mL is considered postpartum hemorrhage. The following conditions intensify the risk of excess bleeding: retained placental fragments or membranes, unrecognized lacerations, hematoma, infection, blood coagulation defects such as a vitamin K deficiency, or a hyperthyroid condition, uterine inversion, and—most significantly—uterine atony. Uterine atony is most likely if there has been an overdistended uterus from a large baby, multiparity, or hydramnios, precipitate or prolonged labor, uterine tumors, maternal exhaustion, poor nutritional state, dehydration, deep general anesthesia, a traumatic operative delivery, or obstetrical mismanagement of the third stage.

Assessment

1. Observe and record amount of vaginal bleeding (pad count, weigh pads). Dark blood would likely be venous, for example, from varices or lacerations. Bright blood would likely be arterial, perhaps from a deep cervical laceration. Lack of clotting might indicate a coagulation problem.
2. Inspect external genitalia for lacerations, hematomas.
3. Client may complain of persistent pain, fullness in vagina, backache; she may show restlessness and/or a wide range of emotional responses (calm to a state of panic.)
4. Monitor vital signs, check for bladder distention.
5. Review laboratory results (Hgb, Hct, prothrombin time).

Revised Outcomes

1. Hemorrhage will be controlled.
2. Client's blood pressure and pulse will be in expected range of normal; cardiovascular status will be supported.
3. Client will be aware of her own health status and plan of management.

Interventions

1. For nursing management of the client in shock, see Chapter 48.
2. If uterus is not displaced by full bladder, massage uterus or apply bimanual compression.
3. In collaboration with physician, determine site of bleeding and intravenous fluid and/or blood replacement.
4. Administer oxytoxic agents or other medications as ordered.
5. Prepare for such tests as blood type, crossmatch for additional units of blood as per policy of agency. (See Table 18-3.)
6. Prepare client for actual or potential plans for surgery. Explain all procedures, provide com-

fort and reassurance as appropriate to the situation. Do not leave client alone if she is actively bleeding.

7. Keep family members and significant others informed of client's progress. Provide necessary support.
8. Provide for the baby's father or other family member to be involved in baby's care until mother recovers.

Reevaluation and Follow-up

1. Uterus remained firmly contracted, and repaired lacerations have healed.
2. Blood pressure and pulse were stabilized.
3. Involutional process and lochial characteristics according to an acceptable pattern.
4. Hemoglobin maintained at a minimum of 12 g/dL and hematocrit at 37 percent.
5. Client has complied with plan of follow-up care.

PUERPERAL INFECTION

This condition exists when the client's temperature is over 38°C (100.4°F) in consecutive readings for 48 h, after the first 24 h. In the initial recovery period, a slight temperature may indicate excitement, anxiety, dehydration, beginning lactation, or the start of morbidity. Assessment of potential causes of temperature changes is a key team effort. A client's predisposition to developing an infection arises from anemia, maternal exhaustion, stress, or trauma that allows her own bacteria to become virulent. In addition, poor nutrition, multiple or aggressive manipulations during labor or birth—with or without poor aseptic technique—or prolonged rupture of membranes can lead to infection. Some evidence suggests that increased use of internal electronic fetal monitoring may also increase the infection rate.

Bacteria are of three main types: hemolytic streptococci, mixed anaerobic bacteria normally present in the vagina, or anaerobic bacteria present in the GI tract (*Clostridium* or *Escherichia coli* infections). Infection may originate at any site of the reproductive tract. It may be localized or become generalized. For example, it may be present as endometritis and remain as endometritis until resolution; or, an infected perineum may lead to endometritis, which in turn may lead to pelvic cellulitis, ultimately resulting in peritonitis.

Assessment

1. Client may or may not complain of pain or discomfort.
2. Abdominal incision or episiotomy appear red, edematous, warm to touch. Tissue of repaired lacerations may appear swollen.
3. Wound discharge may or may not be present plus separation of wound along incision line.
4. WBC count may be normal (10,000 to 15,000 per millimeter) or may be elevated.
5. Causative agent must be identified through culture of body orifice, wound, or blood.
6. Urine culture must be done to rule out a urinary tract infection.
7. With an infected perineum, discomfort on voiding may be present when urine touches the affected area.
8. Severe infections may be characterized by the following conditions.
   a. Lochia ranges from normal appearance to foul-smelling, copious brown.
   b. Chills, fever from 101 to 103°F., often spiking.
   c. Anorexia, vomiting, malaise, diarrhea, lethargy may be present.
   d. Client may complain of severe afterpains or abdominal tenderness; abdomen may be rigid; in this case lochia suppression may occur.

Revised Outcomes

1. Client health will be promoted and spread of infection will be prevented.
2. Fluid and electrolyte balance will be maintained.
3. Vital signs will remain within normal limits.
4. Involution will progress within normal rate.
5. Client will know signs and symptoms to report immediately.
6. Client and family will understand her condition and will cooperate with plan of care.
7. Maternal-infant bonding will be fostered within limits of expected separation due to institution policy.

Intervention

1. Usually use isolation technique for gown, linen, pads, dressings if organism is identified in isolation category. (See Table 12-2.)
2. Monitor intake and output. Urge liberal fluid intake of 2,000 mL/day, plus IV fluids. Provide appealing foods that are high in vitamin C and protein.
3. Administer antibiotics, analgesics, and antipyretics as ordered. Observe for expected and untoward effects. IV intermittent antibiotic therapy is usual.
4. Apply local heat: sitz bath, lamp.

5. Monitor vital signs every 4 h.
6. Observe and report any changes in incision, lochial characteristics, client's level of comfort, ability to rest.
7. To stimulate milk production if breastfeeding, help client to manually stimulate breasts or to use electric breast pump.
8. Review self-care and teach reportable signs and symptoms.

Reevaluation and Follow-up

1. Client responded to therapy and became free from infection.
2. Client understood reportable signs and symptoms of recurrence and engaged in positive self-care activities, such as proper cleanliness, good diet, keeping appointments.
3. Involution progressed at a normal rate.
4. Vital signs were stabilized within normal limits.
5. Fluid and electrolyte balance was maintained.
6. Any adverse effects arising from mother/infant separation were resolved.

BREAST INFECTION

This condition occurs in 1 percent of recently delivered women, usually after the fifth postpartum day to the third week, but may occur any time during lactation. Entry of bacteria through cracked or fissured nipple tissue is possible. Handwashing by those assisting the mother with early feeding may prevent initial episodes. Primiparas are especially vulnerable, as inexpert breastfeeding may lead to incomplete emptying of the breast ducts.

Causative organisms are gram-positive cocci, many of which are resistant to commonly used antibiotics. The antibiotic of choice would be one that does not pass into breast milk easily, such as Keflex, but many of the newer semisynthetic antistaphylococcal penicillins are prescribed.

Assessment

1. Mild local pain, tenderness in breast, swollen axillary glands.
2. Red, swollen area on breast is usually unilateral.
3. Fever and chills plus headache, malaise.
4. Diffuse cellulitis may localize into an abscess.
5. Positive culture of discharge from open abscess drainage or needle aspiration.

Revised Outcomes

1. Infection will abate.
2. Breastfeeding will resume.

Interventions

1. Reinforce careful handwashing techniques by mother and hospital personnel.
2. Reinforce principles of breast care, such as hygiene, firm supportive bra.
3. Administer prescribed antibiotic, analgesic. Interpret drug action to reduce mother's fears of harm to infant.
4. Local application of heat q 3 h with special attention to swollen areas.
5. If institution policy permits, have client continue breastfeeding, with frequency of at least q3h. If client is at home, encourage her to continue breastfeeding unless breasts are too sore; if so, suggest use of breast pump for several feedings.
6. Reinforce techniques of breastfeeding, such as changing baby's mouth position (Figure 9-5). Massaging from breast toward nipple over any swollen areas during nursing, without disturbing baby's sucking, will empty the ducts.
7. Reassure client that this is a temporary condition, that successful breastfeeding can be achieved and she need not become discouraged.

Reevaluation and Follow-up

1. All signs and symptoms of infection disappeared within a week.
2. Subsequent examinations revealed no recurrence.
3. Mother demonstrated proper techniques of breast care.
4. Successful breastfeeding reestablished.

URINARY TRACT INFECTION

Cystitis is a relatively common postpartum complication. Symptoms are fever, frequency, urgency, dysuria, and costal-vertebral angle tenderness. The offending organisms usually are from the coliform family. Clients predisposed to cystitis are those who have a history of bladder infections, who have sustained trauma to the bladder or urethra during delivery, or who had frequent or improper catheterization or general or conduction anesthesia. Administration of large volumes of intravenous fluids during labor without subsequent bladder care often leads to bladder distention and bacteriuria. Detailed treatment is presented in Chapter 32.

THROMBOPHLEBITIS

An inflammation in the deep pelvic or femoral veins may appear as late as 7 days after giving birth. Both blood fibrinogen content and the platelet count increase in the puerperium; therefore, there is increased danger of thrombophlebitis developing. Risk increases with maternal age over 30, multiparity, operative delivery, obesity, previous history of thrombophlebitis, or thromboembolic disease. Further, women on estrogen for suppression of lactation or those who need bed rest are at greater risk for clot formation. In the presence of thrombophlebitis, the affected extremity may feel tender and warm and may become progressively edematous; conversely, the extremity may feel pale and cool. Homan's sign is positive in 20 percent of cases. Should a thrombus become dislodged, cardiac or pulmonary embolism may result. Treatment of thrombophlebitis is discussed in Chapter 30.

PSYCHOLOGICAL DISORDERS

Giving birth and coping with the stress of motherhood (and fatherhood) are not causes of emotional breakdown but may be precipitating factors. Having "the blues" or "the weepies" is a common, transient experience during the first 10 days post partum; 10 percent of new mothers may have a period of true depression. Despondency may be intensified to a feeling of helplessness if complicated by anxiety, exaggerated fatigue, and poor nutrition from anorexia. Apathy, lack of interest in the newborn, and a total absence of tears are all serious danger signs. With a previous history of long-term depression the prognosis is poor. The usual expectation, however, would be for a complete recovery if the woman and her family receive needed help. For a discussion of treatment, see the discussion of psychiatric depression in Chapter 36.

REFERENCES

Bowlby, J.: "The Nature of a Child's Tie to His Mother," *International Journal of Psychoanalysis,* **39**:350–373, 1958.

Campbell, S. B. G., and Taylor, P. M.: "Bonding and Attachment: Theoretical Issues," in P. M. Taylor (ed.), *Parent-Infant Relationships,* Grune and Stratton, New York, 1980, p. 12.

Kennell, J. H., and Rolnick, A. M.: "Discussing Problems in Newborn Babies with Their Parents," *Pediatrics,* **26**:832–838, 1960.

Klaus, M. S., and Kennell, J. H.: *Maternal Infant Bonding,* Mosby, St. Louis, 1976, p. 14.

BIBLIOGRAPHY

Bowlby, J.: "Nature of a Child's Tie to His Mother," *International Journal of Psychoanalysis,* **39**:350–373, 1958.

Cannon, R. B.: "The Development of Maternal Touch During Early Mother-Infant Interaction," *Journal of Obstetric, Gynecologic, and Neonatal Nursing,* **8**:2:28, March/April 1977. A research study providing a useful assessment tool.

Cogan, R.: "Postpartum Depression." *I.C.E.A. Review,* **4**:2, August 1980. A six-page abstract of a number of articles with commentary by Niles Newton.

Cohen, N. W.: "Minimizing Emotional Sequellae of Cesarean Childbirth," *Birth Family Journal,* **4**(3):114, 1977. C/SEC, Inc., recommends changes for cesarean parents that will lead to promotion of positive feelings regarding their childbirth experience.

Curry, M. A. H.: "Contact During the First Hour with the Wrapped or Naked Newborn: Effect on Maternal Attachment Behavior at 36 Hours and Three Months," *Birth Family Journal,* **6**(4):227, 1979. Gives a range of options for infant contact with new mothers in a variety of circumstances and readiness for intimacy.

Donaldson, N. E.: "The Postpartum Follow-up Nurse Clinician," *Journal of Obstetric, Gynecologic, and Neonatal Nursing,* **10**(4):249, July/August 1981. Excellent coverage of the common stressors in the fourth trimester, with theory and practice for intervention.

Duncan, M., et al.: *Maternity Care: The Nurse and the Family,* 2d ed., Mosby, St. Louis, 1981. Comprehensive, modern textbook, dealing with the most up-to-date art and science and philosophy of nursing practice in obstetrics.

Ezrati, J. B., and Gordon, H.: "Puerperal Mastitis: Causes, Prevention, Management," *Journal of Nurse-Midwifery,* **24**(6):3 November/December 1979. A comprehensive presentation of this subject, aiming to decrease pathologically based breastfeeding failure.

Gray, J. D., et al.: "Prediction and Prevention of Child Abuse," *Seminars in Perinatology,* **3**(1):85, January 1979. Perinatal assessment provides accurate predictive information leading to intervention that significantly improves infants' chances of escaping physical harm.

Hawrylyshyn, P. A., et al.: "Risk Factors Associated with Infection Following Cesarean Section," *American Journal of Obstetric and Gynecologic,* **139**(3):294 February 1981. Duration of labor, number of preoperative vaginal examinations, time of membrane rupture, and postoperative anemia effects on infection rates, with recommendations regarding the pros and cons of prophylactic antibiotic use.

Howley, C.: "The Older Primipara." *Journal of Obstetric, Gynecologic, and Neonatal Nursing,* **10**(3):182 May/June 1981. Addresses the particular physical and psychological needs of the older couple.

Jenkins, R. L., and Westhus, N. K.: "The Nurse Role in Parent-Infant Bonding," *Journal of Obstetric, Gynecologic, and Neonatal Nursing,* **10**(2):114 March/April 1981. An overview of parent-infant bonding, with recommendations regarding intervention under an assortment of conditions.

Kennell, J. H., and Rolnick, A.: "Discussing Problems in Newborn Babies with Their Parents," Pediatrics, **26:**832–838, 1960.

Kirkly-Best, E., and Kellner, K. R.: "Grief at Stillbirth: An Annotated Bibliography," *Birth and the Family Journal,* **8**(2):91 1981. A particularly valuable resource for both parents and professionals.

Leander, K., and Grassley, J.: "Making Love after Birth," *Birth and the Family Journal,* **7**(3):181, 1980. Reviews major physical and emotional changes affecting sexual functioning after giving birth, with suggestions for health care professionals in counselling couples.

Marut, J. S.: "The Special Needs of the Cesarean Mother," *Maternal Child Nursing,* **3**(4):202, July/August 1978. Recognizing the distinctive condition of the woman who had an unexpected surgical birth, and how to help her cope with feelings of failure and establish a bond with her newborn.

Miller, D. L., and Baird, S. F.: "Helping Parents to be Parents," *Maternal Child Nursing,* **3**(2):117 Mar/Apr 1978. Parents themselves started a center devoted to helping new parents do their job well. Nursing added expertise to the provision of something special to suit the needs of each one seeking aid.

Pridham, K. F.: "Infant Feeding and Anticipatory Care: Supporting the Adaptation of Parents to Their New Babies," *Maternal Child Nursing,* **10**(2):111, 1981. Using problem-solving skills to learn to synchronize care techniques with the infant's capacities and need for care.

Riordan, J., and Countryman, B. A.: "Basics of Breastfeeding." *Journal of Obstetric, Gynecologic, and Neonatal Nursing,* **9**(4):5, 6, July/August, September/October, November/December 1980. A six-part invaluable series of articles to promote breastfeeding success and avoid potential problems.

Taylor, P. M. (ed.): *Parent-Infant Relationships,* Grune and Stratton, New York, 1980. Monographs describing basic developing processes, influences of professional practices, and relationships at risk for both practitioners and researchers.

Zepeda, M.: "Selected Maternal-Infant Care Practices of Spanish-Speaking Women," *Journal of Obstetric, Gynecologic, and Neonatal Nursing,* **11**(6):371, November/December 1982. Gives a background in variations in Hispanic customs to facilitate health-care intervention and teaching.

10

The Full-Term Infant

Elaine Muller Morris

THE NORMAL FULL-TERM INFANT

DESCRIPTION

The delivery of comprehensive services to the newborn infant and the family represents a unique challenge for neonatal and perinatal health practitioners. As the family awaits the birth of the baby, there may be ambivalence. Parents may have anticipated the numerous changes the birth of the baby will bring, but they often are unprepared for the reality of those changes.

The level of preparation, confidence, and enthusiasm demonstrated by the parents as they assume their new role affects the quality of their interaction with the newborn and thus the infant's emotional well-being. Support by professionals during the critical adjustment period following delivery will assist the parents as they assume the role.

The full-term infant's emergence into the world marks the culmination of an intricate process of fetal growth and development. The 266 ± 8 days of development, plus birth conditions and the baby's inate ability to integrate and modify extrauterine stimuli, will govern the quality of early development. Researchers have confirmed what mothers have known for centuries: a healthy full-term newborn, despite size and inexperience, demonstrates significant physical and emotional abilities. Shortly after birth, the infant is able to see, hear, and respond to stimuli and to interact with the immediate environment and with significant caretakers. For such an aware newborn, the quality of care and early stimuli are factors that influence the future well-being of the infant.

The response of the neonate is especially influenced by his or her state of consciousness. There are six infant states: *quiet sleep, active sleep, drowsy, quietly awake*(alert), *actively awake*(alert), and *crying*. (See Chapter 4 for growth and development and Table 10-1 for descriptions of these states.) Parents need to learn these states in order to understand their infant's behavior. Parent education is at the core of quality family-centered nursing, and the nurse who does not participate in promoting such parenting skills is missing an essential aspect of neonatal care.

PREVENTION

Health Promotion

1. Education for a healthy outcome to pregnancy.
2. Media use to communicate information about toxic substances.
3. Early prenatal evaluation and care.
4. Avoidance of exposure to environmental teratogenic agents.
5. Genetic counseling and screening in cases of potential carriers of genetic diseases.
6. Promotion of general health before conception and during pregnancy.

Population at Risk

1. Young unwed mothers receiving poor care or support during pregnancy.

TABLE 10-1 INFANT STATES

State	Characteristics
Quiet sleep	Regular respirations and heart rate; absence of body or eye movements; very little will disturb infant in this phase.
Active sleep (REM sleep)	Phasic limb movements; irregular respiration; eye movement; startles spontaneously; infant can be awakened, usually to cry.
Drowsy	Activity level varied; infant appears to be dozing; delayed neurologic response if being tested; responds to repeated stimuli by becoming more awake.
Quietly awake	Quiet motor activity of arms and legs; opens and closes eyes; reacts to noises with startles; intermittent fussing.
Actively awake	Alert; focuses attention on stimuli; interested in communication with care given.
Crying	Tachycardia; flushed; active motion of all limbs; infant does not pay much attention to attempts to soothe.

SOURCE: Adapted from Prechtl, H. F. R., et al: "Behavioral State Cycles in Abnormal Infants," *Developmental Medicine and Child Neurology*, **15**:606, October 1973.

2. Mothers with high-risk conditions preceding the pregnancy, such as hypertension.
3. Women who are substance abusers.
4. Women who have or develop infections during pregnancy.
5. Women who have poor parenting skills or an inadequate support network.

Screening

1. Prenatal care and counseling.
2. Screening tests with maternal serum or urine or with amniotic fluid for testing fetal condition.
3. Ultrasound evaluation of fetal size and condition.
4. Rubella titer for all prepregnant women; immunization if not already immune.

ASSESSMENT

Maternal and Paternal History

1. Review available medical data and determine maternal and paternal history of heart disease, diabetes, hypertension, and pre- and postconception health problems, especially those involving genetically transmitted problems.
2. Obtain history of prior pregnancies and their outcomes.
3. Ascertain the age of the parents, occupation, level of education, and level of preparation for childbirth and parenting.
4. Determine who are the support persons for this family (see Chapter 5).

Maternal Prenatal Course

1. Check parity and EDD. Note results of special tests and procedures: ultrasound, nonstress tests, oxytocin challenge tests, and amniocentesis.
2. Note prenatal medical problems and interventions. Were there any infections?
3. Note medications taken during pregnancy, especially during first and last trimester. Is there any history of drug abuse?
4. Note results of laboratory tests: maternal blood type, and Rh factor. Coombs' titers if Rh negative, rubella titers, toxoplasmosis titer, serology, hemoglobin, hematocrit in last month, serial estriol levels, urinalysis.

Course and Outcome of Labor and Delivery

1. Determine length of labor in each stage. Was there presence of fetal distress?
2. Note the time of membrane rupture and quality of fluid. Note if there were any signs of maternal infection during labor. More than 4 h of membrane rupture may allow ascending infection, especially for active herpes.
3. What was the type of delivery? Was there any

mechanical manipulation, any delay in descent?

4. Note medications administered during labor and delivery, including time-dose interval. Note especially amount of pitocin, dosage of analgesia.

Physical Assessment at Delivery

1. Note general condition.
2. Take Apgar score at 1 and 5 min (Table 10-2). This score should be reflected in infant's condition upon transfer to nursery. An Apgar score that is lower at 5 than at birth indicates progressive acidosis (Table 10-3).
3. Observe for adequacy of respirations and airway patency.
   a. Rate should be not less than 20 to 30 per minute with good exchange. Crying or deep breaths should result in a pink, oxygenated color within 1 min of birth. There may be some bluish color to hands and feet (acrocyanosis) during the first 24 h of life.
   b. Note any changes in color such as pallor, which is usually associated with low hematocrit, or a ruddy plethoric color, which is usually associated with polycythemia and is often seen in large infants of diabetic mothers.
   c. Cry should be vigorous. Weak or high-pitched cry may indicate CNS damage or depression.
   d. Activity depends on birth stress and levels of maternal medication. Note any results of intrauterine stress such as hypotonia, poor sucking, excessive tremors.

TABLE 10-3 CORRELATION BETWEEN APGAR SCORE AND BLOOD pH

Apgar Score (1 min)	pH
1–3	6.9–7.0
4–7	7.0–7.20
8–10	≥7.25

SOURCE: Adapted from Dawes, P. A. M.: "Resuscitation of the Newborn," *American Journal of Nursing*, **74**(1):68, January 1974.

The baby should be awake and alert for 30–40 min after birth.

4. Assess for gestational age within the first few hours to determine maturity of development.
   a. Defer neurologic assessment for gestational age until after 24 h to allow time for complete recovery from birth.
   b. Plot assessed size and characteristics on graph to determine if infant is within norms for age (Figure 10-1):
      AGA—appropriate for gestational age.
      SGA—small for gestational age, below the 10th percentile.
      LGA—large for gestational age, above the 90th percentile.
   c. Use Figure 10-2, the Brazie-Lubchenco chart, to assess characteristics or use the abbreviated chart in Figure 11-1 that is adapted from the work of Dubowitz. Report any discrepancies.

TABLE 10-2 APGAR NEWBORN SCORING SYSTEM

	Score		
Sign	0	1	2
Heart rate	Not detectable	Below 100	Above 100
Respiratory effort	Absent	Slow, irregular	Good, crying
Muscle tone	Flacid, limp	Some flexion of extremities	Active motion
Reflex irritability	No response	Grimace[a]	Cough, sneeze[a]
Color[b]	Blue, pale	Extremities blue, body pink	Completely pink

[a] When stimulated by suction in nose.

[b] If the natural skin color of the child is dark, alternative tests for color are applied, such as the color of mucous membranes of the mouth and conjunctiva, the color of the lips, palms, and soles of the feet.

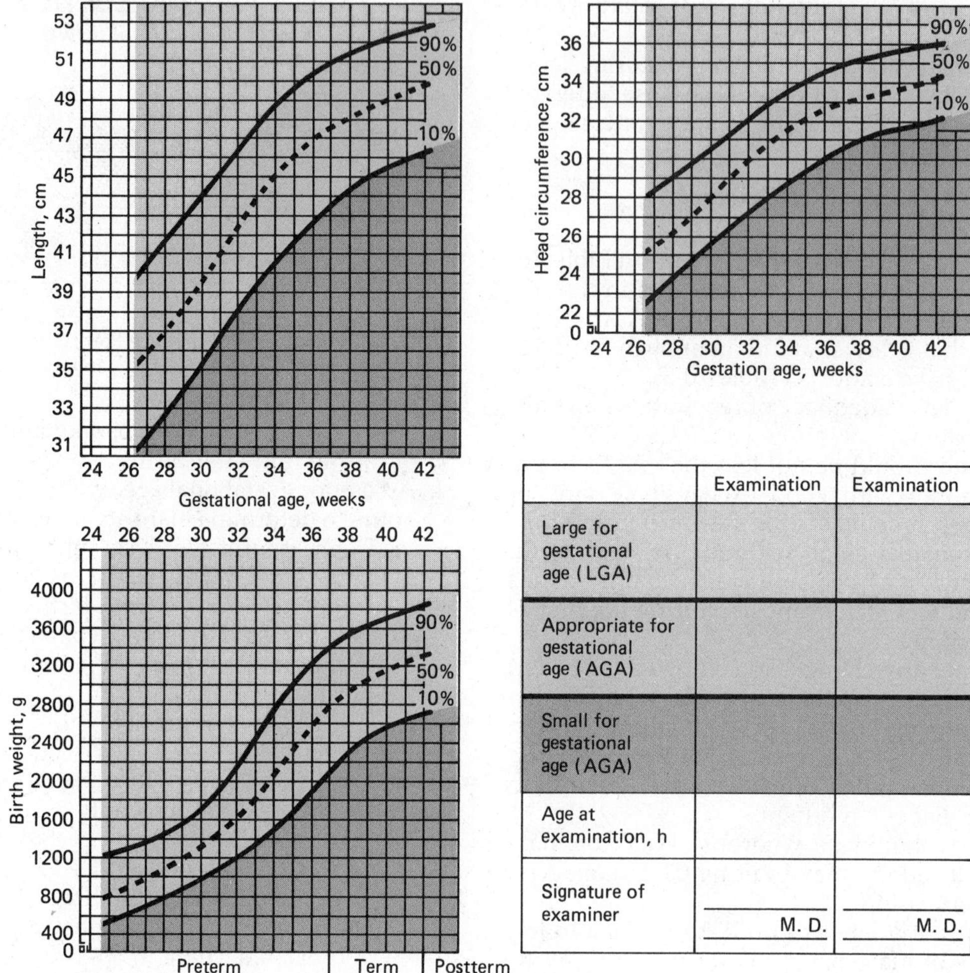

	Examination	Examination
Large for gestational age (LGA)		
Appropriate for gestational age (AGA)		
Small for gestational age (AGA)		
Age at examination, h		
Signature of examiner	M. D.	M. D.

Figure 10-1 Classification of newborns based on maturity and intrauterine growth. (After Lubchenco, L. O., Hansman, C., and Boyd, E., *Pediatrics* **37**:403, 1966; and Battaglia, F. C., and Lubchenco, L. O., *Journal of Pediatrics*, **71**:159, 1967.)

5. Examine infant to determine the presence of normal variations and anomalies. Measure height, weight, and head and chest circumference. See Table 10-4 for normal measurements.
   a. *Head*. Head may be round or molded, depending upon mode of delivery. Should be symmetrical, but there may be edema of the presenting part (caput succedaneum).
      (1) Caput may overlie both occiput and parietal bones, be spongy, and contain some capillary bleeding. Edema resolves usually within 36 h after delivery.
      (2) Cephalhematoma may begin 12 h after birth, especially in infants that are large or are delivered through borderline pelvic bones. Bleeding usually occurs between the parietal bone and the periosteum. Blood is contained within this space, and the swelling does not cross suture lines. In rare instances it is associated with skull fracture; therefore, x-rays may be ordered. Complete resolution occurs within 6 weeks to 2

months. There may be an elevation of bilirubin levels as RBC are reabsorbed.

(3) Molding is apparent at birth as a result of the shifting of fetal skull bones to provide smallest presenting diameter. Head returns to oval position if infant is placed prone to sleep with the head turned to right or left side. Bones are still soft; therefore, early positions in crib influence head shape.

(4) Suture lines may be overriding when there is molding. Anterior fontanelle should be open and flat and measure 1–3 cm by 1–3 cm. Posterior fontanelle should be flat and about 1 cm by 1 cm in size. Bones should be slightly softer at the edges.

(5) Skin should be intact; sometimes a puncture wound of internal monitor electrode is seen and precautions must be taken against infection.

(6) Hair is silky; strands are single and fine. Hair may lie flat to head, be curly or sometimes stand out from head.

b. *Ears.* Exterior canals should be patent (auditory meatus). The insertion of the ear pinna should be level with the inner canthus of the eye, not low set, which suggests renal or chromosomal abnormalities. The presence of skin tags or preauricular pits (sinuses) should be reported as unusual signs. Ear pinna should be well curved to lobe of ear and demonstrate good cartilage development. It should not be rotated posteriorly.

c. *Eyes.* Both eyes should be the color of dark, slate grey blue, or slate brown. There should be no spots or interruption in the iris.

(1) PERRL (*p*upils should be *e*qual, *r*ound, and *r*eactive to *l*ight).

(2) An epicanthal fold or narrow palpebral fissure may indicate possibility of chromosomal abnormality.

(3) Lens and cornea should be clear.

(4) There should be a positive red reflex in both eyes that indicates the absence of cataracts.

d. *Nose.* Patent nares with catheter passing through to pharynx on both sides shows no choanal atresia.

(1) Normally the bridge of the nose is flattened; a very depressed bridge (saddle nose) suggests congenital syphilis.

(2) There may be milia, closed epidermal cysts that appear as whitish pimples on nose, chin, and forehead. These will exfoliate and disappear within a few days.

e. *Mouth.* Mucosa is pink and moist. There are no teeth. There should be no clefts in soft or hard palates and no swellings, masses, lacerations, or abrasions.

(1) Tongue and uvula should be in midline and of appropriate size.

(2) There should be symmetrical movement of lips while crying, no facial palsy.

(3) There may normally be midline inclusion cysts on hard palate (Epstein's pearls).

(4) Tooth buds may be seen on labial surfaces of gums.

f. *Face.* There should be no evidence of chromosomal abnormalities, such as widely spaced eyes, smaller than normal chin (micrognathia), or smaller than usual face. (For characteristics of fetal alcohol syndrome see section on *Infant of a Substance-abusing Mother* later in this chapter.) There may be bruises from forceps marks or reddened areas from birth pressure.

g. *Neck.* The neck should be supple with trachea in midline, with no extra skin or webbing. There should be no swelling or masses, and clavicles should be intact.

h. *Chest.* Bony thorax should be symmetrical with sternum showing no evidence of pectus excavatum (sinking in). There should be no retractions.

(1) Nipples should be appropriate distances apart, with no accessory, extra nipple tissue. Size should be consistent with gestational age; full-term infant has 5–10 mm of breast tissue.

(2) Breast tissue may be swollen due to maternal hormones.

(3) Lungs should sound clear to auscultation with equal expansion noted.

(4) The chest should expand symmetrically with no increase in the AP diameter. (Table 10-4)

(i) *Heart.* No murmurs. The PMI (point of maximal impulse) should be at the mid-

Physical findings		Weeks of gestation																												
		20	21	22	23	24	25	26	27	28	29	30	31	32	33	34	35	36	37	38	39	40	41	42	43	44	45	46	47	48
Vernix		Appears				Covers body, thick layer														On back, scalp, in creases		Scant, in creases		No vernix						
Breast tissue and areola		Areola and nipple barely visible, no palpable breast tissue														Areola raised		1-2 mm nodule		3-5 mm	5-6 mm	7-10 mm				?12 mm				
Ear	Form	Flat, shapeless														Beginning incurving superior		Incurving upper two-thirds pinnae			Well-defined incurving to lobe									
	Cartilage	Pinna soft, stays folded												Cartilage scant, returns slowly from folding				Thin cartilage, springs back from folding				Pinna firm, remains erect from head								
Sole creases		Smooth soles without creases												1-2 anterior creases			2-3 anterior creases	Creases anterior two-thirds of sole		Creases involving heel				Deeper creases over entire sole						
Skin	Thickness and appearance	Thin, translucent skin, plethoric, venules over abdomen, edema												Smooth, thicker, no edema				Pink			Few vessels	Some desquamation, pale pink		Thick, pale, desquamation over entire body						
	Nail plates	Appear												Nails to fingertips										Nails extend well beyond fingertips						
Hair		Appears on head			Eyebrows and lashes					Fine, woolly, bunches out from heat									Silky, single strands, lays flat					?Receding hairline or loss of baby hair, short, fine underneath						
Lanugo		Appears	Covers entire body												Vanishes from face					Present on shoulders				No lanugo						
Genitalia	Testes									Testes palpable in inguinal canal								In upper scrotum				In lower scrotum								
	Scrotum									Few rugae								Rugae, anterior portion				Rugae cover		Pendulous						
	Labia and clitoris											Prominent clitoris, labia majora small, widely separated						Labia majora larger, nearly covered clitoris				Labia minora and clitoris covered								
Skull firmness		Bones are soft								Soft to 1 in. from anterior fontanelle							Spongy at edges of fontanelle, center firm			Bones hard, sutures easily displaced				Bones hard, cannot be displaced						
Posture	Resting	Hypotonic, lateral decubitus 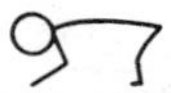						Hypotonic 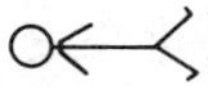				Beginning flexion, thigh 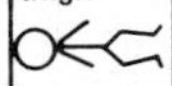		Stronger hip flexion 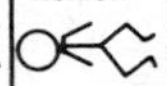		Frog-like 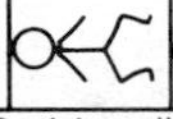		Flexion, all limbs 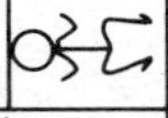		Hypertonic 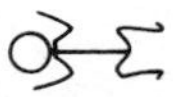				Very hypertonic 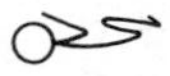						
	Recoil Leg	No recoil 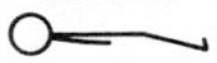												Partial recoil 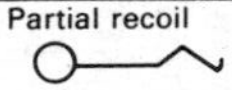						Prompt recoil 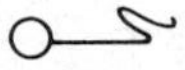										
	Arm.	No recoil 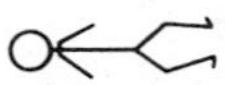														Begin Flexion, no recoil 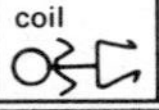		Prompt recoil, may be inhibited 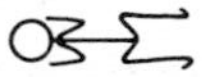				Prompt recoil after 30 s inhibition 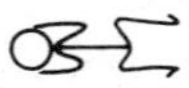								
		20	21	22	23	24	25	26	27	28	29	30	31	32	33	34	35	36	37	38	39	40	41	42	43	44	45	46	47	48

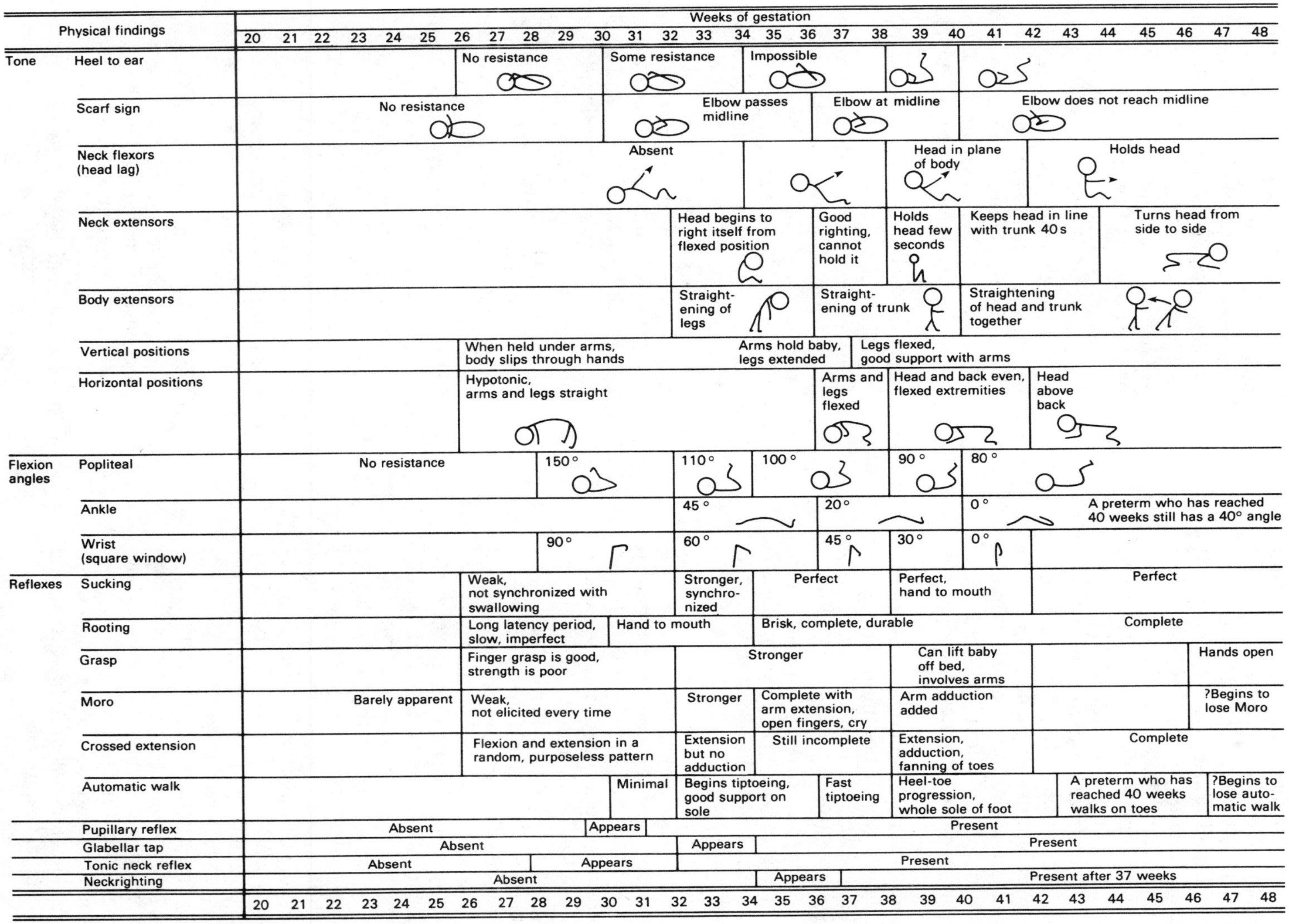

	Physical findings	Weeks of gestation																												
		20	21	22	23	24	25	26	27	28	29	30	31	32	33	34	35	36	37	38	39	40	41	42	43	44	45	46	47	48
Tone	Heel to ear							No resistance				Some resistance				Impossible														
	Scarf sign	No resistance										Elbow passes midline						Elbow at midline				Elbow does not reach midline								
	Neck flexors (head lag)	Absent																		Head in plane of body				Holds head						
	Neck extensors													Head begins to right itself from flexed position				Good righting, cannot hold it		Holds head few seconds		Keeps head in line with trunk 40 s				Turns head from side to side				
	Body extensors													Straightening of legs				Straightening of trunk				Straightening of head and trunk together								
	Vertical positions							When held under arms, body slips through hands								Arms hold baby, legs extended			Legs flexed, good support with arms											
	Horizontal positions							Hypotonic, arms and legs straight										Arms and legs flexed		Head and back even, flexed extremities				Head above back						
Flexion angles	Popliteal	No resistance								150°				110°		100°				90°		80°								
	Ankle													45°				20°				0°				A preterm who has reached 40 weeks still has a 40° angle				
	Wrist (square window)									90°				60°				45°		30°		0°								
Reflexes	Sucking							Weak, not synchronized with swallowing						Stronger, synchronized		Perfect				Perfect, hand to mouth				Perfect						
	Rooting							Long latency period, slow, imperfect				Hand to mouth				Brisk, complete, durable											Complete			
	Grasp							Finger grasp is good, strength is poor						Stronger						Can lift baby off bed, involves arms								Hands open		
	Moro	Barely apparent						Weak, not elicited every time						Stronger		Complete with arm extension, open fingers, cry				Arm adduction added								?Begins to lose Moro		
	Crossed extension							Flexion and extension in a random, purposeless pattern						Extension but no adduction		Still incomplete				Extension, adduction, fanning of toes				Complete						
	Automatic walk											Minimal		Begins tiptoeing, good support on sole				Fast tiptoeing		Heel-toe progression, whole sole of foot					A preterm who has reached 40 weeks walks on toes				?Begins to lose automatic walk	
	Pupillary reflex	Absent										Appears	Present																	
	Glabellar tap	Absent												Appears		Present														
	Tonic neck reflex	Absent								Appears				Present																
	Neckrighting	Absent														Appears			Present after 37 weeks											
		20	21	22	23	24	25	26	27	28	29	30	31	32	33	34	35	36	37	38	39	40	41	42	43	44	45	46	47	48

Figure 10-2 Clinical estimation of gestational age. Top: examination to be completed in first hours after birth; bottom: confirmatory neurological examination to be completed 24 hours after birth. (From Brazie, J. V., and Lubchenco, L. O., "The Estimation of Gestational Age" in C. H. Kempe, H. K. Silver, and D. O'Brien, eds., *Current Pediatric Diagnosis and Treatment*, 7th ed., Lange Medical Publications, Los Altos, Calif., 1982, with permission.)

clavicular line, at the fourth left intercostal space. The mediostinum does not shift unless there is pneumothorax. (See Chapter 11) Heart sounds should not be muffled or distant. Pulses should be equal at the brachial and femoral points.

j. *Abdomen.* Skin should be intact. Cord should be central with two arteries and one larger vein and thick with Wharton's jelly. (The small-for-date cord is shriveled. See Chapter 11.)
   (1) Bowel sounds may be heard in all four quadrants; the liver may be palpated up to 2–3 cm under the right costal margin; spleen tip may be palpated.
   (2) The lower poles of the kidneys, especially on the right, may be palpable.
   (3) Dilated loops of meconium- and/or air-filled bowel may be felt before passage of meconium.
   (4) Linea nigra, a darkened line up the abdomen, may be observed on darker-skinned infants in response to maternal hormones.

k. *Genitalia.*
   (1) For males: Testes should be descended on both sides and the scrotum filled. Scrotum is covered with wrinkles (rugae) and may be pendulous. The urethral meatus should be at the tip of the penis. In case of *hypospadius* (opening of meatus is on underside of shaft), circumcision is not done and evaluation is made regarding need for plastic surgery.
   (2) For females: The clitoris is completely covered by the labia majora. There may be a vaginal (hymenal) tag of skin. There may be an increase in white mucus (pseudomenstruation) in response to maternal hormones.
   (3) Both male and female genetalia may appear enlarged and darker in color due to maternal hormonal stimulus.

l. *Extremities.* There should be five digits on each. There should be full range of motion (ROM), no edema, and symmetrical development and movement.
   (1) There should be no hip click when checking for congenital hip dislocation (Ortolani's sign).
   (2) The hands should show no simian creases (single palmar crease) and should have normal creases, which become deeper with increasing gestational age. There should be a positive grasp reflex that is strong enough to allow infant's arm and shoulder to be lifted.
   (3) There may be sucking blisters on hand or wrist due to intrauterine sucking.
   (4) Fingernails extend to the fingertips.
   (5) The soles of the feet should show creases to the heel that deepen with increasing gestational age. There should be no abnormal single lines or whorls in prints (Down's syndrome). There should be a positive Babinski sign in the curling of the toes (plantar grasp) in response to pressure on the ball of the foot.
   (6) Deep tendon reflexes should present at patellar, calcaneal, and brachial areas.

m. *Back.* The back should be straight with no deviations and or defects (spina bifida or sacral agenesis).
   (1) Birthmarks may appear; for Mongolian spots, or nevus simplex (see Table 23-1). Mongolian spots appear on 90 percent of Indian, Oriental, and black infants as a result of the infiltration of melanocytes deep into the dermis.
   (2) There should be no hair tufts, pits, sinuses, or dimples.

n. *Skin.* Vernix will be found in the creases in a full-term infant. Skin should be pink and clear with few vessels seen. There may be dry skin (desquamation) but there should be no meconium staining. (See *The Postmature Infant* in Chapter 11.)

o. *Central nervous system* (CNS). There should be brisk reflex responses of Moro, suck, rooting, swallowing, gagging, grasping, tonic neck, and crying. Glabellar tap will cause blinking. (See Table 10-5)
   (1) When evaluated for neck flexion and extension the infant should show minimal head lag and should be able to lift head and turn from side to side when prone.
   (2) Infant should be able to respond to noise with startle and then to block sound.
   (3) Infant should be able to follow a light,

TABLE 10-4 NORMAL NEWBORN MEASUREMENTS

Measurement	Normal Values	Comments
Temperature Core (rectal) Skin (axillary)[a]	36.5–37°C, not below 36°C (97.7–98.6°F, not below 97°F) 36.1–36.5°C (97–97.6°F)	Readings may vary, depending on environmental temperatures, presence of infection, or respiratory, neurologic problems.
Pulse (apical rate)	*Average:* 110–130 beats per minute *Range:* 90 when asleep to 180 when crying	A low pulse should accelerate with stimulation. Slight early murmurs are common until cardiovascular changes are complete.
Respiratory rate During 1st hour	40–50 breaths per minute	May have some periodic breathing, short apnea intervals; later these decrease.
Later	*Average:* 30–50 breaths per minute *Range:* 20–60 breaths per minute	A rising rate after first hour; retractions, grunting, flaring nostrils, circumoral cyanosis, or Pa_{O_2} below 50 mmHg indicates distress.
Blood pressure	*Range:* Depends on weight and hour of life. 3 kg = 65/40–80/60.	Varies depending on age, body size, and amount of placental transfusion. If held above placenta too long, may be hypovolemic; if held below, hypervolemic. Hypovolemia is associated with RDS; hypervolemia will cause hyperbilirubinemia and high hematocrit will be seen.
Weight	*Range:* 2500–4000 g *Mean:* 3400 g (7.5 lb)	Term infants above the range are LGA; below, SGA.
Length	*Range:* 44–55 cm *Mean:* 50 cm (20 in)	Crown-heel measurements. Allow for caput and/or cephalhematoma. Measure when infant is drowsy or asleep.
Head circumference	*Range:* 32–38 cm *Mean:* 33 cm (13 in)	Allow for changes in head shape (from moulding) and remeasure before discharge from unit.
Chest circumference[b]	There is a wide range usually 2 cm less than head.	Allow for breast engorgement; measure just below nipple line.

[a] 0.4–0.5°C (0.8–1.0°F) below core temperature.

[b] Ranges from 7 cm less to 5 cm more than the head circumference.

a face, or a bright object when it is brought within range of visual focus of 8–10 in.

(4) Infant should demonstrate definite sleep states (see Table 10-1).

Diagnostic Tests

See Table 10-6.

NURSING DIAGNOSIS: ACTUAL OR POTENTIAL

1. Altered adaptation to extrauterine life due to maternal analgesia or anesthesia during labor, to fetal distress, to physical or neurologic defects or physiologic adjustment.
2. Altered growth pattern—small for gesta-

TABLE 10-5 DEVELOPMENTAL REFLEXES

Reflex	Testing Technique	Normal Response	Indications of Abnormality	Disappearance of Reflex
Moro reflex	Lift the head of the crib about 2 in and drop it. This method is less traumatic on the baby's back and neck than lifting the head and shoulders and dropping them. (Making a loud noise to elicit this reflex tests hearing.)	Abduction and extension of the arms; extension of at least fingers 3–5 followed by adduction and flexion of upper extremities. Lower extremities may be extended. Infant may be startled and cry.	Asymmetrical reaction may indicate hemiparesis, fractured humerus or clavicle, or brachial plexus injury. Sluggish reaction may indicate hypotonia.	After 4 months of age.
Tonic neck reflex (fencing position)	Turn the infant's head to the left.	The left arm and leg will show extension and increased tone; right arm and leg will flex and show a decrease in tone.	The infant who is not able to break this posture a few seconds after it is elicited is exhibiting an obligatory response (abnormal).	After 4 months of age.
Stepping reflex	Hold the infant upright and place one foot in contact with the bed.	The leg in contact with the bed extends while the other leg flexes.	Hypertonia may be indicated if both legs are held in extension. Hypotonia may be indicated if the infant is not able to bear any weight.	After 3 months of age.
Palmar grasp	Apply pressure to the palm of the hand.	Flexion of the fingers and grasp of the object. The grasp is strong enough to allow the arm and shoulder to be lifted from the bed.	Lethargy: illness will cause hypotonia.	3 months of age.
Plantar grasp	Press your thumb to the infant's sole just below the toes.	The toes should flex around your thumb.	Absence of this reflex is seen in infants with hypotonia, spinal cord injury, or injury to the lumbosacral plexus.	After 10 months of age.
Rooting reflex	Touch the infant's cheek.	Infant will turn head toward the stimulus and begin to suck.	Weak in infants with decreased alertness or in those just fed.	After 6 months of age.

SOURCE: Adapted from Silverman, B.: "Assessment of the Newborn," in E. J. Dickason and M. O. Schult (eds.), *Maternal and Infant Care*, 2d ed., McGraw-Hill, New York, 1979, chap. 14.

TABLE 10-6 DIAGNOSTIC TESTS FOR NEWBORN INFANTS

Laboratory Tests	Normal Results	Comments
CORD BLOOD		
Blood type	A, B, AB, O.	Potential for incompatibility, especially if infant is type A or B with a type O mother.
Rh factor	Negative or positive.	Potential for incompatibility if mother is type Rh negative and infant is Rh positive.
Direct Coomb's test	Negative.	Detects sensitized RBCs. Does not define blocking agent.
Bilirubin	1.0–1.8 mg/dL.	Elevated level indicates that fetal hemolysis is present.
Serology-antibody titers		
Syphilis	Negative.	If mother has been treated during pregnancy, newborn serology may still be positive but should decrease by 3 months.
IgM	Negative.	If present, indicates maternal infection during pregnancy with transfer of IgM antibodies to fetus. Specific antibody titers of mother and infant are compared to rule out infections such as TORCH (see Chapter 12).
IgG	Negative.	Formed in infant in response to antigen and does not cross placenta. If found, indicates that infant responded to maternal infection.
HEEL-STICK CAPILLARY BLOOD		
Glucose	Range: 45–90 mg/dL.	If Dextrostix below 45 mg/dL take venous sample for lab analysis. Should be done on all newborns during first 4 h of life. Infants of diabetic mothers, infants over 8 lb and stressed infants need additional testing.
Bilirubin	At 3–4 days normal elevation of 4–6 mg/dL.	For infant with levels elevated above normal, expect q 12 h tests, extra oral fluids, infant to receive phototherapy if over 10–14 mg/dL.
Thyroid screening		
T_4 level	Less than 6 μg/dL at 3 days is abnormally low.	Done on all infants at 2–3 days, especially important for those with wide open suture lines and large fontanelles, thickened

TABLE 10-6 *(continued)*

Laboratory Tests	Normal Results	Comments
TSH on suspected hypothyroid	TSH level >20 μU/dL at 3 days is diagnostic of hypothyroidism.	tongues. Signs of thyroid deficiency develop by the first week.
Inborn errors of metabolism:		
Phenylketonuria (PKU)	Blood levels of 4 mg or more by 48 h indicate a problem.	PKU needs to be repeated by pediatrician if infant discharged early, before adequate milk intake. Ferric chloride reaction in urine will turn specimen green.
Histidinemia		Ferric chloride reaction will turn urine blue-green
Glucose-6-phosphate dehydrogenase	Elevated indirect bilirubin if infant affected by maternal drug intake.	Consult list of drugs causing hemolysis that may be excreted in breast milk and affect infant.
Sickle cell trait		Usually no initial problems. Watch for reduced oxygen tension.
MECONIUM		
Cystic fibrosis	No elevated albumin in meconium.	Test strip changes to deep blue if positive. Sweat test done to measure sodium and cloride concentrations of collected sweat.
PERIPHERAL CULTURES		
Cord, anorectal, ear canal, nasopharyngeal Any lesion	Negative.	Use varies. Done especially if mother had premature rupture of membranes or if nursery epidemic occurs.
URINE		
Urinalysis Culture may be ordered.	1.004–1.018 specific gravity. Uric acid crystals, no protein or RBCs.	Urobilinogen associated with jaundice in infant.

tional age, premature, or both; or large for gestational age or postmature (see Chapter 11).

3. Altered family-infant attachment—delay or disruption due to chronic medical, psychologic, or surgical problems of the mother or to alterations in infant's adaptation to extrauterine life.
4. Alteration in family dynamics due to addition of infant to the family.

EXPECTED OUTCOMES

1. The infant will recover from the process of birth without any residual difficulties.
2. Weight and maturity will be assessed promptly and altered growth patterns will be recognized.
3. Body temperature will be maintained within the normal range.
4. Normal bowel and bladder function will be established.
5. Adequate fluid and caloric needs of the infant will be provided for and parents will understand how to maintain infant's fluid and nutrient needs at home.
6. Parent-infant bonding will be initiated and will develop.
7. Parents will receive anticipatory guidance re-

garding infant care and will demonstrate initial parenting skills.

INTERVENTIONS

1. Interventions in the delivery room.
   a. Stimulate and maintain respirations.
      (1) Position infant in moderate Trendelenburg's position in warmed crib or on mother's abdomen.
      (2) Suction oropharynx and nose gently with bulb syringe. Deeper tracheal suction may be necessary using wall suction unit at 40–60 cm H_2O pressure or with a DeLee trap. Distressed infants may need gastric suctioning to reduce pressure on diaphragm and to reduce regurgitation of swallowed fluids.
      (3) Resuscitate if respiratory function is poor or when infant is depressed because of maternal medication during labor and delivery. Laryngoscope with suction used by physician. Then provide humidified oxygen with mask to apply intermittent positive pressure. Have narcotic antagonist (Narcan) readily available. Use sodium bicarbonate to reverse increasing acidosis if hypoxemia continues.
   b. Maintain body temperature.
      (1) Dry infant thoroughly with warm blanket.
      (2) Care for infant under radiant warmer with probe attached to infant or place infant on skin of mother's abdomen.
      (3) Monitor temperature. Maintain skin or axillary temperature in this early period as high as 36.5 to 37°C; later averages are seen in Table 10-4.
   c. Maintain safety.
      (1) Initiate identification procedures. Footprint and band infant before either mother or infant leaves delivery area.
      (2) Band mother's wrists, making certain numbers on bands are identical and recorded on mother and infant charts.
   d. Monitor adaptation and prevent infection.
      (1) Observe careful asepsis while providing initial care.
      (2) Provide prophylactic eye care for prevention of opthalmic gonorrheal conjunctivitis. 1% silver nitrate, one drop in each eye, is still required in many states. Others use antibiotic ointment, such as Achromycin, or intramuscular administration of an antibiotic. Delay instillation until maternal-infant acquaintence has been initiated. (Instillation is recommended in the nursery rather than in delivery room.)
      (3) Observe newborn for signs of infection. Extramural deliveries and infants born after premature rupture of membranes should have cultures of each body orifice done and, until cultures prove negative, should be isolated from other infants but not isolated from the mother.
      (4) Administer 1 mg vitamin K IM to prevent potential of low prothrombin levels. Milk intake is essential for bacteria in intestinal tract to begin forming endogenous vitamin K.
      (5) Monitor vital signs, color, cry, activity.
         (a) Observe for rising heart rate, respirations, developing signs of respiratory distress.
         (b) Observe for difficulty in regulation of temperature.
         (c) Observe for tremors that may be a sign of hypoglycemia, hypocalcemia, or drug withdrawal.
   e. Initiate parent-infant attachment process.
      (1) After initial suctioning and assessment, if the mother is awake and aware she should have the first opportunity to "claim" her baby before eye drops are instilled.
         (a) Comment positively about baby to parents.
         (b) Place baby skin-to-skin on mother's abdomen for warmth.
         (c) Encourage father to be close to mother and baby and to hold baby himself during this initial contact.
         (d) If mother desires, baby may be put to breast. This requires that the mother be in a semisitting position on the delivery table or birthing bed.
         (e) Delay eye prophylaxsis until after initial period of infant's "eye-to-eye" gazing with mother and father.
         (f) Encourage father to accompany baby to nursery for admission care. Ask father to observe care.
         (g) After the mother is moved to the

recovery room plan at least 45 min for the mother, father, and infant to have a getting-acquainted period when mother's condition permits a leisurely visit (Klaus and Kennell, 1982).

(h) Note any difficulty parents may be having with infant's sex or appearance. Alert the nursery when there are signs of delayed or negative responses.

(2) If mother is physically unable to hold infant, such as after a cesarean section, or if the father is not present, ensure earliest possible time for contact during the first 24 h.

(3) Units with birthing rooms may not find it necessary to separate infant and mother during the first hour after birth.

2. Interventions in the Nursery
   a. Support the infant's transition to extrauterine life.
      (1) Monitor vital signs, every 15 min for the first hour and then qlh until stable.
      (2) Place infant in crib with overhead radiant warmer, attach skin probe for continuous temperature monitoring, and observe.
      (3) Delay bathing until core temperature stabilizes at 37°C or above.
      (4) Observe for hypoglycemia. Check glucose level q1h four times then q4h on any large infant (8 or more pounds) and for any distressed infant or infant of a diabetic mother. Initiate an early feeding schedule for newborns that are prone to hypoglycemia.
   b. Assess adequacy of growth and development.
      (1) Note weight at birth and check daily. Calculate any weight loss. Maximum acceptable loss is 10 percent if not fed early or if infant is breastfeeding.
      (2) Loss should be kept to 2 to 3 percent by starting early feedings.
   c. Provide for fluid and caloric needs (see Table 10-7)
      (1) Newborns are often kept NPO for the first 2 h of recovery except for initial attempts at breastfeeding. During the first transitional sleep there may be oropharyngeal mucus.
      (2) Sips of sterile water are usually given first to evaluate sucking, swallowing, and gag reflexes and to facilitate removal of excess mucus from the stomach. This test feeding is followed with glucose water, up to 15–30 mL.
      (3) Begin formula feeding or breastfeeding within 4–6 h of birth to prevent weight loss. (See Appendix for complete nutrient requirements for infants.)
   d. Assist mother in establishing breastfeeding.
      (1) Assist in initial contact just after birth when infant does exploratory sucking.
      (2) Plan with mother for demand feeding, which is best facilitated by rooming-in. Mother may come to nursery in between regular scheduled feedings when rooming-in not available.
      (3) Usually offer glucose water after each early nursing period. Glucose is used in the conversion of bilirubin from indirect to the direct form. Some mothers may refuse, having been told that glucose reduces the infant's desire to suck.
      (4) Adequacy of volume of milk is evaluated by weight pattern and condition of mucous membranes and other signs of fluid balance. Infant may have slightly elevated temperature if dehydrated. Offer glucose water as necessary between feedings.
      (5) Assess mother's knowledge of feeding techniques and supplement as neces-

TABLE 10-7 INFANT FLUID AND NUTRIENT REQUIREMENTS

Requirements	Birth to 6 months	6 months to 1 year
Kilocalories	117 kcal/kg	108 kcal/kg
Protein	2.2 g/kg	2.0 g/kg
Fluid intake	165 mL/kg	150 mL/kg

NOTE: Formula and breast milk provide 20 kcal/oz.

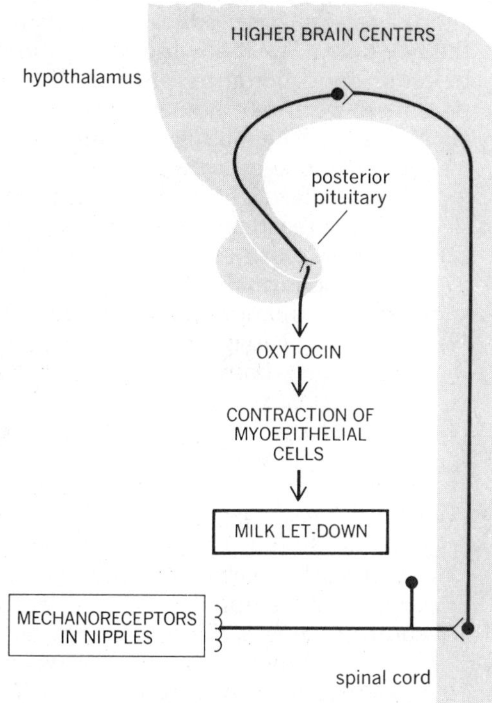

Figure 10-3 The let down-reflex. Sucking stimulates oxytocin secretion and milk let-down. (From Vander, A., et al., *Human Physiology*, McGraw-Hill, New York, 1980.)

sary. Include:

(a) Anatomy and physiology of lactation (Figure 10-3)

(b) Advantages—especially, additional antibodies for infant, easy accessibility for mother, easy digestion for baby.

(c) Schedule—Once lactation is well established, suggest offering one breast until it seems "empty" of milk before offering other side. Next feeding teach mother to start with last breast that was used.

(d) Discuss what feeding on demand means at home, following infant's pattern of hunger. Discuss need to encourage infant to suck to empty breast. Stomach empties in about 1½–2 h in breast-fed babies, so early feedings may be every 2 h; gradually the interval will lengthen.

(e) Once nursing is well established, water or formula may be used for one bottle feeding each day.

(f) Instruct about usual treatment for breast engorgement (see Chapter 9).

(g) Provide written instructions. Acquaint mother with activities of local groups that support breastfeeding mothers.

e. Assist the mother in establishing bottle feeding if she chooses not to breastfeed.

(1) Begin with ½–1 oz and progress within first week to 3–4 oz per feeding, depending on weight and frequency of infant demand.

(2) Feed every 3–4 h. Discuss the meaning of "demand" feeding. Caution against waking infant for a feeding. Discuss home schedule.

(3) In nursery, offer glucose water between feedings if infant is hungry, jaundiced, or receiving phototherapy.

(4) Assess mother's knowledge of technique of feeding and her interest.

(a) Teach preparation of formula, usually using concentrated liquid formula.

(b) Discuss fluid and caloric needs and expected weight-gain pattern. Caution against overfeeding, but teach signs of adequate intake.

(c) Demonstrate all burping techniques and positions after feeding.

f. Observe bowel and bladder function.

(1) Voiding should be initiated within the first 24 h; 30–60 mL during the first 48 h is normal, depending on blood volume and whether infant voided in the delivery room.

(2) Admission urinalysis—Use plastic urine bag to collect urine. Expect low specific gravity, 1.004 to maximum of 1.018. No protein or RBC should be present. Uric acid crystals may appear as "brick dust," a peach-colored residue on the diaper.

(3) Stools depend on milk intake; first meconium stool is usually passed by 24 h.

(a) Delayed passage must be investigated by physician because there may be enterohepatic recycling of bilirubin and there may be obstruction.

(b) Time of transitional stool depends on volume of milk. Breastfed infants must await the "let down" of mother's milk before stool is completely transitional.

(c) A meconium plug may suggest the presence of cystic fibrosis.

g. Maintain skin integrity.

(1) Bathe infant only when core temperature is stabilized at 37°C (98.6°F) or above.

(2) Use warm water only, or water with very mild soap.

(3) Teach mother how to sponge-bathe infant until the cord is dried and removed.

(a) Teach appropriate positions and handling for bathing.

(b) Teach cord care at home. Use alcohol with diaper changes until the cord falls off.

(c) Teach methods of caring for simple diaper rashes.

(i) Dry skin care—Do not use elaborate ointments; soap removes protective bacteria. Plain water is best for diaper changes.

(ii) Do not use plastic diaper covers.

(iii) Change diapers often, or expose buttocks to air.

(iv) Rash often gets infected with Candida; have physician check.

h. Care of circumcision.

Many parents do not understand that there is a choice to be made about circumcision. A careful explanation by physician is needed before consent is signed.

(1) Following use of the Gomco clamp procedure, petroleum gauze is wrapped around penis and left in place for 24 h.

(2) Plastic ring is left in place after the Hollister bell procedure.

(a) Instruct mother that ring will detach within 3 to 5 days.

(b) Instruct mother to observe for any problems in voiding and any bleeding.

(c) Vitamin A and D ointment may be applied over penis for period of early healing.

(d) Position infant only on back or side immediately following procedure.

3. Discharge planning.

a. Planning should begin early. Parents should receive basic education in care of the newborn. The following topics should be taught and literature provided for the parents to peruse at home.

(1) *Nutrition.* The timing and amount of feedings; use of extra fluids, expected patterns of weight gain, formula preparation, breastfeeding skills.

(2) *Output.* Color, consistency, and frequency of normal output. Signs of diarrhea, constipation, and dehydration.

(3) *Skin care.* Diapering and diaper rash prevention. Bathing, skin and hair care, cord care.

(4) *Sleep patterns.* Timing of sleep cycles; signs of infant fatigue, boredom, and frustration.

(5) *Activity and stimulation.* Some information should be given to parents about early learning ability and the rate of development of visual and auditory senses. Emphasize the need for touching, holding, rhythmic movements, conversation. (See Chapter 4.)

(6) *Safety.* Identify need for car seats and safe toys and furniture. Warn against placing infant on surfaces, leaving unattended, and propping bottle in mouth or putting infant to sleep with bottle.

(7) *Signs of illness.* Teach how to take infant's temperature. Give list of symptoms that should be reported to doctor.

(8) *Equipment.* Indicate basic essentials for infant care.

b. Specific referrals should be made to the visiting nurse services, social services, and food supplement programs, such as WIC—Women, Infant, and Childrens' Food Program—when the parents evidence psychosocial problems that may affect infant care.

c. Pediatrician and clinic appointments should be confirmed.

d. Reassess infant to ascertain current status before discharge.

(1) All lab screening is completed (see Table 10-6).

(2) Bilirubin levels within normal limits; higher levels should be resolving after treatment.

(3) Feeding is established; infant is not losing weight and is not dehydrated.

(4) Neurologic responsiveness is within the normal range.
(5) Gestational age parameters are at term or post term.
(6) Minor deviations are showing resolution where possible.

e. The nurse discharging the infant should help the mother think about infant care. Although excitement may not promote good planning, note signs of poor understanding. Make referrals or engage other members of the family in immediate care. Give mother telephone numbers to call for questions regarding care that may arise at home.

EVALUATION

Outcome Criteria

1. Adaptation to extrauterine life completed with no residual difficulties, as evidenced by beginning weight gain and good feeding established. Infant has ability to maintain temperature when dressed in an open crib. Neurologic responses, vital signs and sleep patterns are within the normal ranges.
2. Infant assessment shows normal findings. The infant is average for gestational age and all responses are elicited.
3. Family interactions are being established in a positive direction, as evidenced by behavior that indicates acquaintance and attachment processes have been started.
4. Parents are able to describe or demonstrate basic infant care and know when and how to get assistance.

COMPLICATIONS

INHIBITED OR DISRUPTED BONDING

The development of the maternal-infant-paternal bond is still only partially understood. The concept of a critical period during the first hours of life is related to the quiet alert state that is observed in many infants for 45–60 min after birth. In this period, the infant will gaze and follow objects and look at the parents (Klaus and Kennell, 1982) Most observers of a normal delivery agree that this is a vulnerable period for the parents. The process of "taking in" the reality of the baby and giving up the idealized infant must be recognized as well and allowed for by nurses who are caring for the mother. When a mother is separated from the infant because of illness, recovery complications, or infant disease, she will have an image of sickness, trouble, and disease in caring for the infant. Hospital customs that separate or inhibit the bonding process must be rigorously reexamined in light of the current studies.

When, in spite of all support, family relationships are so disturbed that it is necessary for the infant to be placed for foster care or adoption, the quality and quantity of "mothering" provided by the staff during the mother's absence takes on an additional importance. The infant should be observed for deviations from normal developmental patterns whenever the hospital stay is prolonged. Stimulation by touching, holding, and rocking plus visual and auditory stimulation must be provided. Finally, and most importantly, a consistent person on each shift should be assigned to care for the infant. These nurses must be prepared for the feelings of grief related to separation from the infant when the baby is finally placed. The depth of those feelings may be one measure of the quality of interaction provided for the baby.

Assessment

1. Maternal responses are expressed as tension or detachment.
2. The mother remains aloof from the infant.
3. The mother becomes angry at prolonged separation from her infant and projects the anger inappropriately.
4. Maternal illness, especially infection, severe preeclampsia, or delayed recovery from cesarean section prevents normal contact with the infant.
5. The infant needed special care and was removed from easy access by the mother (see Chapter 12).

Revised Outcomes

1. Beginning with acquaintance, the attachment process will be initiated before discharge from the hospital.
2. When attachment is delayed, referral will be made to a visiting nurse service to continue home assessment and support.
3. The mother will be referred to social service

TABLE 10-8 FIMI: THE FUNKE-IRBE MOTHER INFANT INTERACTIONAL ASSESSMENT[a]

Activities	Column I[b]	Column II	Column III	Column IV[b]
Feeding	Force feeds baby. Disrupts feeding pattern of baby. Stops feeding before baby's need is met. Withdraws and then offers repeatedly.	Feeds baby only after several minutes of baby's crying.	Wakes baby for scheduled feeding. Hurries baby while feeding. Displays neutral affect during feeding. Occupies time more with observer than with baby once feeding has begun.	Maintains eye contact with baby. Feeds baby immediately upon demand. Spends most of time looking at baby. Responds to baby's behavior by changing own behavior, i.e., withdraws nipple when baby spits out milk on side of mouth.
Moving Holding	Restrains or controls baby's movements.	Changes baby's position only after baby has cried for 3 to 4 min. Does not change baby's position; is unaware of baby's need for positional comfort.	Displays inconsistent awareness of baby's need for positional comfort; at times changes baby's position to meet baby's needs and other times does not. Enfolds baby in arms with some rigidness.	Rocks baby gently. Enfolds baby close to body. Changes baby's position gently. Responds to baby's need for positional comfort.
Cleaning Diapering	Wipes baby compulsively, disruptively. Cleans roughly. Displays verbal or facial displeasure at and rejection of cleaning activity. Does not respond to baby's need for cleaning or change of clothing.	Delays cleaning 4–5 min when baby is in need of cleaning. Changes baby's diapers only after baby fusses for 3–4 min.	Delays cleaning slightly, 1–2 min, when baby is in need of cleaning. Does not interact during cleaning activities; is task-oriented.	Responds immediately to baby's need for cleaning. Keeps baby well groomed.

Touching	Touches baby roughly. Does not touch baby.	Touches baby only after 3–4 min of baby's demands.	Touches baby infrequently, only 3–4 times during specific activity. Displays protective touching only.	Kisses. Fingers. Strokes. Gently pats.
Nonverbal and verbal communication	Commands the baby. Voices negative criticism. Angrily voices disapproval. Displays angry facial expression. Makes no eye contact. Refers to baby as "it."	Speaks to baby but withholds affect. Makes eye contact only 3 to 4 times. Is inconsistently pleasant and harsh in voice.	Refers to baby as "he" or "she." Speaks to baby casually. Displays inconsistent eye contact.	Calls baby by name. Speaks with affection. Empathizes. Maintains eye contact. Uses a warm vocal tone.

SOURCE: With permission from *Journal of Obstetric, Gynecologic, and Neonatal Nursing*, 7(5):21, 1978.

[a] For characteristics of interaction observed during early acquaintance and attachment periods.

[b] Column I, poor adaptation; column IV, competent function.

if difficulties seem deep-rooted; a conference with the health care team will precede any final plan for the care of the infant.
4. The mother who must give up her infant will do so only after careful, supportive interaction with appropriate members of the health care team.

Interventions

Whenever possible initiate acquaintance in the delivery room during the first hour of life.

1. Maintain warmth for infant, but do not interfere with natural exploratory curiosity of parents to examine all parts of infant's body.
2. Encourage additional attempts at breastfeeding in the recovery area.
3. Extend feeding periods in room if the mother is having difficulty; encourage rooming-in for any new mother.
4. Assess and document quality of observed early attachment behavior (see Table 10-8). Reassess before mother goes home.
5. When there is separation, keep mother informed of infant's progress (see Chapters 11 and 12).
6. Assist mother in caring for infant so as to foster her confidence in her own ability to provide care.

Reevaluation and Follow-up

1. Mother named the baby and made plans for care at home. She demonstrated willingness to look after basic needs.
2. Parents have verbalized knowledge of infant care and can list ways of obtaining help when/if needed.
3. Parents have understood and appear to have accepted reasons for any delay in contact with infant. They took steps to obtain information as they desired.
4. Anticipatory grieving has been minimized (see Chapter 12), as evidenced by mother's positive comments about her baby and her interest in the infant's progress.
5. Any mother who has given up her infant has been followed by a social worker to reduce the possibility of delayed development of difficulties.

JAUNDICE IN THE FULL-TERM INFANT

Most full-term infants develop physiologic hyperbilirubinemia. Within the first week levels rise to 6–8 mg/dL and may rise to 12 mg/dL. As the liver matures to metabolize the bilirubin load more effectively, unconjugated bilirubin returns slowly to adult normal levels of 1.8–2 mg/dL.

BREAST-MILK JAUNDICE

In some cases higher than normal levels of bilirubin are still considered to be nonpathologic and transient. Some women secrete the steroid pregnanediol in amounts sufficient to slow the reduction of indirect bilirubin into the excretable water-soluble, direct form. In these cases, levels will rise by 3 or 4 days and peak at 10 to 15 days, with the usual levels reaching 15–20 mg/dL bilirubin unless intervention is started. Treatment is usually conservative. Breastfeeding is discontinued for 2 to 3 days to allow levels to fall. The mother may resume breastfeeding when levels reach 10–12 mg/dL. The infant should receive formula and extra glucose water in the interim and the mother should use a breast pump to maintain flow of milk. The mother may be upset by the change in breastfeeding routine as well as feel that her milk is somehow injurious to the infant.

When jaundice is greater than expected, the infant should be assessed for factors such as polycythemia, hemolytic anemia due to abnormality of hemoglobin structure, metabolic or endocrine deficiencies, obstructive disorders, sepsis, or blood-type incompatibility (see Table 11-5).

BLOOD INCOMPATIBILITY

When incompatibility exists between the maternal and fetal blood types, an antigen-antibody reaction may occur that leads to hemolysis of fetal red blood cells. Added to an already present load of unconjugated bilirubin, the extra bilirubin may raise levels into the pathologic range. The result may be *kernicterus,* which is unconjugated bilirubin deposits in the basal ganglia and hippocampus of the brain. Kernicterus may occur when levels reach 20 mg or more in the full-term infant but has occurred at much lower levels in the preterm infant or the distressed infant.

The most frequently seen incompatibility is that between a mother with type O blood who bears an infant with type A or B blood. Maternal serum contains anti-A and anti-B antibodies (agglutinins), and these may cross into fetal circulation during later pregnancy to cause hemolysis of the fetal RBCs. The onset of hemolysis with subsequent jaundice is evident within the first 36 h of life. Cord bilirubin levels may be elevated and concentrations may increase by more than 5 mg/dL per day. Treatment with phototherapy may start when levels are ≥ 12 mg and levels will be evaluated q12h. Only in unusual cases of ABO incompatibility will levels become high enough to threaten kernicterus, and evaluation before such high levels occur may lead to the decision to do an exchange transfusion. (See Hyperbilirubinemia in Chapter 11.)

Jaundice may develop with other cell group incompatibilities such as with anti-c, anti-E, or anti-Kell, and treatment is as above.

Rh INCOMPATIBILITY

The Rh-negative mother may develop an isoimmunologic response as a result of a prior infusion of Rh-positive fetal RBCs during a previous pregnancy, after an abortion or ectopic pregnancy, or during a poorly typed blood transfusion. As little as 0.5 mL of fetal blood may cause the antigen-antibody response with the formulation of IgG antibodies against the Rh_oD antigen. Unless there is prompt intervention with passive immunization using Rh-immune globulin, the maternal system will form antibodies during every subsequent pregnancy where there is an Rh-positive fetus. The goal of prevention and treatment is to make early diagnosis of the potential for sensitization and to use appropriate doses of immune globulin within 72 h of any insult.

Currently, Rh_oD immune globulin is administered to every susceptible woman (indirect Coombs' test, negative) as follows:

1. After an elective or spontaneous abortion or an ectopic pregnancy.
2. At 28 to 32 weeks of pregnancy.
3. After an amniocentesis.
4. After the delivery of an Rh-positive infant whose Coombs' test is negative.

Recently, some neonatologists are administering Rh_oD immune globulin to Rh-negative female infants born to Rh-positive women because it has been found that some Rh-negative persons have developed Rh-positive antibodies although never pregnant or transfused with blood. The premise is that small amounts of maternal blood entered the fetal circulation at the time of birth, causing the formation of antibodies in these babies.

PREVENTION

Health Promotion

1. Careful type and cross match procedures prior to any transfusion.
2. Early identification of incompatibility risk in a newly pregnant couple.
3. Administration of Rh-immune globulin without exception after potential insult with Rh-incompatible blood.
4. Routine administration of immune globulin at 28 to 30 weeks of gestation in Coombs' negative but susceptible women.

Population at Risk

1. Rh-negative women whose sexual partners are Rh positive.
2. Potentially, Rh-negative female infants of Rh-positive women.
3. Women who have type O blood and deliver a type A or B infant.

Screening

1. Indirect Coombs' test on initial visit to prenatal clinic, repeated at 24 and 28 weeks.
2. Cord bilirubin levels on all infants.

Diagnostic Tests

For Rh-negative women who have become immunized through prior insult, serial measurements of bilirubin optic density ΔOD_{450} in amniotic fluid samples (Queenan, 1982) to determine trends:

1. Decreasing trend equals a favorable outcome to the pregnancy.
2. Horizontal or rising trend after 31 weeks indicates early delivery.
3. Rising trend before 31 weeks may indicate need for intrauterine transfusion, as infant fetal hemolysis is progressing at a rapid rate.

NURSING DIAGNOSES/ INTERVENTIONS

See *Hyperbilirubinemia* in Chapter 11.

INFANT OF A SUBSTANCE-ABUSING MOTHER

DRUGS

The newborn of the maternal drug abuser will have special problems in adjustment to extrauterine life. Unfortunately, in every area there may be women addicted to several drugs; combinations of barbiturates, tranquilizers, and alcohol complicate recovery for the infant. Use of cocaine is rising but still is not very common in the childbearing population. The majority of severely drug-addicted women are addicted either to heroin or methadone, and management of the infants of these women is an important part of neonatal nursing, especially in large urban areas.

Care of the infant will be determined by the signs present during the first days of life, and depends upon the type of substance causing these signs. The severity of withdrawal depends on the degree of addiction and the level of dosage in the maternal system at the time of birth. The time that signs will appear is a factor of the half-life of the drug in the infant's body and is related to the rate at which metabolites of the drug are excreted. Heroin and alcohol are examples of drugs excreted rapidly, while methadone and barbiturates are excreted slowly. In these cases onset of signs may be discovered after discharge from the hospital unless drug use has been identified by careful maternal history and detailed newborn observation.

1. *Heroin.* There is a high incidence of intrauterine growth retardation and prematurity associated with heroin but no anomalies. Accompanied by effects of multiple maternal problems, withdrawal begins before 72 h and is relatively short in duration.
2. *Methadone.* If doses have been regular and diet adequate, there should be no growth retardation. Withdrawal may be severe however, and there is a 20 percent chance of seizures in infants whose mothers received high doses. Woman would have received daily dose on day of delivery; therefore, withdrawal onset may vary. It begins by 72 h if dose is as much as 20 mg or more, and 90 percent of infants will demonstrate symptoms; onset begins later if dose is less than 20 mg, and only 50 percent demonstrate symptoms. Infant may relapse at 2 to 4 weeks, or symptoms may develop only after 2 to 3 weeks of life.
3. *Barbiturates.* Depressed responses are noted at birth, and withdrawal period is delayed until after 5 days. There is a high incidence of seizures.
4. *Diazepam, Chlordiazepoxide.* CNS depression may be present at birth, indicated by hypotonia, poor sucking, listlessness; may cause hypothermia.
5. *Propoxyphene* (Darvon). Infant drug level may be higher than mother's at birth. Onset of withdrawal occurs within 3 to 14 h. Infant becomes drug-free by 5 days.

ALCOHOL

The fetal alcohol syndrome (FAS) should be assessed in any infant of an alcohol-abusing mother. FAS may or may not show obvious signs. Craniofacial signs are a small head, eyelids with small palpebral fissures, and an epicanthal fold. The bridge of the nose is depressed, and there is a small chin and long, thin upper lip. There may also be growth retardation, mental retardation, and prematurity. Other defects may be cardiac or limb defects.

Structural defects are usually caused by ingestion of alcohol in the period of organogenesis, the first trimester, and growth retardation results from alcohol abuse in the second and third trimesters. If there is abstinence and careful prenatal care during pregnancy, growth retardation may be prevented and a better developmental outcome may be gained (Lindor, 1980). Signs of withdrawal from alcohol will begin only if the mother has been recently addicted (Bartlett, 1980). Supportive care is similar to that listed for other addictive drugs.

SMOKING

Cigarette smoking does not cause a withdrawal effect but does have documented effects on the developing infant. Smoking more than half a pack a day increases the risk of spontaneous abortion (1.4 times), low birth weight (1.9 times), and perinatal mortality (1.2 times) (Bottoms, 1982). Smoking decreases the oxygen delivery to the fetus because hemoglobin combines with carbon monoxide (COHb) and nicotine and thiocyanate decrease uterine blood flow. Currently reports about marijuana smoking indicate that there may be an effect on the immunologic development in the fetus. No withdrawal effects have been noted in the infant.

PREVENTION

Health Promotion

1. Mother should avoid smoking during pregnancy to prevent adverse effects on fetal growth.
2. Mother should abstain from alcoholic beverages, especially in the first trimester. Later in pregnancy 1 oz of absolute alcohol (2 drinks) per day substantially reduces birth weight.
3. Public should be educated about adverse effects of habituating substances such as: nicotine, alcohol, marijuana, amphetamines, tranquilizers, sleeping pills.
4. Educational and social programs that contribute to the reduction in addiction to street drugs should be encouraged.

Population at Risk

1. Mild to heavy smokers.
2. Mild to heavy alcohol users.
3. Persons growing up in areas of high drug use, alcohol abuse.
4. Teenagers and young adults within a culture increasingly tolerant of multiple drug use.
5. Depressed persons seeking substance-induced elevation of mood.
6. Persons who use stimulants to treat weight problems.
7. Persons with increased dependency needs (see Chapter 38 for maternal treatment).
8. Certain women who do not seek prenatal care before labor begins.
9. Women who want to sign out of hospital shortly after delivery.

Screening

1. Analysis for specific drug: thin-layer chromatography, gas chromatography.
2. Detection of presence of venereal diseases that often accompany addiction to street drugs: syphilis, gonorrhea, herpes.
3. Hepatitis antibody screening; hepatitis is more frequent if parenteral route is being used.
4. Nonstress tests during later pregnancy do not elicit good fetal activity.
5. Blood estriols are tested because estriols in 24-h urine may be diminished in women receiving methadone or may be inaccurately measured as a result of poor specimen collection by mother.
6. In detoxification centers, early identification of any pregnant client should be followed by mandatory prenatal care.

ASSESSMENT

Health History of Mother

1. The examiner is usually unable to determine accurate history of drugs. Note evidence of paresthesias, needle marks, poor nutrition.
2. Determine, if possible, daily dosage and when dose was last taken.
3. Determine if woman is on methadone maintenance and level of dosage.
4. Determine probable health maintenance patterns: smoking patterns, alcohol intake, nutritional intake.
5. Ascertain if client has already had episodes of heroin withdrawal. Such episodes are damaging to fetus and should be prevented by methadone maintenance.
6. Note mother's level of interest in fetal health, ability to cooperate with fetal assessment testing.
7. Determine if there are accompanying medical problems; occurrence rate is high: syphilis, 18%; gonorrhea, 5%; urinary tract infection, 15%; anemia, 24%; and premature rupture of membranes, 21% in one sample urban setting (Zuspan, 1982).
8. After baby is born, determine dosage mother received in her daily dose of methadone and if narcotics or analgesia were used in labor.

Physical Assessment of the Infant

1. Reduced fetal movements that change during labor into hyperactive movements will indicate withdrawal may have begun in utero; there may be meconium aspiration.
2. There may be intrauterine growth retardation; infant may be SGA. Infant may be preterm if there was premature labor.
3. After delivery there usually will not be respiratory distress syndrome as the stress of addiction tends to facilitate lung maturity.
4. There will be decreased muscle tone if drug is a CNS depressant.

5. Withdrawal signs will begin at varying times, depending on type of drug and maternal dosage and presence of other drugs.
   a. CNS signs: hyperactivity, irritability, high-pitched cry, excessive crying, interrupted sleep cycles, difficult to console, poor persistence in sucking, poor coordination of sucking and swallowing, tremors, hypertonicity, and convulsions (6 to 10 percent of methadone cases).
   b. Gastrointestinal signs: weight loss due to vomiting, diarrhea; infant appears very hungry.
   c. Respiratory signs: nasal congestion, tachypnea, hyperpnea leading to respiratory alkalosis; in severe cases, cyanosis and periods of apnea.
   d. Signs related to autonomic nervous system: sneezing, lacrimation, yawning, hiccoughs, hyperpyrexia, sweating.
   e. Integumentary signs: abrasions on knees, toes, elbows, heels from rubbing on sheets; sores on fists from excessive sucking.

Diagnostic Tests

1. Infant's first urine for drug levels; should be refrigerated and sent to lab promptly; subsequent urines may be needed to determine rate of excretion of drug.
2. Sepsis workup if mother has been identified as having infection during labor.
3. Blood gasses if baby has any respiratory difficulty or if the possibility of metabolic imbalance exists because of diarrhea and vomiting.
4. Frequent tests of glucose levels and calcium levels in order to differentiate hypocalcemia from signs of withdrawal.

NURSING DIAGNOSES: ACTUAL OR POTENTIAL

1. Inadequate growth and development—growth inhibited by maternal environment.
2. Alteration in adjustment of body systems due to drug withdrawal.
3. Mother-infant bonding disrupted or inhibited because of maternal problems or infant recovery problems.
4. Potential for poor parenting; possible foster care or adoption may be necessary.

EXPECTED OUTCOMES

1. The infant's gradual adjustment to nontoxic drug levels will be controlled by early recognition and treatment of withdrawal syndrome.
2. Any deviations from normal growth patterns will be identified.
3. The mother will agree to begin detoxification.
4. Counseling for related psychosocial problems will be available for the mother.
5. Parents will receive support as they cope with feelings of anxiety, guilt, and separation from their infant.

INTERVENTIONS

1. Identify addictive drug and the toxicity levels in mother and infant.
2. Maintain close observation of infant in nursery; especially relate expected time of appearance of signs with current ongoing assessment of infant.
3. Provide safe, protective environment. For a hyperactive infant:
   a. Swaddle, pad sides of crib; cover hands with mitts.
   b. Use prone position as much as tolerated.
   c. Soothe agitated infant with alternate means—chair swing, rocking motion, pacifier; sometimes soothing music may help.
4. Decrease unnecessary environmental stimuli—loud noises; talking may set up agitation. Try darkening area around crib to promote sleep.
5. Maintain careful record of intake and output. Prevent dehydration. Give more frequent feedings. Prevent excoriation of perineum.
6. Medicate to reduce CNS signs during withdrawal period. Phenobarbital is the drug of choice although some units use pargoric, tincture of opium, or chlorpromazine. The infant should be comfortable but not evidencing symptoms. Doses are titrated and gradually tapered over 2 to 6 weeks.
7. Facilitate bonding if parent is to assume infant care.
8. After social service evaluation and decision by public agency such as Bureau of Child Welfare, help formulate a plan for homegoing. Most states have laws that require re-

porting withdrawal in infant as a case of child abuse.

Risk factors—length of maternal habituation, place of residence, lifestyle, history of successful treatment in rehabilitation center and, finally, maternal interest.

EVALUATION

Outcome Criteria

1. Signs of withdrawal have ceased without causing residual trauma to infant.
2. Normal physiological patterns have been established; especially for sleep, feeding and output.
3. The family with social service has decided on who will care for the infant.
4. The mother has agreed to undergo detoxification.

Complications

Family relations remain disrupted; once the infant reaches full-term weight and performance and is free of symptomatology, he or she will be placed for foster care or adoption.

REFERENCES

Bartlett, D., and Davis, A.: "Recognizing Fetal Alcohol Syndrome in the Nursery," *Journal of Obstetric, Gynecologic, and Neonatal Nursing,* **9**(4):223, July/August, 1980.

Bottoms, S.: "Smoking," in J. T. Queenan and J. C. Hobbins (eds.), *Protocols for High-Risk Pregnancies,* Medical Economics, Oradell, N.J., 1982, chap. 3.

Klaus, M. H., and Kennell, J. H.: *Parent-Infant Bonding,* 2d ed., Mosby, St. Louis, 1982.

Lindor, E., McCarthy, A. M., and McRae, M. G.: "Fetal Alcohol Syndrome: A Review and Case Presentation," *Journal of Obstetric, Gynecologic, and Neonatal Nursing,* **9**(4)222, July/August, 1980.

Queenan, J. T., and Hobbins, J. C., (eds.): Protocols for High-Risk Pregnancies, Medical Economics, Oradell, NJ, 1982.

Zuspan, R. P.: "Drug and Alcohol Addiction", in J. T. Queenan and J. C. Hobbins (eds.), *Protocols for High-Risk Pregnancies,* Medical Economics, Oradell, NJ, 1982, chap. 1.

BIBLIOGRAPHY

Avant, K. C.: "Anxiety as a Potential Factor Affecting Maternal Attachment," *Journal of Obstetric, Gynecologic, and Neonatal Nursing,* **10**(6):416, November/December 1981. This small study demonstrates that anxiety decreases attachment behavior. Highly anxious mothers had low attachment scores (using modified tool as developed by Klaus and Kennel). Nursing interventions for anxiety may favorably increase attachment scores.

Buckley, K., and Kulb, N. W.: *Handbook of Maternal-Newborn Nursing,* Wiley, New York, 1983. Clinical details of management of newborn care makeup 3 of 23 chapters. There is a listing of drugs that might adversely affect the newborn in the transitional period.

Cloherty, J. P., and Stark, A. R. (eds.): *Manual of Neonatal Care,* Little, Brown, Boston, 1980. Very usable handbook for care of the neonate. Each condition is reviewed. Contains a useful listing of drug therapy.

Gay, J.: "A Conceptual Framework of Bonding," *Journal of Obstetric, Gynecologic, and Neonatal Nursing,* **10**(6):440, November/December 1981. Provides a framework for the conceptualization of parent-infant acquaintance and attachment as components of bonding process. Defines terms carefully.

Glass, L.: "The Neonate in Withdrawal: Identification, Diagnosis, and Treatment," *Pediatric Annals,* **4**:25, July 1975. Basic care illuminated.

Greenberg, M., and Morris, N.: "Engrossment: The Newborn's Impact on the Father," *American Journal of Orthopsychiatry,* **44**(4):520, July 1974. A study corroborating the work of earlier investigators that the father can enter bonding as intensely as the mother if given the opportunity of early contact.

Kantor, G.: "Addicted Mother, Addicted Baby: A Challenge to Health Care Providers," *MCN: American Journal of Maternal Child Nursing,* **3**:281, 1977.

Klaus, M. H., and Kennell, J. H.: *Parent-Infant Bonding,* 2d ed., Mosby, St. Louis, 1982. Updates and clearly describes the work of various investigators of attachment, bonding, and grieving in the early parenting period. Intersperses content with comments from dissenting or contrasting views.

Lozoff, B., et al.: "The Mother-Newborn Relationship: Limits of Adaptability," *Journal of Pediatrics,* **91**(1):1, July 1977. Lead article by several of the associates of Kennell, describes the boundries around bonding/attachment.

National Foundation-March of Dimes, "Early Parent-Infant Relationships," Module Three of *The First Six Hours of Life,* 1978. Free from National Foundation-March of Dimes, an excellent set of three slide-tape programs to encourage nursing personnel in the promotion of quality time for parents and infant interaction.

Silverman, B., and Dickason, E. J.: "The Full-term Infant," in E. J. Dickason, and M. O. Schult (eds.), *Maternal and Infant Care,* McGraw-Hill, New York, 1979. Detailed guide to basic physical assessment of the newborn.

11

The High-Risk Infant

Bonnie Silverman and Laurie Weintraub

THE PREMATURE INFANT

DESCRIPTION

Premature labor continues to be the major cause of infant mortality. The health of a baby born before 37 completed weeks of gestation depends in large measure on the management of the intrapartum period by the perinatal team. Therapy to delay premature labor may allow a few more hours or days for the maturation of body systems, and careful delivery management will further protect the fragile infant. It is important to differentiate between weight and maturity; these two parameters influence birth outcome in different ways. A *low-birth-weight infant* is an infant whose weight at birth falls between 500 and 2500 g. A *premature infant* is any infant born after the beginning of the twentieth week of gestation and before the end of the thirty-seventh week. Within the parameters of weight and age further distinctions are necessary. By means of the graph in Figure 11-1 an infant who is plotted below the 10th percentile in expected weight will be identified as being *small for gestational age* (SGA). The infant whose weight is plotted above the 90th percentile is termed a *large for gestational age* infant (LGA). All infants should be described in terms of gestational age and their growth plotted in relation to age because morbidity/mortality may be estimated.

The infant's maturity at birth will affect every system and all physiologic functions. Especially at risk are respiratory, metabolic, hematologic, immunologic, neurologic, and gastrointestinal functions. Infants born with less than 30 weeks of gestation are termed "very small prematures;" mortality in this group may be 30 to 100 percent. Prematures of 30 to 40 weeks gestation have a mortality rate of 10 to 40 percent; for those over 34 weeks of gestation the rate drops to 5 to 10 percent. Quality pre- and intrapartum management can lower the risks of prematurity, and the establishment of regional perinatal intensive care centers has reduced mortality and morbidity.

PREVENTION

Health Promotion

1. Prenatal care with emphasis on nutrition.
2. Identification of mothers at risk for premature birth.
3. Postponement of delivery when possible for cases of premature labor to allow for maturation of processes necessary to support extrauterine life. (See Chapter 8.)
4. If preterm labor occurs, administration of steroids (betamethasone) to certain mothers at 12–24 h before delivery to stimulate maturation of fetal lung development when the fetus is less than 34 weeks gestational age.
5. Careful delivery management to avoid hypoxia and birth trauma.

Population at Risk

1. Mothers younger than 18 or older than 35 years of age.
2. Mothers of low socioeconomic class, as af-

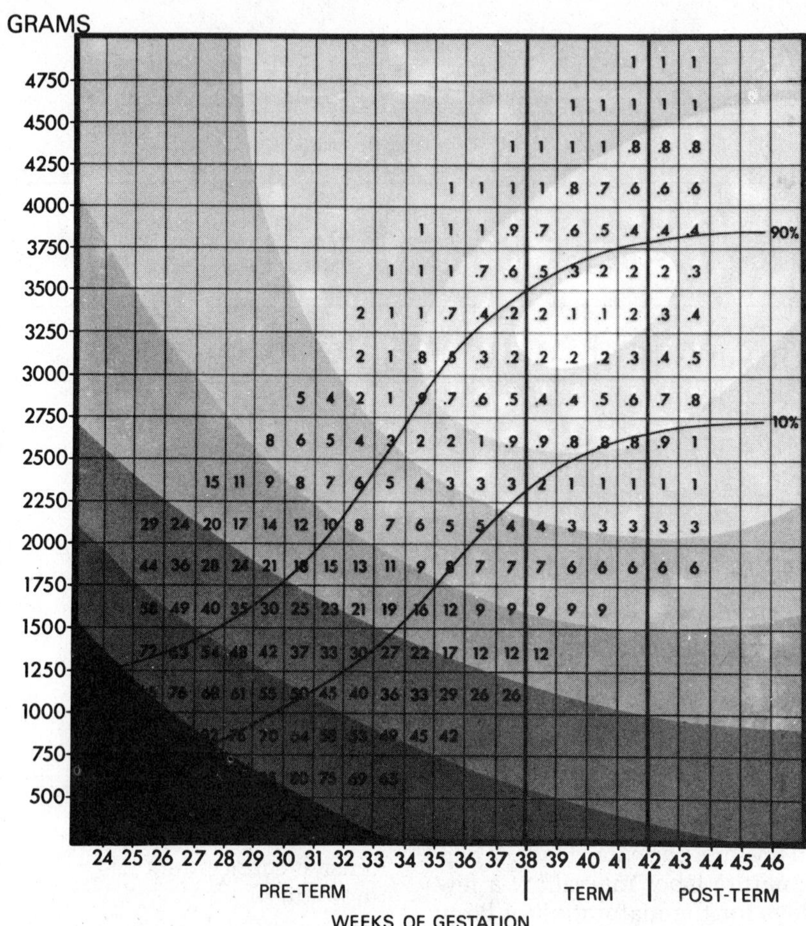

Figure 11-1 Neonatal mortality risk based on birth weight and gestational age (Colorado data, 1958 to 1968). LGA, AGA, SGA represent large, appropriate, and small for gestational age, respectively. (From Lubchenco, L. O., et al., *Journal of Pediatrics*, **81**:814, 1972, with permission from C. V. Mosby Co., St. Louis.)

fected by poverty for nutritional and health standards.

3. Mothers with a history of spontaneous abortion, premature labor, or closely spaced pregnancies.
4. There is some evidence that multiple voluntary abortions may contribute to the incidence of prematurity in later pregnancies; the cause is possible injury to cervix, resulting in early dilation.
5. Women with an incompetent cervix.
6. Mothers with reproductive tract anomalies such as septated uterus.
7. Multiple pregnancy with uterine overcrowding.
8. Complications of pregnancy that, although not contributing to prematurity, may necessitate elective premature delivery (e.g., maternal diabetes mellitus, preeclampsia, Rh isoimmunization, premature rupture of the membranes, severe maternal cardiac disease).

Screening

Prenatal identification of women at risk.

ASSESSMENT

Health History

Factors contributing to premature delivery (see *Population at Risk* above).

Physical Assessment

1. The modified Dubowitz examination is performed to assess gestational age. The gestational age is then plotted against the birth weight to identify the large or small for gestational age infant (see Figure 11-2). (See Figure 10-2 for Brazie-Lubchenco exam.) Refer to Table 11-1.
2. *Head.* Usually round, less molded than full-

	0	1	2	3	4	5
Neuromuscular maturity						
Posture						
Square window (wrist)	90°	60°	45°	30°	0°	
Arm recoil	180°		100°–180°	90°–100°	<90°	
Popliteal angle	180°	160°	130°	110°	90°	<90°
Scarf sign						
Heel to ear						
Physical maturity						
Skin	Gelatinous, red, transparent	Smooth, pink; visible veins	Superficial peeling and/or rash; few veins	Cracking, pale area; rare veins	Parchment, deep cracking; no vessels	Leathery, cracked wrinkled
Lanugo	None	Abundant	Thinning	Bald areas	Mostly bald	
Plantar creases	No crease	Faint red marks	Anterior transverse crease only	Creases anterior two-thirds	Creases cover entire sole	
Breast	Barely perceptible	Flat areola; no bud	Stippled aerola; bud, 1–2 mm	Raised areola; bud, 3–4 mm	Full areola; bud, 5–10 mm	
Ear	Pinna flat; stays folded	Slightly curved pinna; soft; slow recoil	Well-curved pinna; soft; ready recoil	Formed and firm; instant recoil	Thick cartilage; ear stiff	
Genitals (male)	Scrotum empty; no rugae		Testes descending; few rugae	Testes down; good rugae	Testes pendulous; deep rugae	
Genitals (female)	Prominent clitoris and labia minora		Majora and minora equally prominent	Majora large; minora small	Clitoris and minora completely covered	

Score	5	10	15	20	25	30	35	40	45	50
Weeks	26	28	30	32	34	36	38	40	42	44

Figure 11-2 Estimation of gestational age by maturity rating. (Adapted from Dubowitz, et al., *Journal of Pediatrics*, 77:1, 1970, and reproduced with permission from Klaus, M. H., and Fanaroff, A. A., *Care of the High Risk Neonate*, 2nd edition Saunders, Philadelphia, 1979.)

TABLE 11.1 NOTES ON ASSESSMENT TECHNIQUE OF NEUROLOGICAL CRITERIA FOR USE WITH FIGURE 11-2

1. *Posture*
   Observe infant in supine position at rest.
   Score: 0—arms and legs extended.
   1—slight flexion of hips and knees, arms extended.
   2—increased flexion of hips and knees, arms extended.
   3—abduction of flexion of legs, arms slightly flexed.
   4.—flexion of arms and legs.
2. *Square Window*
   Apply pressure to infant's hand (without rotating wrist) to obtain as much flexion toward forearm as possible. Score is graded according to angle obtained.
3. *Arm Recoil*
   With infant in supine position, fully flex arms for 5 s, then fully extend by pulling on hands and then releasing. Score is determined by measuring flexed angle of arm upon release, with absence of recoil scoring 0.
4. *Popliteal Angle*
   With infant in supine position, place legs in knee-to-chest position with pelvis remaining flat on table. Support knee with one hand while gently extending leg by holding ankle with the other hand. The greater the degree of extension, the less mature the infant.
5. *Scarf Sign*
   With infant in supine position and head in midline, take infant's hand and bring it across body to opposite shoulder as far as possible. Assist maneuver by lifting elbow across body. Note how far across body elbow reaches and score accordingly.
6. *Heel-to-Ear Maneuver*
   With infant in supine position, draw foot as close to head as it will go by gently extending leg without forcing it. The closer the foot is to the head, the less mature the infant.

NOTE: This exam should be done within the first 24 h and then again on the following day. Note that the outcome may be affected by use of drugs, asphyxia, and any other problems causing hypotonia or hypertonia.

term baby but may show more edema (caput succedeneum) and may have a cephalhematoma.

a. Suture lines may be widely spaced and fontanelles larger than full-term measurements of anterior 1 × 3 cm, posterior 1 × 1 cm.
b. Edges of bones are springy (spongy) to touch and are moveable.
c. Hair appears wooly and bunches together, sticking out from head. Single strands are not silky to feel.

3. *Ears.* Pinna is slightly incurved; curving increases with gestational age. Cartiledge has not developed; the ear may appear as a flap of thicker skin. It does not spring back when pinna is folded down.
4. *Eyes.* Color remains slate gray or brown. Pupillary reflex appears at 28 to 30 weeks.
5. *Nose.* Usually no milia. Passageway has narrow diameter.
6. *Face.* Lanugo can be seen on forehead and cheeks. Eyebrows become more distinct with increasing age.
7. *Neck.* Head may be rotated past shoulder. Does not show tonic neck reflex. Head lag prominent, as neck flexors and extensors are not strong.
8. *Chest.* Appears less stable than full-term infant's. Ribs may seem pliable. Sternum is more flexible with decreasing age. Bony landmarks are prominent due to lack of subcutaneous tissue. Nipples are completely flat with very little color to areola.
9. *Heart.* Patent ductus arteriosus murmur may be heard. Heart rate decreases as baby matures. Pulses may be difficult to palpate. Blood pressure increases with maturity. Cir-

culating blood volume approximates 10 percent of body weight in grams.

10. *Abdomen.* Hepatosplenomegaly may be present because these organs are sites for blood production in prematures. Dilated loops of bowel may be seen through the abdominal wall. Peristalsis may be observed.
11. *Genitalia.*
    a. Male—Testes may be undescended or in inguinal canal. Testes should descend by 37 weeks. Size of scrotum with wrinkled skin (rugae) becomes larger with increasing age.
    b. Female—Fatty deposits in labia majora are inadequate. Clitoris appears large and labia minora prominent.
12. *Extremities.* Lack of subcutaneous fat evident, poor muscle tone. Sole creases appear by 30 to 32 weeks and progress posteriorly, deepening with increasing age. Nails do not reach fingertips.
13. *Skin.* Skin is thin, reddened, and appears gelatinous in very young infants; becomes more opaque with age. Vessels may be seen clearly, and areas of vasoconstriction/vasodilatation often lead to appearance of mottling. Lanugo is present in varying degrees, as well as vernix that covers the body between 20 to 36 weeks. Vernix gradually diminishes, to be absent or remain only in creases by 42 weeks.
14. *Central nervous system.* All reflexes are sluggish to absent (see Table 10-5). Suck and swallow are not coordinated until after 34 weeks. Muscle tone varies with gestational age.
15. *State.* Sleeps more; shorter periods of awake state and not well differentiated. Any interaction is costly in terms of energy expenditures. Easily disorganized by too much stimuli.
16. Physical examination will identify emerging problems such as difficulties with respiration and thermoregulation.

Diagnostic Tests

1. Prenatal.
    a. No testing will positively identify the mother who will deliver prematurely.
    b. Ultrasonic examination can identify intrauterine growth retardation.
    c. Analysis of amniotic fluid for lecithin/sphingomyelin (L/S) ratio, Nile blue stain for fetal epithelial cells, and creatinine levels is recommended before all but emergency delivery of a premature infant. These will reflect the potential for fetal lung maturity, adequate fat stores, and kidney function. (See Figure 11-3.)
2. For the infant.
    a. Routine metabolic screening for inborn errors of metabolism.
    b. Shortly after birth, ethanol shake or foam test as a predictor of lung maturity; use amniotic fluid obtained by neonatal gastric aspiration.
    c. Blood testing to identify complications of prematurity.
        (1) CBC with white cell differential and platelet count to identify anemia or polycythemia and to aid in the early de-

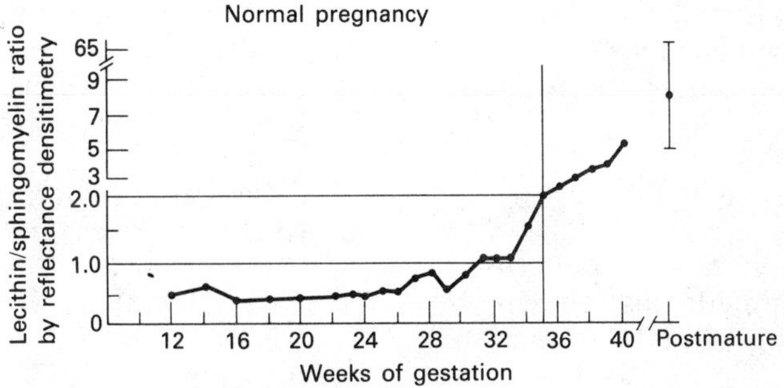

Figure 11-3 Expected ratios of lecithin and sphingomyelin as the fetus matures during pregnancy. (From Gluck, L., and Kulevich, M. V., "Lecithin/spingomyelin ratios in amniotic fluid in normal and abnormal pregnancy," *American Journal of Obstetrics and Gynecology,* **115**:541, 1973.)

tection of sepsis or red cell abnormalities.
(2) Serum bilirubin determination; the immature liver will be less able to metabolize bilirubin. (See Hyperbilrubinemia later in this chapter.)
(3) Glucose and calcium levels usually lower in the preterm infant.
(4) Electrolytes, especially if birth asphyxia has occurred or if intravenous fluids are necessary.
(5) Cord blood pH at birth or blood from scalp sample in late labor may normally be 7.28.
(6) Blood gases—Pa_{O_2} and Pa_{CO_2} done at regular intervals.

d. Chest x-ray.

NURSING DIAGNOSES: ACTUAL OR POTENTIAL

1. Altered growth and development due to difficulty with adaptation to extrauterine environment.
2. Altered thermoregulation due to immaturity of the CNS, increased surface area in proportion to body weight, and body position of extension rather than flexion.
3. Respiratory dysfunction due to immaturity of respiratory system.
4. Altered nutrition due to immature neurologic, gastrointestinal, and metabolic functions.
5. Altered hematologic status due to immaturity of erythropoetic function, immunologic function, and difficulty in metabolizing bilirubin.
6. Delayed attachment process due to early, prolonged separation, parental anxiety, or infant's potential for complications.
7. Altered response to infection due to inadequate body defenses.

EXPECTED OUTCOMES

1. The infant will exhibit normal patterns of growth and development, as shown by weight gain, maturing of reflexes, and responsive behavior.
2. The infant will maintain a normal temperature in a neutral thermal environment. (See *Hypothermia* later in this Chapter.)
3. The infant will be able to sustain respirations in room air without mechanical assistance.
4. The infant will take milk by nipple and retain oral feedings starting at 34 weeks of gestational age.
5. The family will have access to their child and will exhibit progressive attachment behavior. There will be minimal anticipatory grieving.
6. Parents will be prepared for the infant's discharge and for infant care.

INTERVENTIONS

1. Maintain infant in a thermoneutral environment in which heat production, as measured by oxygen consumption, is minimal yet core temperature is within the normal range. (See *Hypothermia*.)
   a. Hourly, monitor temperature of infant and environment until condition is stable and then monitor q4h.
   b. Control radiant heat or temperature, airflow, and humidity in controlled environment of incubator. Use skin temperature probe for continuous monitoring.
   c. Prevent more than 2 or 3 degrees of temperature gradient between infant and walls in incubator. Within incubator place plastic shield over small preterm infant.
   d. Use stockinette cap to reduce heat loss through scalp.
2. Monitor and support respiratory status.
   a. Look for early signs of respiratory difficulty. (See *Respiratory Distress Syndrome* later in this Chapter.)
   b. Prevent *hypoxia* (Pa_{O_2} below 50 mmHg) and *hyperoxia* (Pa_{O_2} over 110 mmHg.
3. Daily assess weight, weekly assess length and head circumference to identify deviations from normal.
   a. Weight beginning by 1 week should follow fetal pattern of gain until infant reaches 40 weeks.
   b. Gain is delayed by difficulty in adaptation.
4. Assess at regular intervals the infant's neurologic reflexes and behavioral responses using Denver Developmental Screening Test (DDST) or Brazelton exam after 40 weeks.
   a. Before 40 weeks gestational age compare the infant's characteristics and neurologic responses with fetal developmental milestones; for example, suck and swallow reflexes should be present after 34 weeks gestation.
   b. Teach parents that the infant will "catch

up" by 2 years of age, barring complications, and that at the time of reaching 40 weeks in physical development and 2500 g in weight, regardless of extrauterine age, the baby should be considered a newborn.

5. Provide visual and tactile stimulation for the infant and teach parents to do the same.
6. Maintain fluid balance.
   a. Calculate fluid needs daily after assessment of infant's condition and environmental factors, such as assisted ventilation or phototherapy. An overhead radiant warmer may cause insensible water loss. Fluid requirements are as follows:

      80 mL/kg 1st 24 h,
      100 mL/kg 2d 24 h,
      120 mL/kg progressing to
      150 mL/kg thereafter.

   b. Measure urine output whenever possible for infants in fragile balance. Normal hydration will yield a urine volume of 1–3 mL/kg with a specific gravity of 1.005 to 1.012. Urine volume increases as the infant gains weight to the normal newborn volume of 15–60 mL/kg.
   c. Recognize dehydration by weight loss, elevation of temperature, poor skin turgor, decreased urine output, increased specific gravity.
7. Maintain adequate nutrition.
   a. Maintain infant NPO (usually) during critical period of recovery or during respiratory distress episodes.
   b. Use parenteral feedings when infant is too immature to be fed orally or complications such as necrotizing enterocolitis (NEC) occur. Begin peripheral alimentation after the initial adjustment period.
   c. Use gavage feedings for infants of less than 34 weeks gestation to prevent aspiration due to immaturity of suck, swallow, and gag reflexes.
      (1) Intermittent gavage feedings are usually tolerated well.
      (2) The smaller infant may require continuous naso/orogastric or jejunal feedings. (See Table 11-2.)
   d. Begin with and progress as tolerated:
      (1) Weight less than kg: 2 mL every 2 h.
      (2) Weight 1–1.5 kg: 2 to 3 mL every 2 h.
      (3) Weight over 1.5 kg: 7–10 mL every 3 h. (see Table 11-3)
   e. Supplement with IV fluids if infant is not able to take adequate amounts (Figure 11-4).
   f. Feeding volumes depend on infant responses to last feeding.
      (1) Check gastric residuals before each feeding; should not be greater than the hourly intake of formula or breast milk for continuous feedings or more than 25 percent of the intermittent feeding.
      (2) Subtract the amount of the residual from the next feeding and refeed it to the infant.
      (3) Stop oral feedings if there are large residuals, abdominal distention, vomiting (especially if bile stained), diarrhea, failure to pass stool, or bloody stool. (See *Necrotizing Enterocolitis* later in this chapter.)
   g. Feeding choices (see Table 11-2).
      (1) Breast milk is tolerated best by the small infant.
      (2) Formula in ratio of 20 kcal/oz or 67 kcal/dL is tolerated best but does not provide enough calories for the rapidly growing infant; 24 kcal/oz or 87 kcal/dL may be selected.
   h. There are varying regimens for vitamin administration.
      (1) Vitamin K given IM after birth, repeated weekly if infant on parenteral therapy or nutrition.
      (2) Commercial multivitamin preparation 0.5 to 1.0 ml given daily
      (3) 25 IU water-soluble vitamin E given daily until 2 or 3 months of age. Iron interferes with intestinal absorption of tocopherol; if inadequate amounts of vitamin E are present red cell fragility may be increased in the baby (Klaus and Fanaroff, 1978).
   i. After baby is 2 months old, iron fortified formula is used to prevent anemia of prematurity.
   j. Total parenteral nutrition (TPN) through peripheral intravenous line may be necessary for small infants who cannot tolerate milk (see Necrotizing Enterocolitis). TPN may be initiated after 72 h of age when oral feedings are not being tolerated.
8. Support normal bowel and bladder function.

TABLE 11-2 SOME ADVANTAGES AND DISADVANTAGES OF THE VARIOUS METHODS OF ENTERAL FEEDING

	Advantages		Disadvantages	
Method	Intermittent	Indwelling	Intermittent	Indwelling
Orogastric	Can use larger diameter catheter than with nasogastric.	No vagal stimulation.	Danger of tracheal intubation and possible aspiration.	
Nasogastric	Less chance of aspiration. Can aspirate for residual before feeding. Can use with endotracheal tube in place. Conserves energy and prevents fatigue. Easy and quick to pass catheter. Can be quickly taught.	No vagal stimulation.	Vagal stimulation. Gagging and possible vomiting on introduction catheter. Vagal stimulation with rapid infusion.	Nasal erosion. Nasal airway obstruction. Rhinorrhea. Otitis media. Conjunctivitis.
Nasojejunal	Less chance of aspiration. Less nursing time for feeding. Conserves energy and prevents fatigue. Possibly greater fluid and calorie intake in early neonatal period.		Danger of perforation with polyvinyl and polyethylene catheters. Can use only isosmolar or hypoosmolar feedings. Causes change in duodenal microflora. It may take hours for tube to pass pylorus. Vomiting and/or diarrhea. Gagging on introducing catheter. Clogging of catheter.	
Gastrostomy	Less chance of aspiration. Not for routine neonatal feeding.			Utilizes calories. Infection.
Dropper	No vagal stimulation. ?Allows baby to use some swallowing function.		Staphylococcal enterocolitis. Considerable skill required. Aspiration, gagging, vomiting, air swallowing.	
Nipple	Physiologic (32–34 weeks). No vagal stimulation.	Utilizes calories. Aspiration, gagging, vomiting, air swallowing.		

SOURCE: From Dweck, H. S.: "Feeding the Prematurely Born Infant," *Clinics in Perinatology*, **2**(1):194, 1975.

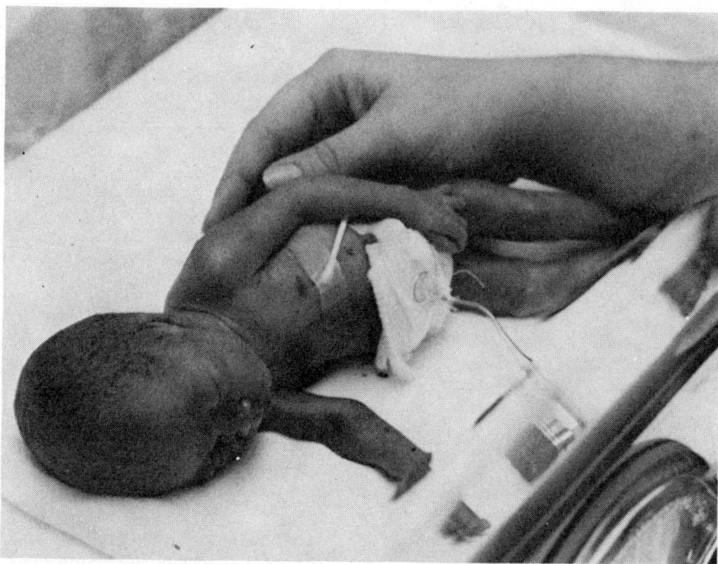

Figure 11-4 A 1300 g infant with estimated gestational age of 31 weeks. (Courtesy of Schneider Children's Hospital of Long Island Jewish–Hillside Medical Center, New York.)

a. The preterm infant usually voids within 12–16 h after birth. The quantity is dependent upon early or late cord clamping, which affects blood volume. Check the birth record for observation of any voiding at the time of delivery.
b. The first meconium stool will be expelled within 12–16 h for about 65 percent of infants. Most infants pass stool by 36 h.
c. Because of critical condition, if stool is delayed beyond 36–48 h there may be enterohepatic recycling of bilirubin and slightly higher jaundice levels.

9. Maintain skin integrity; the smaller infant has translucent, fragile skin. Abrasions, pressure areas, and skin breakdown occur easily.
   a. Position infant in correct body alignment, protecting skin surfaces.
   b. Turn every 2–3 h, as a minimum, to prevent pressure areas, stasis.
   c. Use protective lamb's wool for vulnerable spots.
   d. Keep bathing to a minimum; use nondrying soaps or plain water.
10. Prevent infection, as host defenses are not mature.
    a. There is limited phagocytosis and delayed inflammatory response.
    b. Depending on age at birth, there is incomplete transfer of placentally acquired immunoglobulins.
    c. There is immaturity of intestinal tract with vulnerability to gastrointestinal infections.
    d. Follow infection control policy of hospital, but do not keep parents away from infant.
    e. Check umbilical catheter site for signs of infection. There is a higher potential for infection with use of catheters for infusions.
11. Support maternal-paternal attachment process.
    a. Perform interventions similar to those implemented when an anomalous child is born (See Chapter 12), as the family must align the image of the expected and the now realized child. Premature delivery denies parents those experiences in the last trimester that prepare a family for delivery.
    b. Note parental reactions to initial contacts. Encourage touching; observe for en face position, for instance.
    c. Involve parents from the outset; provide knowledge of prognosis, treatments, and daily progress. Answer all questions and

TABLE 11-3 TWENTY-FOUR HOUR NUTRIENT NEEDS OF LOW-BIRTH-WEIGHT INFANTS

Nutrient	First Week	Period of Active Growth
Calories	50–100 kcal/kg.	120 kcal/kg (110–150 kcal/kg[a]).
Protein	Amount depends on intake and concentration of formula (parenteral amino acid hydrolysate may be ordered).	2.5–3.5 g/kg (using modified whey: casein ratio). Breast milk.[b]
Fluids	60–100 mL/kg (80–120 mL/kg). Often provided intravenously as 5–10% dextrose in water for first 48 h.	150 mL/kg (150–200 mL/kg per day).[c] 1.8% NaCl in 4.3% dextrose and water, or 2% NaCl in 5% dextrose and water, given intravenously to make up total fluid requirements.
Fat	Amount depends on intake of formula, unsaturated fats are absorbed best.	40–50% caloric intake with at least 3% made up of linoleic acid.

SOURCE: Adapted from Cox, M. A.: and Thrift, M. C.: *Nutrition*, Chapter 27 in Cloherty, J. P.: and Stark, A. R.: (eds) Manual of Neonatal Care, Little Brown, Boston, 1980.

[a] SGA infants have a higher basal metabolic rate than AGA infants of the same weight and may need more calories.

[b] With adequate intake, the lower protein of breast milk may still support desired growth because of the unique distribution of amino acids. Breast milk also confers other benefits because of ideal protein and fat quantity and quality, immune factors, and osmolar factors suited to human infants.

[c] Higher fluid needs are present when the infant is under a radiant heater, receiving phototherapy, or has diarrhea, vomiting, or cold stress.

provide reports by telephone when parents are unable to visit.

d. Involve both parents in care of infant as soon as possible.
e. If possible encourage mother to express breast milk. Work out procedure to supply milk to infant.
f. Observe clues to poor adjustment to preterm infant.

12. Make referrals and prepare parents for discharge.
    a. On admission begin process by outlining expected time parameters.
    b. Teach routine care when parents attend infant. Be sure they know infant is considered developmentally a "newborn" when discharged home.
    c. Explain growth patterns during first few months. Explain the expected "catch-up" process. (Brazelton, 1973)
    d. Alert them to the infant's vulnerability to infection.
    e. With parents, neonatologist, social worker, and nurses, plan a discharge conference to summarize infant's progress and to make follow-up plans.

EVALUATION

Outcome Criteria

1. After initial weight loss, the infant has gained 20–30 g per day and has increased head circumference by 0.5–1 cm/week.
2. Developmental milestones are being reached within a schedule that relates to degree of immaturity.
3. The infant maintains a core temperature of 37°C and a surface temperature of 36.5°C when dressed and in an open crib.
4. The infant has progressed to oral feedings without complications. Normal glucose, calcium, and electrolyte balances are being maintained.
5. Adaptation of all systems have reached a full-

term newborn infant level of functioning before discharge to the home.

6. The family has begun to exhibit normal parenting roles and attachment behavior. They are prepared for discharge and show competence and enjoyment when caring for their child.

COMPLICATIONS

RESPIRATORY DISTRESS SYNDROME

Respiratory distress syndrome (RDS) or hyaline membrane disease, is a life-threatening syndrome characterized by decreased exchange of oxygen and carbon dioxide in the lung. This is caused primarily by a decrease or absence of the substance secreted in the alveoli, *surfactant*. Surfactant contributes to surface tension, preventing the alveoli from collapsing at the end of each expiration. This altered production of surfactant leads to atelectasis and reduced residual capacity, requiring greater inflation pressures and therefore increased effort on the part of the infant to reexpand the lungs after each expiration.

In addition, there may be a persistent high pulmonary vascular resistence that inhibits the development of neonatal circulation. There may be a persistent right-to-left shunt through a patent ductus arteriosus (PDA), a condition that commonly may occur in infants of less than 34 weeks gestation. A PDA complicates RDS in about 30 to 50 percent of the cases. The result is reduction of oxygenation in spite of tachypnea and adequate supplemental oxygen supply.

RDS is the major cause of death in the preterm infant, although its incidence and mortality have decreased over the past two decades. Earlier diagnosis, improved perinatal intensive care, and transport to regional centers have contributed to the reduction. Infants weighing below 1200 g have the highest mortality rate (50 to 80 percent). Half of the infants below 2000 g will develop some respiratory difficulty; the syndrome occurs in about 10 percent of all infants weighing between 2000 and 2500 grams.

Additional factors such as maternal diabetes, second-born twin, and male sex as well as perinatal asphyxia and hypovolemia will add to the risk of RDS in the preterm infant. It is believed that such factors as maternal preeclampsia, prolonged rupture of membranes, stress in utero, plus the administration of glucocorticoids before delivery may decrease the incidence. The explanation may be an accelerated maturation of lung function in response to stress-induced hormones. (Fawcett and Gluck, 1977).

Signs of RDS usually appear within the first 8 h but may become evident in the delivery room. The degree of intervention depends on the severity of the signs. Most infants with RDS require supportive oxygen therapy in order to maintain adequate tissue oxygenation. Therapy may be accomplished with bag and mask, oxyhood, CPAP (continuous positive airway pressure), or mechanical ventilation.

1. Bag and mask—Use intermittently when P_{CO_2} is rising and P_{O_2} is within normal limits.
2. Oxyhood—Use as long as infant has spontaneous respirations. Switch to CPAP if it requires 40 to 60 percent fraction of inspired oxygen ($F_{I_{O_2}}$) to maintain arterial Pa_{O_2} of 50 to 80 percent.
3. CPAP—Infant must still have spontaneous respirations. Use nasal prongs or endotracheal tube, depending on condition. Provides a steady flow of oxygen at a pressure of 5–6 cm H_2O to prevent alveolar collapse at the end of the expiration.
4. Mechanical ventilation—Use if condition worsens, Pa_{CO_2} levels rise rapidly, P_{O_2} levels fall, severe apnea occurs, or if spontaneous respirations cease.

Ventilatory assistance must be carefully used as it produces changes in intrathoracic pressure that may interfere with cardiac functioning and contribute to intracranial bleeding and circulatory insufficiency in very low birth weight infants. See Table 11-4 for complications that may occur with RDS.

Assessment

1. Lecithin/sphyngomyelin (L/S) ratio is usually less than 2:1 (see Figure 11-3).
2. The following signs may be present.
   a. Grunting respirations—audible sounds made by exhaling against a partially closed glottis in an effort to distend collapsing alveoli.

TABLE 11-4 COMPLICATIONS OF RDS

Acute	Long-Term
Complications associated with umbilical vessel catheterization: Infection Thromboemboli Air emboli Hemorrhage Air leak: Pneumothorax Pneumomediastinum Interstitial emphysema Pneumopericardium Pulmonary hemorrhage Patent ductus arteriosus (may complicate or be the result of RDS)	Bronchopulmonary dysplasia Retrolental fibroplasia Tissue necrosis caused by: CPAP nasal prongs Nasotracheal tubes Endotracheal tubes Neurological impairment Infections due to respiratory equipment Intracranial hemorrhage (related to RDS, asphyxia, prematurity)
Impairment of parent-infant interaction, distancing by equipment, anxiety	Possible long-term impairment of parent-infant interaction[a]

[a] Incidence of child abuse is said to be increased in premature and ill newborns as opposed to normal newborns.

b. Tachypnea—respiratory rate greater than 60 per minute, counted over a full 60 s. Rate may be rising.
c. Chest retractions—depression of the sternum, suprasternal, substernal notch, intercostal spaces and subcostal margin indicating the use of accessory muscles of respiration.
d. Cyanosis—progressing from circumoral, periorbital, and nail beds to become generalized as hypoxemia increases. Usually becomes visible at Pa_{O_2} of less than 50 mmHg.
e. Nasal flaring on inspiration.
f. Rales and decreased breath sounds upon auscultation.
g. Apnea as condition worsens.
h. Hypothermia (see *Hypothermia—Cold Stress*).
i. Cardiac murmur due to presence of right-to-left shunting.
j. Hypotension and hypovolemia.
k. Increasing acidosis and hypoxemia.

3. Chest x-ray film shows haziness (ground glass) in all lung areas and poor expansion.
4. Transcutaneous (TC) Po_2 monitoring shows poor TC Po_2 in room air. (<50 mmHg).
5. There may be a rapidly deteriorating condition due to pneumothorax (relatively common).
   a. Deteriorating respiratory status; increased O_2 requirements, respiratory rate, grunting, cyanosis, retractions.
   b. Increase anterior-posterior chest diameter; unilateral chest bulging with mediastinal shift. Heart sounds will shift toward the affected side.
   c. Decreased breath sounds on affected side.
   d. Shock because of decreased venous return to the right side of heart.
6. There may be progressive opening of PDA.

Revised Outcomes

1. Respiratory distress will be reduced and adequate oxygenation maintained to prevent tissue damage. Arterial levels of oxygen and carbon dioxide will be within normal range:
   Pa_{O_2}: in range of 50 to 80 mmHg.
   Pa_{CO_2}: in range of 35 to 45 mmHg.
   pH: in range of 7.35.
2. Infant will not develop complications due to:
   a. *Hyperoxia*—With Pa_{O_2} over maximum of 100 mmHg for prolonged periods resulting in retrolental fibroplasia (RLF), oxygen toxicity to immature retinal tissues, or bronchopulmonary displasia (BPD), injury to fragile lung alveolar tissue.

b. *Hypoxia*—Pa_{O_2} under 50 mmHg resulting in oxygen deprivation to body cells.
3. Infant will be free of infection from sources dependent on aseptic procedures. The infant is especially vulnerable when umbilical catheters or endotracheal tubes are used.
4. The infant will be stressed by treatment modalities as little as possible and normal physiologic function will return.
5. Parent-infant interaction will be maintained.

Interventions

1. Observe closely for signs of deteriorating condition and complications such as pneumothorax, shock, right-to-left shunting.
2. Check that emergency equipment is available and in working order, such as:
   a. Intubation equipment, including Ambu bag.
   b. Equipment needed for needle aspiration of pneumothorax, including underwater seals.
   c. Umbilical vessel catheterization tray.
3. Continuous cardiac and respiratory monitoring. Vital signs at frequent intervals until stable. Range of blood pressure is dependent on weight and age: 60/30 to 80/60.
4. Dextrosix monitoring of glucose levels to keep level above 20 mg/dL for small prematures, above 30 mg/dL for term infants, and below 130 mg/dL for both.
5. Disturb infant as little as possible to avoid increased stress and therefore increased oxygen consumption. Organize care to keep handling at a minimum.
6. Deliver prescribed amount of oxygen to keep blood gases in the optimal range.
   a. Check oxygen analyzer; calibrate with room air and 100 percent oxygen at the beginning of each shift.
   b. Arterial or arterialized capillary blood gasses should be monitored at least every 4 h and within 20 min of a change in Fi_{O_2}. Place blood on ice until sent for analysis.
7. Deliver warmed humidified oxygen.
   a. Temperature should be within 2 or 3 degrees Fahrenheit of environmental temperature to prevent alterations in body temperature.
   b. Warming can be done by using humidity with a nebulizer; too large a discrepancy between ambient and oxygen tempera-

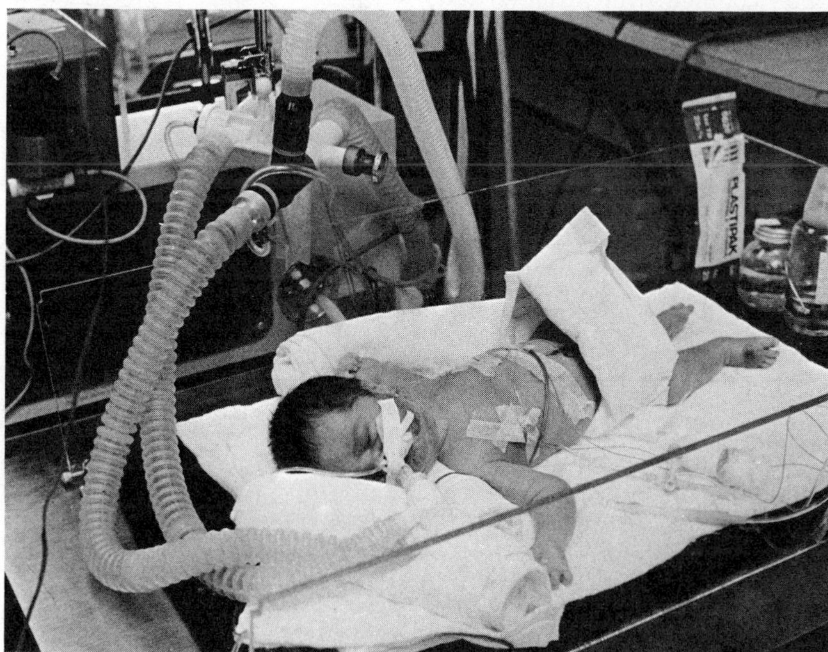

Figure 11-5 Infant on respirator. (Courtesy of Schneider Children's Hospital of Long Island Jewish–Hillside Medical Center, New York. Photograph by Herbert Bennett.)

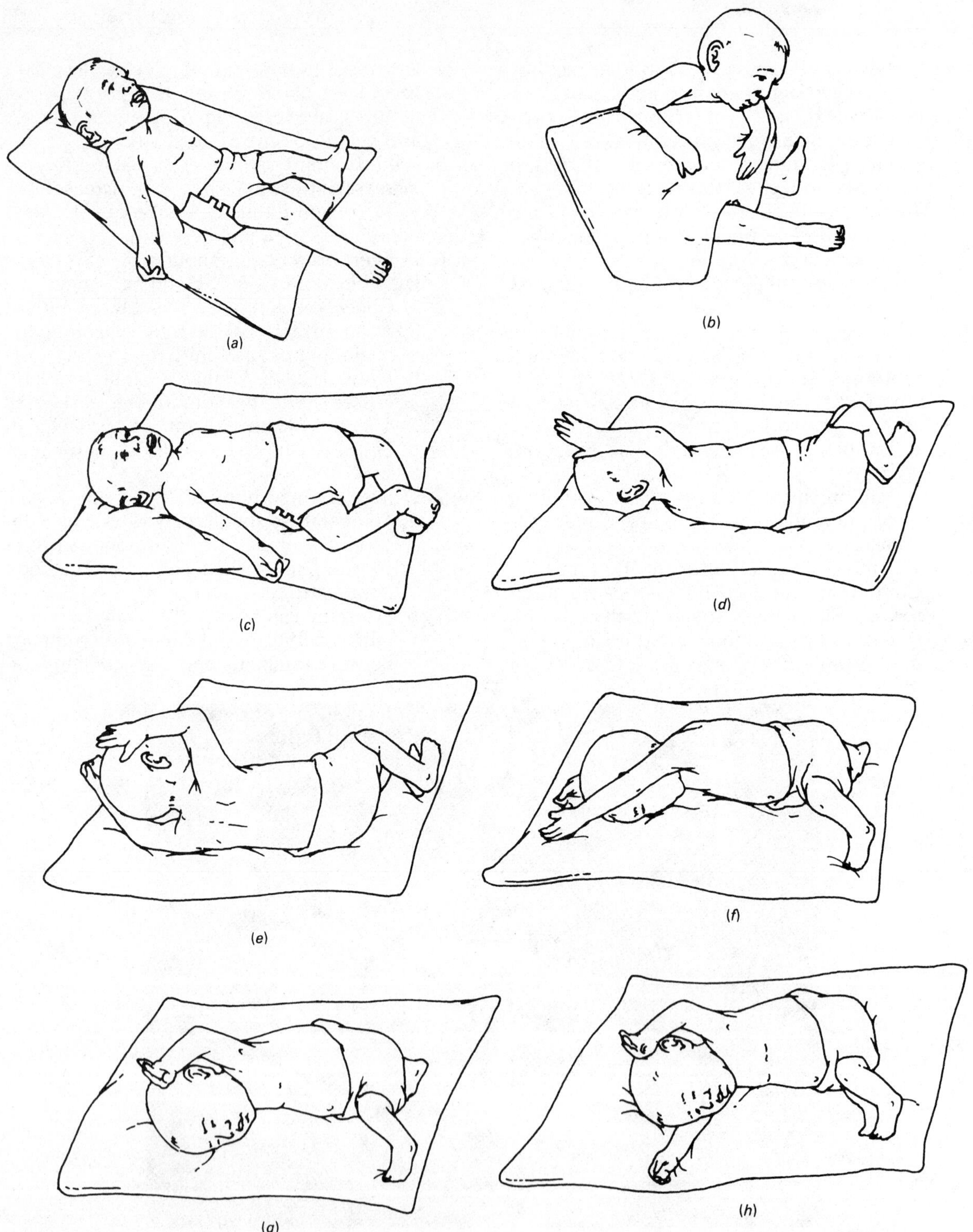

Figure 11-6 Chest physical therapy. Positions for percussion. (To drain upper lobes, infant should be tilted slightly by raising head of surface on which it is lying by 30 degrees. To drain lower lobes, infant should be tilted slightly by lowering head of surface on which it is lying by

ture will result in condensation within the oxyhood or tubing used with CPAP or ventilator.

c. Check that oxyhood is flush with bed surface to reduce leakage.

8. Maintain proper CPAP control at 5–6 cm H_2O (or at whatever pressure is ordered).
   a. Gently suction nasopharynx and mouth q2h or as necessary to prevent build-up of secretions, being very gentle to prevent injury to mucus membranes.
   b. Position infant with CPAP tubing carefully and reposition q2h.
   c. Maintain slight extension of neck while infant is in supine position.
   d. Intubated infants may also be placed in prone position.
9. Frequently check infant on mechanical ventilation.
   a. Auscultate for equal breath sounds to check proper placement of endotracheal tube.
   b. Observe for sudden changes in color.
   c. Observe for signs of complications, especially pneumothorax.
10. Suction endotrachial tube q2h to prevent plugging. Maintain strict asepsis.
   a. Bag infant for 20 s with 100 percent oxygen before suctioning with pressure-regulated bag.
   b. Instill 0.5–1.0 mL normal saline into tube to loosen secretions. Insert suction catheter into end of tube; suction briefly with vacuum set at 40–80 cm H_2O. If suctioning is done too long, infant may become temporarily hypoxic. Allow infant to recover after suctioning. Replace ventilator tubing carefully.
11. Chest physical therapy is prescribed for infants on mechanical ventilation or CPAP (see Figure 11-6). Include percussion, vibration, and gentle suctioning. Use cupped fingers, small rubber infant oxygen mask, or a rubber nipple for percussion. Use fingertips or an electric toothbrush with a soft rubber adapter (covered by gauze) for a tip. Vibration is done just after percussion. Chest physical therapy may be replaced by positional rotation for infants under 1000 g.
12. Maintain infusion into umbilical vessel catheter and prevent complications in technique.
   a. Withdraw blood by means of a three-way stop cock.
   b. Secure all connections with tape.
   c. Prevent injection of air or clotted blood into line.
13. Regulate and administer IV fluids through umbilical vessel catheter.
   a. Check infusion rate q1h. Use electric infusion pump.
   b. Avoid fluid overload to prevent congestive heart failure in infants who have or might develop PDA. An extra 20 mL of fluid constitutes approximately 25 percent of total blood volume for a 1000 g infant.
14. Administer blood transfusion through peripheral intravenous line. Use umbilical *arterial* catheters only for blood sampling or measurement of arterial blood pressure. Some institutions add heparin to arterial line to keep catheter open. Calculate daily amount of blood withdrawn for sampling and analysis to prevent hypovolemia, which will need blood replacement.

Reevaluation and Follow-up

1. Weaning off assisted respiration proceded without relapses, apnea, or cyanosis.
2. Respiratory rate, depth, rhythm assumed normal characteristics.
3. No complications related to IV therapy occurred.
4. Postdischarge follow-up revealed no BPD or RLF as results of oxygen toxicity.

30 degrees.) Place infant in proper positions to drain all lobes. *Percuss* using cupped hand, small rubber nipple, or small rubber infant oxygen mask. Follow by *vibration* over each lobe with fingertips or electric toothbrush with soft adapter. *Suction* follows percussion and vibration. (*a*) Percuss over nipple area on both sides of chest. (*b*) Percuss over scapula on both sides of chest. (*c*) Supine position: percuss over nipple area on both sides of chest. (*d*) $\frac{1}{4}$ turn on left side: percuss over armpit and nipple on right side. (*e*) $\frac{1}{4}$ turn more toward front on left side: percuss over scapula on right side. (*f*) Prone: percuss over each scapula. (*g*) $\frac{1}{4}$ turn toward back on right side: percuss over scapula on left side. (*h*) $\frac{1}{4}$ turn more toward back on right side: percuss over armpit and nipple on left side.

APNEA

DESCRIPTION

Apnea is the cessation of respiration for at least 20 s accompanied by bradycardia of less than 100 beats per minute. Most very small premature infants of less than 30 weeks gestation and about 20 percent of those less than 1800 g and 34 weeks gestation will have apneic episodes. For the premature, apnea usually presents during the first 2 days of life and may recur up to 21 days of life. It is therefore strongly recommended that all infants of less than 34 weeks gestation be monitored continuously for cardiorespiratory status.

Factors that predispose an infant to apnea in the early days of life include hypoxemia and respiratory center depression due to electrolyte or metabolic imbalance, drug effects, sepsis, or intracranial hemorrhage. In addition, vagal stimulation from the presence of suction catheters or upper airway fluid, increases in environmental temperature, obstruction due to passive neck flexion, and immaturity of the central nervous system may cause apnea. All infants demonstrating more extended periods of periodic breathing (PB) and apneic periods should be investigated for precipitating causes, especially when those infants are more than 34 weeks of gestational age. (Lewak, et al., 1979)

Apnea occurring later in the neonatal period or during early infancy is associated with the sudden infant death syndrome (SIDS). By postmortem exam, SIDS has been associated with tissue changes resulting from chronic hypoxemia and chronic hypoventilation (hypoxia).

The rate of SIDS is about 0.2 percent each year. Innumerable potential causes have been investigated; to date not one cause can be used as a predictor. There is no reliable screening method; each method has many false positives (Valdez-DaPena, 1980). However, periodic breathing and apnea have been used as a warning of susceptibility, and apnea monitoring is used fairly widely for known "at special risk" infants.

Several prospective studies are in progress, funded by the National Institute of child Health and Human Development. The Sudden Infant Death Syndrome Act of 1974 provided government funding for education of the public and for health practitioners. Correct support in the crisis period for a SIDS family may prevent subsequent unresolved guilt, anger, and grief (Smialek, 1978).

PREVENTION

Health Promotion

1. Increased public awareness of potential warning signs.
2. Increased health professionals' understanding and support for parents of susceptible infants.
3. Avoidance of precipitating factors during early days of life of premature infant.

Population at Risk

1. Some infants who have experienced birth asphyxia, perinatal stress.
2. Certain infants with erratic sleep states; more crying and higher than usual respiratory rates while at rest.
3. Certain infants who become pale during the quiet sleep state.
4. Certain infants who demonstrate an unusual cry; weaker, breathy, or very high pitched, with abrupt pitch changes.
5. Infants who continue to demonstrate increased periodic breathing, often more than 2 percent of 100 min, continuing into the infancy period.

Screening

None of the following are discriminatory as screening criteria (Lewak et al., 1979) but are useful to keep in mind.

1. History of heavy maternal smoking.
2. Young mother with no prenatal care.
3. Short interpregnancy intervals.
4. Infant under 40 weeks gestational age.
5. Birth weight under 3000 g.
6. Mother from lower socioeconomic status.
7. Infant of male sex.
8. Previous SIDS infant as sibling.

ASSESSMENT

Health History

1. Maternal status related to potential screening criteria.
2. Record of birth management.
3. For later apnea: record of cardiorespiratory adaptation in nursery.

Physical Assessment

1. Apnea of as much as 20 s or more with bradycardia.
2. Cyanosis followed by pallor and hypotonia if apnea continues as much as 20–45 s or more.
3. No response to stimulation if duration is 45 s or greater.
4. Episodes of periodic breathing or apnea during feeding periods.
5. Some infants have statistically significant higher heart rates at 10 to 14 weeks than does the normal average infant.
6. Presence in some cases of mild respiratory illness.
7. Five percent of later apneic infants (SIDS) may have infant botulism (Arnon et al., 1978).

Diagnostic Tests

1. Continuous transcutaneous oxygen monitoring in susceptible immature infants.
2. Arterial blood gas levels.
3. Culture of or isolation of organisms, sepsis workup.
4. Cardiopulmonary monitoring.

NURSING DIAGNOSIS: ACTUAL OR POTENTIAL

1. Altered rhythm of sleep states due to unknown causes, due to immaturity.
2. Respiratory dysfunction due to unknown causes, due to perinatal stress, due to immaturity.
3. Parental anxiety about susceptible infant at risk for prolonged apnea.

INTERVENTIONS

1. Neonatal apnea.
   a. Control for large swings in environmental temperature.
   b. Position correctly to prevent neck flexion and airway obstruction.
   c. Suction carefully, briefly.
   d. Stimulate respirations by touch, flicking feet, rubbing back; use cardiopulmonary monitoring.
   e. Correct any anemia by blood transfusion to raise hematocrit $\geq$ 45 percent.
   f. Analyze progress in diminishing episodes of periodic breathing during quiet sleep. Evaluate infant states.
   g. If PB episodes are frequent, administer theophylline to decrease frequency. Check infant's heart rate before administering. Observe for and prevent toxic levels shown by tachycardia, GI problems.
   h. Terminate any oxygen supplement gradually to prevent cyanosis.
   i. If infant progresses beyond 20-s apnea and does not respond to stimulation, assess heart rate then begin ventilation by bag and mask. Begin mechanical ventilation, if necessary.
   j. In severe cases, evaluate and begin cardiac resuscitation while continuing bag breathing.
2. Later apnea.
   a. For parents of "near miss infants" who are brought to SIDS centers, cardiopulmonary resuscitation for the infant should be taught in detail.
   b. Evaluate parents' ability to manage the anxiety of apnea monitoring over extended periods of time.
   c. Provide for and encourage special support for parents during the higher risk periods between 10 and 14 weeks of age (3 to 4 months)
   d. Encourage methods of anxiety reduction in parents and other siblings; counseling, parent sharing groups, close contact with SIDS center.
   e. Teach parents health care of infant to promote optimum health during high-risk period.

EVALUATION

Outcome Criteria

1. Treatment has stabilized the immature infant or perinatally stressed infant. Respiratory rates are within normal ranges.
2. Infant in susceptible category is managed at home until the high-risk period has passed.

SEPSIS

Neonates are subject to infection from various sources—prenatally from transplacental transfer of organisms, intrapartally from contamination of the birth canal or via ascending infection, and postnatally due to contamination from the environment. Over the years, major causative organisms have varied from group A β-hemolytic streptococci prior to the 1940s, to *Staphylococcus aureus* in the 1950s, to gram-negative organisms in the 1960s, and currently to group B β-hemolytic streptococci. There are also differences in causative organisms in primary and secondary infection. Primary sepsis is usually caused by organisms such as *Escherichia coli, Klebsiella,* enterococci, and β-streptococci that are contracted in the birth canal or from ascending infection after PROM. Contamination during the nursery stay with *Staphylococcus aureus* and pseudomonas is responsible for secondary sepsis. (See Table 12-3 for infectious diseases.) Despite these differences, the incidence of neonatal septicemia has varied between 1:500 to 1:1600 live births for the past 40 years. However, the mortality rate has dropped from over 90 percent before the advent of antibiotics to the current rate of 13 to 14 percent. Immaturity of the immune system, specifically decreased levels of complement, inadequate phagocytosis, and opsoninization, makes the newborn especially vulnerable to sepsis.

There are many warning signals that should alert the nurse to the possibility of infection. Prenatally, prolonged rupture of membranes—over 12 h—increases the possibility of ascending infection. During the intrapartum period, maternal fever of unknown origin, foul-smelling, cloudy, brownish, or meconium-stained amniotic fluid, or low Apgar scores place the neonate at risk for infection. After birth, the signs of infection are subtle and can be easily mistaken or overlooked. They may include:

1. Respiratory distress
2. Shock
3. Temperature instability
4. Metabolic acidosis
5. Gastrointestinal symptoms: poor feeding, abdominal distension, diarrhea, vomiting
6. Lethargy—baby is "just not doing well"
7. Omphalitis
8. Seizures
9. Hepatomegaly
10. Petechiae or purpura

Treatment of sepsis varies with the causative organism. Most often, a combination of antibiotics effective against both gram-positive and gram-negative organisms will be used. After all appropriate cultures (blood, surface, urine, and cerebrospinal fluid) have been obtained, penicillin or ampicillin plus one of the aminoglycosides are given intravenously for 24–48 h to achieve adequate blood levels. If staphylococcus infection is suspected, a penicillinase resistant penicillin such as oxacillin is used. Routes of administration may be changed to intramuscular depending upon results of the cultures and the infant's clinical condition. As such drugs are excreted by the kidneys and aminoglycosides may be toxic to the kidneys, voiding patterns, urinalysis, and BUN and creatinine levels should be monitored.

NECROTIZING ENTEROCOLITIS

Necrotizing enterocolitis (NEC) is a disease seen primarily in premature and low-birth-weight infants who have suffered some severe perinatal stress. It is precipitated by problems causing hypoxia or ischemia of the bowels. Respiratory distress syndrome, apnea, low Apgar, metabolic acidosis, or hemodynamic changes due to exchange transfusion, umbilical vessel catheters, plus infected amniotic fluid may predispose the neonate to NEC. Because NEC is almost never seen in infants that have not been fed, it is believed that in some way hyperosmolar formula may initiate the damage, due perhaps to a direct effect of the hypertonic fluid on the mucosal cells. In addition, episodes of asphyxia that trigger the redistribution of cardiac output cause reflex vasoconstriction of the intestinal vasculature, leading to bowel ischemia and mucosal damage. During these episodes, blood is shunted away from mesenteric, renal, and peripheral beds to protect the brain and heart—a state referred to as the "diving reflex."

Furthermore, during the first 2 to 3 weeks of life the neonate has an absence of intestinal immunities due to the lack of local antibodies. The intestine, therefore, has an increased susceptibility to microorganisms during this time, and these organisms may gain access to and proliferate in the bowel wall. Following an asphyxic episode, a portion of the bowel may become ischemic and necrotic. Perforation of the bowel wall may occur with multiplication and colonization of bacteria. The final result can be overwhelming sepsis and death.

The frequency of NEC in premature intensive care nurseries is 1 to 10 percent. The onset is usually seen within the first week of life but may appear as late as the second or third week. Infants suspected of having NEC may present the following symptoms: abdominal distension, poor feeding, vomiting, residuals from previous feeding, apnea, bradycardia, lethargy, tachypnea, temperature instability, jaundice, blood in the stool, and decreased bowel sounds. Upon abdominal x-ray, intramural air may be seen.

As soon as NEC is suspected, gastrointestinal feedings are discontinued and parenteral nutrition is begun. An abdominal x-ray taken immediately will rule out perforation of the bowel, which would require emergency surgery. A nasogastic tube is placed and connected to low suction and the infant examined frequently, especially to note abdominal girth and the presence or absence of bowel sounds. A sepsis workup is done and a broad spectrum of antibiotics administered. Special attention is paid to fluid and electrolyte balance. Close observation and prompt action are essential in preventing bowel perforation. (See Chapter 22 for detailed outline of treatment.)

HYPOGLYCEMIA

DESCRIPTION

When serum glucose levels in the first 3 days of life are below 30 mg/dL in the full-term infant and 20 mg/dL in the preterm infant, a state of hypoglycemia exists. Thereafter, levels below 40 mg should be cause for concern. Hypoglycemia is commonest at 24–72 h of life but will occur early if there is any perinatal stress, such as birth trauma, low Apgar score with acidosis, respiratory distress, or neonatal sepsis. Glycogen stores are quickly depleted and the infant shows signs as early as 2–4 h. Preterm infants are often in distress with hypothermia or respiratory difficulty and may commonly demonstrate hypoglycemia in the early adjustment period.

Infants who are small for gestational age can become hypoglycemic because of chronically low glycogen and fat stores as well as the increased incidence of perinatal stress associated with being SGA. Of special concern is the infant of a diabetic mother (IDM) (see Chapter 7). This infant may be LGA due to increased overall growth and extra fat stores plus visceromegaly—hepatomegaly, pancreatic hyperplasia, and cardiac septal hypertrophy, especially. Hypoglycemia is precipitated by pancreatic beta cell hyperplasia and resultant hyperinsulinemia. When maternal circulating glucose is abruptly cut off by delivery, pancreatic activity continues into the first hours after birth and hypoglycemia may be profound. In addition, hypocalcemia, polycythemia, and hyperbilirubinemia are also seen more commonly. Respiratory distress may stress the infant and cause further utilization of available glycogen stores.

There is an increased incidence of congenital anomalies in these infants; as the mother's disease progresses in severity, more defects are seen. Cardiac defects—ventricular septal defect (VSD) and transposition of great arteries (TGA)—caudal regression syndrome (sacral agenesis), and renal anomalies are the most frequent. If maternal disease is very severe, the infant may suffer from intrauterine growth retardation due to placental dysfunction. In all cases, hypoglycemia is a primary factor in morbidity.

PREVENTION

1. Well-monitored low-risk delivery.
2. Stabilized pregnancy and delivery for diabetic women.
3. Early monitoring for all neonates at risk.
4. Early feedings for all newborn infants.

Screening

Dextrostix (Ames) done for any infant weighing 8 or more lb, for any high-risk infant, and for any infant in the 90th or more percentile for weight regardless of gestational age.

ASSESSMENT

Health History

1. Maternal status—diabetes, drug addiction, intrapartum stress.
2. Record of course of labor and delivery; monitoring record, fetal scalp sampling results.
3. Apgar score at 1 and 5 min of life.

Physical Assessment

1. Assessment for gestational age.
   a. Infant may be preterm yet appear average in weight.
   b. Infant may be postmature.
   c. Infant may be LGA even without maternal history of diabetes. Mother may later be

shown to be a latent diabetic, or to have had a nutritional surplus.
   d. Infant may be SGA.
2. Infant may have been stressed during labor and delivery, with a lower than expected Apgar score.
3. Infant demonstrates signs of jitteriness, refusal to feed, limpness, irritability, periods of apnea and, when very severe, seizures.
4. Signs may be confused with those of hypocalcemia, sepsis, results of withdrawal from maternal drug of abuse or may be attributed to unknown causes.
5. Cry may be high-pitched or weak.
6. Labile temperature, tends toward hypothermia.
7. Other signs of poor adjustment occur, respiratory distress, acidosis, hypoxemia.

EXPECTED OUTCOMES

The infant's glucose balance will be returned to the normal range.

INTERVENTIONS

1. Evaluate blood glucose at capillary level every 1–2 h until stable and above 45 mg/dL:
   a. *Birth:* mean 55 mg/dL.
   b. *2–4 h:* mean 51 mg/dL.
   c. *By 72 h:* mean 70 mg/dL.
2. Confirm low results by lab analysis of true blood glucose.
3. Begin early oral or gavage feedings of 10% glucose water if possible at 1–2 h for any IDM, low-birth-weight infant, or high-risk infant. If oral feedings are not possible, begin parenteral glucose.
   a. Give at least 200 mg/kg 25% dextrose and water by IV push at rate of 1 mL/min. Occasionally up to 1 g/kg is needed to restore balance.
   b. Follow with steady infusion of 10% dextrose and water to provide about 4–8 mg/kg per min.
   c. Higher concentrations can cause rebound hypoglycemia when discontinued; hyperosmolar solutions may cause tissue damage if infiltration occurs.
   d. If glucose level cannot be maintained, increase concentration slowly to 12.5 or 15 percent to maintain requirements.
   e. Maintain constant infusion rate by IV pump. Never abruptly discontinue solution. Wean infant off IV after oral feedings are well established.
   f. Maintain temperature and humidity control during period of hypoglycemia.

EVALUATION

Outcome Criteria

Infant is progressing to taking oral feedings and is maintaining normoglycemia.

Complications

Persistent Hypoglycemia. Glucagon and glucocorticoids may be ordered, and a workup for alternate causes of the problem will be done.

HYPOCALCEMIA

DESCRIPTION

Hypocalcemia is defined as a serum calcium level below 7 mg/100 mL for the infant. Low levels of serum calcium commonly follow a drop in glucose, partially because glucagon is activated, which in turn promotes calcium excretion. Premature infants are particularly at risk as a result of low calcium stores at birth; however, other infants may also be at risk for developing hypocalcemia: infants of diabetic mothers, asphyxiated infants (especially those resuscitated with sodium bicarbonate), infants of preeclamptic mothers, and infants who have been exchange-transfused with citrated blood (calcium binds to citrate). In some infants a calcium phosphate imbalance may develop several days after formula feedings have been established. Symptoms are nonspecific and frequently confused with those of other problems (e.g., hypoglycemia). The most common signs are irritability, jitteriness, cyanosis, vomiting and, if severe, seizures.

Hypocalcemia is usually treated parenterally or orally with 10% calcium gluconate. Infants receiving parenteral calcium should be monitored carefully for IV infiltration, as severe tissue necrosis results. Vital signs should be monitored carefully, especially for heart rate; bradycardia may result from too much calcium. For infants suffering from calcium-phosphorous imbalance, a low-phosphorous formula such as PM 60/40 (Ross) should be ordered.

HYPOTHERMIA

DESCRIPTION

Neonates produce most of their body heat by metabolic processes, by nonshivering thermogenesis. Hypothermia—cold stress—is common in neonates because there is a large skin surface to body weight ratio, varying degrees of subcutaneous fat, and no shivering response to cold, and in the early hours of adjustment there may be a lack of calories in quantities sufficient for heat production. A full-term infant has an additional source of fat, BAT or *brown fat*, deposited around certain organs, around the neck and the trachea, and under the scapula (Davis, 1980). This BAT may produce additional calories in response to hypothermia. The preterm infant is deficient in BAT as well as in glycogen stores and subcutaneous fat and thus is much more likely to have difficulty with temperature control. Any respiratory distress or disturbance in endocrine or neurologic function will further delay body temperature adjustment.

When an infant suffers moderate to severe cooling, there is a series of responses that ultimately lead to anaerobic metabolism and acidosis. Even under normal delivery room conditions without special precautions, body temperature may fall 2 to 3 degrees. As temperature drops, oxygen consumption and glucose utilization increase and the infant may become hypoglycemic.

The goal of preventive care is to keep the infant within the neutral thermal environment (NTE) and thereby minimize heat loss. The NTE is defined as the "thermal condition at which heat production, as measured by oxygen consumption, is minimal, yet core temperature is within the normal range" (Cloherty, 1980). NTE varies with age in hours and with the weight of the infant.

Heat may be lost by *convection*—loss of heat from skin to moving air—and especially may be lost because of the difference in temperature of incubator air and ambient room air. Heat lost by *conduction* is transferred from skin to a colder surface such as a scale or examining table. Heat lost by *radiation* is lost into the air of a colder environment or to colder incubator walls; heat is especially lost from the head by radiation. *Evaporation* is the loss of heat from wet skin. Measures taken to prevent heat loss begin in the delivery room with every infant.

PREVENTION

Health Promotion

1. Correct adjustment of heat sources in delivery room.
2. Reduction of potential heat loss at delivery through:
   a. Convection—close all doors to delivery room.
   b. Conduction—warm crib pad, blankets; use skin-to-skin conduction when with mother.
   c. Radiation—increase delivery room ambient temperature; carefully control overhead radiant heater.
   d. Evaporation—dry the infant at once.
3. Use of overhead radiant heater for any treatments or handling of potentially hypothermic infant. Use of overhead source of heat if early acquaintance periods are in the cooler recovery room when infant is full term.
4. Serial measurements of nursery ambient temperature in comparison with incubator wall and air temperature.

Population at Risk

1. Any infant at birth.
2. Small infants in nursery or incubators.
3. Any infant having an extramural delivery.
4. Infants cared for in homes without adequate heat regulation.
5. Infants exposed to cold as the result of ignorance or carelessness of the care provider.

ASSESSMENT

Health History

1. Control of environmental and body temperature before admission.
2. Maternal history of exposure to cold, for example, delivery enroute to hospital.

Physical Assessment

1. Core temperature below 37°C; may fall as low as 35°C.
2. Skin cold to touch, especially extremities.

3. Grunting; periods of apnea; slow, shallow, irregular breathing.
4. Bradycardia proportionate to degree of temperature drop.
5. Cyanosis, or pallor, or infant may be bright red in color due to dissociation of oxyhemoglobin at low temperatures.
6. Infant feeds poorly, is lethargic.
7. CNS depression, poor reflexes.
8. Edema of extremities and face and, very late, *sclerema*, hardening of skin.

Diagnostic Tests

1. Blood glucose levels.
2. Blood gasses to determine level of hypoxemia.
3. Constant monitoring of temperature.
4. Electrolytes; hyperkalemia; elevated BUN may occur.

NURSING DIAGNOSES: ACTUAL OR POTENTIAL

1. Alteration in body temperature due to exposure, to very small body size, or to asphyxia, RDS, or hypoglycemia.
2. Potential for cold injury.
3. Alteration in tissue oxygenation; in glucose metabolism as a result of increased metabolic activity.

EXPECTED OUTCOMES

1. A skin temperature of 36 to 36.5°C will be maintained after rewarming.
2. Weight loss will be kept to a minimum by providing supplemental calories.
3. Respiratory distress will be corrected.
4. Metabolic balance will be recovered.
5. Infant will resume thermoregulation within normal infant parameters in the correctly controlled environment of nursery or home.

INTERVENTIONS

1. Rewarm the infant slowly. Set control for air temperature at 1.5°C above skin abdominal temperature on admission. Change subsequent settings of radiant warmer after infant's temperature has equilibrated.
   a. Do not rewarm too rapidly as it will cause apnea.
   b. Check skin temperature every 15 min.
   c. Use radiant warmer only until up to reaching 36°C, then transfer infant to incubator to prevent heat loss through convection. Continue to use skin probe to maintain temperature of skin at 36.5°C.
   d. Check incubator wall temperature; a clear plastic shield may be needed as a double wall if more than 2 to 3 degrees of difference are found.
2. If the infant is later removed from incubator, double wrap.
3. Apply stockinette cap to prevent heat loss from scalp.
4. Monitor blood glucose qlh.
   a. Feed glucose PO or IV for hypoglycemia.
   b. Do not nipple feed until skin temperature of 36°C is reached.
5. Monitor blood gasses.
   a. Administer warmed, humidified oxygen as needed.
   b. Administer sodium bicarbonate as needed.

EVALUATION

Outcome Criteria

1. Infant temperature control center is maturing to provide adequate newborn control.
2. Infant is being maintained in fluid and electrolyte balance; no damage from hypoglycemia or hypoxia.
3. Weight loss has been minimized; infant is gaining weight.

HYPERBILIRUBINEMIA

DESCRIPTION

Jaundice is one of the most common problems seen during the neonatal period. The newborn infant has a normal increase in bilirubin after birth due to the rapid breakdown of extra fetal hemoglobin that the immature liver is slow to metabolize. The extra bilirubin produced as fetal hemoglobin is broken down and remains in a fat-soluble, unconjugated, indirect form until further metabolized into water-soluble, direct bilirubin. Levels will rise normally in a newborn during the first 3 days of life but should peak before reaching 15 mg/dL in the preterm and 12 mg/dL in the full-term infant. The average rise for a mature infant is 4–8 mg/dL. Jaundice becomes evident at 5 mg/dL. (Maisels, 1980).

Treatment is initiated in the preterm and term infant if levels appear to be rising steadily and there are factors accentuating the delay in bilirubin metabolism. Prevention of *kernicterus*, deposit of bilirubin in the gray matter of the brain, especially in the basal ganglia, is essential. The degeneration of these cells may result in varying degrees of neurologic defects; deafness, mental retardation, cerebral palsy are severe effects. In less severe cases "minimal brain dysfunction" may develop.

Factors such as acidosis, asphyxia, perinatal distress, prematurity, and low birth weight may allow kernicterus to develop at lower than expected levels; small infants have developed kernicterus at 6–10 mg bilirubin.

In unusual cases when direct, conjugated bilirubin levels are more than 2 mg/dL, it is due to a failure to excrete conjugated water-soluble bilirubin. This may be a result of biliary atresia, neonatal hepatitis, sepsis, intrauterine infections (TORCH), galactosemia, cystic fibrosis, and alpha-antitrypsin deficiency. Such infants are not treated with phototherapy as there is a risk of producing the "bronze baby" syndrome, that is, the skin takes on a bronze color. Although such pigmentation has not yet been proved harmful, the reason for its presence is not clear.

Table 11-5 presents the main causes of hyperbilirubinemia in infants. See Chapter 10 for a description of blood incompatibilities leading to elevated bilirubin.

PREVENTION

Health Promotion

1. Avoid any prenatal intake of drugs that affect metabolic cycle of bilirubin.
2. Monitor mothers for TORCH and associated infections.
3. Prevent sensitization in cases of blood incompatibility (see Chapter 10).

Population at Risk

1. Premature, immature infants.
2. Infants with perinatal stress, asphyxia, polycythemia.
3. Infants of diabetic mothers.
4. Some infants of breastfeeding mothers.
5. Infants with certain inborn errors of metabolism.
6. Infants with blood incompatibilities (see Chapter 10).

TABLE 11.5 SELECTED CAUSES OF HYPERBILIRUBINEMIA

Blood group incompatibilities—hemolysis:
- ABO—mother type O, infant type A or B with positive direct Coombs'
- Rh—mother Rh negative, infant Rh positive with positive direct Coombs'
- Minor groups—Duffy, Kell, etc.

Enclosed hemorrhage:
- Birth trauma—cephalhematoma, vacuum extraction
- Cerebral or pulmonary hemorrhage
- Ecchymosis—face presentation

Polycythemia (central hematocrit ≥ 60%); jaundice appears after 48 h
- Delayed cord clamping, infant held below placenta for too long a time
- Twin-to-twin transfusion
- Maternal-fetal transfusion
- SGA, LGA, IDM

Infections—intrauterine and neonatal:
- TORCH diseases
- Hepatitis
- Sepsis

Respiratory distress

Metabolic deficiencies:
- Prematurity
- Hypothyroidism
- Drug inhibition of bilirubin metabolism: diazepam, erythromycin, apresoline, sulfonamides
- Lucy Driscoll syndrome
- Some breast milks: inhibition by pregnanediol

Nonhemolytic anemia—familial, Criqler-Najjar syndrome

Hemolytic anemia:
- Glucose-6-phosphate dehydrogenase plus drug inducement
- Pyruvate kinase deficiency
- Thalassemias

Increased enterohepatic circulation:
- Meconium ileus
- Swallowed blood
- Intestinal atresia
- Hypoperistalsis

Obstruction in bile passage:
- Biliary atresia
- Alpha-antitrypsin deficiency
- Cystic fibrosis

Screening

1. Cord blood for direct, indirect, and total bilirubin levels.
2. Cord blood for type and Coombs' test.

ASSESSMENT

Physical Assessment

1. Any of the problems listed in Table 11-5 are present.
2. Infant's skin and possibly sclera are yellow. Jaundice becomes visible at 5 mg/dL and is observed on face and central trunk, progressing distally as levels rise.
3. There is a darker color to stool, urine.
4. Toxic signs are varied. Apneic periods may be only sign in immature infants.
   a. Diminished neurologic responses.
   b. Poor sucking.
   c. Hypotonia.
   d. Vomiting.
   e. High-pitched cry.

Diagnostic Tests

1. Blood type and Coombs' test.
2. Cross match of blood with mother's serum to identify incompatibility when both are of same major blood type.
3. Hematocrit and reticulocyte count; hemolysis—hematocrit falls, reticulytes may be higher than normal.
4. Peripheral blood smear, hemoglobin electrophoresis. Rule out structural problems due to defects in hemoglobin.
5. Sepsis workup.
6. Cord bilirubin—direct, indirect, total. Total should be less than 2 mg/dL at birth.
7. Albumin ratios—normal 3–3.5 g/dL.

NURSING DIAGNOSES: ACTUAL OR POTENTIAL

1. Altered adaptation to extrauterine life related to cause of hyperbilirubinemia.
2. Potential: altered fluid volume due to increased insensible water loss with treatment.
3. Potential for injury due to toxic effects of bilirubin.

EXPECTED OUTCOMES

1. Toxic effects will be avoided by early detection of rising bilirubin levels, with appropriate intervention taken.
2. Parents will understand why treatments are done and the possible outcome.
3. The infant will return to normal bilirubin levels for age.

INTERVENTIONS

1. Note and report any maternal drugs that may occupy albumin binding sites and thus displace protein-bound bilirubin (see Table 11-5).
2. Evaluate meconium passage (time and amount), as a delay in stooling will result in increased enterohepatic reabsorption (recycling) of bilirubin.
3. Evaluate any enclosed hemorrhage; cephalhematoma, intracranial, or serious bruising.
4. Feed infant adequate amounts of fluids to prevent dehydration in the first recovery period.
5. Evaluate bilirubin levels on all high-risk infants. Initiate capillary evaluation of bilirubin on infants showing jaundice.
6. Choice of phototherapy or exchange transfusion depends on onset and rate of increase, birth weight, and condition.
   a. Phototherapy—photodegrades bilirubin into water-soluble readily excretable form. It is used when:
      (1) Levels of 5–9 mg/dL are present in the first 24 h of life.
      (2) Levels of 10–14 mg/100 mL occur in 24–72 h.
      (3) Levels of 15–19 mg/100 mL occur in 48–72 h. Exchange may be considered for infants weighing less than 2500 g at these levels. It is suggested that phototherapy begin at 8 mg/100 mL in sick preterm infants.
   b. Exchange transfusion is usually planned when:
      (1) Levels over 10 mg/100 mL occur in first 24 h.
      (2) Levels of 15–19 mg/100 mL in 24–48 h.
      (3) All levels over 20 mg/100 mL. Regimen is modified whenever respiratory distress, acidosis, hypothermia, immaturity, and low serum albumin are present and exchange is indicated earlier (Klaus and Fanaroff, 1978).
7. Support infant during phototherapy.
   a. Lights must be monitored for wave-

length, not brightness. "Brightness of light is not the key, but rather the amount of energy output at wavelengths close to 460" (Klaus and Fanaroff). Energy output must be monitored by hospital engineer.

b. Side effects of diarrhea and increased insensible water loss can be treated with lactose-free formula and extra fluid intake. Careful observation of intake and output is important, as there is a 300 percent greater insensible water loss and greater than twice as much water loss via stools in infants weighing less than 2500 g. (Seligman, 1977).
c. Some infants develop a rash for which there is no specific treatment.
d. Skin must be uncovered as much as possible while correct ambient temperature is maintained. Monitor temperature. Do not allow hypothermia or hyperthermia to develop.
e. Eyes must be completely covered with an opaque mask over soft cotton eye patches (Figure 11-7). Remove for feeding to observe eyes, allow blinking and prevent sensory deprivation. Often, isotonic eye drops may be prescribed.
f. Careful explanation to parents about reasons for and progress of treatment. Mother should feed infant wherever possible.

8. Support infant during exchange transfusion. Klaus and Fanaroff (1978) describe the basic technique. Important points are:
   a. Correctly cross-matched blood, depending on cause of hemolytic disease.
   b. Initial transfusion of 1 g/kg albumin may be used $\frac{1}{2}$–1 h before exchange to bind with and reduce serum bilirubin.
   c. Use of warmed donor blood, fresh if possible.
   d. Infant kept NPO, with IV fluids containing glucose.
   e. Use of overhead radiant warmer to prevent chilling.
   f. Resuscitation equipment at hand.
   g. Oxygen, humidified.
   h. Cardiac and respiratory and temperature monitors in place.
   i. Strict sterile technique, exchange via umbilical vein if possible.
   j. Blood pressure checked at specified intervals.
   k. Careful check for hypocalcemia, calcium gluconate provided as necessary.
   l. Use of first and last sample to check of bilirubin, hematocrit, other blood counts.
   m. Protamine sulfate may be needed if heparinized blood must be used.
   n. Calcium gluconate 100 mg may be given for every 100 mL blood to prevent hypocalcemia. When citrated blood is used, the citrate bonds with calcium, thus lowering serum calcium levels. Heart rate should be monitored while the calcium is administered slowly. This procedure varies from institution to institution.

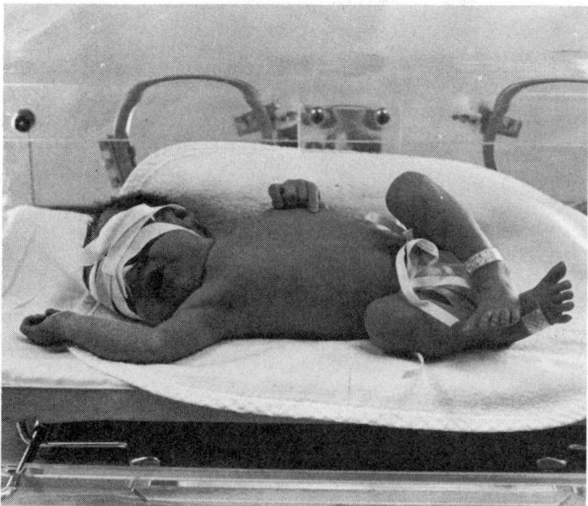

Figure 11-7 Infant under phototherapy light.

OUTCOME CRITERIA

Bilirubin levels are returning to the normal range for age in response to therapy.

THE POSTMATURE INFANT

Postmaturity is defined as gestation lasting beyond 42 weeks. The incidence of postmaturity varies with its causes. Prolonged pregnancy may be a normal variant, as some women routinely deliver as much as 2 to 3 weeks after their EDD; however, it may also be associated with trisomy 16-18 or Seckel's dwarfism and anencephaly (where the absent pituitary-adrenal axis delays initiation of labor).

The infant who has the "postmaturity syndrome" is an infant whose length and head circumference are normal but who has lost weight in utero. This weight loss is due to malnutrition as a result of poor placental function after 42 weeks. There are three stages of postmaturity as classified by physical assessment.

Stage 1: Dry, cracked peeling, loose, wrinkled skin.
Malnourished appearance.
Decreased subcutaneous tissue.
Skin too big for baby.
Open-eyed, alert, hungry baby.

Stage 2: All features of stage 1.
Meconium staining of cord and nails.
Birth asphyxia in some cases.

Stage 3: All features of stages 1 and 2.
Peeling skin, especially on palms, soles, often in large patches.
Many fetal, intrapartum, and neonatal deaths.

Mothers who have delivered one postmature infant must be observed carefully during subsequent pregnancies. A good menstrual history and early serial ultrasonic examination of the fetus will yield accurate pregnancy dating. Fetal status is also monitored by use of estriols and nonstress testing. Delivery is planned when the fetus is mature.

MECONIUM ASPIRATION SYNDROME

Postmature infants should be observed during the intrapartum period for signs of asphyxia and meconium aspiration syndrome (MAS). Meconium aspiration occurs when the fetus passes meconium in utero, possibly in response to a period of hypoxia or stress, and then hypoxic gasps deeply pull the meconium-stained amniotic fluid into the respiratory tree. Meconium is a tenacious material that obstructs large and small airways, thus causing air to be trapped within the areoli; it is also an excellent medium for growth of organisms. Signs of an infant with MAS include rupture of membranes with meconium-stained fluid, postmaturity, and/or var-

TABLE 11-6 SIGNS OF THE POSTMATURITY SYNDROME

Head.	No lanugo on face, edges of skull bones are hard, fontanelles small. Hair is smooth but may be receding from forehead.
Ears.	Pinna incurved to lobe, firm with cartilage.
Eyes.	Appears very alert; eyes wide open, gazing at objects.
Face.	Appears thin, "little old man" look.
Chest.	May show retractions if perinatal asphyxia with MAS. Bony prominences may be evident. Loss of weight clearly evident.
Abdomen.	May be flattened if infant has passed meconium; appears sunken in, not protuberant. Cord may be thin with little Wharton's jelly, may be meconium-stained.
Heart.	Check for distant heart sounds as air leaks (pneumomediastinum and pneumothorax are more common).
Genitalia.	Very pendulous scrotum with descended testes. Labia cover clitoris but may show loss of fatty tissue.
Extremities.	Loss of subcutaneous tissue makes legs and arms look wasted. Nails are long and may be meconium-stained. There are very deep creases over soles of feet and ankle flexion easily assumes a zero angle.
Skin.	Degrees of dry peeling skin evident, may be peeling off in sheets. No lanugo or vernix. May have poor skin turgor.
Central Nervous System.	Hypertonic. All reflexes readily elicited. Vigorous suck, often appears hungry. Tremors of hypoglycemia or hypocalcemia are frequent.

iable or late decelerations with poor variability. MAS can be prevented or its severity lessened by immediate suctioning of the naso/oral pharynx upon delivery of the infant's head, followed by intubation and suction of the trachea. Postpartum polycythemia secondary to stress and hypoglycemia secondary to decreased glycogen stores are common.

Postmature infants who progress without complication through the immediate recovery period usually show rapid weight gain, good appetite, and visual alertness. If the infant was not subjected to fetal distress and anoxic insult, the parents usually can be assured that brain tissue was selectively protected during the period of fetal weight loss (see Table 11-6).

TRANSPORT TO A REGIONAL CENTER

DESCRIPTION

The improvement in survival rate and the quality of survival of the high-risk and ill neonate is partially due to improvements in regionalization of care. Approximately 10 percent of all live births require specialized neonatal intensive care that can be provided at tertiary-level hospitals with neonatal intensive care units or secondary hospitals with neonatal special care units (Ferrara and Harin, 1980). Although primary-level smaller hospitals usually need to transport high-risk neonates to larger hospitals, in any obstetrical unit it is essential that there be personnel who are trained to perform resuscitation of the newborn and provide support to stabilize the infant until a transport team arrives.

Classification of different level hospitals and efficient transport systems are the trend around the country. A well-equipped transport facility is important to the tiny neonate during the period when early extrauterine adjustment is taking place. To reduce the risks of delay involved in transport of a very sick preterm infant, some institutions are now planning to deliver all high-risk mothers in regional tertiary centers (Figure 11-8).

ASSESSMENT

1. High-risk mother with impending delivery at primary-level hospital.
2. Low-birth-weight, preterm, or other high-risk infant is delivered at primary-level hospital.
3. Infant needs intensive care because of anomalies, RDS, or other life-threatening disease.
4. Parents are anxious and may be upset and confused about what is happening to their infant.

EXPECTED OUTCOMES

1. High-risk mother will be taken to a regional center for delivery if hospital is ill-equipped to care for baby.
2. Infant will be given prompt attention and will be stabilized before transport team arrives.
3. Infant will not be unnecessarily stressed by treatments and diagnostic tests before transfer.
4. Infant will be in thermoneutral state before and during transport and upon arrival.
5. Parents will have understanding about transport requirement and will see their infant before transfer; father will accompany infant when possible.

INTERVENTIONS

1. Notify transport team of impending high-risk delivery that will require transfer (e.g., very premature births or cases of known genetic or congenital defects.)
2. Arrange for transport team to arrive at sending hospital before delivery, if possible.
3. Support infant before arrival of transport team.
   a. Obtain vital signs, attach monitors.
   b. Dextrostix upon admission to nursery and q1h thereafter.
   c. Maintain neutral thermal environment by means of overhead radiant heater.
   d. Support infant's condition as necessary.
      (1) Provide oxygen via oxyhood, or do bag breathing via bag and mask. In severe distress, use endotracheal tube (if experienced personnel available to intubate) with mechanical ventilator or with bagging if mechanical ventilator not available.

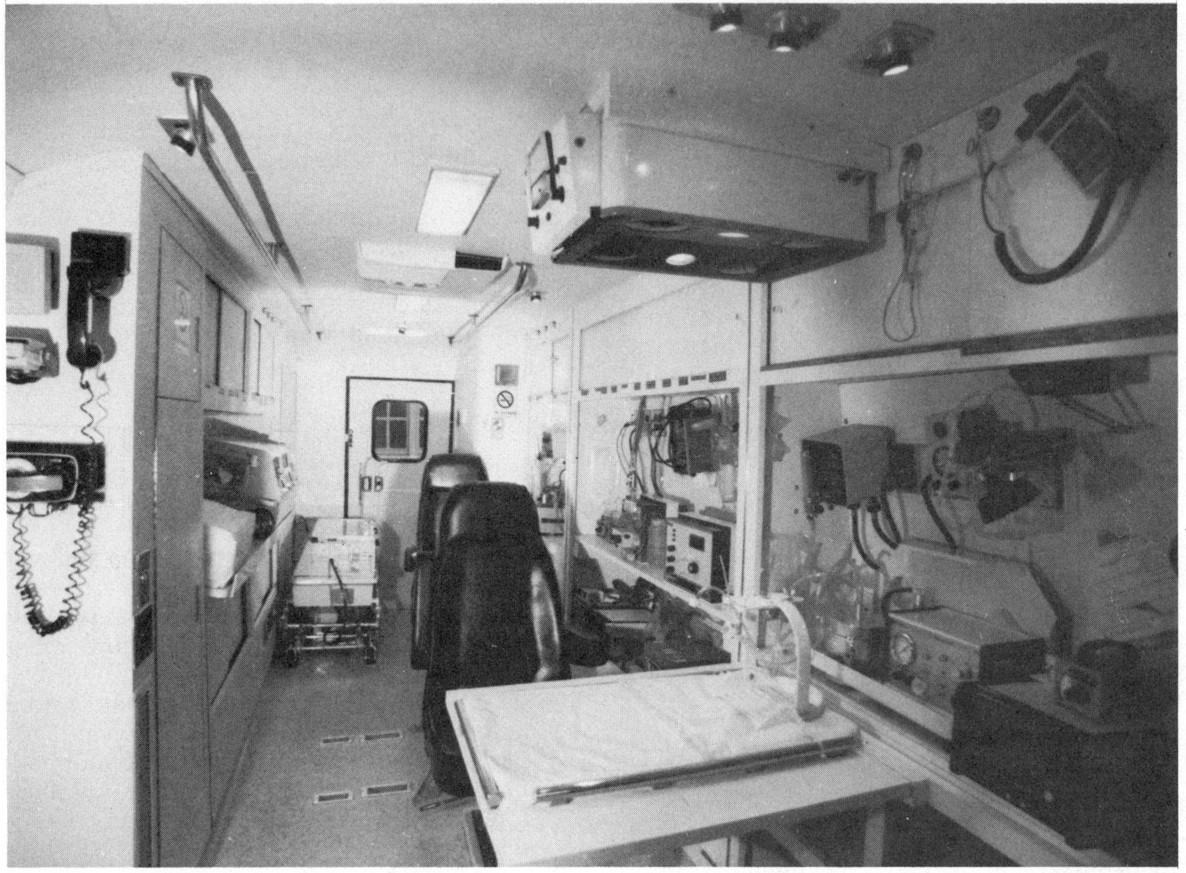

Figure 11-8 Interior of high-risk transport bus. (Courtesy of Perinatology Center, The New York Hospital–Cornell Medical Center.)

(2) Begin peripheral intravenous infusion with 10% dextrose and water.
(3) Obtain portable chest x-ray.

e. Obtain blood samples for baseline lab evaluations of electrolytes, hematocrit, CBC, and blood gasses.

4. Prepare records before the transport team arrives.
   a. Prepare copies of prenatal and labor records and immediate recovery records of the mother.
   b. List names, addresses, and telephone numbers of physicians responsible for prenatal care, delivery, and follow-up.
   c. Provide record of initial infant responses (Apgar score, respiratory efforts, temperature) and initial treatment in the delivery room.
   d. Note if vitamin K and eye prophylaxis were omitted due to unstable condition.
   e. Provide copies of nurse's and doctor's recording during nursery stay.
   f. Provide laboratory reports of acid-base status during labor and after delivery; indicate serial glucose levels, electrolytes, blood gases, pH.
   g. Have tubes of maternal blood and cord blood ready (and the placenta is required in some cases). In some instances placental fetal blood is extracted by the blood bank and prepared for autotransfusion, if deemed necessary.
   h. Provide chest x-ray films if respiratory difficulty, pneumothorax are suspected.
   i. Note if baptism was administered.
   j. Provide copies of consent for transfer, and

obtain consents for treatment. If a parent was not able to sign before transport, ensure that father arrives promptly at regional center.

5. Before taking baby the transport team will:
   a. Evaluate temperature stability and current glucose level.
   b. Evaluate continuing needs of baby for respiratory stabilization; for example, whether oxygen, intubation, or bag breathing is necessary.
   c. Secure the cardiac monitor.
   d. Call center and report findings and stability of infant and report approximate time of departure.
6. Prepare the parents for expected sequence of care.
   a. Check identification and verify information as to address, which persons are to be considered immediate relatives (in cases of single parent).
   b. Take baby in transport incubator to see mother. Encourage both parents to touch and hold infant if condition permits.
   c. Explain plan of care at the center. Review telephone and visiting opportunities.
   d. Ask father to come with the ambulance. If not possible, ask him to visit center as soon as possible. Encourage father to photograph child, if possible. Otherwise, referring hospital should provide photograph for the parents.
7. Admission to center.
   a. Report infant status and any unusual findings during transit.
   b. Check identification of infant with primary nurse receiving infant.
   c. Determine vital signs once infant is placed in warm environment. Place on cardiorespiratory monitoring.
   d. Obtain complete lab work as ordered, but do not let infant become extremely fatigued.
      (1) Tests should include a CBC with differential, platelets, reticulocytes, hemoglobin, hematocrit, and bilirubin (if not already done).
      (2) Acid-base tests should indicate pH, Pa_{CO_2}, Pa_{O_2}, base deficit.
      (3) Include septic workup if membranes were ruptured for more than 12–24 h before birth and culture of throat, blood, urine, cord, skin, and stool.
   e. X-ray location of umbilical line, of position of any tubes in place, and of lung should be done if indicated. Protect infant from chilling.
   f. Communicate infant status to obstetrician and referring hospital. Report any new findings after workup.

Safe transport will allow the best possible chance for the infant to begin recovery and growth.

REFERENCES

Arnon, S. S., Midura, T. F., and Damus, K.: "Intestinal Infection and Toxin Production by *Clostridium Botulinum* as One Cause of Sudden Infant Death Syndrome," *Lancet* **1**:1273, 1978.

Brazelton, T. B.: Neonatal Behavioral Assessment, National Spastics Society Monographs, *Clinics in Developmental Medicine*, #50, London, William Heinemann and Sons, 1973. Distributed in the United States by Lippincott, Philadelphia.

Cloherty, J. P.: "Temperature Control," in J. P. Cloherty and A. P. Stark, (eds.), *Manual of Neonatal Care*, Little, Brown, Boston, 1980, p. 350.

Davis, V.: "The Structure and Function of Brown Adipose Tissue in the Neonate," *Journal of Obstetric, Gynecologic, and Neonatal Nursing*, **9**(6):368, November/December, 1980.

Fawcett, W. A., and Gluck, L.: "RDS in the Tiny Baby," *Clinics in Perinatology*, **4**(2):411, September 1977.

Ferrara, A., and Harin, A.: *Emergency Transfer of the High Risk Neonate*, Mosby, St. Louis, 1980.

Klaus, M. H., and Fanaroff, A.: *Care of the High Risk Neonate*, Philadelphia, Saunders, 1978, p. 66.

Lewak, N., Van Den Berg, B. J., and Beckwith, J. B.: "Sudden Infant Death Syndrome Risk Factors: Prospective Data Reviewed," *Clinical Pediatrics*, **18**:404, 1979.

Maisels, M. J.: "Neonatal Jaundice," in G. B. Avery (ed.), *Neonatology: Pathophysiology and Management of the Newborn*, Lippincott, Philadelphia, 1980, p. 357.

Seligman, J. W.: "Recent and Changing Concepts of Hyperbilirubinemia and Its Management in the Newborn," *Pediatric Clinics of North America*, **24**(3):509, August 1977.

Smialek, Z.: "Observations on Immediate Reactions of Families to Sudden Infant Death," *Pediatrics*, **62**(2):160, 1978.

Valdez-DaPena, M. A.: "Sudden Infant Death Syndrome: A Review 1974–1979," *Pediatrics*, **66**(4):597, 1980.

BIBLIOGRAPHY

Avery, G. B. (ed.): *Neonatology: Pathophysiology and Management of the Newborn*, Lippincott, Philadelphia, 1980. Comprehensive text with contributions by leading authorities.

Cloherty, J. P., and Stark, A. R. (eds.): *Manual of Neonatal Care*, Little, Brown, Boston, 1980. Concise but thorough review of neonatology in manual form.

Ferrara, A., and Harin, A.: *Emergency Transfer of the High-Risk Neonate*, Mosby, St. Louis, 1980. Excellent reference for preparation for transfer of the newborn.

Harper, R. G., Sia, C. G., and Kierney, M. B.: "Kernicterus 1980: Problems and Practices Viewed From the Perspective of the Practicing Clinician", *Clinics in Perinatology*, **7**(1):75, March 1980. Changing concepts in causes and therapy concerning the control of bilirubin level and development of kernicterus.

Klaus, M. H., and Fanaroff, A. A.: *Care of the High Risk Neonate*, Saunders, Philadelphia, 1978. Text includes many case studies in question-and-answer form.

Korones, S. B.: *High Risk Newborn Infants*, 2d ed., Mosby, St. Louis, 1981. Classic textbook of neonatal nursing care.

12

Birth Defects: The Grieving Family

Bonnie Silverman and Elizabeth J. Dickason

DESCRIPTION

Birth defects are the result of disturbances during the formation or growth of the fetus. These disturbances may be divided into three categories: (1) genetic disorders caused by chromosomal, single-gene, or polygenic defects; (2) congenital disorders resulting from teratogenic or disease interference with the growth and development of the fetus in utero; (3) disorders caused by birth injuries such as anoxic or drug insult during labor or trauma during the birth process.

Birth defects may disturb structural or biochemical function and may cause growth retardation and behavioral effects lasting a lifetime. A defect may be apparent at birth or may show up in gene or chromosome function in later years. Fortunately, in the surviving infants most disorders are minor in nature or are correctable by surgery. However, mental retardation continues to be a severe uncorrectable result of genetic or teratogenic insult to the fragile human fetus.

CHROMOSOMAL DEFECTS

MONOSOMY

Monosomy is the absence of one of a pair of chromosomes.

1. Autosomal chromosome monosomy—mortality 100 percent.
2. Sex chromosome monosomy—Turner's syndrome, 45,XO.
   a. Incidence—1:2,500 plus 15 to 20 percent of abnormal abortuses in the first trimester.
   b. Characteristics—short stature, shield chest, web neck, infertility, lack of secondary sex characteristics, mild mental retardation.
   c. Mortality—98 percent abort spontaneously, 2 percent survive.

TRISOMY

Trisomy is the presence of a third chromosome in a grouping. Trisomy is usually the result of nondisjunction at either the first or second *meiotic* division. Translocation can also occur to cause some of the same effects, if one or more chromosomes break and recombine in various ways. Translocation is more commonly seen in babies of younger clients, whereas nondisjunction appears to be related to maternal age and the "aging" ovum. (See also Mosaicism, below.)

1. Autosomal Trisomy.
   a. Trisomy 21—Down's syndrome, 47,XX or XY, +21. Nondisjunction, 95 percent; mosaicism, 2 to 3 percent; translocation (D/g or G/G), 2 percent.
      (1) Incidence—1:600 but 1:100 in women over 40 and 1:50 in women over 45.

(2) Characteristics—mental retardation, multiple organ defects (especially cardiac), macroglossia, low-set ears, epicanthal fold over inner aspect of eyelid, flat bridge of nose, simian crease in palm, and abnormal finger- and footprints.
(3) Mortality—30 percent die in first month from respiratory difficulty, failure to thrive, defects. 60 percent die by 10 years of age.

b. Trisomy 18—Edward's syndrome: 47,XX or XY, +18.
   (1) Incidence—1:4,500.
   (2) Characteristics—cardiac defects, severe mental retardation, small chin, low-set ears, strangely flexed fingers, failure to thrive.
   (3) Mortality—90 percent die by 1 year of age.

c. Trisomy 13—Patau's syndrome, 47,XX or XY, +13.
   (1) Incidence—1:5,500.
   (2) Characteristics—mental retardation, microphthalmia, cleft lip and palate, polydactyly, rocker-bottom feet.
   (3) Mortality—rare survival after infancy.

d. Trisomy is also possible at chromosome pairs 8, 9, and 22.

2. Sex chromosomal trisomy.
   Most commonly linked with increased maternal age, sex chromosomal trisomy does not accentuate sexual characteristics but may contribute to mental retardation and systemic malfunctions.
   a. Triple-X syndrome—47,XXX.
      (1) Incidence—1:1,200.
      (2) Characteristics—fertility is unaffected, abnormality may be passed to offspring; mild mental retardation may occur, but more severely with tetrasomy (XXXX) or pentasomy (XXXXX).
   b. Klinefelter's syndrome—47,XXY.
      (1) Incidence—1:600 to 1:1,000.
      (2) Characteristics—IQ is affected to varying degrees, sometimes there is mild mental retardation; because of low testosterone levels and lack of testicular growth in puberty there will be infertility but not usually impotence; lack of development of secondary sex characteristics in puberty may be the first indication of the syndrome (Gerald, 1976).
   c. XYY syndrome—47,XYY.
      (1) Incidence—1:1,000.
      (2) Characteristics—no mental retardation, fertility, above-average height, aggressiveness, acne may continue into adulthood, appearance normal otherwise.

POLYPLOIDY

This defect occurs when an entire extra set (23) of chromosomes are present; triploidy (69) and tetraploidy (92) are seen most frequently in aborted embryos.

MOSAICISM

As a result of *mitotic nondisjunction* there occurs a mixed karyotype with some normal and some abnormal cells. Symptoms of the above disorders are muted by the presence of cells with normal chromosome configurations. Gonadal dysgenesis may occur, resulting in infants who appear to have a male-female phenotype with ambiguous genitalia, even though most cells are predominantly XX or XY. Often mosaicism occurs with Turner's syndrome.

DOUBLE FERTILIZATION

This condition is also called true hermaphroditism. The "origin is probably double fertilization of a binucleate egg since such patients have two distinct sets of blood groups". Of those affected, 50 percent have only XX cells present, 25 percent have only XY cells present, and 25 percent are mosaics. At birth, the infant is seen to have ambiguous genitalia or cryptorchidism, hypospadius, and failure of labioscrotal fusion.

1. Assignment of sex of rearing for these infants is crucial. Whenever there are ambiguous genitalia, there is an immediate need for complete evaluation of cause, for there are many possible reasons, including the following: congenital virilizing adrenal hyperplasia, maternally induced masculizing hormones, testicular feminization, and congenital adrenal hyperplasia. The latter condition may become life-threatening because of an adrenal failure.

Chromosomal analysis, studies for cell Barr body-indicating presence of X chromosomes in body cells, and steroid excretion patterns will be done on all such infants. There may be a delay in diagnosis, one that causes intense emotional difficulty for the family. Determination of gonad structure is all important, for puberty will see the development of secondary sex characteristics of the gonads that are present, no matter how the initial external visual structure of the infant's genitalia appears. (Porter, 1976).
2. Sympathetic, supportive nursing and medical care is necessary for the family during the waiting period and during any subsequent hospital admission for surgery.

ABNORMAL STRUCTURE

Abnormal structures of chromosomes or deletions of parts of chromosomes may lead to extensive effects in an infant, especially if genetic material is lost. Mental retardation is universal and cardiac disease often occurs.

1. Cri-du-chat syndrome—46,XX or XY,5p− (broken arm of chromosome 5). Characteristics are mental retardation, weak "cat cry," cardiac defects, failure to thrive, short stature, low-set ears, simian crease on palm, and many more possible anomalies.
2. Deletions are also possible at chromosomes 4, 9, 13, 18, 21, and 22.

SINGLE-GENE DEFECTS*

Single-gene defects present on autosomal chromosomes affect males and females with equal frequency. (Figure 12-1)

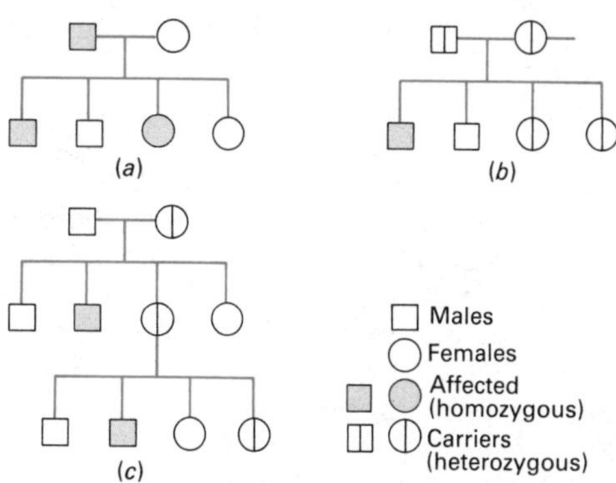

Figure 12-1 Patterns of genetic transmission. (*a*) Pattern of dominant inheritance; there is a 50% chance of overt disease with inheritance from only one percent. (*b*) Recessive inheritance pattern shows a 50% risk of carrying the trait (heterozygous) and a 25% risk of overt disease (homozygous) and 25% chance of being completely free of either trait or disease. (*c*) A sex-linked pattern of inheritance. When the disease is carried as a defective gene on the X chromosome, overt disease is shown in a son inheriting that X since there is no partner X to "lyonize" or compensate for the defect.

AUTOSOMAL DOMINANT

Dominant gene defects need be (and usually are) carried by only one partner and, following Mendel's inheritance pattern, have a risk of 50 percent for any offspring. Passed directly to the next generation, a child therefore has a 1:2 chance of inheriting the disease. Most dominantly inherited autosomal gene defects are not lethal, but unfortunately several of the severe diseases become evident only in adulthood, for example, Huntington's chorea. There are over 1,200 dominant-gene defects, among them:

1. Genetic hyperlipidemia—contributes to premature coronary artery disease.
2. Gastrointestinal polyposis—predisposes to cancer of the gastrointestinal tract.
3. Multiple neurofibromatosis (von Recklinghausen's disease)—multiple skin tumors, CNS involvement, hypertension.
4. Retinoblastoma—tumor of eye in young infants.

AUTOSOMAL RECESSIVE

Recessively carried traits for autosomal defects are common in the population. It is estimated

* All reports of incidence are from Porter (1976).

that each person carries five to eight recessive deleterious genes. It is only when both parents carry the same defective autosomal recessive gene that there is a 1:4 chance of overt signs of the disease appearing in the child. Early diagnosis with amniocentesis or genetic screening has become possible, and several diseases may be modified by prenatal treatment or diet modification. There are more than 900 recessive-gene defects, which tend to follow racial lines. Intermarriage and migration have, somewhat reduced chances that specific groups will contain individuals with the genes needed for passage of such diseases. The following conditions are a few of those resulting from recessively carried traits.

1. Inborn errors of metabolism—These defects result from a deficiency of one enzyme of the metabolic cycle. Those that may be diagnosed prenatally are a potentially large number, but many are rare. More commonly occurring problems may be categorized into the following five groups:

   Mucopolysaccharide metabolism—Hurler's syndrome and Gluronidase deficiency.

   Carbohydrate metabolism—glycogen storage disease, galactosemia, and glucose-6-phosphate dehydrogenase deficiency.

   Lipidoses—Tay-Sachs disease, Gaucher's disease, and Niemann-Pick disease.

   Amino acid deficiencies—histidinemia, maple sugar urine disease, and phenylketonuria.

   Miscellaneous—cystic fibrosis, hypothyroidism, and muscular dystrophy of certain types. (See Chapter 22.)

   a. Phenylketonuria (PKU)—1:10,000 incidence in those of northern European ancestry. Diet restriction can allow normal growth and development. Dietary precautions must again be taken during an affected woman's childbearing period.
   b. Tay-Sachs disease—1:6,000 incidence in those of eastern European Ashkenazi Jewish ancestry. Carriers occur with a frequency of 1:30. Infants with Tay Sachs disease do not survive infancy.
   c. Lactose intolerance–Not yet diagnosed prenatally, incidence 10:100 in people of Hispanic ancestry. An intolerance to milk develops early in the newborn period. Treatment is to remove the foods containing lactose and provide formula such as Isomil.
2. Cystic fibrosis—1:2,000 incidence in newborns of middle or northern European ancestry. Life expectancy now extends past puberty. Newly introduced early testing of meconium for excess mucus allows early diagnosis. (See Chapter 20.)
3. Sickle cell anemia—Incidence 1:600 in newborns of African or Mediterranean area ancestry. Genetic screening for hemoglobin SS is required for all newborns in susceptible populations. (See Chapter 18.)

SEX-LINKED DEFECTS

A normal X chromosome can dominate ("Lyonize") an abnormal gene on a second X chromosome; therefore, females can carry a trait without having the disease or having only mild to moderate symptoms. Males always show the disease if they have the abnormal X chromosome, as the Y chromosome does not counterbalance the effect. The most common sex-linked diseases include:

1. Glucose-6-phosphate dehydrogenase (G-6-PD)—predisposes individuals to hemolytic disease on exposure to certain foods and drugs. 12:100 incidence among black males, 1:140 incidence among black females, 24:100 black females are carriers. G-6-PD follows the same worldwide geographic distribution as to sickling diseases but is very common in people of the Mediterranean area: Greece, Cypress, Italy, and Sicily.
2. Duchenne's muscular dystrophy—1:10,000 incidence among males; those affected rarely survive teenage period.
3. Hemophilia—1:8,000 incidence among males, mostly from northern European ancestry; only recently have they survived the teenage period.
4. Red-green color blindness—10:100 incidence among males of Arab, Caucasian, or Ashkenazi Jewish ancestry. Lower rates exist in other groups studied, but the disorder is very widespread throughout the world.

POLYGENIC DEFECTS: MULTIFACTORIAL DISORDERS

A combination of genes and environment affects all inherited characteristics. Polygenic inheritance underlies the predisposition for certain diseases passed on in families. This predisposition, when combined with unfavorable environmental factors, may result in overt signs of the disease. The risk of inheritance is difficult to calculate and is much smaller than with single-gene defects, as risk does not follow Mendel's patterns of predictability. Among the major disorders thought to be caused by polygenic inheritance are those listed below, categorized as appearing either at birth and in infancy or later in childhood and adult life (Erbe*).

Infancy

1. Anencephaly.
2. Spina bifida.
3. Congenital dislocation of the hip.
4. Congenital heart disease (some types).
5. Cleft lip, plus cleft palate (some types).
6. Pyloric stenosis.
7. Hydrocephalus.
8. Club foot.

Childhood and Later

1. Coronary artery disease.
2. Diabetes mellitus (?).
3. Gout.
4. Hypertension.
5. Schizophrenia.
6. Allergies.
7. Asthma.

CONGENITAL DISORDERS: ENVIRONMENTAL FACTORS

TERATOGENS

Teratogenic agents (teratogens) are "one or more mechanisms that cause cells to die, change their rate of proliferation or biosynthesis, or otherwise fail to follow their prescribed course in development" (Wilson, 1977). Genetic susceptibility, dosage level and duration, and the specific day of embryonic development that coincides with drug intake are major factors influencing drug effect. In addition, maternal health and nutrition, placental functioning, and numerous other factors will be influential in whether or not a specific teratogenic agent does in fact have an injurious effect on the developing human. Such agents are thought to be the cause of 2 to 3 percent of birth defects and to contribute to a large number of unknown causes for disability or dysfunction in the developing human (see Table 12-1).

* All reports of incidence are from Erbe (1976).

VIRUSES OR BACTERIA

Teratogenic agents also may be viruses or bacteria. Table 12-2 identifies problems caused by infections during pregnancy and suggests infection control in the newborn period. The group of infecting agents most commonly seen has been labeled *TORCH*, an acronym for a group of diseases that are capable of causing similar congenital malformations and/or illness in the newborn. These diseases are *to*xoplasmosis, *r*ubella, *c*ytomegalic inclusion disease, and *h*erpes simplex. Maternal exposure to these agents may come from various sources. Toxoplasmosis is contracted by eating undercooked meat or through contact with cat feces. Infection with *Toxoplasma gondii*, parasitic protozoans, is much more common than expected, and signs in the adult are often clinically unrecognizable or "flulike." If the protozoan infects the mother during the second trimester, especially destructive inflammation of the retina (chorioretinitis) and brain malformations in the fetus may develop. Diagnosis during pregnancy is by means of comparative toxoplasma titers. Treatment is not recommended during the first half of pregnancy as the drug, pyrimethamine, may be teratogenic.

Rubella is spread by droplet contamination. Immunization of susceptable women of childbearing age and children has lowered the incidence in recent years. It is recommended that any woman with a rubella titer of less than 1:20 be vaccinated during the immediate postpartum period, with the precaution of abstaining from pregnancy for 3 months after the vaccination. (See Table 12-2 for effects of selected infections during pregnancy.)

Cytomegalic inclusion disease (cytomegalo-

TABLE 12-1 ENVIRONMENTAL AND PHARMACOLOGIC TERATOGENS

Agents	Potential Adverse Effects
Radiation:	
Low dose	Increased incidence of leukemia in prepubertal child, genetic mutations
High dose	Early abortion, microcephaly
Antimetabolites:	
Alkylating agents Folic acid antagonists	Inhibited cell proliferation, early abortion, multiple anomalies
Antibiotics:	
Streptomycin	Injury to VIIIth cranial nerve
Tetracycline	Long bone and tooth deposits, some bone growth inhibition
Steroid hormones:	
Androgenic agents	Masculinization of female fetus
Estrogenic agents	Abortion (high doses)
Nonsteroid hormones:	
Estrogenic agents (DES)	Vaginal adenosis with possibility of adenocarcinoma when female approaches puberty; effect on male shows higher rate of gonadal dysfunction
Heavy metals:	
Lead Mercury	Abortion, multiple deformities

SOURCE: Wilson, J. G.: "Environmental Effects on Developmental Teratology," in N. Assali and C. R. Brinkman (eds.), *Pathyphysiology of Gestation: Fetal Disorders*, vol. 2, Academic Press, New York, 1972.

virus infection) is more severe in effect if the infection occurs during fetal life. Symptoms in the adult are mild, somewhat like flu symptoms, with a low fever, and antibodies are formed. As the illness is rather common in childhood, it is the woman who was not exposed then who might acquire the virus during pregnancy. Effects on the fetus are in the brain: underdevelopment, mental retardation; in the newborn, jaundice, liver and spleen enlargement, and purpura may be seen. Ten to eighteen percent of all women have antibodies against CMV and antibody titers can be followed during pregnancy to diagnose exposure.

Herpes simplex virus type 2 (HSV-2) or genital herpes, is a venereally disseminated disease, now listed as the nation's second most frequent venereal disease (Bahr, 1978). It is seen as recurrent vesicular eruptions on the genitalia that may progress to shallow painful ulcers. Burning sensation in the affected areas and then extreme pain may occur, with dysuria. Because there is no real cure, the disease runs its course and then recurs, throughout the lifetime. There is some evidence of HSV-2 as a cause for spontaneous abortion and premature delivery, but the more serious concern is for the neonate: severe disseminated viral infection currently shows a mortality rate of 80 percent. There may be CNS and eye damage as a residual of milder disease. Symptoms appear in the first week of life, but may do so after discharge from the hospital. To prevent contamination of the neonate by active lesions in the birth canal, most physicians choose cesarean section as the method of delivery (see Chapter 9).

Prenatal detection of the TORCH group is possible by measurement of maternal serum antibody titers, which should be assessed at least twice during the pregnancy. Any large rise in titer may indicate the presence of active infection. Stable titers can indicate past exposure with previous mobilization of the immune system.

Diagnosis of infectious disease in the newborn is made through physical examination and

TABLE 12-2 INFECTIOUS AGENTS ASSOCIATED WITH FETAL OR NEONATAL PROBLEMS

Organism	Fetal Problems	Neonatal Precautions
Candida albicans	Does not affect infant in uterus.	Observe for thrush infection in mouth or GI tract.
Varicella-zoster virus (chickenpox)	Crosses placenta; incubation 10–18 days, 2% defects if in first trimester; fetus may develop chickenpox in utero; may cause hypoxia, fetal death.	Isolate infected mother and child together; room air must be strictly controlled. Neonatal varicella if maternal infection occurs late in pregnancy.
Coxsackie virus B	Infection of fetal cardiac tissue; anomalies of heart.	
Cytomegalovirus (cytomegalic inclusion disease)[a]	Microcephaly, cerebral calcification, jaundice, stunted growth; both mother and infant may shed virus.	Mother and infant may be isolated together in single rooming in.
Neisseria gonorrhoeae (gonorrhea)	Does not affect fetus in utero unless generalized severe infection in mother.	Prophylaxis for infection of conjunctiva, 1% silver nitrate in each eye or opthalmic antibiotic treatment.
Hepatitis virus B	May cross placenta or be transferred through colostrum milk.	Infant should be bottle fed. Isolate both mother and infant with usual hepatitis precautions for serum or infectious hepatitis.
Herpes hominis type 2 (herpes simplex virus)[a]	Disseminated infection, residual CNS damage if infected in utero. If virus is picked up at birth: necrotizing lesions in lungs, liver, brain, and vesicular skin erruptions.	Gown and glove isolation for infant; mother may feed in nursery.
Mumps virus	Sometimes early abortion. Some question of endocardial fibroelastosis in infant when mother has mumps in first half of pregnancy.	Observe mother and infant for current signs of illness—See Appendix E.
Rubella virus[a]	Cardiac defects, cataracts, deafness, microcephaly, mental retardation, depending on week of infection during first 4 months. Shedding of virus for up to a year, if infected later in pregnancy.	Isolate infant showing any signs of current infection with rubella. Isolate on any subsequent admission within first year.
Smallpox (variola) Vaccinia (smallpox vaccination)	Fetal smallpox, fetal death. Fetal infection, death (?).	Now rare in the United States and Worldwide; vaccination during pregnancy not recommended.

TABLE 12-2 *(continued)*

Organism	Fetal Problems	Neonatal Precautions
Treponema pallidum (syphilis)	During first 16 weeks, does not cross placenta; after, may cause bone and tooth deformities, progressive CNS damage, stillbirth, or neonatal syphilis.	Untreated primary or secondary syphilis; wear gown, gloves; for latent or tertiary: no precautions. Treatment of mother cures fetus but serology may be slow to return to negative.
Toxoplasma gondii (toxoplasmosis)	Parasitic protozoan infection during pregnancy may cause microcephaly, cerebal calcifications, chorioretinitis. Maternal symptoms are confusing; follow titers.	No vaccine; medication not recommended during early months of pregnancy. Breastfeeding contraindicated, if infection current in mother.

[a] Viruses identified in the TORCH group, plus the parasite *Toxoplasma gondii*. Isolation precautions based on recommendations in "Infection Control for the Obstetric Patient and Newborn Infant," NAACOG Technical Bulletin, no. 9 March 1981.

serum testing. Specific congenital anomalies such as microcephaly, intracranial calcifications, intrauterine growth retardation, cataracts, cardiac lesions, and signs such as petechiae and hepatosplenomegaly are suggestive of congenital viral disease. the infant's antibody titers can be measured and compared with the maternal levels. Although passive transfer may cause newborn-maternal titers to be similar, any subsequent rise in newborn titers is suggestive of infection. In addition, serum levels of IgM can contribute to the diagnosis of infection. The infant forms IgM, one of the immunoglobulins, in response to viral transmission across the placenta. IgM is too large a molecule to cross the placenta from maternal circulation; therefore, higher levels in the neonate can indicate a specific fetal response.

BIRTH INJURIES

DRUG EFFECTS

The transitional period before birth is a highly sensitive one as any drugs in the maternal system usually reach the fetus at the maternal blood drug concentration. After birth, without the maternal excretory mechanisms, the infant must metabolize and excrete dosages near to or higher than the maternal levels. Immaturity of body functions will result in extended periods before the drug is finally excreted from the infant's body. Drugs used during labor are especially implicated, but chronic drug use (addiction) or drugs given for maternal disease may also have adverse effects. All resulting effects of maternal drugs in the newborn should be thought of as "withdrawal" effects, and careful monitoring of signs and symptoms will be necessary during the extended period before the infant is drug free (see Chapter 10).

It is essential to understand the concept of the drug's time-dose interval before birth. The rate of metabolism and excretion of the drug from the maternal system affects whether it will be present in amounts high enough to adversely affect the infant. The half-life of the drug is the time in which half of the absorbed dose is metabolized in order to be excreted from the body. Any delay in metabolism or recycling or difficulty in excretion would extend the drug's effect in the maternal system. Examples of drugs with a short half-life are oxytocin (3 to 5 min) and Demerol (IV) (1–1½ h); a drug with a long half-life is phenobarbital (8–12 h).

When the newborn is affected by a high maternal dose that equilibrates across the placenta,

TABLE 12-3 TRANSITIONAL DRUGS USED DURING LABOR

Drug	Maternal Precautions	Fetal or Neonatal Precautions
PRETERM LABOR		
Ethyl alcohol (IV): 100 mL 95% alcohol in 900 mL D_5W; up to 15 mL/kg/per h; tritrated dosage.	Metabolized at 7 g/h, blood levels of 0.09–0.16% needed for effect. Watch interaction with other drugs. Side effects: confusion, slurred speech, headache, vomiting. May cause postinfusion "hangover." Recovery takes up to 12 h.	Half-time for metabolism is twice that of mother due to immature hepatic function. Elevated blood levels at birth lead to hypotonia, CNS depression, hiccups, hypothermia, hypoglycemia. Small infants more vulnerable. Used infrequently in the United States.
Ritodrine (IV): Not to exceed 0.35 mg/min; titrate with body response; PO dosage up to 120 mg/day.	Acts on $beta_2$ receptors of sympathetic system: relaxes uterine, bronchial smooth muscle. Peripheral vasodilation with increased heart rate, contractility, increased pulse pressure. Adverse effects: restlessness, anxiety, pulse above 140, increased blood sugar, free fatty acids, reduced excretion of water.	Fetal and neonatal tachycardia. If rate above 180, reduce infusion rate. May cause hypoglycemia and increased blood volume but reduces incidence of RDS.
INDUCTION		
Oxytocin (IV): 20 U diluted in 500 or 1000 mL D_5W; IV pump.	Watch for myometrial hypertonus. When given in high doses for late abortion, stillbirth, watch for water intoxication due to mild antidiuretic effect; effect reduced when in presence of other vasodilating drugs, smooth muscle relaxants.	Watch for fetal bradycardia in response to hypertonic contractions and impaired uteroplacental circulation or extreme pressure on presenting part. Watch for neonatal hyperbilirubinemia and fluid and electrolyte imbalance after prolonged maternal infusion.
ANALGESICS IN LABOR (See Table 8-2)		
Scopolamine: 0.2–0.4 mg with analgesic and tranquilizer	Still being used in some settings in spite of discomfort to mother: flushed skin, tachycardia, extreme dry mouth, amnesia; large doses inhibiting voiding. When not calculated correctly and analgesic dose reduced, hyperactivity, delirium in presence of pain will result.	Elevates fetal heart rate, erases variability, marks fetal distress.
ANTIHYPERTENSIVES		
Phenobarbital: 30–60 mg PO tid.	Half-life is 8–12 h in mother; therefore dose may still be present even if d/c before labor. Observe dose-to-delivery time and report to nursery/pediatric staff. Usually delay breastfeeding if significant doses are needed during recovery.	Potent inducer of microsome enzyme systems. May change newborn responses to other drugs. Excreted up to 7 days after birth. Watch for CNS depression, feeding response and, in severe cases, withdrawal symptoms beginning at about 5 days.

TABLE 12-3 *(continued)*

Drug	Maternal Precautions	Fetal or Neonatal Precautions
Magnesium sulfate: 4 g loading dose, 1 to 2 g/h IV to maintain 4–8 mEq blood level.	Inhibits transfer of electrical impulses at myoneural junction. Depresses smooth muscle. Uterine function may be diminished by large doses. Watch output carefully: low doses have antidiuretic effect; large doses, osmotic diuretic effect. Increase cerebral blood flow and peripheral vasodilation thus reducing BP somewhat while improving cerebral circulation.	Fetal blood levels equal mother's. Cord blood levels may be 3 to 4 times normal, but infant will show various signs. Observe hypotonia, respirations, and urinary output. Excessive doses may lead to marked neonatal depression requiring cardiopulmonary support. Careful infusion of calcium gluconate or exchange transfusion in very severe cases.
Hydralazine	Direct relaxation of arterioles, thus reduces BP but may cause tachycardia, postural hypotension. Chills, fever, headaches, palpitations, dizziness, nausea, vomiting may occur. Potentiates many drugs, especially anesthetics, MAO inhibitors. May be given with thiazide to block side effects.	Watch for effect of maternal hypotension on fetal oxygenation. Watch neonate's vital signs.
OTHER DRUGs		
Insulin	Regular insulin given SC only, to cover in labor. Follow with blood glucose levels. Expect normoglycemia or lability in recovery. Avoid acetonemia.	Insulin does not cross placenta but newborn glucose levels must be monitored every 1–2 h by Dextrostix, and if below 45 mg/% by more accurate blood glucose samples.
Betamethasone, IM	To mother 24 h before delivery unless in preeclampsia or receiving drugs that may have already potentiated maturation of fetal lung.	Speeds maturation of fetal lung, with surfactant production as a stress response.

the infant, because of the immaturity of metabolic function, will need two or three times the maternal period for metabolism and excretion. Newborn body systems are affected in approximately the same ways as the adult by the drug; for example, sedatives depress the CNS and respiratory and temperature control centers. In addition, certain metabolites of drugs may not be excreted or may be excreted very poorly by the immature kidneys. For example, the metabolites of Demerol have been noted up to 1 month after birth in infants whose mothers received large doses during labor (Brackbill et al., 1974).

The nurse shares the responsiblity for dose-time interval for any drug administered during labor (see Table 8-2). If the interval can be spaced correctly to allow the maternal metabolism to excrete the drug before delivery, the infant will be relatively free of effect. For example:

1. No Demerol should be administered IV within 1–1½ h of birth to allow the time needed for excretion.

2. When possible, oxytocin drip should be discontinued by the time second stage begins. Extended oxytocin use has been correlated with higher levels of neonatal jaundice.
3. Long-acting sedatives such as secobarbital should never be administered once active labor has started. (See Table 12-3 for common drugs with maternal and newborn precautions.)

ANOXIA

Anoxia during labor must be prevented by careful observation for any signs of fetal distress. Persistent late decelerations or variable decelerations that increase in intensity and recover to baseline more slowly indicate developing hypoxemia. Decreased beat-to-beat variability indicates acidosis developing with rising CO_2 levels. Special indications are fetal pH levels, using capillary blood samples obtained during labor after membranes have ruptured:

Normal = value over 7.25.
Borderline = value of 7.2 to 7.25.
Acidosis = value less than 7.2.

Special problems in labor warn of anoxic trauma to the fetus:

1. The second twin with the potential of partial placental separation before birth.
2. Traumatic breech delivery with compression of the cord.
3. Cord prolapse, partial or complete.
4. Placenta previa or abruptio placentae.
5. Chronic fetal distress with placental insufficiency.
6. Precipitate delivery.
7. Injudicious use of oxytocin with speeded labor. Uterine tonus rises, and there is incomplete refilling of placental tissue when contractions are too frequent and very strong.

Injury from hypoxia causes varying degrees of brain injury from minimal brain dysfunction to cerebral palsy (CP); it may be the cause of 20 to 30 percent of CP. In many cases such injury is due to inadequate assessment of fetal status, as early warning signs are now more easily discerned.

After the birth, trained personnel must be skilled in resuscitation procedures. A nursing staff must carefully assess its potential for adequate care for these special clients and ensure that inservice education is provided to keep skills proficient. Currently, the wisest choice in any case expected to be high-risk for anoxia is to transfer the mother while in early labor to a tertiary obstetric care unit where a high-risk team is available and neonatal intensive care is readily at hand (see Chapter 11).

TRAUMA

Mechanical injuries are less common today than previously because the choice of cesarean section is being made for any potentially mechanically difficult delivery, for example, primary breech, borderline CPD. However, every neonate should be assessed in the nursery for mechanical trauma. Evaluation for body symmetry, presence of nerve damage, fractures or contusions, and cephalhematoma must be done.

PERINATAL GRIEVING

DESCRIPTION

The birth of any imperfect infant will percipitate a crisis for a family. Perinatal grieving stems from the bereavement that may occur during the prepartum, intrapartum or postpartum periods. It may be prompted by situations other than death of the fetus, for example, spontaneous abortion, birth of a premature infant, or birth of an infant with a congenital anomaly. Bereavement can also be seen in families whose otherwise healthy infant differs greatly from the imagined, ideal infant. These differences can be of sex or such minor factors as hair color or familial traits. Perinatal grieving, therefore, occurs to some degree in many families. In all cases, lack of realignment of the conflicting images of the fantasy child and the real child is the basis for this grieving. Perinatal grieving differs from grieving in other situations because of the lack of recognition the problem has received until very recently. In addition, when an expected healthy outcome changes to one causing grieving, most health professionals experience extreme discomfort while interacting with a family facing the impact of the outcome.

An example in which grieving is the primary nursing diagnosis is given below:

> A 3400-g male infant with a 3 inch by 4 inch lumbar meningomyelocele was born after a 12-h labor. Several diagnostic tests were done and the infant showed loss of sensation at the level of L4 and below, anal relaxation, and hypotonia of lower extremities. With subsequent CAT scan (computerized axial tomography) to identify hydrocephalus, surgery for closure of the spinal defect was scheduled 24 h after birth.
>
> The mother had worked as a high school teacher until the thirty-eighth week. There were no prenatal health problems or prior history in the family of this primigravida. At birth the infant was shown briefly to the parents and taken to the NICU for "stabilization." The obstetrician explained that there was a spinal defect that would cause varying degrees of problems but that the immediate danger was of infection. The importance of prompt closure of the defect was explained as the surgical consent was obtained.
>
> Early signs of grieving were seen in both parents; the mother began to cry and express shock, the father showed no external reactions at all, another expression of shock. Both parents expressed anger; she toward God for "doing this" to her baby, he toward the obstetrician for reassuring them that the pregnancy was normal.
>
> Five hours after birth the parents and grandparents saw the baby for a more extended period. The parents touched the baby; the mother commented that "he is so beautiful"; she talked to the baby and positioned herself en face. The father did not comment about the baby except to ask about the time of surgery. The grandparents said "doctors can fix anything nowadays." Intervention began with the assignment of one primary nurse who first evaluated her own feelings about this family, as her desire to reassure them that "everything will be all right" would only discourage further verbalization by the parents. She sat with the parents, allowing the mother to cry and the father to be silent; she progressed at the family's own pace, taking cues from them. After the parents' conference with the neurosurgeon, she clarified any misunderstandings about the plan of care.
>
> When the mother had difficulty sleeping that night she was given a mild sedative, but strong, emotion-blunting drugs were avoided. Because she was anorexic, she was offered light nourishing foods instead of the regular diet.
>
> The infant's defect was closed the next day, and he returned in good condition, but unable to move his legs. The parents made frequent visits to see him. The father became upset with the nursing staff, claiming that they were not observing the infant carefully enough.
>
> During conference the staff recognized the grief phase of a father who was angry, disappointed, and suffering from loss of self-esteem. They also noted the mother's denial, shown by her preoccupation with the cuteness of the baby. The grandparents' reactions were also discussed and plans for further assessment of their grieving phase were agreed upon. It became evident that the parents were not grieving in synchrony and that their reactions, although part of the grieving process, were preventing them from adjusting together.

PREVENTION

Health Promotion

1. Prenatal care with emphasis on nutrition and avoidance of exposure to teratogenic agents.
2. Identification of families at high risk (e.g., those with an increased incidence of congenital anomalies, loss of the pregnancy, or unusually high expectations), followed by referral to an appropriate high-risk obstetric service.
3. Once the situation stimulating perinatal grieving has occurred, nursing intervention can be instrumental in the prevention of pathological grieving (Klaus and Kennell, 1982).

Population at Risk

1. Mothers less than 18 years old or more than 35 years old, especially primigravidas.
2. There is some evidence that increased paternal age may also contribute to birth anomalies.
3. History of previous spontaneous abortions, infants with congenital anomalies, and/or stillbirths.
4. History of genetic disease in the family.
5. Racial or geographic disposition to congenital anomalies or genetic disease, (i.e. Tay-Sachs disease in Ashkenazi Jews, sickle cell anemia in blacks from north and central Africa, neural tube defects more common in Great Britain, or PKU in fair-skinned children of northern European ancestry).
6. Maternal or paternal exposure to teratogens.
7. Women with diabetes mellitus, hypertension.
8. Families demonstrating unusually rigid and unreasonable expectations of the neonate.

Screening

1. Prenatal identification of population at risk.
2. Specific diagnostic testing to be performed on selected high-risk families.

ASSESSMENT

Health History

1. Factors contributing to a high-risk pregnancy (see *Population at Risk* above).
2. Families not prepared for or expecting an infant other than the ideal infant.
3. Families without previous knowledge of the situation that prompts grieving.
4. Families with unreasonable expectations of the pregnancy.

Physical Assessment

Signs of perinatal grieving are psychophysical and can occur in both parents.

1. Excessive crying or lack of crying.
2. Anger directed at spouse, staff, infant, or at God.
3. Denial of the situation.
4. Lack of appetite or other physical complaints.
5. Sleep disorders.
6. Disintegration of normal family roles (see Chapter 4).

Diagnostic Tests.

1. Prenatal.
   a. Blood testing of parents at risk.
      (1) Maternal and paternal metabolic tests to identify carriers of disorders such as Tay-Sachs disease.
      (2) Maternal and paternal karyotyping to identify carriers of certain chromosomal defects such as translocations.
      (3) Maternal TORCH titers may be obtained to determine the presence of either active infection or prior exposure to several viral diseases: toxoplasmosis, rubella, cytomegalic inclusion disease, and herpes simplex virus.
      (4) Maternal alpha-fetoprotein levels (AFP) after the tenth week of pregnancy if elevated above the normal curve can indicate the presence of open neural tube defects (NTD) in the fetus (may also be normally elevated in multiple gestations). (Cowchock, 1976)
   b. Tests performed on amniotic fluid for mothers at risk. Amniocentesis may have been refused by a family that does not accept the option of abortion (see Figure 12-2).
      (1) Metabolic analysis to diagnose inborn errors of metabolism in the fetus.

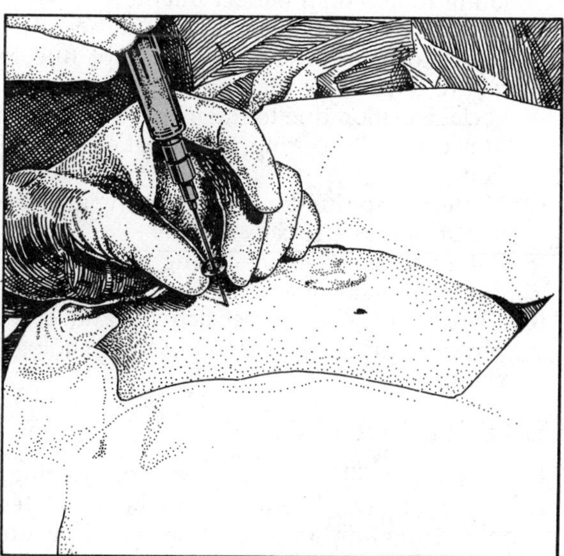

Figure 12-2 Amniocentesis. (Redrawn, courtesy of Bernard Mandelbaum, M.D.)

(2) Karyotyping of fetal cells to diagnose specific chromosomal aberrations in the fetus.
(3) Identification of fetal sex in cases of severe sex-linked disorders where there is no other method of identification of affected fetuses (such as hemophilia and Duchenne's muscular dystrophy).
(4) Measurement of AFP levels in amniotic fluid can confirm the presence of open NTD when the mother also has an elevated serum level of AFP (incidence: 0.2 percent).

c. Ultrasonic and/or radiographic studies to confirm specific conditions such as achondroplasia, NTD, micro- or hydrocephalus.

2. Postnatal tests.
   a. Routine screening of newborns.
   b. Appropriate metabolic, genetic, ultrasonic, and/or radiographic testing as indicated by the condition of the newborn.

NURSING DIAGNOSES: ACTUAL OR POTENTIAL

1. Parents lack of knowledge of genetic disorders and birth defects; confusion about long-term implications.
2. Grieving due to loss of imagined, ideal infant.
3. Alterations in parenting due to difficulty relating to less than perfect infant.
4. Role disturbance, especially for father.
5. Alterations in parents' self-concept due to failure to produce the perfect infant.
6. Social isolation due to the inability of others to accept grief during the childbearing period.
7. Matters of spirituality—questioning in an attempt to find a reason "why."
8. Potential: maladaptive coping patterns.
9. Potential: inadequate family processes.
10. Disruption of sleep-rest activity and other physical processes because of psychologic stress.

EXPECTED OUTCOMES

1. The family will exhibit evidence of grieving.
2. Psychosomatic disorders will be exhibited only temporarily and the family will show understanding of the relation of such symptoms to perinatal grieving.
3. The family will communicate feelings with friends and relatives. Parents will share feelings with each other.
4. The parents will seek out spiritual counseling in accordance with their beliefs.
5. The family will become knowledgeable about the child's condition.
6. The mother and father will be able to separate the creation of an affected child from their own self-image.
7. The family will align the images of imagined child and realized child and then proceed with parenting.
8. The family will be able to identify maladaptions in individual or family coping mechanisms and seek help as needed.

INTERVENTIONS

1. To avoid confusion, assign a primary nurse to interact with family.
   a. The nurse must become aware of own feelings and reactions to this family in order to provide effective intervention.
   b. Essential are identification of one's feelings, a thorough knowledge of grieving theory, and a desire to help.
   c. Arrange support persons for this nurse.
2. Provide a comfortable, flexible atmosphere for the family. Encourage them to verbalize freely, even if they are hostile at first.
3. Recognize stages of grief being expressed. Allow for time and do not preempt these by anticipatory descriptions that may cut off processes.
4. Maintain communication with other health professionals and seek help as needed from chaplain and perinatal bereavement team.
5. Encourage frequent family-infant interactions and provide support for the family before, during, and after contact with the child.
6. Facilitate communication with friends and relatives.
   a. Encourage family visits at any time and interpret infant's status freely.
   b. Provide suggestions for friends about support they can offer.
7. If infant dies, assist family in any details pertaining to contact of chaplain, changes in discharge planning.
8. Provide family with telephone number to

call back if they need additional help at home.

9. Make appropriate referrals to other health professionals and lay support groups, especially if family identifies maladaptive coping or dysrhythm in grieving.
10. Some perinatal grieving teams make arrangements to see family at 3-, 6-, and 12-month anniversaries. (Drotar, et al, 1975)

EVALUATION

Outcome Criteria

1. Each of the stages of grieving follows a reasonable expectation in terms of intensity and length (see Figure 12-3). (Refer to Chapter 36.)
2. The family members offer mutual support to each other.
3. The parents are able to describe their infant's condition accurately.
4. The family is becoming attached to the child and is beginning to provide a nuturing relationship.
5. The parents are aware of any lingering guilt and seek counseling appropriately.
6. Supportive social relationships with family members and friends are being reestablished.

Complications

FAILURE TO GRIEVE NORMALLY

Assessment

1. Fixation at one stage of grieving.
2. Lack of one or more stages.
3. Asynchrony—parents are grieving at different rates. This is most often seen in families whose members fail to share feelings. Emotional separation of the family and eventually even divorce can result.
4. Continuation of psychosomatic symptoms.

Revised Outcomes

The family will accept extended professional help.

Interventions

A mental health professional should be involved at this time.

Reevaluation and Follow-up

1. Grief work is proceeding.
2. The infant and parents have developed a relationship that is positive.

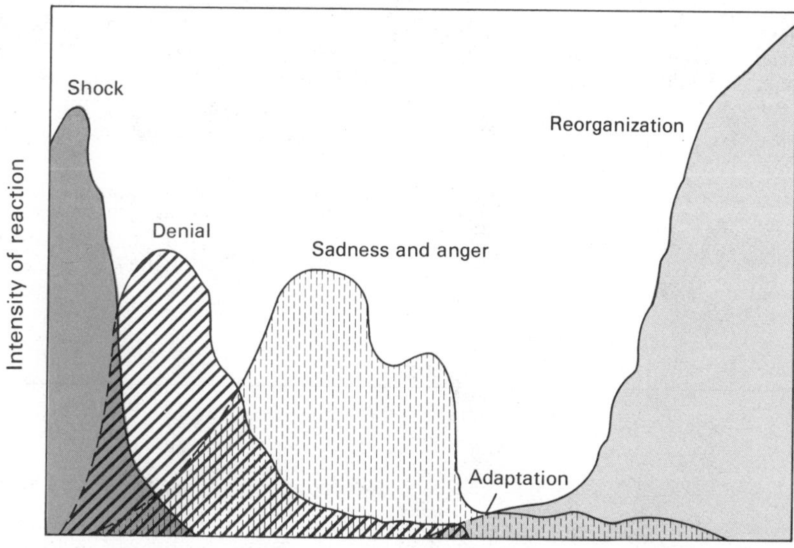

Figure 12-3 Hypothetical model of sequence of normal parental reactions to birth of a child with congenital malformations. (After Drotar, D., Baskiewicz, A., Irvin, N., Kennell, J. H., and Klaus, M. H., *Pediatrics* **56:**710, November 1975. Copyright American Academy of Pediatrics 1975.)

REFERENCES

Bahr, J. E.: "Rising Perinatal Infections: Herpes Virus Hominus, Type 2 in Women and Newborns," *MCN: Maternal and Child Nursing,* **3**:16, 1978.

Brackbill, et al.: "Obstetric Meperidine Usage and Assessment of Newborn Status," *Anesthesiology,* **40**:116, February 1974.

Cowchock, F. S.: "Use of Alpha Fetoprotein in Prenatal Diagnosis," *Clinical Obstetrics and Gynecology,* **19**(4):871, December 1976.

Drotar, D., Baskiewicz, A., Irvin, N., Kennell, J. H., and Klaus, M. H.: "The Adaptation of Parents to the Birth of an Infant with a Congenital Malformation: A Hypthetical Model," *Pediatrics,* **56**(5):710, November 1975.

Erbe, R. W.: "Principles of Medical Genetics," *New England Journal of Medicine,* **294**:281,480, 1976.

Gerald, P. S.: "Sex Chromosome Disorders," *New England Journal of Medicine,* **294**:706, 1976.

"Infection Control for the Obstetric Patient and the Newborn Infant," *NAACOG Technical Bulletin,* No. 9, March 1981.

Klaus, M. H., and Kennell, J. H.: *Parent-Infant Bonding,* 2d ed., Mosby, St. Louis, 1982, p. 85.

Porter, I. H.: "The Clinical Side of Cytogenetics," *Journal of Reproductive Medicine,* **17**(1):3–15, July 1976.

Wilson, J. G., and Frazier, F. C. (eds.), *Handbook of Teratology,* New York, Plenum, New York, 1977.

BIBLIOGRAPHY

Bartlett, D., and Davis, A.: "Recognizing the Fetal Alcohol Syndrome in the Nursery," *Journal of Obstetric, Gynecologic, and Neonatal Nursing,* **9**(4)223, July/August, 1980. Suggests nursing care plan for identified infants.

Eppink, H.: "Genetic Causes of Abnormal Fetal Development and Inherited Disease," *Journal of Obstetric, Gynecologic, and Neonatal Nursing,* **6**(4):14, September/October 1977. A review of the principles of genetics with basic terms defined and genetic history (pedigree) illustrated and explained.

Floyd, C. C.: "A Defective Child is Born: A Study of Newborns with Spina Bifida and Hydrocephalus," *Journal of Obstetric, Gynecologic, and Neonatal Nursing,* **6**(4):56, September/October 1977. A study of 11 mothers during the process of grieving in the first week, with suggestions for intervention.

Miller, K. L.: *Before We are Born: Basic Embryology and Birth Defects,* Saunders, Philadelphia, 1974. Well-illustrated explanation of origins of birth defects.

Pirani, B. B. K.: "Smoking During Pregnancy," *Obstetrical and Gynecological Survey,* **33**(1):1–11, 1978. Review of effects of smoking on fetal health. Excellent bibliography.

Queenan, J., and Hobbins, J. C. (eds.): *Protocols for High-Risk Pregnancies,* Medical Economics, Oradell, N. J., 1982. Testing and management for 63 different high-risk problems that may impinge on fetal health.

Witti, R. P.: "Alcohol and Birth Defects," *FDA Consumer,* HEW publication No. 78-1047, May 1978. Overview of current recommendations regarding alcohol and pregnancy.

Young, R. K.: "Chronic Sorrow: Parents' Response to the Birth of a Child with a Defect," *MCN: Journal of Maternal and Child Nursing,* **2**:38, January/February, 1977. Describes the continuing support needed by such a family.

13

The Family Unready for Childbearing

Cynthia S. Luke

ADOLESCENT AND ADULT ABORTION

DESCRIPTION

Elective abortion is a voluntary means to terminate an unwanted pregnancy. The choice comes either in the early period, the first trimester, or in the late period, after 16 weeks gestation. The early second trimester has been a waiting period because methods currently used for uterine evacuations have not been thought safe in this intermediate period when amniotic fluid supply is inadequate for amniocentesis and the fetal size and uterine wall status make suction or curettage more difficult. However, most recently some physicians do use dilatation and evacuation during the intermediate period.

The United States Supreme Court decision in 1973, based on the due process clause of the 14th Amendment, stated that:

1. For the stage prior to approximately the end of the first trimester, the abortion decision and its effectuation must be left to the medical judgment of the pregnant woman and her attending physician.
2. For the stage subsequent to approximately the end of the first trimester (12–13 weeks) the state, in promoting its interest in the health of the mother may, if it chooses, regulate the abortion procedure in ways that are reasonably related to maternal health.
3. For the state subsequent to viability (24 weeks) the state, in promoting its interest in the potentiality of human life may, if it chooses, regulate, and even proscribe abortion except where it is necessary in appropriate medical judgment for the preservation of the life or health of the mother (Osofsky and Osofsky, 1973).

Much controversy now surrounds the issue of women's rights to choose versus the fetal right to life. During the decade of the seventies, abortion laws focused on the health and social welfare of women and their existing families. States established policies and procedures in accordance with the Court ruling; some states, being more restrictive than others, required parental consent for minors and a waiting period between request and procedure. Pressure on legislatures and hospital administrators now most acutely limits availability and accessibility of services for young, poor rural or urban women (Cook, 1978). Social changes and attitudes of professionals are evolving. In late 1977, Congress passed the Hyde Amendment restricting government financing for abortions through Medicaid. The Supreme Court upheld the Hyde Amendment as constitutional in June 1980. The effect seen in 1978–1979 was a drop in abortion rate for women on Medicaid to a rate that was 1 percent of the previous rate in 1977. In 1978 there were 33 percent fewer federally funded abortions (Forrest et al., 1979).

Recognizing that there threatens to be a return to the high rate of self-induced or criminal abortions that preexisted the 1973 ruling, some states provide funding for these services to poor women. In this current transitional time, the development of improved techniques to decrease procedural time and to minimize side effects can result only in improved safety and efficacy.

The incidence of reported statistics for women having abortions has changed with the ruling, but it is unclear how these numbers compare with earlier decades as illegal abortions were only estimated. Statistics have not separated abortions by the woman's age, or gestational age since 1975, but one can infer from Table 13-1 that the percentage of adolescents seeking abortions is relatively the same. The current incidence is 213,000 births to adolescents 17 years old or less and abortions in this group are recorded as 135,000. Of these numbers 11,000 births and 13,000 abortions occurred in girls younger than 14 years of age. (*Morbidity & Mortality*, 1980).

Despite efforts of many communities, schools, and programs to provide adolescents with sex education and contraceptive information, one-third of all the women receiving abortions were in their teens. It is hypothesized that adolescents have greater difficulty in achieving effective contraceptive usage as a result of the coercive and unsatisfying nature of many of their sexual relations as well as because of the immaturity of their phase of growth in responsibility for self (see Chapter 5). For many adolescents, the decision to have an abortion may be the first major control issue in the care of their own bodies (Steinhoff et al., 1979). They are confronted with considering future goals. When adolescents make the decision with parents, there may be intense conflict between parental and teen value systems, as well as many issues relating to the need to assert independence and manage affairs. With support, adolescents and parents have reported that this experience can be growth producing, both individually and in their relationship. Others find it a crisis event that may result in distancing or separation.

A nurse can expect a vacillation between dependence and independence typical of the adolescent's stage of development. Such behavior ought not to be identified by health care providers as decision ambivalence. The information and skills acquired during this experience will contribute toward shaping the girl's future interactions with the health care system. Therefore, preventive management, instructive self-care concepts, informed decision making, and assertive, questioning behavior are to be encouraged.

PREVENTION

Health Promotion

1. Contraception information aimed at selection of method(s) acceptable to both woman and partner in terms of lifestyle, belief system, and health needs (see Chapter 6).
2. Decision making for choosing to parent—when an individual's criteria are unrealistic, or circumstances are overwhelming, termination may be the choice. Assistance *before* such a choice is available from Planned Parenthood and other groups.
3. Education about sexuality—ways of forming, maintaining, and ending relationships should be included in education by families, schools, and religious groups. Education about developing sexuality and ways to act and not act on one's feelings will help young people to choose from a variety of options based on their own developing values. Pa-

TABLE 13-1 ABORTION RATIOS FOR ADOLESCENTS: 1972 TO 1977

	1972	1973	1974	1975	1976	1977
Percent below 19 years old	32.6	32.7	32.6	33.1	32.1	31.3

SOURCE: *Family Planning Perspectives*, 1978, 1979.

rental and religious values need to be made clear by the family in order to counteract the intense sexual emphasis in the media.

4. Values clarification must be promoted for the teenager to recognize if her values differ from parental or others' values. Teenagers need assistance in anticipating choices, and decision making can be clearer if this activity has occurred in a secure setting.
5. Job and lifestyle options for women have opened choices other than parenting. Presenting realistic options, ways to attain them, and role models may encourage choices other than early parenting.
6. Follow-up services for adolescent health care are functioning in many areas, with peer counseling, role modeling, and adult involvement to help the adolescent sort out issues.

Populations at Risk

1. Adolescents today begin sexual activity at an earlier age, use birth control less frequently, and often do not understand method usage. Services for adolescents may not be accessible or acceptable for early identification of problems. Adolescents are at risk when they:
   a. Feel uncared for by others, "want someone to love."
   b. Have limited opportunity to explore ideas and feelings with adults.
   c. Identify with the portrayed media values of sexual involvement.
   d. Identify with family patterns and desire to repeat negative patterns.
   e. Desire escape from family conflicts.
2. Poor women because of difficulty in obtaining adequate health care or because of lack of knowledge about options are at risk.
3. Women with preexisting illnesses such as severe insulin-dependent diabetes, hypertension, leukemia, or sickle cell disease.
4. Women with infectious or genetic diseases affecting fetal health.
5. Women with repeated voluntary abortions; *recidivism* is correlated with medical complications (Howe et al., 1979).

Screening

1. Tools to identify adolescents at risk already are in place in school, community agencies, individual families and church groups. Behavioral clues can be identified and validated with the adolescent.
2. Health teachers, school nurses, counselors, clergy, social and community workers, parents, concerned adults, and peers make assessments and can refer high-risk persons for further interventions (Gedan, 1972).

ASSESSMENT

Health History

1. Ask client about own beliefs about abortion and knowledge of procedure. Explore previous experiences with the health care system.
2. Examine expectations of self—motivations for pregnancy, perception of reality of pregnancy, situational supports, coping methods, financial resources, impact of abortion choice on concerns for self, and future pregnancies (Bracker et al., 1978).
3. Assess prior obstetric experiences—outcome of prior pregnancies and any previous abortions.
4. Discuss use of contraceptives, failures and reasons.
5. Assess for any condition affecting anesthesia method—respiratory problems, renal, cardiovascular or metabolic problems. Discover if there are any cervical disorders that may affect dilatation.
6. Assess drug usage and allergic or sensitivity reactions to drugs.

Caseworker Assessment of Psychosocial Status

1. Assistance in decision-making process: "Is this your own decision? Is it compatible with your religious values, ethical beliefs? Which important people support and/or disagree with your decision? What alternative decisions did you consider?"
2. Previous reactions to loss—as termination of pregnancy usually is perceived as a loss event, even if it is undesired, coping mechanisms with recent loss experiences will help manage these feelings (Cherazi, 1979).

Physical Assessment

1. Determination of gestational size by palpation of the uterus, estimating age from LMP and observing signs of pregnancy in vaginal and cervical tissue. If the woman's statements and physical exam are incongruent, a clear explanation is necessary and expectations will have to be adjusted.

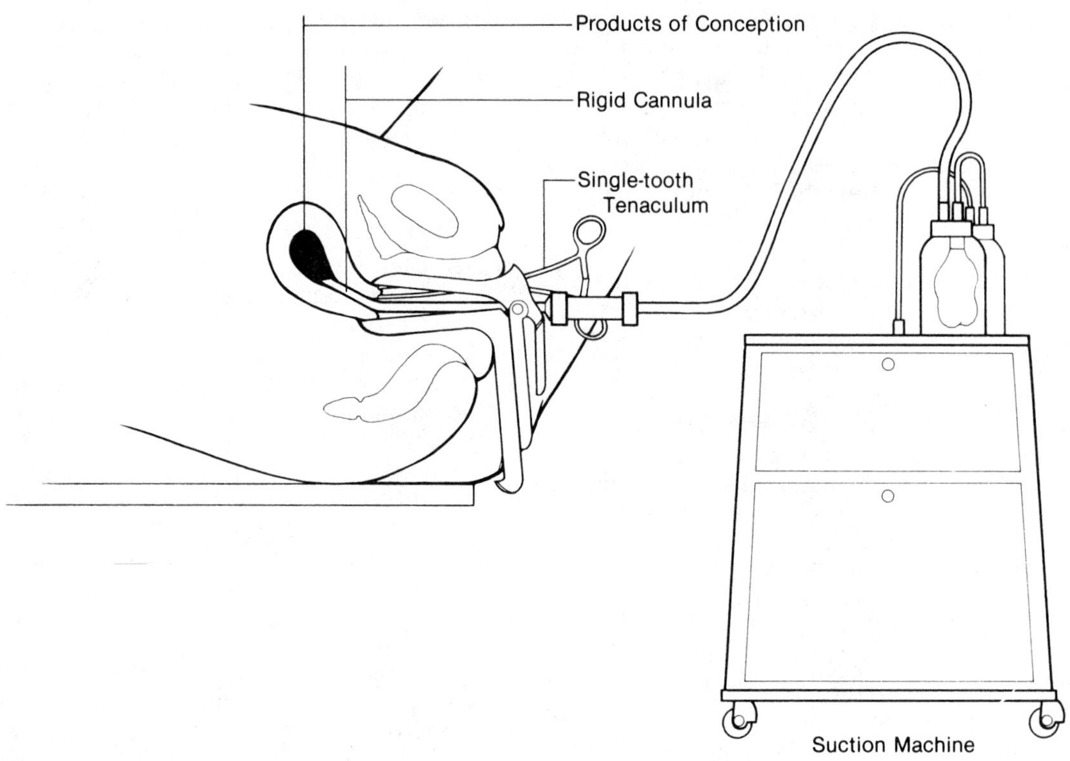

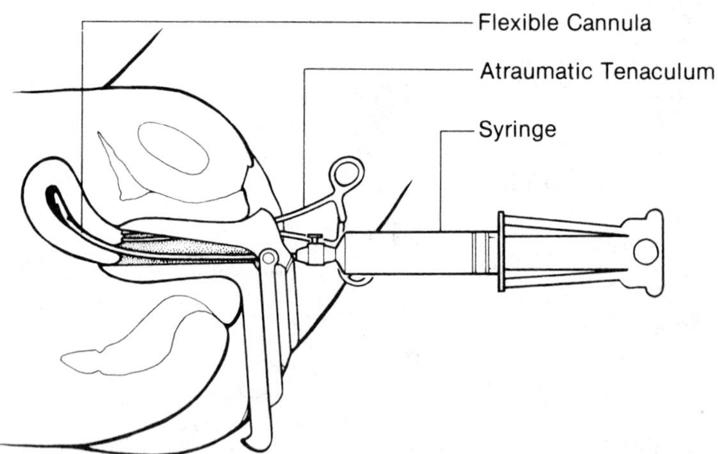

Figure 13-1 (*a*) The tenaculum steadies the cervix during the abortion procedure. Local anesthesia numbs the cervix. Metal dilating rods are used to widen the cervical canal. A vacuum tube draws the amniotic sac out of the uterus. (b) Early menstrual extraction may be done by syringe suction during the period of the fifth to seventh weeks. (See Table 13-2.) (From Butnarescu, G. and Tillotson, D., *Maternity Nursing: Theory to Practice,* John Wiley & Sons, Inc., New York, 1983, used with permission.)

2. Assessment of cervix and vagina by palpation and visualization. Note any swelling of Skene's glands, Bartholin's glands, and any vaginal discharge of mucus.

Diagnostic Tests

1. Pregnancy test—positive tests by 6 weeks post LMP using the presence of urinary HCG as a marker. By urinary/radioimmunoassay 10–24 days after ovulation.
2. General health screening:
   a. Papanicolaou smear of cervical tissue.
   b. Smear or culture of any discharge from cervix, rectum, throat to check on gonorrheal infection, depending on sexual practices.
   c. Serologic study for syphilis.
   d. Complete blood count; urinalysis for glucose, bacteria.
3. Antibody screening for maternal Rh-negative isoimmunization—explanation of Rh_0D immune globulin to prevent isoimmunization if Coombs' test is negative. Rh_0D gamma globulin should be administered if gestation is greater than 52 days or if any early bleeding has occurred.

NURSING DIAGNOSES: ACTUAL OR POTENTIAL

1. Spiritual distress—potential for unresolved guilt.
2. Potential disturbance in self-concept.
3. Anxiety about future ability to parent or conceive.
4. Potential: knowledge deficit about self-care, family planning.

EXPECTED OUTCOMES

1. Client will identify ambivalent feelings and make best decision for herself at this time.
2. Client will explore fears or anxieties related to dying, disgrace, or physical punishment, future deformed child, or fears about withdrawal of love or retaliation from significant others.
3. Client will explain steps of procedure and expected outcomes to counselor (see Table 13-2 and Figure 13-1).
4. Client will show evidence of complete uterine evacuation by lochia discharge limited to saturating one pad every 2 h for first day only and diminishing each hour, without large clots.
5. Client will exhibit evidence of health after procedure; she will be free from elevated temperature, chills, foul-smelling lochia, and uterine cramping for 1 week.
6. Client who demonstrates psychosocial problems will be referred to counselor before procedure.
7. Client will choose and use a contraceptive following the recovery period (10 days).

INTERVENTIONS

1. Assist in decision-making process. Refer as necessary.
2. Provide information about procedure. Description of likely physical sensations is effective in reducing stress. Nonprofessional counselors have proved effective (see Table 13-2).
3. Enhance effectiveness of support persons by preparing them. Plan a group counseling session (Gordon and Kilpatrick, 1977).
4. Instruct client in use of contraceptive method of choice. Assess client's receptivity to instruction before procedure; anxiety may interrupt learning.
5. After procedure:
   a. Monitor physical and immediate psychologic responses.
   b. Instruct on management and observations for complications—fever; chills; abdominal pain; lochia, bleeding persists or has odor.
   c. Instruct on self-care activities during recovery. Advise her to:
      (*1*) Rest more than usual for following 3 days.
      (*2*) Eat nutritional foods and drink 6 glasses of water each day for 1 week.
      (*3*) Resume sexual activity when desired after 10 days, unless discharge persists.
      (*4*) Use only perineal pads during recovery.
   d. Make referral for continuing concerns. Discuss follow-up appointment. Two weeks is preferred for continuity of health care. Revisit includes evaluation of experience, pelvic examination, reinforcing contraceptive instructions.

EVALUATION

Outcome Criteria

1. Client is clear about options and has made an informed decision.

TABLE 13-2 METHODS OF ABORTION WITH NURSING INTERVENTIONS

Method	Side Effects/Problems	Nursing Interventions
FIFTH TO SEVENTH WEEKS		
Menstrual extraction (endometrial aspiration, menstrual regulation, miniabortion, and EUE): Contents of the uterus are removed by syringe suction. May or may not require positive pregnancy test depending on practitioner. *Procedure*: 1–3 min. Cervical anesthesia may or may not be used (5–10 mL 1% lidocaine) *Blood loss*: 5–30 mL.	Expect mild cramping, minimal vaginal bleeding. Systemic and allergic reactions (vertigo, pruritis, hypotension). In rare instances incomplete removal of tissue. Repeat pregnancy test at follow-up visit as there is a chance of missing an ectopic pregnancy.	Client fasts for 4 h before procedure and empties her bladder. Assist in lithotomy position; cleanse vulva with antiseptic solution. Repeat explanation about procedure. Assist with relaxation techniques when tenaculum is applied to cervix for dilation. Observe supine for 10 min. Monitor vital signs and feeling response. Encourage rest and fluids for 15–30 min.
SEVENTH TO TWELFTH		
Vacuum aspiration (suction curettage): Contents of uterus removed by suction. Performed in clinic, hospital, or physician's office with local or general anesthesia. *Procedure*: 10–20 min. May be followed by curette exploration of uterine cavity. *Blood loss*: 30–100 mL (See Figure 13-1)	Mild cramping during procedure. Minimal bleeding, mild cramping after.	As for menstrual extraction, above, except extend rest period to 1–2 h. Less chance of missing ectopic pregnancy, and pathology specimen will indicate presence of fetus. Offer analgesia for cramping.
Dilatation and Evacuation (D & E): Contents of uterus scraped out. Performed in clinic or physician's office with local cervical or general anesthesia. *Procedure*: 10–30 min. *Blood loss*: 30–100 mL.	Trauma to uterus and cervix, particularly if cervix is rigid. Incomplete evacuation, infection. General anesthesia associated with higher rates of uterine hemorrhage, perforation, intraabdominal hemorrhage, cervical injury.	As above. Depending on type of anesthesia, postanesthesia care. Client must be fully responsive for 1–2 h before discharge. Encourage food and rest.

THIRTEENTH TO FIFTEENTH WEEKS		
Dilatation and evacuation (D & E): Becoming more widely used (73% of all abortions for this gestational age in 1977). Lower complication rates than saline or PGF_2 alpha; quicker, cheaper than other types. Less difficult for client, but more difficult for physician	The following procedures are more difficult to perform and involve a 10 times greater complication rate when begun in this trimester. Cervical injury and uterine perforation in rare instances.	As above. Analgesia may be more necessary since there has been increased dilation of cervix and manipulation of uterus. Oxytoxic drug to assist in contracting uterus. Monitor IV fluids.
Prostaglandin suppository (PGE_2): Suppository inserted in vagina, resulting in mechanical as well as hormonal dilating effect on cervix. Laminara vaginal suppository may be inserted 24 h before procedure to ripen cervix for dilation and to reduce trauma to cervix. Cervical polymer plugs to dilate cervix with minimal stress are in the research stage.	Vomiting and diarrhea, temperature elevation (CNS reaction). Contractions indicate uterus is emptying.	Instruct to use no aspirin as it inhibits natural prostaglandin activity. Give Lomotil ½ h before insertion. Administer prochlorperazine if vomiting occurs (not very effective, as the cause is prostaglandin activity on smooth muscle).
SIXTEENTH TO TWENTY-FOURTH WEEKS		
Prostaglandin extra amniotic gel or suppository: Suppository inserted in vagina. Causes less trauma to cervix than other methods. *Procedure*: Mean abortive time is 12–16 h. May be supplemented with IM injection.	GI symptoms most frequently at 3 h after administration.	Observe for symptoms. Emergency drugs include bronchial dilator and O_2. Monitor IV fluids and vital signs.
Prostaglandin intra-amniotic injection (PGF_2 alpha, 25–40 mg, or methyl PGF_2 alpha, 5 mg): Administered via amniocentesis after test dosage. Contractions may begin within 15 min. *Procedure*: Mean abortive time 12–48	Vomiting and diarrhea, temperature elevation (CNS reaction). Contractions indicate uterus is emptying. During procedure: allergic reaction to test done with erythematous wheals at site, fever, shivering, bronchial con-	Monitor IV fluids. Assist with relaxation and breathing techniques. Administer analgesia. Prepare for expulsion of fetus when contractions increase in intensity and frequency. Prepare container for fetus and suture clamp, scissors for cord. Inform client of expulsion

TABLE 13-2 *(continued)*

Method	Side Effects/Problems	Nursing Interventions
h. Safer and faster than saline. Repeat dosage of prostaglandin may be necessary if aborting has not occurred within 48 h and membranes are intact. If several hours elapse between rupture of membranes and aborting, IV oxytocin may be started (50 U in 1,000 mL) Ringer's lactate at 20–30 gtt/min). Suture repair is necessary if cervix is lacerated.	striction (mostly with asthmatics). Greater GI effects than with saline: vomiting and diarrhea, plus headache. Rupture of membranes may occur before or with fetus expulsion. May have live fetus in rate 5 to 40 times greater than with saline. After procedure: Disruption of normal coagulation; fever may occur. Hypotonic uterus. In case of retained placenta removal by manual exam or D & E is necessary. Retained placenta more common than with saline. Cervical lacerations.	and sex of fetus, if desired. Placenta expulsion may occur with fetus or up to 4 h later. Seek medical consultation after 1 h. As placenta may be expelled and lying in vagina, check with sterile glove. Oxytocin may be used IM or IV to hasten expulsion and assist in uterine contractions. Encourage fluids, food and rest. Discharge client after vital signs have been stable for 2–6 h. Explain follow-up care.
Urea intraamniotic injection (80 g/200 mL solution): Administered via amniocentesis. *Procedure*: Mean abortive time 12–48 h. May be used with oxytocin or PGF_2 alpha, but less commonly used.	Dehydration, disruption of normal coagulation factors may occur. Note fibrinogen levels (normal range: 160–415 mg/100 mL) and platelet count changes (normal range: 140,000–400,000/mL by Brecher-Cronkite method).	Prepare for amniocentesis. Start IV fluids. Obtain baseline vital signs.
Hypertonic saline injection Administered via amniocentesis. Withdrawal of 250 mL amniotic fluid, test dosage, then injection of 30–40 g NaCl diluted in 200–350 mL amniotic fluid. *Procedure*: Average abortive time 10–48 h. May be used with oxytocin to enhance contractions.	During instillation phase: Client experiences stinging like a bee sting, filling up, feeling full, bloated. During latency and labor phase: Severe cramps constant and becoming constantly stronger, feeling of pressure moving from the naval downward. Placental phase: Cramping. With infiltration into tissue, hypernatremia is evidenced by increased thirst shortly thereafter. Leakage of solution into vas-	Observe for symptoms. Emergency drugs include bronchial dilator and O_2. Monitor IV fluids and vital signs. Accurate infusion rate and observation and recording of hourly urinary output. Observe for signs of uterine bleeding with uterine tenderness and rigidity and abdominal pain. Observe for fibrinogen changes. Be prepared for fibrinogen changes. Be prepared to administer blood or blood products. Record vital

	cular system causes abdominal pain, severe headache, backache, tachycardia, confusion, drowsiness, seizure. Coagulation defects leading to hemorrhage. With uncontrolled amounts of oxytocin infusion may have water intoxication, confusion, drowsiness, headache, cervical tear.	signs on flow sheet and increase frequency of monitoring. An emergency hysterotomy may be necessary.
Hysterotomy Same procedure as cesarean section: Uterine contents removed by abdominal surgery under general or regional anesthesia. Used if other procedures are unsuccessful in completing abortion.		Postoperative care following abdominal surgery. Infection can occur whenever membranes are ruptured over 12 h. Observe for signs, request cervical culture.

2. Client recognizes that ambivalent feelings are usual and is able to identify own feelings.
3. Client can describe after-abortion self-care and signs of complications.
4. Client can state which contraceptive method she will use for subsequent period until choosing to parent.
5. Client has been referred in case unresolved problems continue.

Complications

TRAUMA TO CERVIX

Cervical trauma may occur from rapid, forceful dilatation of a rigid cervix and result in laceration of the cervix. Trauma to uterus may occur from difficulty or incomplete emptying of uterus. Uterine perforation, retained tissue, and hemorrhage may result. Trauma is the main cause of additional medical care in cases of abortion. Retained tissue and perforation account for 68 percent of the mortality rate (Benditt, 1980). With local cervical anesthesia fever and convulsions may occur due to accidental high level of absorption.

At the time of the procedure, hemorrhage or perforation should be noted by changes in vital signs. Disruption of normal blood coagulation may occur, evidenced by petechiae and altered platelet count.

Assessment

1. Bleeding after procedure.
2. Subsequent bleeding after first day that does not subside with 2 h of rest.
3. Bleeding accompanied by unusual uterine cramping or unusual odor.

Revised Outcomes

1. Bleeding will diminish with effective uterine contractions augmented by oxytocin.
2. Retained products will be removed by physician.
3. Any perforation will be discovered and repaired.

Interventions

1. Use oxytocic drug for 24–48 h (Methergine PO 0.2 mg three to four times daily); or, if client admitted to hospital for observation, establish and monitor IV fluids with oxytocin.
2. Increase rest, fluids, nutrition; reduce stressors by identifying sources and facilitating supports.
3. Teach self-care again.

Reevaluation and Follow-up

Client needs more intense follow-up with screening for anemia, residual effects.

INFECTION (ENDOMETRITIS)

Infection may be introduced into the uterus from instruments used or from bacteria resident in the vagina and carried to the uterus during procedure, or it may be introduced during recovery period. The main causative organisms are *Escherichia coli, Pseudomonas*, hemolytic streptococci A and B, *Clostridium*, and *Staphylococcus aureus*. Septic abortion is a variant of postpartum endometritis and is treated in similar manner (see Chapter 9).

FUTURE RISK

The harmful effect of abortion on subsequent pregnancies has been found to be minimal in recent research. There appears to be no association between previous first abortions and subsequent stillbirth, ectopic pregnancy, complications of delivery, low birth weight in newborn, or ill health in newborn. However, repeated abortions may increase the likelihood of future spontaneous abortions, premature births, and low-birth-weight infants (Dating et al., 1981). This increase in incidence rises with maternal age and parity. Future reproductive health depends, therefore, on preventive care, with family planning, and then careful observation when a pregnancy is desired. (Benditt, 1980; Grimes and Cates, 1979).

DELAYED GRIEVING

Because abortion is often perceived by women to be a loss event, reactions of depression, grief, mourning, and relief are to be expected. These reactions are short-lived and tend to reflect the circumstances and attitudes of those involved with the woman in the decision making and during the procedure itself. When distress occurs there is a high correlation with lack of partner support. Initial counseling assumes significant importance in a population that shows a high rate of unresolved grief. Assessment of the client's previous reactions to loss and the degree of support during decision making will help to identify those who may be suffering from religious conflicts, loss of self-esteem, alienation from others, and beginning symptoms of depression. (See Chapter 38 for assessment of the person in crisis.)

Studies have been done to follow up reactions to the abortion choice (Levin et al., 1980; Freeman et al., 1980). A random sample of 393 women from two abortion clinics revealed that very few women suffered negative psychological aftereffects. The woman's emotional reactions were related to her satisfaction with her decision, the degree of intimacy between her and the male partner, and how anxious or angry she was when the pregnancy was first discovered (Schusterman, 1979). Women having repeated abortions have a significantly higher emotional distress score regarding interpersonal relationships (Freeman, 1980) Such information is useful for assessing potential problems and providing necessary nursing interventions for this crisis time.

REFERENCES

Benditt, J. "Second Trimester Abortion in the U.S.," *Family Planning Perspectives,* **12**(2):112, 1980.

Bracker, M., Klerman, L., and Bucken, M.: "Abortion, Adoption, or Motherhood: An Empirical Study of Decision-Making During Pregnancy," *American Journal of Obstetrics and Gynecology,* **130**(3):251, 1978.

Cherazi, S.: "Brief Communication: Psychological Reaction to Abortion," *Journal of Medical Women's Association,* **34**(6):287, 1979.

Cook, R. J., and Dickens, B.: "A Decade of International Change in Abortion Law: 1967–77," *American Journal of Public Health,* **68**(7):637, 1978.

Dating, J., Spadoni, S., and Emanuel, I.: "Role of Induced Abortion in Secondary Infertility," *Obstetrics and Gynecology,* **57**(1):59, 1981.

Forrest, J. D., Sullivan, E., and Tietze, C.: "Abortion in the United States 1977–78," in *Family Planning Perspectives,* **11**(6):329, 1979.

Freeman, E., Rickels, K., Huggins, G., Garcia, C. R., and Palin, J.: "Emotional Distress Patterns Among Women Having First or Repeat Abortions," *Obstetrics and Gynecology,* **55**(5):630, 1980.

Gedan, S.: "Pre-Abortion Emotional Counseling," in *ANA Clinical Sessions,* Appleton-Century-Crofts, New York, 1972.

Gordon, R. H., and Kilpatrick, C.: "A Program of Group Counseling for Men Who Accompany Women Seeking Legal Abortions," *Community Mental Health Journal,* **13**(4):291, 1977.

Grimes, D. A., and Cates, W.: "The Comparative Efficacy and Safety of Intraamniotic Prostaglandin/Hypertonic Saline for Second Trimester Abortion," *Journal of Reproductive Medicine,* **22**(5):248, 1979.

Howe, B., Kaplan, H., and English, C.: "Repeat Abortions: Blaming the Victims," *American Journal of Public Health,* **69**(12):1242, 1979.

Levin, A., Schoenbaum, S., Nearson, S., and Phillips, R.: "Assessment of Induced Abortion with Subsequent Pregnancy Loss," *Journal of American Medical Associates,* **243**(24):2495, 1980.

Morbidity & Mortality Weekly Report, 29(14):157, 158, April 11, 1980.

Osofsky, H. J., and Osofsky, J. D.: *The Abortion Experience: Psychological and Medical Impact,* Harper & Row, New York, 1973.

Schusterman, L.: "Predicting the Psychological Consequences of Abortion," *Social Science and Medicine,* **13A**:683, 1979.

Steinhoff, S. S., Palmore, J., Diamond M., and Chung, C. S.: "Women Who Obtain Repeat Abortions: A Study Based on Record Linkage," *Family Planning Perspectives,* **11**(1):38, 1979.

BIBLIOGRAPHY

Anders, R.: "Program Consultation by a Clinical Specialist," *Journal of Nursing Administration,* **7**(11):34, 1978. Describes consultation to nurses developing an abortion counseling program. Includes health education about the procedure, opportunity for clients to talk about their feelings concerning their decision, and birth control information.

Anderson, C., Clancy, B., and Hassanein, R.: "Psychoprophylaxis in Mid-trimester Abortions," *Journal of Obstetric, Gynecologic, and Neonatal Nursing,* **5**(6):29, November/December 1976. Study comparing abortion experiences between women utilizing modified LaMaze techniques and those receiving routine nursing care.

Barlow, P.: "Abortion 1975: The Psychiatric Perspective: With a Discussion of Abortion and Contraception in Adolescence," *Journal of Obstetric and Gynecologic Nursing,* **5**(1):41, January/February 1976. Discusses behavioral reactions based on developmental needs of adolescents.

Beazley, J. M.: "The Prostaglandin," *Nursing Times,* **72**(16):1800, November 18, 1976. Review of prostaglandins and their physiologic effects on various body systems.

Bracken, M., and Kasl, S. V.: "Delay in Seeking Induced Abortion: A Review and Theoretical Analysis," *American Journal of Obstetrics and Gynecology,* **121**:1009, April 1975. Examines reasons for delay by women seeking abortions.

Easterbrook, B., and Rust, B.: "A New Role for Nurses," *The Canadian Nurse,* **73**(1):28, January 1977. Nursing model for pre- and postabortion care utilizing group counseling techniques.

"Further Ethical Considerations in Induced Abortions," *Journal of Obstetric, Gynecologic, and Neonatal Nursing,* **7**(3):53, 1978. A statement policy from the Executive Board of the American College of Obstetricians and Gynecologists reflecting moral and humane concerns and offering review of ethical issues involved.

Gordon, R. H., and Kilpatrick, C.: "A Program of Group Counseling for Men Who Accompany Women Seeking Legal Abortions," *Community Mental Health Journal*, **13**(4):291, 1977. Describes short counseling sessions with questions assisting men to increase their understanding and support ability.

Kaminsky, B. A., and Sheckter, L.: "Abortion Counseling in a Generalist Hospital," *Health and Social Work*, **4**(2):93, 1979. Describes a counseling program by nonprofessionally trained social workers oriented toward crisis intervention and prevention.

Luke, C.: "Sexuality and Abortion," in N. F. Woods, *Human Sexuality in Health and Illness*, 2d ed., Mosby, St. Louis, 1979, p. 215. Considers antecedents to abortion. Assists practitioner in dealing with feelings concerning abortion. Reviews questions at end of chapter.

Muldoon, M.: *Abortion: An Annotated Indexed Bibliography*, Edwin Mellon, New York, 1980. Contains 3397 entries arranged in general topics.

National Organization of Women, "A Brief Chronology" and "Abortion: Federal Staus" in *Reproductive Rights Kit*, NOW, Washington, D.C., 1982. Reviews federal and state bills and committee actions as well as Supreme Court and lower court decisions.

14

The Infertile Family

Elizabeth J. Dickason and Carol Ann McKenzie

Reproductive failure is a complex life crisis that is psychologically threatening, financially expensive, emotionally stressful, and often physically painful. It involves an individual's self-image and self-esteem and feelings about sexuality. It necessitates the exploration and assessment of a very sensitive area of a couple's relationship. Approximately 1:6, or 15 percent, of the couples of childbearing age are involuntarily childless. Because of career goals many families delay childbearing and when ready may find that they cannot conceive. When conception does not occur, the emotional crises for these couples can be intense. The treatments they undergo and the supportive care during the prolonged crisis period constitute a subspecialty of health care that requires sensitive and highly qualified care by health professionals. An overview of such care is presented here. Nurses may play a crucial part in the quality of treatment such families receive.

GENERAL INFERTILITY FACTORS

DESCRIPTION

Infertility is a relative term that indicates that a particular couple has difficulty achieving conception. In contrast, *sterility* indicates the inability of an individual to produce functional gametes and may be the final diagnosis of the male or female partner in the infertile dyad. *Primary infertility* is the inability of a couple to conceive after at least 1 year of unprotected intercourse; normally 80 percent of couples having regular intercourse will conceive during this time. *Secondary infertility* indicates that a couple has already conceived one or more times (regardless of outcome) but that further unrestricted efforts have failed to achieve another conception. *Idiopathic*, or *unexplained, infertility* may be the diagnosis when no medical cause for infertility can be determined. The treatment of infertility may have multiple protocols. The success rate declines with the duration of infertility and with increasing age; 50 to 60 percent of couples seen promptly will become pregnant after varying lengths of treatment (Table 14-1).

Requisites for fertility in the female are:

1. Normal ovulation with adequate gonadotropin secretion.
2. Unobstructed mechanism for pickup of ovum by fimbria of fallopian tube.
3. Patent tube with adequate cilia and tubal fluids so that sperm has access to ovum and fertilized ovum may descend to the uterus.
4. Normal implantation and maintenance of corpus luteum until placental hormones are adequate.
5. Normal uterine structure, cervical competence, and penetrable mucus.

NOTE: The author acknowledges the contributions of Nancy Reame, Ph.D.

TABLE 14-1 CAUSES OF INFERTILITY

Genetic

Chromosome deletions or trisomy:
- Turner's syndrome 45,XO
- Klienfelter's syndrome 47,XXY

Mosaicism of sex chromosomes

Production of pathologic deformed sperm or ova

21-hydroxylase deficiency (chromosome 6)

HSD-3_{β}Hydroxysteroid deficiency

Testicular feminization

Hormonal

Female:
- Ovarian or adrenal hypersecretion:
  - Stein-Levanthal syndrome—polycystic ovarian disease (PCOD)
  - Excess androgen production
  - Luteal Phase defects
- Hypogonadotrophic conditions:
- Amenorrhea, anovulation
- Premenopausal, menopausal states
- Post-pill amenorrhea
- Hypo- or hypersecretion from pituitary, thyroid, adrenals

Male:
- Hypgonadotrophic conditions causing reduced testosterone secretion or changes in FSH, LH levels.

Mechanical Obstruction

Female:
- Adhesions due to endometriosis or surgery, salpingitis
- Ectopic pregnancy with repair
- Uterine myomata or polyps

Male:
- Retrograde ejaculation
- Vasectomy repair (vasovasotomy)
- Spinal cord injury or disease

Genetic or Developmental

Agenesis of reproductive organs, streak gonads

Dysgenesis of reproductive structures:
- Male factors: hydrocele, phimosis, Hypo- or epispadius, cryptorchidism (undescended testes)
- Female factors: cervical stenosis, malformations of the uterus, ambiguous genitalia

Drug Effects in utero: DES syndrome

Inflammatory

In female reproductive tract: tuberculosis, gonorrhea

Mycoplasmas
- Chlamydial tracheomatis
- Other salpingitis causes: postabortion sepsis, puerperal or IUD infection
- Endometriosis

In male reproductive tract: prostatitis, mumps orchitis, diseases with high fevers, epididymitis

Immunologic responses: antisperm antibodies in female, sperm agglutinins in semen

Environmental, Drug-induced

Overexposure to extremes of heat

Strenuous excercise (athletes)

Tight male undergarments

Exposure to chemicals, radiation, or heavy metals

Certain drugs: phenothiazines, reserpine, drug addiction, especially in women

Reduced testosterone levels as a result of alcoholism

Possible reduced motility and number of normal sperm due to nicotine

Psychogenic

Chronic physical or mental stress, high anxiety:
- In female, results in anovulation, amenorrhea
- In male, may result in impotence, sham ejaculation, retrograde ejaculation, or oligospermia

Inadequate sexual understanding with use of poor techniques

Anorexia nervosa:
- Excessive weight loss

Chronic Disease

Nutritional deficiencies

Metabolic disease, especially severe diabetes

Cardiac disease

Renal disease

Hypertension

Cancer

Chronic fatigue, anemia

Requisites in the male are:

1. The ability to have intercourse with vaginal penetration and ejaculation.
2. Production of an adequate number of sperm with normal shape and motility that are free of hinderances in moving into the cervix.
3. Adequate quantity and quality of seminal fluids, without immunologic inhibition.

Infertility is almost equally divided between male and female factors. Any underlying chronic disease should be evaluated and treated before any expectation of fertility enhancement. Occupational factors must be assessed and any adverse social customs should be identified and discontinued during treatment. Any inflammation in the acute stage in either partner will be treated with antibiotics and later adhesions or scarring with surgery. Exciting new developments have identified a group of causative agents such as *Mycoplasma* and *Chlamydia* infections, which are amenable to antibiotic therapy.

Immunologic infertility in either partner may occur in about 5 percent of infertile couples. Difficult to diagnose and treat, autoimmunization or antispermatozoan antibody formation may require extensive evaluation and finally artificial insemination with donor sperm or in vitro fertilization with embryo transfer.

The most common causes of female subfertility and the ones most amenable to treatment are the endocrine disturbances underlying amenorrhea, organ maturation, anovulation, and repeated early spontaneous abortions. Included in this group are polycystic ovarian disease (PCOD), luteal phase defects, endometriosis, and hyperandrogenemia. These endocrine disturbances may be amenable to drug therapy with gonadotropics, steroid stimulants, or suppressants such as bromocryptine or danocrine.

Structural or obstructive defects of the reproductive tract such as genetic and congenital defects or adhesions resulting from endometriosis or salpingitis may be repaired by surgery.

Male reproductive failure accounts for 40 to 50 percent of diagnosed infertility. Male infertility is influenced by genetic and hormonal factors and especially by stress, occupational hazards, and urologic problems. The major cause is inadequate production of sperm with vigorous motility. Many factors besides hormone imbalance will affect sperm function; variocele, alcoholism, and excessive smoking will affect motility, and hyposecretion of gonadotropins and reproductive tract defects will affect production.

Because causes may be very difficult to pinpoint and frustration and stress accompany the prolonged evaluation, it may become more stressful to go through infertility procedures than to remain childless. A couple's motivation, support systems, finances, and marriage bonds can be severely tested in the process. Grieving, anger, and disappointment may be the outcome after all, and these couples especially need understanding and support from the health team.

PREVENTION

Health Promotion/Men and Women

1. Good health habits with adequate rest, nutrition; avoidance of excessive alcohol, smoking, and any use of drugs unless prescribed.
2. Avoidance of undue stress; use of coping mechanisms.
3. Reduced exposure to venereal diseases.
4. Proper safety precautions with occupational health hazards (heat, radiation, poisons, metals, dyes).
5. Prompt health care during illness.
6. Adequate sex education and information for any sexual dysfunction.

Additional Health Promotion for Women

1. Early assessment of underlying causes for menstrual irregularities or the development of hirsutism.
2. Avoidance of steroid contraceptives if there are irregular menstrual cycles or within 2 years of menarche.
3. Early detection of IUD-related infections, cervical infections.
4. Avoidance of multiple elective abortions.
5. Avoidance of infections that may lead to abortion, such as toxoplasmosis, for example, use of caution while caring for cats or gardening if cats are about.
6. Avoidance of hyperthermia during pregnancy, especially in the first 3 months.

Additional Health Promotion for Men

1. Early detection of undescended testicles or hyposecretion of gonadotropins related to genetic or developmental disturbances.
2. Prevention of mumps orchitis or infections with high fevers, such as diptheria, or typhoid by double-checking on childhood immunizations.

3. Avoidance of constrictive underclothing, hot tubs, saunas.
4. No unusual lubricants with intercourse.

Population at Risk

1. Men.
   a. For reduced sperm quality, structure and motility:
      (1) Firemen, workers in steel plants or boiler works, those exposed to hazardous wastes, radiation.
      (2) Variocele, or undescended testicles.
      (3) Exposure to DES in utero, some cases.
      (4) Strenuous exercise (e.g., some athletes).
      (5) Hypogonadotropin secretion.
      (6) Diagosed venereal disease, *Mycoplasma* infection.
   b. For reduced ejaculation:
      (1) Spinal cord injuries or disease.
      (2) Metabolic disease, diabetes.
      (3) Use of antihypertensive agents.
      (4) Chronic emotional stress, chronic fatigue.
   c. For passage occlusion:
      (1) Reversal of vasectomy (vasovasotomy).
      (2) Genetic malformations of urogenital tract.
2. Women.
   a. For reduced ovulation and disorders of menstrual cycle:
      (1) Dramatic loss or gain in weight.
      (2) Prolonged contraceptive steroid use (1 percent of users).
      (3) Drug abuse, multiple sexual partners.
      (4) Fatigue, chronic stress affecting central catecholamines.
      (5) Strenuous exercise (athletes).
   b. For inability to maintain pregnancy after conception:
      (1) Multiple elective abortions with cervical scarring.
      (2) DES exposure in utero, some cases.
      (3) Hypogonadotropin secretions.
   c. For tubal occlusion or malfunction:
      (1) Untreated salpingitis, postabortion or puerperal infections causing adhesions and scar tissue. Post pelvic surgery adhesions.
      (2) Prior ectopic pregnancy and repair.
      (3) Endometriosis.
3. Both sexes.
   a. Chronic systemic illness.
   b. Genetic chromosomal or single-gene defects, especially sex chromosome aberration.
   c. Brain tumors, cancer.
   d. Those nearing physiologic menopause and aging.

ASSESSMENT

Initial Health History/Men and Women

1. Duration of infertility.
2. Reasons couple ascribe to their infertility and motivation for childbearing.
3. Support systems available during this crisis.
4. Ages, occupations, lifestyles, stress levels.
5. General medical history, including hereditary disorders.
6. Gynecologic, obstetric, contraceptive, and urologic histories.
7. History of previous tests or therapy for infertility.
8. Any history of fertility with a different partner.
9. Sexual knowledge and practices influencing fertility.
   a. Coital frequency, two to three times a week is optimal for achieving conception.
   b. Coital timing with midcycle ovulation.
   c. Coital techniques—Does ejaculation leave pool of semen at cervical opening?
   d. Adverse practices (Use of nonphysiologic lubricants such as petroleum jelly or douching too soon after intercourse).
   e. Multiple sexual partners; oral or anal intercourse (may lead to development of immunologic problems).
10. Sexual libido, feelings about fertility testing.
11. Sociocultural beliefs and values about children.

Physical Assessment

1. General physical stature and indications of secondary sex characteristics.
2. Size, position, and condition of reproductive organs.
3. Signs of infection in the reproductive tract.
4. Evidence of chronic disease.
5. For specific assessment see the conditions following in this chapter.

Diagnostic Tests/Men and Women

1. Genetic screening. (see Chapter 12)
   a. Karyotype, H-Y antigen.
   b. Screening for certain inborn errors of metabolism that may affect general health.

2. Screening for venereal disease, infections.
3. Skull x-ray for sella tursica enlargment, possible tumor if prolactin levels are elevated.
4. Hormone assays.

NURSING DIAGNOSES/ INTERVENTIONS

Refer to the following specific conditions.

FEMALE INFERTILITY FACTORS

HYPOGONADOTROPIC SECRETION

Amenorrhea may be primary or secondary. *Primary amenorrhea* with delayed onset of menarche usually is due to genetic causes or to malformation of the genital tract. *Secondary amenorrhea,* after menses pattern is well established, may often be psychogenic during adolescence or during periods of high stress or may be due to hyposecretion of gonadotropins, luteal phase defects, or androgen excess. Amenorrhea may be divided into four groups (Table 14-2), and the usual infertile client seeking fertility assistance falls into the category of secondary amenorrhea. Poor ovulatory function may stem from hypothalamic pituitary or ovarian causes. It may also be a phenomenon after steroid contraceptive usage and may be only temporary. The availability of potent physiologic and pharmacologic agents to induce ovulation has led to a high degree of success in these cases of infertility. (See Table 14-3)

ASSESSMENT

Health History

1. Dramatic weight fluctuations; anorexic women have amenorrhea.
2. Use of stimulants or sedatives, chronic lack of sleep, depression.
3. Chronic strenuous exercise, especially with athletes.
4. History of drug intake that influences menses (see Table 14-1).
5. Family history of subfertility, late onset of menarche.
6. Precocious or delayed onset of menarche
   a. Normal range: 11–12.4 ±1.4 years.
   b. In 99 percent of females menarche occurs within 5 years of onset of breast growth.
7. Menstrual cycles may be irregular and unpredictable, ±5 or more days difference from cycle to cycle.
8. Menstrual cycles may be associated with breakthrough bleeding, spotting, and absence of premenstrual symptoms (breast tenderness, edema, cramping). Obtain date of last period and description.

TABLE 14-2 CAUSES OF AMENORRHEA

Level I—Disorders of Reproductive Tract or Uterine Response to Hormones
- Evaluate structure and patency of tract.
- Test for withdrawal bleeding with Provera, or add estrogen and Provera to obtain withdrawal bleeding.
- Endometrial biopsy during luteal phase to evaluate response.

Level II—Disorders of the Ovary
- Assay of gonadotropins, FSH, LH, prolactin levels.
- Elevated levels of FSH alone require karyotype for Y chromosome unless woman is premenopausal.
- Elevated LH and low FSH may be found in POCD.
- Low LH, low FSH may indicate pituitary failure.

Level III—Disorders of the Anterior Pituitary
- Elevated prolactin, often with galactorrhea, indicates study for microadenoma; polytomography of sella turcica.
- Thyroid screening.

Level IV—Disorders in the CNS (Hypothalmus)
- Psychologic stress
- Rapid weight loss, anorexia
- Decreased response to GnRH
- Increased circulating androgens

SOURCE: Adapted from Speroff, L., Glass, R. H., and Kase, N. G.: *Clinical Gynecologic Endocrinology and Infertility,* 2d ed., Williams & Wilkins, Baltimore, 1978.

9. History of any pelvic surgery for cysts.
10. Any prior evaluation for menstrual irregularity.
11. History of any prolonged use of steroid contraceptives especially for those with prior irregular menses.

Physical Assessment

1. Most amenorrheal clients appear normal in body build.
2. Weight may be inappropriate for body build, marked weight loss must be evaluated.
3. Body contours may show more masculine characteristics and/or hair distribution, and breast size may have decreased.
4. Acne may have increased.
5. Voice may be deeper than expected, in rare cases.
6. Thyroid will be palpated for enlargement.
7. There may be a milky discharge from the breasts (galactorrhea).
8. Pelvic exam may show any of the following:
   a. Small and smooth or large and cystic ovaries.
   b. Ovaries fixed in position.
   c. Closed cervical os at midcycle.
   d. Cervical erosion, chronic infection.
   e. Clitoral hypertrophy.
   f. Pale vaginal mucosa.

Diagnostic Tests

1. Endogenous estrogen evaluation is abnormal if the following appear:
   a. Vaginal smear—few cornified epithelial cells, many intermediate and basiphillic (blue-staining) cells.
   b. Cervical mucus—scant, opaque, or tacky at midcycle, pH lower than expected.
   c. Endometrial biopsy—during midluteal cycle does not show adequate build up.
   d. Progesterone challenge test—medroxyprogesterone 10 mg for 5 days or 100–200 mg IM does not result in withdrawal menses.
2. Various hormones are evaluated by radioimmunoassay (RAI):
   a. Luteinizing hormone (LH)—Presence of LH surge at midcycle is detected by obtaining daily assay for 4 to 5 days at midcycle. Mean interval of peak to time of ovulation is less than 48 h in all cycles and less than 24 h in 75 percent. New methods of rapid assay are being developed. FSH and FH may be abnormally low or elevated, depending on the site of the endocrine dysfunction (Figure 14-1).
   b. Gonadotropin-releasing hormone (GnRH) (hypothalamic origin)—Injection of GnRH will cause a release of LH and FSH into plasma similar in nature to midcycle ovulatory surge. When anovulation occurs in secondary ovarian failure due to hypothalamic dysfunction, GnRH may be used when exact timing of ovulation is desired, but hCG is more widely used.
   c. Estrogen—Serum estradiol (E_2) peaks 1 day before LH surge and 37 h before ovulation. Serial assay may be done at midcycle by serum or urinary assay.
   d. Progesterone.
      (1) Serum progesterone less than 1 ng/mL in follicular phase and rises sharply with the LH surge to peak at more than 10 ng/mL at 8 days after peak. Two samples will be obtained at day 8 and day 21 of cycle, an increase to more than 5 ng/mL presumes formation of corpus luteum.
      (2) Urinary pregnanediol levels of 4–6 mg/24 h in the midluteal phase are normal.
   e. As evaluation becomes more detailed and more difficult, further investigation into hormonal levels of testosterone, prolactin, thyroid hormones—T_3, T_4 and TSH—and adrenal steroids will be done.
3. Basal body temperature (BBT), obtained through course of cycle for several months is necessary to chart the regularity of biphasic temperature (Figures 14-2 and 14-3). BBT obtained correctly will show an abnormal monophasic anovulatory pattern or normally a reduced temperature at midcycle with elevation in secretory phase. A short luteal phase may indicate luteal defects. Mean BBT in the first phase should be 97.48° $\pm$0.22° and in the second phase should remain elevated until progesterone levels fall below 4 ng/mL. The characteristic change in temperature is evidence of ovulation 2 to 3 days after it has occurred.
4. Characteristics of cervical mucus are shown in Figure 14-4. Sperm penetration is possible only when estrogen-supported mucus at midcycle develops the following properties:
   a. Spinnbarkeit—ability to be stretched apart into a thin continuous thread of at least 5 to 8 cm in length.

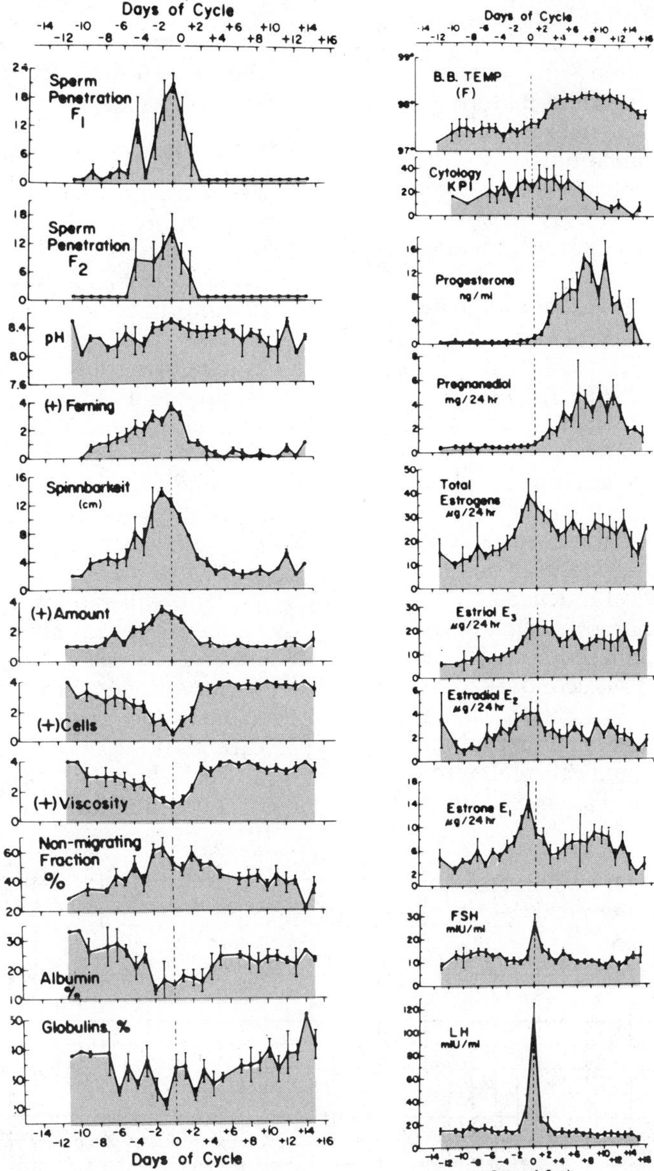

Figure 14-1 Composite profile of sperm penetration, gonadotropin and progesterone, urinary estrogens and pregnanediol, basal body temperature (B. B. T.), karyopyknotic index (KPI) of vaginal cytology, and cervical mucus properties throughout the menstrual cycles of 10 normal women. Day 0, day of luteinizing hormone (LH) peak (dotted line). The vertical bars represent 1 SEM. F_1 and F_2 indicate the number of sperm in the first and second microscopic fields ($\times 200$) from interface 15 minutes after the start of the in vitro sperm-cervical mucus penetration test. FSH, follicle-stimulation hormone. (From Moghissi, K. S., in E. E. Wallach, and R. D. Kempers, eds., *Modern Trends in Infertility and Conception Control,* Vol. I, William and Wilkins, Baltimore, 1979.)

b. Ferning (arborization—the crystalization of mucus into a fernlike pattern (due to increased NaCl) when airdried on a slide. The degree of branching (1°, 2°, 3°) indicates the extent of estrogenic influence.
c. Appearance—lowered viscosity, clear, odorless, increased amount, lowered proteins, no cells, pH above 7.5.

5. Postcoital Test—see evaluation of semen.

NURSING DIAGNOSES: ACTUAL OR POTENTIAL

1. Altered reproductive function, as evidenced by:
   a. Monophasic BBT profile associated with irregular menstrual cycles.
   b. Poor quality cervical mucus.
   c. Anovulatory pattern of plasma hormones.
2. Loss of self-esteem, altered body image, and increased martial stress secondary to reduced ability to conceive.
3. Knowledge deficit about menstrual and sexual physiology and medical treatments.
4. Potential for noncompliance by one partner due to extensive infertility testing and invasion of privacy.

EXPECTED OUTCOMES

1. Physical and psychosocial problems influencing fertility will be identified.
2. Rapport between the couple and health team will be established in order to promote open communication and expression of feeling.
3. Couple will understand purposes, costs, and course of fertility investigation.
4. Couple will understand information and discuss all means of becoming natural parents.
5. Couple will attend counseling sessions to explore impact of infertility on marriage and effect on emotional status of each partner.
6. Couple will maintain decision-making ability and sense of self-control.
7. Woman will exhibit biphasic BBT pattern, enhanced ferning, spinnbarkeit, and adequate midcycle mucus within 6–12 months after treatment is begun.
8. Woman will give evidence of complying with care plan by:
   a. Recording daily BBT and bringing in charts for evaluation.

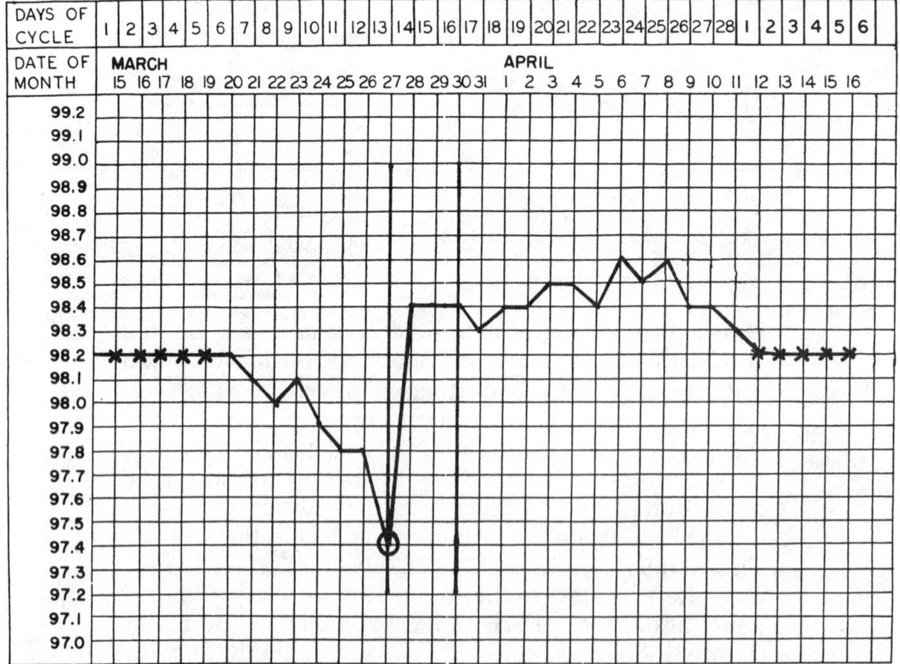

Figure 14-2 Basal body temperature chart illustrating the thermal shift indicative of ovulation in a normal cycle. X, menstruation; O, ovulation.

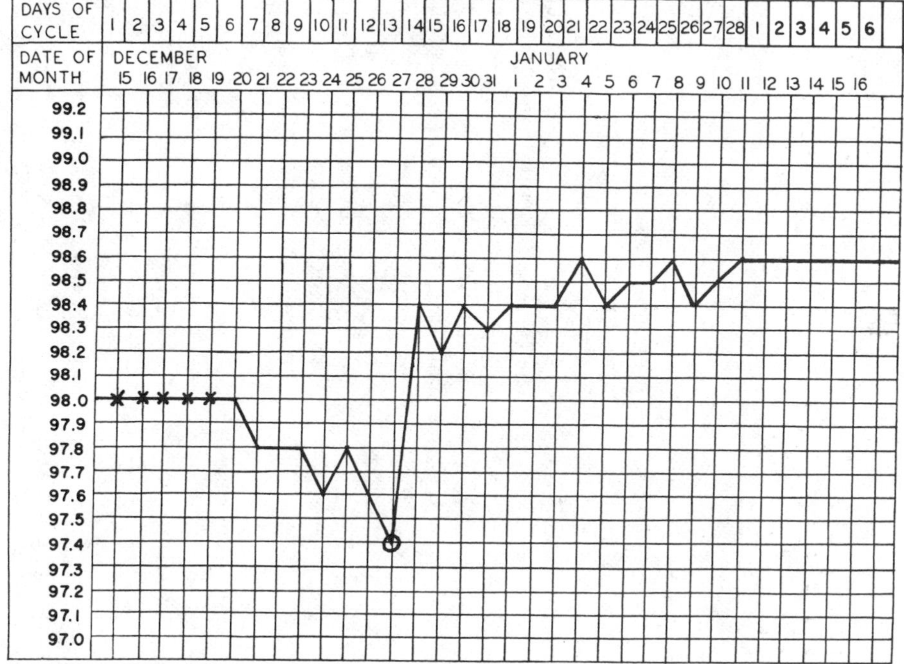

Figure 14-3 Basal body temperature chart illustrating an ovulatory cycle with persisting elevation indicating conception.

b. Adhering to vaginal intercourse schedule as indicated by BBT.
c. Adhering to medication regimen. (See Table 14-3.)

INTERVENTIONS

1. Provide therapeutic setting where sexual questions, practices, misinformation may be discussed in a nonthreatening manner.
2. Provide anticipatory guidance about the feelings, physical sensations, and emotions that the woman may experience during the assessment of amenorrhea or anovulation.
3. Teach woman to prepare reports of menstrual changes during treatment—BBT patterns, characteristics of cervical mucus.
4. Provide thorough explanations of specimen-collecting techniques.
5. Reinforce understanding of timing of intercourse with ovulatory period. Be sure client understands medication dosage and timing.
6. Answer questions about diagnostic tests. Prepare couple for each procedure. Follow up with telephone reminders as necessary.
7. Plan teaching to build on current understanding. Suggest readings, provide literature. (See Guide for Partners later in this chapter.)
8. Encourage couple to verbalize feelings about evaluative process. Recognize when referral for counseling may be advised. Intake interviews may have explored expressed conflicts arising from religious beliefs, marital stress, ambivalence, or poor communication, but in the course of evaluation and treatment other problems may surface and opportunity should be provided for exploration.

EVALUATION

Outcome Criteria

1. Woman is complying with care regimen.
2. Woman can recall verbally the content of each teaching session and follows directions in obtaining BBT or specimens.
3. Communication stays open between partners and between partners and health team.
4. Couple identifies purposes, costs, and expected course of fertility investigation.
5. Couple attends marital counseling sessions when indicated.
6. After diagnosis and therapy, BBT character-

TABLE 14-3 DRUG THERAPY FOR INFERTILITY

Drug	Dosage	Uses	Precautions
Clomiphene Clomid	Start with 50 mg qd for 5 days beginning the fifth day LMP for three cycles. Raise to 100 mg qd for 5 days for three cycles, to a maximum of 200 mg.	Nonsteroid estrogen antagonist modifies hypothalamic activity resulting in a release of GnRH that causes an increase of FSH and LH and thus develops Graafian follicle. Ovulatory surge should begin 5–10 days after last pill is taken. Advise coitus every other day for 1 week beginning 5 days after clomiphene tabs are stopped.	Always evaluate BBT, plasma progesterones, and estrogens. Endometrial biopsy may be done in the third week. *Side effects:* Flushing, abdominal distention, bloating, breast tenderness, nausea, vomiting, visual disturbances, dryness of hair, hair loss; symptoms cease at end of treatment. *Adverse effects:* Ovarian enlargement. Drug not reused if visual disturbances occur. Multiple pregnancy risk is 6–18%.
hCG	10,000 IU IM 7–10 days after last clomiphene tablet has been taken.	Added to clomiphene regimen if there is no effect at the 200-mg level or there is a short luteal phase. Used to trigger ovulation from a ripe follicle. May be used in lower, more frequent doses for men with hypogonadotropic hypogonadism (lack of secondary sex characteristics) or for those with low sperm production.	May use ultrasonography to measure follicle development of 1.8–2.5 cm before administration of hCG. Intercourse is planned for evening of first day after injection and for next 2 days. *Side effects:* Contributes to hyperstimulation syndrome with hMG. *Adverse effects:* Multiple pregnancy risk at 20–40% with hMG.

hMG, menotropins Pergonal	Purofied gonadotropins contain 75 IU of FSH, 75 IU of LH given IM for 1 day or 2 ampules qd for 7–14 days.	Primary ovarian failure 9–12 days only to effect maturation of follicle, must be followed by hCG, 10,000 IU for ovulation, when estrogen and cervical mucus show readiness. May be used for women who do not ovulate with clomiphene.	Maturation of follicle must be closely followed to avoid overstimulation. *Side effects:* Not given if FSH or LH is already elevated or if thyroid or adrenal problems or ovarian cyst present. Client may have febrile reaction. *Adverse effects:* After treatment is finished, overstimulation of ovary may occur. Abdominal distension; pain, from mild to severe. High multiple pregnancy risk (20–40%) with 5% in triplets or quadruplets.
	For men: Pretreatment with hCG 5000 IU three times a week may be necessary for 4 to 6 months then add Pergonal 1 ampule three times a week plus hCG 2000 IU twice a week for 4 more months.	For primary or secondary hypogonadotropic hypogonadism. Given to stimulate testosterone. Pergonal with hCG may stimulate spermatogenesis or induce development of secondary sex characteristics; given to induce more active, numerous sperm production.	*Side effects:* Gynecomastia may occur. Treatment is expensive, time-consuming.
Danocrine Danazol	200 mg up to 800 mg in 4 divided doses daily for 3–9 months.	Synthetic weak androgen suppresses gonadotropins FSH, LH so that endometriosis is inhibited and tissue regresses and atrophies. Stimulates menopausal effect on endometrial tissue. Results in monophasic BBT. Sometimes used in fibrocystic breast disease to relieve pain, tender nodules.	Accompanying symptoms related to reduced gonadotropins: amenorrhea, weight gain, some acne and skin oil increase, plus vasomotor flushing. Vaginal tissues may need lubrication. 60–90 day return of ovulation; take care to maintain BBT as drug is not to be used during pregnancy—may cause clitoral hypertrophy, labial fusion in female infants. *Side effects:* Fluid retention; conditions aggravated by this will preclude use.

TABLE 14-3 *(continued)*

Drug	Dosage	Uses	Precautions
Bromocryptine Parlodel	2.5–10 mg qd	An ergot alkaloid: nonhormonal nonestrogenic dopamine antagonist (receptor agonist); inhibits prolactin in clients with elevated levels that may be associated with pituitary tumors. Used in amenorrhea-galactorrhea syndrome. When prolactin is suppressed the normal ovulatory cycle usually begins in 2 months.	Observe any woman with elevated prolactin for pituitary tumors. *Side effects:* Hypotension, nausea, headache, dizziness, abdominal cramps, vomiting, nasal congestion, constipation, or diarrhea.
	2.5 mg bid for 10 days. Must begin within 12 h after delivery for suppression of lactation.	Woman must be informed that she will ovulate by 30 days because of suppression of prolactin. Drug also used in Parkinson's disease.	*Side effects:* As above. There may be rebound engorgement when drug is stopped. Woman may, however, initiate breastfeeding after drug is stopped if she changes her mind.

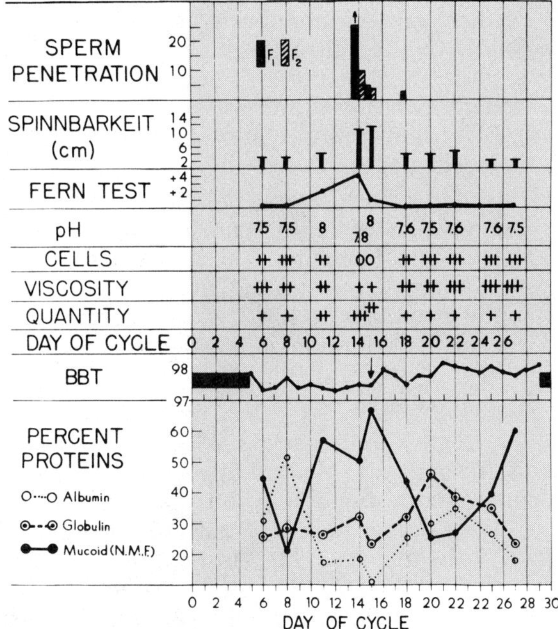

Figure 14-4 Correlation of basal body temperature (BBT) with cervical mucus properties and sperm penetrability in vitro. F_1 and F_2 indicate the number of spermatozoa in the first and second microscopic fields (×200) from interface, 15 minutes after the start of the in vitro sperm-cervical mucus penetration test. The arrow shows the probable time of ovulation. N.M.F., non-migration fraction. Note the significant sperm penetrability is evident only on the day of ovulation. (From Moghissi, K. S., in E. E. Wallach, and R. D. Kempers, eds, *Modern Trends in Infertility, and Conception Control*, Vol. I, William and Wilkins, Baltimore, 1979.) (See Figure 14-2, p. 288.)

istics show biphasic profile and gonadotropins have resumed normal levels.

7. Conception has occured. Client has been referred for obstetric care.

Complications

MULTIPLE OVULATION

Ovulation induction may induce multiple ovulation and multiple pregnancy occurs more often (see Chapter 7). The risk rate depends a great deal on the cause of amenorrhea or anovulation, as well as on the particular drug and the extent of treatment required. The World Health Organization classification for clients requiring induction of ovulation is as follows.

Group One—Those women with low levels of endogenous gonadotropins and poor endogenous estrogen activity. These women require a higher dose of gonadotropin and a longer period of therapy.

Group Two—Those women with anovulation who have evidence of endogenous estrogenic activity and need smaller doses over shorter periods. These women are more susceptible to overstimulation and multiple ovulation.

The incidence of multiple ovulation and conception is highest with the use of combined hMG-hCG therapy (20 to 40 percent). Careful estrogen monitoring before the use of the drugs will reduce risk. Clomiphene alone carries a risk of 6 to 18 percent. Combinations of clomiphene with hCG, hMG, or GnRH have been reported to cause a rate of 8 to 34 percent. (Speroff, 1979)

POLYCYSTIC OVARIAN DISEASE (PCOD)

Persistent high estrogen with elevated LH levels inhibit FSH so that the follicles are stimulated but are not completely developed and ovulation does not occur. The ovary is often enlarged and appears smooth and pearly with a thickened capsule. The endometrium demonstrates the effect of a steady state of estrogen. (See chapter 28.)

Assessment

1. Elevated steady state of LH with low FSH and no peaks.
2. Elevated estrogens and androgens.
3. Endometrial biopsy indicates poor progesterone effect, indicating overstimulation of endometrium by estrogen.
4. Client complains of irregular heavy bleeding (20 percent) because estrogen is unopposed by progesterone, or
5. Client may complain of amenorrhea (55 percent).
6. Hirsuitism may develop, or acne, seborrhea, and weight gain.

Revised Outcomes

1. The woman who wishes to become pregnant will have a successful medical induction of ovulation.
2. Cyclic hormonal patterns will be restored.

Interventions

1. Interventions are mainly pharmacologic. The addition of a form of progesterone, such as Provera, or the use of an oral contraceptive potent enough to reduce LH levels will be chosen.

2. For clients who wish to become pregnant, clomiphene is tried first, then a combination of hMG and hCG may be prescribed.
3. If there is hyperprolactinemia, bromocriptine may be prescribed.
4. Support, teaching, and interaction as previously described.

Reevaluation and Follow-up

1. The problem of reoccurrence of disease is present with PCOD after drug therapy is discontinued.
2. When a client has hyposecretion of FSH and has been on contraceptive steroids for some time, postpill amenorrhea may occur.
3. The client should be followed at regular intervals during the months after therapy has been started in order that hormonal levels may be evaluated.

HYPERSTIMULATION OF OVARIES

With hMG and hCG induction of ovulation, hyperstimulation of the ovaries may occur as an adverse effect when estrogen levels rise too high. The condition usually resolves within 1 or 2 weeks with supportive care but may be life-threatening if recognized too late.

Assessment

1. Excessive sudden weight gain of more than 20 lb within 3 to 4 days.
2. Hemoconcentration with hematocrit over 50 percent, fluid shift into abdominal cavity (acites).
3. Hypovolemia with oliguria, hypotension, electrolyte imbalance.
4. Enlarged, fragile ovaries.
5. Abdominal pain, bloating.

Revised Outcomes

1. Fluid and electrolyte balance will be returned to normal.
2. Intravascular pressure will be restored and diuresis will occur.
3. Careful monitoring during resolution will include evaluation for possible pregnancy.

Interventions

1. Give no pelvic or abdominal exams, as manipulation may rupture ovary.
2. Give no diuretics as problem is not at level of kidney. Measure specific gravity of urine.
3. Carefully check intake and output, with careful evaluation of IV fluid balanced with urine output to avoid overload.
4. Frequently measure vital signs.
5. Perform cardiac monitoring at intervals,
6. Follow by diagnostic tests:
   a. Serial hematocrit to detect resolution of hemoconcentration.
   b. BUN, A-G ratio, total proteins.
   c. Electrolytes.

Reevaluation and Follow-up

1. Estrogen levels have been monitored carefully and have resumed normal levels.
2. A woman demonstrating this failure to respond positively to hMG will probably need to consider adoption as an alternative.

LUTEAL PHASE DEFECTS

Some women demonstrate a low secretion of progesterone and subsequently a short phase of corpus luteum function. The result is a 6- to 9-day phase after the LH peak and then rapid onset of the menses. This short phase is usually an insufficient period for implantation and establishment of the placental tissue and results in infertility, despite fertilization of the ovum.

Assessment

1. Estradiol levels and FSH surge before ovulation are lower than normal.
2. Prolactin levels may be abnormal.
3. Endometrial biopsy shows tissue development more than 2 days out of phase.
4. BBT shows a rise in temperature lasting less than 10 days, or a very slow rise in temperature.
5. Pregnancy is not achieved.

Revised Outcomes

1. By use of supportive therapy, ovulation will occur and the corpus luteum will be maintained.
2. The woman will continue to measure BBT carefully and to report signs of the cycle.

Interventions

1. Elicit the woman's cooperation in ongoing evaluation of BBT and timed coitus.
2. Progesterone vaginal suppositories (50 mg) daily may be advised after the midcycle rise in temperature.
3. hCG injection may be attempted, beginning 2 to 3 days after the rise in temperature and continued every other day for 4 days.
4. Explain to the woman that the luteal phase defect is difficult to treat because the cause is confusing. Client should be informed that treatment may not be successful.

Reevaluation and Follow-up

1. If pregnancy results, progesterone suppositories may be ordered at regular intervals, especially in the first trimester.
2. If pregnancy does not occur, regulation of a normal biphasic cycle will be attempted over 6 months to a year.

OCCLUSION OF THE OVIDUCTS

DESCRIPTION

Tubal defects account for 20 to 30 percent of the cases of infertility in women. The oviduct is a complicated, delicate structure. Each section has a different purpose, and tubal fluids and cilia are essential for optimal egg transport. In one survey 75 percent of the clients with tubal causes of infertility had a history of previous pelvic surgery, such as a myomectomy, appendectomy, ovarian cyst or wedge resection, or tubal repair after an ectopic pregnancy. Infection in the tubes, *salpingitis,* may occur after abortion or delivery or because of gonorrhea or pelvic tuberculosis. Adhesions and scarring may result because of these conditions or may be the result of occlusion by endometriosis.

There are many methods of attempting tuboplasty. Some appear still experimental, but microsurgery offers a new possibility of repair of this most delicate tissue. Postsurgical fertility rates are not yet very encouraging, and the client must be prepared for a negative outcome.

PREVENTION

Health Promotion

1. Careful pelvic diagnosis before indiscriminate surgery or unnecessary appendectomy.
2. Limit to numbers of elective abortions because of the risk of endometritis or salpingitis. Careful preabortion assessment of infection potential.
3. Early diagnosis of endometriosis.
4. Venereal disease prevention measures.

Population at Risk

1. See general risk factors.
2. Clients subjected to poor procedures in pelvic surgery.

ASSESSMENT

Health History

1. Exposure to gonorrhea, tuberculosis.
2. Previous pelvic surgery.
3. History of IUD use with subsequent infection.
4. Degree of dysmenorrhea that is indicative of endometriosis.
5. Method of a prior tubal ligation.
6. In spite of ovulation and demonstration of a good biphasic temperature chart, inability to become pregnant.
7. Prior obstetric history, postpartum complications.
8. History of attempted tubal repair or other fertility evaluations, treatments.

Physical Assessment

1. All procedures are medical evaluations for tubal patency.
2. Hysterosalpingography (HSG) with contrast media for visualization of the passageway through the cervix, uterus, and tubes.
   a. Performed 2 to 6 days after the end of menses to avoid flushing out endometrial tissue into peritoneum (one probable origin of endometriosis). Timing avoids chance of flushing out fertilized ovum.
   b. Spillage of dye into peritoneal cavity should occur at 10–15 min. Observation by image-intensive fluoroscopy, with three films taken—before, at expected time of spillage, and a delayed film at 24 h.
   c. Client needs no preparation if Ethiodol is used (Speroff, 1978).
   d. There may be a beneficial side effect of clearing a blocked tube by the mechanical lavage of the dye. Pregnancies have resulted after use of HSG as a diagnostic procedure.
3. Laparoscopy permits direct visualization of the surface of the reproductive organs for assessment of ovarian cysts, endometriosis, tubal adhesions, tumors, or other abnormalities.
   a. Done only after other diagnostic tests have yielded poor results or have shown that surgery may be necessary. There is usually a delay of 6 months after HSG to allow for possible conception.
   b. Done under general or local; laparoscope inserted into small incision near umbili-

cus. Peritoneal cavity insufflated with carbon dioxide to enhance visualization.

c. A second stab wound may be made above pubic area to insert instrument to manipulate organs for view of undersurface.

d. Overnight hospitalization is usually planned. Complications are rare but include reactions to anesthesia, pelvic infection, bleeding, intestinal perforation, and reactions to any dye that might be used simultaneously to observe tubal patency.

NURSING DIAGNOSES: ACTUAL OR POTENTIAL

Altered reproductive function as evidenced by findings on HSG or laparoscopy.

EXPECTED OUTCOMES

1. Tubal patency will be reestablished by HSG or by surgical intervention.
2. Client and partner will be prepared emotionally and will understand the procedures to be undergone.
3. There will be a normal recovery from surgical interventions.

INTERVENTIONS

1. Medical or surgical interventions predominate in these cases. Types of tuboplasty:
   a. Salpingolysis—the separation of peritubal adhesions may lead to a 40 percent chance of pregnancy.
   b. Salpingostomy—opening of the occluded distal end of the tube or, if there are badly occluded fimbria, a fimbrioplasty is done. If no fimbria can be freed, the prognosis is poor.
   c. Midsegment reconstruction.
   d. Resection and reimplatation into the uterus.
2. Provide explanations of surgical procedures, pre- and postoperative care, and expected physical sensations and emotional responses to the surgery.
3. Prepare client for abdominal surgery.
4. Teach client the signs and symptoms of adverse reactions; ectopic pregnancy may occur.
5. Provide information about postoperative physical activity, especially in relation to fertility enhancement.
   a. Review with woman the BBT and mucus testing to determine fertile period.
   b. Review positional and timing criteria for intercourse. (See Guide for Partners later in this chapter.)
6. Provide accepting support for expression of anxieties, fears about failure of surgical intervention.
7. Be sure partners have complete information about their alternatives in the event of failure. (See Artificial Insemination and In Vitro Fertilization in this chapter.)

EVALUATION

Outcome Criteria

1. Tubal patency is surgically accomplished when HSG does not effect opening of tubes.
2. Client and partner successfully cope with surgery and postoperative anxieties.
3. Client has an uneventful recovery period.

Complications

1. Endometriosis is diagnosed, adhesions are removed surgically, but drug therapy must be prescribed before fertility is possible. Some physicians place the client on hormones preoperatively to cause the ectopic endometrial tissue to atrophy. Conservative surgery includes lysis of adhesions, removal of endometriomas or implants, with the uterus suspended in the correct position, and the removal of the appendix. "Chocolate cysts" may be found if tissue in the ovary has been affected. Conservative surgery has been followed by success rates of about 50 percent. The addition of drug therapy has increased fertility by reducing ectopic tissue. (See Table 14-3 and Endometriosis in Chapter 34.)
2. Fertility is not returned after surgery. As surgery is the last modality to be used in an infertility protocol, when there is no conception in the next 1 or 2 years, the couple should be prepared to accept the alternatives of adoption or in vitro fertilization and embryo transfer—the last chance for having their own child. (Garner, 1983).

MALE INFERTILITY FACTORS

DESCRIPTION

In almost half of the cases of infertility, a male factor is implicated. Most commonly there is inadequate sperm production, sperm motility, or morphology. A sperm count of more than 30 million per milliliter is thought to provide the best potential for fertilization of the ovum. (See Table 14-4 for all characteristics of the semen.) At least 50 percent of the sperm must be motile, "only straight swimmers fertilize the ovum" (Amelar, 1982). Sperm with abnormal shapes, or which swim erratically, do not ascend as far as the fallopian tube.

Once analysis has been done for semen quality, other reasons such as structural impairment, genetic or environmental abnormalities, or infection must be ruled out. For instance, in some cases, colonies of the mycoplasma *Ureaplasma urealyticum* may be observed. Attached to the neck of the sperm such colonies cause sperm to swim in tight circles. Treatment with antibiotics may restore normal motility for these men.

Because it is not generally known that infertility is often found in men, when a man is told that his semen is inadequate in some way severe anxiety may be felt. Special supportive health care will be important to this person as he works through the implications of infertility.

PREVENTION

1. See general factors for men and women.
2. See factors for men and the male population at risk.

TABLE 14-4 NORMAL VALUES IN SEMEN ANALYSES

Characteristics	Description	Comments
Color	Opaque.	
pH	7.2–7.8	Sperm movement is inhibited by lower pH levels.
Consistency	Fluid; quickly gels and then liquifies before 20 min.	
Volume	3–6 mL; mean volume: 3.2 mL.	Over 6 mL causes low concentration of sperm at cervical os.
Count	≥20 million to 100 million mL.	Count may depend on frequency of ejaculation.
	>30 million is more frequent.	Allow 48–72 h abstinence before specimen is obtained.
Motility	≥50–60% with good forward progression; evaluated at grade 2+ to 4 is normal.	Graded on a scale of 0–4 measured 2 h after ejaculation.
Morphology (structure)	≥60% normal, oviform.	Higher percentage of tapering forms and spermatids is associated with varicocele.
Viability (Eosin)	≥50%	
Cells (WBC and others)	None to occasional.	Increased WBC indicates infection.
Agglutination	None.	If persistent, *E. coli* infection or sperm antibodies are present.

ASSESSMENT

Health History

1. History of earlier chromosome evaluation.
2. Exposure to environmental poisons or radiation.
3. History of mumps orchitis—episodes of testicular hyperthermia swelling and pain with subsequent areas of testicular atrophy.
4. History of epididymitis or infections causing high body temperatures.
5. Venereal disease.
6. Hypothalamic or pituitary disease resulting in hypogonatotropic state.
7. Thyroid, adrenal, or testicular problems of hormone secretion.
8. Any hernia repair with potential of interferance with blood supply to testes.
9. History of therapy with androgens during puberty to promote growth of testicles or for body growth, any androgen use to improve athletic strength. Androgens may be detrimental to seminiferous epithelium.
10. History of chemotherapy.
11. Current temporary or chronic exposure to heat; short-term causes reversible, long-term causes irreversible damage to seminiferous epithelium.

Physical Assessment

1. Scrotal sac palpated for presence of descended testicles. Unilateral cryptorchidism may cause decreased sperm count.
2. Testicle size:
   a. Normal diameter: 4.7 ± 0.2 cm.
   b. Smaller than usual size is associated with azoospermia, oligospermia.
3. Presence of varicocele—incidence is 15% in the general population and much higher in populations attending infertility clinics.
   a. Left unilateral is most common.
   b. Large: scrotal mass visible, palpable.
   c. Moderate: dilated tortuous vein that enlarges with Valsalva maneuver.
   d. Small: single convoluted supratesticular vein.
4. External genitalia assessed for structural defects.

Diagnostic Tests

1. Semen analysis (Table 14-4)
   a. Collect three samples at 2- to 3-week intervals, each obtained after 48–72 h abstinence.
   b. Collect specimens in glass jar by means of ejaculation after masturbation. Do not use condom.
   c. May need split ejaculate; place first one-third in first jar, remainder in second, to evaluate sperm count and motility in first portion. Split ejaculate is used in AIH, and is the basis of using withdrawal as a technique to place the most sperm-rich portion in contact with the cervix.
2. Urinalysis—sperm in urine may indicate retrograde ejaculation.
3. Postcoital test of cervical mucus for evaluation of cervical mucus—sperm interaction. If 21 or more sperm per high-powered field, correlated with sperm count over 20 million.
4. Microscopic evaluation of motility and morphology.
5. Testicular biopsy—azoospermia with normal spermatogenesis indicates obstruction of the duct.
6. Serum levels of:
   a. TSH—sensitive test for primary hypothyroidism.
   b. LH, FSH levels.
   c. Testosterone.
   d. Prolactin—if elevated, evaluation for presence of pituitary tumor.
7. X-ray—with contrast material to evaluate patency of vas deferens.

NURSING DIAGNOSES: ACTUAL OR POTENTIAL

1. Altered reproductive function as evidenced by findings of semen analysis.
2. Altered self-esteem associated with guilt or sexual conflicts about pursuing diagnosis of infertility.
3. Potential for noncompliance due to psychosexual conflicts about pursuing diagnosis of infertility.
4. Potential for disruption of interpersonal relationships with sexual partner due to inadequate understanding of evaluative process.
5. Impotence secondary to being required to have intercourse according to a schedule.

EXPECTED OUTCOMES

1. After treatment there will be adequate numbers and forms of sperm in the semen.
2. Man and woman will understand and coop-

erate with sequence of diagnostic tests and treatments.
3. Potentially infertile man will be able to maintain a sense of control and self-esteem during evaluation.
4. Other goals as stated in general infertility evaluation.

INTERVENTIONS

1. Give thorough explanations of procedures and appropriate timing of coitus. (See *Guide for Partners* later in the chapter.)
   a. Often modification of withdrawal technique may be tried. Early part of ejaculate contains more sperm. There is benefit to a "split ejaculate," depositing first third at opening of cervix and immediately withdrawing penis. Technique reduces sexual pleasure and is therefore often thought of as a "treatment."
   b. Note timing suggestions when woman is being treated with Clomid or hMG (Table 14-3).
2. With partners, evaluate if sexual techniques or health practices have been inadequate or inhibiting of best sperm production or deposit near cervix.
3. Counseling about impotence or psychogenic factors may need more extensive work and referral to therapist.
4. Explain medication or surgical procedures when there is an obstruction—varicocele. (See Reproductive System, Chapter 34.)
5. If infection is identified, antibiotic treatment will be ordered:
   a. Gonorrhea—Ampicillin and probenecid.
   b. *Ureaplasma urealyticum*—Vibramycin (doxycyline) (Moghissi and Wallach, 1983).
6. When count and structure are normal but motility is poor some physicians order:
   a. Low-dose androgen therapy.
   b. hCG biweekly for 10 weeks or weekly, which may result in improved motility within 3 months. Many clients note improved libido with this treatment.
7. When there is reduced sperm count, 25 mg Clomiphene for 25 days PO may be ordered.

EVALUATION

Outcome Criteria

1. Reproductive function is restored and semen analyses are within normal limits.
2. Client and partner maintain a sense of adequate control and self-esteem during the process of evaluation.

Complications

IMMUNOLOGIC INFERTILITY

Assessment

When a couple has persistent infertility after passing all the first-level assessment of hormonal and sperm criteria for fertility, they will be evaluated for immunologic infertility, which is thought to be present in up to 40 percent of these refractory cases. There are many antigens in semen, and sperm have antigens in the acrosome (head), midpiece, and tail. Men may produce autoantibodies against any of the seminal components and sperm may be coated with antibodies and be agglutinated before reaching the cervix. In certain instances, when a vasectomy has been done, immunologic factors may have developed to the level of preventing fertility when the man seeks to have the vasectomy reversed. Sperm are still produced in the presence of a vasectomy and must be reabsorbed. In that process autoantibodies may be developed.

The cervix is a site of local immunologic activity that may prevent sperm penetration of mucus. Antibodies may occur only in the cervical mucus or may be present in the female serum and mucus (Moghissi and Wallace, 1983). There is some thought that nonvaginal routes of coitus may increase the development of serologic antibody formation. This area of analysis is still incomplete, and many ongoing studies may shed light on immunologic causes of infertility.

Revised Outcomes

1. Positive tests for agglutinating antibodies will be negative after treatment.
2. If no response, couples will accept alternate means such as artificial insemination in their attempt at parenthood.

Interventions

1. Separation of sperm from cervical mucus for up to 12 months by means of careful use of a condom may allow woman's antibody titer to diminish, in some cases.
2. Couple should avoid anal or oral coitus.
3. Some physicians use immunosuppressants for women, but this is not universal.
4. "Washed" spermatozoa from husband may be used for insemination into cervical canal,

avoiding vaginal and cervical mucus. Sperm are put through a process with a physiologic buffer.

Reevaluation and Follow-up

1. The process of evaluation and testing is time consuming and frustrating. Many couples become discouraged at this point.
2. Some couples may have to accept incompatibility causing infertility.
3. If unsuccessful, couple should be encouraged to begin considering AID, donor insemination.

THE FUTURE IN INFERTILITY

There have been many new developments in the last few years that indicate a better outcome for infertile couples. Micro-surgery for tubal repair, developments in immunologic treatments, laser laparoscopy to remove adhesions and plaques of endometriosis are all becoming possible. Artificial insemination (AI) particularly, either with husband-donated sperm (AIH) or with donor sperm (AID) is a well-established method circumventing low fertility. In vitro fertilization with embryo transfer (IVF/ET) is the newest area becoming affordable to couples who have gone the route of all other treatments. Through all the evaluations and treatments, the psychological cost continues to be high as couples deal with an area that often results in low self-esteem and marital stress. Nurses participate in this highly technological area of assessment and treatment by providing counseling, education, support, and follow-up for these families.

ARTIFICIAL INSEMINATION

1. Semen used for insemination may be fresh or frozen, preferably fresh.
   a. Frozen semen is mixed with a cryopreservative and stored at -80 to -196.5°C in a liquid nitrogen tank.
   b. Before insemination, frozen semen is thawed for approximately 30 min and sperm are checked for count and motility.
2. Fresh semen is collected by masturbation into a sterile glass container.
3. Methods of artificial insemination:
   a. Cervicovaginal or intracervical: Approximately 0.5 mL of semen is slowly injected into the cervical canal under direct vision. The remainder is allowed to spill onto the cervix and vaginal vault.
   b. Intravaginal: The entire semen specimen is injected into the vaginal vault.
   c. Cap technique: Semen is placed in a plastic cap that is fitted over the cervix and left in position for at least 8 h.
   d. Intrauterine: Approximately 0.1 mL of semen is introduced directly into the uterus. This method is generally reserved for instances when the cervix must be bypassed.
4. AI is carefully timed to coincide with ovulation as indicated by BBT and spinnbarkeit. If the menstrual cycle is significantly irregular, ovulation may be drug-induced and ultrasonic measure of graafian follicle may be used.
5. Two or three inseminations are often done per cycle, usually over a period of time not longer than 12 months.
6. Ninety percent of women who will become pregnant via AI do so within 6 months, the rest within 12 months.
7. AI practices should be held carefully confidential, and the professional staff should take precautions to ensure confidentiality.
8. The couple is advised not to discuss AI with family and friends.
9. Also, it must be noted that artificial insemination is morally unacceptable to many people.
10. The infertility examination, specifically the semen analysis, determines whether *homologous* or *heterologous* insemination is indicated.
    a. Artificial insemination via husband (AIH)—homologous insemination.
    (1) AIH may be recommended in cases where normal coitus is not possible, as with severe vaginismus, vaginal narrowing, marked obesity of partner(s), deformities produced by injury or accident, hypospadius, premature or retrograde ejaculation, impotence, or union of long vagina and short penis.

(2) AIH is indicated if the sperm count is adequate but the volume of ejaculate is low.

(3) If the sperm count is low normal, but the volume of ejaculate is adequate, AIH is performed for several cycles before considering AID.

b. Artificial insemination via donor (AID)—heterologous insemination.

(1) AID is recommended to couples with infertility secondary to azoospermia or after unsuccessful AIH with oligospermia; to couples in which the male is a carrier of a serious hereditary disease; and to couples with Rh immunologic incompatibility.

(2) Potential donors must be carefully screened and tested with particular attention to inheritable traits, medication and drug habits, blood type and Rh factor, relevant infections, and semen analysis.

(3) Ethnic background and physical characteristics are matched to those of the husband as closely as possible.

(4) The same donor is used, whenever possible, until pregnancy occurs.

(5) The donor and recipient remain anonymous to each other.

(6) There are approximately 10,000 AID children born each year in the United States.

(7) Some believed advantages of AID over adoption for the infertile family include: the full experience of parenthood, a normal pregnancy, a more private process with less people aware, elimination of the fear that the natural parents might reclaim the child, and donor matching with improved chances that the child will resemble the parents.

(8) The infertile couple must sign a contract indicating that they understand the procedure and its goal and that any resulting offspring are legitimate legal heirs.

(9) Successful couples should be referred elsewhere for obstetric care to avoid conflict of interest and legal problems (such as perjury with regard to legitimacy in signing the birth certificate).

IN VITRO FERTILIZATION AND EMBRYO TRANSFER

1. Mature ova are removed from the graafian follicle and fertilized in a culture medium:
   a. With fresh or frozen husband-donated sperm.
   b. With fresh or frozen donor sperm.
2. Embryo is transferred to woman's uterus 40–44 h after sperm contact in culture medium.
3. In vitro fertilization (IVF) and embryo transfer (ET) are chosen when all other methods are unsuccessful. It is costly and may require repeated tries. There is a low success rate (overall 15 to 20 percent) (Garner, 1983).
4. Usually a protocol is worked out that includes:
   a. Screening laparoscopy.
   b. Stimulated cycle with ovulation induction by clomiphene or hMG.
   c. Exact timing of ovulation may be obtained by GnRH or hCG.
   d. Ultrasound monitoring of graafian follicles, plus estrogen and LH levels indicate time of ovulation.
   e. Aspiration of ovum from the follicle using laparoscope.
   f. There is better success if there is multiple ovulation and recovery of several ova.
5. Couples need intensive support during the period of waiting and embryo transfer.
6. Grief reactions may occur if IVF/ET fails, as it is usually done as the last resort for those whose tubal transport has failed (Garner, 1983).

GUIDE FOR PARTNERS

Many times lack of information on the part of the couple may be the reason for delayed fertility. Health professionals can assist by providing education, referring to special organizations, or suggesting readings that will inform and reduce anxious feelings.

Couples should realize that the cost for an infertility workup may be between $500 and $1500 to begin with and up to $6000 for an in vitro fertilization. Thus, if misinformation has been one reason for infertility, education may reduce costs for the couple. General helpful points are listed below.

1. The average couple takes 6 to 9 months of unprotected intercourse to achieve pregnancy.
2. Women who ovulate regularly do so 14 days ±2 before the *next* menstrual period. Distinctive changes in the woman's early morning temperature (BBT) will indicate that ovulation has probably happened.
3. This BBT chart will be very important to the evaluation and must be kept strictly while going through the evaluation.
4. The woman may be asked to keep a record of distinctive changes in the cervical mucus. This, clear, abundant mucus precedes the day of ovulation and provides a transport medium for the sperm. If these changes do not occur, the physician will evaluate hormonal levels.
5. The normal fertile man needs 30–40 h to return to his usual sperm production levels after an ejaculation. A man with low sperm count may need as long as 48 h.
6. With a typical menstrual cycle of 28 days (remember, there are many variations in cycle length), intercourse should occur in the following pattern when a woman is trying to conceive:
   a. Nights 9 and 12,
   b. Morning 14,
   c. Night 15, and
   d. No times in between.

   This schedule allows the pituitary gland to stimulate sperm production and provides time for return to sperm production at peak levels. It also maintains active sperm in the female reproductive tract.
7. Intercourse should occur three to four times per week during the month to stimulate sperm production.
8. Positions are important. The superior (man above) position is best for intercourse aimed at fertility. The woman's hips should be elevated on a small pillow to facilitate sperm collection (the seminal pool) near the opening of the cervix.
9. At penetration time, the deepest penetration is advised. The woman may fold her knees on her chest and spread them as far apart as possible.
10. At ejaculation, the man should penetrate as deeply as possible and stop thrusting so that ejaculation occurs as near the cervix as possible. Withdrawal should occur just after ejaculation.
11. When female orgasm occurs during or after ejaculation, the cervix is allowed to dip into the seminal pool.
12. The woman should remain in bed for 1 h after ejaculation to hold the seminal pool near the cervix.
13. No artificial lubricants should be used. Saliva, egg white, or olive oil are physiologic and will not hinder sperm mobility.
14. No douching should be used before or after.
15. Remember, because intercourse on "demand" or on a "medical schedule" may seem artificial, care should be taken that technique and timing do not destroy an atmosphere of making love. Some men experience temporary impotence. Talking this over with the fertility nurse or physician may lessen tension and promote appropriate function.

GROUPS THAT CAN HELP

American Fertility Society
1801 Ninth Avenue South
Birmingham, Ala. 35205

RESOLVE, Inc.
PO Box 474
Belmont, Mass. 02178

BOOKS FOR COUPLES WHO WANT TO BE PARENTS

Deckee, A., and Loebl, S.: *Why Can't We Have A Baby?* Warner, New York, 1978. A paperback that answers questions and provides information about infertility.

Kaufman, S. A.: *You Can Have A Baby*, Bantam, New York, 1978. A paperback that provides a positive approach to infertility treatment.

Menning, B. E.: *Infertility: A Guide for the Childless Couple*, Prentice-Hall, Englewood Cliffs, N.J. 1977. A paperback written by the person who started the Resolve Groups. This book has heavy emphasis on emotional support for couples and is excellent.

REFERENCES

Amelar, R. D., Dubin, L., and Schoenfeld, C.: "Sperm Motility," in E. E. Wallach and R. D. Kempers (eds.), *Modern Trends in Fertility*, vol. II, Harper & Row, Philadelphia, 1982.

Garner, C. H.: "*In Vitro* Fertilization and Embryo Transfer," *Journal of Obstetric, Gynecologic, and Neonatal Nursing*, **12**(2):75, March/April 1983.

Moghissi, K. S., and Wallach, E. E.: "Unexplained Infertility," *Fertility and Sterility*, **39**(1):5–19, January 1983.

Speroff, L., Glass, R. H., and Kase, N. G.: *Clinical Gynecologic Endocrinology and Infertility*, 2nd ed., Williams & Wilkins, Baltimore, 1978.

BIBLIOGRAPHY

Amelar, R. D., Dubin, L., and Schoenfeld, C.: "Sperm Motility" in E. E. Wallach and R. D. Kempers (eds.), *Modern Trends in Infertility*, vol. II, Harper & Row, Philadelphia, 1982.

Garner, C. H.: "*In Vitro* Fertilization and Embryo Transfer," *Journal of Obstetric, Gynecologic, and Neonatal Nursing*, **12**(2):75, March/April 1983.

Kapstrom, A. B.: "Does the Career Woman Face Infertility?" *Supervisor Nurse*, July 1981, pp. 54–60. Interesting article about delaying childbearing. Explores all possible areas.

Kistner, R. W.: "Endometriosis and Infertility," *Clinical Obstetrics and Gynecology*, **22**(1):101, March 1979. Good overview of latest information and treatment of endometrosis.

McCormick, T. M.: "Out of Control: One Aspect of Infertility," *Journal of Obstetric, Gynecologic, and Neonatal Nursing*, **9**(4):205–206, July/August, 1980. Good overview and reminder that clients feel out of control when infertile. Article suggests nursing assistance.

Menning, B. E.: "The Psychosocial Impact of Infertility," *Nursing Clinics of North America*, **17**(1):155–163, March 1982. An overview article of the psychosocial needs of the infertile couple. Well done.

Moghissi, K. S.: "Basic Work-Up and Evaluation of Infertile Couples," *Clinical Obstetrics and Gynecology*, **22**(1):11–25, March 1979. Good overview article of the basic workup for infertile couples.

Moghissi, K. S., and Wallace, E. E.: "Unexplained Infertility," *Fertility and Sterility*, **39**(1):5–19, January 1983. Review of methods to use in evaluation of the couple who have not conceived after usual treatment.

Rutledge, A. L.: "Psychomarital Evaluation and Treatment of the Infertile Couple," *Clinical Obstetrics and Gynecology*, **22**(1):255–267, March 1979. Excellent article on treating the marital and psychologic well-being of infertile couples.

Silber, S. J.: *How to Get Pregnant*, Scribner, New York, 1980. Popular, *excellent* book for professionals and lay persons with good solid information.

Wallach, E. E.: "Evaluation and Management of Uterine Causes of Infertility," *Clinical Obstetrics and Gynecology*, **22**(1):43–59, March 1979. Good update article on uterine causes of infertility and treatment.

Wallach, E. E., and Kemper, R. D.: *Modern Trends in Infertility and Conception Control*, vol. I, William & Wilkins, Baltimore, 1979. Each volume contains 36 review articles from *Fertility and Sterility*. They cover the current clinical developments in infertility, reproductive endocrinology, and conception control.

Wallach, E. E., and Kemper, R. D.: *Modern Trends in Infertility and Conception Control*, vol. II, Harper & Row, Philadelphia, 1982. Each volume contains 36 review articles from *Fertility and Sterility*. They cover the most current clinical developments in infertility, reproductive endocrinology, and conception control.

THE NURSING CARE OF CHILDREN AND ADOLESCENTS

PART III

PART III CONTENTS

CHAPTER 15
THE NERVOUS SYSTEM 311

Abnormal Cellular Growth 311
Spina bifida occulta and spina bifida cystica 311
Hydrocephalus 316
Arnold-Chiari malformation 318
Encephalocele 319
Microcephaly 319
Craniosynostosis 319
Arteriovenous malformations 319
Intracranial tumors: cerebellar astrocytoma, medulloblastoma, ependymoma, brainstem glioma, and craniopharyngioma 320
Extracranial tumors: neuroblastoma and intraspinal tumors 324

Hyperactivity and Hypoactivity 325
Seizures: febrile convulsions; epilepsy (grand mal, petit mal, psychomotor, and focal seizures); infantile spasms 325

Trauma 328
Concussions, contusions, lacerations, skull fractures, and hematomas 328
Spinal cord injury 331

Inflammations 331
Meningitis 331
Encephalitis 333
Reye's syndrome 334

Metabolic Disorders 334
Lead poisoning 334
Phenylketonuria 336
Maple syrup disease 336
Tay-Sachs disease 336

Developmental Disorders 336
Mental retardation 336
Cerebral palsy 338
Minimal brain dysfunction 339
Hearing impairment 340
Visual impairment 341

CHAPTER 16
THE MUSCULOSKELETAL SYSTEM 345

Abnormal Cellular Growth 345
Torticollis 345
Clubfoot (talipes equinovarus) 346
Congenital dislocation of the hip 348
Osteogenesis imperfecta (brittle bone disease) 350
Osteogenic sarcoma and Ewing's sarcoma 352

Inflammations 355
Osteomyelitis and septic arthritis 355
Juvenile rheumatoid arthritis 357

Hyperactivity and Hypoactivity 359
Legg-Perthes disease 359
Structural scoliosis 361

Degenerative Diseases 364
Duchenne's muscular dystrophy 364

Traumatic Injuries 366
Epiphyseal plate fracture 366
Slipped upper femoral epiphysis 368

CHAPTER 17
THE ENDOCRINE SYSTEM 371

Hyperactivity and Hypoactivity (Anterior Pituitary Gland) 371
Gigantism 373
Giantism 374
Precocious puberty 375
Dwarfism 377
Addison's disease, Sheehan's syndrome, and Simmonds' disease 379
Gonadotropin deficiency 380

Hyperactivity and Hypoactivity (Posterior Pituitary Gland) 381
Diabetes insipidus 382

Hyperactivity and Hypoactivity (Thyroid Gland) 383
Graves' disease 384
Cretinism 384
Acquired hypothyroidism 386

PART III CONTENTS (*continued*)

Hyperactivity and Hypoactivity (Adrenal Glands) **387**
Cushing's disease 387
Cushing's syndrome 388
Addison's disease 388
Adrenogenital syndrome or adrenocortical hyperplasia 388

Hyperactivity and Hypoactivity (Pancreas) **391**
Hypoglycemia 392
Diabetes mellitus 392

Hyperactivity and Hypoactivity (Chromosomal Aberrations Affecting Gonadal Hormones) **399**
Turner's syndrome 399
Klinefelter's syndrome 401

CHAPTER 18
THE HEMATOLOGIC SYSTEM 405

Hyperactivity and Hypoactivity **405**
Aplastic anemia 405
Fanconi's anemia 411
Acquired hemolytic anemia 412
Polycythemia of cyanotic heart disease 413
Diamond-Blackfan syndrome 414
Megaloblastic nutritional anemias (vitamin B_{12} and folic acid deficiency anemias) 415
Iron deficiency anemia 417
Glucose 6-phosphate deficiency (G6PD) 419
Neutropenia 420
Disorders of phagocytosis (chronic granulomatous disease and Chédiak-Higashi syndrome) 424
Thrombocytopenia (idiopathic and acquired) 425
Immune thrombocytopenia 427
Wiskott-Aldrich syndrome 428
Hemophilia 429
Von Willebrand's disease 433
Immunoglobulin deficiency 434

Abnormal Cellular Growth **435**
Sickle cell anemia (hemoglobin SS disease) 435
Sickle cell trait (hemoglobin AS disease) 439
Additional hemoglobinopathies (hemoglobin SF disease, hemoglobin CC disease, hemoglobin SC disease) 439
Beta-thalassemia major (Cooley's anemia, Mediterranean anemia) 440
Hereditary spherocytosis (chronic familial jaundice) 442
Hereditary elliptocytosis (hereditary ovalocytosis) 444
Leukemia 444
Histiocytosis 454

Inflammations **455**
Henoch-Schönlein purpura (anaphylactoid purpura) 455

Metabolic Disorders **456**
Storage diseases (Niemann-Pick disease and Gaucher's disease) 456

CHAPTER 19
THE CARDIOVASCULAR SYSTEM 459

Hyperactivity and Hypoactivity **459**
Congestive heart failure 459

Abnormal Cellular Growth: Care of the Child Requiring Cardiovascular Surgery **466**
Closed-heart surgery 466
Open-heart surgery 470

Abnormal Cellular Growth: Congenital Heart Defects **472**
Patent ductus arteriosus 472
Aorticopulmonary window 475
Coarctation of the aorta 475
Congenital aortic stenosis 479
Vascular rings 481
Atrial septal defect 482
Ventricular septal defect 484

PART III CONTENTS (*continued*)

Endocardial cushion defects 486
Tetralogy of Fallot 489
Pulmonary valvular stenosis and atresia 493
Tricuspid atresia 494
Transposition of the great vessels 495
Truncus arteriosus 500
Total anomalous pulmonary venous return or connection 501
Hypoplastic left-heart syndrome 502

Inflammations **502**
Rheumatic heart disease 502

CHAPTER 20
THE RESPIRATORY SYSTEM 505

Abnormal Cellular Growth **505**
Diaphragmatic hernia 505
Laryngotracheal malacia 510

Obstructions **511**
Foreign body aspiration 511
Foreign body in the ear 513
Bronchiolitis 514
Croup 516
Epiglottitis 518
Bronchial asthma 519
Cystic fibrosis 524

Inflammations **527**
Bronchopulmonary dysplasia 527
Bronchopneumonia 529
Chemical pneumonia 530
Tonsillitis 531
Otitis media 533

CHAPTER 21
THE URINARY SYSTEM 537

Abnormal Cellular Growth **537**
Polycystic disease 537
Vesicoureteral reflux 541
Exstrophy of the urinary bladder 543
Posterior urethral valves 544
Hypospadias and epispadias 546
Undescended testicles (cryptorchidism) 547
Wilms' tumor (nephroblastoma) 548
Benign tumors 550

Inflammations **550**
Urinary tract infection 550
Acute poststreptococcal glomerulonephritis (nephritis, nephritic syndrome) 551
Nephrotic syndrome (nephrosis) 553

Obstructions **554**
Neuropathic (neurogenic) bladder 554
Renal vein thrombosis 556
Renal artery thrombosis 558

Traumatic Injuries **558**
Renal injury 558

Hyperactivity and Hypoactivity **558**
Acute renal failure 558
Chronic renal failure 560

Metabolic Disorders **564**
Renal tubular acidosis 564

CHAPTER 22
THE GASTROINTESTINAL SYSTEM 567

Obstructions **567**
Pyloric stenosis 567
Malrotation and volvulus 569
Intussusception 570
Meckel's diverticulum 572
Inguinal hernia 573
Umbilical hernia 575

Inflammations **575**
Necrotizing enterocolitis 575
Appendicitis 577
Gastroenteritis 577

Trauma **578**
Ingestion of corrosive substance 578

Abnormal Cellular Growth **580**
Cleft lip and palate 580

PART III CONTENTS *(continued)*

Esophageal atresia and tracheoesophageal fistula 581
Omphalocele and gastroschisis 585
Hirschsprung's disease (congenital aganglionic megacolon) 587
Imperforate anus 589

Metabolic Disorders **591**
Cystic fibrosis 591
Celiac disease 591

Other Gastrointestinal Disorders **593**
Dental caries 593

CHAPTER 23
THE INTEGUMENTARY SYSTEM 597

Abnormal Cellular Growth **597**
Vascular nevi (birthmarks) 597
Pigmented nevi (mongolian spots) 599

Inflammations **600**
Diaper dermatitis 600
Urticaria (hives) 601
Poison ivy and poison oak 602
Eczema (atopic dermatitis) 604
Seborrhea 606
Miliaria rubra (prickly heat) 607
Acne 607

Infectious Dermatitis **609**
Candidiasis (moniliasis) 609
Impetigo pyoderma 610
Herpes simplex type 1 612
Herpes zoster (shingles) 613
Slapped cheek syndrome (fifth disease, erythema infectiosum) 613
Pityriasis rosea 613
Tinea capitis (ringworm of the scalp) 614
Tinea corporis (tinea circinata, body ringworm) 616
Tinea pedis (athlete's foot) 616
Pediculosis (lice) 617
Scabies ("itch") 618

CHAPTER 24
COMMUNICABLE DISEASES 621

Infections **621**
Diphtheria 621
Tetanus ("lockjaw") 625
Pertussis (whooping cough) 628
Rubeola (measles, "red measles") 630
Rubella (German measles) 632
Mumps 634
Chickenpox (varicella) 636
Poliomyelitis (polio, infantile paralysis) 638
Tuberculosis 641
Gonorrhea 644
Syphilis 646
Cat-scratch disease 648
Rocky Mountain spotted fever 649
Infectious mononucleosis 651
Cytomegalic inclusion disease 652

Parasitic Infestations **654**
Enterobiasis (pinworm disease, oxyuriasis) 654
Hookworm disease 655
Ascariasis 656
Trichuriasis (whipworm infestation) 658

15

The Nervous System

Beverly A. Bowens

ABNORMAL CELLULAR GROWTH

SPINA BIFIDA OCCULTA AND SPINA BIFIDA CYSTICA

DESCRIPTION

Spina bifida occulta is the congenital failure of closure of the vertebral column without protrusion or displacement of intraspinal contents. This defect is found in 25 percent of hospitalized children and in 10 percent of the general pediatric population. It most frequently involves the posterior arches of the fifth lumbar and first sacral vertebrae. Spina bifida occulta is generally asymptomatic and discovered accidentally on routine spinal films. The appearance of dimples, tufts of hair, and small fatty masses along the spinal column may be indicative of this defect. Sphincter control may be difficult.

Spina bifida cystica is a far more serious defect in which the inadequately closed vertebral column is accompanied by displacement of intraspinal contents into a saclike structure on the exterior surface of the spine (Figure 15-1). The incidence is estimated to be 0.2 to 4.2 per 1,000 live births. These defects are of two types—meningoceles and myelomeningoceles. The meningocele, accounting for 25 percent of the cystic type, contains spinal fluid and meninges in the saclike mass. The myelomeningocele, making up the remaining 75 percent, contains these elements plus neural tissue. These defects may be covered by a very thin membrane, by meninges, by dura, or by normal skin. Approximately 80 percent of myelomeningoceles are located in the lumbar and lumbosacral regions.

About three-fourths of the infants with myelomeningocele also have hydrocephalus. Early surgery to correct the spinal defect and the hydrocephalus in these infants results in a survival rate of approximately 65 percent. Ninety percent of these newborns have associated malformations and infections of the urinary tract.

The treatment of children born with myelomeningocele continues to be hotly debated in the neurosurgical community. Management protocols vary from one extreme to the other, with some physicians recommending surgical intervention for *every* child and others advocating that *none* of these defects be surgically repaired. Of course, the opinions of most physicians are somewhere between these two extremes. The quality of life for the children who survive has been a large part of the debate, since many of them are left with significant mental retardation and neurological defects, including paraplegia. Many have locomotor problems due to associated musculoskeletal anomalies, such as clubfoot, dislocated hips, contractures, and scoliosis. Special education is eventually required for many of these children, and personality and disciplinary problems are common. These facts provide some insight into the impact of the birth of such a child on the family, the health care system, and society as a whole.

PREVENTION

Health Promotion

No preventive measures are known.

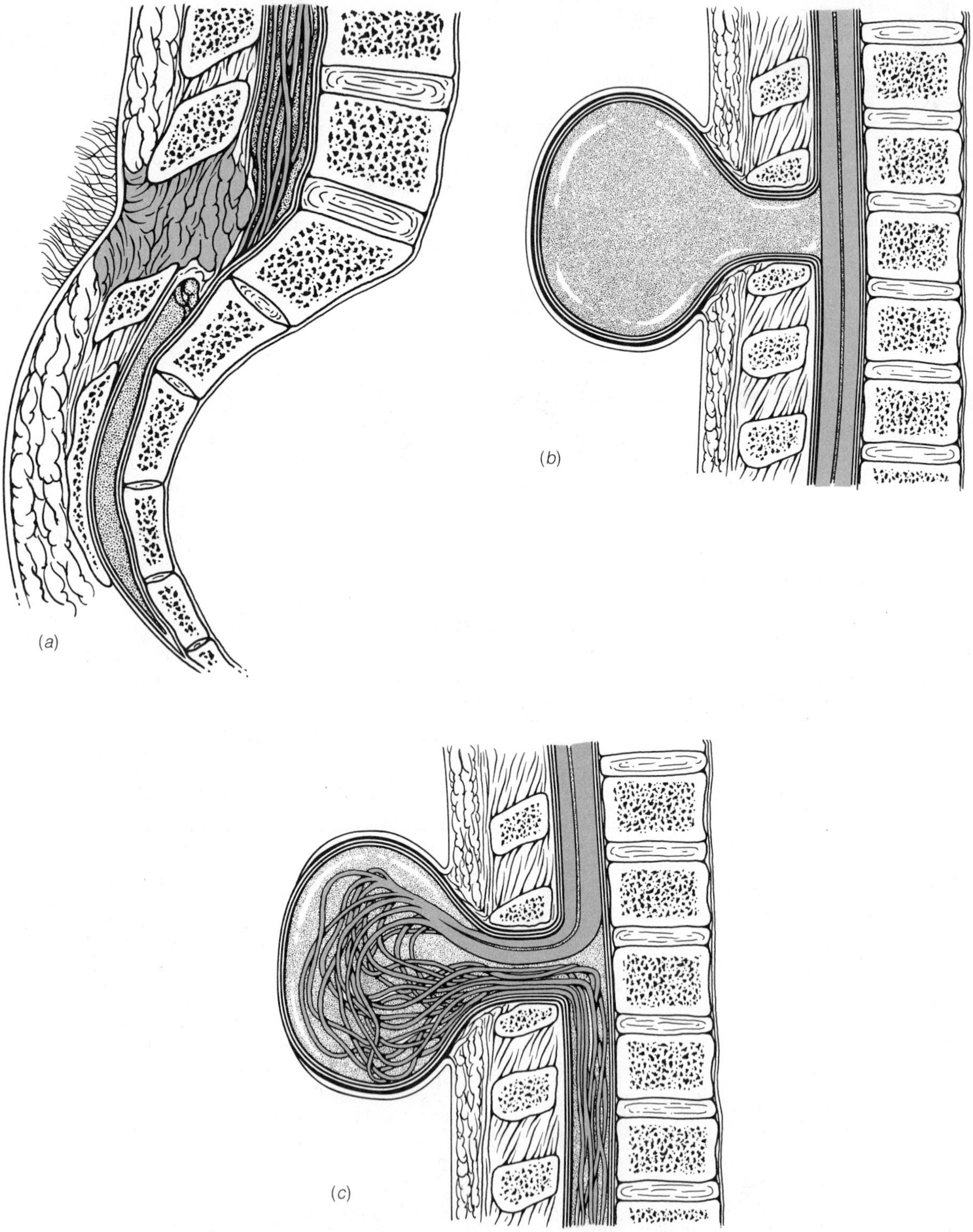

(*b*)

(*a*)

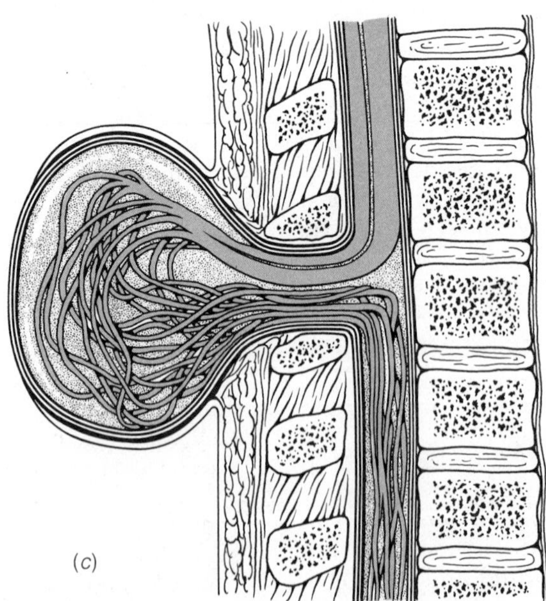

Figure 15-1 Congenital malformations of the spine: (*a*) spina bifida occulta, (*b*) meningocele, (*c*) myelomeningocele.

Population at Risk
Neonates.

Screening
Physical examination.

ASSESSMENT

Health History

1. Symptoms of increased intracranial pressure (hydrocephalus is often an associated finding): increasing lethargy, seizures, anorexia and weight loss, vomiting, headaches, and irritability.
2. Delay in toilet training.
3. Frequent urinary tract infections.
4. Delay in walking.

Physical Assessment

1. Flaccid or spastic lower extremities.
2. Defects in spinous processes.
3. Dimples, tufts of hair, fatty masses, or a cystic mass along the spinal column.
4. Curvature of the spine.
5. Constant dribbling of urine.
6. Flaccid anal sphincter.
7. Signs of increased intracranial pressure (increasing head circumference; tense, bulging fontanels; separated suture lines; increased resonance on percussion; delayed developmental milestones).
8. Clubfoot.

Diagnostic Tests

1. Spine and skull x-ray films.
2. Computerized axial tomography (CAT scan) (see *Hydrocephalus*).
3. Pneumoencephalogram (see *Hydrocephalus*).

NURSING DIAGNOSES: ACTUAL OR POTENTIAL

1. Loss of skin integrity associated with rupture of the sac secondary to trauma.
2. Risk of infection secondary to loss of skin integrity.
3. Altered level of consciousness secondary to increased intracranial pressure.
4. Parents' knowledge deficit regarding the defect, diagnostic tests, and pre- and postoperative routines.
5. Parental anxiety regarding the surgical outcome.
6. Ineffective family coping secondary to the birth of a defective child and extreme expense of child's therapy.
7. Alteration in nutritional status secondary to vomiting and anorexia.
8. Fluid and electrolyte imbalances secondary to vomiting.
9. Impairment of mobility secondary to paralysis of lower extremities.
10. Alteration in bowel elimination secondary to impaired neurological functioning.
11. Alteration in urinary elimination secondary to impaired neurological functioning.
12. Impairment of skin integrity secondary to incontinence and limited movement.
13. Delayed development.

EXPECTED OUTCOMES

1. Sac will remain intact.
2. Central nervous system infection will not occur.
3. The child will have adequate neurological functioning (within the limits imposed by the defect) as evidenced by
   a. Being awake and alert.
   b. Vital signs within normal limits for age.
   c. Absence of seizures.
   d. Maintenance of baseline neurological functioning.
4. Parents will be able to describe the anatomy and physiology of the defect and be able to state specifics of diagnostic tests and pre- and postoperative routines.
5. Parental anxiety will be within expected, tolerable limits.
6. The family will be able to maintain their decision-making ability regarding the child and the child's care and will cope with the financial burdens.
7. The family will maintain intrafamily communication.
8. The child will ingest and retain nutrients and fluids sufficient to maintain current weight and gain at an expected rate.
9. The child's lower extremities will be free of contractures.
10. The child will have regular bowel movements and will be clean at all times.
11. The child will have adequate urinary functioning as evidenced by
    a. Absence of urinary tract infections.
    b. Clear urine free of foul odor.
    c. Output compatible with intake.
    d. Serum electrolyte values within normal limits.

12. The child will be free of skin breakdown.
13. The child will demonstrate optimal development within limits of disability.

INTERVENTIONS

1. Position child on abdomen. Bradford frame can be used if available.
2. Protect defect from contamination by feces or urine (see Figure 15-2).
3. Assess vital signs, pupils, and level of consciousness every 4 hours, or as ordered.
4. Assess fontanels for fullness and measure head circumference daily.
5. Monitor fluid intake carefully—generally, the child is kept mildly dehydrated in order to decrease intracranial pressure.
6. Assess parents' current knowledge level and readiness to learn.
7. Teach basic information through the use of charts, books, pictures, and other written material at parents' level of understanding.
8. Give information about hospital routines, how child will look and behave after surgery, and the parents' role.
9. Provide time for questions.
10. Allow the family to grieve.
11. Provide time and quiet place for the parents to talk about the child's condition with the nurse and/or other health team members.
12. Be honest in responding to questions.
13. When the parents visit the child, remain nearby to answer questions and provide emotional support.
14. Involve parents in the care to the extent that they are able—physically and emotionally—to participate.
15. Provide verbal and written information about available financial assistance.
16. Refer family to state crippled children's agency and to social worker.
17. Feed child slowly and allow frequent rest periods.
18. "Bubble" baby during and after feeding.
19. Teach parents effective methods of feeding baby.
20. Assess electrolyte values as laboratory reports become available.
21. Weigh child daily.
22. Give passive range-of-motion exercises to lower extremities every 8 hours or more frequently.

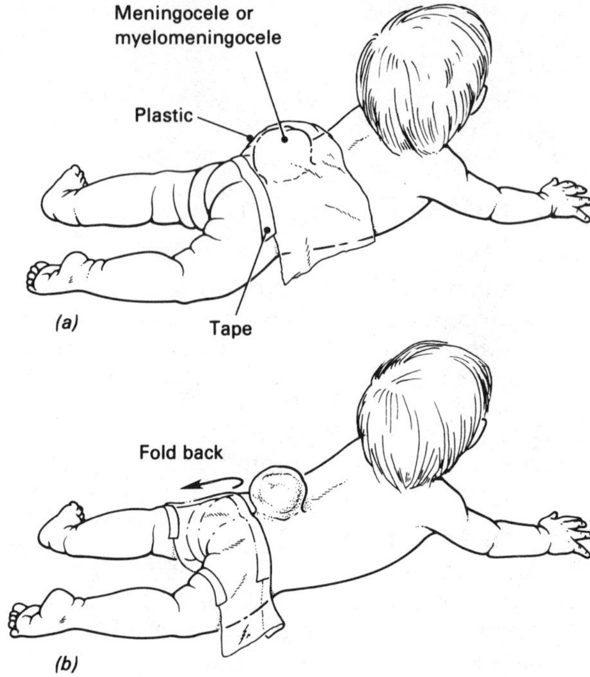

Figure 15-2 Application of plastic wrap to protect spinal defect from contamination by urine and feces. (*a*) Plastic wrap (ordinary kitchen variety) is taped to skin. (*b*) Plastic wrap is folded back over the tape applied in (*a*) and secured to the thighs.

23. Release restraints on upper extremities and exercise at least once during every shift.
24. Teach bowel training regimen once child is old enough for toilet training.
    a. Check rectum for impaction every other day.
    b. Insert a suppository against the wall of the rectum every other day at the same time each day.
    c. Give a stool softener, if indicated.
    d. Provide dietary instruction regarding bulk, avoidance of foods likely to cause diarrhea, importance of fruits and vegetables, and so forth.
25. Encourage drinking of juices that acidify the urine (e.g., grape, apple, cranberry).
26. Teach bladder training techniques when child is old enough for toilet training.
27. Teach use of external urinary collection device for boys.

28. Teach signs and symptoms of urinary tract infection.
29. Teach importance of keeping child clean and dry to protect skin and discourage infection.
30. Teach self-catheterization when child is old enough.
31. Teach family to provide frequent skin care with particular attention to pressure points: knees, toes, ankles, elbows, and ears.
32. Apply petroleum jelly to perineal area.
33. Keep linens clean, dry, and wrinkle-free.
34. Encourage parents to cuddle, stroke, and talk to child, even during acute phase of illness.
35. Provide continuity in staff assignment to the extent possible.
36. Provide appropriate toys and bright objects for visual stimulation.
37. Include specifics of developmental stimulation in plan of care.
38. Provide parents with written information about play and developmental stimulation.
39. Surgical intervention is generally indicated in the treatment of myelomeningocele. Specific postoperative nursing interventions are listed below:
    a. Protect dressings from urinary and fecal contamination (see Figure 15-2).
    b. If dressing becomes soiled, change, using strict aseptic technique.
    c. After dressing is removed, keep suture line clean.
    d. Do not use diapers until suture line is completely healed.
    e. Avoid pressure and traction on suture line.
    f. Provide diet high in protein, calories, and vitamins.

EVALUATION

Outcome Criteria

1. Absence of drainage from the sac.
2. Neurological functioning is normal, within limits of disability.
3. Parents verbalize basic facts about the anatomy and physiology of the defect and describe diagnostic tests and pre- and postoperative routines accurately.
4. Parents verbalize their feelings of anxiety.
5. Absence of signs of excessive parental anxiety, such as constant, repetitive questions; crying, depression, and irrational behavior; withdrawal.
6. Parents verbalize feelings of grief.
7. Parents exhibit mood appropriate to stage of grief process.
8. Both parents visit and care for child.
9. Parents show affection toward child.
10. Parents verbalize willingness to take advantage of financial assistance.
11. Parents correctly verbalize methods of obtaining financial assistance.
12. Baby retains formula and gains weight.
13. Electrolyte values remain within normal limits.
14. Parents handle infant in a comfortable manner.
15. Parents verbalize plans for feeding (i.e., formula and solid food).
16. Child's joints are movable through full range of motion.
17. Child exhibits regular bowel movement pattern.
18. Family verbalizes understanding of fecal incontinence and bowel training regimen.
19. Child is free of signs and symptoms of urinary tract infection.
20. Family verbalizes understanding of urinary incontinence.
21. Skin is free of redness, rashes, and breakdown.
22. Parents verbalize understanding of the importance of developmental stimulation.
23. Parents correctly demonstrate techniques taught.
24. Child exhibits development appropriate for age.

Complications

MENINGITIS SECONDARY TO RUPTURE AND CONTAMINATION OF SAC

Assessment

1. Drainage from the sac.
2. Temperature higher than 38.5°C.
3. Irritability, nuchal rigidity, and lethargy.
4. Tense, bulging fontanels.
5. Increasing head circumference.

Revised Outcomes

1. Infection will be promptly and adequately treated.
2. Further infections will not occur.

Interventions

1. Immediately report assessment findings listed above.

2. Administer antibiotics as ordered.
3. Assess fontanels and measure head circumference daily.
4. Assess vital signs and level of consciousness every 4 hours, or as ordered.
5. Use strict aseptic technique when changing bandage.
6. Keep perineal area scrupulously clean at all times.
7. Do not use diapers.
8. Use plastic sheeting, such as ordinary kitchen wrap, to keep urine and feces away from the bandaged area (see Figure 15-2).
9. See *Meningitis*.

POSTOPERATIVE WOUND INFECTION

Assessment

1. Temperature higher than 38.5°C.
2. Drainage from incision.
3. Redness, warmth, and swelling around wound.

Revised Outcomes

Same as for meningitis, immediately above.

Interventions

Same as for meningitis, immediately above.

COMPLICATIONS ASSOCIATED WITH THE TREATMENT OF ACCOMPANYING HYDROCEPHALUS

(See *Hydrocephalus*, below)

DEVELOPMENTAL DELAYS

Reevaluation and Follow-up

Parents verbalize understanding of need for long-term follow-up and willingness to seek this care.

HYDROCEPHALUS

DESCRIPTION

Hydrocephalus is characterized by an increased amount of cerebrospinal fluid and consequent increased intracranial pressure. In young children whose skull sutures have not yet fused, characteristic enlargement of the head is seen. Hydrocephalus is usually classified as either communicating or noncommunicating. In the communicating type, there is unobstructed flow of cerebrospinal fluid (CSF) through the ventricular system. The defect lies along the absorptive surfaces of the brain—the subarachnoid space. The fluid cannot be absorbed due to a thickened arachnoid, most often secondary to meningitis or intracranial hemorrhage. In the noncommunicating type, there is a block to CSF flow within the ventricles. The blockage may be a result of tumor, hematoma formation, or malformation of the ventricular system. Surgery is generally indicated in the treatment of hydrocephalus. If there is a blockage within the ventricles the surgeon will attempt to remove it in hopes of establishing normal CSF flow. Communicating hydrocephalus is treated by the insertion of a shunt (ventriculoatrial or ventriculoperitoneal).

PREVENTION

Health Promotion

This disorder is most often idiopathic, hence specific preventive measures are not known. Other causes include neoplasia and trauma and infection involving the central nervous system. Trauma and infection are often preventable and in all instances should have prompt treatment.

Population at Risk

Neonates and infants primarily; when noncongenital factors are involved (e.g., tumor), anyone may be affected.

Screening

Head circumference measurements at all well-child assessments until at least age 3 years. A child whose head is large or whose head circumference crosses percentile channels on the growth grid requires referral to a physician.

ASSESSMENT

Health History

1. Trauma, with associated intracranial hemorrhage, can predispose to communicating hydrocephalus.
2. History of febrile illness: meningitis is a frequent cause of hydrocephalus.
3. Increasing lethargy.
4. Seizures.
5. Anorexia and weight loss.
6. Vomiting, often a sign of increased intracranial pressure.
7. Headaches.
8. Irritability.

Physical Assessment

1. Primarily directed toward identifying signs of increased pressure.

a. Increasing head circumference or a measurement out of proportion to the chest.
b. Increased resonance on percussion of the skull.
c. Tense, bulging fontanels and separated sutures.
d. "Sunset" eyes (late sign of hydrocephalus): eyes sit low in the palpebral fissure so that the iris is partially hidden by the lower lid, like a setting sun partly hidden by the horizon.
e. Delayed developmental milestones.
f. Decreasing level of consciousness.
g. Disturbances in balance and coordination.
h. Changes in movement and strength of extremities.
i. Dilated scalp veins.
j. Papilledema, if skull sutures have closed.
k. Vital sign changes: these occur late in progression of disease. Look for increased blood pressure, decreased pulse, and changes in respiratory pattern.
l. Unequal, sluggish pupils (late change).

2. Presence of other congenital anomalies. Myelomeningocele (discussed above) is frequently associated with hydrocephalus.

Diagnostic Tests

1. *Skull x-ray films.* Useful in evaluating condition of fontanels and suture lines.
2. *CAT scan.* A radiological procedure that provides photographs of various transverse "slices" of the brain. Useful in demonstrating dilated ventricles.
3. *Subdural taps.* To rule out the presence of chronic subdural hematomas.
4. *Pneumoencephalogram or ventriculogram.* The injection of gases (air or oxygen) into the ventricular system through a lumbar puncture or a ventricular tap; shows changes in ventricular size, shape, and placement.

NURSING DIAGNOSES: ACTUAL OR POTENTIAL

1. Altered levels of consciousness secondary to increased intracranial pressure.
2. Nutritional deficit secondary to vomiting and anorexia.
3. Fluid and electrolyte imbalance secondary to vomiting.
4. Parents' knowledge deficit regarding diagnostic tests and pre- and postoperative routines.
5. Parental anxiety secondary to implications of test results and surgical outcomes.
6. Delayed developmental milestones.
7. Risk of skin breakdown on scalp overlying pumping chamber of surgically implanted shunt valve.

EXPECTED OUTCOMES

1. The child will have adequate neurological functioning as evidenced by
   a. Being awake and alert.
   b. Equal movement and strength of extremities.
   c. Pupils equal and briskly reactive.
   d. Vital signs within normal limits.
   e. Absence of seizures.
2. The child will ingest and retain nutrients and fluids sufficient to maintain or increase current weight.
3. Parents will be able to state specifics of diagnostic tests and pre- and postoperative routines.
4. Parental anxiety will be within expected tolerable limits.
5. The child will exhibit development appropriate for age.
6. Skin will remain intact.

INTERVENTIONS

1. Assess vital signs, pupils, level of consciousness, and movement of extremities every 4 hours, or as ordered.
2. Assess fontanels for fullness, and measure head circumference daily.
3. Elevate head of bed 20–30 degrees.
4. Monitor fluid intake carefully: generally, the child is kept mildly dehydrated in order to decrease intracranial pressure.
5. Insure patent airway: increased level of CO_2 in the blood leads to increased intracranial pressure.
6. Weigh child daily.
7. Investigate food preferences.
8. Offer small, frequent feedings.
9. If child vomits, allow rest period and then feed again.
10. Obtain dietary consultation.
11. Assess current knowledge level and readiness to learn.
12. Provide information about tests. Use pictures, tell what to expect after tests are com-

pleted and when the results will be available.

13. Give information about hospital routines, how child will look after surgery, and the parents' role.
14. Provide time for questions.
15. Encourage parents to cuddle, stroke, and talk to child, even during acute phase of illness.
16. Provide continuity in staff assignment to the extent possible.
17. Provide appropriate toys and bright objects for visual stimulation.
18. Include specifics of developmental stimulation in plan of care.
19. Provide parents with written information about play and developmental stimulation.
20. Protect shunt and overlying skin.
    a. Turn child frequently.
    b. Avoid positioning child directly on shunt site.
    c. Discourage manipulation of pump chamber unless pumping has been ordered by physician.
    d. Provide discharge teaching about signs and symptoms of shunt malfunction.

EVALUATION

Outcome Criteria

1. Neurological functioning is within normal limits: child is awake and alert, moves all extremities with equal strength, has equal and readily reactive pupils, has normal vital signs, and is free of seizures.
2. Child retains foods.
3. Weight is the same as or greater than upon admission.
4. Parents verbalize importance and understanding of developmental stimulation.
5. Parents verbalize pre- and postoperative routines accurately.
6. Parents' anxiety is not excessive for the situation.
7. Parents accurately demonstrate developmental stimulation techniques they have been taught.
8. Child is at developmental level appropriate for age.
9. Scalp is free from pressure sores.
10. Parents accurately describe signs and symptoms of shunt malfunction.
11. Parents accurately demonstrate skills to protect shunt site.

Complications

POSTOPERATIVE INFECTION (WOUND INFECTION OR MENINGITIS)

Assessment

1. Temperature higher than 38.5°C (101°F).
2. Wound red and swollen.
3. Nuchal rigidity, restlessness, irritability, and lethargy.
4. Increasing head circumference.
5. Tense, bulging fontanels.
6. Purulent drainage from suture line.

Revised Outcomes

1. Infection will be promptly and adequately treated.
2. Further infections will not occur.

Interventions

1. Immediately report assessment findings listed above.
2. Administer antibiotics as ordered.
3. Keep bandage clean and dry.
4. Use strict aseptic technique when changing soiled bandage.
5. Assess vital signs and level of consciousness every 4 hours, or as ordered.
6. Assess fontanels and measure head circumference daily.
7. See *Meningitis*.

PARALYTIC ILEUS AFTER VENTRICULOPERITONEAL SHUNT

Assessment

1. Absence of bowel sounds.
2. Vomiting.
3. Abdominal distention.

Reevaluation and Follow-up

1. Family is referred to community health nurse and/or state crippled children's agency.
2. Parents verbalize understanding of need for long-term follow-up care.

ARNOLD-CHIARI MALFORMATION

DESCRIPTION

Arnold-Chiari malformation is frequently associated with obstructive hydrocephalus and spina bifida cystica of the lumbosacral region.

The most common type has (1) malformations at the base of the skull and upper cervical region with hydrocephalus which exerts a downward pressure, and (2) spina bifida cystica which tethers the cord in the lumbosacral region resulting in downward traction. The pons and medulla may be kinked and malpositioned. The only treatment for this condition is surgical. Frequently, a shunting procedure is done to relieve symptoms of increased pressure. The problems and nursing care are the same as for a child with hydrocephalus.

ENCEPHALOCELE

DESCRIPTION

Encephalocele occurs when the bones of the fetal skull fail to unite properly, resulting in protrusion of brain tissue through the defect. Treatment is aimed at protection of the sac until surgical closure of the defect is accomplished. Nursing care is the same as for spina bifida cystica.

MICROCEPHALY

DESCRIPTION

Microcephaly is characterized by a head circumference at least two standard deviations below the mean. There are many causes for this abnormally—genetic, chromosomal, radiation, infectious, or chemical. Maternal infections that have been implicated in the occurrence of microcephaly are toxoplasmosis, cytomegalovirus, and the rubella virus. Nursing care is directed toward the management of mental retardation, which is usually severe, and of seizures or other related problems.

CRANIOSYNOSTOSIS

DESCRIPTION

Craniosynostosis is the premature closure of one or more cranial sutures. This defect interferes with normal skull expansion and thus results in impaired brain growth. Depending on which sutures are closed, there may be various deformities of the skull and face. The incidence is less than five per 10,000 births, and the exact etiology is unknown. The treatment is early surgical opening of the prematurely closed suture. Surgery carries an excellent prognosis for normal appearance and neurological and intellectual function. Nursing care is directed toward early diagnosis and care of the child and family through the surgical episode.

ARTERIOVENOUS MALFORMATIONS

DESCRIPTION

Arteriovenous malformations (AVM) result from a failure of capillary development during embryonic growth, which leads to abnormal veins and dilated, tortuous arteries. Arteriovenous malformations are the most common vascular abnormalities found in children. Symptoms generally develop between the ages of 10 and 30 years, with 10 percent of cases presenting during the first 10 years of life and 45 percent by the end of the third decade. Most often the condition is recognized in association with an intracranial bleed—intraventricular, subarachnoid, intracerebral, or subdural. Other presenting symptoms can include seizures, intractable headaches, and mental deterioration.

The prognosis varies, depending on the location of the malformation. The mortality rate for intracranial hemorrhage in the neonatal period is nearly 100 percent; it drops to 80 percent in infancy and drops further, to about 50 percent, in older children (Swaiman and Wright, 1975). Arteriovenous malformations can be treated by artificial embolization and/or surgical ligation.

Preoperatively, nursing care is directed toward the prevention of a massive intracranial hemorrhage and increased intracranial pressure. Following surgery, the nurse is intensively involved in the management of fluid and electrolyte balance, drug therapy, and maintenance of optimal respiratory function. All of these are, of course, crucial in the control of postoperative cerebral edema. The nurse also plays the primary role in teaching and providing emotional support for the child and the family both pre-

and postoperatively. Long-term follow-up for rehabilitation may be indicated.

INTRACRANIAL TUMORS: CEREBELLAR ASTROCYTOMA, MEDULLOBLASTOMA, EPENDYMOMA, BRAINSTEM GLIOMA, AND CRANIOPHARYNGIOMA

DESCRIPTION

Intracranial tumors are the second most frequently occurring neoplasm in infants and children, preceded only by leukemia. Since 75 percent of all brain tumors in children are gliomas, the chances of finding a benign tumor at operation are quite small. In children, 50 to 60 percent of brain tumors are found below the tentorium, as opposed to 25 to 30 percent in this location in adults.

The signs and symptoms of brain tumor vary considerably, based on location, tissue type, and other factors. These symptoms are often so varied and nonspecific that they can easily be mistaken for an everyday, harmless childhood malady. The tumors generally manifest themselves as increased intracranial pressure and/or focal neurological deficit. The signs and symptoms most frequently seen are headache, impaired consciousness, cranial enlargement, vomiting, diplopia, strabismus, papilledema, nystagmus, impaired vision, cranial nerve involvement, personality changes, ataxia, seizures, and hypothalamic and endocrine dysfunction.

The discussion of such terms as benign and malignant becomes complex when related to brain tumors. Malignancy depends less on the histological assessment of the mass than on such factors as its accessibility to chemotherapy, irradiation, or surgery, the extent of its interference with brain function and CSF circulation, and the amount of increase in intracranial pressure.

Cerebellar astrocytomas, peak incidence at ages 5 to 8 years, account for approximately 25 percent of all brain tumors in children. These tumors occur almost exclusively in childhood and early adolescence and are the most benign type. They arise from either the vermis or the cerebellar hemispheres, are almost always well circumscribed, and have a tendency toward cyst formation. The treatment of choice is surgical since these tumors are not sensitive to radiotherapy. The prognosis is good, with about 90 percent of the patients surviving from 5 years to several decades. Approximately 90 percent of these survivors have no permanent significant neurological disturbances.

Medulloblastoma, the peak incidence of which occurs during the first decade of life, is a malignant, invasive tumor accounting for 20 percent of all childhood and adolescent brain tumors. Approximately 40 percent of the posterior fossa tumors in children are of this type. It arises from the roof of the fourth ventricle, involves the vermis, and can extend to fill the fourth ventricle, thus blocking the flow of CSF. Medulloblastoma is different from other tumors in that it frequently "seeds" to other parts of the central nervous system (CNS) via the CSF pathways.

The treatment for this tumor is often threefold—surgical excision, radiotherapy, and chemotherapy. Radiotherapy generally includes the head, as well as the total spine, to destroy the tumor cells that have "seeded" to other areas. In spite of the fact that the tumor is highly radiosensitive, the outlook for long-term survival remains poor, with only 30 percent of patients surviving longer than 3 years.

Ependymomas arise most frequently from the floor of the fourth ventricle, fill the ventricle with tumor, and interfere with the flow of CSF, thus producing signs and symptoms of obstructive hydrocephalus. Children with this tumor may present with persistent vomiting (due to direct pressure on the emetic center) as an early manifestation of the disease. Total surgical removal is impossible since the tumor is inseparable from the floor of the fourth ventricle. Therefore, the aim of surgery is to clean out the ventricle and establish free flow of CSF. Radiotherapy can also be directed to the posterior fossa postoperatively. The survival rate varies from several months to 10 years or longer.

Brainstem gliomas are malignant, invasive tumors that most often arise from the pons. They account for about 10 percent of all intracranial childhood tumors and have an average age of onset of approximately 6 years. Brainstem gliomas present with cranial nerve involvement and vomiting, with increased intracranial pressure as an infrequent finding. Surgical intervention is seldom, if ever, indicated, since these tumors are such an integral part of vital brain structures. Even with radiotherapy, the child rarely survives longer than 12 months.

Craniopharyngiomas, constituting 5 to 13 percent of all intracranial tumors in childhood, are of congenital origin and are believed to be a remnant of embryonic squamous cells. As the tumor grows, it may compress the optic chiasm and the pituitary gland and extend into the third ventricle, interfering with the flow of CSF. Thus, the presenting symptoms are almost classically those of increased intracranial pressure, visual disturbances, and endocrine and hypothalamic dysfunction.

The treatment of choice is surgical since these tumors are relatively resistant to radiotherapy. Response to treatment is generally good if careful consideration is given to endocrine balance before, during, and after the surgical procedure. Even with subtotal removal, the interval between surgery and recurrence is several years.

PREVENTION

Health Promotion

No preventive measures are known.

Population at Risk

Brain tumors occur in both sexes and at all ages, but the peak incidence is about 6 years.

Screening

None.

ASSESSMENT

Health History

1. Developmental—any deterioration in child's gross motor and fine motor skills, language, or school performance.
2. Seizures.
3. Headaches: Note time of day. (Headache upon awakening is suggestive of increased intracranial pressure.)
4. Vomiting.
5. Any change in temperament or behavior.

Physical Assessment

1. *Height and weight.* Abnormalities may point to endocrine imbalances resulting from tumor in the area of the pituitary.
2. *Head.* Assess for rapidly increasing circumference; tense, bulging fontanels; and separated sutures, all of which are indicative of increased intracranial pressure.
3. *Cerebral function.* Level of consciousness, overall behavior, orientation, intellectual performance.
4. *Cranial nerves.* Abnormalities are frequent in brain tumors of childhood (Table 15-1).
5. *Cerebellar function (balance and coordination).* Disturbance of cerebellar function is a common finding since 50 to 60 percent of childhood tumors are located below the tentorium.
6. *Motor function.* Look for asymmetry in movement and strength of extremities.
7. Babinski reflex.

Diagnostic Tests

1. Skull x-rays films.
2. CAT scan.
3. Pneumoencephalogram.
4. Endocrine workup.

NURSING DIAGNOSES: ACTUAL OR POTENTIAL

1. Altered level of consciousness secondary to increased intracranial pressure.
2. Inadequate nutritional status secondary to persistent vomiting.
3. Fluid and electrolyte imbalance secondary to vomiting and pituitary involvement (especially diabetes insipidus).
4. Anxiety about diagnostic procedures, pre- and postoperative routines, treatment regimen (chemotherapy), surgery, and prognosis.
5. Potential for injury secondary to vision, gait, and coordination disturbances and seizure activity.
6. Alteration in comfort (headache).
7. Knowledge deficit regarding diagnostic tests and pre- and postoperative routines.
8. Parental grieving secondary to a potentially fatal diagnosis.
9. Anger and frustration (child) secondary to vision, gait, and coordination disturbances.
10. Altered self-esteem and/or embarrassment secondary to loss of hair.

EXPECTED OUTCOMES

1. The child will have adequate neurological functioning.
2. The child will ingest and retain nutrients and fluids sufficient to maintain current weight.
3. The child will receive appropriate drug therapy to control endocrine imbalances.

TABLE 15-1 CRANIAL NERVE CONSIDERATIONS IN THE ASSESSMENT OF CHILDREN

1. Cranial nerve I (olfactory).
   a. Rarely affected in neurological diseases of childhood.
   b. Loss of smell (anosmia) most often due to upper respiratory infections, frontal lobe tumors, and fractures of cribriform plate.
2. Cranial nerve II (optic).
   a. May have varying patterns of visual field loss with tumors impinging on optic chiasm.
   b. Optic nerve gliomas are not uncommon in children.
   c. Papilledema may occur with increased intracranial pressure.
3. Cranial nerves III, IV, VI (oculomotor, trochlear, abducens).
   a. Involvement of these nerves can be an invaluable clue to the location of lesions.
   b. Involvement of third nerve may indicate impending uncal herniation.
   c. Diplopia, strabismus, and nystagmus may be symptoms of brain tumor.
4. Cranial nerve V (trigeminal) may be involved in trauma, brainstem tumors, and cerebellar pontine angle tumors.
5. Cranial nerve VII (facial).
   a. Bilateral peripheral facial palsy may be congenital, as with Möbius' syndrome.
   b. Brainstem and cerebral infections may lead to facial nerve palsy.
   c. Acoustic neuromas may affect facial nerve function.
6. Cranial nerve VIII (acoustic) may be affected by tumors, such as neurofibromas.
7. Cranial nerves IX and X (glossopharyngeal and vagus) may be affected by tumors in the posterior fossa.
8. Cranial nerve XI (spinal accessory) involvement indicates lesion in foramen magnum.
9. Cranial nerve XII (hypoglossal) involvement may be due to vascular, neoplastic, or congenital lesions in posterior fossa.

4. The child will be free of injury.
5. The child will be maximally comfortable and rested.
6. The child and/or family will be able to state the specifics of the diagnostic procedures, pre- and postoperative routines, and postoperative treatment regimen.
7. The child will be able to cooperate during the procedures.
8. The family and child will be able to verbalize and cope with their anxiety.
9. The family will be able to verbalize their feelings and effectively cope with guilt.
10. The child will be able to cope with limitations imposed by the neurological condition and with the loss of hair.

INTERVENTIONS

1. Assess level of consciousness, vital signs, pupils, and movement of extremities every 4 hours, or as ordered.
2. Weigh child daily, and keep a record.
3. Take a careful dietary history upon admission, paying special attention to likes and dislikes.
4. Provide high protein, between-meal feedings.
5. Provide light meal in mornings (the time vomiting most frequently occurs).
6. If vomiting occurs, allow rest time and feed again.
7. Accurately record all foods eaten.
8. Avoid performing frightening, painful procedures near mealtime.
9. Make tray and food as attractive as possible.
10. Record intake and output every 8 hours, or as ordered.
11. Measure urine specific gravity with each voiding.
12. Review electrolyte values as they become available from the laboratory.
13. Administer steroids as ordered.
14. Elevate head of bed 30 degrees to assist with venous drainage.

15. Keep room dim and quiet when headache begins.
16. Give pain medications as ordered.
17. Keep side rails up at all times.
18. Provide soft toys.
19. Be sure foods and liquids are of a safe temperature.
20. Keep walkways uncluttered.
21. Teach parents child's limitations and how to help child protect self.
22. Remain with child and protect during seizure activity.
23. During seizure, turn child's body or head to side to avoid aspiration.
24. Give parents and child explanation of seizure activity.
25. Provide preprocedure teaching compatible with developmental level. Use dolls, toys, and pictures as teaching media.
26. Provide playtime and materials before and after procedures to help work out anxieties.
27. Remain with child during procedures when possible.
28. Carefully assess child's abilities and limitations.
29. Allow child to perform those self-care tasks, social roles, and family activities of which he or she is capable.
30. Teach parents and significant others the importance of child's maintaining independence.
31. Provide playtime to ventilate frustrations.
32. Discuss with child the rationale for cutting hair.
33. If possible, avoid cutting hair until immediately before surgery (preferably after child is asleep in operating room).
34. Plan with child ways of covering head postoperatively (e.g., hats, wigs, colorful scarves).
35. Provide quiet place and time for family to talk.
36. Provide information that might help dispel guilt.
37. Support in grief as appropriate to stage of grieving.
38. Promote intrafamily communication.
39. Refer to mental health professional or clergy, as indicated.
40. Engage physician's aid in correcting misconceptions regarding surgical outcome.
41. Provide family with explicit details about postoperative course—exactly how child will look, frequent vital signs, medications, how long the surgery can be expected to take, when they can expect to talk with the physician, and so on.
42. Administer chemotherapeutic agents as ordered. Until recently, chemotherapy for brain tumors of childhood was employed mainly as palliative treatment of recurrent malignancies after maximal amounts of radiation have been used. There are still relatively few chemotherapeutic agents that have been proved effective in the treatment of childhood brain tumors. The drugs currently being employed are methotrexate (for medulloblastoma), vincristine, vinblastine, the nitrosureas (BCNU, CCNU, and an investigational drug—MeCCNU). These drugs are generally part of a combined treatment approach—surgery, radiation therapy, and chemotherapy.
43. Provide nursing interventions appropriate for a child receiving chemotherapy and/or radiation, emphasizing recognition and relief of adverse effects, parental education, and rehabilitation.

EVALUATION

Outcome Criteria

1. Neurological functioning maintained or improved within limits imposed by tumor.
2. Child retains food.
3. Weight the same as or greater than upon admission.
4. Urine specific gravity within normal limits.
5. Serum blood values within normal limits.
6. Child demonstrates adequate energy levels and willingness to perform activities of daily living.
7. Absence of complaints of pain.
8. Absence of cuts, scrapes, bruises, and burns.
9. Parents verbalize understanding of protective measures.
10. Child complies with and understands protective measures.
11. Parents able to verbalize correctly facts about procedures and pre- and postoperative routines.
12. Absence of excessive overt signs of anxiety (constant crying, short attention span, irritability, excessive repetitive questions).
13. Parents able to make rational decisions about child's care.
14. Absence of blame placing.

15. Absence of parental behavior designed "to make up for" failure in preventing disease (excessive gift buying, planning elaborate trips, no limitations on behavior).
16. Child participates in planning and providing care and maintains social activities appropriate for developmental stage and health status.
17. Absence of withdrawal (parents and child).

Complications

POSSIBLE DISCIPLINARY PROBLEMS

Revised Outcome

Parents will be able to set limits on child's behavior.

Interventions

1. Discuss importance of limits in contributing to child's sense of security.
2. Support family's attempts to set limits.
3. Assist nurses in implementing plan for limit setting.
4. Provide quiet time and place for parents to discuss concerns.

Reevaluation and Follow-up

1. Increased instances of controlling unacceptable behavior.
2. Decreased anxiety regarding discipline.
3. Increased participation by child in "normal" activities.
4. Follow-up care is indicated to evaluate child's condition and identify signs of deterioration. The parents need support and information about anticipated changes in the child's condition.

EXTRACRANIAL TUMORS: NEUROBLASTOMA AND INTRASPINAL TUMORS

DESCRIPTION

Neuroblastoma is a malignant tumor of early life. It is probably the most common solid, malignant tumor of childhood, accounting for about half of malignant tumors in the neonate. It is an embryonal tumor that arises from neural crest ectoderm. Incidence is highest during the first 5 years of life, with a peak incidence before age 3 years.

Most commonly, neuroblastoma arises from the adrenal medulla or along the sympathetic chain in the chest or abdomen. However, it can be found anywhere in the body where sympathetic nervous tissue is located. It is difficult to discover neuroblastoma in the early stages because the beginning symptoms are so nonspecific—weight loss or failure to gain, abdominal pain, feeding problems. These tumors metastasize early by vascular and lymphatic spread to a variety of body areas, typically to lymph nodes, bones, bone marrow, or liver. Consequently, most children have extensive disease by the time they come to medical attention.

The most common presenting symptom is an abdominal mass that may be discovered by the parents during bathing or by the nurse or physician during a routine physical exam. Other indications may be subcutaneous nodules, periorbital swelling due to a retro-orbital tumor, bone pain, limp, paresis of lower extremities, anemia, and irritability.

The nurse's first responsibility involving neuroblastoma is for case finding and referral. Once the child is hospitalized, nursing care involves pre- and postoperative preparation and care. Due to the poor prognosis for the majority of these children, the nurse must be prepared to be supportive to both the terminally ill child and the family.

Intraspinal tumors occur approximately one-fifth as often as intracranial tumors. The most common intraspinal tumors are lipomas, dermoid and teratoid tumors, neuroblastomas, and intramedullary gliomas.

It is imperative that these tumors be diagnosed in the early stages because (1) irreversible neurological dysfunction can occur when the diagnosis is delayed; (2) most tumors, even gliomas, can respond dramatically to surgical excision and radiation therapy; (3) intraspinal tumors may be associated, even after only partial excision, with prolonged relief of signs and symptoms. The occurring signs and symptoms most frequently are disturbances of gait and posture, pain, weakness, reflex changes, impaired bladder and bowel function, sensory impairment, and cutaneous and skeletal changes.

Treatment depends on tumor type and location, but it primarily includes surgical decompression, radiation therapy, and corticosteroid and/or other chemotherapy. Nursing care is directed primarily toward the following areas:

1. Case finding and referral.

2. Prevention of deformities and maintenance of bodily functions during hospitalization.
3. Teaching for child and family.
4. Play therapy to help child cope with anxiety.
5. Planning for rehabilitation.

HYPERACTIVITY AND HYPOACTIVITY

SEIZURES: FEBRILE CONVULSIONS; EPILEPSY (GRAND MAL, PETIT MAL, PSYCHOMOTOR, AND FOCAL SEIZURES); INFANTILE SPASMS

DESCRIPTION

"A seizure is an episodic involuntary alteration in consciousness, motor activity, behavior, sensation, or autonomic function" (Swaiman and Wright, 1975). Paroxysmal neuronal discharge within the CNS can best be viewed as a symptom of a disease rather than as the disease entity itself. Convulsions during childhood result from a variety of conditions: congenital defects, trauma, metabolic disorders, fluid and electrolyte imbalance, temperature elevation, intracranial tumor, epilepsy, and invasion of the CNS by microorganisms, drugs, or toxins.

Febrile convulsions occur with a sudden rise in temperature above 39°C (102°F) during acute febrile diseases, primarily upper respiratory disorders, such as tonsillitis, pharyngitis, and otitis. These seizures occur in approximately 8 percent of infants and children between the ages of 6 months and 3 years. Some authors feel that there are factors, such as age, degree of temperature elevation, nature of illness, genetic makeup, and rate of fever rise, that contribute to a predisposition for febrile seizures.

Epilepsy can be defined as recurrent, paroxysmal, neuronal discharges leading to disturbances in consciousness or in autonomic, motor, or sensory function. It is not one specific disease, but rather a group of recurrent seizure patterns. Accurate figures on the incidence of epilepsy are not available, since this is not a reportable condition. The most common estimate is that one in 100 individuals in the United States suffers with epileptic seizures (about 2 million persons). Other investigators feel that the number is much higher, possibly as high as one in 50.

The epilepsies have been classified over the years using a variety of systems, such as clinical, anatomical, electroencephalographic, and etiological. The etiological system that divides these patterns into two broad patterns appears frequently in writings on the subject. Children who develop seizures without any demonstrable cerebral damage are said to have *idiopathic* or *genetic* epilepsy. Epilepsy is identified as *organic* or *symptomatic* when it develops subsequent to cerebral change or damage.

A *grand mal seizure* (convulsion) is the type of epilepsy most commonly found during childhood. Classically, there is an aura followed by loss of consciousness and rolling up of the eyes. There is generalized tonic contraction of body musculature leading to the emission of a sharp cry and a period of apnea and cyanosis. During the clonic phase, the trunk and extremities alternately contract and relax. This activity may cause biting of the tongue and urinary and fecal incontinence. The seizure can last from a few seconds to a few minutes. Usually the child will sleep for a time following the seizure and, upon awakening, may continue to be drowsy and confused. There may be some transient neurological deficit that may be helpful in pinpointing the origin of the seizures.

Petit mal seizures are often described as "staring" or "absence" episodes. These are transient losses of consciousness that may be accompanied by lipsmacking, fluttering of the eyelids, eye-rolling movements, drooping of the head, or slight clonic contractions of the limb and trunk muscles. These attacks are so brief that they may not be noticed until their occurrence begins to interfere with school performance and behavior. Petit mal seizures may be precipitated by flashing light or hyperventilation.

Psychomotor seizures are periods of abnormal but apparently purposeful behavior that the patient is not able to remember after the seizure is over. Children frequently experience an aura of intense fear before the seizure. An aura of epigastric discomfort, smelling a bad odor, or buzzing in the ear may also precede the attack. There are a variety of motor symptoms that can appear as manifestations of the seizure. Some of the most common are jerking of the mouth and face, aphasia, tonic posturing, and repetitive coordinated but inappropriate movements (walking or running in circles, swallowing, smacking, chewing).

Focal (Jacksonian) seizures, as the name implies, involve a specific, localized part of the brain. The Jacksonian type of focal seizure originates in one area of the cortex and progresses to involve the entire motor strip. Quite often this seizure escalates to a grand mal attack.

Infantile (myoclonic) spasms are seizures peculiar to infancy. Generally, the EEG shows a characteristic pattern known as hypsarrhythmia. In approximately 50 percent of cases, the etiology is unknown. The other 50 percent arise from a variety of causes—developmental anomalies, birth trauma, anoxia, postnatal birth trauma, meningitis, and encephalitis. Most frequently, the attacks are characterized by sudden, forceful contractions of the musculature of the trunk, extremities, and neck. The child is noticed to suddenly adduct and flex the limbs and drop the head. The prognosis for these children is rather bleak, since development is arrested or regresses with the onset of seizures. As the attacks continue, there is further deterioration of motor and mental abilities. Eventually, approximately 10 to 15 percent of the children die. Of those that survive, more than 90 percent are mentally retarded.

The first step in the management of epilepsy is to document the occurrence of seizures and obtain an accurate description of the seizure pattern. The second step is to rule out an organic cause for the seizures which would be amenable to medical or surgical intervention. Generally, the child is admitted to a hospital for this phase of management. If no organic cause can be found, the child begins a drug regimen to bring the seizures under control. See Table 15-2 for a list of drugs used most often to control seizures.

PREVENTION

Health Promotion

1. Febrile convulsions are usually preventable.
   a. Provide adequate hydration and make judicious use of antipyretics and cooling baths during febrile illnesses.
   b. Avoid severe environmental conditions, such as leaving child closed in a hot automobile.
   c. Prevention is important not only because seizures place the child at risk for injury or aspiration but also because repeated or prolonged febrile seizures can induce permanent brain damage that may lead to temporal lobe seizure disorders (Bresnan, 1978).
2. Epilepsy is sometimes preventable.
   a. Prevent brain insults: birth trauma, including hypoxia; CNS infections; head injury; intoxications (e.g., pesticides).
   b. Prevent, where appropriate (by genetic counseling), inherited metabolic and degenerative diseases associated with seizures.
   c. Most epilepsy is of unknown causes; accordingly, preventive measures are not understood.

Population at Risk

1. Febrile convulsions.
   a. Children under 5, particularly those between 6 and 36 months.
   b. Boys are more often affected than girls.
   c. Family history of febrile convulsions contributes to risk.
2. Epilepsy.
   a. About 90 percent of all epileptics develop their initial symptoms before age 20.

TABLE 15-2 DRUGS USED IN THE CONTROL OF EPILEPTIC SEIZURES

Grand Mal	Petit Mal	Psychomotor	Myoclonic
Phenobarbital	Zarontin	Tegretol	Valium
Mysoline	Tridione	Mysoline	ACTH
Dilantin		Dilantin	Corticosteroids
			Ketogenic diet

b. Epilepsy can begin at any time in childhood, but the commonest ages are before 2 years, between 5 and 7 years, and (especially for females) at puberty.
c. Family history of epilepsy increases risk. The 1 to 3 percent incidence in the general population is approximately doubled among children who have one epileptic parent and doubled again for those whose parents both have epilepsy.

Screening

None

ASSESSMENT

Health History

1. Family history of seizures, mental retardation, movement disturbances, cerebral palsy, dementia, or mental illness.
2. Prenatal history: illness, accidents, or surgery.
3. Labor and delivery history: length of labor, forceps, breech or unusual presentation, type of anesthesia, delay in respirations or cry (Apgar score), baby's need for oxygen.
4. Postnatal history: cyanosis, jaundice, infections, seizures.
5. Age at appearance of developmental milestones.
6. School performance.
7. History of childhood illnesses and injuries.

Physical Assessment

1. Cerebral function: level of consciousness, overall behavior, orientation, intellectual performance, cortical sensory interpretation, cortical motor integration, and language.
   a. Developmental tests, such as the Denver Developmental Screening Test (DDST), are good measures of cerebral function.
2. Cranial nerves (see Table 15-1).
3. Cerebellar function: balance, coordination, nystagmus, hypotonia.
4. Motor function: size, tone, symmetry, and strength of muscles; presence of abnormal movements.
5. Reflexes: superficial, deep, and pathological reflexes.

Diagnostic Tests

1. Skull x-ray films.
2. CAT scan, done to rule out organic basis for seizures.
3. Electroencephalogram (EEG).

NURSING DIAGNOSES: ACTUAL OR POTENTIAL

1. Anxiety secondary to unfamiliar surroundings and diagnostic tests.
2. Social isolation and feelings of embarrassment (child and parents) secondary to occurrence of seizures and societal reaction.
3. Altered self-concept (child).
4. Risk of injury or aspiration secondary to seizures.
5. Noncompliance with medication regimen.

EXPECTED OUTCOMES

1. The child and parents will be able to describe hospital routines and specifics of diagnostic tests.
2. The child will be able to cooperate during the procedures.
3. The child and parents will be able to recognize and express feelings about epilepsy.
4. The child will be free of injury and aspiration.
5. Medication will be taken as ordered.

INTERVENTIONS

1. Encourage parents to bring toys and other familiar objects from home.
2. Provide continuity in staff assignments to the extent possible.
3. Assess current knowledge level and readiness to learn.
4. Before diagnostic tests, provide child with explanations compatible with developmental level (use dolls, toys, and pictures).
5. Provide playtime and materials before and after procedure to work out anxieties.
6. Provide time and a quiet place for parents to discuss concerns about epilepsy with nurse and/or other health team members.
7. Provide written information about epilepsy.
8. Provide structured play situations to help child express and work through feelings.
9. If appropriate, put family in contact with other families in the community who also have a child with epilepsy.
10. Place padded tongue blade at bedside. Instruct family in its use.
11. Keep bed rails up at all times.
12. Remove toys and other potentially injurious objects from bed if seizure activity occurs.
13. Position child on side or turn head to side during seizure activity.

Remain with child during seizure. Do not restrain.
Teach parents and child importance of drug therapy.
16. Provide written instructions about when to take drugs.
17. Investigate financial resources for securing drugs.
18. Teach family importance of keeping drugs out of reach of other children.

EVALUATION

Outcome Criteria

1. Parents correctly verbalize facts about procedures.
2. Absence of signs of excessive anxiety.
3. Child sleeps well, without nightmares.
4. Parents verbalize anxiety. Child expresses anxiety verbally or through play activities.
5. Parents verbalize plans for informing others about seizures as appropriate (e.g., school, friends, family).
6. Child is free of bruises and abrasions.
7. Child has normal respiratory function (no aspiration).
8. Following implementation of medication regimen, child is free of seizures.
9. Child has adequate blood levels of drug.

Complications

TOXIC EFFECTS OF THE DRUG THERAPY

Revised Outcome
Early prevention and recognition of toxic symptoms.

Interventions
1. Provide written list of toxic symptoms.
2. Give written instructions regarding measures to be taken if toxic symptoms occur.
3. Caution against changing drug dosage unless instructed to do so by physician.

Reevaluation and Follow-up
Child needs periodic medical follow-up to check blood levels of drugs, to assess for toxic symptoms, and to adjust drug dosages as indicated.

TRAUMA

Accidents are the leading cause of death in children between the ages of 1 and 15 years. Central nervous system (CNS) trauma occurs in a large percentage of fatal injuries, particularly if the injuries resulted from a motor vehicle accident. Head injuries account for about 15 percent of all admissions to pediatric wards.

Head injuries can be classified as major or minor. Major injuries include contusions, lacerations, skull fractures, and hematomas. Although concussion is generally considered a minor injury, the child often exhibits alarming symptoms, such as irritability, confusion, lethargy, and vomiting. Older children and adolescents may also exhibit the postconcussion syndrome, characterized by headache, dizziness, irritability, and poor concentration, which may persist for days or weeks following the injury.

CONCUSSIONS, CONTUSIONS, LACERATIONS, SKULL FRACTURES, AND HEMATOMAS

DESCRIPTION

Concussion is a type of injury that is still not completely understood. With this injury, transient neuronal dysfunction occurs, resulting in a temporary loss of consciousness without any permanent damage to brain tissue. There is amnesia for the accident itself and for varying periods of time preceding the injury (retrograde amnesia).

Contusions and *lacerations* are more severe types of injuries with hemorrhagic lesions and tears of brain tissue. Damage is often accompanied by cerebral edema, which worsens the condition.

Ninety percent of pediatric head injuries are of the closed type, but skull fractures *do* occur. The skull of the child is more pliable, thus accounting for the low incidence of fractures. *Linear fractures* are classified as simple fractures without displacement of bone and are the most common type in childhood. These fractures generally do not require any special treatment or observation *unless* they cross the path of major vessels or enter the paranasal sinuses. *Basilar skull fractures* are those that extend through the base of the skull; they are rare in children. Basilar fractures may be accompanied by CSF rhinorrhea or otorrhea, by bleeding from the nasopharynx or middle ear, and/or by postauricular ecchymosis (Battle's sign). *Depressed fractures* are those with displacement of the bony fragment. These may be accompanied by contusion of the brain and laceration of the dura.

An *epidural hematoma* is a collection of blood between the dura and the skull, usually resulting from the tearing of an artery (Figure 15-3). Since the bleeding is arterial, the hematoma accumulates rapidly. Characteristically, the child is unconscious only briefly, or not at all, followed by a lucid period and then by progressively deteriorating neurological functioning over a period of minutes to several days. Though this is the classic chain of events with epidural hematoma, it does not always hold true for children. Rather, they may present with headache, vomiting, irritability, unequal pupils, hemiparesis, and stupor or coma. These symptoms must be recognized early in order to prevent permanent brain damage and death.

A *subdural hematoma* is the collection of blood between the dura and the brain substance itself (Figure 15-3). In children subdural hematomas usually result from damage to the cortical bridging veins that drain into the dural sinus. Since these hematomas are a result of venous bleeding, accumulation and subsequent symptoms develop very slowly. The symptoms, as they develop, are those of increased intracranial pressure.

PREVENTION

Health Promotion

Prevention of falls and head injuries (e.g., by use of car seat restraints); prevention of child neglect and abuse.

Population at Risk

All children and adolescents, but especially those at highest risk for falls (infants and toddlers); automobile passenger accidents (unrestrained infants, children, and adolescents); pedestrian or bicycle accidents (preschoolers and school-age children); motorcycle and automobile operator accidents (teenagers); and neglected and abused children.

Screening

None.

ASSESSMENT

Health History

1. Explanation of how injury occurred.
2. Posttrauma clinical course.
   a. Unconsciousness: duration.
   b. Level of consciousness after the injury.
   c. Seizure activity.
   d. Vomiting.

Physical Assessment

1. Vital signs: look for changes indicating increased intracranial pressure (increasing blood pressure, decreasing heart rate).

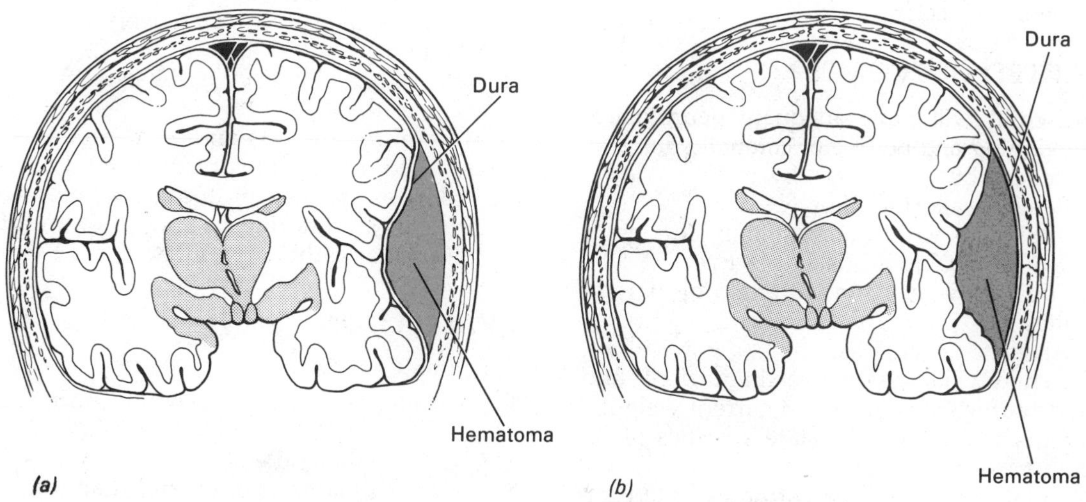

Figure 15-3 (*a*) Epidural and (*b*) subdural hematomas.

2. Check for ecchymotic areas on head and face.
3. Note clear or bloody drainage from ears or nose.
4. Cerebral function: level of consciousness, overall behavior, orientation.
5. Cranial nerve function: make special note of pupil size and reactivity (cranial nerve III).
6. Cerebellar function: balance and coordination.
7. Motor function: movement and strength of extremities.

Diagnostic Tests

1. Skull x-ray films.
2. Echoencephalogram. An ultrasonic technique useful in detecting a shift of midline brain structures.
3. CAT scan. Useful in demonstrating cerebral edema, shift of brain structures, and hematomas.

NURSING DIAGNOSES: ACTUAL OR POTENTIAL

1. Altered level of consciousness secondary to increased intracranial pressure.
2. Inadequate nutritional status secondary to vomiting.
3. Fluid and electrolyte imbalance secondary to vomiting and fluid restriction.
4. Parental knowledge deficit regarding diagnostic tests and their implications.
5. Parental anxiety regarding the possibility of brain damage.
6. Disturbance in parenting leading to child abuse or neglect.

EXPECTED OUTCOMES

1. The child will have adequate neurological functioning and be free of cerebral edema as evidenced by
   a. Being awake and alert.
   b. Vital signs within normal limits for age.
   c. Pupils equal and briskly reactive.
   d. Equal movement and strength of extremities.
   e. Absence of seizures.
2. The child will ingest and retain nutrients and fluids sufficient to maintain current weight.
3. Parents will be able to state specifics of diagnostic tests.
4. Parental anxiety will be within expected tolerable limits.
5. Abuse or neglect, if they exist, will be detected and interventions begun.

INTERVENTIONS

1. Assess vital signs, pupils, level of consciousness, and movement of extremities every hour, or as ordered.
2. Insure patent airway (elevated carbon dioxide levels lead to increased cerebral edema and, thus, to increased intracranial pressure).
3. Elevate child's head 30 degrees to promote venous drainage.
4. Monitor fluid intake carefully—the child is generally kept mildly dehydrated in order to decrease intracranial pressure.
5. Weigh child daily.
6. Check pillow and sheets for signs of possible CSF drainage.
7. If drainage is present on bedding, note whether there is a "double ring" pattern. Such a pattern would indicate that the drainage contains both blood and CSF.
8. If possible, collect some of the drainage from the ear or nose in a test tube to check for the presence of glucose. A test positive for glucose may be indicative of CSF.
9. Report the presence of drainage from ear or nose to the physician immediately.
10. Provide the parents with information about tests.
11. Provide time for questions.
12. Be honest in answering parents' questions about child's condition.
13. Teach usual pattern of recovery from cerebral injury.
14. Refer to social agency if abuse or neglect is suspected.
15. Administer steriods and/or mannitol as ordered to prevent or control cerebral edema.
16. Follow established protocols for intracranial pressure monitoring by means of an intraventricular catheter or subarachnoid screw.

EVALUATION

Outcome Criteria

1. Neurological functioning within normal limits.
2. Child retains food.
3. Weight the same as or greater than upon admission.

4. Parents verbalize information about diagnostic tests accurately.
5. Parents' anxiety is not excessive for situation.
6. Appropriate social agency referral completed if abuse and neglect cannot be ruled out.

Complication

1. Meningitis, secondary to CSF rhinorrhea or otorrhea (see *Meningitis*).
2. Possible developmental delays, secondary to head injury.

Reevaluation and Follow-up

Children demonstrate a remarkable ability to recover, even after a significant head injury. Elaborate rehabilitation is generally not necessary, except in case of severe deficits.

SPINAL CORD INJURY

Spinal cord injury generally results from hyperextension or hyperflexion of the neck or from vertical compression of the spine by falls on the head or buttocks. The most common sites for childhood cord injuries are vertebrae C5 to C6, T12 to L1, and C2 to C3. The most common type of injury leading to cord damage is fracture dislocation.

Since trauma to the vertebral column and spinal cord is fairly uncommon in children, accounting for less than 5 percent of childhood injuries, it will not be discussed in detail here. The interested reader is referred to a more complete discussion of this condition in Chapters 25 and 27. Principles of nursing management are essentially the same for children and adults.

INFLAMMATIONS

MENINGITIS

DESCRIPTION

Meningitis is inflammation of the meninges, the coverings of the brain and spinal cord. There are numerous organisms, both bacterial and viral, that cause meningitis. These organisms may reach the meninges through any of several routes: through the bloodstream from a focus of infection elsewhere in the body, by invasion from structures that adjoin the CNS, or through direct introduction into the CNS (e.g., traumatic injuries of the skull or birth defects, such as myelomeningocele).

Bacterial meningitis occurs more frequently during childhood than at any other time in the life cycle and is one of the most serious types of infection that a child can contract. Meningitis is particularly lethal during the first year of life because the signs of meningeal irritation may be less distinct and the sequelae more frequent when bacterial agents attack the immature brain. Although almost any bacterium is capable of causing meningitis, certain age groups seem predisposed to meningitis caused by particular organisms.

Before the age of 2 months, gram-negative organisms and group B beta-hemolytic streptococci are the most frequent offenders. The most common cause of meningitis between the ages of 4 months and 3 years is *Hemophilus influenzae.* Pneumococci and meningococci are the most common organisms causing meningitis in children over the age of 4 years (Swaiman and Wright, 1975).

The signs and symptoms of bacterial meningitis vary, depending upon the age of the child, the infecting organism, and the duration of illness. The most common symptoms are irritability, vomiting, lethargy, anorexia, fever, signs of meningeal irritation, headache, confusion, and seizures. It is imperative that antibiotic treatment be started *immediately* in these children, since delays drastically increase mortality and sequelae.

PREVENTION

Health Promotion

1. Viral meningitis.
   a. Immunization against mumps, which is the most common cause of viral meningitis (Chapter 24 contains immunization schedules).
2. Bacterial meningitis.
   a. Prevention of injuries that can introduce bacteria into the CNS (spinal and skull trauma).
   b. Adequate treatment of bacterial infections, especially otitis media and pneumonia.

c. Avoidance of contact with persons known to have bacterial meningitis or other infections with *H. influenzae,* group B beta-hemolytic streptococcus, pneumococcus, or meningococcus.
d. Prophylactic antibiotic treatment of family members, hospital staff, and other contacts of children with meningitis (especially meningococcal meningitis) is recommended by some physicians.

Population at Risk

1. Viral meningitis.
   a. Everyone, but particularly children recovering from viral infections, especially mumps.
2. Bacterial meningitis.
   a. Everyone, but especially children with cyanotic heart disease, otitis media, pneumonia, recent head or spine trauma, or midline defects, such as spina bifida.

Screening

None.

ASSESSMENT

Health History

1. Explore time and sequence of symptom development—a disease that peaks in a day to several days may be due to an infectious process rather than some other cause (see Table 15-3).
2. Any recent injuries to head or spinal column.
3. Any recent febrile illnesses.

TABLE 15-3 PROBABLE SIGNIFICANCE OF THE RAPIDITY WITH WHICH NEUROLOGICAL SIGNS AND SYMPTOMS DEVELOP

1. Diseases that develop acutely over a period of minutes to hours are usually of a vascular or traumatic nature.
2. Diseases that peak in a day to several days are usually a result of a toxic process, an electrolyte imbalance, or an infectious process.
3. Diseases that develop insidiously over many days, weeks, or months are usually associated with neoplastic, inborn metabolic, or degenerative processes.

4. Sudden, severe headaches.
5. Signs and symptoms of increased intracranial pressure (lethargy, seizures, vomiting, headache, irritability, increased blood pressure with decreased heart rate).

Physical Assessment

1. Rapidly increasing head circumference.
2. Tense, bulging fontanels.
3. Nuchal rigidity (neck stiffness), a sign of meningeal irritation.
4. Detailed neurological assessment.
   a. Cerebral function: level of consciousness, overall behavior, orientation, intellectual performance, cortical sensory interpretation, cortical motor integration, and language. Developmental tests, such as the Denver Developmental Screening Test (DDST), are good measures of cerebral function after acute illness has passed.
   b. Cranial nerves (see Table 15-1).
   c. Cerebellar function: balance, coordination, nystagmus, hypotonia.
   d. Motor function: tone, symmetry, and strength of muscles, presence of abnormal movements.
   e. Reflexes: superficial, deep, and pathological reflexes.

Diagnostic Tests

1. Lumbar puncture—done to measure CSF pressure and obtain fluid for laboratory analysis. Cerebrospinal fluid will be tested for glucose, protein, cell count; a Gram's stain and cultures will be done.
2. Blood cultures to identify or rule out systemic infection.
3. Urine cultures to rule out infection of genitourinary (GU) system.

NURSING DIAGNOSES: ACTUAL OR POTENTIAL

1. Altered homeostasis (elevated temperature).
2. Alteration in comfort: head, neck, and back pain secondary to meningeal irritation.
3. Nutritional deficit and metabolic imbalance secondary to nausea and vomiting.
4. Parental anxiety regarding child's immediate and long-term prognosis.
5. Risk of infecting other persons (principally with meningococcus).
6. Sensory deprivation secondary to isolation and restricted movement.

EXPECTED OUTCOMES

1. Child's fever will be reduced as rapidly and safely as possible.
2. Child will be as comfortable as possible.
3. Child will maintain admission weight and will be free of signs and symptoms of metabolic disturbance.
4. Parental anxiety will be within expected tolerable limits.
5. Other persons will not become infected.
6. Child will be free of signs of sensory deprivation.

INTERVENTIONS

1. Administer antipyretics as ordered.
2. Keep room cool and child lightly clothed.
3. Sponge with tepid or cool wet towels.
4. Avoid overchilling, since shivering elevates the temperature.
5. Place child in private room if possible (imperative for meningococcal meningitis).
6. Limit visitors.
7. Perform nursing activities and treatments together to allow uninterrupted rest periods.
8. Keep lights dim.
9. Ask parents to bring a favorite toy.
10. Avoid moving child unnecessarily during the acute phase of the illness.
11. Offer small amounts of clear liquids frequently. Gelatin and popsicles are often well accepted.
12. Weigh child daily if condition permits.
13. Monitor intake and output carefully.
14. As child improves, try to obtain favorite foods to stimulate appetite.
15. Administer intravenous (IV) antibiotics as ordered.
16. Teach parents and child necessity and importance of IV antibiotics.
17. Encourage family to talk to and touch child while awake.
18. As condition improves, provide play activities compatible with age and within constraints imposed by IV fluids.
19. Provide time and a quiet place for parents to discuss concerns with nurse and/or other health team members.
20. Explain difficulties in making predictions about future development during the acute phase of illness.
21. Make developmental assessment before discharge.
22. Teach parents methods of developmental stimulation.
23. Investigate family contacts and staff members for need of prophylactic antibiotics.

EVALUATION

Outcome Criteria

1. Temperature less than 38.5°C (101°F).
2. Parents verbalize understanding of restrictions.
3. Child has decreasing episodes of restlessness and irritability.
4. Child has increased periods of rest and sleep.
5. Child maintains or increases admission weight.
6. Child has serum electrolyte values within normal limits.
7. Child is free of signs of sensory deprivation.
8. Parents verbalize anxieties.
9. Parents describe and demonstrate developmental stimulation.
10. No new cases of meningitis develop.

Complications

1. Hydrocephalus (see *Hydrocephalus*).
2. Developmental delays.

Reevaluation and Follow-up

A community health nurse referral is indicated to evaluate development in the home environment and to observe for symptoms of developing hydrocephalus.

ENCEPHALITIS

Encephalitis is an inflammatory process of the brain, most often of viral origin. Pathological changes are generally cellular infiltration, proliferation of microglial cells, arteritis, and/or other changes in the blood vessel walls. Encephalitis may appear in children as complications of other disease processes, such as chickenpox, mumps, measles, and herpes simplex.

Encephalitis may begin insidiously or have an abrupt, explosive onset. The most common signs and symptoms are changes in level of consciousness, fever, headache, vomiting, ataxia, seizures, and nuchal rigidity. The treatment and nursing care are symptomatic and supportive.

REYE'S SYNDROME

Reye's syndrome is a disorder with an obscure etiology that was first described in 1963. Recent research shows a correlation between the use of aspirin (and antiemetics) for viral infections and the occurrence of Reye's syndrome. Some physicians now recommend that neither aspirin nor acetaminophen be given to children unless fever exceeds 30°C (102°F). The incidence of Reye's syndrome has been relatively low. However, recent epidemiological data seem to indicate that this syndrome is one of the most common neurological complications of viral infections in childhood. It is characterized by fever, seriously impaired consciousness, hypoglycemia, seizures, and impaired hepatic function. Mortality has been reported to be as high as 85 percent. Treatment is primarily of a supportive nature.

METABOLIC DISORDERS

LEAD POISONING

DESCRIPTION

Lead poisoning may result from either ingestion or inhalation of lead. In children, it results most frequently from repeated ingestion of inorganic lead compounds. Chronic lead poisoning, with an insidious onset, is the most common type in children. Ninety percent of these children present with overt signs of lead encephalopathy. The tragedy of this statistic becomes apparent when it is realized that 30 to 40 percent of the children who receive treatment after the onset of neurological involvement suffer severe, irreversible brain damage—that is, spasticity, quadriplegia, hemiparesis, blindness, deafness, convulsions, and mental retardation.

Although early detection is crucial, the task seems almost impossible because the initial symptoms are nonspecific. The child may be more irritable, less active, more sleepy, may have diarrhea, constipation, nausea and vomiting, and incoordination. Such symptoms may be passed off by the family—as well as by the physician—as everyday childhood illness. Lead poisoning is generally detected once the child develops seizures and symptoms of increased intracranial pressure.

PREVENTION

Health Promotion

Children ingest lead by chewing wood (e.g., window ledges, porch rails) coated with lead-based paint or by eating crumbling plaster, putty, or paint flakes. Lead paint was mostly used in homes before the 1950s. Although federal law now prohibits the use of such paints inside dwellings, there are no laws requiring removal of old paint containing lead from preexisting homes. Community health and school nurses can be invaluable in educating the public about lead poisoning and in case finding.

Population at Risk

1. Children 1 to 5 years of age, with the highest incidence occurring between ages 1 and 3 years.
2. Toddlers with pica (the practice of eating nonfood substances, such as paint chips or dirt) who live in dilapidated pre-World War II homes are at highest risk (Chisholm, 1975; Piomelli, 1978; Toy, 1978).

Screening

Since symptoms of lead poisoning are difficult to recognize and are often not detected until irreversible brain damage has taken place, screening is exceedingly important. Blood sampling for free erythrocyte porphyrin (EP) is simple and inexpensive and is highly recommended at 3- to 6-month intervals for asymptomatic children at risk.

EP screening accurately identifies children who *do not* have lead toxicity; children with positive EP tests require follow-up blood lead analysis to differentiate between porphyrin elevation due to lead poisoning and porphyrin elevation due instead to iron deficiency or some other cause.

ASSESSMENT

Health History

1. Explore sequence of symptom development.
2. Type (especially age) of family dwelling.
3. Family history of neurological disease.
4. Developmental milestones attained. Any regression.

5. Gastrointestinal (GI) problems—nausea, vomiting, diarrhea, constipation.

Physical Assessment

1. Assess for symptoms of increased intracranial pressure (lethargy, seizures, vomiting, headache, irritability, bulging fontanel, high blood pressure with slowed pulse).
2. Cerebral function—level of consciousness, overall behavior, orientation.
3. Assess cranial nerve function (see Table 15-1).
4. Cerebellar and motor function—dysfunction is common with lead poisoning.

Diagnostic Tests

1. Skull x-ray films, EEG, and CAT scan to rule out other neurological disorders.
2. Urine and serum analysis for lead levels.

NURSING DIAGNOSES: ACTUAL OR POTENTIAL

1. Altered level of consciousness secondary to increased intracranial pressure and lead poisoning.
2. Risk of injury secondary to intractable seizures.
3. Parental knowledge deficit regarding treatment regimen.
4. Ineffective family coping secondary to guilt about poisoning.
5. Separation anxiety secondary to hospitalization at young child's level of development.

EXPECTED OUTCOMES

1. The child will have adequate neurological functioning.
2. The child will be free of injury and aspiration during seizure.
3. Parents will be able to discuss correctly basic points of treatment.
4. Parents will be able to cope with feelings of guilt and maintain intrafamily communication.
5. The child will be able to cope effectively with hospitalization.

INTERVENTIONS

1. Administer osmotic diuretics (urea or mannitol) as ordered.
2. Monitor intake and output carefully.
3. Assess and record neurological status every hour. Report deterioration to physician immediately.
4. Administer anticonvulsants as ordered.
5. Keep bed rails up at all times.
6. Remove toys and other potentially injurious objects from bed if seizures occur.
7. Remain with child during seizures. Position child on side or turn head to side to prevent aspiration.
8. If seizure activity persists, notify physician immediately.
9. Provide parents with information about drugs used and expected results.
10. Notify physician of unrealistic parental expectations and misconceptions regarding treatment.
11. Provide time for questions.
12. Provide family with facts about lead poisoning.
13. Emphasize difficulty in recognizing early symptoms.
14. Provide parents with a place to discuss concerns together.
15. Notify clergyman, if indicated.
16. Teach family and staff how to identify and prevent separation anxiety.
17. Encourage parents to bring familiar objects from home.
18. Encourage parents to stay with child, if feasible.
19. Provide continuity in nursing assignment.

EVALUATION

Outcome Criteria

1. Absence of deteriorating neurological status.
2. Decreased severity and incidence of seizures.
3. Absence of injury and aspiration.
4. Parents correctly verbalize basics of treatment regimen.
5. Parents verbalize realistic outcomes of therapy.
6. Parents verbalize feelings about poisoning and do not engage in "blame placing."
7. Parents able to involve themselves in child's care to a realistic degree.
8. Child free of withdrawal and apathy.
9. Child relates to staff as appropriate for developmental level.
10. Child maintains relationship with parents.

Complications

1. Possible toxic effects of anticonvulsant therapy.
2. Possible recurrence of poisoning following discharge.
3. Possible delayed developmental milestones.

Reevaluation and Follow-up

1. Refer to local social service and public health agencies for assistance in identifying poison source.
2. Teach parents methods of developmental stimulation.
3. Community health nurse visits for periodic developmental assessment.

PHENYLKETONURIA

Phenylketonuria (PKU) is an inborn error of metabolism that affects the conversion of phenylalanine to tyrosine. Phenylketonuria is genetically transmitted as an autosomal recessive trait. It occurs about once in 10,000 live births. Mental retardation is the primary result of the disorder and is the basis for concern about early diagnosis and treatment. Although still a topic of much controversy, a low phenylalanine diet is the treatment of choice. Nurses are generally involved in case finding, in family teaching regarding dietary management and in family support.

MAPLE SYRUP DISEASE

Maple syrup disease is a familial cerebral degenerative disease caused by a defect in amino acid metabolism. The disease is characterized by the passage of urine with an odor of maple syrup. This disorder is transmitted as an autosomal recessive trait. The only known treatment is dietary restriction of specific amino acids.

TAY-SACHS DISEASE

Tay-Sachs disease results from a disorder in lipid metabolism involving one of the lysosomal enzymes. It is inherited as an autosomal recessive trait and occurs almost exclusively in Jews of Eastern European origin. There is no known effective treatment.

By the age of 6 months, children with Tay-Sachs disease generally exhibit irritability, apathy, lack of visual fixation, and unusual sensitivity to noise. The child has delayed developmental milestones. As the disease progresses, the child develops seizures, blindness, macular cherry-red spots, spasticity, decerebrate posturing, and dementia. Death usually occurs between the ages of 2 and 4 years.

DEVELOPMENTAL DISORDERS

MENTAL RETARDATION

DESCRIPTION

Mental retardation is a label traditionally attached to those individuals who perform two standard deviations below the mean on a standardized psychological test. Such a definition might prove useful in certain circumstances but serves little purpose in the planning and provision of health care. The American Association on Mental Deficiency defines mental retardation as subaverage intellectual functioning that originates in the developmental period and is associated with impairment in adaptive behavior. In the final analysis, the primary concerns for the individual are the ability to *adapt* to the environment and to compete successfully in society.

Mental retardation is one of the most serious conditions in our society today because of the major health, social, and economic problems that it encompasses. Approximately 3 percent of the population is mentally retarded. There are more than 6 million retarded individuals in the United States, with more than one-third of these under the age of 20 years. Of those under age 20, approximately 75 percent are mildly retarded, 15 percent are moderately retarded, 8 percent are severely retarded, and 2 percent are profoundly retarded (unable to care for themselves).

A discussion of etiology is somewhat unrewarding since, in a large percentage of children, the cause is not known. The most frequently used system for classification is based on causative factors. The system proposed by Baker and Barton (1975) is based on the development of the child when the condition occurred. See Table 15-4 for an outline of the most common conditions in their classification system.

The IQ score has been used, rightly or wrongly, to group retarded individuals into three major categories:

1. Educable mentally retarded.
   a. IQ between 50 and 75.
   b. Can reach third- to fifth-grade level of academic achievement.
   c. Independent in activities of daily living.
   d. As adult, generally functions independently.
   e. Able to work as unskilled or semiskilled laborer.
2. Trainable mentally retarded.
   a. IQ between 25 and 50.
   b. Rarely learns to read or write.
   c. Can learn self-care activities.
   d. Can learn social skills, such as acceptable behavior, table manners, and acceptable means of communication.
   e. Requires assistance as adult.
   f. Can learn simple job skills and function within a sheltered workshop or the home environment.
3. Severely or profoundly retarded.
   a. IQ between 0 and 25.
   b. Acquires no academic skills.
   c. Requires assistance with essentially all activities of daily living.
   d. Can learn the tasks of infancy (i.e., to sit, stand, relate to others, play with toys).
   e. As adult, requires continual care and protection.

The beginning of effective nursing care is to view mentally retarded children first as children who have the basic needs of all children. Having accomplished this, the nurse must try to assess the child and design care in terms of functional level rather than chronological age. This can be quite a task indeed when, for example, the child is a big 10-year old functioning at toddler level.

The nursing care of children who are mentally retarded cannot be discussed in detail here. The following sections are included to alert the nurse to some important considerations. Refer to the bibliography for additional assistance.

TABLE 15-4 CLASSIFICATION OF MENTAL RETARDATION

Prenatal period
- Chromosome anomalies
  - Down's syndrome (trisomy 21)
  - Klinefelter's syndrome
- Errors of metabolism
  - Phenylketonuria (PKU)
  - Hypothyroidism (cretinism)
  - Hurler's disease (gargoylism)
- Malformation of the cranium
  - Microcephaly
  - Hydrocephaly
- Maternal factors
  - Rubella (German measles)
  - Some other viral illnesses of mother
  - Syphilis
  - Anoxia
  - Blood type incompatibility
  - Malnutrition
  - Toxemia

Neonatal or perinatal period
- Anoxia
- Intracranial hemorrhage
- Birth injury
- Kernicterus
- Prematurity

Postnatal period
- Infections
  - Meningitis
  - Encephalitis
- Poisoning
  - Insecticides
  - Medications
  - Lead
- Degenerative disease
  - Tay-Sachs disease
  - Huntington's chorea
  - Niemann-Pick disease
- Physical injury
  - Head injury
  - Asphyxia
  - Hyperpyrexia
- Brain tumors
- Social and cultural factors
  - Deprivation
  - Emotional disturbance
  - Nutritional deficiency

SOURCE: Baker, A., and Barton, P.: "The Mentally Retarded Child," in G. Scipien et al. (eds.), *Comprehensive Pediatric Nursing*, McGraw-Hill, New York, 1975. Reproduced with permission.

PREVENTION

Health Promotion

Because mental retardation can result from such a wide range of causes, prevention is highly variable.

1. Genetic counseling is helpful for prospective parents known to be at risk for producing a retarded child (e.g., persons with family histories of familial disorders, such as Tay-Sachs disease or phenylketonuria.)
2. Amniocentesis is useful in identifying fetuses with some conditions that are associated with mental retardation (e.g., Down's syndrome). After indicative amniocentesis, abortion may be elected.
3. Good prenatal and perinatal care are critical to the prevention of retardation by promoting good gestational nutrition and oxygenation to the infant's brain.
4. Brain injury must be avoided at all stages of growth and development by
   a. Prevention of accidents and abuse.
   b. Prevention of poisoning.
   c. Prevention of central nervous system infection.
   d. Prevention of hypoxia.
5. Nonstimulating environments, such as households in which all persons are mentally retarded, foster environmental deprivation and a low level of intellectual functioning.

Population at Risk

1. Children with family histories of inherited retardation.
2. Children with histories of brain damage (e.g., birth injury, head trauma at any age, lead poisoning, encephalitis, or hypoxia from any cause).
3. Children from nonstimulating social environments.

Screening

1. Developmental milestone attainment.
2. Developmental screening tests.
3. IQ tests.
4. School achievement.

NURSING DIAGNOSES: ACTUAL OR POTENTIAL

1. Alteration in parenting: parental grief (including possible fixation in the denial stage of grieving).
2. Alteration in parenting: ineffective limit setting associated with guilt, overprotection, or rejection.
3. Alteration in parenting: lack of confidence about ability to bring up a "special" child.
4. Inadequate family coping: real or perceived inattention to siblings.
5. Inadequate family coping associated with conflict between parents about the care and management of the child.
6. Inadequate family coping associated with overwhelming financial burden of child's care.
7. Inadequate family coping associated with pressures from professionals and relatives to institutionalize child.
8. Alteration in child's development: delayed developmental milestones.
9. Self-care deficit secondary to cognitive and motor limitations.
10. Alteration in self-esteem: poor self-concept secondary to experiences with social disapproval.
11. Knowledge deficit (parents, health care workers) about stimulation, self-care training, education, and other special needs of child.

CEREBRAL PALSY

DESCRIPTION

"Cerebral palsy is a nonspecific, descriptive term pertaining to disordered motor function, beginning in early infancy, characterized by spasticity and/or involuntary movements of the limbs. The dysfunction is caused by brain impairment and is not episodic or progressive" (Swaiman and Wright, 1975). Cerebral palsy occurs in approximately one to six children per 1,000 live births. The incidence in the United States population is estimated to be about 0.2 percent.

Cerebral palsy is most often classified according to neurological signs and symptoms: (1) spastic, (2) choreoathetotic, (3) ataxic, (4) dystonic, (5) ballismic, and (6) mixed. The spastic forms account for 60 to 70 percent of the affected children. These categories may be further refined as to limb(s) involved, suspected cause, and functional capacity. In addition to motor impairment, the child may have other associated problems, such as hearing and vision impairment, mental retardation, learning disabilities, and seizures.

Nursing is one member of the multidisciplinary team that provides services to the child and the family. Some of the common nursing diagnoses are listed below.

PREVENTION

Health Promotion

There are a number of factors occurring before, during, and shortly after birth that can cause cerebral palsy. Accordingly, health promotion measures cover a broad scope.

1. Adequate nutrition of the pregnant woman.
2. Avoidance of fetal or infant trauma.
3. Avoidance of fetal or infant infection.
4. Avoidance of fetal radiation.
5. Avoidance of prematurity.
6. Avoidance of asphyxia or hypoxia during or immediately after birth.
7. Avoidance of kernicterus.

Population at Risk

1. Premature and low-birth-weight babies.
2. Infants born after difficult or prolonged labors.
3. Infants with low Apgar scores.
4. Infants with maternofetal blood incompatibility.
5. Infants with CNS infections.

Screening

1. Physical examination.
2. Developmental screening.

NURSING DIAGNOSES: ACTUAL OR POTENTIAL

1. Alteration in parenting: parental grief over disabled child.
2. Alteration in family coping: social isolation associated with overprotectiveness or with real or perceived social rejection of child and family by others.
3. Knowledge deficit (parents, health care workers) about self-care training and other special aspects of child's habilitation (speech therapy, bracing, physical therapy, etc.)
4. Nutritional deficit secondary to difficulty with eating and high caloric expenditures for involuntary motor activity.
5. Perceptual, sensory, motor, language, and cognitive deficits secondary to brain insult.
6. Self-care deficit secondary to poor motor control.
7. Impaired self-concept associated with speech and motor problems.

MINIMAL BRAIN DYSFUNCTION

DESCRIPTION

Minimal brain dysfunction (MBD) is a descriptive term applied to

> children of near average, average, or above average intellectual capacity with certain learning and/or behavioral disabilities ranging from mild to severe, which are associated with deviations of function of the central nervous system. These deviations may manifest themselves by various combinations of impairment in perception, conceptualization, language, memory, and control of attention, impulse or motor function. These aberrations may arise from genetic variations, biochemical irregularities, perinatal brain insults, or other illnesses or injuries sustained during the years critical for the development and maturation of the central nervous system . . . (Clements, 1966).

Minimal brain dysfunction may be the most common cause of chronic behavior problems in children. The incidence in the pediatric population is estimated to be between 5 and 10 percent, with boys affected four to five times as often as girls. Therapy is generally directed toward family education and counseling, and medication, educational management, and psychotherapy for the child (Figure 15-4). Nurses most frequently called upon to work with these children and their families are those engaged in community settings, such as schools, health departments, physicians' offices, mental health clinics, and other outpatient clinic settings. Children are rarely hospitalized with MBD as a pri-

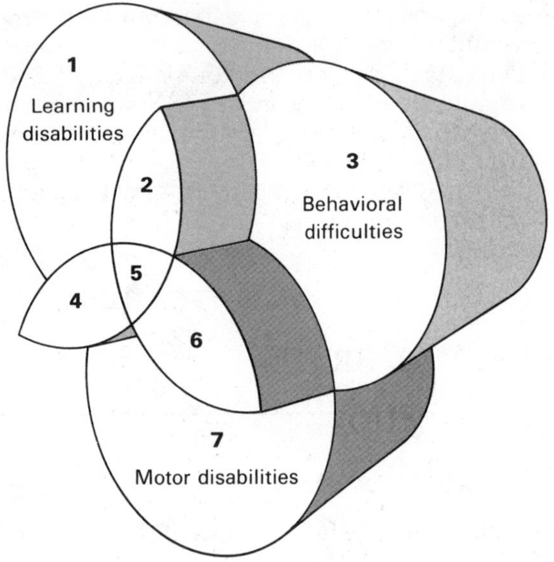

Figure 15-4 Venn diagram depicting three major target symptoms and possible symptomatic combinations in minimal brain dysfunction: (1) learning disabilities, no motor disabilities, no behavioral difficulties; (2) learning disabilities and behavioral difficulties; (3) behavioral difficulties, no motor disabilities, no learning disabilities; (4) learning disabilities and motor disabilities; (5) learning disabilities, behavioral difficulties, and motor disabilities; (6) behavioral difficulties and motor disabilities; (7) motor disabilities. [Redrawn from Wright, F. S., Schain, R. J., Weinberg, W. A., and Rapin, I., "Learning Disabilities and Associated Conditions," in Kenneth F. Swaiman and Francis S. Wright (eds.), *The Practice of Pediatric Neurology*, 2d ed., Mosby, St. Louis, 1982; courtesy Dr. Kenneth F. Swaiman.]

mary diagnosis. However, children hospitalized for other reasons who display "behavior problems" may well have MBD as a coincidental difficulty.

Nursing diagnoses frequently associated with MBD are listed below.

NURSING DIAGNOSES: ACTUAL OR POTENTIAL

1. Alteration in parenting associated with guilt about child's out-of-bounds behavior and uncertainty about how to guide and discipline child.
2. Alteration in family coping associated with child's disruptive behavior and conflict among family members about child-rearing practices.
3. Alterations in child's development: short attention span, easy distractability, hyperactivity, poor motor control, emotional lability, poor impulse control, delayed language development, learning deficits, and disorders in perception of space, time, form, and movement.
4. Alteration in self-concept: poor self-esteem, secondary to experiences with social disapproval.
5. Risk of injury, secondary to judgment errors, impulsiveness, and hyperactivity.

HEARING IMPAIRMENT

DESCRIPTION

Profound deafness occurs about once per 1,000 live births. It is estimated that approximately 25 out of 1,000 newborns have a moderate to severe hearing loss. There are approximately 39,000 school age children in the United States who either were born deaf or lost their hearing before speech and language patterns were developed.

Deafness is often associated with syndromes involving other organ systems, such as kidney disease, thyroid disease, disorders of pigmentation, bone diseases, conductive defects in the heart, and eye anomalies.

There are different methods of classifying hearing impairment based on anatomical factors, severity of hearing loss, and onset and course. Usually, the impairment is referred to as either a conductive loss or a sensorineural loss. A conductive loss is most often due to eustachian tube obstruction or dysfunction, which results from serous otitis media or mucoid otitis media. This type of loss may be associated with external ear and/or facial anomalies and with renal anomalies. In children, a conductive loss can usually be treated with a hearing aid. A sensorineural loss is related to cochlear pathology, damage to the acoustic nerve (cranial nerve VIII), or damage to hearing centers in the brain. This type of loss is still poorly understood.

Hearing loss is difficult to detect in very young children. However, it is imperative that these defects be identified early in order to provide the special training and support needed by such children. This disorder is frequently overlooked in children who are retarded, emotionally disturbed, or who have visual or motor handicaps.

The care of a hearing-impaired child requires a multidisciplinary approach, especially when deafness is paired with other disabilities. The nursing care for children with hearing disorders cannot be discussed in detail here, but nursing diagnoses that commonly apply are listed below.

PREVENTION

Health Promotion

1. Genetic counseling for prospective parents with family histories of heritable forms of deafness.
2. Good prenatal and perinatal care.
3. Prevention and early treatment of childhood ear infections and other infections involving the central nervous system or cranial nerves.
4. Avoidance of ototoxic drugs, such as streptomycin, or careful monitoring of child while such drugs are in use.
5. Immunization against childhood communicable diseases.
6. Avoidance of excessive noise levels.

Population at Risk

1. Children with cerebral palsy.
2. Children with otitis media, especially if recurrent.
3. Children who were born prematurely.
4. Children from families with heritable deafness.
5. Children who have had mumps, measles, or meningitis.
6. Children whose mothers had rubella, syphilis, toxoplasmosis, or cytomegalovirus during pregnancy.
7. Children exposed to high noise levels (especially adolescents who listen to extremely loud music).
8. Children who have taken ototoxic medications.
9. Children who had hyperbilirubinemia as neonates.
10. Children with multiple congenital anomalies or external ear malformations.
11. Children with cleft palate.

Screening

1. Delayed or impaired speech development.
2. Failure to awaken from sleep when called without being touched.
3. Failure to respond to speech or to name being called.
4. Tilting head or assuming unusual postures when listening.
5. Poor school performance.
6. Poor scores on verbal intelligence tests.
7. Constantly spends time alone, even in presence of other children.
8. "Self-stimulation" or other "autistic-type" behaviors.

NURSING DIAGNOSES: ACTUAL OR POTENTIAL

1. Alteration in parenting, associated with guilt, overprotection, perceived inability to parent a handicapped child, overpermissiveness, grief, or rejection.
2. Knowledge deficit about implications of genetic influence (if any) on child's deafness.
3. Alteration in speech and language development: language delays and articulation disorders secondary to impaired hearing.
4. Alteration in self-esteem: low self-concept secondary to altered appearance (hearing aids), peer teasing, and poor school performance.
5. Alteration in learning: delays or deficits in socialization, school achievement, and other forms of learning that require hearing.

VISUAL IMPAIRMENT

DESCRIPTION

The critical period for developing acute vision is between 1 and 6 years of age; there are approximately 16 million children in the United States between the ages of 3 and 6 years. Of this number, only about 500,000 (3 percent) are tested annually for visual disturbances. It is estimated that one child in 20 has visual problems of one kind or another.

Blind children require complex education and care from a multitude of specialists. They need special training in routine activities of daily living, as well as special opportunities for educational and social experiences. The nursing care of children with visual deficits cannot be addressed in detail here, but common nursing diagnoses are listed below.

PREVENTION

Health Promotion

1. Genetic counseling for prospective parents who have a family history of heritable visual defects.
2. Prevention of rubella during pregnancy.
3. Prevention of congenital syphilis by screening and treating infected pregnant women.
4. Prevention of eye, cranial nerve, and brain trauma.
5. Prevention of eye infection acquired during birth by prophylaxis for gonococcal infection.
6. Prevention of retrolental fibroplasia by keeping oxygen administered to premature infants at the minimum required to maintain adequate blood gases.
7. Early treatment (before age 4 or 5 years) of strabismus.
8. Prompt treatment of eye infections.

Population at Risk

1. Children with a family history of visual defects.
2. Children whose mothers had rubella, gonorrhea, or syphilis during pregnancy.
3. Children with untreated strabismus.
4. Children born prematurely and treated with oxygen.

Screening

It is imperative that formal screening be performed before the child is 4 years of age. The Snellen charts are the most commonly used screening tests. Informal screening observations include the following:

1. Infant does not reach for toys or bottle and does not smile responsively at mother.
2. Toddler or older child walks into furniture.
3. Child rubs eyes frequently.
4. Child holds objects very close to the eyes to examine them.
5. Child blinks, squints, or frowns excessively.
6. Eyes are watery, inflamed, or highly sensitive to light.
7. School-age child or adolescent has difficulty reading, seeing the blackboard, or doing close work.

NURSING DIAGNOSES: ACTUAL OR POTENTIAL

1. Alteration in parenting associated with uncertainty about ability to bring up a handicapped child, guilt, grief, overprotection, permissiveness, or rejection.
2. Inadequate family coping associated with overwhelming financial burden of child's care, disagreement about child-rearing practices, and concerns about who will care for the child in later years.
3. Sensory deprivation secondary to severe visual impairment.
4. Alteration in learning: delays or deficits in socialization, schooling, and other forms of learning that require vision.
5. Self-care deficit due to visual impairment.
6. Altered parent–child interaction: prolonged dependency of child secondary to self-care deficit.
7. Low self-esteem secondary to dependency and limited social experience.

REFERENCES

Baker, A. S., and Barton, P. H.: "The Mentally Retarded Child," in G. Scipien et al. (eds.), *Comprehensive Pediatric Nursing*, McGraw-Hill, New York, 1975.

Bresnan, M., "Convulsive Disorders," in R. A. Hoekelman et al. (eds.), *Principles of Pediatrics: Health Care of the Young*, McGraw-Hill, New York, 1978.

Chisholm, J., "Plumbism," in W. K. Frankenburg and B. W. Camp (eds.), *Pediatric Screening Tests*, Charles C Thomas, Springfield, IL, 1975.

Clements, S. D.: *National Project on Minimal Brain Dysfunction in Children: Terminology and Identification*, monograph No. 3, Public Health Service publication No. 1415, U.S. Government Printing Office, Washington, D.C., 1966.

Piomelli, S.: "Screening for Lead Poisoning," in R. A. Hoekelman et al (eds.), *Principles of Pediatrics: Health Care of the Young*, McGraw-Hill, New York, 1978.

Swaiman, K. F., and Wright, F. S.: *The Practice of Pediatric Neurology*, vols. I and II, C. V. Mosby, St. Louis, 1975.

Toy, H. S.: "Poisoning," in R. A. Hoekelman et al. (eds.), *Principles of Pediatrics: Health Care of the Young*, McGraw-Hill, New York, 1978.

BIBLIOGRAPHY

Alexander, M. M., and Brown, M. S.: "Physical Examination, Parts 17 and 18: Neurological Examination," *Nursing 76*, **6**:38, June 1976; **6**:50, July 1976. These two articles present a method for performing a neurological assessment on a child. The first article gives a brief review of the anatomy of the nervous system and presents assessment of cerebral and cranial nerve function. The second article reviews cerebellar, motor, sensory, and reflex functions; there is a discussion of reflexes during infancy.

Barnard, K. E., and Erickson, M. L.: *Teaching Children with Developmental Problems: A Family Care Approach,* 2d ed., C. V. Mosby, St. Louis, 1976. This book is directed to the care of handicapped infants and preschoolers who live at home. Child development concepts are presented and used as the rationale for nursing interventions in work with the mentally retarded child and the family. Specific instructions are given for designing a plan for helping the child progress. Although the book is intended for use with retarded children, the same principles are useful in stimulating development in any child.

Chard, M. A., and Woelk, C. G.: "The Mentally Retarded Child and His Family," in G. Scipien et al. (eds.), *Comprehensive Pediatric Nursing,* 2d ed., McGraw-Hill, New York, 1979. The retarded child is viewed as having the same needs as ordinary children, although at a different rate and chronological age. Nursing for the child and family is discussed for home, community, institution, and general hospital settings.

Conway, B. L.: *Pediatric Neurologic Nursing,* C. V. Mosby, St. Louis, 1977. This book was designed as a supplement for nurses who already have beginning knowledge in basic neurological nursing care. Therefore, little space is given to step-by-step descriptions of nursing management. The first two chapters deal quite extensively with embryology and physiology and provide a good foundation for the neurological disorders discussed later in the book.

Passo, S.: "Outcomes of Neurosurgical Care for the Myelomeningocele Child and His Family," *Journal of Neurosurgical Nursing,* **6**(2):122, December 1974. This article presents a clinical evaluation tool for the care of children with myelomeningocele and their families. The use of the tool is demonstrated with a newborn whose myelomeningocele has been surgically repaired. Nursing objectives, patient outcomes, and family outcomes are specified by the tool.

Scipien, G., and Chard, M. A.: "The Special Senses," in G. Scipien et al. (eds.), *Comprehensive Pediatric Nursing,* 2d ed., McGraw-Hill, New York, 1979. Embryology, anatomy, and physiology of the eye, the ear, and the sense organs of smell, taste, and touch are summarized. Assessment of children for visual and auditory acuity is presented. The bulk of the chapter is a discussion of specific nursing care for a comprehensive range of childhood eye, ear, and nose problems.

Stewart, C.: "Current Concepts of Chemotherapy for Brain Tumors," *Journal of Neurosurgical Nursing,* **12**(2):97, June, 1980. Chemotherapeutic agents attack the tumor cell during its reproductive cycle; the cell cycle is discussed in conjunction with the actions of specific chemotherapeutic agents. The author outlines basic nursing interventions helpful in planning care for patients receiving these drugs.

Swaiman, K. F., and Wright, F. S.: *The Practice of Pediatric Neurology,* 2d ed., vols. I and II, C. V. Mosby, St. Louis, 1982. The book is divided into three sections. Section I places emphasis upon the historical, physical, and laboratory examinations. Section II attempts to develop differential diagnoses based on the chief complaint. This enables the reader to consult the text utilizing the child's signs and symptoms as a guide. Section III is designed to provide the reader with a detailed description of the diseases that affect the nervous system during childhood.

Wender, P. H.: "Minimal Brain Dysfunction in Children—Diagnosis and Management," *Pediatric Clinics of North America,* **20**(1):187, February, 1973. Presents MBD as highly responsive to minimal treatment. Recognizable characteristics of MBD are described (motor, attentional, cognitive, learning, impulsive, interpersonal, emotional, family, and neurological phenomena; and congenital stigmata and psychological test performance). Discusses diagnosis and management. Good bibliography.

Zeidelman, C.: "Increased Intracranial Pressure in the Pediatric Patient: Nursing Assessment and Intervention," *Journal of Neurosurgical Nursing,* **12**(1):7, March, 1980. This article reviews the basic mechanisms of increased intracranial pressure, current medical treatments, and nursing interventions for each of these treatments. Specific therapies presented are (1) continuous ICP monitoring, (2) drug therapy (steroids, mannitol, Pavulon), (3) controlled ventilation, and (4) hypothermia. These sophisticated mechanical treatments are used in conjunction with nursing assessment and intervention—the key to a successful outcome for brain-injured children.

16

The Musculoskeletal System

Sherrilyn DeJean Coffman

ABNORMAL CELLULAR GROWTH

TORTICOLLIS

DESCRIPTION

Torticollis is an abnormality, usually congenital, in which the head is flexed and rotated by a shortening of the sternocleidomastoid muscle on one side of the neck. The etiology is uncertain; however, the defect is seen more frequently following difficult deliveries. At birth the degree of deformity is slight, but after a few weeks a large, firm tumor appears in the sternocleidomastoid muscle. The swelling probably results from hypertrophy of fibrous tissue in the muscle. Without treatment, the muscle remains shortened, and facial asymmetry gradually develops.

PREVENTION

Health Promotion

No preventive measures are known. Early recognition and sustained treatment are required to prevent progression of the deformity.

Population at Risk

Infants, particularly those with a history of difficult birth.

Screening

All newborns and infants should be examined for sternocleidomastoid shortening or swelling.

ASSESSMENT

Health History

The disorder is seen most frequently following difficult deliveries by primiparas and those involving abnormal presentations (e.g., breech).

Physical Assessment

1. Swelling of the sternocleidomastoid muscle, most noticeable after the second or third week of life.
2. Head is tilted toward the affected side and rotated toward the opposite side.
3. Older child may have facial asymmetry.

NURSING DIAGNOSES: ACTUAL OR POTENTIAL

1. Disturbed body image secondary to deformity (in inadequately treated older child).
2. Disturbed family relationships secondary to stress of treatment and uncertain prognosis.
3. Disturbed peer relationships secondary to body image disturbance and decreased self-esteem (in inadequately treated older child).
4. Decreased ability to perform self-care activities if the child is in a shoulder spica cast, traction, or brace.

EXPECTED OUTCOMES

1. Defect will be detected in the first month of life, and treatment will be started at that time.

2. Parents and older child will understand the problem and its management upon initiation of treatment.
3. Family relationships will be supportive of well-being of all family members.
4. Child will have normal peer relationships.
5. Child will develop good self-esteem.
6. Parents and child will comply with the treatment program.
7. Outcome of treatment will be to achieve complete correction or maximal correction of deformity.
8. Recurrence of the deformity will be prevented or detected early.

INTERVENTIONS

1. Preoperative or conservative treatment.
   a. Detect deformity and refer patient for diagnosis and treatment before one month of age.
   b. Counsel parents and child, if old enough, about the nature of the deformity, its prognosis, and family adaptation to treatment.
   c. Teach parents to perform daily stretching exercises with child to correct deformity.
   d. Discuss other simple measures, such as moving the child's bed, so that child must turn away from the affected side.
   e. Prepare child and parents preoperatively when surgery is required.
2. Postoperative treatment.
   a. Maintain dressing, shoulder spica cast, or head-halter traction.
   b. Carry out stretching exercises when ordered, with premedication for pain.
   c. Inform physician if child will not comply with exercises.
   d. Observe for respiratory distress indicating damage to the thoracic duct (see *Complications*).
   e. Teach parents to do postoperative exercises with child at home or plan for cast or brace care.

EVALUATION

Outcome Criteria

1. Parents and child maintain home therapy program, and family copes adequately with daily therapy.
2. Complete correction or maximal correction of deformity is achieved.
3. Recurrence of deformity is prevented or detected early.
4. Child demonstrates good self-concept and normal peer relationships for developmental stage.
5. Complications and unnecessary stress associated with surgery are absent.

Complications

Damage to the thoracic duct, which can occur during surgical correction on the left side of the neck.

Assessment

Signs of respiratory distress: increased respiratory rate, retractions, anxiety.

Revised Outcomes

Damage to the thoracic duct will be repaired.

Interventions

Prepare the child to return to surgery for surgical repair of the thoracic duct.

Reevaluation and Follow-up

1. Teach parents to recognize recurrence of the deformity and seek medical attention immediately.
2. For the child in a cast, arrange for cast removal approximately 6 weeks postoperatively, followed by stretching exercises and wearing of a neck collar or brace.

CLUBFOOT (TALIPES EQUINOVARUS)

DESCRIPTION

Clubfoot is a congenital foot disorder of mixed genetic and environmental origins. The deformity can be classified as *rigid,* in which the talus bone is abnormal at birth but no primary abnormalities of muscles, tendons, nerves, or blood vessels exist; or *flexible,* in which abnormal bony relationships are present at birth but are not severe. In either type, deformities progress, contractures worsen, and the clubfoot becomes more rigid unless treatment is instituted. Treatment should begin during the first week of life. Casts or splints correct most cases with early treatment; later diagnosis usually requires surgery. The incidence of this deformity is estimated at one to four cases per 1,000 live births. An equinovarus deformity may be present at birth in association with other defects, such as myelomeningocele; however, management of clubfoot due to paralysis differs from treatment of talipes equinovarus as an isolated deformity.

PREVENTION

Health Promotion

Genetic factors are implicated in about 10 percent of cases. Persons with a family history of clubfoot should receive genetic counseling.

Population at Risk

1. Newborns.
2. Boys are affected twice as often as girls.
3. Infants with spinal defects or hydrocephalus.

Screening

Newborn physical examination (assessment of the feet).

ASSESSMENT

1. Routine screening of all newborns is essential to identify abnormal angulations or deformities of the feet.
2. Assess for equinus, adduction, and inversion of the hind part of the foot and adduction and inversion of the forward part of the foot.

NURSING DIAGNOSES: ACTUAL OR POTENTIAL

1. Risk of delay in motor development (weight bearing or walking) due to deformity or immobilization.
2. Risk of complications from cast (skin breakdown, impaired circulation, altered sensation or movement).
3. Risk of body image disturbance secondary to persistent deformity, abnormal gait, or casting.
4. Anxiety and ineffective family coping or noncompliance, due to frequent cast changes, hospitalization, uncertainty of prognosis, and potential deformity in future children.

EXPECTED OUTCOMES

1. Child will begin treatment during the first week of life, before deformities become more rigid.
2. Child will demonstrate normal posture, mobility, and range of motion by the end of the treatment program.
3. Family will maintain normal family functions and cooperate with the therapy program.
4. Complications of casting or surgery will be prevented or corrected early.

INTERVENTIONS

1. Refer child for treatment within the first week of life.
2. Explain treatment regimen and need for follow-up to parents.
3. If surgery is to be performed, prepare child and parents.
4. Teach parents (and child if old enough) about preoperative care.
5. Teach family to care for cast at home.
   a. Check circulation, sensation, and skin condition.
   b. For young infant, soak off cast in vinegar water solution before each cast change.
6. Clarify mobility limits for the child in a cast.
7. Teach care of child who has Denis Browne splint (i.e., skin care, application of splint, times to be worn, and use of splint key).

EVALUATION

Outcome Criteria

1. Treatment is begun within 1 week of birth.
2. Parents accurately describe the treatment regimen and their role in it.
3. Parents demonstrate compliance with treatment.
4. Satisfactory correction of the deformity is attained.
5. Complications of casting or surgery do not occur.
6. Child has normal gait, foot form, and range of ankle motion at end of treatment program.
7. Family is free of excessive anxiety, demonstrates normal interpersonal relationships, and performs its functions adequately (see Chapter 5).

Complications

NEUROVASCULAR IMPAIRMENT SECONDARY TO CASTING OR SURGERY

Assessment

1. Circulation: pale or cyanotic toes, cold to touch, excessive swelling.
2. Nerve function: excessive pain, decreased sensation or movement in toes.

Revised Outcomes
Adequate neurovascular function will be restored to the foot.

Interventions
1. Administer therapeutic dose of prescribed analgesic.
2. Elevate the extremity on pillows.
3. Contact the physician immediately to bivalve or split the cast.

Reevaluation and Follow-up
1. The child may wear the Denis Browne splint for several months after the last cast is removed.
2. Parents are taught the importance of seeking help immediately if they notice recurrence of the deformity.
3. Some children need follow-up for 4 to 5 years to assess for recurrence of the deformity.

CONGENITAL DISLOCATION OF THE HIP

DESCRIPTION

Congenital dislocation of the hip is an abnormality of the joint in which the femoral head is completely outside the acetabulum. Less severe forms of congenital hip disease include the unstable hip, which is not dislocated but can become subluxed or dislocated upon manipulation, and the subluxed hip, in which the femoral head rides on the edge of the acetabulum. The origins are unknown, but laxity of the ligaments around the hip joint, malposition *in utero,* and environmental factors after birth have been suspected. If the femoral head remains outside the acetabulum, bony development of the acetabulum becomes progressively abnormal, and contractures develop. Therefore, the earlier treatment is begun, the better the prognosis for normal hip function. Congenital dislocation and subluxation of the hip are quite common disorders, occurring in 1.5 per 1,000 live births. The deformity is bilateral in more than half of the afflicted children, and girls are affected eight times as often as boys.

PREVENTION

Health Promotion

Parents should be cautioned against swaddling infants with their hips extended and adducted. A more common practice that should also be discouraged is that of grabbing the infant by the ankles and pulling the legs upward during diaper changes.

Population at Risk

1. Newborns and young infants, especially girls.
2. Hip dislocation is found more frequently among cultures that customarily swaddle or tightly wrap blankets around the newborn, forcing the hips into the positions of extension and adduction.
3. Familial patterns exist, so that infants with a family history of hip dislocation are at increased risk.

Screening

Part of routine physical examination for all neonates and infants (see *Assessment*, below).

ASSESSMENT

Health History

1. Cultural practice of swaddling infant.
2. Delayed gross motor development, especially delayed walking.
3. Abnormal ambulation patterns, such as a limp or waddling gait.
4. Family history of hip deformity.

Physical Assessment

1. Newborn: Ortolani test.
   a. With the infant supine, the flexed hip is moved into adduction while pressing the femur downward.
   b. A click is elicited as the hip is moved into abduction and becomes located in the acetabulum.
2. Newborn to age 3 months (refer to Figure 16-1):
   a. There is limited abduction of the hip.
   b. The femur appears shortened when infant lies supine with knees and hips flexed.
   c. There are abnormal gluteal and thigh creases (more or deeper creases on the affected side).
3. After 1 year of age:
   a. A ducklike waddle or "sailor's gait" is noticeable.
   b. Trendelenburg's test is positive. When child stands on leg of affected side, pelvis drops on normal side.

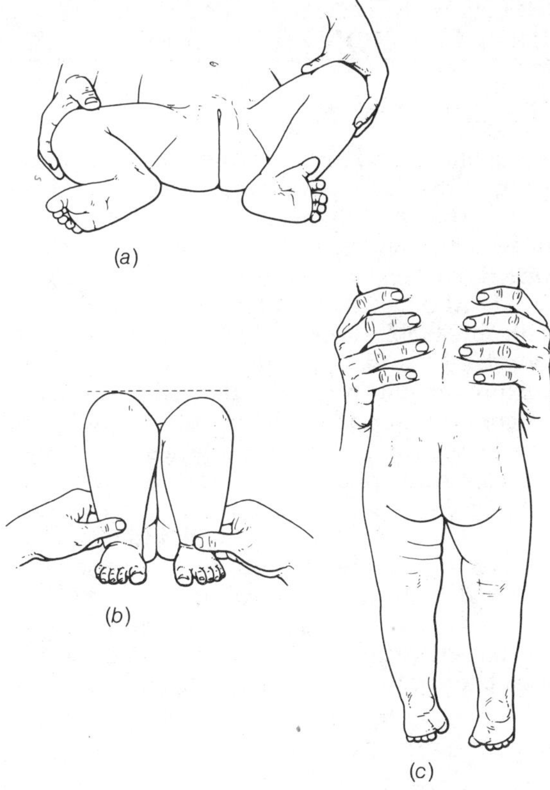

Figure 16-1 Signs of congenital dislocation of the left hip: (*a*) limitation of abduction of left hip, (*b*) apparent displacement of femoral head from the acetabulum and resultant left knee lower than right knee (both soles must be on the same level), and (*c*) asymmetry of gluteal and thigh folds. [Adapted from G. Scipien et al. (eds.), *Comprehensive Pediatric Nursing*, 2d ed., McGraw-Hill, New York, 1979. Used with permission.]

Diagnostic Tests

X-ray examination of the hip shows characteristic changes in the acetabulum and the femoral head, as well as displacement of the joint.

NURSING DIAGNOSES: ACTUAL OR POTENTIAL

1. Impairment of mobility secondary to deformity and abduction devices (i.e., splint, traction, or cast).
2. Risk of impairment of neurovascular function secondary to cast or traction.
3. Ineffective family coping due to demanding treatment regimen, uncertainty of prognosis, and stress of surgery and hospitalization.
4. Alterations in comfort of the child secondary to treatment devices, surgery, and hospitalization.
5. Alterations in body image and self-concept of child secondary to treatment devices, immobility, gait disturbances, or residual hip deformity.

EXPECTED OUTCOMES

1. Congenital deformity will be detected and treatment initiated during the first month of life.
2. Treatment will produce a normal hip joint or keep residual deformity to a minimum.
3. Child's motor development will progress normally or catch up to normal after the treatment period.
4. Complications of casting, traction, or surgery will be prevented or detected early.
5. Child and family will cope successfully with the stresses of illness, hospitalization, and the treatment regimen.

INTERVENTIONS

1. Newborn to 2 months:
   a. Teach parents to apply Frejka pillow or other abduction splint.
   b. Handle infant so that hips remain in abduction.
   c. Discuss modifications in bathing, dressing, and diaper changes with parents.
   d. Discuss appropriate activities for child in splint.
2. After 2 months of age:
   a. Maintain traction.
      (1) Bryant's traction is commonly used in children under 2 years of age or under 30 pounds.
      (2) Buttocks should just clear the bed, so that a hand can pass under.
      (3) Posey restraint maintains child's position in bed, and bandages encircling the legs and feet should be checked daily and rewrapped as necessary to prevent circulatory complications.
   b. Explain purpose of traction and limitations on child's activity while in traction to parents and older child.
   c. Preoperative and postoperative explana-

tions for preschooler or older child can include play in which the child applies cast to doll, using small basin of water and roll of orthopedic plaster.

d. Provide care for child in spica cast. Turn child every 2 hours, check skin and circulation, and prevent cast soilage.
e. Special care is necessary for an incontinent child in a spica cast.
   (1) A Bradford frame allows urine and feces to drain into a bedpan below. If the child is placed directly on bed, the bed can be raised at the head to promote drainage away from the cast.
   (2) Petal cast as soon as dry, apply plastic wrap around edges in perineal area, fasten plastic wrap with tape, and change as necessary.
   (3) A folded diaper or pad is tucked under cast edges and changed frequently. Another diaper is fastened around the cast.
f. Include parents in cast care and discuss modifications for home.
g. Provide age-appropriate activities for child.

EVALUATION

Outcome Criteria

1. A normal hip joint is attained, or residual deformity is minimal.
2. Parents and child comply with treatment program, including follow-up care.
3. Complications of casting, splinting, or traction are avoided.
4. Child's development proceeds at age-appropriate level.
5. Family relationships are normal, and family functions are carried out effectively (see Chapter 5).

Complications

1. Neurovascular impairment of lower extremities secondary to traction or hip spica cast.
2. Residual deformity causing a limp or degenerative hip disease in adult life (see *Total Hip Replacement* in Chapter 27.)

Reevaluation and Follow-up

The time intervals at which reevaluation should be conducted vary with the severity of the deformity and the specific treatment requirements. Physical examination and x-ray films of the hip are used to detect recurrence of dislocation.

OSTEOGENESIS IMPERFECTA (BRITTLE BONE DISEASE)

DESCRIPTION

Osteogenesis imperfecta is a hereditary disorder affecting the connective tissues, particularly the bones. The underlying pathology is failure of collagen to mature; instead of normal compact bone, a coarse, immature type of bone is produced. Manifestations of the disease include easily breakable bones, thin skin and sclerae, poor teeth, and hypermobility of the joints. Fractures result in growth deformities, including curvature or abnormal angulation of limbs, growth retardation due to injuries to the epiphyses, and kyphosis or scoliosis as a result of compression fractures of the vertebral bodies. Fractures may be associated with little pain, especially if they are incomplete. The disease is classified as the *congenita type,* in which multiple fractures are sustained *in utero,* or the *tarda type,* which is characterized by the occurrence of fractures later in infancy or during childhood.

PREVENTION

Health Promotion

People who have this disease and parents who have an affected child should receive genetic counseling. The more severe form, osteogenesis imperfecta congenita, is apparently an autosomal recessive disorder, whereas the tarda form is transmitted by an autosomal dominant gene (Hecht, 1978); however, the inheritance patterns vary more than would be expected from straightforward recessive or dominant transmission (Fialkow, 1980).

Population at Risk

1. Newborns, infants, and young children.
2. Those with a family history of the disorder.

Screening

None.

ASSESSMENT

Health History

1. Family history of other individuals with easily fractured bones.
2. Delayed walking.
3. Multiple, recurrent fractures, occurring at

birth (congenita type) or later in infancy or early childhood (tarda type).

Physical Assessment

1. Signs and symptoms of fractures (same as in a normal child).
   a. Swelling.
   b. Deformity.
   c. Redness.
   d. Heat.
   e. Pain (may not be a complaint when soft tissue injury is minimal).
2. Fractures occur more frequently in lower limbs since they are more prone to trauma.
3. Growth deformities.
   a. Torsional deformities of limbs secondary to fractures and tendency of bones to bend as a consequence of repeated microscopic fractures.
   b. Growth retardation due to abnormal bone development.
   c. Kyphosis or scoliosis as a result of compression fractures of the vertebral bodies.
4. Thin skin.
5. Marked joint laxity.
6. Blue sclerae.
7. Poor teeth secondary to incomplete calcification.
8. Deafness.

NURSING DIAGNOSES: ACTUAL OR POTENTIAL

1. Risk of injury secondary to fragility of bones and teeth.
2. Body image disturbance secondary to growth deformities and treatment measures requiring immobilization for fractures.
3. Impairment of mobility and self-care activities secondary to casts, traction, bone deformities, and susceptibility to fractures.
4. Disturbed peer relationships secondary to frequent hospitalizations and casting that disrupt school and social activities.
5. Alterations in self-concept due to body image disturbance, social isolation, developmental delay, deafness, fear of future fractures, and potential for genetic recurrence of disease.
6. Disturbed family relationships due to guilt and fear of genetic recurrence of disorder, stress caused by frequent fractures and hospitalizations, and dependency of child on others for care.

EXPECTED OUTCOMES

1. Fractures will be prevented or detected and treated early to allow more complete healing.
2. Growth disturbances will be prevented or minimized by appropriate treatment.
3. The child and family will gain a feeling of safety and security from hospital staff.
4. Schooling and social activities will be maintained in hospital and at home.
5. Child's development will proceed as normally as possible, and independence in self-care activities will be maximized.
6. Dental problems (decay, broken teeth, loss of fillings) will be prevented or treated promptly.
7. Hearing impairment will receive appropriate treatment.
8. Parents and child will understand and cope effectively with genetic implications of disease and with chronic condition.

INTERVENTIONS

1. Teach family and child (when old enough) reasonable precautions to avoid fractures (e.g., low bed rather than crib for toddler to minimize injury caused by climbing or falling out of bed).
2. Teach patient and family the signs of fractures and early treatment measures, including splinting the fracture site before bringing child to the hospital.
3. Handle child gently in the hospital to prevent further fractures.
4. Monitor child's condition in traction or cast.
5. Maintain traction or provide cast care.
6. Teach patient and family how to care for the cast at home.
7. Modify clothing, diapering or toileting, bathing, and feeding activities according to the child's needs and self-care capability.
8. Maintain schooling and social activities while the child is hospitalized, and plan with the child and parents for continuing these at home.
9. Discuss realistic activity allowances and limits with child and parents.
10. Plan for preventive and therapeutic dental care; teach proper dental hygiene.
11. Refer parents and older patient for genetic counseling.
12. Refer child for evaluation of suspected hearing impairment.

EVALUATION

Outcome Criteria

1. Fractures from preventable trauma are avoided.
2. Present fracture is corrected satisfactorily.
3. Growth deformities are prevented or treated to achieve maximal correction.
4. Follow-up orthopedic, pediatric, nursing, dental, and audiology care are maintained.
5. Complications of traction and casts are avoided.
6. School and social activities are maintained to meet the child's developmental needs.
7. Parents and child are planning realistically for the future, according to the limitations of the disease and the strengths of the child.

Complications

Osteoporosis secondary to prolonged immobility in casts or traction, which complicates the preexisting osteoporosis. This leads to a vicious cycle of refracture and further atrophy of the bone.

Revised Outcomes

1. Prolonged immobilization during healing of a fracture will be avoided.
2. Fractures will heal at a normal rate and without complication.

Interventions

1. Assist child in use of a walking cast or brace.
2. Provide pre- and postoperative care for the child undergoing insertion of intramedullary metal rods. These rods correct deformity and provide support to prevent further fractures and deformity.

Reevaluation and Follow-up

1. Provide long-term guidance and support for the child and family as they cope with chronic illness.
2. Schedule appointments for evaluation of fracture healing and growth deformities as necessitated by the child's condition.

OSTEOGENIC SARCOMA AND EWING'S SARCOMA

DESCRIPTION

Osteogenic sarcoma is a malignant tumor that arises from the osteoblasts (bone-forming cells) in the metaphysis of a long bone. Hence it appears at sites of active epiphyseal growth, especially the distal end of the femur and the proximal end of the tibia and humerus. Pain begins intermittently at the tumor site and becomes more intense and continuous. Joint function is reduced. Because this neoplasm is highly vascular, swelling over the tumor site is warm to the touch, and overlying veins are dilated. Metastasis to the lungs commonly occurs early in the course of the disease. Pathologic fractures may take place after the bony cortex is eroded. Between 75 and 95 percent of patients die within 5 years.

Ewing's sarcoma is a malignant tumor that arises in the bone marrow. Shafts of the long bones, including the femur, tibia, and humerus are common sites, as are the metatarsals and ileum. The lesion extends longitudinally in the involved bone. Rapidly growing tumor cells soon perforate the cortex of the bone to form a large, palpable, tender soft-tissue mass. Pain at the site becomes increasingly severe. As the central areas of the lesion outgrow their blood supply and degenerate, toxic products enter the bloodstream and cause fever and leukocytosis. Early metastases develop in the lungs, lymph nodes, and other bones. Ninety-five percent of the children die within a few years.

PREVENTION

Health Promotion

No preventive measures are known.

Population at Risk

1. Osteogenic sarcoma is most common (75 percent of cases) in children, adolescents, and young adults.
2. Ewing's sarcoma usually occurs between the ages of 10 and 20 years, but younger children are sometimes affected.
3. For both diseases, boys are affected twice as often as girls.

Screening

None.

ASSESSMENT

Health History

1. Pain at the tumor site that becomes increasingly severe.
2. Development of swelling or a soft tissue mass over the bone.
3. Development of limited movement in the affected joint.

Physical Assessment

1. Pain at tumor site.
2. Swelling or presence of a soft tissue mass over tumor site.
3. Warmth at the site and dilatation of overlying veins.
4. Limitation of motion if the lesion is located at a joint.
5. Pathological fractures.
6. Fever.

Diagnostic Tests

1. X-ray films of bone, lungs, and other sites.
2. Computerized axial tomography (CAT scan) of lungs.
3. Surgical biopsy: results confirm the diagnosis.
4. Hematological tests.
5. Renal function tests.
6. Bone scan.
7. Bone marrow test.
8. Urine tests.
9. Liver function studies.

NURSING DIAGNOSES: ACTUAL OR POTENTIAL

1. Alterations in comfort due to pain, immobility, anxiety, potential pathological fracture, fever, amputation, and potential complications of chemotherapy or radiation therapy.
2. Alteration in body image secondary to presence of mass, amputation, alopecia, or weight loss.
3. Impairment of mobility due to tumor growth, possible amputation, pain, potential fracture, and intravenous chemotherapy.
4. Nutritional deficit and weight loss secondary to illness and side effects of chemotherapy or radiation therapy.
5. Maladaptive coping patterns of the child due to anxiety about prognosis and treatment measures, body image disturbance, hospitalization, disruption of family and peer relationships, immobility, and pain.
6. Ineffective family coping due to potentially fatal prognosis, anxiety about treatment measures, hospitalization, and disruption of family relationships.

EXPECTED OUTCOMES

1. Child's comfort will be maintained as well as possible.
2. Child and family will cope effectively with anxiety about illness, prognosis, and treatment measures.
3. Changes in body image will be incorporated by the child, and a normal image will be maintained through the use of prostheses, wigs, and so forth.
4. Family and peer relationships will be maintained during hospitalization.
5. Alternative methods of mobility will be provided to allow independence in self-care activities.
6. Nutritional status will be maintained as evidenced by height and weight within normal limits for age on a growth chart.
7. Complications of amputation, chemotherapy, and radiation therapy will be prevented or minimized.

INTERVENTIONS

1. Diagnostic period.
   a. Administer analgesics, decrease movement, and use other comfort measures to decrease pain.
   b. Provide alternative means of mobility, such as crutches, wheelchair, or stretcher.
   c. Explain to child and parents what will be done during diagnostic tests and when and where tests will be administered.
   d. Provide pre- and postoperative care associated with surgical biopsy.
   e. Detect and treat complications of illness, such as pathological fracture.
   f. Formulate a consistent approach to be used by all team members during diagnostic period.
   g. Clarify what the child, parents, and siblings have been told and what terms were used.
   h. Be available to listen to misconceptions, concerns, or fears and other feelings regarding diagnosis.
   i. Clarify misconceptions and provide appropriate information about illness and therapy.
2. Treatment period.
   a. In collaboration with team members, provide overall view of therapy program and specific preparation for chemotherapy, radiation therapy, or amputation.
   b. Chemotherapy.
      (1) Monitor patient for drug side effects (Table 16-1).
      (2) Provide nursing measures to control side effects (Table 16-1).

TABLE 16-1 SIDE EFFECTS AND TOXICITY OF DRUGS USED IN TREATMENT OF OSTEOGENIC SARCOMA AND EWING'S SARCOMA

Drug	Side Effects and Toxicity	Special Nursing Measures
Adriamycin (doxorubicin hydrochloride)	Oral ulcerations, anorexia, esophagitis, nausea and vomiting, diarrhea, abdominal pain, alopecia, cardiac toxicity.	ECG should be obtained periodically. Causes red urine (not hematuria) up to 12 days after dose.
Actinomycin D (Dactinomycin, Cosmegen)	Bone marrow depression, diarrhea, nausea and vomiting 4–5 h after dose, oral ulcerations, alopecia, injection site extravasation causes induration.	Observe for skin hypersensitivities, especially at site of radiotherapy.
BCNU	Delayed bone marrow depression (3–5 weeks), nausea and vomiting 6 h after dose, pain along course of vein during administration.	Prevent contact with skin, which causes brown spots. Skin flush and vertigo during administration are due to alcohol diluent.
Bleomycin sulfate (Blenoxane)	Fever, chills, nausea and vomiting, anorexia, mucosal ulcerations, skin hyperpigmentation, induration and erythema of fingers and hands or in areas of radiation therapy, pulmonary toxicity after cumulative dose.	Fever may begin 30 min after infusion and lasts up to 6 h. Treat with acetaminophen and routine nursing measures.
Cis-platinum (CPDD, Cis-Diamminedichloro-Platinum LL)	Nausea and vomiting, mild bone marrow depression, kidney toxicity, hearing loss above the speech range, impaired liver functions.	Hydrate 2–3 times maintenance fluids to avoid renal complications. Serum creatinine and/or creatinine clearance must be normal before drug is given.
Cytoxan Cyclophosphamide)	Bone marrow depression 7–14 days after dose, hemorrhagic cystitis, alopecia, nausea and vomiting 3–4 h after dose, inappropriate ADH secretion, sterility, amenorrhea, aspermia.	Force fluids, 2,000–5,000 ml per day for average child. Empty bladder every 4 h. Hematest urine.
Methotrexate (high dose)	Bone marrow depression, oral mucositis 3–5 days after dose, GI ulcerations, hepatotoxicity, alopecia, osteoporosis, renal involvement.	Have citrovorum factor on hand before giving drug. Serum creatinine and/or creatinine clearance must be normal. Avoid vitamins during administration (folic acid antagonist).
Citrovorum factor (Folinic acid, Leucovorin calcium)	Other than rare allergic reactions, no specific toxicity.	Administer 2 h after high-dose methotrexate to rescue normal cells from much of the toxicity of methotrexate.
Vincristine (Oncovin)	Neurotoxicity, jaw pain, paresthesias, loss of deep tendon reflexes, constipation, abdominal pain, ptosis, hoarseness, alopecia, injection site extravasation causes induration, inappropriate ADH secretion.	Avoid extravasation. Use stool softeners and dietary measures to prevent or manage constipation.

SOURCE: Adapted from a drug information sheet by Morse, M., R.N., M.S.N., P.N.P., and Flummerfelt, P., R.N., M.S.N., P.N.P.; James Whitcomb Riley Hospital for Children, the Division of Pediatric Hematology-Oncology, Indianapolis, IN, July, 1980.

(a) Good oral hygiene for oral ulcerations.
(b) Antiemetics for nausea and vomiting.
(c) Stool softeners for constipation.
(d) High fluid intake to prevent kidney toxicity.
(e) Take precautions to prevent infections.
(f) Discuss obtaining wig or other prostheses.

c. Radiation therapy.
(1) Monitor for side effects: general malaise, anorexia, skin breakdown, and decreased resistance to infection.
(2) Provide nursing measures to control side effects.
(a) Rest to counteract lethargy.

(b) Diet changes for anorexia.
(c) Antiemetics to attempt to control nausea and vomiting.

d. Amputation.
   (1) Give extra support to adolescent already dealing with normal concerns about body changes, body image, and sexual identity.
   (2) Provide general nursing care as described in Chapter 27.
e. Provide continuity of care in hospital and outpatient department to support child in grieving process.
f. Support family members through continuity of care and counseling about child's needs.

EVALUATION

Outcome Criteria

1. Pain is eradicated by treatment of tumor.
2. Child, parents, and siblings understand and cope effectively with illness, prognosis, and plan of treatment.
3. Body image changes are incorporated by the child as he or she works to maintain a healthy image of body and self.
4. Family relationships are strengthened as they cope effectively with stress.
5. Child returns to school or normal activities and supportive peer relationships after hospitalization.
6. Maximum mobility is achieved to allow independence in self-care activities despite limitations.
7. Child's height and weight are within normal limits for age.
8. Complications of treatment are prevented or minimized by early detection.

Complications

METASTASES CAN OCCUR, ESPECIALLY TO THE LUNGS

Reevaluation and Follow-up

1. Maintain long-term follow-up to detect recurrence of tumor or metastases.
2. Assist child in adapting to prosthesis and grieving the loss of amputated body part.
3. When a fatal prognosis is confirmed, support child and family in their grieving.
4. In the period after child's death, provide support for family members to help them continue to resolve grief.

INFLAMMATIONS

OSTEOMYELITIS AND SEPTIC ARTHRITIS

DESCRIPTION

Osteomyelitis is a bacterial infection of bone; septic arthritis is bacterial infection of a joint. Common causative agents are staphylococcus and streptococcus. *Proteus* and *Pseudomonas* also are frequently the causes of osteomyelitis. Bacteria typically enter the body through skin infections, mucous membrane infections of the nose or throat, or open fractures or other wounds. Bacterial access to the bone or joint may be through the bloodstream or by direct extension from the focus of infection. Infection may spread from septic arthritis to neighboring bone, and vice versa. Traumatized bone seems particularly susceptible to bacteria, especially at the metaphysis, which has a sluggish blood flow.

Osteomyelitis most often involves the long bones that are growing rapidly—femur, tibia, humerus, and radius, for example. (Refer to Chapter 27 for more information.) Septic arthritis most often involves the hip joint, with the knee and elbow following in frequency. More than one joint may be affected. The inflammation begins in the synovial membrane. Pus forms in the synovial fluid, and the articular cartilage is rapidly destroyed. Osteomyelitis of the underlying bone may follow. Pathological dislocation and necrosis of the epiphysis and epiphyseal plate can complicate the disease and produce growth disturbances in the affected limb.

PREVENTION

Health Promotion

1. Reinforce safety measures during play to prevent a portal of entry for bacteria through scratches, abrasions, or wounds.
2. Encourage prompt medical treatment of wounds, boils, and upper respiratory tract infections.

Population at Risk

1. Boys are afflicted four times as often as girls, possibly because they have a higher incidence of trauma.
2. In the presence of a bacteremia, a traumatized area of bone is more likely to be affected.
3. Infants and children of one or two years have the highest incidence of septic arthritis.

Screening

None.

ASSESSMENT

Health History

1. Recent occurrence of a wound, boil, or upper respiratory tract infection.
2. Early signs and symptoms reported by parents: pain, unwillingness to move the limb, irritability, weakness, lack of appetite, fever.

Physical Assessment

1. There is pain in the involved joint or limb.
2. Child is unwilling to move the limb and guards it against movement.
3. Patient is irritable and weak.
4. There is soft tissue swelling, with redness and heat.
5. Muscle spasms are present around the joint in septic arthritis.
6. Fever is present.
7. Child has poor appetite.

Diagnostic Tests

1. White blood cell count is elevated.
2. Positive culture of wound or aspirate, plus sensitivity to drugs.
3. X-ray examination reveals destruction of bone after several days.

NURSING DIAGNOSES: ACTUAL OR POTENTIAL

1. Alterations in comfort secondary to pain, immobility, fever, and intravenous therapy.
2. Impairment of mobility due to pain, swelling, muscle spasms, traction, splint or cast, and intravenous therapy.
3. Nutritional deficit due to anorexia, immobility, and strange environment.
4. Sensory-perceptual alteration secondary to immobility, boredom, and social isolation.
5. Ineffective family coping associated with long-term illness and therapy, hospitalization, and unknown prognosis.

EXPECTED OUTCOMES

1. Illness will be diagnosed and appropriate treatment begun within the first few days of onset of signs and symptoms.
2. Child will comply with immobilization of limb to decrease pain, prevent movement that spreads infection, and prevent contractures in soft tissues.
3. Child will cope successfully with stresses of illness and hospitalization.
4. Nutritional requirements will be met.
5. Age appropriate developmental needs of the child will be met.
6. Family members will cope successfully with stresses of child's illness and hospitalization.

INTERVENTIONS

1. Refer child suspected of having either of these disorders to a physician for immediate diagnosis and treatment.
2. Place child on bed rest and maintain immobilization of limb or joint in traction, splint, or cast.
3. Pre- and postoperative care following surgery for decompression of the infected bony area or exploration of the joint.
4. Monitor and maintain system for closed infusion and drainage, if used, including accurate intake and output records.
5. Monitor and protect intravenous line.
6. Plan for age-appropriate activities, including schooling, play, and group activities; activities can be brought to the child, or patient can be taken to them in bed or wheelchair.
7. Provide alternative means of mobility for child, such as wheelchair or stretcher, when possible.
8. Involve parents in care, explaining illness and therapy program and needs of the child during long-term hospitalization.

EVALUATION

Outcome Criteria

1. Infection is eradicated by early and complete treatment.
2. Child's comfort needs are met as completely as possible.
3. Child's nutritional status is adequate.
4. Child is at an appropriate developmental level.
5. Complications of therapy are prevented.
6. Parents and child cope adequately with long-term illness.

Complications

CHRONIC OSTEOMYELITIS DUE TO INADEQUATE TREATMENT OF THE ACUTE PHASE

Assessment

1. Residual painful lesion in the involved long bone.
2. Swelling, tenderness, and loss of function of the limb.
3. There may be draining sinuses in the area.
4. X-ray film reveals obvious sequestra (separated and infected areas of dead bone).
5. Persistent anemia and elevation of the sedimentation rate reflect the chronic infection.

Revised Outcomes

1. Areas of dead bone will be removed surgically.
2. Infection will be eradicated by additional intravenous antibiotic therapy.
3. Residual defects in the bone and soft tissues will be prevented or corrected.

Interventions

1. Pre- and postoperative care of the patient undergoing sequestrectomy (surgical removal of dead bone).
2. Monitor and maintain intravenous antibiotic therapy and continuous infusions to the infected area.
3. Assist physician with reconstructive procedures, such as bone grafting and skin grafting for residual defects.

NECROSIS OF THE EPIPHYSIS FROM SEPTIC ARTHRITIS, WHICH RESULTS IN GROWTH DISTURBANCE OF THE LIMB

(See *Epiphyseal Plate Fracture*)

Reevaluation and Follow-up

Follow-up must be maintained to detect complications of these disorders. Appointments are scheduled at intervals of a few months to detect growth disorders of the affected limb; follow-up may need to be continued for several years. Parents are taught to recognize and report signs and symptoms of major complications.

JUVENILE RHEUMATOID ARTHRITIS

DESCRIPTION

Juvenile rheumatoid arthritis (JRA) is a childhood disease characterized by inflammation of one or more joints. It is estimated that between 150,000 and 250,000 children are affected by the disease in the United States. The etiology is unknown; however, evidence suggests that the primary problem is either a hypersensitivity response in which normal immune mechanisms are exaggerated or a reaction to presently unknown infectious agents.

Juvenile rheumatoid arthritis is classified into three types: (1) systemic onset, including fever, rash, and organ involvement; (2) polyarticular onset, characterized by involvement of five or more joints during the first 6 months of disease and excluding systemic signs, and (3) pauciarticular onset, with involvement of four or fewer joints in the first 6 months of disease. In an affected joint, inflammation of the synovial membrane leads to edema and cellular proliferation. Granulation tissue infiltrates the synovial membrane, producing swelling. Scar tissue replaces the granulation tissue, causing joint contractures. Secondarily, muscles are affected by inflammation and joint immobility. Other body systems and organs may be affected by inflammation. The clinical course for children with JRA involves many exacerbations and remissions.

PREVENTION

Health Promotion

No preventive measures are known.

Population at Risk

1. Girls are afflicted four times as frequently as boys.
2. Preschool and school-age children are the principal victims.
3. Familial patterns (possible genetic predisposition) have been suggested but not proved.

Screening

None.

ASSESSMENT

Health History

1. History of systemic signs and symptoms: Fever, rash, generalized discomfort, abdominal pain.
2. Localized signs and symptoms: joint swelling and pain, limited movement, limp.
3. Family history of rheumatic disease.

Physical Assessment

1. Peripheral involvement (present in one joint for longer than 6 weeks).
   a. Joint swelling.
   b. Mild warmth over joint.
   c. Tenderness and pain.

   d. Limitation of motion (particularly morning stiffness).
   e. Limp.
2. Systemic involvement.
   a. Fever, persistent for 2 or more weeks and characterized by daily spikes.
   b. Rheumatoid rash; a salmon pink, macular rash on the chest, axillae, buttocks, and to a lesser extent, on the extremities.
   c. Malaise.
   d. Subcutaneous nodules (usually on fingers, toes, wrist, elbow).
   e. Lymphadenopathy.
   f. Hepatosplenomegaly.
   g. Pericarditis.

Diagnostic Tests

1. Rheumatoid factor (positive in 20 percent of affected children).
2. Erythrocyte sedimentation rate (elevated).
3. Complete blood cell count (mild anemia may be present).
4. Immunological studies.
5. Synovial fluid analysis (documents inflammation in joint fluid).
6. X-ray examination (articular changes).

NURSING DIAGNOSES: ACTUAL OR POTENTIAL

1. Alteration in comfort due to joint pain, immobility, fever, malaise, or skin rash.
2. Impairment of mobility secondary to joint stiffness.
3. Alteration in self-care activities secondary to loss of movement and function in extremities.
4. Risk of side effects associated with drug therapy regimen.
5. Alteration in body image secondary to joint swelling, immobility, skin rash, and subcutaneous nodules.
6. Noncompliance associated with long-term therapy.
7. Disturbed family relationships due to uncertain prognosis, long-term illness, and requirements of therapy program.
8. Disturbed peer relationships due to frequent hospitalizations with severe disease, social isolation, architectural barriers restricting mobility, disruption of schooling, and body image disturbance.

EXPECTED OUTCOMES

1. Child's comfort will be maintained during exacerbations of disease.
2. Range of motion and maximum function will be maintained in affected joints.
3. Drug complications will be prevented or noted early.
4. Child and parents will comply with the program of therapy.
5. Schooling, social activities, and age-appropriate self-care will be maintained in the hospital and during active disease states.
6. Child and family will cope adequately with the stresses of illness and therapy.

INTERVENTIONS

1. Maintain bed rest or immobilize joints with splints during acute, painful exacerbations.
2. Position the involved joints in extension to prevent stiffness and contractures.
3. Provide passive range of motion, if tolerated, during acute, painful episodes.
4. Reinforce active exercise program as tolerated by patient.
5. Assist with warm baths, showers, or hot packs to overcome morning stiffness.
6. Refer patient to occupational therapy or physical therapy.
7. Encourage diversional activities that involve movement, when tolerated, and that are directed toward child's developmental level.
8. Discuss disease, its course, and therapy program with child and parents.
9. Observe for side effects of prescribed drugs (see Table 16-2) and administer drugs as ordered.
10. Arrange for school and peer activities when child is hospitalized.
11. Assist child and family in coping with long-term disease.

EVALUATION

Outcome Criteria

1. Signs and symptoms of disease respond to treatment.
2. Full range of motion and functional movement are maintained in affected joints.
3. Child's comfort is maintained as much as possible during acute episodes of disease.
4. Blood levels of drugs are maintained at therapeutic levels.
5. Child maintains age-appropriate developmental skills.
6. Parents and child follow treatment program and seek regular medical follow-up.
7. Family relationships are normal, and essen-

TABLE 16-2 DRUGS USED IN TREATMENT OF JUVENILE RHEUMATOID ARTHRITIS

Drug	Specific Action	Route of Administration	Side Effects or Toxicity
Salicylates	Antipyretic, analgesic, anti-inflammatory	PO, IV	Abdominal pain, gastric bleeding (occult blood in stool), hyperventilation in the small child, tinnitis in the older child.
Gold	Unknown	IM	Skin rashes, nephritis with hematuria or albuminuria, thrombocytopenia, neurotoxicity
Steroids	Anti-inflammatory	PO, IV, IM, intra-articular	Masking of infection, peptic ulcer, vascular disorders, hypertension, increased intraocular pressure (blurry or dim vision), osteoporosis with pathological fractures, euphoria or other mental disturbance, glycosuria, weight gain secondary to water retention, appetite stimulation

SOURCE: Scipien, G., et al. (eds.): *Comprehensive Pediatric Nursing*, 2d ed., McGraw-Hill, New York, 1979. Used with permission.

tial family functions are carried out (see Chapter 5).

Complications

1. Joint deformities (subluxation, dislocation, contractures).
2. Growth disturbances (leg length discrepancy, small stature).
3. Iridocyclitis (inflammation of the iris and ciliary body).

Assessment

1. Approximately 80 percent of the iridocyclitis that occurs in JRA occurs in girls with pauciarticular arthritis (Lindsley, 1977).
2. Antinuclear antibodies are frequently elevated in the presence of chronic iridocyclitis.
3. Early signs of disease can only be detected by a special slit-lamp ophthalmology exam.
4. Iridocyclitis leads to diminished vision and ultimately to blindness.

Revised Outcomes

Diagnosis of eye complications will be made early, when treatment will be more effective.

Interventions

Drug treatment does not cure iridocyclitis but can slow its course and prevent the secondary complication of glaucoma. Drugs used include 1% atropine administered topically, 10% phenylephrine topically, and systemic or topical corticosteroids.

Reevaluation and Follow-up

1. Follow-up appointments are scheduled at intervals of a few months to assess the progress of rheumatoid arthritis and check blood levels of drugs.
2. A slit-lamp examination by an ophthalmologist should be scheduled every 3 to 6 months to detect iridocyclitis.
3. Family history of osteochondroses.

HYPERACTIVITY AND HYPOACTIVITY

LEGG-PERTHES DISEASE

DESCRIPTION

Legg-Perthes disease is one of a group of disorders called the *osteochondroses*, which share the common pathology of idiopathic avascular necrosis of the epiphysis. In this disease, the hip is the involved joint. The cause is unknown, but physical activity or trauma may play a part.

The disease progresses through four phases. In phase one, there is spontaneous interruption of the blood supply to the upper femoral epiphysis, and epiphyseal cells die. In phase two, there is revascularization in the area of dead bone. Pathological fractures occur because of bone weakness and are associated with pain and limited hip motion. In phase three, healing takes place, and new bone replaces the dead bone. In the fourth phase, healing is complete but the hip joint may show residual deformity. The disease process may continue for 2 to 8 years.

PREVENTION

Health Promotion

No preventive measures are known.

Population at Risk

1. Boys are affected four to five times as often as girls.
2. Age of onset is 3 to 11 years, usually between 4 and 7.

Screening

None.

ASSESSMENT

Health History

1. Parents report signs and symptoms: pain, decreased leg movement, limp.
2. History of trauma preceding signs and symptoms.

Physical Assessment

1. There is pain in the hip or pain referred to the knee or inner thigh.
2. A protective limp is present.
3. Movement is limited in the hip joint.
4. Muscles of the upper thigh atrophy from disuse.

Diagnostic Tests

X-ray examination demonstrates characteristic changes in the hip joint.

NURSING DIAGNOSES: ACTUAL OR POTENTIAL

1. Alterations in comfort secondary to pain and immobility.
2. Impairment of mobility secondary to defect and treatment devices.
3. Body image disturbance due to immobility and necessity of wearing immobilizing device, such as cast or brace.
4. Disruption of peer relationships secondary to hospitalization, immobility, body image disturbance, and interruption of school and social activities.
5. Disturbed family relationships due to anxiety about hospitalization, stress of chronic illness, and requirements of treatment program.

EXPECTED OUTCOMES

1. Defect will be detected by early in phase two, and treatment will be initiated.
2. Pain will be decreased by immobilization.
3. Immobilization will be successfully maintained to prevent complications and allow healing.
4. Child will accomplish age-appropriate developmental tasks despite treatment restrictions.
5. Child and family will cope successfully with illness and therapy.

INTERVENTIONS

1. Refer child with suspicious symptoms for early diagnosis.
2. Maintain child on bed rest, in traction, or in cast during hospitalization.
3. Administer analgesics for relief of pain.
4. Explain nature of disease and treatment regimen to child and family.
5. Provide pre- and postoperative care for the child and family, if surgery is performed.
6. Plan for home care of the child in an immobilizing device.
7. Plan for continuing school and social activities in the hospital, and discuss plans for home activities with parents.
8. Emphasize importance of following the treatment regimen over a long time period to help prevent residual deformity and promote healing.

EVALUATION

Outcome Criteria

1. Contour of hip joint allows normal function after resolution of disease.
2. Child is at appropriate developmental and educational level.

3. Child and family cope adequately with stress of illness and long-term immobilization; family relationships are constructive, and essential family functions are carried out (see Chapter 5).

Complications

1. Pathological fractures (refer to Chapter 27 for treatment of client with hip fracture).
2. Residual deformity, such as subluxation or flattening of the epiphysis.

Assessment

1. Limitation of motion in hip joint.
2. Deformity shown on x-ray films.

Revised Outcomes

Correction of deformity will be achieved, leading to a more normal joint contour.

Intervention

Surgical treatment by open reduction or osteotomy to correct deformity. Osteotomy and realignment of the femur may be done prophylactically to prevent deformity.

Reevaluation and Follow-up

Follow-up appointments are scheduled periodically to check for progression of the disease.

STRUCTURAL SCOLIOSIS

DESCRIPTION

Structural scoliosis is lateral curvature of the spine caused by structural changes of the spine. Scoliosis may develop as a result of paralysis, neurofibromatosis, or other disease entity, or it may be idiopathic. The structural features of scoliosis include rotation of the vertebral bodies in the area of the greatest curve. The curvature increases as the child grows, causing secondary changes in the ribs and in the vertebrae, which become wedge-shaped in the middle of the curve from pressure on one side of the epiphyseal plate. In idiopathic scoliosis of adolescence, a right thoracic curve is most common. The prognosis for children with idiopathic scoliosis is best when (1) the curve is mild at the time of diagnosis and initial treatment, and (2) the curve begins at an older age and growth is near completion. Untreated scoliosis leads to degenerative joint disease of the spine in adulthood. Respiration may be compromised, and pain may be progressive.

PREVENTION

Health Promotion

No preventive measures are known.

Population at Risk

1. Children with bony defects of the spine (e.g., spina bifida).
2. Children with neuromuscular disorders conducive to curvature (e.g., poliomyelitis, cerebral palsy, muscular dystrophy).
3. For idiopathic scoliosis:
   a. Girls are affected about twice as often as boys.
   b. Curvature may develop at any age but most commonly appears in early adolescence.
   c. Children with a family history of spinal curvature are at special risk; idiopathic scoliosis tends to recur in families, apparently because of a genetic factor.

Screening

Mass school screening programs are recommended (see *Physical Assessment*, below).

ASSESSMENT

Health History

1. An uneven hemline is noticed.
2. One shoulder blade is higher than the other.
3. One hip is more prominent.
4. Spinal curve is noted.
5. History of spinal curvature in other family members.

Physical Assessment

Scoliosis screening program:

a. Population—all children in grades 5 through 8 (ages 10 through 13) should be screened yearly.
b. Setting—physical education class.
c. Procedure—boys strip to the waist; girls may wear a bra or halter top or a bathing suit. The examiner conducts a simple, systematic examination of each child's back, as described in Table 16-3.

Diagnostic Tests

Full length spinal x-ray film reveals the curvature.

NURSING DIAGNOSES: ACTUAL OR POTENTIAL

1. Alterations in body image and self-concept secondary to spinal deformity, Milwaukee

TABLE 16-3 EXAMINATION OF THE BACK: ROUTINE SCOLIOSIS SCREENING

Position of Child	Observations by the Examiner[a]
1. Standing erect, feet together, arms hanging straight down[b]	a. Shoulder level unequal? b. Hip level unequal? c. Waistline uneven? d. Spine curved? e. One shoulder blade more prominent f. than the other? Distances between arms and body unequal?
2. Bending forward at the waist, back parallel to floor, feet together, knees unbent, arms hanging freely, palms together[c]	a. Difference in level between the two sides of the back? b. Hump on one side of the upper back? c. Compensating hump on the other side of the lower back?

SOURCE: Adapated from the film, "Scoliosis Screening for Early Detection," Multi Video International, Inc., Minneapolis, 1975.
[a] If findings are positive, there is a possibility of scoliosis.
[b] Examiner seated, observing child from the rear.
[c] Examiner seated, observing child from front and rear.

brace, Risser cast, back stiffness due to rod, periods of immobility, and decreased independence.
2. Alterations in comfort due to preoperative anxiety and postoperative pain and immobility.
3. Impairment of mobility both pre- and postoperatively secondary to treatment devices and surgery.
4. Disturbed family relationships due to genetic recurrence of disease, stress of complying with treatment measures, anxiety of hospitalization and surgery, and increased dependence of adolescent during postoperative immobilization.

EXPECTED OUTCOMES

1. Spinal curvature will respond to treatment, either conservative or surgical, as indicated.
2. Anxiety of child and parents will be reduced as they learn about the treatment program and comply with it.
3. Discomfort due to pain and immobility will be kept at a minimum level.
4. Adolescent will continue to meet most developmental tasks, despite postoperative immobility and dependence.
5. Spinal curvature, if present in other family members will be detected.
6. Family members will cope effectively with adolescent's illness.
7. Treatment for associated disorders will be maintained (e.g., cardiopulmonary compromise secondary to decreased vital capacity, neurological deficits).

INTERVENTIONS

1. General adolescent care.
   a. Provide opportunities for expression of concerns about body image and changes.
   b. Provide privacy.
   c. Facilitate independence but recognize need for dependence.
   d. Provide health education, including sexuality.
   e. Allow for appropriate socialization.
2. Psychosocial needs complicated by illness.
   a. Provide information that supports medical plan before initiating plan.
   b. Involve patient in scheduling of activities.
   c. Expose patient to others who have achieved positive outcomes after similar therapy.

3. Family involvement and teaching. Include family in planning and counseling.
4. Care of secondary problems related to associated disorders.
   a. Develop nursing care plan and interventions for each specific physical deviation.
   b. Evaluate needs for teaching and follow-through care.
5. Milwaukee brace.
   a. Monitor fit of brace; refer to orthotist for adjustments as needed.
   b. Monitor condition of skin; teach patient to remove brace at first signs of skin breakdown and gradually increase wearing time after area is healed.
   c. Assess patient's compliance with program; offer incentives to reinforce compliance.
6. Cotrel traction.
   a. Monitor traction setup, and teach patient proper use.
   b. Assess skin condition; apply lamb's wool to potential pressure areas at pelvis and mandible.
   c. Supervise activity periods in traction and rest periods out of traction.
7. Halo-femoral traction.
   a. Monitor traction setup.
   b. Monitor patient for complications.
   c. Discuss appropriate activity and movement in traction.
   d. Teach leg exercises: dorsiflexion and plantar flexion of ankle, flexion-extension of knee, quadriceps-setting exercises.
   e. Prevent skin breakdown by preapplication of Betadine shampoo, cleansing of pin sites with hydrogen peroxide and Betadine, and frequent turning and skin care.
   f. Encourage breathing exercises, and turn to prevent respiratory compromise.
   g. Provide stimulation through peer interaction, conversation, radio, television, and use of prism glasses in activities.
8. Harrington rod insertion or Dwyer instrumentation and fusion.
   a. Preoperatively instruct patient and family about surgery and postoperative therapy, such as logrolling, breathing exercises, and use of fracture bedpan.
   b. Postoperative care.
      (1) For immobilization, logroll in bed or use Stryker frame or Circolectric bed.
      (2) Keep patient as comfortable as possible, and administer analgesics for pain.
      (3) Observe for complications by measuring vital signs and intake and output, and by observing wound, skin at pressure points, neurological function in lower extremities, bladder function, and bowel function.
      (4) Have patient perform breathing exercises: blow bottles and perhaps intermittent positive pressure breathing machine.
      (5) Maintain skin integrity by turning every 2 hours, give skin care with each turning, and use sheepskin to pad pressure points.
      (6) Minimize boredom. Establish daily schedule; provide for interactions with peers; arrange activities of interest; resume schooling; and provide prism glasses, bedboard, and easels.
9. Risser jacket application and care.
   a. Prepare patient and accompany during application.
   b. Maintain integrity of cast by careful handling when wet, petaling when dry.
   c. Observe patient for complications by monitoring circulation, respirations, abdominal distress, and skin condition.
   d. Assist patient to develop safe methods for activities and for mobility in cast, if allowed.
10. Alterations needed in home. Plan with patient and family for home care alterations in mobility, activities of daily living, school, and social activities.
11. Recommend scoliosis screening of family members. (Anderson and D'Ambra, 1976)

EVALUATION

Outcome Criteria

1. Therapy program is effective in preventing curve from progressing or brings about correction of curve.
2. Associated problems are controlled.
3. Patient and family discuss and demonstrate knowledge and compliance with home care instructions.
4. Patient and family cope adequately with disease and therapy program.

5. Home environment is adapted to patient's needs.
6. Patient achieves developmental tasks appropriate for age.
7. Family members are screened for scoliosis, and plans are made for future screening of growing children.

Complications

1. Milwaukee brace.
   a. Skin breakdown from improper fit.
2. Cotrel traction.
   a. Skin breakdown at pressure points, especially chin and pelvis.
   b. Fatigue.
3. Halo-femoral traction.
   a. Skin breakdown.
   b. Footdrop.
   c. Contractures.
   d. Nerve compression causing diminished reflexes.
   e. Organ displacement.
   f. Thrombophlebitis.
   g. Pin tract osteomyelitis.
   h. Respiratory compromise.
   i. Motor, sensory, and social deprivation.
4. Spinal fusion and Harrington rod or Dwyer instrumentation.
   a. Shock.
   b. Urinary retention.
   c. Respiratory compromise.
   d. Skin breakdown.
   e. Wound bleeding, dehiscence, or infection.
   f. Neurological deficits.
   g. Paralytic ileus.
   h. Displacement of the rod or instrument.
   i. Motor, sensory, and social deprivation.
   j. Thrombophlebitis.
   k. Constipation.
5. Risser jacket cast.
   a. Circulatory compromise.
   b. Skin breakdown at pressure points.
   c. Discomfort and difficulty sleeping.

UNTREATED SCOLIOSIS

1. Cardiopulmonary compromise.
2. Progressive pain.
3. Degenerative joint disease of the spine.

Reevaluation and Follow-up

1. The adolescent will need to be seen at intervals of 2 to 3 months postoperatively for cast changes and to check for complications.
2. Instructions and suggested activities should be given about mobility limits in the postoperative cast period and later, when patient will experience a stiff back due to the Harrington rod.
3. Because spinal curvature may increase during pregnancy and in the middle years, long-term follow-up should be maintained in adulthood.

DEGENERATIVE DISEASES

DUCHENNE'S MUSCULAR DYSTROPHY

DESCRIPTION

Duchenne's muscular dystrophy is a progressive muscle disorder characterized by muscle weakness. It usually becomes manifest during the preschool years and progresses until death occurs in young adulthood. The common form is found only in boys and is a sex-linked recessive trait. Other types of muscular dystrophy that occur later in life and progress more slowly include facioscapulohumeral and limb-girdle dystrophies.

Because of specific enzyme elevations, a biochemical defect in the muscle tissue is suspected to be the underlying pathology. Progressive muscle wasting is accompanied by *pseudohypertrophy*, in which excessive fibrous tissue and fat cause the muscles to appear to grow larger. The disease runs a relentless course without remissions, and few boys survive beyond age 20 years. Causes of death include respiratory infection, respiratory acidosis, and cardiac failure.

PREVENTION

Health Promotion

Genetic counseling is indicated to inform parents about the risks that future sons will also inherit the disease. The risk that daughters may be carriers of the disorder should also be explained.

Population at Risk

Sons (usually) of female carriers.

Screening

None.

ASSESSMENT

Health History

1. Boy between 2 and 7 years of age.
2. Tires easily and cannot keep up with his playmates.
3. Delays in motor development, such as difficulty in running or climbing stairs.
4. Frequent stumbling and falling.

Physical Assessment

1. Early signs.
   a. Flat feet.
   b. Symmetrical weakness of the pelvic muscles, particularly the gluteus maximus.
   c. *Gowers' sign.* In getting up from the floor, child must "climb up his legs" with his hands.
   d. Pseudohypertrophy of muscles, characteristically in the calf muscles, due to excessive fibrous tissue and fat.
2. Later signs.
   a. Lordosis.
   b. Waddling gait.
   c. Walking on toes.
   d. Scoliosis due to weakness of the trunk and shoulder girdle.
   e. Contractures of the elbows, feet, knees, and hips.

Diagnostic Tests

1. Elevated enzyme levels of creatine phosphokinase (CPK).
2. Abnormal electromyogram (EMG).
3. Abnormal muscle biopsy specimen.

NURSING DIAGNOSES: ACTUAL OR POTENTIAL

1. Altered mobility patterns secondary to progressive weakness and deformities.
2. Disturbed peer relationships secondary to physical limitations, chronic illness, and prognosis.
3. Disturbed family relationships secondary to familial disease, child's disability, care requirements, and prognosis.
4. Altered ability to perform self-care activities.
5. Altered nutritional requirements, excretory patterns, and cardiorespiratory efficiency due to inactivity.
6. Altered self-concept secondary to disability.

EXPECTED OUTCOMES

1. Accidents due to gait instability will be prevented.
2. Anxiety of child and family about diagnostic tests will be minimized by preparation.
3. Parents and older child will understand disease and its course.
4. Child and family will feel supported in their grieving.
5. Appropriate modifications will be made in the home and daily routines to encourage child's independence and socialization.
6. Preventive measures will be taken to decrease complications of immobility.
7. Child and family will receive continuous support and assistance with decision making during terminal stage of illness.

INTERVENTIONS

1. Diagnostic period.
   a. Provide for child's safety needs, which will be increased due to gait and movement disturbances.
   b. Prepare child for EMG according to developmental age (e.g., needle play or other dramatic play).
   c. Preoperative preparation for child and family is necessary (e.g., dramatic play of surgery and discussion of postoperative appearance).
   d. Postoperative care after muscle biopsy will include vital signs, bed rest, and observation of wound.
   e. Explain, clarify, and reinforce parents' knowledge of nature of disease, expected course, and how parents can help their child.
   f. Support family in beginning stages of grieving.
   g. Provide information on genetic transmission and/or refer for genetic counseling.
2. Treatment period.
   a. Refer child to physical therapy, occupational therapy, and social service.
   b. Teach child and family about special treatment measures, such as drugs or bracing.

c. Discuss general care needs, including activity, diet, and rest.
d. Plan for modifications needed at home to promote child's independence.
   (1) Remove architectural barriers.
   (2) Modify clothing.
   (3) Change daily routines of bathing, dressing, feeding, unrinating, and defecating.
   (4) Reorganize school, social, and recreational activities according to level of disability.
e. Teach proper positioning of child in wheelchair to prevent complications, such as contractures.
f. Provide long-term support to help child cope with grieving and fears of death.

3. Terminal period.
   a. Support and assist parents in their grieving and decision making about care of the child in terminal stage.
   b. Provide family with an opportunity to discuss feelings and concerns after child's death.

EVALUATION

Outcome Criteria

1. Parents understand nature of illness, prognosis, and genetic recurrence risks.
2. Child and family cope effectively with diagnostic and surgical procedures.
3. Parents plan realistically for care of child at home.
4. Child functions at maximal potential throughout course of illness.
5. Unnecessary complications are prevented.
6. Child deals effectively with fears and grief.
7. Family able to resolve their grief after child's death.

Complications

1. Respiratory insufficiency and infection (see Chapter 20).
2. Cardiomyopathy, possibly due to replacement fibrosis of the myocardium, and manifested by cardiac arrhythmias and congestive heart failure (see Chapter 19).

Reevaluation and Follow-up

The child should be seen at regular intervals (every few months) to assess the progress of the disease and occurrence of complications. The services of a variety of health professionals are necessary for successful management. The nurse focuses on the child within the context of his family and community, considering both physical and psychosocial needs.

TRAUMATIC INJURIES

EPIPHYSEAL PLATE FRACTURE

DESCRIPTION

The epiphyseal plate lies between the shaft of the bone and its epiphysis. The plate is the part of the bone from which new bone is produced when children grow. The epiphyseal plate can be separated from the bone shaft by trauma, with or without associated bone fracture, as shown in Figure 16-2. Disruption of the vessels to the epiphysis causes both the epiphysis and the plate to become necrotic (*avascular necrosis*), and growth of the bone ceases.

PREVENTION

Health Promotion

Teaching childhood safety measures, such as the use of child restraints in automobiles and bicycle safety rules, is one means of decreasing accidents and, therefore, fractures in children.

Population at Risk

Everyone.

Screening

None.

ASSESSMENT

Health History

Describe the mechanism of injury, including type and severity of force and location of impact on the body.

Physical Assessment

Signs of a fracture:
   a. Swelling.
   b. Deformity.
   c. Redness and heat.
   d. Pain.

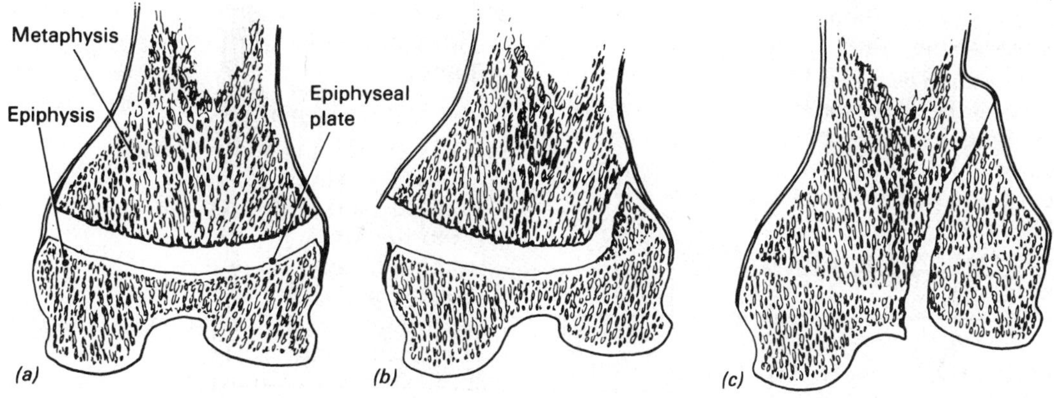

Figure 16-2 Common types of epiphyseal plate fracture: (*a*) complete separation of the epiphysis, (*b*) partial separation of the epiphysis and fracture through the metaphysis, and (*c*) fracture across the epiphyseal plate and the metaphysis.

Diagnostic Tests

X-ray examination demonstrates the fracture line. Diagnosis may be difficult because the epiphyseal plate itself may be mistaken for a fracture line.

NURSING DIAGNOSES: ACTUAL OR POTENTIAL

1. Alterations in comfort due to injury and unfamiliar environment.
2. Ineffective coping of the child and family with the injury and treatment program.
3. Impairment of mobility due to the injury and the cast or traction used for treatment.
4. Risk of neurovascular dysfunction in the affected limb secondary to the cast or traction.

EXPECTED OUTCOMES

1. The fracture will be reduced satisfactorily, immobilization will be maintained, and adequate healing will take place.
2. Child and family will cope successfully with hospitalization, surgery, and immobilization.
3. Child's comfort will be maintained as much as possible.

Interventions

1. Support child and family pre- and postoperatively.
2. Monitor child's condition, and care for child in traction or cast.
3. Teach parents and child about traction and/or cast.
4. Prepare parents for home care of child in cast.
5. Discuss activity limits for hospital and home.

EVALUATION

Outcome Criteria

1. Adequate healing of the fracture has taken place.
2. Child and family cope adequately with the stresses of illness and hospitalization.
3. Parents and child are able to care for cast at home and maintain activity within set limits.

Complications

Growth disturbance, such as limb length discrepancy in the affected limb.

Assessment

1. Disturbance is manifested as shortness of the affected limb or an angular deformity.
2. To measure true leg length, measure from the anterior superior iliac spine to the medial malleolus of the ankle. Compare affected and normal leg lengths.

Revised Outcomes

The deformity will be detected within a few months of onset, and appropriate measures will be taken for therapy.

Interventions

The nurse provides pre- and postoperative care around the following surgical procedures: epiphyseal plate stimulation, epiphyseal plate arrest, epiphysiodesis (bone grafting), or epiphyseal plate stapling (with metal staples).

Reevaluation and Follow-up

1. Reinforce the importance of follow-up appointments to detect growth disturbance.
2. Monitor child for growth disturbance over a 1-year period or, in some cases, longer.

SLIPPED UPPER FEMORAL EPIPHYSIS

DESCRIPTION

This disorder is a displacement of the femoral head from the neck of the femur. The etiology is not known, but hormonal influences and trauma are thought to play a part. Involvement can be unilateral or bilateral. The slippage of the epiphysis downward and backward is most often gradual and leads to a progressive coxa vara deformity of the femoral neck. If separation of the epiphysis from the femur is complete, the blood supply is likely to be interrupted, and avascular necrosis of the femoral head is probable. After the epiphyseal plate closes by bony union, slipping can no longer take place, but residual deformity may lead to degenerative hip disease in adulthood.

PREVENTION

Health Promotion

1. Prevention of obesity.
2. Prevention of hip trauma.

Population at Risk

1. Boys are affected more often than girls.
2. The disorder most commonly occurs in obese, inactive children with underdeveloped sexual characteristics and in very tall, thin, rapidly growing children.
3. It is most likely to develop in older children and adolescents, from the age of 9 years until growth ceases.

Screening

None.

ASSESSMENT

Health History

1. Growth characteristics described above.
2. History of trauma involving the hip joint.
3. Fatigue.
4. Hip pain.
5. Limp.

Physical Assessment

1. Early symptoms and/or signs.
   a. Fatigue after walking or standing.
   b. Mild pain in the hip that may be referred to the knee.
   c. Slight limp.
2. Later signs and/or symptoms.
   a. Progressive external rotation deformity in affected limb.
   b. Restriction of movements of internal rotation, flexion, and abduction.

Diagnostic Tests

X-ray examination confirms the diagnosis by demonstrating the slippage.

NURSING DIAGNOSES: ACTUAL OR POTENTIAL

1. Alterations in comfort due to pain, fatigue, immobility, and anxiety.
2. Body image disturbance resulting from obesity or tallness and thinness, immobility, and progressive rotation deformity of the leg.
3. Immobility secondary to defect and devices used in treatment, such as traction or cast.
4. Alteration in excretory patterns (constipation or urinary retention) as a result of immobility.
5. Nutritional disturbance in the child who is obese or extremely thin.
6. Disturbed peer relationships due to interruption in school and social activities, body image disturbance, and anxiety about illness.
7. Disturbed family relationships secondary to anxiety about illness, potential for bilateral involvement, stresses of hospitalization and surgery, and restrictions due to treatment measures.

EXPECTED OUTCOMES

1. Disease will be detected in early slippage stage.
2. Pain will be reduced by immobilization measures.
3. Immobilization will be effective in preventing further slippage.
4. If surgery is required, child and parents will be able to state accurate description of the procedure and postoperative care.

5. Alterations will be made in home care and activities to allow the child to meet developmental tasks.
6. Parents and child will comply with special diets at home, if needed.
7. Complications from immobility, such as excretory problems, will be prevented.

INTERVENTIONS

1. Refer child to physician when signs and symptoms are detected.
2. Instruct child to avoid unnecessary weight bearing by remaining on bed rest with the affected leg in an internally rotated position.
3. Maintain traction for further immobilization in hospital.
4. Prepare patient and family for surgical procedures, including reduction of separation and stabilization of the epiphyseal plate and subtrochanteric osteotomy of the femur to reduce bony deformity.
5. Care for child in cast, and teach patient and family about home care.
6. Provide hospital activities and stimulation according to age-group needs.
7. Clarify child's mobility limits.
8. Plan with child and family for changes in home routines, activities, and schooling.
9. Begin weight reduction diet for the obese child in the hospital, and plan with parents and child for diet at home.
10. Help child to accept body image by supportively listening to concerns, correcting misconceptions, and providing additional information about body structure and function.

EVALUATION

Outcome Criteria

1. Reduction of slip is obtained and maintained.
2. Pain is reduced by early treatment.
3. Child and family are knowledgeable about disorder and treatment regimen.
4. Changes that are appropriate to child's development needs are made in home and school activities.
5. Successful weight reduction occurs in obese child.
6. Patient becomes more accepting of own body with a more positive body image.

Complications

Residual displacement of the femoral head due to incomplete reduction of the slippage. This can lead to degenerative hip disease in adult life.

Assessment

1. Impaired mobility in the hip, causing changes in ambulation.
2. Residual rotation deformity of affected leg.
3. X-ray examination demonstrates the deformity.

Revised Outcomes

Residual deformity will be corrected surgically to allow more normal joint contour and function.

Interventions

1. Most likely surgical procedure is a subtrochanteric osteotomy of the femur to correct the deformity of the head and neck, as well as the abnormal relationship between the femoral head and the acetabulum.
2. Operation in the region of the epiphyseal plate is contraindicated due to the risk of producing iatrogenic avascular necrosis.

Reevaluation and Follow-up

1. Follow-up care to detect further slippage or deformity in the affected limb must continue at least until the epiphyseal plate has closed in late adolescence.
2. Teach patient and parents the importance of early reporting of signs and symptoms indicating bilateral involvement. There is a 30 percent chance that slippage will occur in the opposite femur before growth is complete.

REFERENCES

Anderson, B., and D'Ambra, P.: "The Adolescent Patient with Scoliosis: A Nursing Care Standard," *Nursing Clinics of North America*, **11**:699, December, 1976.

Fialkow, P. J.: "Disorders of Connective Tissue," in K. J. Isselbacher et al. (eds.), *Harrison's Principles of Internal Medicine*, 9th ed., McGraw-Hill, New York, 1980.

Hecht, F.: "Genetic Diseases," in R. A. Hoekelman et al. (eds.), *Principles of Pediatrics: Health Care of the Young*, McGraw-Hill, New York, 1978.

Lindsley, C.: "The Child with Arthritis," *Issues in Comprehensive Pediatric Nursing* **II**(4):23, November–December, 1977.

BIBLIOGRAPHY

Alexander, M., and Brown, M. S.: *Pediatric History Taking and Physical Diagnosis for Nurses,* 2d ed., McGraw-Hill, New York, 1979. Each chapter of this book relates to an area of the body and presents an anatomical description of the area, guides for assessment, and specific normal and abnormal findings. A very thorough chapter is included on the musculoskeletal system.

Flynn, I., Schwetz, K., and Williams, D.: "Muscular Dystrophy: Comprehensive Nursing Care," *Nursing Clinics of North America,* **14**:123, March, 1979. A comprehensive discussion of physical and psychosocial problems encountered by the child with muscular dystrophy and his family is presented. Nursing approaches for these problems are described.

Hilt, N., and Schmitt, E. W.: *Pediatric Orthopedic Nursing,* C. V. Mosby, St. Louis, 1975. The value of this orthopedic nursing textbook is its emphasis on pediatrics. The common orthopedic diseases and disorders that occur in children are presented, along with extensive discussion of nursing care for the child in casts, traction, and other orthopedic devices.

Lindsley, C.: "The Child with Arthritis," *Issues in Comprehensive Pediatric Nursing* **II**(4):23, November–December, 1977. An overview of JRA is presented in this article. Topics discussed are causes, pathology, clinical manifestations, diagnosis, and treatment. The article is written by a physician, from a medical point of view.

Nathan, S.: "Body Image of Scoliotic Female Adolescents Before and After Surgery," *Maternal-Child Nursing Journal* **6**(3):139, Fall, 1977. Described are the reactions of 25 adolescent girls undergoing surgery for scoliosis. Topics include how teens of different ages and anxiety levels perceived body image changes postoperatively. The effect of limited mobility on the girls' body image is also presented.

Scipien, G. et al. (eds.): *Comprehensive Pediatric Nursing,* 2d, ed., McGraw-Hill, New York, 1979. This comprehensive textbook of pediatric nursing presents information about the nursing process; growth and development; the effects of illness; the development, function, and pathophysiology of each body system; nursing care for specific conditions of each system; and future trends in pediatric nursing.

17

The Endocrine System

Diana W. Guthrie

HYPERACTIVITY AND HYPOACTIVITY (ANTERIOR PITUITARY GLAND)*

The anterior pituitary gland was once thought to be the master gland of the body. It produces stimulating hormones that control the function of the thyroid gland, adrenal glands, and gonads. In addition, it produces growth hormone, the target organ of which is bone, and prolactin, which stimulates lactation. The pituitary gland is now known to be under the control of the hypothalamus, which produces regulator hormones that control pituitary secretions. For most pituitary hormones, the hypothalamus produces a releasing hormone that stimulates the pituitary gland to release a specific hormone that, in turn, stimulates hormone release by the target gland. Hormone from the target gland in turn suppresses the releasing hormone in the hypothalamus, completing the arc. An example of this arc is the hypothalamic-pituitary-thyroid axis. The hypothalamus produces a hormone called thyrotropin-releasing hormone (TRH) that causes the pituitary to release its hormone called thyroid-stimulating hormone (TSH) that, in turn, causes the thyroid gland to release its hormone called thyroxine (T_4). Thyroxine then exerts its effect on every bodily cell to stimulate metabolism. Thyroxine also suppresses TRH production, causing TSH to decrease, thus causing the thyroid gland to decrease its own production. Reduced production of T_4 then allows TRH to increase, and the cycle continues. This control cycle is called a feedback arc and resembles the thermostatic control mechanism of a furnace.

Certain hormones, such as growth hormone, have no target gland to produce a hormone to complete the feedback arc. For these hormones, the hypothalamus produces not only a stimulating or releasing hormone but also an inhibitory hormone to prevent oversecretion.

1. Disease states can be produced by
   a. Increased or decreased hypothalamic hormone secretion.
   b. Increased or decreased pituitary hormone secretion.
   c. Increased or decreased hormone secretion of the target gland.

* Endocrine disorders can arise from any of several causes. Diabetes mellitus, for example, may be genetic or may be due to pancreatitis or pancreatectomy; hypothyroidism may be caused by congenital absence of the thyroid gland, metabolic disorder due to insufficient dietary iodine, inflammation, surgical removal of the gland, or tumor. The essential features of endocrine diseases result from hormone imbalances, regardless of the original cause of the problem. Accordingly, the disorders discussed in this chapter are all placed in the category *hyperactivity and hypoactivity*, even though they might also fit appropriately into one or more of the other major categories used throughout the book. Diseases associated primarily with a particular gland (in this case, the anterior pituitary gland) are presented together, although at times this classification becomes arbitrary since malfunction of any gland can result either from a disorder of that gland or from pathology of the hypothalamus or the anterior pituitary gland, the functions of which affect those of the entire endocrine system. Table 17-1 lists endocrine disorders by etiology.

TABLE 17-1 CLASSIFICATION OF CHILDHOOD ENDOCRINE DISORDERS BY ORIGIN

Disorders of genetic origin
- Gigantism
  - Beckwith's syndrome of giantism, exophthalmos, and macroglossia
- Congenital hyperpituitary function
- Pituitary dwarfism
- Cretinism (congenital hypothyroidism)
- Congenital hypoparathyroidism
- Congenital hyperparathyroidism
- Diabetes mellitus
- Delayed puberty and hypogonadism
- Precocious puberty
  - Hypothalamic origin (constitutional)
  - Due to extrapituitary disease, e.g., adrenogenital syndrome
- Adrenogenital syndrome
- Cushing's and Addison's diseases

Disorders of rate of growth
- Giantism—excess growth hormone secretion
- Dwarfism—lack of growth hormone secretion or unresponsiveness to growth hormone
- Hypothyroidism—congenital or acquired
- Diabetes mellitus—poorly controlled diabetes can result in growth failure (also, diabetes mellitus often arises during the preadolescent growth spurt and is known as "growth onset diabetes")

Disorders of environmental origin
- The infant of a diabetic mother
- The infant of a hypercalcemic mother
- Hyperthyroidism
- Hypothyroidism, acquired
- Ambiguous genital development secondary to maternal hormones
- Diabetes insipidus
- Hypopituitarism due to trauma or destruction of hypothalamus and/or pituitary gland
- Diabetes mellitus secondary to tumor, surgery, trauma, or pancreatectomy
- Addison's and Cushing's diseases
- Hypoparathyroidism with tetany secondary to surgical destruction of the parathyroid or tumor
- Hypogonadism due to destruction of the ovaries and testes by tumors, surgery, or chemical suppression
- Deficient growth hormone due to malnutrition or deprivation
- Growth and menstrual disorders due to eating disorders (anorexia nervosa, exogenous obesity, or bulimia)

Disorders caused by infections
- Thyroiditis with hypothyroidism
- Addison's disease
- Diabetes mellitus (?)
- Graves' disease (hyperthyroidism) (?)

2. States of increased or decreased hormone secretion anywhere in the cycle can be caused by
   a. Genetic inheritance.
   b. Metabolic factors.
   c. Trauma.
   d. Tumors.
   e. Infections.
   f. Drugs.
   g. Unknown (idiopathic) causes.
3. Regardless of origin, the end result is usually the same: the symptoms or signs are those of increased or decreased hormone secretion of the target gland hormone. *Example:* Deficiency of hypothalamic TRH or anterior pituitary TSH results in the same physical problems as failure of the thyroid gland itself, due to lack of T_4. The difference is that TRH and TSH levels will be high if the defect is in the thyroid gland, whereas TRH, but not TSH, will be elevated in pituitary disease, and all will be low in hypothalamic disease. These differences can be used to determine the location of the lesion or disease.
4. Disease of the hypothalamus and/or pituitary can involve a single hormone or several hormones.
   a. Diseases of genetic or congenital origin tend to affect a single hormone, for example, isolated growth hormone deficiency.
   b. Diseases of destruction, such as tumors, surgical ablation, trauma, and so forth, tend to show multiple deficiencies (panhypopituitarism, which causes deficiencies of hormones from all the target organs—thyroid, adrenals, and gonads—as well as deficiencies of growth hormone and prolactin). *Example:* An example of a lesion producing multiple endocrine deficiencies is a craniopharyngioma that destroys the hypothalamus and/or pituitary gland and causes deficiency of all of the hormones.

As far as is now known, there are six clearly defined hormones of the anterior pituitary gland:

1. *Thyroid-stimulating hormone* (TSH), which is controlled by thyroid-releasing hormone (TRH) from the hypothalamus and causes the release of thyroxine (T_4) by the thyroid gland.
2. *Follicle-stimulating hormone* (FSH) and *luteinizing hormone* (LH), which are controlled by LH-releasing hormone (LH-RH) from the hypothalamus and in turn control gonad functions (spermatogenesis, ovogenesis, and the production of estrogen, progesterone, and testosterone).
3. *Adrenocorticotropic hormone* (ACTH), which is controlled by an as yet undefined releasing factor from the hypothalamus (ACTH-RF*) and controls the hormonal secretions of the adrenal cortex (primarily cortisol and small amounts of estrogens, progesterone, and testosterone). Aldosterone is also produced by the adrenal cortex but is not controlled by ACTH.
4. *Human growth hormone* (HGH), which is controlled by both a hypothalamic-stimulating hormone (HGH-RH) and an inhibiting hormone—HGH-releasing hormone-inhibiting hormone (HGH-RH-IH, or somatostatin).
5. *Prolactin*, which is controlled only by an inhibiting hormone factor (PrIF) from the hypothalamus. This inhibiting hormone, PrIF, can be inhibited by a neuroendocrine arc from the breast nipples to the hypothalamus. Sucking at the breast thus allows prolactin production and lactation.

GIGANTISM

DESCRIPTION

Gigantism is a congenital disorder of newborns of unknown etiology. It is characterized by exomphalos, macroglossia, and giantism. Gigantism is also known as Beckwith's syndrome or the E.M.G. syndrome. Also, the infants often have hypoglycemia and omphalocele. Since the disease is not, strictly speaking, an endocrine disease, although the infants do have hyperinsulinemia, it will not be discussed further here.

* Hypothalamic hormones that have been identified are known as releasing or inhibitory hormones, abbreviated RH or IH. Hypothalamic hormones known to exist but as yet not identified are called releasing or inhibitory factors (RF or IF).

GIANTISM

DESCRIPTION

Giantism is a disease of overproduction of HGH and is characterized by excessive growth. When the disease occurs in childhood before epiphyseal closure, very large stature of normal proportions results, and the condition is termed *giantism*. If the condition occurs after puberty and epiphyseal closure has occurred, only those areas with open epiphyses (jaw, hands, and feet) grow, and the face, hands, and feet become excessively large in proportion to the rest of the body. This condition is known as *acromegaly*. Both giantism and acromegaly can be caused by a variety of conditions of the hypothalamus or pituitary gland, but most commonly they result from an adenoma of the pituitary gland.

PREVENTION

Health Promotion

1. Avoidance of injury to the pituitary gland.
2. Good nutrition (as a preventive measure for infections).
3. Use of drugs only as prescribed by a physician.

Population at Risk

1. Children with a family history of giantism (adults taller than usual).
2. Children with tumors involving the pituitary gland.
3. Children who ingest drugs, resulting in direct or indirect effect on the anterior pituitary gland.

Screening

Clinical observation for signs described below, under *Assessment*.

ASSESSMENT

Health History

1. Height has rapidly increased.
2. Family history of occurrence.
3. Health maintenance patterns: frequent infections, poor nutrition practices, use of medications.

Physical Assessment

1. Taller than expected for age.
2. Rapid increase in height as noted on growth chart.
3. Disproportionate growth of the lower jaw, hands, and feet present with acromegaly.
4. Head circumference larger than normal but in proportion to height.
5. Advanced bone age of wrists and hands in both acromegaly and gigantism.

Diagnostic Tests

1. *Growth hormone.* Elevated growth hormone secretion on stimulation by arginine, insulin, or glucagon stress test.
2. *Bone age films.* In either condition, X-ray films of the wrists and hands reveal advanced bone age; X-ray films of the skull may show an enlarged sella turcica (the bony crater that houses the pituitary gland).

NURSING DIAGNOSES: ACTUAL OR POTENTIAL

1. Anxiety secondary to abnormal height and (after puberty) acromegalic features.
2. Ineffective coping secondary to anxiety.
3. Diminished self-esteem due to abnormal height and appearance.
4. Knowledge deficit related to treatment and its outcomes.

EXPECTED OUTCOMES

1. Child and family will be referred for immediate medical diagnosis (skull x-ray films, computerized axial tomography (CAT scan), growth hormone assay, etc.) and treatment (surgical or radiological ablation of tumor).
2. Child and family will be prepared for surgery, if indicated.
3. Child will adjust adequately to tall stature and altered features.
4. If the excessive growth is genetic rather than hormonal (constitutional tall stature is usually considered a problem only in girls, rarely in boys), then the girl and her family will be prepared for sexual development that will result if sex hormone therapy is used to hasten epiphyseal closure and stop growth.

INTERVENTIONS

1. Prepare and support child and family during hospitalization and diagnostic procedures.
2. Prepare child and family for surgery and the surgical outcome if surgery is planned.
3. Preparation for radiation therapy and its outcome will be necessary if radiation is indi-

cated. Surgical removal or radiological ablation of a pituitary tumor usually results in destruction of the pituitary gland with subsequent hypogonadism, hypothyroidism, and hypoadrenalism, all of which must be treated with the appropriate replacement hormones to sustain life.
4. Prepare child and family for hormonal therapy to induce epiphyseal closure if no organic lesion is found.
5. Help child and family with emotional adjustment to excess height, awkwardness, and incoordination.
6. Child and family may need help adjusting to derogatory remarks from others.
7. Help child and family prepare for and adjust to signs of sexual maturation when hormonal therapy is used; emphasize that appropriate behavior is that which fits chronological age, not necessarily sexual developmental stage.

EVALUATION

Outcome Criteria

1. Parents and child (depending on age) can accurately describe what to expect if child is to be hospitalized.
2. Parents and child (depending on age) are knowledgeable about the diagnostic tests that are to be performed.
3. Family understands the possible side effects of radiation.
4. Both parents and child adjust adequately to the child's height, appearance, and/or sexual maturation as evidenced by healthy family relationships (see Chapter 5) and normal child development and social relationships for age (see Chapter 4).

Complications

NAUSEA, DIZZINESS, HAIR LOSS, AND/OR ABDOMINAL DISCOMFORT SECONDARY TO RADIATION THERAPY

Assessment
1. Vomiting.
2. Elevation of temperature.
3. Skin turgor poor.

Revised Outcomes
1. Hydration and comfort will be maintained.
2. Others, as stated in *Expected Outcomes,* above.

Interventions
1. Small, frequent, high-calorie feedings.
2. Intravenous (IV) fluids, as directed.
3. Prescribed medication for nausea.

PSYCHOLOGICAL DISTURBANCES RELATED TO ABNORMAL GROWTH

Assessment
1. Stays alone.
2. Unable to socialize, poor affect.
3. Describes self in degrading terms.

Revised Outcomes
1. Child and family will demonstrate positive regard for child.
2. Child and family will receive professional counseling, if needed.

Interventions
1. Work with child and family in the development of a positive attitude (see Chapters 36 and 40).
2. Assist family and child in looking realistically at other, positive parts of the child's life.
3. Assist child in expressing feelings regarding negative thoughts.
4. Refer child and family to psychiatric nurse specialist or other mental health professional.

ABNORMAL RESPONSE TO SURGERY

Assessment
1. Motor deficits.
2. Increased intracranial pressure (see Chapter 15).
3. Symptoms related to other pituitary hormonal abnormalities (see other pituitary disorders described throughout this chapter).

Revised Outcomes
1. Child will receive care, including self-care instruction, as physical condition requires.
2. Others, as stated in *Expected Outcomes,* above.

Interventions
1. Monitor vital signs for any change.
2. Monitor neurological status.
3. Monitor laboratory values.
4. Support life processes.
5. Prevent injury.
6. Increase counseling and information as to child's response to surgery.
7. See Chapter 15 for care of the child following brain surgery.

PRECOCIOUS PUBERTY

DESCRIPTION

Precocious puberty is the premature maturation of the genital tissues and reproductive organs (Figure 17-1). It may be due to tumor of the hy-

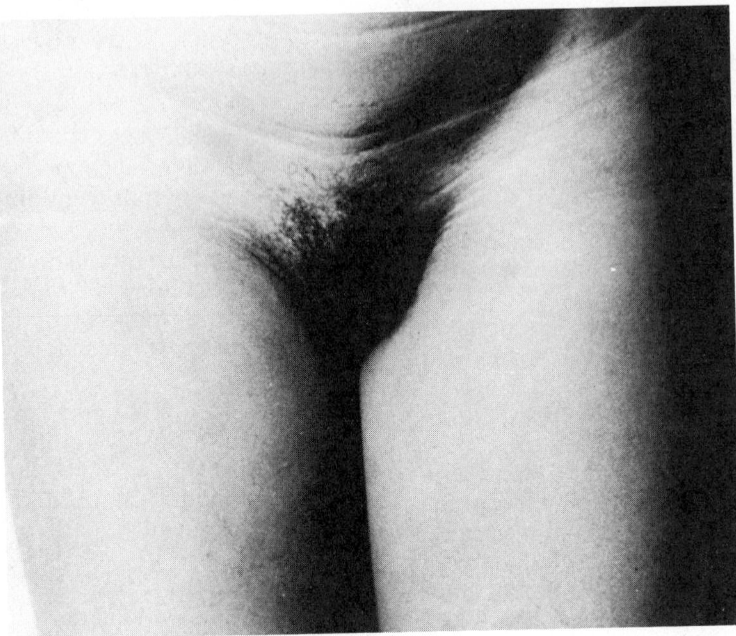

Figure 17-1 Precocious puberty, age 6 years.

pothalamus, pituitary or gonads, and, occasionally, the adrenal glands. Precocious puberty due to ovarian or testicular tumors or adrenal malfunction will be discussed under the specific organs. There are also a few rare syndromes associated with precocious puberty. The most common of these syndromes is the McCune-Albright syndrome, in which precocious puberty is associated with skin and bone lesions; this is probably a genetically transmitted defect.

The most common cause of precocious puberty is simply the so-called early alarm clock, or early puberty due to unknown causes without evidence of organic disease, called constitutional precocious puberty. Puberty can begin at any age (even in infancy) and is called precocious if menstruation occurs before age 8 years or if there are signs of maturation before age 10 years in boys. The major danger, especially for the constitutional type of precocious puberty, is early epiphyseal closure with short stature. If tumors are found they should, of course, be removed. Recently, an experimental program for treatment of constitutional precocious puberty by an analog of LH-RH was initiated. Preliminary results are encouraging. Treatment can now reverse the sexual changes without inducing premature cessation of growth.

PREVENTION

Health Promotion

1. Maintain good health habits: nutrition, avoidance of infections, and so on.
2. Use medication only as prescribed by a health professional.

Population at Risk

1. Children with a positive genetic history, especially early menarche in female relatives.
2. Children with continued exposure to drugs or illnesses affecting the anterior pituitary gland.

Screening

Clinical observation for signs described below, under *Assessment*.

ASSESSMENT

Health History

1. A careful history of the sequence of appearance of early sexual development.
2. Maturation history of family members.
3. Vaginal bleeding in the female patient or spontaneous erection and ejaculation in the male patient.

Physical Assessment

1. Assessment of sexual maturation according to the Tanner scale of pubescent changes (Tanner, 1962).
2. Overdevelopment of internal and external genitalia.
3. Presence of pubic and/or axillary hair.
4. Short stature.

Diagnostic Tests

1. CAT scan.
2. X-ray examination of epiphyseal areas of extremities.
3. Hormone assays.

NURSING DIAGNOSES: ACTUAL OR POTENTIAL

1. Anxiety of parents and child secondary to child's physical appearance (secondary sex characteristics) and sexual feelings.
2. Family coping problems secondary to physical appearance and actions of the child.
3. Diminished self-concept of child secondary to appearance in comparison with peers.
4. Alterations in patterns of sexuality secondary to appearance and sexual feelings.

EXPECTED OUTCOMES

1. Child will obtain medical care to determine the cause of precocious development and to prescribe therapy.
2. Child and family will be well informed about the child's sexual development and what further changes to expect.
3. Family and child will be free from excessive anxiety about the child's sexual development and will cope adequately.
4. Child will not become involved in sexual abuse.

INTERVENTIONS

1. Refer to physician for diagnosis and medical treatment if these have not been done.
2. Instruct and counsel parents and child.
   a. Teach about physiology of sexual maturation and the fundamental normality of the process even at an early age.
   b. Assist with planning for special hygienic needs if these have not already been dealt with by family (e.g., menstrual hygiene, use of underarm deodorant).
   c. Advise that child will be tall for age initially but that adult height will be short or normal (depending on type of treatment).
   d. Explain to family that child's behavior and interests are generally compatible with chronological age rather than with level of sexual development, that is, activities may seem childish in comparison with appearance.
   e. Parents will need to realize that early sexual development is neither "bad" nor calamitous, although it does have inherent problems.
   f. Advise that adolescent adjustment can be expected to be normal.
3. Other persons (teacher, pastor, perhaps close friends) may need instruction and guidance. The teacher may be asked to intervene in specific instances when attention is drawn by classmates to the child's early sexual development or when difficult situations appear to be arising from the child's school contacts.
4. Explain to parents that precocious development places the child (especially if a girl) at risk for sexual exploitation from other children and sexually abusive adolescents and adults; advise preventive, protective surveillance, but caution against extremism or alarm.

EVALUATION

Outcome Criteria

1. Physician's diagnosis and treatment are obtained.
2. Child, family, and involved community members cope adequately.
3. Child's psychosocial development is adequate.
4. Child's advance in sexual development is arrested or slowed.
5. Sexual abuse does not occur.

Complications

1. Early epiphyseal closure and resultant short stature.
2. Psychological illness secondary to sexual abuse and/or self-concept.

DWARFISM

DESCRIPTION

Dwarfism is the failure of growth in height to keep pace with norms. It is generally defined as a growth rate of less than 2 inches per year and an attained stature more than two standard deviations below the mean. There are many causes of dwarfism, of which lack of growth hormone is only one. Insufficient nutritional intake, central nervous system damage, heart or lung disease, gastrointestinal disease causing malabsorption, chronic infection, inborn errors of metabolism, hypothyroidism, uncontrolled diabetes mellitus, and a host of rare congenital syndromes are some of the causes in addition to pituitary failure. Only dwarfism due to growth hormone deficiency will be discussed here, but in the assessment of a patient with short stature all the above must be looked for and ruled out before the endocrine evaluation is started.

By far the commonest cause of short stature, particularly in males, is delayed development. This condition goes by various names, including *constitutional dwarfism, constitutional delayed growth, delayed development,* and *delayed adolescence.* All these terms refer to the child who has no organic disease but simply grows slowly. These children ultimately attain their predetermined height and reach puberty but usually 2 to 3 years later than their peers. Adolescence can be accelerated in these children, making them more like their peers in body size and appearance (pubic hair, beard, etc.), by the use of sex steroids, but with the sacrifice of some adult height because of early epiphyseal closure.

Pituitary dwarfism can be an isolated growth hormone deficiency, for which treatment is the replacement of growth hormone by every-other-day injections of human growth hormone; or it may be a part of multiple pituitary deficiencies or even panhypopituitarism, in which all pituitary function is lost. In panhypopituitarism there are multiple endocrine deficiencies affecting the gonads, adrenals, and thyroid. All must be recognized and treated.

PREVENTION

Health Promotion

1. Maintenance of good health habits: rest, nutrition, and so on.
2. Use of medication only as prescribed by a health professional.

Population at Risk

1. Positive genetic history.
2. Children with continued exposure to drugs or illnesses affecting the anterior pituitary gland.

Screening

Maintenance of growth chart for every child.

ASSESSMENT

Health History

1. Careful health history to determine if cause of dwarfism is nonendocrine related (e.g., malabsorption diarrhea).
2. Family history of parental and family heights, growth patterns, and ages of attaining puberty (most short stature is genetic or constitutional, so history is very important).
3. History of the pattern of the child's growth (height and weight at various ages plotted on a growth chart) can be very helpful, because different causes of short stature produce different patterns of growth. For example, cretins grow slowly from birth, whereas growth hormone-deficient children grow normally for the first 1 to 2 years and then begin to slow down and fall below the curve.

Physical Assessment

1. Clinical observation.
2. Careful taking, plotting, and evaluation of height and weight. The most important element of nursing assessment is the evaluation of the height and weight. Standing height and sitting height should be measured in order to determine the ratio of the upper and lower segments (some conditions, such as achondroplasia and cretinism, produce fairly normal trunk length but short extremities so the upper segment exceeds the lower, whereas genetic dwarfs and pituitary dwarfs have proportional growth with nearly equal upper and lower segments).
3. Head circumference and arm span should also be measured and recorded. (Achondroplasia will present a head size out of proportion to body size—usually enlarged; cretinism will present a head size somewhat smaller than body size; dwarfism will present a head in proportion to body size.)

Diagnostic Tests

1. Bone age films.
2. Skull X-ray films.
3. Growth hormone stimulant test.

NURSING DIAGNOSES: ACTUAL OR POTENTIAL

1. Anxiety in child and parents in regard to child's size.
2. Altered family coping secondary to anxiety or guilt about child's size.
3. Developmental deviations (especially psychosocial) secondary to short stature.
4. Diminished self-esteem secondary to short stature.
5. Knowledge deficit about delayed growth and its treatment.

EXPECTED OUTCOMES

1. Child will receive medical care to
   a. Find and correct organic lesions, if any.
   b. Find and correct metabolic problems, if present.
   c. Identify deficiency of growth hormone, if present, and treat with supplemental growth hormone.
   d. Determine the value or desirability of sex hormone treatment if short stature is constitutional.
2. Child and family will become well informed about child's short stature (origin, treatment, expected outcome, etc.) and able to carry out their role in the treatment regimen.
3. Child and family will be free of signs of excessive anxiety.
4. Child's developmental level (interests, activities, peer relationships) and family relationships will be unimpaired.
5. Child will have positive self-esteem.

INTERVENTIONS

1. Refer to physician if this has not been done.
2. Counsel on good nutrition to be sure intake is adequate to achieve full potential growth.
3. Instruct child and family about underlying cause of short stature and expected outcome of treatment.
4. Instruct child and family about treatment and their part in it.
   a. Growth hormone is given every other day by injection, so teach child or parent injection technique.
5. Counsel as to positive adjustment of a short person in a tall person's world to prevent or treat psychosocial adjustment problems.

EVALUATION

Outcome Criteria

1. Physician referral and follow-up care are obtained.
2. Depending on specific cause of short stature, family can complete food records and prepare diet plans.
3. Parents (or child if old enough) can give injections or oral medications.
4. Parents can take accurate height measurements and keep records of them.
5. Parents and child can discuss their feelings about size and cope and adjust adequately.

Complications

1. Dwarfism is nonresponsive to therapy.
2. Epiphyseal closures have occurred so that growth hormone therapy is not possible.
3. Psychological illness has developed to the extent that psychiatric intervention is necessary.

ADDISON'S DISEASE, SHEEHAN'S SYNDROME, AND SIMMONDS' DISEASE

DESCRIPTION

Addison's disease is a deficiency of adrenocorticosteroids from the adrenal glands. It may be due to hypothalamic or pituitary deficiency but is usually caused by destruction of the adrenal glands themselves. The symptoms and signs are the same in any of the three situations except that the skin pigmentation characteristic of adrenal gland failure does not occur with ACTH deficiency. In adrenal gland failure, ACTH from the pituitary gland is elevated, along with melanophore-stimulating hormone (MSH), because of lack of cortisol feedback. These hormones cause increased pigmentation of the skin, especially of skin creases (palms and soles) and of normally hyperpigmented areas, such as the breast areola and nipples. In pituitary deficiency, ACTH and MSH are deficient, and no pigmentation occurs. Isolated ACTH deficiency is rare in children. It usually appears along with other pituitary hormone deficiencies as a result of hypothalamic or pituitary destruction by a tumor or as a result of infarction of the pituitary gland during periods of profound hypotensive shock and is known as Sheehan's syndrome or Simmonds' disease. Simmonds' disease (panhypopituitarism of vascular origin) is rare in children but has occasionally been seen following profound shock.

Since ACTH deficiency is rare and Addison's disease more commonly results from primary adrenal failure, care of the child with Addison's disease will be discussed in the later section on the adrenal glands.

GONADOTROPIN DEFICIENCY

DESCRIPTION

The gonadotropins—*follicle-stimulating hormone* (FSH) and *luteinizing hormone* (LH)—are responsible for stimulation of the ovaries or testicles to produce sex hormones and reproductive cells. Deficiency of FSH and LH results in poor development of the gonads, lack of sexual development, lack of secondary sex characteristics, and infertility. Lack of sexual development may be due to failure of the gonads, in which case FSH and LH will be elevated. This condition is known as *hypogonadism* and has many causes. Deficiency of FSH and LH can be caused by hypothalamic or pituitary deficiency and is called *hypogonadotropic hypogonadism.* This condition may be genetic but more commonly is due to destruction of a portion of the hypothalamus or pituitary by trauma, infection, tumor, and so forth. Gonadotropin deficiency may be an isolated deficiency or may be a part of multiple pituitary or panpituitary deficiencies. The primary sign of this disease is delayed or absent puberty and infertility.

PREVENTION

Health Promotion

1. Maintenance of good health habits: avoidance of infection and trauma, good nutrition, and so forth.
2. Use of medications only as prescribed by a health professional.

Population at Risk

1. Positive genetic history.
2. Children being treated indiscriminately by drugs that might affect the hypothalamus, pituitary, or gonads.

Screening

Clinical observation for delayed puberty.

ASSESSMENT

Health History

1. Family history of delayed pubescence.
2. Lack of developing sexual characteristics at expected ages.

Physical Assessment

1. Secondary sexual hair (pubic hair, axillary hair, beard) is absent.
2. Penis and testicles are small.
3. Voice deepening in the male does take place.
4. External genitalia in the female are infantile.
5. Female's body contours remain boyish, without breast development.
6. Pelvic examination reveals small ovaries and an infantile uterus.
7. Menstruation is absent.
8. NOTE: Puberty is not considered delayed unless there are no signs of development by age 16 in the male and age 14 in the female.

Diagnostic Tests

1. Bone age x-ray films.
2. FSH and LH levels in blood.

NURSING DIAGNOSES: ACTUAL OR POTENTIAL

1. Delayed pubertal development due to hormonal deficiency.
2. Poor self-esteem secondary to delayed development of primary and secondary sexual characteristics.
3. Alterations in relationships due to differences in physical appearance from peers.
4. Alterations in patterns of sexuality secondary to delayed development.

EXPECTED OUTCOMES

1. Adolescent and parents will obtain medical diagnosis of the origin of the problem, medical treatment of any existing lesions (e.g., tumor removal), and replacement therapy with sex steroids (testosterone for a boy, estrogens and progesterone for a girl).

   NOTE: FSH and LH cannot be given since they are in short supply, expensive, and must be injected. Sex steroids can be given orally.
2. The client will adjust well to both delayed

puberty and the marked change that results from hormone therapy.
3. The adolescent will be psychologically sound and ultimately sexually functional even though he or she may remain infertile.

INTERVENTIONS

1. Refer to physician if this has not been done.
2. Give encouragement about the normalization of physical development following treatment.
3. If no treatment is instituted or if little change in maturation is expected, intervention is directed toward self-image and self-acceptance.
4. If the expected outcome is normal sexual function but continued infertility, child and parents should be given opportunities to express their feelings about infertility, to explore the possibilities of child adoption, and so forth.

EVALUATION

Outcome Criteria

1. Medical evaluation and follow-up treatment are obtained.
2. Adolescent is psychologically well adjusted (see Chapter 4 for developmental expectations for adolescents).
3. Adolescent is sexually adjusted and functional (in accordance with own wishes and circumstances).
4. Adolescent is normal in appearance.

Complications

PSYCHOLOGICAL MALADJUSTMENT

Assessment

1. Child is not socializing with peers.
2. Behavior is behind chronological age.
3. Withdrawal is noted.

Revised Outcomes

1. Adolescent will receive counseling.
2. Family and significant others will be involved as appropriate.

Interventions

1. Refer to psychiatric mental-health nurse specialist or other counseling professional.
2. Increase counseling for family as well as client.
3. Educate and reassure client and family as to expected physical changes.

ADOLESCENT DOES NOT ADEQUATELY RESPOND TO HORMONAL THERAPY

Assessment

1. Expected physiological changes do not occur.
2. History of failure to follow prescribed treatment.

Revised Outcomes

Adolescent will participate cooperatively in the therapeutic regimen.

Interventions

Involve community nurse to assist in the administration of medication and/or closer monitoring of administration of medication.

HYPERACTIVITY AND HYPOACTIVITY (POSTERIOR PITUITARY GLAND)

The posterior pituitary gland is actually an extension of the neural tissue of the hypothalamus of the brain but sits in the bony depression called the sella turcica behind the anterior pituitary gland. Though it exists in anatomical proximity to the anterior pituitary gland, it is completely separate and has totally different functions.

The posterior pituitary gland produces several hormones:

1. The most important is antidiuretic hormone (ADH), which regulates water retention and loss by the kidney.
   a. Increased ADH results in water retention. ADH excess is usually temporary and is seen in diseases of the central nervous system and other conditions. It will not be discussed here.
   b. ADH deficiency results in marked water loss, a condition known as diabetes insipidus.
2. Oxytocin, which is important for uterine contractions.
3. An active blood pressure agent.
4. A let-down hormone important in breastfeeding.
5. Melanophore-stimulating hormones important in pigmentation.

Except for ADH, these hormones have not been linked to childhood illnesses and will not be discussed here.

DIABETES INSIPIDUS

DESCRIPTION

Diabetes insipidus (DI) is a state of chronic and severe water loss resulting from a deficiency of antidiuretic hormone (ADH). The disease, which is fatal unless treated, can result from trauma, infection, atrophy (genetic), vascular infarct, or tumor of the hypothalamic-pituitary axis. In children, diabetes insipidus is commonly associated with a tumor known as *eosinophilic granuloma*. This condition is part of the reticuloendothelial system malignancy called *histiocytosis* X. When an eosinophilic granuloma of the skull and diabetes insipidus exist together, the condition is known as *Hand-Schüller-Christian syndrome*.

Symptoms of diabetes insipidus are excessive urination (polyuria) followed by a compensatory thirst (polydipsia). The condition is differentiated from diabetes mellitus in that, in diabetes insipidus, the urine is very dilute and does not contain sugar. DI, although usually due to a deficiency of ADH, can be of renal origin (nephrogenic DI). This condition is due to inability of the kidney to respond to ADH and is characterized by the presence of DI with elevated ADH levels.

PREVENTION

Health Promotion

1. Maintain adequate health care in order to decrease the possibility of an infection that might affect the posterior pituitary gland.
2. Wear adequate protection when involved in contact sports.
3. Use medication only with guidance of a health professional.

Population at Risk

1. Participants in contact sports.
2. Victims of an infection that affects the brain.
3. Children with a family history of diabetes insipidus.

Screening

None.

ASSESSMENT

Health History

1. A careful history of sequence of drinking and urination (in psychogenic water drinking, the drinking comes first; in DI, the urination comes first, followed by polydipsia).
2. History of no sugar in the urine.
3. Passing of large amounts of nonconcentrated urine (the urine is clear to slightly yellow in color).
4. History of other family members with this condition.
5. Past cerebral infection.
6. Trauma to head from contact sport.
7. Irritability, especially with water deprivation.
8. Enuresis.

Physical Assessment

1. Normally developed at or below expected weight for height.
2. Turgor of skin is diminished; mucous membranes are dry, especially if child has been without water for a period of time.
3. Hyperthermia and other associated signs and symptoms, especially in a more acute state of dehydration (e.g., lowered blood pressure or rapid, thready pulse).

Diagnostic Tests

1. Specific gravity less than 1.010 even with water deprivation; if specific gravity is 1.010 or greater, the child does not have DI.
2. Water deprivation test (ordered by physician). In this test the child is deprived of water for 4 to 12 hours, and the specific gravity of the urine is tested against the osmolarity of the blood. In a child with psychogenic water drinking rather than DI, the osmolarity of the blood stays the same and urine specific gravity goes up as water is conserved. In DI, the osmolarity of the blood goes up and urine stays dilute as water continues to be lost.

   NOTE: During a water deprivation test, the child should be under continuous nursing observation. The child with DI cannot conserve water and can become dehydrated and go into shock if not observed very carefully.

3. Electrolytes, especially to note imbalance of salts or falling BUN.
4. Serum osmolarity to document dehydration.

NURSING DIAGNOSES: ACTUAL OR POTENTIAL

1. Fluid volume deficit (severe) due to hormone-induced diuresis.
2. Fear or anxiety of child and parents secondary to administration at home of frequent injections of medication.
3. Maladaptive child and family coping patterns secondary to injection administration.

EXPECTED OUTCOMES

1. Child will receive early medical diagnosis and treatment.
2. Parents (and child if old enough) will administer medication and regulate medication dose and water intake.

INTERVENTIONS

1. Assist in rapid diagnosis by urine testing and referring suspect children for medical evaluation.
2. Teach self-adjustment of medication by measuring urine output, specific gravity, and weight gain.
   a. If medication dose is too high, water will be retained, specific gravity will increase, and body weight will go up.
   b. If dose is too low, urine volume will increase as will water intake, specific gravity will decrease, and body weight will drop.
3. Teach parents (and child if old enough) to administer the medication. Treatment is by intramuscular injection, usually daily, of ADH in the form of vasopressin tannate in oil. An alternative form of therapy is the inhalation of an analog of vasopressin called DPDV Pasa powder into the nose for absorption through the nasal mucosa.

EVALUATION

Outcome Criteria

1. Medical evaluation and follow-up are obtained.
2. Child and/or family are skilled in injection or insufflation procedure.
3. Patient and/or family carry out proper weighing and urine testing procedures (for specific gravity).
4. Parents (and child if old enough) are able to describe the course, signs, symptoms, and side effects of the disease and treatment.
5. Parents (and child if old enough) can describe the danger signals of dehydration and know when they need to call the health professional.

Complications

1. Oliguria due to a too high dose of medication that will cause retention of body water.
2. Dehydration and weight loss due to insufficient amount of medication.
3. Increase in body weight more rapidly than expected for age due to retention of body fluids.
4. Psychological maladjustment related to route of administration and/or enuresis.

Assessment

1. Withdrawn child who has difficulty in communicating fears.
2. Child and/or parents forget or omit medication administration.

Revised Outcomes

Parents and/or child will administer medication under close supervision.

Interventions

1. Reassess and revise educational program, giving extra consideration to individualization.
2. Refer to psychiatric mental health nurse specialist or other professional if increased counseling results in no change or worsened psychosocial response.

HYPERACTIVITY AND HYPOACTIVITY (THYROID GLAND)

The thyroid gland, located in the lower neck, can be felt by gentle palpation even in normal children. The gland is composed of three kinds of tissue: (1) tissue for the secretion of the thyroid hormones, *thyroxine* (T_4) and *triiodothyronine* (T_3); (2) tissue for the secretion of *calcitonin;* and (3) the *parathyroid glands.* Calcitonin from the thyroid and *parathormone* from the parathyroids are involved in calcium metabolism.

The hypothalamic-pituitary-thyroid axis has already been explained (see *Anterior Pituitary Gland*). When the thyroid gland is stimulated by thyroid-stimulating hormone (TSH) from the anterior pituitary, a series of biochemical reactions for the metabolism of iodine occur.

Inorganic iodine is trapped by the gland, converted to iodide, and hooked to tyrosine to form a mono- or diiodotyrosine. The iodinated tyrosine molecules then condense into a double molecule called thyronine containing two, three, or four iodines. Diiodothyronine is not biologically active. Triiodothyronine (T_3) is the most potent of the thyroid compounds, but very little is produced by the thyroid gland. Most of the T_3 is produced peripherally in the blood or tissue by the deiodination of T_4.

T_3 or T_4, once manufactured by the gland, is stored in the thyroid follicles attached to a binding protein. When it is needed, T_4 is unbound and secreted into the bloodstream where it is again bound to a protein, *thyrobinding globulin* (TGB), and transported to the tissues. In the tissues, T_4 is converted to T_3 and unbound from TGB to have its desired effect on the cells. *The major effect of T_3 or T_4 on the tissues is to stimulate the rate of metabolism.*

Thus, in thyroid hormone *deficiency,* metabolism slows down markedly, and all bodily processes are slowed. In thyroid *excess,* all bodily processes are speeded up.

Deficiency of thyroid hormone can occur due to

1. TRH (hypothalamus) or TSH (anterior pituitary) deficiency.
2. Lack of a thyroid gland (athyrotic cretinism).
3. Destruction of the gland (acute, subacute, or chronic thyroiditis).
4. Tumors.
5. Enzyme deficiencies at any of the steps in the formation of thyroxine, its storage, release, peripheral binding, T_3 formation, or peripheral release.

The signs and symptoms produced by these five defects are the same and are the direct result of the slowing of all metabolic processes.

Increased thyroid secretion (hyperthyroidism) can be caused by

1. TRH or TSH excess.
2. Tumors ("hot" nodules) of the thyroid gland.
3. Inflammation of the thyroid.
4. Graves' disease (the most common cause).

GRAVES' DISEASE

Graves' disease, the only cause of hyperthyroidism that is not rare in childhood, is nevertheless more commonly seen in adults. Because the nursing care of children with Graves' disease is like the care of afflicted adults, information about this disorder is presented in Chapter 28.

CRETINISM

DESCRIPTION

Cretinism (congenital hypothyroidism) is a congenital thyroid hormone deficiency due to lack of a thyroid gland (athyreotic cretinism) or, rarely, lack of one or more of the enzymes needed for the manufacture or release of thyroxine. Lack of a thyroid gland or of the necessary enzymes causes slowing of all metabolic processes, including brain development. The most important consequence of cretinism is permanent mental retardation. Because some T_4 is passed from the mother to the fetus through the placenta, the infant may not show signs of hypothyroidism at birth. *Early diagnosis, however, is of critical importance in the prevention or minimization of brain damage.* For this reason many states now require T_4 screening for all newborn infants so that treatment can be started soon after birth.

Progressive, permanent mental retardation will occur unless thyroid replacement therapy is started promptly. Maximal brain growth and development are completed by 6 months of age. For every day treatment is delayed, some intellectual capacity is irretrievably lost. All other problems (dry skin, bradycardia, constipation, growth, etc.) will respond to therapy and correct themselves. Growth, if long neglected, may not reach maximal genetic potential, but if treatment is started in the first year or so of life, growth should ultimately be normal.

PREVENTION

Health Promotion

1. Proper health practices for the mother while the baby is *in utero*, so that the infant will not be stressed with thyroid inhibiting factors, antithyroid drugs, cobalt treatments, para-aminosalicylic acid, and so forth.
2. T_4 screening program for every institution in which babies are born.
3. Breast-feeding for the first 6 to 12 months of life for the infant to receive sufficient thyroid hormone to reduce or prevent the tragic consequences of mental retardation if not previously screened and treated.

Population at Risk

1. Infant of mother who, during pregnancy, received treatment for cancer, tuberculosis (TB), or hyperthyroidism.
2. Infant with family history of cretinism.
3. Infant from an area of the country with an inadequate supply of iodine in water or food.

Screening

1. Clinical observation for inactivity and appearance of cretinism.
2. A "too good" baby.
3. Prolonged jaundice, constipation, or poor feeding.
4. Laboratory data by T_4 screening of all neonates.

ASSESSMENT

Health History

1. A "good" baby who sleeps much of the time.
2. A baby who is a poor feeder.
3. Documented low level of activity.
4. Prolonged jaundice or constipation.
5. Family history of cretinism.
6. Family living in "goiter belt."
7. Mother with history of treatment that might affect the infant while *in utero* (e.g., medication for TB, cancer, hyperthyroidism).

Physical Assessment

1. Poor feeding with obesity and puffiness (myxedema).
2. Signs of slow metabolism are
   a. Dry scaly skin.
   b. Slow heart rate and low blood pressure.
   c. Slow neurological development (behind in the developmental milestones).
   d. Blank look and lack of playfulness.
   e. Constipation.
3. Large, thick tongue may be present.
4. Facial features are coarse.
5. Umbilical hernia may be present.
6. Growth is poor, especially in height.

Diagnostic Tests

1. T_4 will be depressed.
2. THS will be elevated in classic athyreotic cretinism and depressed or absent in hypothalamic hyperthyroidism.

NURSING DIAGNOSES: ACTUAL OR POTENTIAL

1. Risk of severe, progressive neurological deficit associated with delay in recognizing and treating cretinism.
2. Alterations in level of consciousness secondary to decreased metabolic rate (infant sleeps most of the time).
3. Delayed growth secondary to deficiency in thyroid hormone.
4. Developmental delays (motor, social, and intellectual) secondary to deficiency of thyroid hormone.
5. Knowledge deficit (parents) about child's condition, prognosis, and treatment regimen.

EXPECTED OUTCOMES

1. Child will receive early medical diagnosis and prompt institution of thyroid replacement (within hours or days of birth).
2. Euthyroid state will be established and maintained throughout life.
3. Child will conform to developmental and growth norms for age.
4. Parents will be informed about child's condition and required care (thyroid replacement will be mandatory throughout life) and will follow the recommended treatment plan.

INTERVENTIONS

1. Screen all newborns and assess all infants for cretinism; refer suspect babies for immediate medical diagnosis and hormone replacement therapy.

   NOTE: Even if diagnosis is delayed, thyroid replacement should begin as soon as cretinism is diagnosed.

2. Educate parents about the prescribed medication and expected outcomes of treatment.
3. Educate parents about the consequences of discontinuing the medication (occurrence of hypothyroidism at any age).
4. Teach parents to recognize signs of hyperthyroidism, too much medication, (e.g., irritability, diarrhea).
5. If diagnosis is delayed, evaluate child's neurological development.
6. Monitor to maintain euthyroid state.

EVALUATION

Outcome Criteria

1. Newborn's hypothyroidism is promptly recognized and treatment begun.
2. Mental development and physical growth (see Chapter 4) are within expected norms.
3. Parents understand and participate cooperatively in the treatment regimen.
4. Euthyroidism is achieved and maintained for life.

Complications

MENTAL RETARDATION DUE TO DELAYED DETECTION OR LACK OF PARENTS' COOPERATION WITH MEDICAL MANAGEMENT

Assessment

1. Decreased or decreasing neurological response.
2. Increased or increasing obesity and accompanying edema.
3. Poor suck reflex.
4. Poor or worsening performance on developmental assessment test (e.g., Denver Developmental Screening Test).

Revised Outcomes

1. Child will receive replacement hormone as recommended, beginning as soon as difficulty is recognized.
2. Child and family will participate in special education program, such as infant stimulation program.
3. Parents and child will adjust to remedial programs.

Interventions

1. Find out why thyroid hormone replacement regimen has not been followed, if it has not.
2. Institute appropriate action to promote compliance with medication program (e.g., counseling, teaching) depending upon reason for noncompliance.
3. Refer to infant stimulation program or other developmental remediation program.
4. Refer to community health nurse for follow-up.

ABNORMAL APPEARANCE IN ADVANCED STAGES OF CONDITION

CARDIOVASCULAR CHANGES ACCOMPANIED BY LOW METABOLIC RATE AND EXERTIONAL DYSPNEA

Assessment

1. Slowed pulse rate.
2. Labored respirations with decreased respiration response.
3. Decreased pulse pressure.

Revised Outcomes

Child's respiratory exchange will be unimpaired.

Interventions

1. Maintain airway through positioning of infant, or as directed.
2. Administer oxygen as indicated.
3. Administer medication as prescribed (dosage will be adjusted in accordance with laboratory values).
4. Administer oral feedings carefully to avoid respiratory distress and aspiration.

ACQUIRED HYPOTHYROIDISM

DESCRIPTION

Acquired hypothyroidism can have many causes, such as iodine deficiency, destruction of the gland by tumor, infection, inflammation (thyroiditis), or surgical extirpation. Iodine deficiency goiter with hypothyroidism is now rare in the United States but was, at one time, the commonest cause of goiter. Iodination of salt, bread, and other foods has practically obliterated iodine deficiency. Acquired hypothyroidism in children is now most commonly a result of chronic thyroiditis (Hashimoto's thyroiditis) or subacute thyroiditis. Hashimoto's disease is thought to be an autoimmune disorder. Subacute thyroiditis is a viral disease. In chronic lymphocytic thyroiditis (Hashimoto's), antithyroid antibodies can often be found in the serum. As the gland begins to fail, TSH is released in increased amounts, and the gland hypertrophies to form a goiter. Untreated Hashimoto's disease can result in complete destruction of the gland and permanent hypothyroidism. Treatment should be instituted before hypothyroidism occurs. Treatment is aimed at suppression of TSH in order to put the thyroid gland at rest; thyroxine is the treatment of choice. After 1 to 3 years of suppression the problem may remit and the client be normal. If hypothyroidism of even a mild degree has occurred, however, lifelong treatment with thyroxine is necessary.

Nursing assessment, diagnoses, expected outcomes, interventions, and evaluation are no different for these conditions than for congenital hypothyroidism (above) except that the clients are older (usually preteen girls) and the mental slowness is reversible once medication is begun. For additional care of clients with acquired hypothyroidism, see Chapter 28.

HYPERACTIVITY AND HYPOACTIVITY (ADRENAL GLANDS)

An adrenal gland sits atop each kidney like a three-cornered hat. Each gland consists of an inner part called the *medulla* and an outer layer called the *cortex*.

The medulla secretes *epinephrine* and *norepinephrine*. Tumors of the medulla do occur in children (*neuroblastoma*) but are not hormone producing. Hormone-producing tumors of the medulla (*pheochromocytomas*) have very seldom been reported in children. Disorders of the adrenal medulla will not be discussed here further.

The cortex consists of several layers of cells involved in various stages of steroid hormone production. The adrenal cortex is controlled by the hypothalamus and anterior pituitary gland through the secretion of a releasing hormone from the hypothalamus and adrenocorticotropic hormone (ACTH) from the anterior pituitary in a biological feedback mechanism similar to the hypothalamic-pituitary-thyroid axis previously described (see *Anterior Pituitary Gland*). Consequently, diseases of adrenal steroid excess or deficiency may be due to excess or deficiency of either hypothalamic ACTH-releasing hormone or ACTH or may result from disorders of the adrenal gland itself. All causes will be discussed together since symptoms are similar.

When stimulated by ACTH, the adrenal cortex takes up cholesterol and begins a synthesizing process ending with cortisol (hydrocortisone) and aldosterone. A variety of intermediate products, including estrogen, progesterone, and testosterone, are also produced and reach the bloodstream in small quantities. There are basically five steps in the synthesis of cortisol or aldosterone from cholesterol. Each step is catalyzed by an enzyme. Deficiencies of any one of these enzymes block synthesis and result in deficiency of cortisol and/or aldosterone. Such blocks are known and are genetic disorders often appearing in siblings (adrenocortical hyperplasia or the adrenogenital syndrome).

Disorders of the cortex hormones take four forms:

1. An *excess of cortisol* produces Cushing's disease.
2. A *deficiency of cortisol* produces either Addison's disease or adrenogenital syndrome (AGS).
3. An *excess of aldosterone* produces hyperaldosteronism with salt and water retention and hypertension. This is primarily an adult disease and is discussed in Chapter 28.
4. A *deficiency of aldosterone* produces salt loss and addisonian crisis.

CUSHING'S DISEASE

DESCRIPTION

Cushing's disease or *hypercortisolism* is due to excess secretion of cortisol by the adrenal cortex. The disease can result from an excess of ACTH from a pituitary tumor or from a tumor of the adrenal cortex. The two causal conditions are differentiated from each other by measurement of the serum ACTH level. When a pituitary tumor is present ACTH is elevated, whereas with adrenal tumors it is low. ACTH suppression tests with dexamethasone may be helpful in identifying hypothalamic problems until such time as an assay is developed for ACTH-releasing factor. When surgical removal of a tumor can be done without destroying the glands, the result will be complete reversal of signs and symptoms and return to normal life. Surgical ablation, however, produces Addison's disease and results in a lifelong need for replacement hormone therapy to sustain life; close medical follow-up is required for dosage adjustments. Cushing's disease in children does not differ from Cushing's disease in adults except that short stature is an important assessment factor, the alterations in appearance that accompany the disease (obesity, acne, hirsutism, and shortness) may present special psychosocial adjustment difficulties for children and adolescents, and of course parents or other family members are involved in the child's care. See Chapter 28 for detailed information about Cushing's disease.

CUSHING'S SYNDROME

DESCRIPTION

Cushing's syndrome is a group of signs and symptoms resembling Cushing's disease, but due to administration of exogenous adrenocorticosteroids rather than to their excessive production within the body. The syndrome is frequently seen when large doses of steroids are given in the treatment of such diseases as leukemia, nephrosis, and collagen diseases. Though Cushing's syndrome is reversed by discontinuation of the steroids, this treatment is often not possible because of the underlying disorder for which the steroids were given. Nursing intervention then takes the form of helping the child and family to adjust to the problems created by the drug—altered appearance and body image, susceptibility to infection, poor growth, and so on, as outlined in Chapter 28 under *Cushing's Disease*.

ADDISON'S DISEASE

DESCRIPTION

Addison's disease is a general term for adrenal insufficiency (lack of secretion of adrenocortical hormones). Adrenal insufficiency usually involves failure of production of both cortisol (a glucocorticoid) and aldosterone (a mineralocorticoid). (See *Adrenal Gland*, above). Of these deficiencies, the loss of aldosterone is more important. The function of this hormone is to facilitate the retention of sodium by the kidney. In the absence of aldosterone there is marked loss of sodium in the urine, resulting in serum sodium reduction (hyponatremia), which causes nausea and vomiting and, with further salt loss, convulsions, vascular collapse, shock, and death. This severe state of salt depletion is known as *addisonian crisis*.

Addison's disease can be caused by a deficiency of hypothalamic-releasing factor or of ACTH but more commonly is due to destruction of the adrenal gland by tumor, trauma, hemorrhage, or infection. In the past, the most common cause of Addison's disease was destruction of the gland by tuberculosis. Histoplasmosis is still a common cause of gland destruction. A recently described cause of adrenal destruction is an autoimmune response similar to that of thyroiditis and indeed often occurring concurrently with it. Autoimmune adrenal and thyroid disease occurring with diabetes is called *Schmidt's disease*.

Addison's disease is less common now than formerly, since the incidence of tuberculosis has decreased, but it should be watched for in children with diabetes and/or thyroiditis since an addisonian crisis is potentially fatal.

Nursing care of children with Addison's disease does not differ appreciably from that of afflicted adults, which is outlined in Chapter 28.

ADRENOGENITAL SYNDROME OR ADRENOCORTICAL HYPERPLASIA

DESCRIPTION

There are three basic biochemical pathways of steroid synthesis:

1. *Mineralocorticoid synthesis,* the end product of which is aldosterone.
2. *Glucocorticoid synthesis,* which produces cortisol.
3. *Sex steroid synthesis,* which produces testosterone and, from it, estrogen.

Several steps are involved in the final synthesis of each compound. Each step requires an enzyme to catalyze the chemical reaction. Any one of these five or so enzymes may be congenitally lacking, resulting in a block of that step. Since some early steps are common to all three pathways, a block at a later stage in synthesis of the final compounds, especially of cortisol and aldosterone, will result in shunting of synthesis into alternate pathways, particularly toward testosterone synthesis. There are some enzymes involved in early stages of steroid synthesis that block all three pathways and consequently produce feminization (from lack of testosterone) and severe salt loss (from lack of aldosterone). Unless recognized and treated within the first few hours of life, this severe form of the disease is fatal.

The most common enzymatic blocks occur later in the pathway of cortisol and aldosterone synthesis and do not involve the testosterone pathway. When this happens, cortisol and aldosterone deficiencies cause failure of the normal suppression of ACTH. Under continual ACTH stimulation, the adrenal glands, in an attempt to make cortisol, hypertrophy (*adrenocortical hyperplasia*). Since cortisol and aldosterone still cannot be manufactured in spite of the glandular hypertrophy, ACTH continues to rise, which causes an increase in that synthesis which *can* occur, namely testosterone production. Increased testosterone during fetal life causes masculinization of the fetus of either sex. If the child is male, the genitalia become hypertrophied (*macrogenitalia precox*). If the condition is not treated in the male there will be continued masculinization, causing precocious puberty (Figure 17-2). In the female fetus, masculinization results in ambiguous genitalia. The external genitalia show fusion of the labia and an enlarged clitoris, and the infant may mistakenly be thought to be male with severe hypospadias. Early differentiation is necessary both for proper gender identification and for prompt treatment of possible salt loss that could otherwise lead to addisonian crisis.

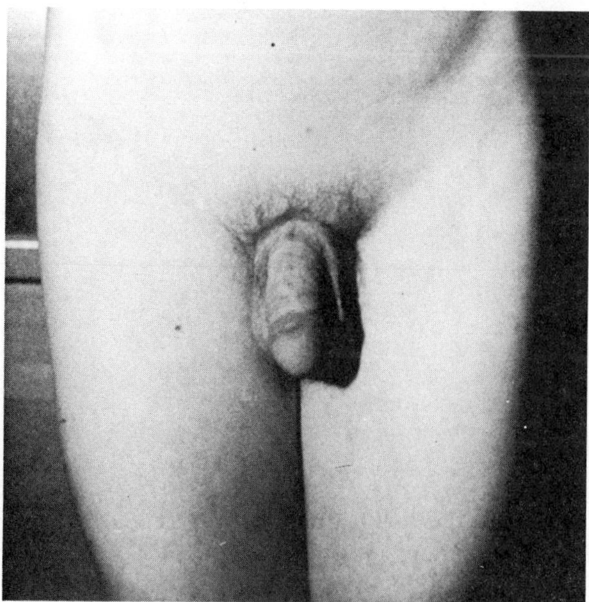

Figure 17-2 Non-salt-losing adrenogenital syndrome, age 5 years.

Some infants have blocks only in cortisol synthesis and are not salt-losers. Especially if these children are male, the problem may not be discovered until precocious puberty results. If there is a block in aldosterone production as well as cortisol, as there often is in the common form of the disease (21-hydroxylase enzyme deficiency), then salt loss is the main problem and must be detected early to prevent death from hyponatremia and shock (addisonian crisis).

The adrenogenital syndrome (AGS), or adrenocortical hyperplasia (ACH), is inherited as an autosomal recessive disorder. It is a complex process, requiring prompt diagnosis and institution of treatment with salt, glucocorticoids, hydrocortisone, and mineralocorticoids, to correct or prevent salt loss and stop the masculinization of the child. Careful follow-up to adjust dosages of the replacement steroids is necessary, and later surgery may be necessary to correct the abnormal appearance of the female's external genitalia. The labia must be separated, the vagina opened, and the clitoris resected to decrease its size.

PREVENTION

Health Promotion

Genetic counseling for persons with a family history of this autosomal recessive disorder.

Population at Risk

Infants and children with a family history of early virilization.

Screening

Clinical observation for signs and symptoms (see *Assessment*, below) in all neonates and other infants, and children below the usual age of puberty.

ASSESSMENT

Health History

1. Family history of this disorder.
2. Inability to withstand heat-producing activi-

ties or above-normal environmental temperatures.

Physical Assessment

1. AGS can usually be recognized at birth by genital examination.
   a. The male infant's penis is usually much larger than normal, and the testes are very small.
   b. The female's genitals are masculinized and may look like those of a male with severe hypospadias, but close inspection will reveal the absence of testicles in the labia, a vestibule rather than complete labial fusion, a perineal urethra in the vestibule, and a phallus that is really a large clitoris rather than a small penis. X-ray or ultrasonographic examinations of the genitals will reveal a vagina and uterus.

      NOTE: A careful examination of the external genitalia should be part of the nurse's evaluation of every infant at birth, preferably in the delivery room or transitional care nursery. *Proper assessment at this time may prevent salt loss and addisonian crisis and may be lifesaving.* Also, correct sex identification is important for naming the child and orienting the parents.
2. Children who have escaped diagnosis in infancy develop early pubertal changes, often during the preschool or early school-age period.
   a. Children of both sexes demonstrate
      (1) Accelerated growth in height for their age, although ultimate adult height may be below normal because pubertal hormonal changes close the epiphyses and terminate linear growth.
      (2) Advanced bone age.
      (3) Masculine physique (well-developed musculature, broad shoulders, etc.).
      (4) Axillary, pubic, and facial hair.
      (5) Deepening of the voice.
      (6) Adolescent skin changes, including acne.
   b. Girls do not menstruate or develop breasts (in contrast with precocious puberty, discussed earlier in this chapter).

Diagnostic Tests

1. Elevated plasma levels of 17-hydroxyprogesterone and other intermediates of testosterone metabolism.
2. Electrolyte levels (especially serum sodium less than normal and elevated serum potassium).
3. 24-hour urine for absence of 17-hydroxysteroids and excess of 17-ketosteroids.
4. Advanced bone age (even at birth) by x-ray examination.

NURSING DIAGNOSES: ACTUAL OR POTENTIAL

1. Alteration in physical development due to abnormal hormonal influence on tissues: ambiguous genitalia in female infant, exaggerated genital growth in male infant, or precocious pubertal changes in child of either sex.
2. Family coping difficulty associated with uncertainty over sex of child or early pubertal development.
3. Alterations in self-concept, secondary to physical changes making child different from peers, or to genital surgery, or to responses of family or others.
4. Risk of severe, life-threatening fluid and electrolyte imbalance (salt-losing syndrome producing addisonian crisis—see Chapter 28) secondary to faulty hormonal control of renal sodium excretion.

EXPECTED OUTCOMES

1. Child will receive prompt and correct identification of gender.
2. Child will receive prompt medical diagnosis and prompt and long-term medical treatment (salt intake, which is initially high, and steroid management must be adjusted as child grows).
3. Child will not experience addisonian crisis.
4. Child's genitals will become normal-appearing and functional.
5. Family and child will cope adequately with child's condition as evidenced by
   a. Normal family relationships (described in Chapter 5).
   b. Normal psychosocial development of child (described in Chapter 4).
   c. Cooperative participation in long-term treatment regimen.
6. Parents will accurately adjust child's medication dosage during periods of illness or other stress.

INTERVENTIONS

1. Ensure that every newborn receives a skilled physical examination for prompt and correct gender identification.
2. *Alert the medical staff for possible salt-losing syndrome.*
3. Ensure absolute accuracy in specimen collection (e.g., 24-hour urines, blood samples to be drawn at specified times).
4. Carefully observe weight, feeding, blood pressure, and urinary output in response to medications.
5. Teach and counsel parents about
   a. Child's gender.
   b. Potential psychological problems related to abnormal genital appearance.
   c. Adjustment of medication doses (hydrocortisone, perhaps Doca) by physician as child grows.
   d. Regulation of salt intake and medication dose by parents during periods of illness or other stress.
   e. Need for long-term medical follow-up (lifelong medication and dosage adjustment).
   f. Signs and symptoms of abnormal salt loss and impending addisonian crisis (see Chapter 28).
   g. When to call for medical or nursing help.

EVALUATION

Outcome Criteria

1. Gender identification is prompt and correct.
2. Addisonian crises are avoided.
3. Parents understand, cooperate in, and cope well with plan of care.
4. Child adjusts well and is free of problems related to gender.

Complications

ABNORMALITIES RELATED TO GENDER ARE OVERLOOKED OR NOT BROUGHT TO THE ATTENTION OF PROPER HEALTH PROFESSIONALS

PSYCHOLOGICAL ADJUSTMENT IS POOR, RELATED TO INCORRECT GENDER IDENTIFICATION

Assessment

1. Child is being reared in a gender role that does not match the external genitalia.
2. Laboratory tests show that incorrect sexual determination was made.

Revised Outcomes

Family will select and reinforce the sexual role that appears to be most functional.

Interventions

1. Support parents in choosing sex role in conformity with physiological manifestations.
2. If child is old enough (about 2 years), refer to psychologist to identify child's perception of sexual identity to assist in choice of sex role assignment.

NONCOOPERATION OF PARENTS IN ADMINISTRATION OF MEDICATION AS DIRECTED

Assessment

1. Genital changes are not progressing as expected.
2. Laboratory values are not being corrected as anticipated by changes in medication dosage.

Revised Outcomes

1. Parents will follow prescribed regimen.
2. Other expected outcomes as previously stated.

Interventions

1. Involve community nurse, especially if distance to health care facility is a problem.
2. Reeducate parents as to importance of medications and methods of measuring and administering them.
3. Reeducate parents to recognize causes of addisonian crisis (e.g., vomiting, fever) so that adequate alterations in dosage may be made to prevent crisis.

ADDISONIAN CRISIS

See Chapter 28

HYPERACTIVITY AND HYPOACTIVITY (PANCREAS)

Pancreatic endocrine disorders are characterized by insufficient, absent, or excessive insulin. The hormone *insulin* is responsible for keying glucose into muscle and fat cells, preventing fat mobilization, and promoting protein synthesis by increasing the permeability of cell membranes to amino acids as well as to glucose. Pancreatic diseases can be inherited or may be caused by trauma, infection, or tumor. *Congenital disorders,* due to mutation or other alteration in the genes, result in inadequacy of the insulin-making process, especially in the presence of stress, such as viral infection, severe illness, or prolonged emotional strain. *Trauma* can lead to partial or total removal of the pancreas, causing loss of the number of cells necessary to produce adequate amounts of insulin. *Infection* of the pancreas can lead to an alteration of the insulin-making cells (the beta cells in the millions of islets of Langerhans scattered throughout the acinar tissue of the gland), setting up an antibody response that can then lead to autoimmune action against the beta cells. *Tumors* cause either increased or decreased functioning of cells.

HYPOGLYCEMIA

DESCRIPTION

Excessive secretion of insulin occurs as a result of islet cell hyperplasia in infants (a disease known as *nesidioblastosis*) or, in older children, as a result of islet cell tumors. Both of these conditions are sufficiently rare as to warrant only minimal discussion here. Both disorders cause severe *hypoglycemia,* usually accompanied by convulsions, and are diagnosed by confirmation of the hypoglycemia by blood sugar measurement and documentation of the hyperinsulinism by measurement of serum insulin levels. Treatment of both conditions is with a drug called diazoxide or surgical removal of the tumor or pancreas.

DIABETES MELLITUS

DESCRIPTION

Diabetes mellitus is an insulin-dependent or non-insulin-dependent disorder resulting from inadequate functioning of the beta cells of the islets of Langerhans in the pancreas. It is characterized by frequent urination, thirst, and weight loss in the insulin-dependent state known as *juvenile* or *type I* diabetes mellitus. Fatigue, slow healing of infections, obesity, and blurred vision are more frequently seen in the non-insulin-dependent state, called *maturity onset* or *type II* diabetes mellitus. Type II diabetes is discussed in Chapter 28.

Of the 11.6 million people in the United States with diabetes mellitus, 15% are dependent on insulin injections. One of every 600 school-age children has this disease. Children can develop the disease in infancy, early childhood, late childhood, or adolescence, but the commonest time is during the preadolescent growth spurt.

Type I diabetes mellitus is associated with lack of insulin production. During early treatment the diabetes may appear to go into a partial remission, and the client needs little external insulin to maintain normal metabolism. The beta cells evidently continue to decrease in number, however, and almost all diabetic youths become totally dependent on exogenous insulin for life.

The severest manifestation of this disease is *diabetic ketoacidosis,* which results in nausea, vomiting, dehydration, oliguria, abdominal pain, coma, and even death. Besides hyperglycemia (blood glucose levels higher than the normal 110 mg/dL—often above 800 mg/dL), the client also has ketones in the urine as a by-product of the body's effort to burn fats when glucose is not available *to the cells* because of insufficient insulin. Severe polyuria results and, without compensatory fluid intake, produces dehydration and electrolyte imbalance.

Juvenile diabetes is a disorder in which client education is a major part of treatment. An essential overall goal is that the child adjust to a lifetime disease and attain the level of control over the disease that will prevent or delay complications. Learning must be continually emphasized throughout the patient's life, both to enhance understanding as the child's developmental capacity expands and to inform the child and family about periodic advances in treatment. Hope must be given continually to motivate the child and family to attain the best control possible.

Like other hormone-deficiency diseases, type I diabetes is treated with hormone replacement, by insulin injection. For 24-hour coverage of glucose levels, many professionals now recognize that multiple doses of insulin increase the flexibility of the client's lifestyle (diet and exercise regimens, for example) and also improve the control of the disease. Informing clients and their families of this kind of new development, as well as other ongoing changes in the field of diabetes (self-blood glucose monitoring, HbA_1C, insulin pumps, pancreas transplants, and so forth) are an important part of the continuing support of children with diabetes.

PREVENTION

Health Promotion

1. Genetic counseling for people with a family history of diabetes mellitus.
2. Good nutrition: carbohydrates, protein, and fats in proper balance; vitamin A and C; niacin, thiamine, iron, and calcium.
   a. Avoid fad diets.
   b. Avoid empty calorie foods, especially concentrated sweets.
   c. Avoid intake of more calories than are needed for daily activity.
3. Use steroids only as necessary.
4. Maintain good health habits: this will not prevent type I diabetes but may prevent complications of the disease.
   a. Brush and floss teeth at least twice daily.
   b. See the dentist twice yearly.
   c. Have a complete physical examination every 1 to 2 years.
   d. Have an eye examination every 2 years (yearly for client who wears glasses).
   e. Bathe at least three to five times weekly; shampoo hair at least once a week.
   f. Manicure nails to prevent ingrown toenails or other sites of infection.
   g. Have regular exercise (as child grows beyond the age of full activity in spontaneous play, adequate exercise should be planned as part of daily activity).

Population at Risk

1. Children with a family history of diabetes mellitus.
   a. Forty to 60 percent of the children of parents who both have type I diabetes develop the disorder (recent genetic findings indicate that inheritance is most often by autosomal recessive gene with some environmental interaction).
   b. Genetic probabilities for children of one parent with type I diabetes or children with other kinship patterns are not yet clear.
2. Children with a history of pancreatic tumor, injury, or infection.
3. Persons who take stress drugs (steroids), including oral contraceptive agents.
4. Children whose birth weight was over 9 pounds (and their mothers).
5. Children who contract certain viral illnesses, such as mumps, Venezuelan equine encephalitis, or other Coxsackie B4 viruses.

Screening

1. Fasting blood glucose (this test misses 85 percent of those with impaired glucose tolerance or mild diabetes).
2. Two-hour postprandial or postglucose test.
3. Four- to 6-hour glucose tolerance tests, preferably with insulins.

ASSESSMENT

Health History

1. Family history of diabetes.
2. Frequent urination (bed-wetting).
3. Increased thirst.
4. Increased appetite with weight loss.
5. Delayed growth and/or maturation.

Physical Assessment

1. Evaluate level of consciousness and behavior as compared with child's usual behavior.
2. Labored respiration may be noted (Kussmaul respiration—deep, rapid breathing).
3. Check for dehydration.
   a. Hypotension.
   b. Poor skin turgor.
   c. Soft eyeballs.
   d. Rapid, thready pulse.

Diagnostic Tests

1. Hyperglycemia.
   a. Blood glucose levels elevated (fasting values over 110 mg/dL: suspicion; over 140 mg/dL: diagnostic).
   b. Two-hour postprandial (greater than 150 mg/dL considered suspicious; over 200 mg/dL, diagnostic).
   c. Glucose present in urine.
2. Diabetic ketosis.
   a. Blood glucose levels elevated.
   b. Glucose present in urine.
   c. Ketones present in blood.
   d. Ketones present in urine.
   e. Some dehydration may be present.
3. Diabetic ketoacidosis.
   a. Blood glucose levels elevated.
   b. Glucose present in urine.
   c. Ketones present in blood.
   d. Ketones present in urine.
   e. Dehydration.
   f. Abnormal electrolytes.

(1) Sodium decreased.
(2) Serum potassium increased (or decreased).
(3) Total potassium decreased.
(4) HCO_2^- decreased.

4. Glycosylated hemoglobin (A_1C or A_1 hemoglobin)—the glycosylation of glucose to amino acids, as measured in red blood cells, measures mean blood glucose levels over the last 2 to 3 months.

NURSING DIAGNOSES: ACTUAL OR POTENTIAL

1. Alteration in urinary elimination: polyuria secondary to glycosuria or (if allowed to progress) oliguria secondary to dehydration.
2. Fluid volume deficit secondary to polyuria and, possibly, also to vomiting and diarrhea.
3. Alteration in fluid intake: increased intake secondary to polyuria.
4. Respiratory dysfunction, mild to severe (Kussmaul respirations) secondary to ketoacidosis.
5. Nutritional deficit: weight loss in spite of increased food intake, due to insufficient insulin for cellular metabolism.
6. Nutritional deficit secondary to nausea and vomiting in acidotic state.
7. Impaired growth: sporadic or delayed growth in both height and weight, or only in weight, secondary to insulin deficiency and resulting interference with cellular metabolism (see Figure 17-3).
8. Impaired integrity of subcutaneous tissue: lipodystrophy (atrophy, shown in Figure 17-4, or hypertrophy) secondary to repeated injection of insulin into same site (knowledge deficit).
9. Alteration in comfort: discomfort associated with hypoglycemic or hyperglycemic states.
10. Anxiety secondary to hypoglycemia and catecholamine response and secondary to chronic illness.
11. Impaired thought processes secondary to abnormal levels of blood glucose (high or low).
12. Alteration in consciousness, mild to severe, secondary to abnormally high or low blood glucose levels, and/or ketoacidosis.
13. Knowledge deficit (child or family) regarding diabetes and its treatment, secondary to inadequate information, anxiety that interferes with learning, denial, or other forms of unreadiness to learn.
14. Noncompliance with therapy secondary to denial, knowledge deficit, or inadequate coping with chronic illness.
15. Risk of diabetic complications of eyes, kidneys, nervous system, and blood vessels, secondary to delayed or inadequate treatment and control of diabetes.
16. Ineffective coping due to anxiety about chronic illness and due to knowledge deficit.
17. Impaired self-concept secondary to diagnosis of chronic illness, delayed growth, perceived lack of wholeness, and ineffective individual or family coping.
18. Ineffective family coping secondary to diagnosis of chronic, familial illness and secondary to knowledge deficit.
19. Alterations in parenting secondary to guilt for child's illness or reactions to responsibility for child's care.

EXPECTED OUTCOMES

1. Child will receive early medical diagnosis and treatment adequate for growth and developmental stage.
2. Child will maintain fluid volume, electrolyte balance, and blood glucose level within acceptable ranges.
3. Growth in height and weight will be restored to child's preillness growth percentiles.
4. Parents (and child when old enough) will be well informed about diabetes and the child's treatment program.
   a. Will safely and accurately carry out the mechanical aspects of care, such as
      (1) Withdrawal and injection of insulin.
      (2) Mixing of insulins.
      (3) Rotation of injection sites.
      (4) Urine testing.
      (5) Urine and insulin record keeping.
      (6) Meal planning.
      (7) Recognition, treatment, and prevention of insulin reactions (hypoglycemia).
      (8) Good health and exercise practices.
   b. They will know how to adjust dietary intake and/or insulin dosage to maintain acceptable blood glucose level during periods of stress (e.g., illness) or changed activity level.
   c. They will know when to call the physician or other health professional for assistance.

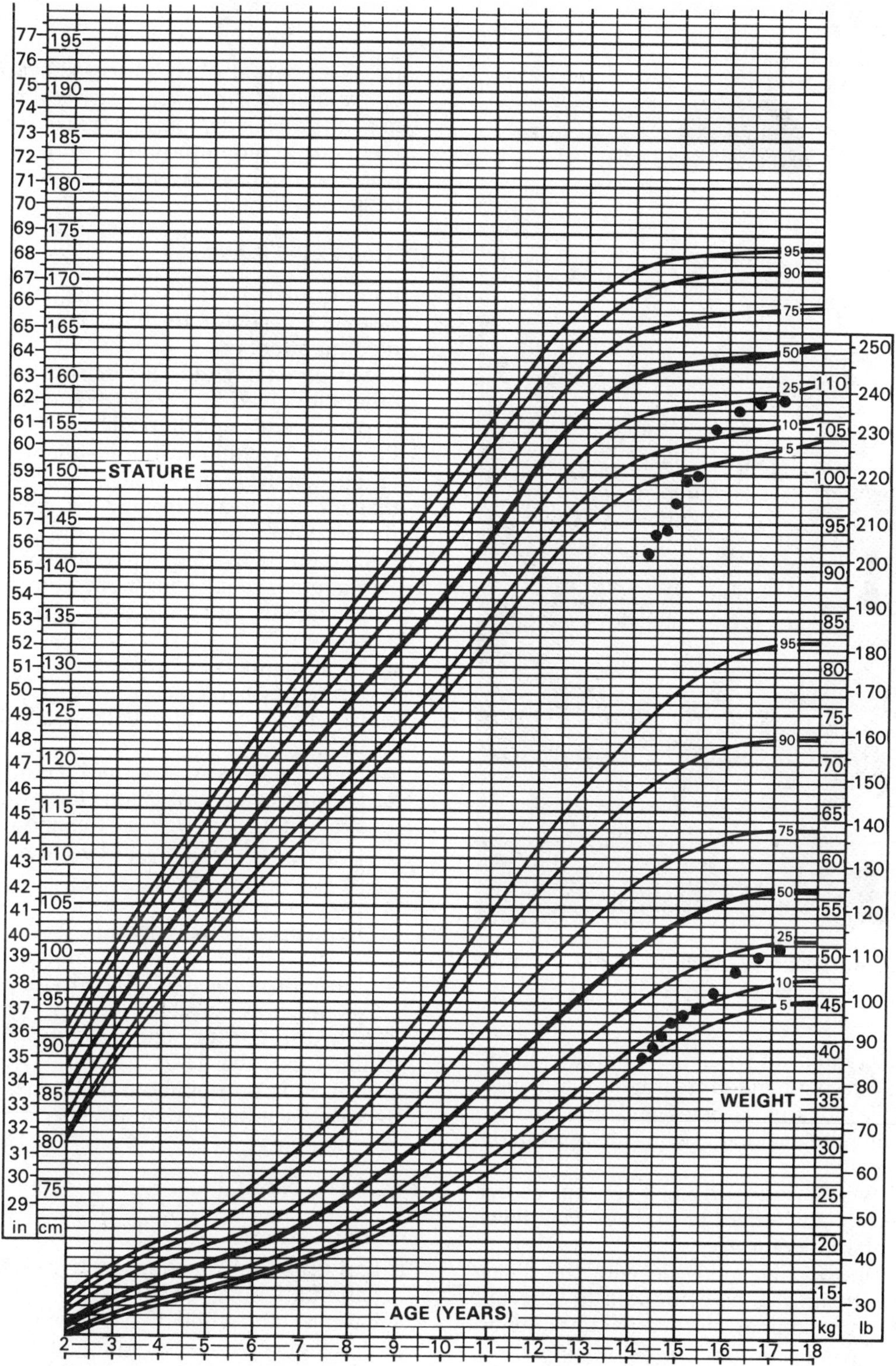

Figure 17-3 Improved growth as a result of improved control of diabetes mellitus. (Adapted from National Center for Health Statistics, NCHS Growth Charts, 1976, Monthly Vital Statistics Report, Health Resources Administration, Rockville, Md., June 1976, vol. 25, no. 3, supp. (HRA) 76-1120. Data from the National Center for Health Statistics. © 1976 Ross Laboratories.)

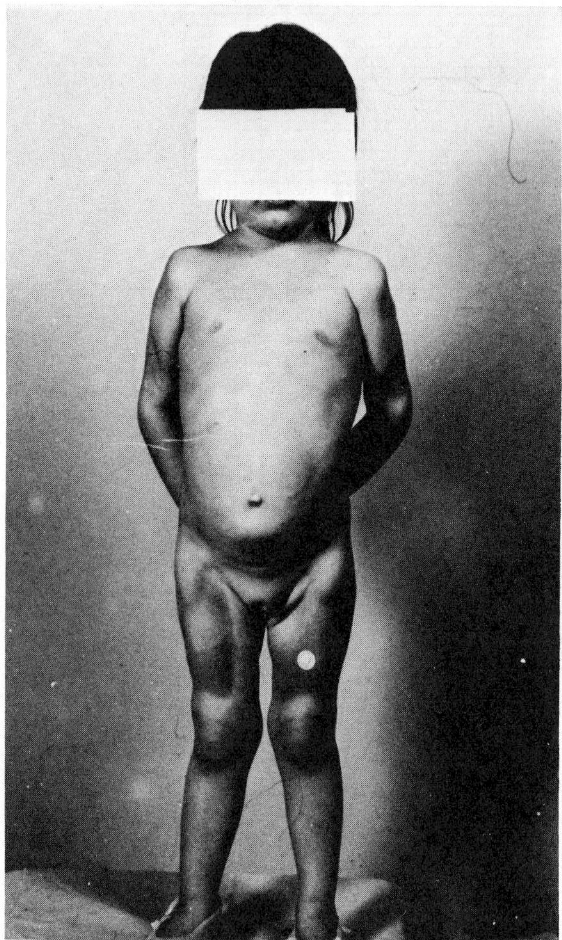

Figure 17-4 Diabetes mellitus with lipoatrophy.

5. Parents (and child when old enough) will follow the recommended treatment regimen.
6. Complications of diabetes and insulin therapy will not develop or will be delayed in development.
7. Child will have positive self-concept as evidenced by attainment of psychosocial developmental tasks for age.
8. Child and family will cope with the illness and its treatment, as evidenced by effective family functioning, normal family interactions (Chapter 5), and normal attainment of developmental tasks for age (Chapter 4).

NOTE: The overall objective in the nursing care of a diabetic child is to enable the boy or girl to function at top capacity with the best possible control of the disease. *This goal can best be attained if diabetes management is designed to fit the child's lifestyle rather than the reverse.* Frequent communication and continual teaching are the best means by which this can be accomplished.

INTERVENTIONS

1. Identify diabetes early by adequate nursing assessment, and help child to get immediate medical attention.
2. Teach parents, child, and school teachers or others involved to recognize and respond to hyperglycemia and hypoglycemia.
3. Promote psychological adjustment by facilitating family's and child's competence to manage the treatment and by emphasizing the normal range of activities and good health that accompany adequate control of diabetes.
4. For avoidance of long-term complications, teach parents and child daily care and management of
   a. Meal planning.
   b. Urine testing.
   c. Injection procedure with good site rotation.
   d. Hygiene of skin, hair, and teeth.
   e. Regular eye examinations for retinopathy.
   f. Prevention (as well as treatment) of hypoglycemia, which can be induced by illness or other stress.
   g. Exercise program.
   h. Regularity in daily living.
   i. Assist family in recognizing the importance of normalizing blood glucose levels as much as possible.
5. Teach duration of action of the various insulins (see Table 17-2).
6. Teach and counsel about maintenance of effective discipline and other aspects of normal family living.

EVALUATION

Outcome Criteria

1. Early medical diagnosis and treatment initiation are obtained.
2. Parents (and child if old enough) demonstrate good understanding of the disease and its course and treatment.
3. Parents (and child if old enough) demonstrate techniques for injection of insulin and testing of urine.

TABLE 17-2 INSULIN ACTIVITY: PEAKS AND DURATIONS OF EFFECTIVENESS OF THE VARIOUS TYPES OF INSULINS

Insulin Type	Peak Action Occurs	Effective Duration of Action
Short acting (Regular, Actrapid, Semilente, Semitard, Humulin-R)	2–4 h after injection	6–8 h
Immediate acting (Protophane-NPH, Insulatard NPH, NPH Monotard, Lentard, Lente, Humulin-N)	8 h ± 2 h after injection	12–18 h
Mixed insulin (Mixtard: 30% short acting and 70% intermediate acting)	3–4 h and 6–8 h after injection	12–16 h
Long acting (Ultratard, PZI, Ultralente)	About 18 h after injection	36–72 h

4. Accurate and complete records (insulin and urine) are kept by the child or parents.
5. Parents (and child if old enough) keep adequate food records when requested and are able to adjust food intake to activity level.
6. Parents (and child if old enough) are able to describe the cause, course, treatment, and prevention of both hyperglycemia and hypoglycemia.
7. Parents (and child if old enough) know when to call the health professional:
   a. When the child's urine tests do not show the kind of control they expect.
   b. When there are ketones in the urine accompanied by elevated urine glucose (2% or higher) more than a few times.
   c. When glucose appears in increasing amounts in the urine or blood.
   d. When a severe insulin reaction occurs.
8. Child accepts the disease and is well adjusted and demonstrates suitable developmental attainment for age.
9. Parents (and child if old enough) recognize and respond correctly to his or her unique individual symptoms of hyperglycemia and hypoglycemia.
10. Child's daily activities are adequately regulated and disciplined to promote general health and development, as well as diabetes control.
11. Episodes of hyperglycemia and hypoglycemia are infrequent and well managed.
12. Growth returns to child's normal percentile track on growth charts.
13. Family functions are carried out, and family relationships are healthful for all family members (see Chapter 5).

Complications

HYPOGLYCEMIA (INSULIN SHOCK, INSULIN REACTION)

Assessment

1. Mild.
   a. Low blood glucose (below normal range by 10–20 mg/dL). Please note, depending on the glucose analysis used, this could be below 60 mg/dL, 70 mg/dL, or 80 mg/dL.
   b. Rapid, strong pulse.
   c. Weakness.
2. Moderate.
   a. Dilated pupils.
   b. Drowsy.
   c. Blood glucose even lower (below normal range by 30–50 mg/dL).
   d. Pulse more rapid and strong.
   e. Profuse perspiration.
3. Severe.
   a. In coma.
   b. Convulsions may occur.
   c. Blood glucose 20 mg/dL or below.

Revised Outcomes

1. Child's blood glucose level will be restored to normal.
2. If convulsions occur, child will not be injured or aspirate.

3. Child, if old enough, and family will accurately describe prevention and early recognition of hypoglycemia.
4. Other outcomes as stated above.

Interventions

1. *Mild insulin reaction.* Give a small amount of food, such as milk; repeat in 10–15 minutes, if needed.
2. *Moderate insulin reaction.* Give simple sugar (20–40 calories) or carbohydrate (10–20 grams), followed by food in 10–15 minutes; repeat simple sugar instead of food if still symptomatic.
3. *Severe insulin reaction.* Give glucagon ($\frac{1}{2}$ mg for children age 3 years or younger; 1 mg for children above age 3 years), followed, when alert (about 15–20 minutes after injection of glucagon), by simple sugar. Follow with food when nausea, if present, subsides.
4. Assess reasons for hypoglycemic episode (e.g., noncompliance, knowledge deficit, denial) and teach, counsel, or refer, as needed.

Reevaluation and Follow-up

1. Develop short- and long-term goals in order to help the child or adolescent to become psychologically well adjusted, as well as socially and metabolically adjusted.
2. Continue to review, reeducate, and counsel the child or adolescent and other family members to assist in adjustment to diabetes and to assist in appropriate decision making.

HYPERGLYCEMIA (DIABETIC KETOSIS, DIABETIC KETOACIDOSIS)

Assessment

1. Hyperglycemia.
   a. Depending on method of glucose analysis: fasting blood glucose greater than 140 mg/dL and 2-hour postprandial greater than 180 mg/dL.
   b. Depending on renal threshold (point at which blood glucose enters into the urine, usually higher than 160–180 mg/dL): $\frac{1}{2}$% or higher.
   c. Cardinal symptoms: polyuria, polyphagia, and polydipsia with weight loss and possible bed-wetting.
2. Diabetic ketosis.
   a. Elevated glucose level in the blood and urine as described above, plus ketones in the urine.
   b. Possible mild dehydration.
   c. Increased irritability and inability to concentrate.
3. Diabetic ketoacidosis.
   a. Elevated glucose, as well as ketones in blood and urine.
   b. Dehydration (usually accompanied by decreased blood pressure), oliguria.
   c. Electrolyte imbalance.
   d. Possible labored respirations (Kussmaul respirations).
   e. Altered consciousness (drowsiness to coma).

Revised Outcomes

1. Child's blood glucose level will be restored to normal.
2. If in coma, child will maintain respiratory exchange and integrity of skin and mucous membranes.
3. Subsequent severe hyperglycemic episodes will be prevented.
4. Other outcomes, as originally stated.

Interventions

1. For hyperglycemia, increase amount of insulin *or* decrease food intake *or* increase amount of exercise; reverse the precipitating illness or other stressor.
2. For diabetic ketosis, decrease food intake (20 percent fewer calories); increase insulin as needed (supplemental insulin may be prescribed); treat precipitating illness or other stressor.
3. For diabetic ketoacidosis, decrease food intake (20 percent fewer calories); administer intravenous (IV) fluids to alter dehydrated state; administer prescribed regular insulin (may be given by IV perfusion, or half the dose IV and half subcutaneously; or may be given in small, frequent doses intramuscularly or subcutaneously); treat precipitating illness or other stressor.
4. Carefully monitor vital signs, electrocardiogram (ECG) readings, fluid intake and output, urine glucose and acetone levels, laboratory values, and insulin administration.
5. Carefully monitor level of consciousness. Children can progress rapidly to ketoacidosis and coma.
6. If child is comatose, maintain airway, prevent aspiration, and provide skin and mouth care. (See Chapter 15 for the care of unconscious children.)
7. Assess reasons for hyperglycemic episode (e.g., noncompliance, knowledge deficit,

denial) and teach, counsel, or refer, as needed.

8. Other expected outcomes as stated above.

HYPERACTIVITY AND HYPOACTIVITY (CHROMOSOMAL ABERRATIONS AFFECTING GONADAL HORMONES)

Only two chromosomal problems, in which endocrine disturbances are important, will be discussed—Turner's and Klinefelter's syndromes. The exact mechanism of chromosomal abnormalities is not known. For the two syndromes discussed here, the problem is thought to involve defective *meiosis* (the cell division phase of the egg or sperm). During meiosis the chromosomes normally divide in such a way as to put one-half of the chromosomes in each daughter cell. When fertilization occurs, the normal number of chromosomes is reestablished. Occasionally during meiosis of the egg or sperm, the chromosomes do not distribute evenly between the daughter cells, so that one cell may contain an extra chromosome and one may be deficient.

TURNER'S SYNDROME

DESCRIPTION

When a sex cell with a missing chromosome combines in fertilization with a normal sex cell, the cells of the resulting fetus lack a chromosome. Most of these situations are incompatible with life, and the fetuses die and are aborted. One such syndrome in which the child can survive is Turner's syndrome, in which there is only one X chromosome, and the other sex chromosome is absent. (This chromosomal configuration is written XO.) Since persons with Turner's syndrome have no Y (male) chromosome, they are females. When only one X chromosome is present, however, sexuality is deficient in that the female has no ovaries and, thus, is sexually infantile even in adulthood.

It is important that Turner's syndrome be recognized before puberty so that estrogen replacement can begin in order to sexualize these girls. Turner's syndrome is suspected from physical examination and confirmed by chromosomal analysis. A presumptive diagnosis can be made in a phenotypic girl by means of a *buccal smear*, which is obtained by scraping the superficial cells of the mucous membrane of the cheek with a flat stick and spreading the cells on a microscope slide. The cells are stained and examined under a microscope for the absence of *Barr bodies*. Whenever two X chromosomes are present in any body cell, one of them is inactivated and deposited as a tight, dark-staining ball (a Barr body) on the edge of the nucleus. Barr bodies can be seen in any cell containing two or more X chromosomes but are easiest to identify in white blood cells or buccal mucosal cells. In the case of Turner's syndrome there is *no* Barr body even though the patient is female and one would be expected.

PREVENTION

Health Promotion

Avoidance by prospective parents of x-rays and chemicals that alter chromosomes.

Population at Risk

1. Girls whose parents were exposed to chemicals or x-ray procedures that might alter chromosomes *in utero* or in the ovary or testis.
2. Girls from families with a history of Turner's syndrome.

Screening

Clinical observation for characteristic signs (described below under *Assessment*).

ASSESSMENT

Health History

1. Positive family history.
2. Abnormal chromosomal analysis.
3. Poor growth progression.
4. Sometimes hearing loss and heart disease.
5. Abnormal physical appearance.
6. If old enough, sexual infantilism.

Physical Assessment

1. Short stature.
2. Webbing of the neck.
3. Low hairline.

4. Wide-spaced nipples and shield-shaped chest.
5. Cubitus valgus.
6. If old enough, sexual infantilism.
7. Sometimes hearing loss, mental retardation, and/or coarctation of the aorta.

NOTE: The physical findings, such as short stature, webbing of the neck, and cubitus valgus, are usually striking enough that girls with Turner's syndrome can be identified from the history and physical examination alone. If the child is below the age of expected puberty, the lack of gonads will not be evident. Often, however, the girl will not be brought in until adolescence, when she comes in because of amenorrhea and lack of sexual development. A buccal smear provides presumptive diagnosis, and a karyotype is diagnostic. The external genitalia show a normal female configuration but are immature and childlike. Examination reveals an infantile uterus and vagina. Ovaries are absent and are replaced by a streaklike gonad that contains no hormonally functional cells and no ova, so females with Turner's syndrome will never be fertile.

Diagnostic Tests

1. Buccal smear showing no Barr body.
2. Chromosomal analysis of blood to show only one female X chromosome.

NURSING DIAGNOSES: ACTUAL OR POTENTIAL

1. Impaired growth and development. Short stature and absence of sexual maturation secondary to chromosomal abnormality.
2. Sensory deficit. Deafness, in about 20 percent of clients, secondary to congenital syndrome.
3. Cognitive impairment. Mental retardation, in about 20 percent of clients, secondary to congenital syndrome.
4. Altered patterns of sexuality. Sexual infantilism (reversible with treatment) and infertility (permanent) secondary to congenital absence of ovaries.
5. Diminished self-esteem secondary to short stature and sexual infantilism.
6. Ineffective coping secondary to poor self-concept and (if present) cognitive impairment and hearing deficit.

EXPECTED OUTCOMES

1. Child's condition will be recognized before the normal age of puberty so that estrogen therapy can be provided to induce sexual maturation at the appropriate time (early or middle adolescence).
2. Client will receive appropriate corrective or supportive care for hearing loss, mental retardation, and other associated problems (e.g., coarctation of the aorta) if these are present.
3. Client will achieve normal sexual function.
4. Client will adjust to continued short stature and infertility, which are not correctable.
5. Client will achieve adequate coping and self-esteem, as evidenced by attainment of age-appropriate psychosocial developmental tasks (described in Chapter 5).

INTERVENTIONS

1. Recognize probable Turner's syndrome by history and physical assessment.
2. Obtain appropriate laboratory confirmation (buccal smear and/or karyotype).
3. Obtain medical consultation for estrogen replacement if approaching pubescent age.
4. Obtain medical assistance for associated medical problems.
5. Refer family for developmental stimulation program or other special education if child has mental retardation.
6. Provide teaching and counseling to promote psychological adjustment to short stature and infertility.
7. Prepare child and family for sexual maturation when estrogen therapy is begun.

EVALUATION

Outcome Criteria

1. Turner's syndrome is recognized before the age of adolescence.
2. Hormonal replacement therapy is provided to induce puberty in early or middle adolescence.
3. Hearing loss, coarctation, and mental retardation have received appropriate referral and follow-up.
4. Client develops normal sexual function.
5. Psychosocial developmental task attainment

is normal for age (allowing for mental retardation, if present).

Complications

BEHAVIORAL ABNORMALITIES RELATED TO SEXUAL IDENTITY OR MATURATION

Assessment

1. Identifies inappropriately with the opposite sex (usually noted at the time pubescence is to occur).
2. Displays exaggeratedly childish, immature behavior for chronological (or if retarded, developmental) age.

Revised Outcomes

Client will achieve acceptance of self as sexually mature female.

Intervention

Referral to sex counselor.

SEXUAL MATURATION DEVELOPS TOO RAPIDLY DUE TO INCORRECT DOSAGE OF ESTROGEN

Assessment

1. Sexual development is ahead of chronological age.
2. Bone age (and epiphyseal closure, terminating linear growth) advancing faster than chronological age.
3. Client is not keeping appointments for dosage adjustments.

Revised Outcomes

1. Client will receive dosage adjustments directed to her developmental rate and stage.
2. Client will comply with treatment regimen.

Interventions

1. Assess reasons why client is not keeping appointments and/or not taking medication as recommended (e.g., financial limitations, knowledge deficit) and teach, counsel, or refer, as needed.
2. Refer to community nurse for assessment of home medication regimen, teaching as needed, and follow-up supervision.

KLINEFELTER'S SYNDROME

DESCRIPTION

The client with Klinefelter's syndrome is a male with one extra X chromosome (occasionally more), usually having an XXY chromosomal configuration. The causative chromosomal nondisjunction is traceable to the mother in about two-thirds of cases and to the father in about one-third. Since a Y chromosome is present, the child is male with male external and internal genitalia. The extra X chromosome, however, exerts an effect and feminizes the individual. The primary effect of the extra X is to suppress the testosterone production and spermatogenesis of the testicles. As a result, feminine physical characteristics become apparent at puberty, and the patient is almost always sterile. Klinefelter's syndrome is suspected by physical appearance and confirmed by laboratory studies.

PREVENTION

Health Promotion

Maintenance of good health habits by prospective parents, including avoidance, where possible, of drugs, other chemicals, or treatments (e.g., x-rays) that can cause chromosomal aberrations.

Population at Risk

1. Male children of men or women who were exposed before pregnancy to radiation or chemicals that induce chromosomal abnormalities.
2. Infertile males (Klinefelter's syndrome is often first diagnosed in infertility clinics).

Screening

Clinical observation for characteristic signs (described below under *Assessment*).

ASSESSMENT

Health History

1. Rapid linear growth with tall stature.
2. Partial or complete failure of sexual development.
3. Possible history of parents' exposure before pregnancy to agents that damage chromosomes.
4. Child may be mentally retarded or have behavior disorder.

Physical Assessment

1. Child is tall in relation to age norms.
2. Child after onset of puberty, has feminine physical characteristics.

a. There is a female fat distribution pattern, including fat around the hips.
b. Breasts are developed (gynecomastia).
3. Masculinization is lacking, if patient is at pubescent age.
a. Penis is small.
b. Testicles are small and sometimes undescended.
c. There may be no pubic, axillary, or facial hair.
d. Voice is high pitched.
4. Indications of mental retardation or behavior disorder may be present.

Diagnostic Tests

1. Buccal smear reveals the presence of Barr bodies. (Buccal smears and Barr bodies are discussed under *Turner's Syndrome,* above).
2. Karyotype shows two or more X chromosomes and one Y.

NURSING DIAGNOSES: ACTUAL OR POTENTIAL

1. Alteration in growth, physique, and sexual maturation secondary to chromosomal influences on hormone regulation.
2. Cognitive impairment (in about 20 percent of cases) associated with chromosomal abnormality.
3. Diminished self-concept secondary to feminine physique, testicular underdevelopment, high voice, and mental retardation, if present.
4. Altered psychosocial development due to poor self-concept and cognitive impairment, if present.
5. Altered patterns of sexuality secondary to alterations in self-concept and physique, lack of secondary sex characteristics, and probable infertility.

EXPECTED OUTCOMES

1. Child's disorder will be recognized before the usual time of puberty and before psychological problems develop.
2. Client will receive testosterone replacement therapy and, consequently, will develop a characteristic male physique and secondary sexual characteristics.

NOTE: Feminine physique that develops without treatment by puberty will reverse with testosterone therapy, but gynecomastia is usually amenable only to surgery.

3. Client with mental retardation or behavior disorder will receive appropriate educational or behavioral interventions (e.g., special education, psychotherapy).
4. Self-concept wil be adequate as evidenced by attainment of normal psychosocial developmental tasks for age (see Chapter 4).
5. Adolescent will develop male gender identity and will become sexually functional.

INTERVENTIONS

1. Routinely screen boys for testicular size, particularly those who are tall for their age. For suspect boys, obtain appropriate laboratory test material (buccal smear for Barr bodies).
2. Obtain medical care for testosterone replacement to masculinize client if at pubescent age.
3. Obtain medical care for plastic repair of gynecomastia.
4. Refer for supportive therapy for mental retardation or behavior disorder.
5. Teach and counsel client about hormone therapy (importance of periodic dosage adjustments, expected outcome of normal secondary sexual development, preparation for physical changes to be expected from testosterone, anticipated normal sexual function, except for probable infertility).
6. Teach and counsel about sexual matters as sexual development progresses.

EVALUATION

Outcome Criteria

1. Klinefelter's syndrome is recognized before the normal age of puberty, and hormone replacement therapy is begun at age of puberty.
2. For client diagnosed later, feminine physique reverses with treatment, and masculine features develop (penis enlarges, body and facial hair develops, voice deepens, sexual interest awakens).
3. Client with cognitive or behavioral problems is in appropriate treatment program and is progressing.
4. Psychosocial developmental task attainment is at chronological age level expectations, or, for client with retardation, at developmental age level (see Chapter 4 for developmental norms).
5. Self-concept is positive and gender-appropriate.

6. Sexual function is normal (client experiences erection and ejaculation), although patient is probably infertile.

Complications

PSYCHOLOGICAL MALADJUSTMENT DUE TO PHYSICAL APPEARANCE AND PEER REJECTION (TEASING) BECAUSE OF BREAST HYPERTROPHY

Assessment

1. Does not wish to participate in gym activities due to embarrassment over shower procedure.
2. Family does not have financial resources for mammoplasty.

Revised Outcomes

1. Mammoplasty will be performed if child and family desire.
2. Client will develop better coping methods and better psychosocial adjustment.
3. Other expected outcomes as previously stated.

Interventions

1. Assess financial resources (Medicaid, community organizations, Red Cross, vocational rehabilitation, or other agency recommended by social worker) for surgery.
2. Refer family for more intensive counseling (should progress from individual to group counseling).

INADEQUATE DOSAGE OF TESTOSTERONE

Assessment

1. Under- or overdevelopment of sexual characteristics.
2. Sexual characteristics not in accordance with chronological age.
3. Client is not keeping appointments for medication dosage adjustments.

Revised Outcomes

1. Client will receive dosage adjustments geared to his developmental rate and stage.
2. Client will comply with treatment regimen.

Interventions

1. Assess reasons why client is not keeping appointments and/or not taking medication as recommended (e.g., knowledge deficit, financial limitations) and teach, counsel, or refer, as needed.
2. Refer to community nurse for assessment of home medication regimen, teaching as needed, and follow-up supervision.

REFERENCES

Tanner, J. M.: *Growth at Adolescence*, 2d ed., Lippincott, Philadelphia, 1962.

BIBLIOGRAPHY

Alsever, R. N., and Gotlin, R. W.: *Handbook of Endocrine Tests in Adults and Children*, 2d ed., Year Book Medical Publishers, Chicago, 1978. A resource book for health professionals discussing tests for determining basal hormone levels, results of stimulation or suppression tests, general considerations, and variations of test results for infants and children as compared with adults.

Chinn, P. L., and Leitch, C. J.: *Child Health Maintenance*, C. V. Mosby, St. Louis, 2d ed., 1979. A pediatric nursing text aimed at expected normal growth and development and the alterations caused by illness, injury, or stress. A useful tool accompanying this text is *A Guide to Clinical Assessment* by the same authors.

Guthrie, D. W., and Guthrie, R. A. (eds.): *Nursing Management of Diabetes Mellitus*, C. V. Mosby, St. Louis, 2d ed., 1982. A collection of subjects and authors representing varying areas of thought, as well as information, in the United States, to assist the health professional in offering the highest quality patient care and professional education.

Kaplan, S. A. (ed.): "Symposium on Pediatric Endocrinology," *Pediatric Clinics of North America*, **26**(1):1, February 1979. Physicians' papers on a range of childhood and adolescent endocrine disorders. Includes many photographs and extensive reference lists.

Scipien, G. M., Barnard, M. U., Chard, M. A., et al (eds.): *Comprehensive Pediatric Nursing*, 2d ed., McGraw-Hill, New York, 1979. Diabetes in children is presented in a compact and organized form as part of an in-depth study of children in various states of health. Nursing management for a range of endocrine disorders is included.

Solomon, B. (ed.): "Endocrine Disorders," *Nursing Clinics of North America*, **15**(3):433, September 1980. Although children's disorders are not emphasized, the discussions of nurses' roles in caring for clients with endocrine problems are generally applicable. Contains a clear presentation of the pituitary and hypothalamus and their functions in endocrine control.

Tanner, J. M.: *Growth at Adolescence*, 2d ed., Lippincott, Philadelphia, 1962. This is the classic, definitive work on physical growth of adolescence.

Whaley, L. F., and Wong, D. L.: *Nursing Care of Infants and Children*, C. V. Mosby, St. Louis, 1979, pp. 1453–1504. A pediatric nursing text covering the developmental framework and the continuum of developmental changes, based on the concept of family-centered care.

18

The Hematologic System

C. Marie Hall Smith and Patricia E. Greene

HYPERACTIVITY AND HYPOACTIVITY

APLASTIC ANEMIA

DESCRIPTION

The bone marrow is the primary producer of erythrocytes, leukocytes, and platelets. Severe hypoplasia or absence of their precursors in the marrow is aplastic anemia. A viral illness can precipitate an aplastic state; the most severe instance occurs after viral hepatitis. Certain drugs, such as chloramphenicol and the sulfonamides, have been implicated as causing aplastic anemia. Toxic chemicals, such as aromatic hydrocarbons, are known causative agents. Aplastic anemia may begin with anemia, infection secondary to leukopenia, or bruising and bleeding secondary to thrombocytopenia. The patient's course is highly variable, and the outcome is closely related to the initial cause and severity of aplasia. Diagnosis is confirmed by a bone marrow biopsy, which shows hypocellularity. Treatment can include steroids, androgens, cytotoxic drugs, and antithymocyte preparations, although the response is unpredicatable. Supportive measures consist of antibiotics and frequent transfusions.

PREVENTION

Health Promotion

Avoid causative agents named above.

Population at Risk

Anyone.

Screening

None.

ASSESSMENT

Health History

1. Recent infection—viral hepatitis is the most common illness associated with the onset of aplastic anemia.
2. Exposure to toxic chemicals, particularly insecticides, toluenes, and aromatic hydrocarbons.
3. Recent doses of toxic drugs, such as chloramphenicol, sulfonamides, or anticonvulsants.
4. Weakness of several weeks' duration.
5. Pallor of several weeks' duration.
6. Fever, which may be low-grade and persistent over several days or high and associated with septicemia.
7. Bleeding from gums or gastrointestinal tract; sometimes hematuria.
8. Recent bruises over trunk.

Physical Assessment

1. Tachycardia secondary to anemia.
2. Mild tachypnea secondary to anemia.
3. Fever, indicative of infection, is of concern since there is a decrease in the pool of white cells.
4. Skin and mucous membranes may have petechial hemorrhages. There may be larger bruises over the trunk as well as extremities.
5. Cardiac exam reveals flow murmur secondary to the anemia.

6. There is no hepatosplenomegaly upon abdominal exam.
7. Adenopathy is rare.

Diagnostic Tests

1. Red blood cell (RBC) count (PCV or Hgb), white blood cell (WBC) count, and platelet count.
2. Bone marrow aspirate and biopsy: the marrow assay ascertains the quantity and quality of early RBCs, WBCs, and platelets.
3. Surface cell marker studies (T- and B-cell quantitation) to characterize the predominant population of lymphocytes; results can give insight as to preferred therapy.
4. Human lymphocyte antigen (HLA) typing—the patient's and family's lymphocytes are examined to evaluate whether a bone marrow transplant is feasible.
5. Mixed lymphocyte culture (MLC) studies—if there is an HLA match between the patient and a family member, MLC studies are done to document further the compatibility of the family member's and patient's blood.

NURSING DIAGNOSES: ACTUAL OR POTENTIAL

1. Decreased ability to fight infections, secondary to leukopenia.
2. Decreased ability to provide for hemostasis, secondary to thrombocytopenia.
3. Decreased exercise tolerance secondary to anemia.
4. Risk of toxicities from therapy:
   a. Androgens.
   b. Steroids.
   c. Cytotoxic drugs.
   d. Antithymocyte derivatives.
   e. Transfusions.
   f. Bone marrow transplant (not discussed in this chapter).

EXPECTED OUTCOMES

1. Client will receive maximum protection from exogenous and endogenous infections for duration of leukopenia.
2. Bleeding will be prevented.
3. Activity will be restricted as appropriate for degree of anemia.
4. Parents (and child if old enough) will be able to recognize and deal with side effects of therapy.
5. Parents (and child if old enough) will avoid reexposure of child to causative agent if it is identified.

INTERVENTIONS

1. Ensure maximum protection from exogenous and endogenous organisms (see leukopenia guidelines under *Neutropenia*).
2. Prevent bleeding. See Table 18-1 for activity guidelines.
3. Modify activity by degree of anemia (Table 18-2).
4. Teach parents (and child if old enough) about side effects of steroid therapy.
   a. Fluid retention with concomitant weight gain and cushingoid appearance.
   b. Hypertension—when hypertension is present, teach about low-salt diet.
   c. Increased diaphoresis and night sweats.
   d. Increased urinary frequency (bed-wetting).
   e. Transient increase in appetite.
   f. Gastrointestinal irritability—suggest giving steroids with milk or meals.
   g. Masked infections.
   h. When steroids are used for more than 3 weeks and then discontinued, it is important to taper dose over a 10- to 14-day period to minimize any addisonian symptomatology.
5. Teach parents (and child if old enough) about side effects of cytotoxic drugs (drug most commonly used is cyclophosphamide).
   a. Potential nausea—recommend small frequent meals, high in calories.
   b. Potential hemorrhagic cystitis (rare—encourage maintenance fluids (1500–1800 $ml/m^2/day$), at least, for the time during which the child is receiving the drug; client may need supplemental parenteral fluids.
   c. Potential alopecia, partial or complete—recommend alternatives, such as wigs, scarfs, caps, or hats.
   d. Further decrease in WBC population—will probably need to augment therapy with WBC transfusions.
6. Teach parents (and child if old enough) about side effects of antithymocyte derivatives (either serum or globulin, lapine or equine).
   a. Potential allergic reaction to the protein, even to the point of anaphylaxis.
      (1) Have resuscitative equipment and drugs at bedside.

TABLE 18-1 ACTIVITY GUIDELINES AND PRECAUTIONS TO BE TAKEN FOR CLIENTS WITH LOW PLATELET COUNTS

Platelet Count Values	Recommendations	Precautions
<10,000	Sedentary activity with bathroom privileges.	Maintain pressure over intravenous and finger sticks until bleeding stops.
10,000–50,000	Light exercise, e.g. walking, swimming (not diving). Consult physical therapist for suggested exercises. Encourage patient not to overexert or sweat, as this may precipitate petechial bleeding. If petechiae develop, stop activity.	Evaluate carefully the need for intramuscular injections. Observe carefully for signs of intracranial bleeding and for altered neurological status. Evaluate the need for gastrointestinal or mucosal irritants (i.e., nasogastric tube, suctioning, catheters). For mouth care, use only soft bristles, cotton swabs, or such products as Toothettes. Monitor stools for occult blood. Observe for and report bleeding from mucosal membranes. Avoid the use of salicylates (aspirin), which interfere with platelet aggregation.
50,000–100,000	Moderate exercise, discourage contact sports, such as football, basketball, soccer, and wrestling. Should not ride bikes, use skateboards, or climb trees.	Monitor stools for occult blood. Observe for and report bleeding from mucosal membranes. Avoid the use of salicylates (aspirin), which interfere with platelet aggregation.
>100,000	Normal activity.	No precautions are necessary.

(2) May premedicate client with drugs (steroids and other anti-inflammatory drugs).

b. Probable febrile response, which can be minimized by premedicating with acetaminophen and repeated at intervals after the administration of the antithymocyte serum (ATS) or antithymocyte globulin (ATG).

c. Potential nausea—recommend small, frequent, high-calorie meals.

7. Provide maximum protection from complications of transfusions (see Table 18-3).
8. Teach parents to avoid reexposure of child to causative agent, if identified.
   a. Counsel parents and others (e.g., schoolteacher) to prevent reexposure of child to causative agent.
   b. Consider obtaining Medic-Alert necklace.
   c. See *Neutropenia*.

EVALUATION

Outcome Criteria

1. Infections are prevented or controlled.
2. Traumatic and/or life-threatening bleeding does not occur.
3. Activity is adjusted to degree of anemia and is well tolerated.
4. Parents (and child if old enough) can describe, recognize, and intervene as necessary regarding side effects of therapy and cope with them.

TABLE 18-2 ACTIVITY GUIDELINES FOR CLIENTS WITH ANEMIA

Hemoglobin Values	Recommendations
<5 g	Bed rest with bathroom privileges. Monitor pulse and respiration every 2 hours; monitor temperature and blood pressure every 4 hours.
5–8 g	Light exercise, e.g., walking, some swimming. Frequent rest periods.
>8 g	Activity as tolerated.

5. Causative agent, if identified, is subsequently avoided.
6. Marrow function returns with or without the therapies mentioned.

Complications

INFECTION, ESPECIALLY SEPTICEMIA

Assessment

1. Fever 101°F (38.3°C) or higher.
2. Malaise and lethargy.
3. Complaint of a particular locus of infection (e.g., earache).

Revised Outcomes

1. Eliminate infection.
2. Other goals, as originally stated.

Interventions

1. Broad spectrum antibiotics.
2. WBC transfusions (antibiotics by themselves cannot ablate bacterial or fungal infections.)

TABLE 18-3 TRANSFUSION REACTIONS

HEMOLYTIC TRANSFUSION REACTION

Prevention

Identify patient and blood product to ensure proper match. Double-check all blood products with another nurse or health professional.

Begin infusion at a slow rate, remain with patient for first 15 minutes. Severe reactions tend to begin soon after initiation of transfusion.

Signs and Symptoms

Immediate onset, usually. Delayed onset may be observed when an Rh incompatibility is involved.

Burning sensation along the vein.

Facial flushing.

Fever, chills. Temperature may be 105°F or higher.

Chest pain; rapid, labored respirations.

Headache.

Low back pain.

Shock.

Nursing Actions

Stop transfusion immediately to reduce further risk. Severity of reaction is related to amount transfused.

Treat shock if present. Administer oxygen, fluids, epinephrine as ordered by physician.

Recheck blood slip with unit of blood and patient to determine if error was made.

Obtain two blood samples from a vein distant from infusion site. One specimen is sent for centrifuge (pink or red plasma indicates hemolysis); other specimen is sent to blood bank with remainder of transfusion.

TABLE 18-3 (*continued*)

Obtain first voided urine to test for hemoglobinuria. Specimen may be red or black, indicating potential renal damage.

With suspected renal involvement, prompt treatment with mannitol is initiated to promote diuresis and prevent renal tubular damage. Monitor fluid and electrolyte balance as soon as diuresis begins.

ALLERGIC REACTION

Prevention

Determine whether patient has history of allergy, particularly a previous allergic reaction to transfused blood products.

Administer antihistamine, for example, diphenhydramine (Benadryl) orally or parenterally 15 to 20 minutes before starting infusion.

Signs and Symptoms

Urticaria (hives), pruritis.

Facial and/or glottal edema (rare).

Asthma (rare).

Pulmonary edema with infiltrates (rare).

Anaphylaxis.

Nursing Actions

Stop transfusion immediately.

Treat life-threatening reactions (edema, anaphylaxis) immediately.

Administer antihistamine parenterally.

FEBRILE REACTION

Prevention

Keep patient covered and warm during transfusion.

Administer antipyretic medication to persons known to have this reaction.

Transfusion with leukocyte-poor red blood cells or frozen washed packed cells may prevent this reaction in persons susceptible to it.

Signs and Symptoms

Chills and fever, usually beginning about 1 hour after start of infusion.

Headache, flushing, tachycardia, and general discomfort may be present.

Symptoms may persist for 8 to 10 hours; most are more transient.

Nursing Action

Stop transfusion immediately.

Treat symptomatically.

BACTERIAL REACTION

Prevention

Maintain aseptic collection techniques.

Change transfusion equipment frequently.

Do not allow blood to stand at room temperature unnecessarily, even while infusing.

Do not use blood that has been heated to above room temperature.

Do not prewarm infusions.

Inspect all blood for evidence of hemolysis.

Signs and Symptoms

Shaking fever.

TABLE 18-3 (*continued*)

Severe hypotension.
Dry, flushed skin.
Pain in abdomen and extremities.
Vomiting and bloody diarrhea.

Nursing Actions

Stop transfusion immediately.
Administer broad-spectrum antibiotics as ordered immediately, by most rapid route.
Treat shock aggressively.
Monitor vital signs, fluid and electrolyte balance.

CIRCULATORY OVERLOAD

Prevention

Give packed cells to persons susceptible to circulatory overload (elderly, infants, persons with cardiac or respiratory disorders).
Administer infusion slowly, with patient in a sitting position.

Signs and Symptoms

Tightness in chest, labored breathing.
Dry cough.
Rales at base of lungs.
Pulmonary edema.

Nursing Actions

Stop or slow transfusion, depending on severity of symptoms.
Have patient sit up.
Monitor vital signs.
Treat severe overload with rotating tourniquets or phlebotomy.
Administer diuretics as ordered.

AIR EMBOLISM

Prevention

Avoid introducing air into system.
If air is introduced, stop the infusion.

Signs and Symptoms

Cyanosis.
Dyspnea.
Shock.
Cardiac arrest.

Nursing Actions

Lower patient's head and turn patient on left side. Air will collect in right atrium, where it can be released gradually to the lungs.
Treat shock and/or cardiac arrest immediately if these should occur.

3. Fever control with acetaminophen, cooling blanket, and so on.

BLEEDING DIATHESIS—INTRACRANIAL

See Chapter 15 for management of intracranial bleeding.

FANCONI'S ANEMIA

DESCRIPTION

Fanconi's anemia is characterized by pancytopenia and a concomitant decrease of precursor blood elements in the bone marrow. It is often associated with a variety of congenital anomalies: skeletal changes (abnormalities of thumb and radius), small genitalia, hyperpigmentation of the skin, kidney abnormalities, and mental retardation. The anemia is usually noticed between the ages of 4 and 12 years. The trait for Fanconi's anemia is autosomal recessive with variable expression and may or may not be clinically apparent in other family members.

The treatment consists of steroids and androgens used separately or together to stimulate the bone marrow. The remainder of the therapy is supportive. (If the child is not responsive to standard treatment, the supportive therapy becomes the maintenance therapy.) If there is poor bone marrow response to the drugs, the patient may be maintained on blood transfusions. Persons with Fanconi's anemia can develop complications secondary to treatment (see *Diamond-Blackfan Syndrome*) of the anemia and have a propensity to develop leukemia later in life.

PREVENTION

Health Promotion

Genetic counseling may prevent birth of future siblings with the autosomal recessive trait; however, there is no known prevention of Fanconi's anemia in the firstborn.

Population at Risk

Children in families with a history of the disorder.

Screening

None.

ASSESSMENT

Health History

1. Presence of other congenital anomalies.
2. Pallor noted after the first 6 months of life.
3. Weakness, fatigue noticed after the first 6 months of life.

Physical Assessment

1. Height and weight are usually below the tenth percentile and may be associated with dwarfism.
2. Skin and mucous membranes: pallor and hyperpigmentation.
3. Head: microcephaly may be present.
4. Eyes: strabismus may be present.
5. Ears: inner and outer ear anomalies.
6. Cardiac exam: possible increased heart size, murmurs associated with decreased cardiac output, decreased stroke volume.
7. Abdomen: possible increased liver and spleen size.
8. Extremities: skeletal changes, thumb and radial abnormalities.
9. Kidneys: malformations in genitourinary tract.
10. Neurological exam: possible neurological deficits, mental retardation.
11. Genitalia: delayed puberty.

Diagnostic Tests

1. Hematocrit, hemoglobin with RBC indices. Fanconi's anemia may be characterized by either a normochromic, normocytic, or slightly hypochromic, microcytic anemia with lowered hemoglobin and hematocrit values.
2. Reticulocyte count will be negligible.
3. Bone marrow aspirate and biopsy. As the bone marrow is the factory for the blood cells, the marrow assay ascertains the quantity and quality of early RBCs, WBCs, and platelets.
4. Chromosomal studies.

NURSING DIAGNOSES: ACTUAL OR POTENTIAL

See *Aplastic Anemia* and *Diamond-Blackfan Syndrome.*

EXPECTED OUTCOMES

See *Aplastic Anemia* and *Diamond-Blackfan Syndrome.*

INTERVENTIONS

See *Aplastic Anemia* and *Diamond-Blackfan Syndrome.*

EVALUATION

See *Aplastic Anemia* and *Diamond-Blackfan Syndrome.*

ACQUIRED HEMOLYTIC ANEMIA

DESCRIPTION

The reduced RBC population in acquired hemolytic anemia may be a result of radiation therapy, chemicals, drugs, or infections. Red blood cells can be destroyed by complement fixation, which is an autoimmune mechanism. The drugs implicated in RBC aplasia are quinidine, quinine, salicylic acid, phenacetin, aminopyrine, streptomycin, penicillin, cephalosporins, methyldopa, and stibophen. Compounds with benzene rings and sulfa and chloro- compounds are the general categories of causative agents. Also implicated in acquired RBC aplasia are Coxsackie virus, measles, varicella, cytomegalovirus, and encephalitis. Although normal RBC production can recover with time, steroids may be used to stimulate marrow activity. The condition should not recur except in the presence of the causative agent.

PREVENTION

Health Promotion

If drug or chemically induced, avoid causative agent.

Population at Risk

Anyone.

Screening

None.

ASSESSMENT

Health HIstory

1. Recent infection: Coxsackie virus, measles, varicella, cytomegalovirus.
2. Recent exposure to chemicals: insecticides, benzene compounds.
3. Recent exposure to drugs: quinidine, quinine, salicylic acid, phenacetin, aminopyrine, streptomycin, penicillin, cephalosporins, sulfa compounds, chloro- compounds, stibophen, methyldopa.
4. Previous history of a similar incident.
5. Weakness of several weeks' duration.
6. Pallor of several weeks' duration.

Physical Assessment

1. Tachycardia secondary to anemia.
2. Mild tachypnea secondary to anemia.
3. Skin and mucous membranes are pale.
4. Possibly palpable spleen tip and liver edge if anemia is severe.
5. Flow murmur on cardiac exam secondary to anemia.

Diagnostic Tests

1. Blood counts to obtain ongoing values as to the RBC count (PCV or Hgb).
2. Bone marrow aspirate and biopsy. As the bone marrow is the factory for the blood cells, the marrow evaluation ascertains the quality and quantity of early RBCs. There are normal numbers of WBC precursors and megakaryocytes; there may be toxic granulation of the marrow elements secondary to the insulting agent.

NURSING DIAGNOSES: ACTUAL OR POTENTIAL

1. Decreased exercise tolerance secondary to anemia.
2. Potential complications from therapy (e.g., steroids or transfusions).

EXPECTED OUTCOMES

1. Activity will be modified as appropriate for degree of anemia.
2. Parents (and child if old enough) will recognize, respond appropriately to, and cope with side effects of therapy.
3. Child and parents will avoid exposure of child to causative agent, if identified.

INTERVENTIONS

1. Modify activity according to degree of anemia (see Table 18-2).
2. Provide maximum protection from complications of transfusions (see Table 18-3).

3. Teach parents (and child if old enough) about side effects of steroid therapy (see *Aplastic Anemia*).
4. Teach parents to avoid reexposure of child to causative agent, if identified (see *Aplastic Anemia*).

EVALUATION

Outcome Criteria

1. Activity is adjusted to degree of anemia and is well tolerated.
2. Causative agent, if identified, is subsequently avoided.
3. Marrow function returns with or without the therapies mentioned.

POLYCYTHEMIA OF CYANOTIC HEART DISEASE

DESCRIPTION

Cyanotic heart disease induces a state of polycythemia, or increased numbers of RBCs, to compensate for hypoxia caused by the heart anomaly. Once hematocrit has exceeded 60 percent, the blood viscosity becomes markedly increased. For example a hematocrit of 60 percent represents an increase in viscosity of four times the viscosity at 40 percent.

Characteristic symptoms are the result of sludging of blood and include headache, irritability, and shortness of breath. Polycythemia of the newborn (with or without heart disease) presents with convulsions, hypoglycemia, hypocalcemia, priapism, decreased platelets, and renal vein thrombosis, all attributable to the increase in RBC mass.

Partial exchange transfusion is one temporary measure used in managing polycythemia. Removal of the blood must be done gradually, as a rapid loss can result in vascular collapse and cerebral insults. Optimally, the lowered hematocrit leads to a lowered peripheral resistance, producing a more efficient, larger stroke volume with an increased oxygen perfusion to tissues. With correction of the heart disease, the polycythemia resolves.

PREVENTION

Health Promotion

No preventive measures are known.

Population at Risk

Children with cyanotic heart disease and newborns.

Screening

None.

ASSESSMENT

Health History

1. Congenital cyanotic heart anomaly.
2. Shortness of breath.
3. Irritability.
4. Headache.
5. Seizures.

Physical Assessment

1. Skin: ruddy complexion in face, cyanotic extremities.
2. Chest: use of accessory respiratory muscles.
3. Cardiac exam: murmurs associated with heart defect.
4. Genitalia: priapism.
5. Neurological exam: neurological deficits.

Diagnostic Tests

Packed-cell volume (PCV) will be above 40 percent and will be in conjunction with a preexisting cardiomyopathy or associated with the newborn period.

NURSING DIAGNOSES: ACTUAL OR POTENTIAL

1. Decreased activity tolerance due to poor tissue perfusion.
2. Risk for complications from phlebotomizing.
3. Susceptibility to bleeding and thrombus formation secondary to the increased viscosity of the blood.
4. Parental knowledge deficit regarding cyanotic heart disease and prevention or detection of thrombosis.

EXPECTED OUTCOMES

1. Child will enjoy maximal activity in view of altered tissue perfusion.
2. Child will not have complications of treatment (exchange transfusions).
3. Bleeding and thromboembolic disease will not occur or will be promptly recognized and treated.
4. Parents will understand potential complica-

tions and promote the child's comfort and safety.

INTERVENTIONS

1. Advise parents and school personnel (and child if old enough) that child should rest as necessary and avoid strenuous activities. (Infants, toddlers, and preschoolers usually restrict their own activity to their level of tolerance; school-age children and adolescents often do not.)
   a. Teach parents, child, and teachers that good hydration is essential to reduce the risk of thrombosis (e.g., child should have free access to school drinking fountain).
2. For care of child having exchange transfusion, see Table 18-3.
3. Teach parents about management of susceptibility to bleeding. See Table 18-1, although the cause is not related to the platelet count.
4. Teach parents about observations to detect thromboembolic disease:
   a. Evaluate for renal vein thrombosis (anuria, uremia).
   b. Observe for signs of cerebral thrombosis (sudden vertigo, headaches, convulsions, nausea and vomiting, fainting, confusion).
   c. Observe for signs of cardiac thrombosis (chest pain).

EVALUATION

Outcome Criteria

1. Activity does not exceed tolerance.
2. Avoidable complications of transfusion do not occur; others are promptly detected and treated.
3. Child is adequately hydrated.
4. Bleeding is avoided as much as possible; bleeding that does occur is properly treated.
5. Thrombosis is detected and properly treated.

DIAMOND-BLACKFAN SYNDROME

DESCRIPTION

Diamond-Blackfan syndrome (DBS) is an apparently congenital aplasia or hypoplasia of RBCs. The anemia is either transient, resolving by puberty (as many as one-third of cases) or, more commonly, will require long-term support. One of the first observable signs is pallor, which becomes apparent by 6 months of age.

If the anemia associated with DBS is severe, compensatory tachycardia and congestive heart failure may result. Liver and spleen size may increase due to the cardiac alterations. As many as one-fifth of the patients have skeletal abnormalities.

Numerous other anomalies become apparent during long-term management of the disease and are related to the therapy. Steroids and androgens may be helpful bone marrow stimulants. Repeated RBC transfusions are necessary during periods of stress or for long-term management of the anemia. As RBCs from transfusions are broken down, the products are excreted, with the exception of iron, which is stored in the bone marrow and components of the reticuloendothelial system. Organs that may evidence deposits of iron during long-term treatment are the kidney, liver, spleen, heart, and gastrointestinal tract. The toxic deposition of iron is called *hemosiderosis*. Other phenomena accompanying the iron deposition are a bronzed dusky skin color, retardation of bone growth (short stature), and eventual cirrhosis. The iron deposits in the heart can alter cardiac function significantly. The hazards of iron deposition are minimized by the administration of an iron-chelating agent, deferoxamine, that binds the iron and aids its excretion.

PREVENTION

Health Promotion

No preventive measures are known.

Population at Risk

Children under 1 year of age.

Screening

None.

ASSESSMENT

Health History

1. Presence of other congenital anomalies.
2. Pallor noticed in the first 6 months of life.
3. Weakness, fatigue.

Physical Assessment

1. Height and weight are usually below the tenth percentile and may be associated with dwarfism.
2. Pallor of the skin and mucous membranes.
3. Child may have microcephaly.

4. Cardiac exam may reveal an enlarged heart and murmurs associated with decreased cardiac output and decreased stroke volume.
5. Abdominal exam may reveal increased liver and spleen size.
6. Extremities may have skeletal changes.
7. Neurological exam may reveal deficits and mental retardation.

Diagnostic Tests

1. Hematocrit, hemoglobin with RBC indices. Diamond-Blackfan syndrome is characterized by a normochromic, normocytic anemia with lowered hematocrit and hemoglobin values.
2. Reticulocyte count will be negligible.
3. Bone marrow aspirate reveals a virtual absence of erythropoietic activity (RBC production) in conjunction with relatively normal leukopoiesis and thrombopoiesis.

NURSING DIAGNOSES: ACTUAL OR POTENTIAL

1. Reduced activity tolerance secondary to erythropoietic failure.
2. Risk of toxicity from steroids, hormonal therapy, and transfusions.
3. Altered self-concept secondary to DBS and its treatment.

EXPECTED OUTCOMES

1. Activity will be restricted as appropriate for degree of anemia.
2. Parents and child will be well informed regarding side effects of therapy (steroids, hormones, and transfusions).
3. Child will develop a positive self-concept and engage in activities appropriate for growth and development.

INTERVENTIONS

1. Modify activity by degree of anemia (Table 18-2).
2. Educate parents (and child if old enough) regarding side effects of therapy.
   a. Steroids (see *Aplastic Anemia*).
   b. Hormones (see *Aplastic Anemia*).
   c. Transfusions (see *Aplastic Anemia* and Table 18-3).
3. Encourage positive self-concept through
   a. Participation in activities, such as school and church groups, that are age and interest appropriate.
   b. Participation in peer support group activities where feasible in conjunction with health care facilities and/or community organizations.

EVALUATION

Outcome Criteria

1. Anemia resolves spontaneously or responds to steroid and hormone augmentation.
2. Activity does not exceed tolerance.
3. Child demonstrates positive self-esteem and interacts with the environment as appropriate for developmental level (see Chapter 4).

Complications

Anemia is persistent and mediated only by transfusion therapy.

Assessment

Anemia is not responsive to steroids and/or hormones.

Revised Outcomes

1. Child and parents will understand and cope well with transfusion therapy.
2. Complications of transfusion will be avoided or promptly recognized and treated.

Interventions

Deferoxamine, an iron-chelating agent, will be medically prescribed with the transfusions, as the child will begin to have deposition of iron in vital tissues. When there is no iron chelation in patients receiving more than 100 transfusions, irreparable damage to tissues occurs. Deferoxamine is commonly given by a portable, constant infusion device inserted subcutaneously.

a. Teach child and parents procedure for infusion and preparation of deferoxamine.
b. Teach child and parents side effects of deferoxamine, such as rust-colored urine from excretion of iron, local erythema, and, occasionally, pruritis from the agent, which can be mediated by antihistamines.

MEGALOBLASTIC NUTRITIONAL ANEMIAS (VITAMIN B_{12} AND FOLIC ACID DEFICIENCY ANEMIAS)

DESCRIPTION

Vitamin B_{12} deficiency anemia is a megaloblastic anemia rarely seen in children and usually associated with neurological sequelae. Vitamin B_{12} absorption is dependent upon an intrinsic factor (IF) secreted by the stomach and then transported to the terminal ilium, where the IF and B_{12} are absorbed into the bloodstream. In conditions where there is little IF available, as in the atrophic gastritis of pernicious anemia, B_{12} deficiency is predictable.

Neurological manifestations are the hallmarks of the deficiency when they occur with anemia. Paresthesias in the extremities, ataxia, irritability, and alterations in sight, smell, and taste are attributable to the lack of B_{12}. Smoking can aggravate visual symptoms so that they progress to amblyopia. The hematologic picture is made up of a megaloblastic hyperchromic anemia with hypersegmented polymorphonuclear cells.

In the juvenile form of the disease, there may be a congenital deficiency of IF. A thorough family history is helpful, as the deficiency can be hereditary. A complete dietary history is another necessary aspect of the assessment. Vitamin B_{12} deficiency is ameliorated by supplemental B_{12}.

Folic acid deficiency anemia is rare among infants born in the United States, as adequate doses of folic acid are contained in cow's milk and commercially available formulas. Goat's milk and dry milk may contain less folic acid.

Folic acid levels are known to decrease with diarrhea, infections, and decreased ascorbic acid (vitamin C) intake. Ascorbic acid is necessary for the utilization of folic acid. Folates are absorbed by bacteria in the gut. Diarrhea does not allow time for absorption of the ingested folates or ascorbic acid. Presence of weakness, pallor, and lethargy with diarrhea or infection should be an indication to examine for nutritional deficiencies, one of them being folic acid. Folic acid deficits are associated with other anemias, such as sickle cell anemia. Findings that support the diagnosis of folate deficiencies are glossitis and mouth or mucous membrane ulceration. Malabsorption, malnutrition, and alcoholism are predisposing factors. Methotrexate therapy, used for various malignancies, can cause a folic acid deficiency.

Folate may be supplemented whenever the production of RBCs is increased, as in sickle cell anemia. Folic acid deficiency has been linked with B_{12} deficiency, as both are megaloblastic anemias; however, only B_{12} deficiency can cause neurological sequelae. With folate supplements, there is observable improvement in a few days.

PREVENTION

Health Promotion

Adequate intake of vitamin B complexes.

Population at Risk

Children and adolescents (and adults) with inadequate dietary intake, reduced absorption for any reason, or increased requirements (e.g., pregnancy or cancer).

Screening

None.

ASSESSMENT

Health History

1. Recent history of diarrhea or evidence of malabsorption.
2. Recent history of decreased B_{12} intake, such as in strict vegetarian diets.
3. Recent history of gastric resection, which would impede absorption of B_{12} due to a decrease of IF (pernicious anemia).
4. Recent history of alcoholism (e.g., a teenager), which would predispose to a poor intake of folic acid rich foods as well as a decrease in vitamin C intake (folic acid deficiency).
5. Recent methotrexate therapy, which would predispose to folic acid deficiency, as methotrexate competitively binds with folic acid.
6. Gastric complaints, such as heartburn, nausea, or hematemesis, related to alcoholism or gastritis of pernicious anemia.
7. Diarrhea or other malabsorption syndrome.
8. Recent protracted antibiotic therapy.
9. Sickle cell crisis or other stress conditions in patients with hemoglobinopathies. The anemia associated with sickle cell crisis increases the demand for RBCs; consequently the need for constituents of RBCs increases, particularly folates.
10. Recent pallor.
11. Recent weakness.

Physical Assessment

1. Mild tachycardia secondary to anemia.
2. Mild tachypnea secondary to anemia.
3. Skin and mucous membranes may show pallor; mouth may reveal ulcers (methotrexate therapy) or the glossitis of pernicious anemia or alcoholism.
4. Cardiac exam may reveal flow murmur secondary to anemia.

5. Neurological exam of client with B_{12} deficiency may reveal irritability, amblyopia, paresthesias, ataxia, and alterations in sight, taste, and smell.

Diagnostic Tests

1. Hematocrit and hemoglobin with RBC indices: the B vitamin deficiencies yield a megaloblastic, hyperchromic anemia with high mean corpuscular volume (MCV), relatively normal mean corpuscular hemoglobin (MCH), and a relatively low mean corpuscular hemoglobin concentration (MCHC).
2. Serum folate level will be decreased in folic acid deficiencies.
3. Reticulocyte count will be variable depending upon the cause of the megaloblastic anemia. In an aplastic crisis of sickle cell anemia, the reticulocyte count will be extremely low. In the nutritional anemia of scurvy the reticulocyte count will be low to normal.

NURSING DIAGNOSES: ACTUAL OR POTENTIAL

1. Altered nutritional status: inadequate B vitamin ingestion or absorption.
2. Decreased exercise tolerance secondary to anemia.
3. Increased risk of injury secondary to altered neurological status in B_{12} deficiency.

EXPECTED OUTCOMES

1. Client's nutritional status will be restored.
2. Activity will be restricted as appropriate for degree of anemia.
3. Client will not be injured.
4. Client will receive counseling or other appropriate assistance for dealing with the underlying cause of the anemia (sickle cell crisis, alcoholism, etc.).

INTERVENTIONS

1. Restore B_{12} stores.
   a. Supplementation: No particular precautions are needed when administering the oral preparation. If giving B_{12} by injection, rotate the sites.
   b. Diet: Educate parents or client about natural sources of B_{12} (meats, cheese, eggs, milk, not vegetables).
2. Restore folic acid stores.
   a. Supplementation: No particular precautions are needed when administering the oral preparation or the parenteral compound (intravenously or intramuscularly). Folic acid supplementation may be contraindicated when the deficiency is secondary to methotrexate therapy.
   b. Diet: Educate parents and child about natural sources of folic acid (deep green vegetables, such as asparagus, broccoli, spinach; kidney, liver, yeast, veal, eggs, and whole grain cereals).
3. Modify activity by degree of anemia (see Table 18-2).
4. Record and report paresthesias, kinesthetic disturbances, ataxia; provide a protective environment as necessary to prevent injury.
5. Counsel or provide other appropriate assistance for dealing with the underlying cause of the anemia, if known.

EVALUATION

Outcome Criteria

1. With appropriate B vitamin therapy, reticulocytosis occurs within a few days of initiating therapy. The reticulocytes will be normochromic and normocytic. The anemia will be corrected within 2 weeks.
2. Activity does not exceed tolerance.
3. Injuries due to altered neurological status are avoided.
4. Client demonstrates understanding of underlying cause of the anemia and states intent to take appropriate action.

IRON DEFICIENCY ANEMIA

DESCRIPTION

Iron deficiency, the most common cause of anemia, occurs as a result of decreased available iron stores. The iron shortage can be caused by insufficient dietary intake, decreased absorption, or by loss of RBCs. Infants who are premature or growth retarded *in utero* may also have a transient iron deficiency. Inadequate dietary intake is the usual cause of iron deficiency anemia. Dietary iron insufficiency is most common between the ages of 6 months and 3 years and is prevalent again in adolescence. Gastrointestinal malabsorption syndromes can produce iron deficiency anemia because iron, although available in the diet, is not absorbed by the gut.

PREVENTION

Health Promotion

1. Balanced diet, rich in foods that contain iron.
2. Early nutritional counseling for parents of babies and young children.
3. Removal of lead-containing house paint from walls, as children's ingestion of the flakes of paint (pica) predisposes them to iron deficiency (the lead from the paint competes for the iron binding site).
4. Counsel about detection of parasitic infestations of the gut, as these precipitate anemia.

Population at Risk

1. Children between the ages of 6 months and 3 years, whose milk intake is excessive for age.
2. Young children in older housing, where walls still have leaded paint.
3. Adolescents, particularly girls (because of self-restricted diet and menstrual RBC loss).
4. Persons living in substandard housing with poor hygiene practices (because of risk of worm infestation).

Screening

1. Hematocrit or PCV.
2. Stool for ova and parasites.

ASSESSMENT

Health History

1. Weakness of several months' duration.
2. Pallor of several weeks' or months' duration.
3. Abdominal cramping and gas.
4. Pica.
5. Cow's milk intolerance resulting in the use of evaporated milk, which has less than 2 percent iron.
6. Predominance of milk in the child's diet and few foods containing iron ("milk babies").
7. Irritability related to the anemia.
8. Similarity of symptoms in other family members that could be related to parasitic infections.

Physical Assessment

1. Tachycardia secondary to anemia.
2. Mild tachypnea secondary to anemia.
3. Skin and mucous membranes: pallor, translucent appearance to skin.
4. Cardiac exam: flow murmur secondary to anemia.
5. Abdominal exam: hepatosplenomegaly. There may also be pain with deep palpation, particularly with pica, or tenderness related to Meckel's diverticulum and esophageal varices.
6. Obesity in infants and toddlers secondary to excessive milk intake. Milk is a very poor source of iron; when taken in large quantities, it displaces iron-rich foods in the diet.

Diagnostic Tests

1. Hematocrit and hemoglobin with RBC indices. Iron deficiency produces a microcytic, hypochromic anemia, low MCV, low MCH, and low MCHC.
2. Serum iron will indicate that the circulating pool of iron is decreased, usually below 30 μg/100 ml.
3. Serum (total) iron binding capacity (TIBC) is markedly elevated. The test is a measure of available transferrin, which is the protein that binds iron from the gut and transfers it to the erythropoietic areas, such as the bone marrow. The body, sensing that there is a decrease of iron, will increase the production and release of transferrin compensatorily.
4. Reticulocyte count will be low as there are not the constituents, namely iron, to make hemoglobin.
5. Bone marrow aspirate (optional) may be stained to ascertain the presence and amount of iron stores. The iron stores are decreased in iron deficiency anemia.
6. Stool guaiac may be positive if iron deficiency is associated with gastrointestinal blood loss; otherwise the test is negative.
7. Stool for ova and parasites is positive in the presence of intestinal parasitic infections.

NURSING DIAGNOSES: ACTUAL OR POTENTIAL

1. Decreased exercise tolerance secondary to anemia.
2. Potential toxicities from iron therapy.

EXPECTED OUTCOMES

1. Restoration of iron stores by supplemental iron therapy, diet modifications, and/or treatment for parasites, Meckel's diverticulum, or other cause of blood loss.
2. Activity will be restricted as appropriate for degree of anemia.
3. Parents and child will be informed about the side effects of iron therapy.

INTERVENTIONS

1. Restoration of iron stores.
   a. Iron therapy—encourage parents to administer iron with fruit juices to promote optimal absorption, which occurs in the presence of acidic pH. Milk and milk products are not conducive to iron absorption.
   b. Diet modification—curtail the amount of formula or milk ingestion, and encourage iron fortified formulas when appropriate. The child younger than 1 year of age should not receive more than one quart (32 ounces) of milk per day. The addition of iron fortified baby foods (e.g., cereals, egg yolk, beef liver) to the diet will help resolve the iron deficiency. Educate parents (and child if old enough) about natural sources of iron (e.g., fortified cereals and breads, green and some yellow vegetables, organ meats, lean meats, egg yolks). Consult dietician for complete list.
   c. Treat primary insults, such as parasites or Meckel's diverticulum. The anemia will resolve once the underlying cause has been treated and diet augmented.
2. Teach parents (and child if old enough) to modify activity as appropriate for degree of anemia (see Table 18-2).
3. Teach about potential toxicities from iron therapy.
   a. If oral iron preparation is prescribed, counsel parents regarding possible side effects: diarrhea, constipation, nausea, black stools. Suggest that iron supplement be given with meals to minimize gastric irritation. Liquid iron preparation can stain teeth if it comes in contact with them: use a straw.
   b. If intramuscular or intravenous preparation is used, counsel parents regarding side effects: soreness at intramuscular injection site, soreness along the vein when given intravenously (rarely necessary), and possibility of stain in skin at injection site. Use the Z-track method for intramuscular administration of iron.

EVALUATION

Outcome Criteria

1. Anemia resolves.
2. Activity is adjusted to degree of anemia and is well tolerated.
3. Anemia does not recur.

Complications

ANEMIA RECALCITRANT

Assessment
Persistent anemia indicative of iron deficiency.

Revised Outcomes
Control of anemia.

Interventions
1. Use of concomitant oral and intramuscular iron preparations (see *Interventions* above).
2. Use of packed RBC transfusions.
   a. See *Aplastic Anemia* for interventions and further evaluation.

ALLERGIC REACTION TO INTRAMUSCULAR PREPARATION

Assessment
Generalized papular rash over injection site; may involve trunk and extremities.

Revised Outcomes
Control of allergic symptomatology; if reaction severe, pursuit of alternative therapy.

Interventions
1. Monitor extent and degree of rash.
2. Administer antihistamines as ordered.

GLUCOSE 6-PHOSPHATE DEFICIENCY (G6PD)

DESCRIPTION

Glucose 6-phosphate deficiency is classified as a nonspherocytic hemolytic anemia and is transmitted genetically as an X-linked recessive trait. The deficiency occurs in black American males (10 percent) and is also found among Mediterranean and certain Oriental populations. The disease is more severe in white and Oriental people. The neonate may present with prolonged jaundice. Later in childhood, the anemia of G6PD does not become apparent except in the presence of a precipitating factor, such as infection, diabetic acidosis, hepatitis, chronic renal failure, the ingestion of fava beans, or exposure to oxidizing compounds, such as sulfonamides, nitrofurans, antipyretics, and analgesics. Transfusions may be required.

PREVENTION

Health Promotion

Genetic counseling about inheritance of the deficiency, for informed family planning.

Population at Risk

Male offspring of carrier women.

Screening

None.

ASSESSMENT

Health History

1. Client or family history of sudden pallor associated with infection and ingestion of oxidant compounds or foods.
2. Stillbirths or early childhood death of boys.
3. Pallor or neonatal jaundice that can be linked to anoxia and subsequent hemolysis of RBCs.
4. Transient weakness or fatigue.
5. Recent or present infection.
6. Recent or present exposure to drugs or chemicals.

Physical Assessment

1. Temperature may be elevated if the recent or present episode of hemolysis is related to infection.
2. Skin and mucous membranes may be pale or jaundiced, depending on the degree of hemolysis.
3. Tachycardia and tachypnea secondary to anemia.

Diagnostic Tests

1. Hemoglobin and hematocrit are slightly lower than normal values for age, unless in the presence of insulting agent or condition, in which case RBC values will fall lower. On peripheral smear, the RBCs will be of varying shapes and sizes.
2. Autohemolysis test, obtained several months after a hemolytic episode, will be increased.
3. G6PD assays may be obtained with such compounds as brilliant cresyl blue, ascorbic-cyanide test, and fluorescent NADP.

NURSING DIAGNOSES: ACTUAL OR POTENTIAL

1. Decreased exercise tolerance secondary to anemia.
2. Potential complications from transfusion therapy.
3. Knowledge deficit regarding crisis prevention.

EXPECTED OUTCOMES

1. Activity will be restricted as appropriate for degree of anemia.
2. Parents and client will recognize indications for transfusions.
3. Complications of transfusions will be avoided or minimized.
4. Parents and client will avoid exposure of child to oxidizing agents and other crisis-inducing situations.

INTERVENTIONS

1. Teach child and parents to modify child's activity as appropriate for anemia (see Table 18-2).
2. Educate parents and client to recognize indications for transfusions (i.e., sudden onset of pallor with associated vertigo, tachycardia, tachypnea, darkening of urine).
3. Provide maximum protection from complications of transfusions (see Table 18-3).
4. Teach parents and client about
   a. Compounds to be avoided by persons with G6PD: sulfonamides, nitrofurans, antipyretics (except acetaminophen), analgesics, fava beans, primaquine, pamaquine, quinine, and quinidine.
   b. Circumstances to be avoided when feasible by persons with G6PD: infection, diabetic acidosis, hepatitis.

EVALUATION

Outcome Criteria

1. Activity does not exceed tolerance.
2. Parents and client seek medical attention for sudden onset of pallor.
3. Preventable transfusion complications do not occur; others are promptly recognized and treated.
4. Parents and client verbalize an understanding of precipitating factors.

NEUTROPENIA

DESCRIPTION

Neutropenia is a deficiency of circulating granulocytes (polymorphonuclear leukocytes). An absolute granulocyte count of less than 1500 per cubic millimeter in older children and adults, and less than 1000 per cubic millimeter in infants 2 weeks to 1 year of age, is considered neutropenia. Granulocytes are active in phagocytosis, a major defense against infection. Therefore, the incidence of infection, particularly bacterial infection, increases in direct proportion to the severity of neutropenia.

Infections result when *exogenous* organisms (those that are not part of the normal flora) enter a receptive site, become established, and multiply. *Endogenous* organisms (normal, harmless residents in the body) can cause severe infection when they are introduced into an area where they are not normally found or when a change in the normal floral balance is favorable to their excessive multiplication.

The most common sites of infection are those to which organisms gain easiest entry: the skin, respiratory tract, mucosa, bloodstream, and bladder and kidneys. Frequent elevations in temperature are usually the major sign. In the absence of neutrophils, purulent exudates are often not formed, and the usual signs of infection may not be seen. If meningitis develops, children may manifest the usual meningeal signs.

Radiotherapy delivered to areas of the body that include large portions of functioning bone marrow and many cancer chemotherapeutic agents have a potentially toxic effect on rapidly dividing cells of the bone marrow and can lead to profound neutropenia. The onset, degree, and duration of neutropenia varies with different agents. Often the dosage and administration of therapy will be adjusted to minimize these effects.

Noncytotoxic drug-induced neutropenia is a syndrome of decreased production of granulocytes often associated with administration of a particular therapeutic agent. The mechanism for the reaction is not clearly understood. The Registry of Blood Dyscrasias of the Council on Drugs of the American Medical Association maintains a list of drugs suspected of causing neutropenia. The onset of neutropenia can be sudden, as with aminopyrine, which produces an immunologically mediated destruction of circulating neutrophils, or may occur days to weeks after institution of drug therapy.

The disease is usually self-limiting. The duration of neutropenia is variable, but death from overwhelming infection can occur.

Cyclic neutropenia is an unusual disease characterized by periodic episodes of neutropenia, fever, and infection, particularly oral ulceration. Serious infections are rare. The duration of the cycle is usually about 3 weeks (range 14 to 30 days). With each cycle there is approximately 1 week of illness followed by a period of well-being. The onset of the disease is usually early in childhood, and it persists, becoming less severe with age.

The most important therapeutic measure is identification and elimination of any agent that may be contributing to the neutropenia. Infections are treated with appropriate antibiotics. Early detection and prompt treatment enhance the effectiveness of therapy.

PREVENTION

Health Promotion

1. General health measures that support good immune-system function (e.g., nutrition and rest).
2. Avoidance of toxins (DDT, other pesticides, toxic paints, etc.).
3. Judicious use of medications that can induce neutropenia, and periodic monitoring of WBC levels in clients who are receiving these drugs.

Population at Risk

1. Children receiving cancer chemotherapy or radiotherapy.
2. Children receiving medications that can cause WBC suppression; these drugs are numerous and include phenothiazines, aminopyrine and its derivatives, chloramphenicol, sulfonamides, propylthiouracil, and phenylbutazone.

Screening

White blood cell count.

ASSESSMENT

Health History

1. Recurrent or recent infections.
2. Exposure to drugs, chemicals, or radiation.
3. Previous drug reactions.
4. Home environment—potential for adequate hygiene, separate sleeping facilities.
5. Family history.

Physical Assessment

1. General: elevated temperature, pulse, respiratory rate, lethargy, malaise, irritability.

2. Skin: cutaneous ulcerations, furunculosis, absence of pus, and usual signs of infection.
3. Mucous membranes: ulceration, stomatitis, perianal abscess, pain, vaginal drainage, redness, and swelling.
4. Lungs: cough, rhonchi, rales, tachypnea, dyspnea, and decreased breath sounds.
5. Neurological: rigidity of neck and spine or irritability.

Diagnostic Tests

1. Complete blood count: total WBC count and absolute neutrophil count are low, compensatory monocytosis and eosinophilia may occur.
2. Bone marrow: variable according to pathogenesis of neutropenia.

NURSING DIAGNOSES: ACTUAL OR POTENTIAL

1. Increased susceptibility to infections secondary to decreased neutrophil count.
2. Risk of reexposure to offending agent (drug induced).

EXPECTED OUTCOMES

1. Client will avoid unnecessary exposure to exogenous and endogenous organisms.
2. Infections that do occur will be promptly recognized and treated.
3. Client will avoid reexposure to offending agent.

INTERVENTIONS

1. Minimize client's exposure to infectious organisms.
   a. Strict handwashing. (There is little evidence that other isolation techniques, such as masks, gowns, or gloves, provide greater protection. These measures may have an adverse effect on the client's emotional state and may discourage needed nursing attention.)
   b. Use iodine skin preparation before any puncture (e.g., intravenous injection, finger puncture).
   c. Protect skin integrity: evaluate carefully the need for punctures, rotate puncture site, use paper tape rather than regular adhesive tape, maintain good hygiene, turn bedridden patient frequently, massage as needed.
   d. Limit rectal manipulation (i.e., temperature, enema, exam, suppositories).
   e. Assist client with mouth care qid.
   f. Screen visitors and staff members carefully for infections.
   g. Plan staff assignments to avoid cross-contamination.
   h. Provide high-calorie, high-protein diet; consider need for vitamin supplementation.
   i. Plan and implement exercise program appropriate for client's condition.
   j. Date and change intravenous infusion tubing daily. Apply antibiotic ointment and sterile dressing to insertion site daily. Scalp vein needles are recommended.
   k. Keep client's fingernails and toenails short, clean, and well manicured.
   l. Ensure that perineal care is performed for postpubescent girls twice daily.
   m. Teach girls proper wiping technique for bowel movement.
   n. Administer stool softeners.
   o. Avoid bladder catheterization; when necessary use smallest possible catheter, strict aseptic technique, and adequate lubrication. Maintain a *closed* sterile drainage system.
   p. Clean and dress wounds as needed (at least bid). Use strict aseptic technique.
   q. Ensure good pulmonary hygiene by coughing, deep breathing, physiotherapy.
   r. Teach client and family to avoid exposure to people with certain infections, particularly herpes zoster, varicella, measles, or bacterial infections.
   s. Teach client and family to notify physician immediately if exposure to varicella has occurred (in some cases zoster immune globulin can be administered within 72 hours of exposure, and the disease can be prevented or attenuated).
   t. Teach client and family about the role of neutrophils in control of infection, the implications of neutropenia, and the rationale for the interventions listed above.
   u. Teach client and family the signs and symptoms of infection and what to do if they are detected.
2. Promptly recognize and control infections.

   a. Observe closely for signs and symptoms of infection (may be masked by absence of pus).
   b. Notify physician immediately if signs and symptoms are detected.
   c. Administer antibiotic therapy as prescribed.
   d. Prevent the spread of infection with strict handwashing and hygiene (removal of drainage from wounds, if present).
   e. Monitor for signs of reaction if granulocyte transfusion is administered.
3. Take measures to avoid recurrence of neutropenia.
   a. Identify and eliminate offending agent, if possible.
   b. Indicate hypersensitivity on medical record.
   c. Arrange for Medic-Alert bracelet, if appropriate.
   d. Instruct client, family, and schoolteacher about hazards of reexposure and methods of avoiding reexposure.

EVALUATION

Outcome Criteria

1. Reexposure to causative agent is avoided.
2. Avoidable infections do not occur.
3. Infections are controlled.

Complications

PERSISTENT FEVER

Assessment

Elevated temperature for longer than 24 hours.

Revised Outcomes

1. Client will be comfortable.
2. Fever will be reduced.
3. Client will avoid complications of hyperpyrexia (febrile convulsions, dehydration, weight loss).

Interventions

1. Administer antipyretics as prescribed.
2. Provide client with appropriate bedclothing.
3. Change bedclothing and linen as needed.
4. Place client on a cooling mattress, if prescribed.
5. Cool room temperature.
6. Sponge client with tepid water.
7. Force fluids.
8. Monitor sodium and potassium loss.
9. Ensure high-protein, high-calorie diet.

SUPERINFECTION AS A RESULT OF ANTIBIOTIC THERAPY

Assessment

1. Oral, vaginal, or rectal fungal lesions.
2. Rash.
3. Urinary tract infection.

Revised Outcomes

Infection will be controlled.

Interventions

Appropriate antibiotic therapy, usually oral suspension, suppository, or creams or ointments; instruct in method of application.

OTOTOXICITY AS A RESULT OF PROLONGED ANTIBIOTIC THERAPY (PARTICULARLY AMINOGLYCOSIDES)

Assessment

1. Abnormal audiometry.
2. Vertigo.

Revised Outcomes

Drug toxicity will be recognized early.

Interventions

1. Monitor serum antibiotic levels.
2. Routine audiometry.
3. Monitor renal function.
4. Notify physician of abnormality of hearing, balance, or urinalysis.

RENAL DYSFUNCTION AS A RESULT OF PROLONGED ANTIBIOTIC THERAPY (PARTICULARLY AMINOGLYCOSIDES)

Assessment

1. Elevated urea nitrogen or creatinine.
2. Decreased urine output.
3. Decreased creatinine clearance.
4. Decreased urine specific gravity.
5. Presence of cells, casts, proteinuria.

Revised Outcomes

Drug toxicity will be recognized early.

Interventions

1. Monitor serum antibiotic levels.
2. Monitor renal function studies.
3. Monitor intake, output, and weight.
4. Notify physician of abnormalities.

OVERWHELMING BACTERIAL INFECTION

Assessment

1. Persistent spiking fever.
2. Shock.

Revised Outcomes

1. Client's perfusion and vital functions will be maintained.
2. Antibacterial therapy will begin promptly.

Interventions
1. Notify physician immediately.
2. See interventions section under *Shock.*

DISORDERS OF PHAGOCYTOSIS (CHRONIC GRANULOMATOUS DISEASE AND CHÉDIAK-HIGASHI SYNDROME)

DESCRIPTION

Chronic granulomatous disease (CGD) is a hereditary disorder of neutrophil bactericidal function. In most cases it is transmitted in a sex-linked recessive pattern, although it can, rarely, be an autosomal recessive disease. Recurrent pyogenic infections are characteristic.

With CGD there are adequate numbers of neutrophils that are capable of phagocytizing but not killing bacteria. Also, there is a defective leukocyte respiratory metabolism that prevents the cell from producing superoxide, an integral part of the normal biochemical response to phagocytized bacteria.

The clinical manifestations of the disease are usually evident before 2 years of age. Infections are treated aggressively with appropriate antibiotics and, if necessary, WBC transfusions. Early detection and identification of the organism causing the infection enhance the effectiveness of treatment, but generally, the prognosis is poor, and patients succumb to infection early in childhood.

Chédiak-Higashi syndrome (CHS) is an autosomal recessive hereditary disorder of leukocytes associated with an unusual group of clinical features: partial albinism, photophobia, nystagmus, hepatosplenomegaly, and cranial and peripheral neuropathies. There is an associated increased incidence of lymphoreticular malignancies. Granulocytes contain characteristic giant cytoplasmic granular inclusions.

The characteristic predisposition to severe bacterial infections is not entirely understood, but it is thought to be caused by the fact that the giant granules fail to release the appropriate enzymes and interfere with the bactericidal reaction.

Clinical features are usually recognized in the first months of life. Treatment is primarily management of infectious episodes with appropriate antibiotics. The use of ascorbic acid is currently under investigation. The prognosis is poor; children can die of sepsis early in life or from a malignancy developed subsequently.

PREVENTION

Health Promotion

Genetic counseling for prospective parents with a family history of the disorder.

Population at Risk

Infants and young children with a family history of the disease.

Screening

1. For CGD: WBC count.
2. For CHS: physical examination for observable signs and WBC count.

ASSESSMENT

Health History

1. Family history of similar disorder.
2. Recurrent or recent infections.
3. Changes in abdominal girth.
4. Abnormalities of gait, bone pain with osteomyelitis (CGD).
5. Changes in bowel pattern: diarrhea, pain with defecation (CGD).
6. Abnormalities of sensorium, gait, fine or gross motor movements, sensory function (CHS).
7. Photophobia (CHS).

Physical Assessment

1. General: elevated temperature, pulse, respiratory rate, lethargy, malaise, irritability.
2. Skin: eczematoid dermatitis, furunculosis, pus present to produce the usual signs of infection (CHS); light pigmentation.
3. Mucous membranes: ulcerations, perianal abscesses.
4. Lymph nodes: enlarged, suppurative.
5. Abdomen: hepatosplenomegaly, tenderness.
6. Skeletal: tenderness, swelling, warmth (particularly hands and feet).
7. Lungs: rales, rhonchi, tachypnea, dyspnea, decreased breath sounds.
8. Neurological: hyporeflexia or areflexia, ataxia, weakness, footdrop, sensory loss, seizures (CHS).

9. Eyes: retinal albinism, horizontal nystagmus, squinting in light (CHS).
10. Hair: gray or light brown in color (CHS).

Diagnostic Tests

1. Chronic granulomatous disease.
   a. Complete blood count: mild to moderate anemia, lymphocytosis.
   b. Erythrocyte sedimentation rate: elevated.
   c. Immunoglobulins: elevated.
   d. Qualitative nitroblue tetrazolium (NBT) dye test: fails to reduce dye from yellow to blue (can be used to detect carrier females).
2. Chédiak-Higashi syndrome: Complete blood count; erythrocytes and platelets are normal, granulocytes contain giant cytoplasmic granular inclusions.

NURSING DIAGNOSES: ACTUAL OR POTENTIAL

1. Increased susceptibility to infection secondary to reduced WBC response.
2. Risk of injury due to neurological deterioration and visual disorders.
3. Impairment of development secondary to neurological deficit.

EXPECTED OUTCOMES

1. Client will avoid unnecessary infections from exogenous and endogenous organisms.
2. Infections that occur will be promptly recognized and treated.
3. Child will engage in normal activities for developmental level insofar as condition permits.
4. Neurological and ophthalmologic problems will be treated; related injury will not occur.

INTERVENTIONS

See *Neutropenia* and Chapter 15 for intervention for neurological problems.

THROMBOCYTOPENIA (IDIOPATHIC AND ACQUIRED)

DESCRIPTION

A reduced number of circulating platelets, fewer than 100,000, characterizes idiopathic thrombocytopenia (ITP). The hematologic abnormality occurs secondary to increased platelet destruction that is caused by platelet antibodies or other humeral factors. The causative agent cannot be specifically identified. The reduced platelet population exists in the presence of a relatively normal bone marrow.

More than one-half of the cases of ITP are preceded by a recent illness, and as many as 85 percent of cases recover after 4 months of observation. A debate exists as to the efficacy of steroid therapy in ITP. Steroids or similar drugs are chosen to minimize the possibility of a serious bleeding episode. For those who do not respond to drug therapy or who do not improve without therapy, splenectomy may be indicated. Platelet transfusions are not helpful, because the mechanism that destroys the host's platelets destroys transfused platelets as well.

Acquired thrombocytopenia (AT) is similar to ITP, but a causative agent is identifiable. Several drugs or chemicals are linked with the disorder (see *Health History*). With infection-induced thrombocytopenia, the agent may be a virus, as in Rocky Mountain spotted fever (RMSF) and Colorado tick fever (CTF) or malarial or bacterial. With either drug-induced or infection-induced thrombocytopenia, the platelet count recovers when the offending organism is removed. In acquired platelet disorders, a health history and titers may be the most helpful data.

PREVENTION

Health Promotion

If drug or chemical induced, avoid causative agent.

Population at Risk

Everyone.

Screening

None.

ASSESSMENT

Health History

1. Recent bleeding: epistaxis, blood in feces, hematemesis.
2. Recent infection.
3. Past history of similar bleeding or bruises.
4. Recent exposure to chemicals (AT), for example, insecticides, paint, kerosene, gasoline.

5. Recent exposure to drugs (AT), for example, diphenylhydantoin, barbiturates, sulfonamides, antihistamines, quinidine, quinine, digitoxin, para-aminosalicylic acid.
6. Recent exposure to or contraction of Rocky Mountain spotted fever, Colorado tick fever, vivax malaria, bacteremia, viral infection (AT).

Physical Assessment

1. Skin: presence of petechiae or purpura on torso, face, and extremities.
2. Mucous membranes: bleeding from orifices (e.g., epistaxis), scabs.
3. Abdominal examination: hepatosplenomegaly may accompany infection-induced purpura, is absent in drug-induced purpura.

Diagnostic Tests

1. Platelet count: significantly decreased, often below 10,000.
2. Bone marrow aspirate: reveals normal to increased numbers of megakaryocytes (platelet precursors), particularly in transient thrombocytopenia.
3. Platelet antibody: will remain elevated during the time of platelet destruction. As the antibody decreases, with the resolution of the infection and/or removal of causative agent, the platelet count is allowed to return to normal.

NURSING DIAGNOSES: ACTUAL OR POTENTIAL

1. Decreased ability to provide for hemostasis, secondary to thrombocytopenia.
2. Risk of toxicities from therapy (steroids).
3. Altered self-concept secondary to ITP or AT and their treatment.

EXPECTED OUTCOMES

1. Bleeding will be prevented or promptly arrested.
2. Parents (and child if old enough) will understand and cope with side effects of therapy.
3. Encourage positive self-concept and activities appropriate for growth and development.
4. Client will not be reexposed to causative agent (AT).

INTERVENTIONS

1. Prevent and immediately treat bleeding (see Table 18-1).
2. Teach parents (and child if old enough) the side effects of steroid or androgen therapy (see *Aplastic Anemia*).
3. Encourage a positive self-image (child and parents), reinforcing activities appropriate for client's development.
   a. Observe for guilt feelings of parents or child.
   b. Observe for depression or poor self-concept of child. Support realistic activities appropriate for growth and developmental age.
4. Protect client from reexposure to offending agent by educating client and family.

EVALUATION

Outcome Criteria

1. Avoidable serious bleeding does not occur; other bleeding is promptly detected and treated.
2. Side effects of therapy are detected early and minimized.
3. Parents (and child if old enough) are well informed about the disease and the side effects of therapy, and they cope well.
4. Development and adjustment are appropriate.
5. Reexposure to causative agent is avoided (AT).

Complications

Persistent thrombocytopenia.

Assessment

1. Persistent low platelet count.
2. Bleeding episodes, such as epistaxis, gastrointestinal bleeding, petechiae, and bruises.

Revised Outcomes

Mediation of platelet destruction.

Interventions

1. Use of drugs that could impede the immunological destruction of platelets, such as vincristine, cyclophosphamide, 6-mercaptopurine.
2. Splenectomy, which causes resolution of thrombocytopenia in approximately 70 percent of the instances of chronic ITP.
   a. See *Hereditary Spherocytosis* for further information about splenectomy.

Reevaluation and Follow-up

Ideally, platelet count will resolve; if not, patient will need to modify activities of daily living to prevent bleeding diatheses.

IMMUNE THROMBOCYTOPENIA

DESCRIPTION

Immune thrombocytopenia results from maternal antibody formation to fetal platelets and subsequent destruction of platelets in the fetus and newborn. Maternal idiopathic thrombocytopenia (ITP, previously discussed) can result, at any point during pregnancy, in platelet antibodies crossing the placental barrier and destroying the fetal platelets.

Signs of thrombocytopenia can include a purpuric rash, jaundice from the absorption of heme products from the purpuric areas, frank bleeding from any orifice, and platelet counts below 100,000. Generally, no therapy is needed. With active bleeding, however, platelet transfusions are indicated. Maternal platelets are often used for the platelet transfusions. Treatment may consist of steroids, which are thought to stimulate the bone marrow's production of precursor cells, particularly platelet precursors. The tapering-off precautions observed with long-term steroid therapy in aplastic anemia and ITP are not applicable to the short-term steroid use in immune thrombocytopenia. Therapy is supportive, as the condition lasts only a few weeks.

PREVENTION

Health Promotion

None.

Population at Risk

Neonates, especially those whose mothers have ITP.

Screening

None.

ASSESSMENT

Health HIstory

1. Maternal history of thrombocytopenia.
2. Prolonged bleeding at birth.
3. Prolonged bleeding from invasive procedures in the newborn period.

Physical Assessment

1. Skin and mucous membranes may have purpuric lesions and jaundice.
2. Mouth, nasopharynx, and cord may have oozing from traumatized areas.

Diagnostic Tests

1. Platelet count will be below normal.
2. Bone marrow aspirate will reveal normal to elevated numbers of megakaryocytes.
3. Platelet antibody will, initially, be elevated, but as the maternal antibody is removed from circulation, the antibody will decline.

NURSING DIAGNOSES: ACTUAL OR POTENTIAL

1. Decreased ability to provide for hemostasis, secondary to thrombocytopenia.
2. Risk for toxicities from therapy (steroids and platelet transfusions).

EXPECTED OUTCOMES

1. Infant will not have serious bleeding.
2. Side effects of therapy will be minimal.
3. Family will be informed about side effects; they will recognize them, respond appropriately to them, and cope adequately.

INTERVENTIONS

1. Prevent and observe for serious bleeding.
   a. See *Aplastic Anemia.*
   b. Postpone elective procedures, such as circumcision.
2. Observe for gastrointestinal irritability (vomiting, hematemesis), particularly with persistent thrombocytopenia.
3. Administer drugs with feedings to decrease gastrointestinal irritability.
4. Consider contraindications if used concomitantly with diuretics or antibiotics.
5. See *Aplastic Anemia* for a complete list of steroid effects.
6. Provide maximum protection against adverse side effects of platelet transfusion (see Table 18-3).

EVALUATION

Outcome Criteria

1. Avoidable bleeding does not occur; bleeding that does arise is detected early and treated adequately.
2. Avoidable side effects of therapy do not occur; family is well informed about inevitable side effects and copes well.

WISKOTT-ALDRICH SYNDROME

DESCRIPTION

Wiskott-Aldrich syndrome is an X-linked recessive condition characterized by thrombocytopenia, eczematous dermatitis, immunoglobulin changes (deficiency of IgM and increase in IgA), decreased lymphocytes, and subsequent susceptibility to a variety of infectious agents. The condition can be diagnosed early in life by means of a family history of the disease and occurrence of thrombocytopenia in a child. The problems associated with the syndrome are varied and include hemorrhage, infections, and the possibility of developing a malignancy. Temporary joint inflammations have been observed.

Symptomatic treatment is the primary intervention. Although splenectomy is used to intervene with idiopathic thrombocytopenia (ITP), it is not advantageous in the thrombocytopenia of Wiskott-Aldrich syndrome, since the removal of the spleen increases morbidity from infection.

A further differentiation between ITP and Wiskott-Aldrich syndrome is that the levels of immunoglobulins and isohemagglutinins in ITP are normal, whereas in Wiskott-Aldrich syndrome they are not.

PREVENTION

Health Promotion

Genetic counseling may prevent birth of future siblings with the X-linked recessive trait; however, there is no prevention per se for Wiskott-Aldrich syndrome in first-born children.

Population at Risk

Male offspring of carrier women.

Screening

None.

ASSESSMENT

Health History

1. Family history: similar symptoms in mother's extended family.
2. Infant deaths in immediate family.
3. Recent or presenting otitis media, meningitis, pneumonia, or generalized sepsis.

Physical Assessment

1. Temperature is increased.
2. Skin reveals eczema on face, arms, hands; petechial lesions, ecchymotic areas.
3. Evidence of infection.

Diagnostic Tests

1. Blood counts: the RBC values are usually within normal limits. The WBC count may be reduced. The platelet count will almost always be below normal.
2. Isohemagglutinins (naturally occurring antibodies to various blood groups) are usually below normal, indicative of the suppression of immunological activity.
3. Immunoglobulins: there is usually a selective aberration of immunoglobulin levels, with lowered amounts of IgM and increased amounts of IgA.

NURSING DIAGNOSES: ACTUAL OR POTENTIAL

1. Increased susceptibility to serious bleeding secondary to thrombocytopenia.
2. Increased susceptibility to infection secondary to altered WBC function.
3. Altered skin integrity—eczema possibly secondary to altered WBC function.
4. Poor self-concept of child and/or parents secondary to disease and treatment.
5. Risk of further incidence of disease in subsequent offspring of this mother and her family members.

EXPECTED OUTCOMES

1. Bleeding will be minimal and will be promptly recognized and treated.
2. Child will receive maximum protection from infectious agents; unavoidable infections will be promptly recognized and treated.
3. Skin integrity will be promoted.
4. Self-concept will be maximized.
5. Family will obtain genetic counseling.

INTERVENTIONS

1. Prevent or minimize bleeding (see Table 18-1); teach parents to do so.
2. Protect against infectious agents; teach parents to do so.
   a. See guidelines of *Neutropenia* with particular attention to detection of infection.

b. Keep skin well lubricated to prevent cracking.
c. Watch for and report erythematous, edematous areas, as skin infections are common.
d. Steroid creams may be used for eczema.

3. Promote self-concept.
   a. Identify strengths and weaknesses of family system and support figures.
   b. Watch for feelings of guilt on part of child or parents.
   c. Reinforce decisions that incorporate normal growth and developmental needs of parents and/or child.
   d. Provide an understanding of disease and treatment and measures client and family can take to prevent complications.
4. Refer family for genetic counseling.

EVALUATION

Outcome Criteria

1. Avoidable bleeding does not occur; other bleeding is promptly recognized and treated.
2. Avoidable infections do not occur; other infections are promptly recognized and treated.
3. Eczema is consistently treated, and complications are promptly recognized and treated.
4. Child's adjustment and development are adequate.
5. Family members avail themselves of genetic counseling.
6. Parents demonstrate understanding of the disease course and therapy and cope adequately.

HEMOPHILIA

DESCRIPTION

Hemophilia is an inherited coagulation disorder. The most common forms of the disease, classic hemophilia (hemophilia A, or factor VIII deficiency) and Christmas disease (hemophilia B, or factor IX deficiency) account for 95 percent of the hemophilias, with classic hemophilia accounting for 84 percent of the total.

Classic hemophilia and Christmas disease are transmitted in a sex-linked recessive manner, generally from an asymptomatic carrier mother to an affected son. The disease is due to deficient activity of the coagulation factor involved. Children with less than 1 percent of the plasma factor activity are considered to be severe hemophiliacs. Children with 1 to 4.9 percent or 5 to 39.9 percent of the factor activity have, respectively, a moderate or mild form of hemophilia. Children with mild to moderate hemophilia may be free of spontaneous bleeding and require replacement therapy only in the event of surgery or trauma.

Severe disease is characterized by recurrent episodes of hemorrhage. The bleeding may be spontaneous or caused by slight injury. The specific manifestations depend on the area involved. Prolonged hemorrhage can occur following circumcision. For the toddler who experiences frequent falls, bleeding into soft tissue and from mucous membranes are common, especially epistaxis and bleeding from the mouth.

Perhaps the most debilitating complication of the disease is hemarthrosis, bleeding into a joint. Early signs are stiffness, warmth, tenderness, pain, and limitation of motion. As bleeding progresses, the joint becomes swollen. Muscle spasms and changes in soft tissue structure occur, resulting in the formation of flexion contractures. Recurrence of bleeding causes further degenerative changes that can lead to permanent joint damage.

The goal of therapy is prevention of morbidity from bleeding episodes. When there is evidence of bleeding, factor replacement therapy should be started immediately. Infusion of appropriate sources of the deficient factor will raise the plasma factor level sufficiently to allow hemostasis. Cryoprecipitate and commercial concentrates of factor VIII are the treatments of choice for classic hemophilia. Cryoprecipitate is easily prepared in the blood bank from fresh plasma but must be stored in the frozen state. Several commercial concentrates are available. They are stored at 5°C to 10°C and are, therefore, more convenient for home transfusion and travel. Hemarthroses may require continuation of replacement therapy for 3 to 4 days. Plasma and commercial factor IX concentrates are used to treat Christmas disease.

In some cases when the disease is severe and frequent transfusions are required to control bleeding, prophylactic infusion programs are instituted. Therapy is administered routinely two or three times a week. The goal of this approach is maintenance of adequate levels of the clotting factor and prevention of bleeding. The prophylactic approach may be used to eliminate the risk of bleeding when the patient is participating in aggressive rehabilitative physical therapy programs and must be able to engage in active exercise.

The cost and inconvenience of frequent infusions have promoted the development of home management programs. In these programs, clients and their families are taught to administer the infusions. Early institution of therapy permits earlier control of bleeding, fewer complications, and less interruption of normal activity. In some situations children as young as 5 and 6 years of age are administering their own factor.

Epsilon aminocaproic acid (EACA or Amicar) may be administered in conjunction with factor replacement to control mouth bleeding. EACA is an inhibitor of the fibrinolytic enzyme system, which is particularly active in mucosal tissue. Suspected renal bleeding usually is a contraindication for administration of Amicar.

Approximately 10 percent of patients with classic hemophilia will develop an IgG antibody to factor VIII. This inhibitor in the patient's plasma results in the inactivation of factor VIII in normal plasma. The development of an inhibitor calls for an alteration of the plan for treatment of bleeding problems. Alternative approaches to management are currently being investigated.

The pyschosocial implications of the disease are great. The genetic aspect has obvious implications. Many mothers feel responsible and guilty. This often leads to overprotection. Two behavior patterns described in hemophiliac children are thought to be related to maternal overprotection: passive dependence and risk taking. Fathers and siblings may resent the child's limitations. The constant threat of hemorrhage interferes with many family activities and stands between the child and his peers who are able to lead active lives. The cost of treatment may create a strain on the entire family. The average cost of replacement therapy for one bleeding episode ranges from $50 to $350, depending on the severity of the bleeding and the weight of the patient.

The team approach to treatment of hemophilia is essential. Ideally, the team should consist of the child and his family, a pediatrician, a hematologist, an orthopedist, a dentist, a physical therapist, a psychologist, a social worker, and a nurse. Coordination of the efforts of all members of the team should provide smooth, comprehensive management of this complex disease and afford the client the opportunity to function as a healthy, independent individual.

PREVENTION

Health Promotion

1. Genetic counseling should be provided to prospective parents with a family history of hemophilia.
2. Prenatal sex determination may be done by amniocentesis when known carrier mothers are pregnant.

Population at Risk

Sons of carrier mothers.

Screening

Partial thromboplastin time (PTT) test and factor VIII activity assay.

ASSESSMENT

Health History

1. Family history of bleeding tendency.
2. History of prolonged bleeding after circumcision, intramuscular injection, laceration, trauma.
3. Bleeding into joints—many patients will describe a pattern of particular joints that are involved.
4. Bleeding into muscles.
5. Gastrointestinal bleeding.
6. Hematuria.
7. Spontaneous bleeding that often occurs in phases or cycles.
8. Maternal overprotection.
9. Parental rejection.
10. Child's passive dependency, risk taking.
11. Sibling rivalry.

Physical Assessment

1. Examine during a bleeding episode.
   a. General: agitated, in pain.
   b. Skin: bruises, soft tissue bleeding with pain, swelling.
   c. Mucous membranes: persistent oozing from lacerations, particularly upper lip frenulum in toddler.
   d. Muscular: pain, warmth, swelling of muscle mass.

   e. Skeletal: stiffness, warmth, pain, limitations of motion, swelling at joints, contractions and ankylosis from previous episodes if therapy was not instituted early.

Diagnostic Tests

1. Bleeding time, fibrinogen concentration, prothrombin time (PT), platelet count, platelet adhesiveness and aggregation, and clot retraction are all normal.
2. Partial thromboplastin time (PTT) is elevated, corrects with administration of factor concentrate.
3. Factor activity assay: decreased (expressed as a percent of a normal standard).
4. Factor antigen: normal.

NURSING DIAGNOSES: ACTUAL OR POTENTIAL

1. Bleeding secondary to clotting defect.
2. Anemia, secondary to bleeding (rarely severe enough to require restriction of activity).
3. Alteration of comfort: discomfort secondary to hemarthroses or bleeding into muscles.
4. Musculoskeletal deformities secondary to hemarthroses or bleeding into muscles.
5. Alterations in parenting: maternal guilt and overprotection, parental rejection.
6. Alterations of lifestyle for family.
7. Lack of knowledge regarding disease and treatment.

EXPECTED OUTCOMES

1. Child will not have unnecessary bleeding; unavoidable bleeding episodes will be promptly controlled.
2. Child will not develop musculoskeletal deformities.
3. Pain will be controlled.
4. Child will receive maximum benefit from iron replacement therapy.
5. Client and family will be well informed about disease and management.
6. Parental guilt will be absent or minimal.
7. Parent–child interaction will be unimpaired.

INTERVENTIONS

1. Prevent bleeding.
   a. Pad crib and playpen for infants.
   b. Remove hazards from environment for toddlers: pacifiers can aggravate frenulum trauma; sharp furniture and throw rugs can facilitate injury.
   c. For toddlers, have mother sew padded patches into the knees and elbows of clothing to protect joints during falls.
   d. Avoid deep intramuscular injections.
   e. Apply pressure for 5 minutes after intravenous puncture or subcutaneous injection for immunizations.
   f. Teach client and family to avoid drugs that interfere with platelet function (aspirin and aspirin-containing drugs, antihistamines).
2. Control bleeding when prevention fails.
   a. Prepare and administer replacement factor as prescribed.
   b. Immobilize affected area and apply ice.
   c. Pack nose or mouth with hemostatic agents as prescribed for mucosal bleeds.
   d. Reassure client and family that bleeding will be controlled.
   e. Encourage client to rest.
3. When bleeding is controlled, encourage active range of motion to the level of pain as prescribed. If mobilization has been restricted, encourage cautious ambulation as prescribed (may begin within 48 hours).
4. Control pain with analgesic as ordered. Aspirin and aspirin-containing drugs will not be used. Encourage client to use relaxation and distraction techniques.
5. Encourage parents to administer iron with fruit juices to promote optimal absorption, which occurs in the presence of acidic pH. Milk and milk products are not as conducive to iron absorption.
6. Teach client and family about life with the disease.
   a. Provide written and verbal information about the nature of the disease, signs and symptoms of bleeding, measures to control bleeding, indications for replacement therapy, and procedure for obtaining medical assistance. Schedule teaching when child is stable and relaxed. Ask family to repeat information to nurse at a later time.
   b. Assess client and family readiness for home transfusion program.
   c. Provide written and verbal instructions about dose calculation and procedure for administration.
   d. Begin preparing family for administering

factor by showing them the techniques involved.
   e. Encourage client and/or parents gradually to attempt procedure; begin by withdrawing factor, applying tourniquet, and so on.
   f. Reassure client and parents as they learn techniques.
   g. Observe client and parents in return demonstration.
   h. Counsel teacher or employer as indicated.
   i. Inform family of summer camps for hemophiliacs if available.
   j. Use resources of (and inform family about) hemophilia groups (Table 18-4).
7. Communicating with parents.
   a. Encourage parents to verbalize feelings of guilt and reassure them that this is a normal reaction.
   b. Encourage parents to identify their strengths as parents and help them develop a plan for allowing child's independence.
   c. Reassure them during stress of allowing independence.
   d. Facilitate communication with other parents of hemophiliac children.

EVALUATION

Outcome Criteria

1. Avoidable bleeding does not occur; bleeding that does take place is adequately treated.
2. Musculoskeletal deformities are minimized.
3. Pain is well controlled.
4. Anemia is corrected with iron therapy.
5. Child's adjustment and development are adequate.
6. Parent's adjustment and parenting styles are adequate.
7. Parents and child, as age permits, understand hemophilia and competently carry out their parts of the treatment regimen.

Complications

DEVELOPMENT OF AN INHIBITOR

Assessment
1. Persistent bleeding after replacement therapy.
2. Elevated factor antibody titer.

Revised Outcomes
Client's bleeding will be controlled.

Interventions
1. Notify physician immediately.
2. Discontinue factor VIII replacement therapy until further notification by physician.
3. Administer alternate therapy as prescribed (may be factor IX).

SKELETAL CONTRACTURE

Assessment
1. Persistent restriction of range of motion.
2. Radiographic changes (i.e., joint degeneration and effusion).

Revised Outcome
Range of motion of joint will be restored.

Interventions
Orthopedic traction: patient may be placed in a quingle cast and undergo gradual reduction of contraction under replacement therapy.

MUSCLE ATROPHY

Assessment
1. Decreased muscle mass.
2. Weakness.

TABLE 18-4 INFORMATION FOR PARENTS AND PROFESSIONALS

Sickle cell
   National Association for Sickle Cell Disease, Inc., 3460 Wilshire Boulevard, Los Angeles, CA 90010. (213) 731-1166

Hemophilia
   The National Hemophilia Foundation, 19 West 34th Street, New York, NY 10001. (212) 536-0211

Leukemia
   American Cancer Society, state divisions (for listings, see *Ca: A Cancer Journal for Clinicians*)
   Candlelighters Foundation, 2025 Eye Street NW, Washington, DC 20006. (212) 659-5136
   Leukemia Society of America, Inc., 800 2nd Avenue, New York, NY 10017. (212) 573-8484
   National Cancer Institute, 9000 Rockville Pike, Bethesda, MD 20205. (800) 638-6694; in Alaska (800) 638-6070; in Maryland (800) 492-1444.

Revised Outcomes
Child will regain muscle function.
Interventions
Child will have a muscle strengthening exercise program.

HEPATITIS

Assessment
1. Elevated liver enzymes.
2. Elevated hepatitis-associated antigens.
3. Skin rash and itching.
4. Arthritis.
5. Fever.
6. Loss of appetite.
7. Nausea and vomiting.
8. Abdominal pain.
(See *Hepatitis.*)

VON WILLEBRAND'S DISEASE

DESCRIPTION

Von Willebrand's disease is a hereditary coagulation disorder with an autosomal dominant pattern of inheritance. It is characterized by a prolonged bleeding time and a deficiency of factor VIII. There is reduction of both the molecular concentration and activity of factor VIII. The prolonged bleeding time is due to a deficiency of a component of the factor VIII molecule involved in platelet adhesiveness and aggregation. The deficiency, therefore, produces a defect in platelet adhesion and aggregation as well as plasma coagulation.

The clinical manifestations of the disease are variable among clients and occasionally in the same client at different times. Bleeding from the skin and mucosa is common. Hemarthroses are rare. Menorrhagia and bleeding following dental extraction, surgery, or trauma may be severe.

Local hemostatic measures are usually effective in controlling nosebleeds. Serious bleeding is treated with transfusions of cryoprecipitate or whole fresh frozen plasma.

PREVENTION

Health Promotion

Genetic counseling should be provided to parents with a family history of bleeding disorders.

Population at Risk

Children of a carrier.

Screening

Bleeding time, PTT, and factor VIII activity assay.

ASSESSMENT

Health History

1. Family history of bleeding tendency.
2. Client history of bleeding tendency (e.g., prolonged bleeding after circumcision, intramuscular injections, lacerations, or trauma).
3. Gastrointestinal bleeding.
4. Mucosal bleeding.
5. Menorrhagia.
6. Easy bruisability.

Physical Assessment

Exam during a bleeding episode.
- a. General: agitated client.
- b. Skin: ecchymoses, petechiae.
- c. Mucous membranes: persistent oozing from nose or gums.

Diagnostic Tests

1. Bleeding time and PTT are both prolonged.
2. Factor VIII activity assay and antigen are both decreased.
3. Platelet adhesion to glass beads is decreased.
4. Platelet aggregation with ristocetin is decreased.
5. Response to transfused factor VIII antigen reveals disproportionate increase in factor VIII activity 12 to 96 hours after transfusion.

NURSING DIAGNOSES: ACTUAL OR POTENTIAL

1. Bleeding.
2. Anemia secondary to bleeding (rarely severe enough to require restriction of activity).
3. Lack of knowledge regarding disease and treatment.

EXPECTED OUTCOMES

1. Client will not experience unnecessary bleeding; unavoidable bleeding will be promptly controlled.
2. Client will receive maximum benefit from iron replacement therapy.
3. Client and family will be well informed about disease and management.

INTERVENTIONS

See *Hemophilia* and *Thrombocytopenia.* Patients with von Willebrand's disease do not require home care transfusions and do not have bleeding into joints. They may, however, require prophylactic treatment for a dental extraction.

EVALUATION

See *Thrombocytopenia*.

IMMUNOGLOBULIN DEFICIENCY

DESCRIPTION

Immunoglobulin deficiency includes disorders of varying severity. Transient hypogammaglobulinemia is a frequently occurring condition in childhood, resolving over a period of months. Isolated deficiencies of IgG, IgA, IgM, IgD, and IgE are also well recognized. A third classification is X-linked agammaglobulinemia, which represents an absence of IgA, IgM, and IgD with an absence of lymphocytes and lowered levels of IgG. Finally, severe combined immunodeficiency (SCID) is a disease incorporating an absence of B- and T-cell lymphocyte function with a deficiency of immunoglobulins. The child may have a history of repeated infections that have not responded to traditional antibiotic therapy. Malabsorption and failure to thrive are often present.

In addition to measuring immunoglobulins to ascertain their decrease or absence, standard medical practice includes testing for the delayed hypersensitivity mechanism through skin tests, such as streptokinase-streptodornase (SKSD) or *Candida*. Titers may be obtained to evaluate the antibody responses to foreign antigens produced by immunizations. Never administer a live attenuated virus or live virus of any kind, as the child can succumb to an overwhelming infection as a result.

Treatment of an immunoglobulin deficiency entails replacement with gammaglobulins, which should be given for symptomatic control in mild cases and regularly for severe deficiencies. If the child does not improve on gammaglobulin therapy, fresh frozen plasma is an alternative. The child should find a "buddy" if possible: a person who can consistently donate plasma. Donor consistency minimizes such complications as hepatitis. The long-term prognosis is variable and depends on the severity of the disease. Prognosis is guarded in the severe combined immunodeficiencies.

PREVENTION

Health Promotion

Genetic counseling for families with X-linked recessive SCID is advisable, as the condition is not compatible with a long life expectancy.

Population at Risk

Most immune deficiency diseases appear in childhood, with the most severe deficiencies being recognized earliest. Boys are affected four times as often as girls.

Screening

None.

ASSESSMENT

Health History

1. History of recent infection.
2. Cough, productive or nonproductive.
3. Skin infections.
4. Malabsorption, diarrhea.
5. Weight loss or poor weight gain.

Physical Assessment

1. Evaluate thoroughly for sites of infection.
2. Height and weight may be below normal due to malabsorption.
3. Skin lesions or inflamed areas, pallor.
4. There may be rhinorrhea.
5. Rhonchi, rales, or cough may be present.
6. Lymph nodes and tonsillar tissue are present.

Diagnostic Tests

1. Immunoglobulin levels. All immunoglobulins may be decreased, or selected immunoglobins may be below normal.
2. Skin testing. Children who have SCID will not produce an inflammatory response to *Candida* or diphtheria-tetanus toxins because the defective B lymphocytes (antibody-forming lymphocytes) and T lymphocytes (lymphocytes involved in attacking and removing foreign antigens) cannot respond to the challenge of a previously seen antigen.
3. Diphtheria and tetanus titers. The titers will be negligible or low despite numerous immunizations.

NURSING DIAGNOSES: ACTUAL OR POTENTIAL

1. Risk of overwhelming infection due to altered immunological defense mechanisms.
2. Alteration in nutritional status: undernutrition due to malabsorption and associated with chronic debilitation and chronic infection.
3. Risk of alteration of homeostasis secondary to gammaglobulin therapy.
4. Altered self-concept secondary to disease.

EXPECTED OUTCOMES

1. Child will not experience preventable infections and will be promptly treated for infection that does occur.
2. Child will receive adequate nutrition to support growth.
3. Complications of gammaglobulin therapy will be promptly recognized and treated.
4. Child will have optimal self-image.

INTERVENTIONS

1. Protect against infection and minimize effects of infection (see *Neutropenia*).
2. Instruct parents in providing a high-protein, high-calorie diet. Consult dietitian regarding specific dietary deficiencies.
3. Take weights, daily if hospitalized and weekly at home.
4. Monitor characteristics and consistency of bowel movement.
5. Promote tolerance of gammaglobulin therapy.
   a. Rotate injection sites.
   b. Observe injection sites for signs of abscess formation.
   c. Use warm compresses after injection of gammaglobulin.
   d. Encourage child to use muscle after injection.

EVALUATION

Outcome Criteria

1. Avoidable infections do not occur.
2. Nutritional status is adequate.
3. Preventable complications of therapy do not occur.
4. Family demonstrates understanding of disease course and therapy and copes well.
5. Child's adjustment and development are adequate.

ABNORMAL CELLULAR GROWTH

SICKLE CELL ANEMIA (HEMOGLOBIN SS DISEASE)

DESCRIPTION

Sickle cell anemia is the most common of the several sickling syndromes. All are characterized by an abnormality of the chemical makeup of the hemoglobin molecule, which predisposes the red cells to assume a sickle (crescent) shape under certain circumstances. The sickled cells obstruct the microvasculature, causing decreased blood flow to the tissues. The lowered oxygen transport produces metabolic acidosis, and the decreased pH, in turn, precipitates sickling of more RBCs. Severe sickling episodes are called *sickle cell crises*.

Crises in sickle cell anemia may be precipitated by dehydration, fever, infection, surgery, prolonged or relative anoxia, such as may occur in underwater swimming or sudden exposure to high altitudes, and sometimes pregnancy. There are four types of sickle cell crisis: aplastic crisis, vaso-occlusive or pain crisis, hyperhemolytic crisis, and sequestration crisis in which blood pools in the viscera with resultant shock and possibly death. Recurrent crises damage the liver, kidneys, eyes, heart, brain, and spleen. Sickle cell anemia decreases life expectancy, but childhood death is not universal and should not be considered the fate of each child with the disease. Death can result from overwhelming infection (due in part to decreased splenic function caused by repeated infarcts), infarction of vital organs, congestive heart failure caused by severe anemia, or the hypovolemia of sequestration crisis. The care of patients with sickle cell anemia is directed at preventing crises by avoiding factors that precipitate them and at effectively treating crises that do occur. Crisis treatment usually consists of controlling pain, providing adequate hydration, giving supplemental oxygen, and transfusing with whole blood or packed red cells.

PREVENTION

Health Promotion

1. Genetic counseling may prevent birth of future siblings with the SS hemoglobin.
2. Parents with sickle trait (hemoglobin AS disease) should also be advised as to the potential inheritance patterns (see *AS Disease*).

Population at Risk

Sickle hemoglobin is found primarily among blacks, but there are numerous instances of the hemoglobin abnormality in other races and occasionally in persons who are phenotypically white. Sickle cell anemia is an inherited homozygous disorder. The incidence among American blacks has been estimated at one in 600.

Screening

Sickling is detectable by simple laboratory screening tests (sickling test, and Sickledex); hemoglobin electrophoresis can be used to differentiate between sickle cell (hemoglobin SS) disease and sickle cell trait (hemoglobin AS disease), the carrier state.

ASSESSMENT

Health History

1. Frequent infections occur in patients who are asplenic because of infarcts; the most common infectious organism is pneumococcus.
2. Jaundice ("yellow eyes," that is, yellow sclerae) may be present, particularly with febrile episodes.
3. History of the disorder in the nuclear or extended family and children who died in infancy or early childhood.
4. Joint, abdominal, or back pain that, if transient, is usually related to stress of exercise. If chronic, it is related to crises-induced damage in the affected joints.
5. Swollen joints, usually transient and related to crises.
6. Frequent headaches that are sharp and transient.
7. Pallor that may be transient or chronic.
8. Decreased exercise tolerance, dyspnea.
9. Hand and foot swelling (due to vaso-occlusion) in infancy.

Physical Assessment

1. Height and weight are usually in the lower percentiles.
2. Skin: pallor (nail beds, mucous membranes), jaundice.
3. Cardiac exam: anemia produces flow murmurs.
4. Abdominal exam: increase or decrease in spleen size; possibly increased liver size.
5. Extremities: joint or bone abnormalities, ulcerations; hand and foot swelling in infants.
6. Funduscopic exam: retinal changes secondary to infarcts, occurring later in life.
7. Neurological exam may reveal some neurological deficits, particularly with intracerebral vaso-occlusive crisis.
8. Delayed puberty.

Diagnostic Tests

1. Blood counts reveal hypochromic anemia with RBCs of varying shapes and sizes. In crisis, there is marked increase in the number of sickle-shaped cells. Leukocytosis (12,000–25,000/mL of blood) accompanies a "normal" picture for persons with sickle cell anemia, as there is thought to be a stimulatory effect on the marrow either by a cross-reactivity to erythropoietin or a parallel stimulatory effect on WBC precursors by leukopoietin. The platelet count is within normal limits.
2. Hemoglobin electrophoresis establishes the diagnosis of the hemoglobinopathy by passing a current through a patch of blood on specially prepared filter paper. The different hemoglobins "migrate" at varying rates depending on the genetic anomaly.

NURSING DIAGNOSES: ACTUAL OR POTENTIAL

1. Knowledge deficit regarding the disease, its inheritance patterns, and its treatment.
2. Risk of infection due to lowered immunocompetence and impaired circulation.
3. Risk of sickling crises and their sequelae.
4. Altered self-esteem of child, associated with activity limitations, growth retardation, and delayed puberty.
5. Altered self-esteem of parents due to heritability of the disease.

TABLE 18-5 STATISTICAL PROBABILITIES FOR GENOTYPE OF OFFSPRING[a]

1. Normal AA mated with carrier AS
   Each child has a 50% chance of being normal and a 50% chance of being a carrier.

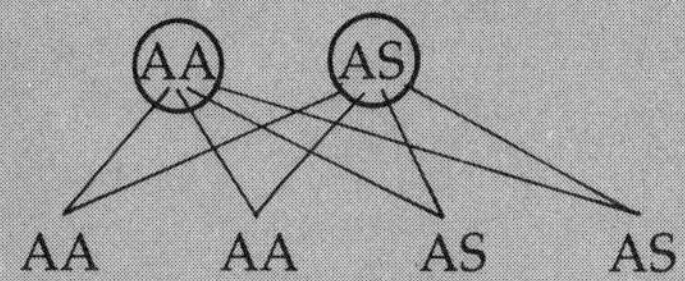

2. Two carriers AS mated together
   Each child has a 25% chance of being normal AA, a 50% chance of being a carrier AS, and a 25% chance of having sickle cell disease SS.

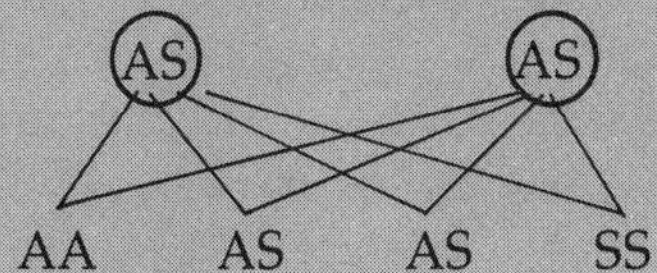

3. People with sickle cell disease SS have reduced fertility. The genetic possibilities for their offspring are as follows:
   a. Person with SS disease mated with normal AA
      All children would be carriers AS.

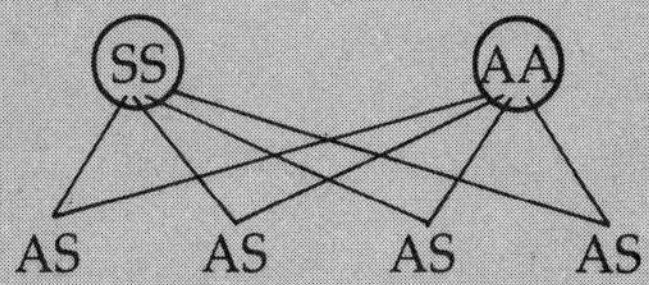

   b. Person with SS disease mated with a carrier AS
      Each child has a 50% chance of being a carrier AS and a 50% chance of having sickle cell disease SS.

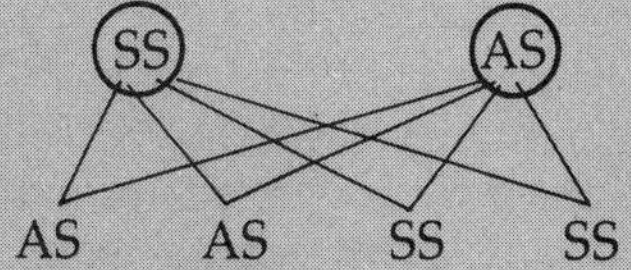

   c. Two persons with sickle cell disease SS mated together
      All children would have SS disease.

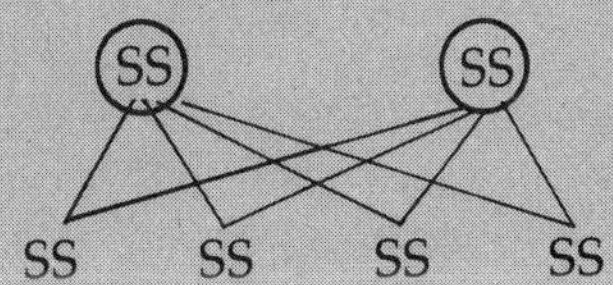

[a] Depending on parents' hemoglobin type: normal AA, sickle cell trait (carrier) AS, or sickle cell disease SS.

EXPECTED OUTCOMES

1. Family members (and child when old enough) will understand inheritance pattern, signs and symptoms, and management of the disease.
2. Infections will be infrequent and, when occurring, will receive prompt and effective treatment.
3. Avoidable sickling crises will not occur.
4. Crises that do occur will be promptly and effectively treated and will not produce unnecessary sequelae.
5. Child will have positive self-esteem.
6. Parents will have positive self-esteem.

INTERVENTIONS

1. Teach family the inheritance pattern of the disease and explain the implications for other offspring in the family (Table 18-5).
2. Teach about the anatomical and physiological alterations that characterize the disease.
   a. Height and weight may be below normal; delayed puberty is common and should not need hormonal supplementation.
   b. Child should receive the usual childhood immunizations.
   c. Child may need folic acid supplements, mostly during crises. Encourage a diet high in folic acid (see *Megaloblastic Nutritional Anemias*).
   d. Child should have regular dental and ophthalmic evaluations.
   e. Observe for unusual urinary patterns (bed-wetting, increased frequency); the disease can precipitate chronic kidney problems.

f. Limit stressful activity, such as football, basketball, soccer, and track, as they cause periods of anoxia and predispose to sickling of red cells.
g. Contact school system regarding child's activity limitations.

3. Teach parents the home management of child to prevent crises and complications (Table 18-6).
   a. Notify doctor about temperature of 101°F or higher for 4 hours or longer.
   b. Encourage the use of acetaminophen (not aspirin) for fever; acetaminophen does not alter blood pH.
   c. If child has acute back pain, abdominal pain, persistent headaches, nausea, or vomiting, notify doctor.
   d. Encourage hydration: suggest a minimum daily hydration of one to one and one-half times maintenance (1500–2200 mL/m^2/24 h). Suggest two times maintenance (3000–3600 mL/m^2/24 h) during extremes in environmental conditions and stressful situations, such as fever or pain.
   e. Avoid infections; seek early treatment for beginning infections.
   f. Emphasize crisis prevention.
4. Minimize sequelae of crisis.
   a. Monitor vital signs, reporting precipitous drops in blood pressure and/or sharp increases in heart rate and respirations indicative of shock.
   b. Maintain pain-free status (pain increases stress and oxygen requirements).
   c. Keep accurate intake and output records.
   d. Encourage oral fluids (if child is vomiting, all fluids must be parenteral).
   e. Administer antipyretics.
   f. Use of humidified oxygen may be indicated, particularly in pulmonary insults, such as pneumonia. The use of oxygen in other crises is controversial.
   g. Use of transfusions as necessary, for aplastic crises and to promote healing of damaged tissues (e.g., in cerebral vascular accidents and chronic leg ulcerations).
5. Encourage a positive self-image of child and parent, reinforcing activities appropriate for child's development.
   a. Observe for feelings of guilt on part of parents or child (see guidelines under *Leukemia*).

TABLE 18-6 GUIDELINES FOR MANAGING SICKLE CELL ANEMIA

Do not take any aspirin or aspirin-containing products. Aspirin can make cells sickle more easily. Aspirin is salicylic acid.

Tylenol and Tempra *can* be used for control of fever, pain, or headache. Tylenol and Tempra are acetaminophen. Be sure to determine the correct dosage (on the side of the bottle or box) for your child or yourself.

If you or your child runs a fever (i.e., 101°F or 38.3°C or greater), you should see a doctor. Before coming to the hospital or clinic, take Tylenol or Tempera. Fever can make cells sickle more easily.

Signs of a sickle cell crisis are

- Pain in arm, leg, abdomen, chest, or head.
- Swelling, most often seen in an arm or leg.
- Jaundice, yellow eyes.
- Dark urine.
- Blood in urine.

What you should do.

- Give Tylenol or Tempra for fever or pain.
- Encourage drinking fluids as they help prevent problems from a sickle cell crisis.
- Rest, try to relax as much as possible.

What about school?

- Client should not participate in strenuous activities, although he or she can engage in moderate exercise. Stressful exercise may cause pain in legs and chest because of cells sickling. If this occurs, drink fluids, take Tylenol or Tempra, and rest.
- Client should have the same scholastic expectations as everyone else. Sickle cell anemia does not affect the ability to read, think, and so forth.
- For fever (temperature higher than 101°F), give Tylenol or Tempra and call the parents so that the child may be seen by a physician.

b. Observe for childhood depression or poor self-concept, and support realistic aspirations and activities. Encourage peer support.
c. Refer family to appropriate agencies for further information (Table 18-4).

EVALUATION

Outcome Criteria

1. Blood relatives of the patient understand the inheritance pattern of the disease. Patient's siblings are tested for the sickling trait. Appropriate genetic counseling is provided.
2. Parents (and child at appropriate developmental level) demonstrate understanding of measures to be taken to avoid crises and of home and hospital care, by conforming to recommendations and by seeking health care at appropriate times.
3. Crises occur infrequently and are promptly treated. Avoidable sequelae do not occur.
4. Child's development, adjustment, and self-concept are appropriate.
5. Parents' adjustment, self-esteem, and coping are effective and appropriate.

Complications

Assessment
Cerebral vascular accident with resultant neurological deficits; chronic site of infection.

Revised Outcomes
Injured area will heal.

Interventions
Provide for monthly transfusions of packed cells that will facilitate optimal oxygen transport to the damaged areas, faciliating healing.

Reevaluation and Follow-up
Resolving neurological deficits; resolution of chronic lesions.

SICKLE CELL TRAIT (HEMOGLOBIN AS DISEASE)

DESCRIPTION

Sickle cell trait is the carrier state of sickle cell anemia (hemoglobin SS disease, previously discussed). Sickle cell trait is a heterozygous condition in which some of the RBCs contain sickling hemoglobin and some contain normal hemoglobin. Persons with the trait are less susceptible to problems and sickling crises than are those with the homozygous (SS) disease. Infections pose no unusual threat. Children with sickle cell trait do not ordinarily demonstrate growth disturbances or delayed puberty. Any of the symptoms described under sickle cell anemia can arise, but the probability of their occurrence is markedly less. *Surgery is one of the common precipitators of crises.* Crisis, when it does occur, is vaso-occlusive (pain crisis) rather than aplastic, sequestration, or hemolytic. Approximately 8 percent of American blacks carry the sickle cell trait. One-fourth of the offspring of two carriers can be expected to have sickle cell anemia and half can be expected to have the trait, on the average. Hence, genetic counseling is highly important for persons with the sickling trait.

Keeping in mind the above distinctions between sickle cell trait and sickle cell anemia, refer to the section on sickle cell anemia for nursing care guidelines.

ADDITIONAL HEMOGLOBINOPATHIES (HEMOGLOBIN SF DISEASE, HEMOGLOBIN CC DISEASE, HEMOGLOBIN SC DISEASE)

DESCRIPTION

There can be multiple abnormalities in synthesis or structure of the hemoglobin molecule. Hemoglobin SF disease, or sickle thalassemia, refers to the heterozygous presence of sickle hemoglobin and elevated fetal hemoglobin characteristic of beta-thalassemia. SF disease is common and one of the mildest sickling hemoglobinopathies. The fetal hemoglobin retards the sickling phenomenon, largely protecting the individual from the sequelae of sickle cell trait or sickle cell disease. Minimal intervention is necessary in the management of the disease. It is important to counsel the individual and family regarding the sickle cell trait (see *Sickle Cell Trait*).

Hemoglobin CC disease is a homozygous, inherited disease that can have manifestations as serious as those of sickle cell anemia (see *Sickle*

Cell Anemia). The sequelae of hemoglobin CC disease are very similar to those of hemoglobin SS disease, although the numbers of crises and problems with management may be somewhat fewer with hemoglobin CC disease. Preventive measures, management of crises, and counseling for CC disease should follow the guidelines of sickle cell anemia.

Hemoglobin SC disease is the second most common expression of sickle cell anemia. The implications and findings of SC disease are the same as for SS disease, although the crises and other manifestations of the disease are fewer, as with CC disease.

The person with sickle cell trait or SF disease experiences fewer side effects than the person with SS disease. The comparison is a generality, and each person possessing any of the hemoglobin abnormalities should be granted maximum benefits of counseling and intervention.

With the above considerations in mind, refer to *Sickle Cell Anemia* for nursing care.

BETA-THALASSEMIA MAJOR (COOLEY'S ANEMIA, MEDITERRANEAN ANEMIA)

DESCRIPTION

Thalassemia is a group of inherited conditions in which there is a decreased production of one or more globin chains. There may be a deficiency of alpha (α) or beta (β) chains. Homozygous alpha-thalassemia is incompatible with life because of the severe anemia. Infants with alpha-thalassemia present with hydrops fetalis and die soon after birth. Heterozygous beta-thalassemia, thalassemia minor, produces mild anemia and mild symptomatology. Homozygous beta-thalassemia, the decreased or absent production of beta chains, may require extensive therapeutic support or may necessitate only periodic intervention. There are a variety of clinical findings usually associated with beta-thalassemia major. Ineffective erythropoiesis results in marrow hyperactivity and produces "bossing" of the forehead. Growth retardation becomes most noticeable by 9 to 10 years of age, with a subsequent delay or absence of secondary sex characteristics. Hyperuricemia, as a result of RBC lysis, predisposes to gallstones and sometimes gout. The liver and spleen become enlarged as they assume some responsibility for erythropoiesis. Diabetes mellitus and altered immunity are associated with thalassemia.

Congestive heart failure is commonly associated with the long-term management of the unremitting anemia. Chronic anemia is a primary causative factor in the heart disease, although the condition may be accentuated by iron deposits in the myocardium. Iron accumulation, which is characterized by hemosiderin deposits, may be detected in the skin, giving a bronzed appearance. The iron deposition also occurs in internal organs, including the heart and brain. The iron is harvested from the bodys' breakdown of excess RBCs that result from the frequent transfusions necessary for management of the disease.

Three avenues of supportive therapy are available to promote optimal activity. The first entails maintaining the hemoglobin level between 7 and 8 grams per 100 mL of blood by regular transfusions. The second alternative uses hypertransfusion therapy, maintaining a hemoglobin level of 10 grams per 100 mL or higher with concomitant deferoxamine therapy. Hypertransfusions are used to help allay growth retardation and repeated pathologic fractures. The transfusions allow for healing. The third alternative includes splenectomy, with continued transfusion therapy. Splenectomy is indicated only when the spleen has enlarged progressively and the transfusion requirements have increased. The spleen begins trapping the transfused RBCs, presumably through an autoimmune mechanism. If the child weathers preadolescence with minimal supportive therapy, the outlook is optimistic that he or she will continue to do well.

PREVENTION

Health Promotion

1. Genetic counseling may prevent birth of future siblings with thalassemia.
2. Parents with thalassemia trait should be advised as to the potential inheritance patterns.

Population at Risk

Italians and Greeks and, to a lesser degree, Orientals and blacks.

Screening

Carriers of the trait can be identified by blood test (hemoglobin electrophoresis).

ASSESSMENT

Health History

1. Occurrence of similar findings in other family members: characteristic facies, anemia, heart problems.
2. Black, Mediterranean, or Oriental origin of family.
3. Jaundice, particularly with febrile episodes.
4. History of pallor and decreased exercise tolerance.
5. Stillbirths or infant deaths in the family.

Physical Assessment

1. Height and weight are usually in the lower percentiles.
2. Skin: pallor or jaundice in early childhood; a bronzed appearance later in life (due to iron deposits).
3. Face: "bossing" of forehead.
4. Cardiac exam: flow murmurs indicative of anemia. In late childhood and adolescence the cardiovascular system may exhibit changes related to enlarged liver and spleen. Myocardial fibrosis results from chronic anemia and iron deposition.
5. Abdominal exam: in later childhood and adolescence, reveals cirrhosis of the liver that may develop from the strain of erythropoiesis and iron deposition. The spleen and pancreas can be similarly affected.
6. Extremities: structural abnormalities, which may or may not be related to pathologic fractures.

Diagnostic Tests

1. Blood counts. The RBCs give evidence of the beta chain deficiency by their microcytic, hypochromic values, and a variability in morphology. The PCV is lower than usual in beta-thalassemia major and may be only slightly lower in beta-thalassemia minor.
2. Hemoglobin electrophoresis. This provides the definitive diagnosis because it will reveal compensatory elevation of hemoglobin F and variable production of A_2 in homozygous beta-thalassemia. In alpha-thalassemia, hemoglobins A_2 and F are normal, and hemoglobin H is demonstrable.

NURSING DIAGNOSES: ACTUAL OR POTENTIAL

1. Knowledge deficit regarding the disease, its inheritance, and medical management.
2. Decreased exercise tolerance secondary to anemia.
3. Altered self-concept secondary to disease and its treatment.

EXPECTED OUTCOMES

1. Client and parents will understand thalassemia and its treatment.
2. Child will modify daily activity according to degree of anemia.
3. Child will have a positive self-image and will engage in activities appropriate to development.

INTERVENTION

1. Teach client and parents about disease, its management, and its effects.
   a. Genetic considerations.
      (1) Explain that beta-thalassemia is an inherited disorder in which the RBCs contain decreased amounts of normal hemoglobin, and anemia results.
      (2) Explain the inheritance pattern of the condition and the prospects for siblings who are heterozygous carriers (same pattern as in sickle cell disease; see Table 18-4).
   b. Therapeutic considerations.
      (1) For transfusion precautions, see Table 18-3.
      (2) Explain and instruct about therapy; it may include client- or parent-administered deferoxamine injections.
   c. Miscellaneous considerations.
      (1) Child may be smaller than peers.
      (2) Child may have more infections, especially if splenectomy has been performed.
      (3) Child should receive appropriate immunizations.
      (4) Child may not be able to tolerate stressful sports, such as football, basketball, soccer.
      (5) Child may have delayed puberty.
2. Modify activity according to degree of anemia (see Table 18-2).
3. Encourage a positive self-image, reinforcing activities appropriate for development.
   a. Observe for feelings of guilt or denial on part of parents and child.
   b. Observe for childhood depression or poor

self-concept. Suggest realistic aspirations and activities.
c. Anticipate delayed puberty.

EVALUATION

Outcome Criteria

1. Family members understand inheritance pattern of the disease and avail themselves of genetic counseling.
2. Avoidable complications of transfusion do not occur; others are promptly recognized and treated.
3. Parents and child demonstrate understanding of and compliance with treatment, including home care.
4. Activity does not exceed tolerance.
5. Development, adjustment, and self-concept are adequate.

HEREDITARY SPHEROCYTOSIS (CHRONIC FAMILIAL JAUNDICE)

DESCRIPTION

Red blood cell membrane abnormalities result in hemolytic anemias, similar to hemoglobinopathies. Hereditary spherocytosis (HS) is a dominantly inherited hemolytic anemia. The syndrome is typified by spherocytes in the peripheral smear and the presence of fragments. The RBCs assume a spherical shape because of a deficiency in membrane lipids that allows for an influx of sodium ions and water. It is difficult for the spherical cells to pass through capillary circulation. The spleen is the site primarily responsible for destruction of the RBCs. The RBCs are normally polished and cleaned by the spleen. Cleaning implies plucking excess membrane from the erythrocytes. The membrane loss further predisposes the spherocytic cells to hemolysis.

Most patients with hereditary spherocytosis are asymptomatic. Infection or stress, however, can stimulate further hemolysis that results in intermittent jaundice, anemia, splenomegaly, and hyperpigmented stools and urine. Supportive transfusions may be required.

Splenectomy is the preferred treatment for management of the hemolysis. Some lysis can still occur after splenectomy, but it is minimal. The child 5 years of age or older is a candidate for splenectomy, as problems with infections are decreased by that age. It is in the child's best interest to wait as long as possible for splenectomy, as the spleen is a useful adjunct in the maturation of immunocompetence. When splenectomy is delayed, however, gallstones can occur secondary to the breakdown products of RBC hemolysis. Leg ulcers, heart murmurs, and radiological findings of thickened parietal and frontal bones may be associated with spherocytic anemia and its course.

PREVENTION

Health Promotion

Genetic counseling as to the inheritance of the anomaly. With optimal management, the condition is compatible with longevity and should not be a contraindication for future pregnancies.

Population at Risk

Children of affected families.

Screening

None.

ASSESSMENT

Health History

1. Familial history of HS or jaundice, yellow sclerae, pallor, decreased exercise tolerance, dark urine, dark stools.
2. Presence of the above signs and symptoms in the child, particularly associated with infections or stressful events.

Physical Assessment

1. Eyes may have yellow sclerae secondary to tissue deposition of unconjugated bilirubin from rapid RBC hemolysis.
2. Mucous membranes may be slightly pale.
3. Skin is usually pale with episodic tinges of jaundice due to periods of rapid hemolysis.
4. Cardiac exam may reveal flow murmurs.
5. Abdominal exam reveals an enlarged firm spleen.
6. Leg ulcers may be present.
7. Urine is dark and clear.
8. Feces are hyperpigmented; client may have constipation.

Diagnostic Tests

Hemoglobin, hematocrit with RBC indices. HS is associated with a lowered hemoglobin and hematocrit with spherocytic cells on peripheral smear that are hypochromic and a mixed population of macrocytic and microcytic cells. The variability is a function of the phagocytic action of the spleen. The majority of cells are macrocytic. The MCH and MCV are low to normal with a relatively high MCHC.

NURSING DIAGNOSES: ACTUAL OR POTENTIAL

1. Decreased exercise tolerance secondary to anemia.
2. Risk of complications from transfusions and splenectomy.
3. Knowledge deficit regarding disease and therapy.

EXPECTED OUTCOMES

1. Child will restrict activity as appropriate for degree of anemia.
2. Parents and client will be well informed about the complications of HS and the need for therapeutic intervention with transfusions or splenectomy.

INTERVENTIONS

1. Modify activity as appropriate for degree of anemia.
   a. See Table 18-2.
   b. Teach parents and child that client must avoid contact sports because of vulnerability to traumatic rupture of the spleen.
2. Teach parents and client about the disease and its treatment.
   a. Fever or other stress will often induce a temporary state of aplasia secondary to increased hemolysis. In such circumstances, the parents should seek medical attention for the child; he or she will likely require a blood transfusion.
   b. Client and parents need to be prepared for blood transfusion of packed RBCs. See Table 18-3.
   c. Provide preoperative preparation for the child and parents as to the specifics of surgery, such as intravenous infusions, abdominal incision, nasogastric tube, and respiratory hygiene after surgery.
   d. Administer pneumococcal vaccine before splenectomy, as studies reveal a more efficient antibody response if given before surgery. Pneumococcal infections are one of the foremost causes of morbidity in splenectomized patients.
   e. Teach parents and client about the use and purpose of prophylactic penicillin therapy, postsplenectomy. Even though the pneumococcal vaccine is given before splenectomy, the vaccine immunizes the individual against only some of the strains of pneumococcus. Penicillin prophylaxis is beneficial for patients under the age of 5 years and individuals who have not shown a definitive antibody response to the vaccine. The side effects of the therapy are minimal gastrointestinal irritability and/or occasional diarrhea.

EVALUATION

Outcome Criteria

1. Activity does not exceed tolerance.
2. Preventable infections and stress are avoided.
3. Patient tolerates splenectomy well.

Complications

NUMEROUS HEMOLYTIC EPISODES

Assessment
Three to four life-threatening episodes per year of brisk hemolysis, often with infection (before splenectomy).

Revised Outcomes
Child and family will be well prepared for and supported during splenectomy.

Interventions
Refer to previous discussion of splenectomy.

RUPTURED SPLEEN SECONDARY TO TRAUMA

Assessment
Signs and symptoms of shock, with rapid blood loss into peritoneal cavity: sudden pallor, increase in pulse and respiratory rates, and decrease in blood pressure.

Revised Outcomes
Tissue perfusion and vital functions will be maintained.

Interventions

1. Supportive care as ordered by physician.
2. Prepare client and family for immediate splenectomy.

HEREDITARY ELLIPTOCYTOSIS (HEREDITARY OVALOCYTOSIS)

DESCRIPTION

Hereditary elliptocytosis is an autosomal dominant, hemolytic anemia. It may be several months before the affected infant manifests elliptocytes. Jaundice may be present secondary to hemolysis with or without clinical anemia. As there is no abnormal hemoglobin in the cell, it is thought that the condition results from a deficient cell membrane. Eventually, elliptical cells may compose 50 percent of the circulating RBC population. Splenomegaly may be present early in the child's life. If rapid destruction of RBCs occurs, splenectomy may be suggested. Transfusions, if indicated, constitute the supportive therapy. See *Hereditary Spherocytosis* for nursing interventions.

LEUKEMIA

DESCRIPTION

Leukemia is a malignancy of unknown origin characterized by a replacement of the normal marrow elements with abnormal leukocytes and their precursors. The disease is subclassified according to the type of WBC that is predominant in the bone marrow and peripheral blood. Approximately 80 percent of the cases of childhood leukemia are classified as acute lymphocytic or lymphoblastic leukemia (ALL). Most of the remaining cases are acute myelocytic or myeloblastic leukemia (AML). Myeloblastic leukemia is less responsive to therapy, and clients suffering from it have a poorer prognosis than do those will ALL. Erythroleukemia, also called Di Guglielmo syndrome, is a variant of acute leukemia, involving *all* cell lines, including erythroid precursors. Promyelocytic leukemia is a variant of myeloblastic leukemia. Disorders of coagulation and some bleeding are a particular problem with this latter disease.

Results of recent investigations suggest that other factors, such as immunological cell surface characteristics and clinical features, should be considered in classifying acute leukemia. Leukemias that possess surface markers suggesting a T- or B-cell origin have a poorer prognosis than those in which the cell of origin cannot be identified (null cell).

The clinical features may be related to the disease process itself or to the therapy used. Anemia results from erythropoietic failure and from blood loss. The complications of anemia experienced by the child with leukemia are similar to those of *Aplastic Anemia*.

Neutropenia is the single most important factor predisposing the leukemic patient to infection. Profound neutropenia can result from the leukemic replacement of normal bone marrow or drug toxicity. Clients with leukemia may also have qualitative defects in neutrophil functions and, consequently, inadequate resistance to infection. Overwhelming infections are the cause of death in 60 to 80 percent of the children who succumb to leukemia.

Hemorrhage is usually the result of thrombocytopenia. Preexisting thrombocytopenia may be worsened by infection. Occasionally, a child with a low platelet count may not manifest signs of bleeding until an infection develops.

Leukemic invasion of any organ system in the body can result in alteration or failure of that organ system. Disease occurring in an organ other than the bone marrow is termed extramedullary. Leukemic infiltration can occur in the liver, spleen, lymph nodes, central nervous system, lungs, kidneys, bones, testicles, and ovaries.

When therapy is instituted and large numbers of cells are rapidly destroyed, large amounts of uric acid are produced. If the uric acid crystalizes in the kidney, obstruction of the renal tubules and impaired renal function can result. Hyperuricemia usually can be effectively controlled with increased fluid intake, alkalinization of the urine with intravenous sodium bicarbonate, and administration of allopurinol.

Untreated leukemia progresses rapidly; death occurs within weeks to months after diagnosis. Utilization of chemotherapeutic agents enables more than 90 percent of children with newly diagnosed ALL to achieve a remission.

A child in remission is free of signs and symptoms attributable to leukemia. As many as 40 to 50 percent of children in remission are maintained in their initial remission states for longer than 5 years. Current recommendations have been to discontinue therapy after 3 years if the child has remained in continuous complete remission. Most children who reach this point will never experience a relapse. Boys have a slightly increased rate of relapse due to testicular recurrence.

In spite of this optimistic outlook for many children, a significant number are not able to experience eradication of their disease. A number of prognostic factors evaluated at the time of diagnosis seem to be predictive of the likelihood of disease eradication: (1) the classification of disease based on cell surface markers, (2) the age of the patient at the time of diagnosis, (3) the initial WBC count, (4) the degree of organomegaly, and (5) the presence of detectable central nervous system leukemia. Generally, a child with null cell leukemia, between the ages of 2 and 10 years, with a WBC count of less than 10,000 per cu mm and no significant extramedullary disease, has a much better prognosis.

If the child's leukemic cells become resistant to the drugs being used or the leukemic cell population is not totally eradicated, the abnormal cells return, and a relapse occurs. Extramedullary relapses are frequently followed by bone marrow relapses. Once relapse occurs, succeeding remissions become more difficult to obtain and are progressively shorter in duration. A child may experience several remissions and relapses before succumbing to complications of the disease.

The goal of therapy is eradication of leukemia cells and restoration of normal marrow function. Numerous drugs can be used in a variety of combinations to induce and maintain a remission. Side effects of chemotherapy are experienced by all children, but the severity of these side effects varies from one child to another. Table 18-7 presents information about drugs used in treatment of children with leukemia.

The *induction* course of therapy is designed to reduce the leukemic cell population sufficiently to achieve a complete remission. Complete remission means that the patient is free of signs and symptoms attributable to leukemia, and that the bone marrow shows evidence of adequate function (reasonable numbers of RBCs, WBCs, and platelets) and less than 5 percent blast cells.

Certain drugs are more effective in inducing a remission than others. The chemotherapy most commonly given in this phase is a three-drug combination of prednisone given daily, vincristine given weekly, and a third agent, such as daunomycin or L-Asparaginase. Generally, after 4 to 6 weeks of induction therapy, a remission is achieved.

It is important to recognize that current methods of evaluation may fail to detect up to 10^9 leukemic cells. This means that a complete remission should not be equated with total eradication of all leukemic cells. Therefore, many treatment programs include a course of *consolidation* or *intensification* chemotherapy designed to further reduce the number of leukemia cells. This can be done by administering single agents, such as methotrexate or L-Asparaginase, in intensive courses or multiple agents in cyclic or combination therapy.

Treatment to prevent central nervous system relapse is administered early in the course of the illness. Generally, therapy consists of cranial irradiation, plus several doses of intrathecal methotrexate administered by lumbar puncture. An alternate approach includes initial intensive intrathecal therapy with methotrexate either alone or in combination with cytosine arabinoside and hydrocortisone followed by intrathecal treatment every 2 months.

The consistent side effect of cranial irradiation is alopecia. The severity and duration of alopecia varies from patient to patient, but, generally children lose all of their hair before the completion of therapy. Hair grows back within several months, but may be of a different color and texture. Episodes of fever, irritability, lethargy, headache, nausea, and vomiting occur less commonly. Preliminary data indicated that prophylactic central nervous system (CNS) radiotherapy in the treatment of acute lymphoblastic leukemia produced no clinically detectable neurological or psychological impairment. More recent studies have contradicted this finding. More investigation is needed, as this question is of extreme importance to growing, developing children.

The goals of *maintenance* or *continuation* chemotherapy are to maintain remission and to continue reducing the residual leukemic cell population toward zero. A combination of 6-mercaptopurine administered daily and methotrexate administered weekly is effective continuation therapy and is associated with minimal complications of drug toxicity.

TABLE 18-7 DRUGS MOST COMMONLY USED TO TREAT LEUKEMIA IN CHILDREN

Drug	Uses	Storage/Stability	Supply/Reconstitution	Administration	Dosage	Side Effects/Toxicity
Vincristine (Oncovin)	Induction, reinforcement	Refrigerate before and after reconstitution, use within 14 days after mixing	1- and 5-mg vials, recon-stitute with 10 ml supplied diluent	IV, avoid extravasation[a]	1.5–2 mg/m^2 (max. 2 mg) IV weekly × 2–6	Alopecia, peripheral neu-ropathy, constipation, hyponatremia, mild myelosuppression, jaw pain.
Prednisone	Induction, reinforcement	Room temp.	2.5-, 5-, 20-, and 50-mg tablets	PO, bitter to taste	40–60 mg/m^2 for 14–28-day course	Cushing's syndrome, fluid retention, muscle wasting, hypertension, hyperphagia, immunosuppression, diabetes, GI tract ulceration, striation, psychosis
L-Asparaginase[b] (Elspar)[b] (Erwinia)[b]	Induction, intensification	Refrigerate, use immediately, discard unused portion	10,000-IU vial, reconstitute with 2–5 ml unpreserved sterile water or sodium chloride	IV or IM, observe for hypersensitivity reaction, have epinephrine and resuscitation equipment available	Various dosage schedules	Hypersensitivity reaction, pancreatitis, nausea/vomiting, lethargy, somnolence, fever, hepatotoxicity, coagulopathy, hyperglycemia, convulsions
Doxorubicin (Adriamycin)	Induction	Store at controlled room temp., discard unused portion	10- and 50-mg vials, reconstitute with 5 or 25 ml normal saline	IV, avoid extravasation[a]	90 mg/m^2 in divided doses (usually 3); total cumulative lifetime dose 400–550 mg/m^2	Nausea/vomiting, alopecia, mucositis, myelosuppression, cardiotoxicity, red urine
Daunomycin (Cerubidine)	Induction	Store at controlled room temp., discard unused portion	20-mg vials, reconstituted with 4 ml sterile water	IV, avoid extravasation[a]	Various dosage schedules; total cumulative lifetime dose 500 mg/m^2	Cardiotoxicity, myelosuppression, nausea/vomiting, abdominal pain, alopecia, fever, skin rash, red urine
Hydrocortisone (Solu-Cortef)	CNS prophylaxis, induction, maintenance	Store at controlled room temp.	100-mg plain (reconstitute with 2 ml sterile water) and 100-, 250-, 500-, and 1000-mg mix-o-vials (as directed)	IT, do not enter vial twice. Should be diluted with preservative-free vehicle.	15 mg/m^2, max. dose 15 mg	See Prednisone

Cytosine arabinoside (Cytosar)	CNS prophylaxis, induction, maintenance. Systemic induction, maintenance	Store at controlled room temp., after reconstitution, store at room temp. for 48 h, discard if haze appears	100- and 500-mg vials, reconstitute with 5–10 ml supplied diluent	IV, IM, SC, or IT, may require premedication with antiemetics. Do not enter vial twice for IT use	IV, IM, SC various dosage schedules; IT once or twice weekly	Nausea/vomiting, myelosuppression, mucositis, hepatotoxicity, immunosuppression
Methotrexate	CNS prophylaxis, induction, and maintenance. Systemic maintenance	Room temp.	2.5-mg tablets, 5-mg and 50-mg/2 ml vials in solution, 20-, 50-, and 100-mg vials of cryodesiccated powder	PO, IV, IM, IT. IT preparations should be diluted with preservative-free vehicle. Do not enter vial twice for IT use	10–15 mg/m^2 IT once or twice weekly $\times$ 6 (max. dose 15 mg). 5–20 mg/m^2 once or twice weekly, IV, IM, or PO	Nausea/vomiting, mucositis, myelosuppression, hepatotoxicity, pneumonitis, osteoporosis, hyperpigmentation
6-Mercaptopurine (Purinethol)	Maintenance	Room temp.	50-mg tablets	PO	50 mg/m^2 daily	Nausea/vomiting, myelosuppression, anorexia, dermatitis, stomatitis, hepatotoxicity, abdominal pain
Cyclophosphamide (Cytoxan)	Intensification, maintenance	Room temp., refrigerate after reconstitution	25- and 50-mg tablets, 100-, 200-, and 500-mg vials, reconstitute with 5–25 ml sterile water	PO, IV, maintain liberal hydration 48 h after weekly dose and continuously when given daily	3–5 mg/m^2 daily PO, various IV dosage schedule	Nausea/vomiting, myelosuppression, alopecia, hemorrhagic cystitis, mucositis, infertility, immunosuppression, hyperpigmentation
Thioguanine (6-thioguanine)	Induction, maintenance	Room temp.	40-mg tablets	PO	80–100 mg/m^2/day	Nausea/vomiting, stomatitis, myelosuppression, liver function abnormalities, dermatitis

SOURCE: Adapted from Greene, T.: "Current Therapy for Acute Leukemia in Childhood," *Nursing Clinics of North America*, **11**(1):8, 1976.

[a] Causes chemical irritation on extravasation. Use different needles to withdraw and inject. Before injection use saline flush to establish that IV line is patent and not infiltrating. Inject with caution observing for signs of infiltration. Follow injection with saline flush.

[b] Investigational agents.

In an effort to increase the duration of remission, some investigators have employed *reinduction* or *reinforcement* therapy. With this approach, prednisone or prednisone plus vincristine "pulses" are given every 3 to 4 months for 2 to 4 weeks.

When a relapse occurs, induction therapy with vincristine and prednisone may be administered. When these agents are no longer effective, L-Asparaginase, cytosine arabinoside, daunomycin, adriamycin, or investigational agents may be used as single agents or in combination. After the remission has been reinduced, maintenance therapy will be administered. Usually, however, the occurrence of a single relapse, whether in the bone marrow or in extramedullary site, means that permanent control of the disease will be impossible.

Unfortunately, AML is less responsive to therapy. Combinations of such drugs as vincristine, prednisone, adriamycin, cyclophosphamide, daunomycin, cytosine arabinoside, 5-azacytidine, and 6-thioguanine are effective for remission induction in approximately 50 to 80 percent of children with AML. Some of these agents, particularly cytosine arabinoside and 6-thioguanine, are used for maintenance also, but the duration of remission is usually short—less than 1 year. Four- to 5-year disease-free survival is seen in only 20 percent of children with AML.

Two other modes of therapy, bone marrow transplantation and immunotherapy, have been used. Because of a number of factors, such as cost, inaccessibility of donors, and technical difficulty of the procedure, bone marrow transplantation is reserved at this time for research settings. Numerous clinical trials of immunotherapy in acute leukemia have failed to support the promising experience reported by Mathé in 1963. Although further investigation is underway, the vast majority of studies to date indicate no benefit when immunotherapy is given for acute leukemia.

Supportive therapy is essential during periods of intensive treatment. Early recognition of infection and prompt institution of appropriate measures can be lifesaving. Antibiotics are used aggressively to combat the infectious process. Transfusion is used to counteract the complications of bone marrow suppression. Packed RBCs are generally transfused in place of whole blood to avoid volume overload. The use of platelet concentrates has helped to control the hemorrhagic manifestations of thrombocytopenia. Granulocyte transfusions have been studied for use during profound neutropenia, but the benefit of their use remains controversial, and the expense and difficulty of preparation limit their use. Another measure used to combat complications of leukopenia is protection in a germ-free, laminar air-flow unit. While such units clearly reduce the infectious complications during intensive treatment, most studies have failed to show that their use improves client survival.

The diagnosis of leukemia has a tremendous emotional impact on the child, the family, and the community. Despite increasing evidence that leukemia is controllable and possibly curable, the initial reaction is to the threat of fatal illness.

There are three possible courses of the illness: (1) treatment and no response, leading to death, (2) temporary control of the disease until recurrence and death, and (3) indefinite control of the disease. The uncertainty of the outcome is perhaps the most difficult aspect to accept. Parents and children are encouraged to return to their normal lifestyle, but treatment regimens often make this an impossibility.

The responsibility of administration of therapy and observation for side effects must be shared by the family. At a time of extreme stress, families are expected to assimilate a new and confusing body of knowledge.

It is well recognized that a multidisciplinary team is best able to appreciate and meet the complex psychosocial and physical needs of the leukemic child and family. Consequently, treatment is usually coordinated through a comprehensive cancer center.

PREVENTION

Health Promotion

1. Avoid exposure to radiation, benzene.
2. Amniocentesis to detect Down's syndrome. (Children with Down's syndrome have an elevated incidence of leukemia.)

Population at Risk

1. Identical twin siblings of children with leukemia.
2. Children with Bloom's syndrome, Down's syndrome, and Fanconi's syndrome.
3. Siblings of leukemic children. (There is a slight risk, one in 720 compared with one in

2880 for white children under 15 years of age without affected siblings.)

Screening

None.

ASSESSMENT

Health History

1. Recurrent or recent infections.
2. Exposure to offending agent, such as benzene or radiation (rare).
3. Anorexia, weight loss.
4. Lethargy, fatigue, malaise.
5. Easily bruised, bleeding from nose or gums.
6. Pain (bone, abdominal).
7. Home environment should include potential for adequate hygiene, separate sleeping facilities (to decrease transmission of infections to the child).
8. Family experience with chronic illness, cancer, death, coping patterns.

Physical Assessment

1. General: elevated temperature, pulse, and respiratory rate; lethargy, malaise, irritability.
2. Skin: petechiae, ecchymoses, cellulitis, furunculosis, absence of pus and usual signs of infection (depending on degree of neutropenia) cutaneous tumor nodules (rare).
3. Lymph nodes: generalized adenopathy.
4. Mucous membranes: bleeding from gums and nose, ulceration, stomatitis, perianal abscess, pain.
5. Abdomen: hepatosplenomegaly.
6. Musculoskeletal: muscle wasting, bone pain, joint pain.
7. Lungs: cough, rhonchi, rales, tachypnea, dyspnea, decreased breath sounds.
8. Cardiac: flow murmur.
9. Neurological: with central nervous infiltration child may have nausea, vomiting, lethargy, headache, irritability, convulsions, cranial nerve palsies, papilledema, pain upon neck flexion, hyperphagia, blindness.
10. Genital: with testicular infiltration boy will have progressive, painless enlargement of one or both testicles; involved testes become nodular and firm.

Diagnostic Tests

1. Complete blood count: total WBC count may be decreased, normal, or elevated; differential usually shows the presence of blast cells and neutropenia; child has thrombocytopenia and anemia.
2. Bone marrow: often hypercelluar with 60 to 100 percent blast cells; megakaryocytes are decreased or absent; bright red Auer rods can be seen on a stained smear of peripheral blood or bone marrow with AML.
3. Serum uric acid: elevated.
4. Intravenous urogram: with renal infiltration, X-ray films show enlargement of kidneys, increase in thickness of renal cortex, distortion of calyceal system (test may be contraindicated in the presence of hyperuricemia).
5. Lumbar puncture: with central nervous system infiltration, centrifugate of cerebrospinal fluid, when Wright-stained, shows mononuclear or blast cells; pressure may be elevated, glucose may be normal or decreased, protein may be elevated.
6. Chest radiograph: mediastinal adenopathy, lung infiltrates.
7. Skeletal radiograph: osteolytic lesions, subperiosteal resorption, rarefaction of the metaphysis.

NURSING DIAGNOSES: ACTUAL OR POTENTIAL

1. Alteration in activity: decrease due to anemia from bone marrow suppression.
2. Increased risk of bleeding and increased susceptibility to infection due to bone marrow suppression.
3. Alteration in respiratory function: respiratory impairment associated with tracheal compression due to mediastinal mass.
4. Nutritional alteration: bulimia due to neurological infiltration; or anorexia and nausea and vomiting associated with intestinal obstruction from abdominal adenopathy.
5. Alterations in comfort and perception: headache, vertigo, and visual disturbances secondary to central nervous system infiltration.
6. Impairment of mobility due to bone pain.
7. Impairment of urinary elimination due to hyperuricemia.
8. Alterations in comfort due to side effects of chemotherapy: nausea and vomiting, anorexia and weight loss, increased appetite and weight gain with prednisone, mucositis, peripheral neuropathies, alopecia, sterile hemorrhagic cystitis, and local tissue irritation due to extravasation of chemotherapeutic agents.

9. Alteration in child development and family function due to seriousness of illness, stressors of treatment, and uncertainty of prognosis.

EXPECTED OUTCOMES

1. Child will modify activity level as appropriate for degree of anemia.
2. Child will not have unnecessary bleeding; bleeding that does occur will be promptly controlled.
3. Child will not have avoidable infections; infections that do occur will be promptly recognized and treated.
4. Child will have adequate O_2–CO_2 exchange.
5. Nutrition and hydration will be maintained.
6. Child will not have unnecessary discomfort from pain, nausea, vomiting, and perceptual disturbances.
7. Mucositis will be prevented insofar as possible; mucositis that does occur will be effectively treated.
8. Child will maintain normal excretory patterns (i.e., no constipation, hemorrhagic cystitis, or uric acid nephropathy).
9. Tissue necrosis due to extravasation of drugs will not occur.
10. Child and parents will understand and cope with the disease, therapy, and side effects of treatment.
11. Family members, individually and as a family, will function adequately at an appropriate developmental level (see Chapters 4 and 5).

INTERVENTIONS

For anemia, bleeding, and infection, see *Aplastic Anemia*, *Thrombocytopenia*, and *Neutropenia*. Also see Chapter 20 regarding airway obstruction, Chapter 22 regarding intestinal obstruction, and Chapter 15 regarding increased intracranial pressure.

1. Pain.
   a. When pain is anticipated, devise a plan for controlling it involving the medical and nursing staff, the patient, and family *before the onset*.
   b. Explain to the patient and family that the plan is made and that comfort measures are available. Do so in positive manner conveying confidence that the pain will be controlled.
   c. Obtain a thorough assessment of the patient's pain, including the location, nature, intensity, and pattern; patient's, family's, and staff's reaction, and measures that have controlled pain in the past.
   d. Explain the nature of the pain experience to patient and family in a language that is understandable.
   e. Provide a comfortable, nonthreatening environment: remove offensive sights, sounds, and smells.
   f. Ensure patient's and family's trust and confidence by demonstrating compassion, knowledge, and competence.
   g. Assist patient to a comfortable position.
   h. Employ measures designed to relieve pain: distraction is useful (e.g., reading, records, movies, games), if appropriate; encourage the patient to imagine pleasant sensations or situations that family can help support with stories, music, pictures, smells, and so on; decrease perception of pain with sensory and tactile stimulation (massage, vibration, heat, cold, motion, gentle scratching) based on gate-control theory.
   i. Administer analgesics as prescribed (those which do not interfere with platelet function).
   j. Evaluate each measure for effectiveness.
   k. Record a detailed description of pain experience, relief measures, and effectiveness.
2. Hyperuricemia.
   a. Ensure adequate hydration (usually twice maintenance) with oral or parenteral fluids.
   b. Administer allopurinol as prescribed (if 6-mercaptopurine is administered concomitantly, adjust dose).
   c. Monitor urine pH (should be 7.0 or greater).
   d. If urine becomes acidic, administer alkalinizing agents as prescribed (sodium bicarbonate, Diamox, Scholl's solution).
3. Nausea and vomiting.
   a. Alert patient and family to the potential for nausea and vomiting in a positive manner, assuring them that there is a plan for managing it (avoid dwelling on the possibility, as the power of suggestion is great).
   b. Allow the patient and family to partici-

pate in making the decision about timing of administration of nauseating agents (often evening administration is preferred).

c. Administer antiemetics, sedatives, or tranquilizers as prescribed *before* administering nauseating agent. Record effectiveness of these drugs.
d. Teach patient and parents about the potential for aspiration and preventive measures.
e. Eliminate offensive sights, sounds, and smells.
f. Assist patient to a comfortable, safe position (elevated upper torso may be best).
g. Have emesis basin within reach but out of sight.
h. Cleanse mouth, particularly after each vomiting episode (some patients are relieved by sucking on a sour ball).
i. Employ measures to decrease anxiety and perception of nausea, such as distraction and imagination.

4. Nutrition.
   a. Obtain a thorough assessment of eating patterns and food preferences.
   b. Offer preferred foods—many patients will tolerate foods that their mother commonly offers during illness.
   c. Encourage family to prepare foods at home or in hospital.
   d. Ensure that environment is conducive to eating at mealtime—that patient is clean (hands and face washed, mouth cleansed), relaxed, rested, and free from pain and fear; offensive sights, sounds, and smells are removed.
   e. Assist patient to a comfortable position.
   f. Suggest that patient eat with other patients or family members.
   g. Use a positive approach when discussing eating.
   h. Offer small portions of food in frequent feedings.
   i. Offer foods high in protein and calories.
   j. Make food tray attractive and appropriate for age.
   k. When appetite is increased, from steroids or hypothalamic disease, limit the amount of food at each feeding rather than the frequency of feedings; offer foods low in salt.
   l. Warn patient and family that fluctuations in appetite and weight may be marked and frequent—requiring a new wardrobe and middle-of-the night snacks.
5. Mucositis.
   a. Examine mouth and perianal area carefully before chemotherapy.
   b. Instruct patient and family in the importance of immediate reporting of stomatitis.
   c. Administer mouth care four times a day. Many approaches are used. A soft-bristled toothbrush should be used unless ulceration or bleeding occurs. Then a sponge or cotton-tipped applicator may be substituted. The mouth may be rinsed with 1:1 solution of hydrogen peroxide and saline. Rinsing with a Water Pik removes food particles and provides the stimulation of the gums that normally occurs with mastication. However, water under pressure can lacerate gums and force bacteria into the bloodstream, causing septicemia. If a Water Pik is used, it must be set on a low pressure.
   d. Notify physician immediately if lesions occur.
   e. Examine area closely for signs of superinfection with opportunistic organisms.
   f. If superinfection occurs, administer antibiotics as prescribed, and instruct patient and family in method of administration.
6. Constipation.
   a. Obtain a thorough assessment of normal bowel pattern.
   b. Ensure a high fluid intake.
   c. Employ natural laxatives, such as prune juice or high roughage foods, and exercise.
   d. Administer stool softeners and cathartics as prescribed.
7. Weakness.
   a. Warn patient, family, and schoolteachers of the potential for weakness.
   b. Assist in the selection of activities that patient can achieve (may be able to ride a bicycle or tricycle but unable to walk long distances or climb stairs; may be able to write with larger diameter pencil, fasten zipper but not button).
   c. Refer to Chapter 15 for additional guidelines.
8. Alopecia.

a. Warn patient, family, and others that alopecia will occur.
b. Make patient and family aware of alternatives, such as wigs, scarfs, caps, and so on.
c. Inform family of financial assistance for purchase of wigs, if available.
d. During period of hair loss, change patient's clothes and bed linen frequently as hair accumulates. Patient may want to cut hair or wear a hair net to catch loose hair.
e. Prepare patient for reactions of others by encouraging expression of feelings through role play, doll play, and so on.

9. Cystitis.
a. Administer cyclophosphamide early in the day to allow patient to keep emptying bladder frequently while metabolites are excreted.
b. If a large dose is given, ensure high fluid intake to ensure diuresis.
c. Ensure continuous high fluid intake with daily dose.
d. Instruct patient and family to report immediately any sign of dysuria, frequency, urgency, or hematuria; discontinue cyclophosphamide until further notice from physician.
e. If bleeding occurs, continue high fluid intake.
f. Monitor urine output (formation of clots may cause obstruction and distension).

10. Extravasation of IV chemotherapy.
a. Do not inject with the same needle used to withdraw medication from the vial.
b. Administer drug through scalp vein needle, using largest available vein.
c. Before injecting drug into any IV line, confirm that the line is patent and not infiltrating by infusing at least 5 mL of normal saline and observing for blood return (more may be needed if the vein is deep in subcutaneous tissue).
d. When patency and integrity of the vein are confirmed, inject the medication slowly. It is safest to inject the drug into the side-arm of a free-flowing IV line.
e. Observe the site of injection continuously for signs of infiltration.
f. Periodically confirm patency of the line with blood return.
g. After the medication is injected, flush the line with at least 5 mL of normal saline.
h. If infiltration occurs
(1) Discontinue the infusion immediately. Contact with a minute amount of the drug is enough to cause severe tissue reaction, necrosis, and sloughing.
(2) Notify the physician immediately. Some doctors prescribe subcutaneous Solu-Cortef to be injected at the site.
(3) Remove the IV.
(4) Apply ice packs and continue to do so intermittently for 24 hours.
(5) Instruct the patient to keep the site of injection elevated.
(6) If swelling subsides, apply warm packs (again, at frequent intervals) until inflammation subsides.
(7) Observe the site frequently for signs of tissue breakdown and infection.
(8) Instruct the patient to notify the physician immediately if complications develop.

11. Patient education.
a. Explain the nature of the disease and treatment in clear terms appropriate for developmental level and degree of stress.
b. Repeat explanations as often as needed.
c. Provide written information about the details of treatment and side effects.
d. Facilitate communication with other patients and parents.

12. Readaptation.
a. Assess the patient's ability to participate in activities.
b. Communicate strengths and limitations clearly to patient and family.
c. Modify activities to degree of limitation (homebound instruction, etc., if needed).
d. Communicate with significant family members and others to clarify objectives.
e. Provide positive reinforcement for involvement in activities.
f. Acknowledge and allow patient's and family's anxiety.

13. Grief and grieving.
In working with the grieving patient and family, the nurse should realize that there is great variety in experiences with and expressions of grief. The nurse's role is to observe and assess the patient's and family's

behavior, support them at any phase, and create an environment that will allow for progression as they are ready. It should be recognized that defense mechanisms are necessary and should not be denied. Possible interventions for each phase include

a. Denial:
   (1) Establish reality of recent past. Relate and discuss illness leading up to diagnosis.
   (2) Have parent or child express what has been done during present hospitalization, establishing further reality of present.
   (3) Clarify feelings of parents ("I know you must feel tired and worn out," etc.).
   (4) With shock or bewilderment, encourage activities, allowing parents and child to hold on to reality, particularly those routines that have been part of the family's routine before diagnosis.

b. Anger:
   (1) Help family identify source of its anger.
   (2) Supply consistent and truthful information.
   (3) Observe for self-directed anger and/or self-inflicted punishment.
      (a) Channel anger away from individuals and redirect energies to the present (i.e., constructive participation in the child's treatment).
      (b) Reassure that the onset of disease was not anyone's "fault."
   (4) Encourage verbalization of feelings.
   (5) Offer family the opportunity to talk with other parents of children with cancer who have accepted disease and treatment.
   (6) Give family decision-making abilities.

c. Bargaining:
   (1) Acknowledge and allow feelings.
   (2) Be aware of signs of guilt, "if only." (see b. (3), above.)
   (3) Encourage intrafamily support. Evaluate family resources (financial, emotional).

d. Depression:
   (1) Encourage consistency of those staying with child.
      (a) Limit visitors.
      (b) Provide scheduled times to relieve family and allow patient to rest or relax and not feel he or she has to entertain.
   (2) Encourage routine self-care activities on part of family and child and permit them to feel productive and worthwhile.
   (3) Offer praise for efforts expended.
   (4) Slowly encourage patient to expand activities of daily living (school, play, etc.).
   (5) Watch out for an abundance of relatives and other visitors, who can be taxing to child and family.

e. Acceptance:
   (1) Continue to provide consistent information to the parents and child, not giving them any opportunity to mistrust.
   (2) Ask the family to help other parents, as this can help keep the family at a level of acceptance and coping with their own child's disease.
   (3) Continue with positive reinforcement and realistic hope.

14. Support the staff.
   a. Provide staff members with opportunities for ventilation.
   b. Provide opportunities for rotation to other areas (e.g., outpatient clinic).
   c. Establish routine patient care planning sessions.

15. Utilize appropriate agencies for information and support (see Table 18-4).

EVALUATION

Outcome Criteria

1. Activity does not exceed tolerance.
2. Avoidable complications of transfusion do not occur; others are promptly detected and treated.
3. Bleeding is minimized.
4. Infections are minimized.
5. Medication regimen is followed; side effects are promptly detected and managed.
6. Signs and symptoms of leukemic invasion of body tissues are recognized and treated.
7. Renal function is maintained.
8. Side effects of therapy are minimized and effectively treated.

9. Family is well informed about the course and prognosis of the disease and copes adequately.
10. Child's adjustment and development are adequate.

HISTIOCYTOSIS

DESCRIPTION

Histiocytosis is a disease category that includes several overlapping syndromes. *Eosinophilic granuloma* (EG) is the mildest disorder and consists of lytic lesions of the bones of the skull. Frequently there are tender, sometimes elevated areas over the radiologically well-circumscribed lesions. EG can progress to more severe syndromes or may resolve, with or without treatment. There is no involvement of skin, viscera, or other soft tissues.

Hand-Schüller-Christian syndrome (HSC) is an eosinophilic granulomatous lesion of the skeleton, viscera, or skin, and carries an optimistic prognosis with treatment. *Letterer-Siwe* disease (LS) is a malignant form of eosinophilic granulomatous disease seen primarily in infants and involving skin, bones, and organs. The outset of LS is marked by systemic symptoms of fever, weight loss, and malaise with apparent skin and/or skeletal lesions. Radiologically, the skeletal lesions of HSC and LS have sharp, nonreactive borders. The liver, spleen, and lymph nodes may or may not show evidence of disease in LS and HSC. Exophthalmos, diabetes insipidus, pulmonary infiltrates, and retarded growth and development can be observed with the more extensive involvement of eosinophilic granulomatous diseases.

Diagnosis is confirmed by surgical excision and histological evaluation of the suspicious area. Eosinophilic granuloma is treated by curettage and/or radiation therapy. For HSC and LS, cytotoxic drugs (steroids, vinblastine, nitrogen mustard, cyclophosphamide, methotrexate, 6-mercaptopurine, chlorambucil) have been used, as well as curettage and radiation. Younger children have the poorest prognosis. Disseminated disease at diagnosis also has a poor prognostic index. In all cases, response to therapy is slow.

PREVENTION

Health Promotion

No preventive measures are known.

Population at Risk

Anyone, but the peak incidence occurs during the neonatal period and the period from age 6 months to 3 years. Male: female ratio is 2:1.

Screening

None.

ASSESSMENT

Health History

1. Recent fever, weight loss, and malaise (HSC, LS) are common.
2. Polyuria, polydipsia (usually LS, although can be HSC as well).
3. Bony lesions (EG, HSC, LS) are usually present.
4. A purpuric or seborrheic skin rash is the most common hallmark of the three forms of histiocytosis.

Physical Assessment

1. Growth retardation, in both height and weight.
2. Skin: presence of maculopapular granulomatous lesions on skin, scalp; pallor.
3. Eyes: exophthalmos (LS, sometimes HSC).
4. Abdomen: increase in liver and spleen size (LS, sometimes HSC).
5. Lymph nodes: presence of palpable, tender, immobile nodes (LS, HSC).
6. Skeletal: bony lesions or nodules (EG, HSC, LS) that may be asymptomatic or may cause local swelling and pain.

Diagnostic Tests

1. Bone marrow aspirate or biopsy. In LS, the marrow is often involved, which results in suppression of normal marrow elements. There are malignant histiocytes in the bone marrow with advanced disease.
2. Blood counts: In LS, there may be anemia, neutropenia, and thrombocytopenia.
3. Biopsy of the skin rash or lesion is diagnostic of histiocytosis. The degree of histiocytosis or category (EG, HSC or LS) is determined by the degree to which other organ systems are involved.

NURSING DIAGNOSES: ACTUAL OR POTENTIAL

1. Knowledge deficit about the disease, its progression, and home management of child's care.
2. Risk for toxicities from therapy (HSC, LS) (e.g., from steroids, myelosuppressive agents).
3. Risk for diabetes insipidus secondary to progressive disease.

EXPECTED OUTCOMES

1. Parents (and child if old enough) will be well informed about the condition, its treatment, and the care and observations the child requires.
2. Diabetes insipidus, if it develops, will be promptly recognized.

INTERVENTIONS

1. Inform client and parents about the specifics of the diagnosed condition (e.g., EG is a mild form of histiocytosis). Include treatment in discussion.
2. If drug therapy is used, teach about side effects. Generally, side effects can include myelosuppression, increased susceptibility to infections, and mild nausea (see *Leukemia*).
3. If radiation therapy is used, teach about side effects.
   a. Temporary loss of hair in radiation field.
   b. Temporarily decreased skin integrity in field of radiation; skin may be more sensitive to sun and other irritants.
   c. If cranial radiation is used, child may have some temporary nausea or vertigo.
   d. Long-range effects can include hypofunction of gland or organ in radiation field, such as loss of salivary gland function when radiating mandibular area.
4. Evaluate urine regularly for specific gravity (to rule out diabetes insipidus); most common in HSC. Obtain a careful history regarding fluid intake and output at regular intervals (to rule out diabetes insipidus). Monitor height and weight.

EVALUATION

Outcome Criteria

1. Evidence of progressive disease or complications is detected promptly.
2. Family verbalizes an understanding of the disease and its treatment; child receives observation and care as instructed; family copes well.

INFLAMMATIONS

HENOCH-SCHÖNLEIN PURPURA (ANAPHYLACTOID PURPURA)

DESCRIPTION

Henoch-Schönlein purpura (HSP) is a syndrome characterized by systemic vasculitis, often precipitated by a recent illness. The basic cause is unknown.

The vasculitis is most apparent on legs, buttocks, and perineal areas; the thorax is clear from obvious lesions. The lesions are urticarial at onset, later developing into hemorrhagic areas. Scattered petechiae may be present. The kidney may have lesions similar to those apparent in the skin, causing hematuria, hypertension, and, sometimes, chronic renal disease. There may be associated edema of the head and neck. Painful joints are common, with the pain arising from periarticular swelling. If the gastrointestinal system is affected, abdominal colic may be present with gastrointestinal bleeding. Often steroid therapy is used to increase the integrity of the endothelium and to minimize the pain associated with swollen joints and the abdominal symptoms.

PREVENTION

Health Promotion

No preventive measures are known.

Population at Risk

Everyone; male:female ratio is 2:1. Renal complications are most common in children over 6 years of age.

Screening

None.

ASSESSMENT

Health History

History of recent infection, febrile episode.

Physical Assessment

1. Skin: diffuse, red, raised, nonblanching rash over lower torso and legs is a hallmark of the syndrome.
2. Head and neck: possibly some edema.
3. Extremities: some observable, palpable swelling.
4. Gastrointestinal: hematemesis, occult blood in stools.
5. Genitourinary: hematuria.
6. Blood pressure: may be elevated, particularly if associated with renal manifestations.
7. Temperature may be elevated.

Diagnostic Tests

1. Platelet count is normal.
2. Urinalysis reveals hematuria, gross and microscopic, secondary to tubular damage. In chronic renal failure, there is loss of albumin and protein in the urine.
3. Antinuclear antibody (ANA): may be elevated in situations of chronic renal failure, where the disorder has become more of an autoimmune phenomenon.

NURSING DIAGNOSES: ACTUAL OR POTENTIAL

1. Altered urinary output: reduced output, hematuria, and proteinuria secondary to vascular changes in the kidney.
2. Altered gastrointestinal function: severe colicky pain, hematemesis, and blood in the stool secondary to vascular changes in the gastrointestinal tract.
3. Alteration in comfort: abdominal pain related to gastrointestinal changes, and joint pain secondary to ischemia from edema.
4. Knowledge deficit: family and client need information about the disease and treatment.

EXPECTED OUTCOMES

1. Urine will become free of blood and protein; urinary output will remain adequate (with maintenance intake of 1500–1800 ml/M^2/day, output will be 400–1000 ml/M^2/day).
2. Hematemesis, abdominal pain, and blood in stool will resolve.
3. Pain will resolve.
4. Client will resume activities of daily living.
5. Client and family will be adequately informed about disease and treatment.

INTERVENTIONS

1. Record intake and output, noting any changes in urinary patterns: report diminished output or diuresis.
2. Observe for hemoglobinuria, hematuria, proteinuria; report any changes.
3. Evaluate stool daily for occult blood.
4. Record consistency, color, and frequency of stools.
5. NPO for hematemesis.
6. Suggest diet modifications if there is blood in the stool. Consult dietitian for low-residue diet.
7. Administer steroids, as ordered, to minimize symptoms of HSP and associated pain.
8. Have alternate pain medications available.
9. Monitor and report complaints of abdominal pain, since infection and intussusception are possible.
10. Encourage activity as tolerated.
11. Teach client and family about course of disease and precautions.
12. Counsel regarding side effects of steroids (see *Aplastic Anemia*).

EVALUATION

Outcome Criteria

1. Aberrations in renal or gastrointestinal function are prevented or detected promptly and treated.
2. Pain is controlled.
3. Family and patient verbalize an understanding of disease and its treatment.

Complications

Chronic renal failure (see Chapter 21).

METABOLIC DISORDERS

STORAGE DISEASES (NIEMANN-PICK DISEASE AND GAUCHER'S DISEASE)

DESCRIPTION

Niemann-Pick and Gaucher's diseases are two examples of conditions in which lipid materials are abnormally stored in various systems. The initial sites of the deposition are generally in the reticuloendothelial system. Although both diseases have various presenting signs and symptoms, Niemann-Pick disease has a psychomotor component, including mental retardation, indicative of storage deposits in the central nervous system, hepatosplenomegaly, and a decreased life span. The earlier the disease manifests itself, the earlier death may occur.

A liver biopsy is performed to confirm the diagnosis and presence of storage cells in the liver. The primary means of differentiating the two diseases is biochemical. The treatment is generally palliative and may include antibiotics and transfusions.

PREVENTION

Health Promotion

Genetic counseling may prevent birth of future siblings with the autosomal recessive trait; however, there is no prevention for Niemann-Pick or Gaucher's disease in firstborn children.

Population at Risk

Predominantly Jews, especially those with a family history of these recessively inherited disorders.

Screening

None.

ASSESSMENT

Health History

1. Presence of similar symptoms in immediate family or extended family.
2. Growth and developmental history: retardation of gross motor, fine motor, language, and psychosocial skills.

Physical Assessment

1. Skin: brown pigmentation.
2. Abdomen: hepatosplenomegaly.
3. Lymph nodes: palpable, nonmobile, sometimes tender.
4. Neurological evaluation: loss of gross motor function, fine motor control, and speech and social interaction skills; hyporeflexia; mental retardation.

Diagnostic Tests

Biopsy of the marrow and/or liver reveals the presence of Niemann-Pick or Gaucher's cells.

NURSING DIAGNOSES: ACTUAL OR POTENTIAL

1. Altered development: developmental delay secondary to neurological damage caused by nervous system storage of abnormal constituents.
2. Risk for reduced activity tolerance, infection, and bleeding secondary to pancytopenia.
3. Parental knowledge deficit regarding the storage disease, side effects, and treatment.
4. Altered family function due to potentially fatal familial disease.

EXPECTED OUTCOMES

1. Child will receive developmentally appropriate care.
2. Infection, bleeding, and side effects of treatment will be minimal and promptly detected and treated.
3. Family members will receive genetic counseling.
4. The family will cope and function adequately.

INTERVENTIONS

1. Encourage tasks achievable and appropriate for development of child, as assessed by Denver Developmental Screening Test (DDST) or Washington Guide.
2. Discuss methods of stimulating child with parents and other care providers.
3. Be prepared to use supportive measures, such as gavage feeding (see Chapter 15 for care of neurologically impaired children).
4. Monitor hematologic status: see *Aplastic Anemia*.
5. Assist family members to receive and understand genetic counseling.
6. Identify and (with parents' agreement) include important support persons in discussions of care (visiting nurse, member of extended family, nursery school teacher).
7. Observe for guilt feelings on the part of parents, and encourage openness in communication among care-givers.
8. Reinforce decisions that incorporate appropriate developmental and mental health needs for parents.

EVALUATION

Outcome Criteria

1. Child receives care appropriate to developmental level (stimulation, protection, and so on).

2. Avoidable complications of neurological disease (e.g., injuries or aspiration during convulsion) do not occur.
3. Avoidable complications of hematologic disorders (e.g., anemia) and treatment (drugs, transfusions, etc.) do not occur. See *Aplastic Anemia*.
4. Parents are well informed about the disease course and therapy.
5. Family members avail themselves of genetic counseling.
6. Family receives the psychosocial supportive services needed to maximize individual coping and family function.

BIBLIOGRAPHY

Beck, W. S. (ed.): *Hematology*, 3d ed., Massachusetts Institute of Technology Press, Cambridge, MA., 1981. This collection of lectures provides an abbreviated explanation and review of blood disorders. Although not as comprehensive as some other texts, it provides a quick reference.

DeAngelis, C., Guthneck, M., Straub, N., and Smith, J.: "Introduction of New Foods into the Newborn and Infant Diet," *Issues in Comprehensive Pediatric Nursing*, **1**:23, April, 1977. This article presents valuable suggestions and guidelines for infant diets with adequate vitamins, minerals, and calories.

Fudenberg, H. H., Stites, D. P., Caldwell, J. L., and Wells, J. V.: *Basic and Clinical Immunology*, 3d ed., Lange Medical Publications, Los Altos, CA, 1980. This book explains basic immunology. It contains concise information about pathophysiology, diagnostic tests, and treatment. Specific immunological phenomena are presented as they pertain to various diseases and body systems.

Greene, T. (ed.): "Cancer in Children," *Nursing Clinics of North America*, **2**(1):1, 1976. These nine papers, written by practicing nurse-specialists in leading cancer treatment centers, address the following issues: therapy for acute leukemia, care of the child on immunosuppressive therapy, outpatient care, bone marrow transplantation, immunotherapy, psychosocial reactions, care of the dying child, and care by parents.

Honig, G. R.: "Sickling Syndromes in Children," *Advances in Pediatrics*, **23**:271, 1976. This excellent article should be required reading for those participating in the care of children with sickling syndromes. Differences are clarified among sickle cell disease, sickle trait, and sickle thalassemia. A lengthy bibliography is included.

Nathan, D. G., and Oski, F. A.: *Hematology of Infancy and Childhood*. Saunders, Philadelphia, 1974. This fine book is both comprehensive and easy to understand. It describes hematological pathophysiology and treatment from infancy through adolescence.

Pearson, H. A., and Robinson, J. E.: "The Role of Iron in Host Resistance," *Advances in Pediatrics*, **23**:1, 1976. Few discussions of iron therapy are this understandable. The authors encourage an analytical evaluation of the use of iron as opposed to flagrant use of iron for anemias and infections.

Rudolph, A. M., et al. (eds.): *Pediatrics*, 17th ed., Appleton-Century-Crofts, New York, 1982. This is the current edition of the earlier text edited by Barnett. It is one of the most comprehensive pediatric texts, and it presents recent statistical data.

Sutow, W. W., Vietti, T. J., and Fernback, D. H.: *Clinical Pediatric Oncology*, Mosby, St. Louis, 1978. This comprehensive text includes discussions of the principles and implications of childhood cancer and its treatment. Illustrations and diagrams are used extensively.

Whaley, L. F., and Wong, D. L.: *Nursing Care of Infants and Children*, Mosby, St. Louis, 1979. An exceptional text containing the basics of pathophysiology with an emphasis on nursing intervention. It contains a solid framework on growth and development. Good indexes and cross references are included.

Wintrobe, M. M., et al.: *Clinical Hematology*, 8th ed., Lea & Febiger, Philadelphia, 1981. A very complete reference, particularly as it pertains to pediatric chapters. Perhaps somewhat more complex than other books listed here.

19

The Cardiovascular System

Mary Fran Hazinski

HYPERACTIVITY AND HYPOACTIVITY

CONGESTIVE HEART FAILURE

DESCRIPTION

Congestive heart failure (CHF) is a term used to describe a set of clinical findings that develop when cardiac output is insufficient to meet the metabolic demands of the body. Congenital heart defects (intracardiac or great vessel structural abnormalities present from birth) are the most common cause of congestive heart failure in children. Surgical repair of these defects often requires myocardial resection, septal reconstruction, or valvular alterations. Even if congestive heart failure is not present preoperatively, changes in blood flow patterns can produce postoperative heart failure. Other causes of CHF in children include arrhythmias, inflammatory diseases of the heart or pericardium, metabolic disorders, and respiratory disease. Arrhythmias can decrease ventricular filling time (e.g., paroxysmal atrial tachycardia) or alter the sequence of cardiac contraction (e.g., congenital heart block). Inflammatory diseases, such as rheumatic, viral, or bacterial carditis can interfere with myocardial or valvular function. Metabolic disease, such as anemia, can be accompanied by an increase in cardiac output; electrolyte imbalance alters myocardial cellular environment and may decrease excitability or contractility of the myocardium. (Please refer to Chapter 30.) Prolonged alveolar hypoxia (e.g., respiratory distress syndrome or cystic fibrosis) can produce severe pulmonary hypertension (high pulmonary vascular resistance with arterial wall thickening) and ultimately result in right ventricular failure (cor pulmonale, see p. 985).

1. Pathophysiology of heart failure: metabolic aspects.
   a. Cardiac output is decreased, and cardiac contraction is less efficient.
   b. Sympathetic nervous system compensatory mechanisms are activated, producing (1) increased heart rate and improved cardiac contractility and (2) increased vasomotor tone (and resultant increased venous return to the heart and peripheral vasoconstriction).
   c. Renal compensatory mechanisms are activated by renal vasoconstriction, and result in increased blood volume.
      (1) Decreased renal perfusion stimulates renin release.
      (2) Sodium and water retention occur as a result of aldosterone secretion.
      (3) Water retention may also be produced by antidiuretic hormone release.
2. Pathophysiology of heart failure: hemodynamic mechanisms.
   a. Sympathetic nervous system response normally produces an immediate increase in heart rate and contractility.
   b. Ventricular diastolic and filling pressures increase, and ventricular hypertrophy

may occur. If cardiac output continues to fall, the heart dilates.

c. Increased circulating blood volume and increased ventricular filling pressures cause venous engorgement.
   (1) Hepatomegaly and, later, peripheral edema result from systemic venous engorgement.
   (2) With pulmonary venous engorgement, the lungs become less compliant, so tachypnea, decreased tidal volume (more shallow respirations), and increased respiratory effort result as respiratory compensatory mechanisms are stimulated.

3. Either ventricle can fail, but in children symptoms of combined ventricular failure usually coexist, so both systemic venous engorgement and pulmonary venous engorgement are present.

PREVENTION

Health Promotion

1. Regular physical examinations should allow early detection of congenital heart defects.
2. Patients at risk for development of CHF should not receive large volumes of fluid over short periods of time and should be monitored closely for earliest signs of cardiac compromise; prompt, early treatment may prevent later decompensation.

Population at Risk

1. Children with congenital heart defects producing increased pulmonary blood flow under high pressures (e.g., large ventricular septal defect) or severe left heart or aortic obstruction (e.g., critical aortic stenosis).
2. Premature neonates, particularly those with birth weights under 1,200 g, have a high incidence of patent ductus arteriosus, which can cause CHF, particularly if high volumes of fluid are administered.
3. Children who have surgical repair of congenital heart defects (particularly muscular ventricular septal defect, endocardial cushion defect, tetralogy of Fallot, truncus arteriosus, or transposition of the great vessels).
4. Children with supraventricular tachycardia (paroxysmal atrial tachycardia, or Wolff-Parkinson-White syndrome), heart block with slow ventricular rate, or ventricular irritability.
5. Children receiving anthracycline agents to treat childhood cancer (particularly adriamycin or daunomycin in high doses).
6. Children with severe anemia (hemoglobin less than 6 g).
7. Children with severe respiratory disease or pulmonary hypertension.

Screening

Physical exam reveals evidence of pulmonary and systemic venous engorgement.

ASSESSMENT

Health History

1. History of events preceding onset of symptoms usually provides valuable information that can help isolate the cause of the CHF.
2. Disposition change: child may take longer naps or be more lethargic or more irritable.
3. Change in feeding behavior: infants usually do not tolerate oral feedings due to tachypnea and air swallowing; increased duration and/or decreased volume of feedings may be reported by mother.
   a. Poor weight gain may be noted due to poor feeding.
   b. Sudden weight gain in older child, despite anorexia, may be due to systemic edema.
4. Respiratory infections may have a prolonged course in children with heart disease. A history of wheezing may be noted in infants.
5. Difficulty breathing, rapid respiratory rate, or early exercise fatigue often is noted by parents (child "can't keep up" with peers).
6. Parents may note that child's chest has appeared "jumpy"—this can indicate evidence of an active precordium (due to tachycardia and more forceful ventricular filling or ejection or turbulent intracardiac blood flow due to a shunt or valvular obstruction).
7. Previous illnesses.
   a. Group A beta-hemolytic strep throat precedes the development of rheumatic fever (and its associated carditis).
   b. Cancer chemotherapy with a known cardiotoxic agent can precipitate cardiomyopathy and CHF.
   c. Bacterial, viral, or protozoan illness may result in cardiac infection and CHF.

Physicial Assessment

1. Four main signs of CHF observed in children are
   a. Tachycardia (see Table 19-1 for normal heart rates).
   b. Tachypnea (see Table 19-2 for normal respiratory rates).
   c. Decreased urine output.
   d. Hepatomegaly.
2. Evidence of cardiovascular sequelae or sympathetic nervous system compensatory mechanisms include
   a. Tachycardia (a gallop rhythm may also be present).
   b. Cardiomegaly: active precordium may be observed, and cardiac silhouette will be enlarged on chest x-ray film.
   c. Decreased urine output (less than 1 mL/kg/h or 25 mL/h in adolescents) or oliguria will occur *despite* adequate fluid intake.
   d. Peripheral vasoconstriction will be noted, and extremities may be cool.
   e. Diaphoresis may be noted, particularly in infants.
3. Pulmonary venous engorgement will produce respiratory symptoms.
   a. Tachypnea.
   b. There will be evidence of increased respiratory effort (retractions will be present in infants, and nasal flaring or use of accessory muscles of respiration may be observed).
   c. Infants will have feeding difficulties because it is difficult to coordinate rapid breathing with sucking and swallowing.
   d. Rales occur only as a late sign of pulmonary venous engorgement in children; they may indicate, however, the presence of concurrent respiratory infection.
4. Signs of systemic venous engorgement will also be noted.
   a. Hepatomegaly will usually be the first symptom observed in children.
   b. Periorbital edema.
   c. Jugular venous distension may exist but is usually difficult to perceive in infants.
   d. Edema of the hands and feet may be noted in infants but is not often seen in older children.
   e. Dependent (sacral) edema and ascites are only *very late* signs of chronic or severe heart failure in children.
5. With continued severe reduction of cardiac output, evidence of severe compromise of systemic perfusion will be apparent. These indicate critical decompensation.
   a. Altered level of consciousness (child may be "fussy" or lethargic).
   b. Weak, thready pulses.
   c. Metabolic acidosis (the result of inadequate tissue oxygenation and shock).
   d. Anuria.

TABLE 19-1 NORMAL HEART RATE RANGES FOR CHILDREN

Age	Range (Beats/ Minute)
Infant	120–160
Toddler	90–140
Preschooler	80–110
School-age child	75–100
Adolescent	60–90

NOTE: Always consider the child's own normal range, and note that heart rate will increase in the presence of fever or stress and decrease during sleep and vagal stimulation.

TABLE 19-2 NORMAL RESPIRATORY RATES IN CHILDREN

Age	Rate (Breaths/ Minute)
Infant	30–60
Toddler	24–40
Preschooler	22–34
School-age child	18–30
Adolescent	12–20

NOTE: Always consider the child's own normal range, and note that respiratory rate will increase in the presence of fever or stress.

Diagnostic Tests

Chest x-ray film, electrocardiogram, echocardiogram, and cardiac catheterization can provide more information to determine cardiac pathology responsible for heart failure.

NURSING DIAGNOSES: ACTUAL OR POTENTIAL

1. Circulatory impairment related to decreased cardiac output.
2. Respiratory dysfunction secondary to pulmonary venous engorgement and perhaps also concurrent respiratory infection.
3. Fluid volume excess secondary to decreased urinary output and continued fluid intake.
4. Nutritional deficit: reduction in caloric intake secondary to dyspnea, anorexia, and, perhaps, increase in metabolic requirements.
5. Anxiety and malaise related to circulatory and respiratory insufficiency, hospitalization, and separation from parents.
6. Parental anxiety, knowledge deficit, anger, or frustration related to child's illness, prognosis, and hospitalization.
7. Parental knowledge deficit regarding home care for child following discharge from hospital.

EXPECTED OUTCOMES

1. Child's heart rate will return to within 10 percent of normal range within 2 days of treatment (see Table 19-1 for norms).
2. Blood pressure will remain in normal range for age (see Table 19-3) throughout hospitalization.
3. Peripheral pulses will be strong and equal within 1 day of treatment, and hepatomegaly will decrease within 5 days.
4. Urine output will be 1–2 mL/kg/h (average) for infants and small children, and 25–30 mL/kg/h (average) for adolescents.
5. Child will demonstrate normal respiratory rate for age (see Table 19-2), with minimal use of accessory muscles, and clear breath sounds to auscultation within 2–5 days of treatment.
6. Child will consume maintenance calories (Table 19-4) and demonstrate adequate subcutaneous tissue and skin integrity.
7. Child and parent(s) will demonstrate (and receive) appropriate communication with health care team and will be able to relate (with 85 percent accuracy) the plan for the child's care following discharge.

INTERVENTIONS

1. Monitor carefully for signs of decreased cardiac output and severe compromise of systemic perfusion. If signs of severe deterioration in child's condition occur, notify physician immediately.
2. Administer digitalis derivative, if prescribed.
   a. Check dosage appropriate for child's age and weight (Table 19-5).
   b. Monitor cardiovascular response to digitalis (heart rate should slow, PR interval should be slightly prolonged, and cardiac output should increase).
      (1) Arrhythmias are usually the first sign of digitalis toxicity in children (vomiting occurs only as a late sign, or in older children). Almost every arrhythmia possible has been linked to digitalis toxicity, so report any arrhythmias to the physician and be prepared to withhold the next dose or send blood sample for drug level if ordered.
      (2) Confer with physician if heart rate

TABLE 19-3 NORMAL PEDIATRIC BLOOD PRESSURE RANGES[a]

Age	Systolic (mm Hg)	Diastolic (mm Hg)
Newborn (age 12 h) (<1,000 g)	39–59	16–36
Newborn (age 12 h) (3 kg)	50–70	25–45
Newborn (age 96 h)	60–90	20–60
Infant	74–100	50–70
Toddler	80–112	50–80
Preschooler	82–110	50–78
School-age child	84–120	54–80
Adolescent	94–140	62–88

[a] Ranges represent the 10th and 90th percentiles determined by the following studies.
1. National Heart, Lung, and Blood Institute's Task Force on Blood Pressure Control in Children, 1978.
2. De Swiet, M., Fayers, P., and Shinebourne, E. A.: "Systolic Blood Pressure in a Population of Infants in the First Year of Life: The Brompton Study," *Pediatrics*, **65**:1028, May 1980.
3. Versmold, H., Kitterman, J. A., Phibbs, R. H., et al.: "Aortic Blood Pressure During the First 12 Hours of Life in Infants with Birth Weight 610–4220 Grams," *Pediatrics*, **67**:607, May 1981.

TABLE 19-4 CALCULATION OF CALORIC REQUIREMENTS FOR CHILDREN

Age	Daily Requirements
High-risk neonate	120–150 Calories/kg
Normal neonate	100–120 Calories/kg
1–2 Years	90–100 Calories/kg
2–6 Years	80–90 Calories/kg
7–9 Years	70–80 Calories/kg
10–12 Years	50–60 Calories/kg

NOTE: Ill children (with disease, surgery, fever, or pain) may require extra calories above the maintenance value, and immobilized children may require fewer calories because of lack of exercise.

slows significantly (consider child's previous rate also).

(a) Fewer than 110 beats per minute (bpm) in infants.
(b) Fewer than 90 bpm in toddlers.
(c) Fewer than 80 bpm in school-age children.
(d) Fewer than 60 bpm in adolescents.

TABLE 19-5 TOTAL ORAL DIGITALIZING DOSES FOR CHILDREN (DIGOXIN)

Child's Age	Dosage of Digoxin[a]
Neonate	0.044–0.066 mg/kg (0.02–0.03 mg/lb)
2 weeks to 2 years	0.066–0.088 mg/kg (0.03–0.04 mg/lb)
2–10 years	0.044–0.066 mg/kg (0.02–0.03 mg/lb)
10 years to adult	0.5–1.0 mg (average)

[a] Intravenous dosage should be two-thirds of given dosages.

NOTE: Above dosages should be given in divided doses approximately as follows (may be slight variation in various institutions): For digitalization: $\frac{1}{2}$ of digitalizing dose given intially; $\frac{1}{4}$ of digitalizing dose given 6–8 h later; last $\frac{1}{4}$ of digitalizing dose given after 6–8 h more. For maintenance: $\frac{1}{8}$ of digitalizing dose given 12 h later and every 12 h thereafter.

c. Teach adolescent, or younger child's primary caretaker, to administer digitalis and provide teaching to ensure detection of digitalis toxicity.
   (1) If caretakers are sensitive and observant, request that they notify physician if child becomes ill or fatigues more easily.
   (2) Some health care facilities require that caretakers be taught to take patient's pulse before administration of digitalis. Focusing on firm range of heart rate must be avoided, however (tell caretaker to allow for rate increase with exercise or decrease during sleep).

3. Monitor electrolyte values (if child is hospitalized), as low serum potassium can make patient more susceptible to digitalis toxicity (ingestion of a glass of orange juice or a banana in the morning should prevent hypokalemia).
4. If child is in moderate distress, attempt to decrease any physical and emotional stress that may increase cardiovascular requirements.
   a. Ensure adequate rest periods without examinations and procedures for child.
   b. Prevent rapid or frequent fluctuations in body or environmental temperature (especially in neonatal period, when thermoregulatory mechanisms are immature).
   c. Ensure adequate nutritional intake.
   d. Provide soothing, sensitive nursing care to reduce child's anxiety.
5. Assess carefully for signs of increased respiratory distress. If severe respiratory distress is present, maintenance of adequate ventilation becomes the priority.
6. Provide adequate pulmonary toilet to a degree appropriate to child's distress.
   a. If oxygen therapy is required to maintain acceptable arterial oxygen tension, monitor inspired oxygen levels carefully (to prevent oxygen toxicity), and monitor child's response to therapy. Note child's tolerance of brief periods away from oxygen.
   b. If oxygen therapy is required, or if there is pulmonary congestion, humidification of inspired air (using hood, high-humidity tent, or home vaporizer) is usually or-

dered; monitor response to and tolerance of humidity.

c. If concurrent respiratory infection is present, provide chest physiotherapy (postural drainage, percussion, vibration, or suctioning) to facilitate removal of respiratory secretions. Enlist child's participation.
   (1) Encourage child to cough vigorously and to take deep breaths.
   (2) *Slight* pressure on the trachea, just above sternum, will usually stimulate cough (if absolutely necessary).
   (3) Ask child to blow inverted paper cup across counter top, blow soap bubbles, or to pretend to blow out birthday candles to provide deep-breathing exercise.

7. Attempt to minimize oxygen requirements. If severe distress is present place child in a comfortable position with head and chest elevated.
8. Monitor child's fluid balance (see Table 19-6).
   a. If there is associated respiratory distress, oral fluid intake may be minimal as appetite or ability to suckle probably is decreased.
   b. If supplemental intravenous therapy is ordered, verify the amount ordered. It should not exceed the patient's daily fluid requirements, and it should be reduced in the presence of decreased urine output

TABLE 19-6 CALCULATION OF DAILY MAINTENANCE FLUIDS IN CHILDREN

Child's Weight	Kilogram Body Weight Formula
Newborn (0–72 h old)	60–100 mL/kg
0–10 kg	100 mL/kg (may increase up to 150 mL if renal and cardiac function adequate)
11–20 kg	1000 mL for the first 10 kg + 50 mL/kg for each kg over 10 kg
21–30 kg	1500 mL for the first 20 kg + 25 mL/kg for each kg over 20 kg

TABLE 19-7 DIURETIC DOSAGES FOR CHILDREN

Drug[a]	Dosage
Furosemide (Lasix)	1–2 mg/kg/IV dose (may be increased if given in oral form)
Chlorothiazide (Diuril)	20–40 mg/kg/day, in one or two doses
Hydrochlorothiazide + spironolactone (Aldactazide)	1.65–3.3 mg/kg/day, in one or two doses

[a] Trade name in parentheses.

and heart failure or if the child begins to resume adequate oral intake.

   c. Daily weights and records of 24-hour intake and output may be necessary to determine fluid balance during hospitalization (rarely needed when child is at home).
   d. Infant's diapers should be weighed before and after infant wears them if accurate measurement of urine output is required (only in hospital): 1 mL weighs 1 g.
   e. Diuretics may be necessary to promote diuresis.
      (1) Ensure appropriate dosage for age and weight (Table 19-7).
      (2) Teach adolescent, or younger child's primary caretaker, how to administer dosage and note renal response.
      (3) If client is receiving concurrent digitalis and diuretic therapy, ensure adequate electrolyte (potassium) replacement, if necessary.
      (4) Monitor for diuretic response; notify physician if there is inadequate urine response following diuretic administration.
   f. A low-sodium diet may be prescribed by physician in order to decrease probability of fluid retention.
      (1) Child and primary caretaker should be taught which salty foods to avoid.
      (2) Attempt to provide palatable, yet appropriate diet; since most "fad" foods (potato chips, pizza, some soft drinks)

are not compatible with a low-sodium diet, school-age child or adolescent may be expected to "test" diet (and break it).

(3) It is *nearly always* physically and emotionally healthier if health team manipulates diuretic dosage and allows child to eat regular diet. (It is usually impractical and unsafe to rely on child's strict adherence to diet.)

g. If fluid restriction is required, discuss this with client and primary caretaker and attempt to formulate the most reasonable distribution of fluids throughout the day.

h. Provide thorough mouth care, particularly if fluids are restricted. Hard candy may provide effective route for caloric intake while relieving dryness of mouth (lemon and glycerine swabs only increase dryness).

i. Provide thorough skin care (keep skin dry, and improve circulation with massage); children usually turn often without being told or assisted.

j. Maintain adequate nutritional intake.

(1) Calculate the daily fluid and nutritional requirements and divide into individual feedings (Tables 19-4 and 19-6).

(2) Small, frequent feedings are usually better tolerated by children with cardiorespiratory distress.

(3) If infant is unable to suck strongly enough to obtain adequate nutrition through the nipple, supplementation of oral intake with gavage or nasojejunal feedings or parenteral nutrition may be required temporarily. Continue to reinforce infant's sucking reflex, however.

(4) Assess weight gain, skin turgor, and hair and fingernail texture to ensure adequate nutritional intake.

9. Provide psychological support for child and parents (for specific interventions, see the section of Chapter 4 that pertains to hospitalized children, pp. 63–71).

10. Teach parents how to assess child's condition at home.

a. Primary caretaker should be aware that child with CHF may have more difficulty getting rid of respiratory infections.

b. Child and family should be urged to seek medical care whenever child demonstrates evidence of respiratory congestion.

c. Cyanotic child should not be allowed to become dehydrated, since fluid deficit can cause hemoconcentration and further increase the child's hematocrit and risk of spontaneous thromboembolus. Parents should be taught to contact the child's physician if child develops gastroenteritis or diminished fluid intake.

11. Teach child and parents about appropriate level of activity for child.

a. In the majority of cardiac conditions, few, if any, restrictions must be placed on activity (child will usually tire long before there is stress on cardiac function).

b. If acute rheumatic carditis is the cause of congestive failure or heart disease, child's activity may be curtailed, although activity restriction is usually reserved for seriously ill children.

c. Adolescents and school-age children may frequently test restrictions on activity due to peer pressure; when children have CHF, they usually tire and limit their own activity before any serious compromise of cardiac function occurs.

EVALUATION

Outcome Criteria

1. Heart rate is decreased or within normal range for child's age.
2. Perfusion is improved with good peripheral pulses.
3. Signs of systemic and pulmonary venous engorgement are reduced or absent.
4. Tachypnea is decreased, or respiratory rate is normal for child's age.
5. Respiratory effort is reduced, and retractions and other use of accessory muscles are minimal.
6. Breath sounds are clear, with no evidence of concurrent respiratory infection.
7. Fluid intake and output are appropriate for age and weight of child.
8. Weight is between the tenth and 90th percentiles for child's age.
9. Skin is warm and dry with no evidence of breakdown.
10. Child and parents are able to discuss child's condition and care plan accurately.
11. Parents (and child if old enough) describe child's medication dosage schedule accurately.

12. Child and family are returning to physician for follow-up visits on schedule.
13. Child is demonstrating appropriate motor and verbal skills for age.
14. Parents relate their ability to manage associated stress and decisions regarding child's health care coherently and appropriately.

Complications

1. Worsening CHF progressing to low cardiac output (shock).
2. Pneumonia (see Chapter 20 for care of child with pneumonia).
3. Increased respiratory dysfunction progressing to respiratory failure.

Assessment

1. With respiratory fatigue child will begin to demonstrate gasping or grunting with slow, labored breathing.
2. Level of consciousness will be affected (child will be more agitated with a high-pitched or breathless cry, then will progress to a more lethargic state with no energy to cry).
3. Child will begin to demonstrate carbon dioxide retention, and, later, respiratory and/or metabolic acidosis will be evident by blood gas measurements.

Revised Outcomes

1. Respiratory exchange will be adequate: ventilation will be conducted mechanically until child is able to resume effective independent ventilation.
2. Child will not demonstrate complications of mechanical ventilation (tracheal stenosis or edema from intubation, respiratory infection, etc.).

ABNORMAL CELLULAR GROWTH: CARE OF THE CHILD REQUIRING CARDIOVASCULAR SURGERY

CLOSED-HEART SURGERY

DESCRIPTION

Closed-heart surgery involves surgery performed on the heart or great vessels *without* use of cardiopulmonary bypass. Such surgery usually involves a thoracotomy incision but may also be performed through a median sternotomy incision. Shunts (abnormal blood flow pathways) may be created (e.g., creation of a Blalock-Taussig shunt to increase pulmonary blood flow for a child with pulmonary atresia) or eliminated (e.g., division of patent ductus arteriosus) during closed-heart surgery. Surgery may be confined to the great vessels (e.g., repair of coarctation of the aorta), or the heart may actually be entered (as in the Blalock-Hanlon septectomy, when an atrial septal defect is created). The common denominator of these procedures, however, is that cardiopulmonary bypass is not necessary. Operative complications include those of a thoracotomy procedure, in addition to specific complications related to location and complexity of the specific surgery performed. A chest tube is often inserted at the end of the procedure.

PREOPERATIVE ASSESSMENT

Please refer to later sections relating to specific heart defects.

POSTOPERATIVE ASSESSMENT

1. Monitor for evidence of CHF (see *Congestive Heart Failure*, p. 459).
2. Monitor heart rate and rhythm for evidence of irregularity that can result in compromise of cardiac output.
   a. If child is on cardiac monitor, watch for arrhythmias.
   b. Monitor electrolyte values, especially potassium and calcium, since imbalance may precipitate arrhythmias.
3. Monitor for evidence of cardiovascular compromise due to hemorrhage (tachycardia, peripheral vasoconstriction, decreased urine output, and, ultimately, hypotension).
4. Monitor chest tube output.
   a. Bleeding more than 3 mL/kg/h for 3 or more hours results in loss of greater than 10 percent of the child's circulating blood volume; therefore, physician should be notified, and blood replacement should be ordered.
   b. Chest tube output greater than 5 mL/kg/h is significant and may require reoperation (particularly if a coagulopathy has been ruled out by appropriate tests of coagulation).

   c. Ensure appropriate function of chest tube and water seal.
   d. Assess for evidence of pneumothorax or hemothorax (decreased breath sounds, hyperresonance or dullness to percussion, increasing oxygen requirements, and increasing respiratory effort).
5. Monitor child's respiratory rate and effort for evidence of distress.
   a. Atelectasis, pneumothorax, or hemothorax can occur.
   b. Assess quality of breath sounds and chest expansion as well as rate and depth of respirations and use of accessory muscles of respiration.
6. Assess wound for evidence of infection (heat, redness, dehiscence, drainage, fever, and leukocytosis).

POSTOPERATIVE NURSING DIAGNOSES: ACTUAL OR POTENTIAL

1. Anxiety of child and parents related to surgical procedure and its risks, as well as complexity of postoperative care.
2. Risk of CHF (and consequent systemic and pulmonary venous engorgement) related to surgical cardiac manipulation and/or alteration in blood pressure and flow patterns.
3. Risk of compromise in cardiac output related to hemorrhage or arrhythmias.
4. Risk of respiratory compromise, related to hemothorax, atelectasis, decreased respiratory effort, chest wall splinting, or malfunction of chest tube (and resultant pneumothorax).
5. Alteration in comfort: pain (mild to moderate) or discomfort due to surgical incision.
6. Risk of infection related to loss of tissue integrity due to thoracotomy incision.
7. Risk of insufficient client respiratory effort and ambulatory effort due to incisional pain or discomfort.
8. Knowledge deficit related to provision of appropriate home care following discharge from hospital.

POSTOPERATIVE EXPECTED OUTCOMES

1. Child and parents will participate in child's care at level with which they appear comfortable.
2. Child and parents will interact in a mutually supportive manner.
3. Child and parents will accurately discuss child's plan of care and schedule of treatments.
4. Child and parents will demonstrate knowledge and skills needed to provide child's home health care.
5. Child's heart rate, blood pressure, and urine output will be within expected range for age (or equal to child's preoperative levels) within 1 postoperative day.
6. Child will demonstrate regular cardiac rhythm with strong peripheral pulses and no evidence of systemic or pulmonary venous engorgement from the immediate postoperative period through discharge.
7. Child will demonstrate no evidence of respiratory deterioration (depressed respiratory rate, gasping or grunting, poor lung aeration, deterioration in blood gases).
8. Child will be free of respiratory infection and atelectasis (with normal respiratory rate and clear, adequate breath sounds to auscultation) within 3–5 postoperative days.
9. Child will demonstrate no evidence of fever, wound drainage, or dehiscence within 3–5 postoperative days.
10. Child will be able to ambulate and raise both arms with minimal pain (tolerable without use of narcotic analgesics) within 3–5 postoperative days.

POSTOPERATIVE INTERVENTIONS

1. Please refer to Chapter 4 for discussion of psychosocial support and preoperative teaching of child and family (pp. 63–71).
2. If evidence of CHF is present, see interventions in *Congestive Heart Failure* (p. 462).
3. If cardiac arrhythmia is present, notify physician, and determine if irregularity is causing compromise of systemic perfusion.
   a. Administer antiarrhythmic drug as ordered (ensure proper dosage, and monitor for therapeutic, side, and toxic effects).
   b. If child has external cardiac pacer wires in place, keep a functioning external pacemaker *at bedside* and ready for use upon physician order. Keep pacer wires dry and covered to prevent electrical hazard.

c. If child has external cardiac pacer *in use*, check function of pacer (ability to "capture" and ability to "sense" child's ventricular activity) and threshold every 8 hours.
d. Determine if any precipitating factors, such as vagal stimulation or electrolyte imbalance, or alleviating factors, such as administration of potassium chloride, exist, so further arrhythmias can be prevented.
e. If child is stable, continue to monitor for arrhythmias, but avoid focusing attention on auscultation of the chest or on observation of the cardiac monitor, as this may magnify child's and family's anxiety.

4. If postoperative hemorrhage is suspected, notify physician, administer blood components as ordered, obtain chest x-ray film (as ordered) to rule out significant hemothorax, and be prepared to institute emergency measures.
5. Administer humidified oxygen or mechanical ventilation as necessary (and ordered by physician).
6. Provide pulmonary toilet.
   a. See also intervention 6 under *Congestive Heart Failure* (p. 463).
   b. Provide vigorous chest physiotherapy, and encourage child to cough and to breathe deeply.
   c. Child may breathe shallowly due to incisional pain. This may cause decreased lung aeration and make the child more susceptible to development of respiratory infection or atelectasis.
      (1) Child may cough more effectively if pain medications are administered (as ordered) before any chest physiotherapy.
      (2) Holding pillow or pressed hands against incision site (to support it) may decrease pain of coughing.
7. Keep incision clean and dry. If infection is suspected, obtain culture of incision area and blood (as ordered), and administer antibiotics as ordered.
8. Administer pain medications as ordered to relieve postoperative discomfort.
9. Provide gentle handling and soothing support to minimize child's anxiety and discomfort.
10. Provide regular schedule of rest and activities to increase the child's security and minimize disorientation.

POSTOPERATIVE EVALUATION

Outcome Criteria

1. Parents and child discuss child's plan of care and anticipated schedule of postoperative treatment with 85 percent accuracy.
2. Child and parents demonstrate supportive interaction and ability to discuss items of concern.
3. Child and parents participate in child's plan of care with requests or choices that coincide with discussed plan of care at least 60 percent of the time.
4. Child's heart rate and blood pressure are within 10 percent of normal values (Tables 19-1 and 19-3).
5. Child's urine output averages 1–2 mL/kg/h (or a minimum average of 25 mL/h for adolescents).
6. Child demonstrates no significant cardiac arrhythmia.
7. Child's lung aeration is adequate and equal bilaterally, with respiratory rate within 10 percent of normal range (Table 19-2) and lungs clear to auscultation.
8. Wound remains clean and dry, and child is afebrile.
9. Child is able to raise both arms above head without use of narcotic analgesics.
10. Child and parents demonstrate knowledge of child's home care (wound care, medications, follow-up appointments, and any diet or fluid restrictions) by the time of the child's discharge from hospital.

Complications

1. Child or parents demonstrate increasing anxiety and distortion, denial, or lack of comprehension of teaching information (see *Evaluation*, p. 71).
2. Congestive heart failure (see *Congestive Heart Failure*, p. 459).
3. Arrhythmias (see *Arrhythmias*, p. 1002).
4. Pneumonia (see *Bronchopneumonia*, p. 529).
5. Pneumothorax (see *Pneumothorax*, p. 1087).
6. Hemorrhage.

Assessment

1. Chest tube output greater than 3 mL/kg/hour of blood.
2. Falling cardiac output (measured by ther-

modilution or other method) and poor systemic perfusion.
3. Falling hematocrit (see Table 19-8).
4. Decreasing urine output (less than 1 mL/kg/h).
5. Coagulation screening profile: If normal, bleeding is probably surgical in origin, and will probably require reoperation to stop. If abnormal, bleeding may be due to coagulopathy. In this case, hemorrhage may be treated successfully with administration of appropriate blood components, vitamin K, or protamine sulfate.
6. Hypotension: *Note that this is a late sign of hemorrhage*. Once hypotension is present, treatment for bleeding must be performed on an emergency basis.

Revised Outcomes
1. Chest tube output will be less than 3 mL/kg/h and will be serosanguineous.
2. Hematocrit will be within normal levels for age (see Table 19-8).
3. Urine output will be 1–2 mL/kg/h or, for adolescents, a minimal total average of 25–30 mL/h.
4. Coagulation screening profile will be normal.
5. Child will have blood pressure not less than 5 percent below normal for age (or the same as preoperative levels for that patient).

Interventions
1. Keep chest tubes drained and free of clots. (Clots can interfere with drainage and measurement of blood.)

TABLE 19-8 NORMAL PEDIATRIC HEMATOCRIT LEVELS

Age	Hematocrit (%)
Newborn (0–72 hours)	
Premature	45–55
Full term	43–65
Infant (3–60 days)	
Premature	27–55
Full term	38–58
Infant (2–6 months)	34–42
Infant (6–18 months)	33–40
Toddler	34–40
Preschooler	36–44
School age	39–47
Adolescent	37–52

2. Notify physician as soon as hemorrhage is observed.
3. Administer blood replacement, as ordered, to prevent hypovolemia. NOTE: 10 mL/kg of packed red blood cells (RBCs) should be sufficient to raise child's hematocrit approximately 10 points.
4. Monitor for evidence of hemothorax. Obtain chest x-ray film, as ordered.
5. Be prepared to institute emergency measures as needed (if hypovolemic shock occurs).

Reevaluation and Follow-up

Child should demonstrate rapid resolution of bleeding, with no clinical sequelae (shock, loss of consciousness, pulmonary complications, etc.), with normal hematocrit within hours, and at the time of discharge from the hospital.

WOUND INFECTION

Assessment
1. Fluctuation of wound edges.
2. Wound drainage, which grows bacteria or fungus when cultured, noted on dressing.
3. Wound edges are reddened and/or warm.
4. Client demonstrates fever and/or leukocytosis.

Revised Outcomes
1. Wound drainage will cease or change to a clear, culture-negative discharge in small amounts within 3 to 5 days of therapy.
2. Wound surface will demonstrate normal granulation healing without redness or fluctuation within 10 to 14 days.
3. Client temperature and white blood cell (WBC) count will return to normal within 3 to 5 days.

Interventions
1. Change wound dressing frequently to keep surface dry.
2. Maintain wound isolation.
3. Administer antibiotics as ordered.
4. Apply topical bactericidal or antifungal ointment or solution to wound as ordered.
5. Once wound infection has been determined to be the cause of the client's fever, administer antipyretics as ordered to promote patient comfort.
6. If wound drainage is copious, client should be encouraged to recline with wound in a dependent position to facilitate wound drainage (and prevent abscess formation).

Reevaluation and Follow-up
No further evidence of infection (including bacteremia) should be found within 3 to 5 days of commencement of treatment of wound infection. Wound should heal completely with no dehiscence within 2 to 3 weeks.

OPEN-HEART SURGERY

DESCRIPTION

Open-heart surgery requires that the patient be supported by cardiopulmonary bypass while cardiac or great vessel repair is accomplished. The heart-lung machine receives venous blood, oxygenates it, removes carbon dioxide, and returns it to the systemic circulation (usually at the ascending aorta). The child is fully heparinized during bypass, and the heparin is reversed at the end of the surgical procedure.

Many congenital heart defects must be repaired or improved by some form of open-heart surgery. While the child must always be watched closely for the "standard" postoperative complications (bleeding, arrhythmias, low cardiac output, CHF, respiratory insufficiency, neurological impairment, renal failure, and infection), the most likely complications to be anticipated depend on the particular surgical procedure performed. If the surgery involves cardiac resection, or the child had significant preoperative cyanosis and polycythemia, bleeding is to be anticipated postoperatively. If surgery is performed near cardiac conduction tissue, it is necessary to watch closely for evidence of arrhythmias and heart block postoperatively. The nurse should watch also for heart failure postoperatively if extensive cardiac manipulation or reconstruction is required during surgery.

Cardiopulmonary bypass can also be used to cool infants to a blood temperature of approximately 20°C (68°F) so that surgery can be performed under complete (hypothermic) circulatory arrest. When surgery is completed, the child is again placed on cardiopulmonary bypass and rewarmed to normothermia. The infant who has open-heart surgery with deep hypothermia must be monitored closely for the "standard" postoperative cardiovascular complications but also must be watched carefully for evidence of neurological sequelae (seizures or evidence of cerebrovascular accident), bleeding, and hyper- and hypoglycemia.

A median sternotomy incision is usually used for open-heart surgery, and mediastinal tubes are placed at the end of the surgical procedure. Temporary pacing wires, arterial line, and central and/or peripheral venous lines are often in place. Some surgeons also place Swan-Ganz, left atrial, or thermistor cardiac output probes to aid in postoperative monitoring of the child.

Because of the complexity of postoperative equipment and care routines, it is especially important that the child (if old enough) and parents receive thorough preoperative instruction. Please refer to hospitalized child section of Chapter 4 for discussion of appropriate assessment, diagnoses, expected outcomes of care, interventions, and evaluations related to preoperative preparation.

POSTOPERATIVE ASSESSMENT

1. Please see postoperative assessment section of *Closed-Heart Surgery* (p. 466) for assessment of:
   a. Congestive heart failure.
   b. Arrhythmias.
   c. Hemorrhage.
   d. Chest tube output.
   e. Respiratory insufficiency.
   f. Wound infection.
2. Monitor child closely for evidence of *cardiac tamponade* (systemic venous engorgement and rising central venous pressures, with fall in cardiac output due to collection of blood in pericardium).
3. Assess child's fluid status at least every hour. (Note total of *all* intravenous fluids, including "flush" for any pressure lines, and output from all drainage tubes and urine catheter.)
4. Monitor for electrolyte imbalances, which may precipitate arrhythmias or digitalis toxicity.
5. Assess evidence of coagulation function. Observe for petechiae and ecchymoses, as well as depressed coagulation factor levels on coagulation screening panel.
6. Assess client level of consciousness, response to command, pupil size, and response to light at frequent intervals.
7. Assess urine quantity (should be at least 1–2 mL/kg/h in children and 25–30 mL/h in adolescents), color (especially for evidence of

hematuria), and specific gravity (this provides information about kidneys' ability to concentrate urine as well as about child's level of hydration).

POSTOPERATIVE NURSING DIAGNOSES: ACTUAL OR POTENTIAL

1. Anxiety of child and parents related to surgical procedure and its risks, as well as complexity of postoperative care.
2. Risk of decreased cardiac function related to surgical cardiac manipulation and/or alteration in cardiac preload, contractility, or afterload; or to tamponade or hemorrhage.
3. Risk of compromise in cardiac output related to tamponade, hemorrhage, or arrhythmias.
4. Risk of respiratory compromise related to hemothorax, atelectasis, decreased respiratory effort, chest wall "splinting," or malfunction of the chest tube (and resultant pneumothorax).
5. Alteration in comfort: pain (mild or moderate) or discomfort due to surgical incision.
6. Risk of coagulopathy (and bleeding or petechiae) related to inadequate reversal of surgical heparinization or to platelet and RBC trauma during cardiopulmonary bypass.
7. Risk of renal impairment or injury related to perioperative hypoxemia, renal thrombus or embolus, or hemoglobinuria.
8. Risk of neurological impairment or injury related to perioperative cerebrovascular accident or cerebral hypoxia.
9. Risk of infection related to chest incision, multiple invasion sites of monitoring lines, or inadequate aseptic technique by health care personnel.
10. Risk of insufficient client respiratory effort and ambulatory effort, due to pain or discomfort.
11. Knowledge deficit related to provision of home care for child following hospital discharge.

POSTOPERATIVE EXPECTED OUTCOMES

1. See postoperative expected outcomes under *Closed-Heart Surgery* (p. 467) for expected outcomes for any child who has cardiovascular surgery.
2. Child will not demonstrate chest tube output of more than 2 mL/kg/h or a fall in hematocrit of more than 15 percent of preoperative value; no petechiae or ecchymoses will be present during the immediate postoperative period or up to the time of discharge.
3. Urine output will be 0.5 mL/kg/h for children and 25–30 mL/h in adolescents in the immediate postoperative period and until discharge. Urine will be clear and free of bacteria.
4. Child will demonstrate no seizure activity, pupil inequality, or inappropriate movement from the immediate postoperative period through discharge.
5. See expected outcomes section pertaining to child's and family's anxiety and learning needs (p. 69).

POSTOPERATIVE INTERVENTIONS

1. Refer to postoperative interventions under *Closed-Heart Surgery* (p. 467) for interventions specific to any child having cardiovascular surgery.
2. Keep mediastinal tubes stripped vigorously, to prevent formation of clots and resultant cardiac tamponade.
3. If urine output is inadequate or hematuria is present, discuss plan of care with physician.
4. If petechiae or ecchymoses are observed, discuss with physician and obtain ordered coagulation screening panel. When results are available, discuss appropriate therapy with physician. If coagulopathy is present, monitor extent of chest tube output carefully, and apply pressure for at least 5 minutes to venous puncture sites and for at least 20 minutes to arterial puncture sites. Handle child gently.
5. Perform neurological examination at least every hour for the first 12 to 24 postoperative hours. Report any abnormalities to physician, and be prepared to institute emergency measures if severe neurological deterioration occurs.
6. Report any fever above 39.5°C (103°F) beyond the first 24 postoperative hours to physician; obtain ordered blood cultures. (These patients are more at risk for postoperative endocarditis or pericarditis with periods of bacteremia, since the mediastinum has been entered in surgery. If prosthetic material has

been placed in surgery, the risk of endocarditis with bacteremia is greater.)

POSTOPERATIVE EVALUATION

Outcome Criteria

1. See postoperative evaluation section under *Closed-Heart Surgery* (p. 468) for evaluation and potential complications for any child who has cardiovascular surgery.
2. Child will demonstrate no petechiae or ecchymoses, and coagulation screening panel will demonstrate coagulation factors within normal limits throughout hospital course.
3. Child's serum electrolyte levels will be within normal ranges throughout postoperative course.
4. Urine output will remain appropriate in quantity (0.5–1 mL/kg/h in children and 25–30 mL/h average in adolescents) and color and specific gravity throughout postoperative hospital stay.
5. Child will demonstrate appropriate movement and sensation for duration of postoperative hospital stay and will remain oriented in time and place (as age-appropriate).

Complications

1. Shock (see *Shock* and *Cardiac and Great Vessel Trauma* in Chapter 48 for assessment and interventions; see also *Cardiovascular Emergencies* in Chapter 49 for additional information regarding resuscitation).
2. Renal failure (see *Acute Renal Failure* in Chapter 21).
3. Status epilepticus (see *Seizures,* in Chapters 15 and 49).

ABNORMAL CELLULAR GROWTH: CONGENITAL HEART DEFECTS

PATENT DUCTUS ARTERIOSUS

DESCRIPTION

The ductus arteriosus is a necessary, normal vessel that provides the pathway for diversion of blood from the pulmonary artery into the aorta during fetal life. The ductus arteriosus normally constricts within 72 hours after birth, and eventually becomes a ligament. It is thought that the most potent stimulus for ductal constriction is the normal rise in the neonate's arterial Po_2 after birth. Patent ductus arteriosus (PDA) is the term applied to persistence of the ductus arteriosus beyond the first days of life (Figure 19-1).

Patent ductus arteriosus usually results in shunting of blood from the aorta into the pulmonary artery (the path of less resistance) once the prenatal pulmonary vascular resistance has fallen. The clinical significance of the patent ductus depends on the size of the ductus (and the size of the shunt) and the general health of the child. Infants who are premature or who have a very *large* PDA may develop CHF, usually in the first months of life, because the ductus provides increased pulmonary blood flow under high (aortic) pressures. These children require closure of the ductus on a semiurgent basis if medical management of CHF is unsuccessful. For children who remain *asymptomatic* with PDA, surgical closure is recommended before school age to eliminate the risk of bacterial endocarditis. Surgical closure of the PDA is accomplished through a left thoracotomy (closed-heart surgery). Postoperative complications include

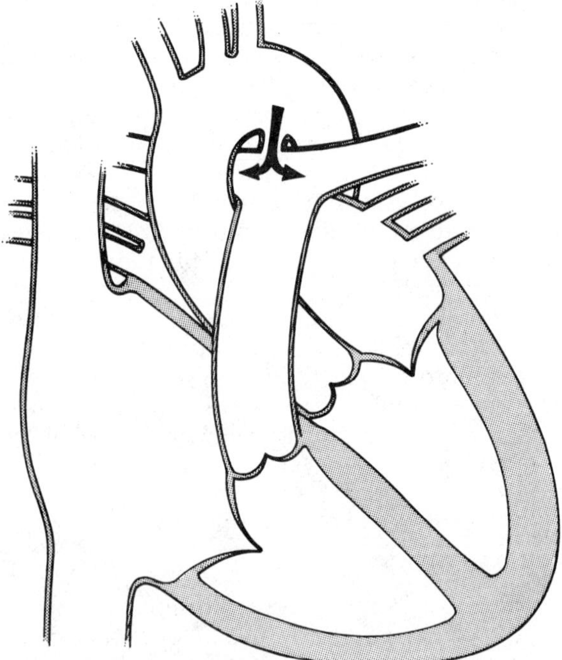

Figure 19-1 Patent ductus arteriosus.

those of a thoracotomy, including hemo- and pneumothorax, and, rarely, injury to the phrenic and recurrent laryngeal nerves. Surgical mortality is very low, although it is somewhat higher for tiny premature infants with CHF and respiratory distress syndrome.

Oral administration of prostaglandin inhibitor (indomethacin) has been found to induce ductus arteriosus closure and eliminate the need for surgery in some premature neonates. Therefore, in symptomatic neonates with PDA who are younger than 14 days old, one to three doses of the indomethacin (0.2 mg/dose, at 8- to 12-hour intervals) may be administered orally before surgery is recommended.

The ductus arteriosus can provide essential pulmonary blood flow for the child with cyanotic heart disease and restricted pulmonary blood flow (e.g., pulmonary atresia). In these children, no attempt is made to close the ductus; in fact, prostaglandin E_1 can be administered (in continuous intravenous doses of approximately 0.05–0.1 μg/kg/min) to prevent ductus closure.

If a large PDA is present for many years, the high pulmonary blood flow under high pressures can cause irreversible pulmonary hypertension.

PREVENTION

Health Promotion

1. Good prenatal care, in an effort to reduce the incidence of premature births, should reduce the incidence of PDA.
2. High daily parenteral fluid administration may increase the incidence of clinically significant PDA in low-birth-weight premature neonates.
3. Perinatal hypoxemia, due to cyanotic heart disease or respiratory distress syndrome, is associated with an increased incidence of PDA. Usually, children with respiratory distress syndrome do not develop symptoms of PDA until their respiratory disease improves (alveolar hypoxia produces pulmonary arterial vasoconstriction and high pulmonary vascular resistance; when the lung disease improves, pulmonary vascular resistance falls, and shunting from the aorta to pulmonary artery occurs).

Population At Risk

1. Premature infants with low birth weight and/or respiratory distress syndrome.
2. Neonates with cyanotic heart disease or other causes of perinatal hypoxemia.
3. Patent ductus arteriosus also occurs in otherwise healthy children.

Screening

The best screening is the physical exam. In addition, an echocardiogram will reveal a left atrial to aortic ratio of greater than 1:1.

ASSESSMENT

Health History

1. A history of prematurity, low birth weight, or perinatal hypoxemia should arouse suspicion of PDA if the child has a murmur.
2. Recent resolution of respiratory distress syndrome, or of rapid (or increased) intravenous fluid administration in the premature neonate, would increase the suspicion of the presence of a PDA.
3. History of symptoms associated with CHF: tachycardia, tachypnea, hepatomegaly, increased respiratory rate and effort, diaphoresis, poor feeding, and increased oxygen requirements (if the neonate is receiving mechanical ventilatory support) may indicate the presence of a large PDA.

Physical Assessment

1. Many children with PDA remain asymptomatic, with a cardiac murmur as their only clinically significant finding. The classic murmur associated with PDA is a continuous, "machinery-like" murmur heard in the second left intercostal space at the midclavicular line.
2. With a large shunt, signs and symptoms of CHF may appear (see assessment section under *Congestive Heart Failure*, p. 460).
3. Peripheral pulses are often bounding (also called water-hammer or "aortic runoff" pulses), and a widened pulse pressure (due to aortic runoff into pulmonary artery) can be noted.
4. Cyanosis is rare.
5. If pulmonary hypertension is present, there may be minimal shunting through the ductus, so a short, systolic murmur may be heard instead of the classical one. If pulmonary hypertension is severe with PDA, there may be reversal of the direction of the shunt (it becomes right-to-left, or blood flows from pulmonary artery to aorta) and cyanosis.

Diagnostic Tests

Echocardiogram and/or cardiac catheterization.

NURSING DIAGNOSES: ACTUAL OR POTENTIAL

1. If child has CHF, see nursing diagnoses (p. 462).
2. If child will be going to surgery, see nursing diagnoses under *Closed-Heart Surgery* (p. 467).
3. For diagnoses related to child's and family's anxiety and learning needs, see the section that addresses the special needs of hospitalized children (pp. 63–71).
4. Risk of cardiac compromise related to increased pulmonary blood flow and possible CHF, bacterial endocarditis, or postoperative hemothorax.
5. Risk of respiratory insufficiency related to postoperative atelectasis, pneumothorax, hemothorax, infection, or diaphragmatic paralysis.
6. Risk of hoarseness postoperatively related to injury of the recurrent laryngeal nerve during surgery.

EXPECTED OUTCOMES

1. If child has cardiac catheterization
   a. Catheterization site will not bleed.
   b. Pulse, warmth, and perfusion of catheterized extremity will be unaffected by the procedure.
2. Refer to expected outcomes section under *Closed-Heart Surgery* (p. 467).
3. Child will demonstrate equal and adequate movement of chest wall and lung aeration following surgery.
4. Child will demonstrate normal voice quality after the first postoperative day.
5. Child will not develop bacterial endocarditis.

INTERVENTIONS

1. If the child has CHF, see interventions listed under *Congestive Heart Failure* (p. 462).
2. Since the child has a cardiovascular defect causing turbulent blood flow, he or she is at increased risk for the development of bacterial endocarditis (beyond the age of 5 years) anytime that bacteremia is present.
   a. If the defect has not been repaired by school age, the child should receive antibiotic prophylaxis before dental or surgical procedures. Penicillin is the prophylactic antibiotic of choice (unless the child has a penicillin sensitivity).
   b. The child and parents should be aware of the need for prophylaxis.
3. If cardiac catheterization is necessary, the child and parents will require precatheterization teaching (see interventions 7 and 8, p. 70).
4. Postcatheterization care.
   a. Monitor cardiac output, as cardiac arrhythmias and irritability may follow angiocardiography. If arrhythmia is present, determine whether it compromises cardiac output, and notify physician.
   b. Monitor urine output: Contrast media can act as an osmotic diuretic (causing increased urine volume as kidneys attempt to excrete hypertonic solution), but children may not void immediately if still sedated. A reaction to the contrast medium can cause hematuria.
   c. *If an artery is used for catheterization*, ensure maintenance of adequate arterial perfusion to extremity distal to catheterization site.
      (1) The patient is usually kept in bed for several hours after catheterization to decrease possibility of hemorrhage.
      (2) Peripheral pulses should be present, and the extremity should remain warm with pink nail beds—notify physician *immediately* if extremity becomes cool, mottled, or pale.
      (3) If artery develops spasms, thrombus formation can occur quickly along length of artery, causing severe compromise of circulation to extremity as pulses decrease in intensity. If this occurs acutely, collateral circulation will not develop rapidly enough to maintain perfusion to extremity, and severe tissue necrosis can result.
         (a) If arterial circulation is compromised, application of heat to the *opposite* extremity may cause reflex arterial vasodilatation to affected extremity. *Do not apply heat to affected extremity,* as that increases metabolic demands of already compromised tissue.
         (b) Intravenous infusion of heparin may arrest progression of thrombus formation, if begun as soon as com-

promise of arterial perfusion is noted.

d. *If a vein is used for catheterization*, ensure maintenance of adequate venous return from extremity.
   (1) Veins used for catheterization can be tied off after the procedure, so venous return from extremity must be accomplished by other veins and by newly developed collateral circulation.
   (2) Bed rest following catheterization usually is less restrictive than if an artery is used.
   (3) The extremity can become edematous and cyanotic, because venous return is impeded (unoxygenated blood remains in capillaries in extremity). Notify physician if edema interferes with arterial perfusion (evidenced by decreased pulse).
      (a) Elevation of the extremity will promote venous return.
      (b) Provide thorough skin care and gentle handling of the extremity, as it can be very painful.
e. Monitor catheterization site for evidence of bleeding or hematoma; apply pressure and ice if bleeding is present, and notify physician immediately if bleeding is prolonged or severe.

5. Postoperative care.
   a. See *Closed-Heart Surgery* Assessment (p. 466) and Interventions (p. 467) sections.
   b. The nurse should monitor especially for evidence of
      (1) Hemothorax or pneumothorax.
      (2) Atelectasis of the left lung (this lung must be retracted during surgery).
      (3) Infrequent, diaphragmatic paralysis or recurrent laryngeal nerve injury.

EVALUATION

Refer to evaluation section of *Closed-Heart Surgery* (p. 468) for outcome criteria and complications.

AORTICOPULMONARY WINDOW

DESCRIPTION

This unusual defect, caused by incomplete division of the common great artery trunk, results in the presence of a hole (and associated shunt) between the aorta and the pulmonary artery at a place where they share a common wall. Hemodynamic consequences and nursing care are the same as those involved in care of a child with large PDA. The surgical intervention carries a slightly greater risk, as cardiopulmonary bypass (open-heart surgery) may be required. Postoperative complications are similar.

COARCTATION OF THE AORTA

DESCRIPTION

In this disorder, narrowing of the aorta occurs as a result of infolding of the inner wall of the aorta. This narrowing (coarctation) most often occurs in the thoracic aorta. Coarctation of the aorta (CoA) can occur as a single defect or in combination with other defects (such as ventricular septal defects). It accounts for approximately 8 percent of all congenital heart defects. The clinical course of the child with coarctation is determined by the location of the narrowing, the extent of any collateral circulation, and the severity of the aortic obstruction (Figure 19-2).

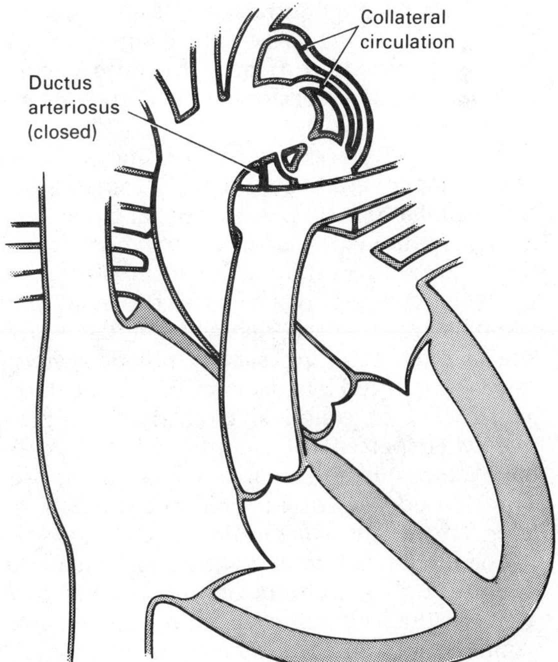

Figure 19-2 Postductal coarctation of the aorta with formation of collateral circulation.

Coarctation of the aorta can be distal to the ductus arteriosus (postductal), proximal to the ductus arteriosus (preductal), or at the ductus arteriosus (periductal).

The most common form of coarctation is *postductal*, in which the aortic narrowing is just distal to the ductus arteriosus (this is also known as "adult" type of coarctation, since clients with this defect may remain asymptomatic until adulthood). In this form of CoA, collateral circulation is thought to develop during fetal life, to provide blood flow around the coarctation (under reduced pressure) to the descending aorta.

A *preductal coarctation* is a narrowing in the aorta proximal to the ductus arteriosus. Aortic arch hypoplasia, or even interruption, may be present (a formerly used term for this defect was "infantile" coarctation, because affected clients usually become symptomatic in infancy). With preductal CoA, the ascending aorta (proximal to the coarctation) is perfused with oxygenated blood from the left ventricle, and the descending aorta (distal to the coarctation) is perfused with venous blood from the right ventricle through the ductus arteriosus. In these clients, there is no stimulus for the development of collateral circulation during fetal life, and severe aortic obstruction and hypoperfusion of the descending aorta usually occur after birth if the ductus arteriosus begins to constrict. This type of coarctation is often associated with early onset of CHF.

A *periductal coarctation* (narrowing at the site of the ductus arteriosus) usually causes symptoms similar to those of a postductal coarctation.

In any child with CoA, CHF will occur within the first months of life if the aortic obstruction is severe enough. Hypertension proximal to the site of coarctation and hypotension distal to the site of coarctation are usually noted, although this is influenced by adequacy of cardiac output and extent of collateral circulation. Approximately 60 percent of children with CoA also have a bicuspid aortic valve, which places them at increased risk for bacterial endocarditis and later, aortic valve calcification and stenosis.

Coarctation is repaired with closed-heart surgery through a left thoracotomy. The narrowed aortic segment is removed, and the remaining segments of the aorta are rejoined directly or with use of a graft. The graft may consist of the proximal portion of the child's subclavian artery, or it may be made of woven material. Potential postoperative complications include those of a thoracotomy (including pneumothorax and hemothorax), residual upper extremity hypertension, mesenteric vasculitis, chylothorax, and, rarely, spinal cord injury.

PREVENTION

Health Promotion

No known prevention.

Population at Risk

No predisposition known except Turner's syndrome.

Screening

Good physical examination.

ASSESSMENT

Health History

Congestive heart failure and extreme cardiorespiratory distress can occur within the first weeks of life if the coarctation is severe, or if an additional cardiac lesion is present. Refer to the assessment of *Congestive Heart Failure*, (p. 460).

Physical Assessment

1. A systolic aortic murmur can be heard at the center of the client's back if sufficient blood is passing through the coarctation. Systolic bruits can be heard over the ribs and chest if large collateral arteries are present (they usually consist of dilated mammary and intercostal arteries). If the child has a bicuspid aortic valve, a systolic aortic valve murmur may be noted.
2. Cyanosis is usually absent, although occasionally children with *preductal* coarctation may demonstrate some lower extremity cyanosis, since their lower extremities are perfused with venous blood (usually the lower extremities are pale).
3. Children with CoA usually demonstrate hypertension of any vessels supplied from the aorta proximal to the coarctation.
   a. Decreased blood pressure to the lower extremities is thought to stimulate the renin-angiotensin-aldosterone system, as well as neural vasopressor secretion, causing hypertension.
   b. If the coarctation is *postductal*, there will be hypertension of both upper extremities.

c. If the coarctation is *preductal*, the hypertension will be present only in those vessels supplied from the aorta proximal to the coarctation; often hypertension will be seen only in the right arm (supplied by the innominate artery—the first branch of the aortic arch).

d. If the child has severe CHF, *all* pulses (and blood pressure) may be depressed due to low cardiac output; once the child's cardiac output improves, the differential hypertension may be appreciated.

4. Hypotension (and decrease in pulses) will be noted in any vessels supplied from the aorta distal to the coarctation.
   a. Hypotension of the lower extremities is usually present.
   b. If the *preductal* coarctation is located proximal to the aortic origin of the left subclavian artery, pulses and blood pressure to the left arm will also be reduced.
5. The child may experience leg claudication with exercise (due to the diminished pressure of lower extremity blood flow).

Diagnostic Tests

Echocardiogram and cardiac catheterization.

NURSING DIAGNOSES: ACTUAL OR POTENTIAL

1. If the child has CHF, see nursing diagnoses for *Congestive Heart Failure* (p. 462).
2. Refer to section on hospitalized children (p. 63) for diagnoses related to child and parent anxiety and learning needs.
3. Child has upper extremity hypertension and lower extremity hypotension (and possible claudication) related to aortic narrowing and renal and neural vasopressor compensatory mechanisms.
4. Risk of bacterial endocarditis and cardiorespiratory compromise related to coarctation of the aorta, its surgical repair, potential residual hypertension, possible chylothorax, and possible associated bicuspid aortic valve.
5. Child may develop abdominal pain, tenderness, or distension as the result of mesenteric vasculitis. While the etiology of postoperative mesenteric vasculitis is unknown, it is thought to be related to friability of the mesenteric arteries and severe postoperative hypertension.
6. Child may demonstrate nutritional or respiratory compromise due to loss of lymph fluid into thoracic cavity (or out chest tube).
7. Child may demonstrate postoperative decrease in movement or sensation to lower extremities related to injury to spinal cord arteries during coarctation repair.

EXPECTED OUTCOMES

1. If the child has CHF, see expected outcomes under *Congestive Heart Failure* (p. 462).
2. Refer to expected outcomes related to child's and parents' anxiety and learning needs (p. 69).
3. Child will not demonstrate any measurable bleeding from the catheterization site.
4. If child has arterial catheterization, child will not demonstrate any decrease in pulse, warmth, or perfusion to catheterized extremity.
5. Refer to expected outcomes under *Closed-Heart Surgery* (p. 467) for the postoperative expected outcomes with the following additions:
   a. Child will demonstrate normal blood pressures in lower extremities immediately after surgery and normal upper extremity blood pressure by the time of discharge.
   b. Child will be free from abdominal pain, distension, and other evidence of mesenteric vasculitis from the time of the immediate postoperative period through discharge.
   c. Child will demonstrate no evidence of chylothorax throughout postoperative course.
   d. Child will demonstrate appropriate movement of and sensation to lower extremities immediately after recovery from anesthesia.

INTERVENTIONS

1. If the child has CHF, see section on *Congestive Heart Failure* (p. 462).
2. Refer to Chapter 4, hospitalized child section, for preoperative and preprocedure teaching, p. 70, interventions 7 and 8.
3. See Chapter 4, hospitalized child section, for interventions to reduce child's and parents' anxiety, p. 69, interventions 1 and 2.
4. Postcatheterization care is described in intervention 4 under *Patent Ductus Arteriosus*, (p. 474).

5. Postoperative care is as described in the section on *Closed-Heart Surgery* (p. 467) with the following additions:
   a. If prosthetic patch material was needed to rejoin aortic segments, child is at increased risk for bacterial endocarditis at the graft site whenever any bacteremia is present. Therefore, if the child has fever higher than 39.5°C (103°F) after the first postoperative day, blood cultures should be obtained to rule out bacteremia.
   b. Monitor blood pressure in upper and lower extremities, and report any decrease in lower extremity blood pressure immediately to physician (a clot or an intimal flap could develop at the site of CoA repair). See Table 19-3 for normal blood pressure measurements in children.
   c. Blood pressure in upper extremities usually remains elevated for a few postoperative hours or days, but report any extreme upper and lower extremity hypertension (systolic blood pressure exceeding 160 mmHg and diastolic pressure exceeding 90–100 mmHg) to physician, as extremely high postoperative blood pressures are thought to be associated with increased risk of mesenteric vasculitis and cerebral and cardiovascular compromise.
      (1) The physician may wish to control hypertension by administration of intravenous antihypertensive medications. The most popular medications for this purpose are intravenous sodium nitroprusside and nitroglycerin. Intravenous antihypertensive medications should not be administered unless an arterial line is in place for continuous monitoring of arterial blood pressure.
      (2) If the client's hospital environment is kept quiet and free of distractions and if pain relief is adequate, the blood pressure may be kept down without use of antihypertensive medications.
   d. Monitor for evidence of abdominal pain, tenderness, or distension, and report their presence to physician.
      (1) Monitor bowel sounds carefully (absent bowel sounds beyond the first 24 postoperative hours may indicate paralytic ileus).
      (2) Check function and patency of nasogastric (NG) tube (usually in place for 24 hours), at least every 2 hours (irrigate and aspirate).
      (3) When adequate bowel sounds are present, begin postoperative feedings very slowly, and monitor for nausea, vomiting, or abdominal distension, which may indicate intolerance of volume or concentration of oral fluids.
   e. While chest tube is in place, monitor for presence of milky drainage (lymph), which can occur due to injury to a large lymphatic vessel during dissection for coarctation repair. If chylothorax is present, chest tube should not be removed until lymph drainage has ceased.
      (1) Since lymph drainage represents loss of fat, some physicians advocate administration of a low-fat elemental diet to the child, to prevent further fat absorption and loss through chylothorax.
      (2) Child should receive supplemental fat-soluable vitamins.
   f. Once the chest tube is removed, monitor carefully for evidence of pleural fluid, which can indicate development of chylothorax. If present, chylous fluid will need to be evacuated by thoracentesis or by means of chest tube insertion.
   g. Check movements and sensation of lower extremities immediately after surgery. If the child does not withdraw legs from painful stimuli once recovered from anesthesia, notify physician, since paraplegia can occur as the result of impairment of spinal cord circulation.

EVALUATION

Outcome Criteria

1. If child has CHF, see evaluation section under *Congestive Heart Failure* (p. 465).
2. Please refer to section on hospitalized children (p. 71) for evaluation of teaching interventions and psychological support of child and parents.
3. See evaluation section under *Closed-Heart Surgery* (p. 468).
4. Child's lower extremity blood pressure will be normal in the immediate postoperative period.
5. Child should demonstrate normal upper extremity blood pressure by the time of discharge.
6. Child is at increased risk of bacterial endo-

carditis if prosthetic material was used to repair CoA or if bicuspid aortic valve is present, so child and parents should receive instruction regarding the need for antibiotic prophylaxis at times of increased risk of bacteremia.

7. Child should have no abdominal pain, tenderness, or distension during the postoperative course.
8. Child should demonstrate normal movement and sensation in lower extremities once recovered from anesthesia.

Complication
Child may demonstrate extreme lower extremity hypotension in the immediate postoperative period due to inadequate resection of coarctation or clot or intimal flap at repair site.

Reevaluation and Follow-up
Surgeon should be consulted immediately, as reoperation may be necessary.

Complication
Child may demonstrate residual hypertension, related to increased plasma renin activity or inadequate resection of coarctation.

Reevaluation and Follow-up
Child and family should receive teaching regarding long-term consequences of hypertension, and child should be followed closely on an outpatient basis. If hypertension does not resolve after the child returns to normal activities, and restenosis of CoA repair site has been ruled out, child should be placed on antihypertensive medications.

Complication
Child may develop extreme tenderness, abdominal distension and pain, vomiting, fever, and elevated WBC count, indicating possible bowel necrosis.

Reevaluation and Follow-up
Physician should be notified immediately, the child should be kept NPO, and an NG tube should be placed. The bowel inflammation may resolve with only supportive care but may require surgical intervention in rare, extreme cases.

Complication
Child may, rarely, demonstrate postoperative paralysis or paresthesia related to interference with spinal cord circulation during CoA repair.

Reevaluation and Follow-up
If injury is permanent, refer to Chapter 27.

CONGENITAL AORTIC STENOSIS

DESCRIPTION

Aortic stenosis refers to several forms of obstruction to left ventricular outflow. There are three main types of congenital aortic stenosis: valvular, subvalvular, and supravalvular.

Valvular aortic stenosis, the most common form, results from incomplete separation of valve leaflets during embryological development. A bicuspid valve is usually present.

Subvalvular aortic stenosis usually results from the formation of a membranous web below the aortic valve. Idiopathic hypertrophic subaortic stenosis (IHSS) is an unusual form of subvalvular stenosis caused by thickening of the left side of the ventricular septum that obstructs left ventricular outflow.

Supravalvular aortic stenosis is the least common form of congenital aortic obstruction. It is usually caused by formation of a fibrous ring just above the aortic valve (may be seen in conjunction with hypertelorism, mental retardation, and unusual facial characteristics).

With all forms of aortic stenosis, the left ventricle must generate higher pressure to maintain blood flow through the narrowed outflow tract, so left ventricular hypertrophy develops. The pressure gradient and degree of left ventricular hypertrophy determine the child's symptoms and prognosis. If the gradient is small, the aortic stenosis is usually well tolerated, and the child may only be monitored for evidence of increasing stenosis. If the gradient is high (above 50–60 mmHg), the left ventricle must generate very high pressures to maintain adequate blood flow through the stenotic area. Clients with valvular and subvalvular stenosis and high gradients are watched very closely for the development of left ventricular strain patterns (ST segment changes) on ECG, syncope, angina, palpitations, or dyspnea. Any of these symptoms indicates that the aortic stenosis is critical; at this point, increased activity or demands on cardiac output can result in sudden death (thought to be caused by myocardial hypoxia and fatal arrhythmias). Children with critical valvular or subvalvular aortic stenosis are usually restricted from vigorous physical activity until the stenosis is surgically relieved.

The development of CHF in children with aortic stenosis (in the absence of any other defect) is unusual and usually indicates severe aortic obstruction.

Many children with congenital aortic stenosis remain asymptomatic except for a murmur and are watched closely. Antibiotic prophylaxis is given at times of increased risk of bacteremia. The stenosis is repaired with open-heart surgery on an elective basis, before evidence of critical aortic stenosis develops. Children with subvalvular stenosis may have surgery earlier than children with valvular stenosis, since the subvalvular surgical resection is often curative. Children who require aortic valvulotomy or valve replacement early in childhood will usually require additional valvular surgery in early adulthood.

If the aortic stenosis is critical in the neonatal period, CHF occurs, and the infant requires vigorous medical management and urgent surgical intervention. Open-heart aortic valvulotomy (with deep hypothermia) is usually the procedure of choice, although it carries a high risk.

Potential postoperative complications include bleeding, heart block, CHF (especially if present preoperatively), and arrhythmias.

PREVENTION

Health Promotion

No known preventative measures.

Population at Risk

1. Children with Williams elfin facies syndrome have an increased incidence of supravalvular aortic stenosis.
2. Most children with CoA have a bicuspid aortic valve and may develop valvular stenosis.

Screening

Physical exam should detect an aortic murmur, and ECG will reveal left ventricular hypertrophy.

ASSESSMENT

Health History

It is extremely important to determine if child has any history of angina, syncope, arrhythmias, palpatations, or dyspnea on exertion. Question child and primary caretaker about child's exercise tolerance, and notify physician immediately of any history of syncopal episodes. Also, determine if any restrictions are placed on activity (and extent of child's compliance).

Physical Assessment

1. The majority of patients with aortic stenosis are asymptomatic.
2. If CHF is present, see *Congestive Heart Failure* (p. 459) for appropriate assessments.
3. Cyanosis is rare.
4. Left ventricular heave may be palpated due to left ventricular hypertrophy. Check ECG for signs of left ventricular strain.
5. Heart sounds.
   a. With all forms of aortic stenosis, an ejection systolic murmur is present and is usually heard best at the aortic area (may be accompanied by a thrill).
   b. With valvular aortic stenosis, a click may be noted in the fourth intercostal space at the left sternal border.
   c. If aortic valvular insufficiency coexists, an aortic diastolic murmur will be present.
6. Peripheral pulses.
   a. Peripheral pulses may be unremarkable if stenosis is mild.
   b. With moderate stenosis, decreased systolic blood pressure and a narrow pulse pressure are usually present (if aortic insufficiency is also present, pulse pressure may be normal).
   c. With severe stenosis and CHF, peripheral pulses may be diminished.
   d. "Streamlining" of blood flow into the innominate artery (first branch off the aortic arch) may cause higher blood pressure measurements in right than in left arm.

Diagnostic Tests

ECG and echocardiogram.

NURSING DIAGNOSES: ACTUAL OR POTENTIAL

1. If child has CHF, see nursing diagnoses under *Congestive Heart Failure* (p. 462).
2. Refer to section on hospitalized children (p. 63) for diagnoses related to child and family anxiety. Note that if child's activity has been restricted by physician because of fear that child is at risk for sudden death, child and parents can be expected to be extremely anxious.
3. Child may experience exercise intolerance, syncope, palpitations, or angina related to se-

vere aortic stenosis, extreme left ventricular hypertrophy and probable decrease in coronary artery perfusion of thickened myocardium, and left ventricular strain.
4. Refer to nursing diagnoses section under *Open-Heart Surgery* (p. 471).
5. Risk of bacterial endocarditis both before and after surgery because of turbulence in blood flow caused by abnormal valve leaflets or supra- or subvalvular membranes.

EXPECTED OUTCOMES

1. Refer to expected outcomes section on hospitalized children (p. 69) for outcomes related to child and parent anxiety and learning needs.
2. If child has cardiac catheterization
   a. Catheterization site will not bleed.
   b. Pulse, warmth, and perfusion of catheterized extremity will not be affected by the procedure.
3. If child has CHF, see *Congestive Heart Failure* (p. 462) for outcomes.
4. Refer to *Open-Heart Surgery* (p. 471) for postoperative outcomes.
5. Child will not develop bacterial endocarditis.

INTERVENTIONS

1. See *Congestive Heart Failure* (p. 462) for related interventions if child has CHF.
2. If child has cardiac catheterization, see interventions 3 and 4 under *Patent Ductus Arteriosus* (p. 474).
3. See section on hospitalized children (p. 69) for interventions to reduce child's and family's anxiety.
4. To avoid bacterial endocarditis, teach parents (and child if old enough) that child requires prophylactic antibiotics before any dental or surgical procedure. Penicillin is the drug of choice unless child is allergic to it.
5. See *Closed-Heart Surgery* (p. 467) and *Open-Heart Surgery* (p. 471) for postoperative interventions. The nurse should especially monitor for postoperative bleeding, arrhythmias, heart block, and CHF. Long-term postoperative complications include potential aortic insufficiency or residual aortic stenosis.
6. If the child has been hospitalized for diagnosis and will be sent home with activity restrictions until surgery at some later time, specific interventions are required to provide the child and family with teaching and support.
   a. Health team should confer with client and parents and determine specific activities child is to avoid.
      (1) If a specific plan of activity restriction is provided by physician, attempt to make this more acceptable by suggesting or supplying quiet, diversional activities.
      (2) Activity restriction will be especially difficult during adolescence, when peer pressure may cause the teenager to test activity restrictions. (Surgery should be scheduled as soon as evidence of stenosis requiring activity restriction is discovered.)
      (3) Family may be comforted to know that health team members are available to answer questions or provide assistance if necessary.
   b. Health care follow-up must be frequent and thorough; physician should be notified immediately if there are any syncopal episodes or further deterioration in health status.
   c. Attempt to help family avoid focusing excessively on child's health status.
7. Usually a digitalis derivative is not helpful in improving cardiac output unless CHF is present, as increased cardiac contractility will not change the amount of resistance offered by the stenotic outflow area of left ventricle or aorta preoperatively. Digitalis is contraindicated if the child has IHSS.
8. Nitroglycerin is not helpful in relieving preoperative angina in clients with aortic stenosis, and it can increase the risk of syncope, so it should be avoided.

EVALUATION

Refer to *Closed-Heart Surgery* (p. 468) and *Open-Heart Surgery* (p. 472) for evaluation criteria and complications.

VASCULAR RINGS

DESCRIPTION

Vascular rings consist of one or several anomalous vessels that encircle or distort the trachea and/or esophagus (Figure 19-3). They can be

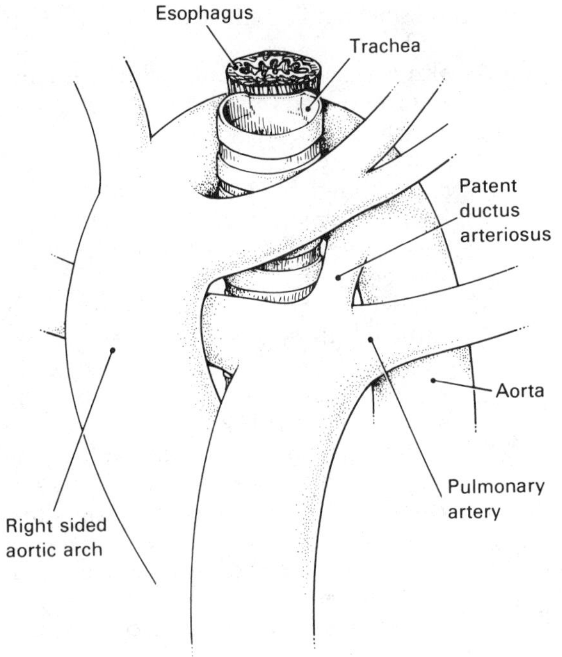

Figure 19-3 Vascular ring.

produced by formation or remnants of a double aortic arch, a right (instead of left) aortic arch with a left ductus arteriosus, or an anomalous subclavian or innominate artery.

Occasionally, the client with a vascular ring remains asymptomatic. Usually, however, symptoms of airway obstruction (and frequent upper airway infections), apnea, or dysphagia develop due to compression of the trachea or esophagus by the vascular ring. The diagnosis should be suspected in the child who has upper airway obstruction (e.g., stridor, frequent infections, increased respiratory infections), and feeding difficulties (including frequent vomiting). It is confirmed by barium swallow and bronchoscopy. An angiogram may not be necessary for diagnosis.

Medical treatment of respiratory infections and (closed-heart) surgical ligation or movement of anomalous vessels is required. Potential postoperative complications are similar to those anticipated following ligation of PDA or repair of CoA.

ATRIAL SEPTAL DEFECT

DESCRIPTION

Atrial septal defect (ASD) is a hole in the atrial septum as a result of inappropriate embryological development (Figure 19-4). Several different types of ASDs exist; together, they represent approximately 12 percent of all congenital heart defects.

The *ostium secundum* defect, the most common form, is located high in the atrial septum. The *sinus venosus* defect is near the junction of the right atrium and the superior vena cava and can be associated with anomalous drainage of some pulmonary veins into the *right* atrium. The *ostium primum* defect (a form of endocardial cushion defect) is located low in the atrial septum and is associated with malformations of the atrioventricular valves and possible ventricular septal defect (refer to *Endocardial Cushion Defects*, p. 486). Reopening of the fetal *foramen ovale* can occur (as an acquired defect) in association with defects causing severe increase in right atrial and/or ventricular volume and increased right atrial pressure. Most commonly, a patent fora-

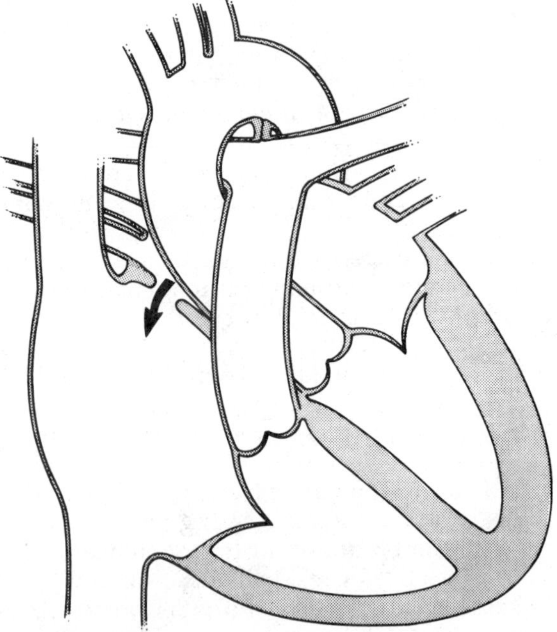

Figure 19-4 Secundum atrial septal defect.

men ovale allows blood to shunt from the right to left atrium.

Children with uncomplicated ASDs are usually asymptomatic. Once pulmonary vascular resistance falls, in the first few weeks after birth, blood flows through the defect from left to right atrium (in the direction of least resistance) causing *increased* pulmonary blood flow. This high pulmonary blood flow is usually well tolerated, because it is under *low* pressure; pulmonary vascular resistance does not increase for decades, if at all. The right ventricle (and both atria, in adults) hypertrophies due to this pure volume load. Congestive heart failure is rare during childhood and only occurs if right ventricular dysfunction is present. In adults, atrial arrhythmias may occur.

The ASD must be surgically closed, using sutures or a patch. This open-heart procedure is usually performed on an elective basis, before the child starts school. Potential postoperative complications include arrhythmias and heart block. Congestive heart failure occurs postoperatively in approximately 2 percent of children with ASD. The incidence of bacterial endocarditis pre- and postoperatively is low but somewhat higher if a prosthetic patch was used to close the ASD.

PREVENTION

Health Promotion

No known method of prevention.

Population at Risk

Occasionally, there is a familial incidence of secundum ASD; however, most children with ASD have no recognized predisposing factors.

Screening

Physical exam is the best method of screening.

ASSESSMENT

Health History

1. The young child may demonstrate some exercise intolerance, but no activity restriction is necessary.
2. The young adult may report some palpitations if atrial enlargement is causing atrial arrhythmias.

Physical Assessment

1. Children with secundum ASD are generally asymptomatic (see *Endocardial Cushion Defects*, p. 487, for discussion of assessment of child with ostium primum defect).
2. Pulmonary congestion and heart failure are rare in childhood.
3. Right ventricular hypertrophy may cause sternal lift, and ripple may be noted along middle of chest as large blood flow enters right ventricle.
4. Heart sounds and rhythm.
   a. Soft, pulmonic systolic murmur is present due to greatly increased pulmonary blood flow; fixed, wide splitting of the S_2 sound occurs (pulmonary valve closes late with high flow).
   b. With a large shunt, a tricuspid diastolic murmur may appear and may be accompanied by a thrill due to large flow through this valve into the right ventricle.
   c. Atrial fibrillation or flutter may appear if the right atrium becomes very large.

Diagnostic Tests

Echocardiogram and cardiac catheterization confirm the diagnosis. Angiocardiogram may be performed to document the presence or absence of associated anomalous pulmonary veins (pulmonary veins that empty into the systemic venous circulation or right atrium instead of the left atrium).

NURSING DIAGNOSES: ACTUAL OR POTENTIAL

1. See section on hospitalized children (p. 69) for diagnoses pertaining to child and family anxiety and learning needs.
2. See *Open-Heart Surgery* (p. 471) for postoperative diagnoses.
3. Child has slight increase in risk for bacterial endocarditis and late-onset pulmonary hypertension related to atrial septal defect.

EXPECTED OUTCOMES

1. See section on hospitalized children (p. 69) for outcomes related to child and family anxiety and learning needs.
2. If child has cardiac catheterization
   a. Catheterization site will not bleed.
   b. Pulses, warmth, and perfusion of cathet-

erized extremity will be unaffected by the procedure.

3. Postoperative expected outcomes are as stated in the section on *Open-Heart Surgery* (p. 471).

INTERVENTIONS

1. Please see section on hospitalized children (p. 69) for general supportive interventions and teaching.
2. If child has cardiac catheterization, see intervention 4 under *Patent Ductus Arteriosus* (p. 474).
3. Postoperative interventions are discussed in the section on *Open-Heart Surgery* (p. 471).
4. Teach parents (and child if old enough) that in order to avoid bacterial endocarditis, child requires prophylactic antibiotics before any dental or surgical procedure. Penicillin is the drug of choice unless child is allergic to it.

EVALUATION

Outcome criteria and complications are as stated in *Open-Heart Surgery* (p. 472).

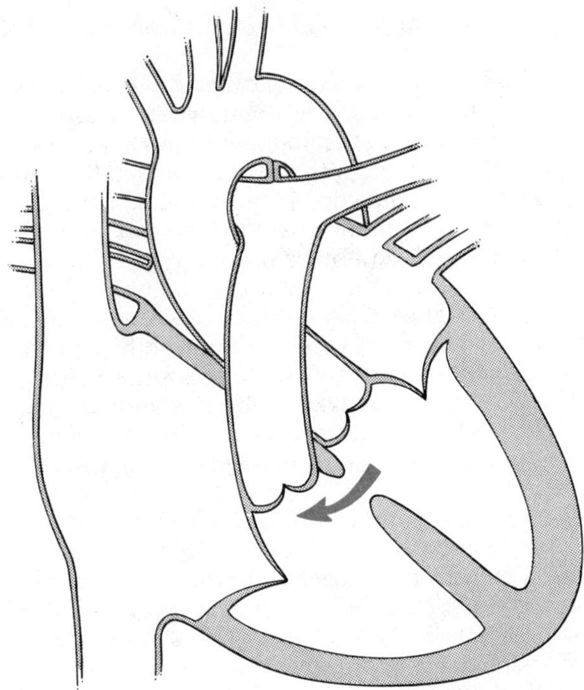

Figure 19-5 Ventricular septal defect.

VENTRICULAR SEPTAL DEFECT

DESCRIPTION

Ventricular septal defect (VSD) is a hole in the ventricular septum that results from improper embryological formation (Figure 19-5). Ventricular septal defect is the most common congenital heart defect, responsible for approximately 30 percent of all congenital heart lesions. The severity of the child's symptoms depends on the size and location of the defect, as well as the child's pulmonary vascular resistance.

With an uncomplicated VSD, little or no shunting of blood occurs during the neonatal period while pulmonary vascular resistance is still high, but left-to-right ventricular shunting will occur once pulmonary vascular resistance drops (at approximately 4 to 12 weeks of age), because the pulmonary circulation then offers the path of less resistance. The amount of pulmonary blood flow is determined by the size of the defect and its location. A *small* defect allows only a small shunt, and this results in only slightly increased pulmonary blood flow under *low* pressures. This low-pressure shunt is usually well tolerated by the child, and there is thought to be no risk of pulmonary hypertension. If the defect is *large*, equalization of pressures between ventricles occurs, and increased pulmonary blood flow under *high* pressures results once pulmonary vascular resistance falls. This high-pressure pulmonary blood flow is usually not well tolerated, and CHF frequently develops at around 1 to 3 months of age. With this high pulmonary blood flow under high pressure, pulmonary hypertension can develop within a few months or years.

Many small VSDs close spontaneously; all become smaller, relatively, as the child grows. As a result, asymptomatic children with small VSDs may be followed closely for several years, with hopes that the defect will close spontaneously. Until the defect closes, these children require antibiotic prophylaxis to prevent bacterial endocarditis at times of increased risk of bacteremia.

When a large defect causes CHF, medical management with digitalis derivatives and diuretics is necessary; if the child remains in severe CHF, surgery is required. Formerly, a closed-heart palliative procedure, *pulmonary ar-*

tery banding, was performed to relieve CHF and reduce high-pressure pulmonary blood flow by placing a tight cloth band around the pulmonary artery, creating pulmonary stenosis. This procedure prevents development of pulmonary hypertension while the child grows. Although there are still occasional indications for pulmonary artery banding in children with complex heart disease, many surgeons prefer early closure of VSDs.

Open-heart closure of the VSD can be performed in conjunction with deep hypothermia in the critically ill infant. It can be done on a more elective basis for the child with a moderate defect and minimal symptoms. The defect is closed with sutures or a patch, through an incision in the atrium (an atriotomy) or ventricle (ventriculotomy). Potential postoperative complications after this repair include arrhythmias, heart block, and CHF (especially if a ventriculotomy was performed). Mortality is low, except in the very ill infant or the child with significant pulmonary hypertension.

PREVENTION

Health Promotion

No preventive measures are known.

Population at Risk

No known predeterminants, except increased incidence in children with trisomy 13 and trisomy 18.

Screening

Physical exam.

ASSESSMENT

Health History

1. Important to determine when the child's murmur was first heard.
2. Inquire about history of feeding difficulty, diaphoresis, tachypnea, or dyspnea (signs of CHF).
3. Any history of cyanosis can indicate that the child has some pulmonary stenosis or severe pulmonary hypertension.

Physical Assessment

1. Child may remain asymptomatic if defect is small or if child is a neonate (and pulmonary vascular resistance is still high).
2. Symptoms of CHF and respiratory distress may be present in infant beyond 4 weeks of age.
3. Cyanosis is unusual; it can occur during crying or late in the clinical course (due to development of increased pulmonary vascular resistance and consequent reversal of shunt).
4. The "classic" VSD murmur is a harsh, systolic murmur heard best at the left lower sternal border and radiating over much of the chest (it may be accompanied by a thrill). If shunt is large, causing *large* pulmonary blood flow, a diastolic mitral murmur may be heard over the apex when large pulmonary venous return passes into the left ventricle.

Diagnostic Tests

Echocardiogram and cardiac catheterization.

NURSING DIAGNOSES: ACTUAL OR POTENTIAL

1. Risk of pulmonary hypertension, if the defect is large, or of bacterial endocarditis due to the presence of the VSD and its effect on blood flow patterns.
2. If child has CHF, see diagnoses listed under *Congestive Heart Failure* (p. 462).
3. Refer to section on hospitalized children (p. 63) for diagnoses related to child and family anxiety and learning needs.
4. If the child requires surgery, see nursing diagnoses sections of *Closed-Heart Surgery* (p. 467) or *Open-Heart Surgery* (p. 471).

EXPECTED OUTCOMES

1. If child has CHF, see expected outcomes under *Congestive Heart Failure* (p. 462).
2. See expected outcomes section (p. 69) for hospitalized child's and family's anxiety and learning needs.
3. Please see expected outcomes sections of *Closed-Heart Surgery* (p. 467) and *Open-Heart Surgery* (p. 471) for postoperative care.

INTERVENTIONS

1. If child has CHF, see interventions listed under *Congestive Heart Failure* (p. 462).
2. Refer to section on hospitalized children (p. 69) for interventions to reduce child's and family's anxiety and for teaching interventions.

3. Please see interventions section under *Closed-Heart Surgery* (p. 467) or *Open-Heart Surgery* (p. 471) for postoperative care. Monitor especially for postoperative arrhythmias and heart block, and for CHF if it was present preoperatively.
4. Teach parents (and child if old enough) that prophylactic antibiotics will be required before any surgical or dental procedures, in order to avoid bacterial endocarditis. Penicillin is the drug of choice unless child is allergic to it.

EVALUATION

See sections of *Closed-Heart Surgery* (p. 468) or *Open-Heart Surgery* (p. 472) for evaluation criteria and complications.

ENDOCARDIAL CUSHION DEFECTS

DESCRIPTION

Endocardial cushion defects (ECD) result from improper fusion of the anterior and posterior endocardial cushions during fetal development and result in some combination of the following defects: an *ostium primum ASD, abnormalities of the atrioventricular valves*, and a *VSD* (Figure 19-6). While endocardial cushion defects represent only 3 percent of all congenital heart defects, they are the most frequent congenital heart lesions seen in children with Down's syndrome (trisomy 21).

There is a wide range in the severity of ECDs. The mildest form of this defect is an ostium primum ASD. This is a defect low in the atrial septum with some deformity of the atrioventricular valves, most often a cleft in a mitral valve leaflet The hemodynamic effects of a primum ASD are similar to those of a secundum ASD (both described under *Atrial Septal Defects* p. 482), preoperatively, although the mitral valve will not be normal, and significant residual mitral insufficiency can cause postoperative problems.

The most severe form of ECD is a *complete atrioventricular (AV) canal*. The AV canal consists of a large atrial or atrial and ventricular septal defect, with a single atrioventricular valve that is usually insufficient. This defect can allow mixing of oxygenated and venous blood at the atrial or ventricular level, although the direction of

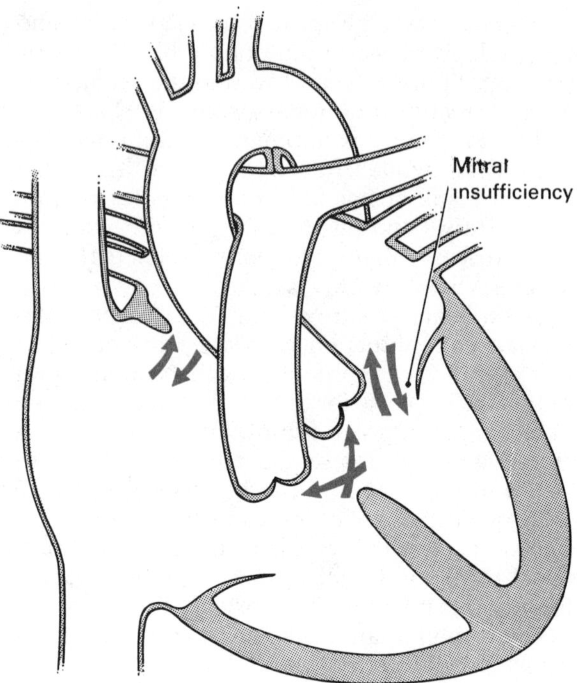

Figure 19-6 Endocardial cushion defect (complete atrioventricular canal shown).

shunting through this defect is still predominantly left to right, if pulmonary vascular resistance is low. The child with AV canal usually develops clinical symptoms similar to those of a child with a large VSD, with additional findings of variable degrees of cyanosis and atrioventricular valve insufficiency.

Preoperative CHF requires aggressive medical management. Pulmonary hypertension can develop rapidly in the child with a complete AV canal.

Pulmonary artery banding may be performed as a palliative (closed-heart) surgical procedure (see *Ventricular Septal Defect*, p. 484, for further discussion) to reduce pulmonary blood flow and relieve CHF in the child with AV canal. Complete "repair" of AV canal is electively performed when the child is more than 6 months of age but may be performed earlier with the aid of deep hypothermia if the child fails to respond to medical management of heart failure. Total "correction" of this defect consists of closure of the central defect with a single prosthetic patch or one pericardial patch and one prosthetic patch. The common atrioventricular valve is divided and sewn to the patch(es). Residual severe mitral insufficiency is usually repaired with placement of some sutures in the cleft of the insufficient mitral leaflet. Although this repair does not make the atrioventricular valves "normal," it reduces postoperative mitral insufficiency and attempts to restore normal blood flow patterns. Postoperative morbidity and mortality are related to the degree of residual mitral insufficiency and the size and function of the left ventricule. Other potential postoperative complications to be anticipated include bleeding, heart block, arrhythmias, heart failure, and low cardiac output. These patients are at risk for bacterial endocarditis whenever they have bacteremia (pre- or postoperatively).

A primum ASD is also repaired with a patch, and the cleft in the mitral valve leaflet is usually sutured. Potential postoperative complications include those following any ASD repair; the nurse should particularly monitor for arrhythmias and heart block. Congestive heart failure or low cardiac output can result if significant mitral insufficiency remains or if the left ventricle is small.

If the child is cyanotic, he or she is at risk for the development of systemic consequences of polycythemia—these are discussed in the description section of *Tetralogy of Fallot* (p. 489).

PREVENTION

Health Promotion

Reduction in incidence of Down's syndrome (trisomy 21).

1. Avoidance of pregnancy by women at risk for having infants with Down's syndrome (those with a family history and those over 35 years of age).
2. Termination of pregnancy if amniocentesis is positive for trisomy 21.

Population at Risk

Children with Down's syndrome, but not all children with ECD have Down's syndrome.

Screening

Careful physical exam, particularly of children with Down's syndrome.

ASSESSMENT

Health History

1. Note any history of feeding difficulties, diaphoresis, tachypnea, or increased respiratory effort (signs of CHF).
2. If the child has a history of cyanosis, the nurse should elicit information about signs of consequences of polycythemia (spontaneous embolus or thrombus, cerebral vascular accident, brain abscess, and postoperative bleeding).
3. While a history of cyanosis may be normal for the defect, it can also indicate development of pulmonary hypertension and reversal of shunt due to increasing pulmonary vascular resistance. Therefore, it is important to note information about onset, severity, and precipitating factors of cyanosis.

Physical Assessment

1. Congestive heart failure may be present (see *Congestive Heart Failure* (p. 460) for assessment factors).
2. Cyanosis.
   a. Cyanosis may be absent, if child's defect consists primarily of an ASD.
   b. Cyanosis will be present in child with complete AV canal, if much mixing of arterial and venous blood occurs or if pulmonary hypertension is present.
   c. With chronic cyanosis, clubbing of tips of fingers and toes will be noted.
   d. If cyanosis is present, check child's hematocrit test results for evidence of polycythemia.
   e. Cyanosis is most readily discernible in nail beds or mucous membranes (e.g., inside the child's mouth).
   f. Because the newborn has fetal hemoglobin present (with an oxyhemoglobin dissociation curve to the left of the normal adult curve), cyanosis is not apparent in the newborn until hypoxemia is more severe (Po_2 less than 50 mmHg).
   g. Cyanosis is less readily apparent if the child is anemic and more apparent if the child is polycythemic.
   h. Note the degree of cyanosis at rest and with activity.
   i. Monitor for any periods of extreme, sudden worsening of cyanosis and loss of consciousness ("tet" spells).
3. Heart sounds.
   a. Atrial septal defect produces soft pulmonic systolic murmur due to greatly increased pulmonary blood flow; fixed, wide splitting of the S_2 sound occurs (pulmonary valve closes late with high flow). With a large shunt, a tricuspid diastolic

murmur may appear and may be accompanied by a thrill due to large flow through this valve into the right ventricle. Atrial fibrillation or flutter may appear if the right atrium becomes very large.
b. Mitral insufficiency will produce a mitral systolic murmur (heard at the apex of the heart).
c. If a VSD is present, the VSD murmur is a harsh, systolic murmur heard best at the left lower sternal border and radiating over much of the chest. It may be accompanied by a thrill. If the shunt is large, causing large pulmonary blood flow, a diastolic mitral murmur may be heard over the apex when large pulmonary venous return passes into the left ventricle.
d. If pulmonary hypertension is present, the pulmonary component of the second heart sound will be loud and slapping.

4. Right bundle branch block and left axis deviation are usually noted on the ECG.
5. The abnormal facies and other signs of Down's syndrome will be noted if the child has trisomy 21.

Diagnostic Tests

ECG, echocardiogram, and cardiac catheterization.

NURSING DIAGNOSES: ACTUAL OR POTENTIAL

1. If child has CHF, see *Congestive Heart Failure* (p. 462) for diagnoses.
2. Refer to section on hospitalized children (p. 63) for diagnoses related to child's and parents' anxiety and learning needs.
3. If cyanosis is present and hematocrit is above 60 percent, child is at increased risk for spontaneous thrombus or embolus formation, brain abscess, or postoperative bleeding related to polycythemia.
4. Risk of bacterial endocarditis pre- and postoperatively (lifelong risk) related to abnormal mitral valve structure.
5. See sections under *Closed-Heart Surgery* (p. 467) and *Open-Heart Surgery* (p. 471) for diagnoses related to surgical intervention.
6. Alterations in respiratory function: progressive dyspnea and cyanosis related to severe pulmonary hypertension and consequent reversal of shunt pathway (Eisenmenger's syndrome).
7. Alterations in parenting due to guilt, anger, or grief associated with child's chromosomal abnormality, if present.
8. Developmental delay secondary to mental retardation associated with trisomy 21, if present.

EXPECTED OUTCOMES

1. See *Congestive Heart Failure* (p. 462) for expected outcomes for child with CHF.
2. Refer to hospitalized child section (p. 69) for expected outcomes for child's and parents' anxiety and learning needs.
3. Child will not develop systemic consequences of polycythemia (cerebrovascular accident, other thromboembolic disorder, or brain abscess).
4. Following cardiac catheterization, child will be free from incisional bleeding and will have normal pulses, warmth, and perfusion of the catheterized extremity.
5. See *Closed-Heart Surgery* (p. 467) and *Open-Heart Surgery* (p. 471) for postoperative client outcomes.
6. If child has incurable pulmonary hypertension, see *Pulmonary Heart Disease* (p. 991).
7. Parenting and child development will be maximized.

INTERVENTIONS

1. If child has CHF, see interventions under *Congestive Heart Failure* (p. 462).
2. Refer to section on hospitalized children (p. 69) for interventions to reduce child's and parents' anxiety and provide appropriate teaching.
3. Teach parents to contact physician if child develops prolonged or recurrent fever, vomiting, diarrhea, or irritability (may cause dehydration and danger of cerebrovascular accident or may be signs of brain abscess).
4. If the child has preoperative cyanosis, or cyanosis due to severe pulmonary hypertension and Eisenmenger's syndrome, some venous blood is passing directly into the systemic circulation. Therefore, *no air can be allowed into any intravenous line*, as it can pass into cerebral circulation and cause cerebral air embolus (stroke).
5. Interventions for child having cardiac catheterization are presented in intervention 4, under *Patent Ductus Arteriosus* (p. 474).

6. See *Closed-Heart Surgery* (p. 467) and *Open-Heart Surgery* (p. 471) for postoperative interventions, and make the following additions:
   a. There is a wide range of surgical morbidity and mortality following complete repair of this defect; if severe mitral insufficiency is present postoperatively or if the left ventricle is small, mortality is higher. Development of low cardiac output, arrhythmias, and CHF are the most frequent postoperative complications.
      (1) Ausculate the chest for mitral insufficiency murmur.
      (2) Ausculate chest and check chest x-ray film for evidence of pulmonary edema.
      (3) Monitor child carefully for the development of CHF (see assessment section under *Congestive Heart Failure*, p. 460) low cardiac output (shock), and respiratory distress.
         (a) If heart failure, pulmonary hypertension, or pulmonary edema are present, scrupulous monitoring of fluid intake and urine output is required.
         (b) Aggressive chest physiotherapy is required.
   b. Monitor for and report arrhythmia: arrhythmias occur frequently following repair of ECD.
   c. Assess child carefully for any evidence of thrombus or embolus formation, especially cerebral or pulmonary emboli.
   d. Watch closely for bleeding: children with cyanotic heart disease and polycythemia often have abnormalities of platelet function and have an increased risk of postoperative hemorrhage.
7. Refer to Chapter 12 (p. 253) for family supportive measures if child has Down's syndrome (trisomy 21).
8. If child has developmental delays and mental retardation, refer family to infant stimulation program or other special education.
9. Teach parents that child requires prophylactic antibiotics before any surgery or dental procedures, to prevent bacterial endocarditis. Penicillin is the drug of choice unless child is allergic to it.
10. If child has severe, irreversible pulmonary hypertension due to increased pulmonary vascular resistance, refer to *Pulmonary Heart Disease* (p. 992).

EVALUATION

1. See *Closed-Heart Surgery* (p. 468) and *Open-Heart Surgery* (p. 472) for evaluation and complications of postoperative care.
2. If child has CHF, refer to *Congestive Heart Failure* (p. 465) for evaluation criteria and complications.
3. If child has severe pulmonary hypertension, see *Pulmonary Heart Disease* (p. 993) for evaluation.
4. See p. 267 for evaluation of supportive measures if child has Down's syndrome.

TETRALOGY OF FALLOT

DESCRIPTION

Tetralogy of Fallot is a cyanotic heart lesion, responsible for approximately 8 percent of all congenital heart defects. It consists of four cardiac abnormalities: pulmonary (infundibular) stenosis, a VSD, right ventricular hypertrophy, and dextroposition of the aorta (the aorta is located to the right of its normal position, so that it is above the VSD) (Figure 19-7).

If the pulmonary infundibular stenosis is mild, pulmonary blood flow can be nearly normal, with a "balanced" shunt: pulmonary stenosis prevents left-to-right shunting through the VSD but is not severe enough to produce right-to-left shunting.

When pulmonary stenosis is more significant and provides more resistance to pulmonary blood flow, more and more right-to-left shunting through the VSD occurs. This causes a decrease in pulmonary blood flow and progressive cyanosis.

If pulmonary hypoplasia or atresia is present, pulmonary blood flow is severely limited, and severe cyanosis and hypoxemia may be present. With pulmonary atresia, the only source of pulmonary blood flow is the PDA and collateral circulation from the descending aorta (see also *Truncus Arteriosus*, type IV, p. 500). The neonate may suddenly deteriorate as the ductus arteriosus (the main source of the child's pulmonary blood flow) begins to close. These children require immediate surgical intervention, although

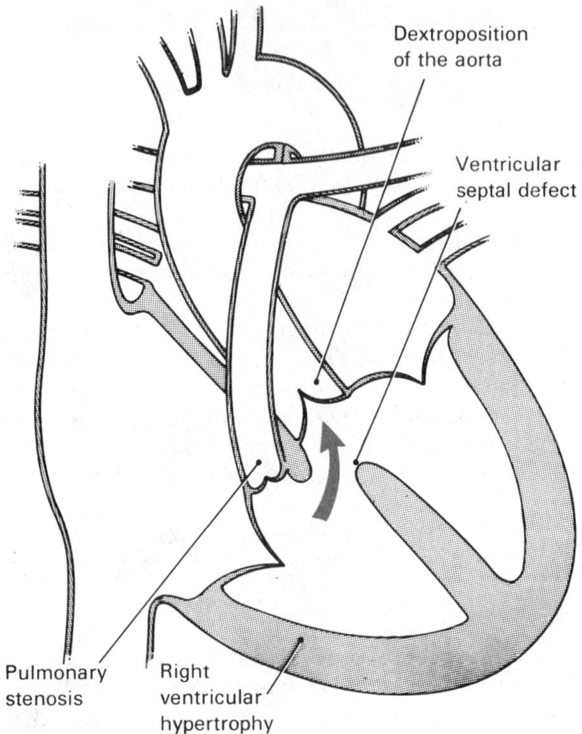

Figure 19-7 Tetralogy of Fallot.

prostaglandin E_1 may be administered temporarily to keep the ductus open (see description section of *Patent Ductus Arteriosus*, p. 472) until catheterization and surgery are performed.

Most children with tetralogy of Fallot are only slightly or moderately cyanotic at birth. During the first months of life, the pulmonary stenosis and resultant cyanosis become more severe. Congestive heart failure is rare. These children usually have elective surgical repair anytime after 6 months of age if pulmonary arteries are of adequate size, but the defect can be repaired earlier if cyanosis or compensatory polycythemia becomes severe, or if "tet" spells develop.

The hypertrophied muscles producing the pulmonary infundibular stenosis can constrict suddenly, causing acute, severe decrease in pulmonary blood flow, with severe cyanosis, hypoxemia, syncope, and possible acidosis. The onset of these "tet" spells indicates the need for urgent surgical intervention. "Tet" spells can be relieved by placing the child in the knee-chest position (this is thought to increase pulmonary blood flow by increasing systemic venous return and systemic arterial resistance). Administration of oxygen and beta-adrenergic-blocking medications or morphine can also terminate the spell.

Surgical treatment for tetralogy can be either palliative or "corrective." All forms of palliative surgery provide increased pulmonary blood flow and decrease cyanosis by creation of a shunt (abnormal route of blood flow) between the aorta and the pulmonary artery. It is hoped that the blood flow through the shunt will also stimulate growth of the main and distal pulmonary arteries, to make later corrective surgery more successful.

The most popular palliative shunt, the subclavian to pulmonary artery (*Blalock-Taussig*) anastomosis, involves attachment of the distal aspect of the subclavian artery to the pulmonary artery. This shunt then carries blood from the aorta to the pulmonary artery through the subclavian artery.

Prosthetic graft material (e.g., polytetrafluoroethylene grafts) can also be used to create a systemic-to-pulmonary artery shunt to increase pulmonary blood flow. Most frequently, shunts of this type are constricted between the subclavian artery or the aorta and the pulmonary artery.

A hole between the posterior wall of the ascending aorta and the right pulmonary artery can also be created (this is called a *Waterston* shunt). This shunt is currently less popular, because pulmonary hypertension and right pulmonary artery distortion have been reported as late complications.

Corrective (open-heart) surgery involves closure of the VSD, resection of pulmonary infundibular stenosis (one or two cloth patches may be required to enlarge adequately the pulmonary artery and right ventricular outflow tract), and closure of any previously constructed palliative shunts. Potential postoperative complications to be anticipated include bleeding, heart failure (especially right heart failure), arrhythmias, heart block, and respiratory insufficiency.

Systemic Consequences of Polycythemia

Most children with chronic hypoxemia develop compensatory polycythemia. As a result, these children have a higher risk of spontaneous thrombus and embolus formation, which can cause a cerebrovascular accident (particularly under the age of 2 years), brain abscess (after the age of 2 years), and postoperative bleeding. Platelet dysfunction can contribute to these problems.

The risk of cerebrovascular accident is thought to increase significantly if the child's hematocrit is above 60 percent. Dehydration, causing a rise in hematocrit due to hemoconcentration, microcytic anemia, and bacteremia can also increase the risk of cerebrovascular accident.

Any child with cyanotic heart disease should have intravenous lines monitored closely to *prevent air infusion, since any intravenous air entering the right ventricle can be shunted into the systemic arterial circulation, causing a cerebral air embolus (stroke).*

PREVENTION

Health Promotion

There is no known prevention for tetralogy of Fallot.

Population at Risk

Newborn infants.

Screening

Physical examination.

ASSESSMENT

Health History

1. History of cyanosis: it is extremely important to obtain information about the onset, severity, precipitating or alleviating factors, and distribution of cyanosis.
2. If the parent feels the child's cyanosis is getting worse or increasing at rest, the physician should be notified, as child may require surgical intervention. The parent should be asked his or her opinion about any deterioration in the child's condition.
3. A history of squatting during play may reflect the child's instinctive attempt to increase pulmonary blood flow to feel better or continue playing. Squatting serves the same purpose as the knee-chest position (see discussion of "tet" spells, above).
4. A history of "tet" spells should be reported to the physician immediately.
5. The development of a brain abscess or septic embolus is often preceded by bacteremia, so recent illness should be investigated, as well as recent history of vomiting, irritability, fever, and headaches.

Physical Assessment

1. The infant with tetralogy may have few signs or symptoms at birth but usually becomes progressively cyanotic during infancy.
2. Development of CHF is unusual preoperatively.
3. Cyanosis is usually present.
   a. Cyanosis is most readily discernible in nail beds or mucous membranes (inside the child's mouth).
   b. Because the newborn has fetal hemoglobin present (with an oxyhemoglobin dissociation curve to the left of the normal adult curve), cyanosis is not apparent in the newborn until hypoxemia is more severe (Po_2 less than 50 mmHg).
   c. Cyanosis is less readily apparent if the child is anemic and more apparent if the child is polycythemic.
   d. Note the degree of cyanosis at rest and with activity.
   e. Monitor for any periods of extreme, sudden worsening of cyanosis and loss of consciousness ("tet" spells).
   f. With chronic cyanosis, clubbing of tips of fingers and toes will be present.
   g. If a palliative shunt has been created, note its effect on the child's color; usually color improves initially but returns or worsens within a few months or years as the child "outgrows" the shunt.
4. Heart sounds.
   a. Child will have a systolic pulmonic murmur caused by turbulent blood flow through stenotic area, with possible precordial thrill.
   b. A harsh, systolic murmur is noted at the left lower sternal border due to ventricular septal defect; it may be accompanied by a thrill.
   c. A right ventricular (sternal) lift may be palpated.
5. Neurological assessment should be performed if there is any suspicion of brain abscess or cerebrovascular accident.
6. Note child's hematocrit. Hematocrit near or above 60 percent, particularly with a microcytic anemia, is associated with increased incidence of spontaneous cerebrovascular accident.

7. Assess child's level of hydration, since hematocrit can rise with dehydration (due to hemoconcentration).

Diagnostic Tests

Echocardiogram and cardiac catheterization.

NURSING DIAGNOSES: ACTUAL OR POTENTIAL

1. See section on hospitalized children (p. 63) for diagnoses related to child and parent anxiety and learning needs. Keep in mind that cyanosis is a very visible reminder of the child's heart disease. This visibility often causes more anxiety for parents and decreases the possibility of normal lifestyle for the child, since schoolmates and all others are aware of the defect.
2. Risk for cerebrovascular accident, brain abscess, and postoperative hemorrhage due to cyanotic heart disease and systemic consequences of polycythemia.
3. Risk for development of bacterial endocarditis, both preoperatively and postoperatively, due to turbulent intracardiac blood flow.
4. Risk for profound cyanosis, loss of consciousness, hypoxemia, and acidosis related to infundibular muscle spasm ("tet" spell).
5. See sections *Closed-Heart Surgery* (p. 467) and *Open-Heart Surgery* (p. 471) for diagnoses related to surgery.

EXPECTED OUTCOMES

1. See section on hospitalized children (p. 69) for expected outcomes of care related to child's and parents' anxiety and learning needs.
2. Child will not develop cerebral air embolus, cerebrovascular accident, or brain abscess.
3. Child will not develop bacterial endocarditis.
4. Child will be placed promptly in the knee-chest position if "tet" spell occurs and will receive prompt administration of oxygen and prompt attention by physician.
5. Following cardiac catheterization, incision will not bleed, and incised extremity will have normal color, warmth, pulses, and perfusion.
6. See *Closed-Heart Surgery* (p. 467) and *Open-Heart Surgery* (p. 471) for expected outcomes.

INTERVENTIONS

1. Refer to section on hospitalized children (p. 69) for interventions to reduce child's and parents' anxiety and meet their learning needs.
2. See section on hospitalized children, intervention 9, for teaching about child's home care; make the following additions:
   a. Until child has correction of tetralogy, parents should be aware of the possibility of "tet" spells, taught to place the child in the knee-chest position, and to contact physician if they occur.
   b. Parents should be taught to contact physician if child develops prolonged or recurrent fever, vomiting, diarrhea, or irritability (may result in dehydration and increased risk of cerebrovascular accident or may be signs of brain abscess).
   c. Teach parents that child requires prophylactic antibiotics before any surgical or dental procedure, in order to avoid bacterial endocarditis. Penicillin is the drug of choice unless child is allergic to it.
3. Monitor carefully for signs of increased cardiorespiratory distress preoperatively:
   a. Watch for deepening of cyanosis.
   b. Monitor heart rate and rhythm—severe hypoxemia can compromise heart function.
   c. Note respiratory rate and effort: tachypnea or hyperpnea can occur.
   d. Increased irritability, lethargy, or fatigue can also indicate increased respiratory distress.
   e. Monitor blood gas values if child's condition warrants. The development of acidosis usually indicates serious deterioration and need for prompt surgical intervention.
   f. Note child's tolerance of activity or vigorous cry; notify physician if increased cyanosis occurs at rest.
4. If child demonstrates a "tet" spell
   a. Place child immediately in the knee-chest position and administer oxygen.
   b. Notify physician immediately, and administer beta-adrenergic blockade medications as ordered.
5. Monitor child's fluid balance carefully. Calculate child's maintenance fluid daily, and discuss with physician if child's fluid intake is inappropriate (see Table 19-6). Monitor level of hydration closely if child is NPO for surgical or medical procedure; it may be necessary to provide intravenous fluids if oral fluids must be restricted for several hours.

6. As long as child's intracardiac right-to-left shunt is present, *absolutely no air can be allowed into intravenous lines*, as it can be shunted into systemic circulation, causing cerebral air embolus.
7. Child will usually not require any activity restriction, since he or she will probably limit own activity based on physical tolerance.
8. See *Patent Ductus Arteriosus* (p. 474) intervention 4, for postcatheterization care.
9. See postoperative care interventions listed under *Closed-Heart Surgery* (p. 467) or *Open-Heart Surgery* (p. 471); make the following additions:
   a. Provide *thorough* neurological assessment for the first 2 postoperative days. Notify physician of any abnormalities that may indicate cerebral thrombus or embolus.
   b. Monitor chest tube output closely, report suspected postoperative hemorrhage immediately, and provide prompt and adequate blood replacement to prevent hypovolemia. (These children are particularly prone to bleeding postoperatively, since with polycythemia platelets are usually abnormal in number and/or function.)
   c. *Monitor closely* for early evidence of CHF (see *Congestive Heart Failure*, p. 460, for assessments). Treatment with digitalis derivative, diuretics, and fluid restriction may be necessary.
   d. Monitor for signs of poor systemic perfusion and low cardiac output: poor peripheral pulses, cool extremities, decreased urine output, possible high rectal temperature, possible acidosis, and (a late sign) hypotension. Report these observations to physician immediately. Child may require treatment with volume expander, sympathomimetic drugs, or vasodilation.
   e. Monitor for arrhythmias or heart block, since surgery was performed in area of conduction tissue. Since a right ventricular incision is made for the repair, right bundle branch block is almost inevitable.
   f. Monitor for right ventricular dysfunction, which may be increased by postoperative pulmonary vasoconstriction. This is thought to occur in some clients with tetralogy due to the presence of preoperative pulmonary microemboli or the development of postoperative alveolar hypoxia, acidosis, or hypothermia.
   g. To avoid respiratory insufficiency postoperatively, pulmonary support must be meticulous.

EVALUATION

1. If child has postoperative heart failure, see evaluation criteria and complications listed under *Congestive Heart Failure* (p. 465).
2. See section on hospitalized children (p. 71) for evaluation of efforts to reduce child's and family's anxiety and to meet their learning needs.
3. See *Closed-Heart Surgery* (p. 468) and *Open-Heart Surgery* (p. 472) for evaluation of postoperative care and complications following surgery.

PULMONARY VALVULAR STENOSIS AND ATRESIA

DESCRIPTION

Pulmonary valvular stenosis results from improper formation of the valve leaflets, causing resistance to right ventricular outflow. Pulmonary valvular atresia results when the valve commissures fail to form, so a membrane totally occludes the pulmonary artery where the valve would normally be located.

With any obstruction to right ventricular outflow, the right ventricle hypertrophies. With severe stenosis or atresia, pulmonary blood flow is drastically reduced, right ventricular end-diastolic pressure increases, and right atrial pressure rises. This can cause the foramen ovale to reopen, resulting in right-to-left atrial shunting and cyanosis.

Pulmonary valve atresia causes severe cyanosis in the first hours of life, and the child may decompensate rapidly if the PDA begins to close, since the PDA is the child's only source of pulmonary blood flow. These infants require immediate surgical intervention, although intravenous prostaglandins can be administered temporarily to keep the ductus arteriosus open. The Brock procedure (a form of closed-heart surgery) involves insertion of a curved blade into the right ventricle to cut open the pulmonary valve (membrane). An open-heart pulmonary valvulotomy under direct visualization can also be performed using deep hypothermia in the neonate.

Most children with isolated pulmonary stenosis do not require urgent surgical intervention. They usually have no cyanosis and remain fairly asymptomatic, with only mild exercise intolerance. If the stenosis is becoming more severe, cyanosis or polycythemia may appear—this is an indication that surgery is necessary. Generally, these children have an open-heart pulmonary valvulotomy electively before school age.

If cyanosis is present, these children are at risk for development of systemic consequences of cyanosis (see discussion of polycythemia in *Tetralogy of Fallot*, description section, p. 490). Their risk of bacterial endocarditis is low.

Potential postoperative complications include bleeding, arrhythmias, and, less frequently, CHF.

TRICUSPID ATRESIA

DESCRIPTION

Tricuspid atresia accounts for approximately 1 percent of all congenital heart disease. It occurs as a result of complete failure of tricuspid valve development; no opening exists between the right atrium and the right ventricle, and the right ventricle and pulmonary outflow tract are hypoplastic (Figure 19-8).

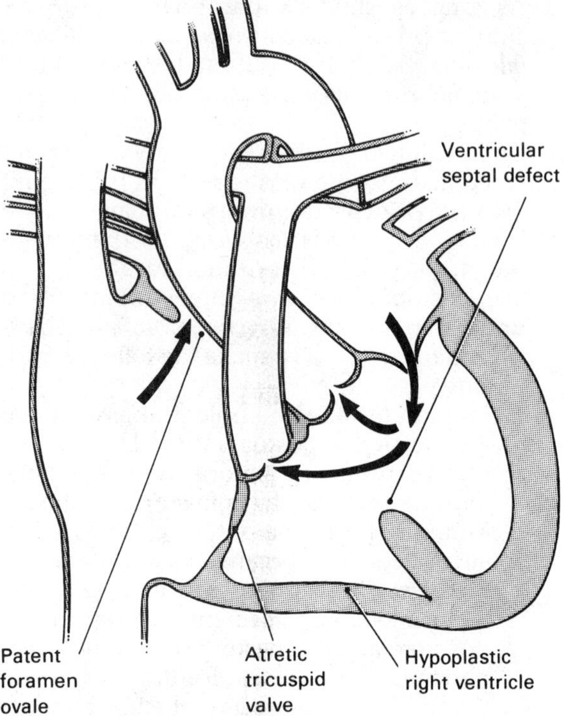

Figure 19-8 Tricuspid atresia with ventricular septal defect.

The child requires the presence of several other congenital cardiac abnormalities to survive; otherwise the infant has no source of pulmonary blood flow. Most commonly, a foramen ovale ASD, a VSD, and some degree of pulmonary stenosis are present (transposition of the great vessels may also be present). The foramen ovale is usually forced open as a result of engorgement of the right atrium; this allows shunting of blood from the right to the left atrium. The VSD allows some blood to return to the right heart and pass into the pulmonary artery, although the amount of this left-to-right shunting is restricted by the size of the VSD and the degree of pulmonary stenosis.

The child with tricuspid atresia may demonstrate a wide variety of clinical signs and symptoms, depending on the quantity of pulmonary blood flow. If pulmonary blood flow is significantly reduced, cyanosis is severe, and the child requires surgical intervention in the first days of life to increase pulmonary blood flow and to improve arterial oxygen saturation. If pulmonary blood flow is excessive, the child may develop CHF and only moderate cyanosis. This child requires careful medical management of the heart failure and may require palliative surgery to reduce pulmonary blood flow (pulmonary artery banding, described under *Ventricular Septal Defect*, p. 484).

The child may have signs of systemic venous engorgement (hepatomegaly, periorbital edema) if the foramen ovale is too small to allow free passage of blood from the right to the left atrium. In this case, a balloon atrial septostomy is performed during cardiac catheterization to enlarge the communication between the right and the left atria. The cardiologist performs the atrial septostomy (called the Rashkind balloon septostomy) by inserting a balloon-tipped catheter through the foramen ovale. Once the tip of the catheter is in the left atrium, the cardiologist inflates the balloon and pulls it back into the right atrium. This tears a larger hole in the atrial septum. The procedure is not painful. If the atrial septostomy does not provide an adequate hole to allow mixing of blood in the atria and free flow of blood from the right to the left atrium, surgical removal of a portion of atrial septum can be performed. This surgery is called the Blalock-Hanlon septectomy and is performed without use of cardiopulmonary bypass.

Palliative systemic-to-pulmonary artery shunts can be created to increase the child's pulmonary blood flow. Most commonly, a communication between the child's aorta and the pulmonary artery is created, utilizing the subclavian artery alone, or utilizing a prosthetic graft between the subclavian and a pulmonary artery, or between the aorta and pulmonary artery.

A Glenn procedure can be performed as a palliative procedure or as the first step in the correction of tricuspid atresia. This procedure is a form of closed-heart surgery. The superior vena cava is detached from the right atrium and sewn to the pulmonary artery (usually to the right pulmonary artery). Thus, all of the venous blood from the superior vena cava will flow directly into the pulmonary artery, bypassing the heart completely. This procedure should improve the child's systemic arterial oxygenation, since only the inferior vena caval blood (approximately one-half of the systemic venous blood) will enter the right atrium and pass to the left side of the heart, mixing with (oxygenated) pulmonary venous blood.

The surgical procedure for repair of tricuspid atresia is called the Fontan procedure and requires open-heart surgery. In the repair, a connection is made between the right atrium and the pulmonary artery. This connection can consist of a valved conduit, a valveless conduit, or a portion of the right atrium. As a result of the procedure, the systemic venous blood that enters the right atrium is conducted to the pulmonary artery. The child's pulmonary vascular resistance must be low for this procedure to be attempted. Occasionally, the right ventricle will also be joined to the right atrium and the pulmonary artery by the connection, so that the right ventricle can be given the opportunity to grow. At the time the Fontan procedure is performed, other systemic-to-pulmonary artery shunts are eliminated, although the Glenn shunt may remain.

Preoperatively, these children are at risk for the development of systemic consequences of polycythemia (these include thromboembolic events and brain abscess, as well as abnormalities of platelet function). These children also have a higher risk of bacterial endocarditis.

Potential postoperative complications include neurological complications (from emboli), CHF, arrhythmias, and bleeding. Often, following the Fontan procedure, the child will demonstrate persistent signs of systemic venous engorgement (including hepatomegaly, periorbital edema, and ascites) for weeks after surgery.

TRANSPOSITION OF THE GREAT VESSELS

DESCRIPTION

Transposition of the great vessels (TGV) is a defect in which the normal relationship of the ventricles to the great vessels is reversed: the aorta arises from the right ventricle, and the pulmonary artery arises from the left ventricle (Figure 19-9). Transposition of the great vessels is often found in combination with other defects; an ASD, a VSD, a PDA, pulmonary stenosis, or tricuspid atresia may be present. Transposition of the great vessels accounts for approximately 4 percent of all congenital heart lesions but is the most common cyanotic heart lesion causing symptoms in the newborn period.

If simple TGV is present, systemic venous return passes through the right heart and back into the systemic arterial circulation from the aorta (without receiving oxygen). Pulmonary venous blood enters the left heart and returns to the pulmonary circulation through the pulmonary artery. If the child has no additional shunt allowing some of the poorly oxygenated systemic venous blood to mix with the oxygenated pulmonary venous blood, the child will display severe distress (cyanosis, hypoxemia, and acidosis) within hours of life.

If a large ASD is present or if the child's foramen ovale is large, fairly good mixing of oxygenated (pulmonary venous) and deoxygenated (systemic venous) blood occurs within the atria; this usually improves systemic arterial oxygenation. An ASD does produce an increase in pulmonary blood flow, but the flow is under low pressure, so development of CHF is unusual. If atrial mixing is very effective, cyanosis is minimal, although the ASD may need to be enlarged by cardiac catheterization or surgery.

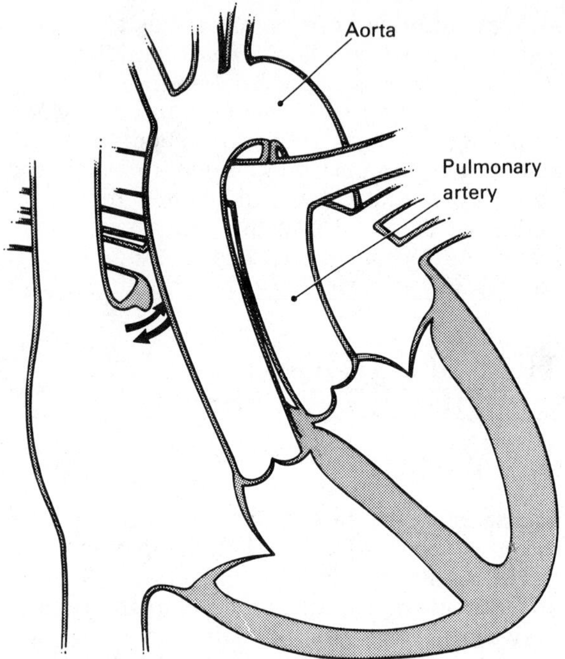

Figure 19-9 Transposition of the great vessels with atrial septal defect. This hemodynamic pattern may exist naturally or occur as a result of Rashkind or Blalock-Hanlon procedures.

During cardiac catheterization of the neonate, a balloon-tipped catheter may be used to produce a large hole in the atrial septum; this procedure is known as a *Rashkind balloon atrial septostomy*. The enlarged interatrial shunt may provide enough mixing of blood (and better arterial oxygen saturation) to postpone further palliative or corrective surgery until the child is several months of age. If the Rashkind procedure does not provide adequate mixing, a *Blalock-Hanlon atrial septectomy* may be performed. This closed-heart procedure is performed through an anterior thoracotomy and involves removal of most of the atrial septum. This procedure usually provides thorough mixing of oxygenated and deoxygenated blood. If either of these procedures is successful, the child should respond with an immediate improvement in arterial oxygen saturation.

A VSD does not usually provide adequate mixing of systemic and pulmonary venous blood and may complicate the child's clinical picture, causing the development of CHF after the first weeks of life. If moderate pulmonary stenosis is present with the VSD, however, it may prevent large pulmonary blood flow (under high pressure) and CHF. In addition, the pulmonary stenosis may promote shunting of oxygenated (left ventricular) blood into the aorta, improving the child's systemic arterial oxygen saturation. The presence of severe pulmonary stenosis, however, would drastically reduce the child's pulmonary blood flow and result in severe hypoxemia and cyanosis.

If pulmonary blood flow is excessive (e.g., due to a large VSD without pulmonary stenosis), the child will develop CHF, in addition to cyanosis, within the first weeks of life. This child will require vigorous medical management of the CHF. If the CHF is not controlled with medical management, surgical intervention is required. Corrective surgery is often performed at this time, although some surgeons may prefer to perform pulmonary artery banding (see *Ventricular Septal Defect*, p. 484).

If severe pulmonary stenosis is causing decreased pulmonary blood flow, CHF will not be present, but cyanosis and hypoxemia will be severe, particularly once the PDA closes. Prostaglandin E_1 is administered intravenously (0.05–0.1 μg/kg/min) to the neonate in an effort to keep the ductus arteriosus patent, increase pulmonary blood flow, and reduce the neonate's hypoxemia. If needed, a permanent shunt is surgically created. A Blalock-Taussig shunt is performed through a thoracotomy and involves joining the subclavian artery to a pulmonary artery. Other shunts between the aorta and the main pulmonary artery or the right or left pulmonary arteries can be created utilizing a prosthetic material (polytetrafluoroethylene or Gore-tex or Impra). These shunts should improve effective pulmonary blood flow and reduce the child's hypoxemia.

Preoperatively, children with TGV are at risk for the development of systemic consequences of polycythemia (thromboembolic phenomena and brain abscess). The risk of cerebrovascular accident or death is particularly high during the period between cardiac catheterization and surgery.

Corrective surgery most frequently is either the Mustard or the Senning procedure; both require open-heart surgery. Both procedures provide redirection of atrial (systemic and pulmonary venous) blood, using an intra-atrial baffle. As a result, systemic venous blood is diverted through the atria to the mitral valve; it then passes into the left ventricle and to the pulmonary artery, so that it enters the pulmonary circulation and receives oxygen. Pulmonary venous blood is diverted to the tricuspid valve; it then enters the right ventricle, then the aorta, and passes into the systemic arterial circulation. These repairs are performed on children of any age; deep hypothermia may be utilized if the repair is required during the neonatal period.

Potential postoperative complications include CHF, bleeding, arrhythmias (especially those originating in the atria), heart block, and potential perioperative cerebrovascular accident. Children who have had these corrective operations are all followed indefinitely postoperatively, since late onset arrhythmias, systemic or pulmonary venous obstruction due to baffle obstruction, and sudden death have been reported. In addition, the long-term function of the right ventricle and tricuspid valve is uncertain.

Recently, attempts to correct TGV by switching the great vessels has received renewed support. The great vessel switch or Jatene procedure requires open-heart surgery. Not only are the great vessels detached from their original inappropriate ventricles, and reattached to the appropriate ventricles, but the coronary arteries must also be reimplanted into the aorta at its new location. The Jatene operation currently has a somewhat higher perioperative risk than the Mustard procedure but is thought to provide better long-term results, since blood flow patterns are more nearly normal afterwards. However, long-term follow-up of children after the Jatene has not yet been accomplished, since the surgery has only recently been performed in a significant number of children. The Jatene operation must be performed in the neonatal period, while the left ventricle is still thick, or else a pulmonary artery banding must be performed so that the left ventricle remains muscular. This preparation of the left ventricle is necessary if the left ventricle is to be able to generate high pressure to supply the systemic circulation following the Jatene repair.

Postoperative complications following the Jatene repair include low cardiac output (shock), CHF, bleeding, arrhythmias, and neurological complications (seizures, cerebrovascular accident, etc.).

PREVENTION

Health Promotion

No known method of prevention.

Population at Risk

There is an increased incidence of TGV in the offspring of insulin-dependent diabetic mothers, although the vast majority of children with TGV have no recognizable risk factors.

Screening

Good neonatal physical exam.

ASSESSMENT

Health History

1. Details of degree and onset of cyanosis are important.
   a. Circumoral cyanosis or acrocyanosis can be normal in neonates.
   b. Cyanosis relieved by crying can indicate that hypoxemia is respiratory in origin: lung aeration improves during crying and causes improved respiratory function and decreased cyanosis.
   c. Cyanosis aggravated by crying can indicate that hypoxemia is cardiac in origin: resistance to pulmonary blood flow is increased during expiratory phase of cry and causes decreased pulmonary blood flow and increased cyanosis.
2. Inquire about history of feeding difficulties, diaphoresis, tachypnea, or increased respiratory effort, which may indicate CHF.
3. Increased risk of brain abscess and septic cerebral emboli is associated with episodes of bacteremia (although some brain abscesses occur with no documented bacteremia), so history of recent illnesses should be investigated, as well as recent history of vomiting, irritability, fever, headaches, or seizures.

Physical Assessment

1. Children with TGV may be minimally or severely cyanotic. They do not have "tet" spells, described under *Tetralogy of Fallot* (p. 489).
   a. Cyanosis is most readily discernible in nail

beds or mucous membranes (inside the child's mouth).

b. Because the newborn has fetal hemoglobin present (with an oxyhemoglobin dissociation curve located to the left of the normal adult curve), cyanosis is not apparent in the newborn until hypoxemia is more severe (Po_2 less than 50 mmHg).
c. Cyanosis is less readily apparent if the child is anemic and more apparent if the child is polycythemic.
d. Note the degree of cyanosis at rest and with activity.
e. With chronic cyanosis, clubbing of tips of fingers and toes will be present.
f. If a palliative shunt has been created, note its effect on the child's color; usually color improves initially, but as the child "outgrows" the shunt within a few months or years the cyanosis returns or worsens.

2. There is no characteristic murmur associated with TGV; the murmurs noted in these children are those characteristic of associated lesions (VSD, pulmonary stenosis, PDA, etc.). Children with TGV do have a loud, single S_2 heard best in the pulmonic area (this sound is actually due to aortic valve closure).
3. The child should be assessed closely for evidence of CHF (see *Congestive Heart Failure*, p. 459) if a VSD is present.
4. Thorough neurological assessments should be performed throughout the child's hospitalization; they should be recorded particularly following cardiac catheterization and surgery, since the child is at risk for development of spontaneous cerebrovascular accident.
5. Note the child's hematocrit, and notify physician if it is near or exceeding 60 percent (this is the level associated with increased risk of spontaneous cerebrovascular accident).
6. Monitor for evidence of dehydration (depressed fontanelle in infants under age 18 months, dry mucous membranes, "tenting" of skin), since the hematocrit can rise due to hemoconcentration.
7. The child's arterial oxygen saturation and Po_2 may be extremely low. The nurse should assess the correlation between the child's appearance (and level of cyanosis) and blood gas values and notify the physician if the arterial Po_2 drops or the child's appearance deteriorates.

Diagnostic Tests

Echocardiogram and cardiac catheterization.

NURSING DIAGNOSES: ACTUAL OR POTENTIAL

1. Please see section on hospitalized children (p. 63) for diagnoses related to child's and parents' anxiety and learning needs. Keep in mind that cyanosis is a highly visible reminder of the child's heart disease. This visibility often causes more anxiety for parents and decreases the possibility of a normal lifestyle for the child since schoolmates and others are aware of the cardiac disease.
2. Risk of cerebrovascular accident, brain abscess, and postoperative hemorrhage due to systemic consequences of polycythemia.
3. Risk of bacterial endocarditis, both pre- and postoperatively, due to turbulent intracardiac blood flow.
4. Risk of profound hypoxemia and metabolic acidosis if there is inadequate mixing of pulmonary venous (oxygenated) blood with systemic venous blood. NOTE: The development of acidosis usually signals decompensation in these infants and the need for urgent surgical intervention.
5. If child has CHF, refer to *Congestive Heart Failure* (p. 462) for additional diagnoses.
6. See *Closed-Heart Surgery* (p. 467) and *Open-Heart Surgery* (p. 471) for diagnoses related to surgery.

EXPECTED OUTCOMES

1. See section on hospitalized children (p. 69) for outcomes expected from care related to child's and parents' anxiety and learning needs.
2. Child will not develop cerebral air embolus, cerebrovascular accident, or brain abscess.
3. If child has CHF, see *Congestive Heart Failure* (p. 462) for expected outcomes of care.
4. Child will not develop bacterial endocarditis.
5. Child will demonstrate no deterioration in color, and there will be no evidence of further arterial oxygen desaturation and acidosis throughout preoperative period; following surgical correction of TGV, child will be free from cyanosis and will have normal arterial oxygen saturation and acid-base balance.
6. Following cardiac catheterization, incision

will not bleed, and pulse, warmth, and perfusion will remain normal in the catheterized extremity.

7. See *Closed-Heart Surgery* (p. 467) and *Open-Heart Surgery* (p. 471) for expected outcomes of postoperative care.

INTERVENTIONS

1. Refer to hospitalized child section (p. 69) for interventions to reduce child's and family's anxiety and to meet their learning needs.
2. See hospitalized child section, intervention 9, for teaching of child's home care, with the following additions:
   a. Before surgical repair: Parents should be taught to contact physician if child has prolonged or recurrent fever, vomiting, diarrhea, or irritability; these signs may indicate brain abscess or may lead to dehydration and increased risk of cerebrovascular accident.
   b. Teach parents that in order to avoid bacterial endocarditis, child requires prophylactic antibiotics before any dental or surgical procedure. Penicillin is the drug of choice unless child is allergic to it.
3. Monitor carefully for signs of increased cardiorespiratory distress preoperatively:
   a. Watch for deepening of cyanosis.
   b. Monitor heart rate and rhythm: severe hypoxemia can compromise cardiac function.
   c. Note respiratory rate and effort: tachypnea or hyperpnea may be seen.
   d. Increased irritability, lethargy, or fatigue can also indicate increased distress.
   e. Monitor blood gas values if child's condition warrants. The development of acidosis usually indicates serious deterioration and the need for prompt surgical intervention.
   f. Note child's tolerance of activity or vigorous cry; notify physician if increased cyanosis occurs at rest.
4. Monitor child's fluid balance carefully. Calculate child's maintenance fluid daily, and discuss with physician if child's fluid intake is inappropriate (see Table 19-6). Monitor level of hydration closely if child is NPO for surgical or medical procedure; it may be necessary to provide intravenous fluids if oral fluids must be restricted for several hours.
5. As long as child's intracardiac right-to-left shunt is present, *absolutely no air can be allowed into intravenous lines*, as it may be shunted into systemic circulation, causing cerebral air embolus.
6. If the child has CHF, refer to interventions listed under *Congestive Heart Failure* (p. 462).
7. See *Patent Ductus Arteriosus* (p. 474) intervention 4, for postcatheterization care.
8. See interventions under *Closed-Heart Surgery* (p. 467) and *Open-Heart Surgery* (p. 471); make the following additions:
   a. Provide *thorough* neurological assessment for the first 2 postoperative days. Notify physician of any abnormalities that may indicate cerebral thrombus or embolus.
   b. Monitor chest tube output closely; report suspected postoperative hemorrhage immediately, and provide prompt and adequate blood replacement to prevent hypovolemia. (Children with cyanosis and polycythemia are particularly prone to bleeding postoperatively, since their platelets are usually abnormal in number and/or function.)
   c. Monitor *closely* for early evidence of CHF (see *Congestive Heart Failure*, p. 460). Treatment with digitalis derivative, diuretics, and fluid restrictions may be necessary.
   d. Baffle obstruction can cause postoperative evidence of pulmonary or systemic venous engorgement—the nurse should monitor for evidence of venous engorgement and discuss with physician. NOTE: Superior vena caval obstruction postoperatively in infants has been associated with development of hydrocephalus and chylothorax in small infants.
      (1) While chest tube is in place, monitor for presence of milky drainage (lymph), which can occur due to injury of large lymphatic during dissection for surgical repair. If chylothorax is present, chest tube should not be removed until lymph drainage has ceased.
         (a) Since lymph drainage represents loss of fat, some physicians advocate administration of a low-fat diet to the child, to prevent further fat absorption (and loss through the chylothorax).
         (b) Child should receive supplemental fat soluable vitamins.

(2) Once chest tube is removed, monitor carefully for evidence of pleural fluid, which can indicate accumulation of chylothorax. If present, chylous fluid will need to be evacuated with chest tube.
   (a) The most likely postoperative arrhythmias are supraventricular arrhythmias or heart block, since extensive suturing in the atria is necessary for the Mustard and Senning procedures.
   (b) Respiratory insufficiency can occur postoperatively and will be increased if any pulmonary venous obstruction due to the intra-atrial baffle is present. Accordingly, pulmonary support must be skilled and meticulous.

EVALUATION

1. See section on hospitalized children (p. 71) for evaluation of efforts to reduce child's and parents' anxiety and to meet their learning needs.
2. Refer to *Congestive Heart Failure* (p. 465) for evaluation of interventions to treat the child who has CHF.
3. See *Closed-Heart Surgery* (p. 468) and *Open-Heart Surgery* (p. 472) for evaluation of postoperative care.

TRUNCUS ARTERIOSUS

DESCRIPTION

Truncus arteriosus is a defect that occurs when the common fetal great vessel fails to divide normally into a pulmonary artery and aorta. As a result, a single great vessel arises from both ventricles, straddling a VSD.

If the pulmonary branches from the trunk are large, pulmonary blood flow can become excessive at approximately 4 to 12 weeks of age (when pulmonary vascular resistance drops), and CHF results from increased pulmonary blood flow under high pressure (Figure 19-10).

If there is no major pulmonary artery branch from the trunk or existing branches are small or stenotic, pulmonary blood flow occurs through the small pulmonary artery(-ies), if they exist, or through development of collateral circulation from enlarged bronchial and mammary arteries from the descending aorta (Figure 19-11). In either case the infant is extremely cyanotic at birth. This defect is also known as pulmonary atresia, or pseudotruncus.

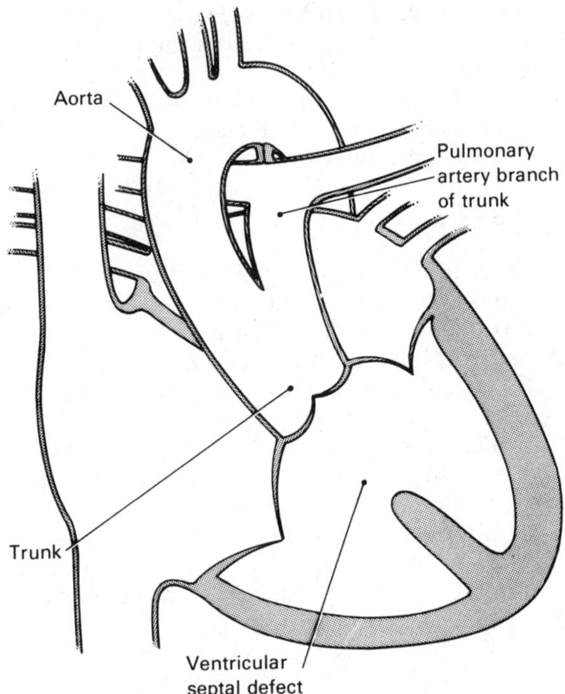

Figure 19-10 Truncus arteriosus, type I.

As systemic *and* pulmonary venous blood enter the trunk, some cyanosis will be present (since systemic arterial blood is mixed with systemic venous blood). Therefore, these children are at risk for development of systemic consequences of cyanosis and polycythemia, discussed under *Tetralogy of Fallot* (p. 490).

If pulmonary blood flow is excessive, causing CHF, banding of the pulmonary artery branch(es) can be performed during infancy (this surgery is described under *Ventricular Septal Defect*, p. 484). If pulmonary blood flow is inadequate, resulting in hypoxemia and severe cyanosis, a Blalock-Taussig or prosthetic systemic–pulmonary artery shunt may be performed (these procedures are described under *Tetralogy of Fallot*, p. 489).

Corrective (open-heart) surgery involves closure of the VSD so the left ventricular outflow

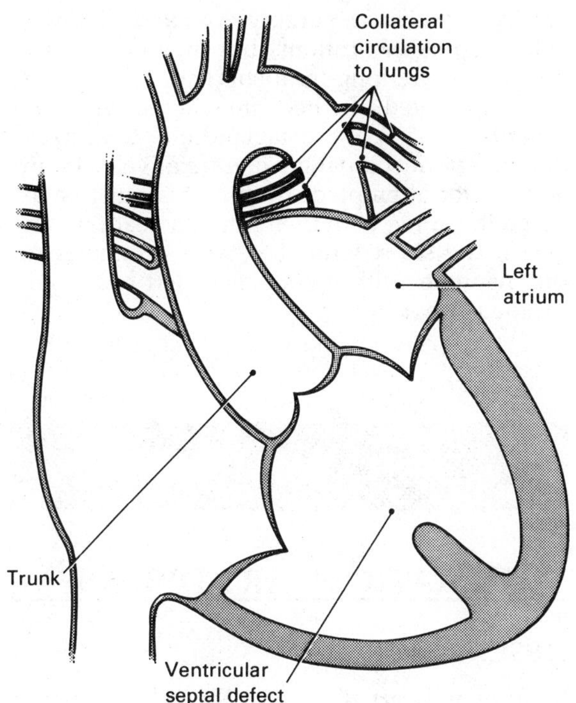

Figure 19-11 Truncus arteriosus, type IV ("pseudotruncus").

enters the trunk. A valved conduit is then placed between the right ventricle and main (or distal) pulmonary artery(-ies).

Potential postoperative complications include bleeding, low cardiac output, CHF, arrhythmias, and heart block.

TOTAL ANOMALOUS PULMONARY VENOUS RETURN OR CONNECTION

DESCRIPTION

Total anomalous pulmonary venous return (TAPVR) also called total anomalous pulmonary venous connection (TAPVC) results from failure of the pulmonary veins to join with the left atrium during fetal development. As a result, pulmonary venous blood returns to the heart through the systemic venous circulation. Thus, no totally oxygenated blood is ever delivered to the systemic circulation, and the child is cyanotic. In addition, all systemic and pulmonary venous blood is returned to the right atrium; some of this mixed venous blood is shunted to the left atrium through an ASD or patent foramen ovale. Right ventricular failure can occur as a result of volume overload, and the left atrium and ventricle may be small, because of reduced flow to the left heart.

In most forms of TAPVR the pulmonary venous blood enters the systemic venous circulation near the heart. These children present with mild to moderate cyanosis and possible heart failure. They also demonstrate evidence of some systemic venous engorgement if the existing ASD (or patent foramen ovale) is too small to allow free flow of blood to the left side of the heart.

If pulmonary venous blood joins systemic venous circulation *below the diaphragm* (infradiaphragmatic TAPVR), the systemic veins will probably provide some resistance to flow. The pulmonary veins usually join the hepatic circulation in TAPVR below the diaphragm. This causes pulmonary venous obstruction and severe pulmonary edema in the first few weeks of life. The child with TAPVR below the diaphragm usually presents in severe distress at this time and requires aggressive medical management and pulmonary care, preceding urgent surgical intervention. The diagnosis is suspected in a child who develops cyanosis and severe pulmonary edema in the first weeks of life, with no significant heart murmur or primary respiratory disease.

Corrective (open-heart) surgery utilizes deep hypothermia in neonates and involves joining of the pulmonary veins to the back of the left atrium (they usually join in a common vessel directly behind the left atrium; this vessel is the one joined to the back of the left atrium).

Potential postoperative complications include bleeding, CHF, and supraventricular arrhythmias. If the infant had the infradiaphragmatic form of TAPVR, respiratory failure and low cardiac output are the most severe postoperative complications. Since these infants often have preoperative pulmonary hypertension, postoperative weaning from respiratory support and postoperative respiratory care must be excellent, since atelectasis, alveolar hypoxia, acidosis, and hypothermia can produce pulmonary vasoconstriction and resultant right heart failure.

Pulmonary venous obstruction can occur as a late complication of surgical repair of TAPVR. The development of this obstruction is thought to be due to scarring and narrowing of the site of anastomosis between the pulmonary veins and the left atrium. This complication is more common after repair of infradiaphragmatic TAPVC and may also be related to anomalies of the pulmonary veins themselves. Signs of this obstruction include the development of respiratory distress and evidence of pulmonary edema on chest radiograph.

HYPOPLASTIC LEFT-HEART SYNDROME

DESCRIPTION

Hypoplastic left-heart syndrome represents a group of congenital heart defects that occur when the left side of the heart and/or the aorta fail to develop completely. Any or all of the left heart structures and the aorta can be extremely small and inadequate to provide systemic perfusion. The neonate with hypoplastic left-heart syndrome may appear normal at birth and during the first days of life, because the right ventricle is perfusing both the pulmonary circulation and the systemic circulation (through the PDA). When the ductus arteriosus begins to close, the neonate usually develops severe CHF and signs of circulatory collapse, unresponsive to medical management. The diagnosis should be suspected in the neonate with no evidence of cyanosis or pallor, who suddenly develops poor peripheral perfusion with decreased peripheral pulses and poor urine output. Signs of CHF may also be present, and pulmonary edema and cardiomegaly are noted on chest radiograph. The electrocardiogram will reveal right ventricular and possibly right atrial hypertrophy, and decreased left ventricular forces. The diagnosis is usually confirmed by echocardiogram, because a diminutive left ventricle is demonstrated with decreased or absent movement of the mitral valve. The ascending aorta and aortic valve may also be very small. Occasionally, cardiac catheterization is necessary to distinguish between hypoplastic left-heart syndrome and severe forms of CoA or critical aortic stenosis.

Since there is currently no method of reconstructing the left heart, particularly the left ventricle, there is currently no corrective surgery available for the infant with this heart defect. Forms of palliative surgery are currently available at some institutions, but they do not necessarily assure long-term survival. If surgery is to be attempted, the neonate will receive a continuous infusion of prostaglandin E_1 to keep the ductus arteriosus patent preoperatively. If surgery is not attempted, the parents must be assisted in coping with their infant's death. In any event, the short- and long-term prognosis for the neonate with hypoplastic left-heart syndrome is poor.

INFLAMMATIONS

RHEUMATIC HEART DISEASE

DESCRIPTION

Rheumatic heart disease is the most common form of acquired heart disease in children; it results from inflammatory changes occurring within the heart in association with rheumatic fever.

Rheumatic fever is most prevalent in children ages 5 to 15 years and follows a group A beta-hemolytic streptococcal infection. Carditis occurs in approximately half of the children during the acute phase of rheumatic fever and involves an inflammatory and, possibly, autoimmune process that causes temporary or permanent damage to any of the three layers of the heart. Myocardial and pericardial involvement are usually transient and mild, although endocardial involvement can produce long-term scarring or fibrosis of valve leaflets and papillary muscles.

The presence of rheumatic carditis is suggested by any of the following symptoms: cardiomegaly, appearance of a *new* cardiac murmur, pericarditis (may be accompanied by a pericardial effusion), onset of CHF, and changes in the ECG indicating chamber hypertrophy. Marked cardiomegaly and/or CHF at the time of acute rheumatic fever are the most consistent precursors of later rheumatic heart disease.

Edema and inflammatory erosion of valve tissue occur acutely, and then scarring of valve leaflets, fusion of valve cusps, or fibrosis and shortening of papillary muscles can produce valvular stenosis or insufficiency. If the acute inflammation progresses or recurs, valvular damage may become permanent. Mitral insufficiency is the most common rheumatic heart lesion in children; aortic insufficiency occurs less frequently.

Rapid treatment of rheumatic fever and minimization of associated inflammation of cardiac tissue may prevent permanent cardiac damage. Penicillin is usually used to treat the streptococcal infection, and antibiotic therapy is continued indefinitely to prevent recurrence of rheumatic fever and repeated risk of cardiac damage. Salicylates (and possible administration of corticosteroids) may be used to decrease the acute inflammatory reaction. Bed rest can be encouraged to reduce cardiac work load (it is sometimes thought that this will decrease extent of cardiac damage), especially if the child has CHF.

Children who have had rheumatic fever should also receive antibiotic prophylaxis for times of increased risk of bacteremia, to prevent development of bacterial endocarditis; however, often the child is still receiving penicillin for long-term prevention of recurrent rheumatic fever. Refer to p. 975 for discussion of *Valvular Heart Diseases*.

BIBLIOGRAPHY

Engle, M. A.: "Pediatric Cardiovascular Disease," in *Cardiovascular Clinics*, Volume 11, Number 2, F. A. Davis, Philadelphia, 1981. This text provides an full range of information about medical and surgical management of the child with cardiovascular disease. The contributors are all well known in their field, and the information in each chapter is covered thoroughly. Several of the chapters deal with long-term results of surgical correction of congenital heart defects.

Fink, B. W.: *Congenital Heart Disease: A Deductive Approach to Its Diagnosis*, Year Book Medical Publishers, Chicago, 1975. Excellent paperback reference that discusses embryology, hemodynamic principles, and clinical presentation for all the major congenital heart defects. Very helpful for nurses. Small bibliography provided.

Fyler, D. C.: "Report of the New England Regional Infant Cardiac Program," *Pediatrics*, **65**(Feb. suppl.):377, 1980. This summary of information obtained from the now-famous regional cardiac program is loaded with facts and figures about the incidence, clinical presentation, natural history and morbidity, and surgical results of most forms of congenital heart disease. The figures are fairly current, and the summaries are based on extensive clinical experience.

Graham, T. P., and Bender, H. W.: "Preoperative Diagnosis and Management of Infants with Critical Congenital Heart Disease," *The Annals of Thoracic Surgery*, **29**:272, March 1980. This recent review summarizes the presentation of infants with common forms of congenital heart disease. It describes catheterization and other diagnostic information required for management decisions and summarizes current trends in medical and surgical care of infants with heart disease.

Hazinski, M. F.: "Congenital Heart Lesions," Bio-Service Corporation, Chicago, 1978 (pamphlet). This six-page, full-color pamphlet presents 16 congenital heart lesions with color-coding to depict various oxygen concentrations within each cardiac chamber. Accompanying each illustration is a brief summary of hemodynamics, clinical signs and symptoms, and medical and surgical treatment. Consequences of CHF and cyanotic heart disease are also summarized. Accompanying slides are available.

Hazinski, M. F.: "Critical Care of the Pediatric Cardiovascular Patient," *Nursing Clinics of North America*, **16**:671, 1981. This article summarizes briefly assessment and treatment of the cardiovascular client with CHF, low cardiac output, arrhythmias, postoperative bleeding, and respiratory distress. Many reference tables are provided.

Linde, L. M., and Linde, S. D.: "Emotional Factors of Pediatric Patients in Cardiac Surgery," *American Operating Room Nurse*, **18**:95, July 1973. Very good article that considers psychosocial factors of heart disease in children (applicable to both surgical and nonsurgical child cardiac clients).

Loomis, J. C.: "Care of the Pediatric Patient Following Cardiovascular Surgery," in A. K. Ream and R. P. Fogdall (eds.), *Acute Cardiovascular Management*, Lippincott, Philadelphia, 1982. This chapter provides an excellent overview of the assessment (including hemodynamic monitoring) and management of the child after cardiovascular surgery. Rationale for therapy is discussed in detail.

Mills, L. J., Newfeld, E. A., Mast, C. P., and Carew, J.: "Cardiothoracic Surgery," in D. L. Levin, F. C. Morriss, and G. C. Moore (eds.), *A Practical Guide to Pediatric Intensive Care*, C. V. Mosby, St. Louis, 1979. This chapter provides a valuable summary of appropriate management of common cardiovascular postoperative complications. The entire text is a handy reference for the pediatric intensive care unit. The authors and editors are outstanding clinicians with thorough knowledge of pathophysiology and current trends in pediatric critical care.

Moss, A. J.: "What Every Primary Physician Should Know About the Postoperative Cardiac Patient," *Pediatrics*, **63**:320, February 1979. This concise, thorough article provides an excellent review of current surgery for congenital heart disease, as well as an outstanding summary of early and late postoperative complications.

Moss, A. J., Adams, F. H., and Emmanouilides, G. C.: *Heart Disease in Infants, Children, and Adolescents,* 2d ed., Williams & Wilkins, Baltimore, 1977. This contributed text is a solid reference book for thorough discussion of common cardiovascular problems in children.

Reif, K.: "A Heart Makes You Live," *The American Journal of Nursing,* **72:**1085, June 1972. Brief, interesting summary describing the progression of a child's concepts about the function of the heart (based on interviews and art from a small group of children).

Wenger, N. K., Hurst, J. W., and Mc Intyre, M. C.: *Cardiology for Nurses,* McGraw-Hill, New York, 1980. This is an outstanding reference book for nurses caring for cardiovascular patients of any age. The authors are internationally known clinicians who have provided complete information needed by the cardiovascular nurse. The chapters on chest x-ray interpretation and arrhythmias are particularly useful.

Whaley, L. F., and Wong, D. L.: "The Child with Heart Disease," in L. F. Whaley and D. L. Wong (eds.), *Nursing Care of Infants and Children,* C. V. Mosby, St. Louis, 1979. This pediatric nursing text has an excellent chapter on nursing care of the pediatric cardiovascular client. Various congenital heart lesions are covered, but the chapter also provides very useful information about the care of the child with CHF or rheumatic fever and the child who has had cardiovascular surgery. A strength of the book is the "quick-reference" nursing care plans included as tables.

20

The Respiratory System

Janet L. Snow

ABNORMAL CELLULAR GROWTH

DIAPHRAGMATIC HERNIA

DESCRIPTION

Diaphragmatic hernia is a congenital free communication between the thoracic and abdominal cavities with the abdominal contents displaced into the chest. Because of the resultant respiratory distress, diaphragmatic hernia is a surgical emergency. The condition occurs approximately once in 2200 live births and shows no predilection for race or sex. The most common site for the diaphragm defect is the posterolateral segment, through the foramen of Bochdalek, which normally fuses by the sixth week of fetal life to separate the pleural cavity from the peritoneal cavity. The defect occurs five times more often on the left side than on the right. The homolateral lung is usually completely collapsed and may be hypoplastic. The mediastinal structures are shifted to the contralateral side of the chest. The contralateral lung is often partially compressed and may be hypoplastic. Respiration is further compromised by distension of the stomach and intestine, which results from swallowing air while crying. The treatment is surgical. The contralateral lung is capable, except in rare cases, of maintaining both ventilation and oxygenation. This disorder carries a mortality rate of 25 to 40 percent; the lower limits of these figures are associated with early diagnosis and treatment. If the infant survives, the affected lung will expand and become functional. There may be some persistent pulmonary hypertension in the affected lung, but this gradually subsides.

PREVENTION

Health Promotion

No preventive measures are known.

Population at Risk

Herniation manifests itself shortly after birth. Newborn infants are the population at risk.

Screening

None.

ASSESSMENT

Health History

1. Respiratory distress is usually present at birth, not necessarily to any greater degree in premature infants.
2. Difficulty feeding because of respiratory distress.

Physical Assessment

1. Large barrel chest in comparison with small abdomen.
2. Tachypnea (respiratory rate may be as high as 120 per minute).
3. Nasal flaring.
4. Severe chest retractions usually becoming more prominent after several hours and with crying.

5. Cyanosis: progressive.
6. Absent breath sounds, particularly on the left side of the chest.
7. Heart sounds may be displaced to the right due to compression from the intestine.
8. Severe respiratory acidosis due to hypoxemia and ineffective ventilation.

Diagnostic Tests

1. Chest x-ray film shows displacement of intestine into chest cavity.
2. Blood gas determination.
   a. pH decreased, usually less than 7.32.
   b. Pco_2 increased, usually above 50 mmHg.
   c. Pco_2 decreased, usually below 60 mmHg.

NURSING DIAGNOSES: ACTUAL OR POTENTIAL

1. Respiratory insufficiency, moderate to severe, secondary to lung compression by the intestine.
2. Activity intolerance (e.g., crying, handling) due to hypoxemia.
3. Nutritional deficit: alteration in food intake due to respiratory distress and possible bowel obstruction.
4. Fluid volume deficit secondary to decreased intake, rapid respirations, and gastrointestinal (GI) losses (vomiting or intubation).
5. Alteration in parenting due to long-term hospitalization and threatened loss of child.
6. Anxiety in the parents due to the disorder and its prognosis.

EXPECTED OUTCOMES

1. Respiratory distress will be partially relieved within a few hours of birth, after intubation. Progressive relief will occur after operative repair. Complete relief will occur before discharge from the hospital.
2. A normal blood pH will be established within the first few hours after birth.
3. Adequate fluids, calories, and electrolytes will be provided, beginning immediately.
4. Complications, such as further respiratory insufficiency and circulatory problems, will be prevented or reduced in incidence.
5. Parents will exhibit bonding to infant; anxiety will be lessened within 3 to 4 days of initial hospitalization.

INTERVENTIONS

1. Preoperative.
   a. Monitor vital signs, especially pulse and respirations (see Tables 20-1 and 20-2 and Figures 20-1 and 20-2).
   b. Monitor child's color.
   c. Monitor breath sounds (Table 20-2) frequently to detect further respiratory compromise.
   d. Monitor blood gases (increased Pco_2 and decreased Po_2 occur with hypoxemia); have a ventilator on standby ready for use; administer sodium bicarbonate as prescribed.
   e. Provide supplemental oxygen and humidity; measure concentration of oxygen every hour; note child's response to oxygen.
   f. Assess child's level of activity: increased restlessness may indicate increasing fatigue. Avoid having child cry.
   g. Position for optimal lung expansion: semi-Fowler's position will help alleviate pressure of the abdominal contents upon the thorax; lying on the affected side al-

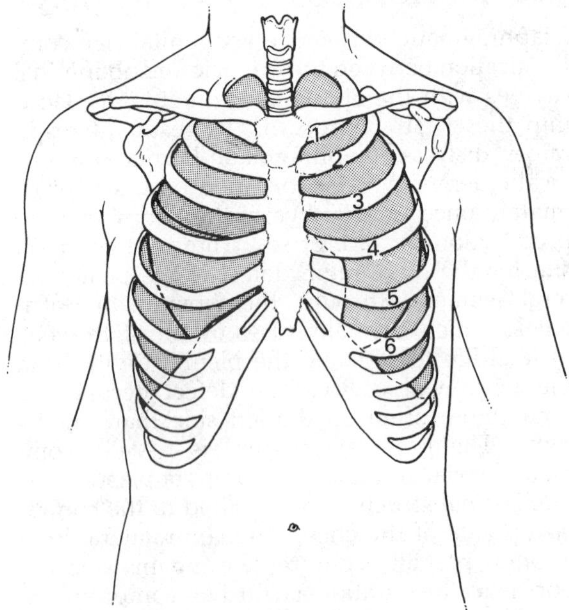

Figure 20-1 Anterior view of the chest showing lung lobes (shaded) in relative location to the ribs (numbered). The right lung has three lobes, the left has two.

TABLE 20-1 ASSESSMENT OF RESPIRATIONS

1. Respiratory rate (can best be assessed when the child is asleep or resting).
   a. Normal rates for age:

Newborn	30–60 per min
Toddler	24–40 per min
Preschooler	22–34 per min
School age	18–30 per min
Adolescent	12–20 per min

   b. Rapid rate (tachypnea) is common in respiratory disorders, particularly lower airway obstruction, fever, anxiety, and heart failure.
   c. Slow rate (bradypnea) suggests central respiratory depression, increased intracranial pressure, or alkalosis of long duration.
2. Depth of respirations: Deep respirations (hyperpnea) indicate anoxia, acidosis, or possible upper airway obstruction.
3. Quality of respirations: Gasping, grunting respirations, as well as dyspnea, orthopnea, and restlessness, may indicate respiratory distress.
4. Breath sounds.
   a. Auscultation can be performed on a crying infant as inspiration can be heard between cries.
   b. Infant's head should be in straight alignment with the body; turning head to one side may cause decreased breath sounds in the opposite side of the chest.
   c. Secure child's cooperation.
      (1) Allow young child to handle stethoscope before its use; grasping the stethoscope during the exam distorts the sounds.
      (2) Older child can listen through stethoscope to alleviate anxiety.
      (3) Deep breathing can be elicited during auscultation by asking child to "take a deep breath and pretend to blow out all the candles on a birthday cake."
   d. Auscultate over each lung lobe (the right lung has three lobes, the left has two). Figure 20-1 shows an anterior view of the lobes (shaded) in relative location to the ribs (numbered). The landmarks are
      (1) Ribs 1 to 6 = upper lobe, left side.
      (2) Ribs 1 to 4 = upper lobe, right side.
      (3) Ribs 4 to 6 = upper middle lobe, right side.
      NOTE: Only a wedge of the lower lobe is present in the anterior chest.
      Posterior chest landmarks are
      (1) Clavicular area to fourth rib = upper lobe, right and left sides.
      (2) Ribs 4 to 10 = lower lobes, right and left sides.
   e. Normal findings of auscultation: Bronchovesicular and even bronchial breath sounds are considered normal in infants and small children. The thin chest wall and lack of muscle mass account for sounds that are louder and harsher than in older children and adults. NOTE: Normal breath sounds are easily transmitted to all parts of the chest. An infant with a pneumothorax may have seemingly normal breath sounds.
   f. Abnormal breath sounds.
      (1) Crackling sounds (rales) may be heard scattered over the chest in infants and children with bronchiolitis, bronchopneumonia, atelectasis, and edema.
      (2) Coarse sounds (rhonchi) may be heard in children with airway obstruction.
      (3) Wheezing may be heard in children with laryngeal edema, foreign body, asthma, or bronchiolitis.
      (4) Inspiratory stridor may be heard without the stethoscope and usually indicates upper airway obstruction.

lows unrestricted respiratory movements on the unaffected side.

h. Use a nasogastric (NG) tube to decrease distension and minimize lung compression.
i. Keep child NPO.
j. Provide mouth care.
k. Provide routine suctioning of endotracheal tube if child is intubated.
l. Help family establish realistic goals in view of high mortality.
m. Monitor intravenous (IV) fluids precisely.
n. Weigh daily.

2. Postoperative.
   a. Monitor vital signs closely.
   b. Maintain water-seal chest suction (usually continued for 2 to 3 days after surgery).
   c. Place in semi-Flowler's position to aid in

TABLE 20-2 SIGNS AND SYMPTOMS OF RESPIRATORY DISTRESS

Signs and symptoms of respiratory distress in infants.

1. Flaring nares—bilateral widening of the nares during inspiratory efforts, which accompanies labored breathing (see Figure 20-2).
2. Head bobbing—observed as a subtle flexion of the head accompanying each inspiratory effort during episodes of increased work of breathing in an infant under 3 months of age.
3. Expiratory grunting—occurs when an infant exhales against a partially closed glottis. This maneuver retards expiratory flow of air, producing a back-pressure that is transmitted from the glottis to the alveoli. This expiratory retard maintains an increased functional residual capacity and, therefore, increases arterial oxygen tension (see Figure 20-2).
4. Abnormal retractions of the chest—the soft tissues of the chest wall are not fully developed in the young child, and ossification of the sternum and anterior ribs is incomplete. These pliable structures readily yield and pull inward when abnormally low intrathoracic pressures are required for ventilation (see Figure 20-2).
5. Intercostal bulging—this sign indicates that an increased muscular effort is required to force air out of the lungs as, for example, in asthma. The result is an exaggeration in intrapleural pressure, causing it to exceed atmospheric pressure, and resulting in flattening or bulging out of the soft tissues of the intercostal spaces.
6. Inability to suckle.
7. Inspiratory stridor—this sign is observed as a high-pitched, harsh sound that is produced by obstruction to the flow of air through the larynx. Obstruction of the larynx or of the epiglottic or hypopharyngeal regions causes stridor during inspiration because the extrathoracic airways normally constrict during inspiration. Any additional reduction of the diameter of the airway results in stridor.

Signs and symptoms of distress in older children.

1. Shortness of breath.
2. Recurrent cough.
3. Lung congestion.
4. Nasal congestion.
5. Orthopnea.
6. Sneezing.
7. Possible chest pain.

Nonspecific signs and symptoms of respiratory distress.

1. Anorexia—often the first sign of illness in a child.
2. Irritability.
3. Vomiting and diarrhea—early sign of an infectious process in a child. Toxins appear to affect the immature nervous system of children by stimulating the medullary area of the brain where the centers for vomiting and defecation are located.

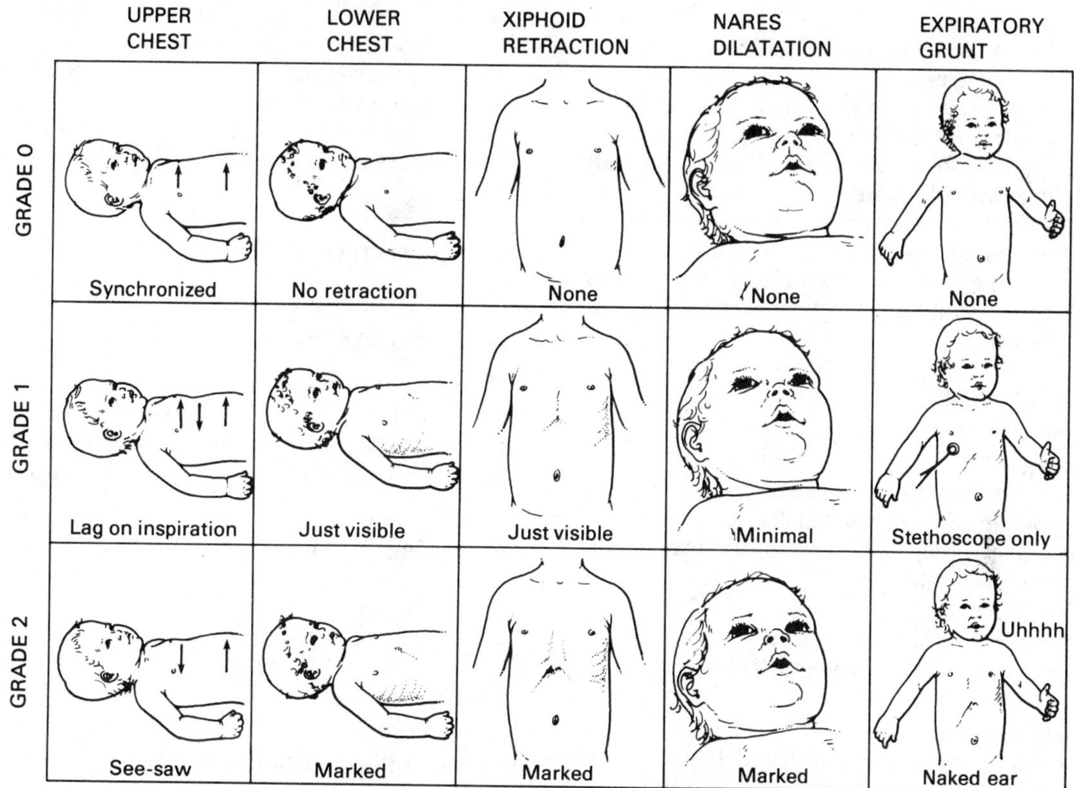

Figure 20-2 Observations indicating presence and severity of respiratory distress. (From Bauman, W. A., "The Respiratory Distress Syndrome and Its Significance in Premature Infants," *Pediatrics*, **24**(2):194–204, August 1959. Copyright American Academy of Pediatrics, 1959.)

ventilatory maneuvers; turn from side to side every hour.

d. Monitor blood gases.
e. Provide supplemental oxygen if necessary.
f. Provide ventilatory assistance if necessary.
g. Use NG tube to prevent gastric distension and respiratory compromise.
h. Keep NPO until peristalsis resumes.
i. Monitor IV fluids carefully.
j. Maintain strict I and O record.
k. Monitor serum electrolyte values.
l. Monitor daily weights.
m. Provide mouth care if NPO.
n. Assess for bleeding or abdominal distension.
o. Provide realistic reassurance and explanations for parents.
p. Encourage parents to visit child often.
q. Assess desire and readiness of parents to participate in child's care.
r. Teach newborn care and feeding techniques before child is discharged.

EVALUATION

Outcome Criteria

1. Preoperative.
   a. Respiratory effort and retractions decrease; respiratory rate stabilizes.
   b. Nasogastric tube works well to decompress GI organs in the chest and prevent vomiting and aspiration.
   c. Proper hydration and electrolyte balance are maintained.
   d. Parents cope adequately and are prepared for infant's surgery.
   e. Normal acid-base balance and hydration are maintained.

2. Postoperative.
   a. No cyanosis or other evidence of respiratory distress.
   b. Water-seal drainage functions properly.
   c. Gastrointestinal function is restored.
   d. Hydration, electrolyte balance, and nutrition are adequate.
   e. A good parent–child interaction exists, as evidenced by parents' freedom from excessive anxiety, participation in child's care, and realistic preparations for discharge.

Complications

Respiratory insufficiency.

Assessment

1. Hypoxemia—decreased Pa_{O_2}.
2. Hypercapnia—increased Pa_{CO_2}.
3. Decreased pH, from respiratory acidosis and/or metabolic acidosis.
4. Restlessness.
5. Shallow, rapid respirations.
6. More severe retractions of the chest.
7. Increased heart rate.

Revised Outcomes

1. Oxygenation will be restored to within normal limits; restlessness, shallow rapid respirations, chest retractions, severe hypotension, and increased heart rate will be corrected.
2. pH will be restored to within normal limits.

Interventions

1. Monitor blood gases to evaluate progression of disease.
2. Suction as needed.
3. Monitor amount of humidified oxygen provided.
4. Monitor heart rate and rhythm to determine cardiac changes.
5. Monitor electrolyte values.
6. Administer any medications ordered for relief of respiratory distress.

LARYNGOTRACHEAL MALACIA

DESCRIPTION

Malacia refers to softening and resultant loss of support in the area. Laryngeal malacia is flabbiness of the epiglottis and/or supraglottic area; tracheal malacia is weakening of a section of tracheal cartilage resulting in collapse of the area during inspiration (the extrathoracic airways normally constrict on inspiration). Noisy respirations may cause concern, but treatment is seldom necessary; the condition is usually self-limiting.

PREVENTION

Health Promotion

No preventive measures are known.

Population at Risk

Any child can be born with the condition. Since the malformation manifests itself at or shortly after birth, newborn infants are the population at risk.

Screening

None.

ASSESSMENT

Health History

1. Neonate.
2. Inspiratory stridor.
3. Feeding difficulty.

Physical Assessment

1. Stridor on inspriation.
2. Retractions of chest wall due to high intrathoracic pressures necessary to overcome the obstruction created when the affected area collapses.

Diagnostic Tests

1. Lateral chest or neck x-ray films may reveal area of collapse.
2. Laryngoscopy will allow visualization of the area.

NURSING DIAGNOSES: ACTUAL OR POTENTIAL

1. Respiratory dysfunction, mild to moderate, due to partial collapse of a portion of the upper airway.
2. Nutritional deficit due to inability to breathe and suckle simultaneously.
3. Failure to gain weight due to inability to suckle.
4. Parental anxiety due to child's distress.

EXPECTED OUTCOMES

1. Respiratory distress will be partially relieved within the first few hours after birth and more fully relieved within 6 months after birth.
2. Adequate fluids and calories will be provided.
3. Parents will exhibit less anxiety related to the disorder with 2 to 3 weeks after birth as they understand the self-limiting nature of the disorder and learn specific interventions to alleviate respiratory distress.

INTERVENTIONS

1. Monitor degree of respiratory distress.
2. Have emergency intubation equipment ready at bedside in case it is needed.
3. Provide humidified air.
4. Maintain semi-Fowler's position during distress.
5. Provide slow, careful feedings.
6. Allow frequent rest periods if distress is present.
7. Weigh daily.
8. Promote parental participation in care of the child.
9. Teach parents:
   a. Health maintenance of the child.
   b. Prevention of respiratory infection.
   c. How to assess degree of respiratory distress.
   d. Feeding techniques.
10. Reassure parents that the disorder is self-limiting.

EVALUATION

Outcome Criteria

1. Respiratory distress is alleviated by normal growth process as the child nears 6 months to 1 year of age.
2. Child receives adequate fluids and calories as evidenced by normal weight gains, tissue turgor, and output.
3. Child's parents are informed about the treatment regimen and the likelihood that the child will outgrow the disorder.

Complications

Respiratory insufficiency. See complications section under *Diaphragmatic Hernia*.

OBSTRUCTIONS

FOREIGN BODY ASPIRATION

DESCRIPTION

Young children are prone to aspiration of food and other objects. The severity and treatment of the resultant respiratory distress depend on the type of object aspirated, the location of the object in the respiratory tract, and the degree of obstruction.

Aspirated objects commonly lodge in the laryngotracheal area, but they can pass into a main stem bronchus or further down into a segmental bronchus. Foreign bodies that pass through the larynx are more likely to enter the right lung than the left one, because the right main bronchus is wider and more directly in line with the axis of the trachea than is the left main bronchus.

The signs and symptoms depend on the degree of obstruction caused by the foreign body and the nature of the object itself. Vegetables, for example, can swell when wet, creating even further obstruction after they become saturated by body fluids. A small object, such as a bead, can cause no symptoms at all. (Emergency treatment of acute airway obstruction is discussed in Chapter 48. See also *Chemical Pneumonia*.)

PREVENTION

Health Promotion

1. Small children should not be allowed access to small objects that they can put in their mouth or nose.
2. Children younger than $2\frac{1}{2}$ years should not be allowed nuts, raisins, popcorn, or whole-kernel corn.
3. Care should be taken when feeding weak, debilitated, or uncooperative children.
4. Solid foods should not be introduced until the child has teeth with which to chew the food.
5. Children should be encouraged to chew food thoroughly and to not talk while eating.
6. Parents should be instructed to teach their children to keep foreign bodies, such as toothpicks, pins, or nails, away from the lips and mouth.

Population at Risk

1. Aspiration can occur at any age but is most common in 1- to 3-year-old children.
2. Weak or debilitated children.

Screening

Neck and chest x-ray films when aspiration is suspected.

ASSESSMENT

Health History

1. Report from child or other that an object has been "swallowed."
2. Discovery of an opened container with small objects (e.g., safety pins, beads).
3. Sudden onset of aphonia (loss of voice).
4. Sudden onset of dyspnea.
5. History of choking may or may not be positive.

Physical Assessment

1. Immediate signs.
   a. Choking may occur suddenly.
   b. Gagging.
   c. Coughing of sudden onset, maybe with hemoptysis.
   d. Sudden aphonia.
2. Later signs.
   a. Hoarseness—muffled voice.
   b. Coughing.
   c. Cyanosis of lips.
   d. Dyspnea with wheezing.
   e. Possible fever.
   f. Retractions of the chest (Figure 20-2).

Diagnostic Tests

1. Posterior and lateral chest x-ray films and lateral neck x-ray films allow visualization of the neck and chest in various views to help identify foreign bodies. Metallic objects will be visible on x-ray examination; objects, such as vegetables, may manifest with an area of swelling only.
2. Direct laryngoscopy allows direct visualization of the area of the airway suspected of harboring a foreign body, and removal of the object. A bronchoscopy may be necessary to remove an object located further down the airway.

NURSING DIAGNOSES: ACTUAL OR POTENTIAL

1. Respiratory dysfunction, mild to severe dyspnea secondary to obstruction.
2. Alterations in comfort: discomfort secondary to edema and obstruction.
3. Fluid and nutritional deficit: decreased intake secondary to respiratory dysfunction.
4. Decreased activity tolerance secondary to respiratory dysfunction.
5. Anxiety, mild to severe, in the child and parents secondary to dyspnea.

EXPECTED OUTCOMES

1. Respiratory distress will be partially relieved within the first hour after admission and fully relieved within 2 days after removal of the object.
2. Adequate fluids and calories will be provided.
3. Complications, such as further airway obstruction, will be prevented.
4. Child and parents will exhibit less anxiety related to child's condition within the first several hours after admission.
5. Teaching regarding safety in the home and prevention of recurrence will occur before discharge from the hospital.

INTERVENTIONS

1. Immediate.
   NOTE: Emergency treatment of acute respiratory obstruction is presented in Chapter 48.
   a. Monitor vital signs.
   b. Assess degree of respiratory distress (see Table 20-2) and oxygenation.
      (1) Check color, note any cyanosis.
      (2) Note retractions of chest.
      (3) Note loss of voice and drooling of secretions.
   c. Provide a quiet, nonstimulating environment.
2. After removal of object.
   a. Monitor vital signs, especially respiratory status.
   b. Observe closely for postoperative edema formation at the site of foreign body.
   c. Provide liquids and diet when awake.
   d. Counsel about prevention of recurrence.

EVALUATION

Outcome Criteria

1. Respiratory distress is alleviated.
2. Child is reciving adequate fluids and calories.

3. Anxiety level is significantly reduced in both child and parents.
4. Family member describes methods to be used to prevent recurrence.

Complications

Increased dyspnea.

Assessment

1. Increased restlessness.
2. More severe retractions of chest.
3. Increased heart rate.
4. Cyanosis.

Revised Outcomes

1. Oxygenation will be restored within normal limits.
2. Restlessness, respirations, and increased heart rate will return to normal limits.

Interventions

1. Notify physician of any change immediately.
2. Provide humidified air and, possibly, oxygen, as ordered.
3. Monitor heart rate and rhythm.
4. Prepare for possible laryngoscopy or tracheostomy if obstruction is located high in the airway.

Reevaluation and Follow-up

Continue to reinforce preventive measures.

FOREIGN BODY IN THE EAR

DESCRIPTION

Foreign bodies, such as beads, stones, food, and insects, may be pushed into the external auditory canal by young children. An object may be hygroscopic (attracts water and swells) or rough-edged and cause damage within the ear. Objects can remain in the ear canal for weeks before their presence is known. A foreign body in the ear canal can cause obstruction, infection, and possible deafness in the affected ear.

PREVENTION

Health Promotion

See *Foreign Body Aspiration.*

Population at Risk

See *Foreign Body Aspiration.*

Screening

Visualization of the external ear canal with an otoscope.

ASSESSMENT

Health History

1. Report from child or other that an object has been placed in the ear.
2. Discovery of an open container containing small objects, such as beads or dry beans.
3. Constant rubbing or pulling at the ear.

Physical Assessment

1. Discomfort or pain in affected ear.
2. Hearing loss.
3. Inflammation and edema of ear canal.

Diagnostic Tests

Direct visualization of ear canal.

NURSING DIAGNOSES: ACTUAL OR POTENTIAL

1. Temporary hearing loss, mild to severe, secondary to obstruction of ear canal.
2. Alterations in comfort: discomfort or pain due to edema of the ear canal.
3. Anxiety in child due to discomfort or hearing loss.

EXPECTED OUTCOMES

1. Object will be removed as soon as possible.
2. Discomfort and pain will be relieved within 1 day after object is removed.
3. Parents will receive information concerning safety in the home and will be taught that if an object accidently or deliberately is placed in the canal, a skilled person should remove it.
4. Hearing will be restored.

INTERVENTIONS

1. Reassure parents and child.
2. Place the child in a quiet environment immediately.
3. Identify the object before removal, as different objects require different methods of removal.
4. Instill prescribed irrigant or lubricant solution (except for a hygroscopic object, which should have no irrigant (lest it swell further): (e.g., removal of wax is facilitated by hydrogen peroxide instillation; beads can be lubricated with an oil or a soap solution).
5. Assist child (teach, reassure, hold) while physician removes the object.
6. Consider that the child may have a temporary

hearing deficit; approach the child with this in mind.
7. Assess external ear for edema and/or break in the skin.
8. Monitor for signs of infection: fever, exudate, redness.
9. Provide parents and child with information about foreign body removal and prevention of recurrence.

EVALUATION

Outcome Criteria

1. Foreign body removed without complications.
2. Residual infection, if any, responds to treatment.
3. Child's hearing has been restored.
4. Parents and child state methods to be used to prevent recurrence.
5. No discomfort is present.

Complications

Hearing loss after removal of object.

Assessment

1. Loss of hearing in affected ear.
2. Headache.
3. Possible intermittent hearing loss.

Revised Outcomes

1. Parents and child will receive reassurance that the deafness may persist but is most likely to be only temporary.
2. Teaching regarding coping with hearing in one ear will begin before hospital discharge if the hearing loss persists.

Interventions

1. Administer medication as ordered (e.g., steroid preparation, pain medication).
2. Provide constant realistic reassurance to the child and family.
3. Teach the child and parents precautions that should be followed if the deafness persists.

Reevaluation and Follow-up

Continue to reassess need for preventive teaching concerning safety in the home and with small children.

BRONCHIOLITIS

DESCRIPTION

Bronchiolitis is an acute viral illness that is usually caused by the respiratory syncytial or parainfluenza viruses. The condition can also, in rare instances, be caused by adenoviruses or *Mycoplasma pneumoniae*. It is characterized by widespread lower airway obstruction. Bronchioles become partially or totally occluded by the inflamed, edematous bronchiolar mucosa. The tenacious exudate, made up of mucus and cellular debris, causes hyperinflation and atelectasis of the alveoli. The inflammation is primarily confined to the smaller bronchioles. Bronchiolitis occurs almost exclusively in children ages 2 to 18 months. The peak incidence is around 6 months of age. Several factors contribute to the occurrence at this age:

1. The short distance between the upper and lower airway, which facilitates rapid spreading of the viral infection and inflammation from the upper airway along the continuous respiratory membrane to the lower airways.
2. Low levels of antibodies during the first year of life (prenatally acquired antibodies are largely destroyed by the third month of life).
3. Very small lumen diameters of the bronchioles.
4. Rapid respiratory rates produce more turbulent airflow, increased airway resistance, and increased effort for breathing.

PREVENTION

Health Promotion

Avoid exposure to individuals with upper respiratory infections.

Population at Risk

1. Children ages 2 to 18 months.
2. Children living in densely populated areas.
3. Increased incidence in children born prematurely.
4. Peak incidence occurs at about 6 months.

Screening

None.

ASSESSMENT

Health History

1. Vulnerable age group: 2 to 18 months.
2. Exposure to recent upper respiratory infection.
3. Sudden onset of mild to moderate respiratory distress stemming from a simple upper respiratory infection.
4. Little or no response to sympathomimetics and corticosteroids.
5. Hacking cough.

Physical Assessment

See Tables 20-1 and 20-2.

1. Expiratory wheezing may be auscultated.
2. Nasal flaring.
3. Overdistended chest.
4. Retractions of the chest.
5. Cyanosis.
6. Restlessness.
7. Hacking cough.
8. Tachypnea, respiratory rate up to 60–80 per minute.
9. Fever may or may not be present.
10. Emphysema with barrel chest and palpable liver and spleen from depressed diaphragm may be present.
11. Fine rales with scattered consolidation may be present.
12. Hyperresonance over the chest with percussion.
13. Signs of dehydration may be present.

Diagnostic Tests

1. Chest x-ray film reveals pulmonary hyperinflation and scattered infiltrates.
2. Viral cultures: positive in up to one-half of infections with bronchiolitis.
3. Arterial blood gases: early gases reveal hypoxemia, later hypercapnia.

NURSING DIAGNOSES: ACTUAL OR POTENTIAL

1. Respiratory dysfunction: mild to severe distress secondary to inflammatory reaction in the lower airway and subsequent obstruction.
2. Increased body temperature due to viral infection and possible dehydration.
3. Fluid volume deficit due to decreased intake, fever, and rapid respirations.
4. Altered acid-base balance due to hypoxemia and viral invasion of lung tissue.
5. Alteration in comfort due to fever, cough, and dyspnea.

EXPECTED OUTCOMES

1. Respiratory distress will be partially relieved within the first day after treatment is initiated and fully relieved within 4 to 6 weeks after the peak of the illness.
2. A normal blood pH will be established within the first 24 hours of treatment.
3. An environment will be provided that promotes maximum rest within the first 24 hours after admission.
4. A normal body temperature will be established and maintained within the first 2 to 3 days after diagnosis.
5. Adequate fluids and calories will be provided; signs of dehydration will disappear.
6. Parents will exhibit less anxiety relating to child's condition and hospital environment within 3 days of initial hospitalization.
7. Irritability and other signs of discomfort will resolve within 2 days of admission.

INTERVENTIONS

1. Provide humidified oxygen.
   a. Monitor concentration of oxygen.
   b. Note child's response to a given amount of oxygen.
2. Monitor arterial blood gases if child is in severe distress.
3. Reposition frequently to allow increased ventilation of affected lung.
4. Continually assess degree of respiratory distress.
5. Provide chest physiotherapy as ordered.
6. Reduce stressors in the environment.
7. Provide frequent rest periods.
8. Observe for cardiac arrhythmias—most cardiac arrhythmias are the result of hypoxia.
9. Monitor intake and output.
10. Assess for signs of dehydration—daily water loss may be increased because insensible water loss (that lost through skin and lungs) increases with increased respiratory rate.
11. Parenteral fluid therapy when in severe distress.
12. Encourage oral intake of fluids when not in acute distress.
13. Prevent overhydration.
14. Monitor temperature.
15. Administer antipyretic agent as prescribed.
16. Sponge with tepid water as needed.
17. Observe for febrile convulsions.
18. Keep parents informed of progress.
19. Welcome parents to stay with child as much as possible.
20. Parents and staff provide reassurance and comfort measures for child (holding, touch, etc.).

EVALUATION

Outcome Criteria

1. Respiratory distress resolves totally by 4 to 6 weeks after peak of disease.

2. A normal blood pH is established.
3. A normal body temperature is maintained.
4. Child is receiving adequate fluids and calories and tolerating them well.
5. Parents are informed and kept up to date with treatment regimen and nursing care.
6. Child is comfortable and resumes activities appropriate for developmental stage.

Complications

Respiratory insufficiency. See complications Section under *Diaphragmatic Hernia*.

CROUP

DESCRIPTION

Croup is a general term that refers to the clinical syndrome of laryngitis and laryngotracheobronchitis (LTB). The vocal cords, subglottic tissue, trachea, bronchi, and bronchioles can be involved. The infectious type of croup can be of either viral or bacterial origin. Viral croup (85 percent of reported cases) occurs mostly in children between the ages of 3 months and 4 years. Bacterial croup (caused by *Hemophilus influenzae* type B) occurs in children aged 2 to 7 years. Croup caused by *Corynebacterium diphtheriae* is rare but is always a possibility in a child who has not received the series of DTP (diphtheria-tetanus-pertusis) immunizations. Noninfectious croup can result from asthma or may follow endotracheal intubation or foreign body aspiration. There is often a positive family history for croup.

In response to either mechanical or infectious processes occurring in the laryngeal area, the tissues become inflamed and edematous, and partial or total obstruction of the airway results. With the child under 2 years of age, the glottic opening is small, and the mucous membrane of the laryngeal airway is highly vascular and apt to become rapidly edematous in response to inflammation.

PREVENTION

Health Promotion

1. Avoid contact with others with respiratory infections.
2. Maintain immunizations, especially the DTP series.

Population at Risk

1. Children between ages 3 months and 7 years.
2. Children who have had croup before.
3. Children living in densely populated areas.

Screening

None.

ASSESSMENT

Health History

1. Recent or concurrent upper respiratory infection.
2. Family history of croup.
3. Past history of croup in this child.

Physical Assessment

See Table 20-2.

1. Hoarse, barking cough.
2. Inspiratory stridor due to inflammation and obstruction of the laryngeal area.
3. Restlessness, anxiety.
4. Chest retractions due to increased transmural pressure in the airway.
5. Diminished breath sounds with rales and rhonchi.
6. Intermittent cyanosis.
7. Possible fever.
8. Possible hypercapnia and hypoxemia.
9. Tachycardia.

Diagnostic Tests

1. Lateral x-ray film of neck shows a normal epiglottic area and an area of density below the larynx caused by swelling of the tracheal soft tissues.
2. Viral cultures may be positive for parainfluenzae, influenza, and adenoviruses.

NURSING DIAGNOSES: ACTUAL OR POTENTIAL

1. Respiratory dysfunction, moderate to severe, secondary to inflammation.
2. Fluid and nutritional deficit: decreased intake due to respiratory distress and increased fluid loss secondary to fever.
3. Altered body temperature due to infectious processes.
4. Decreased activity tolerance secondary to respiratory dysfunction.
5. Anxiety of parents and child secondary to respiratory distress.

EXPECTED OUTCOMES

1. Respiratory distress will be partially relieved within the first few hours after initial treatment and almost completely within 7 days after peak of disease.
2. An environment conducive to maximum rest will be provided immediately for the child.
3. Normal body temperature will be reestablished within 2 to 4 days after treatment initiation.
4. Adequate fluid and calories will be provided.
5. Teaching regarding recurrence will begin before discharge.
6. Child and parents will demonstrate relief from anxiety within a few hours of initial treatment.

INTERVENTIONS

1. Provide humidified oxygen.
2. Continually reassess degree of airway obstruction.
3. Monitor respiratory rate, depth, pattern, presence of retractions, and nasal flaring. Observe for hoarseness, stridor, cough. Monitor heart rate and rhythm.
4. Monitor blood gases as ordered.
5. Administer antibiotics as prescribed.
6. Have intubation and tracheostomy equipment of the proper size ready at bedside for possible use.
7. Provide reassurance to child and parents.
8. Explain nursing actions before care.
9. Assist the older child in communicating his or her needs.
10. Anticipate the child's needs.
11. Provide a quiet environment that allows for physical and emotional rest.
12. Try not to disturb the child except for necessary nursing care.
13. Monitor temperature.
14. Administer prescribed antipyretic agents.
15. Administer sponge bath with tepid water as necessary.
16. Keep child NPO during acute distress to prevent aspiration.
17. Provide adequate fluid and calories by intravenous feeding in acute phase of the disease.
18. Encourage high-calorie liquids when no longer in danger of aspiration.
19. Progress to regular diet as condition improves.
20. Check specific gravity of urine.
21. Maintain accurate intake and output records.
22. Teach parents to prevent, recognize, and treat recurrence of croup.
    a. See health promotion guidelines, above.
    b. Early signs of recurrence include hoarseness, cough, and respiratory congestion.
    c. Attacks often occur during the night.
    d. Humidification in the early stages may arrest the attack.
        (1) A bedside humidifier is very helpful for families with a child who has croup.
        (2) A bathroom can be converted into a steam chamber by closing the door and running a hot shower; an adult can hold the child in the shower, if precautions are taken against burns, or can simply remain with the child in the steamy room.
    e. Worsening or acute distress in spite of humidification must be treated by a physician.

EVALUATION

Outcome Criteria

1. Respiratory distress is alleviated.
2. Normal body temperature is maintained.
3. Child is receiving adequate fluids and calories and maintaining weight.
4. Parents are informed and kept up to date about treatment regimen and nursing care.
5. Parents are familiar with signs of distress and are able to recognize signs of recurrence; they know how to treat croup at home and when to call the physician.
6. Parents are skilled in tracheostomy care if child is discharged with a tracheostomy tube in place.
7. Child resumes activities of daily living at preillness level.

Complications

Increase in respiratory insufficiency (see Table 20-2).

Assessment

1. Hypoxemia.
2. Increased restlessness.
3. Increased chest retractions.
4. Increased heart rate.

Revised Outcomes
1. Oxygenation will be restored within normal limits; restlessness, retractions, and tachycardia will cease.
2. Other expected outcomes, as originally stated.

Interventions
1. Administer oxygen as needed.
2. Administer mild sedation as ordered.
3. Monitor blood gases.
4. Monitor for source of attack (e.g., cold air).

Reevaluation and Follow-up
Establish a specific individualized plan to ensure that complications are overcome. Also establish a long-term plan if child is discharged with a tracheostomy tube in place.

EPIGLOTTITIS

DESCRIPTION

Epiglottitis is an inflammatory response to an infectious agent; it causes swelling of the epiglottis, false cords, and aryepiglottic folds. The bacterial agents most often responsible are *H. influenzae* type B, pneumococci, *Staphylococcus aureus,* and beta-hemolytic streptococci. The epiglottis is a long, narrow structure that closes off the narrow glottis during swallowing. Edema of the epiglottis and surrounding tissues can completely occlude the laryngeal airway in a matter of minutes or hours.

PREVENTION

Health Promotion
1. Avoid contact with others with respiratory infections.
2. Maintain immunizations, especially the DTP series.

Population at Risk
1. Occurs chiefly in children ages 3 to 7 years but can occur in younger or older children.
2. Children living in crowded conditions.

Screening
None.

ASSESSMENT

Health History
1. Exposure to an upper respiratory infection or a recent respiratory infection.
2. Sudden onset of respiratory distress.

Physical Assessment
1. Severe inspiratory stridor.
2. Marked retractions of the chest and supraclavicular area (see Table 20-2); abrupt onset and usually rapidly progressing.
3. Acute anxiety.
4. Hoarseness, muffled voice.
5. Restlessness.
6. Abrupt onset of high fever; 39–40°C (102–104°F).
7. Dysphagia and drooling can occur. The client usually prefers a sitting position with mouth open, tongue protruding—tripod position (seated but leaning back on hands with arms extended).
8. Cyanosis.
9. Breath sounds may be diminished.
10. Possible hypercapnia and/or hypoxia.
11. Cherry-red epiglottis, throat red, inflamed (see note under Diagnostic Tests section, below).
12. Fatigue.
13. Impaired consciousness.

Diagnostic Tests
1. Visualization of a cherry-red epiglottis. NOTE: Visualization of the epiglottis in a child suspected of epiglottitis should be done only by a skilled person prepared to perform immediate tracheotomy. Placing a tongue blade in the child's throat is very dangerous. It can induce laryngospasm or cause increased swelling of the epiglottis or both. Either of these can result in sudden and complete obstruction of the airway.
2. Lateral neck x-ray film. The epiglottis is seen as a large, rounded, soft tissue density in the hypopharynx. It can be seen obstructing the entrance to the trachea.

NURSING DIAGNOSES: ACTUAL OR POTENTIAL

See *Croup.*

EXPECTED OUTCOMES

See *Croup.*

INTERVENTIONS

See *Croup.*

EVALUATION

See *Croup.*

BRONCHIAL ASTHMA

DESCRIPTION

Bronchial asthma is a recurrent, reversible generalized airway obstruction characterized by dyspnea and wheezing that, in the early stages, are paroxysmal and reversible. A severe form, status asthmaticus, exists in which the client deteriorates in spite of treatment.

A complex disorder, biochemical, immunological, infectious, endocrine, and psychological factors are involved. Asthma can be allergic or nonallergic. Common irritants that can cause bronchial asthma include pollen, mold spores, feathers, house dust, certain foods, air pollutants, psychological or emotional factors, cold weather and exercise, and respiratory infections. Most children have the allergic type, but bronchial compression from external pressure can cause a nonallergic type of asthma.

An attack of allergic asthma begins with an antigen-antibody reaction that causes the release of histamine and the slow-reacting substance of anaphylaxis (SRS-A). The result is dilatation of blood vessels, excess production of mucus, accumulation of secretions, development of edema, and contraction of small muscles in the airways. The lungs become emphysematous because inspired air cannot be fully exhaled.

PREVENTION

Health Promotion

1. For children with history of asthma.
   a. Modify environment to reduce contact with offending allergen.
      (1) Remove causative allergen from home.
      (2) Avoid excessive cold, wind, smoke, and sprays.
      (3) Eliminate offending foods from diet.
   b. Provide emotionally stable environment.
   c. Take asthma medications as prescribed.
   d. Avoid contact with others with respiratory infections.
   e. Practice breathing exercises regularly and correctly.

Population at Risk

1. Asthma is rare in infancy but increases in incidence in children over 2 years of age.
2. Approximately 75 percent of children with asthma have a positive family history.
3. Asthmatic children also frequently have a history of eczema in infancy or early childhood.

Screening

None.

ASSESSMENT

Health History

1. Past history of atopic dermatitis (eczema) or allergic rhinitis in child or history of familial allergic disease.
2. Onset between ages 3 and 8 years.
3. Emotional status should be evaluated.

Physical Assessment

1. Early signs and symptoms.
   a. Gradual onset with nasal congestion and sneezing.
   b. Wheezing on expiration.
   c. Anxiety and restlessness.
   d. Altered vital signs: increased heart and respiratory rates.
   e. Diaphoresis.
   f. Coughing.
2. Late signs and symptoms.
   a. Increased wheezing.
   b. Thick, tenacious mucus, ineffective cough.
   c. Nasal flaring.
   d. Use of accessory muscles of respiration.
   e. Hyperresonance on percussion.
   f. Cyanosis.
   g. Extreme fatigue.
   h. Coarse rhonchi on auscultation of chest.
   i. Altered blood gases.
   j. Vomiting.
   k. Change in facial appearance.
      (1) Flattened malar bones.
      (2) Circles under eyes.
      (3) Narrow nose and prominent upper teeth.
   l. Color of mucosa—pale, boggy nasal mucosa occurs in children with allergies.
   m. The "allergic salute" (a characteristic gesture of rubbing the nose) may cause a crease across the bridge of the nose and is commonly found in children with allergies.

Diagnostic Tests

1. Skin testing to identify allergens.
2. Pulmonary function studies show
   a. Increased airway resistance.

b. Decreased forced expiratory volume within 1 second.
c. Increased total lung volume.
d. Increased functional residual capacity.
e. Uneven ventilation/perfusion ratios.
3. Chest x-ray films are used to rule out other diseases.
4. Sputum may show large numbers of eosinophils.
5. White blood cell (WBC) count: eosinophils may reach 30 to 40 percent in severe disease.

NURSING DIAGNOSES: ACTUAL OR POTENTIAL

1. Respiratory dysfunction, mild to severe, secondary to antigen-antibody reaction, swelling, bronchospasm, and mucus production.
2. Alteration in comfort: discomfort secondary to respiratory distress.
3. Nutritional deficit: decreased intake secondary to respiratory distress.
4. Decreased activity tolerance secondary to respiratory distress.
5. Altered self-concept and social development secondary to chronic illness.
6. Anxiety secondary to respiratory distress.
7. Knowledge deficit about self-care and treatment regimen.
8. Noncompliance with recommended treatment due to knowledge deficit.

EXPECTED OUTCOMES

1. Respiratory distress will be reduced immediately after initiation of medical regimen.
2. Nutrition and fluid intake will be adequate as evidenced by normal weight and hydration and report of diet, including the four food groups.
3. Ventilatory capacity will increase steadily weekly as evidenced by decreased fatigue after activity.
4. Self-concept and social adjustment will be adequate as evidenced by normal social skills and relationships for developmental stage (see Chapter 4).
5. Stressors in the environment will be reduced within 1 month of initial diagnosis of asthma.
6. Psychological counseling for child and family will be secured within 2 weeks, if necessary.
7. Client will understand information presented in teaching sessions as evidenced by 80 percent accuracy on paper and pencil tests.
8. Client will give evidence of compliance with care plan by
   a. Avoiding environmental irritants and pollutants.
   b. Removing offending substances from the home environment before discharge from the hospital, if possible.
   c. Adhering to medication regimen as demonstrated by a medication chart maintained by the client.
   d. Establishing and maintaining an effective exercise regimen.

INTERVENTIONS

1. Monitor vital signs, especially during an attack and when drugs are being administered.
2. Assess degree and progression of respiratory distress.
   a. Observe for nasal flaring or chest retractions (see Table 20-2 and Figure 20-2), wheezing, and cyanosis.
   b. Note any increase in restlessness or anxiety, or both.
3. Place child in Fowler's position with arms extended over bed table to allow for maximum lung expansion.
4. Administer oxygen, and provide mist tent.
5. Monitor blood gases—treat acidosis if present.
6. Administer medications and vaporized inhalations as prescribed (Table 20-3); observe for drug toxicity.
7. Reduce stressors in environment, and give sedation if necessary.
8. Teach chest physiotherapy and proper breathing habits.
   a. General considerations:
      (1) Breathing exercises provide for maximum use of the respiratory muscles, especially the diaphragm.
      (2) Have the child remove secretions from nasal passages before beginning exercises.
   b. Abdominal breathing (Figure 20-3*a*):
      (1) Have child lie on back with knees bent and feet flat on the floor.
      (2) Have child inflate lungs by taking a series of short inspirations through nose without allowing chest to rise.
      (3) Then have child exhale through mouth with pursed lips very slowly and completely until all the air is out.

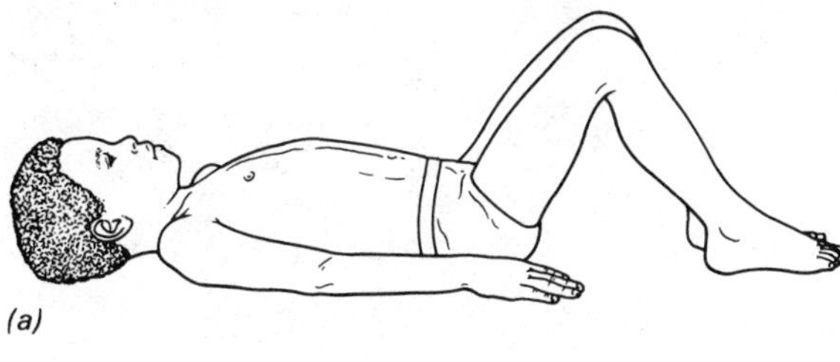

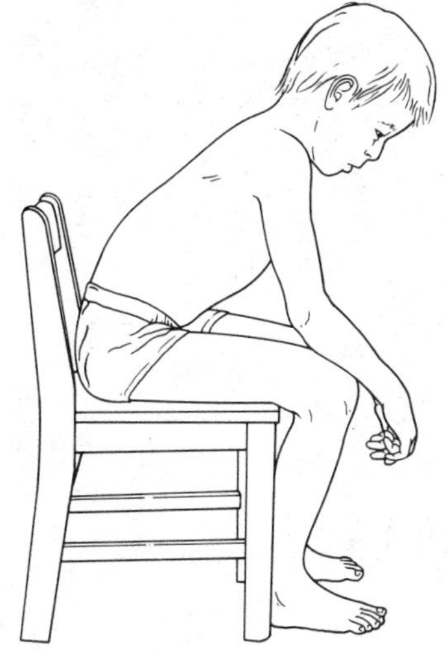

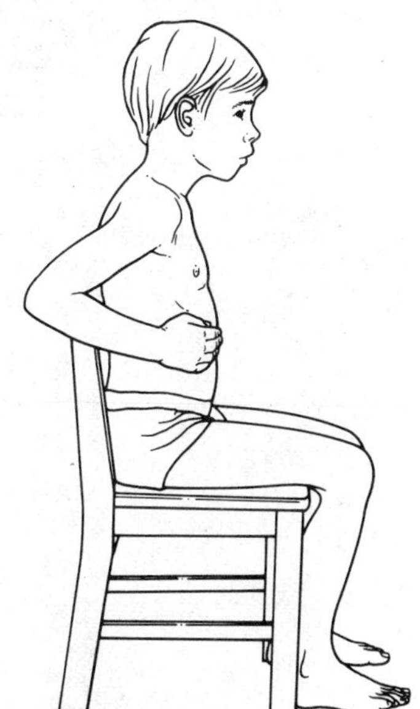

Figure 20-3 (*a*). Abdominal breathing position. (*b*). Forward-leaning position. (*c*). Side expansion position.

(4) Repeat 10 times.

c. Forward bending (Figure 20-3*b*):
   (1) Sit, leaning forward with a straight back and arms resting on the knees.
   (2) Breathe in through nose, expanding upper abdomen, and blow all the air out slowly through the mouth while keeping the chest still and remaining erect.
   (3) Repeat 10 times.
d. Side expansion (Figure 20-3*c*):
   (1) Sit in a chair with palms of hands on each side of the lower ribs.
   (2) Inhale, expanding lower ribs, then exhale through mouth, contracting upper part of the thorax and lower ribs.
   (3) Compress hands against ribs, and expel air from the base of the lungs.
   (4) Repeat 10 times.

9. Assess response to present therapy, including drugs.
10. Assess need for further hyposensitization.
11. Maintain parenteral fluid administration in acute phase.
12. Encourage oral fluid intake.
    a. Determine fluid preferences.
    b. Avoid iced fluids as they can stimulate bronchospasm.
13. Observe for signs of dehydration.
    a. Lack of tears.
    b. Dry mucous membranes.
    c. Poor skin turgor.
    d. Decreased urinary output.
14. Monitor intake and output.
15. Return to normal diet as soon as feasible.
16. Provide opportunity for parents to discuss their frustrations.
17. Avoid overprotection and dependence.
18. Encourage child to manage for him- or herself.
19. Promote an open, accepting atmosphere at home and in the hospital.
20. Encourage peer interactions by arranging or suggesting shared activities with other children whose development and physical activity levels are compatible with child's.
21. Help family and child to view asthma as only one of the child's many characteristics.
22. Assess child's level of anxiety.
23. Provide child maximal reassurance.
24. Provide a quiet, clean environment.
25. Evaluate need for sedation.

TABLE 20-3 DRUGS USED BY ASTHMATIC CHILDREN

Drug	Rationale	Action	Method	Dosage	Side Effects
Aminophylline[a]	Relief of paroxysm when ephedrine has failed	Slow; prolonged; bronchodilation	Suppository: drug is unevenly distributed in suppository, so fractional doses are unreliable Oral IV in a 2.5% solution *slowly* to avoid cardiac arrythmias or hypertension	3–4 mg/kg every 8 h (total daily dose by all routes should not exceed 12 mg/kg)	Initial signs of toxicity: increasing restlessness, irritability, and vomiting Life-threatening signs of toxicity; increasing excitement or delirium, vomiting of blood, convulsions, and hypotension
Beclomethasone	Used for chronic, perennial asthmatics who (*a*) cannot be controlled on any medication or (*b*) cannot be weaned from steroids	Controls symptoms of asthma by steroid action; is not a bronchodilator and is not to be used for acute asthma attack	Aerosol	Begin with 2 "puffs," 3 times a day; severe asthmatics may use 9 puffs per day; with exacerbation, may use up to 16 puffs per day	Bronchospasm that can interfere with inhalation, skin rashes, eosinophilic pneumonia, monilial infections of the mouth, pharynx, or larynx
Cromolyn sodium	Pretreatment (prophylaxis) of severe, recurrent asthma	Inhibits production of SRS-A and histamine; decreases frequency and severity of attacks; is not a bronchodilator and is not to be used for acute asthma attack	Inhalation	One capsule (20 mg) inhaled 4 times per day with a turboinhaler; restricted to children 5 years of age and over; drug is not effective if swallowed	Same as beclomethasone

Ephedrine	Prophylactic relief of nocturnal paroxysms and wheezing induced by exercise	Slow; prolonged duration; bronchodilation	Oral	Varies from 8 mg for preschooler to 25 mg for older children	Tachycardia, central nervous system stimulation, vomiting
Pseudoephedrine	Same as ephedrine	Same as ephedrine	Oral	About twice the dose of ephedrine	Relatively free of side effects
Epinephrine	Severe asthma: relief of paroxysm	Rapid; short duration; bronchodilation	1:1000 solution subcutaneously(SC) 1:1000 solution by inhalation; *never used for injection*	Small doses at 20- to 30-min intervals: 0.05 mL for infant; 0.01 mL/kg or 0.3 mL/m^2 to a maximum of 0.5 mL for older child	Pallor, tachycardia, and palpitation
Epinephrine aqueous suspension	Relief of paroxysms, especially frequent ones	Rapid; sustained (8–10 h)	1:200 aqueous suspension SC	Maximum single dose 0.15 mL (0.005 mL/kg)	Anxiety, restlessness, tremor, headache, dizzines, pallor, respiratory weakness, and palpitation
Ethylnorepinephrine	Same as epinephrine	Same as epinephrine	SC or IV	Same as epinephrine	Relatively free of side effects
Isopropylnorepinephrine	Relief of paroxysm	Same as epinephrine	Aerosol: Use must be supervised by an adult	1–2 "puffs" or sprays at $\frac{1}{2}$- to 1-h intervals (4–6 *total* daily "puffs")	Status asthmaticus with prolonged use: overdose (hypotension and cardiac arrest) with daily use

SOURCE: Adapted from Chard, M., and Scipien, G. M.: "The Respiratory System," in Scipien, G. M. et al (eds.): *Comprehensive Pediatric Nursing* 2d ed., McGraw-Hill, New York, 1979, p. 618–619. Used with permission.

[a] *Never* given in conjunction with epinephrine or ephedrine *unless aminophylline dosage reduced*. Otherwise toxic effects are potentiated.

26. Arrange for psychiatric counseling if necessary.
27. In hospital, organize care so as not to disturb child.
28. Discuss plan of care with child and parent.
29. Assess child's and parents' knowledge of drugs used in treatment.
30. Teach child and parents action, dosage, and side effects of drugs used in the treatment of asthma.
31. Encourage child and parents to administer only drugs prescribed by the physician.
32. Avoid any physical exertion or irritant that causes wheezing or dyspnea.
33. Teach child and parents to avoid offending antigens.
34. Encourage parent and child to keep physician's or clinic follow-up appointments.

EVALUATION

Outcome Criteria

1. Breath sounds are clearing to clear; wheezing is absent.
2. Physiological status is optimized; nutrition, hydration, rest, and acid-base balance are within normal limits.
3. Child is taking appropriate medications at correct times as indicated by a medication chart that the child or parent keeps.
4. Child, if age appropriate, and parents can recall either verbally or in writing (with 80 percent accuracy), the content presented in teaching sessions.
5. Child is able to participate in most play activities without dyspnea.
6. The offending antigen has been removed from the environment.
7. The child and family are coping adequately with the illness and following the recommended treatment regimen.
8. The child and family are receiving psychological counseling if necessary.

Complications

Respiratory insufficiency (see complications section under *Diaphragmatic Hernia*): need to evaluate if cause of insufficiency is progression of the disease, noncompliance with therapy, inappropriate drug dosages, or need for revision of a drug being given.

CYSTIC FIBROSIS

DESCRIPTION

Cystic fibrosis is a recessive hereditary disorder of the exocrine glands. The affected child inherits defective genes from both parents; on the average, one in four children in an affected family has the disease. The incidence is approximately one in every 2000 live births, in predominately white populations, with males and females equally affected. About 50 percent of children with cystic fibrosis survive to the age of 10 years; approximately 20 percent may live to be 30 years of age.

Five to 10 percent of children with cystic fibrosis have meconium ileus as newborns. With pancreatic insufficiency present in about 80 percent of children with cystic fibrosis, symptoms of intestinal malabsorption arise as the pancreatic ducts become clogged with abnormally tenacious mucus and are unable to secrete essential digestive enzymes. Pulmonary involvement is progressive as the thick secretions cause obstruction and permanent dilatation of the smaller airways. The result is lobar atelectasis, fibrotic changes, hypoxemia, pulmonary hypertension, and possible cor pulmonale. Pulmonary complications constitute the most serious threat to life.

PREVENTION

Health Promotion

Genetic counseling for parents known to be carriers of the disease.

Population at Risk

There is an overall one in four incidence in children whose parents both are carriers.

Screening

1. At present, it is not possible to isolate carriers. It is estimated that the number of carriers might be 1:20 to 1:50.
2. Sweat test in children with recurrent respiratory infections to rule out cystic fibrosis.

ASSESSMENT

Health History

1. Parent or sibling with the disease.
2. Meconium ileus in the newborn.
3. Repeated or chronic respiratory infections.

4. Failure to gain weight.
5. Bulky, foul-smelling stools.
6. Easy fatigability.

Physical Assessment

1. General characteristics.
   a. May be irritable.
   b. Thin extremities and protruding abdomen.
2. Pancreatic insufficiency.
   a. Slow weight gain in spite of voracious appetite.
   b. Increase in frequency of bowel movements.
   c. Massive, foul-smelling stools with fatty deposits (steatorrhea).
   d. Abdominal distension.
   e. Rectal prolapse.
   f. Abdominal cramps.
   g. Fat-soluble vitamin deficiency with anemia.
   h. Intestinal obstruction with or without intussusception in advanced stages.
3. Pulmonary manifestations—onset may be within weeks or years after birth.
   a. Dry, nonproductive cough progressing to a productive cough.
   b. Cyanosis.
   c. Barrel chest.
   d. Chest retractions.
   e. Clubbing of fingers and toes.
   f. Chronic hypoxemia.
   g. Recurrent respiratory infections.
   h. Bronchial rales.
   i. Lowered diaphragmatic arch.
   j. Dyspnea.
   k. Signs of cardiac insufficiency.

Diagnostic Tests

1. Sweat test: Increased sweat electrolytes, particularly chloride (normal = less than 60 mEq/L).
2. Pancreatic enzymes: Duodenal enzymes are absent or diminished. Trypsin is absent in more than 80 percent of children with cystic fibrosis.
3. Fat absorption tests: Large volumes of fat excreted in stool. A 5-day stool collection is usually the best way to detect fat.
4. Radiographs: Chest x-ray film shows general obstructive emphysema, patchy atelectasis, and a disseminated infiltrate pattern of bronchopneumonia.
5. Pulmonary function tests.
   a. Increased airway resistance.
   b. Uneven ventilation/perfusion ratios.
   c. Increased residual lung volume.

NURSING DIAGNOSES: ACTUAL OR POTENTIAL

1. Progressive respiratory dysfunction, moderate to severe, due to accumulation of mucus and plugging of terminal airways.
2. Alteration in comfort: discomfort secondary to respiratory changes.
3. Nutritional deficit secondary to absorption problem and loss of appetite with respiratory distress.
4. Diminished activity/exercise tolerance secondary to chronic hypoxemia and muscle wasting.
5. Noncompliance with therapy regimen due to knowledge deficit and/or denial of chronicity of disease.

EXPECTED OUTCOMES

1. Child will cough productively as evidenced by (a) removal of mucus from lungs after coughing and chest physiotherapy and (b) arrest of lung disease on x-ray film.
2. Ventilatory capacity will remain stable or increase weekly as evidenced by decreased fatigue after a selected activity.
3. Client and parent will understand information given in teaching sessions as evidenced by 80 percent accuracy on written or verbal tests.
4. Client will demonstrate gradual weight gain over a specified period of time.
5. Client and family will give evidence of compliance with care plan by
   a. Adhering to medication and chest physiotherapy regimen as indicated by chart maintained by the client and/or parents.
   b. Demonstration of a gradual weight gain.
   c. Avoiding respiratory irritants and pollutants.
   d. Maintaining good general health habits.

INTERVENTIONS

1. Provide prescribed pancreatic extracts, such as Cotazym or Viokase. The dosage is dependent on the preparation selected and the child's response. It can be sprinkled on the

food directly or ingested as a tablet. The preparation is given with each meal and snack in a dose appropriate to the amount of food taken.

2. Medium-chain triglycerides may be given as a dietary supplement.
3. Administer supplemental fat-soluble vitamins (A,D,E, and K) as prescribed. (Children with cystic fibrosis require a water-miscible vitamin preparation, usually administered in double the usual recommended dose because of poor absorption by the intestine.)
4. The child may require sodium chloride tablets in hot weather when perspiring excessively.
5. For an infant, Progestimil formula may be recommended.
6. Use clapping, cupping, deep breathing, assisted coughing, and vibration techniques as part of chest physiotherapy (techniques are described in Chapter 31).
7. Use aerosol therapy to hydrate bronchial secretions.
8. A mist tent is helpful; mucolytic agents can be given via mist treatment.
9. Give expectorants as prescribed.
10. Employ bronchial lavage.
11. Prevent and treat respiratory infections.
    a. Teach avoidance of contact with infection.
    b. Administer prescribed antibiotic therapy (drug of choice depends on the organism).
    c. Perform pulmonary lavage.
12. Administer oxygen therapy.
13. Provide emotional support to the child and family with the assistance of other health team members.
    a. Provide an opportunity for the family to discuss concerns and frustrations.
    b. Promote growth and development.
14. Educate family in
    a. Use of equipment.
    b. Exercises.
    c. Diet.
    d. Administration of drugs.
    e. Genetic counseling.
    f. Preventive measures (i.e., infection control).
    g. Home care.
15. Help family acquire medications and equipment.
16. Arrange for follow-up appointments or care.
17. Assist family in problem solving.
18. Assist family with appropriate referrals.
    a. Social worker.
    b. Psychologist.
    c. Community resources (e.g., American Lung Association, state crippled children's services, home health agency).
    d. Genetic counseling.

EVALUATION

Outcome Criteria

1. Cough becomes more productive and remains productive as secretions are removed.
2. Child begins to gain weight within 2 weeks of initial dietary therapy.
3. Child is taking medications at appropriate times and in correct amounts as indicated by a chart the child or parent keeps.
4. Child and/or adult will recall with 80 percent accuracy, either verbally or in writing, the content presented in teaching sessions.
5. Child is able to participate in appropriate play activities without undue fatigue.
6. Child and parents understand and cooperatively participate in treatment regimen, including home care as evidenced by charts kept.
7. Child and family are coping and adjusting adequately to the chronic state of the disease.
8. Family members are informed about genetic transmission risks.

Complications

RESPIRATORY INSUFFICIENCY

See complications section under *Diaphragmatic Hernia*.

COR PULMONALE

Assessment

1. Progressive dyspnea.
2. Progressively increased heart rate.
3. Enlarged liver.
4. Possible edema of eyes and/or extremities (in an older child).
5. Progressive cyanosis.
6. Progressive acidosis with hypoxemia and hypercapnia.

Revised Outcomes

1. Oxygenation will be restored to within normal limits, dyspnea will cease, and respiratory and heart rates will return to normal.

2. pH will be restored to within normal limits.
3. Cardiac function will be restored to normal limits.

Interventions

1. Administer oxygen as ordered.
2. Monitor blood gases.
3. Administer digoxin and diuretic as ordered.
4. Administer bronchodilators as ordered.
5. Monitor ECG. There is an increased incidence of arrhythmias in these clients.
6. Administer antibiotics as ordered to treat underlying respiratory infection.

INFLAMMATIONS

BRONCHOPULMONARY DYSPLASIA

DESCRIPTION

Bronchopulmonary dysplasia (BPD) is a syndrome of infancy similar to adult pulmonary oxygen toxicity. Bronchopulmonary dysplasia occurs in some infants who survive respiratory distress syndrome (RDS, discussed in Chapter 11). The cause is postulated to be a combination of high oxygen concentrations during treatment for RDS and respirator therapy.

Physiological features include

1. Hyalin membranes form in proximal bronchioles.
2. Areas of pulmonary hemorrhage and fibrosis develop.
3. Capillaries and alveolar membranes sustain damage and show evidence of increased permeability.
4. The infant suffers chronic hypoxia, decreased pulmonary perfusion, pulmonary vascular disease, pulmonary hypertension, and resultant cor pulmonale (right-sided heart failure as blood cannot enter the pulmonary system as well due to the fibrosis).
5. Pulmonary damage is reversible, but healing can take months or years.

PREVENTION

Health Promotion

See prevention section of RDS, Chapter 11.

Population at Risk

1. Appears primarily in children who have had RDS.
2. Appears to be associated with high concentrations of oxygen administered during treatment phase of RDS.
3. Infants who have received positive pressure ventilation with or without continuous positive airway pressure (CPAP).
4. Infants who have had prolonged endotracheal intubation.
5. Seldom seen in infants who were administered negative pressure ventilation without intubation.

Screening

None.

ASSESSMENT

Health History

1. Development of RDS after birth.
2. Long-term treatment for RDS, consisting of endotracheal intubation, high concentrations of oxygen, and use of positive pressure ventilation.
3. Prematurity at birth.
4. Decreased activity tolerance.
5. Poor appetite.

Physical Assessment

The child with BPD has, essentially, chronic lung disease. The specific findings are general to all children with a chronic lung disorder.

1. Signs of increased work of breathing.
   a. Tachypnea.
   b. Cyanosis.
   c. Shortness of breath.
   d. Irritability.
   e. Barrel-shaped chest from lung hyperinflation.
2. Chronic hypoxemia.
3. Possible hypercapnia.
4. Clubbing of fingers and toes.
5. Possible delayed physical development.
6. Chronic respiratory infection.
7. Signs of heart failure (see Chapter 19).

Diagnostic Tests

1. Chest x-ray film: shows characteristic cystlike pattern of fibrosis.
2. Arterial blood gases: estimates the progression of the disease (as the fibrosis increases,

P_{CO_2} increases to levels usually 60–70 mmHg).

NURSING DIAGNOSES: ACTUAL OR POTENTIAL

1. Respiratory dysfunction, mild to severe, secondary to fibrosis and development of cor pulmonale.
2. Nutritional deficit: failure to gain weight and weight loss secondary to chronic respiratory dysfunction.
3. Decreased activity tolerance secondary to chronic respiratory dysfunction.
4. Alteration in comfort: discomfort and orthopnea secondary to respiratory changes.
5. Potential right-sided heart failure secondary to pulmonary vascular changes.
6. Parental frustration and anxiety due to chronic iatrogenic disease.

EXPECTED OUTCOMES

1. Degree of respiratory distress will decrease over time as evidenced by a decrease in the obvious signs of distress, progression towards clean lung sounds, and increased activity tolerance.
2. Degree of oxygenation will improve as evidenced by arterial blood gases that are nearer normal levels.
3. Child will demonstrate steady weight gain over a specified period of time.
4. Child will remain as free from recurrent respiratory infections as possible.
5. Child will remain free from secondary heart failure (cor pulmonale).
6. Parents will understand the treatment regimen regarding home care and demonstrate competence in carrying out the necessary therapies.
7. Parents will be able to express frustrations that they may have related to the chronicity of the disease.
8. Parents will demonstrate less anxiety about the care and prognosis of the disease process.

INTERVENTIONS

1. Administer oxygen and humidity therapy.
2. Chest physiotherapy methods should be used (see Chapter 31).
3. Clear out respiratory secretions.
4. Use bronchodilators and antibiotics as prescribed.
5. Tracheostomy may be necessary to provide pulmonary toilet.
6. Assisted ventilation may be necessary.
7. Advise parents to keep child away from others with infections.
8. Encourage regular medical follow-up.
9. Monitor growth and development—take weekly weights during infancy; keep a growth chart.
10. Provide rest periods for child during day, depending on level of activity.
11. Encourage parents to treat child as normally as possible.
12. Monitor for signs of heart failure.
    a. Hepatomegaly.
    b. Anorexia.
    c. Abdominal pain.
    d. Edema.
    e. Decreased urine output.
    f. Diaphoresis.
    g. Tachypnea.
    h. Tachycardia.
13. Instruct parents in home care:
    a. Oxygen therapy.
    b. Chest physiotherapy and removal of secretions.
    c. Diet therapy: furnishing a diet high in protein and calories.
    d. Importance of prevention of respiratory infections.
    e. Monitoring for complications.
        (1) Respiratory infections.
        (2) Heart failure.
14. Assist parents to develop a realistic attitude toward the child's illness.
15. Encourage parents to ask questions and discuss frustrations.
16. Assist with referrals.
    a. Home health nurse.
    b. Social service.
    c. American Lung Association.
    d. State crippled children's agency.

EVALUATION

Outcome Criteria

1. Respiratory distress becomes progressively less obvious, and activity tolerance is increased.
2. Breath sounds are clearing to clear; adventitious sounds are absent.

3. Chest percussion and vibration are yielding few, if any, secretions.
4. Child has remained free from recurrent respiratory infections.
5. Child has demonstrated a steady weight gain and is within normal weight range for age.
6. Parents are following the daily therapeutic regimen outlined by the physician.
7. Child has demonstrated no signs of heart failure.
8. Parents are more comfortable with the home care regimen and prognosis.

Complications

1. Cor pulmonale.
2. Recurrent respiratory infections.
3. Respiratory insufficiency.

Assessment

1. Hypoxemia: decreased Po_2.
2. Hypercapnia: increased Pco_2 levels.
3. Lowered pH: respiratory acidosis or metabolic acidosis related to severe hypoxemia.
4. Increase in severity of other signs of respiratory distress.

Revised Outcomes

1. Arterial blood gases will return to near normal levels.
2. Signs of respiratory distress will lessen or cease.

Interventions

1. Administer humidified oxygen (as needed).
2. Assist ventilation (as needed).
3. Monitor arterial blood gases to evaluate progression of disease.
4. Monitor cardiac function to assess impending heart failure.

Reevaluation and Follow-up

Revise plan of care to ensure that complications are overcome, and continue with close surveillance of respiratory and cardiac status.

BRONCHOPNEUMONIA

DESCRIPTION

Bronchopneumonia is an inflammation of the lungs in which there are scattered areas of consolidation and inflammation of the interstitial mucosa. Bronchopneumonia can be caused by a viral or bacterial agent. Affected areas of the lung cannot be ventilated properly, and ventilation/perfusion mismatching occurs. The alveoli become congested with red blood cells (RBCs) and fibrin exudate.

Bronchopneumonia is prevalent in children in the first 4 years of life. It differs from the kind of pneumonia that older children or adults get, in which only one or more lobes are involved.

PREVENTION

Health Promotion

1. Avoid crowded living conditions, if possible.
2. Avoid exposure to individuals with upper respiratory infections.
3. Maintain good health habits (rest, nutrition, etc.).

Population at Risk

1. Persons living in densely populated areas.
2. Children exposed to individuals with respiratory infections.
3. Infants and children up to 4 years of age.

Screening

None.

ASSESSMENT

Health History

1. Upper respiratory infection of several days' duration before pneumonia.
2. Decrease in appetite before diagnosis.
3. Possible vomiting and diarrhea.
4. Fatigability.

Physical Assessment

1. Abrupt onset of fever.
2. Nasal flaring (Table 20-2).
3. Retractions of chest (Table 20-2).
4. Cough.
5. Tachypnea and tachycardia.
6. Rales.
7. Possible chest pain.

Diagnostic Tests

1. Chest x-ray film shows areas of consolidation or disseminated infiltration.
2. Leukocytosis (normal values are age dependent).
3. Sputum culture is positive for the organism if bacterial.
4. Blood culture may be positive.
5. Antistreptolysin O titer level may be elevated in streptococcal pneumonia.

NURSING DIAGNOSES: ACTUAL OR POTENTIAL

1. Respiratory dysfunction, mild to severe: dyspnea secondary to infiltrates that form in lung.
2. Alteration in comfort: discomfort secondary to fever and respiratory changes (cough, chest pain).
3. Nutritional deficit: decreased intake secondary to respiratory dysfunction; vomiting.
4. Fluid volume deficit secondary to fever, vomiting, diarrhea, and decreased intake.
5. Decreased activity tolerance due to respiratory dysfunction (dyspnea, cough).

EXPECTED OUTCOMES

1. Respiratory distress and status of oxygenation will improve as evidenced by physical assessment and arterial blood gases.
2. Body temperature will return to normal within 2 to 5 days of treatment initiation.
3. Child will be able to ingest adequate fluids and calories within 3 to 5 days of treatment initiation.
4. Level of fatigue will lessen within 5 to 7 days as evidenced by child's involvement in play and the environment.
5. Child will not exhibit signs of complications.

INTERVENTIONS

1. Monitor vital signs closely.
2. Assess degree of distress (see Table 20-2).
3. Provide humidified oxygen.
4. Remove respiratory secretions.
5. Provide frequent position changes.
6. Provide chest physiotherapy (see Chapter 31).
7. Administer antibiotic therapy as prescribed.
8. Administer antipyretics as prescribed.
9. Give sponge baths as necessary.
10. Observe for febrile convulsions.
11. Administer parenteral therapy when in acute distress.
12. Keep accurate intake and output records.
13. Encourage oral fluid intake.
14. Offer child small, frequent feedings except when in acute distress.
15. Provide quiet, restful environment.
16. Allow for frequent rest periods.
17. Try not to disturb child unless necessary.

EVALUATION

Outcome Criteria

1. Degree of respiratory distress is reduced or absent within 2 to 5 days after treatment initiation.
2. Breath sounds are clear to clearing; adventitious sounds are absent.
3. Body temperature has returned to a normal level.
4. Child is eating a general diet and taking in adequate fluids; vomiting and diarrhea are absent.
5. Child is able to resume play and interest in the environment.

Complications

1. Aspiration of feeding due to severe respiratory distress.
2. Development of a tension pneumothorax.
3. Development of a paralytic ileus.
4. Development of constipation.
5. Respiratory insufficiency.

Assessment

1. Hypoxemia: decreased P_{O_2}.
2. Hypercapnia: increased P_{CO_2}.
3. Lowered pH: respiratory acidosis.
4. Restlessness.
5. Increased signs of respiratory distress.

Revised Outcomes

1. Oxygenation will be restored to within normal limits; all other signs of respiratory distress will cease.
2. Other outcomes, as originally stated.

Interventions

1. Administer humidified oxygen (as needed).
2. Monitor arterial blood gases to evaluate disease.
3. Suction as necessary.
4. Administer nebulized bronchodilator as ordered to increase bronchial dilation.

CHEMICAL PNEUMONIA

DESCRIPTION

Ingestion (as well as direct aspiration) of lipid and hydrocarbon substances can cause chemical pneumonia, depending on the amount and type of material ingested. Common agents include kerosene, gasoline, turpentine, and vegetable oils. Oil aspiration results in chronic fibrosis of the affected lung tissue. Ingested petroleum distillates (kerosene, charcoal starter, gasoline, etc.), because of their low surface tension, easily spread along the esophageal mucosa to enter the respiratory tract where they can set up a stubborn pneumonia. Petroleum distillate ingestion and aspiration are serious and potentially fatal, both because of the pulmonary sequelae and because of their metabolic and neurological consequences. Emergency treatment is dealt with in Part VII.

PREVENTION

Health Promotion

1. Solvents, lighter fluid, and other hydrocarbon substances should be kept well out of reach of all children.
2. Kerosene, gasoline, and other potential poisons should never be stored in soft drink bottles or other containers that may encourage ingestion.
3. Oil-base vitamins or nosedrops and other orally or nasally administered oily substances must never be forced upon a resisting or crying child because of the danger of aspiration.
4. Oily foods that are easily aspirated (e.g., nuts, sunflower seeds, bacon) should not be given to children under $2\frac{1}{2}$ years of age.

Population at Risk

1. Aspiration can occur at any age but is most common in 1- to 3-year-old children.
2. Ingestion of inedible substances, such as hydrocarbons, is most common in children between 1 and 3 years of age and in hyperactive and impulsive children and those with a history of other ingestion accidents (e.g., aspirin poisoning, corrosive burns of the mouth).
3. Weak or debilitated children who receive oil-base liquid vitamins or other oily preparations.

Screening

None.

ASSESSMENT

Health History

1. A weak or debilitated state.
2. One to 3 years of age.
3. Use of an oil-base medication.
4. History of choking may or may not be positive.

Physical Assessment

See *Bronchopneumonia.* Additional considerations may be warranted by neurological status.

Diagnostic Tests

1. Chest x-ray film.
2. Sputum culture.

NURSING DIAGNOSES: ACTUAL OR POTENTIAL

See *Bronchopneumonia.*

EXPECTED OUTCOMES

See *Bronchopneumonia.* Additional considerations may be warranted by neurological status.

INTERVENTIONS

See *Bronchopneumonia.* Emergency treatment measures are presented in Part VII. Additional considerations may be warranted by neurological status.

EVALUATION

See *Bronchopneumonia.* Additional considerations may be warranted by neurological status.

TONSILLITIS

DESCRIPTION

Also referred to as *pharyngitis,* tonsillitis is an infectious invasion of the lymphatic tissue called the *faucial tonsils* located on either side of the pharynx. An acute as well as a chronic form of the condition exists. About 85 percent of all cases are caused by viruses, while 15 percent are caused by group A beta-hemolytic streptococcus.

The faucial tonsils are part of Waldeyer's ring, a circle of lymph tissue that surrounds the pharynx. The tissue filters microorganisms and protects against infection of the respiratory and GI tracts. Invasion by microorganisms causes the tissues to swell and, potentially, to obstruct the airways. The lymphoid tissues are normally largest in children under 5 years of age and gradually decrease in size until puberty. Chronic tonsillitis may require tonsillectomy.

PREVENTION

Health Promotion

1. Avoid close contact with individuals with upper respiratory infections.
2. Maintain good health habits (e.g., rest, nutrition).

Population at Risk

1. The peak incidence is between ages 4 and 6 years.
2. Children exposed to an individual with an upper respiratory infection.

Screening

None.

ASSESSMENT

Health History

1. Exposure to an individual with an upper respiratory infection.
2. A member of the age group at risk.
3. Sore throat.
4. Difficulty in swallowing.
5. Sneezing.
6. Cough.
7. Sometimes vomiting and diarrhea, especially in younger children.
8. Sometimes headache in older children.
9. Irritability and malaise.
10. Muscles may ache.
11. History of previous tonsillitis is common.

Physical Assessment

1. A fever up to 40°C (104°F) orally is likely to be present when the organism is streptococcus; in viral infections the fever is slight to moderate.
2. The child is likely to exhibit generalized malaise and uninterest in the environment.
3. Pharyngeal erythema and exudate may or may not be present.
4. Cervical lymph nodes may be enlarged.
5. In chronic tonsillitis, the child may have offensive breath odor.

Diagnostic Tests

1. Throat culture: Most cases will be viral, but a culture will rule out beta-hemolytic streptococcus.
2. The WBC level may be elevated to 40,000 per cubic millimeter.

NURSING DIAGNOSES: ACTUAL OR POTENTIAL

1. Alteration in comfort: discomfort secondary to sore throat, cough, headache, muscular aches, malaise, and fever.
2. Nutritional deficit secondary to sore throat and difficult swallowing.
3. Fluid volume deficit secondary to fever, decreased intake, vomiting, and diarrhea.
4. Decreased activity secondary to discomfort and fever.

EXPECTED OUTCOMES

1. Patency of airway will be maintained at all times.
2. Body temperature will return to normal within 2 to 5 days of treatment initiation.
3. Any reaction to penicillin will be immediately detected and the medication discontinued.
4. Nutritional intake and fluid balance will be restored.
5. Child and family will be prepared for surgery if surgical intervention is planned.
6. Child and family will receive effective postoperative care if surgery is performed.

INTERVENTIONS

1. Immediate.
   a. Give warm saline gargles.
   b. Apply hot or cold packs to neck area.
   c. Give aspirin as prescribed for pain.
   d. Avoid hot foods or liquids—administer cool, bland liquids only.
   e. Administer antipyretic agent as prescribed.
   f. Give client sponge bath with tepid water as needed for fever.
   g. Have client drink fluids as tolerated.
   h. Observe for signs of penicillin allergy: increased heart rate, increased respiratory rate, decreased blood pressure, skin rash, difficulty breathing.
   i. If surgery is planned, prepare child and parents.
2. Postoperative.
   a. Keep in semiprone position until recovered from anesthesia (to facilitate drainage and detection of bleeding).

b. Observe for excessive bleeding (frequent swallowing, bloody emesis, vital signs changes, postanesthetic restlessness).
c. Give fluids and a soft diet.
d. Apply ice collar (if tolerated), and give aspirin as prescribed for pain.
e. Instruct parents regarding home care (give soft diet, avoid overactivity, and observe for bleeding, all for 1 week).

EVALUATION

Outcome Criteria

1. Sore throat and pharyngeal erythema will be absent.
2. Cervical lymph nodes will diminish in size.
3. Child will be active and consume adequate fluids and calories.
4. If surgery is indicated, the outcome will be uneventful.

Complications

1. Development of chronic tonsillitis.
2. Reaction to penicillin.
3. Postoperative hemorrhage.

OTITIS MEDIA

DESCRIPTION

Otitis media is an infection of the middle ear that usually occurs secondary to a recent upper respiratory infection. About two-thirds of cases are of viral origin, and one-third are bacterial. Common bacterial pathogens are pneumococci, *H. influenzae*, beta-hemolytic streptococcus, *S. aureus*, and *Escherichia coli*. The microorganisms that infect the middle ear usually are transmitted from the pharyngeal area via the eustachian tube.

PREVENTION

Health Promotion

Avoid contact with an individual with an upper respiratory infection.

Population at Risk

1. Infants and young children are at greatest risk because
   a. Their eustachian tubes are wide, short, and straight, and thus allow pathogens easy access to the middle ear; as the child grows, the tubes become longer, more twisted, and narrow, providing anatomical protection against infection.
   b. The eustachian tubes are more distensible and more likely to open inappropriately.
   c. The abundant lymph tissue normally present in the airway of a child readily obstructs the eustachian tube opening in the nasopharynx.
   d. The humoral defense mechanisms are still immature.
2. Incidence is higher in low socioeconomic groups.
3. Children with cleft palate are highly susceptible.
4. Those with a history of otitis media are at risk for recurrences.

Screening

None.

ASSESSMENT

Health History

1. Exposure to an individual with an upper respiratory infection.
2. Member of the population at risk.
3. Irritability and restlessness.
4. Pulling or rubbing ear, especially infant.
5. Older child may have headache and dizziness.
6. Earache is not present in all cases.
7. Poor appetite.
8. Diarrhea, especially infant.

Physical Assessment

1. Irritability and restlessness.
2. Fever (not present in all children with otitis media).
3. Eardrum may be bulging or retracted and red or yellow in color instead of normal pearl-gray.
4. If tympanic membrane has ruptured, there may be discharge from the ear (i.e., pus or serous fluid).
5. There may be hearing loss.

Diagnostic Tests

1. Otoscopy reveals a bright red or yellow, bulging or retracted tympanic membrane.
2. Tympanometry, measurement of the tympanic membrane compliance, reveals loss of mobility of the membrane.

NURSING DIAGNOSES: ACTUAL OR POTENTIAL

1. Alteration in comfort: discomfort secondary to inflammation in the ear, headache, dizziness.
2. Sensory deficit: diminished ability to hear secondary to fluid-filled middle ear compartment and edematous tympanic membrane.
3. Nutritional deficit: decreased food intake or absorption secondary to pain, vomiting, and diarrhea.
4. Fluid volume deficit secondary to fever and decreased intake.
5. Decreased activity tolerance due to discomfort.

EXPECTED OUTCOMES

1. Pain and discomfort will be relieved within 2 to 5 days after treatment initiation.
2. Body temperature will return to normal within 2 to 3 days after treatment initiation.
3. Signs of infection will be resolved within 7 to 10 days after treatment initiation.
4. Child will return to normal activities and food and fluid intake within 7 days.

INTERVENTIONS

1. Administer prescribed antibiotic (penicillin for 10 days is the drug of choice for streptococcal or pneumococcal otitis).
2. Give analgesic as prescribed to reduce discomfort.
3. Administer prescribed decongestant to shrink mucous membranes.
4. Apply heat over the affected ear by using a hot water bottle or a heating pad.
5. Surgery (myringotomy) is indicated when there is inadequate response to antibiotic.
6. Monitor temperature closely.
7. Administer antipyretic as prescribed.
8. Encourage oral fluids.
9. Give sponge bath with tepid water if necessary.
10. Observe for perforation of eardrum, febrile convulsions, and development of chronic otitis media, mastoiditis, brain abscess, and reaction to penicillin.
11. Provide follow-up evaluation for hearing loss.

EVALUATION

Outcome Critera

1. Discomfort and pain in ear cease.
2. Temperature returns to normal.
3. Hearing, if affected, is restored.
4. Activities of daily living are resumed.
5. Nutrition and fluid balance are restored.
6. If surgery is performed, the outcome is uneventful.

Complications

1. Perforation of eardrum.
2. Mastoiditis.
3. Brain abscess.
4. Chronic otitis media.
5. Febrile convulsions.
6. Residual hearing loss.

BIBLIOGRAPHY

Avery, M. E.: *The Lung and its Disorders in The Newborn Infant*, 4th ed., W. B. Saunders, Philadelphia, 1981. This monograph is specifically devoted to the lung and its disorders in the newborn infant. Normal development and physiology of the fetal and neonatal lung, disorders of respiration, and artificial respiration are described in detail.

Kendig, E.: *Disorders of the Respiratory Tract in Children*, vol. 11, W. B. Saunders, Philadelphia, 1979. This book serves as a complete reference for anatomy, physiology, development, and diseases of the respiratory system in children.

Levison, H.: "Symposium on the Chest," *Pediatric Clinics of North America*, vol. 26, no. 3, August, 1979, pp. 467–701. Levison edits this edition consisting of current therapies and management. Each chapter is written by a specialist in the particular field. Topics range from medical and surgical respiratory problems to radiology of the chest. An excellent bibliography is located at the end of each chapter.

Lough, M., Doershuk, C., and Stern, R.: *Pediatric Respiratory Therapy*, 2d ed., Year Book Medical Publishers, Chicago, 1979. Written for nurses, respiratory therapists, physical therapists, and physicians interested in pulmonary diseases in children. Lough and other contributors present development and physiology of the respiratory system, respiratory diseases in the newborn, respiratory therapy techniques, respiratory physical therapy, and pulmonary function testing. A bibliography follows each chapter. A useful variety of diagrams and photographs accompanies the text.

Scipien, G. M., Barnard, M. U., Chard, M., et al. (eds.): *Comprehensive Pediatric Nursing*, 2d ed., McGraw-Hill, New York, 1979. This comprehensive and current pediatric textbook includes chapters on the nursing process and an extensive chapter dealing in detail with the care of children with respiratory problems.

Smith, M. J., Goodman, J. A., Ramsey, N. L., et al. (eds.): *Child and Family: Concepts of Nursing Practice*, McGraw-Hill, New York, 1982. This new textbook includes respiratory disorders of infancy and childhood, with many tables and illustrations supplementing a clear presentation of nursing care for clients with these disorders. Detailed care plan for infant with croup is given.

Whaley, L., and Wong, D. (eds.): *Nursing Care of Infants and Children*, C. V. Mosby, St. Louis, 1979. An excellent respiratory section with comprehensive nursing care plans is presented. The chapter includes physiological principles, diagnostic tests, disease entities, and nursing care. An extensive bibliography is included in the chapter.

21

The Urinary System

Annette Crosby Frauman and Cyrena M. Gilman

ABNORMAL CELLULAR GROWTH

POLYCYSTIC DISEASE

DESCRIPTION

Polycystic disease begins in fetal life. The ureteric bud gives rise to the ureters, pelvis of the kidneys, and lower collecting ducts. The metanephrogenic cap gives rise to the glomeruli, tubules, and upper collecting ducts. If these upper and lower ducts fail to join properly in fetal life, polycystic kidneys result. The disease is divided into two types. The infantile type is autosomal recessive, and 25 to 90 percent of the renal tubules are cystic. It usually becomes apparent in the neonatal period and can result in death in the first 2 months of life. In the adult type, which is autosomal dominant, symptoms may not occur until the fourth decade of life, as less than 10 percent of the tubules are affected. Approximately 10 percent of individuals with the adult form manifest symptoms as children or adolescents. Medical treatment consists of medication for pulmonary and cardiac complications, shunting for portacaval hypertension, and dialysis and transplantation for end-stage renal disease.

PREVENTION

Health Promotion

Genetic counseling for prospective parents with a family history of the disorder.

Population at Risk

1. Persons with known family history of polycystic disease.
2. Persons with family history of childhood deaths from "kidney trouble."

Screening

None.

ASSESSMENT

Health History

1. Infantile type.
   a. Born after prolonged labor due to infant's enlarged abdomen.
   b. Respiratory and circulatory problems at birth.
2. Adult type.
   a. Pain in both flanks.
   b. Polyuria.
   c. Headaches.
   d. Recurrent urinary tract infections.

Physical Assessment

1. Infantile type.
   a. Large bilateral flank masses that are tense and symmetrical and do not illuminate.

b. Variable urinary output; oliguria is common.
c. Hypertension.
d. Congestive heart failure (CHF): tachycardia, tachypnea, hepatomegaly.
e. Respiratory distress due to large kidneys, pneumothorax, or pneumomediastinum.

2. Adult type.
a. Bilateral flank masses.
b. Growth failure in clients whose disease began to manifest itself in childhood or adolescence.
c. Hypertension.
d. Hypersplenism and splenomegaly.
e. Esophageal and gastric varices and resultant hematemesis due to portacaval hypertension.
f. Decreasing renal function, shown by elevated BUN and creatinine, leads to osteodystrophy and anemia.

Diagnostic Tests

1. Abdominal ultrasonography.
2. Intravenous pyelogram (IVP).
3. Renal angiography.

NURSING DIAGNOSES: ACTUAL OR POTENTIAL

1. Impairment of urinary elimination: oliguria secondary to glomerular damage.
2. Alteration in cardiac output: CHF secondary to fluid retention.
3. Alteration in fluid volume: hypertension due to fluid overload and renal hormonal response to damage.
4. Respiratory dysfunction due to pneumothorax or pneumomendiastinum that may be associated with polycystic disease.

EXPECTED OUTCOMES

1. Infantile type.
a. Urinary output will be accurately monitored.
b. Hypertension will be detected and controlled.
c. Congestive heart failure will be prevented or quickly detected and treated.
d. Respiratory distress will be quickly detected and treated.

2. Adult type.
a. Child will attain maximum growth possible.
b. Hypertension will be detected and controlled.
c. Bleeding will be prevented, especially when thrombocytopenia is present.
d. End-stage renal disease will be detected and treated.
e. When dialysis and transplantation become necessary, the child and family will be prepared for them.

INTERVENTIONS

1. Infantile type.
a. Strict monitoring of intake and output. If necessary, weigh diapers to estimate urinary output (1 mL of urine weighs approximately 1 g).
b. Frequent blood pressure readings. Nurses may certainly monitor blood pressures as often as they may deem necessary; a physician's order is not needed. Indications of irritability, lethargy, headache, or CHF warrant frequent blood pressure readings.
c. Frequent vital signs and abdominal palpation for hepatomegaly if cardiac or respiratory rates are increased. Tachypnea, tachycardia, and a lower-than-normal liver margin are cardinal signs of CHF in the infant or young child. (See *Congestive Heart Failure* in Chapter 19.)
d. Report any signs of CHF immediately. Digitalization, antihypertensive agents and low-sodium feedings may be ordered; such orders are to be followed scrupulously.
e. Observe for and immediately report any respiratory distress. Pneumothorax and pneumomediastinum are not infrequent complications. Oxygen by hood, intubation, or ventilator may be required.

2. Adult type.
a. Provide high-calorie meals within the framework of any dietary restrictions of protein, sodium, and potassium. Child, family, and personnel need to be aware of child's restrictions, since children find many ways of obtaining forbidden foods, even in a hospital.
b. Monitor blood pressure frequently. Give antihypertensive medication as directed.
c. Immediately report any bleeding, especially if hard to control (hypersplenism can lead to thrombocytopenia).

d. Monitor BUN and creatinine values (Table 21–1). Rising values indicate onset of end-stage renal disease; this can come about quickly or slowly.
e. Provide parents opportunities to discuss their child's defect and hemodialysis and transplantation. Provide as much information as they are ready to hear about both procedures.
f. Prepare child for hemodialysis and transplantation by visiting the dialysis unit, playing with dolls who have "similar problems," telling stories, and drawing pictures. Be honest about possible discomforts.

EVALUATION

Outcome Criteria

1. Intake and output are strictly monitored.
2. Blood pressure is taken frequently, certainly

TABLE 21-1 SELECTED LABORATORY PROCEDURES AND THEIR NORMAL VALUES

CHEMISTRIES	
Blood urea nitrogen (BUN)	5–20 mg per 100 mL
Creatinine	0.05–0.5 mg per 100 mL
Electrolytes	
Sodium	135–145 mEq/L
Potassium	3.2–6.0 mEq/L
Carbon dioxide	21–28 mEq/L
Chloride	94–106 mEq/L
Creatinine clearance—a measure of renal function, reflecting the ability of the kidneys to clear creatinine from the blood.	85–125 mL/min (males) 75–115 mL/min (females)

24-hour clearance: A 24-hour specimen is obtained, measured, and analyzed for amount of creatinine. A plasma creatinine is determined, and the following formula is used:

$$C_{cr} = \frac{U_{cr}V}{P_{cr}}$$

where C_{cr} = creatinine clearance
U_{cr} = urine creatinine
V = volume
P_{cr} = plasma creatinine

6-hour creatinine clearance is a miniature version of a 24-hour clearance.

HEMATOLOGY: (normal values vary among laboratories)	
Complete blood count (CBC)	
Red blood cells (RBC)	4½ million to 5 million per cubic millimeter. NOTE: anemia may be indicative of renal impairment.
White blood cells (WBC)	5,000–10,000 per cubic millimeter. NOTE: WBC may be lowered in immunosuppressive therapy, elevated in infection.
Hematocrit (Hct)	43 percent. NOTE: Low Hct may indicate renal impairment; elevation may indicate dehydration.
Hemoglobin (Hb)	13 g. NOTE: Low Hb may indicate renal impairment.
Platelets	200,000–400,000 per cubic millimeter.

each time child is irritable, complains of headache, or shows signs of CHF.
3. Antihypertensive agents are given on schedule.
4. Vital signs are taken frequently. If tachycardia and tachypnea are present, liver margins are palpated, and level is recorded in nursing notes. NOTE: Children on antihypertensive medication must be monitored carefully for hypotension.
5. Respiratory distress or cyanosis is quickly noted and treatment begun.
6. The child takes in an adequate number of calories for size daily, yet remains within dietary restrictions.
7. Spontaneous bleeding does not occur.

TABLE 21-2 METHODS OF OBTAINING URINE SPECIMENS

1. Urine for urinalysis
   a. If the child is not toilet trained, bagging is necessary.
   b. Use equipment to which the child is accustomed, if possible. For example, a potty-chair may be used instead of a toilet.
   c. It may be very difficult to get a boy toddler to void in a urinal in bed. Having the mother explain that it is necessary and not a "bad" behavior may help.
2. Clean catch
   a. Infant: Scrub perineum well with Betadine or other antiseptic, dry with sterile sponge, and apply sterile bag. Be sure to retract foreskin when cleaning penis.
   b. Toddler to 4-year-old: Need to adapt approach to the individual child. Most in this age group are uncooperative with either bagging or adult method.
   c. Five-year-old or older: Use same method as for adult, assisting only as necessary.
3. Twenty-four–hour urine
   a. Void at beginning of 24-hour period and dispose of urine. Save all urine thereafter. Have child void as near the 24-hour mark as possible and include this specimen with total collection.
   b. It is important to impress the older child with the need to save all urine (a toilet-trained youngster may void in the toilet without telling anyone).
   c. An infant should be bagged with a bag that can be emptied while left in place. Removal and rebagging with each voiding lead rapidly to skin breakdown.
   d. Most 24-hour urine collections should be kept on ice or in preservatives. Check with the laboratory if unsure.
4. Catheterized specimen: Rarely done on children unless no alternative is available, then usually done by a physician.
5. Suprapubic tap: Often done in infants and small children instead of catheterization to obtain a sterile specimen. Nursing responsibility in this procedure is restraint of child, maintenance of sterile technique, and comforting of child after procedure.
6. Stoma catheterization (to obtain a sterile specimen). A prepackaged kit called Double Lumen Catheterization Kit is manufactured by Mentor Co. An alternative method, illustrated in Figure 21-1, is performed as follows:
   a. Remove bag from stoma, and clean area with Betadine on sterile 4 by 4 inch square of gauze.
   b. Wearing sterile gloves, gently insert the dropper end of a sterile plastic eyedropper. The bulb portion should have been cut off using sterile technique.
   c. If the child is old enough, a deep breath, slowly exhaled, relaxes the stoma. This makes passage of the eyedropper much easier.
   d. When eyedropper is in place, gently guide a sterile no. 5 to 12 French infant feeding tube through it.
   e. Aspirate urine through the tube with a sterile syringe.
   f. Remove dropper and feeding tube from stoma simultaneously.

8. The onset of end-stage renal disease as shown by rising serum BUN and creatinine is quickly noted.
9. The parents understand hemodialysis and transplantation before these treatments are instituted for their child.
10. The child is prepared for hemodialysis and transplantation if they are imminent. The child understands what is to happen and why and is given opportunities to resolve anxieties verbally or in play.

Complications

1. Urinary tract infections.
2. Hypertension; it is crucial that this be well controlled, since cranial aneurysms are frequently associated with polycystic disease.

Reevaluation and Follow-up

1. Clinic visits should be regular (about every 3 months) through the early part of the disease.
2. As the child approaches and enters end-stage renal disease, clinic visits should increase in frequency until the child attends weekly just before beginning dialysis.
3. At each clinic visit blood tests for BUN, creatinine, and electrolyte values should be done, as well as urinalysis and urine culture. See Table 21–1 for normal laboratory values and Table 21–2 and Figure 21–1 for urine collection procedures.

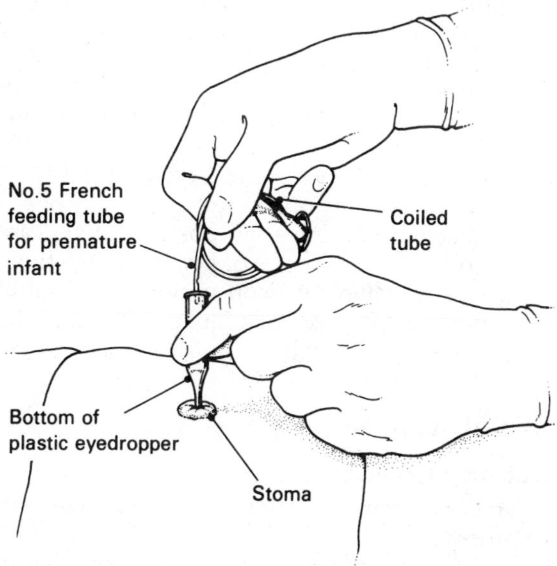

Figure 21-1 Catheterization of urinary stoma. Use sterile technique. Have patient exhale slowly if possible. Procedure is fully described in Table 21-2.

VESICOURETERAL REFLUX

DESCRIPTION

Vesicoureteral reflux is characterized by backflow of urine from the bladder into the ureters. The backflow is due to incompetence of the distal portion of the ureter, which forms a valve as it joins the bladder wall (Figure 21–2). The valve may be congenitally incompetent or it may be incompetent as a result of repeated infections. Continued backflow can result in dilatation and damage to the ureters and kidneys. Surgical reimplantation of the ureters into the bladder, forming a vesicoureteral valve, may be necessary. Prognosis depends on correction of the physical defect and prevention of urinary tract infection.

PREVENTION

Health Promotion

1. No preventive measures are known for congenital valve incompetence.
2. Prevention of urinary tract infections or prompt, adequate treatment eliminates or reduces the risk of valve damage.

Population at Risk

Children with frequent urinary tract infections.

Screening

None.

ASSESSMENT

Health History

1. History of frequent urinary tract infections.
2. History of frequent or constant urinary incontinence.

Physical Assessment

1. Observe voiding, noting stream, straining, dribbling, and quantity.
2. Percuss and palpate for bladder above the symphysis.

Diagnostic Tests

1. Clean catch urine specimen for protein, bacteria, and hematuria (see Table 21–2 for urine collection procedures).
2. Voiding cystourethrogram.

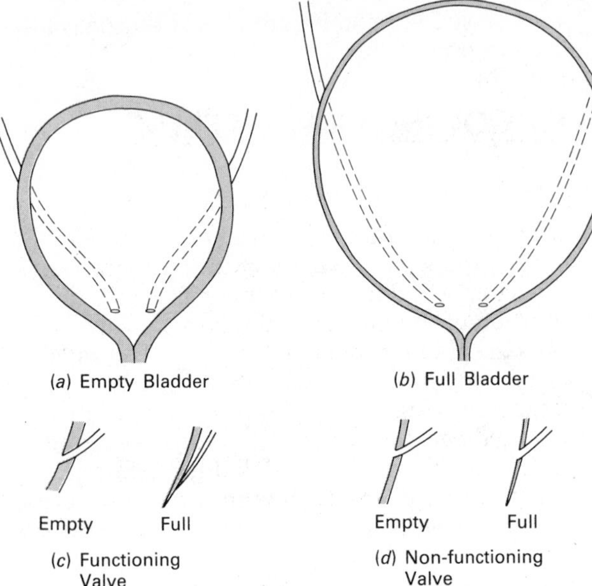

Figure 21-2 Vesicoureteral reflux is due to incorrect implantation of ureters in the bladder wall. (*a*) Empty bladder; (*b*) full bladder; (*c*) functioning valve; (*d*) nonfunctioning valve. Correctly placed ureters are occluded as bladder fills (*c*); the only direction for urine to go is down the urethra as the bladder contracts. Incorrectly implanted ureters do not pass through the bladder wall at an oblique angle (*d*). As a result they do not occlude as the bladder fills, and urine can reflux back toward the kidney as well as pass down the urethra during voiding.

NURSING DIAGNOSES: ACTUAL OR POTENTIAL

1. Alterations in comfort: postoperative pain or pain of urinary tract infection.
2. Impairment of urinary elimination secondary to urinary stasis and/or infection.
3. Alteration of self-concept secondary to frequent voidings and incontinence.

EXPECTED OUTCOMES

1. The child will remain continent if old enough to have been toilet trained.
2. The child will remain free of urinary tract infection.
3. The child will be free of pain or complications after surgery.
4. The child will demonstrate, through verbalizations or play, an integrated self-concept.

INTERVENTIONS

1. Promote drainage postoperatively.
   a. Keep catheters patent.
   b. Prevent dependent loops in drainage tubing.
   c. Change child's position frequently (every 1 to 2 hours).
   d. Monitor intake and output accurately.
   e. Empty drainage bag at least every 8 hours.
2. Prevent or treat infection.
   a. Use careful catheter technique: avoid irrigations, and change drainage bag and tubing every day.
   b. Administer antibiotics and urinary antiseptics on schedule.
   c. Encourage high fluid intake.
3. Prevent dislodging of "stints" (ureteral catheters, sometimes incorrectly called "splints") and urethral or suprapubic catheter.
   a. Restrain judiciously.
      (1) Avoid using restraints insofar as possible.
      (2) Apply night restraints only as needed.
      (3) Fully explain all restraints to child and family.
      (4) When child is restrained, provide routine respiratory toilet every 2 hours, or as necessary.
      (5) When child is restrained, provide sensory stimulation and mental diversion.
   b. Tape catheters well to prevent dislodging.
4. Conduct directed play sessions.
   a. Allow expressions of anger.
   b. Teach techniques of postoperative care and prevention of urinary tract infection.
   c. Correct child's misconceptions (e.g., guilt) and feelings of inadequacy that may be disclosed in play.

EVALUATION

Outcome Criteria

1. The child remains dry if developmentally appropriate.
2. Child is free of symptoms of urinary tract infection.
3. Renal failure due to damage by infection is not impending.
4. Self-concept is adequate as demonstrated by

psychosocial development (see Chapter 4 for developmental norms).

Complications

1. Infection.
2. Renal damage.

EXSTROPHY OF THE URINARY BLADDER

DESCRIPTION

Exstrophy of the urinary bladder actually consists of a group of congenital defects, of which the open bladder is the most obvious. The other defects include failure of the symphysis pubis to fuse and lack of urethral tubularization. Surgery to repair the defect is often unsuccessful, and a diversionary procedure with cystectomy is sometimes the treatment of choice.

PREVENTION

Health Promotion

No preventive measures are known.

Population at Risk

1. Neonates.
2. Boys are affected more often than girls.
3. Family history of this disorder is rarely positive.

Screening

None (defect is obvious).

ASSESSMENT

Health History

1. History of possible teratogens during mother's pregnancy.
2. Possible positive family history (rare).

Physical Assessment

1. Assess for associated anomalies: undescended testicles, epispadias, inguinal hernia.
2. Test pelvic mobility for involvement of the symphysis.
3. Assess stability of gait if child is walking.
4. Assess condition of skin and mucous membrane around and in defect.

Diagnostic Tests

Cystogram to determine extent and size of the defect.

NURSING DIAGNOSES: ACTUAL OR POTENTIAL

1. Impairment of urinary elimination: constant urine drainage through abdominal defect.
2. Impairment of skin integrity due to constant urinary drainage onto skin.
3. Increased risk of urinary tract infection due to open bladder.
4. Impairment of mobility due to associated defect of the pelvis.
5. Alterations in parenting due to difficulty accepting child's defect.
6. Alterations in self-concept due to permanent ileal conduit (if child has this kind of urinary diversion), anomalies of the penis (if they are present), and alterations in parenting.

EXPECTED OUTCOMES

1. Urinary tract infection will not occur.
2. Urinary obstruction will be avoided or promptly recognized and corrected.
3. Skin will remain free of excoriation and infection.
4. The defect will be surgically repaired to the maximum extent possible, or alternative drainage measures will be instituted.
5. Child will be free of pain or complications after surgery.
6. Normal mobility will be achieved.
7. Parents will demonstrate bonding and acceptance of their child verbally and in physical interactions.
8. Through play or projective techniques, the child will demonstrate an integrated self-concept.

INTERVENTIONS

1. Protect against fecal contamination of bladder by careful diapering, positioning infant on back (elevated frame with canvas lying surface and hole for fecal drop-through may be helpful), and maintaining scrupulous cleanliness. Provide high oral fluid intake to "flush" bladder.
2. Watch for possible obstruction of urine flow. Diaper should be constantly wet; if dry for a period of time, obstruction has probably occurred. Reposition infant and, if urine outflow does not occur immediately, notify physician.
3. If accurate intake and output is necessary,

weigh diapers (1 mL urine weighs approximately 1 g).

4. Bagging of defect must not be done, as it will result in severe skin breakdown.
5. Change diapers frequently. Advise parents to wash and rinse well and sun-dry periodically to reduce ammoniacal bacteria. Use karaya rings or powder around defect.
6. Advise parents that child may be slower to walk, may require more practice with support, and may fall more often than other children. Normal mobility is to be expected except for temporary delays.
7. Protect from falls in hospital. Pad crib sides as necessary.
8. Assist family in accepting malformed child. Demonstrate acceptance; promote resolution of grief; as parents become ready to learn, teach care of the child.
9. Provide play therapy to enhance child's self-esteem, body image, and understanding of altered appearance, function, treatments, appliances, or other areas of concern.

EVALUATION

Outcome Criteria

1. Urinary tract infection does not occur.
2. Obstruction is avoided or promptly recognized and relieved.
3. Skin and mucous membrane remain intact.
4. Urinary continence is achieved after surgery.
5. Normal mobility is achieved.
6. Child is developing normally (see Chapter 4) and receiving appropriate support from parents.

Complications

1. Renal failure due to hydronephrosis and infection.
2. Injury or falls due to abnormal pelvic structure.
3. Social isolation due to parental rejection or poor self-image.

POSTERIOR URETHRAL VALVES

DESCRIPTION

Posterior urethral valves are anomalous folds of mucosal tissue in the male urethra, which act as one-way valves. Unfortunately, the valves open in toward the bladder, not out. This creates obstruction, usually so severe that without surgical intervention it leads to hydroureter, hydronephrosis, and, ultimately, renal failure. Because urine is produced in fetal life, damage begins *in utero*. For some children permanent urinary diversion (e.g., ileal conduit) is necessary. Prognosis depends on the extent of renal and lower tract damage.

PREVENTION

Health Promotion

No preventive measures are known.

Population at Risk

Newborn and infant boys; rarely the disorder is discovered somewhat later.

Screening

None.

ASSESSMENT

Health History

1. History of incontinence.
2. History of dribbling or straining to void.
3. In older babies and children, history of recurrent urinary tract infection.

Physical Assessment

1. Palpation or percussion of the bladder above the symphysis.
2. Costovertebral angle tenderness from back-pressure or infection.
3. Flank mass or abdominal mass (hydronephrotic kidneys).

Diagnostic Tests

1. Voiding cystourethrogram.
2. Cystometrogram (study of bladder capacity and pressures).
3. BUN, creatinine, electrolyte values (see Table 21–1).
4. Intravenous pyelogram.
5. Creatinine clearances (see Table 21–1).

NURSING DIAGNOSES: ACTUAL OR POTENTIAL

1. Impairment of urinary elimination due to urethral obstruction.
2. Fluid volume excess due to impaired elimination of fluids.
3. Alteration in comfort: pain following surgery.

EXPECTED OUTCOMES

1. The child will be free of urinary tract infection.
2. The defect will be repaired as soon as possible to avoid further renal damage.
3. The child will be free of fluid and electrolyte imbalances.
4. The child and family will manage drainage devices in the home, unassisted by health care workers.
5. The child will be free of pain and complications after surgery.

INTERVENTIONS

1. Preoperative.
   a. Prepare child and family for surgery; provide teaching and comfort.
   b. Maintain intake and output before surgery.
      (1) Observe for clinical signs of overhydration.
      (2) Use careful catheter technique; avoid irrigations, and change tubing and drainage bag each day.
2. Postoperative.
   a. Keep catheter patent by "milking" tube as needed.
   b. Prevent dependent loops in drainage tubing.
   c. Change child's position every 2 hours.
   d. Accurately measure intake and output; empty drainage bag at least every 8 hours.
   e. Use careful catheter technique: avoid irrigations, and change tubing and drainage bag each day.
   f. Administer antibiotics and urinary tract antiseptics on schedule.
   g. Force fluids (as tolerated by renal function).
   h. Monitor laboratory values (see Table 21–1 for normal values).
   i. Provide skin care for overhydrated child.
      (1) Avoid pressure.
      (2) Immediately treat any small break in skin.
      (3) Prevent friction in intertriginous areas by use of cornstarch, powder, or lubricants.
   j. Prevent catheter or "stint" (ureteral catheter) from dislodging (see interventions described for postoperative care under *Vesicoureteral Reflux*, above).
   k. Promote mobility in spite of drainage tubes. Use leg bag with harness (Figure 21–3).
   l. Help parents and child become comfortable about drainage appliances and competent in their care.
      (1) Cleaning and care of skin.
      (2) Proper fitting and sealing of appliance.
      (3) Sterile technique.

EVALUATION

Outcome Criteria

1. Urinary drainage is established.
2. Renal impairment is limited.
3. Urinary tract infection does not occur.
4. Parents (and child if old enough) demonstrate knowledge and comfort in caring for drainage appliances and stoma.

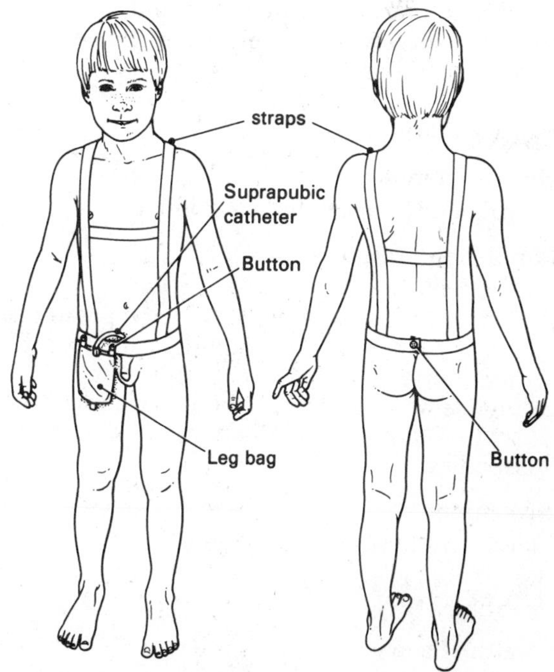

Figure 21-3 Harness for securing "leg bag" to suprapubic catheter. Buttons for drainage bag may be placed anywhere on the hip band. Straps are muslin. If a short catheter is used, the catheter loop does not interfere with drainage. Harness can also be used for child with nephrostomy tube, in which case the hip-level band pictured here can be raised to the waist.

Complications

1. Infection due to stasis.
2. Continued drainage impairment.
3. Progressive renal disease.
4. Poor adjustment associated with external urinary diversion.

HYPOSPADIAS AND EPISPADIAS

DESCRIPTION

Hypospadias is a misplaced urethral meatus at any point along the underside (ventrum) of the penis. Epispadias is a misplaced meatus on the upper side (dorsum) of the penis. Either of these congenital defects can be associated with chordee (flexion deformity of the penis), ambiguous genitalia, or cryptorchidism. Plastic surgery is done (sometimes in stages) to extend the urethra to place the meatus in the glans and to release chordee; surgery is usually done during the child's second or third year.

PREVENTION

Health Promotion

No preventive measures are known.

Population at Risk

1. Newborn boys.
2. Risk of hypospadias appears to be greater in infants with a positive family history for the deformity.
3. Infants with exstrophy of the bladder (described earlier in this chapter) often have epispadias.

Screening

Newborn physical examination.

ASSESSMENT

Health History

1. History of any prenatal teratogen or fetal insult.
2. History of misdirected urinary stream or dribbling.
3. Family history of hypospadias.

Physical Assessment

1. Carefully inspect male neonates to locate the site of the meatus: retract the foreskin, and look at the perineum. If any evidence is found of either hypospadias or epispadias, *circumcision should not be done*, since the prepuce will be needed for reparative plastic surgery.
2. Inspect for possible associated deformities, such as ambiguous genitalia, cryptorchidism, or chordee.

Diagnostic Tests

Voiding cystourethrogram.

NURSING DIAGNOSES: ACTUAL OR POTENTIAL

1. Alteration in comfort due to postoperative pain.
2. Impairment in self-concept due to abnormal genitalia.
3. Alterations in parenting associated with child's abnormal genitalia.

EXPECTED OUTCOMES

1. Abnormal placement of the meatus will be surgically corrected.
2. Child will experience normal psychosocial development.
3. Parents will exhibit acceptance and functional parenting of the child through verbal and nonverbal interactions.

INTERVENTIONS

1. Provide and interpret factual information for parents (and child if old enough).
2. Explore and help resolve parents' and child's attitudes toward anomaly.
3. Prepare child for surgery.
   a. Provide cognitive-psychological preparation appropriate for age.
   b. Clear up any diaper rash or other skin breakdown in the operative area.
4. Provide postoperative care.
   a. Take precautions to prevent pulling or dislodging the urethral catheter or otherwise traumatizing the surgical repair. Restrain child if necessary (see restraining under postoperative interventions, under *Vesicoureteral Reflux*, earlier in this chapter).
   b. Keep careful records of intake and output.
   c. Empty drainage bag at least every 8 hours.
   d. If drainage slows or stops, tube may be milked to achieve patency, but *irrigation should be done only as a last resort* because

of the danger of disturbing the surgical repair of the urethra.

EVALUATION

Outcome Criteria

1. Normal placement of the urinary meatus after surgery is completed.
2. Unimpaired wound healing after surgery.
3. Normal self-concept, as evidenced by psychosocial development at norms for age (see Chapter 4).
4. Parental acceptance of child and normal parent–child relations (see Chapter 5).

Complications

1. Damage of the plastic repair due to postoperative infection or trauma.
2. Abnormal sex-role behavior due to impaired self-concept.
3. Disturbed sexual functioning due to associated defect (e.g., chordee interfering with erection).

UNDESCENDED TESTICLES (CRYPTORCHIDISM)

DESCRIPTION

Cryptorchidism is a condition in which one or both testes do not descend from their fetal origin on the urogenital ridge in the upper abdomen to the lower abdomen, and down through the inguinal ring to the bottom of the scrotum. This descent, which normally occurs during the eighth month of gestation, may be prohibited by an abnormality in the testis itself, lack of endocrine stimulation, or structural defects in the inguinal canal or scrotum. The descent of the testis may be interrupted at any level, so it may be found in the inguinal canal or in the abdomen. Spontaneous descent usually occurs in early childhood; 10 percent of newborn boys are cryptorchid, but only 0.3 percent of men are. If surgical correction (orchiopexy or, rarely, orchiectomy) is necessary, it is usually done between the ages of 5 and 9 years.

PREVENTION

Health Promotion

No preventive measures are known.

Population at Risk

Boys, especially premature neonates.

Screening

Scrotal palpation to ascertain the presence of both testes is a routine part of the physical examination of all male infants and children.

ASSESSMENT

Health History

1. Empty scrotal sac.
2. Child may have inguinal pain. Pain in testis usually indicates onset of complications (e.g., circulatory compromise).
3. Child may have inguinal hernia.

Physical Assessment

1. Scrotal rugae are absent: they do not develop unless the testes have been in the scrotum.
2. Scrotal sac is empty on one or both sides. Differentiate from pseudocryptorchidism in which testes will descend when child is relaxed and warm.
3. Testis may be palpated in inguinal canal.
4. Inguinal hernia may be palpated.

NURSING DIAGNOSES: ACTUAL OR POTENTIAL

1. Alterations in comfort: discomfort secondary to testis in the inguinal canal, traumatic orchitis, torsion of the testicle, or inguinal hernia.
2. Alterations in self-esteem due to empty scrotal sac.
3. Alterations in patterns of sexuality of the older child or teenager due to self-consciousness about empty scrotal sac or knowledge (or presumption) of sterility.

EXPECTED OUTCOMES

1. Cryptorchidism will be found before the child reaches the age of 4 years.
2. Preoperatively, child will be free of pain due to injury or complication of the condition.
3. If surgery is to be done, child and family will be prepared.
4. Child will be free of postoperative complications.
5. Child will verbalize or demonstrate through play an integrated self-image.

INTERVENTIONS

1. Include palpation for testes in physical assessment of all boys.
2. Any boy with undescended testes who complains of pain or shows signs of inguinal hernia or inflammation must be referred to a physician.
3. Provide preoperative preparation for child and family if surgery is planned. Detect and deal with castration anxiety.
4. Prevent postoperative complications.
   a. Provide pulmonary toilet, and see that child moves about in bed during period of bed rest.
   b. Encourage mobility as soon as permitted.
   c. Observe for signs of ischemia in testes.
   d. Maintain traction apparatus (Figure 21–4).
   e. Observe for recurrent hernia.
5. Foster integrated body image and self-esteem. Encourage child to discuss his concerns.
6. Postoperatively, teach child and/or parents to perform testicular examination at monthly intervals.
   a. Palpate for masses or irregularities.
   b. Detect changes in size of testicle, either hypertrophy or atrophy.
   c. Seek prompt medical attention if above examinations are positive.
7. Instruct child and family that postoperative trauma should be avoided by child's wearing a rigid athletic supporter.

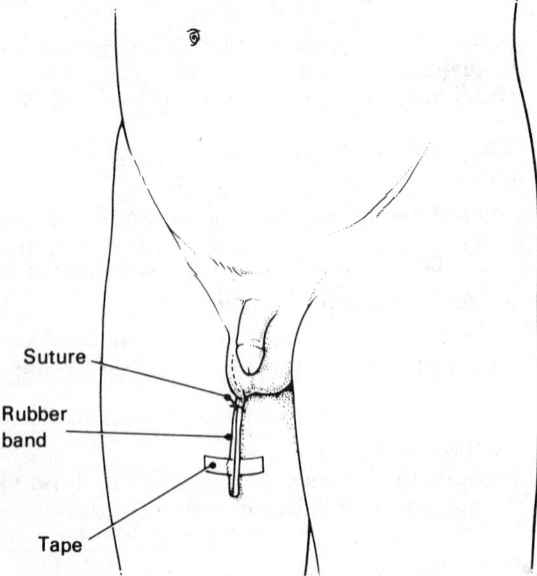

Figure 21-4 Traction apparatus used following orchlopexy.

EVALUATION

Outcome Criteria

1. Child has testes in scrotum.
2. Rugae form.
3. Child and parents do not manifest abnormal levels of anxiety (e.g., refusal to look at operative area, continuous touching of penis).
4. Spermatogenesis occurs after puberty.
5. Orchiectomy is not necessary.

Complications

1. Hematocele.
2. Trauma to the testis.
3. Malignancy of testis.

Reevaluation and Follow-up
See intervention 6, above.

WILMS' TUMOR (NEPHROBLASTOMA)

DESCRIPTION

Nephroblastoma is a malignant tumor arising from embryonic renal tissue. The most pronounced early symptom is an abdominal mass, often discovered by parents in bathing or dressing the child. Usual treatment is excision followed by chemotherapy and irradiation. Using this regimen, prognosis has improved dramatically in recent years, and more than 75 percent of children survive 5 or more years after diagnosis.

PREVENTION

Health Promotion

No preventive measures are known.

Population at Risk

The peak incidence is between 6 months and 4 years, although younger or older children may also be affected.

Screening

Abdominal palpation for renal tumor is part of the routine physical examination for all children.

ASSESSMENT

Health History

1. Sudden appearance and rapid growth of abdominal mass.
2. Abdominal pain may be reported.

Physical Assessment

1. Abdominal mass. *Do not palpate unnecessarily,* since palpation can rupture the renal capsule and release malignant cells.
2. Hematuria may be present.
3. Abdominal pain may be induced by examination.

Diagnostic Tests

1. Intravenous pyelogram.
2. Abdominal ultrasound.
3. Open biopsy.

NURSING DIAGNOSES: ACTUAL OR POTENTIAL

1. Alterations in comfort: pain due to tumor preoperatively, incisional discomfort postoperatively.
2. Nutritional deficit due to anorexia, nausea, and vomiting resulting from chemotherapy or radiotherapy.
3. Anxiety associated with discomfort and fear of the unknown outcome of the disease process on the part of both child and parents.

EXPECTED OUTCOMES

1. Pain from both the tumor and the surgery will be controlled.
2. Postoperative complications, such as bleeding and pneumonia, will be prevented.
3. Nausea and vomiting will be controlled.
4. Nutritional and fluid intake will be adequate.
5. The child and family will cope constructively with their anxiety and feelings about the malignancy, surgery, and chemotherapy or radiation.
6. The child will adapt to the change in body appearance resulting from therapy.

INTERVENTIONS

1. Assist family in discussion of concerns, both separately and together. Provide information and assistance with grief.
2. Prepare child and family for surgery.
3. Pain may be controlled by medications, positioning, diversion, and other comfort measures. Be alert to effective pain-relieving measures for each child.
4. Observe carefully for changes in color, breathing patterns, and body language. Obtain vital signs as necessary.
5. Provide respiratory toilet. Small infants may need to be allowed to cry to aerate their lungs (this needs to be explained carefully to parents). Older children should be taught before surgery to cough and splint wound, then assisted to cough and deep breathe after surgery. Other useful devices include blow glove, blow bottle, and inflatable party favors.
6. Provide foods liked and tolerated by child; avoid greasy foods. Small, frequent portions, attractively served, are better tolerated. Carefully record intake and output to be sure adequate fluids are taken. Distractions may help to prevent nausea. Avoid noxious odors; do not keep emesis basin in sight. Room temperature should be cool. Rinse mouth after vomiting. Medication may be necessary.
7. Carefully explain necessity for intravenous (IV) therapy to child at his or her developmental level. Explain reasons for therapy to parents. Explain what will be done and how. Provide exercise for other extremities in bed. Walking can be done with IV pole on wheels.
8. Allow child to ventilate feelings about loss of hair and weight loss. Drawing a picture of self may be helpful or engaging in play therapy with doll that "gets chemotherapy." Carefully explain cause and time span of changes at child's developmental level. Wigs, scarves, and caps may be welcome.

EVALUATION

Outcome Criteria

1. The family, including the child, has a realistic view of the disease and its prognosis. They are able to state facts about the disease and treatment accurately.

2. Pain is relieved by medication and nursing interventions.
3. Postoperative bleeding, if any, is promptly detected and controlled.
4. Postoperative pneumonia and/or atelectasis do not occur.
5. Vomiting secondary to chemotherapy or radiation is controlled.
6. The child's nutritional intake is adequate for age and weight.
7. Intravenous lines are maintained for therapy without causing undue immobility.
8. Child recognizes that therapy-induced body changes are temporary, and that he or she is essentially the same person.

Complications

1. Incomplete removal of tumor, especially if tumor is metastatic before surgery.
2. Malnutrition secondary to nausea and vomiting.
3. Bone marrow depression secondary to chemotherapy or radiation.
4. Death, although survival rate is steadily climbing.
5. End-stage renal disease and its complications if bilateral nephrectomy is necessary (see *Chronic Renal Failure* later in this chapter).

Reevaluation and Follow-up

1. Follow-up clinic visits should be weekly, then monthly during the 24 months of therapy.
2. Monthly chest x-ray films should be obtained during the first 2 years.
3. Intravenous pyelograms should be obtained every 6 months during the first 2 years.
4. After the 24 months of therapy, checkups should be done every 3 months for 2 years, then annually.

BENIGN TUMORS

DESCRIPTION

Benign tumors of the kidney are extremely rare in children. One type of benign tumor is associated with tuberous sclerosis, and hemangiomas of the kidney can occur, rarely, in infants and children. Treatment is usually surgical, and nursing care is essentially the same as for any surgery on the kidney (see *Wilms' Tumor*, immediately above).

INFLAMMATIONS

URINARY TRACT INFECTION

DESCRIPTION

At one time urinary tract infections were described in terms of the part of the tract exhibiting the most striking symptoms, for example, cystitis or nephritis. The accepted terminology at the present time is simply urinary tract infection. Infections are more common in boys during the first year of life, due to seeding from septicemia. After the first year, infections are far more common in girls, at least partially due to the short urethra.

PREVENTION

Health Promotion

1. General hygienic methods to prevent sepsis in infants: good nutrition, childhood immunizations, avoidance and prompt treatment of infections.
2. Front-to-back wiping by girls in order to avoid carrying fecal contaminants to the urethra.
3. Avoidance by girls of chemicals that irritate the urethra (e.g., bubble baths, deodorant sprays).
4. Avoidance and treatment of pinworm infestation in girls (see *Enterobiasis* in Chapter 24).
5. Avoidance of dirty kiddie pools and prolonged contact with wet swim suits.
6. Drinking adequate fluids, especially in warm weather.
7. Voiding before and after sexual intercourse flushes bacteria from the urethral meatus.
8. Avoidance of nonessential catheterization and application of immaculate aseptic technique when catheterization is required.

Population at Risk

1. Females, especially when sexually active.
2. Males or females with incomplete emptying of the urinary tract for any reason: acquired or congenital obstructions or neurogenic bladder.
3. Males or females with structural defects of the urinary tract or renal damage.

4. Males or females after catheterization or instrumentation of the urinary tract.

Screening

1. Some authorities believe periodic screening urine cultures are advisable for girls and for all sexually active females.
2. Infants with unexplained fever should be checked for urinary tract infection.

ASSESSMENT

Health History

1. Burning or pain on urination.
2. Discolored or bloody urine.
3. Foul-smelling urine.
4. Anorexia, vomiting, and fever of recent onset.
5. Frequency or urgency of urination.
6. Past history of urinary tract infection.
7. Recent catheterization or other instrumentation of the urinary tract.

Physical Assessment

1. Palpation may reveal guarding and tenderness of the lower abdomen.
2. Child may have fever.
3. Costovertebral angle tenderness may be present.

Diagnostic Tests

1. Clean catch urinalysis for culture and sensitivity (see Table 21–2).
2. Intravenous pyelogram to rule out contributing obstruction or abnormality.

NURSING DIAGNOSES: ACTUAL OR POTENTIAL

1. Alterations in comfort secondary to pain of inflamed tissue and secondary to fever.
2. Impairment of urinary elimination due to inflammation.
3. Nutrition and fluid deficits secondary to anorexia, nausea, vomiting, and fever.

EXPECTED OUTCOMES

1. The present urinary tract infection will be successfully treated, with relief of all symptoms.
2. Future urinary tract infections will be prevented.
3. Nutrition and fluid balance will be restored to normal.

INTERVENTIONS

1. Teach girls and their parents prophylaxis (see prevention section, above).
2. Administer prescribed medications accurately.
3. Reduce fever, if it occurs, by tepid sponging, administering prescribed medication and adequate fluids, and reducing room temperature.
4. Encourage fluid intake and adequate diet (basic four food groups—see Appendix F) when nausea is relieved.

EVALUATION

Outcome Criteria

1. Urinary tract infection clears, producing relief of symptoms.
2. Further infections do not occur.

Complications

1. Renal damage.
2. Dehydration due to fever and vomiting.

ACUTE POSTSTREPTOCOCCAL GLOMERULONEPHRITIS (NEPHRITIS, NEPHRITIC SYNDROME)

DESCRIPTION

Poststreptococcal glomerulonephritis is an acute condition that follows an infection with a streptococcal organism, usually group A beta-hemolytic, and is thought to be an immunological reaction to the organism. Treatment is largely supportive, with steroid treatment not usually indicated. The great majority of these patients recover.

PREVENTION

Health Promotion

1. Avoidance of exposure to streptococcal infections.
2. Early detection and immediate treatment of streptococcal infections contracted.
3. Complete compliance with prescribed antibiotic regimens.
4. Maintenance of good health habits (e.g., rest, nutrition).

Population at Risk

1. Persons with untreated or incompletely treated streptococcal infections.
2. Peak incidence is 6 to 10 years of age.

Screening

None.

ASSESSMENT

Health History

1. History of streptococcus infection in past 14 days, especially strep throat or impetigo (history of infection is not discernible in all clients).
2. No treatment, or incomplete treatment, of infection.
3. Acute onset of symptoms.

Physical Assessment

1. Hematuria (brownish or red).
2. Periorbital edema.
3. Hypertension.
4. Fever may be present.
5. Oliguria or anuria.

Diagnostic Tests

1. Serum BUN, creatinine, and electrolytes.
2. Creatinine clearance.
3. Kidney biopsy.

NURSING DIAGNOSES: ACTUAL OR POTENTIAL

1. Impairment of urinary elimination: oliguria or anuria due to glomerular insult.
2. Alteration of fluid volume: hypertension and fluid overload due to kidney damage.
3. Nutritional alteration due to restrictions that are part of dietary management.
4. Alterations in electrolyte balance due to decreased kidney function.
5. Decreased activity tolerance associated with weakness, headache, and, perhaps, nausea.

EXPECTED OUTCOMES

1. Complications of hypertension will be avoided.
2. Adequate nutrition and any prescribed dietary restrictions will be maintained.
3. Adequate recreation and stimulation will be provided without overtiring the child.
4. Complications of fluid and electrolyte imbalance will be prevented or controlled.

INTERVENTIONS

1. Monitor closely blood pressure, being as consistent as possible (same arm, same position, same size cuff).
2. Observe for headache, restlessness, lethargy, convulsion, tachycardia, cardiac gallop.
3. Administer antihypertensive agents as ordered.
4. Monitor carefully IV fluids as ordered.
5. Maintain bed rest if indicated for elevated blood pressure.
6. Diet should be planned after discussion with child and parents. Compliance will be more consistent if dietary plan is as near as possible to child's normal diet. Explain that restrictions are probably temporary. Sodium should not be restricted unduly, as this often results in not eating with a consequent inadequate caloric intake. Provide frequent small, attractive, meals using foods the child likes. For example, peanut butter provides protein, and popsicles provide fluid and calories. These may be well tolerated by the anorexic child.
7. Provide activities that are interesting without being tiring. Assist with care, having child do some parts of the care each day, as physical condition permits.
8. Observe for symptoms of fluid and electrolyte imbalance. Monitor laboratory test results (see Table 21–1).
9. Weigh daily.

EVALUATION

Outcome Criteria

1. Blood pressures are frequently and accurately monitored.
2. Any hypertensive encephalopathy or cardiac decompensation is noted and reported immediately.
3. The child consumes an adequate diet that is within dietary restrictions.
4. The child rests as necessary but receives sufficient stimulation from quiet activities.
5. Fluid overload and electrolyte imbalances are prevented or controlled through fluid and dietary restrictions.

Complications

1. Pulmonary edema secondary to fluid overload.
2. Congestive heart failure secondary to fluid overload.
3. Stroke secondary to hypertension.

Reevaluation and Follow-up

1. A mild case can last only 10 to 14 days; severe disease can take months or years to resolve. Clinic visits should occur on a regular basis; the frequency depends on the severity of the symptoms.
2. When both clinical symptoms and laboratory values have returned to normal, yearly follow-up is sufficient.
3. Recurrent disease following another streptococcus infection is not unheard of.

NEPHROTIC SYNDROME (NEPHROSIS)

DESCRIPTION

Nephrotic syndrome is not a disease entity but a collection of symptoms that include proteinuria, hypoproteinemia, edema, ascites, hyperlipidemia, and sometimes oliguria, all due to increased permeability of the glomerular membrane and loss of serum protein into the urine. The origin is obscure. The course is characterized by remissions and exacerbations. Medical treatment usually consists of steroids and IV administration of salt-poor albumin.

PREVENTION

Health Promotion

No prevention is known except thorough treatment of acute poststreptococcal glomerulonephritis (described earlier in this chapter), which is occasionally followed by nephrosis.

Population at Risk

1. The peak incidence is 2 to 5 years.
2. Children who have had glomerulonephritis.
3. Children with a range of metabolic, immune, and allergic disorders: diabetes, systemic lupus erythematosus, mercury poisoning, bee sting, and others.

Screening

None.

ASSESSMENT

Health History

1. There is usually nothing particularly notable in the health history of children experiencing a first episode of nephrotic syndrome.
2. A respiratory illness, either viral or bacterial, often precedes recurrent episodes.
3. Edema develops gradually, first in the feet and legs, then involving the genitals and abdomen (ascites); periorbital edema may be noted in the morning in the early stages of nephrosis, then becomes persistent and conspicuous.
4. Decreased urinary output.

Physical Assessment

1. Proteinuria.
2. Edema, including ascites (may be very pronounced).
3. Skin lesions secondary to edema.
4. Dyspnea secondary to ascites.

Diagnostic Tests

1. Urinalysis.
2. Serum protein.

NURSING DIAGNOSES: ACTUAL OR POTENTIAL

1. Alteration in fluid volume: edema secondary to spillage of serum protein in the urine (and resultant loss of capillary osmotic pressure so that intravascular fluid seeps into the intracellular space).
2. Loss of skin integrity associated with edema.
3. Alteration in comfort associated with edema.
4. Alteration in cardiac output due to edema and hypotension.
5. Impairment of body image associated with edema.
6. Decreased activity tolerance associated with edema and hypotension.
7. Nutritional alteration: increased protein need due to albumin excretion in the urine.
8. Respiratory dysfunction due to ascites.
9. Decreased urinary elimination due to decreased vascular fluid volume and hypotension.
10. Increased risk of infection due to suppressed immune response associated with steroid therapy.

EXPECTED OUTCOMES

1. Skin breakdown will be prevented.
2. Child will be as comfortable as possible.
3. Problems associated with hypotension (e.g., weakness, activity intolerance) will be minimized.

4. Complications of immobility will be avoided.
5. Child will cope adequately with changes in body appearance.
6. Child will receive adequate rest with appropriate diversion.
7. Child will receive adequate nutrition and fluids.
8. Respiratory exchange will be adequate.
9. Infection will be prevented.

INTERVENTIONS

1. Avoid pressure and abrasion injuries to skin (sheet burns, bedpan abrasions, tape burns, etc.). Support edematous scrotum with Bellevue bridge, shown in Figure 21–5.
2. Prevent friction in intertriginous areas with baby powder or cornstarch.
3. Promote activity as tolerated. Enjoyable activities will be met with the best cooperation.
4. Explore child's body image (e.g., through art work). Tell child the changes in appearance are temporary. If cognitive development permits, explain edema and Cushing's stigmata in simple terms.
5. Plan care to provide times for resting.
6. Give frequent attractive, small feedings of preferred high-protein foods.
7. Monitor carefully IV protein infusions. Regulate rate accurately; prevent clogging of tube by rinsing with normal saline; use filter to remove crystals and sediment of protein.
8. Provide pulmonary toilet for inactive child.
9. Do not allow contact with staff members, visitors, or other patients who show signs of infection.

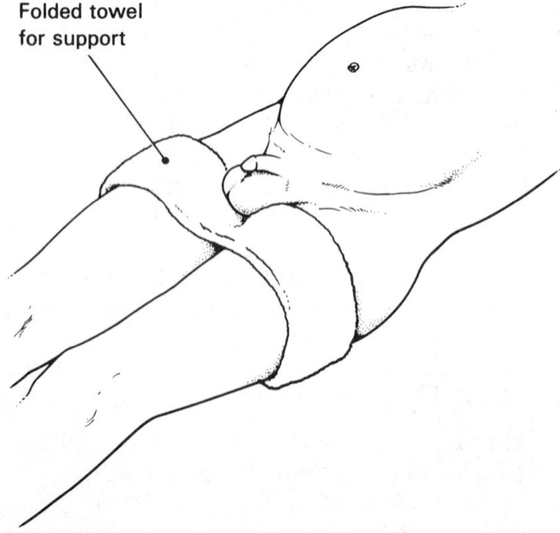

Figure 21-5 Bellevue bridge for scrotal support.

EVALUATION

Outcome Criteria

1. Edema is markedly reduced with therapy.
2. Skin breakdown is prevented.
3. Crying, irritability, and cranky behavior are minimal or nonexistent.
4. Complaints of fatigue and indications of boredom are decreasing or absent.
5. Child verbalizes or demonstrates in play and social interaction acceptance of the changes in body appearance and understands that they are temporary.
6. Therapeutic diet and prescribed IV fluids are administered as ordered and are well tolerated.
7. Indications of respiratory distress or infection are absent.
8. Infections are prevented or controlled.

Complications

1. Sepsis.
2. Hypovolemic shock secondary to loss of intravascular fluid into the interstitial space.
3. Respiratory distress secondary to thoracic fluid collections or ascites.
4. Hypertension secondary to steroid therapy.
5. Nonresponse to steroid therapy.
6. Progression of the disease to end-stage renal disease needing dialysis and transplantation.

Reevaluation and Follow-up

1. Frequency of clinic visits for checkups and IV albumin administration depends on severity of symptoms and the progress of the disease. Monthly visits are most common; weekly visits may be necessary.
2. With resolution of the disease, yearly follow-ups are sufficient.

OBSTRUCTIONS

NEUROPATHIC (NEUROGENIC) BLADDER

DESCRIPTION

Neuropathic bladder is a condition caused by impairment of the motor and/or sensory nerve supply of the bladder. Urinary incontinence and/or retention result. If uncorrected, neuropathic bladder leads to infection, reflux, and, possibly, renal failure. The social problems stemming from incontinence are also of great concern. The cause is most commonly a congenital spinal defect, such as myelomeningocele, but spinal cord injuries can also be responsible.

PREVENTION

Health Promotion

1. No preventive measures are known for birth defects of the spinal cord except avoidance of irradiation and other teratogens during pregnancy.
2. Spinal cord injuries are preventable by provision of good supervision for young children and safety instruction for older children and adolescents (safety is addressed in Chapter 5).

Population at Risk

Children with congenital or acquired abnormal bladder innervation.

Screening

None.

ASSESSMENT

Health History

1. Constipation: hard, infrequent stools.
2. Malodorous, discolored urine.
3. Urinary incontinence with dribbling.
4. Congenital spinal defect or spinal injury.

Physical Assessment

1. Redness and irritation of the perineal area.
2. Bladder palpated or percussed above the symphysis.
3. Increased or decreased rectal tone.
4. Urine leakage observed on clothing or genital area.

Diagnostic Tests

1. Cystometrogram
2. Intravenous pyelogram

NURSING DIAGNOSES: ACTUAL OR POTENTIAL

1. Impairment of urinary elimination due to abnormal innervation of the bladder.
2. Risk of urinary tract infection due to incomplete voiding (urinary stasis).
3. Risk of renal tissue injury due to back pressure or infection.
4. Impairment of skin integrity due to constant dribbling of urine.
5. Alteration in self-concept and social interaction due to incontinence.

EXPECTED OUTCOMES

1. The child will achieve continence through the use of prosthesis, diversion procedure, or clean catheterization.
2. Urinary tract infection will be prevented.
3. Renal tissue damage will not occur.
4. Skin will remain intact.
5. Child will demonstrate good psychosocial development.

INTERVENTIONS

1. Continence may be achieved in several acceptable ways, and the specific method selected by the physician depends on many factors, such as sex, age, and the presence of reflux or renal damage. The nurse is involved in all these methods in teaching the parents and/or client how best to perform the procedures.
   a. The Credé method of manually compressing the bladder to empty it has in the past been used for infants who had no ureteral reflux. Current thinking is that Credé is contraindicated because it can induce reflux even in children with competent ureterovesicular valves. Upper tract damage is more frequent in children who have had Credé, especially boys, than in those whose voiding is initiated in other ways (Bauer, 1983; Klauber, 1983).
   b. Self-catheterization, a clean (not sterile) technique, may be selected for a client old enough to learn it. The client, usually a girl, carries with her a clean catheter, sometimes of a soft metal, and uses this as often as necessary (about every 2 hours) to empty the bladder while sitting on the toilet.
   c. Most frequently, however, an ileal conduit is created surgically.
      (1) The single most important aspect of conduit nursing care, because this is a permanent procedure, is teaching the parents and the child how to manage the care after the child is discharged. This should be kept in mind while the

nurse is performing care, and some part of teaching should be done each time.

(2) Another important part of the care of the client with an ileal conduit is the incorporation of the stoma into the child's body image. Young boys may fear greatly the loss of their penis now that it is no longer used for voiding. The nurse's acceptance of the stoma in a matter-of-fact way and straightforward approach to teaching and answering questions go a long way toward helping the client accept the stoma.

(3) Clean rather than sterile technique should be used.

(4) The type of appliance most commonly used consists of a faceplate, a bag, and a belt. The faceplate is covered with an adhesive substance that creates a watertight seal with the skin around the stoma. The belt gives further support to the appliance when the container is heavy with urine. However, the appliance should be emptied frequently to avoid undue stress on the seal.

(5) Skin breakdown around the stoma, a continuing problem for most clients, can be easily cared for by substituting a special karaya-containing seal on the faceplate. If the appliance is properly sealed, the client can swim, shower, or take a tub bath without leakage.

2. Fluid intake must be adequate according to body size, especially in summer because of increased insensible loss. Recommend fluids liked and tolerated by the patient.
3. Bladder should be kept as empty as possible. Methods used for emptying should avoid injuring or bruising bladder walls.
4. Diet should include fruits, fruit juices, and leafy vegetables to stimulate bowel peristalsis.

EVALUATION

Outcome Criteria

1. The child remains dry.
2. The child and/or parents safely and comfortably manage the procedure used to achieve continence.
3. Skin shows no evidence of excoriation.
4. Urinary tract infection is infrequent and well controlled.
5. The child verbalizes or demonstrates through play an integrated self-concept and is at appropriate level of psychosocial development (see Chapter 4).

Complications

1. Infection due to stasis.
2. Renal failure secondary to back pressure or infection.
3. Child avoids social contacts due to continuing incontinence.

RENAL VEIN THROMBOSIS

DESCRIPTION

Renal vein thrombosis is a condition in which thrombi form in the arcuate, interlobular, and main renal veins. One or both kidneys may be affected. The child (usually a neonate) then develops acute manifestations of renal failure, hematuria, fever, and a palpable flank mass. Medical management of the problem consists of (1) correcting underlying problems, such as electrolyte imbalance or sepsis, (2) hydration, (3) administering heparin intravenously to treat disseminated intravascular clotting, and (4) surgical excision of thrombi. The mortality rate has been as high as 60 percent, usually due to sepsis or uncorrected fluid and electrolyte imbalance, but the prognosis has improved in recent years.

PREVENTION

Health Promotion

Avoidance or adequate treatment of predisposing factors (see following section on the population at risk).

Population at Risk

1. Predisposing factors are numerous and include the high hematocrit characteristic of the neonatal period, dehydration, severe hypoxia, a diabetic mother, shock, septicemia, cyanotic heart disease, renal anomalies, pyelonephritis, and nephrotic syndrome.
2. Seventy percent of victims are infants under 1 month of age.

Screening

None.

ASSESSMENT

Health History

1. Predisposing condition (see preceding section on population at risk): typically the client is a newborn with hyperviscous blood (e.g., secondary to dehydration, polycythemia of cyanotic heart disease, or sepsis), or a newborn whose mother has diabetes.
2. Sudden decline in child's condition.
3. Oliguria.

Physical Assessment

1. Dehydrated, shocky, gravely ill child.
2. Hard flank mass on affected side(s).
3. Gross or microscopic hematuria.
4. Fever.
5. Vomiting.
6. Flank pain.

Diagnostic Tests

1. Intravenous pyelogram.
2. Abdominal ultrasound.
3. Selective renal venograms.

NURSING DIAGNOSES: ACTUAL OR POTENTIAL

1. Impairment of urinary elimination: oliguria secondary to renal shutdown.
2. Alterations in electrolyte balance due to decreased kidney function.
3. Alterations in fluid volume associated with dehydration and shock.
4. Alterations in comfort: pain secondary to ischemia or necrosis of kidney.
5. Nutritional alterations associated with vomiting and dietary restrictions of therapy.

EXPECTED OUTCOMES

1. Adequate hydration will be maintained as evidenced by body temperature, skin turgor, and fontanel fullness.
2. Adequate nutrition for size and age will be maintained.
3. Signs of shock will be eliminated as evidenced by restoration of normal vital signs and normal hydration.
4. Pain will be relieved.

INTERVENTIONS

1. Maintain IV line by careful taping or splinting of site. This will provide adequate route for IV nutrition and hydration.
2. Keep strict records of intake and output. Weigh diapers if necessary to estimate urinary output (1 mL urine weighs approximately 1 g).
3. Test urine for blood and protein.
4. Monitor skin turgor, fontanels, eyes, and temperature for signs of dehydration.
5. Take blood pressure frequently to determine if child is hypertensive or hypotensive.
   a. Elevate feet and keep warm, if hypotensive.
   b. Also reassess hydration if hypotensive; suspect hypovolemia as well as shock.
6. Give pain medication as needed. Help child assume position of comfort. Encourage turning frequently (every 1 to 2 hours) to prevent pulmonary stasis.

EVALUATION

Outcome Criteria

1. The IV line is kept patent; infiltration is prevented.
2. The child is well nourished and in electrolyte balance.
3. The child's urinary output is monitored. The occurrence of oliguria, anuria, hematuria, or proteinuria is noted and reported.
4. The child is adequately hydrated. The fontanels, eyes, skin turgor, and temperature are used as indicators of hydration.
5. The child's blood pressure is closely monitored.
6. If shock occurs, it is promptly noted and treated.
7. The child's discomfort, as evidenced by irritability or restlessness, is relieved with medication.

Complications

1. Extension of thrombi into venous system.
2. Hypertension several months after acute state.
3. Nephrotic syndrome.
4. Infection.
5. Tubular dysfunctions, proximal or distal.
6. Necrosis of papillae or medulla.
7. Renal insufficiency or failure.

Reevaluation and Follow-up

1. Resolution of the acute phase can take as long as a month, if it is going to occur at all.
2. Due to the rather high incidence of late complications, follow-up visits should be every 2 to 4 weeks.
3. If residual symptoms warrant, weekly clinic visits may be necessary.

RENAL ARTERY THROMBOSIS

DESCRIPTION

Renal artery thrombosis is an extremely rare condition that, until recently, was usually diagnosed at autopsy. Causative factors are external trauma such as surgical manipulation of the kidney, embolism from bacterial endocarditis or thrombosed ductus arteriosus, prolonged umbilical artery catheterization, or renal artery aneurysm. The child develops sudden, severe, unremitting flank pain, fever, and shock. If medical diagnosis is made promptly, surgical embolectomy followed by heparinization can give good results. If the disease is not treated promptly, however, complete or partial nephrectomy may be necessary. Nursing care of the child with renal artery thrombosis is directed at

1. Pain relief by administering prescribed analgesics and by assisting the child to a position of comfort.
2. Monitoring blood pressure very carefully, since the client may become hypotensive from shock or hypertensive as a renal response to ischemia.
3. Monitoring fluid and electrolyte balance and renal output (including urine checks for blood and protein).
4. Maintaining nutrition, hydration, and electrolyte balance in spite of the child's nausea and vomiting.

Hypertension can be a late complication. End-stage renal disease can occur if thromboses are bilateral and do not resolve (see *Chronic Renal Failure*, later in this chapter). If the thrombosis responds to treatment, follow-up is the same as for renal vein thrombosis (described above).

TRAUMATIC INJURIES

RENAL INJURY

DESCRIPTION

The kidneys are particularly susceptible to childhood injury because of the child's level of activity, lack of perirenal fat deposits, and the relatively larger size of the kidneys. Most injuries are the result of blunt trauma from falls, blows, contact sports, and sledding. Degree of injury can range from contusions to cortical laceration and tearing of the collecting system to complete fragmentation and maceration of the kidney. Medical management, usually drainage and immobilization, is most commonly used for the less severe degrees of injury. Partial or total nephrectomy is performed only as a last resort to control hemorrhage or extravasation of urine. Renal injury is most frequent in boys during the second decade of life. Care of clients with kidney trauma is presented in Chapter 32.

HYPERACTIVITY AND HYPOACTIVITY

ACUTE RENAL FAILURE

DESCRIPTION

Acute renal failure is a syndrome characterized by decrease or cessation of renal function, over a period of days or weeks, due to compromise of the renal blood flow, injury or disease of the kidney or its vessels, obstruction of the urinary tract, or exposure to nephrotoxic substances. It may be called acute tubular necrosis, because in many instances the cells lining the kidney tubules die and slough. Medical treatment depends on the severity of the disease and may range from management by medication and dietary restriction to hemodialysis. The prognosis for remission is favorable if the child's general condition is good, if the blood chemistries are not severely disordered, and if the oliguric phase does not last long. The recovery phase is usually heralded by a period of diuresis.

PREVENTION

Health Promotion

1. Prevention or adequate treatment of the widely varied disorders that can lead to acute renal failure.
   a. Causes of severe hypovolemia and inadequate kidney perfusion: burns, sepsis, hemorrhage.
   b. Toxicity due to renotoxic chemicals: heavy metals, carbon tetrachloride, numerous drugs.
   c. Obstructions of the major vessels: renal vein or artery thrombosis (discussed earlier in this chapter).
   d. Kidney disorders, such as acute poststreptococcal glomerulonephritis (discussed earlier in this chapter)
   e. Hemolysis, for example, from blood transfusion reaction.
   f. Many others.

Population at Risk

Children exposed to causal factors mentioned above.

Screening

None.

ASSESSMENT

Health History

1. Exposure to known cause of acute renal failure (see section on Prevention).
2. Many children have had previous good health.
3. Sudden onset of symptoms.
   a. Edema, shortness of breath.
   b. Headache, lethargy, drowsiness.
   c. Seizures or coma.
   d. Nausea and vomiting, diarrhea.
   e. Oliguria or anuria.

Physical Assessment

1. Edema.
2. Shortness of breath.
3. Lethargy or coma.
4. Pallor.
5. Hypertension.
6. Bruising, easy bleeding, prolonged clotting time.

Diagnostic Tests

1. Accurate weight and vital signs.
2. Serum BUN, creatinine, electrolyte values, calcium, phosphorus, hematocrit, and white blood cells (WBC) (see Table 21–2).
3. 24-hour urine collection (see Table 21–2).
4. Intravenous pyelogram, if carefully done; if performed when child is dehydrated or shocky, IVP will aggravate the renal failure.
5. Renal biopsy.

NURSING DIAGNOSES: ACTUAL OR POTENTIAL

1. Impairment of urinary elimination: oliguria or anuria due to tubular shutdown.
2. Excess fluid volume: overload due to decreased kidney function.
3. Alteration in electrolyte balance: acidosis, hyperkalemia, and hypernatremia due to diminished renal function.
4. Hypertension secondary to fluid overload.
5. Altered level of cognition and perception due to blood chemistry imbalances (azotemia).
6. Decreased activity tolerance due to altered level of consciousness and anemia.
7. Increased risk of injury associated with altered level of consciousness.
8. Increased risk of bleeding associated with platelet malfunction due to azotemia.
9. Increased risk of infection due to friable skin and mucous membranes associated with azotemia, and due to immunosuppression associated with azotemia.

EXPECTED OUTCOMES

1. Volume overload will be prevented or controlled.
2. The degree of acidosis will be kept to a minimum.
3. The degree of electrolyte imbalance will be kept to a minimum.
4. Any central nervous system (CNS) changes will be detected and reported promptly.
5. Hypertension will be detected and controlled.
6. Child will not be injured (e.g., from convulsion or confusion).
7. Activity level will not exceed tolerance.
8. Bleeding will be minimized or absent.
9. Child will not become infected.

INTERVENTIONS

1. Keep a strict record of intake and output. Measure everything in exact milliliters. Oral fluids are usually restricted; divide allotted fluids into three 8-hour portions, with amounts based on projected needs and desires for an 8-hour period. Be sure to consider fluids needed to take medications as part of restriction.
2. Monitor diet carefully. With renal failure, a low protein, low potassium, low to moderate sodium diet is typical. Buildup of end products of protein metabolism is one cause of acidosis. Hyperkalemia causes cardiac arrhythmias, including ventricular standstill. Forbidden high-potassium foods are bananas, oranges, tomatoes, molasses, and potatoes.
3. Inform child, family members, and hospital personnel of child's dietary restriction. A reasonably intelligent child will find an amazing variety of food sources, even in the hospital.
4. Monitor the child's affect, alertness, and energy levels. Central nervous system depression may be a sign of approaching seizure activity.
5. Keep padded tongue blade in a handy place for immediate use if seizure activity begins.
6. Monitor blood pressure frequently. If child complains of headache or visual disturbances, monitor blood pressure and notify physician. Administer ordered antihypertensive agents on time.
7. Prevent trauma as much as possible. Coordinate with laboratory to keep blood drawn for tests to absolute minimum. If bleeding occurs, apply ice and direct pressure for 7 to 10 minutes to control bleeding.
8. Avoid exposure to infectious disease. Thoroughly clean any breaks in skin. Administer ordered antibiotics. Use scrupulous aseptic technique.

EVALUATION

Outcome Criteria

1. Intake and output are charted accurately.
2. Signs of volume overload, such as CHF or pulmonary edema, or of dehydration, such as decreased skin turgor, are detected and reported immediately, and progressively decrease until absent.
3. Diet is carefully followed. Dietary changes are initiated as laboratory results indicate that modifications are appropriate.
4. Parents appropriately set limits on child's dietary behavior.
5. Serum potassium levels are between 4.0 and 6.0. An elevated potassium level is incompatible with good cardiac function.
6. The child's level of consciousness is restored to normal level of cognition and perception.
7. Activity level does not exceed energy level; activities are increased as child's condition permits.
8. Blood pressure returns to normal or nearly normal.
9. Signs and symptoms of anemia are reduced; hematocrit is maintained at optimal level (all clients with azotemia are anemic).
10. Injury does not occur.
11. Spontaneous bleeding is prevented or controlled immediately.
12. Exposure to contagious diseases is prevented.
13. Child does not develop infections.

Complications

1. Hyperkalemia leading to cardiac malfunction or arrest.
2. Stroke, CHF, or pulmonary edema due to fluid overload.
3. Convulsions due to fluid overload, hyponatremia, hypocalcemia, or too rapid a dialysis.
4. Sepsis with a fatal outcome in as many as one-third of the clients with acute renal failure.
5. Decreased renal function when recovery is complete in about 50 percent of the clients.
6. Chronic renal failure (i.e., no recovery of function at all).

Reevaluation and Follow-up

1. This depends on the symptoms and their degree of severity at the completion of the recovery phase.
2. Follow-up may be required as frequently as three times a week (for dialysis of those with no return of function) or as infrequently as once a year evaluations of those with apparently complete return of function.

CHRONIC RENAL FAILURE

DESCRIPTION

Chronic renal failure differs from acute renal failure in that it develops over a period of months or years. It usually passes through three stages. In the first stage, *decreased renal reserve*, the function of the kidney is slightly impaired, but the body's chemistry is maintained at essentially normal levels. The second stage, *renal insufficiency*, is usually reached when the glomerular filtration rate falls below 50 percent. Wastes are beginning to accumulate in the blood, and the body is slow in coping with electrolyte and fluid volume changes. The final stage, in which kidney function is minimal or nonexistent, is called *uremia, azotemia, or end-stage renal disease*. If left untreated, chronic renal failure ends eventually in death. The medical treatment of choice in children is dialysis, (peritoneal or hemodialysis), and eventual kidney transplant.

The cause of chronic renal failure in children up to 5 years of age is most often a birth defect, such as hypoplastic or dysplastic kidneys. From 6 to 12 years old the cause is most likely to be urological, whereas at 13 and beyond the most frequent cause is some form of glomerulonephritis. Whatever the basic disease process, once chronic renal failure has progressed to end-stage renal disease (ESRD), the symptoms and treatment are the same for all clients.

PREVENTION

Health Promotion

Although ESRD cannot be prevented entirely, it is possible to slow the progress of some of the diseases that cause chronic renal failure.

1. Aggressive treatment of urinary tract infections in children with a history of urinary tract anomaly.
2. Early and careful treatment of glomerulonephritis.
3. Early treatment of hypertension.

Population at Risk

1. Children with other birth defects have an increased incidence of renal or genitourinary birth defects that may eventuate in renal failure.
2. Children with streptococcal infections are at risk to develop glomerulonephritis, which can produce chronic renal failure.
3. Some other diseases, such as lupus erythematosus, can lead to chronic renal failure.
4. Children with acute renal failure can develop the chronic form of the disease.

Screening

1. Blood pressure.
2. Urinalysis.
3. Serum BUN, creatinine, and electrolyte values.

ASSESSMENT

Health History

1. No clear-cut history of distinct change from health to illness.
2. History of risk factors (see preceeding section on population at risk).
3. Fatigue, lethargy.

Physical Assessment

1. Polyuria, oliguria, or anuria may be present.
2. Hypertension.
3. Poor growth.
4. Delayed sexual maturation.
5. Dry skin and severe itching are rare in children.
6. Paresthesias are rare in children.
7. Pallor, anemia.
8. Tendency to bleed easily; rapidly variable clotting time.
9. Bone pain is unusual in children.
10. Muscle loss.
11. Assess for cardiac murmurs and PMI to monitor CHF and degree of anemia.
12. Assess frequently (with every vital signs check) for rales.

Diagnostic Tests

1. Accurate weights and vital signs.
2. Serum BUN, creatinine, electrolyte values, calcium, phosphorus, alkaline phosphatase, hematocrit, WBC (see Tables 21–1 and 21–2).
3. 24-hour urine for creatinine clearance.
4. Renal biopsy.

NURSING DIAGNOSES: ACTUAL OR POTENTIAL

1. Excess fluid volume due to decreased kidney output.
2. Alteration in electrolyte balance: acidosis, hyperkalemia, and hypernatremia due to diminished renal function.
3. Altered level of cognition and perception due to blood chemistry imbalances (azotemia).
4. Decreased activity tolerance due to malaise, muscle atrophy, and anemia.

5. Increased risk of bleeding associated with platelet malfunction due to azotemia.
6. Impairment of skin integrity associated with intractable itching.
7. Alteration in comfort: headache, bone pain, nausea, and muscle cramps associated with azotemia.
8. Knowledge deficit about treatment for chronic renal failure.
9. Alteration in parenting associated with chronic, life-threatening illness.
10. Increased risk of infection due to depressed immune response associated with azotemia.
11. Alteration in self-concept due to growth retardation and chronic illness.

EXPECTED OUTCOMES

1. Child will achieve and maintain fluid and electrolyte balance.
2. Child will achieve and maintain normal level of consciousness.
3. Child will maintain a sufficient hematocrit for comfort, and activity level will be adjusted to level of tolerance.
4. Skin will remain intact and free from infection.
5. Child will experience optimal growth and development.
6. Optimal level of comfort will be achieved and maintained.
7. Traumatic bleeding will not occur.
8. The child and family, with the health care team, will choose a method of treatment (form of dialysis) that is least disruptive for their situation and best promotes physical well-being for this child.
9. Child and family will understand the treatment method and will carry out their roles in the therapy.
10. Child will remain free of infection.
11. The family will maintain as normal a lifestyle as possible.
12. Child will demonstrate (through verbalization or play) an integrated self-concept.

INTERVENTIONS

FOR THE CHILD ON PERITONEAL DIALYSIS: CONTINUOUS AMBULATORY PERITONEAL DIALYSIS (CAPD) OR CONTINUOUS CYCLE PERITONEAL DIALYSIS (CCPD)

1. Encourage adequate nutrition; diet should be *high* in protein and moderate in potassium, sodium, and fluids. The child should manage the dietary pattern as much as is developmentally appropriate.
2. Avoid exposure to contagious disease. Thoroughly clean any breaks in skin. Administer ordered antiobiotic; use scrupulous aseptic technique.
3. Prepare the child and family for hemodialysis by showing them the dialysis unit, introducing them to the staff, and having them meet children who are already on dialysis and their families. Encourage questions. Be honest in your answers. Allow younger children the opportunity to work through their anxieties through play or by drawing pictures. Allow older children and parents the opportunity to talk about their anxieties.
4. Teach the family and child the techniques of CAPD, tailoring teaching methods to the needs of the individual child and family.
5. Reinforce this teaching on repeat clinic visits, emphasizing measures to prevent peritonitis.
6. Help parents to verbalize their frustrations and, if necessary, arrange for alternative care when parents need a break.
7. Prepare the child and family for renal transplantation by talking about the operation, showing pictures for the procedure, discussing postoperative changes in lifestyle, and introducing them to the intensive care unit (ICU) staff and transplant staff. Again, provide many opportunities for all involved to work through their anxieties.

FOR THE CHILD ON HEMODIALYSIS

1. Keep a *strict* record of intake and output. Measure everything in exact milliliters. Oral fluids are usually restricted; allocate fluids according to anticipated needs and desires of individual child at various times of the day. Be sure to consider fluids needed to take medications as part of intake.
2. Monitor diet carefully. With renal failure a low-protein, low-potassium, and low-to-moderate sodium diet is typical. Buildup of end products of protein metabolism is one cause of acidosis. Hyperkalemia causes cardiac arrhythmias, including ventricular standstill. Forbidden high-potassium foods are bananas, oranges, tomatoes, potatoes, and molasses.
3. Inform child, family members, and hospital personnel of child's dietary restriction. A

reasonably intelligent child will find an amazing variety of food sources, even in the hospital.

4. Avoid exposure to infections. Use scrupulous aseptic technique. Thoroughly cleanse any skin breaks. Administer ordered antibiotics.
5. Monitor blood pressure frequently. If child complains of headache or visual disturbances, monitor blood pressure and notify physician. Administer ordered antihypertensives on time and in the correct amount.
6. Coordinate with laboratory to keep venipunctures to absolute minimum. Prevent trauma as much as possible. If bleeding occurs, apply ice and direct pressure for 7 to 10 minutes to control bleeding.
7. Prepare the child and family for hemodialysis by showing them the dialysis unit, introducing them to the staff, and having them meet children who are already on dialysis and their families. Encourage questions. Be honest in your answers. Allow younger children the opportunity to work through their anxieties through play or by drawing pictures. Allow older children and parents the opportunity to talk about their anxieties.
8. High-calorie diets are helpful in promoting growth. High-calorie carbohydrate supplements should be taken if adequate calories are not otherwise consumed. Dietary restrictions on protein, fluids, potassium, or sodium should not be relaxed in the effort to increase calories.
9. Encourage frequent, liberal use of hand lotion to keep skin moisturized. Use of bath oils or moisturizers should also be recommended.
10. Ensure that calcium and aluminum hydroxide are taken as recommended to prevent or control osteodystrophy. Magnesium aluminum hydroxide is not a substitute for aluminum hydroxide in patients with chronic renal failure.
11. Allow the child and parents to talk as needed about the inconvenience of dialysis. Transportation to the nearest dialysis center suitable for children and the large amount of time expended in dialysis and en route are common problems.
12. Prepare the child and family for renal transplantation by talking about the operation, showing pictures of the procedure, discussing postoperative changes in lifestyle, and introducing them to the ICU staff and transplant staff. Again, provide many opportunities for all involved to work through their anxieties.

EVALUATION

Outcome Criteria

1. Child is free of fluid volume overload (shows no signs of CHF or pulmonary edema) and is not dehydrated. Hypertension is controlled. Intake and output are accurately recorded. Serum potassium remains between 4.0 and 6.0 meq/L (elevated potassium is incompatible with good cardiac function).
2. Child is comfortable and moderatively active. Nausea, cramps, headache, and bone and joint pains are absent or minimal.
3. Hematocrit is stable. Spontaneous bleeding does not occur.
4. Height and weight (exclusive of edema) are increasing. Appetite is good, and child is adhering to prescribed diet, including sufficient calories for growth.
5. Behavioral development is appropriate for age (see Chapter 4). School-age child or adolescent attends school. Child shows evidences of favorable self-concept.
6. Infection does not occur or is promptly treated. Unnecessary exposure to infections is avoided. Child takes antibiotics as prescribed and applies skin moisturizers. Skin is intact.
7. Child who is about to begin dialysis, and family members, can describe simply what will happen; they talk about their concerns and ask questions. All are actively and adequately coping.
8. Child who is to receive a kidney transplant, and family members, are well prepared. They can describe simply what will happen; they talk about their concerns and ask questions. All are adequately and actively coping.
9. Family lifestyle is as normal as possible. Parents set limits on child's behavior. Adults maintain employment. Individuals and family together have recreation.

Complications

1. Hyperkalemia leading to cardiac malfunction or arrest.
2. Stroke, CHF, or pulmonary edema due to fluid overload.

3. Convulsions due to elevated BUN, fluid overload, hyponatremia, hypocalcemia, or too rapid a dialysis.
4. Sepsis.

Reevaluation and Follow-up
The course of chronic renal failure is progressive and relentless. The child will require follow-up indefinitely by the health team, eventually including dialysis and transplant teams. Children are generally quite readily accepted as transplant candidates.

METABOLIC DISORDERS

RENAL TUBULAR ACIDOSIS

DESCRIPTION

Renal tubular acidosis is a disease in which the kidney is unable to excrete sufficient hydrogen ion and loses too much bicarbonate ion in the urine. In addition, sodium, calcium, and potassium are lost in large amounts along with the bicarbonate ion. Generally, the loss of calcium and sodium is responsible for most symptoms. Most authorities divide this disease into two types. The first, called classical or persistent primary renal tubular acidosis, is thought to be a disease of the distal convoluted tubules. It is familial (autosomal dominant) and occurs mainly in 2-year-old girls. The second type, transient or proximal renal tubular acidosis, is rare. It occurs mainly in boys in the first year of life; the origin is unknown. Medical treatment of both types of renal tubular acidosis consists of administration of alkali (sodium bicarbonate, sodium citrate, or both) as well as high doses of vitamin D.

PREVENTION

Health Promotion

Genetic counseling for prospective parents with a family history of this disorder.

Population at Risk

Infants and young children, especially those with a positive family history.

Screening

None.

ASSESSMENT

Health History

1. Recurrent dehydration with polyuria, thirst, polydipsia, constipation.
2. Irritability.
3. Mental confusion.
4. Labored respirations.
5. Frequent urination.
6. Anorexia, vomiting.

Physical Assessment

1. Kussmaul respirations.
2. General appearance of failure to thrive, including retarded growth, retarded bone age, low weight, lethargy, and irritability.
3. Rickets, bone pain, deformity, and pathologic fractures due to loss of calcium from bones.
4. Costovertebral angle tenderness.
5. Muscular hypotonia and cardiac arrhythmia due to loss of serum potassium.
6. Renal colic as a consequence of high serum calcium leading to nephrocalcinosis and nephrolithiasis.

Diagnostic Tests

1. Serum electrolyte values may be normal or abnormal, except chloride, which will always be increased.
2. Serum BUN and creatinine are within normal limits (see Table 21–2).
3. Urine is relatively alkaline.

NURSING DIAGNOSES: ACTUAL OR POTENTIAL

1. Nutritional deficit due to anorexia and vomiting.
2. Fluid volume deficit (dehydration) due to polyuria.
3. Loss of skin integrity: diaper area lesions associated with continual wetness from polyuria.
4. Alteration in electrolyte balance: acidosis, hypercalcemia, and hypokalemia due to renal tubular malfunction.
5. Alterations in cardiac output: arrhythmias due to hypokalemia.
6. Alterations in comfort: Kussmaul respirations due to acidosis, bone pain due to loss of calcium from bones, and renal colic due to

stones associated with elevated serum calcium.

7. Increased risk of injury associated with bone fragility.

EXPECTED OUTCOMES

1. Good nutrition will be maintained.
2. Adequate hydration will be maintained.
3. Pathologic fractures will be prevented.
4. Cardiac arrhythmias will be promptly detected and treatment quickly begun.
5. Stone formation will be prevented or rapidly treated.

INTERVENTIONS

1. Provide several small, light meals each day as long as anorexia or vomiting persist. Offer favorite foods as much as possible.
2. Offer fluids frequently; give fluids as often as requested by child. Monitor skin turgor, fontanels, eyes, and temperature for signs of dehydration.
3. Change diaper frequently to prevent skin irritation due to polyuria.
4. Give medication as prescribed, in spite of child's dislike of taste, to combat acidosis, bone disease, and stone formation.
5. If bone disease is advanced, handle child as little as possible and discourage strenuous activities to prevent pathologic fractures. Provide for quiet diversion and sensory stimulation.
6. If laboratory results show hypokalemia, maintain child on cardiac monitor to detect cardiac arrhythmias as quickly as possible. Notify physician immediately of hypokalemia or arrhythmia.
7. Test all urine for hematuria; strain for calculi. Observe for symptoms of renal colic. Notify physician if any of these are present.

EVALUATION

Outcome Criteria

1. Child is taking and retaining an adequate diet and is growing and gaining weight.
2. The child shows no signs of dehydration.
3. The child's skin in the diaper area remains intact.
4. The child takes medication on schedule in sufficient amounts; as a consequence, acidosis is corrected, and rickets is improving.
5. Pathologic fractures are prevented or healed.
6. If the child is on bed rest, sensory deprivation is prevented.
7. Cardiac arrhythmias are detected quickly and treatment begun rapidly.
8. Urinary tract stone formation is prevented.

Complications

1. Pathologic fractures leading to deformity.
2. Cardiac arrest due to hypokalemia.
3. Obstructive uropathy due to stone formation.
4. Chronic renal failure, if renal damage due to stone formation is severe.

Reevaluation and Follow-up

1. Frequency of follow-up depends on severity of symptoms when disease initially presents.
2. Child's compliance with medication regimen and the resulting decrease in symptoms is also a factor in frequency of follow-up.
3. Daily examinations and treatment may be required in the face of severe symptoms. With good medication compliance and control of the disease, only quarterly visits are necessary.

REFERENCES

Bauer, S. B.: "Indications for Antireflux Surgery," *Dialogues in Pediatric Urology*, **6**(1):4, January 1983.

Klauber, G. T.: "Nonsurgical Therapy," *Dialogues in Pediatric Urology*, **6**(1):3, January 1983.

BIBLIOGRAPHY

Charny, C. W., and Wolgin, W.: *Cryptorchism*, Paul B. Hoeber, Inc., Harper & Brothers, New York, 1957. Although not recent, this is a comprehensive treatise covering the embryology, etiology, pathology, symptoms, complications, diagnosis, and treatment of cryptorchidism. Written in a readily understandable style, it combines a review of the then-current literature with the authors' own experiences. It is referred to by many authors as a primary source.

Harrington, J. O., and Brener, E. R.: *Patient Care in Renal Failure*, W. B. Saunders, Philadelphia, 1973. This is a very complete explanation of the anatomy, physiology, pathology, and treatment of renal failure, along with descriptions of treatment modules available. Nursing care is emphasized. This is a useful book for student and practitioner alike.

Kelalis, P. P., King, L. R., and Belman, A. B.: (eds.): *Clinical Pediatric Urology*, vols. I and II, W. B. Saunders, Philadelphia, 1976. This comprehensive book is invaluable to the nurse who wishes to understand the surgical management and goals of care for the pediatric patient with a urological problem.

Lieberman, E. (ed.): *Clinical Pediatric Nephrology*, J. B. Lippincott, Philadelphia, 1976. A truly comprehensive work by 21 contributors that covers the workup and medical management of a wide range of nephrological conditions in the pediatric client. Written for physicians.

Netter, F. H.: *The Ciba Collection of Medical Illustrations, Volume 6, Kidneys, Ureters, and Urinary Bladder*, CIBA Pharmaceutical Company, Summit, NJ, 1979. A classic work that details anatomy, physiology, embryology, diagnostic techniques, diseases, congenital and hereditary disorders, and therapeutics of the kidneys and urinary tract. An invaluable aid to illustrate lectures to students as well as explanations to clients.

Rubin, M. I., and Barratt, T. M. (eds.): *Pediatric Nephrology*, Williams & Wilkins, Baltimore, 1975. A comprehensive book by 51 contributors that provides great detail about assorted specific aspects of pediatric nephrology. It would be most useful to the nurse with a background in nephrology or urology.

Scipien, G. M., Barnard, M. U., Chard, M., et al. (eds.): *Comprehensive Pediatric Nursing*, 2d ed., McGraw-Hill, New York, 1979. This outstanding textbook includes chapters on the urinary and reproductive systems in which embryology, anatomy, and physiology of the systems are discussed; nursing care for children with a wide range of health care disorders is presented. The nursing process and growth and development are given extensive treatment elsewhere in the book.

Vaughn, V. C., McKay, R. J., and Nelson W. E., (eds.): *Nelson Textbook of Pediatrics*, 11th ed., W. B. Saunders, Philadelphia, 1979. This widely used book, although written for medical students, is an invaluable reference for nurses seeking detailed information about children's diseases and their medical treatment.

Vander, A. J.: *Renal Physiology*, McGraw-Hill, New York, 1975. This is a well-written comprehensive text designed primarily for medical students. It is easily understood by those with some background in anatomy and physiology. Study is guided by learning objectives printed at the beginning of each chapter and test questions at the end of the book. There is also a list of suggested readings for each chapter.

22

The Gastrointestinal System

Catherine Kneut

OBSTRUCTIONS

PYLORIC STENOSIS

DESCRIPTION

Pyloric stenosis is the progressive hypertrophy of the pyloric muscle at the gastric outlet (see Figure 22–1). The cause is unknown. The highest incidence occurs in firstborn Caucasian males, and familial tendencies do exist. The main symptom is vomiting after feedings, which soon becomes projectile. The vomitus is not bile stained, because the obstruction is proximal to the ampulla of Vater, where bile enters the intestinal tract. Weight loss and dehydration are evident. The infant sucks eagerly even after vomiting. The treatment for nearly all babies is surgery to incise the hypertrophied pylorus—Ramstedt pyloromyotomy. Pyloromyotomy is curative and carries an extremely low operative risk. A very small number of infants (usually those who have other problems that make them poor surgical candidates) are treated nonsurgically, with antispasmodics and varied feeding thicknesses and positions. This therapy can take several months and is not always successful.

Acknowledgment is made to Elizabeth Butler Marren and Linda M. Burton, whose chapter for the first edition of this work was adapted for this revision.

PREVENTION

Health Promotion

No preventive measures are known.

Population at Risk

Infants from early neonatal period to 4 months of age. The usual age at onset is 3 to 4 weeks. Eighty percent of patients are boys.

Screening

None.

ASSESSMENT

Health History

1. Feeding history: usually takes bottle eagerly after vomiting.
2. Projectile vomiting.

Physical Assessment

1. Observable peristaltic waves passing left to right during or immediately after feeding.
2. Palpable olive-sized mass (pylorus) in right upper quadrant.
3. Dehydration.
4. Weight loss accompanied by reduced body fat and muscle mass.

Diagnostic Tests

Medical diagnosis is made by history (characteristic vomiting followed by hunger) and physical examination (palpation of pyloric mass and observation of peristaltic waves). Upper gastrointestinal (GI) x-ray films with contrast media may or may not help clarify an uncertain diagnosis.

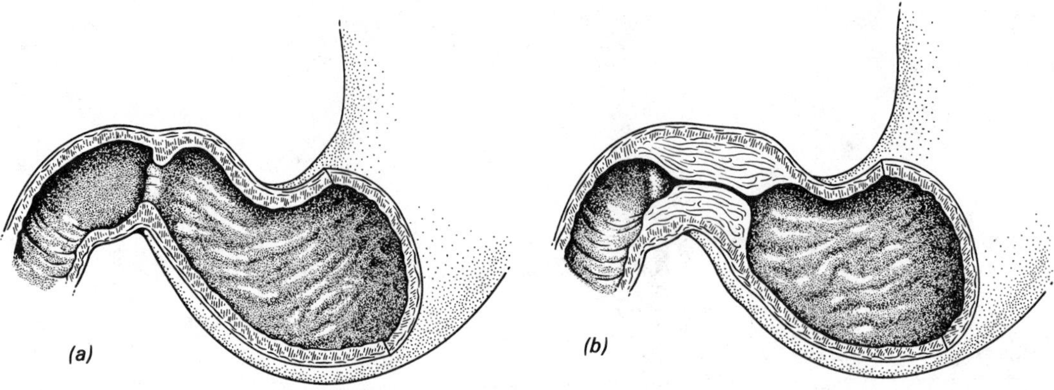

Figure 22-1 (*a*) Normal pylorus. (*b*) Pyloric stenosis. Notice the hypertrophied muscle mass and narrowed lumen.

NURSING DIAGNOSES: ACTUAL OR POTENTIAL

1. Alteration in fluid volume due to vomiting.
2. Alteration in comfort: discomfort due to vomiting and dehydration.
3. Alteration in family dynamics due to ill infant.
4. Electrolyte imbalance secondary to vomiting (hypochloremia).
5. Risk of aspiration due to vomiting.

EXPECTED OUTCOMES

1. Preoperative.
   a. Infant's fluid volume will be within normal limits 24 to 48 hours after admission.
   b. Parents will demonstrate knowledge of infant's physical problem.
   c. Parents will understand the need for surgical intervention.
   d. Electrolyte values will be within normal limits.
   e. Infant's lung sounds will be clear on auscultation.
2. Postoperative.
   a. Infant will retain oral feedings of increasing strength and amount.
   b. Parents will feed infant postoperatively.
   c. Wound will heal without complications.

INTERVENTIONS

1. Preoperative.
   a. NPO.
   b. Observe and record amount of vomitus.
   c. Monitor patency of nasogastric (NG) tube.
   d. Measure abdominal girth.
   e. Regulate flow of intravenous fluids.
   f. Monitor intake and output; measure urine specific gravity.
   g. Keep accurate record of daily weights.
   h. Position infant on side or in chalasia chair to prevent aspiration.
   i. Note electrolyte values.
   j. Reassure parents that infant's problem is not related to feeding practices. Provide support and information about surgery.
2. Postoperative.
   a. NPO for 12 hours.
   b. Pulmonary toilet and humidity.
   c. Chart NG tube output.
   d. Monitor flow of parenteral fluids.
   e. Monitor intake and output; measure urine specific gravity.
   f. Institute oral feedings (half-strength glucose water) and gradually increase amount and type of formula.
   g. Burp infant frequently during feedings.
   h. Have parents feed infant and involve them in other aspects of care.
   i. Include visual and tactile stimuli for infant.
   j. Discharge teaching: Make sure parents understand wound care and feeding techniques. Parents may need help with routine newborn care. Home nurse referral.

EVALUATION

Outcome Criteria

1. Preoperative.
   a. Infant is well hydrated, skin turgor is good, and specific gravity is within normal limits.
   b. Nasogastric tube relieves discomfort.
   c. Breath sounds remain clear.
   d. Parents can state the reasons for surgery.

2. Postoperative.
   a. Infant retains full-strength formula before discharge.
   b. Parents exhibit correct feeding skills and are comfortable in providing care.
   c. Wound is clean, dry, and intact at time of discharge.

Reevaluation and Follow-up

Full recover is expected. Feeding and growth and development should be normal.

MALROTATION AND VOLVULUS

DESCRIPTION

Malrotation is an abnormality of intestinal rotation that occurs during embryological development. The cecum and terminal ileum fail to rotate across the peritoneal cavity to lie in the right lower quadrant. Instead, the process is arrested, and they are positioned in the right upper quadrant. The duodenum may be compressed by bands from the cecum or ascending colon, which can produce obstruction. Because the mesentery is not firmly attached to the abdominal wall, twisting of the small intestine (volvulus) can occur. The volvulus may wrap around the mesentery, causing bowel strangulation. Symptoms usually occur in the first 3 weeks of life and include vomiting, abdominal distension, and failure to pass stools. Treatment is surgical correction of the malposition and resection of ischemic bowel.

PREVENTION

Health Promotion

No preventive measures are known for this congenital defect.

Population at Risk

Newborns.

Screening

None.

ASSESSMENT

Health History

1. Bile-stained vomitus.
2. Absence of stool, particularly within the first 24 hours of life.
3. Bloody, mucoid drainage from the rectum.

Physical Assessment

1. Abdominal distension.
2. Signs of shock or toxicity may be present.

Diagnostic Tests

Barium enema and upper GI series will differentiate malrotation and volvulus from other intestinal obstructions.

NURSING DIAGNOSES: ACTUAL OR POTENTIAL

1. Loss of fluid volume due to vomiting and bleeding.
2. Alteration in electrolyte balance due to vomiting (bile, pancreatic enzymes, and GI fluids are lost in vomitus).
3. Alteration in oxygenation: decrease, due to blood loss and abdominal distension.
4. Alteration in comfort: discomfort due to vomiting, distension, and respiratory distress.
5. Disruption in parent–infant bonding due to critical illness.
6. Risk of aspiration due to vomiting.

EXPECTED OUTCOMES

1. Preoperative.
   a. Client will be hydrated as evidenced by physical exam and laboratory data.
   b. Electrolyte values will be within normal limits as evidenced by laboratory data.
   c. Oxygen/carbon dioxide gas exchange will be within normal limits as documented by arterial blood gases.
   d. Abdominal distension will decrease as measured by abdominal girths.
   e. Lung sounds will be clear on auscultation.
   f. Parents will make physical contact with child and participate in care.
2. Postoperative.
   a. Fluid and electrolyte balance will remain within normal limits.
   b. Infant maintains adequate oxygenation as measured by arterial blood gases.
   c. Infant retains formula feedings in increasing concentration and amount.
   d. Normal bowel elimination will occur within 7 to 10 days postoperatively.
   e. Wound will remain clean and intact.
   f. Parents will participate in infant's care.

INTERVENTIONS

1. Preoperative.
   a. Monitor vital signs and abdominal girth every 1 to 2 hours.

b. Record type and amount of vomitus.
c. Record type of stools, as well as absence.
d. Maintain patency of NG tube, and record output.
e. Regulate and monitor flow of parenteral fluids.
f. Record intake, output, and urine specific gravity.
g. Note electrolyte and blood gas values.
h. Position infant to prevent aspiration.
i. Note changes in skin color (duskiness, cyanosis, paleness).
j. Provide parents with information about surgery and the infant's condition. Encourage them to touch the child and provide support and reassurance.

2. Postoperative.
   a. Maintain flow rate of intervenous (IV) fluids.
   b. Measure intake, output, and urine specific gravity.
   c. Ensure patency of NG tube, and chart output.
   d. Provide pulmonary toilet, and position to prevent aspiration.
   e. Measure abdominal girth every 2 to 4 hours.
   f. Auscultate abdomen for return of bowel sounds.
   g. Observe and chart type of stool.
   h. Begin oral feedings with clear liquids when peristalsis returns, and gradually increase in amount and strength (this is a longer process than for pyloric stenosis).
   i. Observe for vomiting and/or distension after feedings are initiated.
   j. Observe wound for redness, drainage, or swelling.
   k. Provide visual and tactile stimuli for infant.
   l. Encourage parental contact with infant. Have parents feed child and perform other aspects of care. Prepare parents for home care.

EVALUATION

Outcome Criteria

1. Preoperative.
   a. Fluid and electrolyte values are within normal limits.
   b. Oxygen/carbon dioxide gas exchange is adequate according to arterial blood gases.
   c. Abdominal distension decreases.
   d. Lung sounds are clear; aspiration is prevented.
   e. Parents comprehend need for surgery as evidenced by verbal feedback.
2. Postoperative.
   a. Full-strength formula feedings are tolerated.
   b. Stool assumes normal consistency and color.
   c. Wound is clean, dry, and intact.
   d. Parent–infant relationship is established, and parents feel capable of providing care.

Reevaluation and Follow-up

1. Normal growth and development are to be expected.
2. Dietary modifications may be required if extensive bowel resection was necessary (because of circulatory compromise before surgery).

INTUSSUSCEPTION

DESCRIPTION

Intussusception is the invagination, or telescoping, of a portion of the intestine into a more distal segment (Figure 22–2). A barium enema may succeed in reducing the intussusception by hydrostatic pressure. Surgery is performed when barium enema is unsuccessful.

PREVENTION

Health Promotion

No preventive measures are known.

Population at Risk

Children, especially whites, between 6 months and 2 years of age. Boys are affected three times more often than girls.

Screening

None.

ASSESSMENT

Health History

1. Sudden onset of severe colicky abdominal pain.
2. Bile-stained emesis.
3. "Currant jelly" stools (brown, bloody, mucoid).

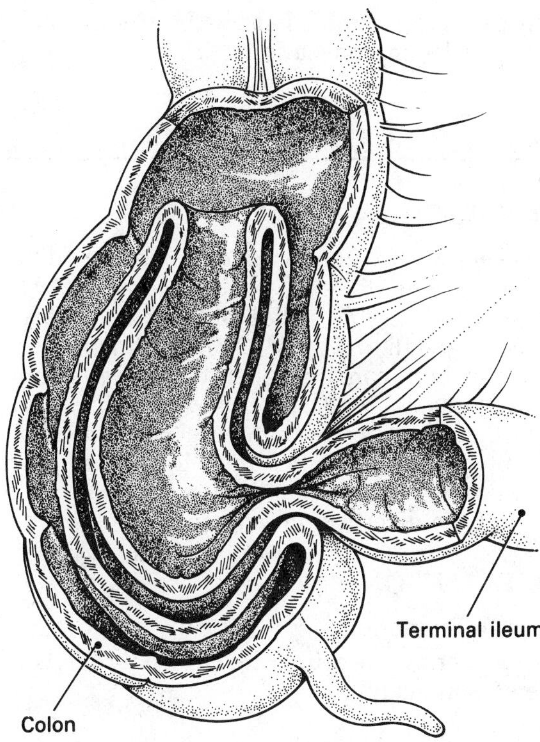

Figure 22-2 Intussusception. Small bowel is invaginated and passed by peristalsis into the cecum. Bowel obstruction and ischemia result.

Physical Assessment

1. Palpable sausagelike mass along the transverse or ascending colon.
2. Rectal examination reveals blood and mucus.

Diagnostic Tests

Barium enema (contraindicated in the presence of peritonitis).

NURSING DIAGNOSES: ACTUAL OR POTENTIAL

1. Alteration in comfort: discomfort due to abdominal pain and vomiting.
2. Loss of fluids and electrolytes due to vomiting.
3. Potential risk of bowel rupture and peritonitis.

EXPECTED OUTCOMES

1. Nonoperative.
   a. Barium enema will reduce intussusception.
   b. Oral feedings will be tolerated.
   c. Child will have a normal bowel movement.
   d. Child will be discharged within 48 hours after barium enema reduction.
   e. Parents will state signs of intussusception (will recognize recurrence).
2. Preoperative.
   a. Fluid and electrolyte balance will be within normal limits.
   b. Pain will abate as evidenced by assuming position of comfort.
   c. Bowel rupture and peritonitis will not occur.
3. Postoperative.
   a. Fluid and electrolyte balance will be within normal limits.
   b. Child will tolerate feedings.
   c. Normal bowel movement will occur 3 to 5 days postoperatively.
   d. Wound will heal without complications.

INTERVENTIONS

1. Nonoperative.
   a. Prepare child for barium enema.
   b. Observe child for signs and symptoms of recurrence of intussusception.
   c. Monitor intake and output; note type of stools.
   d. Note tolerance of normal diet.
   e. Teach parents signs of recurrence (intussusception is more likely to recur after barium enema reduction than after surgery.
2. Preoperative.
   a. NPO.
   b. Monitor rate of IV fluids.
   c. Maintain patency of NG tube.
   d. Position child to prevent aspiration.
   e. Administer analgesics as prescribed.
   f. Record type and amount of vomitus.
   g. Record type and number of stools.
   h. Monitor vital signs frequently (take axillary temperatures).
   i. Measure abdominal girths every 2 to 4 hours.
   j. Report any increase in the severity of symptoms that may indicate shock and peritonitis (increased heart rate, increased respirations, decreased blood pressure, increased or decreased temperature, lethargy, pallor, increased abdominal girth).
3. Postoperative.
   a. Administer IV fluids at the prescribed rate.

b. Maintain patency of the NG tube, and record output.
c. Measure intake, output, and urine specific gravity.
d. Auscultate abdomen for return of peristalsis.
e. Institute and increase feedings as ordered.
f. Observe type and number of stools.
g. Inspect wound for healing.
h. Incorporate parents in the plan of care.
i. Prepare parents for discharge by teaching them wound care, diet, and the need for outpatient follow-up.

EVALUATION

Outcome Criteria

1. Nonoperative.
   a. Barium enema reduction of intussusception is successful.
   b. Child tolerates normal diet without pain or vomiting.
   c. Child has a normal bowel movement.
   d. Parents are aware of signs to observe child for.
   e. Child is discharged within 48 hours.
2. Preoperative.
   a. Hydration and electrolyte balance are restored and maintained by administration of parenteral fluids.
   b. Pain is relieved by medication and positioning.
   c. Vital signs are stable, and signs of bowel rupture are not evident.
3. Postoperative.
   a. Child tolerates normal diet without pain or vomiting.
   b. Bowel elimination is of normal color and consistency.
   c. Wound is clean, dry, and intact.
   d. Parents participate in their child's care and can state the reasons for follow-up outpatient care.

Complications

Peritonitis (see discussion in Chapter 33).

Reevaluation and Follow-up

Recurrence takes place in about 5 to 10 percent of children whose intussusception is reduced by barium enema, and in a smaller percentage of those who have had surgery. Parents need to know signs and symptoms of recurrence (same as for initial attack) and must know the importance of seeking immediate medical help if these signs and symptoms arise.

MECKEL'S DIVERTICULUM

DESCRIPTION

Meckel's diverticulum is an outpouching on the terminal ileum, a result of the incomplete obliteration of the yolk stalk that feeds the embryo in early gestation (Figure 22-3). The lining of the diverticulum contains aberrant acid-secreting gastric mucosa that can produce massive, painless bleeding; however, Meckel's diverticulum is often asymptomatic. Intestinal obstruction can occur. Surgical intervention involves resection of the diverticulum and anastomosis.

PREVENTION

Health Promotion

No preventive measures are known for this congenital anomaly.

Population at Risk

Symptoms can arise at any age but most commonly occur during childhood, especially before age 2 years. Males are more often affected than are females.

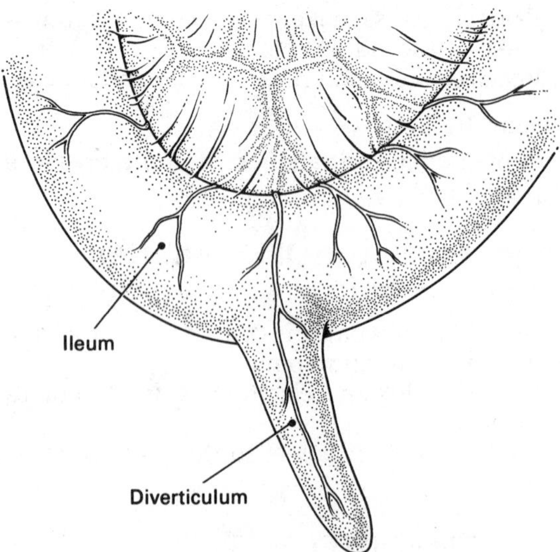

Figure 22-3 Meckel's diverticulum, a blind pouch resulting from incomplete closure of an embryonic duct.

Screening

None.

ASSESSMENT

Health History

1. Painless rectal bleeding that can be massive.
2. Abdominal pain may be present.
3. Brick red stools.

Physical Assessment

Shock can occur secondary to blood loss.

Diagnostic Tests

Barium enema, upper GI series, and proctoscopy are used for diagnosis.

NURSING DIAGNOSES: ACTUAL OR POTENTIAL

1. Alteration in fluid volume: decrease, due to bleeding.
2. Alteration in comfort: discomfort, due to pain and bleeding.
3. Mild to moderate anxiety due to pain and bleeding.
4. Parental anxiety due to child's bleeding and hospitalization.
5. Danger of obstruction and peritonitis.
6. Risk of shock secondary to hemorrhage.

EXPECTED OUTCOMES

1. Preoperative.
   a. Child's blood volume will stabilize as documented by hematocrit and hemoglobin values.
   b. Same as for other GI surgery.
2. Postoperative.
   Same as for other GI surgery.

INTERVENTIONS

1. Preoperative.
   a. Monitor vital signs frequently.
   b. Monitor IV fluids and any infusions of blood or plasma.
   c. Record amount of rectal bleeding.
   d. Monitor for signs and symptoms of shock and peritonitis.
   e. Same as for other GI surgery.
2. Postoperative.
   Same as for other GI surgery.

EVALUATION

Outcome Criteria

1. Preoperative.
   a. Child's hematocrit and hemoglobin are stable according to laboratory data.
   b. Same as for other GI surgery.
2. Postoperative.
   Same as for other GI surgery.

Reevaluation and Follow-up

Normal growth and development, and normal diet and elimination, are to be expected.

INGUINAL HERNIA

DESCRIPTION

The testicle normally descends into the scrotum, preceded by the peritoneal sac, during the seventh month of gestation. If this sac does not close off, there is a potential for the intestine to descend into the inguinal canal, producing a hernia. A comparable phenomenon involving the round ligament and processus vaginalis occasionally produces inguinal hernias in females. If the intestine becomes trapped and cannot be reduced, the hernia is said to be incarcerated. Strangulation (obstruction and circulatory compromise of intestine) is fairly common in children with hernias. Hernias can be either unilateral or bilateral. Herniorrhaphy is the surgical treatment.

PREVENTION

Health Promotion

No preventive measures are known for childhood hernias.

Population at Risk

Boys exceed girls by a ratio about 9 to 1. Hernia can occur at any age, but during childhood about half are present by the first birthday and most of the rest by age 5 years.

Screening

Examination for hernia is a routine part of every physical examination.

ASSESSMENT

Health History and Physical Assessment

Palpable mass in the inguinal region, particularly with straining or crying.

Diagnostic Tests

None required.

NURSING DIAGNOSES: ACTUAL OR POTENTIAL

1. Mild to moderate anxiety due to hospitalization and surgery.
2. Risk of strangulation.

EXPECTED OUTCOMES

1. Preoperative.
   a. Child's hernia will remain reducible.
   b. Child's and parents' anxiety will decrease as evidenced by actions and verbal feedback.
2. Postoperative.
   a. Lung sounds will be clear on auscultation.
   b. Child will eat a normal diet within 24 hours postoperatively.
   c. Wound will heal without complications.

INTERVENTIONS

1. Preoperative.
   a. Prevent straining (comfort child if crying).
   b. Observe for obstruction.
   c. Prepare parents and child for surgery.
   d. Answer questions that child and parents may have.
2. Postoperative.
   a. Pulmonary toilet.
   b. Institute feedings of clear liquids and advance to normal diet.
   c. Ambulate child early (day of surgery).
   d. Observe incision line for redness or drainage.
   e. Discharge teaching: child must avoid straining and strenuous play for 1 month; teach parents to observe wound for signs of infection; arrange for follow-up care.

EVALUATION

Outcome Criteria

1. Preoperative.
   a. Hernia remains reducible.
   b. Parents and child are prepared for surgery.
2. Postoperative.
   a. Breath sounds are clear.
   b. Child ambulates by self.
   c. Normal diet is tolerated.
   d. Discharge teaching is understood (regarding wound care and activity restrictions, if any).

Complications

PARTIAL OR COMPLETE BOWEL OBSTRUCTION

Assessment

1. Symptoms of partial bowel obstruction include
   a. Fretfulness.
   b. Anorexia, vomiting.
   c. Pain and tenderness in inguinal area.
   d. Irreducible mass.
   e. Decreased bowel sounds.
2. Symptoms of complete bowel obstruction include
   a. Shock.
   b. High temperature.
   c. Absent bowel sounds.
   d. High white blood cell count.
   e. Bloody stool.

Revised Outcomes

1. Fluid and electrolyte balance will be within normal limits.
2. Pain will decrease as evidenced by child's actions, position, and verbal feedback.
3. Temperature will be within normal limits.
4. Parents' and child's anxiety will decrease as demonstrated by actions.

Interventions

1. Preoperative.
   a. NPO.
   b. Monitor vital signs frequently; keep child quiet—sedation prn, as ordered.
   c. Monitor flow of IV fluids.
   d. Place child in Trendelenburg's position.
   e. Apply ice to scrotum to decrease edema; do not attempt to reduce the hernia, as perforation can occur.
   f. Control fever with sponge baths and antipyretic agents as ordered.
   g. Provide preoperative teaching to relieve anxiety.

Reevaluation and Follow-up

1. Hernia is manually reduced by the physician.
2. Surgery is performed 1 to 2 days after manual reduction when scrotal edema has decreased.
3. Signs of bowel obstruction are detected early so that further complications are avoided.
4. Parents are informed about home care (activity restrictions, if any, and wound care).

UMBILICAL HERNIA

DESCRIPTION

An umbilical hernia is a protrusion of the small intestine at the umbilicus due to imperfect closure of the umbilical ring. Spontaneous closure usually occurs before the fourth year. Strangulation is rare in children. The incidence of umbilical hernia is increased in blacks, premature infants, and in infants with hypothyroidism.

Abdominal binders are contraindicated as they do not correct the defect and can cause skin breakdown and umbilical infection. The home remedy of taping a coin over the hernia is decidely dangerous. Surgery is indicated only if the hernia is very large and increasing in size.

Nursing care is similar to that for inguinal hernia. Peristalsis is delayed, and the child is NPO until bowel activity resumes. The diet is gradually increased from clear liquids to normal. Vomiting is a frequent postoperative manifestation. A large pressure dressing is applied over the abdominal incision. Evaluation is the same as for inguinal hernia.

INFLAMMATIONS

NECROTIZING ENTEROCOLITIS

DESCRIPTION

Necrotizing enterocolitis (NEC) is a condition of premature newborns characterized by ischemic necrosis of the small bowel. The etiology is poorly understood, but it is suspected that hypoxia causes a protective shunting of blood from the mesenteric vascular bed to vital organs (heart, brain, kidneys). The intestinal cells are consequently damaged so that their protective mucus secreting function is severely impaired, and autodigestion ensues. Bowel perforation and overwhelming sepsis often occur, and mortality can be high. Studies have linked early enteral feedings of hypoxic infants with NEC. Fresh (not frozen) breast milk may protect against this disease through the induction of passive enteric immunity. Medical treatment includes GI decompression and broad-spectrum antibiotics, as well as other supportive measures. Surgical intervention involves bowel resection with colostomy or ileostomy. This is done only when the condition of the infant deteriorates under medical measures or when free intraperitoneal air is evident on x-ray examination.

PREVENTION

Health Promotion

Prenatal care, good maternal nutrition, avoidance of tobacco and alcoholic beverages, and other efforts to prevent premature birth. Umbilical catheters and early feedings, except fresh breast milk, have been associated with NEC, but these relationships are not yet understood.

Population at Risk

Premature infants with birth weight under 2500 g are the principal victims, especially those who have intestinal ischemia for any reason (birth asphyxia, respiratory distress syndrome, patent ductus arteriosus). Symptoms can begin any time during the first month of life but most commonly arise during the first week.

Screening

None.

ASSESSMENT

Health History

1. Low Apgar scores.
2. Perinatal or neonatal stress.
3. Perinatal or neonatal hypoxia.
4. Birth weight below 2500 g.

Physical Assessment

1. Abdominal distension.
2. Delayed gastric emptying.
3. Vomiting.
4. Lethargy.
5. Temperature instability.
6. Apnea.
7. Guaiac positive stools.
8. Jaundice can be present.
9. Bloody diarrhea can occur.

Diagnostic Tests

Abdominal flat-plate x-ray films.

NURSING DIAGNOSES: ACTUAL OR POTENTIAL

1. Alteration in fluid and electrolyte balance due to vomiting, diarrhea, and blood loss.
2. Alteration in digestive ability due to compromised bowel integrity.
3. Alteration in oxygenation due to apnea and abdominal distension.
4. Risk of aspiration due to vomiting.
5. Increased susceptibility to infection due to immature immune system, debilitated state, and loss of bowel integrity.
6. Inability to stabilize temperature due to immature physiological state and multiple stressors.
7. Potential disruption in parent–infant bonding process due to critical condition of infant.
8. Parental anxiety due to critical condition of infant.

EXPECTED OUTCOMES

1. Fluid and electrolyte balance will be within normal limits as evidenced by laboratory data and physical exam.
2. Oxygen/carbon dioxide gas exchange will be adequate as evidenced by arterial blood gas measurements.
3. Infant will gain weight on hyperalimentation and intralipids.
4. Hematocrit and hemoglobin levels will be within normal limits as documented by laboratory data.
5. Abdominal distension will decrease as documented by abdominal girth measurements.
6. Parents will make physical contact with their infant.
7. Parental anxiety will decrease as demonstrated by actions and verbal communication.
8. Infant will gradually tolerate enteral feedings.

INTERVENTIONS

1. Observe newborns, especially prematures and those with breathing difficulty, for inability to absorb glucose or formula feedings. Check food absorption by aspirating stomach contents through the NG tube before feeding. Record amount of aspirate and stage of digestion. Return to stomach and subtract this total from present feeding.
2. Observe and report symptoms of NEC as noted in the assessment.
3. Note number, frequency, and length of apneic periods.
4. Monitor vital signs every hour, or more frequently, as needed.
5. Report any of the following:
   a. Abdominal girth increase of 1 cm or more.
   b. Elevated axillary temperature.
   c. Increased or decreased pulse, low blood pressure.
   d. Respiratory distress.
   e. Absent bowel sounds.
   f. Abdominal tenderness.
   g. Involuntary rigidity of abdominal wall.
6. Maintain patency of NG tube, and attach to low intermittent suction.
7. Measure intake, output, and urine specific gravity.
8. Regulate flow of IV fluids, hyperalimentation solution, and intralipids.
9. Continually assess respiratory status; provide oxygen and humidification as ordered; ventilatory assistance may be necessary.
10. Obtain urine, stool, and blood cultures; administer antibiotics as orderded.
11. Note electrolyte and arterial blood gas values.
12. Provide skin care to buttocks to prevent excoriation and breakdown. Expose to air, and apply zinc oxide as needed.
13. Support parents through this ordeal by giving frequent explanations and information. Have parents touch infant and provide care. Encourage them to call and visit whenever they wish.
14. Surgical intervention involves the creation of a temporary colostomy or ileostomy.
15. Stoma care.
    a. Cover stoma with petroleum jelly gauze until resumption of stool.
    b. Use karaya gum sheet over abdomen (not over incision).
    c. Use urine bags over the stoma, or collect stool on a 4 by 4 inch pad secured with gauze wrapped around the abdomen.
    d. Use zinc oxide or aluminum paste around the peristomal area to protect against excoriation.
    e. Record amount, color, and consistency of stool.
16. Prepare parents for the appearance of the ileostomy or colostomy. Explain the purpose of this surgical procedure.

17. Gradually reintroduce enteral feedings, and observe the infant for recurrence of symptoms. Fresh breast milk is used whenever possible.

EVALUATION

Outcome Criteria

1. Signs and symptoms of NEC are detected early.
2. Acid-base balance is maintained.
3. Sepsis is controlled by antibiotic therapy.
4. Infant's temperature stabilizes.
5. Infant gains weight on hyperalimentation and intralipids.
6. Parents are able to express their fears about diagnosis and prognosis.
7. Parents make contact with their child and are involved in care.
8. The peristomal area remains intact, and the incision heals without complications.
9. Feces assumes normal color and consistency.
10. Enteral feedings are tolerated in increased concentration and amount.

Reevaluation and Follow-up

Infants who survive NEC remain at risk for long-term sequellae of prematurity (respiratory disease, neurological consequences of hypoxia, disturbances of parenting, etc.). The extent of surgical resection of bowel can affect diet and nutritional status. Obtain home nursing referral.

APPENDICITIS

DESCRIPTION

Appendicitis with perforation can be a life-threatening problem in younger children. Although it is rare in the first 2 years of life (peak incidence is 15 to 21 years), the younger child is most seriously affected. This is because the omentum is very short; consequently, the infection is not well walled off and spreads quickly to generalized peritonitis. Early diagnosis is essential but difficult due to the nonspecificity of presenting symptoms.

Appendicitis is discussed at length in Chapter 33.

GASTROENTERITIS

DESCRIPTION

Gastroenteritis is an inflammation of the GI tract that can be either viral or bacterial in origin. The incidence and severity are highest in infancy and early childhood. Vomiting and diarrhea can produce life-threatening dehydration. Antidiarrheal medications are not usually effective.

PREVENTION

Health Promotion

Good health habits (e.g., rest, nutrition, environmental cleanliness, and hygiene).

Population at Risk

Everyone, but particularly those who are in contact with infected people and those who are debilitated.

Screening

None.

ASSESSMENT

Health History

1. Vomiting (may be projectile).
2. Frequent, loose watery stools.
3. Crampy abdominal pain.

Physical Assessment

1. Dehydration.
2. Fever may be present.
3. Abdominal distension.

Diagnostic Tests

Stool culture may be ordered to identify causative organism.

NURSING DIAGNOSES: ACTUAL OR POTENTIAL

1. Alteration in bowel elimination: increase in number and frequency of stools.
2. Alteration in fluid and electrolyte balance: loss of fluids and electrolytes due to vomiting and diarrhea.
3. Increased temperature due to dehydration.
4. Mild to moderate anxiety due to separation and hospitalization.
5. Potential disruption in skin integrity due to diarrhea.

EXPECTED OUTCOMES

1. Number and frequency of stools will decrease to normal within 5 to 10 days.
2. Fluid and electrolyte values will be within normal limits within 48 hours after admission as evidenced by laboratory data.
3. Temperature will return to within normal limits within 5 days.
4. Child's anxiety will decrease as evidenced by actions and verbal communication.
5. Skin around buttocks will remain intact.

INTERVENTIONS

1. NPO; give mouth care often.
2. Administer IV fluids at prescribed rate.
3. Monitor laboratory values (particularly sodium and potassium values).
4. Measure intake, output, and urine specific gravity.
5. Weigh child daily (maybe more often if child is severely dehydrated).
6. Monitor vital signs (axillary temperatures).
7. Assess activity and level of consciousness.
8. Observe and record amount and type of vomitus.
9. Observe and record number, frequency, color, and odor of stools. (Clinitest, Hemetest, and guaiac tests of stools may also be done).
10. Obtain stool culture.
11. Change diapers frequently, and apply zinc oxide. If area becomes excoriated, leave diapers off and apply ointment.
12. Institute isolation procedures with careful handwashing to prevent spread of infection.
13. Institute oral feedings as follows:
    a. Electrolyte solution.
    b. Clear liquids.
    c. Bananas, rice cereal, applesauce, dry toast, and clear liquids (referred to as the BRAT diet).
    d. One-quarter strength formula progressing to full strength.
14. Meet child's developmental needs; provide toys and stimulation.
15. Involve parents in care, and meet their needs for support.

EVALUATION

Outcome Criteria

1. Fluid and electrolyte values are within normal limits.
2. Client demonstrates good skin turgor, normal specific gravity.
3. Stools decrease and gradually assume normal color and consistency.
4. The buttocks do not become excoriated.
5. Child gradually tolerates oral feedings and regular diet.
6. Child develops well; parents cope and manage effectively.

Reevaluation and Follow-up

Recovery is expected to be complete and without sequelae.

TRAUMA

INGESTION OF CORROSIVE SUBSTANCE

DESCRIPTION

The ingestion of caustic materials (lye and other alkaloids, or acids) typically results in severe burns of the mouth and esophagus. Esophageal scarring produces strictures. Emergency care required at the time of ingestion is presented in Chapter 49. Gastrostomy and/or tracheostomy may be necessary in severe burns. Esophageal dilatations are performed on a short- or long-term basis, depending on the severity of the strictures.

PREVENTION

Health Promotion

Accidental ingestions are, in theory, 100 percent preventable. Household safety practices, including "child proofing" the environment and supervising young children, need to be taught to all parents of infants, toddlers, and preschcol children.

Population at Risk

All children who have access to corrosives but lack judgment about what is and is not edible. One- through 3-year-olds are at greatest risk. Other high-risk groups are impulsive or hyperactive children and those with histories of previous ingestion accidents (e.g., aspirin poisoning, hydrocarbon ingestion).

Screening

None.

ASSESSMENT

Health History

History of ingestion.

Physical Assessment

1. Child with recent injury.
   a. Burns in oral cavity.
   b. Degree of respiratory distress.
   c. Level of consciousness.
   d. Ability to swallow.
   e. Degree of pain.
2. Child with old injury and esophageal stricture.
   a. Ability to swallow.
   b. Psychological adjustment.
   c. Speech development.

Diagnostic Tests

Usually none at the time of injury, but some physicians do an esophagoscopy to assess the extent of tissue injury.

NURSING DIAGNOSES: ACTUAL OR POTENTIAL

1. Alteration in respiratory function due to burns.
2. Alteration in comfort: discomfort due to burns.
3. Dysphagia due to scarring/strictures.
4. Parental guilt and anxiety due to child's accident.
5. Potential alteration in nutritional intake: decrease due to esophageal strictures.
6. Potential development of speech problems.

EXPECTED OUTCOMES

1. Oxygenation will be within normal limits as evidenced by arterial blood gases.
2. Child's pain will decrease as demonstrated by actions.
3. Nutritional intake will be adequate for age.
4. Child's esophageal scarring will be minimal as evidenced by ability to swallow solid foods.

INTERVENTIONS

1. Monitor vital signs frequently, particularly respiratory status.
2. Provide humidification and oxygen as necessary.
3. Administer pain medication as prescribed.
4. Position for salivary drainage if unable to swallow.
5. Have tracheostomy set at bedside.
6. Medicate as prescribed with steroids and neutralizers of ingested substances.
7. Have parents participate in child's care; provide parental support, and assist them in coping with guilt feelings.
8. Institute feedings as ordered (either oral or gastrostomy), and note child's tolerance to them.
9. Pave the way for parental cooperation with follow-up care that may be needed (dilatations, speech therapy, psychological assistance).
10. Facilitate child's psychological adjustment to long hospitalization and painful procedures and treatments.
11. Observe child for edema, respiratory distress, and bleeding after dilatation procedures.

EVALUATION

Expected Outcomes

1. Respiratory distress is minimized, detected promptly, and/or dealt with effectively.
2. Skin complications are avoided (face, gastrostomy).
3. Feedings as prescribed are well tolerated.
4. Parents cope well with guilt and fear.
5. Child demonstrates good adjustment and developmental progress for age.
6. The child is able to cooperate during the dilatation with sedation or restraints.
7. The parents "child proof" their house before discharge.
8. On discharge the parents state their understanding of need for follow-up care.
9. On discharge the parents demonstrate proper method of feeding, either oral or gastrostomy.

Reevaluation and Follow-up

1. Esophageal dilatations may be required for months or years on an outpatient basis.
2. Speech therapy and psychotherapy may be indicated.

ABNORMAL CELLULAR GROWTH

CLEFT LIP AND PALATE

DESCRIPTION

These conditions are abnormal developments of the upper lip and palate and can be extensive, involving premaxilla, maxilla, and tissues of the soft palate and uvula. Arrested embryonic fusion of premaxillary and maxillary processes results in a cleft lip; failure of the palatal process to fuse results in cleft palate. The two defects can occur separately or together. Genetic factors are contributory, but clefts can occur without a familial history.

Cleft lip repair by a qualified plastic surgeon usually is done at 1 to 2 months of age with sufficient weight gain and absence of oral, respiratory, or systemic infections. Revisions are done later at age 4 to 5 years. Palate surgery is postponed until the child is 12 to 18 months old, depending on the degree of deformity: if it is done too early, it can damage tooth buds; if it is done too late, the child may develop poor speech patterns. Subsequent revisions and reconstructions are delayed until adolescence and are done when there is no infection present. Prognosis can be very good using the excellent skills of a competent plastic surgeon and with overall management for long-term care utilizing the multidisciplinary team. Parental acceptance and involvement are essential.

PREVENTION

Health Promotion

Some forms of oral clefts show familial inheritance patterns. Genetic counseling may be useful for prospective parents who have clefts or relatives with clefts.

Population at Risk

Newborns, especially those with relatives who have clefts.

Screening

Neonatal physical examination.

ASSESSMENT

Health History

Possible family history of oral clefts.

Physical Assessment

1. Deformity of upper lip.
2. Opening in palate.

Diagnostic Tests

None.

NURSING DIAGNOSES: ACTUAL OR POTENTIAL

1. Alteration in facial/oral integrity.
2. Parental shock and anxiety due to child's obvious defect.
3. Increased susceptibility to infection (children with cleft palate are prone to otitis media).
4. Potential for decreased nutritional intake.
5. Potential for development of speech defects secondary to mouth malformation and/or secondary to hearing loss.

EXPECTED OUTCOMES

1. Child will acquire facial/oral integrity through plastic surgery.
2. Parent–infant bonding will occur.
3. Child will consume adequate calories and gain weight.
4. Hearing ability will remain intact.
5. Speech will develop normally.

INTERVENTIONS

1. Immediately after birth and before repair.
   a. The nurse should show acceptance of infant and support parents in immediate grief and guilt about having a deformed child.
   b. Because baby may not be able to suck due to inability to create a vacuum, consider different feeding devices:
      (1) Lamb's nipple.
      (2) Nipple for premature infants with holes enlarged.
      (3) Asepto syringe with rubber tubing attached.
      (4) Brecht feeder.
   c. Hold baby upright during feeding, feed slowly, and burp often.
   d. Prevent baby's contact with people who have colds or other infections.
   e. Team members usually include plastic surgeon, primary nurse, speech therapist, orthodontist, and ear, nose, and throat physician. The primary nurse should coordinate their efforts.
   f. Discharge teaching should include

(1) Feeding technique.
(2) Avoidance of infection.
(3) Early recognition and prompt treatment of otitis media.
(4) Equipment to use at home.
(5) Visiting nurse referral, if necessary.

2. Following cleft lip repair.
   a. Elbow and limb restraints may be necessary to prevent damage to the surgical repair.
   b. Do not allow child to lie face down or rub face on bed or pillow; position in infant seat or on side.
   c. Observe for respiratory distress.
   d. Give gentle suction of mouth and nose if ordered.
   e. Avoid stress on suture line, including that caused by crying.
   f. Care of suture line.
      (1) Use of Logan bow.
      (2) Cleansing with half-strength solution hydrogen peroxide on cotton swab after feeding.
      (3) Application of antibiotic ointment as prescribed.
   g. Feedings should be by dropper or rubber-tipped syringe. *Do not allow baby to suck.* Generally, the child is on clear liquids until sutures are removed—3 to 14 days after surgery.
3. Following cleft palate repair.
   a. Observe for respiratory distress.
   b. Use elbow and limb restraints.
   c. *Do not put anything into the mouth—no straws or nipples.*
   d. If packing is inserted, observe for bleeding, and position on side to allow bloody mucus to drain.
   e. Humidify the environment.
   f. Feeding techniques: Give clear liquids, gradually increasing to a soft diet by cup. Use a rubber-tipped syringe, and rinse mouth with clear water after feedings.
   g. Weigh daily.
   h. Administer pain medicine as prescribed.
   i. Encourage and assist parents to care for and comfort child.
   j. Discharge instructions for parents should include
      (1) Normal growth and development of child, emphasizing the tendency to put things in the mouth. Parent should use elbow restraints at home to prevent this.
      (2) Full liquid or soft diet should be continued at home.
      (3) Do not permit child to suck or blow.
      (4) Avoid infections and injury to operative site.
      (5) Stress the importance of close follow-up with surgeon, speech therapist, dentist, and audiologist.
      (6) Acquaint parents with financial aid available, as well as with any parent groups or published material that may help them.
      (7) Support the parents, and reinforce the expectation that the child can lead a normal life. Give positive reinforcement for parents' continued efforts.

EVALUATION

Outcome Criteria

1. The parents are able to care for the child at home as demonstrated by feeding, positioning, and oral hygiene. Parents can describe the need and discuss means to prevent infection.
2. The child gains weight.
3. The temperature does not go above 38°C.
4. Asphyxia and aspiration pneumonia do not occur.
5. The suture line remains clean and intact.
6. The child develops a good self-concept and socialization.

Reevaluation and Follow-up

1. Long-term care can include orthodontia for malpositioned teeth, speech therapy, periodic hearing evaluation, and serial surgeries (for stage repairs, scar revisions, correction of associated nasal deformities, and myringotomy).
2. Self-esteem and social development may be facilitated by counseling.

ESOPHAGEAL ATRESIA AND TRACHEOESOPHAGEAL FISTULA

DESCRIPTION

Esophageal atresia is abnormal embryonic development of the esophagus, resulting in the formation of a blind pouch or inadequately sized lumen preventing normal passage of materials (secretions and foods) from pharynx to stomach. Tracheoesophageal fistula is the abnormal development of a sinuslike passage between the esophagus and trachea. Several variations and combinations of the defect occur (see Figure 22-4).

Esophageal atresia and tracheoesophageal fistula, alone or in combination, are life-threatening. Pneumonia and atelectasis or massive airway obstruction result from overflow of feedings and saliva from the blind upper esophageal pouch into the trachea and/or reflux of gastric secretions through the fistula into the respiratory tract. Surgical intervention is undertaken as soon as possible after the diagnosis is confirmed but may be delayed if the infant is premature or critically ill, or if other major anomalies are present. Ligation of fistula is done immediately in most cases. End-to-end anastomosis of the esophagus is performed if parts are sufficiently long. Anastomosis may be deferred to allow for growth of the esophageal ends; in this event measures are taken to prevent pneumonia and provide nourishment. Construction of an esophagus by insertion of a colon segment may be done at 6 months to 2 years of age.

The prognosis for these defects depends upon early diagnosis, degree of prematurity, and coexistence of other serious defects. The survival rate for premature infants is 35 to 40 percent; that for full-term infants is 80 to 85 percent.

PREVENTION

Health Promotion

No preventive measures are known for these congenital defects. Early recognition is critical to prevent complications.

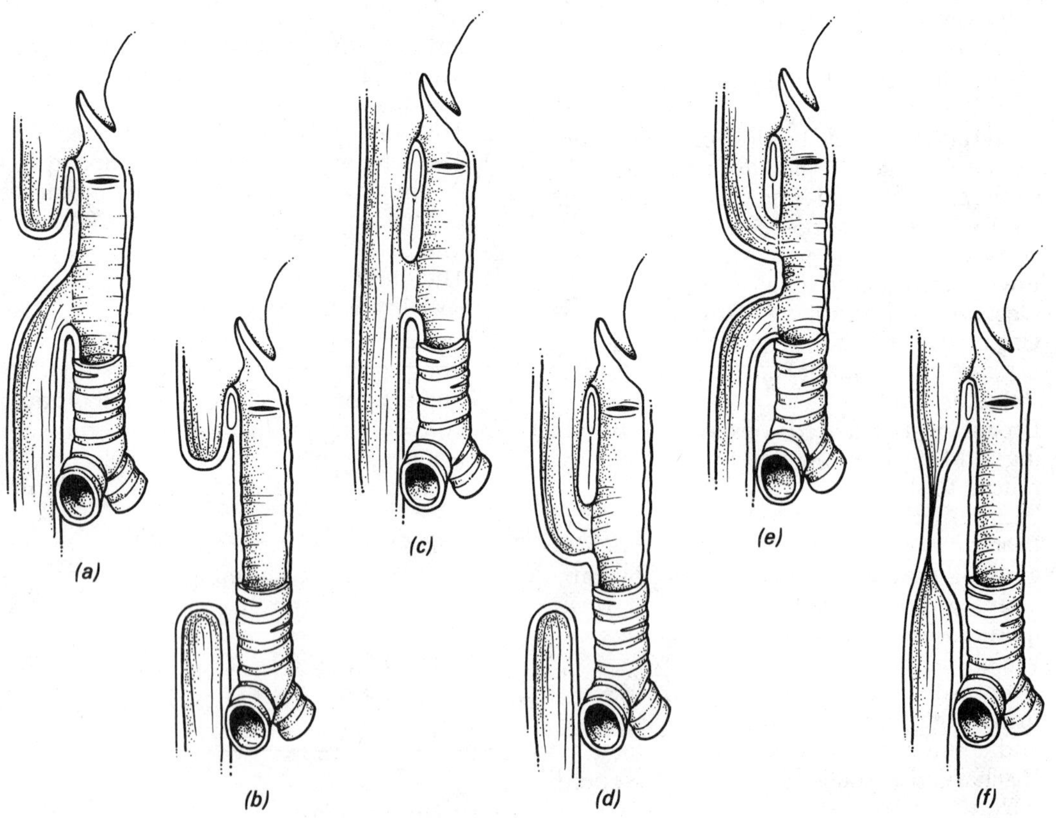

Figure 22-4 Esophageal atresia and tracheoesophageal fistulas. (*a*) Esophageal atresia with distal fistula. (*b*) Esophageal atresia without fistula. (*c*) Tracheoesophageal fistula without atresia. (*d*) Esophageal atresia with proximal fistula. (*e*) Esophageal atresia with proximal and distal fistulas. (*f*) Esophageal stenosis.

Population at Risk

Newborns, especially those whose mothers had hydramnios with the pregnancy.

Screening

None.

ASSESSMENT

Health History

Maternal hydramnios may have been present (15 percent of babies with atresia).

Physical Assessment

NOTE: Astute observation is imperative for early diagnosis in the newborn. Signs and symptoms of atresia and/or fistula appear soon after birth.

1. Excessive mucal secretion and hypersalivation.
   a. Continuous drooling.
   b. Frothing from nose and mouth.
2. Respiratory distress.
   a. Intermittent or circumoral cyanosis.
   b. Nasal flaring.
   c. Tachypnea.
   d. Retractions.
   e. Coarse or diminished breath sounds.
   f. Rales or rhonchi heard on auscultation.
3. Distended or scaphoid abdomen.
4. Dysphagia and inability to retain first feedings.
   a. Coughing and choking after first few swallows.
   b. Return of fluids through nose and mouth.
   c. Infant anxious and irritable.
   d. Cyanosis developing with above symptoms.
5. Fever or subnormal body temperature.
6. Inability to pass tubing through esophagus to stomach—stops in blind pouch at atretic site.
7. Evidence of esophageal stenosis in an older infant often may not appear until chopped or solid foods are started.
   a. Child chokes and gags with solids.
   b. Occasionally vomits undigested foods.
   c. "Fussy eater."
   d. Unable to pass NG tube through to stomach.

Diagnostic Tests

1. Neck and chest x-ray films show the placement of a radiopaque NG tube in the atretic pouch.
2. Abdominal x-ray films showing gastric or intestinal gas in an infant with atresia are diagnostic of tracheoesophageal fistula: the air cannot have been swallowed and has to have entered the GI tract from the trachea.

NURSING DIAGNOSES: ACTUAL OR POTENTIAL

1. Decreased oxygen/carbon dioxide gas exchange due to excess nasopharyngeal secretions and reflux of gastric secretions into the tracheobronchial tree.
2. Inability to take fluids orally secondary to tracheal and esophageal structural defect.
3. Parental anxiety due to illness of neonate.
4. Inability to stabilize temperature due to respiratory distress and immature physiological state.
5. Risk for alteration in fluid and electrolyte balance.

EXPECTED OUTCOMES

1. Immediate and preoperative.
   a. Oxygenation status will be within normal limits as evidenced by acceptable arterial blood gas values.
   b. Lung sounds will be clear on auscultation.
   c. Fluid and electrolyte values will be within normal limits.
   d. Parents will participate in their infant's care.
   e. Temperature will stabilize.
2. Postoperative.
   a. Child will maintain adequate oxygenation as evidenced by acceptable arterial blood gas values.
   b. Nutritional intake will be adequate as demonstrated by weight gain.
   c. Fluid and electrolyte values will be within normal limits according to laboratory data.
   d. Parent–infant bonding will occur as demonstrated by involvement in their child's care.

INTERVENTIONS

1. Immediate and preoperative.
   a. NPO.
   b. Suction infant frequently, and position with head and chest elevated 20 to 30 degrees.
   c. Monitor vital signs frequently; auscultate

breath sounds and note increase or decrease in air exchange.
d. Monitor flow of parenteral fluids.
e. Place infant in incubator or on warming bed to stabilize temperature.
f. Provide oxygen and humidity as ordered.
g. Measure intake, output, and urine specific gravity.
h. Keep tracheostomy set at bedside.
i. Provide support to parents; prepare them for child's surgery; encourage them to touch infant and participate in care.

2. Postoperative.
a. Monitor vital signs every 30 to 60 minutes.
b. Auscultate chest for lung sounds.
c. Change infant's position every hour, and stimulate to cry every 2 hours.
d. Keep equipment for intubation at bedside if infant does not have a tracheostomy.
e. Monitor accessory apparatus, such as cardiac monitor and/or ventilator.
f. Suction secretions taking care not to disturb or disrupt the operative site (usually the suction catheter is inserted only a designated number of inches).
g. Monitor flow of parenteral fluids (NPO for 7 to 10 days).
h. Measure intake, output, and urine specific gravity.
i. Record daily weights.
j. Provide oxygen and humidity as prescribed.
k. Position as ordered—may vary.
(1) Usually head and chest elevated 20 to 30 degrees.
(2) Flat (supine) with anastomosis.
(3) Prone in semi-Fowler's position with palliative treatment.
(4) To the left with cervical esophagostomy.
l. Care of chest tube with water-seal drainage if left thoracotomy done.
m. Gastrostomy care.
(1) Tube care.
(a) Fixation of tube to prevent displacement and continuous irritation to skin.
(b) Irrigate with 2 mL normal saline every 3 hours while open to gravity drainage.
(c) Connect to intermittent low suction after first 24 hours.
(2) Skin care.
(a) Keep skin clean and dry.
(b) Observe for signs of excoriation.
(3) Initiation of feedings as prescribed (withhold if vomiting or abdominal distension occurs).
(a) Tube is suspended from top of Isolette not more than 6 inches above abdomen and attached to a 10-mL syringe.
(b) Before feeding, measure gastric residual and return.
(c) Maintain patency of tube by instilling 5–10 mL of dextrose and water every 2 hours.
(d) Tube is not clamped until infant tolerates full feedings.
(e) Give pacifier at same time gastrostomy feedings are given.
(f) Begin teaching parents to administer feedings.
n. Cervical esophagostomy care.
(1) Suction at frequent, regular intervals during initial 2 to 3 days.
(2) Avoid hyperextension of neck when positioning, and keep neck to left to promote drainage.
(3) Prevent excoriation of skin by putting a thin layer of petroleum jelly around skin edges.
(4) Soft, thick, absorbent dressings should be secured appropriately to absorb drainage.
(5) Teach parents ostomy care and how to prevent excoriation. Teach suctioning.
o. Following esophageal reconstruction.
(1) Astute monitoring of water-seal chest drainage is needed.
(2) Care for NG tube, with regular, frequent suctioning for 2 to 3 days postoperatively.
(3) Continue gastrostomy feedings and care until tube is removed—usually with resumption of peristalsis.
(4) Observe for complications of anastomotic leaks, perforations, or strictures.
(a) Continuous monitoring of vital signs is necessary.
(b) Notify physician at first indication of respiratory distress.
(c) Observe and note dysphagia or vomiting during months after initial repair.
(d) Instruct parents to observe for

symptoms of complications and persistence of bowel odors from oral cavity.

p. Infant's emotional and developmental needs.
   (1) Meet needs for gratification and security.
      (a) Use pacifier to meet sucking need and to coincide with gastrostomy feedings.
      (b) Talk to, cuddle, and hold the child.
      (c) Provide with comfortable, safe environment.
      (d) Institute care plan to consistently meet and anticipate needs.
   (2) Developmental assessment and provision for developmental needs.
      (a) Care plan should change as infant's needs change.
      (b) Verbal and tactile stimulation are needed.
      (c) Mobility—active/passive range of motion.
      (d) Socialization associated with mealtime.

q. Parents' needs.
   (1) Encourage earliest possible parental involvement in care when readiness assessed.
   (2) Teach care of cervical esophagostomy and gastrostomy.
   (3) Emphasize infant's developmental needs, teaching and anticipating to avoid needless developmental delays.
   (4) Plan with parents for immediate and continuing care utilizing community resources and multidisciplinary team approach—refer for community nursing service if necessary.
   (5) Provide parents with support.
      (a) Allow ventilation of feelings.
      (b) Keep in contact by phone calls immediately following discharge, and refer to the visiting nurse.
      (c) Demonstrate acceptance of child.

EVALUATION

Outcome Criteria

1. Preoperative.
   a. Arterial blood gases are within normal limits; aspiration and chemical pneumonia do not occur.
   b. Fluid and electrolyte balance is maintained.
   c. Temperature is stabilized.
   d. Parents become involved in child's care, and the bonding process is initiated.
2. Postoperative.
   a. Patent airway is maintained; lung sounds are clear.
   b. Fluid and electrolyte balance is within normal limits.
   c. Infant gains weight on either oral or gastrostomy feedings.
   d. Parents can care for child and feel comfortable and competent.

OMPHALOCELE AND GASTROSCHISIS

DESCRIPTION

Omphalocele is the protrusion or herniation of abdominal viscera into the base of the umbilical cord. The visceral mass is covered by a transparent avascular membrane that ruptures easily (sometimes at birth or *in utero*). The defect is located centrally on the abdomen and includes the umbilicus. Sac size depends upon visceral contents and can range from a slight enlargement at the base of the cord to a large sac containing colon, liver, and spleen. At birth, measures are taken to avoid rupture of an intact membrane.

Gastroschisis is a congenital full-thickness anterior abdominal wall defect with varying degrees of eviscerating bowel. It is due to failure of the embryological tissues to mature in the abdominal layers. There is no membranous sac covering the thickened, edematous abdominal contents. The defect is located below, to the right, and separate from the umbilicus, which is in its normal position. The herniated viscera consist mainly of small and large bowel. Associated problems can include atresia of the small intestine, some degree of intestinal malrotation, and prematurity.

Mortality rates for both of these problems is highest during the first few days of life. Surgical intervention and nursing care are similar for both of these congenital defects. For large defects, Silastic sheets or silos are used to cover the viscera, and gradually these organs are forced back into the enlarging abdominal cavity.

Another method, not widely employed, involves the application of antibiotics and coagulating agents to unruptured omphaloceles until sufficient granulation and epithelialization occur to allow for skin flap closure.

PREVENTION

Health Promotion

No preventive measures are known for these congenital defects.

Population at Risk

Newborns.

Screening

None.

ASSESSMENT

Defect described above is visible at birth.

NURSING DIAGNOSES: ACTUAL OR POTENTIAL

1. Increased heat loss due to exposed viscera.
2. Alteration in fluid and electrolyte balance due to heat loss and vomiting.
3. Increased susceptibility to infection due to exposed abdominal contents.
4. Alteration in oxygenation due to respiratory distress.
5. Parental anxiety due to neonate's critical condition and prognosis.

EXPECTED OUTCOMES

1. Immediate and preoperative.
   a. Infant's temperature will stabilize at 38°C.
   b. Fluid and electrolyte values will be within normal limits as documented by laboratory data.
   c. Local and/or systemic infection will not occur.
   d. Oxygen/carbon dioxide gas exchange will be within normal limits as documented by arterial blood gas values.
   e. Parents will begin bonding process and participate in child's care.
2. Postoperative.
   a. Infant will tolerate oral feedings and gain weight.
   b. Parents will provide care to infant and state that they are comfortable in doing so.
   c. Infection does not occur.
   d. Same as for other GI surgery.

INTERVENTIONS

1. Immediate and preoperative.
   a. Cover exposed viscera immediately with sterile towels or sponges saturated with normal saline solution.
   b. Moisten sponges at regular intervals, never allowing them to dry.
   c. Cover moist sponges with dry sterile towels.
   d. Maintain sterile technique.
   e. Immediately place baby in incubator.
   f. Monitor and record vital signs at frequent, regular intervals.
   g. Handling and exposure must be minimal.
   h. Reduce distension and edema by inserting an NG tube and monitoring function.
   i. Prevent aspiration by removing nasopharyngeal secretions by suction prn and at regular intervals.
   j. Administer and monitor IV medications and fluids as ordered.
   k. Measure intake and output.
   l. Provide oxygen and humidity as prescribed; ventilator assistance may be necessary.
   m. Provide support to parents and encourage them to touch their infant.
2. Postoperative.
   a. Maintain incubator care.
   b. Continue monitoring of vital signs.
   c. Suction nasopharyngeal area when necessary.
   d. Monitor functioning of NG and gastrostomy tubes.
   e. Wound care.
      (1) Exercise extreme caution in positioning and covering to prevent tension on sutures.
      (2) Observe and record appearance of wound edges for signs of infection or necrosis.
      (3) Maintain sterile technique until healing of wound occurs.
   f. Record intake and output accurately.
   g. Administer parenteral fluids and medications as prescribed.
   h. Administer hyperalimentation feedings as prescribed and monitor.

i. Oral feedings begin with returned peristaltic activity, after two to three stools.
   (1) Begin oral feedings with caution.
   (2) Initial feedings are given usually with sterile water or Pedialyte.
   (3) Note and record infant's tolerance of feedings.

j. Infant's needs.
   (1) Utilize pacifier for sucking.
   (2) Frequent verbal and tactile stimulation are important.

k. Parental involvement.
   (1) Assess parents' reactions and methods of coping to determine their readiness and ability to become involved with the child.
   (2) Encourage participation in care when appropriate.
   (3) Begin and continue teaching about condition and effect of treatment, emphasizing infant's growth and developmental needs.
   (4) Individualize care continuously (e.g., use baby's name).
   (5) Evaluate needs for continuing care by involving parents in early discharge planning and ongoing care.

EVALUATION

Outcome Criteria

1. Immediate and preoperative.
   a. Local and systemic infections are absent.
   b. Body temperature is maintained at normal level.
   c. Absent or minimal abdominal distension with diminishing edema in extruding bowel.
   d. Nasopharyngeal secretions are removed adequately: aspiration pneumonia does not develop.
   e. Adequate hydration and nutrition are attained without complications: insertion sites are free of infection and infiltration.
   f. Infant's general condition remains stable, or changes are noted with appropriate, immediate intervention.
2. Postoperative.
   a. Routine postoperative care is provided with accurate observations of complications or changes, and progress is recorded.
   b. Gastric decompression is maintained, and air swallowing is prevented.
   c. There is adequate wound healing: no dehiscence of wound edges, Silastic nondisplaced, no infection, no abnormal drainage.
   d. Adequate hydration and nutrition are maintained.
      (1) Hyperalimentation feeding is accurate and without complications.
      (2) Successful oral feedings are achieved with infant learning sucking, tolerating feedings, and gaining weight.
   e. Infant thrives.
      (1) Learns sucking of pacifier.
      (2) Responds to verbal and tactile stimulation.
      (3) Develops normally.
   f. Parents adapt.
      (1) Respond to encouragement and form attachment with infant.
      (2) Take part in providing care.
      (3) Visit frequently rather than avoiding.
      (4) Show ability to work through feelings of guilt without blaming selves or each other for infant's condition or suffering.
      (5) Demonstrate openness to teaching and plan realistically for immediate and future needs of infant.

HIRSCHSPRUNG'S DISEASE (CONGENITAL AGANGLIONIC MEGACOLON)

DESCRIPTION

Hirschsprung's disease is the congenital absence of parasympathetic ganglion nerve cells in the mesenteric plexus of the descending colon, resulting in absence of peristalsis in the affected colonic segment. The aganglionic area remains persistently contracted, and the proximal colon becomes distended with gas and feces. Chronic constipation and abdominal distension ensue. The distended bowel may ulcerate. A temporary colostomy is usually created during the neonatal period. Definitive surgery involves resection of the aganglionic segment and anastomosis of the normal colon to the anus. This is postponed until the child is 6 to 12 months of age, as mortality for abdominal pull-through procedures is fairly high in neonates.

PREVENTION

Health Promotion

No preventive measures are known.

Population at Risk

Newborns and infants, especially white males with a family history of Hirschsprung's disease.

Screening

None.

ASSESSMENT

Health History

1. Family history of Hirschsprung's disease is positive in about 10 percent of cases.
2. In the neonatal period.
   a. Failure to pass meconium for 24 to 48 hours.
   b. Reluctance to eat.
   c. Bilious vomiting.
   d. Constipation with overflow diarrhea.
   e. Irritability.
3. Later in infancy.
   a. Obstinate constipation, only minimally and temporarily relieved by enema.
   b. Stools have an offensive odor and ribbon-like shape.
   c. Progressive abdominal distension.

Physical Assessment

1. In the neonatal period.
   a. Abdominal distension.
   b. Rapid breathing and grunting.
   c. Worried, frowning look, often with thin facial features.
   d. Irritability.
   e. Failure to thrive.
2. Later in infancy.
   a. Abdominal distension.
   b. Prominent veins over abdomen.
   c. Visible peristaltic activity.
   d. Palpable fecal masses and impactions.
   e. Failure to thrive.
   f. Hypochromic anemia and hypoproteinemia.

Diagnostic Tests

1. Barium enema to rule out other causes of obstruction.
2. Rectal biopsy: absence of ganglionic cells confirms the diagnosis.

NURSING DIAGNOSES: ACTUAL OR POTENTIAL

1. Alteration in nutrition: decrease due to distension and poor absorption of nutrients.
2. Alteration in oxygenation due to compression of lungs by distended abdomen.
3. Alteration in elimination: constipation due to aganglionic bowel.
4. Alteration in fluid and electrolyte balance due to vomiting and poor oral intake.

EXPECTED OUTCOMES

1. Preoperative.
   a. Infant will take in adequate calories to gain weight.
   b. Oxygenation will be adequate as measured by arterial blood gases.
   c. Abdominal distension will decrease as documented by girth measurements.
   d. Infant will eliminate stool.
   e. Fluid and electrolyte values will be within normal limits.
2. Postoperative.
   a. Colostomy will function.
   b. Infant will gain weight and tolerate oral feedings.
   c. Skin around colostomy will remain intact.
   d. Same as for other GI surgery.
   e. Parents will care for colostomy.

INTERVENTIONS

1. Preoperative.
   a. Evacuation and preparation of bowel for surgery.
      (1) Give enemas as prescribed (solution, frequency, medications).
         (a) Observe for water intoxication.
         (b) Note return and degree of distension.
         (c) Siphon if no return.
      (2) Constantly monitor characteristics and frequency of stool.
      (3) Take *axillary temperature only*.
   b. Feedings and nutrition.
      (1) Give diet as ordered—usually low-residue.
      (2) Offer frequent small feedings.
      (3) Have client in upright position.
   c. Observe for respiratory distress—position with head and chest elevated.

d. Observe for abdominal tenderness and visible peristalsis.
e. Note extent and degree of distension before and after colonic irrigation.
f. Assure functioning of NG tube.
g. Encourage parents to visit as often as possible.
h. Hold the child frequently, and give tactile and verbal stimulation during alert periods.
i. Encourage age-appropriate play activities.

2. Postoperative.
   a. Routine postoperative care—continue axillary temperature procedure.
   b. Care of temporary colostomy.
      (1) Provide good skin care to surrounding area.
         (a) Frequent nonabrasive cleansing.
         (b) Change dressing prn, or as ordered.
         (c) Apply protective agents to skin.
         (d) Expose to air periodically.
      (2) Observe for signs of obstruction.
         (a) Irritability, vomiting, fever.
         (b) Abdominal tenderness.
         (c) Decreased colostomy output.
      (3) Assure proper functioning; position; record characteristics of output.
   c. Abdominal wound care.
      (1) Observe for signs of infection (local, systemic).
      (2) Maintain sterile technique with dressing change.
      (3) Reposition at regular intervals with care not to dislodge tubing.
   d. Nasogastric tube—maintain patency.
   e. Begin oral feedings as ordered before NG tube removal.
      (1) Have child sit in upright position.
      (2) Bubble frequently.
      (3) Avoid overfeeding.
      (4) Observe tolerance.
   f. Emotional and developmental needs of child.
      (1) Promote parent–child interaction.
      (2) Play activity as tolerated.
      (3) Frequent holding with stimulation during alert periods.
   g. Parents' needs.
      (1) Facilitate discussion of feelings toward disease and treatment.
      (2) Begin teaching colostomy care, and encourage earliest possible participation.
      (3) Teach parents growth and developmental levels and tasks child needs to attain and how to achieve.
      (4) Encourage them to treat child as normally as possible.

EVALUATION

Outcome Criteria

1. Preoperative.
   a. Relief of constipation is achieved; there is absence or decrease of distension, absence of water intoxication, and absence of respiratory embarrassment.
   b. Infant tolerates feedings and gains weight.
   c. Infant or child remains calm, and parents demonstrate acceptance by participating in care.
2. Postoperative.
   a. Respiratory problems are absent.
   b. Colostomy functions appropriately without excoriation of surrounding tissues.
   c. Local and systemic infections are absent.
   d. Feedings are tolerated, and there is no recurrence of distension after removal of NG tube.
   e. Child's emotional reactions and development attain and remain within normal range.
   f. Parents assume responsibility for care, interact maturely with child, and provide for ongoing and comprehensive health care.

IMPERFORATE ANUS

DESCRIPTION

Imperforate anus is the congenital absence of a patent anal opening. The severity of the defect varies, as shown in Figure 22–5. Associated fistulas are common. In boys, there may be rectovesicular, rectourethral, or rectoperineal fistulas. In girls, rectovaginal and rectoperineal fistulas can occur. Surgical intervention is essential and is determined by the type and extent of the anomaly.

1. *Stenosis* can be treated with digital dilatations continued for several months.
2. A thin *membrane* with visible meconium and no other anomaly can be treated by surgical perforation of membranous tissue.
3. For *low agenesis*, surgical correction is done through the perineum.

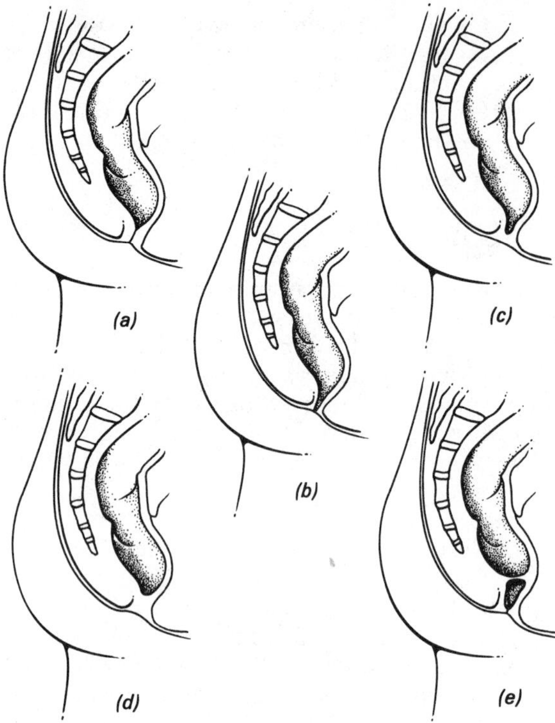

Figure 22-5 Imperforate anus. (*a*) Stenosis of otherwise well-formed tract. (*b*) Membrane occludes anal opening. (*c*) Low agenesis (less than 1.5 cm). (*d*) High agenesis (greater than 1.5 cm). (*e*) Anal atresia.

4. For *high agenesis* and *atretic* types.
   a. Transverse colostomy is done immediately.
   b. Sacroabdominoperineal pull-through is delayed until child is 6 to 12 months old.

The prognosis depends on the birth maturity of infant and the severity of other associated anomalies. The overall mortality rate is 20 percent but increases to 55 percent for premature infants and infants with severe associated anomalies. In less severe types 1 and 2, the prognosis is good with few functional problems. Problems with fecal continence increase with the severity of the anomaly.

PREVENTION

Health Promotion

No preventive measures are known for this congenital defect.

Population at Risk

Newborns.

Screening

None.

ASSESSMENT

Health History

1. Absence of meconium stool.
2. Meconium-stained urine (if fistula to urinary system exists).
3. Progressive abdominal distension.

Physical Assessment

1. Absence of anal opening.
2. Inability to insert thermometer or small finger into rectum.

Diagnostic Tests

None required.

NURSING DIAGNOSES: ACTUAL OR POTENTIAL

1. Inability to eliminate stool.
2. Potential alteration in fluid and electrolyte balance.
3. Potential alteration in respiratory function due to abdominal distension.

EXPECTED OUTCOMES

1. Preoperative.
   a. Abdominal distension will decrease as evidenced by girth measurements.
   b. Fluid and electrolyte balance will be within normal limits as documented by laboratory data.
2. Postoperative.
   a. Parents will perform anal dilatations or colostomy care.
   b. Same as for Hirschsprung's disease.

INTERVENTIONS

1. Preoperative.
   a. NPO.
   b. Maintain patency of NG tube.
   c. Monitor flow of parenteral fluids.
   d. Keep parents informed of infant's condition.
   e. Observe for possible associated problems:
      (1) Stool from fistula.

(2) Meconium-stained urine.
(3) Symptoms of tracheoesophageal fistula (a frequently related anomaly).

2. Postoperative.
   a. Give routine postoperative care, and intervene at first indication of complications.
   b. Colostomy care.
      (1) Appropriate care and precautions are necessary.
      (2) Assure parents that colostomy is a temporary measure until infant has definitive surgery.
         (a) Instruct parents in care.
         (b) Refer to visiting nurse.
   c. Perianal anoplasty.
      (1) Keep perineum exposed to air.
      (2) Position infant as recommended by physician:
         (a) Supine with legs extended and at 90-degree angle to trunk.
         (b) Prone.
      (3) Keep area meticulously clean.
         (a) Irrigate from syringe with warm saline solution.
         (b) Dry gently with absorbent cotton.
   d. Care of abdominal-perineal pull-through.
      (1) Nasogastric or gastrostomy tube is connected to suction or gravity drainage as ordered.
      (2) Urethral catheter care.
         (a) Anchor catheter to avoid displacement.
         (b) Connect to sterile collection system.
         (c) Measure and record output every 8 hours.
      (3) Observe and report complications of respiratory distress, perineal bleeding, or abdominal distension.
      (4) Teach anal dilatation to parents to prevent stricture at anastomotic site.
   e. Encourage parents to become involved in care as soon as they are able.
      (1) Reinforce teaching that colostomy is a temporary measure.
      (2) Provide parents with supportive professional help at home, and keep in contact.
      (3) Review the physical, emotional, and developmental needs of infant with parents.
      (4) Listen to parents, and allay anxieties.

EVALUATION

Outcome Criteria

1. Preoperative.
   a. Stable condition maintained.
   b. Anomalies or complications noted and appropriately cared for.
2. Postoperative.
   a. Complications are avoided or are promptly recognized and treated.
   b. Colostomy functions properly without excoriated tissues.
   c. There is no infection of perineal area.
   d. Urethral catheter functions adequately.
   e. Infant is well hydrated and gains weight adequately.
   f. Parents participate actively in care and overcome their anxieties.

METABOLIC DISORDERS

CYSTIC FIBROSIS

See Chapter 20.

CELIAC DISEASE

DESCRIPTION

Celiac disease (also called gluten-induced enteropathy or sprue) is a chronic disorder with a symptom complex characterized by intestinal malabsorption resulting in malnutrition. The exact cause is unknown, but the disease is thought to result from an inborn error of metabolism exacerbated by ingestion of wheat or rye gluten. Fats and sugars are poorly absorbed from the intestine. As a result, the child passes huge, frothy, malodorous, floating stools and suffers from wasting and from fat-soluble vitamin deficiencies and their consequences, such as osteoporosis and bleeding. Symptoms appear insidiously in the first 2 years of life. Dietary restriction of glutens effectively reverses the intestinal cellular abnormalities, although response to diet therapy takes 6 to 8 weeks. Most children eventually outgrow their intolerance of glutens. Prognosis is good but depends on good management and parents' and child's cooperation with the dietary regimen.

PREVENTION

Health Promotion

No preventive measures are known.

Population at Risk

Children under 5 years of age, mainly those between ages 12 and 24 months.

Screening

None.

ASSESSMENT

Health History

1. Diarrhea, chronic or recurrent.
2. Stools are foul smelling, bulky, greasy, and floating.
3. Developmental delays.
4. Notable mood changes: child is irritable, passive, withdrawn, and has tantrums.

Physical Assessment

1. Signs of wasting and malnutrition.
   a. Flattened buttocks with loosely hanging skin folds.
   b. Progressive abdominal distension.
   c. Round, plump cheeks with saddened facial expression.
   d. Growth retardation (below the third percentile).

Diagnostic Tests

Small-intestine biopsy.

NURSING DIAGNOSES: ACTUAL OR POTENTIAL

1. Alteration in physical growth and development due to poor absorption of nutrients.
2. Alteration in elimination: increase in number and frequency of stools.
3. Alteration in digestion due to malabsorption of fats and sugars.
4. Alteration in personality: irritability and withdrawal.

EXPECTED OUTCOMES

1. Child will gain weight by adhering to diet regimen.
2. Diarrhea will cease, and stools will assume normal color and consistency.
3. Child will absorb nutrients by adherence to diet free of gluten.
4. Child will engage in socialization with peers.

INTERVENTIONS

1. Diet regimen.
   a. NPO during initial period of severe illness or crisis.
   b. Initial diet given is high protein, low fat, and starch free. *No wheat or rye products.*
      (1) Sweeten milk protein or skim milk with sucrose or banana powder.
      (2) Add individual foods one at a time at 2- to 3-day intervals or as prescribed (lean meats, cottage cheese, egg white, raw ground apples).
      (3) Starchy foods (bread and potatoes) added last.
      (4) Vitamin supplements as prescribed.
   c. Begin with frequent feedings of small portions.
      (1) Do not force-feed.
      (2) Feed slowly.
      (3) Socialize.
   d. Note child's reaction to meals and behavior changes during or after mealtime.
   e. Eliminate foods that precipitate recurrent symptoms.
   f. Take measures to prevent ambulatory child from obtaining restricted foods.
      (1) Alert all staff.
      (2) Older pediatric patients may assist by not taunting and tempting and may help supervise.
      (3) Enlist parents' cooperation to avoid bringing snacks.
   g. Discuss diet with parents, and arrange for meeting with nutritionist or dietitian.
2. Regressive behavior.
   a. Be patient.
   b. Avoid exhaustive play for severely ill child.
   c. Play introduced should be age-appropriate.
   d. Encourage social interaction and play involving other children gradually and consistently.
   e. Accept regressive behavior in recurrent episodes or crisis.
   f. Consider play therapy.

g. Allow child to express feelings—listen to older child and console toddler.
h. Note and avoid situations that are emotionally disturbing or upsetting to child.
i. Individualize care plan to assure consistency of effective behavior approaches.
j. Make routine care a pleasant socializing time.

3. Promote a good parent–child relationship.
   a. Encourage parents to visit frequently, and involve them in care and play activities.
   b. Allow parents time to discuss feelings.
   c. Provide genetic counseling (disease tends to recur in the family).
   d. Emphasize need for parents to set limits for child at home and avoid emotionally upsetting situations in child's presence.
   e. Encourage parents to keep ill child's needs in perspective in relation to their needs and needs of other family members.
   f. Refer to social worker to intervene with known social problems or anticipated difficulty with family interrelationships.
4. Infections and celiac crisis.
   a. Observe for and teach parents signs and symptoms of celiac crisis:
      (1) Large, watery stools.
      (2) Restless sleep.
      (3) Excessive perspiration.
      (4) Cold extremities.
   b. Treat and manage as ordered.
      (1) NPO.
      (2) Parenteral therapy.
      (3) Observation of changes.
   c. Instruct parents to seek immediate medical care if child develops an upper respiratory infection.
   d. Urge continued regular medical follow-up.

EVALUATION

Outcome Criteria

1. Improved physical and psychological condition is demonstrated with weight gain, adherence to diet, improved disposition.
2. Child interacts sociably with diminished regressive behavior.
3. Parents exhibit understanding and acceptance and are able to deal effectively with child in routine daily procedures.
4. Absence of crisis and infections, or immediate appropriate care provided.
5. Continuous follow-up management.

OTHER GASTROINTESTINAL DISORDERS

DENTAL CARIES

DESCRIPTION

Dental caries is a disease of the teeth that is characterized by a progressive destructive lesion of the calcified dental tissues eventually involving the pulp. Caries is chiefly a bacterial disease with the principal causative organisms being streptococci and *Lactobacillus acidophilus*. Organisms form and adhere to gelatinous plaque on the tooth surface. Action of the organism and substrates from foodstuffs, mainly carbohydrates (sucrose), produce acids that rapidly decalcify tooth enamel, with destruction of the tooth the end result. Untreated caries results not only in pain and tooth loss but in consequent malocclusion, weakening of the muscles of mastication, and cosmetic defects that can be damaging to the person's self-concept. Abscesses can lead to bone destruction and bony or systemic infection. Children with congenital or rheumatic heart disease are at risk for bacterial endocarditis secondary to dental decay. Caries is the principal oral problem of children and adolescents, affecting more than 90 percent.

Factors contributing to tooth decay include lack of fluoride, lack of oral hygiene, poor state of general health, and poor dietary practices. Decay of the primary (deciduous) teeth is encouraged by the practice of giving milk or other sugar-containing fluids in a nursing bottle at naps and bedtime because of the continuous flow of sugars over the teeth while the child sucks during sleep.

PREVENTION

Health Promotion

Brushing and flossing, fluoridated water or fluoride applications, mixed diet with minimal sugar.

Population at Risk

Everyone who has teeth, especially
1. Babies and children who take a bottle of milk or other sugar-containing fluid to bed.
2. Adolescents.

3. Children with faulty oral hygiene.
4. Children with high dietary sugar intakes, especially sticky substances that cling to the teeth.

Screening

Annual dental checkup beginning at age 18 to 30 months.

ASSESSMENT

Health History

1. Poor dietary practices.
   a. Excessive weight loss or gain.
   b. Excessive intake of refined sugar.
   c. Dislike of chewable foods.
2. History of congenital heart disease or rheumatic heart disease (clients with a positive history require prophylactic antibiotics before having dental work because bacteria introduced into the circulatory system may cause endocarditis in people with abnormal intracardiac blood flow patterns).
3. Developmental difficulties.
   a. Speech and language problems of dental origin.
   b. Withdrawal and isolation secondary to dental disfigurement.

Physical Assessment

1. Decayed areas of teeth, with pitting and fissures.
2. Excessive plaque on tooth surfaces.
3. Accumulation of food debris between teeth.
4. Inflammation and tenderness of gums.
5. Missing or misaligned teeth.

Diagnostic Tests

Dental x-ray films.

NURSING DIAGNOSES: ACTUAL OR POTENTIAL

1. Alteration in mastication due to dental decay.
2. Potential alteration in speech due to dental problems.
3. Potential alteration in self-concept due to poor oral/facial appearance.
4. Alteration in comfort: pain due to dental decay.

EXPECTED OUTCOMES

1. Child will receive dental treatment.
2. Parents and child will comprehend the necessity of dental care as evidenced by dental care and oral hygiene practices.
3. Parents and child will understand the role of nutrition in preventing caries as demonstrated by verbal communication and dietary practices.

INTERVENTIONS

1. Provide treatment.
   a. Discuss need for immediate treatment, and refer to appropriate source.
   b. Assess current oral hygiene practices, parental supervision, and dietary practices.
2. Teach principles of good oral hygiene.
   a. Assess knowledge and current practices.
   b. Instill understanding of need for early and regular visits.
      (1) Begin at 18 to 30 months for checkup and cleaning so child becomes familiar with dentist without necessarily associating pain with treatment.
      (2) Adolescent should have regular visits every 3 to 6 months.
3. Teach proper brushing and care.
   a. Toothbrush appropriate size for age of child.
   b. Up-and-down technique.
   c. Daily brushing after meals and at bedtime.
   d. Flossing between teeth regularly.
4. Explain the effectiveness of fluoridation on strengthening calcification of tooth enamel.
5. Seek parental assistance and guidance with younger children to assure frequent and proper brushing.
6. Individualize teaching plan.
   a. No bottles of milk at bedtime after eruption of teeth. Substitute water, or discontinue bedtime bottle.
   b. Encourage early weaning, as the purpose of the teeth is mastication.
7. Teach nutrition.
   a. Assess and evaluate current dietary habits.
   b. Teach improvement and preventive measures.
      (1) Decrease between-meal snacks to improve appetite at mealtime.
      (2) Substitute fresh fruits and vegetables for refined sugar snacks.
      (3) No milk or milk products before bedtime without rinsing or brushing.
      (4) Evaluate speech. Refer to speech ther-

apist for continued evaluation and therapy.

(5) Developmental and personality concerns.
   (a) Assess in cooperation with parents initially, and note if there is any change after treatment.
   (b) Review needs of child during various stages of development.

EVALUATION

Outcome Criteria

1. Care is obtained early with appropriate treatment done and primary teeth functional until eruption of permanent teeth. No infections.
2. Parents demonstrate understanding of good oral hygiene by supervising child's habits and seeking early care if decay begins again.
3. Parents demonstrate understanding by adhering to dietary recommendations with resultant improvement in nutritional status and reduction of dental caries.
4. Speech problems resolved.
5. No evidence of personality problems or developmental delays.

BIBLIOGRAPHY

Bishop, W. S., and Head, J. H.: "Care of the Infant with a Stoma," *Maternal Child Health Nursing,* **1**:315, September-October, 1976. Because of the client's small size and delicate skin, the most important aspect of stoma care in infants is preventing wound contamination and skin breakdown. The nurse must also be aware of the impact on the family of a sick baby with a stoma.

Bliss, V. J.: "Nursing Care of Infants with Neonatal Necrotizing Enterocolitis," *Maternal Child Health Nursing,* **1**:37, January-February, 1976. Necrotizing enterocolitis often has an insidious onset, and the nurse is in a unique position to detect and intervene in this disease. The article deals with etiology, nursing care, and other treatment.

Brueggemeyer, A.: "Omphalocele: Coping with a Surgical Emergency," *Pediatric Nursing,* **5**:54, 1979. Care of child and parents is discussed.

Filler, R. M.: "Total Parenteral Feeding of Infants," *Hospital Practice,* **9**:79, June, 1976. Review of hyperalimentation procedure and its hazards. The child with a hyperalimentation line requires scrupulous nursing observation and care.

Given, B. A., and Simmons, S. J.: *Gastroenterology in Clinical Nursing,* C. V. Mosby, St. Louis, 1979. General exposition of nursing care for clients with gastrointestinal disorders.

Gross, L.: "Ostomy Care, A Letter to Parents," *American Journal of Nursing,* **74**(8):1427, August, 1974. In order to deal with their child's ostomy surgery and care, parents must first face their own feelings and overcome any guilt or fear. The author points out ten ways to support the child.

Gryboski, J.: *Gastrointestinal Problems in the Infant,* W. B. Saunders, Philadelphia, 1979. Specialized text on diagnosis and treatment of infant gastrointestinal disorders of all causes.

Shannon, R. M.: "The Gastrointestinal System," in Scipien, G. M., Barnard, M.U., Chard, M., et al. (eds.), *Comprehensive Pediatric Nursing,* 2d ed., McGraw-Hill, New York, 1979. Comprehensive discussion of embryology, physiology, anatomy, and disorders of the gastrointestinal tract in children; nursing care is emphasized.

23

The Integumentary System

Patricia Harris

ABNORMAL CELLULAR GROWTH

VASCULAR NEVI (BIRTHMARKS)

DESCRIPTION

Nevi (singular: nevus) are colloquially called birthmarks, even though not all are present at birth. The category nevus generally includes both the vascular and pigmented nevi, including "moles," but some of the professional literature subsumes only the vascular *or* the pigmentary defects under the term (i.e., there is not a uniform usage of the word *nevus*). Nevi, particularly the vascular ones, are also categorized as involuting (self-correcting) or noninvoluting. Clinical findings are frequently less clear-cut than the following discussion suggests, because two or more histological types can be mixed in a single nevus. Etiology is unknown, but heredity evidently plays a role. For a description of specific vascular nevi, see Table 23-1.

PREVENTION

Health Promotion

No preventive measures are known.

Population at Risk

Newborns and infants; family history for vascular nevi is sometimes positive.

Screening

None.

ASSESSMENT

Health History

1. Determine whether nevus was present or absent at birth.
2. Note rate of growth or involution.

Physical Assessment

1. Inspect for
   a. Size.
   b. Color.
   c. Elevation.
   d. Texture.
   e. Blanching.
   f. Compressibility.
   g. Location.

Diagnostic Tests

None.

NURSING DIAGNOSES: ACTUAL OR POTENTIAL

1. Alterations in self-esteem and interpersonal relationships (parent–infant bonding in young babies) due to atypical appearance.
2. Risk of secondary infection associated with trauma or surgery.
3. Predisposition to bleeding or ulceration due to vascular abnormalities of skin lesion.
4. Knowledge deficit and associated risk of unnecessary treatment due to family's eagerness to secure prompt resolution of nevus.

TABLE 23-1 VASCULAR NEVI

Names	Identifying Characteristics	Prognosis
Telangiectatic nevi (those consisting principally of capillaries).		
Nevus simplex, erythema nuchae, salmon patch, stork bite.	This is a flat, pink to red nevus found on the upper eyelids, nape, lip, or forehead of perhaps 30 to 60 percent of newborns. The color becomes redder when the infant cries, which causes concern to parents.	The marks gradually fade as the child grows older and the skin becomes thicker. The majority disappear during infancy or early childhood.
Nevus araneus, spider nevus.	Named for its shape, the spider nevus consists of a tiny flat or very slightly elevated central arteriole with capillaries radiating from it. Approximately 50 percent of children develop one or more spider nevi, usually during the school-age years and usually on the hands, neck, or face.	They blanch with pressure and refill from the center outward. Many disappear spontaneously, particularly after puberty.
Nevus flammeus, port-wine nevus.	This flat, purple-red lesion is composed of a dilated, congested capillary mass under the epidermis. It is always present at birth, blanches only slightly with pressure, and becomes darker with crying. It frequently involves the face and is sometimes associated with neurological disorders (e.g., the Sturge-Weber syndrome).	The port-wine nevus does not involute and does not become larger except to maintain its distribution as the child grows.
Angiomatous nevi (those consisting principally of blood vessels larger than capillaries).		
Hemangioma simplex, nevus vasculosus, capillary hemangioma, strawberry nevus.	This sharply circumscribed, elevated, red or purplish nevus is not present at birth. It appears, usually during the first month of life, as a red macule. The strawberry nevus may be present on any part of the skin. It blanches little if at all.	From the original macule the nevus grows for 6 to 18 months and then gradually recedes over a period of months or years. Most disappear entirely without treatment.
Cavernous hemangioma.	This vascular tumor, present at birth, consists of large venous pools and channels and may include arteriovenous shunts. It may be an elevated, circumscribed red mass or, if the deeper tissues of the skin are involved, a poorly circumscribed bluish mass covered by normal skin and causing some distortion of the affected body area. Either type may become more deeply colored or larger with crying. Cavernous hemangiomas are usually partially compressible but refill when pressure is removed.	These lesions usually do not grow except in proportion to the baby's growth and, after a few months, decrease in size.

EXPECTED OUTCOMES

1. The child will be accepted by family and others.
2. The child will develop a good self-concept.
3. Bleeding, infection, and scarring will be absent or minimal.
4. Family will wait an appropriate length of time for nevus to achieve maximum spontaneous involution rather than subjecting child unnecessarily to the risks of active treatment.

INTERVENTIONS

1. Teach parents about the excellent prognosis for involution (except for port-wine mark). A family history can be quite helpful, since family incidence of vascular nevi is common, and most of the relatives' nevi will have regressed or disappeared.
   a. Prepare family for the fact that the nevus is expected to grow before involuting.
   b. Keep accurate measurements or photographs by which progress of involution can be gauged and demonstrated.
   c. Teach use of cosmetic covering creams, if desired.
   d. Help the child and others keep the skin problem in perspective as just one among the child's qualities.
   e. Search for misconceptions about origin that may contribute to guilt or blame.
2. Support child's self-esteem.
3. Teach skin care and protection as necessary to decrease risks of trauma and infection of the nevus.
4. Refer to physician if indications for active treatment are present:
   a. Alarming growth of lesion—nevus doubles or triples in size in less than a month.
   b. Encroachment on organs; for example, eye orbits, nares, or pinna of ear.
   c. Lesions are atypical, with unusual growth patterns.
   d. Considerable cosmetic objections may be a problem after the end of the preschool period.

EVALUATION

1. Child–parent relationship is satisfactory.
2. Child's social patterns are normal for age.
3. Child's self-esteem is adequate despite skin problem.
4. Local skin problems (bleeding, infection, ulceration) are avoided or adequately treated.
5. Unnecessary active treatment is avoided.

PIGMENTED NEVI (MONGOLIAN SPOTS)

DESCRIPTION

Pigmentary lesions are rarely noted in infants except for mongolian spots, which are discussed below. Café au lait spots (flat tan or brown irregularly shaped areas in otherwise normal skin) are of no consequence unless they are cosmetically disturbing, or unless they are present in numbers of six or more, in which case they suggest the medical diagnosis of neurofibromatosis (von Recklinghausen's disease), a rare neurological disorder.

PREVENTION

Health Promotion

No preventive measures are known for mongolian spots.

Population at Risk

Neonates, especially blacks, Orientals, and Mediterraneans.

Screening

None.

ASSESSMENT

Health History

Mongolian spots are present at birth.

Physical Assessment

Flat, grayish blue areas resembling bruises, usually on the lumbosacral region but occasionally on the back, shoulders, and extensor surfaces of the arms and legs.

Diagnostic tests

None.

NURSING DIAGNOSES: ACTUAL OR POTENTIAL

1. Risk for disturbed parent–child relationship due to skin discoloration.
2. Knowledge deficit about cause, significance, and prognosis of spots.
3. Risk of mistaking lesions for bruises.

EXPECTED OUTCOMES

1. Bonding occurs normally; parent–child interaction is adequate.
2. Parents will be well informed about mongolian spots.
3. Parents and others will not mistake lesions for bruises.

INTERVENTIONS

1. Teach family that the pigmented areas are of no medical significance, are common in babies, and disappear in a year or so, although they may become darker in the first several weeks of life.

NOTE: Mongolian spots have no relationship to Down's syndrome, formerly called mongolism.

2. Distinguish (and clarify for parents if they are uncertain) between mongolian spots and bruises indicative of nursery accident or child abuse; the difference should be clear from history (discoloration present since birth, characteristic location, and absence of swelling, abrasion, and other signs of trauma).

EVALUATION

Outcome criteria

1. Parent–child relationship is adequate.
2. Parents consider spots clinically insignificant and expect them to fade in a year or so.
3. Incorrect suspicions of abuse or accident are not perpetuated.

INFLAMMATIONS

DIAPER DERMATITIS

DESCRIPTION

Diaper dermatitis is composed of erythematous lesions in the diaper area that result from friction of a wet or soiled diaper against wet skin. Without intervention, the rash spreads throughout the diaper area and progresses from macules and papules to eroded, moist, or crusted lesions. Secondary bacterial and/or yeast infection can occur (see also *Candidiasis*, later in this chapter).

PREVENTION

Health Promotion

Keep infant's skin dry and clean by frequent diaper changes and cleansing of irritating substances (urine, feces).

Population at Risk

Infants and children who wear diapers; use of rubber pants reduces ventilation and increases risk.

Screening

None.

ASSESSMENT

Health History

Obtain history of present skin care methods.

Physical Assessment

Inspect diaper area for presence and type of rash.

Diagnostic Tests

None.

NURSING DIAGNOSES: ACTUAL OR POTENTIAL

1. Interruption of skin integrity due to inadequate hygiene.
2. Risk of secondary infection due to skin breaks.
3. Risk of urinary meatus stenosis secondary to scarring.
4. Knowledge deficit about infant skin care.

EXPECTED OUTCOMES

1. Rash will clear, and skin integrity will be restored.
2. Secondary infection will be avoided.
3. Meatal stenosis will not occur.
4. Parents will correctly modify infant skin care practices.

INTERVENTIONS

Teach parents effective skin care methods:

1. Diapers must be changed frequently.
2. Area must be washed thoroughly at each dia-

per change, using water or mild soap with water.
3. Diaper area should be exposed to air during naps.
4. Disposable diapers and rubber pants should not be used.
5. Apply cornstarch to minimize friction.

EVALUATION

Outcome Criteria

1. Skin clears; rash does not recur.
2. Parents demonstrate or describe care methods they have been taught.

Complications

SECONDARY INFECTION

Assessment
Moist, purulent, sometimes fiery red lesions

Revised Outcomes
1. Infection (and rash) will clear.
2. Scarring will not occur.

Interventions
1. Bacteriostatic or mycostatic ointment.
2. Good skin care, as described in Interventions section above.
3. Hydrocortisone cream may be necessary in severe cases (Leyden, 1982).

MEATAL STENOSIS

Assessment
Infant strains to urinate; stream is small, intermittent, or deviates in direction.

Revised Outcomes
Child will maintain normal renal and urinary function.

Interventions
Promptly refer to physician.

URTICARIA (HIVES)

DESCRIPTION

Hives are intensely pruritic, erythematous, confluent, raised lesions that are often accompanied by a noticeable swelling of the face. They can appear suddenly on face and total body surface or may be sparse (see Figure 23-1). Hives are often an allergic reaction.

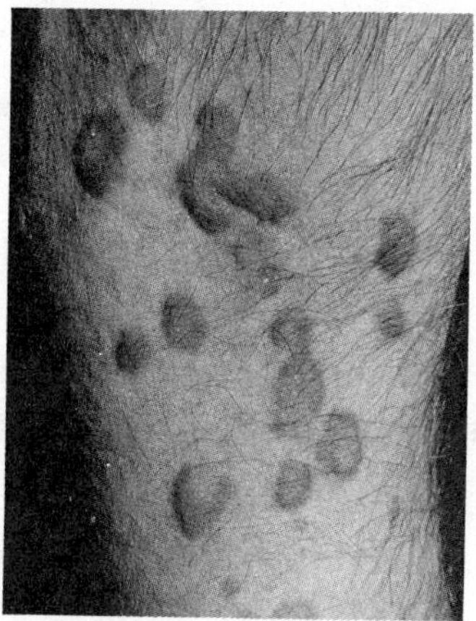

Figure 23-1 Wheals, the lesions of urticaria. Welts are elevated and have pale centers with erythematous margins. Wheals are transient, lasting from a few minutes to a day or so. (From Fitzpatrick, T. B., et al.: *Dermatology in General Medicine,* 2d edition, McGraw-Hill, New York, 1979. Used with permission.)

PREVENTION

Health Promotion

Avoidance of known allergens.

Population at Risk

Everyone, particularly people with allergies.

Screening

None.

ASSESSMENT

Health History

1. New drugs.
2. New foods.
3. Inhalants.
4. Insect bite or sting.
5. Emotional stress.

Physical Assessment

Inspect for characteristic lesion (see Description, above).

Diagnostic Tests

None.

NURSING DIAGNOSES: ACTUAL OR POTENTIAL

1. Alteration in comfort: intense itching secondary to hives.

2. Risk of impending generalized anaphylactic response.
3. Knowledge deficit about causes of attack and ways to avoid or treat subsequent attacks.

EXPECTED OUTCOMES

1. Client will obtain relief from itching.
2. Anaphylaxis, if it occurs, will be promptly recognized and treated.
3. Child and family will know how to avoid subsequent exposure to allergen and how to manage attacks that do occur.

INTERVENTIONS

1. For mild cases, an antihistamine and cool baths will relieve itching.
2. For severe, intense pruritus, aqueous epinephrine is given subcutaneously with one or two subsequent doses 1 or 2 hours later. Short-term oral steroids may be prescribed.
3. Observe client closely for wheezing, shock, or other signs of anaphylaxis, including worsening of urticaria; report such signs immediately.
4. For urticaria after insect stings, client should carry insect sting kit and be referred to allergist for desensitization. Teach child and family how to use kit.

EVALUATION

Outcome Criteria

1. Itching is relieved, and no complications (e.g., excoriation, secondary infection) arise.
2. All reasonable precautions are taken to avoid subsequent exposure to offending allergen.
3. Family (and child if old enough) demonstrate skill in recognizing serious allergic manifestations and in using insect bite kit if anaphylaxis occurs.

POISON IVY AND POISON OAK

DESCRIPTION

Linear streaks of vesicles appear where the plant has touched the skin surface. Lesions first appear as discrete annular papules with mild erythema a few hours to a few days after contact (Figure 23-2). They then become very pruritic with vesicles and weeping. The inflammation usually occurs asymmetrically on exposed body areas.

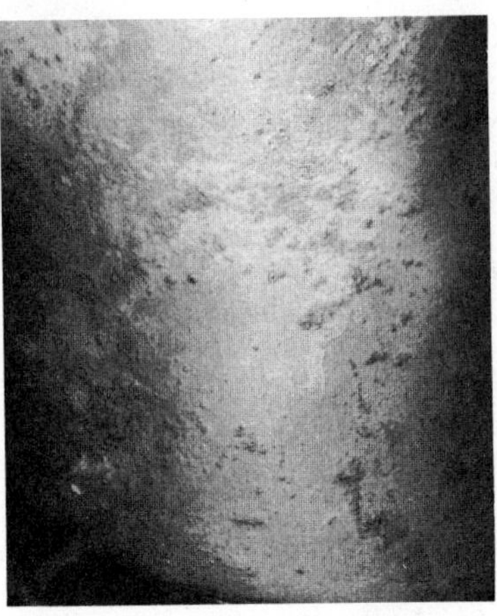

Figure 23-2 Plant-induced contact dermatitis (poison ivy or poison oak). Note the vesicles in linear patches. (From Fitzpatrick, T. B., et al.: *Dermatology in General Medicine,* 2d edition, McGraw-Hill, New York, 1979. Used with permission.)

PREVENTION

Health Promotion

1. Teach children to recognize poison ivy and poison oak so that they can avoid contact with it.
2. When in areas where the plants grow, people should wear protective clothing (shoes and stockings, long sleeved shirts, and trousers) and avoid touching the face with possibly contaminated hands.
   a. Hands should be washed thoroughly with soap.
   b. Clothing should be laundered, as the offending oils from the plants can retain their irritant properties for several days.
3. Inhalation of smoke from bonfires containing these plants can result in severe respiratory tract inflammation.

Population at Risk

Everyone, theoretically, but people vary widely in their susceptibility and the severity of their response.

Screening

None.

ASSESSMENT

Health History

1. Exposure to plants several hours to several days before skin eruption (e.g., wooded play area, camping trip).
2. Dermatitis occasionally results from indirect exposure; plant resins, which can be transferred to the child, can be carried on the coats of household pets.

Physical Assessment

Inspect for characteristic papular rash with distribution described above.

Diagnostic Tests

None.

NURSING DIAGNOSES: ACTUAL OR POTENTIAL

1. Alteration in comfort: intense itching of rash.
2. Risk of secondary infection due to loss of skin integrity caused by scratching.
3. Noncompliance with treatment due to inconvenience (e.g., child cannot draw or write while hands are soaking or covered with cream).
4. Knowledge deficit: risk of recurrence due to continuing sensitivity to the offending plants.

EXPECTED OUTCOMES

1. Itching will be decreased.
2. Secondary infection will not occur.
3. Child and family will carry out recommended treatment.
4. Recurrence will not take place.

INTERVENTIONS

1. Soak the affected area for 20 minutes four times daily in Burow's solution or normal saline.
2. Apply calamine lotion.
3. Oral antihistamines and gel type topical steroids may be prescribed for pruritus.
4. For severe cases, short, tapered courses of corticosteroids may be needed.
5. See Table 23-2 for further interventions to reduce itching and encourage compliance.
6. Instruct child and family in preventive measures (see Prevention, above).

EVALUATION

Outcome Criteria

1. Dermatitis clears in 7 to 14 days.
2. Child and family follow recommended therapy.
3. Child and family recognize and avoid further contact with the offending plants.

TABLE 23-2 GENERAL SUPPORT MEASURES FOR CHILDREN WITH ITCHING OR UNPLEASANT TREATMENTS

1. To decrease itching and scratching
   a. Divert the child (and teach parents the diversion techniques) to age-appropriate activities that require two hands, such as finger painting, water play, block building, or model construction.
   b. Restrain sparingly, allowing for comfort and thumbsucking.
   c. Children who receive antipruritic medications need periodic reevaluation for therapeutic and side effects: Is itching under control? Is the child too sleepy to progress with schoolwork or too active to concentrate?
2. To assist child and family to carry out treatment regimens that are time-consuming or messy or extend over prolonged periods of time
   a. Divert child's attention to age-appropriate activities that can be conducted during treatments. For example, read a story or arrange for the child to hear a favorite record or television show during a 20-minute soak.
   b. Allow child to have as much control over the treatment as possible: child may be permitted to decide whether treatment is done before or after dinner, for example, and should be allowed to perform as much of the treatment as is feasible and desired, such as gathering the equipment, running the water, and measuring and adding the chemical.
   c. Children should be appropriately rewarded and acknowledged for their cooperation and participation, particularly after painful procedures.

ECZEMA (ATOPIC DERMATITIS)

DEFINITION

Eczema is a generally symmetrical, reddish, slightly raised, rough-feeling inflammation, beginning as early as the first weeks after birth. The lesions often develop weeping crusts. Rubbing against bedding or baby clothes exacerbates lesions (see Figure 23-3 for characteristic distribution). The stratum corneum of the skin usually sheds, leaving patchy hypopigmentation. The skin then heals, leaving normal pigmentation without scarring. Many children outgrow infantile eczema at around 2 years of age.

Older children have intense itching, which is then rubbed or scratched, often leading to secondary infection. In persistent dermatitis, the skin takes on areas of hyperpigmentation as well as areas of paler skin. Lichenification and thickening are also common in older children.

1. *Etiology*. The cause is unknown. Eczema is often the earliest manifestation of an allergic tendency. The infant's skin is more easily irritated than normal skin. This triggers the itch-scratch cycle, which then causes more irritation to the skin.

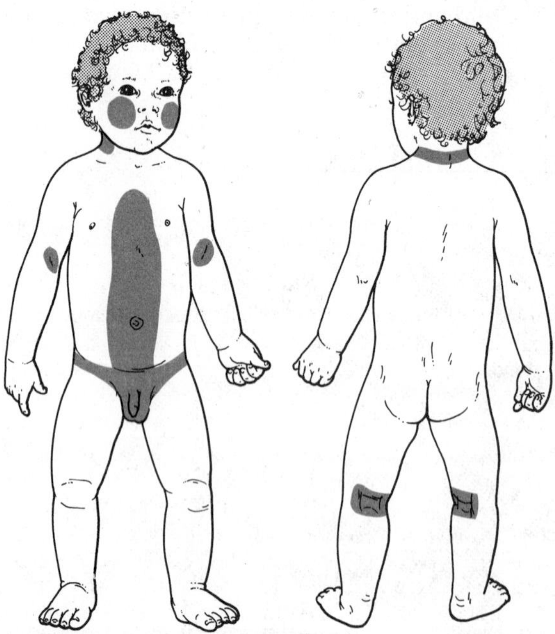

Figure 23-3 Distribution of eczema. Rough, dry, erythematous lesions progress to weeping and crusting.

2. *Itch-scratch cycle*. Dry, pruritic skin results in scratching, which produces excoriation, eczematization, and secondary infection. The dry skin then changes from discrete papules to confluent patches with thickening. This cycle presents a difficult management problem.
3. *Normal course*. About one person in five demonstrates some form of atopic dermatitis at some time. Eczema in many infants clears up by the age of 2 years. However, many continue to have flare-ups. Some develop asthma or hay fever as older children or adults.

   Atopic dermatitis often occurs in children whose parents have allergies, asthma, or atopic dermatitis.
4. *Contributing factors*. During cold winter months when air and skin are dry, extreme temperature changes exacerbate skin lesions and pruritus.

   During emotionally stressful times and during boredom, flare-ups often occur. Flare-ups also occur with excessive sweating after exercise.

   Eczema may be an allergic response to foods, perfumes, soaps, or drugs. Although the part that diet plays in atopic dermatitis is unclear, some children develop eczema with new foods.

   With systemic illnesses, especially viral infections, flare-ups may occur.

PREVENTION

Health Promotion

There is no definitive prevention for eczema, but exacerbations can often be avoided or minimized when the conditions that cause flare-ups for a particular client are identified and avoided.

Population at Risk

Infants over 2 to 3 months of age, children, and adolescents, especially those from families with allergies.

Screening

None.

ASSESSMENT

Health History

1. Note recent changes in diet or type of clothing.
2. Family history of allergic manifestations.

Physical Assessment

1. Characteristic rash and distribution pattern (see Description, above, and Figure 23-3).
2. Assess for excoriation and secondary infection.

Diagnostic Tests

None.

NURSING DIAGNOSES: ACTUAL OR POTENTIAL

1. Alteration in comfort: discomfort and irritability associated with itching.
2. Disturbance of sleep-rest pattern due to discomfort.
3. Alteration in self-concept and social relationships, including parent–child interaction, secondary to altered appearance associated with skin changes.
4. Loss of skin integrity secondary to rash and scratching.
5. Risk of secondary infection associated with loss of skin integrity.
6. Impaired family functioning secondary to time-consuming treatment regimen.
7. Noncompliance due to inconvenience of treatment regimen and child's displeasure with it.

EXPECTED OUTCOMES

1. Itching will be diminished.
2. Sleep pattern will be restored.
3. Self-concept and social interactions will be adequate.
4. Skin integrity will be protected.
5. Secondary infection will not occur.
6. Family will follow recommended treatment regimen and function and cope adequately.

INTERVENTIONS

1. Identify and eliminate allergen or other irritant, if possible.
   a. An elimination diet has been effective for some children. The role of milk allergy is still unclear.
   b. Avoid wool; cotton is preferable. Don't overdress babies.
   c. Humidification in the winter is important.
   d. Child's bedroom should be as dust-free as possible.
   e. Avoid extreme temperature changes.
2. Antihistamines or, rarely, barbiturates may be given.
3. Baths may be given using Aveeno or cornstarch.
4. Topical steroids are applied after compresses during acute phase. Caution must be used due to systemic absorption of steroids, which can lead to fat atrophy, telangiectases, and possible adrenal dysfunction.
5. Help child and family see the skin condition as just one of the child's many characteristics. Teachers and other involved persons should be informed that the condition is not contagious.
6. Encourage parents to treat child normally, (i.e., hold, play with, and stimulate infant). Parents often need support to set reasonable limits, since stress and emotion can cause skin flare-ups. Help parents realize that the eczema must not be a dominant force in childrearing practices and family lifestyle.
7. Elbow restraints, mittens, long pajamas, and/or occlusive dressings are sometimes necessary, especially at night, to prevent further excoriation and secondary infections (see Figure 23-4 for arm restraints).
8. Trim fingernails.
9. The skin should be cleansed with lotion. Bathing should be infrequent, no more than once a week (this protects natural skin oils). For the weekly bath, tepid water should be used with mild soap. After the bath, mild lotion should be applied while the skin is damp. Tar preparations and emollients are helpful.
10. See Table 23-2 for further suggestions about interventions for children with pruritus and for ways to facilitate compliance with therapy.

EVALUATION

Outcome Criteria

1. Itching is greatly decreased; exacerbations occur less often.
2. Child's sleep is not disrupted by itching.
3. Self-concept is favorable; interpersonal interactions are normal for age (see Chapter 4).
4. Parent–child relationship is good; parental discipline is appropriate for child's age.
5. Scratching is controlled.
6. Secondary skin infections do not occur.
7. Treatment regimen is followed.

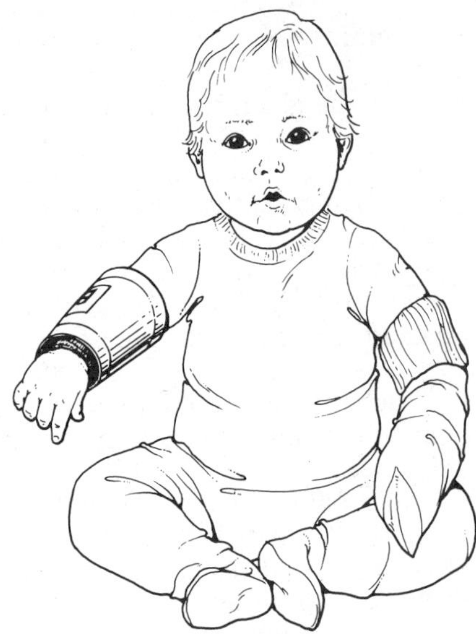

Figure 23-4 A bleach bottle cut into a cylinder and applied over longsleeved pajamas is effective as an elbow restraint to prevent scratching of face, head, trunk, and upper extremities. Mittens may also be quite helpful; adult-size cotton stockings make ideal mittens (avoid wool).

8. Family members cope with the demands of the child's treatment; activities of family, both as individuals and as a group, are indicative of good functioning (see Chapter 5).

SEBORRHEA

DESCRIPTION

Seborrhea (called cradle cap in infancy) consists of oily, scaly lesions with yellowish crusts and white particles, beginning on the scalp. Distribution usually extends to forehead and eyelids. Seborrhea is sometimes found in the axillae and in the diaper area (see Figure 23-5). It is usually self-limiting. Seborrhea can also occur mixed with eczema and bacterial infections.

PREVENTION

Health Promotion

No preventive measures are known.

Population at Risk

People whose sex hormones are in fluctuation—babies in the first weeks of life and adolescents during puberty. Stress may precipitate or exacerbate this skin disorder (Guinter, 1978).

Screening

None.

ASSESSMENT

Health History

1. Complains of itching.
2. Inquire about skin care and shampooing practices.

Physical Assessment

Inspect skin for characteristic lesions and distribution pattern (see Description, above, and Figure 23-5).

Diagnostic Tests

None.

NURSING DIAGNOSES: ACTUAL OR POTENTIAL

1. Loss of skin integrity associated with scaling and scratching.
2. Risk of secondary infection due to loss of skin integrity.
3. Alteration in comfort: discomfort due to itching (often mild).
4. Alteration in self-concept and social relationships secondary to altered appearance.

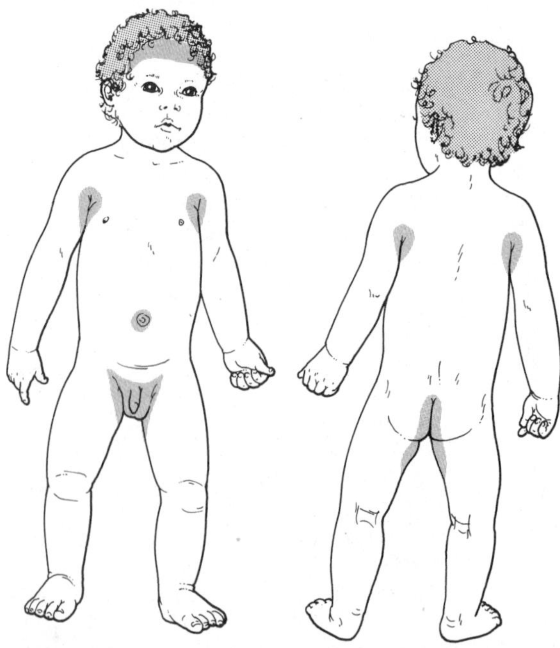

Figure 23-5 Distribution of lesions of seborrhea (intertriginous areas and scalp are primarily affected).

EXPECTED OUTCOMES

1. Skin integrity will be restored.
2. Secondary infection will not occur.
3. Itching will be minimal or absent.
4. Self-concept will be adequate; social interactions will be normal for developmental level.

INTERVENTIONS

1. Explain general principles of well-child hygiene, and assure caretaker that bathing the scalp is beneficial.
2. For mild cases, apply baby oil to scalp, then loosen yellowish crusts and white particles with a fine-tooth comb; shampoo biweekly. Generally, once the scalp clears, the forehead and eyebrows do also.
3. More involved cases respond to a tar shampoo (Sebulex) biweekly. Ointments containing sulfur and salicylic acid may be prescribed for use following shampoo. Topical steroids may be used.
4. Loose-fitting mittens may be used to prevent baby from scratching.
5. Help adolescent and family view seborrhea as just one among many of the young person's characteristics.

EVALUATION

1. Caretaker (or adolescent) demonstrates (or describes) recommended shampooing and skin care procedure.
2. Infant's lesions do not spread to axillae or diaper area.
3. Skin clears, partially or completely.
4. Secondary infection is avoided.
5. Itching and scratching are controlled.
6. Self-esteem is adequate; social activities are normal for developmental level.

MILIARIA RUBRA (PRICKLY HEAT)

DESCRIPTION

Miliaria rubra is a fine, red, papular rash that results from occlusion of the sweat gland pores. The torso, neck, and skin folds are most often affected. This inflammation is caused by hot weather or by being dressed too warmly.

PREVENTION

Health Promotion

Keep child from becoming overly warm.

Population at Risk

Infants, primarily, but also older children with sensitive skin.

Screening

None.

ASSESSMENT

Health History

1. Rash appears during warm weather or other warm conditions.
2. Baby is irritable.

Physical Assessment

Inspect for fine, red, papular rash in skin folds (especially neck and axillae) and on trunk.

Diagnostic Tests

None.

NURSING DIAGNOSES: ACTUAL OR POTENTIAL

Alteration in comfort: discomfort and irritability due to rash.

EXPECTED OUTCOMES

1. Rash will clear.
2. Discomfort will resolve.

INTERVENTIONS

1. Keep baby cool. Dress lightly, and give frequent, cool baths in warm weather.
2. Apply baby powder, cornstarch, or calamine lotion.

EVALUATION

Skin clears, and discomfort is alleviated.

ACNE

DESCRIPTION

Acne is a common, chronic disorder of adolescence and young adulthood characterized by papules, pustules, comedones (blackheads and whiteheads), and in severe cases cystic lesions.

Lesions usually involve large sebaceous follicles distributed over the face, neck, back, and chest. The precise etiology has not been pinpointed, but it is evident that the hormonal fluctuations of adolescence are one causative factor. Skin hygiene, diet, emotional stress, and a family history of acne are among other causal factors that have been implicated. Another causative factor is presence of *Propionibacterium acnes*, aerobic coagulase-negative *Staphylococcus* group II, and *Pityrosporon ovale* (yeast).

PREVENTION

Health Promotion

No preventive measures are known.

Population at Risk

Adolescents and young adults, especially those with a family history of acne.

Screening

None.

ASSESSMENT

Health History

1. Possible causes of flare-ups.
2. Previous methods of treatment and their success.
3. Skin care methods.
4. Cosmetic use.
5. Family history of acne.

Physical Assessment

1. Inspect skin for characteristic lesions.
2. Monitor blood pressure: occasionally hypertension develops when taking systemic antibiotics (Stuart, 1978).

Diagnostic Tests

None.

NURSING DIAGNOSES: ACTUAL OR POTENTIAL

1. Altered skin integrity secondary to inflammatory and pustular changes.
2. Risk of scarring, especially with secondary infection.
3. Altered self-concept secondary to altered appearance.

EXPECTED OUTCOMES

1. Number of lesions will diminish.
2. Scarring will be minimal or absent.
3. Client will have positive self-esteem.

INTERVENTIONS

1. Teach client to manage the treatment plan.
   a. Clean skin with a mild soap once or twice daily (use cleaning pads for midday, to accommodate daily schedule). Avoid abrasive soaps.
   b. Use peeling agents, such as benzyl peroxide or retinoic acid cream (increased pigmentation and redness often occur initially).
   c. Sunshine and/or ultraviolet light exposure may be helpful.
   d. A balanced diet, with particular attention to meeting protein and vitamin C requirements, is important.
   e. Discourage manipulation of the lesions and mannerisms, such as touching the face or resting the head on the hands.
2. Additional treatment may include steroid injection of lesions (fat atrophy is a potential side effect) or incision and comedo extraction. Tetracycline or minocycline may be prescribed, in which case a baseline complete blood cell count and urinalysis are needed, and side effects must be watched for. Monilial vaginitis is a common side effect, particularly among young women who are taking birth control pills.
3. Assist the young person in dealing with stress, which often contributes to acne flare-ups. Help client label feelings, identify alternative courses of action, set reachable goals, communicate with others, and improve peer relationships.
4. The nurse is often instrumental in providing telephone support to the client and overall supervision of the complicated treatment plan.
5. Cosmetics, appropriately used, may decrease the emotional impact of the condition.
6. Help the young person to see the skin condition as but one of a great many of his or her characteristics.

EVALUATION

Outcome Criteria

1. The lesions are clearing within 1 month of treatment.
2. Scarring is minimal or absent.
3. Client demonstrates skill in following the treatment plan and in managing treatment during flare-ups.
4. Client demonstrates adequate self-concept;

social activities are normal for developmental level (see Chapter 4).

Complications
Scar formation.

INFECTIOUS DERMATITIS

CANDIDIASIS (MONILIASIS)

DESCRIPTION

The yeastlike fungus *Candida albicans* (formerly called *Monilia albicans*) is commonly present among the vaginal microorganisms of healthy women and may infect the mouths of infants during birth. Oral lesions (thrush) result and appear as white patches on the tongue, soft palate, and mucous membranes. These lesions resemble milk curds but cannot be rubbed off without revealing reddened areas. Untreated thrush can be transmitted through the gastrointestinal (GI) tract to produce a severe diaper dermatitis characterized by fiery red, sharply demarcated, raw, moist lesions with peripheral islet lesions, that do not respond to usual methods of treatment for diaper rash (see Figure 23-6). Older infants can develop *Candida* infections if the organism is transmitted to them by infected persons or if some systemic condition (diabetes mellitus, for example, or disturbance of the normal microorganism ecology following a course of antibiotics) causes overgrowth of *Candida*.

PREVENTION

Health Promotion

No preventive measures are known. The causative organism is part of the normal flora of healthy people.

Population at Risk

1. Overgrowth of *Candida* occurs
   a. In people who lack competitive flora to keep the *Candida* population down (e.g., neonates and people whose bacteria have been diminished by antibiotics, to which *Candida* is not sensitive).

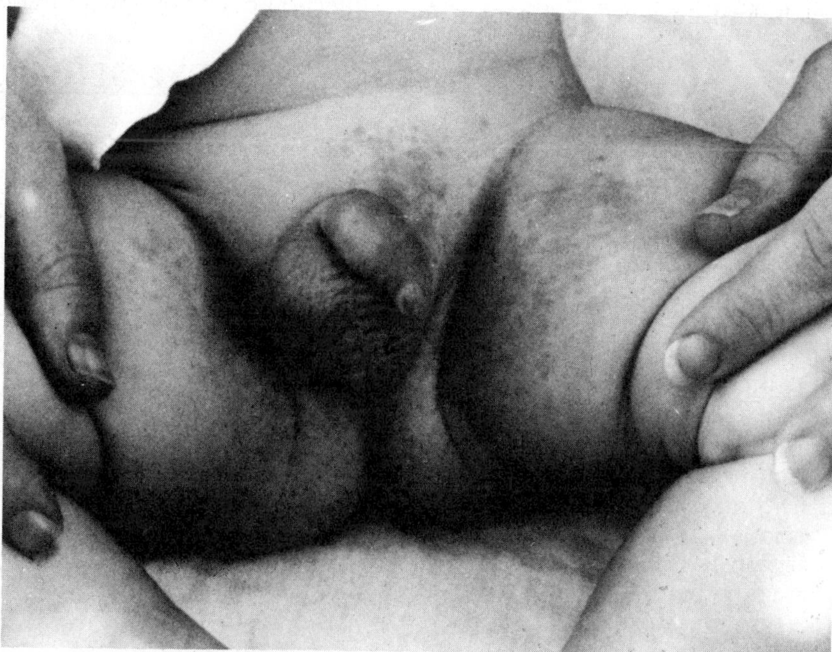

Figure 23-6 Early monilial diaper rash. Islet lesions at the periphery of the confluent, bright red rash are typical. Note the presence of the rash mainly in the body folds, which distinguishes it from a contact type of diaper dermatitis.

b. In those whose body chemistry has been altered in a way that supports *Candida*, notably diabetics and women who take birth control pills.
c. In people with immune deficiency diseases.
d. In people who are debilitated.

Screening

None.

ASSESSMENT

Health History

1. Does infected child or caretaker have diabetes mellitus? (Diabetics are prone to *Candida* infections, which can then be transmitted).
2. Has patient undergone a recent course of antibiotics?
3. Has there been known recent exposure to other children or adults with candidiasis? (Thrush is easily transmitted in newborn nurseries or other infant care group settings).

Physical Assessment

1. Inspect for the white lesions in the mouth and the perineal lesions described above.
2. Assess for indications of immunodeficiency (see Immunoglobulin Deficiency in Chapter 18).

Diagnostic Tests

1. Sabouraud's medium culture (of limited value due to 7- to 10-day wait for results).
2. Potassium hydroxide preparation and Wright's stain and microscopic examination provide immediate confirmation.

NURSING DIAGNOSES: ACTUAL OR POTENTIAL

1. Loss of skin integrity due to infection of oral mucous membranes and skin of diaper area.
2. Risk of secondary bacterial infection in diaper region secondary to skin breakdown.
3. Nutritional deficit: decreased intake secondary to mouth lesions.
4. Risk of transmission to other babies and to nipples of nursing mother.

EXPECTED OUTCOMES

1. Lesions will clear; secondary infection and eating problem will thereby be eliminated.
2. Infection will not spread to others.

INTERVENTIONS

1. Nystatin oral suspension is used for oral lesions, nystatin cream or Mycolog cream for diaper area. Very mild cases of oral thrush may respond to $\frac{1}{8}$ tsp. baking soda in $\frac{1}{2}$ cup water swabbed on oral lesions after each feeding.
2. Expose diaper area to air; do not use rubber pants or disposable diapers.
3. Wash nipples, pacifier, and toys thoroughly; isolate toys and bottles from other children. Insist on careful hand washing by all caretakers.
4. The mother breastfeeding an infant with thrush should apply baking soda solution, nystatin, or Mycolog to nipples after each feeding.
5. Treat any underlying disorder, such as diabetes, monilial vaginitis of the mother, or immune system deficiency of child.
6. Lesions not responding well to above-named drugs may be treated with gentian violet.

EVALUATION

Outcome Criteria

1. Lesions are eliminated in 1 week.
2. Infection does not spread to other persons.

IMPETIGO PYODERMA

DESCRIPTION

Impetigo is an infectious skin disorder caused by streptococci or staphylococci and characterized by pruritus, vesicles, and pustules that weep and develop thick, yellowish crusts. The initial lesions develop adjacent satellite lesions and spread (see Figure 23-7). Impetigo follows some interruption in skin integrity, commonly scabies or insect bites that have been scratched. Besides being a progressive, annoying, contagious disorder that predisposes to other bacterial infections and frequently carries some degree of social stigma, impetigo is important because it places the child at risk for acute glomerulonephritis (a sequela of streptococcal infections).

PREVENTION

Health promotion

Prevent pruritic skin irritations and minor skin breaks insofar as possible (poison ivy, insect

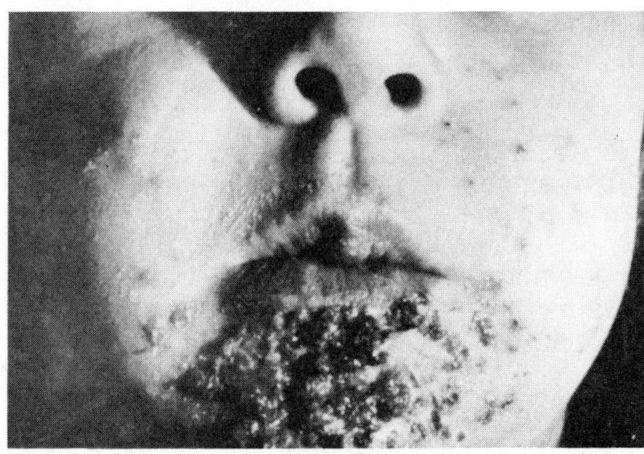

Figure 23-7 Impetigo. Note crusting and developing satellite lesions spreading out from the parent lesion. (From Stewart, W. D., Danto, J. L., and Maddin, S.: *Dermatology: Diagnosis and Treatment of Cutaneous Disorders*, 4th ed., C. V. Mosby, St. Louis, 1978.)

bites, etc.); cleanse and apply antiseptic to abrasions and lacerations; discourage scratching.

Population at Risk

Everyone, especially children who are often exposed to biting insects. Impetigo is highly contagious and readily infects siblings and playmates of infected children.

Screening

None.

ASSESSMENT

Health History

1. History of insect bite at site of lesion.
2. Recent contact with another person who has a suspicious lesion.

Physical Assessment

Inspect skin for characteristic lesion (see Description, above, and Figure 23-7).

Diagnostic Tests

None.

NURSING DIAGNOSES: ACTUAL OR POTENTIAL

1. Loss of skin integrity: open lesion secondary to infection.
2. Risk of scarring unless adequate treatment is imposed.
3. Altered self-concept and altered social interaction associated with disfiguring lesion.
4. Risk of transmitting infection to other sites and other people due to high degree of communicability of impetigo.
5. Risk of acute glomerulonephritis as a sequela to streptococcal infection.

EXPECTED OUTCOMES

1. Lesions will heal without permanent scarring.
2. Self-esteem and social development will not be damaged.
3. Infection will not spread.

INTERVENTIONS

1. Culture lesions to identify organism and sensitivity.
2. Treat with appropriate antibiotic. Child may return to school 48 hours after oral antibiotic is begun.
3. Cut child's fingernails to discourage scratching.
4. Clean lesions thoroughly with soap and water, and apply bacitracin. Instruct family so they will be able to provide this treatment at home.
5. Antihistamines may be used for itching.
6. If child or parent is embarrassed about lesions, reassure that this bacterial infection can happen to anyone, that the offending organism commonly comes from one's own nose or other orifice (Koblenzer, 1978), that the infection is not readily transmitted after 48 hours of antibiotic therapy, and that cure is expected to be quick and complete.
7. Identify and treat impetigo in siblings or other contacts.
8. Instruct family in hygienic measures to avoid transmitting infection from lesion to other body sites (hand washing, avoidance of cross-contamination, cleaning of tub or basin after cleansing lesions, etc.).
9. Instruct family to recognize and immediately report signs of glomerulonephritis if streptococcus is the infecting organism (dark urine, puffy eyes).

EVALUATION

Outcome Criteria

1. Treatment regimen is followed; lesions begin to clear within 2 to 4 days.

2. Spread to other sites is prevented; spread to other people is avoided or promptly treated.
3. Glomerulonephritis, if it occurs, is promptly recognized and treated. (Acute glomerulonephritis is discussed further in Chapter 21.)

HERPES SIMPLEX TYPE 1

DESCRIPTION

The herpes simplex type 1 inflammation is caused by the herpesvirus hominis. The incubation period is 3 to 5 days. Vesicular lesions occur on the mucous membranes and skin. Acute gingivostomatitis usually presents with soreness of the mouth and salivation, fever, and malaise, and lasts 1 to 3 weeks. Vesicles break, then grayish ulcerations form. The gums appear inflamed and swollen, and they bleed. The submandibular lymph nodes are enlarged. Factors promiting recurrence are stress, physical trauma, sunlight, and fever. Vesicles and ulcers often recur around the vermilion border of lips. Herpes is chronically recurrent throughout life.

PREVENTION

Health Promotion

Avoid contact with infected persons (active lesions).

Population at Risk

Everyone. Herpetic stomatitis is most common in children ages 1 to 4 years.

Screening

None.

ASSESSMENT

Health History

1. History of recent exposure to someone with cold sores or other herpesvirus type 1 skin lesions.
2. History of previous flare-ups of cold sores (recurrence is unusual in children).

Physical Assessment

Inspect mouth and skin for characteristic lesions—a group of vesicles or vesicopapules with the surrounding skin showing edema, tenderness, and erythema.

Diagnostic Tests

None.

NURSING DIAGNOSES: ACTUAL OR POTENTIAL

1. Loss of skin integrity due to virus invasion.
2. Alteration in comfort: pain associated with lesions.
3. Alteration in nutrition and hydration: decreased intake due to painful oral lesions.
4. Alteration in body temperature: fever secondary to viral infection.
5. Risk of spreading infection to other people.

EXPECTED OUTCOMES

1. Lesions will heal.
2. Pain will be controlled.
3. Body weight and fluid balance will be maintained.
4. Fever will be controlled.
5. Infection will not spread to others.

INTERVENTIONS

1. Spontaneous healing takes place in 5 to 7 days; supportive measures (hydration, prevention of secondary infection) assist recovery.
2. Relieve pain and fever with acetaminophen.
3. Apply topical anesthetics (viscous lidocaine) to lips and mouth to decrease discomfort and consequently increase fluid intake.
4. Give mouth washes with a tetracycline base to prevent secondary infections.
5. Offer frequent small meals of preferred, soft, nonacid foods; offer nonacid liquids (food acids are not harmful but induce pain).
6. Soak skin lesion to remove thick crust.
7. Apply zinc oxide ointment to skin lesion.
8. Isolate from persons with burns or eczema. Instruct family to avoid spreading infection by kissing while mouth lesions are active.

EVALUATION

Outcome Criteria

1. Lesions clear in 5 to 7 days.
2. Child is afebrile and free of pain.
3. Weight and hydration are maintained.
4. Infection does not spread to other people.

HERPES ZOSTER (SHINGLES)

DESCRIPTION

Shingles is a painful infection of the nerve structure. It is caused by the same virus that causes chickenpox. There is vesicular eruption unilaterally along the dermatomes of the infected nerve root, which is thought to be a secondary manifestation of infection by the virus. Herpes zoster often occurs in newborns 2 or 3 weeks of age whose mothers were exposed. Children who are not immune to chickenpox may develop it after exposure to someone with herpes zoster, and adults can develop shingles after contact with a child with chickenpox. *Children receiving corticosteroids or immunosuppressive therapy (e.g., children with rheumatoid arthritis, leukemia, or nephrosis) are highly susceptible to the virus of chickenpox and herpes zoster, and the infection can be fatal for them.*

SLAPPED CHEEK SYNDROME (FIFTH DISEASE, ERYTHEMA INFECTIOSUM)

DESCRIPTION

This mild, self-limiting infection is caused by a filtrable virus. The incubation period is 7 to 28 days. It is often confused with atypical measles, drug rashes, and lupus erythematosus.

PREVENTION

Health Promotion

No prevention is known; the infection is presumably spread by droplets.

Population at Risk

1. School children (epidemics are not rare).
2. Toddlers and preschoolers.
3. Family members (including adults) of infected children.

Screening

None.

ASSESSMENT

Health History

1. Child is active and apparently healthy before the appearance of an intensely flushed face ("slapped cheeks").
2. Symptoms are absent or mild (headache, coryza, pharyngitis, and GI upset).

Physical Assessment

1. Erythematous, coalescent, maculopapular rash on malar prominences lasts 1 to 4 days.
2. About a week later, a coalescent, then ribbonlike rash forms on buttocks, thighs, arms, chest, abdomen, and neck. Rash may be pruritic.
3. Rash disappears and returns, often brought on by bathing, exercise, or emotion.

Diagnostic Tests

None.

NURSING DIAGNOSIS: ACTUAL OR POTENTIAL

Knowledge deficit about the course of the illness.

EXPECTED OUTCOMES

Child, if old enough, and parents will be adequately informed about the illness.

INTERVENTIONS

1. Teach family.
   a. There is no treatment for this infection; it must run its course.
   b. Prognosis is excellent: the condition resolves spontaneously and without complications, although transient rash may be noticeable for a few weeks.
   c. No isolation is necessary.

EVALUATION

Outcome Criteria

Child, if old enough, and parents demonstrate understanding of the disease course and prognosis.

PITYRIASIS ROSEA

DESCRIPTION

This acute but mild and self-limiting inflammatory disease is probably of viral origin. Involvement is limited to the skin. A prodromal period of slight malaise can precede the first sign of skin eruption, the so-called herald patch, a pink to brown round or oval lesion with a slightly raised border and a fine, branny scale at its edges. The herald patch may become large (10 cm) and resembles ringworm. Several days after the appearance of the herald patch, a generalized, symmetrical, pink papular rash appears on the trunk and proximal limbs; other parts of the body are sometimes involved. Itching can be minimal or intense. The disease resolves spontaneously, but the rash may last for several weeks or a few months. There are no sequelae.

PREVENTION

Health Promotion

No preventive measures are known.

Population at Risk

Anyone, but particularly school-age children and adults approximately 20 to 40 years old.

Screening

None.

ASSESSMENT

Health History

1. Child usually is asymptomatic except for rash. Herald patch may have gone unnoticed.
2. Possible history of slight sore throat or malaise.
3. History of recent exposure to a person with the disease.

Physical Assessment

Inspect skin for characteristic eruption (see Description, above).

Diagnostic Tests

None.

NURSING DIAGNOSES: ACTUAL OR POTENTIAL

1. Knowledge deficit about nature, course, and prognosis of infection.
2. Alteration in comfort: discomfort associated with itching.
3. Risk of skin breakdown and secondary infection due to scratching.

EXPECTED OUTCOMES

1. Parents (and child if old enough) will understand that the disease has no medical significance and will resolve in several weeks without treatment.
2. Itching, if present, will be resolved.
3. Secondary infection will not occur.

INTERVENTIONS

1. Teach child and family as described in Expected Outcomes section, above.
2. An antihistamine, such as Benadryl, is useful to reduce itching. Discourage hot baths; they increase itching. Decreased scratching will decrease danger of secondary infection.
3. Sunlight tends to hasten resolution of the disease.

EVALUATION

Outcome Criteria

1. Itching is minimal or absent.
2. Secondary infection is absent.
3. Rash clears in 2 to 6 weeks.

TINEA CAPITIS (RINGWORM OF THE SCALP)

DESCRIPTION

See Table 23-3.

PREVENTION

Health Promotion

Good personal hygiene and avoidance of infected people, pets, and fomites (combs, hats, etc.).

Population at Risk

1. School-age children, primarily.
2. Family members of infected school-age children.
3. People who live in overcrowded housing.
4. People whose hygiene is poor.
5. Boys are infected more often than girls.

Screening

None.

ASSESSMENT

Health History

History of exposure to infected person or animal.

TABLE 23-3 COMMON FUNGAL INFECTIONS

Tinea capitis (ringworm of the scalp)	Ringworm of the scalp is caused by several species of fungi. Some (*Microsporum audouini* and *Trichophyton tonsurans*) are human-borne and, hence, can pass from child to child, and some (*M. canis*) can be contracted from infected cats and dogs. Lesions consist of rounded, slightly reddened, scaly patches of alopecia and broken hair shafts. Boggy, crusted lesions (kerions) may also be present.
Tinea corporis, tinea circinata (body ringworm)	Body ringworm is a fungal infection usually produced by *M. canis*. It is carried by infected cats and dogs and produces characteristic lesions, generally on the face, hands, or arms. The lesion is a raised, erythematous, scaly patch that assumes a ringlike shape as it spreads outward and clears up in the center. Mild itching is common.
Tinea pedis (athlete's foot)	This familiar fungal infection of the feet (occasionally the hands) is characterized by itching, papules, blisters, scaling, and fissures between the toes or on the soles and sides of the feet. Fungal infections of the nails may be associated. It is most commonly seen in postpubertal males.

Physical Assessment

Characteristic lesion (see Table 23-3) on the scalp.

Diagnostic Tests

1. Wood's lamp (black light) examinations show fluorescence of infected hair shafts, except when *T. tonsurans* is the infecting agent.
2. Microscopic examination using potassium hydroxide or Wright's stain confirms the diagnosis.

NURSING DIAGNOSES: ACTUAL OR POTENTIAL

1. Impaired self-concept due to stigma associated with the infection and to embarrassment over the treatment.
2. Noncompliance due to knowledge deficit (medication must be continued for several weeks, even after symptoms abate).
3. Risk of transmitting the infection to other people or of reinfection from an untreated source.
4. Risk of side effects of treatment medication.

EXPECTED OUTCOMES

1. Child's self-esteem will be maintained.
2. Recommended treatment regimen will be carried to completion; lesions will resolve.
3. Tinea will not spread to others.
4. Side effects, if they occur, will be promptly recognized and reported.

INTERVENTIONS

1. Promote self-esteem by explaining that anyone can become infected and that the hair will regrow, and recovery is expected to be complete if treatment is carried out.
2. Explain treatment to family and encourage them in carrying out their parts of therapy.
3. Clip hair short around the lesion.
4. Scrub scalp with nonfat synthetic soap every day.
5. Administer a topical antifungal agent as prescribed.
6. Give oral griseofulvin as prescribed, sometimes for 4 to 6 weeks.
   a. Instruct family to observe for side effects and to report them promptly: GI upsets, headache, urticaria.
7. Inspect household members and pets, and treat if infected.
8. Teach family to avoid sharing of hats, combs, brushes, wigs, towels, and so forth.
9. Provide school authorities and other involved persons with accurate information about the risk of contagion for the particular fungus involved.

EVALUATION

Outcome Criteria

1. Child evidences positive self-esteem; social interaction is normal for developmental level (see Chapter 4).
2. Family continues recommended treatment.

3. Spread of infection to other people is avoided.
4. Side effects of drug, if they occur, are quickly recognized and reported.
5. Infection responds to treatment after 3 to 4 weeks.

Reevaluation and Follow-up

Children on long-term griseofulvin or those who develop side effects should have periodic lab work to screen for leukopenia.

TINEA CORPORIS (TINEA CIRCINATA, BODY RINGWORM)

DESCRIPTION

See Table 23-3.

HEALTH PROMOTION

See *Tinea Capitis*, above.

ASSESSMENT

Health History

History of exposure to infected person or animal.

Physical Assessment

Characteristic lesion (see Table 23-3).

Diagnostic Tests

1. Direct microscopy (KOH preparation).
2. Culture.

NURSING DIAGNOSES: ACTUAL OR POTENTIAL

1. Alteration in comfort: discomfort associated with pruritus.
2. Risk of secondary infection due to loss of skin integrity associated with lesions and with scratching.
3. Risk of transmission of infection to others and of reinfection from untreated source.
4. Risk of side effects of treatment medication.

EXPECTED OUTCOMES

1. Lesions will resolve.
2. Secondary infection will be prevented.
3. Infection will not spread to others.
4. Infected family members and pets will be identified and treated.
5. Side effects of medication, if they occur, will be promptly recognized and reported.

INTERVENTIONS

1. Scrub lesions with soap and water.
2. Administer topical and systemic (oral) antifungal medications as prescribed.
3. Discourage scratching; trim child's fingernails short.
4. Identify and treat infected household members and pets.
5. Instruct family in preventive hygiene: avoidance of clothing exchange between infected child and other family members without laundering, provision of separate bed for infected child, and soon.
6. Instruct family to observe for and immediately reported signs of side effects of griseofulvin: GI upsets, headache, urticaria.

EVALUATION

Outcome Criteria

1. Lesions clear in 2 to 3 weeks.
2. Child does not develop secondary skin infection.
3. Tinea does not spread to others.
4. Infected pets and household members are treated.
5. Drug side effects, if any, are promptly identified and reported.

TINEA PEDIS (ATHLETE'S FOOT)

DESCRIPTION

See Table 23-3.

PREVENTION

Health Promotion

1. Avoid contact with the fungus: wear rubber or wooden sandals at public showers and public swimming pools.
2. Discourage growth of fungus.
   a. Wear stockings to absorb moisture and help aerate shoes.
   b. Dry thoroughly between toes after bathing.

Population at Risk

Adolescents and adults, primarily; males more often than females.

Screening

None.

ASSESSMENT

Health History

1. Use of public pools or locker rooms.
2. History of previous infection with athlete's foot.

Physical Assessment

Inspect interdigital spaces for characteristic lesions (see Table 23-3).

Diagnostic Tests

1. Direct microscopy.
2. Culture.

NURSING DIAGNOSES: ACTUAL OR POTENTIAL

1. Alteration in comfort: discomfort associated with itching and burning.
2. Risk of secondary infection due to loss of skin integrity.
3. Risk of transmission to others and of reinfection.

EXPECTED OUTCOMES

1. Lesions will clear; itching will stop.
2. Secondary bacterial infection will be prevented.
3. Adolescent will not infect others.
4. Adolescent will take precautions against reinfection.

INTERVENTIONS

1. Soak with Burow's solution for 20 minutes twice a day, then apply antifungal agents as prescribed; oral griseofulvin may also be prescribed (if so, note precautions and instruct client).
2. Instruct client in methods of preventing transmission and reinfection (see Prevention, above).

EVALUATION

Outcome Criteria

1. Infection heals in 4 weeks.
2. Spread to others is prevented.
3. Adolescent is exercising preventive methods to avoid reinfection.

PEDICULOSIS (LICE)

DESCRIPTION

Infestation by lice is readily transmissible to others by personal contact or by contact with articles that harbor the lice or their eggs (nits). Lice are bloodsuckers, and their bites are intensely pruritic. There are three types of louse infestation, as described in Table 23-4. Lice are vectors for typhus.

PREVENTION

Health Promotion

1. Lice are associated with poor hygiene and overcrowding.
   a. Body lice are transmitted in clothing and bedding.
   b. Head lice are transmitted by combs, caps, and other such fomites, as well as by close contact (e.g., sharing a bed).
   c. Pubic lice are spread primarily by sexual contact but also by clothing or bedding.

Population at Risk

1. All people are susceptible.
2. Public lice infest mainly adolescents and young adults.

Screening

None.

ASSESSMENT

Health History

1. History of recent exposure to an infected person.
2. Complaints of itching.

Physical Assessment

1. Inspect for lice, nits, and macular rash, possibly with excoriation and secondary infection from scratching.
   a. Lice are oval and gray, about 2–4 mm long, wingless, and six-legged.
   b. Nits (eggs) are white, oval, translucent, just visible to the unaided eye (0.5 mm long), and are firmly attached to the hair shafts near the skin or to clothing. Nits su-

TABLE 23-4 THE THREE TYPES OF PEDICULOSIS

Type and Site of Infestation	Distinguishing Characteristics
Pediculosis corporis (body lice)	Nits (that resemble dandruff) and lice are found in the clothing but seldom on the body. The bite produces erythematous macules with red or slate-colored petechial centers, most common on the upper back and in areas where clothes are tight. Itching is intense, and long scratch marks are usually present.
Pediculosis capitis (head lice)	These lice primarily infest the scalp but on occasion are found in the brows, lashes, beard, or pubic hair. As the lice themselves are highly mobile and short-lived, they are seldom seen. The white nits are found clinging to hair shafts, particularly in the occipital region and over the ears; nits resemble dandruff but are difficult to dislodge. Itching is severe.
Pediculosis pubis (crabs)	These short, broad, crab-shaped lice infest the public hair and, occasionally, axillae, beards, or eyelashes. Their bites are found as red or slate-colored macules in the hairy region and on abdomen, thighs, or upper arms. Itching is intense. Nits cling to hair shafts.

perficially resemble dandruff, but they cannot be readily dislodged. Low power microscopic examination aids in their identification.

c. Louse bites contain a punctuate hemorrhagic center that is initially red but sometimes turns slate colored from the chemical action of the animal's saliva on bilirubin.

Diagnostic Tests

None.

NURSING DIAGNOSES: ACTUAL OR POTENTIAL

1. Alteration in comfort: intense itching, burning, and pain associated with insect bites.
2. Loss of skin integrity secondary to scratching.
3. Risk of secondary infection due to skin breaks.
4. Risk of transmission to others.

EXPECTED OUTCOMES

1. Nits and lice will be destroyed and removed; itching will cease.
2. Skin lesions will clear.
3. Secondary infection will be avoided or treated.
4. Others will not become infected; those already infected will be identified and treated.

INTERVENTIONS

1. Have patient bathe and wash both underclothing and outer clothing.
2. Nits must be manually removed with a fine-tooth comb.
3. Use benzyl benzoate emulsion or gamma benzene hexachloride (Kwell) lotion, cream, or shampoo.
4. Dust personal articles and clothing with DDT after boiling.
5. Use calamine lotion for itching.
6. All family members and close contacts should be treated.

EVALUATION

Outcome Criteria

1. Lice are killed; rash clears without secondary infection.
2. Client or family describes effective ways to prevent spread of infection to others.
3. Household members and other intimates are examined and, if infected, are treated.

SCABIES ("ITCH")

DESCRIPTION

Scabies is a rash caused by a tiny crab-shaped mite, *Sarcoptes scabiei*, the itch mite. Transmission of scabies is by direct skin contact and, rarely, by contaminated bedding and undergarments. Pruritus, which is intense, is usually worse at night. The primary lesion is a burrow, made in the skin, by the impregnated female mite, in which she lays her eggs.

PREVENTION

Health Promotion

Avoidance of skin contact with persons known to have scabies.

Population at Risk

Persons of all ages.

Screening

None.

ASSESSMENT

Health History

1. History of exposure to someone with scabies.
2. Severe itching of skin lesions.

Physical Assessment

1. The mite's burrow is a grayish brown, threadlike, often tortuous line or dotted line several millimeters long. It is often difficult to see with the naked eye. Inflammation results in the formation of papules, vesicles, excoriation, and crusting.
2. Lesions are distributed in the interspaces of the fingers, the flexor surfaces of the wrists, the nipples of postpubertal females, the belt line, buttocks, and male genitalia. In infants and children the head, neck, and legs are commonly involved.

Diagnostic Tests

1. Diagnosis is made by opening a burrow with a sewing needle and examining it in mineral oil under low-power magnification or with a lens in order to identify the mite or ova.
2. Microscopic examination of skin scrapings may reveal the mite or her eggs.

NURSING DIAGNOSES: ACTUAL OR POTENTIAL

1. Alteration in comfort: severe itching secondary to intradermal mites.
2. Loss of skin integrity secondary to scratching and to mite infestation and local reaction to the mite.
3. Risk of secondary infection due to loss of skin integrity.
4. Risk of transmission to others.

EXPECTED OUTCOMES

1. Offending organism will be destroyed.
2. Irritated skin will be cleaned and soothed; client will experience relief of itching.
3. Secondary infection will be prevented or treated.
4. Infection will not spread to others; contacts already infected will be identified and treated.

INTERVENTIONS

1. Have client bathe thoroughly with soap and water.
2. Apply gamma benzene hexachloride (Kwell) cream or lotion, benzyl benzoate lotion, or crotamiton (Eurax) cream or lotion *strictly* according to manufacturer's directions.
3. Triamcinolone ointment may be prescribed for pruritus.
4. Discourage scratching; keep child's fingernails clipped short.
5. Clothing that the client has worn should be washed in hot water and ironed to kill the mites.
6. Teach family fundamental hygiene for preventing further transmission (avoidance of sharing clothes until they have been laundered and ironed, avoidance of unnecessary skin contact with infected person, importance of handwashing, etc.).
7. Examine and treat household members, playmates, and other close contacts.

EVALUATION

Outcome Criteria

1. Lesions respond to treatment in 1 or 2 weeks.
2. Secondary infection is prevented or adequately treated.
3. Spread of infection to others is prevented or minimized; contacts are treated as necessary.

REFERENCES

Kahn, G.: "Seborrheic Dermatitis," in R. Hoekelman, S. Blatman, P. Brunell, et al. (eds.), *Principles of Pediatrics: Health Care of the Young*, McGraw-Hill, New York, 1978, p. 1360.

Koblenzer, P. J.: "Infections of the Skin," in R. Hoekelman, S. Blatman, P. Brunell, et al. (eds.), *Principles of Pediatrics: Health Care of the Young*, McGraw-Hill, New York, 1978, p. 1370.

Leyden, J.: "Diaper Dermatitis," in S. Maddin (ed.), *Current Dermatologic Therapy*, W. B. Saunders, Philadelphia, 1982.

Stuart, B. H.: "Tetracycline-associated Intracranial Hypertension in an Adolescent: A Complication of Systemic Acne Therapy," *Journal of Pediatrics* **92**(4):679, April 1978.

BIBLIOGRAPHY

Campbell, C.: *"Integument," Nursing Diagnosis and Intervention in Nursing Practice,* John Wiley, New York, 1978, Chapter 19. This includes nursing goals and interventions that are helpful once the diagnosis has been made.

Chalker, D. K., and Smith, J. G.: "Acne Vulgaris: Causes and Preferred Regimens", *Medical Times,* June 1977, p. 57. This article includes explanations and illustrations of treatment regimens and useful bibliography.

Chow, M. P., Durand, B. A., Feldman, M., and Mills, M. A.: *Handbook of Pediatric Primary Care,* John Wiley, New York, 1979, p. 457. This provides a bibliography and quick reference for treatment.

Fitzpatrick, T. B., Arndt, K. A., Clark, W. H., et al.: *Update One: Dermatology in General Medicine,* McGraw-Hill, New York, 1971. An in-depth resource on skin disorders.

Jacobs, A. H. (ed.), "Symposium of Pediatric Dermatology," *Pediatric Clinics of North America* **25**(2), May 1978, pp. 191–386. Common and exotic skin disorders of childhood.

Kopf, A. W., et al., *Atlas of Tumors of the Skin*, W. B. Saunders, Philadelphia, 1978. This atlas contains color photographs listed alphabetically to assist in identifying skin tumors.

Larrow, L.: "Port Wine Stain Hemangiomas," *American Journal of Nursing* **82**(5):786, May 1982. This article deals with nursing care related to laser treatment.

Maddin, S. (ed.): *Current Dermatologic Therapy*, W. B. Saunders, Philadelphia, 1982. This comprehensive text includes descriptions and treatments for common skin conditions and references for further study.

Malkiewicz, J.: "The Integumentary System," *RN* **44**(12):55, December 1981. This article discusses assessment of the skin, including history.

O'Keen, M. R., and Edelstein, L. M.: *Gross and Microscopic Pathology of the Skin* Vols. 1 and 2, Dermatolopathology Foundation Press, Boston, MA, 1976. This provides pictorial documentation of skin findings, which can be quite helpful in identifying skin problems.

Siegel, S. C., Rachelefsky, G., and Katz, R. M.: "Pharmacologic Management of Pediatric Allergic Disorders," *Current Problems in Pediatrics,* **9**(10):60, August 1979. This discusses eczema in detail, including problems, management, and treatment rationale.

Whaley, L. F., and Wong, D. L.: *Nursing Care of Infants and Children,* C. V. Mosby, St. Louis, 1979, p. 657. This describes children's skin problems and nursing care for them; it also includes diagrams helpful for client teaching.

24

Communicable Diseases

Helen L. Farrell

INFECTIONS

DIPHTHERIA

DESCRIPTION

Diphtheria is an acute respiratory disorder caused by *Corynebacterium diphtheriae*. The infection usually occurs in late autumn, winter, and spring. It is most common in children from 1 to 5 years of age; the incidence is increasing in older children and adults. Diphtheria can be seen in crowded areas, such as migrant farm camps and city slum areas. The major sources of the infection are asymptomatic carriers and people who are incubating the disease. The incubation period is 2 to 4 days. Diphtheria is transmitted by direct contact with an infected person or by indirect contact with contaminated articles. Medical treatment includes antibiotics and diphtheria antitoxin. (Caution: persons must be tested for sensitivity to horse serum before antitoxin is administered.) Mortality is low and can be predicted by (1) virulence of the organism, (2) severity of the disease and portion of the respiratory tract affected, (3) immunization status of the client, and (4) quality of nursing care. Complications account for the greatest cause of mortality and morbidity.

PREVENTION

Health Promotion

1. Begin immunization at 2 months of age (see Tables 24-1 and 24-2, and Figure 24-1.)
2. Educational measures to inform the public about the necessity and advantages of active immunization.

Population at Risk

1. Newborns whose mothers have diminished immunity (see Table 24-3).
2. Unimmunized children.

Screening

1. Historically, the Schick test was used to define the susceptibility of populations as well as individuals. The use of the Schick test has diminished since the decline of diphtheria and the advent of a safe, reliable immunizing agent.
2. Immunization history should be determined at the time of well-child visits and immunizations given as necessary.

ASSESSMENT

Health History

1. Exposure to a client with diphtheria or to a carrier.
2. No history of previous immunization to diphtheria.

Physical Assessment

Manifestations: determined by the part of the respiratory tract affected by the disease.

1. Nasal diphtheria.
   a. Rhinorrhea.
      (1) Nasal discharge may be thick and purulent or serosanguineous.
      (2) There is a foul odor to discharge.
      (3) Discharge may excoriate the upper lip.
   b. Nasal diphtheria accounts for a significant

TABLE 24-1 RECOMMENDED SCHEDULE FOR ACTIVE IMMUNIZATION OF NORMAL INFANTS AND CHILDREN

Recommended Age	Vaccine(s)	Comments
2 mo	DTP,[a] OPV[b]	Can be initiated earlier in areas of high endemicity
4 mo	DTP, OPV	2-mo interval desired for OPV to avoid interference
6 mo	DTP (OPV)	OPV optional for areas where polio might be imported (e.g., some areas of southwest United States)
12 mo	Tuberculin test[c]	May be given simultaneously with MMR at 15 mo
15 mo	Measles, mumps, rubella (MMR)[d]	MMR preferred to single vaccines
18 mo	DTP, OPV	Consider as part of primary series—DTP essential
4–6 yr[e]	DTP, OPV	
15–16 yr	Td[f]	Repeat every 10 years for lifetime

SOURCE: *Report of the Committee on Infectious Diseases*, 19th ed.; copyright American Academy of Pediatrics, 1982.

AUTHOR'S NOTE: Immunization schedule for premature infants. The current recommendation is that prematurely born babies be immunized at the same chronological age (disregarding gestational age) as other infants *except* that hospitalized infants should not receive trivalent OPV because of the possibility that virus shed in the stool may create a hazard to other infants in the nursery (Fulginiti, 1982).

[a] DTP—Diphtheria and tetanus toxoids with pertussis vaccine.

[b] OPV—Oral, attenuated poliovirus vaccine contains poliovirus types 1, 2 and 3.

[c] Tuberculin test—Mantoux (intradermal PPD) preferred. Frequency of tests depends on local epidemiology. The Committee recommends annual or biennial testing unless local circumstances dictate less frequent or no testing.

[d] MMR—Live measles, mumps, and rubella viruses in a combined vaccine

[e] Up to the seventh birthday.

[f] Td—Adult tetanus toxoid (full dose) and diphtheria toxoid (reduced dose) in combination.

For all products used, consult manufacturer's brochure for instructions for storage, handling, and administration. Biologics prepared by different manufacturers may vary, and those of the same manufacturer may change from time to time. The package insert should be followed for a specific product.

spread of the disease due to its mild signs and symptoms.

c. A membrane may be present on the nasal septum.

2. Pharyngeal diphtheria.
   a. Sore throat.
   b. Headache.
   c. Malaise.
   d. Low-grade fever.
   e. Rapid pulse that is out of proportion to the fever.
   f. Foul odor to breath.
   g. A membrane forms and may extend to the nose and larynx.
   h. Cervical lymph nodes may be enlarged and tender.
   i. Edema may be present in the neck ("bull neck").
3. Laryngeal diphtheria.
   a. The laryngeal form occurs as a downward extension of pharyngeal diphtheria.
   b. Breathing is noisy, and there is progressive stridor.
   c. Client has harsh cough.

TABLE 24-2 RECOMMENDED IMMUNIZATION SCHEDULES FOR INFANTS AND CHILDREN NOT INITIALLY IMMUNIZED AT USUAL RECOMMENDED TIMES IN EARLY INFANCY

	Recommended Schedules				
		Alternatives			
Timing	**Preferred Schedule**	**#1[a]**	**#2[b]**	**#3[c]**	**Comments**
First visit	DTP[d] #1, OPV[e] #1, Tuberculin test (PPD)[f]	MMR[a], PPD	DTP #1, OPV #1, PPD	DTP #1, OPV #1, MMR, PPD	MMR should be given no younger than 15 mo old.
1 mo after first visit	MMR	DTP #1, OPV #1	MMR, DTP #2	DTP #2	
2 mo after first visit	DTP #2, OPV #2	—	DTP #3, OPV #2	DTP #3, OPV #2	—
3 mo after first visit	(DTP #3)	DTP #2, OPV #2	—	—	In preferred schedule, DTP #3 can be given if OPV #3 is not to be given until 10–16 mo.
4 mo after first visit	DTP #3 (OPV #3)	—	(OPV #3)	(OPV #3)	OPV #3 optional for areas of likely importation of polio (e.g., some southwestern states).
5 mo after first visit	—	DTP # 3 (OPV #3)	—	—	
10–16 mo after last dose	DTP #4, OPV #3 or OPV #4	DTP #4, OPV #3 or OPV #4	DTP #4, OPV #3 or OPV #4	DTP #4, OPV #3 or OPV #4	—
Preschool	DTP #5, OPV #4 or OPV #5	DTP #5, OPV #4 or OPV #5	DTP #5, OPV #4 or OPV #5	DTP #5, OPV #4 or OPV #5	Preschool dose not necessary if DTP #4 or #5 given after fourth birthday.
14–16 yr old	Td[h]	Td	Td	Td	Repeat every 10 yr.

SOURCE: *Report of the Committee on Infectious Diseases*, 19th ed.; copyright American Academy of Pediatrics, 1982.

[a] Alternative #1 can be used in those more than 15 months old if measles is occurring in the community.

[b] Alternative #2 allows for more rapid DTP immunization.

[c] Alternative #3 should be reserved for those whose access to medical care is compromised by poor compliance.

[d] DTP = Diphtheria and tetanus toxoids with pertussis vaccine.

[e] OPV = Oral, attenuated poliovirus vaccine contains types 1, 2, and 3.

[f] Tuberculin test = Mantoux (intradermal PPD) preferred. Frequency of tests depends on local epidemiology. The Committee recommends annual or biennial testing unless local circumstances dictate less frequent or no testing.

[g] MMR = Live measles, mumps, and rubella viruses in a combined vaccine.

[h] Td = Adult tetanus toxoid (full dose) and diphtheria toxoid (reduced dose) in combination.

For all products used, consult manufacturer's brochure for instructions for storage, handling, and administration. Biologics prepared by different manufacturers may vary, and those of the same manufacturer may change from time to time. The package insert should be followed for a specific product.

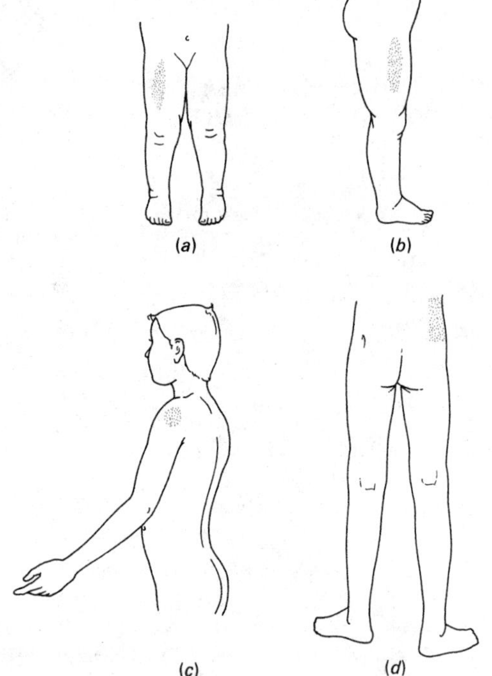

Figure 24-1 Recommended intramuscular injection sites in children under 6 years of age are (*a*) the middle third of the anterior thigh and (*b*) the middle third of the lateral thigh. For children 6 and over, (*c*) the central portion of the deltoid or (*d*) the upper outer quadrant of the buttock can be substituted. NOTE: DTP is given intramuscularly; MMR is given subcutaneously. The anterior or lateral thigh is the recommended subcutaneous injection site.

d. Hoarseness is present.
e. There are suprasternal and substernal retractions.
f. Cyanosis occurs as obstruction progresses.

Diagnostic Tests

Culture lesion for bacteriological examination.

NURSING DIAGNOSES: ACTUAL OR POTENTIAL

1. Respiratory dysfunction secondary to excessive secretions.
2. Impairment of skin integrity secondary to excessive secretions.
3. Alteration in food intake: anorexia secondary to sore throat, secretions, and odor.
4. Alteration in fluid balance: dehydration secondary to sore throat, fever, and excessive secretions.

EXPECTED OUTCOMES

1. Client will maintain patent airway.
2. Area around nose and mouth will be kept free of secretions, thus preventing risk of excoriation and secondary infection.
3. Normal weight will be maintained.
4. Normal fluid balance will be maintained.
5. No complications will develop.

INTERVENTIONS

1. Place client in isolation.
   a. Teach client and all visitors proper disposal of tissues.
   b. Teach client and/or visitors principles of communicability.
2. Keep airway clear by gentle suctioning.
3. Provide ice collar to minimize edema of neck.
4. Provide warm, moist air to relieve airway spasms and to aid in keeping secretions loose.
5. Apply lubricant to nose and upper lip to prevent excoriation.
6. Ventilate room, use room deodorant, and dispose of secretions promptly to minimize odor.
7. Oral hygiene, including the use of cleansing gargles, is necessary for cleanliness and comfort.
8. Offer fluids frequently.
9. Give client frequent, small meals of a consistency easy to swallow.
10. Maintain bed rest for acutely ill client.
11. Observe for complications.
    a. Monitor vital signs.
    b. Monitor amount of secretions.
    c. Observe for presence of edema.
    d. Observe for regurgitation through the nose.
    e. Be alert for evidence of palatal paralysis.
12. Notify physician immediately of signs of respiratory distress or other complications.
13. Administer medications as prescribed.
    a. Antitoxin may be given only after test for sensitivity to horse serum is accomplished.
    b. If horse serum allergy test is positive, desensitization must be done before antitoxin can be given.

EVALUATION

Outcome Criteria

1. Child maintains adequate oxygenation: no cyanosis, no severe respiratory distress.
2. There is no excoriation of nose or upper lip due to excessive secretion.
3. Adequate nutrition and fluid balance are maintained.

Complications

1. Pneumonia (see discussion in Chapter 20).
2. Atelectasis (see discussion in Chapter 20).
3. Cardiac failure (see discussion in Chapter 19).
4. Circulatory failure (see discussion in Chapter 19).
5. Nephritis (see discussion in Chapter 21).
6. Paralysis of palate, phrenic nerve, and ocular muscles.

Assessment

1. Nasal character to the voice.
2. Difficulty in swallowing.
3. Strabismus.
4. Ptosis.
5. Loss of power of accommodation.
6. Intercostal breathing.
7. High diaphragm and scaphoid abdomen.

Revised Outcomes

1. Child will maintain respiratory adequacy and nutrient and fluid intake.
2. Eyes will not be injured.
3. Other expected outcomes, as originally stated.
4. Goals for pneumonia, atelectasis, cardiac failure, circulatory failure, and nephritis are in chapters as noted above.

Interventions

1. Suction as needed.
2. Provide nourishment by tube feeding if unable to swallow.
3. Measure intake and output to ensure adequate hydration.
4. Monitor respirations and assist ventilation as necessary.
5. Protect eyes with eye patches if unable to blink.
6. Interventions for pneumonia, atelectasis, cardiac failure, circulatory failure, and nephritis can be found in chapters related to these conditions.

Reevaluation and Follow-up

1. Ability to swallow returns.
2. There is no regurgitation of fluids through the nose.
3. Fluid balance and nutritional status are maintained.
4. Ventilation is adequate, and normal breath sounds are heard upon asculation.
5. Blinking ability is maintained or restored.

TETANUS ("LOCKJAW")

DESCRIPTION

Tetanus is a life-threatening central nervous system disorder caused by *Clostridium tetani*. Tetanus occurs most often in months of outdoor activity. In the United States, the incidence is higher in the Southeast and among boys. Tetanus most frequently occurs in unimmunized persons and newborn infants of unimmunized mothers. The incubation period is 5 to 20 days, with an average of 10 days. The tetanus organism is introduced into the body during an injury. Puncture wounds, burns, and insect bites are the types of injuries by which the organism most frequently enters the body. The wound may be so slight as to go unnoticed. The organism is found in soil, water, and the intestinal tract of people and animals. For tetanus to develop there must be (1) contact with the organism, (2) anaerobic wound conditions, and (3) a susceptible host. Medical treatment includes tetanus antitoxin (but only after skin testing shows no hypersensitivity to serum), medications to control muscle spasm, antibiotics, and sometimes surgery to remove necrotic tissue. Tetanus immune globulin (TIG) may be given. In unimmunized persons the fatality rate varies from 35 to 90 percent. Prognosis is related to (1) the age of the client (it is poorest in newborns), (2) the number of days required for symptoms to appear (poorest with short incubation period), (3) the extent of muscle involvement, and (4) the degree of fever (prognosis is poor if fever exceeds 38.9°C, 102°F).

PREVENTION

Health Promotion

1. Active immunization with tetanus toxoid should begin in infancy.
2. Early and thorough cleansing of wounds, debridement of any necrotic or nonviable tissue.

Population at Risk

1. Neonates whose births were attended by unqualified midwives.

2. Narcotic addicts account for a large number of cases.
3. Unimmunized people in rural areas where contact with animal excreta is likely.

Screening

1. No specific screening method is available to determine susceptibility.
2. Immunization history should be determined at the time of well-child visits and immunization given as necessary (Tables 24-1 and 24-2 and Figure 24-1).

ASSESSMENT

Health History

1. History of a wound, usually contaminated with soil, animal feces, or dust.
2. No prior history of active immunization.

TABLE 24-3 PRINCIPLES OF IMMUNITY

1. Immunity is
   a. The body's ability to protect itself against foreign proteins (e.g., bacteria, allergens).
   b. The body's ability to build up resistance that prevents being infected a second time by some organisms.

   In response to foreign proteins (*antigens*) the immune system produces protective proteins (*antibodies*) that are carried in the plasma to destroy the offending antigens.
2. Antigen-antibody reactions include
   a. Neutralization.
   b. Precipitation.
   c. Agglutination.
   d. Opsonization.

   (a–d) All render the antigen susceptible to white blood cell (WBC) phagocytosis.

   e. Lysis (rupture and destruction of the invading organism).
3. There are several types of immunity:
   a. Natural: inborn, species-specific nonsusceptibility to certain infections because of the presence of naturally occurring antibodies.
   b. Acquired.
      (1) Active immunity: results from the body's production of antibodies in response to exposure to the antigen, either by invasion of the organism or by therapeutic introduction of the organism or its antigenic by-products. Substances used to induce active immunity include
         (a) Killed bacteria.
         (b) Attenuated live bacteria.
         (c) Denatured toxins of bacteria.
         (d) Dead virus (produces a slow antibody response.)
         (e) Virus vaccines (produced by passing the virus from one animal to another until the virus is nonpathogenic but capable of producing an immune response in humans).
      (2) Passive immunity: results from receiving antibodies that have been produced actively by other humans or animals. Examples include (a) antibodies a fetus receives from its mother, who herself produced them and (b) injection with immune serum.
         (a) Advantage: immediate effect; can be used to increase the immunity of an exposed person within minutes.
         (b) Disadvantage: immunity is temporary.
4. Assessment factors.
   a. Infants whose mothers lack immunity to particular diseases (e.g., tetanus, measles, diphtheria) are born with no immunity to those infections.
   b. Socioeconomic and environmental factors may predispose to those infections.
   c. Travel, especially to areas of epidemic or outside one's own country, increases the risk of some diseases to unimmunized persons.

Physical Assessment

1. Neck and jaw muscles are stiff.
2. Spasms of masseters result in difficulty in opening the mouth and swallowing ("lock-jaw").
3. Client experiences headaches and restlessness.
4. Spasms of other muscle groups occur as the disease progresses.
5. Opisthotonus (extension spasm of trunk and neck) develops.
6. Abdominal rigidity is present.
7. Client experiences apprehension.

Diagnostic Tests

1. Excised wound tissue used for culture studies.
2. Animal inoculation with the client's serum will determine the presence of toxins.

NURSING DIAGNOSES: ACTUAL OR POTENTIAL

1. Risk of injury secondary to seizures, which are precipitated by the slightest stimuli.
2. Respiratory dysfunction secondary to pulmonary complications and excessive secretions.
3. Alterations in nutritional status and fluid balance secondary to inability to swallow either food or fluid.
4. Impairment of skin integrity secondary to incontinence of urine and feces.
5. Severe anxiety secondary to incapacity (sensorium is usually clear).

EXPECTED OUTCOMES

1. Seizures will be absent or infrequent.
2. Client will not develop injury from seizure activity.
3. Airway will remain open.
4. Nutritional status and hydration will be preserved.
5. Anxiety will be minimal.
6. Skin will remain intact.
7. Complications will be avoided or will be mild.

INTERVENTIONS

1. Remain with the client constantly since a life-threatening seizure may develop.
2. Keep room quiet, and avoid any unnecessary stimuli: vocal, tactile, or auditory.
3. Administer sedatives as prescribed to prevent seizures. If sedation is sufficient to render the client unconscious, nursing intervention is the same as for any unconscious person:
   a. Turn frequently.
   b. Maintain body alignment.
   c. Maintain patent airway.
   d. Monitor vital signs.
   e. Monitor intake and output.
   f. Provide meticulous skin care.
   g. Perform oral hygiene measures.
   h. Perform passive exercise for range of motion.
   i. Provide food and fluid by gavage.
4. Nasopharyngeal suctioning of airway if necessary.
5. Give tube feedings if client is unable to swallow.
6. Keep intake and output record.
7. Monitor parenteral fluids.
8. Maintain a weight record, if possible.
9. Explain each procedure to client to allay apprehension.

EVALUATION

Outcome Criteria

1. External stimuli are reduced with resultant lessening of muscle spasm or convulsion.
2. Client does not develop muscle contractures, fractures, or intramuscular hematomas.
3. Full range of motion (ROM) in all joints is maintained.
4. Airway remains patent.
5. Client remains hydrated and maintains normal electrolyte balance.
6. There is no weight loss.
7. Skin remains intact.
8. Apprehension expressed by client is minimal.

Complications

1. Types of complications depend upon the quality of nursing care, the age of the client, and the effectiveness of specific treatment.
2. Pneumonia (see Chapter 20).
3. Atelectasis (see Chapter 20).
4. Pneumothorax (see Chapter 31).
5. Mediastinal emphysema.
6. Oral lacerations (see Chapter 48).
7. Intramuscular hematomas (see Chapter 48).
8. Fractures of the thoracic vertebrae (see Chapter 25).
9. Malnutrition.
10. Fluid and electrolyte imbalance.

Assessment

1. Lowered blood pressure; lowered venous pressure.
2. Poor skin turgor.
3. Dryness of skin and mucous membrane.
4. Elevated skin temperature.
5. Concentrated urine and a specific gravity above 1.030.
6. Loss of weight.
7. Elevated hematocrit.

Revised Outcomes

1. Expected outcomes for pneumonia, atelectasis, pneumothorax, and traumatic injuries are in chapters noted above.
2. Other outcomes as originally stated.
3. Fluid and electrolyte balance will be maintained.
4. Specific gravity of urine will not exceed 1.030.
5. Weight loss will not occur.

Interventions

1. Maintain quiet environment.
2. Administer sedation and muscle relaxants as ordered.
3. Provide fluids and feedings to ensure adequate caloric intake.
4. Interventions for complications listed above can be found in chapters related to those conditions.

Reevaluation and Follow-up

1. Respiratory function remains normal.
2. Seizures and muscle spasms do not occur or are mild.
3. Weight remains stable.
4. Skin turgor is normal.
5. Mucous membrane is moist.

PERTUSSIS (WHOOPING COUGH)

DESCRIPTION

Pertussis is an acute respiratory infection caused by *Bordetella pertussis*. This infection is very contagious for unimmunized persons. Adults are frequently susceptible since immunization during childhood does not produce lifelong immunity. Infants born to mothers with a low immunity level are especially susceptible. Pertussis shows less seasonal variation than other respiratory diseases. There is a high incidence of the disease in developing countries. The incubation period is 7 to 14 days. The infection is transmitted by direct contact with discharges from the laryngeal and bronchial mucous membrane of infected persons; it can also be contracted through indirect contact with contaminated articles. Antibiotics eliminate the organism but do not shorten the paroxysmal phase of the disease. Supportive nursing care is essential. Complications are treated with specific forms of intervention. The mortality rate is as high as 40 percent for infants under 5 months of age.

PREVENTION

Health Promotion

1. Active immunization with DTP (diphtheria-tetanus-pertussis) vaccine is effective in the prevention of pertussis. If a convulsion or other neurological symptom occurs after administration of DTP or other pertussis vaccine, no further pertussis vaccine should be given.
2. Parents need to be educated about the dangers of pertussis and the advantages of immunization.

Population at Risk

1. Susceptibility is general.
2. Children, especially young children, are most often affected. Nonimmunized children should be kept away from school and public gatherings during an outbreak of pertussis.
3. Exposed adults may have second attacks.

Screening

1. No specific screening method is available.
2. Immunization history should be elicited at the time of well-child visits and immunization administered as appropriate (see Tables 24-1 and 24-2 and Figure 24-1).

ASSESSMENT

Health History

1. Child has not been immunized against pertussis.
2. History of exposure to a person with the disease during previous 3-week period.

Physical Assessment

Pertussis occurs in three stages and has a combined duration of several weeks.

1. Catarrhal stage.
   a. Low-grade fever.
   b. Rhinorrhea.
   c. Cough.

2. Paroxysmal stage.
   a. A strangling cough develops with a characteristic whoop upon inspiration at end of coughing.
   b. Cough is accompanied by
      (1) Facial redness or cyanosis.
      (2) Bulging eyes.
      (3) Protruding tongue.
      (4) Anxiety.
   c. Thick mucus is discharged from the nose and mouth.
   d. Sweating and exhaustion occur with coughing attack.
   e. Vomiting often follows coughing attack.
3. Convalescent stage.
   a. Whooping diminishes, and cough becomes less severe and less frequent.
   b. Vomiting diminishes in relation to diminished coughing episodes.

Diagnostic Tests

1. Nasopharyngeal swabs obtained during a paroxysm of coughing and cultured on fresh medium may lead to isolation and identification of the *B. pertussis* organism.
2. Fluorescent antibody staining of pharyngeal secretions will aid in rapid diagnosis.

NURSING DIAGNOSES: ACTUAL OR POTENTIAL

1. Inadequate oxygenation (potential airway obstruction) secondary to excessive, thick mucus.
2. Electrolyte imbalance related to vomiting.
3. Nutritional alteration secondary to vomiting.
4. Impending seizure secondary to prolonged paroxysms of coughing.
5. Anxiety associated with paroxysmal cough.

EXPECTED OUTCOMES

1. Paroxysms of coughing will be infrequent.
2. Airway will remain patent, and oxygenation will be adequate.
3. Weight loss will not occur, and fluid balance will be maintained.
4. Seizures will not result in injury.
5. Anxiety will be minimized.

INTERVENTIONS

1. Isolate client because of communicability of disease.
2. Provide quiet environment since sudden noise and excitement can precipitate paroxysms of coughing.
3. Maintain humidified environment to liquefy secretions.
4. Maintain airway by suctioning as necessary.
5. Administer oxygen for cyanosis.
6. Protect child from injury if convulsions develop.
7. Provide frequent, small meals.
8. If vomiting occurs due to coughing, refeed immediately.
9. Offer fluids frequently to keep client hydrated and to aid in liquefying secretions.
10. Observe for episodes of apnea, especially in the young infant.
11. Remain with child to allay anxiety during coughing episodes.

EVALUATION

Outcome Criteria

1. Paroxysms of coughing are infrequent.
2. Secretions are easily expectorated.
3. There are no episodes of cyanosis or apnea.
4. Client maintains normal weight and fluid balance.
5. Apprehension during paroxysms of coughing is minimal.

Complications

1. Pulmonary infection (see Chapter 20).
2. Otitis media (see Chapter 20).
3. Nutritional disturbance.

Assessment

1. Elevated temperature.
2. Restlessness.
3. Irritability.
4. Holds ear with hand.
5. Decreased or absent breath sounds over affected lung.
6. Weight loss.
7. Daily fluid intake.

Revised Outcomes

1. Temperature within normal limits.
2. No evidence of earache.
   a. Holding of ear subsides.
   b. Appetite restored.
   c. Tenderness is decreased.
3. Breath sounds are normal.
4. No convulsions occur.
5. Normal weight is maintained or restored.

Interventions
1. Encourage increased fluid intake.
2. Handle gently.
3. Administer analgesics as prescribed for pain.
4. Maintain a warm room.
5. Remove as many stresses as possible from environment.
6. Other interventions, as stated above.

Reevaluation and Follow-up
Complications are mild and of short duration.

RUBEOLA (MEASLES, "RED MEASLES")

DESCRIPTION

Measles is an acute systemic disease caused by measles virus. The occurrence of rubeola is worldwide. Epidemics occurred about every 2 to 4 years before the introduction of measles vaccine. Measles is seen most often in unimmunized children. Infants of susceptible mothers have no immunity at birth. Infants of immunized mothers acquire immunity passively from their mothers; it lasts about 6 months. The incubation period is about 10 days from exposure to the initial fever, or about 2 weeks until the rash appears. Measles is transmitted by direct contact with droplets from an infected person. It also can be spread by means of contaminated articles, but this is rare. Prognosis is affected by age (poorest in infants and older adults) and the severity of symptoms. Fatality rates have declined in the United States because of improved socioeconomic conditions and the use of antibiotics to treat complications.

PREVENTION

Health Promotion
1. Immunize at age 15 months.
2. Immunization can be given earlier if an outbreak of rubeola occurs, but it must be repeated when child reaches 15 months of age.
3. Educational measures to inform the public about the necessity and advantages of active immunization.

Population at Risk
1. Infants of susceptible mothers have no immunity and can contract the disease *with* the mother before birth or after the delivery.
2. Unimmunized children are susceptible.

Screening
1. Immunization history should be elicited at the time of well-child visits,and immunization against measles should be administered at the appropriate age (see Tables 24-1 and 24-2 and Figure 24-1).
2. Proof of measles immunization should be required for registration for day care, camp, or school attendance.

ASSESSMENT

Health History
1. Immunization against measles lacking or given before 12 months of age.
2. Exposure to a person with measles.

Physical Assessment
1. Manifestations: measles is characterized by three stages:
   a. Incubation stage, which has few if any symptoms.
   b. Prodromal stage.
      (1) Low-grade fever.
      (2) Slight cough.
      (3) Coryza and conjunctivitis.
      (4) Koplik's spots.
         (a) Koplik's spots appear on buccal mucosa as grayish white dots with a reddish areola.
         (b) They appear during the prodromal stage and disappear within 2 days.
         (c) They tend to occur opposite the lower molars and may spread irregularly over rest of buccal mucosa.
      (5) Photophobia.
   d. Rash stage.
      (1) A fever of 40–40.5°C (104–105°F) is common.
      (2) The rash develops as faint macules on the upper lateral parts of the neck, along the hairline, and on the preauricular part of the cheeks.
      (3) The rash then spreads rapidly over the face, upper arms, and chest. Finally, the rash appears on the back, abdomen, legs, and feet.
      (4) The rash fades in the direction in which it appeared and begins to fade on the face as it reaches the feet.
      (5) A fading rash may produce temporary brownish discoloration of the skin.

Diagnostic Tests

1. Koplik's spots are pathognomonic for rubeola.
2. A hemagglutination inhibition test may be performed using acute and convalescent serum to establish that the patient actually had measles, but it is of no value in making a diagnosis during the acute illness.

NURSING DIAGNOSES: ACTUAL OR POTENTIAL

1. Risk of transmitting virus to others due to ready communicability of the disease.
2. Loss of skin integrity associated with scratching and nasal discharge.
3. Risk of secondary infection due to loss of skin integrity.
4. Risk of injury due to convulsions that can accompany fever.
5. Noncompliance with bed rest order due to child's developmental drive to be active.
6. Alteration in nutrition: decreased intake due to anorexia.
7. Alteration in fluid balance: dehydration due to fever and anorexia.
8. Alteration in sleep and rest pattern: decrease due to cough.
9. Alteration in comfort: discomfort due to photophobia and pruritis.
10. Alteration in body temperature: pyrexia due to viral infection.

EXPECTED OUTCOMES

1. Disease will be limited to the index case, with no spread to other susceptibles.
2. Lip will be gently kept dry, and itching will be controlled, thus preventing secondary infection from breaks in the skin.
3. Fever will remain below 39°C (102°F)
4. Convulsions will not occur.
5. Child will maintain bed rest (or equivalently quiet activities) while fever exceeds 37.8°C (100°F).
6. Dehydration (poor turgor, reduced urine output) and weight loss will not occur.
7. Child will cough productively and intermittently, resting or sleeping between nighttime coughing episodes.
8. Child will experience minimial discomfort due to itching, coughing, or exposure to light.

INTERVENTIONS

1. Isolate infected child from the time measles is diagnosed until 5 days after the rash appears.
2. Teach parents the importance of immunization for other unimmunized and uninfected children.
3. Have child use and properly dispose of tissues to keep nose free of secretions. A paper bag can be pinned to the bedside for this purpose and burned when it becomes full. A lubricant can be used around the nose to prevent excoriation.
4. Keep client in a comfortably warm environment. Clothing should be lightweight and nonirritating to facilitate heat loss and minimize itching.
5. Apply soothing lotion to the skin to reduce itching.
6. Monitor temperature every 2 hours while awake, every $\frac{1}{2}$ hour if over 39°C (102°F), or as otherwise indicated.
7. Administer antipyretics as prescribed.
8. Provide environment conducive to bed rest, and keep febrile child in bed. Quiet activities, such as coloring or having stories read, may help keep client at rest.
9. Offer small feedings served attractively to encourage eating.
10. Maintain hydration by offering water and other fluids, such as fruit juice, frequently.
11. Keep room humidified to minimize cough and keep secretions loose.
12. Keep eyes free of crusts by bathing them with warm water. Keep room dimly lighted, or provide older child with dark glasses.

EVALUATION

Outcome Criteria

1. No other person in family contracts the disease.
2. There is no excoriation around the nose.
3. No secondary infection results from scratching.
4. Fever gradually subsides; convulsions do not occur.
5. Child accepts bed rest or equivalent with minimal resistance.
6. Child remains adequately hydrated and maintains weight.
7. Child sleeps throughout the night with minimal coughing.

8. Eyes are clear of matting and crusts.
9. Rash fades, beginning with the face and proceeding downward in the same sequence as it appeared.
10. Preventable complications do not occur.

Complications

1. Otitis media (see Chapter 20).
2. Pneumonia caused by the measles virus itself (see Chapter 20).
3. Bronchopneumonia due to secondary bacterial infection (see Chapter 20).
4. Encephalitis (see Chapter 15).
5. Laryngitis, tracheitis, and bronchitis (see discussion in Chapter 20).
6. Exacerbation of tuberculosis (see *Tuberculosis*, later in this chapter).
7. Myocarditis occurs infrequently.

Assessment

1. Fever.
2. Earache.
3. Dyspnea.
4. Severe headache.
5. Pain from light glare.
6. Anxiety.

Revised Outcomes

1. Maintain regulating mechanisms and functions of body temperature and acid-base balance.
2. Maintain oxygen to all cells.
3. Achieve comfort.
4. Prevent emotional injury.

Interventions

1. Maintain a comfortable room temperature.
2. Give iced liquids.
3. Approach unhurriedly.
4. Discuss pain-relieving measures, and apply measure of the client's choice.
5. Other interventions, as outlined above.

Reevaluation and Follow-up

1. Body temperature of 38°C (100.4°F)
2. Absence of malaise, fatigue, and weakness.
3. Cessation of complaints of pain.
4. Calm, contented; has relaxed facial expression.
5. Good color to skin and mucous membrane.
6. Vital signs within normal limits.

RUBELLA (GERMAN MEASLES)

DESCRIPTION

Rubella is an acute, mild systemic disorder caused by rubella virus. Epidemics occur approximately every 5 or 6 years. Rubella is more prevalent in winter and spring. It is seen mostly in childhood but affects more adults than does rubeola. Appreciable epidemics occur at military camps and college campuses. In the United States, 80 percent of a population screened will show serological evidence of previous infection. Transplacental immunity is effective for the first 6 months of life. Lifelong immunity is conferred with one attack. In pregnant women, the virus is transferred to the fetus via the placenta during the period of viremia. The risk of congenital anomalies appears to be quite high if the mother contracts rubella during the first 8 to 12 weeks of pregnancy, but it declines as pregnancy advances and is as low as 4 percent in the second and third trimesters. The incubation period is 14 to 21 days, with the average 18 days. Rubella is transmitted (1) by droplet spread or by direct contact with the client, (2) indirectly by contact with articles freshly soiled with discharge from the nose or mouth, and (3) via placenta to the fetus from an infected mother. Treatment is symptomatic unless the disease is complicated by bacterial infection; then treatment is directed toward that specific infection.

PREVENTION

Health Promotion

1. Immunize all children over 1 year of age with a single dose of live attenuated rubella virus vaccine (see Tables 24-1 and 24-2 and Figure 24-1).
2. Immunize women of childbearing age if serological test indicates susceptibility.
   a. Do not give measles vaccine to pregnant women.
   b. Instruct client to avoid pregnancy for 2 months following immunization.
3. It is especially important that girls be immunized before childbearing age.
4. Pregnant women (including nurses) should not come in contact with infants with congenital rubella.
5. An intramuscular injection of immune serum globulin (ISG) may be offered the exposed susceptible person. Effectiveness of ISG is not predictable.
6. In order to protect unborn babies, *all* health care providers (both sexes, all ages) should have evidence of immunity to rubella.
   NOTE: Newly immunized persons do not constitute any risk to pregnant women; ac-

cordingly a woman even in the first trimester can safely have her child immunized.

Population at Risk

1. Unimmunized persons.
2. Infants of susceptible mothers have no immunity and can contract the disease from the mother if she is infected.
3. Epidemics and outbreaks are common in college and military populations.

Screening

1. Serology test to determine immune status.
2. Serology test performed at the time of acute illness and repeated 2 weeks later can be used to confirm a diagnosis of rubella.

ASSESSMENT

Health History

1. Lack of active immunization against measles.
2. Exposure to a person with rubella.

Physical Assessment

1. Mild catarrhal symptoms during prodromal phase may go unnoticed due to mildness and short duration.
2. The characteristic sign is retroauricular, posterior cervical, and postoccipital adenopathy. Nodes are tender for the first 1 or 2 days and are palpable for several weeks.
3. Red spots may appear on the soft palate and may coalesce into a red blush before the eruption of the skin rash.
4. The rash begins on the face and spreads rapidly over the rest of the body.
   a. The maculopapular rash is conspicuous.
   b. There are large areas of flushing, which spread over the entire body within 24 hours after rash appears.
5. Pharyngeal and conjuctival mucosa are slightly inflamed.
6. Fever is slight and, if present, occurs when the rash is at its height. Temperature does not usually exceed 38.3°C (101°F).
7. Polyarthritis may occur with pain, swelling, tenderness, and effusion and generally disappears without consequence.

Diagnostic Tests

1. Serological test using acute and convalescent serum to determine presence of antibodies.
2. Diagnosis must be based on laboratory data, since physical findings are not adequate for making a diagnosis of rubella.

NURSING DIAGNOSES: ACTUAL OR POTENTIAL

1. Risk of transmitting virus to others due to ready communicability of the disease and noncompliance with recommendation to keep child home and away from others until rash has disappeared.
2. Noncompliance with bed rest (recommended for child with arthritis) due to developmental drive to be active.
3. Alteration in body temperature: pyrexia secondary to viral infection.
4. Alteration in comfort: discomfort or pain associated with lymphadenopathy, sore throat, and arthritis.
5. Delinquent immunization: failure to adhere to immunization schedule.

EXPECTED OUTCOMES

1. No new cases of rubella will develop.
2. Child with arthritis or fever over 37.8°C (100°F) will maintain bed rest or equivalent.
3. Fever will not exceed 38.3°C (101°F).
4. Discomfort due to lymphadenopathy and pharyngeal inflammation will be minimal; pain resulting from polyarthritis will be minimal.
5. Parents will ensure that all subsequent immunizations are given as recommended.

INTERVENTIONS

1. Isolate child as soon as diagnosis is established; dispose of tissues properly.
2. Provide environment conducive to rest in bed or equally quiet activity. Coloring books, stories, and other quiet entertainment suitable for developmental level (see Chapter 4) will help.
3. Administer aspirin or acetaminophen to control fever.
4. Administer aspirin or other analgesics as prescribed to relieve arthritic pain. Warm gargles may be used for sore throat.
5. Urge parents to follow up with immunization schedule for all children in the family. The school nurse should initiate an immunization program for all susceptible children in the elementary schools. Parents need to know the expected reaction to the vaccine and how to care for recently immunized children.
   a. Rash develops about 10 days after immunization.

b. Fever may develop.
c. An antipyretic can be given for fever.
d. Warm compresses can be applied to the injection site to relieve tenderness.

EVALUATION

Outcome Criteria

1. Rubella does not spread to others. All susceptible children in exposed population are immunized.
2. Bed rest is maintained during period of fever and arthritic symptoms.
3. Fever does not exceed 38.3°C (101°F).
4. Sore throat is minimal; arthritic symptoms are mild.

Complications

1. Complications are relatively uncommon in childhood rubella.
2. Arthritis occasionally occurs (see discussion in Chapter 16).
3. Encephalitis occurs rarely (see discussion in Chapter 15).
4. Spontaneous abortions occur in about one-third of pregnant women who contract rubella during the first trimester.
5. With the congenital rubella syndrome, the most common defects are
   a. Cataracts.
   b. Cardiovascular anomalies.
   c. Deafness.
   d. Mutism secondary to deafness.
   e. Microcephaly.
   f. Mental retardation.

Assessment

1. Mother has no history of immunization for rubella.
2. Mother has a history of exposure to rubella during the first trimester of pregnancy.
3. Serology test for rubella antibodies indicates recent infection.
4. Virus isolation from the pharynx of the infant reveals presence of rubella virus.

Revised Outcomes

1. Maintain general comfort of infant.
2. Provide for safety of infant.
3. Maintain adequate caloric intake.
4. Parents will achieve awareness of infant's needs.

Interventions

1. Isolate infant until virus can no longer be isolated from pharynx.
2. Parents should stimulate infant by holding, singing, and talking as they would with other infants.
3. Encourage and accept parents' expressions of their feelings.
4. Refer to social agency if parents require assistance for financial help in the prolonged hospitalization and treatment of their child.

Reevaluation and Follow-up

1. No cases of rubella develop as result of exposure to infant.
2. Infant feeds well, and weight gain is acceptable.
3. Parents use healthy coping mechanisms in dealing with their situation.
4. Family receives services for which they are eligible to help meet their financial need.

MUMPS

DESCRIPTION

Mumps is contagious swelling of the parotid salivary glands, caused by mumps virus. Mumps is endemic in most urban populations. It affects males and females equally. The majority of infections occur before adolescence. Epidemics occur at all seasons of the year but are more common in winter and spring. The disease is transmitted by droplets and by direct contact with an infected person. Indirectly, mumps can be spread by articles contaminated with infectious saliva and, possibly, urine. About 30 to 40 percent of cases are subclinical and go unrecognized. The incubation period is 2 to 3 weeks. Treatment is symptomatic. Recovery is usually complete in uncomplicated cases.

PREVENTION

Health Promotion

1. Immunize at age 12 months or older (see Tables 24-1 and 24-2 and Figure 24-1).
2. Educational measures to inform the public about the advantages of active immunization.

Population at Risk

1. Mumps occurs primarily in young school-age children.
2. Unimmunized children are susceptible.
3. About 15 percent of cases occur in adolescents and adults.

Screening

1. No reliable screening method is available to determine susceptibility.
2. A mumps skin test, which uses killed mumps virus, is available but is unreliable in predicting immune status due to the frequency of false-positive as well as false-negative responses.

ASSESSMENT

Health History

1. No history of active immunization with mumps vaccine.
2. History of exposure to a diagnosed case of mumps.

Physical Assessment

1. Prodromal symptoms are not usually present but can include
   a. Fever.
   b. Muscular pain.
   c. Headache.
   d. Malaise.
2. Onset of disease is characterized by pain and swelling in one or both parotid glands.
   a. Swelling begins first between the posterior border of the mandible and the mastoid, then extends downward and forward and is limited by the zygoma.
   b. The swelling may progress rapidly and reach a peak within a few hours after onset, or it may develop over a few days.
   c. The earlobe is pushed upward and outward by the swollen tissue.
   d. Swelling may occur in one gland only but is more often bilateral.
   e. Swollen area is tender and painful.
   f. Fever accompanies the parotid swelling and is usually moderate.
   g. Swelling of submandibular glands frequently accompanies or closely follows parotid swelling.

Diagnostic Tests

1. Routine laboratory tests are nonspecific.
2. Usually there is leukopenia with a relative lymphocytosis.
3. Serum amylase is elevated in most clients with mumps.
4. Medical diagnosis depends on the isolation of the mumps virus from the saliva or urine.

NURSING DIAGNOSES: ACTUAL OR POTENTIAL

1. Risk of transmission to other people due to the communicability of the virus.
2. Alteration in comfort: pain in the neck and jaw, especially upon opening the mouth or chewing, due to parotid swelling.
3. Alteration in nutrition and hydration: decreased intake due to pain.
4. Alteration in body temperature: fever due to viral infection.
5. Loss of skin or mucous membrane integrity associated with dry lips and mouth and diminished oral hygiene.

EXPECTED OUTCOMES

1. Disease will not spread beyond the index client.
2. Pain will be minimal.
3. Adequate nutrition and hydration will be maintained.
4. Fever will not exceed 38.8°C (102°F).
5. Lips and oral cavity will be moist and free of crusts.
6. Complications will be promptly recognized and treated.

INTERVENTIONS

1. Maintain isolation until all swelling has disappeared. Teach parents and other family members preventive measures to protect susceptible persons from getting the disease (prevention of droplet spread, disposal of tissues, immunization for susceptible persons).
2. Provide ice collar to relieve pain in swollen parotid glands.
3. Provide diet that is easy to chew; avoid sour or strongly flavored foods that would cause parotid pain.
4. If fever is present, give antipyretic agents and tepid baths.
5. Maintain bed rest during febrile period.
6. Monitor temperature since a sudden fever may indicate the development of complications.
7. Give frequent oral hygiene.
8. Observe for complications.

EVALUATION

Outcome Criteria

1. Disease does not spread to susceptible persons.

2. Amount of pain due to swollen glands is minimal.
3. Fever remains below 38.8°C (102°F).
4. Adequate nutrition with minimal weight loss.
5. Hydration remains adequate.
6. Lips are free of crusts and cracks.

Complications

1. Meningoencephalomyelitis is the most common complication of childhood mumps (see discussion in Chapter 15).
2. Orchitis and epididymitis are complications seen in male adolescents and adults (see discussion in Chapter 34).
3. Deafness: mumps is considered a leading cause of unilateral nerve deafness. Deafness is permanent.
4. Oophoritis (see discussion in Chapter 34).
5. Pancreatitis (see discussion in Chapter 33).
6. Nephritis (see discussion in Chapter 21).
7. Thyroiditis (see discussion in Chapter 28).
8. Myocarditis (see discussion in Chapter 30).
9. Arthritis (see discussion in Chapter 16).
10. Ocular complications.

Assessment

1. Photophobia.
2. Tearing.
3. Painful swelling of the lacrimal glands.
4. Loss of vision.

Revised Outcomes

1. Discomfort from ocular complications will be minimal.
2. Recovery will be complete and vision restored within 3 weeks of onset.

Interventions

1. Provide a dark room or subdued light to eliminate pain due to light.
2. Handle eye area gently.
3. Instill eye medication as ordered.
4. Reassure client that impairment of vision is temporary.

Reevaluation and Follow-up

1. Recovery is uneventful.
2. Normal vision returns.
3. Swelling subsides.

CHICKENPOX (VARICELLA)

DESCRIPTION

Chickenpox is a highly contagious disease caused by herpesvirus varicella. This infection can occur at any age; the vast majority of children contract chickenpox before the age of 10 years, usually between 5 and 9 years. Chickenpox can occur during the neonatal period. The rate of infection of susceptible household members approaches 100 percent. The disease is most common in winter and early spring. The incubation period is 2 to 3 weeks, most commonly 13 to 17 days. The disease is transmitted (1) by direct contact, (2) by droplet or airborne spread, and (3) indirectly by articles freshly soiled by discharges from the skin and mucous membranes of persons infected with the disease. The treatment is symptomatic: relieve itching, and prevent or combat secondary skin infection. If varicella pneumonia develops, treatment is supportive. The prognosis for chickenpox is good; fatalities occasionally result from complications. *For people with suppressed immune response (e.g., persons who take cortisone), chickenpox can be fatal.*

PREVENTION

Health Promotion

1. Protect clients with immune-deficient conditions against exposure.
2. Zoster immune globulin (ZIG) may prevent or modify disease in close contacts.

Population at Risk

1. Can occur in adults and children; ordinarily a more severe disease for adults than children.
2. Susceptibility is universal among those not previously infected.

Screening

There are no screening tests to identify susceptible people.

ASSESSMENT

Health History

1. Exposure to a person with diagnosed chickenpox.
2. Exposure of a person susceptible to chickenpox to a client with herpes zoster.

Physical Assessment

1. Prodromal symptoms appear at the end of the incubation period:
   a. Slight fever.
   b. Malaise.
   c. Anorexia.

2. Rash appears rapidly:
   a. Rash begins as crops of small red papules on the trunk, then spreads to the face and scalp. Generally, involvement of the distal parts of extremities is minimal.
   b. These papules form into clear vesicles on an erythematous base.
      (1) Vesicles become cloudy in about 24 hours.
      (2) Vesicles break easily, and scabs form.
      (3) Eruption of rash continues for about 3 days.
      (4) Chickenpox is characterized by the simultaneous presence of papules, early and late vesicles, and crusts.
3. Pruritus is constant.
4. Vesicles on mucous membranes become macerated, especially those in the mouth.
5. Generalized lymphadenopathy may be present.

Diagnostic Tests

1. Laboratory data reveal mild leukocytosis.
2. Virus giant cells can be demonstrated in scrapings from fresh vesicles.

NURSING DIAGNOSES: ACTUAL OR POTENTIAL

1. Risk of transmission to others because of high degree of communicability of virus.
2. Alteration in comfort: discomfort due to intense pruritus.
3. Loss of skin integrity and risk of secondary infection due to scratching.
4. Alteration in nutrition and fluid balance: decreased intake due to painful mouth lesions.
5. Alteration in body temperature: fever secondary to viral infection.
6. Alteration in oxygenation: respiratory distress due to laryngeal edema.

EXPECTED OUTCOMES

1. Chickenpox will not be transmitted to adults or to people with suppressed immune response capability.
2. Itching will be relieved.
3. Skin will not be injured by scratching; secondary infection will not occur.
4. Weight and hydration will be maintained.
5. Temperature will not exceed 38.4°C (101°F).
6. Respiratory distress, if it occurs, will be promptly recognized and treated.

INTERVENTIONS

1. Isolate client as soon as diagnosis is established.
2. Separate from general laundry bed linen soiled with drainage from vesicles.
3. Apply lotions, such as calamine, to help alleviate itching.
4. Bathe child in soothing baths to reduce itching and to keep skin clean.
5. Keep child's fingernails clipped.
6. Infants and young children may need mittens to prevent scratching.
7. Keep child's hands scrupulously clean.
8. Avoid breaking vesicles.
9. Change bed linen daily to reduce risk of secondary infection.
10. Provide loose-fitting, cotton clothing, and change clothing at least daily.
11. Offer frequent, small feedings of soft foods and preferred fluids. Avoid pungent or acidic substances and extremes of temperature if child has mouth lesions.
12. Administer antipyretic agents as ordered for fever.
13. Maintain bed rest during febrile period. Provide quiet activity appropriate for developmental level (see Chapter 4).
14. Observe for any sign of respiratory distress: hoarseness, stridor, labored breathing.

EVALUATION

Outcome Criteria

1. Skin lesions become vesicular within 3 to 4 days and dry to a scab with no secondary infection.
2. Constitutional reactions are mild.
3. Recovery is uncomplicated.

Complications

1. Thrombocytopenia can occur, producing hemorrhage into the skin (see discussion in Chapter 18).
2. Internal hemorrhage from ulceration can occur and can be fatal (see discussion in Chapter 33).
3. Varicella pneumonia, more often seen in adult clients than children; see discussion of pneumonia in Chapter 20.
4. Respiratory distress can be precipitated due to laryngeal edema if lesions are present on the larynx.
5. Congenital malformations have occurred in

infants whose mothers had the disease during the first trimester of pregnancy.
6. Postinfectious encephalitis is the most common central nervous system complication (see discussion in Chapter 15).
7. Secondary bacterial infection of skin lesions is the most frequent complication.

Assessment
1. Itching.
2. Pus present in lesions.
3. Burning and redness around lesions.
4. Fever.

Revised Outcomes
1. Infection will be limited to only one small area.
2. Fever will be slight.

Interventions
1. Clean with surgical soap.
2. Apply an antibiotic ointment three or four times daily.
3. Do not allow abraded skin surfaces to touch.
4. Maintain a cool room temperature.

Reevaluation and Follow-up
1. Lesions dry and crust with no spread to unaffected areas.
2. Temperature returns to normal.
3. Itching is controlled, so no new infections result from scratching.

POLIOMYELITIS (POLIO, INFANTILE PARALYSIS)

DESCRIPTION

Poliomyelitis is a central nervous system (CNS) disorder caused by poliovirus types 1, 2, and 3. Outbreaks of clinically recognizable disease occur most often in temperate zones. Outbreaks are most common during warm months. Polio is characteristically a disease of children and adolescents, but all ages can be affected when immunity has not been established. The greatest communicability is during the latter part of the incubation period and the first week of illness. The incubation period is 1 to 2 weeks. Polio is transmitted by direct contact with pharyngeal secretions or feces of infected persons. The virus is detectable for a longer period of time in feces than in throat secretions. No antibiotics are effective against the poliovirus. Human immune globulin is not effective after the onset of illness. Active immunization of all susceptible persons against the three types of poliovirus will prevent catastrophic epidemics, such as have occurred in the past. The prognosis is widely variable. Paralysis is actually very rare but may impair respiration as well as motor function. Case fatalities during epidemics in the United States have been reported at 5 to 7 percent. Deaths usually occur during the first 2 weeks after the onset of the disease. After puberty, there is a higher incidence of fatalities and a higher probability of deformity. The extent of recovery from poliomyelitis is related to the adequacy and promptness of treatment.

PREVENTION

Health Promotion

1. Active immunization against the three types of poliovirus should begin in infancy (see Tables 24-1 and 24-2).
2. Education of the public about the advantages of immunization.
3. Whenever there is a new case of polio, all susceptible persons should be identified and immunized as quickly as possible.
4. NOTE: Newly immunized people shed poliovirus in their stool for up to 2 months, and nonimmune people are susceptible to contract polio from them. Unimmunized grandparents, unimmunized infants, immunosuppressed people (leukemics, renal transplant recipients, etc.), and other unprotected people should not be exposed to infants or others within 2 months after receiving oral polio virus.

Population at Risk

1. Susceptibility is general, and all ages can be affected where there is no naturally or artificially acquired immunity.
2. Characteristically a disease of children and adolescents.

Screening

1. There is no screening method to determine susceptibility.
2. Immunization records should be kept to document that active immunization against polio was accomplished.

ASSESSMENT

Health History

1. Exposure of an unimmunized person to a person with documented polio.

2. No history of prior immunization against the three strains of poliovirus.

Physical Assessment

1. Abortive poliomyelitis.
   a. This diagnosis is applicable during outbreaks of polio, to those persons known to have been exposed to another person with clinical evidence of disease.
   b. Symptoms are mild.
      (1) Generally the fever does not exceed 39.4°C (103°F).
      (2) Anorexia.
      (3) Malaise.
      (4) Vomiting.
      (5) Headache.
      (6) Sore throat.
   c. The person with the foregoing symptoms during an outbreak should be assessed several weeks after the illness for muscular involvement.
2. Nonparalytic poliomyelitis.
   a. The clinical manifestations are similar to but more intense than those for abortive polio.
   b. Constipation is common.
   c. This type of polio occurs in two phases that are referred to as minor and major illness. A short, symptom-free period is common between these two phases.
   d. Nuchal and spinal rigidity are positive diagnostic signs and occur during the major illness.
      (1) Signs of nuchal and spinal rigidity may be obtained either actively or passively.
      (2) The active test for rigidity consists of having the child sit up without assistance. Spinal rigidity is present if undue effort is used, the knees flex upward, and the child rocks somewhat from side to side, then must place the hands behind the body for support.
3. Paralytic poliomyelitis.
   a. Symptoms are identical to those for nonparalytic poliomyelitis with the addition of weakness in one or more muscle groups.
   b. Symptoms may disappear for a period of several days and subsequently recur.
   c. Paralysis is present when symptoms recur.
4. Bulbar poliomyelitis with respiratory insufficiency.
   a. This form of polio presents with bulbar paralysis and coexisting involvement of the respiratory muscles.
   b. Clinical manifestations are
      (1) Inability to speak normally or speaking in breathless sentences.
      (2) Increase respiratory rate.
      (3) Movement of accessory muscles of respiration.
      (4) Inability to cough with full depth.
      (5) Nasal speech due to palatal and pharyngeal weakness.
      (6) Increased pharyngeal secretions.
      (7) Nasal regurgitation of fluids due to palatal paralysis.
      (8) Deviation of the palate, uvula, or tongue.
      (9) Irregular rate, rhythm, and depth of respiration.
      (10) Cardiovascular symptoms.
         (a) Erratic blood pressure.
         (b) Alternate flushing and mottling of the skin.
         (c) Cardiac arrhythmias.
      (11) Rapid changes in body temperature.

Diagnostic Tests

1. Lumbar puncture is of value in making a diagnosis. Absence of organisms on smear and culture, and normal to elevated sugar content, support the diagnosis of poliomyelitis.
2. Viral studies may be undertaken.

NURSING DIAGNOSES: ACTUAL OR POTENTIAL

1. Risk of transmission to others because of the communicability of the virus.
2. Alteration in nutrition and hydration secondary to anorexia and/or inability to swallow.
3. Risk of joint contractures secondary to paralysis.
4. Alteration in oxygenation due to accumulation of oropharyngeal secretions and impaired function of respiratory muscles; fever (and febrile convulsions if they occur) create additional oxygen requirements.
5. Alteration in body temperature: pyrexia due to viral infection and possibly secondary infection (e.g., respiratory or urinary tract).
6. Alteration in excretory patterns: urinary retention secondary to bladder paralysis; constipation and possible impaction.
7. Alteration in comfort: pain due to muscle spasms.

8. Anxiety of child and parents associated with alarming signs, symptoms, and the reputation of the disease.

EXPECTED OUTCOMES

1. Poliomyelitis will not occur beyond the index case.
2. Fluid balance and weight will be maintained.
3. Client will maintain good body alignment and will not develop deformities due to muscle shortening.
4. Patent airway and good O_2–CO_2 exchange will be maintained.
5. Fever will not exceed 39.2°C (102.6°F).
6. Bowel and bladder elimination will be maintained.
7. Urinary tract infection will not occur.
8. Muscle spasm pain will be effectively relieved.
9. Child and parents will receive realistic reassurance about signs and symptoms, therapy, and what they may expect.

INTERVENTIONS

NOTE: Nursing care depends upon the clinical manifestations of the disease, as indicated below.

1. Isolation precautions are taken with any type of polio. Concurrent disinfection of throat discharges and feces is necessary, since polio virus is demonstrable in both throat secretions and stool of infected persons.
2. Approach the child in a calm, reassuring manner, since there may be a high degree of anxiety in the child or parents, especially if respiratory involvement is evident. Explain care procedures and their purposes and expected results.
3. Nonparalytic type of poliomyelitis.
   a. Keep client on bed rest until fever disappears and there is no muscle pain.
   b. Observe for any sign of paralysis.
   c. Give antipyretics as prescribed for fever.
   d. Maintain fluid balance by providing oral fluid.
   e. Provide diet adequate for age.
4. Paralytic poliomyelitis. Nursing measures, in addition to above, include
   a. Maintain good body alignment to prevent deformities.
   b. Apply hot packs to relieve pain due to muscle spasm.
   c. Observe for distended bladder due to transitory paralysis of the bladder.
      (1) Gentle manual compression of the bladder will aid in urination.
      (2) If catheterization is necessary, use meticulous aseptic technique.
   d. Monitor intake and output because of susceptibility to fluid and electrolyte imbalances.
   e. Promote personal hygiene by keeping skin clean and providing oral hygiene. (Client often perspires due to environmental temperature and application of hot packs).
   f. Provide a diet of interest to encourage eating, as anorexia is often a problem in the early stages of polio.
   g. Promote normal bowel function by increasing fluid intake and adjusting diet.
   h. Administer antipyretics as prescribed to control fever. Fans and tepid baths will aid in keeping fever down.
   i. Be alert for any sign of respiratory distress. Be prepared for tracheotomy.
5. Bulbar poliomyelitis with respiratory insufficiency.
   a. Provide quiet, calm environment because of increased anxiety of a client with respiratory insufficiency.
   b. Maintain patent airway by use of gentle suctioning and postural drainage.
   c. Accomplish feeding by gavage and parenteral fluids because of child's inability to swallow.
   d. Observe for signs of respiratory embarrassment, which may necessitate a tracheostomy and use of artificial mechanical respirator. Respiratory difficulty may be due to involvement of the respiratory center in the brain or paralysis of the muscles of respiration.

EVALUATION

Outcome Criteria

1. No skeletal deformities develop.
2. Weight loss is negligible.
3. Adequate fluid and electrolyte balance is maintained.
4. Patent airway is maintained.
5. No urinary infection develops.
6. There is no fecal impaction.
7. Adequate ventilation is maintained.
8. Minimal anxiety.

Complications

1. Erosions in the GI tract (see discussion of GI ulcers in Chapter 33).
2. Gastric dilatation that leads to further respiratory difficulty.
3. Hypertension, especially during the acute stage of illness.
4. Hypercalcemia and renal stones due to immobility (see discussion in Chapter 32).
5. Transitory bladder paralysis (see discussion in Chapter 15).
6. Urinary infection.

Assessment

1. Respirations are labored, and hypoxia may occur.
2. Dimness of vision.
3. Headache.
4. Lightheaded feeling. Above may be regarded as premonitory to a seizure.
5. Diastolic blood pressure consistently above 80 mmHg.
6. Decreased urine output.
7. Bladder distension.

Revised Outcomes

1. Respirations will return to normal, and client will breathe without assistance.
2. Hypertension will be mild, and diastolic blood pressure will remain below 80 mmHg.
3. Urine output will increase, and bladder will empty at each voiding.

Interventions

1. Gastric aspiration and external application of ice bags to alleviate gastric dilatation, which causes respiratory embarrassment.
2. Anticonvulsive medication should be given as ordered.
3. Increased mobilization as soon as possible to correct hypercalcemia and nephrocalcinosis.
4. Increase fluid intake.

Reevaluation and Follow-up

1. Establish a plan, specific to the client, for rehabilitation for the paralytic type of polio.
2. Mobilize the client's and family's resources to assist in a long, difficult period of rehabilitation.

TUBERCULOSIS

DESCRIPTION

Tuberculosis is a serious systemic disease caused by *Mycobacterium tuberculosis*. The infection occurs in all parts of the world; it is most common in underdeveloped countries. The incidence increases with age and is usually higher in urban than rural areas. Epidemics have been reported where people are congregated in enclosed areas, such as classrooms and institutions. The incubation period is about 1 to 3 months from the time of infection to development of a demonstrable primary lesion. Tuberculosis is transmitted by airborne droplets from sputum of infected persons and, infrequently, by indirect contact through articles contaminated with the bacilli. Tuberculosis can occur as a pulmonary or extrapulmonary infection. In either case the specific therapy is antimicrobial drugs, bed rest until there is improvement in the general condition, and a diet that provides a good supply of protein, vitamins, and minerals. Almost any organ or tissue can be involved. Signs and symptoms may simulate many other diseases. The majority of infections in children are intrathoracic. Prognosis of tuberculosis varies. Recovery is the usual outcome of treated primary tuberculosis in children; however, the disease goes unnoticed, undiagnosed, and untreated in the majority of affected children. During the first 2 years of life a high fatality rate is common; otherwise, death rarely occurs except in tuberculosis meningitis or when the disease has progressed rapidly to the terminal stage before it is diagnosed.

PREVENTION

Health Promotion

1. Improve overcrowded conditions.
2. Educate the public about the mode of spread of tuberculosis.
3. People who are contacts to active cases and who have recently converted to a positive skin test should be preventively treated with isoniazid for 1 year.
4. BCG vaccination of uninfected persons provides protection to most individuals.
5. Tuberculosis testing of dairy cattle and slaughter of reactors eliminates milk-borne disease.
6. Pasteurization of milk.

Population at Risk

1. Susceptibility among children is highest under 3 years of age.
2. Undernourished, neglected persons.
3. Persons with partial gastrectomies.

Screening

1. Tuberculin skin testing should be done on all infants at 12 months of age.
2. The frequency of retesting depends on the incidence of tuberculosis in the population and the child's risk of exposure; in high-risk groups skin testing should be repeated at yearly intervals.
3. Periodic chest x-ray films are used to follow up persons with positive skin tests.

ASSESSMENT

Health History

1. Exposure to a household member who has active disease or who was diagnosed as having tuberculosis at the time of death.
2. Travel to an area with a high prevalence of tuberculosis.

Physical Assessment and Additional Features of the History

1. Primary pulmonary tuberculosis.
   a. Child will have a positive skin test.
   b. Symptoms, if present, are usually mild, flulike symptoms and are most often overlooked.
   c. Physical assessment is not remarkable; at most, there may be a slight dullness and slightly diminished breath sounds over the involved area.
2. Progressive primary pulmonary tuberculosis.
   a. Infants are affected more often than older children or adults.
   b. Rapid weight loss.
   c. Infant is apathetic, and appetite is poor.
   d. Examination of the chest reveals dullness upon percussion, and moist rales can be heard over the affected area upon auscultation.
3. Chronic pulmonary tuberculosis.
   a. Uncommon in children; when present, more frequently seen in black than white children and in girls more often than boys.
   b. Slight impairment of the percussion rate.
   c. May be some crepitant inspiratory rales.
4. Cavitary tuberculosis: moderately or far advanced.
   a. Fever.
   b. Night sweats.
   c. Client may complain of malaise and anorexia with subsequent weight loss.
   d. Blood streaked sputum may occur.
5. Acute miliary tuberculosis.
   a. Onset is usually gradual but may be abrupt.
   b. Symptoms are nonspecific and vary widely and may include
      (1) High fever.
      (2) Drowsiness.
      (3) Weight loss.
      (4) Weakness.
      (5) Prostration.
6. Renal tuberculosis.
   a. Symptoms are not specific but may include
      (1) Painless gross hematuria.
      (2) Frequency and urgency in voiding.
      (3) Lumbar pain.
   b. Physical examination that reveals swelling or induration of the epididymides, nodulation along the vas deferens, or a draining sinus are suggestive of tuberculosis.
7. Skeletal tuberculosis.
   a. Tubercle bacilli are sometimes recovered by culture from bone biopsy or from joint fluid.
   b. Pain.
   c. Limp.
   d. Refusal to walk.
   e. Restriction of movement.
   f. Fatigue.

Diagnostic Tests

1. Sputum cultures for acid-fast bacilli.
2. Culture of bronchial secretion and gastric contents.
3. Roentgenographic examination.

NURSING DIAGNOSES: ACTUAL OR POTENTIAL

1. Potential for transmitting disease to others.
2. Noncompliance with long-term medication regimen secondary to lack of motivation, knowledge deficit, expense, or other factors.
3. Knowledge deficit about long-term treatment of disease.
4. Noncompliance with bed rest due to developmental drive to be active.
5. Poor appetite secondary to tuberculous infection.
6. Separation anxiety and impaired development secondary to long-term hospitalization.

EXPECTED OUTCOMES

1. No new cases of tuberculosis will develop as a result of exposure to the index case.

2. Medication will be taken as prescribed.
3. Parents and child will understand the disease and its treatment and will know how to carry out their roles.
4. Child will carry out prescribed activity restrictions.
5. Weight will be maintained; nutrition will be adequate.
6. Hospitalized child will cope with separation with minimal anxiety, and development will proceed normally.

INTERVENTIONS

1. Skin-test all contacts.
2. Isolation is necessary only if child has draining tuberculous lesions.
3. Teach child to use tissue to cover mouth when coughing; tissues must be burned or flushed down the toilet.
4. Assist child and family to secure needed financial assistance (from appropriate agencies) for purchase of medicine; to understand the necessity for continuing medication even when symptoms are gone; or to take other steps necessary to ensure compliance with medication regimen.
5. If child resists medicine because of taste, use flavored liquid medications when available; for other medications it may be possible to disguise taste with fruit juice or fruit, such as applesauce.
6. Teach parents about
   a. The communicability of tuberculosis.
   b. Treatment of the disease.
   c. Prevention of spread to other people.
   d. The importance of long-term chemotherapy, even in the absence of symptoms.
   e. Importance of returning to the clinic for follow-up appointments after discharge from acute care.
7. Provide client with games or other quiet play activities to stimulate development during the time that bed rest is prescribed.
8. Provide a diet high in calories and protein. The older child may be encouraged to eat if given an opportunity to select foods from a menu.
9. Foster parent–child relationship during hospitalization by encouraging visiting, having parents send or bring photographs of family members and other personal mementos, arranging for telephone contact, and so forth.
10. Provide older child with opportunities to keep in touch with friends. A bedside telephone may alleviate boredom and allow contact with peers.

EVALUATION

Outcome Criteria

1. All contacts are found, and treatment is initiated for all those infected with tuberculosis.
2. Client takes medication regularly for length of time it is prescribed.
3. Parents manage home treatment capably.
4. Activity restrictions are followed.
5. Foods from the basic four food groups are ingested daily in quantities appropriate for child's age; weight is within child's usual growth chart "channel."
6. Hospitalized child maintains emotional ties to family as appropriate for developmental age; separation and grief are acted out in play. Family members visit frequently and display attachment to child. Child's development proceeds normally for age (see Chapter 4).
7. Client keeps all follow-up appointments.

Complications

1. Hypersensitivity to antituberculosis drugs.
2. Tubercular meningitis.
   a. Tubercular meningitis is the major cause of death from tuberculosis.
   b. It is always a secondary lesion: the primary lesion is usually in the lung.

Assessment

1. Meningeal symptoms are not present until the terminal stage of the disease.
2. Clinically, the disease can be divided into three stages:
   a. Prodromal stage.
      (1) Onset in gradual.
      (2) A slight fever may be present.
      (3) Mood changes appear.
      (4) Drowsiness is frequent, but sleep is often restless.
      (5) Headache is present.
      (6) There is anorexia.
      (7) Vomiting may occur.
   b. Transitional stage.
      (1) Convulsions occur in many children during this stage.
      (2) Drowsiness becomes deeper.
      (3) Nuchal rigidity is present.

(4) There is stiffness of the back and extremities.
(5) Bulging of the fontanels may occur.

c. Terminal stage.
(1) Paralysis replaces evidence of meningeal irritation.
(2) A comatose state develops.
(3) Pulse and respirations are irregular.
(4) Fever is very high.
(5) Death occurs.

Revised Outcomes

1. Child's comfort will be maximized.
2. Child will receive adequate nutrition.
3. Child will not be injured during seizure or period of altered consciousness.
4. Recovery will be complete.

Interventions

1. Isolate child during febrile stage of illness.
2. Monitor vital signs.
3. Administer antipyretics as prescribed for fever.
4. Approach in an unhurried, calm manner.
5. Offer small feedings at frequent intervals to the child whose appetite is poor.
6. Report to the physician change in the child's mood, level of consciousness, or any signs of nuchal rigidity.
7. Closely observe for seizures.
8. Keep parents informed of child's condition, and allow for as much family interaction as the child's condition will permit.

Reevaluation and Follow-up

1. There is minimal weakness.
2. Muscle spasms, if present, diminish and gradually subside.
3. Personality changes do not persist.
4. The child suffers no permanent paralysis.

GONORRHEA

DESCRIPTION

Gonorrhea is a sexually transmitted disease caused by *Neisseria gonorrhoeae*. This infection is widespread throughout the world; it occurs most frequently among lower socioeconomic groups. Gonorrhea is believed to be the most unreported communicable disease. The incubation period is usually 3 to 5 days. Direct sexual contact accounts for the major transmission of gonorrhea. In gonococcal infection of children, sexual abuse must be considered a possibility and confirmed or ruled out. A child infected with gonorrhea can transfer it to other children if they engage in sex play. Articles contaminated with infected exudate may be a source of infection in young children. Infants can become infected during birth if the mother has the disease. With adequate and appropriate antibiotic treatment, the prognosis for gonorrhea is excellent.

PREVENTION

Health Promotion

1. Educational programs about sexually transmitted diseases should begin no later than the seventh grade.
2. Encourage the use of condoms for sexually active adolescents.
3. Encourage and support responsible sexual behavior.
   a. Rap sessions for adolescents.
   b. Distribute educational literature appropriate to adolescents at public venereal disease and family planning clinics.
4. Routine cultures for gonorrhea in family planning clinics and prenatal clinics will prevent the spread of the disease to newborn babies if the mother receives treatment before the infant is born.
5. Instill prophylactic drops or salve into newborn's eyes at birth.

Population at Risk

1. Susceptibility is general; previous infection confers no immunity.
2. Incidence is greatest in young adult population due to more frequent sexual activity.
3. Newborns whose mothers are infected are at risk.

Screening

1. Routine cultures for gonorrhea on all clients in family planning clinics and prenatal clinics will identify asymptomatic infected women.
2. Cultures for gonorrhea in male sex partners of women who are diagnosed with gonococcal pelvic inflammatory disease.
3. Secure a sexual contact history on female and male clients diagnosed with gonorrhea, and bring all named contacts to treatment.

ASSESSMENT

Health History

1. History of recent sexual contact.
2. Failure to use condom during sexual intercourse.

Physical Assessment

1. Gonorrhea of venereal origin.
   a. In males, a purulent discharge from the urethra appears a few days after exposure to the organism.
   b. Urethral irritation with dysuria occurs, particularly in males.
   c. Urinary meatus is red and swollen, particularly in males.
   d. If untreated, symptoms become worse.
      (1) There is hematuria.
      (2) Headache and malaise sometimes occur.
      (3) If the client had anal sexual intercourse, symptoms can include diarrhea, anal itching, and a purulent discharge adhering to the stool.
   e. Symptoms in the female can include
      (1) Vaginal discharge.
      (2) Frequency of urination.
      (3) Abdominal pain.
      (4) Many females with gonorrhea are asymptomatic.
2. Gonococcal vulvovaginitis.
   a. This form occurs as an inflammatory reaction in prepubescent girls.
   b. There is redness and swelling of the mucous membrane.
   c. Occasionally there is vaginal discharge.
   d. Dysuria is present.
3. Gonococcal ophthalmia neonatorum.
   a. There is acute redness and swelling of the conjunctiva of one or both eyes.
   b. A purulent discharge from the eyes is present.

Diagnostic Tests

1. Smear of the urethral discharge in the male with identification of gram-negative intracellular diplococci.
2. Culture of vaginal or cervical specimens for bacteriological studies.

NURSING DIAGNOSES: ACTUAL OR POTENTIAL

1. Lack of knowledge about sexually transmitted diseases.
2. Risk of transmitting the infection to others.

EXPECTED OUTCOMES

1. Sexually active adolescents will use condoms to decrease chance of reinfection.
2. All contacts will be brought to treatment.
3. Client will have no subsequent reinfections.
4. Recovery will be complete with no complications.

INTERVENTIONS

1. In adolescents and adults.
   a. Educate about the cause, transmission, prevention, and treatment of the disease.
   b. Administer antibiotics as prescribed. Watch for adverse reactions to medications.
   c. Advise client to refrain from having sexual intercourse until cure is established. Reexamination should be done 3 days after treatment.
   d. Advise client not to drink alcohol for a period of 2 weeks after treatment (alcohol can interfere with blood level of penicillin).
   e. Locate, culture, and, if indicated, treat all sexual contacts of the 2 week period before the onset of symptoms.
2. Children and young adolescents for whom sexual abuse cannot be ruled out must be referred to appropriate social agency.
3. All gonococcal infections must be reported to local health authorities for public health investigation.

EVALUATION

Outcome Criteria

1. Reculture is negative after treatment.
2. Client returns to clinic at appointed time for reexamination.
3. All contacts are identified and treated.
4. No complications develop.

Complications

1. Bartholin's gland abscess (see discussion in chapter 34).
2. Proctitis resulting from rectal infection (see discussion in Chapter 33).
3. Urethral stricture (see discussion in Chapter 32).
4. Prostatitis (see discussion in Chapter 32).
5. Gonorrheal arthritis (see discussion in Chapter 16).
6. Sterility (see discussion about infertility in Chapter 14).
7. Acute salpingitis—pelvic inflammatory disease (PID).

Assessment

1. Elevated temperature (above 38.4°C—101°F), chills, rapid pulse.

2. Severe low abdominal pain.
3. Acute tenderness upon cervical palpitation.
4. Elevated white blood cell (WBC) count (20,000–30,000).

Revised Outcomes

1. Pain associated with disease will be controlled.
2. Infection will abate, and temperature and pulse rate will return to normal.
3. White blood cell count will return to normal.
4. No permanent damage (sterility) will result.

Interventions

1. Reduce pain by giving prescribed analgesics.
2. Reduce fever by giving antipyretics and increasing fluid intake.
3. Administer antibiotics as prescribed.
4. Educate the patient about the cause and prevention of gonococcal PID.

Reevaluation and Follow-up

1. Temperature and pulse return to normal range.
2. Pain subsides.
3. White blood cell count returns to normal range.
4. Sexual contacts are identified, and urethral cultures obtained with treatment provided as appropriate.
5. No recurrent infection occurs.

SYPHILIS

DESCRIPTION

Syphilis is a sexually transmitted disease caused by *Treponema pallidum*, a spirochete. Syphilis is a widespread communicable disease. It occurs most frequently in adolescents and young adults. It is more prevalent in urban areas. Males are more often infected than females. The incubation period is 2 to 10 weeks, usually 3 weeks. Sexual contact is the most common mode of transmission. Direct contact (through mucous membrane or break in the skin) with body fluids, such as saliva, semen, blood, and vaginal discharges, of an infected person can result in infection. Transmission also occurs from an infected pregnant woman to the fetus via the placenta after the fourth month of pregnancy. Administration of 2.4 million units of benzathine penicillin is generally effective for primary and secondary syphilis. Congenital syphilis is treated with various doses and types of penicillin, depending on the age of the client. Recovery from syphilis occurs with adequate treatment, but complications and congenital defects that develop before treatment are not reversible. All cases of early infectious syphilis must be reported to the local health authority.

PREVENTION

Health Promotion

1. Education about the cause and spread of syphilis is essential in syphilis control; sex education programs about sexually transmitted diseases should begin no later than the seventh grade.
2. Serological examination for syphilis of all pregnant women.
3. Encourage and support responsible sexual behavior.
   a. Rap sessions for adolescents.
   b. Distribute educational literature appropriate for adolescents at public venereal disease and family planning clinics.
4. Encourage use of condoms for sexually active adolescents.
5. Provide facilities for early diagnosis and treatment, and encourage their use through public education.
6. Conduct intensive case finding programs, investigate contacts for preceding 3 months for primary syphilis and for 6 months for secondary syphilis.

Population at Risk

1. Susceptibility is universal; previous infection confers no immunity.
2. Young adults are infected more frequently than older persons.
3. Males are infected more often than females.
4. Infants born to infected mothers may be infected at birth.

Screening

1. Serological examination for syphilis.
   a. Premarital couples.
   b. Prenatal women.
   c. Persons identified as having any other sexually transmitted disease.
2. Dark-field microscopic examination of any suspicious lesion, especially a lesion on the penis.

ASSESSMENT

Health History

1. Sexually active.
2. Sexual intercourse with a person identified as having a positive serology.

Physical Assessment

1. Primary stage.
   a. A chancre appears at the site of infection.
   b. Swelling of local lymph nodes occurs a few days after the appearance of the chancre.
   c. The chancre is painless and disappears without treatment in a few weeks.
   d. The serological test may be negative up to 8 weeks after infection.
2. Secondary stage.
   a. The client may develop a maculopapular rash that may be so slight as to go unnoticed.
   b. Bald spots may develop on the head.
   c. Coldlike symptoms may develop.
   d. Severe headaches are not uncommon.
3. Tertiary stage.
   a. This stage can develop soon after initial infection or as long as 25 years after infection.
   b. The disease can affect almost any system of the body during this stage.
   c. Symptoms vary according to system or systems affected.

Diagnostic Tests

1. Microscopic examination of scrapings from lesions.
2. Serological examination.
3. FTA-ABS (fluorescent treponemal antibody absorption) test developed in 1949 is treponema specific.

NURSING DIAGNOSES: ACTUAL OR POTENTIAL

1. Lack of knowledge about the cause, transmission, consequences, and prevention of syphilis.
2. Risk of transmitting infection to others.
3. Risk of noncompliance: failure to return for follow-up examination.

EXPECTED OUTCOMES

1. Client will be well informed about sexually transmitted diseases and their prevention and treatment.
2. Pregnant client with syphilis will be treated at the time of diagnosis; child will be born free of disease.
3. Client will not transmit infection to anyone else.
4. Client's recent sexual contacts will be tested and, if infected, treated.
5. Client will complete the recommended course of therapy and follow-up examination for effectiveness of treatment.

INTERVENTIONS

1. Teach client how syphilis is transmitted and prophylactic measures (see Prevention, above).
2. Administer prescribed medication, and observe client for any reaction to the drug.
3. Ensure that all pregnant women have serology test for syphilis.
4. Ensure that articles soiled with discharges from infected lesions do not come in contact with other people.
5. Investigate contacts.
6. Advise client to refrain from sexual intercourse with untreated previous sexual partners.

EVALUATION

Outcome Criteria

1. All contacts are found and treated.
2. Client receives adequate treatment.
3. Client is able to describe how disease is transmitted and verbalizes actions to take to avoid reinfection.

Complications

1. Untreated acquired syphilis can become dormant for many years before complications develop.
   a. Blindness.
   b. Aortic valve incompetence (see discussion in Chapter 30).
   c. Aortic aneursym (see discussion in Chapter 30).
2. Congenital syphilis.

Assessment

1. Positive serology in the mother.
2. Infant may have maculopapular rash.
3. Anemia.
4. Failure to gain weight.
5. Rhinitis.

Revised Outcomes

1. Infant will receive treatment in the first few days of life.
2. Late manifestations will be averted with early treatment.
3. Mother will receive treatment.
4. Other goals, as originally stated.

Interventions

1. Administer antibiotic therapy as ordered.
2. Prevent excoriation of upper lip due to rhinitis.
3. Provide adequate nourishment to correct anemia.

Reevaluation and Follow-up

1. Symptoms disappear after treatment.
2. Infant feeds well and gains weight.
3. Hemoglobin within normal limits.

CAT-SCRATCH DISEASE

DESCRIPTION

The causative agent of this infection is unknown. A virus has been thought to be the cause, although none has been identified. Cat-scratch disease is uncommon but has worldwide distribution. It occurs during all seasons and affects both sexes equally. The infection occurs in young children more often than in other age groups. The incubation period is 1 to 2 weeks from inoculation to the development of the primary lesion. Transmission is from the domestic cat to humans by scratching, biting, or licking. Cats that transmit the disease to people do not appear ill and do not react to the antigen when they receive it by intradermal injection. No specific treatment is known to be helpful. The prognosis is good. The enlarged nodes regress without treatment within 3 months.

PREVENTION

Health Promotion

1. There are no known preventive measures.
2. All cat scratches should be cleaned and treated with antiseptic solution to prevent secondary infections.

Population at Risk

1. Children and young people are most frequently affected.
2. Familial clustering occurs.

Screening

None.

ASSESSMENT

Health History

Association with cats 10 to 30 days before development of symptoms.

Physical Assessment

1. Client generally does not appear acutely ill.
2. Headache and malaise are present.
3. Low-grade fever is present in most clients.
4. Lymph nodes may be strikingly large and tender.
5. There may be swelling and redness at the site of the lesion.

Diagnostic Tests

1. White blood cell count may reveal leukocytosis with a slight shift to the left.
2. Sedimentation rate may be elevated.
3. Skin testing with 0.1 mL of the antigen may have diagnostic significance.
   a. Positive reaction consists of an indurated, raised, erythematous wheal 5 mm or more in diameter 48 to 72 hours after intradermal injection.
   b. Antigen is not available commercially.

NURSING DIAGNOSES: ACTUAL OR POTENTIAL

1. Alteration in body temperature: fever secondary to infection.
2. Alteration in comfort: headache secondary to infection and fever.
3. Alteration in comfort: pain in enlarged lymph nodes.
4. Alteration in nutrition and hydration: decreased intake secondary to anorexia associated with malaise.

EXPECTED OUTCOMES

1. Fever will not exceed 38.9°C (102°F).
2. Headache will be relieved or reduced.
3. Pain in lymph nodes will be relieved or reduced.
4. Child will maintain fluid balance and body weight.

INTERVENTIONS

1. Administer antipyretics as prescribed to control fever.

2. Administer analgesics as prescribed for headache.
3. Keep child at rest until fever and pain subside. Provide child with quiet play activity appropriate for age.
4. Warm, moist compresses may alleviate the tenderness associated with the swollen nodes.
5. Serve small meals at frequent intervals to ensure an adequate intake of food.
6. Offer fluids, such as fruit juice, to keep child hydrated and to aid in control of fever.
7. Observe for and report any sign of central nervous system involvement (see Complications, below).

EVALUATION

Outcome Criteria

1. Fever is low-grade and of short duration.
2. Headache is mild.
3. Normal weight is maintained.
4. Child remains well hydrated.
5. Disease resolves without CNS involvement.

Complications

Encephalitis or encephalomyelitis (see discussion in Chapter 15).

Assessment

1. Fever above 38.5°C (101°F).
2. Restlessness.
3. Irritability.
4. Decrease in level of consciousness.
5. Vomiting.
6. Seizures.

Revised Outcomes

1. Fever will be promptly reduced.
2. Child's comfort will be maintained.
3. Child will remain responsive.
4. Seizures will be controlled.

Interventions

1. Administer antipyretics as prescribed.
2. Administer tepid sponge bath for fever.
3. Maintain cool environment.
4. Approach child unhurriedly and calmly.
5. Monitor intake and output.
6. Provide small, frequent feedings of clear liquids.
7. Administer anticonvulsive medication as prescribed.

Reevaluation and Follow-up

1. Temperature less than 38.5°C (101°F).
2. Decreased periods of restlessness and irritability.
3. Electrolyte values remian within normal limits.
4. Absence of weight loss.
5. Child is alert and responsive.
6. No seizure activity occurs.

ROCKY MOUNTAIN SPOTTED FEVER

DESCRIPTION

This infection is caused by *Rickettsia rickettsii*. The disease occurs throughout the United States. It is seen in the spring and summer and is most prevalent in the southeastern states. Rocky Mountain spotted fever is carried by ticks (generally the wood tick in the western United States and the dog tick in the south) and is transmitted by the bite of an infected tick. Several hours of attachment of the tick are necessary for the organism to infect the human. The disease can also be contracted through contamination of the skin with a crushed tick body or tick feces. Differences in incidence relate to the variations in exposure to infected ticks (e.g., woodsmen and hunters are more often exposed and, hence, more often infected than other groups). Antibiotics have greatly reduced the mortality and morbidity of rickettsial infections.

PREVENTION

Health Promotion

1. Avoid tick-infested areas.
2. Use tick repellent and wear protective (long) clothing.
3. Inspect body at least every 3 hours for ticks when in a wooded area.
4. Remove tick by exerting gentle, steady traction and twisting motion in order to avoid leaving the tick head embedded in the skin.
5. Place tick-repellent collar on family dog or dip dog in liquid tick repellent.
6. Vaccine containing killed *R. rickettsii* is available but is not very effective; it is generally administered only to those at high risk, such as forest rangers.

Population at Risk

1. Susceptibility is general.
2. Those who frequently come in contact with tick-infested areas are at highest risk.

Screening

None.

ASSESSMENT

Health History

1. Exposure to a tick-infested area.
2. Tick bite approximately 3 to 10 days before onset of symptoms.

Physical Assessment

1. There is fever, moderate to high and spiking.
2. Client has poor appetite.
3. Client is restless.
4. Chills occur.
5. A maculopapular rash is observed on about the third day.
   a. Rash begins on the extremities, commonly on wrists and ankles.
   b. It spreads to the palms and soles, then to the entire body.
6. Myalgia is present, especially in calves of legs.
7. Splenomegaly is present in many cases.
8. Severe manifestations include
   a. Central nervous system symptoms.
   b. Edema of the face.
   c. Myocarditis.
   d. Renal involvement.
   e. Thrombocytopenia.

Diagnostic Tests

1. Serological procedures using rickettsial antigens in complement fixation, agglutination, or neutralization test are usually reliable.
2. Rickettsiae may be propagated by inoculating chick embryos, but this procedure is seldom required to diagnose rickettsial infections.

NURSING DIAGNOSES: ACTUAL OR POTENTIAL

1. Alteration in body temperature: pyrexia secondary to infection.
2. Alteration in nutrition and hydration: decreased intake secondary to anorexia and malaise.
3. Risk of neurological, renal, and hemorrhagic complications.
4. Risk associated with continuing exposure to tick-infested environment (e.g., play areas).

EXPECTED OUTCOMES

1. Fever will not exceed 39.5°C (103°F).
2. Child will maintain body weight and hydration.
3. Complications, if any, will be promptly recognized.
4. Family will make a plan for avoiding subsequent tick bites.

INTERVENTIONS

1. Administer medications as prescribed (chloramphenicol, tetracycline); acetaminophen is preferable to aspirin in case the platelet count is low.
2. Monitor temperature and report rising fever. Be alert for febrile convulsions.
3. Keep febrile child in bed and at rest. Provide quiet activities, such as reading, to encourage rest.
4. Provide a diet the child is likely to eat.
   a. Small feedings spaced throughout the day may be better received than three large meals.
   b. Older children may enjoy selecting their own foods.
5. Offer preferred liquids frequently to combat fever and maintain hydration.
6. Monitor intake and output to ensure adequate hydration.
7. Observe and report any sign of CNS disturbance or hemorrhagic disease.
8. Assist family in planning preventive measures to avoid tick bites (see Prevention, above).

EVALUATION

Outcome Criteria

1. Fever is controlled; convulsions do not occur; child is content to rest in bed during febrile period.
2. Body weight and hydration are maintained.
3. Complications do not arise or are promptly recognized, reported, and treated.
4. Family takes measures to reduce risk of tick bite.

Complications

MYOCARDITIS

Assessment

1. Hypoxia.
2. Acidosis.
3. Thrombocytopenia.

Revised Outcomes
1. Oxygenation will be restored to normal levels.
2. Blood pH will return to within normal limits.
3. The infection causing the problem will be treated effectively.
4. Other expected outcomes as stated above.

Interventions
1. Provide humidified oxygen as needed.
2. Obtain ECG to determine cardiac changes.
3. Administer intravenous (IV) medication as prescribed.
4. Monitor arterial blood gases.

Reevaluation and Follow-up
1. Arterial blood gases return to within normal limits.
2. Hypoxia is corrected.
3. Infection is resolved.

Multiple coagulation problems may account for the highest risk of death.

INFECTIOUS MONONUCLEOSIS

DESCRIPTION

Mononucleosis is presumably caused by an Epstein-Barr virus (EBV). The infection has a worldwide occurrence. It is most common in adolescents and young adults in developed countries. In developing countries young children are more commonly affected. In the United States, college students are the main victims. The incubation period is commonly 2 to 6 weeks. The infection is transmitted by direct contact via the oral-pharyngeal route; kissing may be the main means of spread among young adults. Blood transfusions can also transmit the disease. Treatment consists of bed rest, during the febrile period, and supportive therapy; corticosteroids may be used for persons with severe symptoms. The prognosis is good, although there is generally a long convalescence.

PREVENTION

Health Promotion
1. Avoid contact with oral secretions of infected person.
2. Disinfect articles soiled with nose and throat discharges from infected person.

Population at Risk
Susceptibility is general.

Screening
None.

ASSESSMENT

Health History
1. Exposure to droplets from infected person.
2. Recent blood transfusion.

Physical Assessment
1. The onset is usually insidious, but it can be acute.
2. Client experiences malaise.
3. Throat is sore.
4. There is a fever that persists for several weeks.
5. The lymph nodes are enlarged either early or late in the disease. Most commonly, the anterior and posterior cervical nodes are involved and may be enlarged and tender.
6. The appearance of the throat may suggest streptococcal infection or diphtheria.
7. The spleen is usually palpable but is not always tender.
8. A rash is present in a few cases and is most prominent over the trunk.

Diagnostic Tests
1. Heterophile agglutination test that is positive confirms the diagnosis.
2. A titer of 1:56 is considered diagnostic for infectious mononucleosis, and the titer may rise to as much as 1:2028.
3. Lymphocytosis with characteristic changes in the lymphocytes of the peripheral blood.
   a. The lymphocytes are typically larger than mature lymphocytes.
   b. The cell nucleus is frequently placed eccentrically and is irregular in shape or indented.

NURSING DIAGNOSES: ACTUAL OR POTENTIAL

1. Alteration in comfort: sore throat, secondary to disease, and headache, secondary to fever.
2. Alteration in nutrition and hydration: decreased intake due to anorexia and sore throat; accelerated metabolism associated with fever.
3. Noncompliance with bed rest due to com-

pelling need to continue with school activities.
4. Alteration in activity tolerance: fatigue associated with disease and secondary to refusal to rest.

EXPECTED OUTCOMES

1. Throat pain and headache will be relieved.
2. Fever will not exceed 39.2°C (102.6°F).
3. Nutrition and hydration will be maintained.
4. Client will rest as recommended.

INTERVENTIONS

1. Give throat irrigations with warm water several times a day to soothe sore throat. This may be done before meals to lessen pain of swallowing.
2. Administer medications as prescribed to alleviate headache and to minimize fever and sore throat; client may have aspirin or acetaminophen.
3. Offer foods that are soft and easy to swallow.
4. Offer fluids that are not likely to burn or irritate the throat.
5. If there is any doubt that the client is receiving adequate fluids, maintain an intake and output record.
6. Contact appropriate person to assist student in keeping up with studies while in bed.

EVALUATION

Outcome Criteria

1. Complaints of sore throat and headache are minimal.
2. Fever is controlled.
3. Adequate food and fluid intake is maintained.
4. Client remains on bed rest during acute phase.
5. Client keeps pace with schoolwork.

Complications

1. Hepatitis (see discussion in Chapter 33).
2. Rupture of the spleen.
3. Neurological involvement occurs occasionally, generally after the acute phase of the disease.

Assessment

1. Weakness of lower extremities.
2. Weakness progresses to upper extremities and facial muscles usually within 72 hours of onset of lower extremity weakness.
3. Difficulty in swallowing, talking, and chewing.
4. Respiratory failure may occur.

Revised Outcomes

1. Muscular strength will return to normal.
2. Swallowing, talking, and chewing ability will be restored.
3. Respirations will be within normal limits and unassisted.

Interventions

1. Range-of-motion exercises for affected joints.
2. Monitor respirations; use artificial respirator promptly, if indicated.
3. Suction as needed.
4. Approach calmly and reassuringly.
5. Attend the client constantly during any anxiety-provoking procedures.
6. Provide reliable information.

Reevaluation and Follow-up

1. Establish an individualized rehabilitation plan to ensure that complications are overcome.
2. Long-term surveillance must be provided since recovery may take up to 18 months.

CYTOMEGALIC INCLUSION DISEASE

DESCRIPTION

Cytomegalic inclusion disease (CID) is caused by a cytomegalovirus, a member of a group of viruses related to the herpesvirus. The occurrence of CID is worldwide; the prevalence of serum antibody varies from 40 percent in highly developed countries to 100 percent in developing countries. The disease is more common in women than in men. By far the most significant form of the infection is the congenitally acquired form seen in infants. The incubation period is unknown. Infections acquired during birth may be demonstrated 3 to 12 weeks after birth. The mode of transmission is not completely known; the infection may be passed across the placenta to the fetus and may also be transmitted in blood transfusions. There is no known treatment. Seizures have been controlled by anticonvulsant drugs. The prognosis is poor in congenitally acquired infections; the fatality rate is high. Infants who survive may exhibit mental retardation as well as other grave conditions, such as microcephaly, hearing loss, chronic liver disease, and motor disturbances.

PREVENTION

Health Promotion

1. There are no known preventive measures.
2. Infants known to be shedding the virus should be placed in strict isolation.
3. Caretakers of infected infants should be checked often for antibody titer.
4. Women of childbearing age should avoid caring for infected infants.
5. Pregnant women should not care for infants who are shedding the virus.

Population at Risk

1. Infants of infected mothers.
2. Infants cared for in a nursery with undiagnosed infected infants.

Screening

None.

ASSESSMENT

Health History

1. Exposure to a person infected with the virus.
2. Serological studies reveal presence of the virus.

Physical Assessment

1. Low birth weight.
2. Hepatomegaly.
3. Splenomegaly.
4. Icterus.
5. Anemia.
6. Thrombocytopenia.
7. Mental retardation.
8. Deafness.
9. Chronic liver disease.
10. Motor disabilities.

Diagnostic Tests

1. The diagnosis is based on the demonstration of inclusion-bearing cells in the urine, gastric washings, cerebrospinal fluid, and in liver biopsy cells.
2. Inclusion bodies may be present in the cells of the vascular endothelium in older children and adults.

NURSING DIAGNOSES: ACTUAL OR POTENTIAL

1. Alteration in nutritional status: malnutrition secondary to feeding difficulty.
2. Risk of respiratory distress syndrome secondary to low birth weight.
3. Impaired development due to neurological anomalies.
4. Impaired parent–infant bonding secondary to grave illness, anomalies, and parental grieving.
5. Risk of transmitting virus to others.

EXPECTED OUTCOMES

1. Caloric intake will be adequate for growth requirements.
2. Oxygenation will be adequate.
3. Child will receive normal developmental stimulation.
4. Parents will be able to cope with the crisis of having an atypical and gravely ill child.
5. Transmission to others will not occur.

INTERVENTIONS

1. Feed infant by gavage if too weak or too ill to suck.
2. Maintain body temperature to prevent cold stress and resultant increased O_2 requirement; provide supplemental oxygenation, if needed.
3. Stimulate infant by singing, talking, and holding as would be provided other infants. Caution: Pregnant nurses or even nurses who are likely to become pregnant should not care for these babies. Instruct parents in affectionate handling and care of infant.
4. Allow parents to talk about their feelings regarding their child. Promote coping by referral to appropriate agencies (e.g., social service or crippled children's services for financial assistance).
5. Isolate infant if virus is being excreted in urine or saliva.

EVALUATION

Outcome Criteria

1, Infant gains weight.
2. Complications due to secondary infection do not develop.
3. No other cases develop among nursery population.
4. Parents are able to come to terms with their feelings of having a severely ill child.

Complications

1. Mental retardation.
2. Deafness.
3. Chronic liver disease.

4. Motor disabilities.
5. Death.

Revised Outcomes

1. Protect infant from any other infection.
2. Maintain hydration and adequate caloric intake.
3. Safety and comfort of the infant will be maintained.
4. Assist parents in coping and grieving.

Interventions

1. Isolate infant from other infants.
2. Administer anticonvulsants as prescribed.
3. Care for infant unhurriedly.
4. Provide opportunities for parents to discuss their feelings and vent their grief about their infant.

Reevaluation and Follow-up

Establish a plan to meet needs of individual infant according to the degree and type of complications that are present.

PARASITIC INFESTATIONS

ENTEROBIASIS (PINWORM DISEASE, OXYURIASIS)

DESCRIPTION

Enterobius vermicularis is a white, threadlike worm about 4–12 mm long. This intestinal worm infects humans only; pinworms of animals are not transmitted to people. Pinworm infestation occurs worldwide. Children are infected more often than adults, but it is common for an entire family to develop pinworms when one member has them. Pinworms are common in crowded living settings (e.g., institutions). The life span of the worm is 3 to 6 weeks. Infection is usually transmitted by direct transfer of the eggs from the anus to the mouth. This mode of transmission may transfer the infection to other hosts, for example when a mother kisses the infected hands of her child. Eggs can be airborne in dust. They can also be transmitted indirectly by contaminated clothing, food, or any article contaminated with worm eggs. The eggs are ingested and pass into the small intestine, where they hatch. The worms mature in the lower intestine and upper colon; the females migrate to the rectum, crawl out through the anus, and discharge their eggs on the perianal skin. Worms may migrate up the genital tract of females, causing inflammations, such as salpingitis. The specific treatment for pinworm infection is a vermicide such as pyrantel, pyrvinium pamoate, or piperazine citrate. All household members should be treated. Dosage is calculated according to body weight. Control measures include daily bathing, clean bed linen, and good hand washing.

PREVENTION

Health Promotion

1. Education in personal hygiene.
   a. Teach importance of hand washing, especially after defecation and before food preparation or eating.
   b. Discourage nail biting.
   c. Avoid anal scratching.
2. Reduce overcrowded living conditions.
3. Sanitary disposal of feces from infected persons.

Population at Risk

1. Susceptibility is general and universal.
2. Children of school age are infected most often.
3. Mothers of infected children are frequent victims.
4. Prevalence is high among persons in institutions.

Screening

None.

ASSESSMENT

Health History

1. Exposure to household members known to be infected.
2. Severe anal itching, especially at night.
3. Loss of appetite.
4. Weight loss.
5. Insomnia due to severe anal itching.

Physical Assessment

1. Weeping, excoriated skin around the anus.
2. Child may be thin due to anorexia.
3. Child may appear fatigued due to sleep disturbance.

Diagnostic Tests

Cellophane tape test. Female pinworms migrate to the rectum to lay their eggs outside the anus. Cellophane tape pressed firmly against the perianal folds in the early morning hours (before waking, bathing, defecating, or otherwise disturbing the egg deposits) is the best way to obtain a specimen of eggs. The tape is applied to a glass slide and examined under a microscope.

NURSING DIAGNOSES: ACTUAL OR POTENTIAL

1. Nutritional alteration: insufficient intake secondary to anorexia.
2. Self-care deficit: inadequate hygiene (hand washing).
3. Alteration in sleep pattern: wakefulness and restlessness secondary to intense anal itching.
4. Risk of secondary infection caused by scratching.
5. Risk of transmission of worms to others.

EXPECTED OUTCOMES

1. Normal weight will be restored.
2. All household members will be educated in the prevention and control of the infestation.
3. Sleep pattern will be restored to normal.
4. Secondary infection will not develop.
5. All infected household persons will be identified and treated.

INTERVENTIONS

1. Administer prescribed medication (vermicide).
2. Teach family members how the infection is spread.
3. Instruct all family members in good personal hygiene, especially hand washing.
4. Identify by cellophane tape test and medicate all household members who are infected.
5. Assist family to plan well-balanced meals to correct nutritional deficiency.

EVALUATION

Outcome Criteria

1. All infected persons in the household are identified and treated.
2. Family institutes improved hygienic measures as needed.
3. All family members remain free of infection after treatment.
4. Sleep pattern is reestablished.
5. Normal weight is attained.

Complications

1. Appendicitis (see Chapter 33).
2. Reinfection due to nontreatment of contacts.

Assessment

1. Skin around anus is excoriated and weeping.
2. Pain and soreness of area around anus.

Revised Outcomes

1. Skin integrity will be restored.
2. All other expected outcomes, as listed above.

Interventions

1. Treat patient and all infected household contacts.
2. Apply medication as prescribed to excoriated areas.
3. Keep child's hands clean and fingernails clipped short.

Reevaluation and Follow-up

1. Skin heals.
2. Subsequent cellophane tape tests are negative.

HOOKWORM DISEASE

DESCRIPTION

Hookworms are *Necator americanus* and *Ancylostoma duodenale,* roundworms about 9–13 mm long. Hookworm infestation occurs widely in tropical and subtropical countries and also in temperate climates where disposal of human feces is inadequate. Humans initiate the extrinsic phase of the worm's life cycle by discharging stool containing hookworm eggs onto the soil. People in turn become infected by direct contact with the contaminated soil. Older children and adults are more often infected than are infants and young children. The incubation period depends on the intensity of infection and the nutritional status of the host; it may be a few weeks or several months. Transmission is from larvae that hatch and become infective about a week after eggs are deposited in human feces onto the ground. The larvae penetrate the skin of the new host, usually through the sole of the foot. They travel by the bloodstream or lymphatics to the lungs, migrate into the bronchi and into the pharynx, are swallowed, and travel to the small intestine, where they attach to the wall and become mature. The specific treatment is tetrachloroethylene given after an overnight fast. Dosage depends on the weight of the client. The treatment may be repeated in 1 week. Normal hemoglobin is restored by diet rich in iron. The prognosis is good.

PREVENTION

Health Promotion

1. Installation of sanitary disposal systems for human feces.
2. Public education about the dangers of contaminating the soil with human feces.
3. Teach public the importance of wearing shoes.

Population at Risk

1. Populations of underdeveloped areas where disposal of human feces is inadequate.
2. Those who live in warm climates where weather conditions favor development of the infective larvae.

Screening

None.

ASSESSMENT

Health History

1. Exposure to contaminated soil.
2. History of going barefoot.

Physical Assessment

1. Coughing may be present when the larvae are in the lung.
2. Enteritis may be severe.
3. Anorexia.
4. Malnutrition.
5. Patient suffers from chronic fatigue.
6. Anemia.

Diagnostic Tests

Stool examination for the ova or adult hookworm.

NURSING DIAGNOSES: ACTUAL OR POTENTIAL

1. Inadequate knowledge about sanitary disposal of feces.
2. Lack of knowledge about the transmission of the disease.
3. Alteration in nutrition: inadequate intake due to anorexia.
4. Altered exercise tolerance: fatigue secondary to anemia.

EXPECTED OUTCOMES

1. All infected family members will be identified and treated.
2. All family members will wear shoes outdoors.
3. The family will adopt healthful sanitary practices, especially in regard to disposal of feces.
4. After treatment affected family members will regain their appetite and weight and will achieve normal hemoglobin.

INTERVENTIONS

1. Obtain laboratory testing of stool specimens for all household members.
2. Administer prescribed medication (vermicide).
3. Teach family how disease is transmitted and how they can avoid becoming infected.
4. Refer to public health agency for information related to construction of sanitary privy, if the family needs one.
5. Provide anorexic child with small, frequent meals high in iron content.
6. Observe child for symptoms of severe enteritis, and report promptly if they occur.

EVALUATION

Outcome Criteria

1. All family members with the disease are identified and treated.
2. Family demonstrates knowledge about sanitary disposal of feces. Rural families without indoor toilets construct sanitary privies.
3. All family members wear shoes outdoors.
4. Those treated for the disease have a normal hemoglobin count within 1 month after treatment.

ASCARIASIS

DESCRIPTION

Ascariasis is infestation with *Ascaris lumbricoides*, a large roundworm that can be up to 30 cm in length. Ascariasis has a worldwide distribution. It is most common in moist, warm climates; in the United States the disease occurs most often in the South. Children under 10 years of age are most often infected. Rural areas where outdoor toilets are used favor the infestation. The mode of transmission is ingestion of the worm egg, usually from contaminated hands or toys contaminated with soil onto which human feces has been deposited. Children who eat dirt (children with pica) are often infected. The incubation period is about 8 weeks after eggs are ingested. The specific treatment for intestinal infestation is piperazine citrate in two doses given 2 days apart. There is no treatment for the larval stage, during which the young worms live in the lungs.

PREVENTION

Health Promotion

1. Provision of adequate facilities for the sanitary disposal of feces.
2. Prevention of soil contamination in populated areas, especially play areas of children.
3. Education of all persons, especially children, about hand washing after using the toilet.

Population at Risk

1. Children of preschool age and early school age are most frequently infected.
2. Susceptibility is general.

Screening

None.

ASSESSMENT

Health History

1. Exposure to articles contaminated with the eggs.
2. Child has history of eating dirt.
3. Recent travel to area where there is a heavy infestation.

Physical Assessment

1. Atypical pneumonia can occur as the larvae develop in the lungs.
2. Allergic symptoms may be noted.
   a. Urticaria.
   b. Asthma.
   c. Elevated eosinophils.
3. Nausea and vomiting.
4. Anorexia.
5. Weight loss.

Diagnostic Tests

Microscopic examination of the stool for ova.

NURSING DIAGNOSES: ACTUAL OR POTENTIAL

1. Alteration in fluid balance: dehydration secondary to vomiting.
2. Alteration in nutritional status: malnutrition secondary to anorexia.
3. Risk of skin breakdown and secondary infection due to scratching of urticarial rash.
4. Risk of spread of infestation secondary to poor hygiene.
5. Knowledge deficit about the importance of hand washing after eliminating and before handling food.

EXPECTED OUTCOMES

1. Client will maintain adequate hydration, and weight will remain within normal limits.
2. Skin breakdown and secondary infection will not occur.
3. All infected household members will be identified and treated.
4. Family will demonstrate good hand washing practices.

INTERVENTIONS

1. Administer prescribed medication.
2. Prevent dehydration by offering fluids frequently and using prescribed antiemetics.
3. Maintain weight by offering frequent small meals to the anorexic child.
4. Reduce the chance of bacterial infection secondary to scratching by keeping fingernails trimmed.
   a. Apply a soothing antipruritic agent to hives, if present.
   b. Tepid baths with sodium bicarbonate added to the water may reduce itching.
5. Identify all household members who are infected.
6. Teach family members how the parasite is contracted, and instruct them in good personal hygiene, especially hand washing.

EVALUATION

Outcome Criteria

1. Child remains hydrated.
2. Usual weight is maintained.
3. No secondary bacterial skin infection occurs.
4. All infected family members are identified and treated.

5. Family institutes improved hygienic measures, especially good hand washing.
6. Family members remain free of infection after treatment.

Complications

1. Intestinal obstruction can result from a large population of parasites (see discussion in Chapter 33).
2. Intussusception (see discussion in Chapter 22).
3. Paralytic ileus (see discussion in Chapter 33).
4. Appendicitis (see discussion in Chapter 33).

Assessment

1. Pain in abdomen.
2. Vomiting.
3. Change in defecation pattern.

Revised Outcomes

1. All previously stated expected outcomes.
2. Mechanical obstruction will be corrected.
3. Expected outcomes for surgical procedures for above complications will be found in the chapter dealing with the condition.

Interventions

Pre- and postoperative care as outlined in the chapter dealing with the particular problem.

Reevaluation and Follow-up

Child recovers from any surgical procedure.

TRICHURIASIS (WHIPWORM INFESTATION)

DESCRIPTION

The whipworm, *Trichuris trichiura*, can reach 50 cm in length. Trichuriasis is widely distributed, especially in warm, moist climates. The infestation is most common in older children. Whipworms are transmitted by ingestion of worm eggs picked up from contaminated soil. The eggs hatch in the GI tract, and larvae migrate to the cecum and appendix, where they mature. Eggs appear in the feces about 3 months after ingestion. The specific treatment is mebendazole; hexylresorcinol enemas (0.2 percent) may be given hospitalized clients.

PREVENTION

Health Promotion

1. Educate family members, especially children, about the importance of using toilet facilities rather than defecating onto the soil.
2. Provide information about the proper method for building privies for families in rural areas who lack indoor plumbing.
3. Teach families the importance of washing vegetables before eating them.

Population at Risk.

1. Susceptibility is universal.
2. Children are more frequently infected than adults.

Screening

None.

ASSESSMENT

Health History

1. Child is known to eat dirt.
2. Known to live in area of poor toilet facilities.

Physical Assessment

1. Many people harbor the worm without symptoms.
2. In heavy infections there is chronic irritation of the bowel resulting in bloody diarrhea.

Diagnostic Tests

1. Microscopic examination of the feces will demonstrate the ova.
2. Sigmoidoscope will reveal worms in the lower colon.

NURSING DIAGNOSES: ACTUAL OR POTENTIAL

1. Lack of knowledge about adequate, safe toilet facilities and personal hygiene.
2. Alteration in comfort: cramping and tenesmus secondary to heavy infestation of parasites in intestine.

EXPECTED OUTCOMES

1. General hygiene of family will improve.
2. Family will construct adequate, safe toilet facilities if not already available.
3. All infected family members will be identified and treated.

INTERVENTIONS

1. Administer prescribed medication.
2. Examine stool samples from all household members.

3. Teach family good hygiene and proper, safe disposal of feces.

EVALUATION

Outcome Criteria

1. All infected persons are treated and remain free of the disease.
2. Family practices good hygiene.
3. Adequate, safe toilet facilities are constructed when indicated.

Complications

Reinfection with the whipworm.

Assessment

1. Reexamination of the stool from family members reveals reinfection with the parasite.
2. Continuing inadequate hygiene.
3. Inadequate toilet facilities.

Revised Outcomes

1. Family will remain free of disease after retreatment.
2. Family will adopt good hygiene practices.
3. Adequate, safe toilet facilities will be constructed.

Reevalution and Follow-up

1. No ova or parasites are found upon examination of the stool.
2. Other goals, as stated above.

REFERENCE

Fulginiti, V. A.: *Immunization in Clinical Practice*, Lippincott, Philadelphia, 1982, pp. 62–63.

BIBLIOGRAPHY

Benenson, A. (ed.): *Control of Communicable Disease in Man*, 13th ed., American Public Health Association, Washington, D.C., 1981. This is a complete reference manual on communicable disease. It considers every communicable disease known to exist. Its purpose is to provide current information for public health workers and others who are concerned with control of communicable disease. An outstanding reference volume.

Fulginiti, V. A.: *Immunization in Clinical Practice*, Lippincott, Philadelphia, 1982. This excellent reference book is well organized, current, and will be very useful to all professionals who work with vaccine-preventable diseases.

Luckman, J., and Sorensen, K., *Medical-Surgical Nursing: A Psychophysiological Approach*, 2d ed., W. B. Saunders, Philadelphia, 1980. An outstanding textbook for the student as well as the practicing nurse. The section dealing with immunity is an excellent in-depth treatment of the topic. At the beginning of each chapter is a study guide that is most helpful for the reader and aids in providing an overview of what the reader can expect to gain from the particular chapter.

Remington, J., and Klein, J.: *Infectious Diseases of the Fetus and Newborn Infant*, W. B. Saunders, Philadelphia, 1976. An excellent reference book for the reader seeking information about the pathology of certain infectious diseases.

Scipien, G., Barnard, M., Chard, M., et cl.: *Comprehensive Pediatric Nursing*, 2d ed., McGraw-Hill, New York, 1979. This book lives up to its title. It does indeed provide comprehensive coverage. The communicable diseases are found throughout the book and are discussed in relation to the system that is affected. Nursing management is thorough, and the teaching responsibilities of the nurse are discussed.

Vaughn, V. III, McKay, R. J., and Nelson, W., (eds.): *Nelson Textbook of Pediatrics*, 11th ed., W. B. Saunders, Philadelphia, 1979. This latest edition of Nelson's text on pediatrics remains the leader in books of its kind. Comprehensive and complete, it is an outstanding reference book for the health professional.

THE NURSING CARE OF ADULTS

PART IV

PART IV CONTENTS

CHAPTER 25
THE NERVOUS SYSTEM 669

Abnormal Cellular Growth 669
Brain tumors 669
Spinal cord tumors 677
Nerve tumors 680
Pituitary tumors 680

Hyperactivity and Hypoactivity 680
Seizure disorders 680
Abstinence syndromes (withdrawal states) 684
Benign essential tremor (familial tremor) 691
Familial (hypokalemic) periodic paralysis 691
Coma 692

Metabolic Disorders 696
Hypoxic encephalopathy 697
Hypercapnic encephalopathy 698
Hepatic or portal-systemic encephalopathy (hepatic stupor or coma) 698
Uremic encephalopathy 699
Migraine 699
Cerebral edema 700
Increased intracranial pressure 701

Nutritional Disorders 708
Wernicke's encephalopathy (with or without Korsakoff's psychosis) 708
Nutritional polyneuropathy (neuropathic beriberi) 710
Pernicious anemia and pellagra 713

Toxic Disorders 713
Alcohol 713
Opiate and synthetic analgesic 714
Barbiturate 714
Sedative and hypnotic drug 715
Antipsychotic drug 716
Bacterial toxins 717
Heavy metal 718

Inflammations 720
Meningitis (leptomeningitis) 720
Brain abscess 722
Encephalitis (viral) 725
Herpes zoster (shingles) 726
Landry-Guillain-Barré syndrome (acute idiopathic polyneuritis) 728
Neurosyphilis 731
Sarcoidosis 732
Rabies 732
Poliomyelitis 732
Bell's palsy 733
Acute disseminated encephalomyelitis 733
Temporal arteritis 733

Obstructions 734
Cerebrovascular accidents 734
Adult hydrocephalus 742

Degenerative Diseases 742
Neuronal degeneration 742
- Dementia 742
- Amyotrophic lateral sclerosis 747
- Parkinson's disease 751
- Myasthenia gravis 755
- Huntington's chorea 759
- Dyskinesias 760

Myelin degeneration 760
- Multiple sclerosis 760
- Peripheral or cranial nerve degeneration 764

Spinal cord degeneration 765
- Syringomyelia 765

Cervical spondylosis 765
Vascular degeneration 767
- Subarachnoid hemorrhage 767

Traumatic Injuries 770
Blunt (closed) head trauma 770
Open head trauma 771
Cranial nerve injury 776
Spinal cord injury 778

CHAPTER 26
THE SENSORY SYSTEMS 789

Disorders of the Ear 789
The external ear 789
- Otitis externa 789
- External canal blockage 791
- Furunculosis 792
- Perforation of eardrum 792

PART IV CONTENTS *(continued)*

Eustachian salpingitis 794
The middle ear 794
  Acute otitis media 794
  Chronic otitis media and mastoiditis 795
The inner ear 796
  Otosclerosis 796
  Meniere's syndrome 797
  Motion sickness 798
Hearing losses 799
  Sensoneural loss 799
  Conductive loss 799

Disorders of the Eye **800**
Blepharitis 802
Hordeolum 802
Chalazion 803
Dacryocystitis 803
Conjunctivitis 803
Keratitis 804
Corneal ulcer 804
Uveitis 805
Cataracts 806
Glaucoma 807
  Acute (narrow-angle) glaucoma 807
  Chronic (open-angle) glaucoma 808
Detached retina 809
Optic neuritis 810
Malignant melanoma 810
Eye disorders resulting from use of tobacco and alcohol 811
Eye disorders resulting from use of common drugs 811
Eye disorders secondary to systemic diseases 812
  Hypertensive and renal retinopathy 812
  Rheumatoid arthritis 812
  Lupus erythematosus 813
  Anemia 813

Disorders of Taste and Smell **813**
Hypogeusia or ageusia 813
Anosmia, parosmia, and hyposmia 814

Disorders of Sensation **815**
Polyneuropathy 815
Tabetic syndrome 816
Trigeminal neuralgia 817
Thalamic syndrome 818
Parietal syndrome 818
Pain syndromes 819
  Causalgia 819
  Reflex sympathetic dystrophies 819

Disorders of Sleep **820**
Insomnia 820
Hypersomnias 821

CHAPTER 27
THE MUSCULOSKELETAL SYSTEM **823**

Abnormal Cellular Growth **823**
Bone tumors 823
Multiple myeloma 825

Metabolic Disorders **828**
Gout 828
Osteoporosis 830
Paget's disease 832
Osteomalacia 833

Inflammations **834**
Osteomyelitis 834
Ankylosing spondylitis 837
Rheumatoid arthritis 838
Bursitis 838
Tuberculosis of the bones and joints 840

Trauma **841**
Fractures 841
Hip fractures 850
Lower back pain 852

Obstructions **854**
Peripheral vascular disease 854

Degenerative Diseases **858**
Osteoarthritis 858

PART IV CONTENTS *(continued)*

CHAPTER 28
THE ENDOCRINE SYSTEM 865

Abnormal Cellular Growth **866**
Pituitary tumors 866
Thyroid tumors 873
Adrenal medullary tumors 876
Insulinomas 879

Hyperactivity and Hypoactivity **882**
Syndrome of inappropriate ADH secretion 882
Diabetes insipidus 884
Gonadotropin deficiency 886
Diabetes mellitus 887
Hyperthyroidism 892
Graves' disease 893
Hypothyroidism 896
Adrenocortical hyperfunction: hypercortisolism 899
Hyperaldosteronism 904
Hypersecretion of adrenal androgens 907
Adrenocortical hypofunction 907
Hypergonadotropic hypogonadal syndromes 910

Metabolic Disorders **912**
Hyperparathyroidism 912
Hypoparathyroidism 915

Inflammations **917**
Thyroiditis 917

CHAPTER 29
THE HEMATOLOGIC SYSTEM 921

Abnormal Cellular Growth **921**
Leukemia 921
Multiple myeloma 931
Polycythemia vera 935

Hyperactivity and Hypoactivity **936**
Aplastic anemia 936
Agranulocytosis 939
Acquired immune deficiency syndrome 942

Metabolic Disorders **944**
Pernicious anemia 944
Folic acid anemia 948
Iron deficiency anemia 950
Hypoprothrombinemia 954

Inflammations **954**
Infectious mononucleosis 954

Obstructions **955**
Purpura (vascular) 955
Idiopathic thrombocytopenic purpura 956
Disseminated intravascular coagulation 957

Degenerative Disorders **958**
Hemophilia 958
Hemolytic anemias 960

CHAPTER 30
THE CARDIOVASCULAR SYSTEM 967

Abnormal Cellular Growth **971**
Congenital heart disease: coarctation of the aorta 971
Rheumatic heart disease 973
Valvular heart diseases 975
Hypertrophic obstructive cardiomyopathy 982

Hyperactivity and Hypoactivity **984**
Congestive heart failure 984
Pulmonary heart disease 991
Cardiogenic shock 993

Metabolic, Nutritional, and Toxic Disorders **997**
Hypertension 997
Anemia and heart disease 1001
Arrhythmias 1002
Scleroderma 1014
Lupus erythematosus 1016

Inflammations **1018**
Bacterial endocarditis 1018
Myocarditis 1020

PART IV CONTENTS (*continued*)

Pericarditis 1022
Thrombophlebitis 1023

Trauma **1024**
Cardiac and great vessel trauma 1024

Obstructions **1025**
Coronary heart disease 1025

Peripheral Arterial Diseases **1029**
Arteriosclerosis and atherosclerosis 1029
Acute arterial occlusion by arterial embolism 1031
Thromboangiitis obliterans (Buerger's disease) 1034
Raynaud's disease 1036

Degenerative Disorders **1037**
Varicose veins 1037
Aneurysms 1040

CHAPTER 31
THE RESPIRATORY SYSTEM 1045

Abnormal Cellular Growth **1045**
Cancer of the lung 1045
Laryngeal cancer 1049
Sarcoidosis 1054
Polyps 1057

Metabolic Disorders **1059**
Respiratory failure 1059
Cystic fibrosis 1059

Inflammations **1059**
Pneumonia 1059
Tuberculosis 1064
Lung abscess 1071
Pleurisy 1074
Rhinitis 1077
Sinusitis 1079
Tonsillitis (acute) 1083
Acute tracheobronchitis 1083
Pharyngitis (acute) 1085
Laryngitis 1086
Herpes simplex 1087

Trauma **1087**
Pneumothorax 1087
Fractured nose 1093
Epistaxis 1093

Obstructions **1093**
Pulmonary emboli 1093
Bronchiectasis 1097
Deviated septum 1100

Environmental Disorders **1102**
Asthma 1102
Chronic bronchitis 1105
Pulmonary emphysema 1108
Pneumonoconiosis 1111

CHAPTER 32
THE URINARY SYSTEM 1117

Abnormal Cellular Growth **1117**
Renal tumors 1117
Tumors of the urinary bladder 1128
Carcinoma of the prostate 1133

Hyperactivity and Hypoactivity **1135**
Acute renal failure 1135
Chronic renal failure 1140

Inflammations **1149**
Urethritis 1149
Cystitis 1152
Pyelonephritis 1154
Acute glomerulonephritis 1156
Tuberculosis of the urinary tract 1159

Obstructions **1160**
Urethral stricture 1160
Benign prostatic hypertrophy 1160
Nephrolithiasis 1163
Hydronephrosis 1168

Degenerative Diseases **1170**
Chronic glomerulonephritis 1170
Nephrotic syndrome 1170
Polycystic disease of the kidney 1171

Trauma **1172**
Trauma to the kidney 1172
Trauma to the urinary bladder 1174

PART IV CONTENTS (*continued*)

CHAPTER 33
THE GASTROINTESTINAL SYSTEM 1177

Abnormal Cellular Growth 1177
Oral cancer 1177
Leukoplakia 1180
Salivary tumors 1181
Esophageal tumors 1181
Gastric tumors 1182
Small bowel tumors 1182
Colorectal tumors 1182
Tumors of the liver 1183
Pancreatic tumors 1183

Hyperactivity and Hypoactivity 1184
Peptic ulcers 1184
Achalasia 1189
Constipation 1190

Metabolic Disorders 1191
Obesity 1191
Anorexia nervosa 1194
Malabsorption syndromes 1195
Bulimia 1196

Inflammations 1196
Ulcerative colitis 1196
Cholecystitis 1200
Acute pancreatitis 1203
Chronic pancreatitis 1206
Hepatitis 1207
Oral and perioral inflammations 1213
Inflammation of the salivary glands 1213
Esophagitis 1214
Acute gastritis 1214
Chronic gastritis 1214
Regional enteritis 1215
Dysentery 1215
Diverticulitis 1215

Trauma 1216
Esophageal trauma 1216

Obstructions 1218
Intestinal obstructions 1218
Hernias 1222
Hemorrhoids 1223

Degenerative Disorders 1223
Hepatic cirrhosis 1223

CHAPTER 34
THE REPRODUCTIVE SYSTEM 1231

FEMALE REPRODUCTIVE SYSTEM 1231

Abnormal Cellular Growth 1231
Cervical carcinoma 1231
Breast carcinoma 1237
Vulvar carcinoma 1241
Carcinoma of the vagina 1242
Carcinoma of the endometrium 1242
Endometriosis 1242
Choriocarcinoma of the uterus 1244
Carcinoma of the fallopian tube 1244
Ovarian cancer 1245
Benign lesions of the reproductive tract 1245

Inflammations 1246
Vaginitis 1246
Genital herpes 1250
Vulvitis 1252
Cervicitis 1253

Degenerative Changes 1253
Menopause 1253

MALE REPRODUCTIVE SYSTEM 1254

Abnormal Cellular Growth 1254
Benign prostatic hyperplasia or hypertrophy 1254
Prostatic cancer 1254
Testicular neoplasms 1255
Carcinoma of the penis 1255
Hydrocele 1255
Spermatocele 1255
Varicocele 1255

Inflammations 1256
Epididymitis 1256
Orchitis 1256

PART IV CONTENTS *(continued)*

CHAPTER 35
THE INTEGUMENTARY SYSTEM 1259

Abnormal Cellular Growth **1259**
Skin tumors 1259
Warts (verrucae) 1261

Hyperactivity and Hypoactivity **1263**
Psoriasis 1263
Systemic lupus erythematosus 1267
Chronic discoid lupus erythematosus 1269

Inflammations **1269**
Acne vulgaris 1269
Dermatophytosis 1272
Dermatosis: atopic dermatitis 1273
Dermatosis: contact dermatitis 1275
Seborrheic dermatitis 1275
Scabies 1276
Erythema multiforme 1278

Trauma **1279**
Burns 1280

Degenerative Disorders **1286**
Syphilis 1286

25

The Nervous System

Barbara J. Boss

ABNORMAL CELLULAR GROWTH

BRAIN TUMORS

DESCRIPTION

Many types of tumors can be found within the cranium. Such neoplasms are either *primary* tumors composed of nervous system tissue or *secondary* metastatic lesions arising from tissues other than those found within the cranial vault. Both primary and metastatic tumors vary in cell type (see Table 25-1), growth rate, and predilection for growth in specific locations. Some neoplasms, such as glioblastomas, are not encapsulated and thus directly invade normal brain tissues. Other tumors, such as the meningiomas, tend to be encapsulated and are thus predominantly compressive in nature. Tumors normally destroy the immediately adjacent brain tissue and displace more distal tissues and vasculature, producing ischemia, cerebral edema, and increased intracranial pressure. Normal neuronal function is thus impaired. The origins of most primary brain tumors are unclear.

The neurological signs and symptoms associated with a brain tumor are those resulting from the generalized increased intracranial pressure and those specific findings arising predominantly due to the location of the neoplasm. The severity of the signs and symptoms directly relates to tumor size, location, degree of invasiveness, and degree of increased intracranial pressure.

Recognition is given to Gail Barlow Gall, R.N., M.S., who was author of this chapter in the previous edition of this book, and to Laureen Krinsinki, R.N., M.S., and Rosemary Woods, R.N., M.S., who contributed the Prevention sections.

PREVENTION

Health Promotion

1. Other than genetic counseling for those individuals with hereditary tumors, preventive interventions are not possible.
2. Early recognition and surgical intervention for all carcinomas may decrease incidence of metastasis in some instances.
3. Decreasing exposure to hydrocarbons and other pollutants may help.
4. Teaching breast self-examination and other interventions to limit primary cancer sites.

Population at Risk

1. Peak incidence of brain tumors in adults is between the fourth and sixth decade. Males are affected more than females (3:2) except in meningiomas, in which females are affected twice as often as males.
2. Increased incidence of reticulum cell sarcoma has been found in renal transplant recipients (long-time immunosuppressive drug therapy) and in individuals with dysglobulinemia, iridocyclitis, and idiopathic parotitis.
3. Acoustic schwannomas are frequently seen in individuals with von Recklinghausen's neurofibromatosis.
4. Twenty percent of all cancer patients have

TABLE 25-1 TYPES OF INTRACRANIAL TUMOR IN THE COMBINED SERIES OF ZULCH, CUSHING, AND OLIVECRONA EXPRESSED IN PERCENTAGE OF TOTAL (approximately 15,000 cases)

Tumor	Percent of Total
Gliomas	45
Glioblastoma multiforme	20
Astrocytoma	10
Ependymoma	6
Medulloblastoma	4
Oligodendrocytoma	5
Meningioma	15
Pituitary adenoma	7
Neurinoma	7
Metastatic carcinoma	6
Craniopharyngioma, dermoid, epidermoid, teratoma	4
Angiomas	4
Sarcomas	4
Unclassified (mostly gliomas)	5
Miscellaneous (pinealoma, chordoma, granuloma)	3
	100

SOURCE: Adams, R. D., and Victor, M.: *Principles of Neurology*, McGraw-Hill, New York, 1977, p. 586.

brain tumors at autopsy. Primary tumors are most often bronchiogenic and/or breast carcinomas or malignant melanomas. Metastases occur in the 40- to 70-year age group.

5. Inheritance is a known causal factor in development of certain CNS tumors (retinoblastomas, neurofibromas, and hemangioblastomas).
6. Spinal tumors generally occur between 20 and 60 years of age. They are frequently associated with syringomyelia. In addition to primary sites of brain metastases, metastasis often occurs with multiple myeloma, sarcoma, and carcinoma of kidney and prostate.
7. Peripheral nerve tumors occur at any age, are often familial, and may represent metastases from any area, especially those noted for CNS tumors and cancer of face or cervix.
8. Medulloblastomas, polar spongioblastomas (piloid astrocytomas), and pinealomas occur mainly before the age of 20; meningiomas and glioblastomas occur most frequently in the over-50 age group.
9. Exposure to hydrocarbons, nitrosamines, and viruses has resulted in the appearance of gliomas in animals.

Screening

1. Where there is a history of hereditary neurological tumors, family members should be evaluated regularly to facilitate early recognition and surgical intervention. Prevention is not possible for most nervous system tumors.
2. Prevention of metastatic lesions may be aided by regular screening to detect neoplastic disease early. Focus would include yearly x-ray and gynecological exam.

ASSESSMENT

Health History

1. Change in mental function (cognition or affect): such as forgetfulness, diminished insight, difficulty with math calculations, decreased ability to think abstractly, poor judgment, irritability, emotional lability, lack of initiative (apathy), loss of spontaneity, and failure to adhere to acceptable social practices (see Table 25-2).
2. Headache: variable in nature, may be slight and dull in character or severe with either a sharp or dull quality. Initially the head pain may be intermittent. Characteristically the headache associated with a brain tumor is nocturnal in occurrence or occurs on first awakening and has a deep nonpulsatile quality.
3. Vomiting: accompanies the headache and is more common with tumors located in the posterior fossa. The vomiting may occur unexpectedly with no preceding nausea and may be very forceful (projectile vomiting), or both nausea and vomiting may be experienced.
4. Seizures: focal or generalized seizures may occur. Onset of a seizure disorder during adulthood with no history of head trauma is highly suggestive of the existence of an intracranial neoplasm.

TABLE 25-2 CARDINAL PHYSICAL ASSESSMENT FINDINGS ASSOCIATED WITH EACH LEVEL OF BRAIN FUNCTION

Level of Brain Dysfunction	Level of Consciousness	Respiration	Pupils	Movement	Tone Posture	Extensor Plantar Reflex
Cortex	Disorientation Dementia Confusional state Lethargy	Posthyperventilation apnea	Equal and reactive	Roving eye movements present	Paratonia (gegenhalen)	+
Diencephalon	Obtundation Light stupor	Cheyne-Strokes	Small but reactive to light	Bell's phenomenon present	Decortication	+ +
Midbrain	Stupor Semicoma	Central neurogenic hyperventilation	MPF[a]	Doll's eyes present	Decerebration	+ + + + + + +
Pons	Coma	Apneustic	MPF or dilated	Doll's eyes absent	Fading rigidity	+ +
Medulla	Coma	Ataxic	MPF or dilated	Doll's eyes absent	Flaccidity	0

[a] MPF: midposition, fixed to light on testing.

5. Blunted affect, apathy, emotional lability, and loss of spontaneity may be found.

Physical Assessment

1. Diminished cognitive function on examination, particularly regarding memory, proverb interpretation, math calculations, and judgment, may be noted.
2. Unsteady gait may be observed.
3. Papilledema may be noted.
4. Focal signs determined by location of tumor such as nerve palsies, corticospinal tract signs (e.g., hemiparesis or positive Babinski reflex), may be present (see Table 25-3).
5. Other signs and symptoms of increased intracranial pressure; unsteady gait and loss of sphincter control with incontinence.
6. Lapse into an unresponsive state (unconsciousness) is a life-threatening situation indicating presence of a herniation syndrome (see Table 25-4).

Diagnostic Tests

1. Computerized axial tomography (CAT, CT scan) is a noninvasive test that provides direct visualization of intracranial structures. It is particularly useful for identifying mass lesions in the brain in either the supratentorial or infratentorial (posterior fossa) compartments.
2. Skull x-rays and chest x-rays to exclude a primary lung tumor. The skull x-ray may identify a pineal shift, indicating a mass lesion is present, and may show bony erosion, indicating a mass of some type.
3. Lumbar puncture allows measurement of cerebrospinal fluid pressure and provides cerebrospinal fluid for analysis to demonstrate increased protein. (*Done only if there are no indications of increased intracranial pressure.*)
4. Electroencephalogram for localization of cerebral tumors. The closer the lesion to the sur-

TABLE 25-3 DIFFERENTIATION OF CEREBELLAR AND POSTERIOR COLUMN INCOORDINATION

	Cerebellar	Posterior Column
Sensory disturbances	Absent	Always present Loss or impairment of position and vibration senses
Vision	Symptoms not increased by shutting out vision	Symptoms increased by obliteration of vision
Dysmetria	Reaches goal with tremor or overshoots and finally settles on it	Overshoots goal and fails to find it with eyes closed
Tremor	On voluntary movement	Incoordination tremor
Gait	Wide-based, pelvis fixed, trunk and limbs moving asynchronously	Wide-based steppage with eyes watching feet and ground
Station	Romberg's sign not present but unsteadiness in standing with eyes open or closed	Romberg's sign present

SOURCE: Alpers, B. J., and Mancall, E. L.: *Essentials of the Neurological Examination*, Davis, Philadelphia, 1971, p. 80.

face of the cerebrum, the more clear-cut and reliable the localization.

5. Arteriogram to diagnose supratentorial mass lesions. Radiopaque material injected into the cerebral circulation allows identification of alterations in the position of vessels that indicate displacement of brain tissue (see Figure 25-1).
6. Pneumoencephalogram (PEG) for diagnosis of suprasellar (above the sella turcica) and posterior fossa tumors (deep-seated, not easily visualized by other means).
7. Ventriculogram is done if there is risk of herniation from increased intracranial pressure or because of the suspected location of the tumor (in the posterior fossa); a ventriculogram rather than a PEG is done. The same information is obtained from this study as from the PEG, but the risk of herniation is lessened somewhat (see Figure 25-2).
8. In some cases audiograms and vestibular and psychometric tests may be carried out in addition.

NURSING DIAGNOSES: ACTUAL OR POTENTIAL

1. Altered level of cognitive functioning due to fluid volume excess: mild to complete loss,

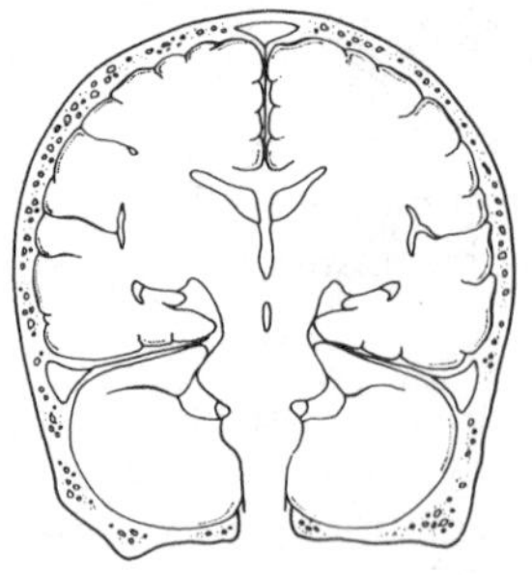

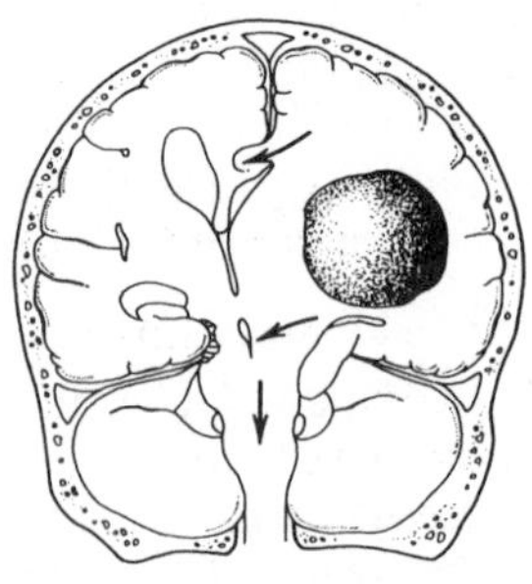

Figure 25-1 Herniation syndromes. Intracranial shifts from supratentorial lesions. On the left is the normal location of structures; on the right various herniation syndromes are demonstrated. (1) Cingulate gyrus is herniating under the falx cerebri. (2) Temporal lobe is herniating downward through the tentorial notch. (3) Compression of the contralateral cerebral peduncle is seen. (4) Downward displacement of brainstem through the tentorial notch is a central herniation syndrome. (Plum, F., and Posner, J. B.: *Diagnosis of Stupor and Coma*, Davis, Philadelphia, 1980, p. 71.)

TABLE 25-4 PROGRESSIVE SIGNS AND SYMPTOMS OF CENTRAL AND UNCAL HERNIATION[a]

	Central Syndrome				
	Early Diencephalon	Later Diencephalon	Midbrain-Upper Pons	Lower Pons-Upper Medulla	Medulla
Pupils	Both small and reactive	→	Not equal in size, but each about midpoint and nonreactive	→	Dilated and fixed
Extraocular signs	May be normal or slightly roving, then difficulty with upward gaze	Difficulty with upward gaze →	And dysconjugate gaze	→	→
Level of consciousness	Difficulty with concentration and becomes agitated or drowsy, then stuporous	Stupor; coma	Deep coma	→	→
Motor	Contralateral hemiparesis to hemiplegia	Plus paratonic rigidity on ipsilateral side that becomes decorticate	Bilateral decerebration	Flaccidity with occasional decerebration	→
Sensory	Progressive deterioration	→	→	→	→
Babinski sign	No Babinski sign	Bilateral positive Babinski sign	→	→	→
Respirations	Cheyne-Stokes	→	And central neurogenic hyperventilation	Shallow	Ataxic, then ceases
Other			Wide variations in temperature (often very high) Many develop diabetes insipidus Bradycardia Elevated systolic blood pressure Widening of pulse pressure	Elevated Pulse erratic (fast and then slow) Blood pressure drops	40.5°C and higher No vital signs

SOURCE: Hickey, J: *The Clinical Practice of Neurological and Neurosurgical Nursing*, Lippincott, Philadelphia, 1981, p. 168.

[a] An important point to keep in mind when observing a client with a possible herniation syndrome is that there is predictable order to the development of signs and symptoms. The neurological deterioration in both central and uncal herniation proceeds in an orderly rostral-caudal scheme; the diencephalon, midbrain, pons, and finally the medulla are affected from the increasing pressure. Signs and symptoms characteristic of each area can be identified. Notice that the last stages of both central and uncal herniation are the same in the medulla.

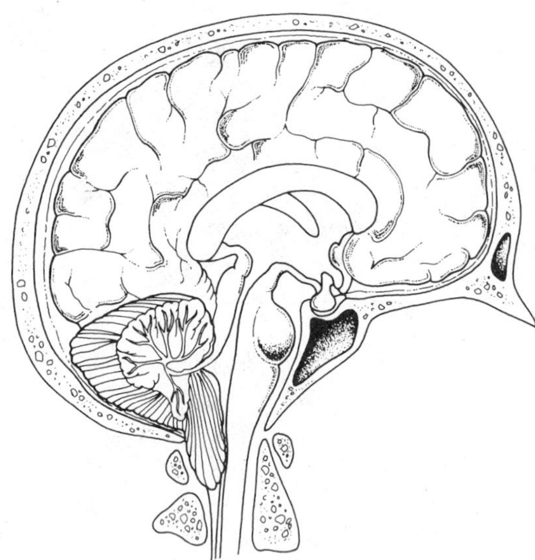

Figure 25-2 Herniation of the cerebellar tonsils into the foramen magnum. (Smith, R. R.: *Essentials of Neurosurgery,* Lippincott, Philadelphia, 1980.)

manifested as an unresponsive (unconscious) state (see Figure 25-3).

2. Alteration in comfort: head pain, mild to severe.
3. Nutritional deficit resulting from vomiting.
4. Potential for injury: secondary to seizures, unsteady gait (if present) or diminished/blurred vision from the papilledema.
5. Alteration in bowel and bladder elimination: incontinence, loss of voluntary control.
6. Impairment of mobility/sensory-perceptual alteration/impairment of communication (verbal and written): possible, depending on the nature of the focal deficits.
7. Knowledge deficit about health status, diagnostic procedures, possible treatment, and hospitalization.
8. Anxiety and fear, mild to severe: due to lack of knowledge and threats to role function, self-concept, and possibly life itself.
9. Role disturbance: related to hospitalization, focal deficits, and therapeutic interventions.
10. Alteration in self-care activities: due to sensory deficits.

EXPECTED OUTCOMES

1. Reduced cerebral edema and intracranial pressure will be evidenced by increased cognition, absence of headache, increased sphincter control, improved gait.
2. Client will be seizure-free within 24–48 h after reduction of cerebral edema and initiation of anticonvulsant therapy (initial).
3. Papilledema will decrease, as evidenced by improvement in visual acuity and decrease in the swelling of the optic disc (initial).
4. Bladder and bowel sphincter control will be evidenced by absence of incontinence within 24–48 h after initiation of measures to control the cerebral edema and the increased intracranial pressure (initial).

INTERVENTIONS

1. Promote establishment of a good rapport and trusting relationship between client, family, and health care providers.
   a. Provide accurate information without false reassurance.
   b. Provide opportunities for client to express fears, anxieties, and feelings about role changes, self-concept, and dependency.

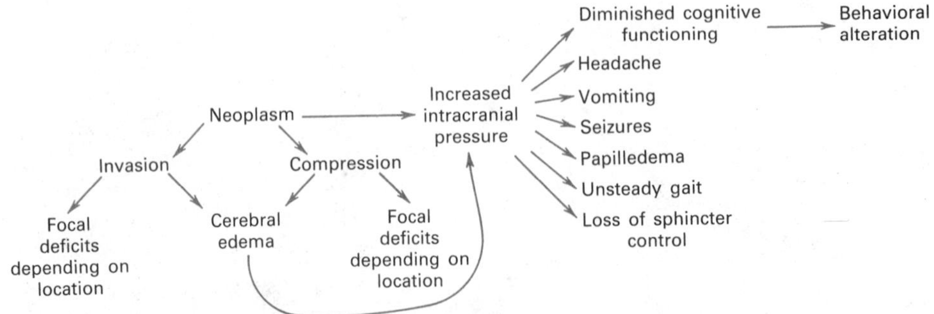

Figure 25-3 Origin of signs and symptoms associated with an intracranial neoplasm.

2. Prepare the client physically and prepare both client and family psychologically for the diagnostic procedures involved in a brain tumor workup.
3. Provide an environment that will optimize the effectiveness of the therapeutic management.
   a. Prepare the client and family for the therapeutic management, whether it be surgery, radiotherapy, chemotherapy, or a combination of these treatments.
   b. Promote the establishment of clear communication between persons participating in the therapeutic regimen.
   c. Promote good nutrition.
   d. Promote skin integrity.
   e. Prevent the hazards of immobility.
   f. Prevent infections with proper Foley, IV, and pulmonary care.
   g. Coordinate needed support services both within the institution and within the client's community.
   h. Assess client to determine response to therapy and the presence of side effects on an ongoing basis.
4. Cranioplasty. Procedure used to correct bony defects in the skull to return the skull contour and integrity for protective and cosmetic purposes; usually follows tumor removal.
   a. A supratentorial approach,
   b. an infratentorial approach, or
   c. transsphenoid approach may be used.

Assessment

See *Increased Intracranial Pressure.*

Revised Outcomes

See *Increased Intracranial Pressure.*

Interventions

See *Increased Intracranial Pressure* with supratentorial approach.

1. Position client.
   a. Elevate head of bed 30 degrees.
   b. Place pillow under client's head and shoulders.
   c. Turn client from side to side once consciousness is regained.
   d. Do not place client on operative side if a large mass has been removed.
   e. With an infratentorial approach:
      (1) Gradually raise the head of the bed to a 30-degree angle over the first postoperative week (10 degrees by day 3, 30 degrees by day 7).
      (2) Place the client's head flat with only a small pillow under the nape of the neck. Avoid flexion of neck.
      (3) Turn client from side to side; usually the client is not placed on his or her back.
   f. With a transsphenoid approach:
      (1) Place client in semi-Fowler's position.
      (2) Turn the client from side to side until consciousness is recovered and swallowing and gag reflexes are intact, then the client may also be positioned on the back.
      (3) Check the nasal drains, nasal packing, and mustache dressing, noting amount and nature of drainage.
      (4) Check dressing on donor site and change dressing as ordered.
      (5) Keep the dressing dry and intact.
      (6) Observe the head dressing frequently for evidence of drainage. Record and report amount and color of drainage. Reinforce a wet dressing immediately.
      (7) Remind the client to avoid touching the dressing. If the client is not alert enough to control pulling or scratching at the dressing, apply mittens to the hands.
2. Maintain client's nutritional and hydration status.
   a. Maintain NPO status for the first 24 h at least or until bowel sounds return.
   b. If no nausea or vomiting is present, test to make sure swallowing and gag reflexes are intact by asking the client to swallow and checking palatal movement.
   c. Usually fluid is restricted until the cerebral edema is resolved and intracranial pressure has returned to normal.
   d. Reassure the client that the loss of taste and smell will return in 2 to 3 weeks.
3. Prevent the detrimental effects associated with arrhythmias.
   a. Monitor ECG continuously.
   b. Administer antiarrhythmic drugs as ordered. Observe for, record, and report signs of therapeutic effectiveness and side effects.
4. Maintain a blood pressure that is *normal for the client.*
5. Institute a pulmonary regimen designed to keep the lungs clear.

6. Promote the maintenance of skin, cornea, and mouth integrity.
   a. See *Coma,* intervention 1a through l, for specific interventions. In addition:
   b. Immediately following surgery, apply cold compresses around the eyes and facial structures to reduce edema formation.
   c. Later in the postoperative period apply warm compresses to the periorbital and other facial areas to help reduce the swelling that may have occurred.
   d. With a transsphenoid approach:
      (1) Remind the client frequently not to blow nose and to avoid sneezing.
      (2) Provide frequent mouth care, as the client is breathing through the mouth.
      (3) *Do not brush the client's teeth* when giving mouth care to avoid trauma to the upper gum.
      (4) Provide frequent oral fluid to help minimize the drying of mucosal tissues.
7. Maintain motor function.
   a. See *Coma,* intervention 3a through g, for specific interventions. In addition:
   b. Begin to get the client out of bed as ordered, usually on the fourth or fifth postoperative day with a supratentorial approach, eighth to tenth day with an infratentorial approach (this delay is due to dizziness, which takes a week or so to resolve), and second to third day with the transsphenoid approach.
8. Institute a bowel evacuation protocol. (See *Coma,* intervention 6a and b, for specific interventions.)
9. Institute a bladder evacuation protocol.
   a. See *Coma,* intervention 5a through d, for specific interventions. In addition:
   b. Observe for signs of diabetes insipidus, for example, excessive thirst, output volume.
10. Assist the client in gaining control over head pain by using medications as needed, positioning, and comfort measures such as back rubs.
11. Determine the status of the gastrointestinal tract.
    a. Listen for bowel sounds to determine the presence of an ileus and watch for abdominal distention.
    b. Maintain the client NPO as ordered until bowel sounds have returned.
    c. Maintain gastrointestinal suction to prevent distention and aspiration of vomitus until gastrointestinal motility returns.
12. Protect client from injury due to decreased cognitive function, seizure activity, and focal deficits.
13. Help client and family assume responsibility for the management of recovery and residual deficits (if any are present).
14. Assist the client in maintaining sexuality functions.
    a. Explore alternate modes of sexual stimuli when sensory impairment exists.
    b. Help the client and spouse to consider alternative means if parenting needs exist.
15. Assist the client and family in learning how to manage the vision problems as well as protect the client from injury due to visual impairment.
16. Help the client and family to learn to protect the client from injury due to impaired tactile sensation. (See *Spinal Cord Tumors,* intervention 4a through c, for specific interventions.)
17. With a pituitary tumor resection or a hypophysectomy, the client and family may need to learn about hormone replacement therapy. (See Chapter 28 for specific discussion of panhypopituitarism.)

EVALUATION

Outcome Criteria

1. Intracranial pressure is reduced to within normal limits.
2. Head pain and vomiting are lessened.
3. Client is seizure-free.
4. Papilledema is decreased. The client's visual acuity is returned to normal.
5. Bowel and bladder are continent.
6. Client and family are able to provide correct information about health status and possible therapeutic regimens.

Complications

1. Brain herniation (see *Increased Intracranial Pressure,* complication 3).
2. Seizures.
3. Blindness.
4. Personality change (see discussion in Chapter 39).

SPINAL CORD TUMORS

DESCRIPTION

A variety of tumors can be found that involve the spinal cord, although they are far less common than those involving the brain. Neoplasms occurring within the spinal canal are classified as (1) *intramedullary,* those arising from within the spinal cord substance, or (2) *extramedullary,* those arising outside of the spinal cord itself either in the vertebrae or epidural tissue (extradural) or in the meninges or nerve roots (intradural).

Although the development of a tumor is occasionally associated with trauma, no known relationship exists between the presence of a primary intraspinal tumor and other specific factors (e.g., the type of tumor and its location within the cord.) The location of the tumor primarily determines the clinical manifestations.

The majority of the intraspinal neoplasms are benign. They produce dysfunction mainly by compressing rather than invading neural tissues. The neurological signs and symptoms associated with an intraspinal tumor are:

1. *Sensorimotor spinal tract syndrome* (cord compression syndrome). Predominantly arising from compression of the spinal cord tracts, an asymmetric impairment in motor function appears and gradually worsens over a period of weeks to months (that is, involves more body parts and becomes more dense). Pain and temperature sensations are often diminished before disturbance in touch, vibration, and position senses. Often the sensory dysfunction is initially contralateral to the motor weakness. Paresthesias may be experienced. Bladder and bowel impairment usually appears as the motor impairment extends.
2. *Radicular spinal cord syndrome* (irritative root syndrome). Knifelike or dull, aching pain with occasional sharp pains is experienced in a sensory nerve root distribution. The pain is intensified by coughing, sneezing, or straining of any kind. Often signs of the cord compression syndrome are also present.

Laminectomy, decompression, excision, and occasionally irradiation are the modes of therapy for intraspinal tumors.

PREVENTION

See *Brain Tumors.*

ASSESSMENT

Health History

1. Radicular pain described as knifelike or dull and aching with occasional sharp pain radiating distally.
2. Subjective sensory symptoms such as tingling, numbness as a heavy sensation that follows a segmental distribution and gradually involves more body parts.
3. Loss of sensation below a certain point may be a complaint.
4. Motor weakness of an asymmetric nature, gradually increasing over a period of weeks to months both in degree of weakness and amount of the body involved is reported (often is the first symptom noted by the person).
5. Incontinence of bladder or bowel may be described.

Physical Assessment

1. Motor deficits ranging from diminished muscular strength and movement (paresis) to paralysis of one or more body parts may be present. Motor deficit may be manifested as spastic weakness of the lower extremities (paraparesis), hemiparesis or hemiplegia, quadriparesis or quadriplegia, or monoparesis or monoplegia, depending on the location of the lesion and the degree of compression.
2. Atrophy of the involved muscles frequently is noted.
3. Fasciculations may be seen and are evidence of increased muscle fiber irritability due to motorneuron dysfunction.
4. Diminished or absent deep tendon reflexes may be seen in the muscles innervated by the segment of the cord directly involved by the lesion.
5. Increased deep tendon reflexes may be seen below the level of the neoplasm due to loss of inhibition from the higher brain centers, and extensor plantar reflexes are frequently seen.
6. Diminished sensation for pinprick and temperature is most commonly found and is in-

itially contralateral to the maximum motor weakness (Brown-Séquard's syndrome).

7. An asymmetrical, segmentally distributed decrease in touch (pressure) sensations may be seen.
8. A diminished position and vibration sense with resultant ataxia may be present.
9. On palpation, tenderness of the spinous process over the tumor may be present.
10. Evidence of a spastic bladder may be found.

Diagnostic Tests

1. X-ray film of the spine: may show calcifications within the tumor, vertebral erosion, widening of the spinal canal due to vertebral erosion, an increase in the size of the interpedicular space, or kyphosis.
2. Lumbar puncture: besides allowing the measurement of cerebrospinal fluid and the analysis of the fluid, the Queckenstedt's maneuver permits the detection of a partial or complete block in CSF circulation.
3. Electromyelogram: demonstrates fasciculations and denervation that result from motor root involvement. These findings assist with the localization of the tumor. Normal EMG activity is found above the lesion; abnormal activity is seen at and below the lesion.
4. Myelogram: clearly demonstrates and localizes the lesion. Dye may be injected below or above the suspected tumor site depending on the location.

NURSING DIAGNOSES: ACUTAL OR POTENTIAL

1. Alterations in comfort: radicular pain, tenderness over the spinous processes (moderate to severe).
2. Potential for injury: secondary to sensory impairments and motor deficits.
3. Impairment of mobility: secondary to motor weakness, possibly spasticity.
4. Alterations in self-care activities: secondary to sensory impairment, motor deficits, diagnostic procedures, and therapeutic interventions.
5. Alteration of urinary elimination: incontinence.
6. Alteration in bowel elimination: incontinence, loss of voluntary control, constipation secondary to immobility.
7. Alteration in patterns of sexuality: secondary to muscle impairment.
8. Anxiety, mild to severe: secondary to lack of knowledge, threats to role function, self-concept, and self-care ability.
9. Alterations in self-concept: secondary to sensory, motor, and reflex deficits, alterations in self-care abilities and role disturbance.

EXPECTED OUTCOMES

1. Tenderness, pain, and spasticity will be reduced. The client will be in control of discomfort as evidenced by verbal statements.
2. Client will report absence of injury.
3. Client will maintain as much self-care and role function as possible in light of sensory, motor, and coordination deficits.
4. Normal pattern of bowel function will be retained, as evidenced by the absence of constipation and/or bowel continence.
5. Client and family will know correct information about health status, therapeutic management, and so on.
6. There will be absence of edema.
7. The family and/or client (if feasible) will make an informed and carefully thought-through decision about the possibility of home management.
8. With a malignant spinal cord tumor, the final goal eventually is that the client will experience a dignified death.

INTERVENTIONS

1. Establish a continued data base with ongoing periodic neurological reassessment.
2. Assist the client to gain control over the pain.
   a. Administer pain medications as ordered.
   b. Provide range of motion exercises every 2–4 h to avoid stiffening in the joints.
   c. Turn client q2h to help avoid stiffening, pressure, and increased spasticity.
   d. Position client so that the spinal cord is not stretched; usually this involves flexing the hips and knees to some degree.
   e. Help client avoid activities that will aggravate the pain, such as coughing, sneezing, or straining to void or at stool.
   f. Provide cutaneous stimulation through touch, temperature, and vibration using such measures as backrubs; the heat available during bathing or showering; application of physiotherapy measures such as ultrasound, diathermy, or dry

heat, as ordered; or stimulation methods such as transcutaneous electrical nerve stimulation, as ordered.

g. Help client to learn to use cognitive pain management strategies such as distraction, imagery, or hypnosis or to use behavioral methods such as relaxation.
h. Maintain an adequate intake of protein in the diet and a sufficient intake of tryptophan.
i. Prepare the client for deep brain stimulation or ablative neurosurgical or radiocoagulation procedures should these become necessary to control the client's pain.

3. Prepare the client physically and prepare both the client and family psychologically for the diagnostic procedures involved in establishing the diagnosis.
4. Assist the client and family to learn how to protect the client from injury due to impaired tactile sensations and motor deficits.
   a. Visually check the position of involved body parts after moving; check often, even when client is at rest.
   b. Visually examine the involved area for signs of trauma or irritation.
   c. Check the temperature of bath water, heating devices, cold applications, food, in order not to cause cold or heat injury.
5. Assist client and family in learning to manage the spasticity. (See *Amyotrophic Lateral Sclerosis,* intervention 3a through f, for specific interventions.)
6. Assist client and family in instituting a skin integrity maintenance program.
7. Assist client and family in instituting a bowel evacuation protocol to prevent constipation and straining at stool.
8. Maintain motor functions through range of motion exercises.
9. Help client and family assume responsibility for the management of the neurological deficits (or for recovery, if the tumor is curable).
10. Maintain urinary tract in the best possible condition if an indwelling catheter is in place.
    a. Administer urinary antiseptic such as methenamine mandelate (Mandelamine) with a urinary acidifier such as vitamin C as ordered.
    b. Force fluid (3,000–5,000 mL/day), if not contraindicated.
    c. Encourage client to drink cranberry juice and apple juice ($2\frac{1}{2}$ qt daily are needed to acidify the urine).
    d. Encourage the client to limit milk and dairy products.
11. Institute an upper motor neuron or mixed bladder training protocol if the urinary function assessment indicates this is appropriate.
    a. Establish a clamping and releasing regimen, starting with clamping for 1 h and then releasing. The time is gradually lengthened until the bladder is holding 300–400 mL, if this can be tolerated. Not all physicians will order this regimen.
    b. Assist the client and family in learning the signs of a full bladder if perception of bladder fullness is diminished (e.g., sweating, restlessness, and abdominal discomfort).
    c. Drugs such as diazepam (Valium) may be used to decrease spasticity in some instances to help control incontinence.
12. Assist the client in maintaining sexual functioning.
    a. Explore alternate modes of sexual stimuli when sensory impairment exists.
    b. If infertility is a problem, help the client and spouse to consider alternative means to meet their parenting needs, if this is realistic for the client's situation.
13. Reduce the client's anxiety through encouraging verbalization of fears and concerns.
14. Provide the client and family with an environment that will optimize the effectiveness of the therapeutic management.
15. If tumor is the result of a primary or secondary malignancy and the client can no longer survive, assist the client and family in the process of grieving. Provide time for them to be together. Assure a dignified death. (See Chapter 45.)

EVALUATION

Outcome Criteria

1. Client is in control of discomfort.
2. Client is free from injury (self-reporting).
3. Client maintains self-care and role function.
4. Normal bowel function is maintained.
5. Bowel continence is restored.
6. Client and family are able to verbalize information about client's health status, di-

agnostic procedures, therapeutic management, and hospital policy and procedures.
7. Skin is intact.
8. Lungs are clear; absence of edema is noted.
9. Absence of urinary retention and infection is reported.
10. Client and family can make an informed decision about home management.
11. Client has a dignified death.

Complications

1. Decubiti.
2. Atelectasis leading to pneumonia (see discussion of pneumonia in Chapter 31).
3. Urinary tract infection (see discussion in Chapter 32).
4. Paraplegia (see *Spinal Cord Injury* for specific discussion).
5. Quadriplegia (see *Spinal Cord Injury* for specific discussion).
6. Severe spasticity or spasms (see discussion under *Multiple Sclerosis*).
7. Chronic pain syndrome.

NERVE TUMORS

An *acoustic neuroma* (schwannoma, neurinoma, or neurofibroma) most commonly occurs in the fifth decade of life and affects both sexes equally. Essentially benign, the tumor almost always originates in the vestibular division of the VIIIth cranial nerve, usually just distal to the junction between the nerve root and the medulla. As the neoplasm grows, it extends into the posterior fossa to occupy the cerebellopontine angle and compress the Vth, VIIth, and less commonly, IXth and Xth cranial nerves. If allowed to grow, the tumor can eventually enlarge to displace and compress the pons and medulla as well as obstruct the flow of cerebrospinal fluid.

Initial symptoms may include hearing loss, headache, impaired balance, unsteady gait, tinnitus, facial weakness, facial pain, and loss of facial sensation on the involved side. Often by the time the client seeks assistance from a health care provider, he or she is experiencing vertigo associated with nausea and vomiting, a sense of pressure in the ear, and moderate to severe unsteadiness with rapid position changes (e.g., turning).

Audiologic evaluation, x-ray studies of the internal auditory meatus, CSF analysis for increased protein, and posterior fossa dye studies help establish the diagnosis. Treatment requires surgical excision using microsurgical techniques via an auditory or intracranial posterior fossa approach.

Nursing diagnoses and interventions primarily focus on lack of knowledge, anxiety and fear, alteration in comfort due to vertigo, nausea, vomiting, and pain, potential for injury due to gait disturbance and balance problems, and alteration in self-concept (potential) if the client is left postoperatively with a motor paresis or paralysis.

Neurinomas (schwannomas) of other cranial nerves, such as the Vth (trigeminal) and IXth (glossopharyngeal) nerves, may occur. These tumors resemble the acoustic neuroma in terms of their nature, location, signs and symptoms, diagnosis, and treatment. Nursing diagnoses and interventions are also similar.

PITUITARY TUMORS

See Chapter 28, The Endocrine System.

HYPERACTIVITY AND HYPOACTIVITY

SEIZURE DISORDERS

DESCRIPTION

A *seizure* is the sudden, explosive, disorderly discharge of cerebral neurons and is characterized by a sudden, transient alteration in brain function, usually involving motor, sensory, autonomic, or psychic signs and symptoms and an alteration in the level of consciousness "responsiveness" (see Table 25-5). Seizure disorders are the second most common neurological disorder and represent a syndrome rather than a specific disease entity. Seizures have a greater tendency to occur in persons with organic brain lesions than in those with a normal central nervous system.

A single seizure or brief outburst of seizures

TABLE 25-5 CLASSIFICATION OF THE EPILEPSIES

1. Partial seizures (seizures begin locally)
   a. Simple (elementary symptomatology, generally without loss of consciousness)
      (1) Motor symptoms present
         (a) Focal (without Jacksonian march)
         (b) Jacksonian
      (2) Sensory symptoms present
         Focal (somatic sensory, visual, auditory, olfactory, vertiginous)
   b. Complex (usually with loss of consciousness, complex symptoms): temporal lobe or psychomotor seizures
      (1) Automatisms present
      (2) Psychosensory symptoms present
      (3) Ideational symptoms present
      (4) Affective symptoms present
      (5) Visceral and autonomic symptoms present
   c. Partial seizure with secondary generalization
2. Generalized seizures (seizures without focal onset, bilaterally symmetrical)
   a. Grand mal (major motor, tonic-clonic) seizures
   b. Absence
      (1) Simple (petit mal)
      (2) Complex (with additional symptoms)
   c. Myoclonic seizures
   d. Tonic or clonic seizures
   e. Atonic or akinetic seizures
   f. Infantile spasms
3. Unclassified seizures
4. Status epilepticus
5. Febrile convulsions

SOURCE: Adapted from G. W. Sypert: "New Concepts on the Management of Epilepsy: Medical and Surgical," in *Clinical Neurosurgery*, The Congress of Neurological Surgeons, 1977, p. 602, Table 46.1.

may accompany a variety of medical illnesses and may be a manifestation of nervous system involvement by the disease process. The onset of a seizure or a series of seizures may be a manifestation of an ongoing primary neurological disease. A seizure disorder that has extended over a long time period with the majority of the episodes being similar may very well represent an old injury that has long ago scarred.

PREVENTION

Health Promotion

Health promotion should focus on removing or correcting the seizure-producing factors when possible and decreasing the individual's susceptibility to seizure activity.

Population at Risk

The seizure activity of most individuals with idiopathic epilepsy begins early in childhood.

1. Cerebral lesions, whether neoplastic, congenital, or vascular may produce seizure activity.
2. Seizures are often sequelae of severe head injuries, especially open-head trauma.
3. Post cortical infarct individuals may have seizures at some time after the stroke.
4. An infectious process (e.g., meningitis) may cause seizure activity in individuals.
5. Decreased oxygen concentration, metabolic disturbances (e.g., hypoglycemia, hypocalcemia) and electrolyte disturbances (e.g., hyponatremia) can be responsible for precipitating seizures.
6. Toxic states (e.g., uremia, drug overdose and/or withdrawl, alcohol withdrawl, heavy metal ingestion) may also precipitate seizure activity.
7. Individuals with a vitamin B deficiency are at risk for seizures.
8. Brain injuries occurring in utero or during the birth process may account for seizure disorders in any age group.
9. Environmental factors (e.g., flickering lights, alterations in smell and taste) also have been known to precipitate seizures. The relation between these factors and seizure activity should be investigated more fully.
10. Any condition that alters the metabolic environment of the brain can cause seizure activity (see Table 25-6).

TABLE 25-6 CAUSES OF RECURRENT CONVULSIONS IN DIFFERENT AGE GROUPS

Age of Onset, Years	Probable Cause
Infancy, under 2	Congenital maldevelopment, birth injury, metabolic disorders (hypocalcemia, hypoglycemia), vitamin B_6 deficiency, phenylketonuria
Childhood, 2–10	Birth injury, trauma, infections, thrombosis of cerebral arteries or veins, beginning of idiopathic epilepsy
Adolescence, 10–18	Idiopathic epilepsy, trauma, congenital defects
Early adulthood, 18–35	Trauma, neoplasm, idiopathic epilepsy, alcoholism, drug addiction
Middle age, 35–60	Neoplasm, trauma, vascular disease, alcoholism, drug addiction
Late life, over 60	Vascular disease, degeneration, tumor

SOURCE: R. D. Adams: "The Convulsive State and Idiopathic Epilepsy," in G. W. Thorn et al. (eds.), *Harrison's Principles of Internal Medicine*, 8th ed., McGraw-Hill, New York, 1977, p. 132, Table 24-1.

Screening

During the health assessment, conditions that are known to induce seizures or precipitating factors should be elicited and recorded. These include:

1. Birth trauma.
2. Head trauma.
3. Stroke history.
4. Metabolic disturbances.
5. Drug and alcohol ingestion.

ASSESSMENT

Health HIstory

1. Presence of any prodromal symptoms.
2. Presence of an aura (e.g., cry).
3. Clinical manifestations noted by the client if conscious or by observers at the onset of the seizure.
4. Sensory or motor manifestations noted during the seizure, including eye movements, body or extremity movement, or changes in consciousness.
5. Description of the postictal state if present, by the client and/or the observers.
6. Presence of any precipitating (risk) factor(s) (e.g., stress).
7. Past personal history related to the seizure etiology.
8. Family history related to the presence of a seizure disorder in other family members.

Physical Assessment

1. Changes in the mental status examination.
2. Changes in cranial nerve function.
3. Changes in muscular tone or strength.
4. Changes in primary or cortical sensations.
5. Abnormal reflexes.
6. Gait changes.
7. Signs of cerebellar dysfunction.
8. Seizure activity may be present during the examination.

Diagnostic Tests

1. Skull x-rays to demonstrate a bony structure abnormality or a pineal shift indicative of the presence of a mass lesion.
2. CAT scan to demonstrate the presence of a tumor, cyst, abscess, hemorrhage, or other brain lesion.
3. Lumbar puncture to demonstrate a normal cerebrospinal fluid pressure and a normal cell count in the cerebrospinal fluid.
4. Electroencephalogram to demonstrate the seizure focus, the location of the focus, and the type of brain waves being produced.

NURSING DIAGNOSES: ACTUAL OR POTENTIAL

1. Potential for injury: due to seizure activity and loss of responsiveness.
2. Altered levels of communication: mild to severe due to changes in consciousness.

3. Anxiety, mild to severe: secondary to seizure activity and potential for injury.
4. Alterations in self-concept: secondary to anxiety and stigma attached to having a seizure disorder.
5. Individual maladaptive coping patterns (e.g., manipulation), mild to severe: secondary to anxiety and stigma attached to having a seizure disorder, modification in lifestyle needed to manage the seizure disorder.
6. Ineffective family coping, mild to severe: secondary to anxiety, stigma attached to having a family member suffer from a seizure disorder and tendency to overprotect the individual.
7. Health management deficit: lack of knowledge about health status, the disorder, diagnostic procedures, and so forth.
8. Potential for noncompliance to therapeutic regimen: due to lack of knowledge, anxiety, individual maladaptive coping.

EXPECTED OUTCOMES

1. Client will be injury-free.
2. Client will be seizure-free within 48–72 h after the initiation of anticonvulsant therapy.
3. Client will report no sensory deficits resulting from the seizure.
4. Client will verbalize fears and concerns (stigma) regarding seizure disorders.

INTERVENTIONS

1. Promote seizure control as well as protect the client from injury.
   a. Observe for, record, and report signs that may be prodroma, an aura, an actual seizure, or a postseizure response.
   b. Institute seizure precautions.
   c. If seizure with unconsciousness occurs, protect the client from injury.
      (1) Prevent or break the client's fall.
      (2) Place the client on the bed or floor.
      (3) If client has chewing mouth movements, place soft, firm object between the client's teeth to prevent injury to the mouth structures. (*Do not force an object between already clenched teeth.*)
      (4) Protect the client from injury by placing the client's head on a pillow or in a person's lap.
      (5) Remove all harmful objects from the client's immediate environment.
      (6) Maintain an open airway by placing client's head in a lateral position to allow drainage of secretions.
      (7) Protect the client from embarrassment and exposure.
      (8) Reorient the client when consciousness is regained.
      (9) Provide a quiet environment and allow the client to rest or sleep until the client recovers from the postictal phase.
      (10) Provide emotional support to the client and significant others.
   d. With the client, determine the possible precipitating factor(s).
   e. Monitor the effectiveness of the therapeutic regimen by noting the blood levels of anticonvulsants and the seizure control achieved.
   f. Observe for signs of side effects and toxic effects of the anticonvulsant medication(s).
2. Teach client about seizures: causes, precipitating factors, and management protocols.
3. Help client assume responsibility for the management for the seizure disorder.
   a. Teach the client and family about the anticonvulsant drugs, their action and effects, and when additional amounts of anticonvulsant may be necessary. Therapeutic blood levels of anticonvulsants must be reached and maintained by daily taking the prescribed dosage. Illness and other physical stresses as well as emotional stress may require an increase in the dosage needed to maintain adequate blood levels.
   b. Teach the client and family how to assess for and recognize side effects such as gum hypertrophy or ataxia from diphenylhydantoin (Dilantin).
   c. Help client and family to avoid the use of other drugs (over-the-counter or "street" drugs) along with anticonvulsants. The physician should be consulted before taking any such drugs. Stimulant drugs (caffeine) may cause a seizure to "break through." Depressant drugs (alcohol) may cause accidental overdose and may lower the seizure threshold when the drug is withdrawn.
   d. Help client and family understand the rationale for lifestyle changes, such as re-

strictions against driving motor vehicles, operating heavy equipment, and using potentially dangerous equipment, and the need to refrain from swimming and possibly tub bathing until the client has been seizure-free for a specified period of time (often 1 to 2 years for licensing purposes).

e. Encourage client and family to participate in structured groups of persons confronted with a similar situation.
f. Encourage client and family to utilize the resources of the local, regional, and national Epilepsy Foundation.
g. If this is a hereditary epilepsy, encourage the client and family to seek genetic counseling.

EVALUATION

Outcome Criteria

1. Client is seizure-free.
2. Client is injury-free.
3. Client and family are able to provide correct information about health status, the seizure disorder, the diagnostic procedures, therapeutic management, and hospital policy and procedures.
4. The client is able to verbalize acceptance of having a chronic health problem and is able to report self-care activities taken to reduce possible onset of seizure activity.

Complications

INJURY

See discussion in appropriate chapter, depending on the nature of the injury.

AFFECTUAL DISORDER

See discussion in Chapter 36.

INTERPERSONAL PROBLEMS

See discussion in Chapter 37.

STATUS EPILEPTICUS

Assessment

Recurrent seizures occurring so frequently that the client does not regain consciousness or normal cognitive function between seizures (Moss et al., 1973).

Revised Outcomes

1. Status epilepticus will be controlled.
2. Other goals will remain as stated previously.

Interventions

1. Administer drug regimen as ordered and carefully monitor its therapeutic effects. Sodium phenobarbital, thiopental (Pentothal sodium), diphenylhydantoin (Dilantin), diazepam (Valium), and paraldehyde are often used to control status. Usually the drugs are given in combinations of two or three drugs. The IV route is often used initially.
2. Administer oxygen as ordered.
3. Maintain patent airway. An airway must sometimes be placed and maintained until the status is controlled.
4. Maintain hydration via IV therapy.
5. Institute measures to protect the client from injury, including heavily padded siderails and headboard.
6. Observe for signs of circulatory collapse, such as persistent tachycardia or hypotension.
7. Monitor temperature and protect the client from hyperthermia by applying appropriate cooling measures.
8. Also see nursing interventions under *coma* for further specific measures related to the decreased consciousness.

Reevaluation and Follow-up

1. Attempt to isolate the factor(s) precipitating the status epilepticus state.
2. Monitor the establishment of therapeutic blood levels of the anticonvulsant drugs.

ABSTINENCE SYNDROMES (WITHDRAWAL STATES)

DESCRIPTION

A period of chronic intoxication with a depressant drug followed by a period of relative or absolute abstinence are the two common factors underlying the development of the four major *withdrawal syndromes,* or states: *tremulousness* (anxiety state), *acute hallucinosis, withdrawal seizures* (known as "rum fits" in an alcohol withdrawal state), and *delirium tremens* (again the name in an alcohol withdrawal state). Only one major state may occur or a combination of the states may appear.

PREVENTION

Health Promotion

1. Health education: should be instituted as early as kindergarten to alert individuals to potential dangers associated with drug use; this may provide the only real source of prevention.

2. Individual instruction: regarding the dangers of withdrawal whenever drugs are to be administered over time.
3. Continued education: via media, printed materials, and health counseling; should focus on dangers of drug use and withdrawal problems associated with use of alcohol and other drugs both legal and illegal. Individuals should be instructed to inform personnel of their drug history whenever a continued drug use may be curtailed.
4. Counseling and controlled drug treatment programs: Alcoholics Anonymous may offer alternatives to drug use. Withdrawal can then be minimized.

Population at Risk

1. Any individual who ingests alcohol, barbiturates, hypnotic sedatives, or opiates is at risk for withdrawal syndrome. The larger the drug dosage and the longer the duration of drug intake, generally the greater the symptom severity, although this may not be the case with the drug "addict."
2. Any individual admitted for emergency or elective surgery may be at risk, and certain factors have been identified that would increase the index of suspicion.
   a. Drug abuse is often associated with psychiatric disorders, especially psychoneurosis and sociopathy, in individuals who begin chronic ingestion patterns and are under 40 years of age.
   b. Drug abuse beginning over 40 years of age is often associated with depression, loss of loved one, or other recent life changes.
   c. Alcohol and opiate abuse are found in most age and ethnic groups. Although no group is totally free from abuse, the incidence is higher in some populations.
   d. Barbiturate, hypnotic, and sedative use necessitates availability, but this is often facilitated by multiple prescriptions. Heavy use is associated with persons experiencing chronic anxiety and/or insomnia.
3. Persons experiencing seizures without any past history may be experiencing early withdrawal from alcohol, barbiturates, or sedative/hypnotic drugs.
4. Addiction to any drug increases the incidence of addiction to other drugs. These individuals are at risk for complicated withdrawal syndrome.

Screening

1. Identifying drug users through nonthreatening interview should identify those individuals with drug-taking history.
2. Risk factors that may lead to alcohol or drug use should be identified early and may actually prevent abuse if alternative therapy is available.

ASSESSMENT: TREMULOUSNESS (ANXIETY) STATE

Health History

1. History of a period of chronic ingestion of a depressant drug that is either a sustained or periodic (spree) intoxication (may be over only a few days).
2. History of a current relative or absolute abstinence from the drug intake (may be as little as overnight while sleeping).
3. Complaint of general irritability by the client or the family.
4. Complaint of gastrointestinal symptoms particularly, anorexia, nausea, and retching.
5. Complaint of insomnia although the person feels a need for rest and sleep.
6. Complaint of being "jittery" or "shaking inside."
7. Mental overalertness apparent, accompanied by inattentiveness and indifference to the environment.
8. Evidence of poor memory for the past few days.

Physical Assessment

1. Mild disorientation to time may be present.
2. A generalized, fast-frequency tremor with a varying degree of severity is present. The tremor increases with motor activity and decreases with quiet and rest. (See Table 25-7.)
3. A flushed facies is seen.
4. Tachycardia is present.

Diagnostic Tests

Electroencephalogram; see diagnostic tests for *Assessment: Delirium Tremens.*

ASSESSMENT: HALLUCINOSIS STATE

Health History/Physical Assessment

1. History of tremulousness preceding this current state.
2. Complaint of "bad dreams."
3. Complaint by the client or family of misinterpretation of sounds and shapes or misper-

TABLE 25-7 TREMORS

Type	Distribution and Rhythm	Rate/ Frequency (Slow–Rapid)	Amplitude (Coarse–Fine)	Effects of Movement and Rest (Resting, Intention, Sustention)
Abnormal Tremors				
Parkinsonian tremor (static tremor)	Tremor is greater distally than proximally	Slow (3–6 Hz) Constant	Coarse but varying, especially augmented by emotion	Resting tremor but disappears with sleep
	Extremity tremor, less frequently involves the jaw, tongue, head; described as "pill-rolling" tremor			
Cerebellar tremor (intention tremor)	Extremity tremor, occasionally rhythmic oscillation of head (titubation) or trunk	Slow (4–6 Hz)	Coarse (jerky)	Intention tremor (action tremor), occurs during movement and is intensified at the termination of movement
Familial tremor, essential tremor, or senile tremor	Most commonly affects the head, less frequently the jaw, tongue, lips, larynx; oc-	Rapid (8–13 Hz) Slow (4–6 Hz)	Coarse but variable, augmented by anxiety	Sustension tremor appears at the initiation of movement or when supporting the extremity

	casionally involves the extremities			or head in a fixed position (when actively maintaining the position); present throughout the movement
Toxic tremor (endogenous: e.g., thyrotoxicosis, uremia; or exogenous: e.g., alcohol or tobacco)		More rapid	Fine	Sustension tremor
In encephalopathy, often referred to as "wrist flapping" or "liver flap"	Seen in the upper extremities on sustension, distal tremor predominantly	Slower (4–6 Hz)	Coarse	Sustension tremor
Wilson's disease tremor	Extremity tremor predominantly	Slow	Coarse	Static (resting) or intention tremor; predominantly resting but aggravated by movement of the extremity
Normal Tremors				
Physiological tremor	All muscles involved	More rapid (8–13 Hz) Slower in children and aged	Fine, is really just an exaggeration of normal muscle fiber movement, just has more amplitude	Action tremor (intention) with some postural (sustension) component

ception of familiar objects. Objects may seem distorted or unreal.
4. Evidence of distorted perception.
5. Hallucinations: visual, auditory, or mixed and occasionally tactile or olfactory in nature; often take the form of human, animal, or insect life.

Diagnostic Tests

See diagnostic tests for *Assessment: Delirium Tremens* below.

ASSESSMENT: WITHDRAWAL SEIZURES

Health History

1. Abstinence following a period of chronic intoxication with a drug.
2. One episode or a burst of seizure episodes in the past, especially during a previous withdrawal state.
3. A seizure disorder.
4. One episode or a burst of seizure episodes that tend to be of the grand mal type during this current withdrawal period.

Physical Assessment

1. A seizure actually occurs.
2. A postictal state exists.
3. Stroboscopic stimulation results in generalized myoclonus or a convulsive seizure.

Diagnostic Tests

See test under *Assessment: Delirium Tremens,* below.

ASSESSMENT: DELIRIUM TREMENS

Health History

1. History of excessive, steady intake of a depressant drug for a prolonged period of time (sometimes years).
2. History of a current abstinence period.
3. History of tremulousness, hallucinosis, or seizure activity during this current abstinence period.
4. A profound confusional state with the presence of delusions and vivid hallucinations.
5. Extreme restlessness and agitation.
6. Sleeplessness.

Physical Assessment

1. Reactive but dilated pupils.
2. Tachycardia.
3. Fever may be present.
4. A profuse diaphoresis.
5. Hyperreflexia and increased muscle tone.

Diagnostic Tests

Electroencephalogram: reflects changes induced by the chronic drug intoxication, that is, decreased brain wave frequency during the chronic intoxication, rapid return to normal after cessation of the drug intake with occurrence of a period of sharp wave activity coinciding with seizure activity.

NURSING DIAGNOSES: ACTUAL OR POTENTIAL

1. With a tremulousness state:
   a. Anxiety, mild to moderate: due to withdrawal from chronic use of depressant drug.
   b. Alteration in cognitive function, mild to moderate: overalertness, impaired memory, disorientation due to impaired memory.
   c. Dysrhythm of sleep-rest activity, mild to severe: secondary to anxiety, and impaired cognitive function.
   d. Nutritional deficit, mild to moderate: due to anorexia and nausea.
   e. Fluid volume deficit, mild to moderate: fluid loss due to anorexia, nausea, and retching.
2. With hallucinosis, *in addition to the above*:
   a. Sensory-perceptual alteration, moderate to severe: secondary to impaired cognitive functioning resulting in illusions, delusions, and hallucinations.
   b. Potential for injury, moderate to severe: secondary to impaired cognitive functioning, anxiety, and hallucinations.
   c. Self-care deficit: due to impaired cognitive functioning, anxiety, and hallucinations.
3. With delirium tremens, *same as the above but*:
   a. Anxiety, severe.
   b. Alteration in cognitive function, severe.
   c. Dysrrhythm of sleep-rest activity, severe.
   d. Fluid volume deficit severe: due to decreased intake and profuse diaphoresis.
   e. Sensory-perceptual alteration, severe.
   f. Potential for injury, severe.
   g. Alterations in self-care activities, severe.
   h. Alteration in cardiac output, moderate to severe: due to overactivity of sympathetic nervous system and volume depletion.

i. Impairment of skin integrity: secondary to trauma, diaphoresis.
j. Altered levels of consciousness: in response to medical management (tranquilization/sedation).
k. Impairment of mobility: in response to medical management (restraints and tranquilization/sedation).
l. Respiratory dysfunction: aspiration and atelectasis secondary to medical management (tranquilization/sedation).
m. Impairment of urinary elimination: incontinence.
n. Alteration in bowel pattern: incontinence; constipation secondary to dehydration.
o. Maladaptive (individual) coping patterns: drug abuse resulting in potential for drug withdrawal state.

4. See additional diagnoses under discussion of *Seizure Disorders*.

EXPECTED OUTCOMES

1. Client will be in control of anxiety, as evidenced by verbal statements, restricted and controlled motor movements, and vital signs within limits *normal for the client*.
2. The client will maintain (or regain) cognitive functions that are currently intact.
3. The client will maintain (or regain) as much self-care as possible.
4. Normal sleep-rest activity pattern will return, as evidenced by verbal report.
5. Nutritional intake of well-balanced diet will be regained, as evidenced by maintenance of body weight and normal hematocrit and hemoglobin.
6. Normal vascular volume will return, as evidenced by normal skin turgor, normal serum electrolytes, and urinary output, 5.0 mL/h.
7. Client will be free from injury.
8. With delirium tremens, *in addition to the above*:
   a. Skin, mouth, and cornea will remain intact.
   b. Vital functions will be maintained within normal limits for the client.
   c. Motor function and coordination will be maintained, as evidenced by normal neurological examination.
   d. Client will verbalize control over drug-abuse problem, as evidenced by abstinence from use of substance.
   e. Normal bowel and bladder patterns will be maintained.

INTERVENTIONS

1. Establish an accurate data base with ongoing periodic neurological reassessment.
2. Reduce the need for the lost mental capacities.
   a. Place orienting measures such as written signs that keep place, date, time, and other such information constantly in the client's environment.
   b. Establish and maintain a constant environment. Orient client to the environment and reinforce the orientation frequently (e.g., label bathroom, bed, and other pertinent objects in the room).
   c. Establish and maintain a constant routine.
   d. Minimize client's exposure to confusing situations and an undue number of simultaneous stimuli.
   e. Avoid transferring the client from one room to another.
   f. Use the same nursing personnel every day whenever possible.
   g. Protect client from needing to make decisions, set priorities, or formulate judgments beyond his or her current cognitive functioning level.
3. Maintain and maximize use of client's remaining capacities.
   a. Place objects familiar to the person in the new environment, such as meaningful objects from home.
   b. Allow a family member or friend to remain with the client.
   c. Maximize the reception of pertinent sensory input.
      (1) Minimize distracting stimuli.
      (2) Initiate and maintain face-to-face contact with the individual.
      (3) Reorient the person to the health care provider with each contact.
      (4) Explain exactly what is going to be done (or is being done) with or for the individual.
      (5) Give simple, specific information or directions.
      (6) Provide new information slowly and in small doses with frequent rest periods.

d. Place prosthetic devices such as glasses and hearing aids on the client if they have been judged to be safe.
e. Remind the client what can be done for himself or herself. Encourage self-care to the extent possible and safe.
f. Focus interpersonal interactions on what is familiar and meaningful to the client.
g. Minimize exposure to emotional stress.

4. Perform appropriate interventions to help reduce the anxiety or give the client a sense of control over anxiety.
   a. Express concern about and caring for the client.
   b. Verbally recognize the client's feelings and fears.
   c. Provide optimistic but realistic reassurance.
   d. Allow the client to maintain rituals that help limit anxiety.
   e. Provide the client with information about what is happening and what can be expected to occur in the future.
   f. Also see *Anxiety* in Chapter 36.
5. Regarding illusions, delusions, and hallucinations, reinforce reality. After recognizing and accepting the client's perception or interpretation, state your perception in a calm, reassuring, and nonargumentative manner.
6. Assist the client in maintaining nutritional and hydration status and personal hygiene.
7. Institute safety precautions.
   a. Control the client's environment; remove all potentially harmful objects.
   b. Provide close or constant supervision.
   c. Limit the extent of the client's mobilization ability, such as restricting movement to only within client's room.
   d. Avoid restraints if possible. If necessary, use mittens and body restraints and give the client repeated explanations for the restraints. *A client should never be placed in wrist and ankle restraints while lying supine and flat in bed, then sedated. The client cannot clear his or her own airway in such a situation.*
8. Administer tranquilizers, sedatives, antiemetics, and other medications as ordered. Observe and record responses.
9. With delirium tremens:
   a. Prevent the detrimental effects associated with arrhythmias.
      (1) Monitor ECG continuously.
      (2) Administer artiarrhythmic drugs as ordered. Observe for, record, and report signs of therapeutic effectiveness and side effects.
   b. Maintain a blood pressure that is *normal* for the client.
   c. If the medical management is directed at placing the client in a light stupor (asleep), the nursing management must include the following interventions.
      (1) Prevent hypoxia and hypercapnia.
         (a) Observe for decreasing respiratory rate, hypoventilation, or cyanosis.
         (b) Maintain a patent airway and improve ventilation.
            (i) Position client so that the lungs may maximally expand; also, prevent aspiration or choking.
            (ii) Turn client q2h.
            (iii) Provide postural drainage as ordered if atelectasis develops.
            (iv) Ventilate client if necessary.
         (c) Treat an elevated temperature with cool environment, cooling sponge baths, and so forth.
      (2) Maintain motor function. (See *Coma*, intervention 3a, d, and e.)
      (3) Promote the maintenance of skin, cornea, and mouth integrity.
         (a) (See *Coma*, intervention 1a and c through i.)
         (b) Turn client from side to side at least q2h to relieve pressure, especially over bony prominences.
      (4) Maintain nutritional and hydration status.
         (a) Maintain IV in place and administer fluids as ordered and monitor (record).
         (b) Maintain the client NPO (usually) throughout the sedation period.
      (5) Maintain the urinary tract in the best possible condition, if an indwelling catheter is in place, by maintaining the closed system drainage. Discontinue catheter when ordered.
   d. When the delirium state has subsided, assist the client in reestablishing a normal bowel pattern by instituting a bowel evacuation protocol. (See *Coma*, intervention 6a and b for specific interventions.)

10. After client recovers, provide nursing interventions to assist with the drug-abuse problem as appropriate. (See discussion in Chapter 37, Interpersonal Problems of Adults, for specific interventions.)

EVALUATION

Outcome Criteria

1. Client is in control of anxiety, as evidenced by verbal reports and an absence of physical symptoms.
2. Client maintains (or regains) cognitive functions that are currently intact or are recoverable.
3. Client maintains (or regains) self-care.
4. Client maintains (or regains) *normal* sleep-rest activity pattern, as evidenced by self-report.
5. Client maintains (or regains) intake of fluids and a nutritionally well-balanced diet, as evidenced by verbal report; weight.
6. Client maintains normal bowel and bladder functions and other motor functions.
7. Client gains control over drug-abuse problem.

Complications

1. Injury (see discussion in appropriate chapter, depending on the nature of the injury).
2. Dehydration (see Evaluation under *Amyotrophic Lateral Sclerosis,* complication 6).
3. Arrhythmia (see discussion in Chapter 30).
4. Hypertension (see discussion in Chapter 30).
5. Atelectasis/aspiration leading to pneumonia (see discussion in Chapter 31).
6. Myocardial infarction (see discussion in Chapter 30).
7. Cerebrovascular accident (see discussion under *Cerebrovascular Accident*).
8. Subarachnoid hemorrhage (see discussion under *Subarachnoid Hemorrhage*).
9. Respiratory arrest (see discussion in Chapter 49).
10. Decubiti.
11. Constipation and impaction (see discussion in Chapter 33).
12. Corneal ulceration (see discussion in Chapter 26).
13. Urinary tract infection (see discussion in Chapter 32).
14. Contractures.

BENIGN ESSENTIAL TREMOR (FAMILIAL TREMOR)

Although the pathology is not understood, essential or familial tremor is an action tremor that is present when the extremities are actively maintained in a certain position. When the tremor occurs as the only neurological abnormality among several family members, it is known as *familial tremor* and is usually inherited as a dominant trait. If there is no evidence of familial inheritance, the tremor is labeled *benign essential tremor*. If the tremor presents only in late adulthood, it is called *senile tremor.*

Nursing diagnoses and interventions center around alteration in self-concept, anxiety, potential for injury, alteration in self-care activities, potential social isolation, and possibly some degree of impairment of verbal communication if the mouth muscles and larynx are involved.

FAMILIAL (HYPOKALEMIC) PERIODIC PARALYSIS

Periodic paralysis is characterized by periodic episodes of muscular weakness (paresis) or paralysis that more severely affect distal extremity muscles than proximal extremity or trunk muscles. The legs often weaken before the arms become involved. Typically the episodes begin during sleep, often after strenuous activity. A high-carbohydrate meal is usually associated with these weakness episodes, also. The weakness lasts from a few hours to several days.

The onset of the disorder generally is in late childhood or adolescence. Paretic or paralytic episodes tend to occur every few weeks. The attacks lessen with age. The ratio between affected males and females is 3:1. There is a strong familial tendency with an autosomal dominant pattern.

Reduced serum potassium levels as low as 1.8 mEq are found during the attack. Potassium is thought to shift from the extracellular compartment into the cell, but as yet unidentified factors must also be present to account for the marked sensitivity to small potassium reductions and to cold, which is often a precipitating factor.

Five to 10 g of potassium chloride daily prevent the episodes in many clients. Persons who are not controlled with this regimen are placed on a low-carbohydrate, low-salt, high-potassium diet, combined with a slowly released potassium preparation. For an episode already in progress, 10 g of a potassium salt is given orally. An additional 5 g may be given in 1–2 h if there is no improvement.

Nursing diagnoses and interventions during an attack center on impairment of mobility, potential for injury, alterations in self-care activities, anxiety, potential impairment of skin integrity, and potential impairment of urinary elimination. When there is no episode of weakness in progress, nursing diagnoses and interventions focus on lack of knowledge related to the disorder, precipitating factors, and therapeutic management of the disorder.

COMA

DESCRIPTION

The ascending reticular activating system (ARAS) controls the amount of central nervous system activity. The exact anatomical boundaries of the ARAS are indistinct. The ARAS nuclei are interpersed throughout the midbrain, hypothalamus, and sensory nuclei of the thalamic and septal regions. The ARAS receives input from the sensory pathways and projects fibers to the thalamus and cerebral cortex. Brainstem centers of the ARAS are responsible for awakeness (arousal). Thalamic and higher cortical centers control mental activity (content of consciousness). Thus consciousness has two components: arousal and content of consciousness.

Impairment of consciousness indicates brain dysfunction and is a symptomatic expression of disease. The common pathophysiology of all impairment of consciousness, despite cause, is either a reduction in cerebral metabolism or a reduction in blood flow. There may be direct interference with the metabolic activities of the neurons in the cerebral cortex, diencephalon, and upper brainstem as in metabolic disorders, intoxications, and nutritional deficiencies. Depressant drugs directly suppress the neuronal activity of the cerebrum, diencephalon, and ARAS, whereas other intoxication states create metabolic disorders such as acidosis or hypoxia. Large, destructive, and space-occupying lesions of the brain may impair consciousness by direct destruction of the midbrain and diencephalon or by herniation. The best indicator of level of brain function is the level of consciousness.

PREVENTION

Health Promotion

1. Health promotion interventions focus on preventing, controlling, or promptly correcting the underlying cause of this altered state of consciousness.
2. Medic alert tags should be worn to identify diabetics and epileptics if they are found unconscious.

Population at Risk

Individuals with:

1. Metabolic disturbances (diabetic acidosis, hypoglycemia, hypoxia, uremia, hepatic dysfunction).
2. Cerebrovascular disease (cerebral hemorrhage, cerebral thrombosis, cerebral embolism).
3. Acute head injuries (severe skull fracture or concussion, brain contusion, subdural hematoma, penetrating wounds).
4. Intoxications (drug intoxication, lead poisoning, carbon monoxide poisoning, and alcoholism).
5. Intracranial masses (brain tumor, brain abscess).
6. Acute brain infections (encephalitis, meningitis).
7. Severe systemic infections (pneumonia, typhoid fever, malaria).
8. Thermal disturbances (hyperthermia, hypothermia).
9. Hypertensive encephalopathy and eclampsia.
10. Idiopathic epilepsy.
11. Circulatory collapse or cardiac decompensation.

Screening

1. Identification of existing abnormality.
2. Environmental hazards that may precipitate coma.
3. Assessment of the levels of perception and coordination through mental status and neu-

rophysical exam is used to determine level of consciousness and functioning.

ASSESSMENT

Health History

1. Lack of initiative, disinterest in work, home, or family, and neglect of routine tasks or hobbies noted by family, friends, or employer.
2. Irritability or apathy is complained of by the family, friends, coworkers, or employer.
3. Distractibility and inattentiveness is noted by family, friends, and employer.
4. Inability to think through a problem or to think clearly is reported.
5. Recent history of poor judgment, poor decision-making ability, and the lack of insight is given.
6. Change in mood, mood shifts, and emotional lability is reported by the family, friends, or employer.
7. Loss of social graces and inattentiveness or indifference to social customs is complained of by the family and friends.
8. Complaint of lethargy by client or family.
9. Complaint of falling asleep by the client or family and of client's not being able to stay awake unless constantly stimulated.
10. Complaint by the family of inability to awaken the client.

Physical Assessment

1. Evidence of distractibility and inattentiveness.
2. Deteriorating mental status is present on examination.
3. Deteriorating ability to use language; that is, varying aphasias in varying degrees may be present.
4. Unkempt, sloppy appearance and dress.
5. Pupil changes may indicate location of cause of coma (see Figure 25-4).

Diagnostic Tests

1. Electroencephalogram to demonstrate the degree of brain wave activity and the type of brain wave activity.
2. Cerebral blood flow studies to demonstrate the areas of compromised blood flow in the brain tissues.
3. See Diagnostic Tests under *Dementia* for specific tests to isolate the cause(s) for the decreased consciousness.

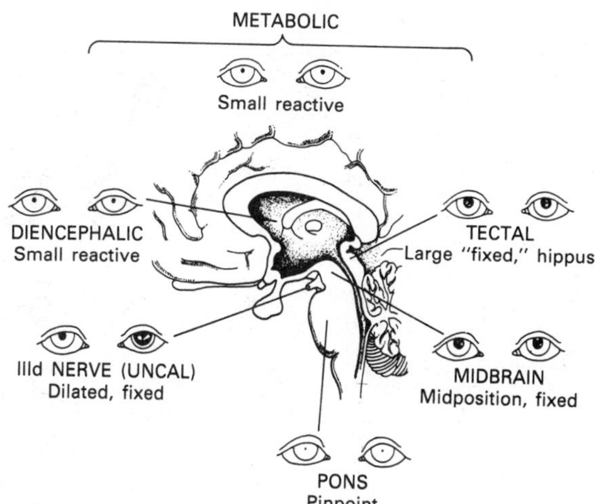

Figure 25-4 Pupils in the comatose client. (Plum, F., and Posner, J. B.: *Diagnosis of Stupor and Coma,* Davis, Philadelphia, 1980, p. 46.)

NURSING DIAGNOSES: ACTUAL OR POTENTIAL

1. Altered level of cognitive functioning, mild to complete loss: manifested as an unresponsive state.
2. Potential for injury: secondary to decreased consciousness.
3. Impairment of mobility, moderate to complete loss: secondary to decreased consciousness (see Figure 25-5).
4. Alterations in self-care activities, moderate to complete loss: secondary to decreased consciousness.
5. Sensory-perceptual deficit: secondary to decreased consciousness and impaired level of brain function.
6. Impairment of verbal or written communication, mild to complete loss: secondary to decreased consciousness.
7. Nutritional deficit, moderate to severe: decreased intake secondary to decreased consciousness.
8. Impairment of urinary function: incontinence secondary to loss of voluntary control and reflex involuntary control.
9. Alteration in bowel patterns, mild to severe:

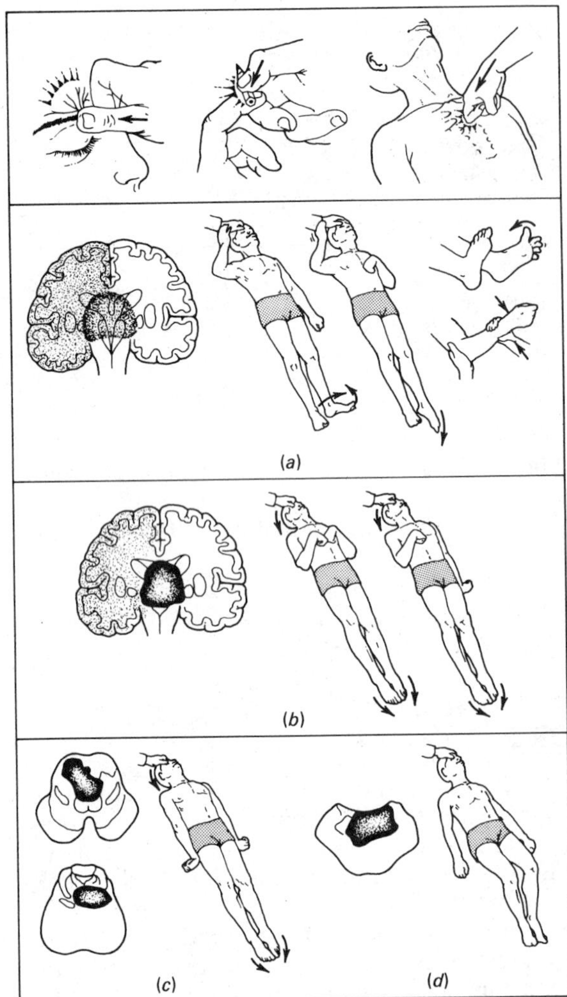

Figure 25-5 Muscle response to noxious stimulation. Motor responses to noxious stimulation in clients with acute cerebral dysfunction. Noxious stimuli can be delivered with minimal trauma to the supraorbital ridge, the nail bed, or the sternum as illustrated at top. Levels of associated brain dysfunction are roughly indicated at left. (*a*) Defensive movement to remove noxious stimulus with an extensor plantar reflex and paratonia. (*b*) Decortication. (*c*) Decerebration. (*d*) Extensor responses in the upper extremities coupled with flexion responses in the lower extremities. (Plum, F., and Posner, J. B.: *Diagnosis of Stupor and Coma*, Davis, Philadelphia, 1980, p. 66.)

incontinence due to loss of voluntary control; constipation secondary to immobility, dietary change, and dehydration; diarrhea secondary to tube feedings.

10. Role disturbance: secondary to decreased consciousness and impaired level of brain function.
11. Knowledge deficit about health status, diagnostic procedures, therapeutic management, and hospitalization.
12. Impairment of skin integrity: secondary to immobility.
13. Respiratory dysfunction: secondary to immobility; aspiration secondary to loss of protective reflexes.
14. Anxiety, mild to moderate: secondary to confusional state.
15. Impaired home maintenance management: secondary to decreased consciousness and impaired level of brain function.

EXPECTED OUTCOMES

1. There will be an absence of reports of injury.
2. Vital functions (ventilation, blood pressure, and pulse) will be supported until the client can self-maintain vital functions within normal limits.
3. Normal vascular volume will be maintained (or slightly decreased vascular volume if intracranial hypertension is present), as evidenced by normal skin turgor, normal serum electrolytes, and a urinary output of 50 mL/h.
4. Potential for motor function will be retained, as evidenced by client's ability to engage in range of motion.
5. Nutritional status will be regained to normal function.
6. Family will make an informed and carefully thought-through decision about the possibility of home management.

INTERVENTIONS

1. Promote maintenance of skin, cornea, and mouth integrity.
   a. Assess skin, mouth, and cornea. Daily, note color, dryness, temperature, and evidence of breakdown.
   b. Turn client from side to side, at least every 2 h to relieve pressure.
   c. Reposition the client by turning and mas-

sage skin over bony prominences and areas subjected to pressure.

d. Use a sheepskin, alternating pressure mattress, or other special pads or turning beds to help diminish pressure.

e. Keep skin clean, dry, and well lubricated, using lotions and bath oils if necessary. Shave male client daily.

f. Protect the skin from excess heat or cold.

g. Keep client's heels from resting on the bed or use heel protectors.

h. Comb client's hair when daily care is given and as necessary throughout the day and wash the client's hair regularly.

i. Trim nails to prevent accidental injury to the client's tissues.

j. Provide mouth care by brushing client's teeth and using suction to remove fluids and debris every 3–4 h. Lubricate the mouth using a moistening agent.

k. Provide eye care. Clean the corners of the eye with cotton balls moistened with normal saline. Irrigate eyes as ordered with normal saline or artificial tears (usually this is done qid).

l. If drying is a problem or there is dysfunction of the IIId or VIIth cranial nerve, tape the eyes closed.

2. Institute a pulmonary regimen designed to keep the lungs clear.

   a. Besides turning the client q2h, perform postural drainage with cupping and clapping q2h. *The client with increased intracranial pressure is not positioned with the head down and may not in severe cases have the head of the bed lowered from the 30 degree angle.*

   b. If client is arousable and able to follow simple commands, mild coughing and deep breathing exercises and IPPB may be instituted if the intracranial pressure is not severe; more vigorous coughing and deep breathing exercises should be done q2h if increased intracranial pressure is not a problem.

   c. When a client is intubated or has a tracheostomy, mouth and tracheostomy care is given at least q4h or more often if needed to assure a patent airway.

   d. An intubated client or a client with a tracheostomy should be suctioned as necessary to maintain a patent airway using appropriate technique.

   e. The respiratory equipment tubing should be changed every 24–48 h as prescribed by hospital policy. The tracheostomy cuff, if not a soft cuff, should be deflated every hour to help prevent tracheal ischemia and erosion.

3. Maintain motor function.

   a. Position client so that the body parts are supported and not dependent.

   b. Bed cradle may be used to keep the bedclothes from resting on the client and thereby applying pressure.

   c. Position a weak or paralyzed body part in a position of functional alignment.

   d. Reposition the client q2h.

   e. Provide an exercise program to prevent contractures, and maintain muscle mass and functional potential. A passive exercise program is instituted for the unresponsive client.

   f. Place the client on a firm mattress; a bedboard may be indicated.

   g. Preserve balancing and sitting through raising the head of the bed, sitting the client on the side of the bed, or getting the client up in a chair as appropriate.

4. Maintain nutritional and fluid intake.

   a. Maintain feeding tubes (Levin, gastrostomy, or jejunostomy) in place and protect surrounding skin tissue by providing skin care and securing tubes so they do not pull on the tissue.

   b. Protect the client from aspiration during or after feedings.

      (1) Check placement of Levin tube before initiating tube feeding.

      (2) Aspirate stomach contents and measure amount of previous feeding still present. If greater than 100 mL, hold the feedings as well as record and report finding. Replace aspirated contents into stomach.

      (3) Place the client in Fowler's position before initiating feeding if not contraindicated.

      (4) Inflate tracheostomy tube cuff, if present, before feeding.

   c. Maintain intake record.

5. Institute a bladder evacuation protocol: In the client being actively treated with osmotic diuretics (volume depletion and steroids) to control intracranial pressure, a Foley catheter will need to be inserted, as an accurate intake and output is essential. In this instance:

a. Maintain a closed system.
b. Provide catheter care.
c. Maintain the urinary tract in the best possible condition.
   (1) Administer urinary antiseptic, such as methenamine mandelate (Mandelamine), with a urinary acidifer, such as vitamin C, as ordered.
   (2) Force fluid (3,000–5,000 mL/day) if increased intracranial pressure is no longer a problem.
   (3) Give the client cranberry juice and apple juice ($2\frac{1}{2}$ qt daily are needed to acidify the urine). Again this is done when increased intracranial pressure is no longer a concern.
   (4) Limit the client's intake of milk and other dairy products.
d. Incontinent male client can be fitted with an external device when hourly urine measurements are not necessary. When removing the catheter:
   (1) Clamp catheter for 1 h and gradually increase the time so that increasing amounts of urine up to 300–400 mL collect in the bladder, thus assisting in reestablishing some bladder tone.
   (2) The catheter can then be removed. Some physicians prefer to discontinue the indwelling Foley catheter. In this case, the client should be checked for bladder distention and intermittently catheterized until able to void on his own.

6. Institute a bowel evacuation protocol:
   a. Stool softeners or a mild laxative is administered, as ordered, to help client regain normal bowel patterns.
   b. If the laxative is not successful, a medicated enema, as ordered, may be given, provided intracranial pressure is not increased at the time.
7. Teach family about the client's health status and therapeutic management.
8. Provide the information, time, and support that the family need to realistically make a decision about home management.

EVALUATION

Outcome Criteria

1. Absence of injury is reported.
2. Vital signs remain within normal limits.
3. During the acute phase, client is slightly volume depleted and nutritionally maintained via IV. During the recovery phase, client is well nourished and well hydrated, as evidenced by stable electrolytes and maintenance of body weight.
4. Skin integrity is maintained and there is an absence of contractures.
5. Bowel and bladder patterns are returned to normal.
6. There is an absence of pulmonary congestion and lungs are clear.
7. Family makes an informed and carefully thought-through decision about home management.

Complications

1. Atelectasis/aspiration leading to pneumonia (see discussion in Chapter 31).
2. Arrhythmia (see discussion in Chapter 30).
3. Hypotension (see discussion in Chapter 30).
4. Decubiti.
5. Constipation and impaction (see discussion in Chapter 33).
6. Diarrhea.
7. Urinary tract infection (see discussion in Chapter 32).
8. Injury (see discussion in appropriate chapter, depending on the nature of the injury).
9. Corneal ulceration.
10. Thrombophlebitis (see discussion in Chapter 30).

METABOLIC DISORDERS

These cerebral disorders occur secondary to visceral dysfunction. Hypoxic-hypotensive encephalopathy, hypercapnia, hepatic failure and portocaval shunting, uremia, hypoglycemia, acidosis due to diabetes mellitus and renal failure, hyponatremia and hypernatremia, hypokalemia and hyperkalemia, Addison's disease, myxedema, and hypercalcemia share a common presentation as encephalopathies in that they manifest clinically as episodic confusional, stuporous, or comatose states (Adams and Victor, 1977).

HYPOXIC ENCEPHALOPATHY

DESCRIPTION

Hypoxic encephalopathy is caused by a lack of oxygen supply to the brain as a result of heart or respiratory failure. The severity of the encephalopathy may vary. Mild degrees of hypoxia result in temporary impairment of mental status and coordination. If anoxia persists, as in a cardiac arrest, permanent damage results, first to the structures with a marginal blood supply, namely the globus pallidus of the basal ganglion, the cerebellum, the parietoccipital lobes, and the hippocampi. With prolonged ischemic anoxia, irreversible damage is done to the cerebrum, cerebellum, and brainstem.

PREVENTION

Health Promotion

1. Counseling may prevent suicide attempt by poisoning.
2. Education should aim at improving physical and environmental safety in home and industry.
   a. Drugs and chemicals should be stored safely.
   b. Protective masks should be used to prevent inhalation of toxic substances in many industries.
   c. Agricultural insecticide spraying should occur under control.
3. All individuals should be immunized against diphtheria and should receive tetanus booster every 10 years. Tetanus toxoid should be given prophylactically for all injuries when threat of tetanus is present.
4. Foods should be properly preserved in homes. Education may decrease or prevent botulism.

Population at Risk

1. Individuals who are depressed or suicidal are at risk.
2. Intoxication with alcohol or barbiturates increases incidence of overdosage (drug automatism).
3. Children frequently ingest drugs or chemicals accidentally.
4. Agricultural workers, miners, industrial workers are at risk for toxicity from a number of sources.
   a. Lead: painting, printing, pottery glazing, lead smelting, and storage battery manufacturing; exposure to tetraethyl lead (gasoline additive).
   b. Mercury: thermometer, mirror, and incandescent light manufacturing; paper, pulp, electrochemical industries; paint and chlorine production; exposure to agriculture fungicide.
   c. Arsenic: insecticide sprays; disinfectant for skins and furs; manufacture of paints, enamels, and metals.
   d. Thallium: rat poisons and depilatories.
   e. Manganese: mining and separating manganese ore.
5. Individuals not properly immunized against tetanus and diphtheria.
6. Exposure to many toxic industrial wastes can occur and may contaminate soil and water sources. Persons living or working near toxic waste sites or potential industrial contaminating sources are at increased risk of developing disorder.

Screening

1. Health history should include safety factors practiced or not practiced in home, especially with children.
2. Routine screening with history and blood levels should be done annually in those industries where there is threat of toxicity.
3. Environmental surveys of industrial waste and disposal should be done routinely.
4. Water sources should be elevated every 6 months to determine content of any toxic substances.

ASSESSMENT

Health History

1. Reported suffocation due to drowning, strangulation, aspiration, or a foreign body in the trachea or due to an iatrogenic cause.
2. Carbon monoxide poisoning.
3. Disorders that impair ventilatory capacity, such as poliomyelitis or Guillain-Barré syndrome, or diffusely damage the central nervous system, such as trauma, vascular disease, or epilepsy.
4. Myocardial infarction, hemorrhage, shock and circulatory collapse, and cardiac arrest.

Physical Assessment

1. For a mild hypoxic episode:
   a. Impaired cognitive functioning manifested as inattentiveness or poor judgment.

   b. Cerebellar dysfunction manifested as motor incoordination.
2. For a moderate hypoxic episode with a good outlook for regaining consciousness:
   a. Presence of an unresponsive state.
   b. Intact pupillary light reflexes and ciliospinal reflexes.
   c. Intact doll's eye response (oculocephalic reflex).
3. For a moderate hypoxic episode with a poor outlook for recovery of consciousness:
   a. Presence of an unresponsive state.
   b. Fixed, dilated pupils.
   c. Absence of brainstem reflexes such as doll's eye response (oculocephalic reflex) and ice water calorics.
4. For a severe hypoxic episode:
   a. Presence of a state of complete unresponsiveness to all stimuli.
   b. Absence of all brainstem reflexes.
   c. Absence of spontaneous respiration.
5. For the common persistent posthypoxic syndromes:
   a. Persistent coma or a stuporous state.
   b. Dementia with or without extrapyramidal signs, that is, rigidity, bradykinesia, and resting tremor.
   c. Presence of a visual agnosia.
   d. An extrapyramidal (parkinsonian) syndrome with mental impairment may be found.
   e. Presence of choreoathetosis.
   f. Presence of cerebellar ataxia.
   g. Presence of intention or action myoclonus.
   h. A Korsakoff's amnesic state.
   i. Presence of a seizure disorder (possibly).

Diagnostic Tests

1. Arterial blood gases to provide evidence of a reduced Po_2 or carbon monoxide intoxication.
2. Blood pressure to provide evidence of hypotension.
3. Electroencephalogram to determine brain wave activity.
4. Cerebral blood flow studies to determine areas of the brain that are still active.

HYPERCAPNIC ENCEPHALOPATHY

PREVENTION

See *Hypoxic Encephalopathy*.

ASSESSMENT

Health History

1. History of chronic emphysema, chronic fibrosing lung disease, or respiratory center inadequacy.
2. History of a secondary polycythemia, cor pulmonale and heart failure, and a possible superimposed pulmonary infection.
3. Complaint of steady, aching headache that tends to be generalized, frontal or occipital in location, and may persist for hours.
4. Complaint by the client or family of client's disinterest in and inattentiveness to one's surroundings.
5. Complaint of intermittent drowsiness.
6. Complaint of forgetfulness.

Physical Assessment

1. Mental dullness and lethargy.
2. A confusional state.
3. Decreasing consciousness progressing into deeper levels of coma.
4. Asterixis ("liver flap") and an action tremor.
5. Reduction in psychomotor activity.

Diagnostic Tests

1. Arterial blood gases to provide evidence of a high Pco_2 and a low Po_2.
2. Lumbar puncture to demonstrate the presence of increased intracranial pressure.
3. Electroencephalogram to demonstrate the presence of slow wave activity.

HEPATIC OR PORTAL-SYSTEMIC ENCEPHALOPATHY (HEPATIC STUPOR OR COMA)

This encephalopathy may complicate all varieties of liver disease.

PREVENTION

See *Hypoxic Encephalopathy*.

ASSESSMENT

Health History

1. History of chronic hepatic insufficiency with portocaval shunting of blood.
2. Complaint by the client or family of client's confusion and drowsiness.
3. History of focal or generalized seizures.

Physical Assessment

1. Decreasing levels of consciousness starting with increasing dullness and progressing into deeper levels of coma.
2. Asterixis (flapping movement of outstretched hands).
3. Truncal and extremity rigidity.
4. Abnormal reflexes, such as the suck or grasp reflex.
5. Grimacing.
6. Exaggerated or asymmetric tendon reflexes.
7. Babinski reflexes (plantar extensor reflexes).

Diagnostic Tests

1. Liver enzyme studies to demonstrate elevated liver enzymes.
2. Liver function studies to evaluate the extent of liver function.
3. BUN to demonstrate a low BUN.
4. Electroencephalogram to demonstrate paroxysms of bilaterally synchronous slow wave activity.

UREMIC ENCEPHALOPATHY

DESCRIPTION

Any form of severe acute or chronic renal disease may result in a uremic encephalopathy presenting as an episodic confusional, stuporous, or comatose state. Neurological syndromes frequently arise as complications of hemodialysis and kidney transplantation. Restoration of renal function completely corrects the neurological dysfunction.

PREVENTION

See *Hypoxic Encephalopathy*.

ASSESSMENT

Health History

1. Complaints of apathy, inattentiveness, and irritability by the client or family.
2. Complaint of fatigue.
3. History of seizures.

Physical Assessment

1. A confusional state.
2. Disturbed sensory perception.
3. Hallucinations.
4. Decreasing level of consciousness into a stuporous or comatose state.
5. Quick, arhythmic, asynchronous muscle twitches that may involve whole muscles or the entire extremity.

Diagnostic Tests

1. BUN and serum creatinine studies to demonstrate accumulation of nitrogenous waste products.
2. Serum electrolytes to demonstrate the exact nature of the electrolyte imbalances.
3. Renal function studies to demonstrate the extent of kidney function.
4. Electroencephalogram to demonstrate EEG abnormalities associated with renal encephalopathy.

MIGRAINE

DESCRIPTION

Migraine is estimated to be found in 5 percent of the general population. Women are slightly more susceptible to migraine than men, and there is a tendency for the head pain to occur during the premenstrual tension and fluid-retention period. Administration of estrogens and progesterone increases the frequency of migraine attacks, but during pregnancy the attacks commonly cease. Occasionally diet is linked to a migraine attack.

Initial vasoconstriction is postulated to be the basis of the neurological symptoms. Cerebral circulation has been shown to slow in early phases of the attack. Release of amines such as norepinephrine, epinephrine, and serotonin (known to be potent vasoconstrictors) are hypothesized to cause the spasm. Vasodilatation and excessive pulsation of branches of the external carotid artery have been observed during the headache.

Several clinical migraine syndromes have been described.

1. *Classic (typical) migraine* frequently occurs soon after waking with vague prodroma. Abruptly clinical symptoms appear that may include a vision disturbance consisting of bright spots or zigzag lines preceding a scotoma; numbness or tingling of the lips, face, and hands; mild confusional state; mild aphasia; weakness of an extremity or extremities. These symptoms last 5–15 min and are fol-

lowed by the onset of a unilateral, throbbing headache that slowly increases in intensity. At its severest point, the client often experiences nausea and vomiting. The headache may last hours to a couple of days. Typical migraine has a familial history in 60 to 80 percent of the cases.

2. *Common (atypical) migraine* is characterized by the sudden onset of generalized head pain with or without nausea and vomiting. A family history is less frequently found.
3. *Cluster headaches* occur predominantly in men and are characterized by a constant, unilateral orbital head pain onsetting during sleep. The intense pain tends to recur nightly for several weeks to a few months and then disappears, sometimes for months to years. Other clinical manifestations associated with the head pain include ipsilateral lacrimation, nasal stuffiness on the ipsilateral side followed by rhinorrhea, miosis, and ptosis of the ipsilateral pupil and eyelid, respectively, and flushing and edema of the ipsilateral side of the face. Cluster headaches are hypothesized to be due to spontaneous release of histamine. They may occur more frequently in times of stress.
4. *Opthalmoplegic migraine* involves a unilateral vascular headache associated with extraocular muscle palsy(ies). Hemiplegic or hemisensory migraine has a motor or sensory deficit respectively associated with the head pain.
5. *"Sick headaches"* vary in severity. Some persons have mild symptoms that allow them to continue their normal activities. Other persons have such severe symptoms that they are incapacitated. With increasing age, the head pain usually becomes less severe.

Inhalation of amyl nitrate during the premonition (aura) has been shown to prevent the attack. Mild analgesics may be sufficient for mild migraine headache. More severe attacks are treated with intramuscular or oral ergot preparations during the vasoconstrictive phase and analgesics during the vasodilatory phase. Individuals with frequent migraine (one to three attacks per week) may be helped by propranolol (Inderal). Recently lithium carbonate has been used with success. Antiserotonin agents such as methysergide (Sansert) have been used also.

Nursing diagnoses include alterations in comfort, anxiety, sensory-perceptual alteration, altered levels of consciousness, alteration in fluid volume, nutritional alteration, impairment of mobility, alterations in self-care activities, role disturbances, lack of knowledge, and maladaptive (individual) coping patterns.

CEREBRAL EDEMA

DESCRIPTION

Cerebral edema is an increase in the volume of brain tissue due to fluid shifts. Three types of brain edema are currently discussed in the neurological-neurosurgical literature (see Figure 25-6).

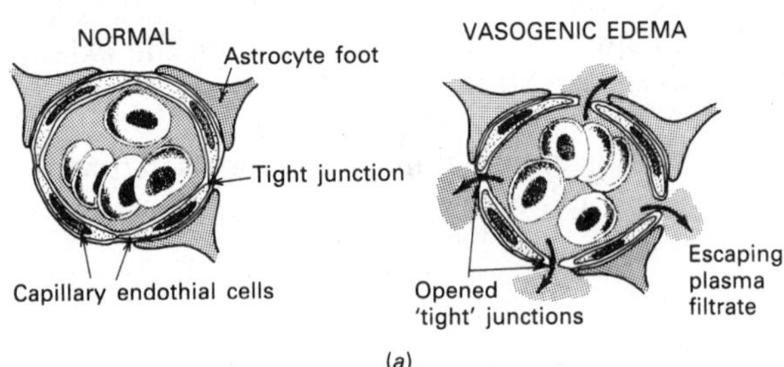

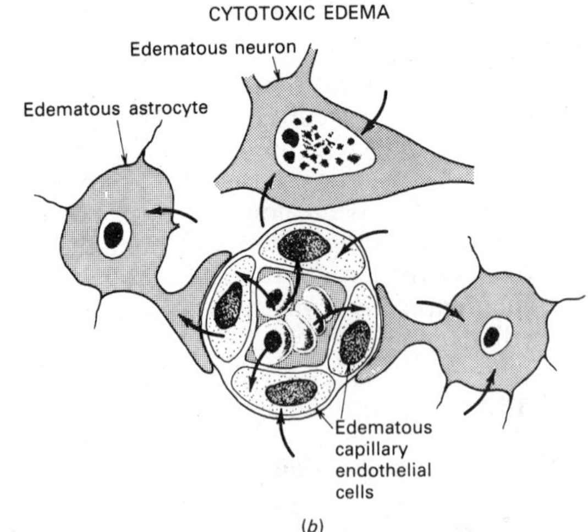

Figure 25-6 Brain edema. (*a*) Schematic representation of the astrocytes and of the endothelial cells and "tight" junctions of the capillary wall in the normal state (left) and in vasogenic edema (right). (*b*) Cytotoxic edema, showing the swelling of the endothelial, glial, and neuronal cells at the expense of the extracellular fluid space of the brain. (Fishman, R.A.: "Brain Edema," *New England Journal of Medicine*, **293**:706, 1975. Reprinted by permission of the *New England Journal of Medicine*.)

1. *Vasogenic edema* is thought to be caused by increased capillary endothelial cell permeability. Plasma is thus allowed to enter the extracellular space. This type of edema is confined to the cerebral white matter. Vasogenic edema is seen in the majority of tumors, in toxic states that injure the blood vessel wall, and in other localized disease processes that damage the blood vessel.
2. In *cytotoxic edema*, all the cellular elements—neurons, glial cells, and endothelial cells—take up water and swell. The ATP-dependent sodium pump within the cell fails because the cell itself can no longer make its own energy. Sodium accumulates in the cell and water is thus drawn into the cell.
3. *Interstitial edema* involves an enlargement of the extracellular fluid space without evidence of vascular or cellular injury.

Brain edema may be localized or generalized. The severity of the edema is generally indicative of the severity of the brain injury. The edema itself compromises the tissue's blood supply and produces pressure on the surrounding tissues, thus compromising that tissue's blood supply and causing further ischemia. With severe edema, brain herniation may occur.

PREVENTION

See *Increased Intracranial Pressure*.

ASSESSMENT

Health History

See Assessment under *Increased Intracranial Pressure* for general symptoms associated with cerebral edema. Focal symptoms are:
1. Complaints of weakness.
2. Complaints of sensory impairment: visual, auditory, or tactile.
3. Complaints of ataxia or clumsiness.

Physical Assessment

See Physical Assessment under *Increased Intracranial Pressure* for physical findings associated with cerebral edema. Focal signs are:
1. Paresis or plegia of the face, arm, or leg.
2. Sensory impairment: tactile, visual, or auditory.
3. Ataxia.

Diagnostic Tests

See Diagnostic Tests under *Increased Intracranial Pressure* for general diagnostic measures that are also associated with cerebral edema. (See Table 25-8.)
1. CAT scan to demonstrate area and extent of brain swelling.
2. Cerebral blood flow studies to demonstrate areas of compromised blood flow within the brain tissues.

NURSING DIAGNOSES: ACTUAL OR POTENTIAL

See Nursing Diagnoses under *Increased Intracranial Pressure* for general nursing diagnoses associated with cerebral edema. In addition:
1. Impairment of mobility, mild to severe: secondary to cerebral edema, producing motor paresis or plegia.
2. Alterations in self-care activities: secondary to paresis or plegia, ataxia, or sensory impairment.
3. Sensory-perceptual alteration: secondary to impaired visual, auditory, or tactile sensations.

EXPECTED OUTCOMES

See Expected Outcomes under *Increased Intracranial Pressure* for general outcomes associated with cerebral edema.

INTERVENTIONS

See Interventions under *Increased Intracranial Pressure* for specific interventions associated with cerebral edema.

EVALUATION

Outcome Criteria

1. The cerebral edema is decreasing. The client has normal intracranial pressure.
2. See also Outcome Criteria under *Increased Intracranial Pressure*.

Complications

See Complications under *Increased Intracranial Pressure*.

INCREASED INTRACRANIAL PRESSURE

DESCRIPTION

The cranial vault is filled with essentially noncompressible contents—brain tissue, blood, and

TABLE 25-8 PHYSIOLOGICAL AND CLINICAL CORRELATION OF PROGRESSIVE, INCREASED INTRACRANIAL ELEVATION

Stage	Intracranial Pressure	Effects
Stage 1	No rise in intracranial pressure is associated with an expanding mass.	*Compensation* phase, no change in vital signs.
Stage 2	Slight increase in the mass of the brain results in great elevations of intracranial pressure.	End stage of *compensation*; changes in vital signs are slight to moderate.
Stage 3	Intracranial pressure can approach arterial blood pressure.	Beginning of *decompensation*, also called the preterminal stage; signs and symptoms that may be observed in the client include deterioration in the level of consciousness, abnormalities in the respiratory patterns, rise in the systolic blood pressure, a widening of the pulse pressure, bradycardia, and cardiac arrhythmias.
Stage 4	The autoregulatory mechanism that normally responds to inceased levels of carbon dioxide by dilating cerebral arteries to supply nutrients and oxygen to the brain is nonfunctional. If the condition is not improved, arterial and intracranial pressure will become equal, resulting in cessation of blood flow and death.	*Decompensation* phase; symptoms as noted in stage 3 continue; death results if there is no immediate reversal of the condition.

SOURCE: Hickey, J.: *The Clinical Practice of Neurological and Neurosurgical Nursing*, Lippincott, Philadelphia, 1981, p. 144.

cerebrospinal fluid. An increase in the volume of any one of the three raises the intracranial pressure, thus necessitating an equal decrease in the volume of one (or both) of the other two volumes. Of the three components, cerebrospinal fluid (CSF), is displaced most readily. If the pressure still remains elevated after CSF displacement, cerebral blood flow begins to be compromised by producing vasoconstriction to further decrease the intracranial pressure. Vasoconstriction, however, cannot be maintained indefinitely. Ischemia results, producing acidosis and CO_2 buildup at the cellular level. This eventually produces vasodilatation with a resultant increase in blood volume, and thus the intracranial pressure is further elevated.

Within the cranial vault, small volume increases can be compensated for more successfully than large volume increases. Also, increased intracranial pressure rising over a long period of time can be more satisfactorily compensated for than can very rapid rises in intracranial pressure.

A dramatic sustained rise in intracranial pressure is not seen until the compensatory mechanisms are exhausted. Once decompensation begins, dramatic rises in intracranial pressure are seen over a very short period of time (Greer, 1974).

PREVENTION

Health Promotion

1. Preventing increased intracranial pressure focuses on correcting or preventing the underlying cause.
2. Avoiding head trauma (see *Traumatic Injuries*) is a primary focus in preventing increased intracranial pressure.

Population at Risk

1. Persons with increased brain mass, such as brain tumor or brain abscess, are at risk for increased intracranial pressure.
2. Head trauma resulting in subdural, epidural, or intracerebral hematoma or contusion or laceration may contribute to increased intracranial pressure.
3. Postoperative and posttraumatic cerebral edema may precipitate increased intracranial pressure.
4. Infectious processes (e.g., encephalitis, meningitis) resulting in edema or swelling of the brain tissue precipitates increased intracranial pressure.
5. Individuals with disturbances of cerebrospinal fluid circulation or absorption (e.g., hydrocephalus) usually have an increased intracranial pressure.

Screening

1. Health history identifying pathological factors contributing to increased intracranial pressure should be elicited and recorded.
2. Clients at risk for neurological problems such as changes in mood and behavior, vital sign changes, or altered pupillary reactions should be monitored carefully.

ASSESSMENT

Health History

1. Complaint of generalized headache that often worsens in the morning upon rising.
2. Unexplained projectile vomiting without nausea.
3. Complaint by client or family of lethargy, mental dullness, or drowsiness.
4. History of neurological problem: head trauma, CVA, mass, drug intoxication, or encephalopathy.

Physical Assessment

(See Table 25-9.)

1. Decreasing consciousness.
2. Changing respiratory patterns.
3. Pupillary changes.
4. Increasing systolic blood pressure (widening pulse pressure).
5. Bradycardia.
6. Papilledema may be seen.

Items 2, 3, 4, and 5 are indications of brainstem dysfunction. These are *not* early changes, and the situation is quite critical.

Diagnostic Tests

1. Continuous intracranial monitoring: intracranial sensors that provide a measurement of intracranial pressure may be placed in the ventricle, subarachnoid space, or epidural space. Changes in pressure are transmitted to a transducer that converts the mechanical impulse to an electric impulse that can be displayed on an oscilloscope or graph paper (see Figure 25-7). Ventricular fluid pressure can be measured by three techniques.
   a. A polyethylene catheter may be implanted via a burr hole into the anterior horn of the lateral ventricle of the nondominant hemisphere.
   b. A hollow screw and transducer may be implanted into the subarachnoid space after a small twist drill hole is placed in the skull and the dura is incised.
   c. A fiberoptic sensor that uses light to measure the movement of a diaphragm in response to external pressure and air may be implanted in the epidural space (see Figure 25-8).
2. Lumbar puncture: pressure can be measured during the procedure; but in the presence of intracranial hypertension, a lumbar puncture is generally contraindicated.
3. Ventriculogram: pressure can be measured during the procedure.

NURSING DIAGNOSES: ACTUAL OR POTENTIAL

1. Impaired thought processes: altered level of cognitive functioning, mild to complete due to unresponsive state.
2. Altered affect: secondary to cerebral edema or intracranial hypertension.
3. Alteration in comfort, mild to severe: head pain.
4. Respiratory dysfunction, mild to severe: due to compression and ischemia of respiratory centers.
5. Alteration in cardiac output, mild to severe: due to compression and ischemia of cardiac and blood pressure centers.
6. Potential for injury: secondary to decreased cognitive function and seizure activity.
7. Potential for skin breakdown: increased due to impaired mobility.
8. Nutritional deficit: secondary to impaired mobility and altered consciousness.

TABLE 25-9 CLINICAL CORRELATES OF COMPENSATED AND DECOMPENSATED PHASES OF INTRACRANIAL HYPERTENSION

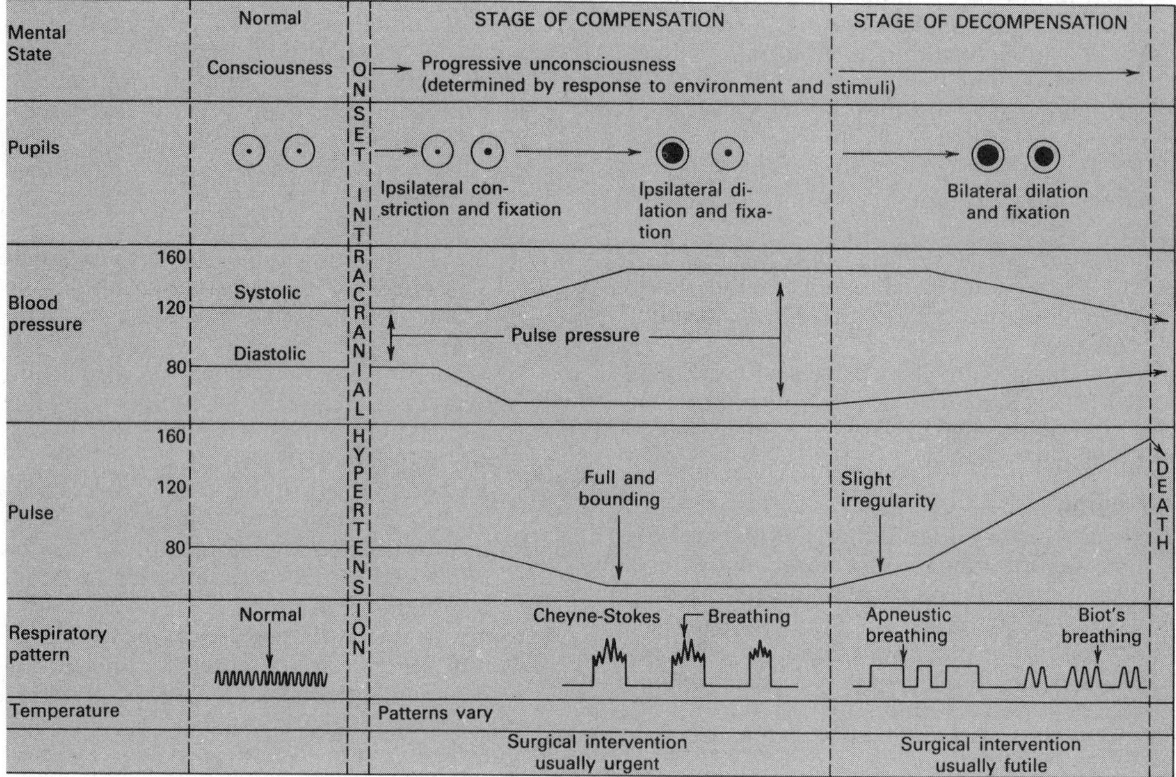

EXPECTED OUTCOMES

1. Intracranial pressure will return to normal level, as evidenced by the reduction or absence of signs and symptoms of increased intracranial pressure (decreased cognition, blunted affect, headache, vomiting, abnormal respiratory patterns, abnormal pupillary responses, abnormal posturing, and vital sign changes) within 3 to 5 days after initiation of treatment to reduce the intracranial pressure is begun.
2. Head pain will be decreased or abolished within 72 h to 5 days after initiation of measures to control the intracranial pressure.
3. The client will be free from injury.
4. The client's vital functions (ventilation, heart beat, and blood pressure) will be maintained until the client is able to resume his or her own maintenance of vital function, as evidenced by P_{O_2}, P_{CO_2}, pulse, and blood pressure.
5. Skin disruptions will be decreased or abolished, as evidenced by skin intactness.
6. Client will have increased mobility; both active and passive range of motion.
7. Client will be able to accept increased nutritional intake.

INTERVENTIONS

1. Establish a continued, accurate data base on motor function.
2. Promote reduction of the cerebral edema and increased intracranial pressure.
   a. Observe for signs and symptoms of increasing intracranial pressure and impending herniation.
   b. Administer osmotic diuretics as ordered. Observe for, record, and report signs of therapeutic effectiveness and side effects. Additionally, monitor intake and output; blood electrolytes, BUN, and so forth.

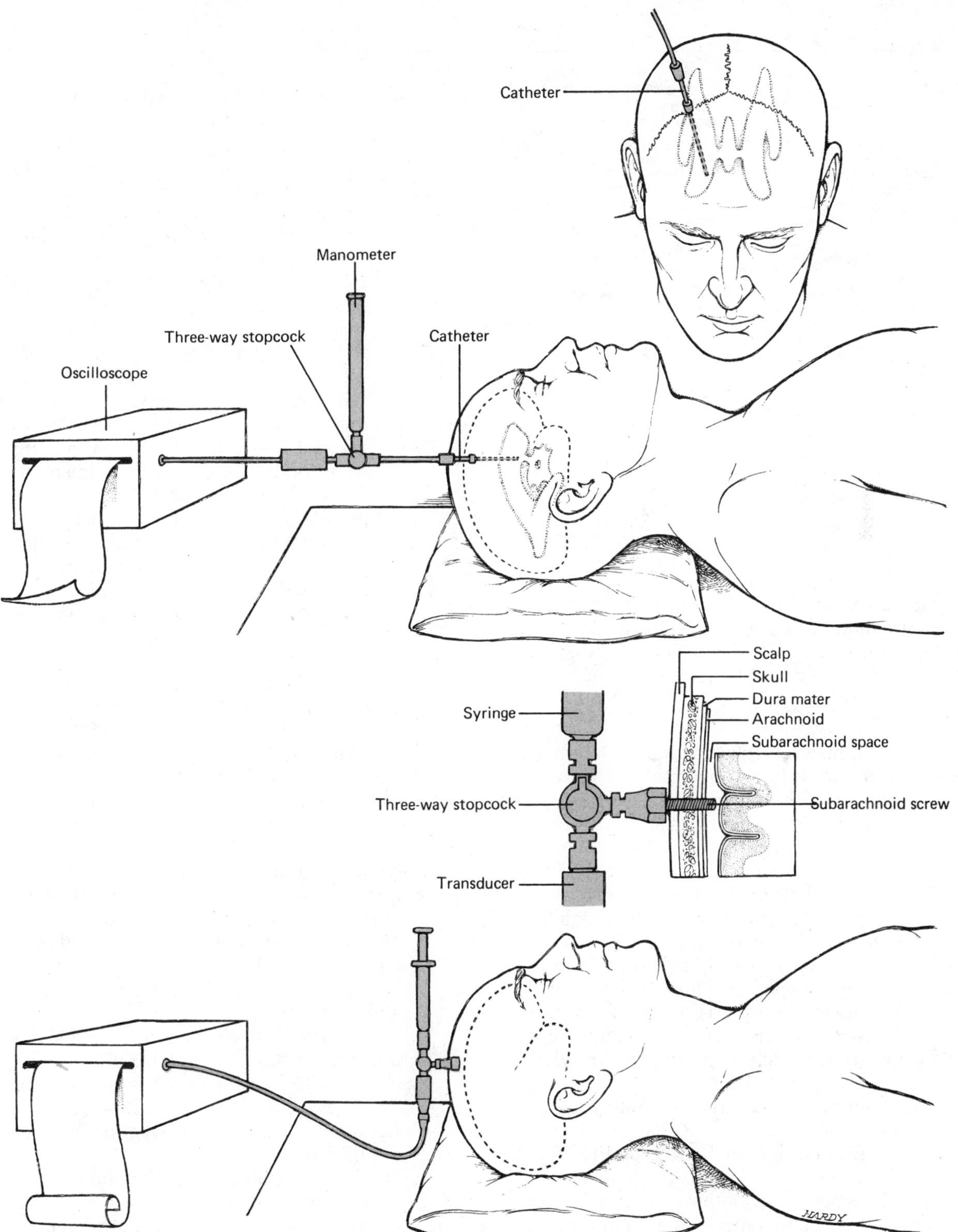

Figure 25-7 Intracranial pressure monitoring. (*Top*) Ventricular catheter. (*Center*) Subarachnoid or hollow screw. (*Bottom*) Monitoring system connected to pressure transducer and display system. (Brunner, L. S., and Suddarth, D. S.: *Textbook of Medical-Surgical Nursing*, Lippincott, Philadelphia, 1980, p. 1187.)

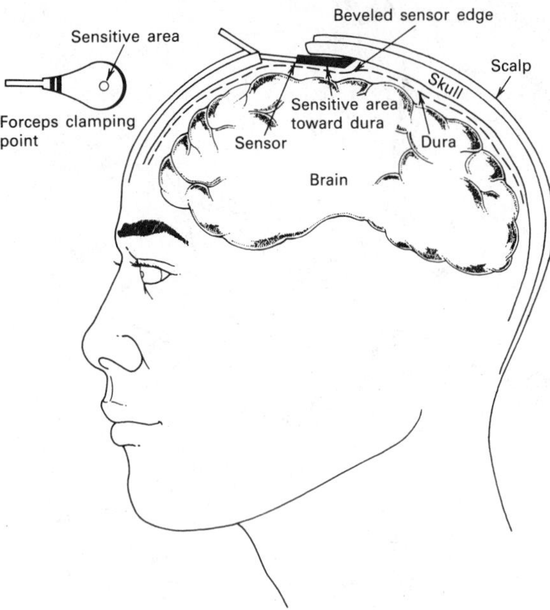

Figure 25–8 Insertion of epidural intracranial pressure monitor, employing a fiberoptic sensor system. (Fein, I. A.: "Cerebral Edema: Prognosis May Be Improved by Monitoring," *Critical Care Monitor*, **1**(4):4, July/August 1981.)

c. Administer corticosteroids with antacid and cimetidine (Tagamet) as ordered. Observe for, record, and report signs of therapeutic effectiveness and side effects. Additionally:
   (1) Check stool, vomitus, or gastric contents for blood.
   (2) Monitor hematocrit and hemoglobin.
   (3) Carefully check for infection at puncture or IV sites; observe urine for signs of an infection and auscultate lungs for increasing congestion, as steroids mask the normal signs of infection such as a temperature elevation.

d. Promote venous drainage from the cranial vault.
   (1) Elevate the head of the bed to 30 degrees.
   (2) Ensure that nothing is snug around the client's neck (e.g., clothing) to impede jugular return.
   (3) Avoid exaggerated neck flexion and rotation, and extreme hip flexion (greater than 90 degrees).

e. Help client avoid activities that raise the intracranial pressure, that is, anything that causes client to perform a valsalva manuever, such as lifting, straining to void or to evacuate the bowel, coughing, sneezing, or blowing the nose. Experiencing anxiety or fear will also raise the intracranial pressure.
   (1) Prevent constipation. Administer stool softeners as ordered. Avoid enemas.
   (2) If the client is able to follow simple instructions, teach the client to exhale when turning or moving.
   (3) Help the client to move in bed. Do *not* ask the client to assist when moving client up in bed or to move himself or herself by pulling up in bed.
   (4) Avoid isometric, active, or active resistive exercises. Only range of motion exercises are instituted until intracranial pressure is controlled.
   (5) Plan activities so that they are spread out as far apart as possible.

f. Maintain the client in a slightly "dry" (slightly dehydrated) state to decrease vascular volume in the cranial vault.
   (1) Monitor fluid intake and carefully regulate IV to the amount prescribed.
   (2) Monitor weight daily.
   (3) Teach the client and the family about the need to diminish fluid volume; establish a fluid plan.

3. Prevent hypoxia and hypercapnia.
   a. Observe for clinical manifestations of increasing ventilatory impairment.
   b. Monitor the arterial blood gases and auscultate the chest to monitor breath sounds. A Po_2 greater than 85 mmHg should be maintained.
   c. Administer oxygen as ordered. Observe and record client's response. *Clients with chronic lung disorders should be given oxygen only in very small quantities*, 2–4 L/min.
   d. Maintain a patent airway and improve ventilation.
      (1) Position client so that the lungs may maximally expand.
      (2) Turn client and encourage mild coughing and deep breathing exercises q2h to improve ventilation.
      (3) If appropriate, suction client as ordered to clear the airway. Hyperin-

flating the lungs with 100 percent oxygen for 1 min before suctioning is desirable. Suction no more than 15 s per catheter insertion. (*See caution above in intervention 3c.*)

(4) Postural drainage with mild cupping and clapping may be appropriate and should be carried out as ordered. In this case, do not position with head dependent.

(5) If required, maintain client on a ventilator. Sigh, or Ambu, the client a few minutes every hour to assure full expansion of the lungs during ventilation.

e. Treat elevated temperature. Depending on cause of the fever:

(1) Administer antipyretic medications as ordered.

(2) Maintain a cool environment with little covering over the client; prevent shivering.

(3) Maintain a cooling system, such as alcohol rubs, sponging briskly with tepid water, ice packs, or a hypothermia blanket, to reduce the fever.

(4) If the hypothermia blanket is used, remove client from the blanket when the body temperature is 1 to 2° from normal.

4. Prevent detrimental effects associated with arrhythmias.
   a. Monitor ECG continuously.
   b. Administer antiarrhythmic drugs as ordered. Observe for, record, and report signs of therapeutic effectiveness and side effects.
5. Maintain normal blood pressure; monitor blood pressure continually; be alert to changes and report accordingly.
6. With intracranial pressure monitoring:
   a. Maintain strict aseptic technique.
   b. Monitor the pressure readings as prescribed.
   c. Administer prophylactic broad-spectrum antibiotics as ordered. Observe for, record, and report side effects.
7. With ventricular drainage:
   a. Place bed flat.
   b. Maintain drainage setup at the prescribed level above the insertion point.
   c. Maintain strict aseptic technique.
   d. Administer prophylactic broad-spectrum antibiotics as ordered. Observe for, record, and report side effects.
8. Promote seizure control as well as protection of the client from injury (refer to Interventions under *Seizure Disorders*).
9. Assist client in gaining control over head pain by using medications as needed, positioning, and comfort measures, such as backrubs and control of the external environment.
10. Protect client from injury. This includes controlling the client's environment predominantly, positioning the client, and controlling the client's ability to mobilize.
11. Teach family how to protect client and how to assist client with activities of daily living.
12. See also Interventions under *Coma*.

EVALUATION

Outcome Criteria

1. The client has normal intracranial pressure.
2. Client's head pain is lessening.
3. Client is injury-free.
4. Client's vital functions remain within normal limits.
5. Client is seizure-free.

Complications

1. Coma.
2. Seizure.
3. Brain herniation. The cranial cavity is subdivided into several compartments by double-layered dural sheets. The falx cerebri separates the right and left hemispheres. The tentorium creates the supratentorial and infratentorial (posterior fossa) compartments and prevents the occipital lobes from resting on and compressing the cerebellum. Increased pressure in one compartment is not evenly distributed among the compartments, and the brain tissue itself shifts (herniates) from the high-pressure compartment to a lower-pressure compartment. The blood supply of the herniating tissue is compromised, causing further ischemia and hypoxia. The herniated tissue puts pressure on the tissues in the adjoining compartment, and this compressed tissue's blood supply is also compromised. Three supratentorial herniation syndromes are commonly seen:
   a. Cingulate herniation.
   b. Transtentorial herniations.
   c. Infratentorial herniation.

Assessment

1. Cingulate herniation signs and symptoms have not at this time been clearly delineated. The recognition of the state occurs when central or temporal lobe herniation ensues or when seen on a diagnostic test such as a CAT scan.
2. See Table 25-4 for clinical manifestations of the various stages of central and temporal herniations.
3. Signs and symptoms of upward transtentorial herniation are also not well delineated.
4. Cerebellar tonsillar herniation.
   a. Initially client may complain of stiff neck and paresthesias over the shoulder area. Evidence of nuchal rigidity may be present, and arching of the neck may appear eventually.
   b. Later coma develops very rapidly, lower brainstem breathing patterns appear, and vasomotor instability is very problematic.

Revised Outcomes

Refer to Outcome Criteria.

Interventions

Refer to those previously stated under Interventions.

Reevaluation and Follow-up

Ongoing neurological assessment is required. Eventually, if the intracranial hypertension cannot be reduced, the question of brain death must be raised. Assessment then focuses on establishing whether the criteria for brain death have been met. Should this be established, interventions to preserve life may be discontinued. Nursing interventions that ensure dignity and a peaceful death are continued.

NUTRITIONAL DISORDERS

WERNICKE'S ENCEPHALOPATHY (WITH OR WITHOUT KORSAKOFF'S PSYCHOSIS)

DESCRIPTION

Wernicke's encephalopathy results from a thiamine deficiency and presents with cortical, motor, and cerebellar deficits. This disease is found predominantly, although not exclusively, among persons who abuse alcohol. Other persons at risk are those who are malnourished or starving and those who have a malabsorption syndrome. The mortality rate associated with the acute phase of Wernicke's disease is due not only to irreversible damage to the neurons but also to liver decompensation and infection. Wernicke's encephalopathy is a medical emergency and must be treated immediately with thiamine. With early treatment, the neurological manifestations are reversible. If treatment is delayed, the person is often left with an irreversible Korsakoff's psychosis that results from damage to the recent memory centers. *Korsakoff's psychosis* refers to a unique mental disorder in which recent memory is impaired out of all proportion to other cognitive function in an otherwise alert and responsive person.

PREVENTION

Health Promotion

1. General health education to include adequate intake of food groups and appropriate vitamin sources may aid in prevention.
2. Adequate nutritional intake provided whenever feasible, especially to high risk population. This may necessitate supplemental vitamin administration (especially thiamine and other B vitamins) to be given to alcoholic individuals or those individuals in whom chronic alcoholism is highly suspect.

Population at Risk

1. Onset is equally distributed between 30 to 70 years of age; both sexes are equally affected.
2. Wernicke's disease occurs mainly in chronic alcoholics. Thiamine deficiency is also seen in chronic malnutritive states associated with gastric carcinoma, other alimentary tract disturbances, and hyperemesis gravidarum and may be present with symptoms of Wernicke's syndrome.
3. Evidence is available, though limited at present, that there is a hereditary factor in the genesis of Wernicke's encephalopathy.

Screening

1. Nursing assessment to include diet history with 24-h recall may aid in uncovering deficiencies.
2. Early recognition of disease is essential to ensure reversal of symptoms.

ASSESSMENT

Health History

1. History of alcohol abuse.
2. History of malabsorption or starvation.
3. History of gastric carcinoma or other gastrointestinal disorders.
4. History of hyperemesis gravidarum.
5. Complaints by client or family of client's apathy, listlessness, inattentiveness, and inability to concentrate.
6. Complaint of drowsiness by the client or family.
7. Complaint of memory impairment by the client or family.
8. Severe impairment of recent memory.
9. A global confusional state.

Physical Assessment

1. Nystagmus in both horizontal and vertical gaze.
2. Weakness or paralysis of the external rectus muscle, indicating impairment of VIth cranial nerve (abducens).
3. Weakness or paralysis of conjugate gaze.
4. Wide-based stance and a slow, uncertain, short-stepped gait (ataxia of gait).
5. Decreasing level of consciousness into a stuporous or comatose state.

Diagnostic Tests

1. Blood transketolase assay: this enzyme requires thiamine pyrophosphate as a cofactor and shows a marked reduction in its activity in a thiamine-deficient state.
2. Electroencephalogram: half the persons with thiamine deficiency show a diffuse decrease in the frequency of brain waves.
3. Cerebral blood flow studies: These demonstrate reduction of blood flow, thus suggesting decreased activity in a certain portion of the brain.

NURSING DIAGNOSES: ACTUAL OR POTENTIAL

1. Altered level of cognitive functioning, mild but rapidly deteriorating into deep coma: due to thiamine deficiency.
2. Impairment of mobility, severe before onset of unresponsiveness: secondary to cerebellar dysfunction.
3. Potential for injury: secondary to decreased cognitive functioning, impaired mobility, and loss of protective reflexes.
4. Sensory-perceptual alteration, moderate to severe: visual impairment, lateral gaze and conjugate gaze impairment.
5. Nutritional alteration, severe: secondary to alcohol abuse, malnutrition, starvation, or malabsorption syndrome.
6. Knowledge deficit: regarding health status, diagnostic procedures, therapeutic management, and hospitalization.
7. Alteration in self-care activities: secondary to impaired memory and decreased mobility.
8. Role disturbance: secondary to residual damage to brain tissue.
9. Impaired home maintenance management: secondary to self-care deficit and behavioral changes.

EXPECTED OUTCOMES

1. Normal blood level of thiamine will be attained within a few hours after treatment is initiated.
2. There will reduced cerebral edema and intracranial pressure to decrease cell ischemia, as evidenced by normal neurological function.
3. Memory will be improved; headaches will diminish or cease altogether.
4. There will be an absence of vomiting; appetite will return.
5. Client will experience increased steadiness in gait; sphincter control will return.
6. Client will be free of injury (initial).

INTERVENTIONS

1. Establish accurate data base with ongoing periodic neurological reassessment.
2. Reduce thiamine deficiency. Administer thiamine immediately and then daily as ordered. When the client regains maximum neurological recovery, the client and family should receive dietary counseling.
3. Prepare the client physically and prepare both the client and family psychologically for the diagnostic procedures involved in establishing a diagnosis.
4. Help the client and family learn about health status and therapeutic management.
5. Protect the client from injury due to ocular palsy.
6. With the other health-related professionals, help the client and family assume responsibility for the management of the recovery and residual deficits (if any are present).
7. If the client recovers, nursing interventions to

assist with the alcohol abuse problem are appropriate if that is the cause of the encephalopathy. (See *Dependent Behavior* in Chapter 37, Interpersonal Problems of Adults.)

EVALUATION

Outcome Criteria

1. Client reports ingestion of a nutritionally well-balanced diet. Weight improves.
2. Client and family report return of neurological function, as evidenced by improved gait; absence of vomiting, return of memory, increased sphincter control.
3. Absence of injuries is reported.
4. Client verbalizes a comprehensive understanding of the disease process.

Complications

KORSAKOFF'S PSYCHOSIS: AN AMNESTIC SYNDROME

Assessment

1. Recent memory is completely lost or seriously impaired.
2. Acute confusional state may be present.
3. Ability to learn new information is seriously or completely impaired.
4. Confabulation is found.
5. Client's behavior is very different from his or her premorbid behavior or personality.

Revised Outcomes

1. The client will maintain present cognitive function, mobility, or sphincter control.
2. The client will maintain as much self-care and role function as possible in light of cognitive functioning and mobility.

Interventions

See Interventions under *Dementia*.

Reevaluation and Follow-up

See Evaluation under *Dementia*.

NUTRITIONAL POLYNEUROPATHY (NEUROPATHIC BERIBERI)

DESCRIPTION

Axonal degeneration with both axon and myelin sheath destruction is the predominant pathological change in nutritional polyneuropathy. Varying degrees of segmental demyelination may also be seen. The most destruction occurs in the distal portions of the longest and largest myelinated nerve fibers. In very severe cases, the anterior and posterior nerve roots may become involved, as can the vagus and phrenic nerves and the sympathetic paravertebral trunks. The precise nutritional factor or factors are not currently defined. Treatment is primarily directed at supplying adequate nutrition with supplemental administration of the B vitamins.

PREVENTION

Health Promotion

1. Nutritional counseling should focus on the need for a balanced and safe diet that meets the nutritional requirements of the individual.
2. B-complex vitamin supplements may be needed for individuals with increased thiamine requirements.
3. In alcoholism, as part of the entire alcohol treatment plan, interventions should include treatment of malnutrition, including probable thiamine deficiency.

Population at Risk

1. The most common reason for thiamine (vitamin B_1) deficiency is inadequate dietary intake of the vitamin. Countries where high-carbohydrate diets are common and where enrichment of rice and wheat is not practiced are at increased risk for beriberi.
2. Vitamin utilization is decreased in individuals with liver disease. In alcoholism, a diminished absorption and utilization of thamine, combined with a deficient dietary intake, places the alcoholic at high risk for nutritional polyneuropathy.
3. Thiamine requirements may increase in pregnant and lactating women and in individuals with hyperthyroidism, fever, and for those in states of increased psychomotor activity.
4. Thiamine absorption is reduced in individuals with gastrointestinal disturbances accompanied by persistent vomiting or diarrhea.

Screening

1. A complete nutritional assessment should be included in the health history.
2. Potential thiamine deficiencies should be identified in the populations at risk.

ASSESSMENT

Health History

1. History of alcohol abuse, malnutrition or starvation, or malabsorption syndrome.
2. Complaint of slowly progressive distal greater than proximal paresthesias in the extremities, such as a feeling of "tightness" in the calves, a bandlike sensation around the legs, a feeling of heat or "burning" of the soles of the feet (less commonly of the dorsum of the feet).
3. Complaint of weakness in an involved extremity or both extremities that is slowly progressive and involves the distal muscles more severely than the proximal.
4. Complaint of muscle cramps in the feet and calves.
5. Complaint of a dull, constant ache in the feet and legs or a sharp lancinating pain in the feet or legs.
6. Complaint of coldness in the extremities.

Physical Assessment

1. A symmetrical loss of sensation or muscular weakness (distal greater than proximal).
   a. Primary superficial sensations: often involving all modalities (touch, pain, and temperature) in the extremities.
   b. Deep sensations: deep pressure, vibration sense, and position sense in the extremities.
   c. Muscular weakness: a wrist or foot drop may be seen.
2. Tenderness of the muscles when pressure is applied.
3. Deep tendon reflexes in the extremities are diminished or absent.
4. Excessive sweating of the soles and on the dorsal aspects of the feet and volar surfaces of the hands and fingers.
5. Hoarseness and weakness of the vocalization muscles may be present if the vagus nerve is affected.
6. Dysphagia may be present with vagal involvement.

Diagnostic Tests

1. Nerve conduction studies to demonstrate the slow and abnormal conduction associated with a nutritional polyneuropathy.
2. Lumbar puncture to demonstrate normal cerebrospinal fluid composition and pressure.

NURSING DIAGNOSES: ACTUAL OR POTENTIAL

1. Nutritional deficit, severe: malnutrition secondary to alcohol abuse, starvation, or a malabsorption syndrome.
2. Sensory-perceptual alteration, mild to severe: diminished or lost sensation resulting from nerve degeneration.
3. Alterations in comfort, mild to severe: paresthesias, aching or pain, coldness, and muscle cramping.
4. Impairment of mobility, mild to severe: secondary to impaired sensations, weakness with footdrop, or pain.
5. Self-care deficit: due to impaired mobility, ataxia, weakness, and pain.
6. Potential for injury: secondary to impaired mobility, ataxia, or weakness.
7. Anxiety: due to fear of unknown; pain, motor deficits, and role disturbance.
8. Knowledge deficit: lack of knowledge about health status, diagnostic procedures, therapeutic management, or hospitalization.
9. Impairment of skin integrity: secondary to immobility and trauma.
10. Potential for suffocation: due to phrenic nerve dysfunction.
11. Impairment of verbal communication: due to vagus nerve dysfunction.
12. Alteration in cardiac output: due to vagus nerve and sympathetic ganglia dysfunction.
13. Role disturbance: secondary to impaired mobility, pain, or anxiety.

EXPECTED OUTCOMES

1. Normal blood levels of the B vitamins will be reached within 2 to 5 days after treatment with vitamins is initiated.
2. Control over the pain and paresthesias will be achieved, as evidenced by verbal statement.
3. The client will maintain as much self-care and role function as possible in light of motor or sensory deficits.
4. Client and family will be able to provide information about health status, diagnostic procedures, therapeutic management, and so on.
5. Client's vital functions (ventilation, heart beat, and blood pressure) will be maintained until the client is able to resume maintenance of vital functions, as evidenced by normal for

the client Po_2, Pco_2, pulse, and blood pressure.

INTERVENTIONS

1. Establish accurate data base with periodic ongoing neurological reassessment.
2. Reduce vitamin deficiencies. Administer B-complex vitamin preparations as ordered.
3. Assist client to gain control over pain and paresthesias. Help client find ways to keep clothing and bed linens from resting on body parts that are experiencing paresthesias. Bed cradles may help.
4. Protect client from further damage to the nerves and the area innervated by the nerves.
5. Maintain motor function.
6. Protect the client from injury due to motor deficits.
7. Assist the client and family to learn how to protect the client from injury due to impaired tactile sensations.
8. Assist the client and family to institute a skin integrity maintenance program.
9. Help client and family learn about health status, diagnostic workup, and therapeutic management.
   a. Explain diagnostic procedures and the preparation for these procedures.
   b. Teach client and family about the polyneuropathy: its causes, clinical manifestations, and therapeutic management.
10. Assist client to maintain adequate nutrition and fluid intake if swallowing is affected.
11. Institute pulmonary regimen designed to keep the lungs clear if immobility and/or respiratory muscle paresis is present.
12. Institute bowel evacuation protocol if the client is moderately immobilized.
13. Prevent hypoxia and hypercapnia.
14. Prevent serious effects resulting from arrhythmias.
    a. Observe for clinical manifestations of arrhythmia (see discussion in Chapter 30).
    b. Monitor ECG continuously and administer antiarrhythmic drugs as ordered.
15. Maintain blood pressure.
    a. Observe for clinical manifestations of hypotension or hypertension.
    b. Administer appropriate hypertensive or antihypertensive medications, as ordered. Observe for, record, and report signs of therapeutic effectiveness and side effects.
16. With the other health professionals help the client and family assume responsibility for the management of neurological deficits and potential recovery.

EVALUATION

Outcome Criteria

1. Nutritional deficiency is gradually corrected.
2. Pain and paresthesias are decreasing as the nerves repair themselves.
3. Client and family can discuss accurately information about the client's health status, diagnostic procedures, therapeutic management, and so forth.

Complications

1. Alcohol withdrawal state.
2. Injury due to faulty balance.
3. Atelectasis/aspiration leading to pneumonia (see discussion in Chapter 31).
4. Respiratory insufficiency/respiratory arrest (see discussion in Chapter 31).
5. Arrhythmias and hypotension (see discussion in Chapter 30).
6. Decubiti.
7. Chronic pain syndrome.

Assessment

1. Identify changes in the paresthesias or pain since treatment was initiated.
2. Identify client's management of paresthesias and pain.
3. Identify other strategies needed to control pain.

Revised Outcomes

Same as those stated under Outcome Criteria.

Interventions

1. Increase emphasis on cutaneous stimulation techniques, especially those that can be applied more frequently or continuously, like transcutaneous electrical nerve stimulation.
2. Administer medications that are ordered to control chronic pain syndromes such as diphenylhydantoin (Dilantin) or carbamazepine (Tegretol). Teach the client and family to observe for the side effects associated with the medication utilized.

Reevaluation and Follow-up

If client is becoming controlled by the pain, referral to a chronic pain management clinic is appropriate.

PERNICIOUS ANEMIA AND PELLAGRA

Vitamin B_{12} deficiency, pernicious anemia, may cause degeneration of the lateral and posterior columns of the spinal cord. See the discussion in Chapter 29, The Hematologic System.

Pellagra has become far less common since the 1940s, probably because of the practice of enriching bread with niacin. But the condition is still seen in persons who abuse alcohol, have a malabsorption syndrome, or suffer from malnutrition or starvation. The nervous system dysfunction involves the cerebrum, the spinal cord, and less frequently the peripheral nerves. The cerebral manifestations include complaints of insomnia, fatigue, nervousness, irritability, and depression and physical findings of mental dullness, apathy, and memory impairment. Manifestations of spinal cord involvement predominantly arise from posterior column dysfunction resulting in loss of position sense and vibration sense with ensuing gait ataxia. Some signs of lateral column disruption such as decreased touch sensations may be seen. Peripheral nerve damage is manifested by sensory, motor, and reflex signs and symptoms similar to neuropathic beriberi. Occasionally a spastic syndrome occurs involving spastic weakness, increased lower extremity reflexes with clonus and extensor plantar reflexes (Babinski reflexes), and loss of position and vibration senses.

Treatment is directed toward correcting the dietary deficiency. Nursing diagnoses and interventions focus on nutritional alteration or impairment of digestion, impairment of cognitive function, sensory-perceptual alteration, impairment of mobility, potential for injury, alterations in self-care activities, anxiety, and role disturbance (potential).

TOXIC DISORDERS

ALCOHOL

DESCRIPTION

Alcohol is a central nervous system depressant. What initially appears to be cortical hyperexcitability is actually due to inhibition of certain subcortical (high brainstem) structures that normally modulate cortical activity. Likewise, the initial hyperactivity of the reflexes is most probably due to the loss of higher inhibitory center control over the spinal motor neurons. With ingestion of increasing amounts of alcohol, the depressant effects not only further involve the cerebral cortex but the brainstem and spinal cord neurons as well. (Refer to the discussion of *Hepatic Cirrhosis* in Chapter 33 for additional information.)

PREVENTION

See *Hypoxic Encephalopathy*.

ASSESSMENT

Health History

1. History of accidents.
2. Decreased productivity, job-related difficulty and absenteeism.
3. History of family disruption.
4. Past medical history of liver disease, gastritis, or pancreatitis.
5. History of past alcohol abuse.
6. History of recent alcohol intake and/or drug use.

Physical Assessment

1. For *mild intoxication* (blood alcohol level under 30 mg/100 mL):
   a. Euphoria evident in client's behavior.
   b. Garrulousness and loss of restraint in client's behavior.
   c. Tendency toward aggressiveness.
   d. Excessive activity.
   e. Reduced attention and concentration ability.
   f. Judgment and decision making are impaired.
   g. Learning process is slowed.
   h. Odor of alcohol.
2. For *mild to moderate intoxication* (blood alcohol level 50 mg/100 mL):
   a. Incoordination of movement and gait appearing as clumsiness and being accident-prone.
   b. Slow and deliberate motor movements.
   c. Slow and deliberate speech.
3. For *moderate intoxication* (blood alcohol level 100 mg/100 mL):
   a. Gait ataxia.
   b. Slurred ataxic speech.

c. Inability to maintain a standing posture unassisted.
d. Extreme motor incoordination.
e. Some degree of drowsiness.
f. Diplopia causing the client visual impairment. Closing one eye is required to see clearly.

4. For *moderate to severe intoxication* (blood alcohol level 200 mg/100 mL):
   a. An acute confusional state with severely impaired recent memory and extremely poor judgment.
   b. Extreme drowsiness.
   c. Extreme ataxia.
   d. Vertigo often accompanied by vomiting.
5. For *severe intoxication* (blood alcohol level 300 mg/100 mL):
   a. Stupor state with response only to noxious stimuli.
   b. Protective reflexes still intact, such as gag, swallowing, cough, and corneal reflexes.
   c. Pupillary reflexes still normal and intact.
   d. Normal respiratory rate.
6. For *potentially fatal intoxication* (blood alcohol level 400 mg/100 mL):
   a. Deep comatose state, with the person unresponsive to all stimuli.
   b. Respiratory depression.
   c. Protective reflexes lost; great danger of aspiration at this point.
   d. Pupillary reflexes sluggish and may be absent.
   e. Bradycardia and hypotension apparent.

Diagnostic Tests

1. Blood alcohol level to determine the presence of alcohol and level of intoxication if alcohol is present.
2. Serum toxicology screen to determine if any other drugs of a depressant nature are contributing to the clinical manifestations.
3. Blood glucose level to determine that hypoglycemia is not the cause of the clinical manifestations.
4. Electroencephalogram to determine the amount of alteration in brain wave activity.

OPIATES AND SYNTHETIC ANALGESICS

DESCRIPTION

Acute opiate poisoning results from suicidal or accidental overdose or from unusual sensitivity to the drugs, such as seen in persons with myxedema, Addison's disease, chronic liver disease, or pneumonia. The most frequent cause of death is respiratory failure. Treatment consists of gastric lavage if the drug was ingested, maintenance of an adequate airway, ventilatory assistance with oxygenation, and administration of naloxone (Narcan).

PREVENTION

See *Hypoxic Encephalopathy*.

ASSESSMENT

Health History

1. History of drug abuse.
2. Medication currently being taken by the client.
3. Description of any available analgesic drugs in the home.
4. Recent alcohol intake.

Physical Assessment

1. Decreasing level of consciousness progressing into stupor or deep coma.
2. Slowing respirations that are shallow in nature.
3. Pinpoint pupils.
4. Bradycardia present with low blood pressure.
5. Hypothermia.
6. With deep coma, protective reflexes such as cough, gag, swallowing, and corneal reflexes are lost.
7. Deep tendon reflexes depressed and often absent.
8. Track marks may be present.

Diagnostic Tests

1. Serum toxicology screen provides a reliable means to identify the drug or drugs.
2. Narcan trial is often done to see if the cause of the coma is an opiate derivative. Improvement will be seen on administration of the drug if an opiate is responsible for the depressed nervous system state.
3. Electroencephalogram to demonstrate the degree of brain wave activity.

BARBITURATES

DESCRIPTION

Acute barbiturate intoxication results from suicidal or accidental overdose. A combination of alcohol and barbiturate intoxication is also frequently seen. Although all parts of the central nervous system are somewhat sensitive to barbiturates, the reticular formation nuclei of the thalami and midbrain are particularly sensitive. Clinical manifestations vary with the type and amount of drug taken. Three grades of severity of acute barbiturate intoxication exist. Treatment depends somewhat on the severity of the intoxication but is directed predominantly at (1) elimination of the drug from the body by such means as gastric lavage if ingestion is recent or dialysis if a large dose has been absorbed, and (2) supportive measures until the drug is metabolized, including ventilatory and circulatory support if necessary.

PREVENTION

See *Hypoxic Encephalopathy*.

ASSESSMENT

Health History

See discussion under *Opiates and Synthetic Analgesics*.

Physical Assessment

1. For *mild* intoxication:
   a. Drowsiness or obtundation (the client is readily awakened by name calling or shaking.
   b. Impaired judgment and slowness of thought.
   c. Slurred speech.
   d. Staggering gait.
   e. Nystagmus.
   f. Lability of mood.
   g. Disorientation or acute confusional state.
2. For *moderate* intoxication:
   a. A state of unresponsiveness except to noxious stimuli such as pain.
   b. Slow but not yet shallow respirations.
   c. Depressed or absence of deep tendon reflexes.
   d. Nystagmus.
   e. Protective reflexes such as cough and gag still intact.
3. For *severe* intoxication:
   a. Completely unresponsive coma state.
   b. Shallow respirations, slow or irregular in rate.
   c. Deep tendon reflexes usually absent.
   d. Protective reflexes often absent.
   e. Pupillary light reflexes retained unless anoxia has been present due to respiratory failure.
   f. Decerebrate posturing and decerebrate rigidity frequently observed initially: if they persist, it is an indication of severe anoxia.
   g. Extensor plantar reflexes (Babinski reflexes) may be seen initially, but again, persistence indicates severe anoxia.
   h. Hyperreflexia with clonus may be seen initially but persistence indicates severe anoxia.

Diagnostic Tests

1. Serum toxicology screen to provide a reliable means of identifying the type and amount of barbiturates in the blood as well as give information as to whether the therapeutic problem can be expected to be short or long in duration.
2. Electroencephalogram to identify the characteristic brain wave patterns that accompany barbiturate intoxication at the three levels of intoxication.

SEDATIVES AND HYPNOTIC DRUGS

DESCRIPTION

This group of drugs includes bromides, chloral hydrate, paraldehyde, chlordiazepoxide (Librium), diazepam (Valium), flurazepan (Dalmane), carbamazepine (Tegretol), meprobamate (Equanil, Miltown), glutethimide (Doriden), and methaqualone (Quaalude) to name a few. A combination of one or more of these with barbiturates and with alcohol can also produce an acute intoxication state. Accidental overdoses of these drugs are as common as deliberate suicidal overdoses.

PREVENTION

See *Hypoxic Encephalopathy*.

ASSESSMENT

Health History

See Chapter 49, Medical Emergencies.

Physical Assessment

1. For *mild* intoxication:
   a. Disorientation or acute confusional state.
   b. Slurred speech.

   c. Incoordination and gait ataxia.
   d. Drowsiness.
2. For *moderate* intoxication:
   a. Decreased level of consciousness progressing into stupor with response only to noxious stimuli such as pain.
   b. Decreased respiratory rate.
   c. Hyporeflexia.
   d. Pupillary light reflexes intact.
   e. Protective reflexes such as cough, gag, swallowing and corneal reflexes still intact.
3. For *severe* intoxication:
   See Physical Assessment under *Barbiturates*, assessment 3a through h.

Diagnostic Tests

1. Serum toxicology screen to provide a reliable means of identifying the drug or drugs and the amount of drug or drugs in the blood.
2. Electroencephalogram to demonstrate the amount of brain wave activity.

ANTIPSYCHOTIC DRUGS

DESCRIPTION

Four categories of antipsychotic drugs exist: (1) the *phenothiazines*, such as chlorpromazine hydrochloride (Thorazine), promazine hydrochloride (Sparine), thioridazine hydrochloride (Mellaril), and trifluoperazine hydrochloride (Stelazine); (2) the *butyrophenones*, such as haloperidol (Haldol) and trifluperidol; (3) the *thioxanthines*, such as chlorprothixene (Taractan); and (4) the *Rauwolfia alkaloids*, such as reserpine. With accidental or suicidal overdose, signs and symptoms of acute intoxication can result.

PREVENTION

See *Hypoxic Encephalopathy*.

ASSESSMENT

The health history, physical assessment, and diagnostic tests are similar to those for acute barbiturate intoxication. Refer to discussion under *Barbiturates*.

NURSING DIAGNOSES: ACTUAL OR POTENTIAL

1. Altered level of cognitive functioning, mild to complete loss manifested as an unresponsive state: due to drug intoxication.
2. Alteration in tissue/fluid volume within the cranial vault (increased intracranial pressure), mild to extreme: cerebral edema due to neuronal cell death from hypoxia and vasodilation.
3. Impairment of mobility, mild to complete loss: secondary to ataxia and drug intoxication.
4. Potential for injury: secondary to inattentiveness, cognitive impairment, vertigo, diplopia, and ataxia.
5. Impairment of communication (verbal and written), mild to complete loss: due to incoordination, decreased consciousness.
6. Sensory-perceptual alteration: due to diplopia and vertigo.
7. Alterations in self-care activities: secondary to impaired cognitive functioning or decreased consciousness, ataxia, diplopia, or vertigo.
8. Respiratory dysfunction: respiratory depression due to drug intoxication; altered respiratory pattern secondary to decreased consciousness; pulmonary congestion or atelectasis secondary to immobility or aspiration.
9. Alteration in cardiac output: due to depression of cardiac and blood pressure centers in the lower brainstem in deep coma.
10. Maladaptive (individual) coping pattern: led to drug abuse.
11. Lack of knowledge about health status, diagnostic procedures, and so forth.
12. Impairment of urinary elimination: incontinence.
13. Alteration in bowel elimination: incontinence due to loss of voluntary control; constipation secondary to immobility, dietary alteration, and dehydration.
14. Impairment of skin integrity: secondary to decreased consciousness, immobility, incontinence, and trauma.
15. Role disturbance: secondary to decreased consciousness or residual damage to brain tissues.
16. Impaired home maintenance management (potential): secondary to neurological deficits.

EXPECTED OUTCOMES

1. The client's vital functions (ventilation, heart beat, blood pressure) will be assisted until the

client is able to resume self-maintenance of vital functions.
2. The client will have normal intracranial pressure (as evidenced by the reduction or absence of signs and symptoms of increased intracranial pressure) within 2 to 5 days after treatment for the drug intoxication and cerebral edema is begun.
3. The client will gain control over drug-abuse problem.

INTERVENTIONS

1. Establish a continued, accurate data base, including periodic neurological reassessment.
2. Promote removal of the drug from the client's body.
   a. Carry out gastric lavage as ordered to remove the drug from the stomach.
   b. Administer naloxone (Narcan) as ordered for diagnostic trial or for treatment.
   c. Administer dialysis as ordered to remove the drug from the blood, if the drug or drugs are dialyzable.
3. Protect the client from injury due to increased cognitive function, ataxia, immobility, or sensory impairment.
4. Help client and family assume responsibility for the management of recovery and dealing with residual deficits (if any are present).
5. Assist the client with drug-abuse problem as appropriate.
6. Provide information, time, and support that the family and client need to realistically make an informed decision about home management.
7. See *Intracranial Hypertension* and *Coma* for other specific interventions.

EVALUATION

Outcome Criteria

1. Client's vital functions remain (or return to) within normal limits.
2. Client no longer experiences neurological deficits.
3. The client is seeking help for drug-abuse problem.

Complications

See Evaluation under *Nutritional Polyneuropathy*, complications 4 through 6.

BACTERIAL TOXINS

The bacteria responsible for tetanus, botulism, and diphtheria produce powerful toxins that primarily affect the nervous system.

Tetanus, caused by the anerobic, spore-forming rod *Clostridium tetani*, is associated in the United States with injuries sustained at home, in gardens, and on farms. Drug addicts are a particular population at risk. The incidence of tetanus is 1 per million per year in the United States. The toxin appears to be disseminated via the blood or lymph system to the nervous system, where it suppresses inhibitory neurons located in the spinal cord and brainstem. Thus, increased activation of the musculature is seen. The incubation time varies, and three forms of tetanus exist—local, cephalic, and generalized.

Local tetanus manifests with stiffness, tightness, and pain in muscles adjacent to the wound progressing to twitching and spasm in the affected muscles. *Cephalic tetanus* may follow wounds of the face and head and presents with weakness or paralysis in the affected muscles, usually the ocular and facial muscles, with tetanic spasms superimposed. Spasms may involve the tongue and throat muscles, resulting in dysarthria, dysphonia, and dysphagia. *Generalized tetanus* presents initially with trismus (spasm of the masseter muscles). Other bulbar musculature is rapidly involved, as are the neck, trunk, and extremity muscles. Consistent muscular rigidity is present in all musculature with superimposed paroxysms of tonic contraction or spasm (tetanic seizures) occurring spontaneously or in response to even slight stimuli. Such a state is extremely painful and spasms of the respiratory, laryngeal, and glottal muscles can result in apnea or suffocation. Death may also occur from heart failure due to the seizuring or from circulatory collapse due to sympathetic nervous system dysfunction.

One dose of tetanus-immune human globulin (antitoxin) is given, and penicillin or tetracycline is administered. Surgical excision or debridement of the wound is necessary, and the wound is infiltrated with antitoxin. Seizure activity is controlled and ventilatory support is given if breathing is compromised.

Nursing diagnoses and interventions center on such problems as alterations in comfort, potential for injury, impairment of mobility, alteration in self-care activities, impairment of verbal communication, and anxiety.

Botulism, caused by the exotoxin of the *Clostridium botulinum*, is more frequently associated with home-preserved foods, particularly vegetables, than with commercially prepared foods. The site of toxin action is at the neuromuscular junction. The toxin interferes with acetylcholine release, thus blocking nerve impulse transmission to the muscles. Clinical manifestations usually appear within 12–36 h after the toxin is ingested. Blurred vision and diplopia (double vision) are the usual initial symptoms. Ptosis, strabimus, and extraocular muscle paralysis appear. Other bulbar signs and symptoms may include vertigo, deafness, nasal voice quality, hoarseness, dysarthria, and dysphagia. Progressive muscular weakness of the neck, trunk, and extremities follows. Signs associated with autonomic nervous system dysfunction may include dilated, unreactive pupils and severe constipation. The sensory system remains intact and consciousness is maintained. Death is related to respiratory failure.

Trivalent antiserum is given intravenously after testing for sensitivity to horse serum has been done. Daily intramuscular injections are continued until improvement begins. Intensive respiratory and circulatory support is frequently required.

Nursing diagnoses and interventions focus on impairment of mobility, impairment of verbal communication, sensory-perceptual alteration, alteration in bowel elimination, impairment of skin integrity.

Diphtheria is an acute infectious disease caused by *Corynebacterium diphtheriae* bacteria. From the inflammatory exudate formed in the throat and trachea, the bacteria elaborate their exotoxin. Approximately 20 percent of persons with diphtheria develop nervous system involvement manifested as paresis or paralysis. Initially, palatal paralysis results in a nasal voice, dysphagia, and regurgitation of fluid or food through the nose when swallowing is attempted. Facial muscle weakness, ptosis, weakness of the jaw muscle affecting speech and chewing, and tongue weakness are seen. Ciliary muscle paralysis then causes the loss of accommodation and blurring of vision. A sensorimotor polyneuropathy or respiratory or cardiac failure may ensue.

Administration of antitoxin is felt to lessen the severity of the clinical manifestations. Supportive treatment is required. Nursing diagnoses and interventions focus on alterations in comfort, nutritional alteration, impairment of verbal communication, sensory-perceptual alteration, potential for suffocation, potential for injury and anxiety.

HEAVY METALS

Lead poisoning (*plumbism*) is most commonly found in children under the age of 5. Developing plumbism in adulthood is usually related to exposure to the dust of inorganic lead salts or to the fumes when lead is heated or burned. At risk are painters, printers, potters, smelters, storage battery manufacturers, and leaded gasoline manufacturers. The common clinical manifestations of plumbism in adults are severe, poorly localized abdominal pain associated with abdominal muscle rigidity, often precipitated by alcohol ingestion or infection (lead colic), mild anemia, and, rarely, peripheral neuropathy with a predominant motor component involving the upper extremities. No or few sensory signs and symptoms are seen. Lead encephalopathy with decreasing consciousness into a stuporous or comatose state is rare in adults and is associated with moonshine ingestion.

Chelating agents, such as 2, 3-dimercaptopropanol (BAL) and calcium disodium edetate (Ca EDTA), will remove lead from soft tissues and are of value except in the case of plumbism from leaded gasoline manufacture. Nursing diagnoses and interventions center on alterations in comfort but may need to be extended to include impairment of mobility, alterations in self-care activities, and potential for injury if a peripheral neuropathy is present. Alterations of cognitive function and altered levels of consciousness must be included if lead encephalopathy is present. (See discussion of lead poisoning in Chapter 15.)

Currently the most common sources of *arsenic* intoxication are suicidal or accidental ingestion of rodenticides containing copper acetoarsenic or calcium or lead arsenate, exposure to insecticides containing arsenic, or use of arsenic in the manufacture of paints, enamels, and metals and as a disinfectant for skins and furs. Arsenic interferes with cellular metabolism. Arsenic poisoning is manifested as an encephalopathy or as a peripheral neuropathy.

Clinical manifestations of acute arsenic encephalopathy include headache, drowsiness, mental confusion, delirium, and seizures. Chronic encephalopathy signs and symptoms include those of an acute encephalopathy and in addition may involve weakness and muscular aching, chills and fever, hemolysis, mucosal irritation, Mees' lines (transverse white lines) in the nails. The peripheral neuropathy associated with chronic arsenic poisoning is a slowly developing sensorimotor distal neuropathy resembling a nutritional polyneuropathy.

Treatment for acute arsenic intoxication includes gastric lavage, fluid replacement, vasopressor agents, and BAL. In chronic poisoning, BAL does not appear to help the polyneuropathy but does lessen the other signs and symptoms. Nursing diagnoses and interventions for the acute encephalopathy center on alterations of cognitive function, altered levels of consciousness, alterations in comfort, impaired thought processes, potential for injury, sensory-perceptual alteration, anxiety, fear, alteration in fluid volume (potential), impairment of skin integrity (potential), and impairment of urinary elimination (potential). For the chronic poisoning, nursing diagnoses and interventions extend to include impairment of mobility, alteration in self-care activities, and role disturbance (potential).

Manganese poisoning occurs among persons who mine manganese ore and who separate manganese from the ore. An acute confusional state may be the initial clinical manifestation. Extrapyramidal signs resembling postencephalitic Parkinson's syndrome, such as expressionless facies, drooling, and so forth, and later retropulsion or propulsion may appear. Additional complaints of progressive weakness, increasing fatigue, and sleepiness are also made. Dystonia and severe axial rigidity may appear rather than a parkinsonian syndrome.

Only symptomatic treatment is available, although L-dopa has been helpful in the chronic "dystonic form" of manganese poisoning. Nursing diagnoses and interventions focus on such things as alteration of cognitive functions, anxiety, impairment of mobility, potential for injury, impairment of verbal communication, and alterations in self-care activities.

Chronic *mercury poisoning* most frequently occurs in persons exposed to large amounts of the metal, which is used in manufacturing thermometers, mirrors, incandescent lights, x-ray machines, vacuum pumps, felt hats, paper and pulp. The presence of mercury in industrial wastes has contaminated water and fish, whose ingestion can cause mercury intoxication. Chronic mercury poisoning may present with a variety of clinical manifestations including tremors of the tongue, lips, and extremities and progressive cerebellar ataxia. Choreoathetosis and a parkinsonian facies may be apparent. Mood and behavior changes that first manifest as complaints of weakness and increased fatigue are seen. These manifestations progress to an extreme lethargy alternating with irritability. Mercury poisoning may also present as a sensorimotor polyneuropathy similar to the nutritional polyneuropathy.

N-acetyl-dl-penicillamine is felt probably to be the drug of choice. Nursing diagnoses and interventions center on such things as self-care deficits, impairment of verbal communication, potential for injury, alterations in self-concept, anxiety, altered levels of consciousness, and lack of knowledge. If the mercury poisoning presents as a polyneuropathy, nursing diagnoses and interventions focus on alterations in comfort, sensory-perceptual alteration, impairment of mobility, potential for injury, and alterations in self-care activities.

Organophosphorous compounds such as triorthocresyl phosphate (TCP) and *inorganic* phosphorous compounds used in rat poisons, roach powder and the manufacture of matchheads are the major cause of phosphate intoxication. Occasional outbreaks come from accidental ingestion of TCP that has contaminated grain or cooking oil stored in the same containers. Organophosphates are powerful cholinesterase inhibitors. Clinical manifestations of phosphorus poisoning predominantly involve signs of a motor polyneuropathy, but the spinal cord, primarily the corticospinal tracts, may be involved.

Supportive care is required until the phosphorus has been eliminated from the body and the anticholinesterase effects have worn off. Nursing diagnoses and interventions center on impairment of mobility, alteration in self-care activities, potential for injury, anxiety, and impaired home maintenance management (potential).

Thallium intoxication may result from accidental or suicidal ingestion of thallium-containing rodenticides. If the acute poisoning is survived, a progressive sensorimotor polyneuropathy accompanied by optic atrophy and occasional ophthalmoplegia appears. With chronic poisoning the progressive sensorimotor polyneuropathy predominates. Potassium chloride by mouth is used to enhance the speed of elimination of the thallium from the body. (See Nursing Diagnoses and Interventions under *Nutritional Polyneuropathy*.)

INFLAMMATIONS

MENINGITIS (LEPTOMENINGITIS)

DESCRIPTION

Common causes of *bacterial meningitis* include meningococcus (*Neisseria meningitidis*), pneumococcus (*Streptococcus pneumoniae*), and *Haemophilus influenzae*. Staphylococcus, streptococcus, gonococcus, and gram-negative bacteria are less frequent causes. Bacterial meningitis is essentially an infection of the pia and arachnoid and of the fluid in the subarachnoid space. Access to the subarachnoid space is gained following a systemic or blood stream infection or by direct extension from an infected area. This bacterial infiltration causes an inflammatory reaction in the pia and arachnoid, the cerebrospinal fluid, and the ventricles. A purulent inflammatory exudate is formed. Changes are found in the small- and medium-sized subarachnoid arteries, veins, choroid plexes, and the spinal and cranial nerve sheaths. Some change in the cortical neuron occurs. Bacterial meningitides can be classied as acute, subacute, or chronic processes.

Fungal meningitis is much less common than bacterial. Although many fungal infections may involve the nervous system, the ones that do so with any regularity are cryptococcosis, coccidioidomycosis, mucormycosis, candidiasis, and aspergillosis. The majority of the time a fungal meningitis arises when there is an impairment of the immune response or alteration in normal body flora. Fungal meningitides develop insidiously over a period of time, from days to weeks. Thrombosis and infarction may result from the arteritis. Diagnosis is difficult, and the antibiotics used to treat the fungus are very toxic.

Aseptic (nonpurulent) meningitis refers to a symptom complex that may be produced by a variety of infective agents, the majority of which are viral. The inflammation is believed to be limited to the meninges. Alteration of consciousness is usually mild. Most common causes of aseptic meningitis are enteroviral infections (echo, Coxsackie, and nonparalytic poliomyelitis), mumps, herpes simplex (type 1), adenovirus infections, and California virus. Other causes of aseptic meningitis include bacterial infections inadequately treated and meningitis mistakenly diagnosed as aseptic but actually caused by syphilis, tuberculosis, or neoplastic meningeal invasion. (See *Meningitis* in Chapter 15.)

PREVENTION

See Prevention under *Meningitis* in Chapter 15.

ASSESSMENT

Health History

1. Violent, generalized, throbbing headache.
2. Neck stiffness and neck pain often severe in nature.
3. Photophobia.
4. Complaint of projectile vomiting.
5. Diplopia.
6. Tinnitus.
7. Generalized or focal seizure disorder recently developing.
8. History of preceding infection.

Physical Assessment

1. Nuchal rigidity with possible head retraction.
2. Fever (may be afebrile with fungal meningitis).
3. Deteriorated mental status with delirium or stupor.
4. Brudzinski's sign, that is, forceful flexion of the neck onto the chest causing flexion of both legs and thighs.
5. Kernig's sign, that is, recumbent leg cannot be extended with the hip joint flexed at a right angle.
6. Papilledema.
7. Petechial or purpuric rash.
8. Focal motor paresis or paralysis especially involving the cranial nerves.

Diagnostic Tests

1. Lumbar puncture to determine if cerebrospinal fluid pressure is elevated. Cerebrospinal fluid analysis shows a high leukocyte cell count, elevated protein level, decreased glucose content, positive cultures. Gram stain helps to identify the organisms.
2. Blood cultures to assist in identifying the organism.
3. Blood studies to gain knowledge of the WBC count and differential WBC count.

NURSING DIAGNOSES: ACTUAL OR POTENTIAL

1. Alterations in comfort, moderate to severe: headache, neck stiffness and pain due to muscle spasm; tinnitus.
2. Sensory-perceptual alteration, moderate to severe: visual impairment due to photophobia, diplopia.
3. Altered levels of consciousness, mild to deep: due to cerebral edema, increased intracranial pressure, seizure activity, or dehydration.
4. Potential for injury: secondary to seizure activity, confusional state, or visual impairment.
5. Alteration in fluid volume, moderate to severe: dehydration secondary to decreased consciousness, fever, and vomiting.
6. Nutritional alteration, moderate to severe: decreased intake.
7. Anxiety, mild to severe: secondary to head pain, confusional state, and visual disturbance.
8. Lack of knowledge about health status, diagnostic procedures and so on.
9. Alteration in self-care activities, moderate to severe secondary to decreased consciousness, pain, and visual impairment.
10. Impairment of skin integrity, diaphoresis, and immobility.
11. Respiratory dysfunction: aspiration secondary to loss of protective reflexes with deep coma; pulmonary congestion and atelectasis secondary to immobility.
12. Impairment of urinary elimination: incontinence secondary to decreased consciousness with loss of voluntary control.
13. Impairment of bowel elimination: constipation secondary to dehydration and immobility; incontinence secondary to loss of voluntary control.
14. Impaired home management maintenance: secondary to nutritional deficits.

EXPECTED OUTCOMES

1. Return of neurological function will be evidenced by normal neurological examination.
2. Client will be comfortable, with both head pain and vomiting controlled, within 48–72 h after initiation of treatment begins. Once the cerebral edema is under control and the client is cognitively intact, direct drug control measures for the head pain, such as pain medication, can be provided.
3. Client will be seizure-free within 48–72 h after treatment and initiation of antibiotic therapy.
4. Papilledema will decrease, as evidenced by improvement in visual acuity and decrease in the swelling of the optic discs (initial).
5. A decrease in vascular volume will be evidenced by slightly decreased skin turgor and serum electrolytes that suggest a slight volume depletion (slightly increased BUN, serum creatinine, slightly increased hemoglobin and hematocrit).
6. Return of bowel function will be evidenced by absence of constipation and diarrhea. (In mild symptomatic meningitis the client will maintain bladder and bowel continence.)
7. Client will retain self-care and role function according to the severity of the meningitis, as evidenced by a return of as much self-care and role function as possible in light of neurological deficits.
8. The client and/or family will report correct information about the client's health status, diagnostic procedures, therapeutic management, and so forth.
9. If severe residual damage is present, family and/or client (if feasible) will make an informed and carefully thought-through decision about the possibility of home management.
10. If recovery is not possible because of the fulminating nature of the meningitis, the client will be able to experience a peaceful and dignified death.

INTERVENTIONS

1. Establish an accurate data base including laboratory data with ongoing periodic neurological reassessment regarding mental status, af-

fectual responses, motor function, sensory function, and incoordination.

2. Promote control of infection.
   a. Administer antibiotics if appropriate for the type of meningitis as ordered. Observe for, record, and report signs of therapeutic effectiveness and side effects.
   b. Maintain administration routes for the antibiotics, especially IV lines and body tissues at the injection or venipuncture site.
3. Reduce fever.
   a. Administer antipyretic medications as ordered.
   b. Maintain a cool environment with little covering over the client.
   c. Maintain a cooling system such as alcohol rubs, sponging briskly with tepid water, ice packs, or a hypothermia blanket to reduce the fever.
4. Prepare client and family for the diagnostic procedures.
5. Maintain client's fluid balance and nutritional status with IV fluids as ordered. *Remember: The client with increased intracranial pressure is kept slightly volume-depleted.*
6. Help client and family to maintain nutrition and fluid intake. Gradually adjust the texture and consistency of the food as the client's swallowing and chewing improve. (See also *Amyotrophic Lateral Sclerosis*, intervention 5a, b, c, and f.)
7. Help client and family assume responsibility for the management of residual deficits (if present).
8. If there are residual deficits, provide information, time, and support that the client and family need to realistically make an informed decision about home management.
9. If the client cannot survive, allow family time to be with the client and time to grieve; ensure a dignified death.

EVALUATION

Outcome Criteria

1. Infection clearing; cerebrospinal fluid WBC count is returning to within normal limits.
2. Skin rash is disappearing and skin integrity is otherwise maintained.
3. Temperature is returning to normal.
4. During acute phase, client is slightly volume-depleted and nutritionally maintained via IV. During the recovery phase, client is nutritionally well-nourished and well-hydrated.

Complications

1. See *Encephalitis*. In addition:
2. Normal-pressure hydrocephalus (see discussion under *Adult Hydrocephalus*).
3. Cerebrovascular accident (see discussion under *Cerebrovascular Accident*).

BRAIN ABSCESS

DESCRIPTION

Brain abscesses generally arise from infections elsewhere in the body, such as in the middle ear, mastoid cells, nasal cavity, or nasal sinuses. *Otogenic* brain abscesses are frequently located in the anterolateral cerebellar hemispheres and in the middle or inferior temporal lobe. *Rhinogenic* abscesses are most frequently located in the frontal and temporal lobes. Bacteria reach the central nervous system by direct extension from an osteomyelitis that develops or by spreading along the vein wall. The other major septic foci are from the lungs or the heart. Occasionally the source is infected pelvic organs, skin, tonsils, abscessed teeth, and osteomyelitis of noncranial bones. Brain abscesses arising from such distant foci most commonly occur in the distal portion of the middle cerebral arteries and are frequently multiple in number. Occasionally, bacteria are introduced by an open head trauma or during neurosurgery. The most common organisms causing brain abscesses are streptococci often found in combination with anaerobes. Staphlococci and fungi have also been found to cause brain abscesses.

Abscesses vary in size. They may be free or encapsulated. Brain abscesses have a predilection to spread or produce daughter abscesses.

Very early antibiotic therapy is highly desirable. Supportive treatment to manage increased intracranial pressure must be instituted. Surgical intervention involving drainage or aspiration of the abscess is required if improvement is not seen.

PREVENTION

Health Promotion

1. Health education should include teaching all persons to seek early treatment for ear, sinus, and dental infections and helping them understand the need and value of such action.
2. General health education should continue to

stress the importance of continuing with the full antibiotic course, even after symptoms improve. Prescriptions should be clearly labeled to indicate when discontinuance is to occur.

3. Early treatment of infection, along with prophylactic use of antibiotics in certain inflammatory processes and in head trauma, will prevent brain abscesses in most instances.
4. Congenital cardiac anamolies should be surgically corrected as soon as advisable to eradicate a source of brain abscess.
5. Aggressive treatment of all brain abscesses may prevent recurrent abscess formation.

Population at Risk

1. Brain abscess is slightly more common during first three decades of life.
2. Recent infectious processes are always present, but not necessarily identified. Most common sources of brain abscess are:
   a. Direct spread from contiguous sources of infection.
      (1) Middle ear.
      (2) Paranasal sinuses.
      (3) Mastoid cells.
   b. Hematogenous spread of infection from:
      (1) Lungs.
         (a) Bronchiectasis.
         (b) Lung abscess.
         (c) Empyema.
         (d) Bronchitis.
         (e) Bronchopleural fistula.
      (2) Heart.
         (a) Congenital defects in children older than 2 (Tetralogy of Fallot, right-to-left shunts).
         (b) Valves (acute bacterial endocarditis).
      (3) Other organs.
         (a) Pelvic organs.
         (b) Skin.
         (c) Teeth.
         (d) Tonsils.
         (e) Bones (extracranial osteomyelitis).
   c. Direct invasion of brain from trauma.
      (1) Penetrating wound.
      (2) Compound skull fracture.
      (3) Lacerated scalp and dura.
      (4) Intracranial surgical procedures.

Screening

1. Source of infections should be determined and evaluated through laboratory and clinical data to ascertain most appropriate antibiotic therapy.
2. Follow-up visits can aid in uncovering infections of resistant organisms.
3. Health history to determine recent infections whenever neurological symptoms are presented will aid in early detection of brain abscesses.

ASSESSMENT

Health History

1. Early *symptoms*.
   a. Headache and neck pain.
   b. Complaint of drowsiness.
   c. History of generalized or focal seizures.
   d. History of ear, nose, lung, or other recent infection.
2. *Late symptoms*.
   a. Complaint of inattentiveness by the client, family or employer.
   b. Complaint of poor memory by the client, family, or employer.
   c. Complaint of decreasing vision.

Physical Assessment

1. *Early signs*.
   a. Confusional state.
   b. Contralateral sensory-motor deficit.
   c. Speech impairment that may be an aphasia, dysarthria, or coordination problem.
   d. Low-grade fever.
   e. Mild nuchal rigidity.
   f. A positive Kernig's sign.
2. *Late signs*.
   a. Deteriorated mental status.
   b. Papilledema nystagmus.
   c. Narrowed visual field.
   d. Weakness of conjugate gaze to the side of the lesion.
   e. Ataxia of the ipsilateral arm and leg.

Diagnostic Tests

1. Chest and skull x-ray films to disclose a possible pulmonary or paracranial source of infection.
2. CAT scan to rule out other types of lesions and to locate the abscess.
3. Electroencephalogram to demonstrate a high-voltage slow (delta) activity over the abscess.
4. Arteriogram to demonstrate the abscess and localize the abscess. (CAT scanning is reducing the need for this.)

5. Lumbar puncture to measure cerebrospinal fluid pressure and permit cerebrospinal fluid analysis as well as culture and gram stains to be done.
6. Ventriculogram to demonstrate abscesses that are deep and not well visualized on arteriogram and possibly on CAT scan.

NURSING DIAGNOSES: ACTUAL OR POTENTIAL

1. Alterations in comfort: headache; neck pain due to muscle spasms; fever.
2. Altered levels of cognitive functioning: decreased mental abilities and memory.
3. Alteration in tissue fluid volume within the cranial vault, mild to moderate: due to the abscess mass.
4. Sensory-perceptual alteration, mild to severe: visual impairment, gaze palsy, cut visual field, or blurring from papilledema.
5. Impairment of mobility, mild to severe: secondary to visual disturbance, impaired sensation, ataxia, motor deficit, or decreased consciousness.
6. Potential for injury: secondary to seizure activity, impaired cognition, ataxia, impaired vision, etc.
7. Impairment of verbal communication, mild to moderate: due to motor aphasia; dysarthria.
8. Self-care deficit, mild to severe: due to impaired cognition or consciousness, impaired vision, ataxia, pain, motor deficits, or sensory deficits.
9. Anxiety, mild to severe: secondary to impaired cognition, motor deficits, communication difficulties, or sensory impairment.
10. Role disturbance: secondary to pain, fever, altered cognitive function, decreased consciousness, visual deficits, motor impairment, impaired communication, and impaired mobility.
11. Knowledge deficit due to lack of information about diagnostic procedures or therapeutic management.
12. Impairment of urinary elimination: incontinence due to loss of voluntary control.
13. Alteration in bowel pattern: constipation due to dietary alterations and immobility; diarrhea.
14. Respiratory dysfunction: pulmonary congestion and atelectasis secondary to immobility; aspiration secondary to loss of protective reflexes with decreased consciousness.
15. Nutritional alteration: decreased intake secondary to motor weakness in chewing or swallowing muscles.
16. Impairment of skin integrity: secondary to immobility, dehydration, incontinence, or trauma.

EXPECTED OUTCOMES

1. See Expected Outcomes under *Meningitis*, outcomes 1 through 5, and then 7 through 10.
2. Client will maintain (or regain) a nutritionally well-balanced dietary intake, as evidenced by maintenance of body weight and a normal hematocrit and hemoglobin.

INTERVENTIONS

1. Establish a continued, accurate data base with periodic neurological reassessment.
2. Promote reduction of the increased intracranial pressure. (See *Increased Intracranial Pressure*, intervention 2, for specific interventions.)
3. Promote the control of the infection. The abscess may well require surgical drainage, and the antibiotics postoperative may be instilled into the ventricular-subarachnoid system via a *ventriculostomy*.
4. Institute additional measures to reduce fever (e.g., ice mattress).
5. Prepare client physically and prepare the client and family psychologically for the diagnostic procedures involved in establishing a diagnosis.
6. Prepare client and family for therapeutic neurosurgical procedure that may be necessary to drain the abscess.
7. Promote seizure control as well as protection of the client from injury. (See *Seizure Disorders* for specific interventions.)
8. Assist client in gaining control over head pain by providing comfort measures such as backrubs, positioning and other cutaneous stimulation, and control of the external environment. Pain medications are used only with alert clients, and then only mild analgesics are utilized.
9. Protect client from injury due to decreased cognitive function, ataxia, immobility, and seizures.
10. Assist client and family in learning how to manage the vision problems as well as pro-

tect the client from injury due to cut visual field, gaze palsy, or nystagmus.
   a. Have client's family and others approach the client from the unaffected or least affected side.
   b. Help the client learn to turn head to compensate for visual deficits.
   c. Assist the client and family in learning to keep environment orderly and uncluttered.
11. Assist the client and family in learning how to protect the client from injury due to impaired tactile sensations.
12. Help the client maintain adequate nutrition and fluid intake.
13. With the other health-related professionals, help the client and family assume responsibility for the management of recovery and residual deficits (if any are present).
14. Nursing interventions to reduce anxiety may be appropriate. (See *Anxiety* in Chapter 36, Anxiety and the Affective Disorders.)

EVALUATION

Outcome Criteria

1. Infection clears.
2. Intracranial pressure returns to within normal limits.
3. Temperature returns to normal.
4. Nutritional pattern returns and is maintained.
5. Neurological deficits diminish in number.

ENCEPHALITIS (VIRAL)

The core of an encephalitis syndrome is an acute febrile illness with evidence of meningeal involvement. Added to this are various combinations of convulsions, delirium, confusion, stupor or coma, aphasia, mutism, hemiparesis with asymmetry of tendon reflexes and extensor plantar reflexes, involuntary movements, ataxia, myoclonic jerks, nystagmus, ocular palsies, and facial weakness (Adams and Victor, 1977). Approximately 20 percent of persons who develop an acute viral encephalitis suffer residua, such as mental deterioration, amnesic states, personality changes, or hemiparesis. There is a wide variation in mortality and occurrence of residua, depending on the specific virus.

The *arthropod-borne (arbo) viral encephalitides* involve widespread degeneration of nerve cells. Eastern equine encephalitis has large degenerative lesions, whereas the others have micro-

TABLE 25-10 VIRAL ENCEPHALITIS

Type	Geographical Incidence	Seasonal Incidence
Arthropod-borne:		
Eastern equine encephalitis	Eastern United States	Autumn
Western equine encephalitis	Uniform distribution throughout the United States	Summer and early fall
St. Louis encephalitis	Widespread distribution, in the far west occurs in rural areas, elsewhere occurs in urban areas	Late summer
Venezuelan equine encephalitis	Southwestern United States	Year round
California virus encephalitis	Midwestern states	Early fall
Herpes simplex encephalitis	No particular geographical distribution	No seasonal incidence
Poliovirus Poliomyelitis	Sporadic distribution where nonimmunized persons cluster	Summer and early fall
Rabies	Sporadic distribution throughout the United States	Bites more common in late spring through the early fall

scopic lesions. These viral encephalitides occur in epidemics except for the California viral encephalitis, which is endemic. Eastern equine encephalitis is the most serious of these viral encephalitides. Two-thirds of the persons who develop this encephalitis die or are left with severe residua. Fortunately, it is also the least commonly occurring (see Table 25-10).

Herpes simplex encephalitis, due almost exclusively to herpes smplex virus type 1, has a predilection for the inferiomedial portions of the frontal and temporal lobes. Hemorrhagic necrotic lesions occur. The mortality rate is unknown because of the extreme difficulty of establishing the diagnosis. Severe mental status deterioration is a common sequela.

Encephalitis may occur as a complication ot systemic viral disease such as poliomyelitis, rabies, or mononucleosis. Also, encephalitis may occur after recovery from some viral infections, such as rubeola or rubella, or postvaccination. Encephalitis is also associated with typhus, trichinosis, malaria, and schistosomiasis.

There is no adequate treatment for viral encephalitis. Supportive therapy to control intracranial hypertension is the major therapeutic focus. (Refer to *Meningitis* for discussion of nursing care and evaluation.)

HERPES ZOSTER (SHINGLES)

DESCRIPTION

This common viral infection of the nervous system is an acute inflammatory reaction occurring in isolated spinal or cranial sensory ganglia, the dorsal gray matter of the spinal cord, and the adjacent meninges. Herpes zoster is thought to be a reactivation of the varicella virus that exists latently in the sensory ganglia from the time of the primary chickenpox infection. The clinical manifestations include radicular pain, vesicular cutaneous eruptions, and possibly segmental sensory loss and motor palsies. The thoracic dermatomes, particularly T5 to T10, are most commonly involved, followed by the craniocervical regions. Herpes zoster is not communicable, occurs sporadically throughout the year, and does not have an increased incidence during chickenpox epidemics.

No specific treatment exists for herpes zoster. Analgesics and corticosteroids may be utilized to provide symptomatic relief from the pain. A persistent postherpetic pain syndrome may develop.

PREVENTION

Health Promotion

1. At present no vaccine exists, although passive immunization with zoster immune globulin is occasionally used.
2. Maintaining optimum health through proper nutrition, adequate rest, and appropriate exercise may decrease the chance of reactivation of virus or at least minimize effects of reactivation.

Population at Risk

1. Although zoster may occur at any age, it is more common in adults over 40 years, and incidence seems to increase with advancing age.
2. Past history of chickenpox is almost always present.
3. Activation of latent virus is almost always attributed to waning immunity (e.g., aging, lymphomas, chronic leukemia and Hodgkin's disease, and administration of immunosuppressive drugs and radiation therapy).
4. Other trigger mechanisms may be in the form of trauma, injection of drugs such as arsenicals, or concommittant debilitating diseases such as tuberculosis.

Screening

1. Screening is not a preventive measure.
2. All persons with zoster should be evaluated, as zoster may be indicative of an internal disease source, especially in persons past middle age.

ASSESSMENT

Health History

1. History of immunotherapy, radiotherapy, or malignancy.
2. Past history of chickenpox.
3. Itching, tingling, or burning sensations in a dermatome or cranial nerve distribution.
4. Malaise.
5. Local pain, sometimes severe, in a dermatome or cranial nerve distribution.

6. Persistent hyperesthesia in a dermatome or cranial nerve distribution.

Physical Assessment

1. Fever.
2. Tense, clear vesicles on an erythematous base that become cloudy after a few days and then become dry, crusted, and scaly.
3. Cutaneous sensations in the affected dermatome(s) may be impaired.
4. Segmental weakness and atrophy.
5. Disuse atrophy and contracturing may be found due to restriction of movement to prevent pain.

Diagnostic Tests

Diagnosis is based on the history and physical findings.

NURSING DIAGNOSES: ACTUAL OR POTENTIAL

1. Alterations in comfort: severe nerve pain.
2. Impairment of skin integrity: due to vesicular skin eruptions.
3. Anxiety: secondary to pain, fear of immobility.
4. Self-care deficits: due to pain and motor palsy.
5. Role disturbance: secondary to pain, motor palsy, or anxiety.
6. Sensory-perceptual alteration, mild to moderate: deminished or lost sensation in the involved area.
7. Knowledge deficit: lack of knowledge about diagnostic procedures, therapeutic management, and hospitalization.
8. Alterations in self-concept: due to the skin disruptions.
9. Maladaptive (individual) coping patterns: secondary to pain.
10. Alteration in bowel elimination: constipation secondary to immobility and pain medication.
11. Nutritional deficit: secondary to pain and anorexia due to pain; swallowing or chewing difficulties secondary to cranial nerve involvement.
12. Alteration in fluid volume, mild to moderate: dehydration secondary to fever and decreased intake due to pain.
13. Respiratory dysfunction: pulmonary congestion and atelectasis secondary to immobility.

EXPECTED OUTCOMES

1. Control of pain will be evidenced by client's verbal statement.
2. Skin intactness will be retained without secondary infection.
3. Client will maintain as much self-care and role function as possible in light of pain and possible sensory and motor deficits.
4. Client will be free of injury.
5. Client and family will verbalize correct information about health status and therapeutic management with 90 percent accuracy.
6. Client will maintain normal pattern of bowel function.
7. Client will report eating a nutritionally well-balanced diet, as evidenced by maintenance of body weight and a normal hematocrit an hemoglobin.
8. Normal vascular volume will be evidenced by normal skin turgor, normal serum, and urinary output of 50 mL/h.
9. Lungs will remain clear.

INTERVENTIONS

1. Assist client to gain control over pain. (See *Spinal Cord Tumors*, intervention 2a, f, g, and h.)
2. Teach the client and family how to promote the reestablishment of skin integrity without the occurrence of a secondary infection in the involved area.
    a. Protect skin from scratching or additional trauma to the affected area.
    b. Wash the skin with mild soap and water and dry thoroughly.
    c. Place a dry protective dressing over unbroken vesicles, if desired.
    d. Apply wet dressings as ordered to broken dried skin lesions.
    e. Apply corticosteroid lotion or sprays to the local lesions as ordered to help relieve discomfort.
    f. Prevent exposure to extremes of temperature in the area involved.
    g. Visually check the involved area for signs of infection.
3. Protect client from further damage to the nerve(s) and area innervated by the nerve(s) by providing rest for the areas involved in the inflammatory process.
4. Maintain motor function.
    a. See *Coma*, intervention 3, for specific interventions. In addition:

b. Provide a range of motion exercise program carried out q2h to prevent contracturing and loss of joint function. (*Active exercise is limited during the acute process.*)
5. Help client and family to find means to avoid contact with the hyperesthetic skin areas.
6. Help client and family to:
   a. Institute a bowel evacuation protocol to prevent constipation.
   b. Maintain adequate nutritional and fluid intake, especially if nerves responsible for chewing and swallowing are affected. (See *Amyotrophic Lateral Sclerosis,* intervention 5a through h, for specific interventions.)
   c. Institute a pulmonary regimen designed to keep the lungs clear.
      (1) Maintain ambulation and activities of daily living to the maximum possible extent; at least have the client get out of bed and sit in a chair several times a day.
      (2) Institute deep breathing and coughing exercise program for the client. Postural drainage with cupping and clapping may be initiated if the lungs begin to become congested.
7. Help client to reduce fever by:
   a. Taking the prescribed antipyretic medication.
   b. Maintaining a cool environment with little covering.
8. Nursing interventions to reduce the dependent behavior, depression, and anxiety may be appropriate. (See *Dependent Behavior* in Chapter 37 and *Anxiety* and *Depression* in Chapters 36 and 38.)

EVALUATION

Outcome Criteria

1. Pain and paresthesias are decreasing as reported by the client.
2. Skin is healing, as evidenced by increased integrity observed on examination.
3. Client is retaining (or regaining) self-care, role function, and socialization patterns.
4. Client and family are able to provide accurate information about the client's health status, therapeutic management, and hospital procedures and policies.
5. Client reports return of normal bowel pattern.
6. Nutritional status is maintained, as evidenced by weight gain and normal hemoglobin and hematocrit levels.
7. Lungs are clear upon ascultation.

Complications

1. Skin infection (see discussion in Chapter 35).
2. Constipation or impaction (see discussion in Chapter 33).
3. Malnutrition (see Evaluation under *Amyotrophic Lateral Sclerosis,* complication 7).
4. Dehydration (see Evaluation under *Amyotrophic Lateral Sclerosis,* complication 6).
5. Atelectasis/aspiration leading to pneumonia (see discussion in Chapter 31).
6. Chronic pain syndrome (see Evaluation under *Nutritional Polyneuropathy,* complication 7).
7. Disuse atrophy and contracturing.

Assessment

1. Decreasing range of joint motion.
2. Increasing joint pain on movement.
3. Atrophy of muscles around the joint(s).

Revised Outcomes

1. Client will regain full range of motion in the joint(s).
2. Muscles will regain normal size and strength.

Interventions

1. Administer prescribed therapy, such as heat vibration, physical therapy, and occupational therapy.
2. Administer range of motion exercises q2h.
3. Administer active exercise, active assistive exercise, or active resistive exercises as ordered.
4. Assist client to maintain the functional positioning of the joint with support and assistive devices as necessary.
5. Use analgesic medications, cutaneous stimulation techniques, and cognitive techniques to control the pain.
6. Encourage the client to use the joint(s) in performing activities of daily living.

Reevaluation and Follow-up

1. Monitor the degree of increase in joint range of motion and in muscular strength.
2. Evaluate the success of pain control measures.

LANDRY-GUILLAIN-BARRÉ SYNDROME (ACUTE IDIOPATHIC POLYNEURITIS)

DESCRIPTION

Landry-Guillain-Barré syndrome is an acute ascending motor paralysis thought to be the result of a cell-mediated immunological reaction involving the peripheral nerves. Lymphocytes infiltrate the involved nerves, and inflammation and demyelination follow. Frequently the syndrome is preceded by a mild viral respiratory or gastrointestinal infection 1 to 3 weeks before the onset of clinical manifestations. Other preceding events have included surgical procedures, viral immunization, and lymphomatous disease. The clinical manifestations vary from involvement, mostly of the legs, to complete quadriplegia, with respiratory insufficiency and autonomic nervous symptom instability.

The disease remits naturally in most cases, and recovery can be complete if the client has received expert care during the paralysis phase. The speed of recovery is variable from weeks to 18 months, depending on the degree of nerve degeneration. The therapeutic management centers on ventilatory support and management of the autonomic nervous system dysfunction, as these two aspects are the predominant causes of mortality from the disorder. Expert nursing care is equally essential. Aggressive rehabilitation must follow after the disease begins to remit. Corticosteroids are often administered during the acute phase.

PREVENTION

Health Promotion

1. Because Landry-Guillain-Barré is of unknown cause, there are at present no preventive measures that health care providers can employ.
2. Health education is limited to recognizing the signs and symptoms of the disease.
3. General health promotion and maintenance may prevent the occurrence of the mild febrile illnesses that precede the disease and that may be related to its occurrence.

Population at Risk

1. The disease occurs in all age groups and both sexes.
2. There is a slight peak in the 16- to 25-year-old age group.
3. A mild febrile illness, usually upper respiratory infectious or gastroenteritis, precedes the disease by days or weeks in approximately 50 percent of the reported cases.
4. Evidence indicates a relation between individuals receiving the influenza vaccine and Landry-Guillain-Barré.

Screening

1. Populations at risk are difficult to identify, as well as precipitating factors, because of the nature of the disease.
2. The development of polyneuropathy with weakness progressing to paralysis should alert health care providers to the possibility of Landry-Guillain-Barré.

ASSESSMENT

Health History

1. History of viral infection, vaccination, surgery, or lymphomatous disease.
2. Complaint of paresthesia that began in the legs and ascended upward (often occurring before the onset of motor weakness).
3. Complaint of progressive motor weakness that began in the feet and is ascending upward.
4. Shortness of breath (air hunger).

Physical Assessment

1. Symmetrical weakness to paralysis involving the trunk, neck, and facial muscles.
2. Impaired position sense and vibration sense.
3. Hypotonia in the involved muscles.
4. Deep tendon reflexes absent.
5. Autonomic nervous system dysfunction, such as sinus tachycardia, hypertension, hypotension, or loss of sweating.
6. Decreased ventilatory capacity.

Diagnostic Tests

1. Lumbar puncture to demonstrate normal pressure with no cells but elevating protein levels that peak in 4 to 6 weeks.
2. Nerve conduction studies to demonstrate slowed velocities soon after the paralysis develops.
3. Electromyelogram denervation potentials (fibrillations) appear later.

NURSING DIAGNOSES: ACTUAL OR POTENTIAL

1. Impairment of mobility, moderate to complete loss: due to motor weakness or paralysis.
2. Alterations in self-care activities: self-care deficit due to motor weakness or paralysis.
3. Potential for injury: due to motor weakness, paralysis, or sensory impairment.
4. Alterations in comfort, mild to moderate: secondary to paresthesias.

5. Anxiety, mild to severe: due to fear of paralysis or impaired body image.
6. Role disturbance: secondary to motor deficits or immobility.
7. Knowledge deficit: lack of information regarding health status, diagnostic procedures, therapeutic management, hospitalization.
8. Sensory-perceptual alteration: impaired sensation.
9. Respiratory dysfunction: due to respiratory muscle weakness.
10. Impairment of written and verbal communication: due to motor deficits and ventilatory impairment.
11. Nutritional deficit: decreased intake due to muscle weakness.
12. Alteration in cardiac output, mild to severe: secondary to arrhythmia, hypotension or hypertension from autonomic nervous system disruption.
13. Alteration in patterns of sexuality: secondary to motor deficits and autonomic nervous system disruption.
14. Impairment of urinary elimination: retention due to motor weakness or paralysis; incontinence due to overflow from retention and impaired voluntary control.
15. Alteration in bowel patterns: constipation due to immobility; incontinence due to impaired voluntary control; diarrhea due to tube feedings.
16. Impairment of skin integrity: due to immobility or incontinence.
17. Alteration in fluid volume: edema secondary to immobility.
18. Impaired home maintenance management: due to neurological and self-care deficits.
19. Respiratory dysfunction: pulmonary congestion and atelectasis secondary to immobility.

EXPECTED OUTCOMES

1. Client will maintain as much self-care, role function, and socialization as possible in light of motor weakness.
2. Client and family will be able to provide correct information about health status, diagnostic procedures, therapeutic management, and so forth.
3. Aching, paresthesias, and contractures will be minimized, as evidenced by client's report of increased comfort.
4. Bowel and bladder will be continent.
5. The skin will remain intact.
6. Normal vital signs will be present and lungs clear.
7. A well-balanced diet and normal dietary intake will be maintained.
8. Normal vascular volume will be maintained.
9. Ventilatory capacity as measured by vital capacity will be greater than 1 L.

INTERVENTIONS

1. Establish accurate data base with ongoing periodic neurological reassessment.
2. Help client and family to learn about client's health status and therapeutic management.
   a. Explain diagnostic procedures and the preparation for these procedures.
   b. Teach the client and family about Landry-Guillain-Barré syndrome: its possible causes, clinical manifestations, and therapeutic management.
3. Protect client from injury.
   a. Provide rest for areas involved in the inflammatory process.
   b. Avoid exposure of denervated areas to extremes of temperature.
   c. Wash skin with mild soap and water and dry thoroughly, applying moistening agents to the skin or bath.
   d. Check skin for trophic changes that occur with denervation states and for signs of irritation.
   e. Check temperature of bath water, heating devices, and so on.
4. Maintain motor function.
   a. See *Coma*, intervention 3a through g. Also:
   b. Provide a range of motion exercise program carried out q2h to prevent contracturing and loss of joint function. (*Avoid active exercise during the acute process.*)
5. Promote maintenance of skin integrity.
6. Institute a pulmonary regimen designed to keep the lungs clear.
   a. Ventilatory assistance is initiated if vital capacity becomes less than 1 L. Intermittent mandatory ventilation (IMV) is used.
   b. An intubated client should be suctioned as necessary to maintain a patent airway; respiratory equipment tubing should be changed every 24–48 h.
7. Institute a bowel evacuation protocol.

8. Help the client to maintain adequate nutrition and fluid intake.
9. With other health-related professionals, help client and family assume responsibility for the management of recovery.
10. Help client to gain control over the discomfort caused by the paresthesias.
    a. Provide cutaneous stimulation through touch, temperature, and vibration, heat and physiotherapy such as ultrasound, diathermy, or dry heat, and stimulation methods such as transcutaneous electrical nerve stimulation.
    b. Help client to learn to use cognitive strategies such as distraction or imagery to control the paresthesias.
    c. Help client maintain an adequate diet to enhance nerve repair.
11. Nursing interventions to reduce anxiety may be appropriate. (See *Anxiety* in Chapter 36, Anxiety and the Affective Disorders.)
12. Prevent serious effects resulting from arrhythmias.
    a. Observe for clinical manifestations of arrhythmia (see discussion in Chapter 30).
    b. Monitor ECG continuously and administer antiarrhythmic drugs as ordered.
13. Maintain a blood pressure that is normal for the client.
14. Institute a lower motor neuron bladder evacuation protocol to prevent retention and overflow incontinence, if appropriate.
15. If appropriate, institute an upper motor neuron or mixed bladder training protocol. (See *Spinal Cord Tumor*, intervention 11.)

EVALUATION

Outcome Criteria

1. See Evaluation under *Amyotrophic Lateral Sclerosis*, outcome criteria 1 through 9.
2. Client's vital capacity is greater than 2 L.
3. Client's vital functions remain within normal limits.
4. Client's nutritional pattern is returning to normal, as evidenced by weight within normal limits.

Complications

1. See Evaluation under *Amyotrophic Lateral Sclerosis*, complications 1 through 8.
2. Arrhythmias (see discussion in Chapter 30).
3. Hypotension (see discussion in Chapter 30).
4. Disuse atrophy and contracturing.

NEUROSYPHILIS

Neurosyphilis occurs in approximately one-fourth of all persons who develop syphilis and exists initially as an asymptomatic meningitis. This asymptomatic meningitis may eventually cause meningeal and parenchymal brain tissue damage. Usually symptomatic meningitis and meningovascular syphilis occur first, then general paresis, tabes dorsalis, optic atrophy, and meningomyelitis appear many years later.

Meningeal syphilis usually manifests clinically within 2 years of the cerebrospinal fluid invasion as a symptomatic meningitis with intracranial hypertension. Meningovascular syphilis usually manifests 6 to 7 years after the original infection. Not only is there infiltration of the meninges but the arteries are inflamed and a fibrotic process causes narrowing and eventual occlusion. The person may then experience repeated cerebrovascular accidents (CVAs).

Paretic neurosyphilis (general paresis, general paralysis of the insane, dementia paralytica, syphilitic meningoencephalitis) is a rare occurrence today. Presenting 15 to 20 years after the original infection, its clinical manifestations include a progressive dementia, dysarthria, development of seizures, presence of hyperreflexia and plantar extensor reflexes, Argyll Robertson pupils, and an action tremor.

Tabes neurosyphilis (tabes dorsalis), developing 15 to 20 years after the first infection, manifests with ataxia due to impairment of vibration and position sense in the foot and legs, lightening pains (sharp, stabbing pain in the legs most frequently), urinary incontinence due to loss of sensation and hypotonia, absent knee and ankle reflexes, paresthesias, and a positive Romberg. In addition, many persons with tabes dorsalis have abnormal pupils, ptosis, ophthalmoplegia, and optic atrophy. Constipation, megacolon, and impotence are also seen. Trophic ulcers and Charcot's joints result from the sensory losses in the lower extremities.

Syphilitic optic atrophy usually presents as a progressive blindness in one eye then extends to involve the other. Visual field constriction occurs due to perioptic meningitis with gliosis and fibrosis of the optic nerve fibers.

In syphilitic meningomyelitis (Erb's spastic paraplegia), bilateral corticospinal tract signs predominate. Spinal meningovascular syphilis presents as a vasculitis with narrowing and occlusion of the spinal arteries.

The cerebrospinal fluid is a sensitive indicator of the presence of active neurosyphilis. Elevated cell counts, an elevated protein level, and positive serology are found. Antibiotic drug therapy is instituted to stop progression of the infection. Supportive therapy is also initiated for the signs and symptoms that the client is experiencing.

In syphilitic meningitis and meningovascular syphilis, nursing diagnoses and interventions focus on alterations in comfort, lack of knowledge, anxiety, nutritional alteration, and altered levels of consciousness (potential). Nursing diagnoses and interventions in late neurosyphilitic conditions such as tabes dorsalis and syphilitic meningomyelitis must be extended to include sensory-perceptual alteration, impairment of mobility, alterations in self-care activities, potential for injury, impairment of urinary elimination, alteration in bowel elimination, role disturbance, and impaired home maintenance management and, with general paresis of the insane, altered cognitive function and impairment of verbal communication.

SARCOIDOSIS

Isolated sarcoid tubercles (granulomas) may involve peripheral or cranial nerves, giving rise to a subacute or chronic asymmetric neuropathy (see *Peripheral or Cranial Nerve Degeneration*). Involvement of the meninges, brain, and spinal cord may occur but is less common. Central nervous system sarcoidosis produces a granulomatous infiltration involving the meninges and underlying parenchyma usually at the base of the brain. Clinical manifestations include visual disturbances, polydipsia, polyuria, somnolence, obesity, seizures, hydrocephalus, cranial nerve palsies, cerebellar signs and symptoms, and signs of corticospinal tract disruption. The spinal meninges and the spinal cord may be infiltrated and produce signs of adhesive arachnoiditis.

The diagnosis is made on the basis of the clinical features and biopsy of other tissues to demonstrate a sarcoid granuloma. Administration of corticosteriods is the current mode of therapy. Some of the nursing diagnoses and interventions center on include sensory-perceptual alterations, anxiety, alterations in fluid volume, altered levels of consciousness, and role disturbance.

RABIES

In practically all instances, the rabies virus is introduced through an animal bite (skunk, fox, bat, racoon, dog, or cat). The virus travels along the peripheral nerves to the central nervous system. The incubation period is usually several months. Initial clinical manifestations include fever, headache, and malaise, followed by severe anxiety and psychomotor overactivity. Dysphagia, spasms of the face, and spasms of the facial muscles then develop. Generalized seizures are seen.

Postexposure prophylactic treatment should be instituted before the infection is established. Once the infection is established and signs and symptoms develop, the disease is usually fatal. Nursing diagnoses and interventions at the time of the bite focus on impairment of skin integrity, anxiety, and lack of knowledge. Fear is the most probable nursing diagnosis during the prophylactic treatment phase. With onset of the disease, nursing diagnoses center on alterations in comfort, altered levels of consciousness, alteration in fluid volume, impairment of mobility, nutritional alteration, respiratory dysfunction, and alteration in cardiac output.

POLIOMYELITIS

Poliomyelitis, a highly communicable viral disease, has its peak incidence from July through September. The virus is found in the human intestinal tract and is transmitted via a fecal-oral route. The incubation period is 1 to 3 weeks. In only a small fraction of infected persons is the nervous system invaded. Most cases today are seen in unvaccinated persons and in adults exposed to a newly immunized infant. Clinical manifestations of nervous system involvement range from an aseptic meningitis (nonparalytic or preparalytic poliomyelitis) to a variety of paralytic forms (paralytic poliomyelitis).

Nonparalytic poliomyelitis presents as a minor illness with listlessness, generalized nonthrobbing headache, fever, stiff aching muscles, sore throat, anorexia, nausea, and vomiting. Although the headache and fever then persist, the muscle tenderness and pain, hamstring tightness, and neck and back pain become the predominant clinical manifestations.

In the paralytic forms, muscle paresis may develop concurrent with the symptoms of generalized illness or after the symptoms abate. The paresis or paralysis may develop rapidly, reaching maximum severity in 48 h, or may develop slowly or in a stuttering pattern for a week or more. In adults, an asymmetric paresis involving all four extremities is the most common presentation. Also in adults, a spinal-bulbar involvement is more commonly seen than the pure bulbar form.

Treatment is supportive in nature with aggressive rehabilitation after the disease has run its course. Nursing diagnoses for nonparalytic poliomyelitis focus on alterations in comfort, alteration in fluid volume, nutritional alteration, impairment of mobility, and alterations in self-care activities. For the paralytic forms, additional nursing diagnoses and interventions focus on respiratory dysfunction, impaired home maintenance management, grieving, role disturbance, and impairment in elimination.

BELL'S PALSY

Bell's palsy is the most common disorder of the facial nerve and is associated with middle-ear infections, meningitis, and hemorrhage. Thought to be due to an inflammatory reaction in or around the nerve, it has an acute onset with paralysis evolving sometimes over a few hours. Most person (80 percent) recover within a few weeks to 2 months. This disorder affects males and females equally and occurs in all age groups. A facial nerve paralysis can also be caused by compression due to tumor or fracture.

Administration of corticosteroids during the first weeks after onset of the paralysis is thought to be of some benefit. Surgical decompression may be indicated for tumors or fractures and is done by some neurosurgeons for idiopathic Bell's palsy. Protection of the eyes, facial splinting, and massage are equally important in the therapeutic management.

Nursing diagnoses and interventions focus on sensory-perceptual alteration, impairment of verbal communication, alterations in self-concept, anxiety, lack of knowledge, social isolation, role disturbance, nutritional alteration.

ACUTE DISSEMINATED ENCEPHALOMYELITIS

Acute disseminated encephalomyelitis is currently viewed as an acute demyelinative and inflammatory process with multiple lesions of varying size scattered throughout the brain and spinal cord. Clinical manifestations suggest diffuse involvement of the brain, spinal cord, and meninges and include an acute onset of confusion, somnolence, and convulsions, accompanied by headache, neck stiffness, ataxia, and abnormal movement such as myoclonus, athetosis, and choreoathetosis. In severe cases, stupor, coma, and possibly decerebrate rigidity may be seen. Spinal cord involvement is indicated by decreased or lost deep tendon reflexes, signs and symptoms of sensory impairment, paraplegia or quadriplegia, or bladder and bowel dysfunction. A predominant encephalitic, myelitic, or encephalomyelitic form of the disorder may be seen concurrently with or shortly following a viral illness (postinfectious encephalomyelitis) with mumps, influenza, and rubella and following vaccination to protect against rabies and smallpox (postvaccinal encephalomyelitis). Mortality and morbidity are high.

Nursing diagnoses and interventions focus on alterations in comfort, altered levels of consciousness, impairment of mobility, alterations in self-care activities, sensory-perceptual alteration, impairment of verbal communication, anxiety, role disturbance, alterations in self-concept, and impairment in bowel and bladder elimination.

TEMPORAL ARTERITIS

The external carotid system, particularly the temporal branches, of an elderly person may become involved in a subacute granulomatous inflammation. The most involved part of the system usually becomes thrombosed.

Head pain, sometimes severe, is the most common clinical manifestation. Systemic signs and symptoms may include aching or painful proximal muscles, stiffness markedly elevated sedimentation rate, fever, anorexia, weight loss, malaise, anemia, and slight leukocytosis. Occlusion of branches of the ophthalmic artery results in blindness. Ophthalmoplegia may occur. Occasionally, occlusion of the internal carotid or vertebral arteries results in a stroke.

Steroid therapy very effectively provides symptomatic relief and prevents blindness. Nursing diagnoses include alterations in comfort, anxiety, lack of knowledge, sensory-perceptual alteration, alterations in self-care activities, and impairment of mobility.

OBSTRUCTIONS

CEREBROVASCULAR ACCIDENTS

DESCRIPTION

Cerebrovascular disease is the most frequently occurring neurological disorder. Over 50 percent of the clients admitted to general hospitals with a neurological problem have cerebrovascular disease. Any abnormality of the brain due to a pathological process in the blood vessels is referred to as *cerebrovascular disease.* Included in this category are lesions of the vessel wall, occlusion of the vessel lumen by a thrombus or embolus, rupture of the vessel, alteration in vessel permeability, or changes in the character of the blood such as viscosity. The brain abnormalities induced by cerebrovascular disease are of two types: *ischemia* with or without *occlusion,* and *hemorrhage* (see Table 25-11).

The common manifestation of cerebrovascular disease is a *stroke*—a sudden, nonconvulsive, focal neurological deficit. In its mildest form, the neurological deficit is so minimal as to go almost unnoticed. In its severest state, hemiplegia and coma result. Cerebrovascular accidents (CVAs) are the third leading cause of death in the United States. The older age group is more affected by CVAs than the younger age group. Men are slightly more affected than women. There is a greater incidence of stroke in the black race. The extent of the neurological dysfunction gives an indication of the size and location of the ischemia, infarction, or hemorrhage.

Transitory neurological deficits, for example, transient ischemic attacks (TIAs) should be thoroughly investigated, especially in persons having identifiable risk factors. Noninvasive diagnostic tests are available to detect cerebrovascular disease, and the client is physically at his or her best before a completed stroke for surgical correction via carotid endarterectomy, extracranial bypass grafting, or intracranial bypass grafting (EC-IC bypass grafting). If the client is not a surgical candidate, controlling risk factors and instituting aspirin therapy may delay the onset of a CVA.

Thrombotic strokes may have an abrupt onset but usually tend to progress slowly, evolving in a step-by-step fashion over minutes to hours. The typical evolution of thrombotic stroke results in the clinical syndrome known as a *stroke-in-evolution.* A stuttering intermittent progression of a neurological deficit over hours to days is considered diagnostic of a thrombotic stroke. Treatment with bed rest, a calm and nonstressful environment, and anticoagulation or aspirin therapy is hoped to be helpful in managing a stroke-in-evolution.

The completed stroke has reached its maximum destructiveness in terms of producing neurological deficits. That is not to say the cerebral edema has reached its maximum state, however. Prognosis for the person who has suffered a thrombotic stroke is guarded. Recovery depends on the extent of neurological damage and the area of the brain involved. Further complicating the situation are the other health problems the person may have, such as hypertension, diabetes mellitus and vascular disease involving other organs and body parts. The more rapidly the neurological function begins to return, the better the prognosis for recovery and rehabilitation.

PREVENTION

Health Promotion

1. Control of hypertension with antihypertensive agents and dietary modifications including limited intake of sodium, cholesterol, and fat are important in the prevention of CVAs (see Chapter 30).
2. Health teaching for women using oral contraceptives should include the possible side effects of specific pills. Follow-up health care is important for these women.
3. Systemic problems, including cardiac impairment/dysfunction that may contribute to a

TABLE 25-11 TYPES OF CEREBROVASCULAR ACCIDENTS

	Occlusion		
	Thrombosis	Embolism	Hemorrhage
Significant history	History of atherosclerosis, diabetes mellitus, hypertension, arteritis History of TIAs Presence of polycythemia	History of heart disease: atrial fibrillation, valvular disease, acute bacterial endocarditis, subacute bacterial endocarditis, myocardial infarction	Family history of aneurysms or AVMs History of head trauma History of hypertension
Prodromal signs and symptoms	TIAs	Presence of embolization in other areas of the body	Seizure onset Presence of head pain: generalized and often very severe, hemiplegia or dementia
Time of onset	Occurs during sleep	Associated with activity and exertion (e.g., getting up to void at night)	Associated with activity and exertion (e.g., sexual activity)
Progression	Intermittent (stepwise) progression over minutes to hours (may be a day or two)	Most rapid onset, seconds to minutes	Steady progression over minutes to hours
Signs	No nuchal rigidity initially; may be seen later with increasing cerebral edema Well-localized neurological deficits		Nuchal rigidity and neck pain Head pain Less well-localized neurological deficits

CVA should be diagnosed and treated promptly.

4. Oversedation in elderly individuals should be avoided, as deep sleep has been cited as a precipitating factor of cerebral ischemia.

Population at Risk

1. Individuals with a history of hypertension or atherosclerotic disease or both are at high risk for CVAs.
2. Individuals with a history of transient ischemic attacks are at risk for CAVs.
3. Diabetes mellitus may predispose individuals for a CVA.
4. Those who have sustained head injuries have a higher incidence of CVA.
5. Individuals with cardiac impairments that may precipitate cerebral emboli, such as chronic atrial fibrillation, myocardial infarction with thrombus, subacute bacterial endocarditis, congenital heart disease, or malfunctioning prosthetic heart valves producing clots, may be predisposed to CVA.
6. Heavy smokers are thought to be at an increased risk for CVA.
7. Elevated blood cholesterol and fat levels may contribute to the occurrence of CVA.
8. Persons with gout and high RBC counts may be at risk for CVA.
9. Women using oral contraceptives may be at a greater risk for cerebrovascular thrombosis, although research is controversial.

Screening

1. Patterns of lifestyle should be assessed to detect populations at risk for cardiovascular disease and CVAs.
2. Blood pressure screening should be included

at each health care visit to detect hypertension. Follow-up health care is imperative when hypertension is suspected.

3. Levels of adherence to prescribed medications, dietary modifications, and follow-up care need to be determined in hypertensive clients.
4. Careful documentation of head injuries and ruptured cerebral blood vessels should be maintained as individuals get older.
5. Changes in perception and coordination including symptoms of transient ischemic attacks should be elicited during the health assessment to detect and promptly treat possible life-threatening problems.

ASSESSMENT

Health History

1. History of risk factors (see above).
2. History of prodromal signs and symptoms.
3. Time of onset, that is, whether the symptoms occur at once or over time.
4. Activity state at time of onset; active or at rest.
5. Temporal pattern of the stroke's progression.
6. Current treatment for other health problems including medications.
7. Headache and neck pain.
8. Varying degrees of consciousness and memory loss.

Physical Assessment

Middle cerebral artery (most common of the stroke syndromes). (See Table 25-12.)

1. *Total occlusion* syndrome.
   a. Contralateral hemiplegia: face, arm, and leg involved; initially, a flaccid state exists.
   b. Contralateral hemianesthesia: face, arm, and leg involved; primary and cortical sensations lost.
   c. Homonymous hemianopsia.
   d. Inability to turn the eyes toward the paralyzed side.
   e. A dull or stuporous state of consciousness.
   f. Dominant hemisphere signs (*left* hemisphere in majority of persons, including 70 percent of left-handed individuals).
      (1) Global aphasia: inability to comprehend either verbal or written language and the inability to communicate by using verbal and written language (Baratz and Norman, 1979).
      (2) *Gerstmann's syndrome*: acalculia (inability to do math calculations), alexia (inability to read), finger agnosia, and right-left confusion; may be seen if the client improves.
   g. Nondominant hemisphere signs (*right* hemisphere in majority of persons).
      (1) Loss of ability to recognize, associate, or interpret sounds including music, voice qualities, bells, horns, and animal or human sounds.
      (2) Inability to recognize musical pieces, scales, and types of instruments.
      (3) Misperception of one's own body parts and inability to orient oneself in space.
      (4) Neglect of involved body parts with denial of disability.
      (5) Auditory agnosia (auditory neglect).
2. *Superior main division* occlusion syndrome.
   a. Contralateral hemiplegia: face, arm, and leg involved; initially, a flaccid state exists.
   b. Contralateral hemianesthesia: face, arm, and leg involved; primary and cortical sensations lost.
   c. Less impairment of alertness than with a total occlusion of the middle cerebral artery.
   d. Dominant hemisphere signs (left hemisphere). Global aphasia present but becoming predominantly a motor aphasia over time with comprehension of verbal and written language returning.
3. *Ascending frontal* branch occlusion syndrome.
   a. Contralateral motor paresis or plegia of the face and arm present; leg only mildly affected or unaffected.
   b. Consciousness not lost; most likely client is generally alert.
   c. Dominant hemisphere signs (left hemisphere). Initial mutism found, but rapidly clears with only a minimal speech disturbance remaining.
4. *Middle branches* (Rolandic branches) occlusion syndrome.
   a. Contralateral hemiplegia: face, arm, and leg involved; initially, a flaccid state exists.
   b. Contralateral hemianesthesia: face, arm, and leg involved; primary and cortical sensations lost.
   c. Severe dysarthria.
5. *Ascending parietal and posterior branches* occlusion syndrome.
   a. Intact sensorimotor system.

TABLE 25-12 NEUROLOGICAL FUNCTIONS AND DEFICITS

Function	Deficit
Dominant Hemisphere (Usually Left)	
Language:	Aphasia: impairment or loss of language, that is, the use of symbols.
Auditory comprehension: recognition or interpretation of the spoken word.	Inability to recognize and associate or express words. Word deafness or Wernicke's aphasia.
Written comprehension: interpretation of the written word (reading).	Wernicke's aphasia or alexia (inability to recognize or comprehend words).
Speech: motor aspects of speaking, word formation.	Broca's aphasia; anomia (inability to name objects or persons).
Written language: motor aspects of writing.	Broca's aphasia; agraphia (inability to write).
Cognitive abilities:	
Logical thinking: reasoning ability, decision-making ability.	Inability to think logically, inductively, or deductively; poor decision-making ability.
Analytical skills, judgment.	Poor judgment; poor ability to abstract.
Mathematical skills.	Impaired performance at math calculations.
Verbal intelligence skills.	Poor performance in manipulating verbal tasks and abstract materials and concepts.
Right-left orientation.	Right-left confusion.
Contralateral sensory interpretation and association areas, including vision: ability to recognize objects and to associate objects through one sense, such as identifying a key by feeling it only.	Contralateral loss or impairment of higher cortical sensations, such as astereognosis (inability to recognize objects by touch), contralateral homonymous hemianopsia (loss of the opposite half of visual field).
Contralateral fine motor skills and fine motor movement.	Contralateral hemparesis or hemiplegia.
Nondominant Hemisphere (Usually Right)	
Nonlinguistic auditory functions:	
Memory, association, and interpretation of nonlinguistic auditory stimuli, including tone, pitch, emotional component of speech.	Loss of ability to recognize, associate, or interpret sounds, including music, voice qualities, bells, horns, animal noises, etc.
Music recognition.	Inability to recognize musical pieces, scales, types of instruments, etc.
Visual-spatial perception, including the ability to orient self or others in space, recognition of geometric figures and shapes, recognition of faces and familiar surrounding, ability to comprehend spatial relationships.	Visual-spatial misperception: inability to recognize and associate familiar environments; inability to orient to new environments; inability to recognize and associate faces; decreased ability to perform nonverbal tasks such as drawing; inability to appreciate anything that has a spatial dimension; loss of artistic abilities and appreciation of art; misperception of own body and body parts; inability to orient oneself in space.

TABLE 25-12 *(continued)*

Function	Deficit
Nondominant Hemisphere (Usually Right) *(continued)*	
	Major self-care deficits and safety hazards result from this visual-spatial deficit. Decreased cognitive abilities lead to concrete thinking and markedly reduced ability to make subtle distinctions, such as the difference between fork and spoon.
Contralateral sensory interpretation and association areas including vision.	Contralateral higher cortical sensations are diminished or lost: Agnosia (inability to recognize objects and symbols by means of the senses, that is, hearing, vision, touch, but primary sensation is intact). Auditory agnosia (auditory neglect). Visual agnosia (visual field neglect). Neglect of involved body parts. Denial of disability or loss of abilities. Contralateral homonymous hemianopsia.
Contralateral fine motor movement and fine motor skills.	Contralateral hemiparesis or hemiplegia.
Conceptualization of the motor movement pattern; how to put the idea of the motor act into operation.	Apraxia (inability to perform purposive movement in the absence of paresis, paralysis, ataxia, or sensory dysfunction).

b. Apraxia.
c. Dominant hemisphere signs (left hemisphere). Conductive aphasia. Spontaneous speech is generally not affected but repetition is seriously affected. Responses to questions may be somewhat disturbed.
d. Nondominant hemisphere signs (right hemisphere).
   (1) Misperception of one's body parts and disability in orienting oneself in space.
   (2) Neglect of involved body parts with some denial of disability.

6. *Inferior main division* occlusion syndrome.
   a. Homonymous hemianopsia.
   b. Dominant hemisphere signs (left hemisphere). Wernicke's aphasia: inability to comprehend verbal or written language.
   c. Nondominant hemisphere signs (right hemisphere).
      (1) Loss of ability to recognize, associate, or interpret sounds, including music, voice qualities, bells, horns, and animal or human noises.
      (2) Inability to recognize musical pieces, scales, and types of instruments.
      (3) Auditory neglect.

Diagnostic Tests

1. Computerized axial tomography shows necrotic tissue within a few days and then demonstrates cavitation; detects hemorrhages of 1.5 cm or more in diameter situated in the cerebral or cerebellar hemispheres; localizes hemorrhage with remarkable accuracy. Also demonstrates coexisting hydrocephalus, tumor, cerebral edema, and displacement of tissue.
2. *Lumbar puncture* detects presence of blood in the cerebrospinal fluid and permits analysis of cerebrospinal fluid to detect infection (both acute or chronic) or other possible nonvas-

cular causes for a bleed. Also gives a pressure measurement.

3. *Arteriogram* is the definitive test for detecting thrombosis or vascular narrowing and identifying collateral blood supply. Allows identification and localization of an aneurysm or arteriovenous malformation.
4. *Cerebral blood flow* study gives an estimate of blood flow and thus an assessment of tissue viability.
5. *Electroencephalogram* gives the amount of brain wave activity present.
6. *Radionuclide brain scan* detects tumor, abscess, or other mass lesions. Takes about two weeks to demonstrate the CVA.

NURSING DIAGNOSES: ACTUAL OR POTENTIAL

1. Alteration in tissue/fluid volume within the cranial vault, mild to extreme: due to ischemia, infarction, or bleeding.
2. Altered level of cognitive functioning due to confusion or unresponsive state or later as a dementia.
3. Alteration in cardiac output, mild to severe: secondary to dysfunction of cardiac or blood pressure regulation centers in the brainstem.
4. Alteration in comfort: head and neck pain, mild to severe.
5. Impairment of mobility, mild to complete loss: secondary to motor weakness or paralysis (later possibly spasticity), loss of tactile and visual sensations and ataxia.
6. Alteration in self-care activities due to decreased consciousness, confusional state, and sensory-motor deficit.
7. Sensory-perceptual alteration, mild to complete loss: visual, auditory, or tactile sensory impairment due to ischemia, infarction, or edema.
8. Potential for injury: due to confusional states, motor deficits, sensory impairments, ataxia, or seizure activity.
9. Impairment of written and verbal communication, mild to complete loss: secondary to aphasia, dysarthria, apraxia, etc.
10. Knowledge deficit: lack of knowledge about health status, diagnostic procedures, therapeutic management, and so forth.
11. Anxiety, mild to severe: fear of sensory-motor loss, pain, and confusional states.
12. Impairment of skin integrity: due to immobility, incontinence, and trauma.
13. Respiratory dysfunction: respiratory pattern change due to aspiration secondary to loss of protective reflexes; pulmonary congestion and atelectasis secondary to immobility.
14. Alteration in fluid volume, mild to severe: dehydration, inability to swallow, nausea, and vomiting.
15. Nutritional deficit: decreased food intake, nausea and vomiting, swallowing or chewing difficulties.
16. Impairment of urinary elimination: incontinence due to loss of voluntary and involuntary reflex control in the frontal lobes and immobility.
17. Alteration in patterns of sexuality: secondary to cognitive deficits, impaired sensation, and motor deficits.
18. Role disturbance: due to decreased cognitive functioning or consciousness and sensory-motor deficits.
19. Alteration in bowel elimination: constipation secondary to immobility, dietary change, and dehydration; diarrhea resulting from tube feedings.
20. Social isolation: impaired communication, mobility deficits, urinary and bowel incontinence, and impaired cognitive functioning.
21. Alteration in self-concept: due to agnosia, continued ischemia, and loss of cognitive functioning.
22. Impaired home maintenance management: secondary to motor deficits, cognitive deficits, or sensory deficits.

EXPECTED OUTCOMES

1. The client will maintain or regain normal intracranial pressure, as evidenced by the reduction or absence of signs and symptoms of increased intracranial pressure (e.g., decreased cognition, blunted affect, headache, vomiting) within 24 h to 5 days after treatment begins.
2. The client will be comfortable with head pain controlled within 5 days after initiation of treatment.
3. The client will be seizure-free.
4. The client's vital functions (ventilation, heart rate, blood pressure) will be maintained until the client is able to resume self-maintenance.

5. The client will retain self-care, role function, and socialization patterns as much as possible in light of the severity of the CVA or residual damage.
6. The client will maintain bladder and bowel continence.
7. The client will retain (or regain) a nutritionally well-balanced dietary intake, as evidenced by maintenance of body weight and normal hematocrit and hemoglobin.
8. The client will maintain vascular volume, as evidenced by normal skin turgor, normal serum and urine electrolytes, and urinary output of 50 mL/h.
9. The client will be comfortable, as evidenced by verbal statement.
10. If severe residual damage is present, the family and/or client (if feasible) will make an informed and carefully thought-through decision about the possibility of home management.
11. If recovery is not possible because of the massive bleed or area of infarction, the client with the family will be able to experience a dignified death.

INTERVENTIONS

For CVAs with evidence of significantly increased intracranial pressure, refer to *Intracranial Pressure*.

1. Establish an accurate data base, including laboratory data with ongoing periodic neurological reassessment.
2. Determine the status of the gastrointestinal tract.
3. Institute a pulmonary regimen designed to keep the lungs clear.
4. Maintain the client's fluid balance and nutritional status with IV fluids as ordered until gastrointestinal function returns. Assist the client and family to maintain adequate nutrition and fluid intake.
   a. Feed the client and assist the family to learn to help the client eat from the side where vision is intact.
   b. With facial paresis or paralysis, turn client's head so that the intact motor side is dependent and place food into the side that can be controlled. Soft foods are often managed better than liquids.
   c. Check the weakened/paralyzed side for food after meals and give mouth care.
5. Prevent skin breakdown.
6. Maintain potential for return of motor function.
7. Maintain the urinary tract in the best possible condition if an indwelling Foley catheter is in place.
8. Protect the client from injury due to motor and sensory deficits. (See *Amyotrophic Lateral Sclerosis*, intervention 4b, c, and d, for specific interventions. Also see *Spinal Cord Tumors*, intervention 4a through c, for specific interventions.)
9. Institute a bowel evacuation protocol.
10. Institute a bladder evacuation protocol.
11. Help the client maintain his or her sexuality.
12. Assist the client in communicating.
13. If the stroke is in evolution, place the client at rest in a calm, nonstimulating environment. Initially provide only passive range of motion. (Active exercise is initiated only after the client has stabilized.) Reduce anxiety by providing information, allowing ventilation of feelings, permitting family to remain. Only absolutely necessary diagnostic procedures and assessments should be carried out.
14. If the CVA is a thrombotic or embolic stroke, administer anticoagulants if ordered. Determine prothrombin time and clotting time. Maintain the heparin lock if one is in place. Observe for signs of therapeutic effectiveness and side effects. Teach client and family how to observe for signs of bleeding.
15. If stroke is of thrombotic origin, measures to improve blood supply may be ordered, such as having the client remain horizontal in bed for 7 to 10 days initially. When mobilization begins, have the client avoid standing still for any period of time and have the client elevate legs when sitting up in a chair. Blood pressure is maintained and not previously diagnosed hypertension is not treated immediately (Baratz and Norman, 1979).
16. If it is a hypertensive bleed, administer antihypertensive medications as ordered. Observe for signs of therapeutic effectiveness and side effects. *Watch for signs of ischemia,* that is, increasing neurological deficits that can result from reducing the blood pressure in diseased cerebral vessels to approaching normal.
17. If it is a ruptured or leaking aneurysm or arteriovenous malformation, administer antifibrinolytic medications as ordered. Ob-

serve for therapeutic effectiveness and side effects.

18. If surgery such as *endarterectomy, bypass graft, embolectomy* or *hematoma removal* is possible:
    a. Prepare the client physically and the client and family pyschologically for the surgical procedure.
    b. Carry out postoperative vascular surgery orders.
    c. See *Brain Tumors* for a complete discussion of postoperative care.
19. Assist the client and family to understand and cope with affectual changes.
    a. Control the number of stressors being experienced by the client.
    b. Accept the behavior, disregard emotional outbursts.
    c. Allow client and family to ventilate their feelings.
    d. Reassure client and family that outbursts or uncontrolled emotional displays are due to illness.
    e. Help the family to learn how to explain the client's behavior to others.
    f. Protect the client from loss of dignity.
20. Help the client and family cope with agnosia (inability to recognize significance of stimuli).
    a. Minimize extraneous stimuli, including keeping the environment quiet and decorations and furnishings simple.
    b. Keep the environment well lighted.
    c. Place client in room so that the unaffected side is toward the doorway.
    d. Break tasks into small segments; encourage client to complete one segment at a time.
    e. For *visual agnosia*:
        (1) Approach the client from the unaffected side. Provide care from the unaffected side.
        (2) Place needed items such as bell cord, water, and the like in the unaffected visual field.
        (3) Place food in the unaffected visual field.
    f. For *auditory agnosia*:
        (1) Make certain you have the client's attention.
        (2) Speak slowly and distinctly.
        (3) Check to make certain the client really has understood verbal instructions, information and the like.
        (4) Break the hearing task into small segments.
    g. For *tactile* agnosia:
        (1) Protect the body parts that are ignored when client is carrying out activities.
        (2) Check these body parts when the client has changed position.
        (3) Remind the client to deliberately focus on these body parts.
    h. For *denial of illness*:
        (1) Do not accept the client's estimate of ability. Recognize that the client is not able to fully comprehend degree of disability. Provide for client's safety with assistance and possibly a posey restraint.
        (2) Do not assume this phenomenon is a denial state reflecting a specific stage of adaptation. Do not treat the client for such a denial state.
        (3) Assist family and significant others in understanding the nature of agnosia and how to assist the client with the problem.
21. Nursing interventions to reduce the client's anxiety may be appropriate.
22. Help the client and family to learn to manage the spasticity. (See *Amyotrophic Lateral Sclerosis*, intervention 3a through f, for specific interventions.)
23. Help the client and family eliminate risk factors, such as smoking, obesity, and various stressors.
24. Assist the client and family in obtaining home care services.

EVALUATION

Outcome Criteria

1. The client has normal intracranial pressure.
2. Head pain is lessening; client is seizure-free.
3. Client is injury-free.
4. Client's vital functions remain within normal limits.
5. Client is free of urinary retention and infection.
6. Client remains well nourished and well hydrated.
7. Client maintains (regains) normal bowel pattern.
8. Client regains self-care, role function, and socialization patterns to the greatest possible extent.

9. Client and family make an informed decision about home management.

Complications

1. Diabetes insipidus (see discussion in Chapter 28).
2. Neurogenic pulmonary edema.
3. Hydrocephalus (see discussion under *Adult Hydrocephalus*).
4. Decubiti.
5. Atelectasis/aspiration leading to pneumonia (see discussion in Chapter 31).
6. Constipation and impaction (see discussion in Chapter 33).
7. Dehydration.
8. Malnutrition.
9. Urinary tract infection (see discussion in Chapter 32).
10. Thrombophlebitis (see discussion in Chapter 30).
11. Ankylosis (see Evaluation under *Spinal Cord Injury*, complication 12, for specific discussion).
12. Contractures (see Evaluation under *Spinal Cord Injury*, complication 13, for specific discussion).
13. Osteoporosis (see discussion in Chapter 27).

ADULT HYDROCEPHALUS

Adults can develop a "noncommunicating" type of hydrocephalus when some abnormality causes the obstruction of cerebrospinal fluid flow within the ventricular system. Mass lesions such as tumors, cysts, and abscesses are the most common cause, although hematomas or malformation of the system may cause obstruction. An acute hydrocephalus that develops in as little as 2 h can occasionally be seen in head trauma victims. The presentation is one of rapidly developing intracranial hypertension.

The more frequent type of hydrocephalus seen in adults is a "communicating" type. One form of this is *hydrocephalus ex vacuo* arising from cerebral atrophy. Cerebrospinal fluid (CSF) fills the unoccupied space, and thus there is an increased amount of CSF present. Another form, *normal- (low) pressure hydrocephalus (occult hydrocephalus)*, most commonly occurs in late middle-age clients. As the name implies, the CSF pressure is normal. The cause is thought to be arachnoid adhesions resulting in obstruction of the subarachnoid space, seen frequently as a complication of head trauma or subarachnoid hemorrhage. This type of hydrocephalus typically has a more chronic presentation slowly developing over a period of time.

The client and family complain of client's deteriorating memory and mental capacity. Reports of an unsteady, broad-based gait with a history of falling is not uncommon. Apathy, inattentiveness, and disinterest in self, family and environment are additional manifestations of this problem. Urinary incontinence may complicate the list of problems already noted. Deteriorated mental status is evident on examination and psychomotor retardation is present.

Diagnostic tests such as the CAT scan, pneumoencephalogram, electroencephalogram, and cerebral arteriogram are done to observe vascular and tissue-related brain changes. A radioisotopic cisternogram is done to observe movement of the radioisotopes as they ascend to the subarachnoid space and cerebral convexities. Instead, with this population, the isotopes flow upward into the ventricular system.

Nursing diagnoses center on problems of impaired cognitive functioning, altered affect, impaired mobility, potential for injury, bowel and bladder incontinence, self-care deficits, social isolation, and altered role and relationship patterns.

Interventions (refer to *Dementia*, interventions 1 through 10) include preparing the client and family, through careful teaching, for treatments and procedures to be performed. In addition, the family can be taught to reduce cerebrospinal fluid by seeing that the client takes diuretics as ordered, equalizing the client's increased CSF accumulation.

Major nursing problems focus on impaired cognitive functioning, impaired mobility, increased potential for injury, impaired respiratory functioning, and alteration in role function.

DEGENERATIVE DISEASES

NEURONAL DEGENERATION

DEMENTIA

DESCRIPTION

The term *dementia* denotes a clinical syndrome involving progressive memory impairment and deteriorating intellectual functions. It may also be viewed as a sociopyschosomatic disorder, as many sociopsychological factors play a significant contributory role (Wells, 1971).

In a dementia syndrome, the brain decreases in mass. Its size and weight are reduced. The cortical areas become relatively thin, and the sulci widen and deepen. The ventricles dilate as cerebrospinal fluid (CSF) increases in amount to fill the additional space. The neuronal cells atrophy, and there is a decrease in the number of nerve fibers. Increased gliosis is present.

Dementia may be labeled *senile dementia* if it presents after the age of 60. *Presenile dementia* presents before age 60, with the age of onset as young as 35 or 40 years of age. Causes of presenile dementias include Alzheimer's disease, Pick's disease, Huntington's chorea, chronic alcohol abuse, head trauma, and normal-pressure hydrocephalus. The most common causes of the senile dementias are senile Alzheimer's disease, arteriosclerotic cerebrovascular disease, and long-standing hypertensive vascular disease. (See Table 25-13.)

Of paramount importance related to the presence of a dementing process is correctly diagnosing a *reversible* (*treatable*) *dementia*. Treatable causes for a dementia include infections, such as syphilitic meningoencephalitis, cryptococcosis, and other fungal meningitides; tumors, either primary or metastatic; toxic encephalopathies due to chronic drug intoxication (bar-

TABLE 25-13 DISEASES CAUSING DEMENTIA

Diffuse parenchymatous diseases of the central nervous system:
- So-called presenile dementias:
  - Alzheimer's disease
  - Pick's disease
  - Creutzfeldt-Jacob disease
  - Kraepelin's disease
  - Parkinson-dementia complex of Guam
  - Huntington's chorea
- Senile dementia
- Other degenerative diseases:
  - Hallervorden-Spatz disease
  - Spinocerebellar degenerations
  - Progressive myoclonus epilepsy
  - Progressive supranuclear palsy
  - Parkinson's disease

Metabolic disorders:
- Myxedema
- Disorders of the parathyroid glands
  - Wilson's disease
- Liver disease
- Hypoglycemia
- Remote effects of carcinoma
- Cushing's syndrome
- Uremia

Normal pressure hydrocephalus

Arteriosclerosis

Inflammatory disease of blood vessels

Aortic arch syndrome

Binswanger's disease

Arteriovenous malformations

Hypoxia and anoxia

Deficiency diseases:
- Wernicke-Korsakoff syndrome
- Pellagra
- Marchiafava-Bignami disease
- Vitamin B_{12} deficiency

Toxins and drugs:
- Metals
- Organic compounds
- Carbon monoxide
- Drugs

Brain tumors

Trauma:
- Open and closed head injuries
- Punch-drunk syndrome
- Subdural hematoma
- Heat stroke

Infections:
- Brain abscess
- Bacterial meningitis
- Fungal meningitis
- Progressive multifocal leukoencephalopathy
- Behçet's syndrome
- Kuru
- Lues
- Encephalitis
- Multiple sclerosis
- Muscular dystrophies
- Whipple's disease
- Concentration-camp syndrome

SOURCE: Haase, G. R.: "Diseases Presenting As Dementia," in C. E. Well, *Dementia*, Davis, Philadelphia, 1971, p. 164.

biturates, bromides); nutritional deficiency states, such as Wernicke's encephalopathy, vitamin B_{12} deficiency, or pellagra; metabolic disorders causing encephalopathy; endocrine disorders, such as hypothyroidism, myxedema, or Cushing's disease; and normal-pressure hydrocephalus and chronic subdural hematomas. With early diagnosis and treatment, the signs and symptoms of the dementia can be reversed. Even if some irreversible neuronal damage has been done, the dementia can be arrested and further progression of clinical manifestations can be stopped.

PREVENTION

See Chapter 39, Disruptions of Perceptual and Cognitive Functions.

ASSESSMENT

Health History

1. Lack of initiative, disinterest in work, home, or family; and neglect of routine tasks or hobbies noted by family, friends, or employer.
2. Irritability or apathy complained of by family, friends, coworkers, or employer.
3. Distractibility and inattentiveness.
4. Inability to think through a problem or to think clearly.
5. Recent history of poor judgments, poor decision-making ability, and lack of insight.
6. Change in mood, mood shifts, and emotional lability.
7. Loss of social graces and inattentiveness or indifference to social customs.
8. History of weight loss and poor nutrition.
9. Loss of spontaneity in speech.
10. History of urinary and bowel incontinence.

PHYSICAL ASSESSMENT

1. Deteriorated mental status present on examination.
2. Deteriorating ability to use language.
3. Unkempt, sloppy appearance and dress; evidence of poor personal hygiene.
4. Abnormal reflexes (frontal lobe releasing signs), such as grasp, suck, snout, palmomental, and plantar extensor reflexes.
5. Muscular rigidity (gegenhalten, paratonia) with passive movement.
6. A frontal lobe gait (Brune's ataxia, slipping clutch gait).
7. Bradykinesia, giving movements a slow, deliberate quality.
8. Fairly continuous mouth movements, often of a chewing or licking nature.
9. Varying degrees of flexion suggestive of decorticate posturing in the upper extremities.
10. Propulsion or retropulsion on walking.
11. Dysarthria and dysphagia.
12. Flexion contracturing of the neck, trunk, and legs.

Diagnostic Tests

1. Skull x-ray to demonstrate the presence of a mass lesion by identifying a pineal shift or bony erosion or by visualizing a calcified mass.
2. Chest x-ray to demonstrate a primary lung tumor, infection, or evidence of chronic pulmonary disease.
3. CAT scan to demonstrate the presence of a mass—tumor, cyst, abscess, hematoma (intracerebral or meningeal)—or evidence of ventricular enlargement.
4. Electroencephalogram to demonstrate a focal lesion or diffuse changes characteristic of encephalopathy or degeneration.
5. Lumbar puncture to demonstrate increased pressure and to enable analysis of the CFS to rule out infection, especially chronic infectious processes.
6. Blood studies to rule out electrolyte imbalance, anemia, vitamin deficiency, renal dysfunction, liver dysfunction, thyroid dysfunction, adrenal dysfunction, drug intoxication, and syphilis.
7. Urinalysis to rule out renal and liver disease.
8. Schilling test to rule out impaired vitamin B_{12} absorption.
9. Arteriogram to demonstrate focal lesions and vascular diseases that may be causing ischemia or compression.
10. Pneumoencephalogram or ventriculogram to demonstrate changes in the ventricular system, to localize deep-seated focal lesions, and to demonstrate atrophy of brain structures.
11. Radioisotopic encephalogram (RISA) to demonstrate circulation abnormality regarding CSF, indicative of normal-pressure hydrocephalus.

NURSING DIAGNOSES: ACTUAL OR POTENTIAL

1. Impaired thought processes: due to altered cognitive function.
2. Anxiety, mild to severe: increased fear regarding cognitive ability.
3. Altered affect: due to cortical neuron degeneration or anxiety.
4. Impairment of mobility: secondary to muscular rigidity, bradykinesia, gait ataxia, and apathy.
5. Potential for injury: due to rigidity and bradykinesia, gait ataxia, flexion posturing, and impaired cognitive function.
6. Alterations in self-care activities: due to dementing process, impaired mobility.
7. Role disturbance: secondary to dementing process and changes in communication patterns.
8. Knowledge deficit: regarding health status, diagnostic procedures, therapeutic management, and so forth.
9. Altered urinary pattern: incontinence due to loss of voluntary and reflex control.
10. Nutritional deficit: malnutrition due to client's inability to buy, prepare, and eat food properly.
11. Alteration in bowel elimination: constipation secondary to immobility and dietary changes; incontinence due to loss of social graces and judgment.
12. Social isolation: due to impairment of verbal and written communication.
13. Impaired home maintenance management: secondary to cognitive impairment, impaired mobility, and impaired self-care.
14. Alteration in patterns of sexuality: due to loss of social graces, poor judgment, and impulsiveness.
15. Respiratory dysfunction, pulmonary congestion, and atelectasis: resulting from immobility and muscular rigidity impairing ventilation.
16. Impairment of skin integrity: secondary to immobility and trauma.
17. Maladaptive (individual) coping patterns: secondary to anxiety.
18. Alterations in self-concept: due to dementing process with loss of cognitive function.
19. Alterations in comfort: pain on flexion.
20. Alteration in fluid volume (potential): dehydration due to impaired fluid intake; edema secondary to immobility and hypoproteinemia.

EXPECTED OUTCOMES

1. A nutritionally well-balanced dietary intake will be restored.
2. Discomfort from stiffness will decrease and flexion contractures will be controlled, as evidenced by the absence of complaint of pain and the absence of motor movements.
3. Normal vascular volume will return, as evidenced by normal skin turgor, normal serum electrolytes, and urinary output of 50 mL/h.

INTERVENTIONS

1. Establish an accurate data base with ongoing periodic physical, psychological, and social reassessment.
2. If the client comes into the hospital setting, remember the following (see Table 25-14):
   a. A person with a dementing process involving recent memory decompensates in an unfamiliar surrounding and may be functional in familiar surroundings.
   b. A person with a dementing process involving recent memory often relies on ritualistic patterns that cannot be maintained in a new environment.
   c. An individual with a dementing process is often more vulnerable to disorientation and confusion at night due to decreased sensory stimulation and decreased tissue perfusion.
   d. Help client's family to understand a, b, and c.
3. Assist family in learning how to maximize the client's cognitive functions.
4. To get optimum results from the therapeutic management of this client:
   a. Improve the client's nutritional status.
   b. Improve client's personal hygiene, if it has deteriorated.
   c. Ensure that client's teeth and gums are in good condition.
   d. Ensure that client is getting exercise.
5. Help family to learn how to optimize the client's therapeutic management.
6. If the client's mobility is seriously impaired, help the family to learn to:
   a. Promote skin integrity
   b. Institute a pulmonary regimen designed

TABLE 25-14 APPROACHES TO CLIENTS WITH COMPREHENSION OR EXPRESSION DEFICITS

Comprehension Deficits	Expression Deficits
What may at first appear to be a problem of comprehension may actually be one of inattention. If a client does not attend to you, that person will have difficulty understanding what you say. To keep distractions at a minimum: Remove unnecessary items from the client's visual field so that the client will attend to only the essentials. Turn off the radio or TV. Have only one person talking to the client at a time. If the client does become distracted, call him or her by name repeatedly until attention is regained. It may be necessary to tap the person on the shoulder or to move into his or her visual field. When the client miscomprehends: Do not raise your voice or shout. The client *can* hear you but cannot understand you. Let the client know there was a misunderstanding. Speak slower than you would ordinarily. Repeat and/or reword your message. Accompany your message with gestures and facial expressions. If the client still fails to comprehend, give the correct response and go on to something else. Teach the family and friends about the nature of comprehension deficits and assist them in using the approaches listed above.	Try to anticipate some of the client's needs, and ask about them, for example, "Do you need the ______?" Encourage the client to talk without forcing. Avoid interrupting. Give the client time to speak. Otherwise, he or she may feel pressured and have even greater difficulty speaking. Discuss topics that are of interest and of immediate importance, such as the client's family, job, or feelings. These kinds of topics are sometimes easier for clients to express. If the client has trouble saying a word, have him or her repeat the word after you say an open-ended sentence for the client to fill in, such as, "I want a cup of ______" (coffee), or write the word down for the client to read out loud. If you are not sure what the client is trying to say, try to guess the word. "Do you mean ______?" You may need to try several possibilities before determining the correct word. Determine if the client can retrieve an alternate word. Can the client use gestures instead? Can the client write it? Some clients' ability to speak is extremely limited. Encourage their nonverbal expressions. For example: They can point to things they need or to what hurts them. They can use gestures and facial expressions to express their ideas. A booklet with pictures of commonly used hospital items can be helpful. The client can point to items needed. Once an item is identified, help the client name it and then repeat the word after you. Teach the family and friends about the nature of expressive deficits and assist them in using the approaches given above.

to keep the lungs clear (see *Amyotrophic Lateral Sclerosis*, intervention 6).

c. Institute a bowel evacuation protocol.
d. Maintain adequate nutritional and fluid intake (see *Amyotrophic Lateral Sclerosis*, intervention 5).
e. Protect the client from injury due to motor deficits (see *Amyotrophic Lateral Sclerosis*, intervention 4).
f. Maintain motor function (see *Coma*, intervention 3).
g. Assist the family in learning to prevent dependent edema.

7. Help the family learn means by which they can assist the client to maintain independence in activities of daily living and to maintain home maintenance.
8. In the early stages of a dementing process,

the client may require nursing interventions to reduce anxiety and maladaptive coping patterns. Often these include those activities that deal with a lack of knowledge and those that help to minimize the need for lost capacities and to maintain or maximize retained cognitive functions. (See *Anxiety* in Chapter 36, Anxiety and Affective Disorders, and Chapter 37, Interpersonal Problems of Adults, for specific interventions.)

9. Help the client and family to institute a bladder evacuation protocol if the client is not continent. A toileting schedule should be established with a frequency that is determined by the client's customary voiding pattern.
10. Ensure client comfort.
    a. Prevent contracturing through proper positioning and use of support and splinting devices.
    b. Avoid flexion positioning by having client lie flat in bed with only a small pillow, elevating feet on a stool so knees are not always flexed when sitting, standing up and walking around frequently, and standing up straight when walking.
    c. Provide range-of-motion exercises every 2–4 h to avoid stiffening, pressure, and increased rigidity.
    d. Provide cutaneous stimulation through touch, temperature, and vibration using such measures as backrubs, heat while bathing or showering and apply physiotherapy measures such as ultrasound, diathermy, or dry heat as ordered.
    e. See that the client moves q2h to help avoid stiffening, pressure, and increased rigidity.

EVALUATION

Outcome Criteria

1. Client maintains present cognitive functions, evidenced by increased mobility of sphincter control, coordinated movements, decrease in mood swings, diminished outbursts, and so forth.
2. Client retains (or regains) self-care, role function, and socialization patterns to the greatest possible extent in view of cognitive function, as evidenced by client's report during interview.
3. Normal bowel and bladder patterns are maintained.
4. Nutritional pattern returns to normal as evidenced by adequate fluid balance, weight balance, and normal hemoglobin/hematocrit levels.
5. Increased social interaction is reported.
6. Family makes an informed decision about home management.

Complications

1. Injury (see discussion in appropriate chapter, depending on the nature of the injury).
2. Constipation or impaction or diarrhea (see discussion in Chapter 33).
3. Decubiti.
4. Atelectasis/aspiration leading to pneumonia (see discussion in Chapter 31).
5. Urinary tract infection (see discussion in Chapter 32).
6. Dehydration (see Evaluation under *Amyotrophic Lateral Sclerosis*).
7. Malnutrition (see Evaluation under *Amyotrophic Lateral Sclerosis*).

AMYOTROPHIC LATERAL SCLEROSIS

DESCRIPTION

Amyotrophic lateral sclerosis (ALS) is a progressive degenerative disorder of the motor neurons in the spinal cord, brainstem, and motor cortex. There is actual loss of the anterior horn cells and motor nuclei in the lower brainstem. The onset is during middle age, and the disease is usually fatal within several years. The mode of onset related to clinical manifestations and the pattern of evolution of the signs and symptoms are highly variable. At least five patterns have been described: *brachial-manual amyotrophy* type, *crural* type, *proximal*, or *shoulder girdle*, type, *hemiplegic* type, and *truncal* type. No specific treatment exists for ALS.

PREVENTION

Health Promotion

1. Adequate nutritional intake, especially vitamin E, may decrease susceptibility.
2. Stress reduction strategies may be helpful.
3. Occupational and environmental safety may play a role in reducing the incidence of ALS, although only hypothetical evidence cur-

rently exists linking ALS to trauma or toxic factors.
4. Genetic counseling should be encouraged once ALS is diagnosed.

Population at Risk

1. Incidence rates are higher during fifth and sixth decades, with men affected more than twice as often as women.
2. Higher incidence is noted in individuals engaged in athletic sports and those persons whose occupation entails heavy work, such as farmers and construction workers.
3. Heredity plays a role in about 10 percent of cases of ALS.

Screening

1. At present, screening does not directly alter course of disease.
2. Full health history may be helpful in identifying possible risk factors (diet, trauma, stress) and may provide for early correction, but it may not directly affect ALS.
3. Early recognition does not alter course of ALS but may facilitate genetic counseling.

ASSESSMENT: BRACHIAL-MANUAL AMYOTROPHY TYPE

Health History

1. Complaint of difficulty with or awkwardness at performing fine motor tasks with the fingers, with later involvement of the hands and the arms.
2. Complaint of cramping in the hand muscles.
3. Complaint of twitching of the forearm or upper arm muscles.
4. Complaint of stiffness of the fingers, with later involvement of the hands and arms.
5. Complaint of swallowing difficulties, choking on fluid and foods, and difficulty eating.

Physical Assessment

1. Loss of fine motor movement.
2. Weakness of the finger abductors, adductors, and extensors, and the thumb, followed by weakness in the finger flexors, progressing to weakness of the hands and forearms.
3. Initial wasting of the hand muscles, especially the dorsal interosseous muscles.
4. Generalized hyperreflexia.
5. Slight spasticity of the lower extremities.
6. Coarse fasciculations in the affected muscles.
7. Wasting and weakness of the upper arm muscles and shoulder muscles spreading to the posterior neck muscles.
8. Weakness and atrophy of the tongue muscles.
9. Fibrillation of the tongue muscles.
10. Weakness of the laryngeal muscles.
11. Weakness of the pharyngeal muscles.
12. Weakness and atrophy of the trunk muscles.

Diagnostic Tests

See Assessment: Other Variants, below.

ASSESSMENT: CRURAL TYPE

Health History

1. Complaint of difficulty with walking and with lower extremity movement leading to falls.
2. Complaint of cramping in the foot and leg muscles.
3. Complaint of twitching of the foot and leg muscles.
4. Complaint of stiffness of the feet and later in the legs.

Physical Assessment

1. Weakness of the muscles of the foot progressing to the lower leg and upper leg.
2. Wasting of the foot muscles and later the leg muscles.
3. Generalized spasticity of the lower extremities.
4. Generalized hyperreflexia.
5. Coarse fasciculations in the affected muscles.
6. Intact sensory system.
7. Evidence of spastic weakness and atrophy extending upward to involve the trunk and shoulder muscles.
8. Evidence of the weakness and atrophy involving the muscles innervated by the cranial nerves.

Diagnostic Tests

See Assessment: Other Variants, below.

ASSESSMENT: OTHER VARIANTS

Health History/Physical Assessment

A proximal or shoulder girdle amyotrophy may be demonstrated to be the presenting clinical manifestation. Early involvement of the thoracic, abdominal, and posterior neck muscles is seen as another variant of the disease. A hemiplegic pattern of arm and leg involvement is occasionally observed.

Diagnostic Tests

1. Skull and spine x-rays to demonstrate abnormalities in the bony encasement that may produce clinical manifestations resembling ALS.
2. Lumbar puncture to demonstrate normal pressure and to rule out possible infectious causes that might account for the signs and symptoms.
3. Electromyelogram and nerve conduction studies to demonstrate that nerve conduction is normal but that there is muscular denervation with fibrillation present.
4. Thyroid studies to rule out thyroid dysfunction.
5. Tensilon test to rule out myasthenia gravis.
6. Myelogram to demonstrate the presence of a spinal cord tumor, intraspinal mass, syringomyelia or other spinal cord pathologies.

NURSING DIAGNOSES: ACTUAL OR POTENTIAL

1. Self-care deficit: due to loss of fine motor movement and muscular weakness.
2. Alterations in comfort: due to twitching, cramping, stiffness, and spasticity.
3. Impairment in written communication: due to loss of fine motor movement and muscular weakness in the upper extremities.
4. Role disturbance: inability to perform due to loss of fine motor movement and muscular weakness.
5. Anxiety, mild to severe: due to fear of loss of body function, pain, and/or role disturbance.
6. Potential for injury: secondary to motor deficits.
7. Knowledge deficit: regarding health status, diagnostic procedures, therapeutic management.
8. Impairment of mobility, mild to severe: secondary to motor deficits in lower extremities and later trunk muscles and spasticity.
9. Impaired home maintenance management: secondary to motor deficits when quadriparesis or quadriplegia exists or ventilatory impairment develops.
10. Alteration in patterns of sexuality: due to motor deficits, discomfort, or anxiety.
11. Impairment of verbal communication, mild to severe: due to laryngeal, pharyngeal, and tongue weakness.
12. Nutritional alteration: due to chewing and swallowing difficulties.
13. Respiratory dysfunction: secondary to swallowing difficulties; pulmonary congestion and atelectasis secondary to immobility.
14. Impairment of skin integrity due to immobility and injury.
15. Impairment of urinary function: incontinence due to loss of voluntary control; urinary retention due to incomplete emptying.
16. Alteration in bowel pattern: constipation due to dietary changes and immobility.
17. Social isolation (potential): secondary to muscular weakness, impaired communication, incontinence, and impaired mobility.

EXPECTED OUTCOMES

1. The client will retain self-care, role function, and socialization in light of motor deficits.
2. The client will be comfortable, as evidenced by verbal statements.
3. Family will be able to manage the client at home. (But when the motor paralysis becomes severe, the goal becomes to make an informed and carefully thought-through decision about home management.)
4. The client's skin will remain intact and lungs will remain clear.
5. The client will retain normal bowel and bladder function.
6. When independent ventilation is no longer possible, the goal becomes: The client with his family will be able to experience a dignified death.

INTERVENTIONS

1. Establish a continued, accurate data base.
2. Help client and family assume responsibility for the management of client's neurological deficits.
3. Help the client and family to learn to manage the spasticity by:
   a. Avoiding precipitating factors that make the spasms worse, such as fatigue, chill or shivering, anxiety, staying in one position too long, or urinary tract infection.
   b. Carrying out passive range of motion exercises q2h while client is awake, espe-

cially when the spasticity has become more severe.

c. Using antispasmodic drugs as prescribed by the physician, such as diazepam (Valium), meprobamate (Equanil), baclofen (Lioresal), or sodium dantrolene (Dantrium), while observing for therapeutic effectiveness and side effects.
d. Using prescribed forms of physiotherapy, such as heat therapy or icing procedures to reduce the spasticity.
e. Using splinting devices to prevent contracturing.
f. Preventing skin breakdown through skin care procedures.

4. Protect the client from injury due to motor deficits.
   a. Assist the client and family in learning how to use equipment to aid in ambulation, such as handrails, assistive devices, braces, or other support devices.
   b. Help client and family to control spasticity.
   c. Help client and family to prevent contracture formation.
   d. Assist client and family in preventing choking and aspiration when the client is eating or drinking.
5. Teach client and family to maintain adequate nutrition and fluid intake by:
   a. Sitting up or at least raising the head to help prevent choking.
   b. Taking small bites and eat slowly.
   c. Providing small feedings as they are better tolerated and less fatiguing to the client.
   d. Gradually adjusting the texture and consistency of the food as the client's swallowing and chewing difficulties increase.
   e. Reviewing the dietary changes with a dietitian, nurse, or other health care personnel to check on the nutritional adequacy of the diet.
   f. Avoiding baby food and pureed foods if possible as this usually undermines the client's self-concept and enhances anorexia.
   g. Providing mouth care after eating to make sure that no food that could be aspirated is still in the mouth.
   h. Keeping a record of the fluid intake to make sure the client is taking in sufficient fluid to flush the kidneys in view of the immobility and possibly voiding problems.
6. Assist the client and family in instituting a pulmonary regimen designed to keep the lungs clear.
   a. Maintain ambulation and activities of daily living to the maximum possible extent.
   b. Institute a vigorous coughing and deep breathing exercise program for the client whose thoracic muscles are not involved or are only minimally involved. If the client's thoracic muscles are weak, intermittent positive pressure breathing (IPPB) treatments should be instituted at least four times a day. If the client becomes bedridden in the final stages of ALS, postural drainage with cupping and clapping as well as the IBBP treatments will be necessary. Each of these regimens as appropriate should be taught to the client and family. Assistance of community agencies in getting the IPPB and oxygen equipment may be necessary.
   c. Teach the client and family tracheostomy care and suction techniques.
7. Help the client and family to institute a skin integrity maintenance program.
8. Help the client and family to institute a bowel evacuation protocol to prevent constipation.
9. Maintain the urinary tract in the best possible condition, if an indwelling catheter is in place. (See *Spinal Cord Tumors*, intervention 10.)
10. Institute an upper motor neuron or mixed bladder training protocol, if the urinary function assessment indicates this is appropriate. (See *Spinal Cord Tumors*, intervention 11.)
11. Nursing interventions to reduce anxiety may be appropriate. (See *Anxiety* interventions in Chapter 36, Anxiety and the Affective Disorders.)
12. When the client can no longer survive, help the client and family to support one another. Allow the family time to be together.

EVALUATION

Outcome Criteria

1. Client maintains self-care, role function, and socialization patterns to the greatest possible extent.

2. Client and family are able to provide information about the client's health status, diagnostic procedures, therapeutic management, and hospital policy and procedures.
3. Client remains well nourished and well hydrated, as evidenced by maintenance weight and hemoglobin and hematocrit levels.
4. Skin is intact.
5. Lungs are clear; vital signs are stable.
6. Client is bowel-continent.
7. Client is free of urinary retention and infection.
8. Client and family make an informed decision about home management.
9. Client has a dignified death.

Complications

1. Injury (see discussion in appropriate chapter, depending on the nature of the injury).
2. Decubiti.
3. Atelectasis/aspiration leading to pneumonia (see discussion in Chapter 31).
4. Constipation and impaction or diarrhea (see discussion in Chapter 33).

DEHYDRATION

Assessment

1. Poor skin turgor, sunken eyeballs.
2. Decreased blood pressure, increased pulse.
3. Decreased urinary output with increased specific gravity or urine osmolality.
4. Complaint of thirst.
5. Elevated serum electrolytes, hemoglobin, hematocrit, BUN, and serum creatinine.
6. Elevated plasma osmolality.

Revised Outcomes

Same as Expected Outcomes stated above.

Interventions

1. Replace fluid volume as ordered with IV fluids, forcing oral fluid, or via a nasogastric tube as necessary.
2. If an adequate oral intake of fluid is not possible:
   a. Prepare the family to manage a nasogastric tube at home.
   b. Prepare the client and family for the surgical procedure to establish a gastrostomy feeding system. Teach the family to use the gastrostomy tube for feeding, how to manage the gastrostomy in general at home, and what fluid to use.
3. Assist the family in learning to manage the diarrhea associated with tube feedings.

Reevaluation and Follow-up

1. Reassess the client's fluid volume status.
2. Evaluate the family's management of the feeding tube.
3. Help the family to manage complications.

MALNUTRITION

Assessment

1. Weight loss and atrophy in areas uninvolved by the disease process.
2. Anemia and hypoproteinemia.
3. Signs and symptoms of vitamin deficiency diseases. (See Chapter 33 for discussion.)

Revised Outcomes

Same as Expected Outcomes stated above.

Interventions

1. Replace dietary deficiency with supplements as ordered.
2. If adequate nutrition cannot be maintained orally, see Interventions under complication 6, Dehydration, above.

Reevaluation and Follow-up

1. Reassess the client's nutritional status on a regular basis.
2. Evaluate the family's management of the feeding tube.
3. Assist the family with managing complications.

URINARY TRACT INFECTIONS

See discussion in Chapter 32.

PARKINSON'S DISEASE

DESCRIPTION

Paralysis agitans is a symptom complex that is associated with loss of pigmented dopamine-containing cells in the substantia nigra and other pigmented nuclei. It occurs in 187 per 100,000 persons. There is also some neuronal loss in the sympathetic ganglia, several lower brainstem nuclei, and the basal ganglia. This results in abnormally low concentrations of the neurotransmitter substance dopamine in the basal ganglia. The causes of the disorder are generally unknown, and it is therefore labeled idiopathic paralysis agitans. A parkinsonian syndrome can be manifested following head trauma, CVA, or other injury to the central nervous system; carbon monoxide poisoning; manganese and other metallic poisoning; neurosyphilis and arteriosclerotic cerebrovascular disease. Tranquilizing drugs, especially the phenothiazides, are known for producing a parkinsonian syndrome as a manifestation of intoxication. A postencephalitic parkinsonian syndrome has been associated with the epidemic of von Economo's disease of 1918–1919.

Usually the onset of clinical manifestations is unilateral and insidious. Initial symptoms are usually associated with rigidity. Occasionally tremor is the initial sign.

PREVENTION

Health Promotion

1. Careful monitoring of individuals on those drugs that may produce parkinsonism-like symptoms may prevent drug-induced parkinsonian syndrome.
2. In settings where individuals are exposed to toxic substances, environmental safety programs should emphasize measures to minimize exposure to these toxins.

Population at Risk

1. The onset of parkinsonism usually occurs in individuals between the ages of 40 and 70 with a peak in the sixth decade.
2. Individuals on phenothiazines, reserpines, and butyrophenones may exhibit drug-induced parkinsonian syndrome.
3. Carbon monoxide or manganese poisoning can place individuals at risk to develop parkinsonian-like syndrome.
4. Postencephalic individuals may exhibit a syndrome clinically indistinguishable from Parkinson's disease.
5. Although some authorities claim the incidence is slightly higher in men, others hold that there is probably no sex difference (Hoehm and Yahr, 1967).

Screening

1. During the health assessment, environmental situations and drug use that may precipitate parkinsonism-like symptoms should be elicited and recorded.
2. Observation and self-report of tremor and changes in posture and locomotion should be further evaluated for Parkinson's disease or other syndromes that resemble parkinsonism.

ASSESSMENT

Health History

1. Complaint of slight stiffness and slowness.
2. Immobility or poverty of movement.
3. Aching or cramps in the neck, shoulders, back, and hips.
4. Complaint of fatigue, excessive sweating, and constipation.
5. Stumbling, tripping, and falling.
6. Complaint of freezing episodes.
7. Complaint of faintness, dizziness, or syncope on sitting up or standing.
8. Complaint of depression.
9. History of von Economo's viral encephalitis, CNS trauma, or carbon monoxide poisoning.
10. Current intake of tranquilizers (phenothiazines).

Physical Assessment

1. Coarse, 4 to 6 per second "pill rolling" resting tremors of the thumbs and fingers that disappear with sleep and are aggravated by anxiety and excitement.
2. Arm, jaw, tongue, eyelid, and foot tremors may appear later in the course of the disease.
3. Akinesia (bradykinesia) with poverty and slowness of voluntary movement.
4. Festinating (petitepes) gait: initially a short-stepped gait gradually becoming a shuffle over time.
5. Soft and monotonous voice becoming only a whisper or inaudible over time.
6. Dysarthria.
7. Infrequent swallowing due to akinesia, resulting in drooling.
8. Slowness of chewing, resulting in altered dietary intake.
9. Masked (expressionless) faces with infrequent blinking.
10. Hypertonus in the flexor muscles of the trunk and extremities; characteristic stooped posture (flexion posture).
11. Rigidity with the presence of a cogwheel phenomenon.
12. Impairment of convergence of the eye muscles due to the rigidity.
13. Oculogyric crises (upward and lateral rotation of the eyes).
14. Reduced or absent arm swing.
15. Micrographia (small handwriting).

16. Loss of postural reflexes with frequent loss of balance; propulsion and retropulsion.
17. An inability to inhibit blinking in response to a tap over the bridge of the nose (Meyerson's sign).
18. Normal or near normal muscle power, especially in the large muscles.
19. Sensory changes not present.
20. Seborrhea.
21. Possible orthostatic (postural) hypotension.
22. Depression.

Diagnostic Tests

1. Serum blood studies to rule out endocrine disorders and metabolic or drug intoxication states.
2. Lumbar puncture to demonstrate normal CSF pressure and normal CSF analysis.
3. CAT scan to rule out tumor or other mass lesion, bleeding, or hydrocephalus.

NURSING DIAGNOSES: ACTUAL OR POTENTIAL

1. Impairment of mobility: due to muscular rigidity, bradykinesia, tremor, loss of postural reflexes, and flexion posturing.
2. Self-care deficits: (levels I–IV) secondary to muscular rigidity, bradykinesia, and tremor.
3. Potential for injury: due to loss of postural reflexes, rigidity, tremor, freezing episodes, dizziness or syncope, and visual impairment.
4. Knowledge deficit: regarding health status, diagnostic procedures, etc.
5. Anxiety, mild to severe: due to impaired self-care, embarrassment about tremor, or role disturbance.
6. Nutritional deficit: due to chewing difficulties from rigidity and bradykinesia.
7. Impairment of written communication: due to rigidity, producing micrographia and secondary to tremor.
8. Impairment of verbal communication: soft and monotonous voice due to dysarthria and impaired ventilation.
9. Role disturbance: secondary to rigidity, bradykinesia, impaired mobility, and impaired communication.
10. Alterations in comfort: aching and cramps due to rigidity and flexion contracturing.
11. Alteration in bowel pattern: constipation due to dietary changes, immobility, and drug therapy.
12. Sensory-perceptual alteration, mild to severe: visual impairment.
13. Alterations in self-concept: secondary to the client's movement, mask facies, and general appearance.
14. Impairment of skin integrity: due to excessive sweating, drooling, immobility, or seborrhea.
15. Impairment of urinary pattern: incontinence due to impaired mobility.
16. Respiratory dysfunction: pulmonary congestion and atelectasis secondary to immobility; aspiration secondary to swallowing difficulties; impaired ventilation due to muscular rigidity.
17. Maladaptive (individual) coping patterns: depression due to motor deficits, impaired self-care.
18. Social isolation: due to impaired communication or depression.
19. Alteration in fluid volume: due to excessive sweating or decreased fluid intake.
20. Self-care deficit: impaired mobility; unable to care for self (levels I–IV).
21. Impaired cognitive function: due to drug therapy or a dementing process.

EXPECTED OUTCOMES

1. The client will maintain self-care, role function, and socialization in light of sensory-motor deficits.
2. The client will be comfortable, as evidenced by verbal statement.
3. The client's skin and cornea will remain intact.
4. The client's bowel and bladder will function within limits of functional ability.
5. Family will be able to manage the client at home or secure additional assistance as needed.
6. Normal vascular volume will be maintained, evidenced by normal skin turgor, normal serum and urine electrolytes, and so forth.
7. Cortical functions that are not lost will be maintained to optimal function.
8. The client will increase social interaction with others.
9. Client and family will learn to communicate more effectively.

10. Coping strategies for reducing stress will be more effective.

INTERVENTIONS

1. Teach client and family about the Parkinson's syndrome: its possible causes, clinical manifestations, and therapeutic management.
2. Help client and family to learn to manage Parkinson's syndrome in order to maintain client's self-care, role function, and socialization through:
   a. Using L-dihydroxyphenylalanine (L-dopa) most commonly with the peripheral utilization blocking agent carbidopa (Sinemet); the anticholinergic agents, such as trihexyphenidyl (Artane), benztropine mesylate (Cogentin), cyrimine hydrochloride (Pagitane), procyclidine hydrochloride (Kemadrin) or biperiden (Akineton); the antihistamines, such as diphenhydramine hydrochloride (Benadryl), chlorphenoxamine hydrochloride (Phenoxene) or orphenadrine hydrochloride (Disipal), or amantadine hydrochloride (Symmetrel) as ordered; observing and recording the extent of therapeutic effectiveness and length of time the drug is effective as well as noting the side effects.
   b. Controlling the side effects of the drug therapy by:
      (1) Taking L-dopa with meals to diminish the gastric irritation and nausea.
      (2) Chewing gum and sucking on hard candy to reduce the dryness of the mouth associated with L-dopa and the anticholinergic agents.
      (3) Rising slowly and not standing still; wearing elastic stockings to reduce the orthostatic hypotension caused by L-dopa.
      (4) Instituting a bowel protocol to avoid the constipation associated with L-dopa.
   c. If using L-dopa, avoiding high protein intake, pyridoxine (vitamin B_6) or multivitamin preparations, and large amounts of alcohol, as all these inhibit the effectiveness of the therapy.
3. Protect the client from injury due to the motor deficits by helping the client and family to:
   a. Learn how to use equipment to aid in ambulation, such as handrails, assistive devices, braces, or other support devices.
   b. Prevent contracture formation.
   c. Prevent choking and aspiration when the client is eating or drinking.
   d. Control the tremor through reducing anxiety, learning to induce a state of relaxation, and creating a nonstressful environment.
4. Maintain adequate nutritional and fluid intake. (See *Amyotrophic Lateral Sclerosis*, intervention 5a through h.)
5. Institute a pulmonary regimen designed to keep the lungs clear. (See *Amytrophic Lateral Sclerosis*, intervention 6.)
6. Institute a skin integrity maintenance program.
7. Manage vision problems as well as protect the client from injury due to visual impairment by:
   a. Teaching the client to consciously blink the eyes and to find ways to remember to blink.
   b. Keeping the eyes clean and using wetting agents if the corneas are becoming dry.
   c. Using an eye patch to stop the diplopia.
8. Improve the client's communication ability.
9. Nursing interventions to reduce anxiety may be appropriate. (See *Anxiety* in Chapter 36.)
10. Institute bladder evacuation protocol, if the client is not continent.
11. Reduce the need for lost mental capacities by labeling frequently used items, phone numbers, for example.
12. Nursing interventions to reduce depression are often appropriate with the client suffering from Parkinson's syndrome. (See *Depression* in Chapter 36.)
13. Assist client and family to maintain home care.
   a. Help the client and family gain insight into their own feelings and behaviors as well as the behavior of others.
   b. Encourage participation in structured groups of persons confronted with a similar situation.
   c. Encourage utilization of resources such as local, regional, and national Parkinson's Disease Foundation.

d. Arrange for home health aide when necessary.

EVALUATION

Outcome Criteria

1. Muscle rigidity and bradykinesia decrease with drug therapy; tremor may increase as the rigidity decreases.
2. Client reports taking medication(s) at appropriate times and in correct amounts without undue side effects.
3. Corneas are intact and vision is not compromised.
4. Bowel and bladder pattern is functional; continence is maintained.
5. Vital functions are within normal limits.
6. Fluid balance is normal, as evidenced by electrolyte balance, hydration, and so forth.
7. Client and family report increased understanding of Parkinson's disease.
8. Client's ability to socialize is reported improved.
9. Client is able to verbalize fears and concerns.

Complications

See *Amyotrophic Lateral Sclerosis,* complications Also:

1. Corneal ulceration (see discussion in Chapter 26).
2. Severe depression (see discussion in Chapter 36).

DRUG SIDE EFFECTS

Assessment

1. Chorea (see discussion under general assessment, dystonias and dyskinesias).
2. Athetosis (see discussion under general assessment, dystonias and dyskinesias).
3. Orthostatic hypotension.
4. Psychotic episodes.

Revised Outcomes

1. Side effects will be eliminated or the effects will be minimized.
2. Other outcomes as originally stated under Expected Outcomes, above.

Interventions

1. Reduce the medication dosage as ordered: either administer more frequently in smaller doses or reduce the dosage altogether to control the abnormal motor movements.
2. With psychotic episodes, L-dopa will have to be discontinued as ordered and other medication initiated.
3. Teach client with orthostatic hypotension to sit up and stand up slowly, not to stand still, and to wear elastic support hose; in some cases start client on volume-expanding drugs such as fludrocortisone acetate (Florinef Acetate), as ordered, if there are no contraindications.

Reevaluation and Follow-up

Continue the assessment for side effects and continue to adjust the medication until satisfactory antiparkinson effects and minimal side effects are achieved. This can be a time-consuming process.

MYASTHENIA GRAVIS

DESCRIPTION

This degenerative disorder, characterized by marked striated muscle weakness and muscle fatigability, is the result of a defect in the transmission of nerve impulses at the myoneural junction. Acetylcholine released from the presynaptic terminals is blocked from reaching and binding with the receptor sites on the motor endplate due to sensitized lymphocytes. Thus the muscle cell is not depolarized. The cause of this sensitization is not known. The prevalence rate is estimated to be 1:10,000 to 1:50,000.

The course of the disease is highly variable. With *ocular myasthenia* (more common in men), the muscle weakness is confined to the eye muscles and the prognosis is good. With *generalized myasthenia*, progression may demonstrate periods of remission, a slowly progressive course, a rapidly progressive course, or a fulminating progression. *Bulbar myasthenia* tends to have a very rapid or fulminating progression. The danger of death is greatest in the first year. The second period of danger in progressive courses is from 4 to 7 years after onset of the disease. After this time, the disease tends to stabilize.

Thymic tumors are found in 15 to 20 percent of persons with myasthenia gravis and are more common in older men. There is an increased incidence of other autoimmune disease such as thyrotoxicosis, rheumatoid arthritis, systemic lupus erythematosus, and polymyositis in persons with myasthenia gravis. Ten to fifteen percent of babies born to myasthenic mothers show transitory signs of myasthenia gravis (*neonatal myasthenia*).

PREVENTION

Health Promotion

1. No preventive measures are currently available for myasthenia.
2. Overall health maintenance may slow the onset and progression of myasthenia: specifically, reduction of stress factors, prevention of respiratory infections, cautious use of drugs during anesthesia, and optimum health practices during pregnancy and puerperium.
3. All drugs should be administered with caution and alternate antibiotics used whenever practical, as it has not been determined in which individuals these drugs are likely to cause a myasthenic syndrome.

Population at Risk

1. Under 40 years of age, women are most often affected; after 40 years, sex distribution is equal.
2. Men between 50 and 70 years have an increased incidence of thymomas, whereas nearly all persons over 40 have follicular hyperplasia of the thymus.
3. There is an above average coincidence of thyrotoxicosis, lupus erythematosus, rheumatoid arthritis, and polymyositis in myasthenic individuals.
4. Familial occurrence is rare and generally of a nonimmunological form.
5. Certain drugs unmask undetected myasthenia (lithium, quinidine, propranolol), whereas others actually produce a myasthenic syndrome (some 30 drugs have been identified, including 18 antibiotics, e.g., kanamycin, neomycin, streptomycin).
6. A special form of myasthenia, Eaton-Lambert syndrome, has been associated with oat-cell carcinoma of the lung and carcinomas of the breast, stomach, prostate, and rectum.

Screening

1. At present, screening is not preventive.
2. Evaluation of lifestyle and health habits may uncover avoidable sources of stress or infection.
3. Early detection is helpful to prevent respiratory arrest or other complications.

ASSESSMENT

Health History

1. Excessive fatigue after exercise.
2. Complaint of diplopia.
3. Inability to chew and history of dietary changes.
4. Swallowing difficulties and episodes of choking (frequently with fluid being expelled from the nose and mouth during the choking episode).
5. Complaint of drooling.
6. Complaint of generalized muscle weakness, especially an inability to raise or keep the arms raised.
7. Easy fatigability.
8. Report of increase in strength after resting.
9. History of weight loss.
10. Shortness of breath (air hunger).
11. History of respiratory tract infections.

Physical Assessment

1. Ptosis.
2. Disconjugate gaze and ocular palsies.
3. Weakness of the orbicularis oculi, thus closure of the eye cannot be maintained on testing.
4. A bilateral facial drop and an expressionless facies; weak muscles of mastication.
5. Weak pharyngeal and esophageal muscles.
6. A high-pitched, soft but nasal speech pattern.
7. Dropping of the jaw so that the mouth is open unless pushed closed by the hand.
8. Weakness of the neck and shoulder muscles.
9. Generalized muscle weakness that is more severe in proximal muscles than distal muscles.
10. Weakness of the diaphragm, abdominal, and intercostal muscles.
11. Intact pupillary reflexes.
12. Normal deep tendon reflexes.
13. Intact smooth muscle function.
14. Sensory function normal on examination.

Diagnostic Tests

1. Tensilon test: there is visible improvement in muscle contractility and strength within 30–60 s after client has been given 10 mg Tensilon IV. Diplopia disappears, ptosis improves, the voice becomes stronger and less nasal, and

generalized muscle strength is increased. The person reports subjective improvement as well.

2. Neostigmine test is similar to the Tensilon test, but improvement takes 10–15 min to appear and persists longer (2–3h).
3. Electromyelogram shows rapid reduction in the amplitude of the muscle action potentials evoked on repetitive peripheral nerve stimulation.
4. Other diagnostic tests to detect the presence of another autoimmune disease or a thymoma are done.

NURSING DIAGNOSES: ACTUAL OR POTENTIAL

1. Self-care deficit: due to easy fatigability, muscle weakness, and shortness of breath.
2. Decreased activity tolerance: due to muscle weakness and shortness of breath.
3. Sensory-perceptual alteration, moderate to severe: visual impairment.
4. Nutritional deficit: due to muscle weakness and swallowing difficulties.
5. Impairment of verbal communication: due to swallowing difficulties and muscle weakness of larynx and pharynx.
6. Potential for injury: resulting from visual impairment and muscle weakness.
7. Anxiety, mild to severe: fear of changes that accompany myasthenia gravis, for example, shortness of breath and visual impairment.
8. Knowledge deficit: regarding health status, diagnostic procedures, and so on.
9. Respiratory dysfunction, moderate to severe: impaired ventilation due to respiratory muscle weakness; swallowing difficulties; pulmonary congestion and atelectasis from immobility and impaired ventilation.
10. Impairment of written communication: secondary to muscle weakness.
11. Alteration in patterns of sexuality: secondary to easy fatigability, muscle weakness, and shortness of breath.
12. Alterations in comfort: cramping from drug therapy.
13. Fear of suffocation, mild to severe: due to respiratory muscle weakness.
14. Impairment of skin integrity: due to immobility and trauma.
15. Social isolation: due to impaired mobility, impaired vision, breathing difficulty, and communication problems.
16. Impaired home maintenance management: secondary to weakness and breathing difficulty.
17. Maladaptive (individual) coping patterns: depression secondary to impaired vision, mobility, role function, and self-care.

EXPECTED OUTCOMES

1. Normal vascular volume will be evidenced by normal skin turgor, normal serum and urine electrolytes, and urinary output of 50 mL/h (initial).
2. Client's ventilatory capacity as measured by vital capacity will be greater than 1 L.
3. Urinary continence will be maintained.
4. The client will be comfortable, as evidenced by verbal statements.
5. Family will be able to manage the client at home.
6. Client will comply with therapeutic plan; lifestyle will be maintained within physical limitations.
7. Client and family will experience improved roles and relationships and increased communication.

INTERVENTIONS

1. During administration of the Tensilon test:
   a. Assess the client for bradycardia, a side effect of the drug; have atropine available for administration if the bradycardia is severe.
   b. Atropine is given before the Tensilon to prevent bradycardia, especially in an elderly person.
   c. Protect the client from injury should the bradycardia result in syncope by positioning the client before the test so that a fall cannot take place.
   d. Have bathroom facilities available for the client during the test or following, as the client may also experience an attack of diarrhea from the Tensilon. Protect the client from embarrassment should this occur or should incontinence result.
2. Assist client and family in learning to manage the fatigue and weakness in order to maintain self-care, role function, and socialization through:
   a. Using the anticholinesterase drugs such

as neostigmine (Prostigmine), pyridostigmine bromide (Mestinon and Mestinon timespan capsules), and ambenonium chloride (Mytelase) as ordered, while observing and recording the extent of therapeutic effectiveness and length of time the drug is effective as well as noting the side effects such as slowed pulse, cramping, fasciculations, diarrheal episodes.
   b. Using anticholinergic drugs such as atropine to control the undesirable side effects of the medication.
   c. Establishing a schedule of activity and rest that allows the client to maintain lifestyle, job, role function, and socialization patterns.
   d. Identifing factors that aggravate the weakness and fatigue, such as sleep deprivation, menses or pregnancy in women, or alcohol ingestion.
3. Help the client and family to learn how to manage the vision problems as well as how to protect the client from injury when the diplopia and ptosis are present by:
   a. Establishing rest periods.
   b. Using an eye patch to stop the diplopia and decrease the risk of injury.
   c. Keeping the eyes clean and using wetting agents if the cornea is dry.
   d. If ptosis is a serious problem causing visual impairment, lifting the lids manually or with tape when mobilizing or carrying out an activity.
4. Assist the client and family in maintaining adequate nutrition and fluid intake by:
   a. Scheduling meals and fluid intake shortly after rest periods and awakening in the morning. Breakfast may become the heaviest meal because the client's strength is best at this time.
   b. Also, see *Amyotrophic Lateral Sclerosis*, intervention 5a through h.
5. Help the client and family to institute a pulmonary regimen to keep the lungs clear. (See *Amyotrophic Lateral Sclerosis*, intervention 6a, b, and c.)
6. Help the client and family to institute a skin integrity maintenance program.
7. Assist the client and family in improving the client's communication ability.
   a. Optimize the client's ability to speak.
      (1) Ensure that dentures fit properly.
      (2) Allow rest periods and plan ahead when the client knows he or she would like to be talking at specific times.
   b. Help the client and family to utilize support devices and assistive devices that will improve writing ability.
   c. Provide alternate methods of communication.
8. Aid the client and family with controlling diarrhea and cramping by administering anticholinergic drugs such as diphenoxylate hydrochloride (Lomotil) and atropine sulfate as prescribed.
9. Institute a bowel evacuation program should the client be constipated.
10. Prevent hypoxia and hypercapnia.
    a. Observe for clinical manifestations of increasing ventilatory impairment, especially increasing hypoventilation, decreasing vital capacity, tachycardia, increasing restlessness, and mental dullness.
    b. Measure the client's vital capacity.
    c. If necessary, maintain client on a ventilator until drug regulation is achieved.
11. Nursing interventions to reduce anxiety may be appropriate. (See *Anxiety* in Chapter 36.)
12. Nursing interventions to reduce the client's depression may be appropriate.
13. Assist client and family in learning to prevent dependent edema.
    a. Position the body parts so that they are supported and not dependent.
    b. Provide an active exercise program to improve venous return without producing undue fatigue.
14. Help the client and family to maintain the home care.
    a. Help the client and family gain insight into their own feelings and behaviors as well as the behavior of others.
    b. Encourage the client and family to participate in structured groups of persons confronted with a similar situation.
    c. Encourage the client and family to utilize the resources of the local, regional, and national Myasthenia Gravis Foundation.

EVALUATION

Outcome Criteria

1. Client is compliant with therapeutic plan, as evidenced by increased muscle strength.

(See Evaluation under *Amyotrophic Lateral Sclerosis*, outcome criteria 1 through 9.)
2. Nutritional pattern is reestablished.
3. There is absence of skin breakdown.
4. Corneas remain intact; visual acuity is retained.
5. Bladder and bowel are continent.
6. There is a decrease to absence of pain.
7. Respiratory function is adequate; vital capacity is greater than 2 L.
8. Client verbalizes fears and concerns regarding myasthenia gravis.
9. Client is able to assume activities of daily living at optimal function.
10. Client experiences increased socialization, improved communication, and increased mobility.

Complications

MYASTHENIC CRISIS

Assessment

1. Extreme weakness (quadriparesis to quadriplegia).
2. Respiratory insufficiency.
3. Extreme swallowing difficulties.

Revised Outcomes

Same as originally stated under Expected Outcomes, above.

Interventions

1. Increase dosages of anticholinergic drugs. Usually neostigmine (Prostigmine) given intramuscularly is used.
2. Provide frequent ventilatory assistance.
3. Maintain the client's pulmonary function and nutritional and volume status while the client is unable to take anything orally.
4. Protect the client from hazards of immobility.

Reevaluation and Follow-up

1. Assess the client's motor strength; ventilatory capacity; fluid volume and nutritional status; and skin, bladder, bowel, and musculoskeletal function.
2. Observe for side effects of the medication and intervene as appropriate to decrease them.

CHOLINERGIC CRISIS

Assessment

Looks identical to myasthenic crisis in terms of motor and pulmonary clinical manifestations (see above) but has the following in addition:

1. Increased intestinal motility, often with episodes of diarrhea and complaints of cramping.
2. Presence of fasciculations.
3. Bradycardia.
4. Constricted pupils.
5. Increased salivation. (Although the client with myasthenic crisis may also appear to have this, in that case it is really due to decreased ability to swallow.)
6. Increase sweating.

Revised Outcomes

1. Drug intoxication will be decreased; toxic effects will decrease.
2. Other goals remain the same as those given under Expected Outcomes, above.

Interventions

1. Withhold drugs as ordered until evidence of cholinergic effects decreases.
2. Gradually restart the client on the anticholinergic drugs and regulate dosage to obtain maximum therapeutic effectiveness without toxic side effects.
3. Also see Interventions under Myasthenic Crisis, above.

Reevaluation and Follow-up

See Reevaluation and Follow-up under complication 1, Myasthenic Crisis, above. See Evaluation under *Amyotrophic Lateral Sclerosis*, complications.

HUNTINGTON'S CHOREA

One of the most frequently seen autosomal-dominant hereditary diseases of the nervous system, Huntington's Chorea (adult chorea, chronic progressive chorea) is a relentlessly progressive disorder. The head of the caudate nuclei and putamen are atrophied, as are the frontal and temporal cortical areas. It is postulated that the abnormal movements seen in Huntington's chorea are due to increased response to dopamine by the striatum receptors. Other neurotransmitters such as γ-aminobutyric acid (GABA) and acetylcholine are probably reduced.

The incidence of chorea is reported to be 2.6 to 6.7 per 100,000 persons. The disease has been found in all races. Both men and women are affected. The usual age of onset is the 40 to 60 age bracket, although occasionally the onset is in adolescence or even childhood.

Mental and mood disturbances ranging from emotional disorders to psychotic behaviors are a predominant feature of the disease. Abnormal choreic movements, at first slight in nature and then becoming progressively worse, may begin at the same time as the mental disturbances or may occur years later. Deterioration of cognitive function eventually appears.

There is no known treatment. Drugs are used to control the motor and mental clinical manifestations. Chronic alcoholism and suicide are common among persons suffering from Huntington's chorea. Nursing diagnoses and interventions center on impaired thought processes, role disturbance, potential for injury, impairment of mobility, impairment of skin integrity, and anxiety.

DYSKINESIAS

Dyskinesias are intermittent, arrhythmic involuntary spasms or continuous spasms that may involve one or more muscle groups (see Table 25-15). If the muscular contractions are frequent and prolonged, pain accompanies the spasm. Dyskinesias worsen under stress and lessen with relaxation and quiet. The dyskinesias generally worsen with time. Facial-cervical and cervical dyskinesias include blepharoclonus and blepharospasm, spastic dysphonia, spastic dysarthria, lingual spasms, facial spasms, spasmodic torticollis, cervicothoracic spasms, and tardive (postphenothiazine) dyskinesia.

Little response to drug therapy is seen. In mild cases, sectioning the muscle or nerve supply may help. Biofeedback is currently being used with some degree of success in certain individuals.

MYELIN DEGENERATION

MULTIPLE SCLEROSIS

DESCRIPTION

Multiple (disseminated) sclerosis, which affects 500,000 persons in the United States today, is a progressive degenerative disease that involves damage to the myelin sheath and thus to the conductive pathway of the central nervous system. It is characterized by episodes of focal deficits that may cuase dysfunction in the optic nerve, spinal cord, and brain interspersed with periods of remission. Onset of the signs and symptoms may be sudden, that is, fully developed in a matter of minutes or hours. In some persons, signs and symptoms may develop more slowly over a day or several days. In still others the clinical manifestations develop over several weeks to months.

Initially the demyelinization is temporary. The location and extent of the demyelinization is variable, but certain clinical syndromes are observed quite frequently. The mixed or generalized type of multiple sclerosis involves signs of optic nerve, brainstem, cerebellar, and spinal cord involvement. A predominant spinal cord form of the disease with ataxia resulting from sensory changes may be seen. A cerebellar or pontobulbar-cerebellar form is occasionally found, as is an amaurotic form.

The rate of progression may be subacute, acute, or fulminating. The time interval between the initial symptoms and the first relapse is highly variable. The relapse generally occurs either within 1 year, 2 years, 5 to 9 years, or 10 to 30 years. Some persons have a steady progressive course, usually resulting in a spastic paraparesis.

As the disease progresses there is usually damage in all areas of the central nervous system. The duration of the disease is equally variable. Some persons die within several months to a few years, but most individuals live an average of over 20 years. Also, a benign form of the disease has been known to exist in some individuals.

Factors associated with the onset of initial symptoms or an exacerbation include infection, vaccination, trauma, fatigue, cold or hot weather, menses, stress and pregnancy, specifically the stress of labor and increased fatigue associated with the postpartal period.

The treatment of multiple sclerosis is supportive in nature—drugs to reduce the signs and symptoms, physiotherapy, rehabilitation, diet and counseling.

PREVENTION

Health Promotion

1. Because the cause is unknown, prevention is not yet available.
2. Promotion of health and wellness in high-risk populations may reduce the incidence of the precipitating factors and might indirectly reduce the incidence of multiple sclerosis.

TABLE 25–15 INVOLUNTARY MOVEMENT DISORDERS

Type	Pattern of Movement	Rhythm	Distribution	Rate	Amplitude	Onset	Duration	Occurrence
Chorea[a] (choreiform movement)	May be simple or elaborate; purposeless, discrete, forcible, jerking movement; if chorea is violent and flailing, it is called *ballismus*	No rhythmicity	Widespread; varies among persons and in the same person; may be limited to one side (hemichorea)	Rapid	Coarse	Sudden	Short	In both awake and sleep states; associated with hypoton
Atheotsis[a] (athetoid movement)	Purposeless, slow, wormlike, sinuous movements that tend to flow into one another; alteration between extension-pronation and flexion-supination of the arm, eversion-inversion of the foot, retraction-pursing of the lips, and twisting of the neck	No rhythmicity	Most pronounced in the digits and hands; may involve face, tongue and throat, foot	Slower than chorea	Coarse		Continuous	Awake state Associated with varying degrees of motor deficits
Dystonia[a] (e.g., torsion spasm, spasmodic torticollis)	Persistent attitude in one or the other extremes of athetoid movement (overextension, overflexion); writhing, bizarre twisting movement of large body parts producing grotesque posturing that is undulant and sinuous in character	No rhythmicity	Disproportionate involvement of large axial muscles (trunk and limb girdles) *Localized Dystonias* Facial-Cervical Dyskinesias 1. Spasm—facial muscles, jaw muscles, lingual muscles 2. Torticollis—trapezius muscle, sternocleidomastoid muscle	Slow	Coarse		Long-sustained	
Myoclonus	Isolated, shocklike muscle contractions	Irregular rhythm	Especially in limbs, also may involve face and oral cavity Asymmetric distribution	Faster than chorea	Irregular	Abrupt	Short-lived	Irregular
Tic (habit spasms)	Recurrent, inappropriate, stereotyped compulsive	No rhythmicity	Involves a small segment of the body	Variable	Variable	Sudden	Brief	Awake state

[a] Distinction often blurs between chorea, athetosis, and dystonia. May see various movement disorders in the same person.

Population at Risk

1. Multiple sclerosis occurs in adults between the ages of 20 and 40 and affects slightly more women than men.
2. The incidence of multiple sclerosis is significantly lower in equatorial areas of the world than in the more temperate (less than 1 per 100,000) and northern latitudes (30 to 80 per 100,000). In addition, individuals who migrate from a high-incidence area to a low-incidence area after the age of 15 years carry the higher risk of developing multiple sclerosis.
3. A familial tendency toward multiple sclerosis has been ascertained, although the exact genetic pattern is yet unknown.
4. The onset of multiple sclerosis is often triggered by a recent episode of fatigue, physical or emotional stress, infection, or trauma.

Screening

1. No specific tests.
2. Populations at risk should be identified through health history and precipitating factors should be reduced if possible.

ASSESSMENT

Health History

1. Fatigue and lack of energy, frequently of weeks to months duration.
2. History of weight loss.
3. Vague muscle and joint pains, frequently of weeks or month duration.
4. Complaint of weakness, often involving the lower extremities.
5. Heaviness, numbness, tingling in the extremities and bandlike sensations around the trunk or extremities.
6. Complaint of foot dragging.
7. Complaint of poor control of one or both legs (ataxia).
8. History of retrobulbar neuritis.
9. Vertigo.
10. Complaint of urinary hesitancy, urgency, frequency, and incontinence.
11. History of impotence in the male.
12. Dull, aching pain in the lower back.
13. Decline in motor function after exposure to heat, such as after a hot shower or bath or after sunbathing (Ulthoff's phenomenon).
14. Declining cognitive function.
15. Apathy or inattentiveness.
16. Depression and slurred speech.
17. History of seizure disorder (late sign).

Physical Assessment

1. Hyperactive deep tendon reflexes.
2. Absence of abdominal reflexes.
3. Plantar extensor reflexes (Babinski reflexes).
4. A tingling, electriclike feeling down the back and, less commonly, down the anterior thighs (Lhermitte's electric sign) induced by passive flexion of the neck.
5. A central scotoma.
6. A visual field deficit.
7. Papillitis on serial fundiscopic examinations.
8. Diplopia, nystagmus, and ophthalmoplegia.
9. Unsteady gait (gait ataxia) with intention tremor of the arms and legs.
10. Scanning speech.
11. Instability of the head and trunk.
12. Incoordination of voluntary movements.
13. Paresis or paralysis, often a spastic paresis or paralysis.
14. Diminished or lost sensations, particularly position sense and vibration sense.
15. Diminished or lost higher cortical sensations.
16. Paraplegia or quadriplegia.
17. Painful sustained spasms.
18. Emotional lability.
19. Impaired memory function.
20. Evidence of a spastic bladder.

Diagnostic Tests

The diagnosis is a diagnosis of exclusion. When all other causes have been ruled out and it can be documented that the lesions have been multiple, occurring at different places in the nervous system and at different times, the diagnosis of multiple sclerosis is made.

1. Skull x-rays to rule out pineal shifts indicative of a mass lesion.
2. CAT scan to rule out defintively a mass lesion of any kind; also to demonstrate any cerebral atrophy.
3. Lumbar puncture to measure CSF pressure and to analyze CSF. Abnormally elevated IgG ratio, elevated or normal protein, and oligoclonal bands on electrophoresis are characteristic of multiple sclerosis.
4. Visual evoked responses (VER), auditory brainstem evoked responses, and somatosensory evoked responses are being used to demonstrate delayed or lost peaks. Such findings are often present when the client is asymp-

tomatic and are suggestive of demyelinating disease.

NURSING DIAGNOSES: ACTUAL OR POTENTIAL

1. Sensory-perceptual deficits: visual impairment, visual paresthesias, and diminished or lost deep or superficial sensations.
2. Alteration in comfort, mild to severe: due to muscle and joint spasms and contractures.
3. Impaired mobility: due to motor deficits, ataxia, pain, or contracture formation.
4. Potential for injury: due to vertigo, visual impairment, ataxia, tremor, motor deficits, or sensory impairment.
5. Self-care deficits due to visual impairment, motor deficits, tremor, or pain.
6. Decreased activity tolerance: due to fatigue and impaired motor activity.
7. Role disturbance: secondary to fatigue, motor deficits, vertigo, impaired vision, impaired communication, incontinence, and altered sexual patterns.
8. Impairment of verbal communication: secondary to motor deficits.
9. Impaired communication: verbal/written due to motor deficits, visual impairment, and tremor.
10. Urinary pattern disturbance: incontinence and/or retention due to spasticity.
11. Knowledge deficit: lack of knowledge about health status, therapeutic management, and so forth.
12. Alteration in patterns of sexuality: due to fatigue, motor deficits, impaired sensation, impotence, or depression.
13. Impaired cognitive functioning: due to cortical neuron loss.
14. Alteration in bowel pattern: incontinence and/or constipation.
15. Impairment of skin integrity: due to impaired sensory perception, immobility, incontinence.
16. Respiratory dysfunction: swallowing difficulties or muscular weakness of respiratory muscles.
17. Maladaptive (individual) coping patterns: depression secondary to self-care deficits, role disturbances, impaired mobility.
18. Impaired home maintenance management: severe motor deficits, severe spasticity and contracturing.
19. Anxiety, mild to moderate: due to fear of the potential health problems.

EXPECTED OUTCOMES

1. The client will be comfortable, as evidenced by verbal statements, decreased spasticity, and decreased pain.
2. Anxiety will decrease, verbalization of fears and concerns will increase.
3. Client and family will verbalize knowledge of the health problem and its course.
4. Bowel and bladder patterns will return to normal, as evidenced by urine and bowel continence, absence of urine retention and infection.
5. Client will verbalize compliance with the therapeutic plan.
6. Nutritional status will improve.
7. Client will maintain cognitive functions that are currently intact.
8. The client's family will be able to manage the client at home.

INTERVENTIONS

1. Protect the client from further damage to the nerve(s) and area innervated by the nerve(s). (See *Landry-Guillain-Barré Syndrome*, intervention 3a through e.)
2. Help the client and family to learn how to manage the vision problems as well as to protect the client from injury due to visual field deficits, diplopia and palsies. (See *Parkinson's Disease*.)
3. Protect the client from injury due to motor deficits. (See *Amyotrophic Lateral Sclerosis*, intervention 4a, b, and c.)
4. Assist the client and family in learning to protect the client from injury due to impaired tactile sensations. (See *Spinal Cord Tumors*, intervention 4a through c.)
5. Maintain motor function. (See *Coma*, intervention 3a through g.) In addition, provide a range of motion exercise program carried out q2h to prevent contracturing and loss of joint function. *The client should not be actively exercised while the acute process is still going on.*
6. Teach client and family about multiple sclerosis: pathology, precipitating factors of an exacerbation, clinical manifestations, and therapeutic management.
7. Assist the client and family in learning to manage the spasticity.

8. Help the client to gain control over the pain.
9. Assist client and family in instituting a skin integrity maintenance program.
10. Help client and family to institute a bowel evacuation protocol to prevent constipation.
11. Help client and family to institute a pulmonary regime designed to keep lungs clear.
12. Maintain the urinary tract in the best possible condition if an indwelling catheter is in place.
13. Institute an upper motor neuron or mixed bladder training protocol if the urinary function assessment indicates this is appropriate.
14. Reduce the need for the lost mental capacities.
15. Maintain and maximize use of the remaining cognitive capacities.
16. Nursing interventions to reduce depression, dependent behavior, and anxiety may be appropriate.
17. Help the client and family to maintain the home care.
    a. Help the client and family gain insight into feelings and behaviors.
    b. Encourage the client and family to participate in structured groups of persons confronted with a similar situation.
    c. Encourage the client and family to utilize the resources of the local, regional, and national Multiple Sclerosis Society.

EVALUATION

Outcome Criteria

1. See *Amyotrophic Lateral Sclerosis*, Outcome Criteria. In addition:
2. The client is continent.

Complications

1. Paraplegia (see *Spinal Cord Injury* for specific discussion).
2. Quadriplegia (see *Spinal Cord Injury* for specific discussion).
3. Severe depression (see discussion in Chapter 36).

SEVERE SPASTICITY OR SPASMS

Assessment

Spasticity has become so severe that activities of daily living are being seriously interfered with at this point.

Revised Outcomes

Same as those originally stated under Expected Outcomes, above.

Interventions

1. Continue measures previously described under managing spasticity, *Amyotrophic Lateral Sclerosis*, intervention 3.
2. Prepare the client physically and the client and family psychologically for administration of chemical blocking agents such as alcohol or phenol intrathecally or directly into a peripheral nerve.
3. Prepare the client physically and the client and family psychologically for surgical or radiofrequency ablative procedures such as tenotomy, myotomy, peripheral neurectomy, or rhizotomy.

Reevaluation and Follow-up

Rehabilitation and retraining to deal with the ablative nature of the procedures and the residual effects.

PERIPHERAL OR CRANIAL NERVE DEGENERATION

DESCRIPTION

In a *mononeuropathy* (mononeuritis), one peripheral or one cranial nerve is affected. The motor, sensory, or reflex changes are confined to the distrbution of one nerve. Generally trauma, compression, invasion of the nerve by a tumor, and damage by systemic disease or toxins are the cause of injury. Varying degrees of paresis and paralysis, with resultant atrophy, may occur. The sensory disturbances may include paresthesias, a pain syndrome, and decreased or lost primary sensations. Reflexes and reflex-mediated functions may be diminished or lost.

Several individual nerves may be affected in a random manner. This is referred to as *mononeuropathy multiplex* (mononeuritis multiplex). The motor, sensory, or reflex changes are confined to the distributions of the affected nerves. Mononeuropathy multiplex is seen in diabetes mellitus, polyarteritis nodosa, leprosy, and occasionally sarcoid. As with mononeuropathies, varying degrees of paresis and paralysis with resultant atrophy may occur. The sensory disturbances, reflex, and reflex-mediated changes are the same as with a mononeuropathy.

When many nerves are affected or the pattern is not that of a single nerve distribution but a stocking-glove distribution, the syndrome is referred to as a *polyneuropathy* (polyneuritis). Polyneuropathies may manifest as syndromes of an acute ascending motor paralysis, a subacute symmetrical or asymmetrical sensory-motor syndrome, and a chronic sensory-motor syndrome. Some genetically determined polyneuropathies exist. In the polyneuropathies several distinct pathological processes are recognized. These are not disease-specific and may exist simultaneously in any one polyneuropathy. In *Wallerian degeneration*, the axis cylinder and myelin distal to the site of axonal interruption degenerate. In *segmental degeneration*, the axon is spared and just the myelin degenerates. In *axonal degeneration*, there is distal degeneration of myelin and axis cylinder as a result of neuronal disease.

SPINAL CORD DEGENERATION

SYRINGOMYELIA

Syringomyelia is a progressive degenerative disorder of the spinal cord characterized by the development of gliosis and central cavitation of the cervical cord. Although its origin is not clearly determined, it is thought to result from imperfect closure of the neural tube. Persistent embryonic rests bring about glial cell proliferation in the central portion of the spinal cord around the central canal. Disturbed hydrodynamics of cerebrospinal fluid is felt to be an important pathogenetic factor (Adams and Victor, 1977). The gliosis and cavitation may extend upward into the medulla oblongata (syringobulbia) or downward into the thoracic and possibly lumbar segments. The central gray matter of the cervical cord is usually affected first, interrupting the pain and temperature fibers crossing in the anterior commissure. Then the posterior and anterior horn becomes involved, and lastly the lateral and posterior tracts are affected.

Symptoms often appear in early adulthood (the 20 to 30 age group). After an initial rapid onset, the disease progression becomes slow and irregular. Clinical features of the disease include initial loss of pain and temperature sensations with touch and deep pressure perserved, wasting of the small hand muscles, and sometime wasting and weakness of the shoulder girdle muscles. Vasomotor and trophic changes in the upper extremities may be seen. A thoracic kyphoscoliosis is characteristically found. The sensory changes predispose the client to burns, injuries, ulcerations, infections, and Charcot's joints. As a result of long motor tract damage, spasticity and ataxia of the lower extremities and disturbed bladder function may appear.

Treatment consists of laminectomy to open the spinal canal and decompression via various techniques, such as needle aspiration or ventriculosubarachnoid shunt (Adams and Victor, 1977). Nursing diagnoses and interventions center on assisting the client to manage the sensory-perceptual alterations, alterations in comfort, impairment of mobility, potential for injury, and alteration in self-care activities.

CERVICAL SPONDYLOSIS

DESCRIPTION

Cervical spondylosis is a slowly and intermittently progressive degenerative disease of the spine, predominantly involving the lower cervical vertebrae. The spinal canal and intervertebral foramina are narrowed, and there is progressive compressive and traumatic injury to the spinal cord, roots, or both. The spinal cord moves over protruding osteophytes. Extruded disc material (often partly calcified) and meningeal thickening may also contribute to the compression. The most characteristic syndrome involves a painful stiff neck, brachialgia, and spastic weakness with ataxia of the lower extremities.

PREVENTION

Health Promotion

1. Avoidance of lifting heavy objects.
2. Proper lifting of heavy items.
3. Exercises to strengthen body musculature and overall mobility.
4. Avoidance of accidents.

Population at Risk

1. Persons working in occupations where lifting heavy objects is routine or where accidental injury may occur (e.g., police).
2. Persons with limited knowledge of good body mechanics.
3. Persons with a history of spinal trauma (e.g., persons involved in automobile accidents).

Screening

1. X-rays may reveal changes in bone structures.
2. Physical examination.

ASSESSMENT

Health History

1. Painful, stiff neck.
2. Pain radiating to an area above the scapula.
3. Stabbing pain in the pre- or postaxial border of the extremity extending to the elbow, wrist, and fingers.
4. Persistent dull ache in the forearm or wrist, sometimes with burning.
5. Paresthesias in one or two digits, in a portion of the palm, or in a longitudinal band along the forearm, and on the soles of the feet and around the ankles.
6. Clumsiness of the hand(s), weakness of the hand(s).
7. Complaint of unsteady gait and history of falling.
8. A feeling of stiffness and heaviness of the leg.
9. Complaint of altered sphincter control (hesitancy or precipitancy of micturition).

Physical Assessment

1. Restriction of lateral flexion and rotation of the neck.
2. Crepitus in the neck.
3. Changes in the deep tendon reflexes.
4. Weakness of the hand, forearm, or leg muscles.
5. Atrophy of the hand and forearm muscles.
6. Sensory impairment particularly related to pain and temperature sensations in the arms.
7. Impairment of vibration, position, and touch sensations in the legs.
8. Plantar extensor reflexes (Babinski reflexes).
9. Gait ataxia.
10. Spasticity in lower extremities.

Diagnostic Tests

1. Cervical spine x-rays to demonstrate degenerative changes in the cervical vertebrae.
2. Lumbar puncture to demonstrate normal cerebrospinal fluid pressure and normal cerebrospinal fliud analysis.
3. Serum blood studies to demonstrate normal blood studies to rule out metabolic or endocrine problems.
4. Nerve conduction study to demonstrate a disturbed conduction that is suggestive of root or cord entrapment.
5. Myelography to demonstrate conclusively the cord or root compression in the cervical cord.

NURSING DIAGNOSES: ACTUAL OR POTENTIAL

1. Alterations in comfort: due to pain; spasticity in the lower extremities; paresthesias.
2. Sensory-perceptual deficit: impaired cutaneous sensations in the hand(s) and deep sensations in the legs.
3. Self-care deficit: incoordination, spasticity, paresthesias, or pain.
4. Potential for injury: secondary to sensory impairment, gait ataxia, weakness, or spasticity.
5. Decreased activity tolerance: secondary to gait ataxia and spasticity.
6. Alteration in urinary elimination: hesitancy, urgency, or incontinence.
7. Anxiety, mild to severe: due to pain and paresthesias, impaired mobility and body image changes, impaired sensation, or altered sexuality patterns.
8. Knowledge deficit: Lack of knowledge about health status, diagnostic procedures, and so on.
9. Alteration in patterns of sexuality: due to pain, incontinence, impaired sensations, spasticity, or weakness.
10. Alteration in bowel pattern: constipation due to pain, medication, and immobility.
11. Maladaptive (individual) coping patterns: due to chronic pain and paresthesias.
12. Role disturbance: secondary to pain and paresthesias, ataxia, incontinence, muscular weakness, or altered sexuality patterns.

EXPECTED OUTCOMES

1. The client will be in control of discomfort, as evidenced by verbal statements.
2. The client will maintain self-care and role function in light of impaired sensation, motor weakness, or incoordination.
3. Client roles and relationships will give evidence of improved interaction.
4. Anxiety and fears will be relieved: client will cope effectively.
5. Client will report compliance with therapeutic plan.

INTERVENTIONS

1. Help client gain control over pain.
2. Help the client and family learn how to protect the client from injury due to impaired tactile sensations.
3. Assist the client and family in learning to manage the spasticity.
4. Protect the client from injury due to motor deficits.
5. Administer drugs as ordered to decrease spasticity to help control incontinence.
6. Assist client in learning signs of a full bladder—sweating, restlessness, and abdominal discomfort—if perception of bladder fullness is diminished.
7. Direct treatment at restricting the anterior-posterior movements of the neck by a cervical collar.
8. Posterior decompressive laminectomy with dendate ligament severance may help to prevent further injury.
9. Removal of localized osteophytic overgrowth through an anterior approach is also employed at times.

EVALUATION

Outcome Criteria

See *Amyotrophic Lateral Sclerosis,* Outcome Criteria 1 through 8.

Complications

1. Constipation or impaction (see discussion in Chapter 33).
2. Urinary tract infection (see discussion in Chapter 32).

VASCULAR DEGENERATION

SUBARACHNOID HEMORRHAGE

DESCRIPTION

In a subarachnoid hemorrhage, blood escapes from a blood vessel into the subarachnoid space. Prodromal signs associated with aneurysms, arteriovenous malformations (AVMs), and hypertension may occur days to weeks before the subarachnoid hemorrhage and may include episodic headache and transitory unilateral weakness, numbness and tingling, or speech disturbance. These are believed to be caused by leakage of blood from the vessel. Frank subarachnoid hemorrhage due to an aneurysm or AVM is often associated with activity and exertion.

Death may occur within minutes to a couple of days in a large bleed. With a small bleed, consciousness may be regained within a few minutes or not lost at all. A confusional state with headache and neck stiffness, however, persists for days. If the hemorrhage is completely confined to the subararachnoid space, there are no lateralizing neurological signs.

Subarachnoid hemorrhages tend to recur. A rebleed is the greatest cause of mortality. Twenty-five to 40 percent of persons surviving the initial bleed suffer a second bleed within the first 4 weeks. This second bleed carries a greater than 40 percent mortality rate. The rebleed most commonly occurs between the third and eleventh days after the first bleed, with the greatest incidence on day 7.

Vasospasm is another serious complication after a bleed. Thirty to 40 percent of the clients with a subarachnoid hemorrhage experience vasospasms during the first 2 weeks after the rupture but not during the first 24 h. The peak time of occurrence is 5 to 6 days after the bleed. These vasospasms may persist for several weeks. Often the vasospasm is in adjacent arteries rather than in vessel that bled. Vasospasms result in ischemia and can cause an infarction. Deterioration in consciousness, hemiparesis, and visual disturbances may be observed.

Treatment for a subarachnoid hemorrhage is aimed at controlling increased intracranial pressure and preventing ischemia and hypoxia, preventing a rebleed, preventing vasospasms, and eventually correcting the primary problem.

PREVENTION

Health Promotion

1. Health promotion cannot prevent aneurysms and is instead focused on minimizing risk of rupture. Hypertension, arteriosclerosis, and atherosclerotic processes, and trauma should be reduced, controlled, or prevented whenever possible (see other sections on health promotion for each risk factor).
2. Malformations may be reduced through genetic counseling and adequate nutrition during gestation.
3. Other factors causing subarachnoid hemor-

rhage, if apparent, should be promptly treated; in the case of trauma, safety factors may be preventive if instituted prophylactically.

Population at Risk

1. Aneurysms occur most often between 35 to 65 years of age, with a peak between 40 to 50 years (berry aneurysm). Women are affected more than men (3:2).
2. An increased incidence of aneurysms is seen in persons with congenital polycystic disease and coarctation of the aorta.
3. Fusiform aneurysms are seen in elderly persons; mycotic aneurysms, seen in younger individuals, occur following sepsis.
4. Arteriovenous malformations are congenital, with symptom onset usually between 10 and 30 years of age. They are more common in males than females.
5. History of trauma, brain tumor, CNS infection, and various blood dyscrasias increases the incidence in other forms of subarachnoid hemorrhage.

Screening

1. Routine physical exam and health history may uncover factors that seem to contribute to aneurysm rupture.
2. Screening may uncover unilateral vision impairment or cranial nerve palsies (IIId and VIth) resulting from compression of aneurysm before rupture.
3. Arteriovenous malformations often include a history of chronic headache and may include focal seizures before hemorrhage. A bruit may be present over eyeball, mastoid, or carotid artery. Consequently, early detection may be possible to prevent hemorrhage, but current treatment options are generally not indicated in clinically silent AVMs. The investigation of low-dose focused proton beams offers future hope in preventing hemorrhage from diagnosed AVMs.
4. Most screening for subarachnoid hemorrhage is aimed at early detection to ensure prompt treatment and prevent complications.
5. Screening for trauma, tumor, and infection are discussed elsewhere.

ASSESSMENT

Health History

1. History of hypertension.
2. Family history of aneurysms or AVMs.
3. Report of head trauma.
4. Report of prodromal signs: episodic headache often associated with exertion, visual disturbances, seizure activity, mental status changes, transitory unilateral weakness, numbness, or speech disturbance.
5. Complaint of a sudden, excruciating, generalized head pain with photophobia and neck stiffness.

Physical Assessment

1. Decreased consciousness.
2. Evidence of irritability and restlessness.
3. Nuchal rigidity and increased tone in the neck muscles.
4. Projectile vomiting.
5. Positive Kernig's sign.
6. Positive Brudzinski's sign.
7. Fever up to 39°C (common during the first week after a bleed).
8. Bilateral extensor plantar (Babinski) reflexes may be present early.

Diagnostic Tests

1. CAT scan to detect a localized blood clot within the brain, ventricular system, or subarachnoid space; also to rule out other possible causes such as brain tumor.
2. Lumbar puncture may reveal grossly bloody CSF. Cerebrospinal fluid pressure is markedly elevated. WBC count may be increased and CSF protein is elevated. Glucose may be low.
3. Arteriogram for definitive diagnostic test to demonstrate an aneurysm or AVM.

NURSING DIAGNOSES: ACTUAL OR POTENTIAL

1. Ineffective cognitive perception; mild to deep: due to altered levels of consciousness.
2. Fluid volume excess within the cranial vault (increased intracranial pressure), mild to extreme.
3. Alterations in comfort, moderate to severe: headache and neck stiffness causing muscle spasm.
4. Sensory-perceptual deficits, moderate to severe: due to visual impairment.
5. Potential for injury: secondary to seizure activity, confusional state, dehydration, or decreased consciousness.
6. Fluid volume deficit due to vomiting and fever.

7. Nutritional deficit: due to decreased food intake, anorexia, and loss of consciousness.
8. Anxiety, mild to severe: secondary to head pain, confusional state, visual impairment; fear of diagnostic procedures and therapeutic management.
9. Knowledge deficit: limited information about health status, diagnostic procedures, and so on.
10. Self-care deficit: due to decreased consciousness, pain, and visual impairment.
11. Impairment of skin integrity: resulting from dehydration, diaphoresis, and immobility.
12. Respiratory dysfunction: aspiration secondary to loss of protective reflexes with deep coma; pulmonary congestion and atelectasis due to immobility and sedation.
13. Alteration in urinary pattern: incontinence due to loss of voluntary control.
14. Impairment of bowel function: constipation due to dehydration and immobility: incontinence due to loss of voluntary control; diarrhea.
15. Impaired home management maintenance: resulting from residual brain damage and sensory-motor deficits.

EXPECTED OUTCOMES

1. Intracranial pressure will return to normal, as evidenced by the reduction or absence of signs and symptoms of increased intracranial pressure and meningeal irritation.
2. Normal level of consciousness will return, with sensory-motor intactness.
3. Client will be comfortable with both head pain and vomiting moderately controlled within 72 h after the initial bleeding episode (initial).
4. The client will be seizure-free.
5. The client will maintain a slightly decreased vascular volume, as evidence by slightly decreased skin turgor and serum electrolytes that suggest a slight volume depletion (initial).
6. Vital functions (ventilation, heart rate, blood pressure) will be maintained until the client is able to resume own maintenance of vital functions.
7. The client will be comfortable, as evidenced by verbal statements.
8. The client will retain (or regain) bowel and bladder continence.
9. The client's nutritional patterns will return to normal.

INTERVENTIONS

1. See *Increased Intracranial Pressure*, for specific interventions associated with a subarachnoid hemorrhage.
2. Maintain strict bed rest with a controlled, quiet environment.
   a. Place client in a private room that is kept dim, blinds drawn. Minimize artificial lighting.
   b. Complete care is provided by the nursing staff.
   c. Eliminate all unessential external stimuli, such as television, radio, and so forth.
   d. Limit visitors to one or two immediate family members or primary significant others for short periods of time.
   e. Modify d. above if the client's anxiety can be reduced by doing so, except allow one family member to remain with the client.
   f. Administer sedatives as ordered. Record therapeutic effectiveness.
3. Maintain client comfort.
   a. Administer analgesics and antiemetics as ordered. Observe, record, and report therapeutic effectiveness and side effects.
   b. Use positioning, massage, and heat to help reduce neck muscle spasms.
   c. Dim lights to reduce the discomfort from photophobia.
4. Prepare the client physically and the client (if possible) and family psychologically for the diagnostic procedures necessary to determine the cause of the bleed.
5. Assist the client (if possible) and family in learning about the client's health status and therapeutic management.
6. Administer aminocaproic acid (Amicar) as prescribed. Observe, record, and report therapeutic effectiveness and side effects.
7. See *Coma*, interventions 1 through 6, for other specific interventions associated with a subarachnoid hemorrhage.
8. If surgery is indicated for a vascular abnormality, see postoperative care under *Brain Tumors*.
9. If hypertension is the cause, see discussion in Chapter 26 and administer antihypertensive medications as ordered. Observe, record, and report therapeutic effectiveness and side effects.

EVALUATION

Outcome Criteria

1. The client has normal intracranial pressure.
2. The client reports increased comfort, as evidenced by lessening of head pain and absence of neck pain.
3. Client's vital functions remain within normal limits, as evidenced by laboratory blood values (e.g., PO_2, PCO_2) within normal limits. Pulse and blood pressure are within normal limits.
4. Client is seizure-free.
5. During the acute phase, client is slightly volume depleted, with normal blood volume returning.
6. Client and family are able to provide accurate information about the client's health status, diagnostic procedures, and so on.
7. Client is bowel and bladder continent.
8. The client is able to gradually engage in sensory motor activities with little impairment.
9. The client's nutritional status has returned to normal, as evidenced by weight within normal limits by charts, and self-report.
10. The client's sleep-rest patterns have returned to normal now that consciousness is returning to pretrauma state.

Complications

1. Rebleed.
2. Brain herniation (see complication 3 under *Increased Intracranial Pressure*).
3. Arrhythmia (see discussion in Chapter 30).
4. Hypotension (see discussion in Chapter 30).
5. Seizure.
6. Atelectasis/aspiration leading to pneumonia (see discussion in Chapter 31).
7. Decubiti.
8. Constipation and impaction (see discussion in Chapter 33).
9. Adult hydrocephalus (see discussion under *Adult Hydrocephalus*).

VASOSPASM

Develops in 35 to 40 percent of persons who have suffered a subarachnoid hemorrhage; peak time is 5 to 6 days after initial bleed; spasms frequently occur in an adjacent vessel and may spread to involve more distant blood vessels.

Assessment

1. Deteriorating level of consciousness.
2. Appearance of a hemiparesis.
3. Presence of a visual disturbance.
4. Seizure activity.

Revised Outcomes

Outcomes are the same as those previously stated under Expected Outcomes, above.

Interventions

1. No widely accepted treatment exists.
2. Administer medications as prescribed: some physicians use papaverine hydrochloride, some order an aminophylline-isoproterenol regimen, and still others recommend and use a prophylactic serotonin antagonist such as reserpine. Observe and record therapeutic effectiveness.

Reevaluation and Follow-up

Ischemia leading to infarction may occur. Unchecked vasospasm may be life-threatening. With permanent damage, an ischemic stroke situation develops (see discussion under *Cerebrovascular Accidents*). If death becomes a real possibility, measures related to death and dying to assist the family are appropriate.

TRAUMATIC INJURIES

BLUNT (CLOSED) HEAD TRAUMA

The most frequently encountered form of head injury is that of minor head trauma that results when the head is struck by a rapidly moving blunt object or the head strikes a hard surface. The person may never lose consciousness, but such blunt trauma often may induce at least a temporary loss of consciousness. Following such an injury, the person may evidence:

1. A delayed traumatic collapse (vasomotor syncopal episode).
2. Immediate drowsiness, headache, and confusion.
3. Immediate traumatic paraplegia (associated with trauma to the top of the head) or blindness (associated with injury to the occiput), thought to be due to a direct, localized concussive effect.
4. Delayed hemiplegia or coma due to a dis-

secting internal or common carotid artery aneurysm, mural thrombus in the carotid that has embolized, acute epidural or subdural hematoma, intracerebral hemorrhage, or cerebral venous thrombosis.

A concussive state (concussion) may have been suffered if the initial period of unconsciousness was less than 5 min and mental clarity returned rapidly. When hours to days pass without the person's fully regaining consciousness, there is almost certainly cerebral bruising (contusion), lacerations, subarachnoid hemorrhage, or scattered intracerebral hemorrhages at the point of injury (coup injury), along the line of force of the injury, and on the opposite side (contrecoup injury). There would also be edema around the injured tissues (see Figure 25–9). In such cases of severe closed head injury, three types of outcomes may be seen:

1. Cerebral damage and other bodily injuries may not be compatible with life.
2. Improvement begins within a few days with eventual recovery although persistent residua may be present.
3. A permanent unresponsive state persists.

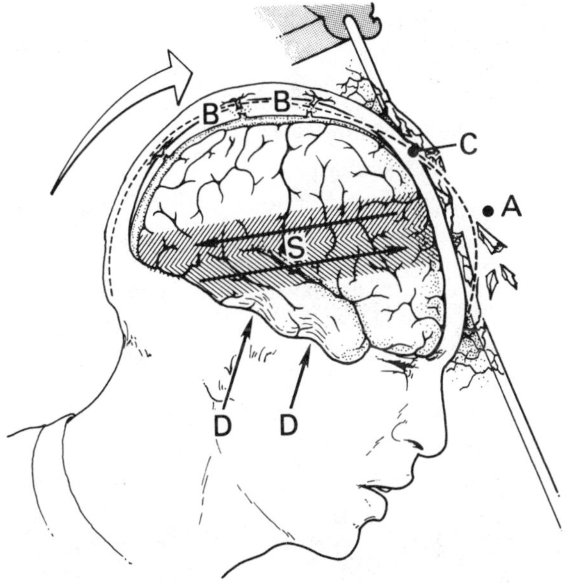

Figure 25-9 Closed blunt injury of head. Skull molding occurs at site of impact. (A) Stippled line: preinjury contour. (C) Contour moments after impact with inbending at point A and outbending at vertex. (B) Subdural veins torn as brain rotates forward. (S) Shearing strains throughout brain. (D) Direct trauma to inferior temporal and frontal lobes over floors of middle and anterior fossa. (Eliasson, S. G., Prensky, A. L., and Hardin, Jr., W. B.: *Neurological Pathophysiology*, Oxford University Press, New York, 1974, p. 293.)

The effects of contusion, hemorrhage, and brain swelling are believed to be worst about 18–36 h after the injury. Beyond 36 h, the risk of dying from the craniocerebral trauma is markedly reduced.

In other cases, persons who have had head trauma, although initially unconscious, regain consciousness shortly after the injury and appear to be recovering well. Surgical intervention, however, soon becomes necessary. Conditions requiring such intervention include:

1. *Acute epidural hemorrhage*: associated with temporal-parietal fractures, the middle meningeal artery is lacerated or a venous sinus is torn open.
2. *Acute or subacute subdural hematoma*: the bridging veins are torn.
3. *Chronic subdural hematoma*: may result from minor head trauma, especially in the elderly or debilitated, malnourished individual.
4. *Subdural hygromas*: the arachnoid is torn and blood and CSF collect in the subdural space.
5. *Acute contusional swelling*: after initial unconsciousness, the client improves but then relapses into an unresponsive state.
6. *Traumatic cerebral hemorrhage*: acute, massive intracerebral hemorrhage may develop as late as a week after moderate to severe head injury; especially seen in the elderly.

OPEN HEAD TRAUMA

DESCRIPTION

In open head trauma, there is a break in (or penetration of) the dura, exposing the cranial vault's content to the environment. A compound or perforating fracture must occur to produce an open head injury.

Open head injury frequently results from penetrating wounds caused by missiles (usually bullets) that are traveling at high velocities, cranial wounds from missiles may be of three types:

1. Tangential injuries involving scalp lacerations, depressed skull fracture(s), and meningeal and cerebral lacerations.
2. Penetrating injuries with impacting material and other debris driven into the brain tissue.
3. Through-and-through wounds (Baratz and Norman, 1979).

Most individuals who have sustained a penetrating head injury do not maintain consciousness. The depth of coma depends on the location and extent of tissue damage and bleeding and the degree of brain edema. If the lower brainstem is penetrated, death occurs immediately due to respiratory and cardiac failure. If vital centers are intact, the threat to life comes from bleeding and swelling that cause intracranial hypertension. With through-and-through injuries, 80 percent of individuals die within a short period of time.

With an open head injury, surgical intervention is normally required and aims at:

1. Debridement to prevent infection, and
2. Removal of blood clots to help reduce intracranial hypertension.

Also, broad spectrum antibiotics are administered along with osmotic diuretics and other dehydrating agents and corticosteroids.

PREVENTION

See Prevention under *Spinal Cord Injury*.

ASSESSMENT: MILD HEAD TRAUMA

This category includes nonconcussive and mild concussive injuries.

Health History

1. Description of the injuring event by the client or observers.
2. History of no loss of consciousness, brief loss of consciousness (less than 5 min), "seeing stars," "being stunned," or confused.
3. Complaint of an initial confusional state that cleared rapidly (within minutes to a few hours).
4. Retrograde pretrauma amnesia.
5. Head pain.
6. Complaint of nervousness.
7. Complaint of "not being oneself."

Physical Assessment

Normal neurological examination is found by the time the person is seen by a health care professional.

Diagnostic Tests

See Assessment: Severe Head Trauma, below

ASSESSMENT: MODERATE HEAD TRAUMA

This category includes severe concussive injuries or contusions.

Health History

1. Description of the injuring event by the client or observers.
2. History of a more prolonged loss of consciousness (greater than 5 min) and, on regining consciousness, persistence of the confusional state (for hours to days).
3. Presence of a retrograde pretrauma amnesia.
4. Head pain.
5. Complaint of nervousness by the client or family.
6. Complaint of "not being oneself."
7. Complaints of nausea, fatigue.

Physical Assessment

1. An unresponsive state (stupor or coma).
2. A motor paresis or paralysis.
3. Cranial nerve palsy (palsies).
4. Signs of intracranial hypertension.
5. Stable vital signs, including temperature.
6. Protective cranial nerve reflexes generally intact.
7. Possible appearance of seizure disorder.

Diagnostic Tests

See Assessment: Severe Head Trauma, below.

ASSESSMENT: SEVERE HEAD TRAUMA

This category includes severe contusion, laceration, and necrosis.

Health History

1. History of a prolonged coma state.
2. Description of injuring event from an observer.
3. History of seizures since the trauma occurred.

Physical Assessment

1. An assessment of the injury site.
2. A state of unresponsiveness (stupor, more likely coma).

3. Signs of severe intracranial hypertension.
4. Increased muscular tone and possible posturing.
5. Motor paresis or paralysis.
6. Cranial nerve palsy (palsies).
7. Poor prognostic signs:
   a. Variable findings related to vital signs, including those evidencing shock.
   b. Signs of brainstem failure with absence of cranial nerve reflexes.
   c. Subnormal temperature.
   d. Flaccidity (hypotonia).
8. Signs that may manifest with the regaining of consciousness:
   a. Aphasia.
   b. A sensory impairment, either primary or cortical.
   c. Acute confusional state.

Diagnostic Tests

1. Skull and cervical x-rays to demonstrate a skull or neck fracture.
2. CAT scan to demonstrate intracerebral or extracerebral bleeds as well as ventricular shift.
3. Echoencephalogram to demonstrate a midline shift indicative of brain tissue shifting.
4. Lumbar puncture may demonstrate increased CSF pressure and presence of blood in the CSF, indicating contusion, laceration, subarachnoid or intracerebral bleed.
5. Electroencephalogram to demonstrate areas of increased or decreased brain wave activity as well as absence of brain wave activity in some instances.
6. Radioisotopic encephalogram (brain scan) to demonstrate an intracerebral or meningeal bleed.

NURSING DIAGNOSES: ACTUAL OR POTENTIAL

1. Altered level of congitive functioning; manifested as an unresponsive state: inability to carry out functions of daily living.
2. Fluid volume excessive within the cranial vault: increased confusion, sleep onset, depressed vital functions.
3. Alterations in comfort, mild to severe: head pain.
4. Anxiety, mild to severe: secondary to pain, confusional state, and circumstances of injury.
5. Increased potential for injury: due to seizure activity, confusional state, motor weakness, and sensory impairment.
6. Impairment of skin integrity: due to trauma or secondary to immobility.
7. Decreased activity tolerance: due to motor deficits, ataxia, or sensory impairment.
8. Self-care deficit, mild to complete loss: secondary to decreased consciousness, motor deficits, ataxia, or impaired sensation.
9. Sensory-perceptual alteration: mild to complete loss of olfactory, visual, auditory, or tactile sensory impairment.
10. Social isolation: due to impairment of verbal or written communication, mild to complete loss.
11. Nutritional deficit, mild to severe: due to nausea and vomiting, swallowing, or chewing difficulty.
12. Respiratory dysfunction: respiratory pattern change due to cerebral edema or increased intracranial pressure; aspiration secondary to loss of protective reflexes; pulmonary congestion and atelectasis secondary to immobility.
13. Alteration in cardiac output, mild to severe: secondary to dysfunction of the cardiac or blood pressure regulation centers in the brainstem.
14. Alteration in roles and relationships: due to hospitalization, decreased consciousness, motor deficits, or sensory impairment.
15. Alteration in urinary elimination pattern: incontinence or retention.
16. Knowledge deficit: due to loss of memory or lack of information about health status, therapeutic management, and so on.
17. Alteration in patterns of sexuality: due to impaired sensation, motor deficits, and incontinence.
18. Alteration in bowel patterns, mild to severe: constipation or diarrhea.
19. Impaired home maintenance management: secondary to decreased cognitive function or decreased consciousness.

EXPECTED OUTCOMES

1. The client will maintain or regain normal intracranial pressure, as evidenced by the reduction or absence of signs and symptoms of increased intracranial pressure within 36 h to 5 days after treatment.
2. Client will be comfortable with head pain

controlled within 5 days after initiation of measures to reduce increased intracranial pressure and cerebral edema.
3. There will be an absence of seizures within 24–48 h after initiation of therapy.
4. Skin integrity will be maintained and will remain intact.
5. Self-care activities, role function, and socialization patterns will be regained, as possible, in light of the severity of the head trauma and/or residual effects.
6. Family and/or client will provide correct information about the client's health status, diagnostic procedures, therapeutic management, and hospital policy and procedures with accuracy.
7. The client's vital functions (ventilation, heart rate, blood pressure) will be maintained until the client is able to resume own maintenance of vital functions, as evidenced by a *normal for the client* Po_2, Pco_2, pulse rate, and blood pressure, or the client will maintain own normal vital signs (if the head trauma is mild).
8. When possible, client will verbalize to the nurse or family fears and concerns about the trauma.
9. If the client has only mild head trauma and is conscious, the client will maintain bladder and bowel continence.
10. Nutritional status will be maintained.
11. If severe residual damage is present, the family and/or client (if feasible) will make an informed and carefully thought-through decision about the possibility of home management.
12. If recovery is not possible because the head trauma was massive, the client and family will experience the client's peaceful and dignified death.

INTERVENTIONS

1. See Interventions under *Increased Intracranial Pressure*. Also:
2. Establish a continued, accurate data base, including ongoing periodic neurological reassessment.
3. Determine the status of the gastrointestinal tract.
   a. Listen for bowel sounds to determine the presence of an ileus.
   b. Maintain the client NPO as ordered until bowel sounds resume.
   c. Maintain gastrointestinal suction to prevent distention and aspiration of vomitus until gastrointestinal motility returns.
4. Maintain the client's fluid balance and nutritional status with IV fluids as ordered until gastrointestinal function returns. *The client with increased intracranial pressure is kept slightly volume depleted.*
5. Prepare the client and family for diagnostic procedures.
6. Prepare the client and family for therapeutic neurosurgical procedures that are necessary to treat bleeds or open head trauma.
7. Assist the client in gaining control over head pain by providing comfort measures such as backrubs and controlling the external environment. Use pain medications only with alert clients and then use only mild analgesics.
8. Promote the control of infection with a basilar skull fracture or other open head injury.
9. Promote the reestablishment of skin integrity without the occurrence of a secondary infection.
   a. Avoid scratching or additional trauma to the affected area.
   b. Wash the skin with mild soap and water and dry thoroughly.
   c. Treat the injury as ordered and apply appropriate dressing as ordered.
   d. Avoid exposure to extremes of temperature in the involved area.
   e. Visually check the involved area for signs of infection.
   f. If surgery has been required and the postoperative head dressing is in place, the neurosurgeon may order no skin care but observation of the dressings and reinforcement should the outside dressing become moist. (See Interventions under *Coma*.)
10. Nursing interventions to reduce anxiety may be appropriate. (See *Anxiety* in Chapter 36.)
11. As the client recovers, the following interventions may become appropriate.
   a. Assist the client and family to maintain adequate nutrition and fluid intake. If taste or smell is diminished or lost, institute measures to enhance food flavors or visual appeal.
   b. With the other health-related professionals, help the client and family assume re-

sponsibility for the management of recovery and residual deficits (if any are present).

c. Help the client and family to learn how to manage the vision problems as well as how to protect the client from injury due to visual impairment.
d. Assist the client and family learning to protect the client from injury due to impaired tactile sensation.
e. Institute an upper motor neuron or mixed bladder training protocol, if appropriate.
f. If there are residual deficits, provide the information, time, and support that the client and family need to realistically make a decision about home management.

EVALUATION

Outcome Criteria

Client's vital functions remain within normal limits.

Complications

ARRHYTHMIA

See discussion in Chapter 30.

HYPOTENSION

See discussion in Chapter 30.

POSTCONCUSSION HEADACHE

Assessment

1. Headache may be initially severe but gradually decreases; may be dull and aching in quality, throbbing or pressurelike.
2. Pain may be paroxysmal in nature, occurring especially with excitement or concentration.
3. Dizziness or vertigo may be present.

Revised outcomes

The client will be in control of head pain.

Interventions

1. Reassure the client that the pain will eventually go away but that takes time and there is nothing seriously wrong.
2. Help the client adjust lifestyle to avoid enhancement of head pain.
3. Assist the client in establishing a medication regimen to aid control of head pain.

Reevaluation and Follow-up

Pain usually disappears within a few weeks but may last 6 months to a year. Reassurance and empathy are of key importance throughout this period of persisting head pain.

POSTTRAUMATIC SYNDROME

Most commonly seen with severe head injuries, especially those injuries where amnesia lasts longer than 24 h:

Assessment

1. Irritability.
2. Unexplainable restlessness.
3. Insomnia.
4. Frequent depression.
5. Apathy.
6. Unexplained euphoria.
7. Loss of social restraint.
8. Marked memory defects.
9. Intellectual defects.
10. Hyperhidrosis.
11. Marked vasomotor instability.

Revised Outcomes

Outcomes are the same as originally stated under Expected Outcomes, above.

Interventions

1. Assist the client and family in establishing an individualized medication regimen of aspirin, antihistamines, phenobarbital, and so on, as prescribed.
2. Help the client and family to verbalize fears and to understand that the client is not losing his or her mind.
3. Emphasize that the clinical manifestations will eventually resolve and that the client is not mentally (psychiatrically) or permanently impaired.
4. Assist the client to resume normal activities as rapidly as possible.

Reevaluation and Follow-up

Ongoing reassurance and empathy is important until the clinical manifestations gradually abate.

POSTTRAUMA SEIZURE DISORDER

Three to 6 percent of persons with nonpenetrating injury develop seizures, whereas 30 to 50 percent of persons with penetrating injuries develop a seizure disorder. Most often the seizures are major motor (generalized) seizures. Seizures are classified according to onset.

1. Early: occurring in the first week.
2. Late: occurring after the first week, the seizure appears and persists. Seizures may develop years after the injury, but the most common time length is 6 to 8 months post injury.

See the discussion under *Seizure Disorders*, earlier in this chapter.

ARTERIOVENOUS ANEURYSM

There is an connection often due to laceration of the internal carotid in the cavernous sinus. There will be an audible bruit, exopthalomos, distended orbital and periorbital veins, extra ocular muscle paresis or paralysis, especially of the lateral rectus muscles (innervated by the VIth cranial nerve). (See the discussion under *Brain Abscess*.)

BRAIN ABSCESS

Usually presents several weeks to months after the head injury as a recurrent meningitis phenomenon. (See discussion under *Brain Abscess*.)

HYDROCEPHALUS

See discussion under *Adult Hydrocephalus*.

POSTTRAUMATIC PERSONALITY DISORDER

See discussion under *Brain Tumors*.

DIABETES INSIPIDUS

See discussion in Chapter 28.

NEUROGENIC PULMONARY EDEMA

See discussion under *Brain Tumors*.

MENINGITIS

See discussion under *Meningitis*.

THROMBOPHLEBITIS

See discussion in Chapter 30.

ATELECTASIS/ASPIRATION LEADING TO PNEUMONIA

See discussion in Chapter 31.

DECUBITI

CORNEAL ULCERATIONS

See discussion in Chapter 26.

URINARY TRACT INFECTION

See discussion in Chapter 32.

CONSTIPATION AND IMPACTION

See discussion in Chapter 33.

CRANIAL NERVE INJURY

DESCRIPTION

Cranial nerves that are especially likely to be traumatically injured are the Ist cranial nerve (the olfactory nerve), IId cranial nerve (the optic nerve), IIId cranial nerve (oculomotor nerve), IVth cranial nerve (trochlear nerve), the first and second divisions of the Vth cranial nerve (trigeminal nerve), VIth cranial nerve (abducens nerve), VIIth cranial nerve (facial nerve), and the VIIIth cranial nerve (vestibular nerve). Damage to the Ist cranial nerve frequently follows when a head injury involving a blow the the occiput causes a contrecoup injury to the nerve or when the trauma results in a basilar skull fracture. This damage often leads to a permanent deficit. Basilar skull fractures and facial fractures may lacerate the cranial nerves IId, IIId, IVth, and VIth cranial nerves. Fractures of the petrous bone may cause damage to the VIIIth cranial nerve. Improvement in hearing occurs in a number of persons with traumatic injury of the VIIIth cranial nerve. Injury to the VIIth cranial nerve is often associated with injury to the VIIIth cranial nerve. The facial nerve (VIIIth) as well as the first and second divisions of the trigeminal nerve (Vth) may be directly injured by a basilar skull fracture or temporal bone fracture. Also, because of the superficial location of the branches, the facial nerve and the trigeminal nerve are frequently injured by stab wounds, cuts, and gunshot wounds. The onset of motor or sensory deficits is usually immediate, although occasionally the onset of the deficit is delayed.

PREVENTION

Health Promotion

Prevention of head injury, especially facial and cranial fractures and severe deceleration impacts, which can cause contrecoup and tearing of the cranial nerve filaments.

1. Use of auto seat and shoulder belts.
2. Avoidance of falls by adherence to general safety precautions.
3. Use of protective headgear for high-impact sports such as boxing, motorcycling, skateboard riding.

Population at Risk

1. Persons with head injuries, especially if a fracture is present.
2. Persons with lacerations, gunshot wounds, and other zygomatic or preauricular tissue damage (facial nerve).

ASSESSMENT

Health History

1. History of a head injury.
2. Complaint of loss of taste and smell.
3. Complaint of blurred or lost vision or diplopia.
4. Numbness and paresthesia over the skin area innervated by the first and second divisions of the trigeminal nerve.
5. Complaint of loss of hearing; vertigo.

Physical Assessment

1. Anosmia.
2. A dilated pupil that is unreactive to direct light but has an intact consensual response; pupils may be dilated and fixed.
3. A pale optic disc; blindness.
4. Internal and vertical movement of the eye may be lost.
5. Sensation on the face may be diminished or lost; facial weakness.
6. Nystagmus.
7. Neurosensory deafness.

Diagnostic Tests

1. Skull x-rays to demonstrate a skull or facial fracture.
2. Radioisotopic cisternogram to demonstrate a basilar skull fracture.
3. Electromyelogram to demonstrate denervation in the affected muscles.
4. Nerve conduction studies to identify decreased conduction time in affected nerves.

NURSING DIAGNOSES: ACTUAL OR POTENTIAL

1. Sensory-perceptual deficit: diminished or lost smell, hearing, facial sensations, and/or visual impairment.
2. Alterations in comfort, mild to severe: facial pain.
3. Potential for injury: secondary to vertigo and visual impairment.
4. Impairment of verbal communication: due to facial muscle weakness.
5. Anxiety, mild to severe: due to fear of motor deficits or sensory loss.
6. Knowledge deficit: expressed lack of information about health status.
7. Nutritional deficit: decreased intake due to anorexia from loss of smell or swallowing difficulties.
8. Self-care deficit: due to visual impairment or blindness, vertigo, or pain.
9. Decreased activity tolerance: due to impaired mobility.
10. Role disturbance: due to impaired vision, vertigo, impaired verbal communication, and altered self-concept.
11. Alterations in self-concept: due to facial droop.
12. Social isolation: secondary to change in self-concept or pain.

EXPECTED OUTCOMES

1. The best possible comfort level will be achieved.
2. Effect of damage will be minimized, as possible.
3. Client will be able to resume self-care and return to pre-injury functions.

INTERVENTIONS

1. Assist the client in gaining control over face pain or paresthesias. (See *Spinal Cord Tumors*, intervention 2a, e, f, and g.)
2. Protect the client from injury due to visual impairment, tactile sensory deficits, hearing loss, and vertigo.
3. If appropriate, help the client and family to learn how to manage the vision problems as well as to protect the client from injury due to visual impairment. In addition, keep eyes clean and use a wetting agent if the cornea is prone to drying or even at risk from client's inability to keep the lid(s) closed when resting or asleep.
4. Assist client and family in maintaining adequate nutrition and fluid intake.
5. If possible, depending on the level of consciousness, assist the client and family in improving the client's communication ability.
6. Promote the maintenance of skin integrity.
7. Help client gain control over vertigo.
   a. Administer prescribed medications to assist in controlling the vertigo.
   b. Help the client identify precipitating factors such as rapid positional changes.
8. Assist the client and family in learning means to regain independence in activities of daily living (bathing, toileting, hair grooming, etc.). This may include:
   a. Ambulation activities and the use of equipment to aid in ambulation.

b. Use of facial support device.
c. Appropriate furnishings and arrangement.
d. Use of specialized equipment to assist the client in bathing, dressing, hair grooming, eating, and brushing teeth.

9. For some clients, training for the blind or deaf may be appropriate.
10. Nursing interventions to reduce anxiety may be appropriate. (See *Anxiety* in Chapter 36.)

EVALUATION

Outcome Criteria

1. Client is in control of pain, paresthesias, or vertigo, as evidenced by expressed level of comfort.
2. Client maintains self-care, role function, and socialization patterns to the greatest possible extent.
3. Client and family are able to return information about the client's health status and therapeutic management.
4. Client's skin is intact upon inspection.
5. Client remains well nourished and well hydrated, as evidenced by physical appearance, weight maintenance, and normal laboratory values.
6. Client's lungs remain clear; vital signs are stable.
7. Client verbalizes fears and concerns about changes in body image.
8. Client gains increased motor function and sensory perception.

Complications

1. Injury due to reduced ability to use affected part.
2. Decubiti on back of scalp, ear.
3. Atelectasis/aspiration leading to pneumonia (see discussion in Chapter 31).
4. Dehydration (see *Amyotrophic Lateral Sclerosis*, complication 5).
5. Malnutrition (see *Amyotrophic Lateral Sclerosis*, complication 6).
6. Chronic pain syndrome (see *Nutritional Polyneuropathy*, complication 7).

SPINAL CORD INJURY

DESCRIPTION

More than 125,000 persons in the United States have a paraplegia or quadriplegia caused by traumatic spinal cord injury. Serious spinal cord injury is sustained by 5,000 to 10,000 persons a year. Four-fifths of these persons are between 15 and 30 years of age, and the majority are men.

Vertebral injuries generally are a result of force(s)—acceleration, decleration, and deformation—applied most frequently at a distance. The forces damage the tissues by compression (pushing tissues together), tension (pulling or exerting a traction force on the tissues), or shearing (sliding or overriding one portion onto another). The mechanisms of injury are hyperflexion, hyperextension, vertical compression, and rotation. *Hyperextension* injuries often fracture and dislocate posterior elements such as spinous processes, transverse processes, laminae, pedicles, or posterior ligaments. *Hyperflexion* injuries fracture or dislocate the vertebral bodies, discs, or ligaments. *Vertical compression* produces shattering fractures. *Rotational forces* rupture supporting ligaments in addition to producing fractures.

Occasionally there is traumatic injury to the spinal cord or nerve roots alone. Hyperextension by a direct force can result in immediate paralysis (e.g., forward fall with face or forehead striking an object). This injury is most commonly seen in elderly persons with osteophytes present in the vertebral canal.

In the majority of cases, the bones, ligaments, and joints of the vertebral column are damaged. These injuries may contribute to or directly cause cord injury. Vertebral injuries are often classified into *fractures, dislocations,* and *fracture-dislocations*. The relative frequency of each type of injury is 1:1:3. The vertebrae fracture easily with either direct or indirect trauma.

Dislocation occurs when the supporting ligaments are torn or ruptured and the vertebra(ae) move out of alignment. The direction of dislocation may be either straight forward from a horizontal force or angulated if a flexed position was present on impact. Dislocation can be due to flexion or extension injuries. Nervous tissue injury may or may not be present.

A head injury often is sustained at the same time as the vertebral and spinal cord injury.

Most vertebral injuries occur at the first to second cervical, fourth to sixth cervical, and eleventh thoracic to second lumbar vertebrae. These are the most mobile portions of the vertebral column. Also the cervical and lumbar cord is enlarged; therefore, the cord occupies most of the canal and is more easily injured.

Injury to the spinal cord may include:

1. *Cord concussion*: results in a momentary disturbance of cord function.
2. *Cord contusion*: the bruising causes swelling and temporary loss of function.
3. *Cord compression*: must be relieved (decompressed) if permanent damage is to be prevented.
4. *Laceration*: may be a reversible injury if only slight damage; may result in permanent loss of function if the spinal tracts are severed.
5. *Transection*: the spinal cord is severed and the loss is permanent.
   a. *Complete* transection: all functions mediated by neurons or carried in tracts below the transection are completely and permanently lost.
   b. *Incomplete* transection: some tracts remain intact and function related to these tracts has the potential to recover.
6. *Hemorrhage*: usually does not cause major loss of function.
7. *Damage or obstruction of spinal blood supply*: causes local ischemia.

With all spinal cord trauma, edema and microscopic hemorrhage develop shortly after injury. Maximal edema and bleeding are at the level of injury and two segments above and below the injury. These compound the functional loss and make it unclear as to what is permanent functional loss and what is temporary loss. Cord edema is life-threatening in the cervical region because of loss of diaphragm innervation and medullary impairment.

Loss of motor and sensory functions depends upon the level of injury. *Paraplegia* refers to paralysis of the lower half of the body with both legs involved. *Quadriplegia* (tetraplegia) refers to paralysis involving all four extremities. In complete quadriplegia the level of injury is above C6 and all upper extremity function is lost. In incomplete quadriplegia, function at or above C6 is preserved, leaving the shoulder, upper arm, and some forearm muscle control intact. Thus the individual has the potential for independent function. Regarding cervical injuries, with acceleration (e.g., rear-end collision) the greatest stress point is C4–5. With a deceleration force (e.g., head-on collision) the greatest stress point is at C5–6 (see Figure 25–10).

Immediately following cord injury, normal activity of the spinal cord cells at and below the level of injury ceases because of loss of the continuous tonic discharge from the brain or brainstem centers. This is referred to as *spinal shock*. All motor, sensory, reflex, and autonomic functions cease below any transected area and may cease below concussed, contused, compressed, or ischemic areas. The duration of the spinal shock stage may be from a few days to months, depending on the severity of the injury. The average duration is 1 to 6 weeks.

Return of spinal neuron excitability occurs slowly. Depending on the degree of damage, either (1) motor, sensory, reflex, and autonomic functions return to normal or (2) autonomic neural activity in the isolated segment will develop. The sequence of hyperactivity phases (which vary in length) may include (1) minimal reflex activity, (2) flexor spasm activity, (3) alternation between flexor and extensor spasm activity, and (4) predominantly extensor spasm activity.

The immediate intervention for a suspected or confirmed vertebral fracture or dislocation with or without spinal cord injury is immobilization of the spine.

PREVENTION

Health Promotion

1. Education of the public to promote safer home environments for individuals of all ages.
2. Families at high risk for child abuse should be identified and supported to prevent physical and emotional trauma in children.
3. Encouraged use of car seats for children, seat belts, helmets for cyclists, and safe paths for bicyclists to promote safety in vehicle use. In addition, avoiding alcohol and drugs while driving should be encouraged.
4. Promotion of student awareness of safety regulations and encouragement of their implementation.
5. Industrial safety programs to emphasize the necessity of wearing hard hats in dangerous areas, safe use of machinery, and general measures to ensure a safe working environment.
6. Encouragement of proper body mechanics and exercises to strengthen back muscles to avoid back injuries.
7. Promotion of neighborhood crime prevention programs.

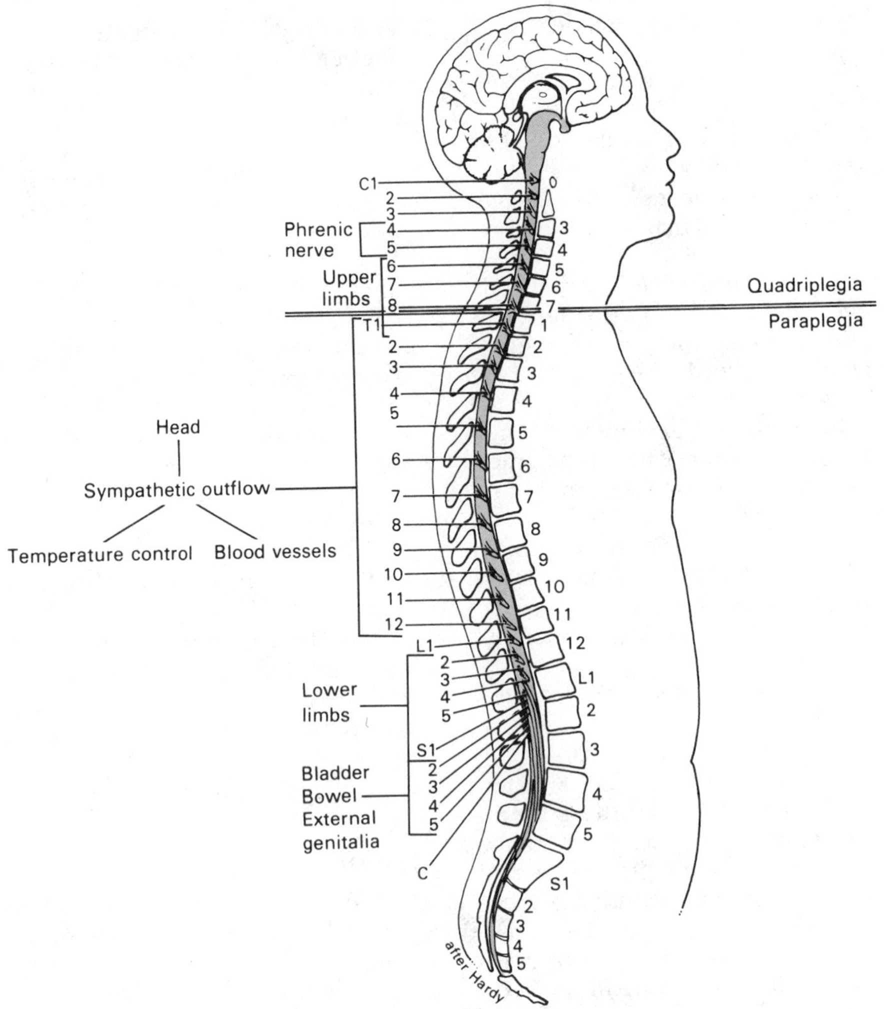

Figure 25-10 Location of cord segments in relation to vertebrae. (Copyright © by Neil Hardy.)

Population at Risk

1. Children between 6 months and 2 years of age are likely candidates for head injuries sustained from falls.
2. Traumatic injuries from physical abuse may occur in children of all ages.
3. Young school-age children are susceptible to head injuries from playground injuries, whereas the older student may sustain head and/or spinal cord injury in sports and recreation. Driving accidents have been reported in many head and spinal cord injuries.
4. Accidents involving transportation vehicles (cars, motorcycles, bicycles) are a major cause of traumatic head and spinal cord injuries in both passengers and pedestrians of all ages. If the driver of any of these vehicles is intoxicated, there may be impaired coordination and judgment that may increase the chance of accidents.
5. Occupational hazards, such as working with

heavy machinery or materials and climbing ladders, may place employees at risk for head and spinal cord injuries.
6. Poor body mechanics in lifting and carrying heavy objects may contribute to extrusion of a portion of the intervertebral disc with impingement on neural tissue.
7. Home hazards, such as unlighted stairways, slippery floors, icy walkways, place household members at risk for falls and injury.
8. Sensory and perceptual impairments that are common with aging along with osteoporosis of age place the elderly at a greater risk for falls and traumatic injury to the head and vertebrae.
9. Individuals living in high crime areas, where guns, knives, and other weapons are used in inflicting bodily harm, are also at risk for head and spinal cord injuries from wounds.

Screening

The health history should include a psychosocial, environmental, and physiological assessment to identify potential hazards and current safety practices.

ASSESSMENT

Health History

1. History of fall, vehicular accident, or sporting accident from client if possible, family member, other accident victim or rescue squad personnel.
2. History of drug or alcohol intoxication.
3. History of cervical spondylosis or osteoarthritis of the spine and other injuries or diseases.
4. Use of prescribed medications.
5. Any known allergies.

Physical Assessment: Spinal Shock Stage—Complete Transection

1. Loss of motor function.
   a. Presence of quadriplegia with lesions of the cervical cord.
   b. Presence of paraplegia with lesions of the thoracic cord.
2. Muscle flaccidity.
3. Loss of all reflexes below the level of injury.
4. Loss of pain, temperature, touch, pressure, and proprioception below the level of injury (see Figure 25–11).
5. Experience of pain at the site of injury due to a zone of hyperesthesia above the lesion.
6. Atonic bladder, bowel.
7. Paralytic ileus present with distention.
8. Loss of vasomotor tone in the lower body parts; low and unstable blood pressure.
9. Loss of perspiration below the level of injury.
10. Loss or extreme depression of genital reflexes, such as penile erection and bulbocavernous reflex.
11. Dry and pale skin; possible ulceration over bony prominences.

Physical Assessment: Spinal Shock Stage—Partial Spinal Cord Transection Syndromes

1. Asymmetrical flaccid motor paralysis below the level of the injury.
2. Asymmetrical reflex loss.
3. Preservation of some sensation below the level of injury.
4. Vasomotor instability less severe than with complete cord transection.
5. Bowel and bladder impairment less than that seen with complete cord transection.
6. Preservation of ability to perspire in some portions of the body below the level of injury.
7. *Brown-Sequard syndrome.* Associated with penetrating injuries (e.g., stab or gunshot wound); arises from a relative hemisection of the cord.
   a. Ipsilateral paralysis or paresis below the level of injury.
   b. Ipsilateral loss of touch, pressure, vibration, and position sense below the level of injury.
   c. Contralateral loss of pain and temperature sensations below the level of injury.
8. *Central cervical cord syndrome.* Associated with hyperextension or interruption of blood supply.
   a. Motor deficit in the upper extremities more dense than in the lower extremities.
   b. Varying degrees of bladder dysfunction.
9. *Anterior cord syndrome.* Compromise of the anterior spinal artery by occlusion or the pressure effect of bone fragments or disc.
   a. Loss of motor function below the level of injury.
   b. Loss of pain and temperature sensations below the level of injury.
   c. Intact touch, pressure, position, and vibration senses.
10. *Horner's syndrome.* Injury to preganglionic

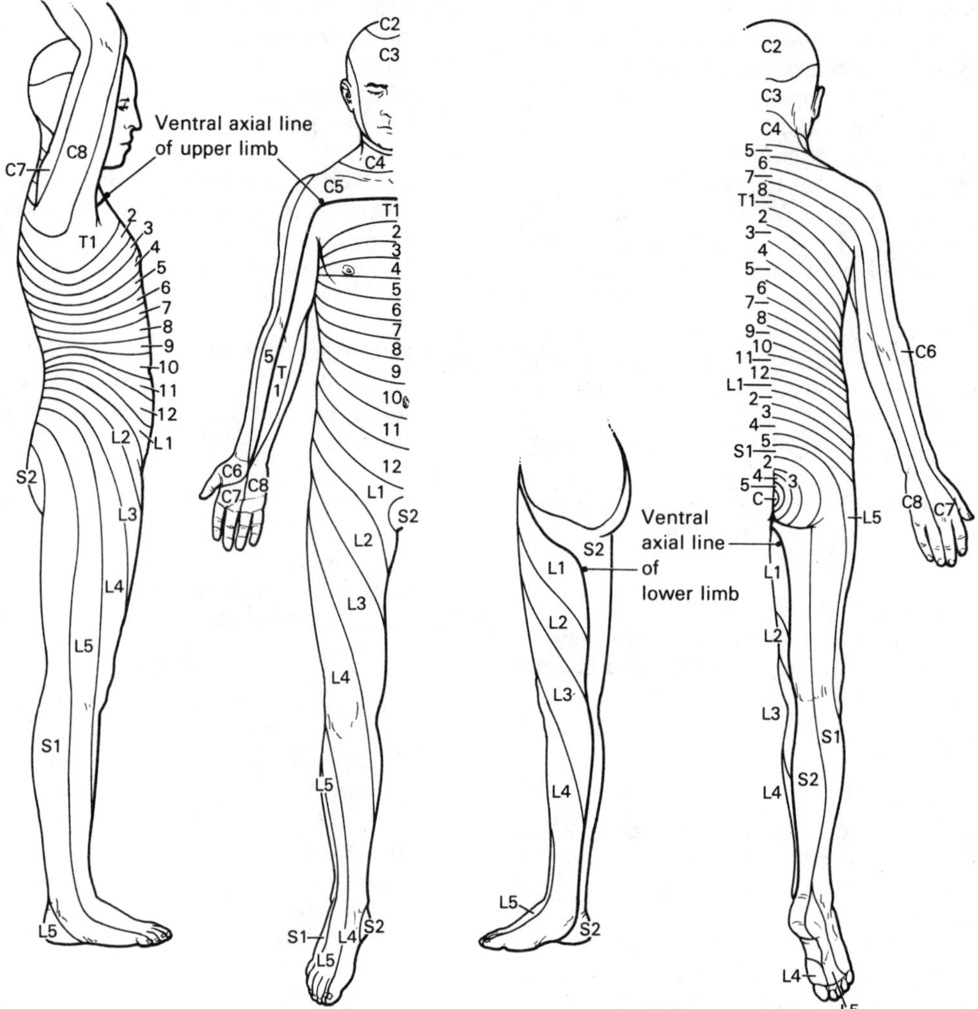

Figure 25-11 Cutaneous distribution of spinal nerves and dermatomes. (Jacob, S. W., and Francone, C.: *Structure and Function in Man,* 4th ed., Saunders, Philadelphia, 1978, p. 236.)

sympathetic trunk or postganglionic sympathetic neurons of the superior cervical ganglion.

a. Ipsilateral pupil smaller than the contralateral pupil.
b. Sunken ipsilateral eyeball.
c. Ptosis of the affected eyelid.
d. Lack of perspiration on the ipsilateral side of the face.

Physical Assessment: Heightened Reflex Activity Stage

1. Emergence of Babinski reflexes, possibly progressing to a triple flexion reflex (i.e., flexion of the foot, leg, and thigh on tactile stimulation); possible development of still later flexor spasms.
2. Reappearance of ankle and knee reflexes; becoming hyperactive.
3. Contraction of reflex detrusor muscle leading to urinary incontinence.
4. Appearance of reflex defecation.
5. Mass reflex with flexion spasms, profuse sweating, piloerection, and automatic bladder and occasional bowel emptying may be evoked by stimulation of skin or from a full bladder.
6. Episodes of hypertension.

7. Defective heat-induced sweating.
8. Eventual development of extensor reflexes, first in muscles of hip and thigh, later in the leg.
9. Possible paresthesias below the level of transection. Dull, burning pain in the lower back, abdomen, buttocks, and perineum.

Diagnostic Tests

1. X-ray films to visualize the vertebrae check for integrity; also, skull films.
2. Epidurogram to visualize any lacerated disc fragments that may have been propelled into the spinal canal at the time of injury or that may have been forced backward into the canal during realignment of the spine by traction.
3. Discogram (sometimes used) to identify a suspected disc laceration in minor spine injuries, whiplash, and simple dislocations.

NURSING DIAGNOSES: ACTUAL OR POTENTIAL

1. Respiratory dysfunction: suffocation due to respiratory muscle paresis or plegia.
2. Alteration in cardiac output, mild to severe: hypotension secondary to autonomic nervous system disruption.
3. Impairment of mobility: paresis or plegia due to transection.
4. Self-care deficit: inability to carry out activities of daily living due to paresis, plegia, or sensory impairment.
5. Alterations in comfort: pain at injury site.
6. Potential for injury: due to sensory-perceptual and/or motor deficits.
7. Alteration of urinary pattern: retention of fluid; later, incontinence due to impaired voluntary control.
8. Alteration of bowel pattern: constipation secondary to immobility or impaired reflex centers; incontinence secondary to impaired voluntary control.
9. Alteration in patterns of sexuality: secondary to motor deficits or damage to reflex centers.
10. Anxiety, severe: secondary to threats to role function, self-concept, and self-care ability.
11. Knowledge deficit: about health status, diagnostic procedures, and so forth.
12. Alterations in self-concept: due to loss of self-esteem, changes in body image, alteration in self-care abilities.
13. Role disturbance: secondary to focal deficits, interruption in lifestyle due to residual deficits.
14. Nutritional deficit: decreased intake and dietary change; eating difficulties and anorexia.
15. Respiratory dysfunction: pulmonary congestion and atelectasis secondary to immobility, respiratory muscle paralysis, and abdominal distention.
16. Impairment of skin integrity: secondary to immobility, incontinence, and impaired vascular tone.
17. Impaired communication due to altered levels of consciousness.
18. Maladaptive (individual) coping patterns: secondary to altered body image.
19. Ineffective family coping: secondary to deficits, hospitalization, and loss of role function.
20. Impaired home maintenance management: secondary to motor deficits, sensory impairment.

EXPECTED OUTCOMES

1. The client's vertebral column (neck and back) will be immobilized.
2. The client will maintain normal vital signs.
3. The client's ventilatory capacity as measured by vital capacity will be greater than 2 L (initial).
4. The client and family will provide correct information about health status, diagnostic procedures, and such.
5. The client will be comfortable, as evidenced by verbal statements.
6. The client will be free of urinary retention and urinary tract infection.
7. The client's skin will remain intact.
8. The client's lungs will remain clear.
9. The client's bowel and bladder patterns will be stabilized.
10. The client will maintain a nutritionally well-balanced dietary intake, as evidenced by maintenance of a normal hematocrit and hemoglobin.
11. The client will maintain normal vascular volume, as evidenced by normal skin turgor, normal serum and urine electrolytes, and urinary output of 50 mL/h.
12. The client will regain as much self-care, role function, and socialization as possible in

light of sensory-motor and coordination deficits.

INTERVENTIONS

1. Continue collection of an accurate data base regarding neurological status.
2. Maintain gastrointestinal suction to prevent vomiting and possible aspiration.
3. Institue bladder drainage via indwelling Foley catheter to avoid overdistention and resultant urinary tract infection.
4. Prevent further injury.
   a. Administer corticosteroids as prescribed to control spinal cord edema. Observe, report, and record therapeutic effectiveness and side effects.
   b. Maintain immobilization.
      (1) For cervical injury, maintain immobilization by skeletal traction.
         (a) Cervical tongs (Crutchfield, Cone Vinke, etc.).
            (i) Explain procedure to client and family; allow verbalizations of fears and concerns; stay with the client and family.
            (ii) Maintain traction: check orthopedic frame and traction at least every shift; check to be sure tongs are secure in the skull at least.
            (iii) Inspect tong sites for infection.
            (iv) Clean and dress tong sites as ordered.
            (v) Administer analgesia as ordered for head and neck discomfort.
         (b) Halo devices.
            (i) Explain procedure to client and family; allow verbalizations of fears and concerns; stay with the client and family.
            (ii) Provide pin care: check pins at least every shift to ensure pins are secure; inspect pin sites every shift; cleanse and dress pin sites as ordered.
            (iii) Provide cast care: check halo jacket for fit and comfort; pedal rough edges of cast; protect cast from soiling and moisture.
            (iv) Maintain client on bed rest as ordered or at least until cast dries.
            (v) Use pad to protect body prominences from pressure while the client is in bed.
            (vi) Provide client and family with reassurance to help with adjustment to the halo device; allow verbalization of feelings.
            (vii) To assist client with ambulation, first sit client on edge of bed ("dangle") while checking vital signs. Due to client's status, you may need to gradually raise the client in bed over time. Once the client is up and standing, gradually ambulate client for longer distances.
            (viii) Have the client accompanied when ambulating, as client is prone to falling; a walker may help to stabilize the ambulating client.
            (ix) Teach the client to deliberately turn his or her eyes to the extreme lateral position to survey the environment while walking.
            (x) Administer analgesics as ordered for head or neck pain from the pins or muscle spasms.
            (xi) When there is cord compression by bony fragments or disc tissues, and often with dislocation injuries, a decompression laminectomy or anterior decompression is necessary.
            (xii) With an anterior decompression, interbody vertebral fusion is done.
            (xiii) Wiring the spinous processes provides additional stabilization with vertebral bony fracture, dislocation, fracture-dislocation, or posterior element fractures.

(xiv) At times Harrington rod implantation is necessary to correct thoracic deformities and stabilize the thoracic spine.

(2) For thoracic or lumbar injury, maintain immobilization by:
(a) Halo device with femoral distraction.
(b) Body cast. (See discussion on cast management in Chapter 31).
(c) Hyperextended position (only usable if there is no permanent spinal cord injury or danger of bony fragment displacement).
(i) With bedboard and footboard in place and using a sponge rubber mattress, gatch the bed to achieve the desired hyperextended position.
(ii) Provide back care given at least q4h by pushing down foam rubber mattress and rubbing the back with lotion to the midline; repeat on the opposite side.
(iii) Turning may be contraindicated: check with the neurosurgeon.
(iv) Do not change bed position except by direct order of the neurosurgeon.
(v) Voiding may be a problem and an indwelling catheter may need to be maintained.

(3) For sacral or coccygeal injury, maintain immobilization by:
(a) Bed rest.
(b) Low girdle or adhesive strapping to injured portion of the spine.
(c) Ensure that client avoids sitting on hard surface.
(d) Assess bladder and bowel function frequently.

5. If surgery to decompress the spinal cord or stabilize the spine is necessary:
   a. Prepare the client physically and prepare the client and family psychologically for the therapeutic neurosurgical or orthopedic procedure(s).
   b. Also, see *Spinal Cord Tumors* for discussion of care.
6. Maintain the client's fluid balance and nutritional status with IV fluids as ordered until gastrointestinal function returns (if lost).
7. Place the client on:
   a. Regular hospital bed with a bedboard and firm mattress.
   b. Stryker frame.
   c. Foster frame.
   d. Rotational bed that changes pressure points.
8. Determine the status of the gastrointestinal tract.
   a. Listen to bowel sounds to determine the presence of an ileus.
   b. Maintain the client NPO as ordered until bowel sounds resume.
   c. Maintain gastrointestinal suction to prevent distention and aspiration of vomitus until gastrointestinal motility returns.
9. Prevent skin breakdown. Turn client q2h from side to back to side. Log roll client, with one nurse stabilizing head and neck and two other nurses turning client as one unit.
10. Institute a pulmonary regimen designed to keep the lungs clear.
    a. Assess vital capacity initially and auscultate at least every shift and later at least every day.
    b. Place suction equipment at bedside (client is especially prone to choking and aspiration with eating and drinking).
    c. Utilize an assistive cough technique to aid the client in clearing secretions.
11. Protect the client from injury due to motor and sensory deficits.
12. Maintain potential for return of motor functions. (See *Coma*, intervention 3 a through g.)
13. Maintain the urinary tract in the best possible condition, if an indwelling Foley is in place.
14. Help the client to maintain adequate nutrition and fluid intake.
15. Institute a bowel evacuation protocol to prevent constipation and straining at stool.
16. Assist the client in maintaining sexuality.
17. Nursing interventions to reduce the client's anxiety may be appropriate.
18. Nursing interventions to reduce the client's and possibly family members' depression may be appropriate. (See Chapter 38).
19. Prepare the client and family for the re-

peated diagnostic reassessments of vertebral column healing.
20. Interventions during the rehabilitative phase:
    a. With the other health-related professional help the client and family assume responsibility for the management of the neurological deficits. Assist the client and family with the grieving process.
    b. Institute an upper motor neuron or mixed bladder training protocol, if the urinary function assessment indicates this is appropriate.
    c. Help the client and family to learn to manage the spasticity.
        (1) See *Amyotrophic Lateral Sclerosis*, intervention 3a through f, for specific interventions.
        (2) Prepare client and family for ablative procedures that are sometimes used to control spasticity of an extreme and incapacitating nature.
    d. Assist the client and family to achieve home care.

EVALUATION

Outcome Criteria

1. Client's vital capacity is greater than 2 L; lungs are clear.
2. Vital functions remain within normal limits.
3. Client has received information regarding health status, diagnostic procedures, therapeutic management, and hospital policy and procedures.
4. Client is free from injury.
5. Client is experiencing increased comfort, absence of pain.
6. There is absence of skin breakdown; skin is intact.
7. Client is free from urinary retention, edema, and infection.
8. *Normal* bowel pattern is maintained.
9. Bowel pattern is regained and stabilized.
10. Nutrition pattern is maintained; client is well nourished and well hydrated.
11. Client regains self-care, role function, and socialization patterns to the greatest possible extent.
12. Client makes informed decision about home management.

Complications

1. Respiratory arrest (see discussion in Chapter 49.)
2. Hypotension (see discussion in Chapter 30.)
3. Decubiti.
4. Atelectasis/aspiration leading to pneumonia (see discussion in Chapter 31).
5. Constipation and impaction (see discussion in Chapter 33).
6. Dehydration (see *Amyotrophic Lateral Sclerosis*, complication 5, for specific discussion).
7. Malnutrition (see *Amyotrophic Lateral Sclerosis*, complication 6, for specific discussion).
8. Urinary tract infection (see discussion in Chapter 32).
9. Thrombophlebitis (see discussion in Chapter 30).
10. Infection or osteomyelitis at tong site (see discussion in Chapter 27).
11. Osteoporosis (see discussion in Chapter 27).
12. Ankylosis (see above).
13. Contractures (see above).

NEUROGENIC HETEROTROPHIC OSSIFICATION

Osteogenesis in a part of the body that does not normally form bone.

Assessment

1. Swelling, either localized or involving the entire extremity.
2. Redness and warmth.
3. Decreased range of motion.
4. Increased serum alkaline phosphatase.
5. Radiographic evidence of osseous formation.

Revised Outcomes/Interventions

Outcomes and interventions as previously stated.

Reevaluation and Follow-up

If ankylosis that limits the client's joint movement to a sufficient degree occurs, surgery is indicated.

AUTONOMIC HYPERREFLEXIA (AUTONOMIC DYSREFLEXIA)

Occurs with cord injuries above T6.

Assessment

1. Pounding headache.
2. Flushing.
3. Profuse sweating.
4. Piloerection above the level of the injury.
5. Nasal congestion.
6. Nausea.

7. Paroxysmal attack of hypertension.
8. Vasodilatation.
9. Chest pain.

Revised Outcomes

1. Client will maintain normal vital signs.
2. Other outcomes as previously stated.

Interventions

1. Remove the stimulus.
   a. Check urinary catheter for patency. Irrigate with no more than 30 mL of normal saline slowly. Replace catheter if patency cannot be reestablished. If catheter is not in place, check for bladder distention and catheterize the client. If distention not the problem, check for urinary tract infection or urinary calculi obstruction.
   b. Check for acute abdominal problem, including hypo- or hyperbowel function.
   c. Check for constipation: ascertain time of last bowel movement, listen to motility, check for rectal impaction. Use dibucaine hydrochloride (Nupercaine) ointment on anus and in rectum to stop reflexes before disimpacting the client or giving a suppository.
   d. Check for pressure on glans penis or elsewhere on the penis in the male. Remove pressure source.
   e. Check for skin lesions below the level of injury: rash, pressure sore, infection, ingrown toenail; apply topical anesthetic to stop stimulation.
2. Administer drugs as ordered if noxious stimulus cannot be removed. Diazoxide (Hyperstat), hydralazine (Apresoline), and ganglionic blocking agents such as phenoxybenzamine (Dibenzyline), guanethidine sulfate (Ismelin), or phentolamine (Regitine) may be used. Observe, record, and report therapeutic effectiveness and side effects.
3. While hypertension and other clinical manifestations are present and for a time following the episode, check vital signs frequently.
4. Assist the client and family in learning the causes, clinical manifestations, and treatment for autonomic hyperreflexia. They must be able to institute treatment as well.

Reevaluation and Follow-up

Assess the management regimen of the client and adjust the regimen to prevent the occurrence of the autonomic hyperreflexia.

REFERENCES

Adams, D., and Victor, M.: *Principles of Neurology*, McGraw-Hill, New York, 1977, pp. 486–488.

Baratz, R. and Norman, S.: "The Management of Patients with Aphasia: A Guide for Nurses," *American Journal of Nursing*, **79**:2136, 1979.

Greer, M.: "Benign Intracranial Hypertension," in P. J. Vinken and G. W. Bruyn (eds.), *Handbook of Clinical Neurology*, North Holland, Amsterdam, 1974, pp. 150–166.

Hoehm, M. M., and Yahr, M. D.: "Parkinsonism Onset, Progression and Mortality," *Neurology*, **17**:427–442, 1967.

Moss, G., Stauton, C., and Stein, A.: "The Centrineurogenic Etiology of Acute Respiratory Distress Syndrome," *American Journal of Surgery*, **126**:37–40, 1973.

Wells, C. E.: *Dementia*, Davis, Philadelphia, 1971.

BIBLIOGRAPHY

Adams, D., and Victor, M.: *Principles of Neurology*, McGraw-Hill, New York, 1977. The phenomenology of neurological disease is presented, followed by an account of the various neurological syndromes. Finally, the diseases that express themselves by each syndrome are considered. A portion of the text discusses neuropsychiatric syndromes.

Chusid, J. G.: *Correlative Neuroanatomy and Functional Neurology*, 17th ed., Lange, Los Altos, Calif., 1979. This book provides a brief and clear discussion of the structural and functional features of the nervous system as they relate to problems encountered in clinical neurology. Illustrations, diagrams, charts, and tables are abundant and helpful. Written for medical students and housestaff.

Cloward, R. B.: "Acute Cervical Spine Injuries," *Clinical Symposia*, **32**(1):2–32, 1980. This symposium provides a discussion of the history of cervical spine injury, classification of injuries, soft tissue injury, treatment at accident site, treatment in the emergency room, and surgical treatment. The illustrations are most helpful. Written for housestaff and neurosurgeons.

Conway-Rutkowski, B. L.: *Carini and Owens' Neurological and Neurosurgical Nursing*, 8th ed., Mosby, St. Louis, 1982. This classic neurological-neurosurgical nursing text follows the traditional neurology text format of general etiological classifications such as infectious diseases, degenerative diseases, metabolic abnormalities, and so on. Chapters on anatomy and physiology, neurological assessment, and diagnostic procedures are presented as well. Chapters on sexual dysfunction, cognitive and behavioral impairment, unconsciousness, rehabilitation, and pain are also included. This text is most useful for persons with some knowledge and experience in neurological and neurosurgical nursing.

Hickey, J. V.: *The Clinical Practice of Neurological and Neurosurgical Nursing*, Lippincott, Philadelphia, 1981. An excellent, well-organized, and comprehensive text covering major areas of neurological-neurosurgical nursing. Illustrations are helpful. Useful as a basic text for nursing students and practicing nurses as well.

Mancall, E. L.: *Alpers and Mancall's Essentials of the Neurological Examination*, 2d ed., Davis, Philadelphia, 1981. This manual provides a guide to the neurological examination, an interpretation of abnormal neurological signs, and a description of commonly employed laboratory techniques. Written for medical students and housestaff as well as medical practitioners.

Merritt, H. H.: *A Textbook of Neurology*, 6th ed., Lea & Febiger, New York, 1979. In this text, diseases are grouped according to etiology. Pathogenesis, incidence, symptomatology, signs, laboratory data, diagnosis, course and prognosis, and treatment are discussed for each disease entity. Written for medical students, housestaff, and practicing physicians.

Petersdorf, R. G., et al.: *Harrison's Principles of Internal Medicine*, 10th ed., McGraw-Hill, New York, 1983. The approach of this medical text centers on an analysis of symptoms to recognize a syndrome and understand the nature of the disease mechanism that may produce the syndrome. Cardinal manifestations of neurological dysfunction are presented initially. Later in the text disorders of the nervous system are discussed.

Plum, F., and Posner, J. D.: *Diagnosis of Stupor and Coma*, 3d ed., Davis, Philadelphia, 1980. This classic text provides a systematic clinical approach to the assessment and diagnosis of states of impaired consciousness. The pathophysiology of altered consciousness, the signs and symptoms associated with different levels of brain function, prognosis, and the approach to management of the unconscious person are presented. Brain death is also discussed.

Rhoton, A. L., Jackson, F. E., Gleave, J., and Rumbaugh, C. T.: "Congenital and Traumatic Intracranial Aneurysms," *Clinical Symposia*, **29**(4):2–40, 1977. This symposium provides a discussion of the pathophysiology of congenital aneurysm, the consequences of rupture and clinical manifestations, specific congenital aneurysm syndromes, diagnostic tests, medical management, and surgical management. Traumatic aneurysms and arteriovenous malformations are also presented. The illustrations are most helpful. Written for housestaff and neurosurgeons.

26

The Sensory Systems

Sue E. Huether

The ability to receive and evaluate information about the external environment is essential for survival. Fortunately, the sensory systems provide an abundance of information for a wide safety margin for our behavior. Because the number of disorders that may occur with the various sensory systems is so extensive, only the relevant aspects of the most common and serious problems are discussed in this chapter. The classification of the disorders is unique to this chapter. Problems are organized from the external to the internal structures of the ear and eye and are mainly hyperactivity and hypoactivity disorders for the other sensory systems. If a sensory problem occurs secondary to a primary disorder in another body system, only the sensory deficits are discussed here with reference to another chapter for the discussion of the primary problem.

Disorders of sleep are difficult to logically place within any particular body system and, therefore, are briefly discussed in this chapter. Although temperature regulation problems may be included in the sensory systems, fever is discussed in Chapter 49, Medical Emergencies, and hypothermia and hyperthermia problems are included in Chapter 48, Traumatic Injuries.

DISORDERS OF THE EAR

THE EXTERNAL EAR

OTITIS EXTERNA

DESCRIPTION

Otitis externa ("swimmer's ear") is an infection often accompanied by inflammation with a bacterial or fungal source and is frequently caused by swimming in contaminated water or extensively chlorinated swimming pools. A trauma to the ear canal can also precipitate the occurrence of this problem. The inflammation may be acute, chronic, or recurrent and generally involves the skin of the external auditory canal.

PREVENTION

Health Promotion

1. Dry ear canal thoroughly after swimming.
2. Avoid traumatic irritation of ear canal.

Population at Risk

1. People who swim regularly.
2. People who routinely traumatize ear during cleaning.

ASSESSMENT

Health History

Itching with the onset of inflammation and progression to mild or severe pain.

Physical Assessment

1. Edema with diminished hearing.
2. Discharge progressing from serious to purulent.
3. Occasional fever.
4. Signs of injury, inflammation, lesions, infection, or bleeding.
5. Because of severe pain and swelling, it may be very difficult to insert the otoscope for assessment.

NURSING DIAGNOSES: ACTUAL OR POTENTIAL

1. Alteration in comfort: discomfort secondary to pain, discharge.
2. Alteration in body temperature: increase secondary to inflammatory process.

EXPECTED OUTCOMES

1. There will be relief of pain within 24–36 h.
2. Infection and edema will be reduced within 2 or 3 days.
3. Permanent tissue damage will be prevented.
4. Recurrence of contact with source of infection will be prevented.

INTERVENTIONS

1. Antibiotic therapy may be necessary.
2. Reduced activity may be necessary.
3. Increase fluid intake to prevent dehydration.
4. Analgesics or codeine may be used to relieve pain (see Figure 26-1).
5. Apply wet or dry heat applications to help soothe discomfort and increase blood supply to the area. Proper instructions for self-applications of heating pad, wet compresses, or hot water bottle should be provided to the client.
6. Remove discharge and debris by gentle suctioning or irrigation with medicated ear drops

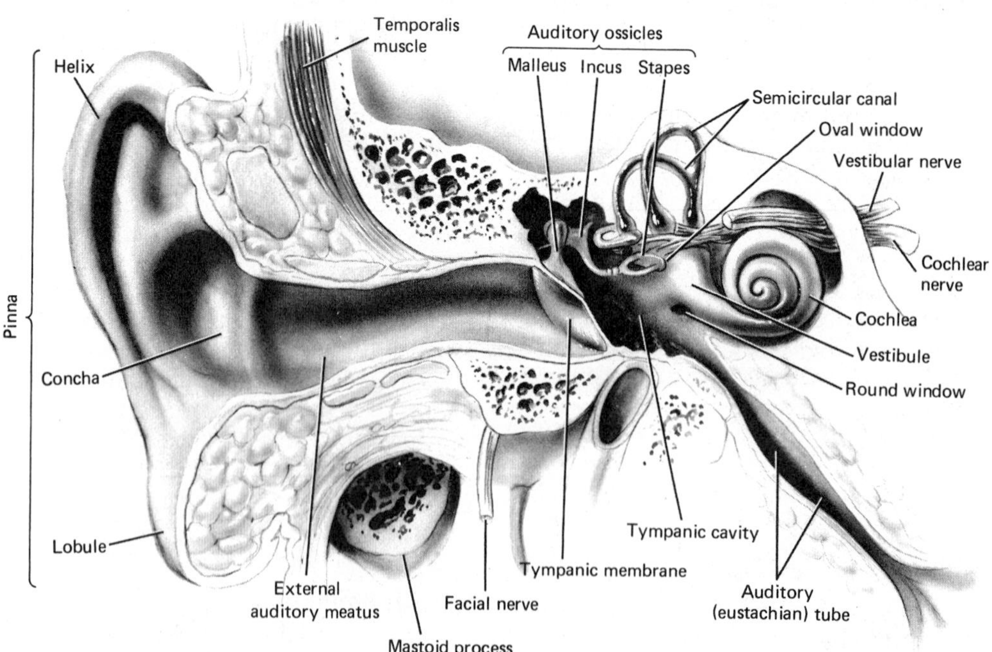

Figure 26-1 The anatomy of the ear. (From Crafts, R. C., *A Textbook of Human Anatomy*, 2d ed., John Wiley & Sons, Inc., New York, 1979, used with permission.)

or instillation of Burow's solution or dilute alcohol.

7. Apply antibiotic eardrops or particular steroid preparations to aid in treating inflammation.
8. If ear canal is not patent, insert a cotton air-wick saturated with antibiotic solution into the auditory canal down to the eardrum.
9. Instruct client to keep ear canal dry, to avoid swimming, showering, or any other source of infection until the condition is eliminated and to avoid use of sharp objects to clean ear canal.

EVALUATION

Outcome Criteria

1. Scaling and discharge resolve.
2. Pain is relieved, and signs of inflammation and edema are eliminated.
3. Ear trauma and contamination with water are avoided.

Complications

Recurrence of problem.

EXTERNAL CANAL BLOCKAGE

DESCRIPTION

The external ear canal may be blocked by a collection of cerumen (wax), foreign bodies, or insects. This may result in reduced hearing, direct tissue damage, or perforation of the eardrum.

PREVENTION

Health Promotion

Keep ear wax soft with eardrops.

Population at Risk

1. Children who place foreign objects in ear canal.
2. People with naturally dry cerumen.

ASSESSMENT

Health History

1. Onset of occurrence with identification of possible cause of the blockage.
2. Increased sensitivity and/or pain.

Physical Assessment

1. Decrease in hearing acuity.
2. Object(s) visible in ear canal.

NURSING DIAGNOSES: ACTUAL OR POTENTIAL

1. Alteration in sensory perception (hearing): secondary to obstruction in ear canal.
2. Sensation of obstruction.

EXPECTED OUTCOMES

1. Blockage will be removed without damage to the external ear canal or eardrum.
2. Infection will be prevented.
3. Hearing will be restored with removal of blockage.

INTERVENTIONS

1. Only skilled and experienced personnel should attempt removal of blockage.
2. In the case of insect blockage, kill insect first with ether or alcohol. Oil drops may be instilled into the external canal so that the insect will float out of the canal in the oil.
3. Soften cerumen with oil before removal.
4. Foreign bodies and other objects:
   a. Remove by instrument if object not beyond isthmus of canal.
   b. Gentle irrigation. (*Caution*: Swelling of some objects may occur with absorption of irrigation solution, rendering removal even more difficult.) Proper technique for irrigation includes:
      (1) Gentle flow.
      (2) Solution at 35 to 40.6°C (95 to 105°F).
      (3) Proper positioning of irrigation device (see Figure 26-2).
5. If irrigation is not helpful, glycerine drops or a saturated solution of sodium bicarbonate may be used two to three times daily for several days.
6. A gentle anesthetic may be required for children or excitable clients.
7. Instruct client and/or family regarding safety precautions to prevent further occurrence.

EVALUATION

Outcome Criteria

1. Auditory canal is patent.
2. Pain is eliminated with removal of blockage.
3. Auditory acuity is restored.

Complications

1. Infection of external canal.
2. Perforation of eardrum with diminished hearing.

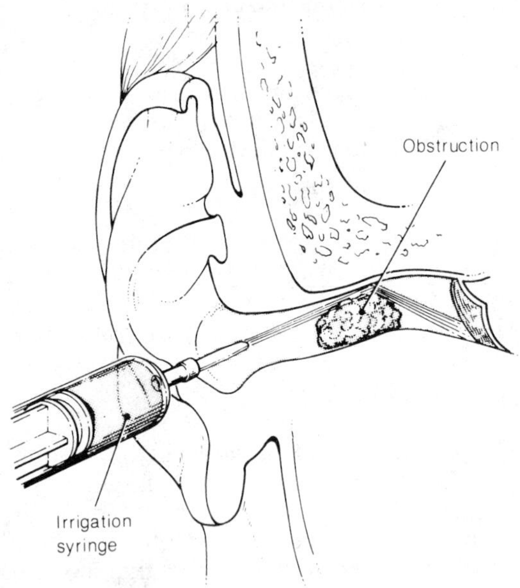

Figure 26-2 Irrigation of the external auditory canal. Note that the solution is directed toward the upper wall of the canal. To gain access to the canal, pull the ear in a superior and posterior direction in an adult, and in a posterior and inferior direction in a child. (Jones, D. A., Dunbar, C. F., and Jirovec, M. M., (eds.): *Medical-Surgical Nursing: A Conceptual Approach*, McGraw-Hill, New York, 1978, p. 1283).

FURUNCULOSIS

DESCRIPTION

Furunculosis, or boils in the ear canal, is usually caused by the entry of staphylococcus via hair follicle or sebacceous gland or via a small crack or a fissure in the skin commonly caused by scratching or trauma of ear canal.

ASSESSMENT

Health History

1. Pain often felt along the jaw as well as in the external canal.
2. Diminished hearing.
3. Feeling of fullness in the ear.

Physical Assessment

1. External ear canal swollen or totally blocked.
2. Adenopathy.
3. Discharge with rupture of furuncle.

NURSING DIAGNOSES: ACTUAL OR POTENTIAL

Pain and inflammation of external canal.

EXPECTED OUTCOMES

1. Pain will be relieved with decreased inflammation.
2. Staphylococcus contamination will be eliminated.
3. Recurrence will be prevented.

INTERVENTIONS

1. Insert cotton pledget saturated with Burow's solution and change every 2–3 h.
2. Give aspirin or apply intermittent heat for relief of pain.
3. Keep ear dry.
4. Administer antibiotic medication, usually penicillin.
5. Instruct client to avoid scratching ear or using any object in the ear, such as bobby pins.

EVALUATION

Outcome Criteria

1. Signs and symptoms are eliminated, and hearing is restored within 10 to 14 days.
2. Problem does not recur.

PERFORATION OF EARDRUM

DESCRIPTION

Perforation of the eardrum may be considered a middle or outer ear problem. The eardrum may be perforated as a result of:

1. Chronic infection, such as acute and/or chronic otitis media.
2. Trauma.
   a. Insertion of toothpicks and bobby pins or careless use of Q-Tips.
   b. Direct blows to the side of the head or a slap with an open palm.
   c. Burns.
   d. High-pressure flow of fluids, such as water.
   e. Blast injury.
3. Postsurgical effect.

PREVENTION

Health Promotion

1. Avoidance of insertion of sharp objects in ear canal.
2. Early treatment of otitis media.

ASSESSMENT

Health History

1. History of trauma or infection.
2. Pain at time of trauma.
3. Diminished hearing.
4. Dizziness, nausea, and vomiting.
5. Hollow, reverberating sound in head.

Physical Assessment

1. Perforation visible with otoscopy.
2. Appearance of blood in ear canal.
3. Serosanguineous or mucopurulent discharge at time of rupture.

NURSING DIAGNOSES: ACTUAL OR POTENTIAL

1. Alteration in comfort: pain may be relieved with perforation secondary to otitis media.
2. Disturbance of coordination: secondary to altered balance.
3. Decreased hearing.

EXPECTED OUTCOMES

1. Immediate.
   a. Cause of perforation will be removed.
   b. Continuity of eardrum will be restored.
   c. Infection will be prevented.
   d. Hearing will be restored.
   e. Pain will be relieved.
2. Postoperative care for myringoplasty.
   a. Infection will be prevented.
   b. Recurrence will be prevented.
   c. Falling due to disturbance of balance will be prevented.

INTERVENTIONS

1. Immediate.
   a. Small perforations will heal spontaneously.
   b. For perforation due to trauma, use cotton in canal to protect from dirt and debris.
   c. Apply trichloroacetic acid qid for traumatic perforation.
   d. Administer antibiotic if secondary to chronic infection.
   e. Give analgesic for relief of pain.
   f. Surgical procedures to close perforation may be necessary:
      (1) Myringoplasty.
      (2) Graft (fashioned from temporal muscle, vein graft occasionally).
2. Postoperative.
   a. Give antibiotic medication for several days; it may be accompanied with application of antibiotic powder to ear canal (Neosporin).
   b. Maintain intact dressing. External dressing may be reinforced.
   c. Usually remove surgical packing 1 week postoperatively.
   d. Do not suction or probe canal. Gentle suction may be used after 2 weeks to remove debris.
   e. Do not use eardrops because of the possibility of dislocating graft.
   f. Assist with early ambulation attempts; client may become dizzy.
   g. Medication may be used for nausea, vomiting, or dizziness.
   h. Instruct client to:
      (1) Avoid immersing head in water, swimming, especially diving.
      (2) Avoid skydiving or flying in unpressurized planes.
      (3) Avoid shampooing or any other contact with water as instructed by physician.
      (4) Continue antibiotic treatment.
      (5) Continue antihistamine medication for approximately 1 month if prescribed.
      (6) Avoid blowing nose with force.

EVALUATION

Outcome Criteria

1. Signs and symptoms, especially pain and signs of infection, diminish.
2. Hearing is restored within 6 months.
3. There is no recurrence of infection.

Complications

Infection and loss of hearing.

EUSTACHIAN SALPINGITIS

DESCRIPTION

Eustachian salpingitis is blockage of the eustachian tube, which connects the postnasal air channel (nasal pharynx) to the middle ear and serves as a safety outlet for secretions from the middle ear as well as an equalizer of air pressure on both sides of the eardrum. Blockage of the tube may be caused by:

1. Early stage of acute otitis media.
2. Inflammation of nasopharyngeal mucosa.
3. Violent blowing of the nose without the mouth open, thereby forcing infected material into the eustachian tube.
4. Enlarged adenoid or tonsils.
5. Cold or allergy attacks.
6. Enlarging tumor mass.
7. Sudden descent in poorly pressurized aircraft.

ASSESSMENT

Health History

1. History of occurrence from common causes.
2. Impaired hearing.
3. Fullness in the ear.
4. Crackling or other noises during swallowing.
5. Sensation of fluid in the ear.
6. Tinnitus.
7. Dizziness.

Physical Assessment

1. Retraction of eardrum without fluid formation.
2. Enlarged tonsils or adenoid or inflammation of pharynx.

EXPECTED OUTCOMES

1. Cause of blockage will be eliminated.
2. Primary disease will respond to treatment.
3. Infection of middle ear will be prevented.

INTERVENTIONS

1. Short course of steroid treatment with decongestants may be given.
2. Fluid is withdrawn by needle placed through anesthetized eardrum. (Children need to be hospitalized and placed under general anesthesia for this procedure.)
3. Fluids may be drained from middle ear by small suction tube via eardrum incision (drainage tube may be left in place for several weeks if drainage is thick.)
4. If chronic condition is accompanied by adenoiditis or tonsillitis, removal of adenoids or tonsils may be appropriate.
5. Antibiotic treatment if acute otitis media.

EVALUATION

Outcome Criteria

1. Signs and symptoms diminish in 7 to 10 days.
2. Hearing is restored with relief of symptoms.

Complications

Recurrence of signs and symptoms indicative of diagnosis or acute otitis media or pharyngitis.

THE MIDDLE EAR

ACUTE OTITIS MEDIA

DESCRIPTION

Acute otitis media is a middle ear inflammation caused by a pathological organism that gains entry through the eustachian tube or via the external auditory canal through a perforated eardrum.

PREVENTION

Health Promotion

1. Avoid putting child to bed with bottle; fluid may enter eustachian tube and cause otitis media.
2. Use decongestants with upper respiratory infections to prevent closure of eustachian tube opening.

Population at Risk

Infants and children.

ASSESSMENT

Health History

1. Severe, painful earache that may be of a stabbing nature and may radiate over involved side of head.
2. Sensation of fullness in the ear that may change with position alteration.
3. Tinnitus.

4. Diminution of hearing.
5. Headache and malaise.

Physical Assessment

1. Tenderness over mastoid bone.
2. High fever, up to 40.6°C (105°F).
3. Increased pulse.
4. Inflamed and/or perforated eardrum.

NURSING DIAGNOSES: ACTUAL OR POTENTIAL

1. Alteration in balance: secondary to inflammation.
2. Alteration in comfort: pain, tinnitus, and headache.
3. Alteration in nutrition: secondary to nausea, anorexia.
4. Decreased hearing.

EXPECTED OUTCOMES

1. Spread of infection to mastoid and brain will be prevented.
2. Pain will be relieved with relief of inflammation.
3. Hearing loss will be restored with prevention of permanent loss of hearing within 6 months.
4. Recurrence will be prevented.

INTERVENTIONS

1. Administer antibiotic therapy appropriate for specific pathological organism (penicillin, ampicillin, and erythromycin are frequently used).
2. Surgical intervention can include myringotomy, an incision through inferior-posterior aspect of eardrum and drainage. Rapid healing usually occurs and does not affect hearing.
3. Instruct client or family, if child, to watch for signs and symptoms of continuation of condition.

EVALUATION

Outcome Criteria

1. Pain is diminished.
2. Tenderness is decreased.
3. Hearing is restored.
4. Appetite is restored.
5. Eardrum is normal.

Complications

Recurrence of signs and symptoms indicative of chronic otitis media, such as bubbles or a fluid level behind eardrum or decreased hearing.

CHRONIC OTITIS MEDIA AND MASTOIDITIS

DESCRIPTION

Chronic serous otitis media (glue ear) may result from reoccurrence of acute otitis media and sustained entry of pathological organisms (that may continue over a period of years) caused by: (1) inadequate treatment of acute otitis media or (2) organisms resistant to antibiotic therapy. Mastoiditis is a complication of otitis media secondary to pus in the middle ear without myringotomy or use of improper antibiotic. The condition may extend to venous sinus, meninges, and labyrinth, or facial nerves.

PREVENTION

Health Promotion

Early treatment of acute otitis media.

Population at Risk

Children recovering from acute otitis media.

ASSESSMENT

Health History

1. Mild hearing loss.
2. Discharge with foul odor.
3. Pain over mastoid bone.

Physical Assessment

1. Signs and symptoms of perforation, including rupture and continued inflammation of eardrum.
2. Collection of soft ball of skin with invasion of eardrum.
3. Signs and symptoms of complication of meningitis (headache, fever, nucchal rigidity, lethargy).
4. Signs indicative of facial nerve involvement include:
   a. Facial paralysis.
   b. Inability to close eyes.
   c. Drooping mouth.
   d. Inability to drink fluid without dripping.
   e. Inability to whistle.
5. Dull or retracted eardrum.
6. Vertigo.

Diagnostic Tests

Mastoid x-rays.

NURSING DIAGNOSES: ACTUAL OR POTENTIAL

1. Fluid level in middle ear with fluctuating hearing loss.
2. Middle ear and/or mastoid pain.

EXPECTED OUTCOMES

1. Immediate:
   a. Fluid will diminish in middle ear.
   b. Source of infection will be eliminated with antibiotics in 10 to 14 days.
   c. Hearing will be restored in 3 to 6 months.
   d. Complications such as mastoiditis, destruction of ossiculor periosteum, and perforation will be avoided.
2. Postoperative for mastoidectomy or placement of myringotomy tubes in eardrum.
   a. Postoperative pain will be controlled.
   b. Complications will be prevented.
   c. Contamination of operative area will not occur.
   d. Recurrence of condition will be prevented.

INTERVENTIONS

1. Immediate.
   a. Antibiotic therapy.
   b. Surgical intervention.
      (1) Tubes are placed inferiorly in eardrum for 3 to 6 months or until they spontaneously come out to drain middle ear.
      (2) Simple mastoidectomy is performed to remove involved mastoid cells.
      (3) Radical mastoidectomy is performed to remove all involved tissues in mastoid and middle ear.
      (4) Posteroanterior mastoidectomy (simple mastoidectomy plus tympanoplasty) is done to repair damaged eardrum and middle ear.
2. Postoperative.
   a. Myringotomy tubes. Instruct client to avoid swimming or any activity by which fluid could enter ear until tubes are removed.
   b. Mastoidectomy.
      (1) Give medication (aspirin, codeine sulfate, sedatives) and use an ice cap for reduction of postoperative pain.
      (2) Observe for complications of facial paralysis, infection, and meningitis.
      (3) Maintain good sterile technique in changing dressings. Packing may be removed third to fourth day postoperatively.
      (4) Instruct client and family regarding:
         (a) Dressing and packing.
         (b) Expected restoration of hearing.
      (5) If stapes and cochlea are uninvolved, expect return of hearing.
      (6) If cochlea or stapes are damaged, client may require hearing aid.

EVALUATION

Outcome Criteria

Signs and symptoms are reduced in 10 to 14 days.

1. Infection is cleared.
2. There is no fluid level.
3. Hearing is restored, with evaluations at 3 months and 1 year.
4. No residual paralysis remains.
5. There is no vertigo.

THE INNER EAR

OTOSCLEROSIS

DESCRIPTION

Otosclerosis consists of ossification of stapes against the oval window with a diminution of sound transmission through the ossicles to the inner ear. Loss of hearing with this condition is associated with development of new spongy bone in the labyrinth. The cause is unknown, with a higher rate of occurrence in females. A hereditary basis may be relevant to this condition.

PREVENTION

Population at Risk

More commonly females, with occurrence after adolescence.

Screening

Yearly evaluation of hearing.

ASSESSMENT

Health History

1. Slow diminution of hearing without middle ear infection.
2. Abnormal bilateral buzzing and ringing noises.

Physical Assessment

Bone conduction is better than air conduction of sound.

Diagnostic Tests

Hearing evaluation.

EXPECTED OUTCOMES

1. Hearing loss will be prevented.
2. Infection will be prevented.
3. Comfort will be maintained.
4. Graft stability will be maintained.
5. Falling due to balance disturbance will be prevented.
6. Information regarding prognosis will be provided.

INTERVENTIONS

1. Immediate.
   a. Surgery.
   b. Stapedectomy for removal of otosclerotic lesions and implantation of prosthesis for restoration of sound conduction.
2. Postoperative.
   a. Observe for signs and symptoms of infection (fever, vertigo, headache, eye pain).
   b. Position client according to physician's preference.
      (1) Upright (ear up) for maximum graft stability.
      (2) Side of operation down to promote drainage.
      (3) Client's preferred position for maximum comfort.
   c. Administer antibiotics, sedative, and pain medication for vertigo, nausea, pain, and nystagmus.
   d. Assist in early ambulation; client may feel dizzy for several days postoperatively.
   e. Instruct client to:
      (1) Avoid blowing nose for a minimum of 1 week.
      (2) Follow instructions for head position.
      (3) Replace soiled cotton padding as necessary.
      (4) Avoid smoking.
      (5) Protect ears when outdoors.
      (6) Avoid crowds and exposure to colds.
   f. Inform client that it may be several weeks before full effects of surgery are known because of tissue edema and surgical pack.
   g. Determine hearing deficit.

EVALUATION

Outcome Criteria

1. Symptoms are reduced.
2. Hearing is restored, with evaluations at 6 months and 1 year.

Complications

1. Graft is not successful.
2. Symptoms recur.
3. Postoperative infection appears.

MENIERE'S SYNDROME

DESCRIPTION

Meniere's syndrome is a dysfunction of the labyrinth resulting in excessive endolymph with swelling of the membraneous labyrinth and effects: variable remissions and loss of equilibrium. This condition may be caused by tumors, infections, leukemia, allergies, arterio- or atherosclerosis, medical toxicity, physical or emotional stress, or genetic factors.

ASSESSMENT

Health History

1. Usually occurs between 20 to 60 years of age.
2. History of associated causes.
3. Attacks primarily characterized by triad of symptoms lasting hours or days.
   a. Dizziness.
   b. Tinnitus with a sense of fullness in the ear.
   c. Diminution of hearing on involved side, a sensorineural loss.
4. Description of other symptoms.
   a. Headaches.
   b. Nausea and vomiting (especially with sudden head motion).
   c. Irritability.
   d. Depression or withdrawn behavior.
   e. Diminution of appetite.
   f. Vertigo.
   g. Feeling of fullness in the ear.
   h. Intolerance to loud sounds.

5. Intermittent attacks, often with abrupt onset, lasting from minutes to hours. Period between attacks may last months or even years.

Physical Assessment

Caloric test: Insertion of fluid below or above body temperature with observation for nystagmus and dizziness after insertion. Dizziness indicates normal functioning of labyrinth. No response indicates presence of acoustic neuroma. Reduced function indicates Meniere's syndrome. Past pointing (inability to place finger on indicated point such as nose, elbow, etc., with eyes closed).

NURSING DIAGNOSES: ACTUAL OR POTENTIAL

1. Sensorineural hearing loss.
2. Dizziness with difficulty maintaining balance.

INTERVENTIONS

1. Immediate.
   a. There is no universally accepted medical or surgical treatment.
   b. Have client comply with diuretic drug and low-sodium diet therapy for reduction of inner ear fluid.
   c. Administer tranquilizers and/or antimotion medication to relieve symptoms.
   d. Administer antihistamines and vasodilators as prescribed.
   e. Explain the reasons for symptoms to the client and provide emotional support.
   f. Surgical procedures are completed.
      (1) Destruction of part or all of inner ear (labyrinthectomy) used only with severe or total deafness for the relief of symptoms.
      (2) Ultrasonic vibrations can be applied to labyrinth.
      (3) Cryosurgery (utilized infrequently).
2. Postoperative.
   a. Instruct client to move slowly and to avoid sudden body movements, jerking, and so on, that may precipitate an attack.
   b. Encourage bed rest for a few days postoperatively.
   c. Provide information regarding possibility of dizziness for 4 to 6 weeks after surgery; it will resolve itself.

EVALUATION

Outcome Criteria

1. Dizziness resolves in 4 to 6 weeks.
2. Hearing is restored, with evaluations at 3 and 6 months.

Complications

Bell's palsy (pain near jaw angle or behind ear).

MOTION SICKNESS

DESCRIPTION

Motion sickness is caused by a disturbance in the nerve receptors of the inner ear resulting from shifting fluid (endolymph) within the semicircular canals. This condition may be caused by any type of transportation such as planes, buses, automobiles, trains, and boats. Individuals with a chronic infection of the eustachian tube, sinus, or the ears are quite prone to this condition. If prolonged, motion sickness may lead to dehydration, acidosis, and profound mental depression.

ASSESSMENT

Health History

1. Nausea and vomiting.
2. Dizziness.
3. Greenish pallor.
4. Cold sweat.
5. Difficulty in breathing.

EXPECTED OUTCOMES

1. Occurrence or recurrence will be prevented with medication.
2. Symptoms will be alleviated within 1 or 2 h after motion ceases.

INTERVENTIONS

1. Prevention: Client should take Dramamine and Bonine (long-lasting but may cause drowsiness), or Marezine (brief duration with no dizziness) before motion exposure.
2. Client should remain in a reclining position with head still.

3. Client should avoid reading and focus on outside static visual reference.
4. Client should avoid alcoholic drinks.
5. Client should suck ice.

HEARING LOSSES

SENSONEURAL LOSS

DESCRIPTION

Sensoneural hearing loss (perceptive hearing loss) occurs when there is damage to the cochlea or VIIIth cranial nerve, which conducts sound from inner ear to the brain. The deafness may be due to hereditary factors, German measles during first trimester of pregnancy, trauma, noise, drug toxicity, tumors, aging, or infection.

ASSESSMENT

Health History

1. History of primary factors causing hearing loss.
2. Difficulty hearing high-frequency sounds, doorbells, telephones.
3. Tinnitus often present.

Physical Assessment

Rinne test indicates air conduction greater than bone conduction.

EXPECTED OUTCOMES

1. Primary causes will be prevented.
2. Early diagnosis and treatment will prevent hearing loss.

INTERVENTIONS

1. Genetic counseling for parents with hereditary deafness.
2. Vaccination for rubella (German measles) before pregnancy.
3. Early treatment of otitis media.
4. Avoidance of use of ototoxic drugs.
5. Protection from prolonged exposure to loud noises, greater than 85–90 dB.
6. Referral to audiologist for diagnostic audiogram.
7. Referral to auditory and speech training.

EVALUATION

Outcome Criteria

Loss of hearing is prevented.

CONDUCTIVE LOSS

DESCRIPTION

Conductive hearing loss (external or middle ear disorders) occurs when sound cannot reach the cochlea due to blockage of the ear canal or disorders of the eardrum or ossicles. The inner ear and VIIIth cranial nerve are normal. Causal factors include foreign body or cerumen impaction, perforated tympanic membrane, exudate in middle ear, otosclerosis, and ossicular adhesions.

ASSESSMENT

Health History

History of causal disorders.

Physical Assessment

1. Weber test indicates better hearing in affected ear.
2. Rinne test indicates bone conduction greater than air conduction.
3. Conduction in affected ear.
4. Difficulty hearing low tones and vowel sounds.

EXPECTED OUTCOMES

1. Primary causes of conductive hearing loss will be prevented.
2. Diagnosis and treatment of otitis media will be initiated early in disease.
3. Correction of otosclerosis or ossicular adhesions will be made surgically.

INTERVENTIONS

1. Removal of foreign body or cerumen.
2. Early diagnosis and treatment of otitis media.
3. Surgical correction of otosclerosis or ossicular adhesions.

EVALUATION

Outcome Criteria

Hearing is maintained.

DISORDERS OF THE EYE

ASSESSMENT

(See Figure 26-3 for location of structures involved in eye disorders.)

Health History

1. Past symptoms of loss, blurred or double vision, floaters, flashes of light, or photophobia.
2. Itching, burning, or excessive tearing or dryness of eyes.
3. Presence of diseases associated with eye pathology, diabetes, and hypertension.
4. Family history of eye disease.
5. Use of drugs that may affect ocular function.

Physical Assessment

1. Visual acuity: Determined by Snellen chart. Yearly evaluation or with change in vision.
   a. Individual stands 20 ft from chart.
   b. Each eye is tested separately with and without glasses.
   c. The large E at the top of the chart is scaled for normal vision at 200 ft from chart.
   d. The rows of letters that follow are scaled to sizes to be read at various distances (20, 40, and 100 ft).
   e. Visual acuity is expressed as a fraction. The numerator equals the distance to the chart, usually 20 ft, and the denominator is the distance the normal eye can read the line. Example: If the individual reads letters of size 40 at 20 ft from chart, visual acuity equals 20/40 vision.
2. Refraction: Determining refractive error and prescribing correction.
   a. Examination is initiated with instillation of

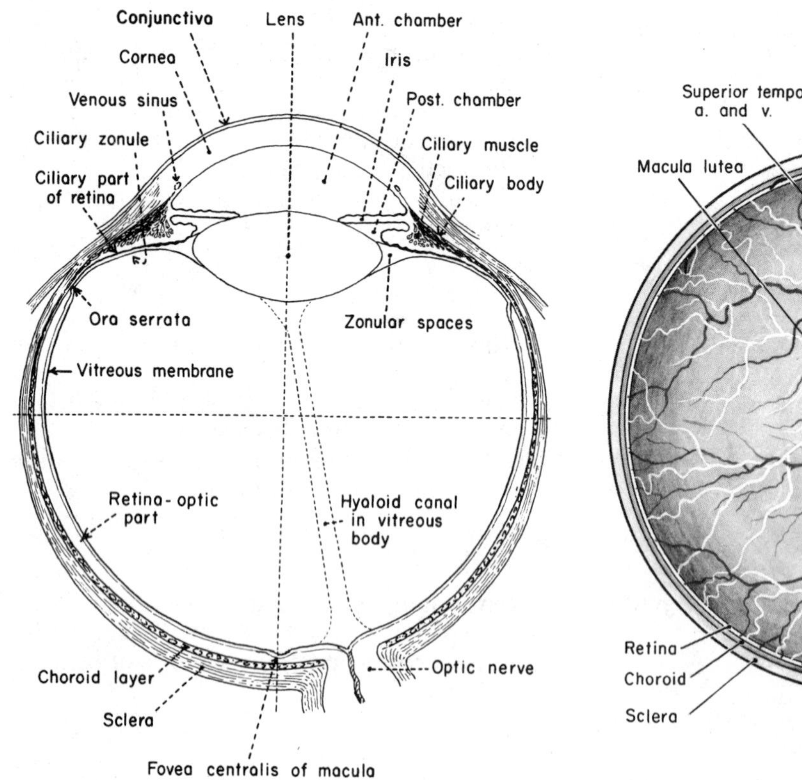

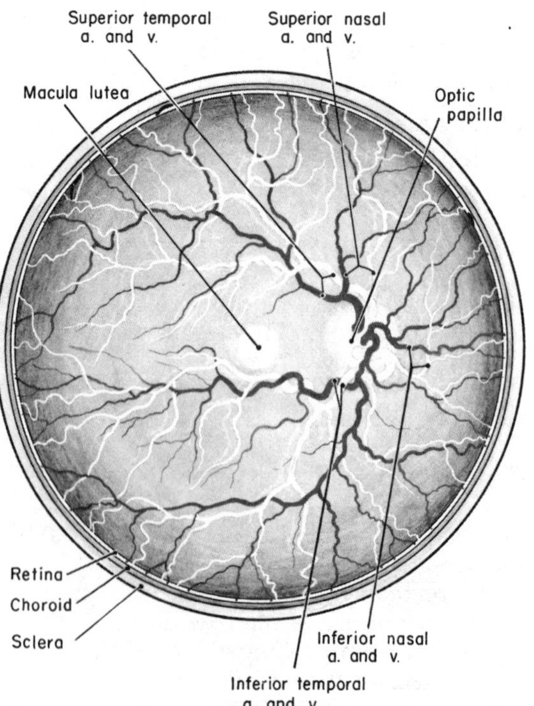

Figure 26-3 The anatomy of the eye. (*Left*) Saggital section. (*Right*) Posterior half. (From Crafts, R. C., *A Textbook of Human Anatomy*, 2d ed., John Wiley & Sons, Inc., New York, 1979, used with permission.)

TABLE 26-1 ERRORS OF REFRACTION

Error	Description	Symptoms	Corrective Lens
Myopia (nearsightedness)	Parallel rays of light focus in *front* of the retina	Blurred distant vision Squinting	Concave (minus) lens
Hyperopia (farsightedness)	Parallel rays of light focus *behind* the retina	Headache Burning sensation of the eye Pulling sensation in the eye	Convex (plus) lens
Astigmatism	Light rays are not refracted equally in all meridians owing to irregular curvature of cornea	Squinting Tilting head to one side	Cylinder lens
Presbyopia	Decrease in accommodative power of the crystalline lens due to aging process	Inability to see comfortably at close range, "arm's length" reading	"Reading glasses": convex lens for near vision; bifocal lenses for near and distant vision

SOURCE: Cullin, I. C., and Holland, N. L., Jones, D. A., Dunbar, C. F., and Jirovec, M. M. (eds.): *Medical-Surgical Nursing: A Conceptual Approach,* McGraw-Hill, New York, 1978, p. 1266.

cyclopegic drug (e.g., atropine) into conjunctival sac. This paralyzes ciliary muscle, thus impeding accommodation process.

   b. Determination of the refractive error is accomplished with sets of trial lenses in an instrument (usually retinoscope) projecting a beam of light into the eye.
   c. Refractive error is identified with observation of light reflex in individual's pupil. (See Table 26-1 for common refractive errors, description, common signs, and corrections.)

3. Visual fields: Examining peripheral and side vision.
   a. Eye is fixed at central point; field is checked with perimeter instrument. Examples of field defects are scotomas with central blind spots in the visual field and hemianopias or peripheral blindness.
   b. Target screen method or confrontation method may also be used.
4. Color vision: Males have a greater genetic tendency to color blindness than females. An individual is asked to identify color patterns in a color plate booklet.
5. Extraocular muscle function: Have individual hold head in one position and follow moving object with eyes.
   a. Check six cardial positions of gaze.
   b. Observe muscle movement, coordination, and alignment.
6. Examination of external and internal eye structures: Lids, vessels, iris, cornea, lens, optic disc, macula, red reflex, scleras, conjunctiva, pupils (reflexes), iris, and chambers. External observation for symmetry, inflammation, and exudates.
   a. Direct opthalmoscope examination: A beam of light is directed through a dilated pupil, permitting visualization of fundus including optic disc, retinal vessels, choroid, and mocula.
   b. The red light reflex is obtained by shining light into the pupil from about 6 in. Red light reflected from vessels of fundus is diminished with cataract or opacities of media.
   c. Indirect ophthalmoscope: Stereoscopic picture of larger area of retina is obtained by use of a binocular, hand-held convex lens, permitting examination of extreme

retinal periphery. A mydriatic agent is used to dilate pupils before examination. This is useful when there are opacities in media.
7. Tonometry: Eyeball tension is measured with use of tonometer. Normal tension equals 11–22 mmHg. A local anesthetic is instilled into the eye before examination.
8. Gonioscopy: The anterior chamber angle (iris-cornea juncture) is examined with a contact glass, illuminator, and hand microscope.

BLEPHARITIS

DESCRIPTION

Blepharitis is an inflammation of eyelid margins, usually bilateral, normally caused by staphylococcus.

ASSESSMENT

Physical Assessment

1. Irritation of eyelid margins.
2. Crusting with scale formation.
3. Ulcers on lid margins causing loss of eyelashes.
4. Burning and itching of eyes.
5. Tearing.
6. Thickened and inflamed eyelids.
7. Feeling of something in the eye.

NURSING DIAGNOSES: ACTUAL OR POTENTIAL

Eyelid pain: secondary to edema and inflammation.

EXPECTED OUTCOMES

1. Inflammation will resolve in 5 to 7 days.
2. Comfort will be maintained.
3. Reoccurrence will be prevented with early treatment.
4. Contamination of other individuals will be prevented.

INTERVENTIONS

1. Use warm compresses to soften and remove crust.
2. Apply an antibiotic or sulfonamide ophthalmic ointment directly to eyelid margins after crust removal.
3. Insert antibiotic and steroid drops to ward off secondary infections.
4. Limit client's use of towels, washcloths, and cosmetics.
5. Instruct client to avoid frequent rubbing of eyelids.

EVALUATION

Outcome Criteria

Symptoms are resolved.

HORDEOLUM

DESCRIPTION

Hordeolum (sty) is one of the most common inflammations of the lid margin. It involves hair follicles and usually is caused by a staphylococcal infection.

ASSESSMENT

Health History

1. Localized redness with swelling on conjunctival side of eyelid.
2. Tenderness at site of infection.
3. Burning, smarting feeling in eye.
4. Feeling of something in the eye.
5. Tearing.
6. Redness, pain, and swelling with appearance of small, hard, red boil at base of eyelash.

NURSING DIAGNOSES: ACTUAL OR POTENTIAL

Pain and swelling of lid margin.

EXPECTED OUTCOMES

1. Pain will be reduced with decreased inflammation.
2. Rupture or resolution of sty will take place in 7 to 10 days.

INTERVENTIONS

1. Instruct client to use warm, moist compresses for 15 min, three to four times a day.
2. An antibiotic ointment may be appropriate to prevent spread of infection.

EVALUATION

Outcome Criteria

Resolution of pain, inflammation, and swelling is accomplished.

CHALAZION

DESCRIPTION

Chalazion is an inflammation with lipogranuloma involving the meibomian gland and the sebaceous eyelid gland. (It often occurrs during pregnancy.)

ASSESSMENT

1. In the acute stage, the assessment is similar to the assessment of a sty.
2. In the later stages, there is a hard, painless lump or cyst on the inner aspect of the eyelid that may continue to increase in size.

NURSING DIAGNOSES: ACTUAL OR POTENTIAL

Pain and swelling at lid margin.

EXPECTED OUTCOMES

Refer to *Hordeolum*.

INTERVENTIONS

1. In the early stage, warm, moist compresses and antibiotic ointments are given.
2. In the later stages, excision by an ophthalmologist may be necessary.

EVALUATION

Outcome Criteria

There is resolution of inflammation and swelling.

DACRYOCYSTITIS

DESCRIPTION

Dacryocystitis is an infection of the lacrimal sac, usually caused by an obstruction of one of the tear canals that lead into the nose.

ASSESSMENT

Physical Assessment

1. Pain and swelling over lacrimal sac.
2. Redness and tenderness below the eye; may extend to the eyelids.
3. Profuse tearing.
4. Purulent discharge.

NURSING DIAGNOSES: ACTUAL OR POTENTIAL

Pain: secondary to obstruction and inflammation of lacrimal duct.

EXPECTED OUTCOMES

1. Inflammation, infection, and obstruction will be reduced in 5 to 7 days with symptomatic treatment and antibiotics.
2. Spread to cornea will be prevented.
3. Patent tear duct with normal tearing will be restored.

INTERVENTIONS

1. Frequent application of hot compresses.
2. Antibiotics may be prescribed.
3. Surgery may be necessary to open a new channel into the nose or to drain an abscess.

EVALUATION

Outcome Criteria

Tear duct is patent.

Complications

1. Spread of infection to cornea.
2. Unresolved obstruction requiring surgical correction.

CONJUNCTIVITIS

DESCRIPTION

Conjunctivitis is an inflammation of the conjunctiva, often caused by bacteria, viruses, allergies, or exposure to irritating chemicals. Classifications may be based on cause, type of exudate, and acute or chronic course of pathology.

ASSESSMENT

Health History

1. History of inflammation or exposure to others with infection.
2. Usually insidious onset, with irritation and exudation.
3. Itching and burning sensation.
4. Blurred vision; feeling that something is in the eyes.

Physcial Assessment

1. Tearing and reddened eye.
2. Serous or purulent discharge.
3. Swollen eyelids.
4. Periauricular adenopathy usually accompanied by pharyngitis.
5. Normal iris, cornea, and pupils.

Diagnostic Tests

Culture and Gram's stain of exudate.

EXPECTED OUTCOMES

1. Inflammation will be reduced within 3 to 5 days.
2. Spread of contamination to other eye or to other people will be prevented.

INTERVENTIONS

1. Warm compresses qid for 15 min.
2. Antibiotic drops.
3. Sulfonamides or steroid drops may be prescribed.
4. Hygienic measures include:
   a. Frequent handwashing.
   b. Separate toweling for infected eye.
   c. No touching or rubbing of eye.

EVALUATION

Outcome Criteria

Inflammatory process is resolved.

KERATITIS

DESCRIPTION

Keratitis is an inflammation of the cornea. *Superficial keratitis* is caused by infection from the external environment. *Deep keratitis* is caused by the spread of an etiological agent through the circulatory system or from neighboring eye structures. It is often caused by viral and/or bacterial infections and is less frequently associated with tuberculosis, syphilis, and other systemic infections.

ASSESSMENT

Health History

1. Photophobia.
2. Impaired vision, blurring, and cloudiness.

Physical Assessment

1. Dilatation of blood vessels around cornea.
2. A cloudy appearance of cornea.
3. Tearing.
4. Increased sensitivity to light.

NURSING DIAGNOSES: ACTUAL OR POTENTIAL

Alteration in vision.

EXPECTED OUTCOMES

1. Inflammation will be reduced.
2. Vision will be restored.

INTERVENTIONS

Immediate use of antibiotics, occasionally cortisone, is necessary.

EVALUATION

Outcome Criteria

Normal visual acuity returns after inflammatory process resolves.

Complications

Scarring of cornea secondary to infectious process.

CORNEAL ULCER

DESCRIPTION

A corneal ulcer arises from loss of corneal epithelium resulting from extension of conjunctivitis to cornea, corneal inflammation, or direct corneal trauma. The pathological organisms involved may be bacterial, viral, or fungal.

ASSESSMENT

Health History

1. History of corneal abrasion.
2. Corneal pain.
3. Photophobia.
4. Tearing.

Physical Assessment

1. Bloodshot appearance to eye.
2. Involvement of iris: purulent discharge and white or yellow deposits behind cornea.
3. Perforated corneal ulcer: prolapse of iris through cornea.
4. Opacity of part or all of cornea.

Diagnostic Tests

1. Culture of corneal swab.
2. Visualization of ulcers with fluorescein or rose bengal corneal stain.

NURSING DIAGNOSES: ACTUAL OR POTENTIAL

1. Alteration in comfort: pain secondary to corneal inflammation or trauma.
2. Alteration in vision: secondary to tearing and photophobia.

EXPECTED OUTCOMES

1. Immediate.
   a. Prevention or resolution of infection will be accomplished with organism-specific antibiotic eyedrops.
   b. Positive agent or accompanying condition will be removed.
   c. Comfort will be promoted.
2. Preoperative for corneal transplant.
   a. Client anxiety will be allayed during waiting period for donor.
   b. Increase of pressure and strain on the eye will be avoided.
3. Postoperative.
   a. Healing will be promoted.
   b. Anxieties will be reduced while awaiting results of surgery.

INTERVENTIONS

1. Immediate.
   a. Patch the eye with corneal abrasion. Regeneration of epithelium occurs in 24–48 h.
   b. Remove foreign bodies.
   c. Instruct client to wear dark glasses.
   d. Administer mydriatics.
   e. Follow examination of eye with medication for relief of pain.
   f. Give antibiotics for specific types of infection.
   g. Apply warm compresses.
   h. Give systemic antibiotics, if appropriate.
   i. Steroid therapy may be prescribed for secondary fungal infections if present.
   j. Corneal transplanatation involves a split-thickness (lamellar keratoplasty) or full-thickness (penetrating keratoplasty) transplant with fresh donor tissue to replace damaged cornea.
2. Postoperative.
   a. Cover both eyes to ensure total rest.
   b. Prepare client for possible failure (88 percent of cases are successful).
   c. Instruct client to wear protective shield over eye for a minimum of 6 weeks after discharge.
   d. Instruct client regarding activities to ensure protection of eyes during healing period.
   e. Assess visual acuity after healing is complete, within 3 to 6 months.

EVALUATION

Outcome Criteria

Ulcer heals with no scar and vision is restored.

Complications

1. Corneal scarring requiring transplant.
2. Rejection of corneal transplant.

UVEITIS

DESCRIPTION

Uveitis is an inflammatory condition of the uveal tract (pigmented vascular layer of the eye including iris, ciliary body, and choroid). If only the iris and ciliary body are involved, the condition is called *iridocyclitis.* When the choroid is involved, the retina will be involved also because of the close proximity of the two structures. This condition is called *chorioretinitis.* Uveitis is a unilateral disease that affects young and middle-aged people. It may be caused by the spread of viral, bacterial, or fungal infection from other structures of the eyes, parasitic invasion, systemic disease, focal infection, or allergic response.

ASSESSMENT: IRIS

Health History

1. Pain (may radiate to temple).
2. Photophobia.

Physical Assessment

1. Sluggish pupil response to light.
2. Irregularly shaped pupil, often constricted.
3. Blurred vision.

Diagnostic Tests

See Assessment: Choroid, below.

ASSESSMENT: CHOROID

Health History

See Assessment: Iris, above.

Physical Assessment

1. Yellowish white lesions on retina.
2. Visual loss in peripheral fields corresponding to lesion locations.
3. Possible decrease in central acuity.

Diagnostic Tests

1. Skin tests to rule out tuberculosis, histoplasmosis, and toxoplasmosis.
2. Tonometry to rule out glaucoma.

NURSING DIAGNOSES: ACTUAL OR POTENTIAL

1. Ocular pain.
2. Diminished vision.

EXPECTED OUTCOMES

1. Conditions with similar symptoms will be ruled out.
2. Inflammation will be reduced.
3. Loss of sight will be prevented by early diagnosis and treatment.
4. Progression to glaucoma will be prevented.
5. Pain will be relieved.
6. Vision will be restored.

INTERVENTIONS

1. Use warm compresses, coating, and/or aspirin.
2. Instruct client to wear dark glasses.
3. Corticosteroids are prescribed early in course of treatment and for recurrence of inflammation.

EVALUATION

Outcome Criteria

1. Symptoms are resolved.
2. Visual acuity is restored.

Complications

1. Development of glaucoma.
2. Permanent loss of vision.

CATARACTS

DESCRIPTION

Cataracts result from slowly growing opaqueness of the eye lens, usually accompanying the aging process, diabetes, eye infection or, rarely, exposure to chemical or physical poisons or secondary to trauma or systemic disease.

ASSESSMENT

Health History

Gradual or painless loss of sight.

Physical Assessment

1. Increased opaqueness of lens with aging or secondary to trauma.
2. Distorted or blurred vision.
3. Irritation from glaring or bright lights.
4. In the later stage, gray or milky white appearance to lens.

NURSING DIAGNOSES: ACTUAL OR POTENTIAL

Gradual blurring and loss of vision.

EXPECTED OUTCOMES

1. Immediate.
   a. Optimal vision will be maintained with periodic refractive correction with glasses.
   b. Client will be reassured and provided with information concerning progression and option of surgery. (Cataract formation is irreversible.)
2. Preoperative.
   a. Comfort and safety will be maintained.
   b. Any infection will be treated.

c. Surgical procedure and postoperative care will be explained.
d. Secondary development of glaucoma will be prevented.
3. Postoperative.
a. Hemorrhage and loss of vitreous humor will be prevented.
b. Increased intraocular pressure will be prevented.
c. Comfort and safety will be maintained.
d. Infection will be prevented.
e. Rehabilitation activities will be planned.

INTERVENTIONS

1. Surgical removal will be performed at appropriate stage of condition, determined by maturation of cataract, occupation, and patient's general health.
2. Preoperative.
a. Provide safety precautions for client's reduced vision. Orient client to surrounding environment by having objects within reach and consistently in same place.
b. Instruct client and family regarding surgery.
c. Administer antibiotics and take conjunctival cultures as prescribed.
d. Instruct client not to touch eyes.
e. Administer mydriatics before surgery, if prescribed.
3. Postoperative.
a. Instruct client to:
(1) Avoid coughing or sneezing.
(2) Avoid rapid movements.
(3) Avoid bending from the waist.
b. Give analgesics for relief of pain.
c. Provide a quiet and safe environment.
d. Notify physician if sudden pain occurs (may be indicative of hemorrhage or ruptured suture).
e. Treat nausea and vomiting immediately.
f. Assist client with early ambulatory activities and perceptual changes from lens removal.
g. Instruct client and family on administration of eyedrops, use of dark glasses, and fitting for corrective lenses.

EVALUATION

Outcome Criteria

1. Cataract is removed and sight is restored with corrective lenses.
2. Client successfully adapts to vision change with planned rehabilitation.

Complications

Postoperative infection or hemorrhage.

GLAUCOMA

DESCRIPTION

Glaucoma is caused by increased intraocular pressure due to increased production of aqueous humor and/or decreased outflow of aqueous humor, occurring in approximately 2 percent of the population over 40 years of age (refer to Nursing Care of the Aged for a discussion of glaucoma in relation to the aged). There are two types of glaucoma in the adult: *acute or chronic congestive glaucoma* (narrow angle) and *chronic simple glaucoma* (open angle). See Figure 26-4 for the route of normal flow of aqueous humor. The increased intraocular pressure causes optic nerve atrophy with loss of vision.

ACUTE (NARROW-ANGLE) GLAUCOMA

DESCRIPTION

In acute (narrow-angle) glaucoma, a dilated or displaced iris prevents drainage of aqueous humor into the canal of Schlemm. This disorder may be an inherited trait.

ASSESSMENT

Health History

1. Severe pain, often unilateral, after prolonged exposure to darkness or with pupil dilation.
2. Cloudy and blurred vision.
3. Progressive (may be rapid) diminution of vision.

Physical Assessment

1. Dilated nonreactive pupils.
2. Nausea and vomiting.
3. Artificial lights around objects.
4. Increased intraocular pressure greater than 18 mmHg.

NURSING DIAGNOSES: ACTUAL OR POTENTIAL

1. Ocular pain with increased intraocular pressure.
2. Loss of visual acuity.

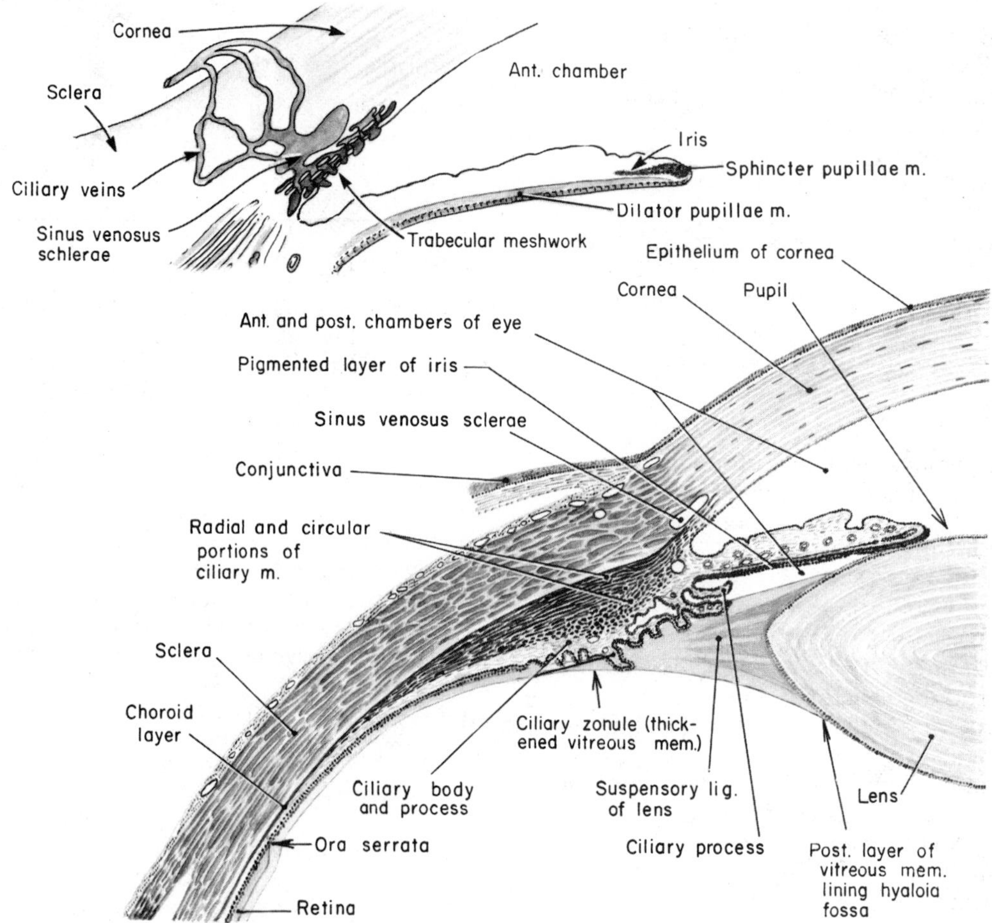

Figure 26-4 Normal circulation of aqueous humor. (From Crafts, R. C., *A Textbook of Human Anatomy*, 2d ed., John Wiley & Sons, Inc., New York, 1979, used with permission.)

EXPECTED OUTCOMES

1. Increasing intraocular pressure will be prevented or reduced.
2. Pain will be controlled.
3. Permanent blindness will be prevented.

INTERVENTIONS

1. Parasympathomimetic drugs are prescribed for miotic action (to draw iris away from cornea for facilitation of drainage of aqueous humor).
2. Eyedrops should not be used as they may increase severity of condition.
3. Treatment needs to be done immediately to prevent permanent blindness.
4. Surgical intervention may be necessary to restore proper drainage.

EVALUATION

Outcome Criteria

Vision is restored, and normal intraocular pressures are maintained.

Complications

Loss of vision.

CHRONIC (OPEN-ANGLE) GLAUCOMA

DESCRIPTION

In chronic (open-angle) glaucoma the intraocular pressure increases over a prolonged period of time, accompanied by cupping and atrophy of the optic disc.

ASSESSMENT

Health History

1. Symptoms usually after 35 years of age.
2. More frequent in near-sighted individuals.
3. Early phase: no symptoms.
4. Tired feeling in eyes.
5. Halos or rainbows around electric lights.
6. Poor night vision.

Physical Assessment

1. Increased intraocular pressure greater than 18 mmHg.
2. Blind spots, slow diminution of peripheral vision.

NURSING DIAGNOSES: ACUTAL OR POTENTIAL

Progressive loss of vision.

EXPECTED OUTCOMES

1. Permanent loss of vision will be prevented if condition is diagnosed early.
2. Compliance with medication will facilitate flow from anterior chamber and decrease formation of acqueous humor.

INTERVENTIONS

1. Miotic eyedrops are prescribed; may cause difficulty seeing in dim light.
2. Close observation is necessary to determine if disease is controlled, along with periodic eye examinations and visual field testing.
3. Surgical intervention may be necessary for proper drainage of aqueous humor.
4. Instruct client to avoid conditions that will increase intraocular pressure, such as:
   a. Emotional stress.
   b. Wearing tight clothing around waist or neck.
   c. Heavy exertion.
   d. Upper respiratory infections.

EVALUATION

Outcome Criteria

1. Intraocular pressure is controlled with medication.
2. Vision is maintained.

Complications

Loss of vision.

DETACHED RETINA

DESCRIPTION

A detached retina is the painless separation of the retina from the choroid. It may be partial at first but may then progress to a complete separation if it is not treated properly. Detachment of the retina is usually due to a break in the retina through which aqueous humor flows into the space between the retina and choroid, producing the separation.

ASSESSMENT

Health History

1. Flashes of light, occasionally followed by a sensation of a curtain drawn across the visual field.
2. Blurred vision.
3. Sensation of particles or dots floating in visual field.
4. Progressive loss of vision.

Physical Assessment

Blind spots.

NURSING DIAGNOSES: ACTUAL OR POTENTIAL

Sudden partial or complete unilateral blindness.

EXPECTED OUTCOMES

1. Preoperative.
   a. Permanent vision loss will be prevented.
   b. Anxiety will be allayed.
   c. Comfort will be maintained.
   d. Surgical intervention will reattach retina.
2. Postoperative.
   a. Retinal reattachment will be maintained.
   b. Permanent visual loss will be prevented.
   c. Comfort will be maintained.
   d. Anxiety will be reduced.

INTERVENTIONS

1. Preoperative.
   a. See that client stays in bed with eyes bandaged.

b. Maintain appropriate head position for area of detachment according to physician's preference.
c. Give support, sedation, and/or tranquilizers to comfort and to allay anxiety.

2. Surgical intervention involves repairing the separation between retina and choroid via:
   a. Diathermy.
   b. Cryosurgery.
   c. Scleral buckling.
   d. Photocoagulation.
   e. Vitrectomy.
3. Postoperative.
   a. Ensure that client stays in bed with eyes bandaged until flattening of retina occurs.
   b. See that safety precautions are observed in client's environment so that client avoids bumping head or making sudden movements.
   c. Supervise client's orientation to immediate surroundings and environment.
   d. Apply cold compresses to relieve local edema; remove crusts and discharge with sterile saline or H_2O with bandage change.
   e. Encourage diversional activities.
   f. Assist client as ambulation progresses.
   g. Support client through waiting period to determine effect of surgery.
   h. Instruct client to limit activity for approximately 6 weeks after surgery.

EVALUATION

Outcome Criteria

Partial or full vision is restored.

Complications

Progressive retinal detachment with loss of vision.

OPTIC NEURITIS

DESCRIPTION

Optic neuritis is an inflammation of the optic nerve resulting from syphilis, acute infectious disease, multiple sclerosis, toxicity, or vitamin B deficiency.

ASSESSMENT

Health History

1. Sudden loss of vision, including blind spots and narrowing of visual field, that may be insidious or acute in onset.
2. Pain with eyeball movement.
3. Loss of color vision.

Physical Assessment

1. Swollen retina.
2. Bleeding from the retina.

NURSING DIAGNOSES: ACTUAL OR POTENTIAL

Loss of vision.

EXPECTED OUTCOMES

1. Signs and symptoms of visual loss will be relieved.
2. Recurrence will be prevented.
3. The underlying cause will be treated.
4. Permanent loss of sight will be prevented.

INTERVENTIONS

1. Immediate steroid therapy.
2. Vitamin B replacement.
3. Treatment of contributing systemic disorders.

EVALUATION

Outcome Criteria

Vision is restored.

Complications

Optic nerve atrophy with permanent loss of vision.

MALIGNANT MELANOMA

DESCRIPTION

Malignant melanoma is the most common malignant intraocular tumor developing in the uveal tract, usually in the choroid, that affects individuals in middle age. It is usually unilateral. (Refer to Chapter 31 for a more complete discussion.)

ASSESSMENT

1. Iris: altered color of iris and size of pupil.
2. Choroid: retinal detachment and sudden pigmented neoplasm in outer layers of choroid or gradual loss of vision.
3. Pain if tumor is large and causing increased intraocular pressure (glaucoma).
4. Macular: blurring of central vision.

NURSING DIAGNOSES: ACTUAL OR POTENTIAL

Gradual or sudden loss of vision.

EXPECTED OUTCOMES

1. Tumor will be removed by ablation or enucleation.
2. Preoperative and postoperative care will be provided according to intervention chosen.
3. Client and family will be supported through progression of diagnosis and treatment.

INTERVENTIONS

1. Photocoagulation or radiation of small lesions.
2. Enucleation of large tumors.
3. Iridectomy when tumor is limited to small portion of iris.
4. Continued evaluation for tumor recurrence.

EVALUATION

Outcome Criteria

All of tumor is removed, with partial loss of vision.

Complications

Progressive growth of tumor with visual loss and metastasis.

EYE DISORDERS RESULTING FROM USE OF TOBACCO AND ALCOHOL

DESCRIPTION

Excessive and/or combined use of alcohol and tobacco may cause vision changes or loss of vision.

ASSESSMENT

Health History

1. Chronic use of alcohol and tobacco.
2. Progressive loss of vision.

Physical Assessment

1. Blind spots in central vision.
2. Disturbances of color vision (especially red and green).
3. Eye muscle palsies.
4. Optic nerve involvement with visual loss.

NURSING DIAGNOSES: ACTUAL OR POTENTIAL

Loss of central and color vision.

EXPECTED OUTCOMES

1. Use of alcohol and tobacco will be decreased or eliminated.
2. Permanent loss of vision will be prevented.

INTERVENTIONS

1. Provide client with information regarding cause and the effects.
2. Encourage a decrease or elimination of tobacco and alcohol.
3. Encourage a balanced diet.

EVALUATION

Outcome Criteria

1. Use of alcohol and tobacco is decreased and eliminated.
2. There is no further loss of vision.

EYE DISORDERS RESULTING FROM USE OF COMMON DRUGS

DESCRIPTION

The occurrence of visual symptoms or loss of vision associated with the utilization of selected common drugs.

ASSESSMENT

1. Aspirin: retinal hemorrhages.
2. Chloroquine: retinal degeneration.
3. Cortisone.
   a. Symptoms of cataracts.
   b. Symptoms of open-angle glaucoma.
4. Digitalis.
   a. Seeing snowflakes or rainbows in visual fields.
   b. Yellow vision.
5. Ethambutol.
   a. Reduced visual acuity.
   b. Reduced green color vision.
6. Tranquilizers.
   a. Blurred or double vision.
   b. Other symptoms of glaucoma.
7. Medications occasionally used for diarrhea:

gall bladder disturbances, Parkinson's disease, motion sickness, gout, and hypertension may also cause eye reactions.

NURSING DIAGNOSES: ACTUAL OR POTENTIAL

Occurrence of symptoms in association with use of specific drugs.

EXPECTED OUTCOMES

1. Associated visual disturbances will be identified.
2. Use of medication will be decreased or eliminated.

INTERVENTIONS

1. Evaluate for visual disturbance.
2. Consult with physician regarding dose reduction or medication change.

EVALUATION

Outcome Criteria

Change or loss of vision is controlled or prevented.

EYE DISORDERS SECONDARY TO SYSTEMIC DISEASES

HYPERTENSIVE AND RENAL RETINOPATHY

DESCRIPTION

Vascular pathology of the retinal vessels that occurs with chronic hypertension and renal disease. See Chapters 30 and 32 for a discussion of hypertension and renal pathology.

ASSESSMENT

Health History

History of chronic hypertension or renal disease.

Physical Assessment

1. Narrowing of retinal arterioles.
2. Increase in capillary permeability with resultant retinal edema, exudates, hemorrhage, and papilledema (refer to Table 26-2 for grades of retinopathy).

NURSING DIAGNOSES: ACTUAL OR POTENTIAL

Impaired vision secondary to retinopathy.

PREVENTION

Health Promotion

1. Provision of information regarding high risk for retinopathy.
2. Periodic funduscopic examination.
3. Compliance with prescribed medical treatment.

EXPECTED OUTCOMES

1. Effect of underlying disease will be reduced.
2. Permanent loss of vision will be prevented.

INTERVENTIONS

1. There is no known ophthalmological treatment for hypertensive retinopathy.
2. Treatment has to be directed toward management of hypertension and chronic glomerulonephritis.

EVALUATION

Outcome Criteria

Vision is maintained through periodic screening and management of underlying disease.

RHEUMATOID ARTHRITIS

DESCRIPTION

See Chapter 27 for a discussion of rheumatoid arthritis.

ASSESSMENT

Health History

1. Episcleritis.
2. Iritis and iridocyclitis.
3. Relapses of symptoms accompanying exacerbation of arthritis.

INTERVENTIONS

1. There is no known satisfactory ophthalmological treatment.
2. Provide supportive measures for client.

TABLE 26-2 GRADES OF RETINOPATHY

Grade	Diabetic Retinopathy	Hypertensive Retinopathy
1	Microaneurysms Dilation of veins	Arteriole narrowing
2	The above plus small distinct exudates	Above plus depression of vein with arteriole crossing (AV nicking)
3	All the above plus cotton wool patches	Cotton wool patches, hemorrhages, exudates silver wire arterioles, severe AV nicking
4	All the above plus small hemorrhages	Above plus papilledema
5	All the above plus new blood vessels and fibrous tissue	

LUPUS ERYTHEMATOSUS

DESCRIPTION

See Chapter 32 for a discussion of lupus erythematosus. Most common ocular involvement is exudates and optic neuritis, although cornea, retina, and sclera may also be inflamed. More common during acute stages of disease.

ASSESSMENT

1. Retinopathy with exudates and hemorrhage.
2. Nystagmus.
3. Occlusion of central retinal artery with loss of vision.

EXPECTED OUTCOMES

Supportive management will be given for complications of underlying disease.

INTERVENTIONS

No known specific ophthalmologic treatment.

ANEMIA

DESCRIPTION

See Chapter 29 for a discussion of anemia.

ASSESSMENT

1. Retinal hemorrhage.
2. A decrease in RBC count (to less than 50 percent of normal).
3. Visual loss if hemorrhage involves macula.

EXPECTED OUTCOMES

1. Permanent vision loss will be prevented.
2. Underlying disease process will be treated.

INTERVENTIONS

Treat anemic process (see Chapter 29 for discussion of anemia).

DISORDERS OF TASTE AND SMELL

HYPOGEUSIA OR AGEUSIA

DESCRIPTION

Disorders of taste may arise from CNS disorders, including lesions of the thalamus or parietal lobe with contralateral loss of taste. Medications, smoking, and alcohol use may diminish or alter taste as well as dental disease, metabolic disturbances of the liver, thyroid, or kidneys, and psychological depression. The VIIth and IXth cranial nerves mediate taste. Loss of smell will also significantly decrease taste.

ASSESSMENT

Health History

1. Alcohol abuse.
2. Smoking.
3. Dental disease.

4. Injury to the VIIth or IXth cranial nerve from trauma, surgery, or disease.
5. Use of drugs, particularly tricyclic antidepressants.
6. Occurrences of olfactory hallucinations in conjunction with other neurological symptoms, including vertigo, tinnitus, or memory loss.

Physical Assessment

1. Inspection of nose, ears, mouth, tongue, and teeth for lesions.
2. Drying of tongue with sloughing of cells.
3. Examination of smell acuity.
4. Taste evaluation with sweet, salty, bitter, and sour stimulants. The VIIth cranial nerve mediates the taste of the anterior two-thirds of the tongue, with the IXth mediating the posterior third.

NURSING DIAGNOSES: ACTUAL OR POTENTIAL

Decrease or loss of taste sensation.

EXPECTED OUTCOMES

1. There will be early diagnosis and treatment of symptoms.
2. Adequate nutritional intake will be maintained.

INTERVENTIONS

1. Encourage client to:
   a. Stop smoking.
   b. Reduce alcohol consumption.
   c. Reduce or alter medication.
2. Refer client for treatment of dental disease.
3. Refer client for medical evaluation with positive cranial nerve findings.
4. Provide education regarding nutrition maintenance when food does not satisfy taste.

EVALUATION

Outcome Criteria

1. Contributing disorders are being effectively treated.
2. Taste sensation is restored.
3. Nutrition is maintained.

ANOSMIA, PAROSMIA, AND HYPOSMIA

DESCRIPTION

The most common cause of anosmia (loss of smell), parosmia (perversion of smell), or hyposmia (reduced smell) is obstruction of the nasal passages, as occurs when the common cold or allergic rhinitis prevents air from reaching the olfactory receptors high in the nasal mucosa. Permanent loss of smell may be precipitated by chronic infection, influenza, or head trauma. Meningiomas and anterior cerebral aneurysms reduce smell with a more gradual progression as the lesions expand. Hysteria should be considered in the absence of other pathology.

ASSESSMENT

Health History

1. Congestion of nares in association with nasal infection, allergy, or influenza.
2. Head trauma, headaches, or visual disturbances.
3. Emotional disturbances.

Physical Assessment

1. Observation of nares for polyps, inflammation, deviated septum, trauma, or discharge.
2. Transillumination of the sinuses.
3. Evaluation of smell acuity with sweet and pungent odors.

Diagnostic Tests

Sinus and skull x-ray films.

NURSING DIAGNOSES: ACTUAL OR POTENTIAL

Decrease or loss of smell acuity.

EXPECTED OUTCOMES

1. There will be early diagnosis and treatment of primary disorder.
2. Smell acuity will be restored.

INTERVENTIONS

1. Fluids, rest, and decongestants for common cold, allergy, or influenza.
2. Antibiotic therapy for infectious conditions.

3. Removal of polyps.
4. Anosmia may be permanent if receptor cells are damaged.

EVALUATION

Outcome Criteria

1. Contributing abnormality is successfully treated.
2. Smell acuity is restored.

DISORDERS OF SENSATION

DESCRIPTION

Disorders of sensation occur when an aberrant sensation is produced in response to a normal stimulus. The sensations may be diminished (hypalgesia), lost (anesthesia), altered or increased (dysesthesia), or morbid or perverted (paresthesia). Many different abnormalities will produce changes in sensation, and lesions may be located at any level of the sensory pathway, including peripheral nerves, spinal cord, thalamus, or cerebral cortex. Symptoms may be symmetrical or asymmetrical and acute or chronic in occurrence.

POLYNEUROPATHY

DESCRIPTION

Polyneuropathy is a pathological process involving many nerve trunks simultaneously, as compared with the more isolated mononeuropathy that involves a single nerve trunk. Both sensory and motor functions may be impaired, with sensory disturbance being acute, subacute, or chronic. Commonly associated conditions include diabetes mellitus, poisoning, alcoholism, vitamin B complex deficiency, and infectious syndromes (hepatitis, Landry-Guillain-Barré) (see Table 26-3). Recovery of nerve function may be incomplete and may require a year or longer. (See Chapter 25 for a detailed discussion of neuropathy disorders.)

ASSESSMENT

Health History

1. Recent illness, for the past 3 to 4 weeks.
2. Character of symptoms: tingling, numbness, pain.

TABLE 26-3 COMMON POLYNEUROPATHIES

Onset	Condition	Distribution	Sensory Change
Acute, usually following an infection	Guillain-Barré Hepatitis Mononucleosis	Distal and proximal limbs and trunk	Numbness and tingling Asymmetrical pain (ascending motor paralysis)
Chronic, over a few months	Alcoholism Vitamin B deficiencies Drug toxicity	Begins distally, progressing to hands and arms	Tingling and numbness Pain and muscle weakness Diminished touch, vibration, and position sense (decreased ankle jerk)
Chronic, over a few years	Diabetes mellitus Hypothyroidism	Symmetrically in feet and legs	Numbness and tingling Decreased ankle jerk Paraesthesias with autonomic disturbance of bowel and bladder in juvenile diabetes

3. Nature of onset and progression of symptoms differentiates cause.
4. Symmetrical or asymmetrical distribution of symptoms.
5. Patterns of exacerbations and remissions of relief.
6. Exposure to toxins.
7. Drug or alcohol use.
8. Dietary intake.

Physical Assessment

1. Evaluation of cranial and peripheral nerves.
2. Map areas of sensory involvement.
3. Evaluation of associated muscle weakness, atrophy, tremor, or spasticity.

Diagnostic Tests

1. Radiological evaluation.
2. Blood and spinal fluid analysis.
3. Electromyography and nerve conduction studies.

NURSING DIAGNOSES: ACTUAL OR POTENTIAL

Change or loss of sensation that may be general or localized and may last for a year or longer with the potential of incomplete recovery.

EXPECTED OUTCOMES

1. There will be diagnosis and treatment with early onset of symptoms.
2. Injury due to sensory deficit will be prevented.
3. Sensory function will be restored, depending on degree of nerve damage.

INTERVENTIONS

1. Control or treat primary disease.
2. Administer dietary and vitamin supplements.
3. Teach client safety measures, that is, to test for hot water, wear protective clothing, inspect skin routinely for trauma, take care in using sharp objects, systematically evaluate if sensation is harmful or safe.
4. Support client with psychological adaptation to function loss by providing information and answering questions, teaching methods of maintaining safety and managing dysfunction, and involving family and friends as resources.

EVALUATION

Outcome Criteria

1. Sensory status is evaluated in regard to treatment response or disease progression every 2 or 3 months.
2. Lifestyle is changed as appropriate for protection of remaining function and prevention of injury.

TABETIC SYNDROME

DESCRIPTION

Tabetic syndrome usually occurs up to 20 years after syphilitic infection and is caused by *Treponema pallidum* or, more rarely, by diabetes mellitus or tumors. The sensory disorder includes loss of proprioception (position sense) with ataxia and a stamping gait and sensations of pain and numbness.

PREVENTION

Health Promotion

1. Avoidance of sexual partners with venereal disease.
2. Sex education regarding prevention and risks of contacting venereal disease.
3. Immediate medical evaluation and treatment if contact suspected.

Population at Risk

People with multiple sexual contacts.

Screening

Serologic examination.

ASSESSMENT

Health History

History of syphilis at a younger age.

Physical Assessment

1. Loss of joint position sense and deep tendon reflexes.
2. Ataxic or staggering gait.
3. Sensation of "shooting pains," pins and needles, numbness, or heat or coldness in leg, or more commonly in feet and legs, and various body parts including abdomen.
4. Loss of bowel or bladder sensation with constipation or incontinence.

5. Swollen joints (Charcot's joints) and skin lesions from multiple trauma due to ataxia and change of sensation.

Diagnostic Tests

1. History of untreated syphilis.
2. Serologic examination of spinal fluid.
3. Clinical presentation of associated neurological symptoms.

NURSING DIAGNOSES: ACTUAL OR POTENTIAL

1. Alteration in sensory functions.
2. Disordered mobility due to sensory deficit.

EXPECTED OUTCOMES

1. Occurrence will be prevented with education and early treatment.
2. Primary disorders will be diagnosed and treated.
3. Client will be protected from physical injury.

INTERVENTIONS

1. Provide or refer client for sex education regarding risks of venereal disease and need for early diagnosis and treatment.
2. Administer penicillin as early treatment of syphilis.
3. Maintain a safe environment by removing objects that may cause tripping or falling.
4. Inspect skin and joints routinely for trauma.
5. Encourage follow-up evaluation after early diagnosis and treatment.

EVALUATION

Outcome Criteria

Symptoms may be relieved with treatment.

TRIGEMINAL NEURALGIA

DESCRIPTION

Trigeminal neuralgia (tic douloureux) is an excruciatingly painful condition involving the sensory component of the Vth cranial nerve. Most clients are middle to older age. The cause is usually unknown.

ASSESSMENT

Health History

1. There may be no significant health history.
2. Sudden onset of unilateral pain radiating over jaw, gum, lips, and maxillary area corresponding to second and third divisions of trigeminal nerve.
3. Attack may be precipitated by stimulation of "trigger zone" by cold draft or touching or may be spontaneous and occur during sleep.
4. Attack may last from seconds to minutes and then subside but recur in paroxysms for weeks or months.
5. No symptoms between attacks.

Physical Assessment

Usually no significant findings.

NURSING DIAGNOSES: ACTUAL OR POTENTIAL

1. Spontaneous severe facial pain.
2. Fear of activities that may precipitate pain, for example, chewing, exposure to cold air, and brushing teeth.

EXPECTED OUTCOMES

1. Occurrence of pain will be prevented.
2. Normal activity and nutrition will be maintained.

INTERVENTIONS

1. Instruct client to avoid stimuli that precipitate attack.
2. Tegretol (carbamazepine), Dilantin, or a combination of the two may provide relief. Instruct client to watch for side effects of drugs. Usual analgesics may not be effective.
3. If medications are not successful, alcohol or phenol blocks or surgical approaches may be tried. Surgery results in a permanent sensory deficit.
4. Assure client that attacks may be self-limiting and controlled in order to relieve fear of attack and promote normal activity.
5. Teach importance of maintaining nutrition and eating during periods of remission if fear of pain prevents normal food intake.

EVALUATION

Outcome Criteria

1. Pain is relieved without recurrence.
2. Side effects of drug treatment are avoided.
3. Normal activity and nutrition are maintained.

THALAMIC SYNDROME

DESCRIPTION

Thalamic syndrome occurs when lesions in the sensory relay nuclei of the thalamus cause loss of sensation on the opposite side of the body.

ASSESSMENT

Health History

1. Symptoms may be aggravated by heightened emotions or diminished by sleep or distraction.
2. Occurrence is characterized by radiation of unpleasant, poorly localized sensations during later stages of the disorder.

Physical Assessment

1. Loss of sensation may be predominantly pain and temperature or proprioception, touch, and vibration on the opposite side from lesion.
2. If proprioception is disturbed, ataxia and astereognosis will be evident.

Diagnostic Tests

X-rays and angiography for tumors or vascular lesions.

NURSING DIAGNOSES: ACTUAL OR POTENTIAL

1. Sensory-perceptual alterations.
2. Potential injury from sensory alteration or loss.

EXPECTED OUTCOMES

1. Primary disease will be identified.
2. Exacerbation of symptoms will be prevented.
3. Sensory function will be restored.

INTERVENTIONS

1. Treat primary disease.
2. Encourage client to avoid situations producing extreme emotions that are known to increase symptoms.
3. Maintain safety and prevent trauma from loss of sensation. (See Interventions under *Polyneuropathy*.)

EVALUATION

Outcome Criteria

1. Sensory function is restored.
2. The client adapts to permanent sensory loss with routine safety precautions.

PARIETAL SYNDROME

DESCRIPTION

Parietal (cortical) syndrome occurs because of lesions in the parietal cortex and is usually not as clearly defined as lesions of the lower sensory pathways.

ASSESSMENT

Health History

Inability to discriminate objects with hand opposite the side of the lesion.

Physical Assessment

1. Loss of fine discrimination, including position sense and two-point discrimination with astereognosis on opposite side of body.
2. Sensations of touch and temperature may not be affected.

Diagnostic Tests

1. Angiography may reveal obstructive vascular lesions.
2. Radiography may demonstrate tumor near parietal cortex.

NURSING DIAGNOSES: ACTUAL OR POTENTIAL

1. Sensory perceptual alteration.
2. Potential injury from sensory alteration.

EXPECTED OUTCOMES

See *Thalamic Syndrome*.

INTERVENTIONS

See *Thalamic Syndrome*.

EVALUATION

See *Thalamic Syndrome.*

PAIN SYNDROMES

CAUSALGIA

DESCRIPTION

Causalgia is constant and severe pain often accompanied by burning following partial or complete transection of a peripheral nerve and may be due to hyperactivity of the remaining pain and temperature fibers. Usually the median, ulnar, or sciatic nerves are involved.

ASSESSMENT

Health History

1. Trauma to the ulnar, medial, or sciatic nerves, usually above the knee or elbow and commonly from a bullet wound.
2. Immediate onset of pain with trauma or within a few days.
3. Pain is burning and located at the periphery of the extremity and is most excruciating in the fingers, toes, palms, or soles of feet.
4. A significant number of clients also describe deep tearing, throbbing pain in the affected limb.
5. Pain may radiate beyond the area innervated by the involved nerve.
6. The pain may be so intense that activity, eating, and sleeping become difficult.
7. Exposure to either heat or cold may exacerbate or alleviate pain.
8. Movement of the affected limb, touching the skin, or extreme sensory input such as loud sounds, bright lights, or emotional disturbances may aggravate the pain.
9. Many clients seek isolation and seclusion as a way of coping with the pain.

Physical Assessment

1. Hyperalgesia of the affected limb.
2. Changes in vasomotion and sweating are common, with vasodilation occurring and vasoconstriction later.
3. In later stages there are haptic changes of the affected skin, muscle, and bone with thinning of the hair and skin and atrophy of underlying tissues.

Diagnostic Tests

Diagnostic sympathetic block with local anesthesia.

NURSING DIAGNOSES: ACTUAL OR POTENTIAL

1. Pain and decreased use of affected limb.
2. Fear of painful sensation.
3. Self-imposed social isolation.

EXPECTED OUTCOMES

1. Pain will be relieved with nerve block or sympathectomy.
2. Normal functioning will be restored.

INTERVENTIONS

1. Sympathetic block with local anesthesia may lead to spontaneous relief of pain if administered within 10 days of symptom onset. It may be necessary to repeat block with recurring symptoms.
2. Surgical sympathectomy will be required if block with anesthesia fails.
3. Protect limb from stimulus that precipitates exaggeration of pain, such as unnecessary touching, movement, or exposure to heat or cold.
4. Support client's ability to cope with pain or fear of pain.
5. Help family and friends to understand the nature of the pain and the client's unusual behavior for coping with it.
6. Encourage client to exercise limb to maintain or restore strength and range of motion.

EVALUATION

Outcome Criteria

1. There is relief from burning pain after sympathectomy.
2. Strength and mobility of affected limb are restored.
3. Normal activities are resumed.

REFLEX SYMPATHETIC DYSTROPHIES

DESCRIPTION

Reflex sympathetic dystrophies include a number of disorders such as posttraumatic pain syndrome, sympathalgia, shoulder-hand syndrome, and posttraumatic edema. Symptomatology is similar to that of causalgia.

ASSESSMENT

Health History

1. Accidental injury including dislocations, sprains, fractures, lacerations, or crushing of extremities, either minor or severe.
2. Iatrogenic complication of surgery or administration of intramuscular medications such as penicillin.
3. Mild, moderate, or severe symptoms.
4. See *Causalgia*.

Physical Assessment

See *Causalgia*.

Diagnostic Tests

See *Causalgia*.

NURSING DIAGNOSES: ACTUAL OR POTENTIAL

See *Causalgia*.

EXPECTED OUTCOMES

1. Pain will be relieved.
2. Function will be restored.

INTERVENTIONS

1. Sympathetic block or sympathectomy.
2. Transcutaneous nerve stimulation.
3. Physical therapy with range of motion and muscle strengthening.
4. Emotional support to relieve fear of pain and encourage use of extremity.

DISORDERS OF SLEEP

DESCRIPTION

Normal sleep consists of a patterned cycle of approximately 70–90 min and is represented by two physiological categories, rapid eye movement (REM) sleep and non-REM sleep. *REM sleep* (also called paradoxical or activated sleep) is characterized by rapid eye movements, increased respiratory and cardiac activity, and flacid muscles of the limbs and trunk. Dreaming most often occurs during this phase of sleep. *Non-REM sleep* consists of four stages distinguished by electroencephalographic patterns. Stage 1 begins with falling asleep, and wave forms have fast frequencies and low amplitude, followed by stage 2, which is a transitional phase leading to stage 3. Progression to stages 3 and 4 occurs with slowing frequencies and higher amplitudes accompanied by deeper sleep.

The sleep pattern begins with the stages of non-REM sleep followed by REM sleep. There are usually four to six complete cycles per night. The amount of sleep required by each person varies, and the quality of sleep with normal progression through the stages of a cycle is as significant as quantity of sleep. Some people are adequately rested after 3–4 h of sleep, whereas others may feel rested only after 8 h of sleep.

INSOMNIA

DESCRIPTION

Insomnia is the most common disorder of sleep and can occur because of a primary disturbance in sleep physiology or secondary to disease with inability to fall asleep or remain asleep. Loss of sleep can affect anyone. Disturbances of sleep may occur with different patterns, including difficulty falling asleep, falling asleep and then awakening in the middle of the night, or falling asleep and waking very early in the morning. The pattern may vary from night to night but generally more time is spent in stage 2 non-REM sleep with increased physiological activity including faster pulse rate, peripheral vasoconstriction, and high body temperature.

PREVENTION

Population at Risk

1. People who chronically use hypnotic drugs or alcohol or overuse stimulants such as caffeine or amphetamines.
2. People who are anxious, stressed, or depressed.
3. People who sleep during the day and exercise infrequently.
4. People with chronic pain or disease.

5. People who are traveling across time zones ("jet lag").

ASSESSMENT

Health History

1. Specific description of patterns of sleeplessness.
2. Symptoms of sleep deprivation, including listlessness, fatigue, aggressiveness, irritability, lack of spontaneity, or feeling "washed out."
3. Inappropriate use of prescription or over-the-counter drugs including hypnotics and stimulants.
4. Excessive intake of caffeine or alcohol.
5. Feelings of anxiety, stress, or depression.
6. Tendency to sleep during the day.
7. Lack of regular exercise.
8. Physical disorders of heart, lung, kidney, or thyroid.
9. History of chronic pain or discomfort.
10. History of recent travel across time zones.

Physical Assessment

1. May have no significant findings.
2. Findings related to underlying disease states.

Diagnostic Tests

EEG recordings in sleep laboratory.

NURSING DIAGNOSES: ACTUAL OR POTENTIAL

Disturbance of sleep-rest cycles.

EXPECTED OUTCOMES

Normal sleep-rest patterns will be restored.

INTERVENTIONS

1. Treat underlying disease conditions.
2. Have client gradually reduce use of hypnotic drugs to prevent rebound insomnia for those with drug dependence.
3. Cautious prescription of hypnotic drugs, usually not longer than 10 to 15 days with shorter duration for the elderly, to establish normal sleep pattern.
4. Instruct client to avoid sleeping during the day.
5. Encourage client to exercise regularly every day.
6. Tell client to avoid going to sleep hungry.
7. Encourage client to establish a routine for going to sleep, for example, brush teeth, undress, read, go to sleep.
8. Teach relaxation exercises to induce sleep; client may use tape recorder with automatic shut-off.
9. Encourage client to discuss anxieties, stress, or feelings of depression.
10. Remind client to allow 2 to 3 days to reestablish sleep-wake cycle when changing time zones.

EVALUATION

Outcome Criteria

1. Normal sleep pattern is restored with sense of being rested on awakening.
2. May help to have client document sleep patterns with a diary to assess effectiveness of interventions.
3. Overuse or dependence on hypnotics is evaluated, with continued symptoms of fatigue and lack of energy. The elderly may paradoxically exhibit excitement or agitation in response to hypnotic drugs.
4. Underlying disease processes, pain, alcoholism, anxiety, or depression is resolved or controlled.

HYPERSOMNIAS

DESCRIPTION

The hypersomnias consist of prolonged states of sleep or an overwhelming desire to sleep (narcolepsy). Prolonged sleep states occur with encephalitis, tumors of the hypothalamus and midbrain, and severe hypothyroidism.

Narcolepsy is an insistent desire to sleep, usually during periods of inactivity and after meals. The period of sleep resembles REM sleep and lasts approximately 15 min, except when the individual is in a recumbent position, in which case the sleep may last an hour or more. The client is easily awakened and initially feels refreshed and energetic. Narcolepsy is often accompanied by catalepsy with sudden loss of muscle tone and excessive emotion such as laughter, crying, or anger. Hallucinations experienced at the onset of sleep (hypnagogic hallucinations) may also occur.

ASSESSMENT

Health History

1. History of hypersomnia or narcolepsy.
2. Possible familial occurrence of symptoms.

Physical Assessment

Symptoms of encephalitis or brain tumor.

NURSING DIAGNOSES: ACTUAL OR POTENTIAL

1. Disturbance of sleep-rest cycle.
2. Impairment of mobility.
3. Anxiety.
4. Safety hazards associated with activities such as driving.

INTERVENTIONS

1. Treat underlying disease states.
2. Narcolepsy is difficult to treat, but encourage client to nap after meals.
3. Inform client that analeptic drugs, amphetamine (Benzedrine), methylphenidate (Ritalin), or pipradrol (Meratan) can be taken to facilitate work and study requirements.
4. Inform client that REM sleep during the day may be diminished with imipramine (Tofranil).

EVALUATION

Outcome Criteria

1. Episodes of sleep are reduced or controlled.
2. Tolerance to drugs develops in 6 to 12 months, requiring that their use be reserved for special occasions when client must not fall asleep, or client is shifted to a different drug therapy.

BIBLIOGRAPHY

Ballenger, J. J.: *Diseases of the Nose, Throat, and Ear*, 12th ed. Lea & Febiger, Philadelphia, 1977. In-depth presentation of the anatomy, physiology, diagnosis, and medical and surgical management of ear, nose, and throat diseases.

Bonica, J. J., Ciebeskind, J. C., and Albe-Fessard, D. G. (eds.): *Advances in Pain Research and Therapy*, vol. 3, Proceedings of the Second World Congress on Pain, Raven Press, New York, 1979.

Braunwald, E., et al. (eds.): *Harrison's Principles of Internal Medicine*. 10th ed., McGraw-Hill, New York, 1983. Excellent source for the generalist in identifying and managing specific disease processes.

De Weese, D. D., and Saunders, W. H.: *Textbook of Otolaryngology*. Mosby St. Louis, 1982. Assessment, anatomy, and medical management of ear, nose, and throat disorders.

Drucker-Cocin, R., Shkurovich, M., and Sterman, M. B. (eds.): *The Functions of Sleep*, Academic Press, New York, 1979. A unique approach to the theoretical, physiological, and clinical implications of the functions of sleep.

Eliasson, S. G., Prensky, A. L., and Hardin, Jr, W. B. (eds.): *Neurological Pathophysiology*. Oxford University Press, New York, 1978. Designed for medical students and generalists, this text presents pathophysiology of neurological problems clearly and simply.

Fraunfelder, F. T., and Hampton Ray, F.: *Current Ocular Therapy*, Saunders, Philadelphia, 1980. A concise outline of approaches to ocular medical management including effects of systemic diseases and specific drug therapy.

Goodhill, V.: *Ear: Diseases, Deafness and Dizziness*, Harper & Row, New York, 1979. Excellent presentation of hearing assessment and management of acquired and degenerative loss of hearing and balance.

Jones, D., Dunbar, C. and Jirovec, M. (eds.). *Medical-Surgical Nursing: A Conceptual Approach*, 2d ed., McGraw-Hill, New York, 1982. The section on perception and coordination offers the reader an in-depth look at neurological disorders, and Chapter 31 presents a good neurological assessment.

Malasanos, L., Barkauskas, V., Moss, M., and Allen, K.: *Health Assessment*, Mosby, St. Louis, 1981. A good resource for examination of the eyes, ears, and nervous system.

Mayo Foundation for Medical Education and Research: *Clinical Examinations in Neurology*, 5th ed., Saunders, Philadelphia, 1981. Excellent source for evaluating problems of the nervous system. Examination techniques and interpretation of results are presented.

Saunders, W. H., Hadener, W. H., Keith, C. F., and Havener, G.: *Nursing Care in Eye, Ear, Nose and Throat Disorders*, Mosby, St. Louis, 1979. Presentation of common diseases of the eye, ear, nose, and throat with descriptions of nursing management.

Smith, J. F., and Nachazel, Jr., D. P.: *Ophthalmologic Nursing*, Little, Brown, Boston, 1980. Review of general and cellular anatomy and pathophysiology of the eye with a section on assessment and techniques useful to nursing in acute and ambulatory care settings.

Taylor, J. W., and Ballenger, S.: *Neurological Dysfunctions and Nursing Intervention*, McGraw-Hill, New York, 1980. A comprehensive consideration of common nursing problems and management approaches for the neurologically impaired client.

27

The Musculoskeletal System

Rosellen M. Garrett

ABNORMAL CELLULAR GROWTH

BONE TUMORS

DESCRIPTION

Abnormal cellular growth in bone produces tumors that may be benign, malignant, or metastatic from other tissues or organs. Local overgrowth of bone, appearing as a benign, tumorlike lesion, may result from a bone injury or fracture.

Osteoclastoma, or benign giant cell tumor, is locally aggressive and destructive but tends not to destroy surrounding tissue or spread to other parts of the body. The tumor occurs in the long bone, later infiltrating the shaft of the bone. Common sites are the distal portions of the femur and radius and the proximal portion of the tibia.

Malignant tumors, or sarcomas, are classified according to the type of tissue formed by the malignant cells, such as osteogenic sarcoma (OS), which is a primary malignant tumor arising from bone cells, most commonly appearing in the distal portion of the femur and the proximal portions of the tibia and fibula.

Metastatic bone tumors, the most common bone tumors, result from metastasis of malignant tumors elsewhere in the body. The common primary sites are the breast, prostate gland, lung, kidney, and thyroid.

Recognition is given to Phyllis Gale, R.N., M.S., who was the author of this chapter for the previous edition of this book.

PREVENTION

Health Promotion

1. Generally, the cause of primary bone tumors is unknown, although some bone tumors are considered to be an aberration of the growth and development of tissue.
2. Other factors have been associated with their formation, including heredity, injury, exposure to sunlight, infection, and metabolic and hormonal disturbances (Powell, 1982).
3. Any exposure to radiation should be avoided.

Population at Risk

1. Giant cell tumors occur primarily between the ages of 21 and 35.
2. Osteogenic sarcomas occur frequently in males between the ages of 10 and 25 and in older persons with Paget's disease.
3. Metastatic bone tumors occur most often in persons over 40 years of age who have a history of carcinoma in one of the primary sites listed above.

Screening

1. X-ray films.
2. Blood serum studies.

ASSESSMENT

Health History

1. Age-specific bone tumors (affect different age groups).

2. Past history that may suggest a primary tumor from which a secondary bone tumor has developed.
3. Limb pain that progressed from mild and intermittent to persistent.
4. Restriction of movement of involved limb.
5. Swelling of involved limb.
6. Generalized weakness.
7. Spontaneous fracture of limb.
8. Decreased nutritional intake.
9. Weight loss.
10. Decreased strength in involved limb.

Physical Assessment

1. Increased body temperature.
2. Increase in skin temperature over tumor.
3. Venous distention of involved area when compared bilaterally.
4. Measurable increase in limb size when compared bilaterally.
5. Decrease in range of motion of limb.
6. Tenderness of limb and/or palpated mass.
7. Pain, which varies according to type of tumor and location and may be either localized or diffuse.
8. Anxiety, which may be manifested in a variety of ways. (Refer to Assessment of *Anxiety* in Chapter 36.)
9. Decrease in strength of limb when compared bilaterally.
10. Atrophy of associated muscles.

Diagnostic Tests

1. X-ray film of involved area (anterior, posterior, lateral, and oblique views) for complete visualization of involved area.
2. Biopsy of lesion via aspiration needle or incision to obtain precise information of tumor type.
3. Bone scan to facilitate early detection of metabolic lesion.
4. Bone marrow biopsy to detect metastasis to the bone marrow.
5. Laboratory tests.
   a. Elevated WBC count.
   b. Elevated sedimentation rate.
   c. Elevated acid phosphatase.
   d. Elevated Bence Jones protein.
6. X-ray film of chest and skeletal radiologic survey to locate additional bone lesions if malignancy or metastasis is suspected.

NURSING DIAGNOSES: ACTUAL OR POTENTIAL

1. Alteration in comfort: pain and local swelling, moderate to severe.
2. Nutritional alteration: weight loss secondary to decrease in food intake.
3. Impairment of mobility: secondary to decreased limb movement.
4. Disruptions of fluid balance: secondary to fever.
5. Alteration in body image: potential amputation.
6. Anxiety, mild to moderate: secondary to fear of surgery.
7. Fear of death.
8. Potential disruption in skin integrity due to surgery.

EXPECTED OUTCOMES

1. Client will adapt to limited mobility initially. Independence will increase as evidenced by self-care activities.
2. Client will achieve and maintain maximal physical comfort.
3. Client will verbalize feelings of self-worth.
4. Client will verbalize fears related to surgery and its consequences.

INTERVENTIONS

1. Administer medications for pain relief (analgesics and narcotics) and chemotherapy. Observe, record, and report drug effects.
2. Reduce fever.
   a. Give antipyretic drugs and force fluids.
   b. Have client under minimal covering; provide a cool external environment.
   c. Give tepid water sponge baths or hyperthermia, as needed.
3. See that client has a high-caloric diet (high carbohydrate, high protein) to maintain the healthy state.
4. Engage in frank discussion with client about disease, treatment, and prognosis and listen for and explore cues (verbal or behavioral) indicating anxiety from underlying stressors.
5. Assist client in working through loss and grief, especially if loss of limb is anticipated.
6. Make referrals for appropriate counseling.
7. Explain all procedures, including biopsy and nature of surgery (refer to *Osteoarthritis* for a complete discussion).

8. Teach client and family about radiation and chemotherapy and common, expected outcomes from these, including:
   a. General malaise.
   b. Weakness.
   c. Alopecia.
   d. Skin integrity disruptions.
   e. Susceptibility to infection.
   f. Stomatitis.
   g. Alterations in blood.
   h. Gastrointestinal disturbances, including anorexia.
   i. Adjustments in work load.
9. Provide supplemental health care, including nutritional counseling, mouth care, planned rest periods, and prevention of upper respiratory and other related infections.

EVALUATION

Outcome Criteria

1. Client reports diminished pain and discomfort.
2. Client gains 2 lb by the follow-up visit; diet intake is optimal.
3. Client reports increased limb movement and diminished impaired mobility.
4. There is absence of fever.
5. Client verbalizes fears and concerns regarding surgery and fear of death.
6. Wound healing is observed.

Complications

1. Secondary infection (refer to Chapter 49).
2. Hemorrhage (refer to Chapter 48).
3. Metastatic progression of primary lesion (refer to discussion under *Abnormal Cellular Growth* as appropriate).

Reevaluation and Follow-up

1. Resolution of complications.
2. Continued follow-up to evaluate health state.

MULTIPLE MYELOMA

DESCRIPTION

Multiple myeloma is an osteocytic malignant disease of the plasma cells that can proliferate throughout the entire skeleton and infiltrate soft tissue. It is the most frequently occurring tumor arising in bone. The bones most commonly affected are those that are the sites of active hematopoietic marrow, such as the vertebrae, skull, ribs, sternum, and pelvis. The lymph nodes, kidneys, liver, and spleen may also become involved in later stages of the disease. Although the disease is fatal, symptoms can be relieved and the disease may be held in abeyance for several years.

PREVENTION

Health Promotion

The cause is unknown.

Population at Risk

1. Multiple myeloma occurs in individuals over 40 years of age, with a peak incidence at about 60 years.
2. Men are affected more often than women.

Screening

1. X-ray films.
2. Blood serum studies.

ASSESSMENT

Health History

1. Age, sex.
2. History of weight loss.
3. Progressive weakness and fatigue; anemia produced when bone marrow is destroyed.
4. Immobility due to bone destruction.
5. Dull migratory pain increasingly more severe and constant; back pain more frequent. Pain due to infiltration of plasma cells into bone marrow.
6. Recurrent infections.
7. Gastrointestinal symptoms (nausea, vomiting, constipation).
8. Leg heaviness and difficulty starting to void.

Physical Assessment

1. Pallor and listlessness.
2. Numbness evident if spinal cord compression present.
3. Diminished visual acuity.
4. Dehydration.

Diagnostic Tests

(Refer to Table 27-1.)

1. Biopsy and bone marrow aspiration will indicate an abnormally high level of plasma cells in aspirate.
2. Bence Jones protein: elevated.

TABLE 27-1 SELECTED TESTS AND PROCEDURES USED TO DIAGNOSE ORTHOPEDIC PROBLEMS

1. Laboratory procedures.
   a. Blood tests.
      (1) Complete blood count: WBC elevated.
      (2) Sedimentation rate: elevated.
      (3) Alkaline phosphatase, total serum: elevated.
      (4) Calcium, serum: elevated.
      (5) Potassium, plasma: elevated.
      (6) Uric acid: elevated.
      (7) Rheumatoid factor: positive.
      (8) HLA-B27: positive.
      (9) Lupus erythematosus (LE) preparation.
   b. Urine tests.
      Bence Jones protein, quantitative (24 h): elevated.
2. Radiography.
   a. *Arteriography:* injection of a radiopaque substance into the arterial system of a given region and the subsequent taking of radiographs to study bone, joints, or bone lesions.
   b. *Arthrography:* introduction of air or a radiopaque material into a joint space, outlining joint structures and detailing views of the joint surface on a radiograph.
   c. *Cineradiography:* radiographic visualization of skeletal movement by utilization of movie camera or videotape recorder.
   d. *Discography:* injection of a radiopaque solution into the nucleus pulposus of an intervertebral disc to view the internal disc structures.
   e. *Electromyography:* insertion of a sterile needle electrode into muscle to evaluate muscular activity.
   f. *Myelography:* injection of air or an opaque material into the subarachnoid space to view filling defects associated with herniated discs and tumors in the spinal column.
   g. *Scintography* (bone scan): intravenous injection of a radioisotope material having a special affinity to bone and emitting penetrating gamma rays to detect, locate, and outline bone lesions.
   h. *Tomography:* body section radiography that focuses on certain tissues, eliminating or blurring surrounding tissue.
   i. *Venography:* intravenous injection of a radiopaque dye to visualize the lower extremity venous system.
3. Special procedures.
   a. *Arthroscopy:* insertion of a lighted instrument, via a small incision, to view the internal structure of a joint.
   b. *Arthrostomy:* temporary opening into a joint for drainage purposes.
   c. *Bone marrow examination:* microscopic examination of bone marrow obtained through needle aspiration or biopsy.
   d. *Joint aspiration:* insertion of a needle into the synovial capsule of the joint for the purposes of withdrawing fluid for microscopic examination.

3. Urine electrophoresis: elevated plasma cells.
4. Total serum protein.
5. X-ray film of the chest and a limited bone survey to determine extent of bone involvement.
6. Quantitative immunoglobulin assay.
7. Blood coagulation studies.

NURSING DIAGNOSES: ACTUAL OR POTENTIAL

1. Alteration in comfort: secondary to bone destruction.
2. Fear of ambulation: due to pain and weakness.
3. Impairment of mobility: reluctance to ambulate; fatigue.
4. Nutritional alteration: deficit-food intolerance due to illness, chemotherapy.
5. Alteration in self-care activities: decreased activity, tolerance, and fatigue.
6. Health management deficit: difficulty adjusting to chronic long-term illness.
7. Increased potential for infection.

EXPECTED OUTCOMES

1. Mobility will increase to level of tolerance. Client will adjust to assistive device (brace, corset) for ambulation.
2. Client will control movements and will be able to participate in self-care activities in 4 to 6 weeks.
3. Client will increase fluid intake daily and maintain that intake after discharge.
4. Client and family will understand the disease and its complications as evidenced by 85 percent accuracy on oral exam.
5. Client will give evidence of compliance with care plan by:
   a. Adhering to medication regimen, as indicated by chart maintained by client.
   b. Establishing and maintaining an effective exercise program.
   c. Taking precautions to avoid infections.
6. Client will verbalize feelings regarding fear of drug addiction and loss of orientation because of constant need for medication.

INTERVENTIONS

1. Administer prescribed medications (analgesic narcotics, muscle relaxants, cytoxic steroids) to relieve pain and promote mobility every 4–6 h until client has achieved a level of pain control while still maintaining orientation to reality.
2. Administer prescribed medication for pain ½ h before ambulation.
3. Involve family in plan of care and coping with disease.
4. Encourage deep breathing and coughing q4h when client is awake along with exercises of extremities and toes.
5. Schedule nursing routines to allow client 2–3 h of rest or play at a time.
6. Reposition client at least q4h at own speed with planned, smooth, supported movements. This should be done to help decrease pain upon movement and to stimulate movement.
   a. Support extremities at joints.
   b. Use turning sheets.
   c. Use jacknife position to provide comfort.
   d. Back brace may be used.
7. Employ safety measures when transferring or ambulating client.
8. Assist with exercise and mobilization.
9. Monitor toes for color, motion, temperature, and sensation and check bilaterally.
10. Provide skin care to area undergoing radiation.
11. Regulate bowel activity by assisting with meals and allowing enough time to eat.
12. Encourage fluid intake and maintain accurate record of fluid intake and output.
13. Assess client for dehydration (monitor urine pH and blood electrolytes).
14. Assess for bleeding (hematomas, ecchymoses, hemorrhagic areas in buccal membrane, and blanching of fingernail beds), especially if client is receiving prednisone. Monitor hemoglobin and hematocrit.

EVALUATION

Outcome Criteria

1. Adequate level of pain control is achieved.
2. Client is able to ambulate and exercise daily (with braces if necessary) and provide self-care.
3. Client remains free from infection.
4. Client maintains appropriate level of fluid intake.
5. Client can verbally report with 85 percent accuracy the nature of the disease and its complications.
6. Client is adjusting lifestyle to disease.

Complications

1. Infections (refer to Chapter 49).
2. Pneumonia (refer to Chapter 31).
3. Anemia (refer to Chapter 29).
4. Hypercalcemia (refer to Chapter 28).
5. Renal failure (refer to Chapter 32).
6. Osteoporosis (refer to *Osteoporosis* later in this chapter).
7. Pathological fractures (refer to *Fractures*).
8. Hemorrhage (refer to Chapter 48).
9. Spinal cord compression (refer to Chapter 25).

Reevaluation and Follow-up

Establish a specific, individualized plan to assist client and family in adapting to periodic visits to hospital to monitor progress of disease. The plan should recognize the terminal nature of the disease.

METABOLIC DISORDERS

GOUT

DESCRIPTION

Gout is a metabolic disorder caused by the overproduction and accumulation of uric acid (increased purine metabolism) in the blood (hyperuricemia) and by the deposition of sodium urate crystals in and around joints, cartilage, epiphyseal bone, and periarticular structures. Physiologically, there is abnormal metabolic degradation of purine (a product of protein metabolism), resulting in reduced urinary secretion of urates and increased accumulation of uric acid in the blood. Because of the low solubility a precipitate forms, depositing masses of crystals, or trophi, at sites where the blood flow is least active, particularly in the large toe, the knuckles, and the ears. *Synovitis* (inflammation of a joint) results, and the cyclic process continues, causing an acute inflammatory process in which there are red, warm, swollen, and painful joints.

Primary gout (gouty arthritis) appears to be a genetic defect in purine metabolism. *Secondary gout* may be associated with multiple myeloma, polycythemia vera, and granulocytic leukemia and with clients who have had prolonged usage of certain thiazide diuretics. Onset of the disease can occur after recent surgery, recent ingestion of purine-rich foods, and excess alcohol intake and with acute infection and emotional trauma.

Pseudogout may present similar symptoms, affecting the larger joints in which calcium pyrophosphate crystals are present in the synovial fluid. Pseudogout does not respond to colchicine.

Gout often begins in one joint and heals within several weeks. However, the problem can return at any time and may affect more than one joint.

PREVENTION

Health Promotion

Predisposition to gout is inherited. An individual with a family history of gout should be encouraged to avoid overindulgence in foods high in purine and in alcoholic beverages.

Population at Risk

1. Gout affects men eight to nine times more than women.
2. Occurs usually between 20 to 60 years of age, with the peak at 40 years of age.
3. Predisposition to gout is inherited.
4. Women can develop gout after menopause.

Screening

1. Increased blood uric acid.
2. Disposition of urate crystals near or in joints.

ASSESSMENT

Health History

1. Age: males above 30, females after menopause.
2. Sex: males affected more; females affected after menopause.
3. Occupation: should be identified, though often not significant.
4. Dietary habits.
   a. Assess recent intake: alcohol may influence the problem.
   b. Assess diet for caloric and protein composition.
5. Recent life experience.
   a. Infection.
   b. Emotional trauma: stress may precipitate problem.

   c. Other illness (e.g., leukemia, polycythemia) or pregnancy.
6. Family history.
7. Health perception.
8. Previous history of gout: note familial tendency.
9. Time of onset of symptoms (usually early morning).
10. Description of pain: usually increased with weight bearing.
11. Anorexia and malaise often common complaints.

Physical Assessment

1. Perform general physical examination, including weight distribution.
2. Agonizing pain is felt in the first joint of large toe (later appears in other joints of foot).
3. Pain may subside or disappear later in day and evening, but returns at night.
4. Joints are swollen, red, warm, tender (appearance remains, although pain may have subsided); decreased range of motion; increased pain with weight bearing.
5. Increased pain is experienced when weight (e.g., linen) is applied.
6. Fever and general malaise may be present.
7. Trophic nodules (deposits of sodium acid urate crystals) may be palpated over bones, joints, and cartilage. Kidneys may also be affected.
8. Tachycardia may be auscultated, palpated.
9. Gastrointestinal disturbances: vomiting, diarrhea, constipation.
10. General appearance: restlessness, anxiety, and stress assessment should be noted.

Diagnostic Tests

1. Elevated serum uric acid above 5 mg/100 mL of serum.
2. Elevated sedimentation rate.
3. Synovial fluid from affected joints: presence of sodium urate crystals.
4. Radiograph findings suggesting gout.
5. Complete blood count: leukocytosis present.
6. Rheumatoid factor test and lupus erythematosus (LE) preparation both negative.

NURSING DIAGNOSES: ACTUAL OR POTENTIAL

1. Alteration in comfort: joint pain.
2. Changes in body temperature: fever.
3. Alteration in nutrition: potential.
4. Impairment of mobility: increased in early morning.
5. Anxiety: mild to moderate.

EXPECTED OUTCOMES

1. Acute discomfort will be reduced.
2. Hyperuricemia and uric acid crystal deposits will be reduced.
3. Effectiveness of treatment will be evaluated.
4. Precipitating causes will be identified (e.g., stress, secondary causes).
5. Recurring gout episodes will be prevented.
6. Development of chronic gouty arthritis, renal calculi, and renal damage will be prevented.
7. Weight will be reduced, if indicated.

INTERVENTIONS

1. Ensure that client has adequate bed rest during acute phase to relax joints and reduce stress on affected body part.
2. Provide quiet environment to help relieve precipitating factor.
3. See that client's bed has foot board or cradle to prevent weight of sheets and blankets on the affected joint.
4. Position involved joints in semiflexion to prevent contractures.
5. Apply heat or cold applications to involved joints to facilitate movement and reduce inflammation.
6. Administer medication for pain: analgesic and narcotics, as well as anti-inflammatory agents (e.g., indomethacin and phenylbutazone). ACTH may be given.
7. Administer medication to reduce hyperuricemia, for example:
   a. Colchicine orally every hour until pain subsides or until onset of gastrointestinal disturbances, and then daily. (Colchicine can be administered intravenously.)
   b. Probenecid (Benemid) or allopurinol (Zyloprim).
8. Maintain client on a low-fat, low-purine diet to help reduce precipitating cause.
9. Ensure a high fluid intake to increase urinary output and prevent the position of urate crystals in the kidney.
10. Observe for gastrointestinal disturbances secondary to medication.
11. Observe for urolithiasis and renal colic. As-

sess the client for flank pain. Teach client to sift urine for crystals (refer to Chapter 32).

12. Discharge planning.
    a. Follow-up care and referrals.
    b. Teaching especially related to:
        (1) Establishing regular habits of eating, exercise, and rest periods.
        (2) Modified dietary regimen, that is:
            (a) Encourage eggs, fat-free milk, cottage cheese, cereals, fruits, and vegetables.
            (b) Limit kidney, liver, sweetbreads, squab, meats, fowl, beans, mushrooms, peas, and spinach.
            (c) Discourage meat extracts, glandular meats, roe, shellfish, sardines, and brain.
13. Teach about medications: Colchicine and other uricosuric agents.
    a. Aspirin in large doses counteracts uricosuric agents.
    b. Gastrointestinal disturbances and bleeding may indicate drug intolerance.
    c. Discourage fasting and ingestion of alcohol, as these changes may stimulate attacks of gout and/or enhance drug reactions.

EVALUATION

Outcome Criteria

1. Client understands the nature of gout and warning symptoms of impending attacks.
2. Client understands the importance of taking prescribed medication even in the absence of symptoms.
3. Client will drink at least eight glasses of water per day to minimize uric acid precipitation.
4. Client tests urine daily to measure urine alkalinity.
5. Client avoids foods high in purine content. If client is obese, weight is reduced at a slow rate. Fasting is to be avoided.
6. Client is symptom-free and the recurrence of acute attacks is reduced.
7. Dosage and side effects of the prescribed medications are explained to the client.

Complications

JOINT DESTRUCTION

1. Deformities secondary to joint destruction and repeat attacks.
2. Cartilage damage (e.g., bony ankylosis).
3. Development of trophic bodies in cartilage.

Assessment

1. Increased pain.
2. Limited mobility.

Revised Outcomes

1. Mobility will be increased.
2. Client will be prepared for surgical intervention.
3. Discomfort will be relieved.

Interventions

1. Surgery may be needed to correct bone deformities that may develop as a result of joint damage (refer to *Osteoarthritis*).
2. Progressive renal dysfunction (refer to Chapter 32).

Reevaluation and Follow-up

1. Evaluate response to medications, as manifested by a decrease in joint swelling, decreased joint pain, and increased mobility.
2. Revise plan with onset of gastrointestinal symptoms or pain relief.
3. Assess compliance concerning medications, activity, diet.
4. Encourage increased mobility and resumption of activities of daily living.

OSTEOPOROSIS

DESCRIPTION

Osteoporosis is a metabolic bone dysfunction in which bone resorption supersedes bone formation, resulting in bone demineralization. The disease is characterized by a reduction in bone density and tensile strength. Defects in osteoplasts result from (1) reduced stress and strain normally caused by physical activity, (2) prolonged immobility, and (3) a decrease in estrogen and androgen levels. Other causes of osteoporosis are liver disease; deficiencies of calcium, phosphorus, and protein; hyperthyroidism; hyperparathyroidism; Cushing's disease; and bone marrow disorders. Prevention of physical trauma may help prevent further damage.

PREVENTION

Health Promotion

1. Preventive aspects relate only to complications resulting from osteoporosis.
2. There is no known means to control or prevent the process.
3. Clients with long-term recumbency should

have adequate hydration (adult: 3,000 mg/day), dietary measures to ensure acid urine, and careful handling of extremities during repositioning and other procedures. Return to mobility and active exercise should be encouraged as soon as physically feasible.

Population at Risk

1. Osteoporosis is most common in postmenopausal women because of a decreased concentration of blood estrogen.
2. Osteoporosis is part of "disease phenomenon"-related immobilization and atrophy of muscles surrounding bone (Hilt and Cogburn, 1980).
3. The disease can occur in older men, approximately 50 to 70 years of age.

Screening

1. X-ray film taken for the purpose of diagnosing and treating an orthopedic condition such as a fracture.
2. Health history of back pain out of proportion to any history of trauma.

ASSESSMENT

Health History

1. Health history often reveals changes presented by older individuals, most frequently fair-skinned, lightweight females.
2. Complaints include difficulty in walking and pain (usually low back pain) induced specifically by lifting or bending.
3. There is a susceptibility to fractures, especially of the proximal femur, ribs, vertebrae, and distal radius (refer to *Fractures*).
4. History regarding diet and activity.

Physical Assessment

1. Joint pain elicited by palpation over an affected area.
2. Loss of body stature.
3. Instability and unsteady gait.
4. Pain elicited by activities (e.g., bending).
5. Changes in individual's self-concept related to musculoskeletal changes may also be apparent.

Diagnostic Tests

1. Radiography shows thin, porous, but otherwise normal bone (radiolucent bone).
2. Blood serum calcium, phosphorus, and alkaline phosphatase levels are normal.
3. Bone is biopsied to rule out malignant disease.

NURSING DIAGNOSES: ACTUAL OR POTENTIAL

1. Impaired physical mobility: secondary to joint swelling and pain.
2. Potential for injury (fracture): unsteady gait, trauma.
3. Alteration in comfort: due to pain.
4. Disturbance in self-concept: altered because of loss of maturity, change in lifestyle.

EXPECTED OUTCOMES

1. The client will increase mobility to carry out activities of daily living.
2. The client will report decrease to absence of bone discomfort.
3. Client will verbalize concerns related to changes in body function.
4. Client will comply with therapeutic plan, including medication, nutrition, and routine physical therapy program.

INTERVENTIONS

1. Encourage physical activity, increasing over a planned period of time, but avoiding severe fatigue.
2. Instruct client to continue exercise regimen established in physical therapy or to consult with physical therapist about appropriate exercises.
3. Provide ambulatory assistance (crutches, canes, walker, brace, or corset, as needed).
4. Teach techniques to avoid possible falling and trauma, heavy lifting, and twisting of spine. Teach client effective body mechanics.
5. Explore verbal and nonverbal cues of self-image, dependence, and other stresses.
6. Ensure adequate diet with increased calcium, phosphorus, proteins, vitamins, and minerals.
7. Administer hormone therapy. This may be done only after careful assessment of each individual's health status.
8. Observe for and warn about possible occurrence of vaginal bleeding with estrogen therapy; report to physician.
9. Supplemental vitamin D may be advantageous.
10. See that client takes frequent rest periods and sleeps on a firm supporting mattress.
11. For specific relief of pain, administer analgesics and muscle relaxants as ordered.

12. Include information about all the above in discharge planning.

EVALUATION

Outcome Criteria

1. Client reports gradual resumption of daily living.
2. Client reports measures taken to prevent fractures.
3. Diminishing to absence of bone pain is reported upon palpation and walking.
4. Increased mobility is achieved as client performs range-of-motion activities.
5. Client reports adherence to therapeutic plan, as evidenced by nutritional log, maintenance of body weight, and adherence to daily exercise plan.

Complications

REFER TO *FRACTURES*

Assessment

1. Deformities of excessive kyphosis.
2. Increased instability.
3. Decreased mobility leading to loss of weight.
4. Increased loss of self-concept.
5. Increased potential for injury.
6. Increased pain.

Revised Outcomes

Discomfort will be controlled.

Interventions

1. Continue teaching to prevent injury.
2. Increase strategies to reduce discomfort (e.g., Medication, heat).
3. Teach client use of assistive devices (e.g., walker).

Reevaluation and Follow-up

1. Continue to monitor client's progress.
2. Assess mobility; evaluate calcium level and adherence to therepeutic plan.
3. Enlist support of family members to assist client and protect him or her from injury.
4. Follow-up is essential.

PAGET'S DISEASE

DESCRIPTION

Osteitis deformans, or Paget's disease, is a metabolic health problem associated with aging. The disease develops insidiously. Physiologically there is hypertrophy and bowing of the long bones and marked thickening and irregular deformities of the flat bones. The process usually begins in the skull, pelvis, femur, tibia, or vertebral column and may eventually involve the entire skeleton. Pain is usually experienced first in the shins and is often attributed to the aging process. The problem may be associated with cardiovascular and pulmonary disorders. Progressive bone dysfunction accompanied by fracture is not uncommon.

PREVENTION

Health Promotion

The cause of Paget's disease is unknown.

Population at Risk

1. The disease usually affects men, although women can become ill also.
2. It is more common in persons over the age of 40.

Screening

The problem is often found accidentally on radiographic examination.

ASSESSMENT

Health History

1. The client complains of pain, usually in the shins, varying in type and intensity, ranging from an ache to a severe intractable pain.
2. A cardiovascular or pulmonary disorder may also be identified.
3. History of fracture is not uncommon.
4. Deafness and defective sight may also be noted (Roaf and Hodkinson, 1980).

Physical Assessment

1. A reduction in stature and an increase in head size is revealed (client usually becomes aware that a hat no longer fits).
2. There is marked enlargement of the cranium.
3. The face appears small and triangular in shape, although its normal configuration is retained.
4. Involvement of spine, thorax, trunk, and legs may be manifested by a noticeable change in posture and stature (up to 30 cm), giving the person an "apelike" appearance.
5. The gait becomes labored and waddling.
6. Complaints of weakness are not uncommon.
7. Although the involved bones become mas-

sive, they are extremely brittle, and fractures occur frequently.
8. There is pain and tenderness on pressure in affected bones.
9. There is increase in skin temperature overlying the bone from increased vascularity of the bone.

Diagnostic Tests

1. Radiography shows areas of opacity and radiolucency in affected bones.
2. An elevated serum alkaline phosphatase level is often seen.
3. Microscopic exam of bone section stains in a mosaic pattern.
4. Urine hydroxy proline excretion is increased.
5. A bone scan may be performed that will denote irregularities in structure.

NURSING DIAGNOSES: ACTUAL OR POTENTIAL

1. Altered self-concept and increased pain.
2. Physical mobility becomes impaired as disease progresses.

EXPECTED OUTCOMES

1. Increased mobility to complete activities of daily living.
2. Decreased to absence of pain and/or discomfort.
3. Increased verbalization of fears and concerns regarding changes in bodily appearance.

INTERVENTIONS

1. Instruct client to follow a modified exercise regimen to prevent additional bone trauma.
2. Encourage promotion of self-care in activities of daily living.
3. Provide assistive devices for ambulation (e.g., cane).
4. Ensure continuity of therapy established by physical and occupational therapists.
5. Administer pain medications such as analgesics and salicylates as ordered.
6. Focus teaching plans on planning careful movements (body mechanics), recognizing increased possibility of fractures (refer to *Fractures*), and managing medication at home.
7. Listen to client's verbal and nonverbal cues about self, health problem, family, finances, and independence, and explore these with the client.
8. Discuss with the client and family the possibility of seeking counseling regarding alterations in body image and other stresses.

EVALUATION

Outcome Criteria

1. Decreased report of pain.
2. Increased mobility evidenced by improved ability to complete activity of daily living.
3. Improved self-concept evidenced by verbal report.

Complications

1. Severe compression.
2. Cardiorespiratory difficulties due to skeletal damage (e.g., thoracic compression).
3. Pathological fractures and potential sensory deficits are not uncommon.

OSTEOMALACIA

DESCRIPTION

Adult rickets, or osteomalacia, is a disorder of calcium and phosphorus metabolism caused by a deficiency in vitamin D. Although the condition is rare today, it can be caused by insufficient exposure to sunlight necessary for the metabolism of vitamin D. Poor absorption of vitamin D in the intestine or inability of the kidney to produce vitamin D in the presence of renal tubular damage are other causes. The disease process is usually manifested through the skeleton and results from the failure of calcium salt deposition in the bone matrix. Bones become soft, flattened, and deformed.

PREVENTION

Health Promotion

1. Maintenance of good dietary intake and avoidance of excessive intake of "junk food."
2. Sufficient exposure to sunlight.

Population at Risk

1. Osteomalacia is rare in the United States in comparison with those countries in which the culture dictates diets deficient in vitamin D (Hilt and Cogburn, 1980).
2. The health problem occurs in women between 20 and 30 years of age, many of whom

have had frequent, repeated pregnancies and lactation.
3. It also appears in clients with gastrointestinal disorders in which calcium and phosphorus are inadequately absorbed. These disorders include sprue, celiac disease, chronic biliary tract obstruction, and pancreatitis, as well as small bowel resections or shunts.
4. Renal disorders and hyperparathyroidism may also cause osteomalacia.

Screening

X-ray radiographic exam.

ASSESSMENT

Health History

1. Extreme tenderness in the areas of the pelvis, back, or hips.
2. Progressive muscular weakness.

Physical Assessment

1. Pain in affected bones.
2. Deformed postures associated with softening of bone structures (these changes may contribute to fractures).
3. Possible alterations in body image.
4. Waddling or limping gait.
5. Bowed legs due to body weight and muscle pull.

Diagnostic Tests

1. Radiography.
2. Serum phosphorus: reduced.
3. Serum calcium: reduced.
4. Serum alkaline phosphatase: increased.
5. Biopsy: microscopically the bone shows a lack of mineral salts.
6. Urine calcium: decreased.

NURSING DIAGNOSES: ACTUAL OR POTENTIAL

1. Alteration in comfort: pain and swelling.
2. Impairment of mobility: unsteady gait, decreased joint mobility.
3. Nutritional alteration: decreased vitamin D intake and absorption.
4. Alteration in body image: secondary to physical changes.
5. Increased potential for injury: due to unsteady gait.

EXPECTED OUTCOMES

1. There will be a decrease or absence of pain.
2. Mobility will increase so that client can carry out activities of daily living.
3. There will be absence of further injury due to bone degeneration.
4. Client will experience an improved self-concept, as evidenced by the individual's willingness to discuss the impact of changes in physical appearance on lifestyle.

INTERVENTIONS

1. Encourage careful, active exercise to counteract atrophy and disease.
2. Ensure adequate diet, including protein, calcium, phosphorus, and dietary supplements of calcium salts, phosphates, and vitamin D.
3. Do cesarean section in pregnant client.
4. Discourage lactation in the postpartum period.
5. Teaching plan should include:
   a. Diet (high calcium, protein, phosphorus).
   b. Planned, less frequent pregnancies.
   c. Protection from trauma, with body exercise and planned activity periods.
6. Encourage exposure to sunshine.
7. Instruct client in how to prevent pathological fractures.

EVALUATION

Outcome Criteria

1. Client adheres to therepeutic plan and reports maintaining a diet containing phosphorus and dietary supplements.
2. Client verbalizes concerns regarding changes in physical appearance.
3. Client participates in planned activity program and reports engaging in exercises daily.
4. Physical mobility is increased.
5. There is absence of physical injury.

Complications

Pathological fractures (refer to *Fractures*).

INFLAMMATORY DISORDERS

OSTEOMYELITIS

DESCRIPTION

Osteomyelitis is an acute or chronic infection in or around bone, usually caused by *Staphylococcus aureus*. The infection is often blood-borne from another infection point or can develop directly as a result of a contaminated, compound fracture. The infection tends to remain medullary, progressing to cancellous and cortical bone. When the suppurative process reaches the periosteum, erosion occurs and a soft-tissue abscess forms. If the infection invades the bone itself, the bone undergoes necrosis and has a tendency to retain the infection, resulting in retardation of the healing process. The necrotic area can become a potential focal point for reinfection. The sequestrum, or necrotic bone, can be surgically separated from normal bone and, following this procedure, new bone begins to form as the body attempts to repair itself. However, some remaining sequestrum may be covered by new bone and, although healing seems to occur, the remaining sequestrum becomes chronically infected and is susceptible to repeated abscess formation. Prevention of this problem is the most critical factor in eliminating osteomyelitis (refer to Chapter 28).

PREVENTION

Health Promotion

1. Maintenance of body's resistance.
2. Careful attention to any type of skin lesion.

Population at Risk

Osteomyelitis occurs most frequently in children in rapidly growing bones on the metaphyseal side of the bone plate.

Screening

1. History of symptoms.
2. Serum laboratory tests.

ASSESSMENT

Health History

1. Age.
2. History of recent health problems (e.g., compound fracture, debilitating disease, infection).
3. Complaints of fever, headache, and malaise not uncommon.
4. Immobility of the affected limb.

Physical Assessment

1. There is local pain and tenderness upon palpation.
2. There is swelling of affected area; if the extremities are involved, bilateral measurements are unequal.
3. Area involved is red and warm to the touch.
4. Client will have an elevated temperature with chills and malaise.
5. Tachycardia may be present.
6. Signs of dehydration may be apparent.
7. There is immobility of the affected limb.
8. Wound odor may be present if the lesion is open.
9. There may be a protective muscle spasm with client holding the affected area in a flexed position (in order to relax muscle).

Diagnostic Tests

1. Leukocytosis: elevated leukocyte count.
2. Elevated sedimentation rate.
3. Blood cultures may grow out of the affecting pathogen.
4. X-ray film of the affected limb is usually normal for a week to 10 days after initial symptoms. Shows area of necrotic bone.
5. Aspiration of suspect bone tissue: biopsy or culture confirms diagnosis.

NURSING DIAGNOSES: ACTUAL OR POTENTIAL

1. Alteration in comfort: pain.
2. Impairment of mobility: secondary to bone pain and infection.
3. Impairment of skin integrity: potential.
4. Disruption in bone integrity: potential.
5. Elevation in body temperature: secondary to infection.
6. Behavioral changes (e.g., anxiety, boredom): secondary to long-term immobility.
7. Alteration in self-image: due to prospect of scars, deformity, and limitation of motion.

EXPECTED OUTCOMES

1. The cause of infection will be identified.
2. Body temperature will be reduced.
3. Anxiety will be relieved.
4. Pain discomfort will be relieved.
5. Infection site will be treated and improved.
6. Client will be allowed to verbalize feelings.
7. The client's individualized needs will be respected.
8. Support network will be established with family to ensure supportive care during and after hospitalization.
9. Complete skin integrity will be regained.
10. There will be complete healing of fracture and of inflammatory site.
11. Recurrence of the problems will be prevented.

12. Complete mobility will be regained within a defined period of time.

INTERVENTIONS

1. During the acute phase, place client in isolation to prevent spread of infection to others and to protect the individual from introduction of additional pathogens (Jones et al., 1982).
2. Ensure adequate bed rest to reduce stress on extremity.
3. Administer antipyretics to reduce inflammation.
4. Maintain a cool environment to help relieve body temperature.
5. Apply cast traction or splint to affected body part to control fracture site and to provide rest for the bone.
6. Support extremity, especially at joints, above and below the affected part, to reduce stress on the affected part.
7. Maintain proper body alignment to reduce deformity; reposition frequently.
8. Apply heat to affected areas to increase circulation to the affected area and to hasten removal of pathogen (warm, moist packs elevate local erythema).
9. Administer antibiotics. Be sure that a culture is done and that sensitivity is tested so that the correct drug will be used. Observe for side effects and allergic reactions to drugs used. In acute cases, intravenous administration is initiated during the first week to 10 days. Oral antibiotics are given for 6 to 8 weeks to maintain adequate blood levels.
10. Apply nonstick dressings (Telfa or Vaseline) using aseptic technique.
11. Wound precautions may or may not be necessary depending upon the presence of wound drainage; drain culture if necessary.
12. Keep irrigation system operational (if initiated) by regulating the flow of solution at proper rate and placing extra pads around the area being irrigated.
13. Include scheduled rest periods in between nursing care routines.
14. Encourage fluids q3h along with a well-balanced diet.
15. Assist client in adapting to the disease and its prolonged recovery and rehabilitation period.
16. Elevate extremity to promote venous return.
17. Use air freshener, if necessary.
18. Provide skin care as necessary and continuously. Observe for other infected sites (e.g., abscess and necrosis).
19. Provide sensory stimulation during prolonged mobility and create diversional activities for the client.
20. Evaluate care on daily basis and revise nursing care plan, if indicated.
21. Allow for client's expression of fear and anxiety.
22. Be supportive and explain things to the client.
23. Follow up health care referrals.

EVALUATION

Outcome Criteria

1. There are decreased reports of pain.
2. Mobility is increased; the bone is healing.
3. There is absence of inflammation; skin integrity and normal body temperature are restored.
4. Client makes verbal reports of intact self-concept and restoration of self-confidence.
5. Client makes verbal reports of diminished anxiety due to improved mobility.

Complications

BONE NECROSIS

Assessment

1. Increased pain and discomfort.
2. Decreased mobility.
3. Increased temperature.
4. Further impairment of skin integrity.

Revised Outcomes

1. Bone destruction will be decreased by isolating the cause.
2. Optimal health will be restored by reducing inflammatory process.

Interventions

1. Massive antibiotic therapy.
2. Surgery may be necessary (e.g., amputation) if blood vessels are involved (refer to *Peripheral Vascular Diseases*).
3. Medication for pain (narcotics may be needed).
4. Skin grafts may also be necessary.

SEPTICEMIA

Refer to Chapter 49.

PATHOLOGICAL FRACTURES

Refer to *Fractures*.

Reevaluation and Follow-up

Essential follow-up program should be planned to evaluate client's health state.

ANKYLOSING SPONDYLITIS

DESCRIPTION

Ankylosing spondylitis, or Marie-Strümpell disease, is a chronic, progressive inflammatory disease of the intervertebral, sacroiliac, and costovertebral joints. As the disease progresses, there is ossification and ankylosing, or fixation, of the joints and spine. The course of the disease is variable, ranging from minimal involvement to severe disability.

PREVENTION

Health Promotion

The cause of ankylosing spondylitis is unknown.

Population at Risk

1. This disease is more common in men than in women.
2. It is seen most frequently between 15 and 30 years of age and appears to have a hereditary predisposition.

Screening

Varying degrees of both pain and stiffness, depending on stage of disease progression at the time of examination.

ASSESSMENT

Health History

1. Spinal stiffness in morning.
2. Pain in lower back radiating into hips, buttocks, or lumbosacral region.
3. Mild fatigue; decreased activity tolerance.
4. Weight loss.

Physical Assessment

1. Pain may or may not be present.
2. Deformity of spine and thorax, decreased respiratory excursion.
3. Limitation of functional movement.
4. Alterations in body image.
5. Continuation of disease process.
6. Tenderness in joints upon palpation.

Diagnostic Tests

1. Radiographic examination may not reveal the disease process during its early stages. Later stages show varying degrees of joint erosion and narrowing with sacroiliac involvement.
2. Blood sedimentation rate is elevated.
3. Rheumatoid blood factor is absent.

NURSING DIAGNOSES: ACTUAL OR POTENTIAL

1. Alteration in comfort: pain, morning stiffness.
2. Decreased activity tolerance: fatigue, immobility.
3. Nutritional deficit, weight loss.
4. Alteration in body image: secondary to physical changes.
5. Decreased respiratory function: secondary to thoracic deformities.
6. Decreased mobility: alteration in functional movement.

EXPECTED OUTCOMES

1. The spine will be maintained straight and erect throughout the disease.
2. Pain will be relieved.
3. The disease process will be retarded to prevent spinal deformity.
4. Client will make a psychological adaptation to having pain, disability, and deformity during prime of life.

INTERVENTIONS

1. Administer medications: indomethacin, phenylbutazone.
2. Teach client to maintain erect posture.
3. Continue prescribed exercises established by physical therapist.
4. Use a firm mattress, small cervical neck roll, and bed board to maintain posture.
5. Establish specific rest periods to be spent on flat, firm surface in prone position.
6. Teach and provide adaptation for activities of daily living.
7. Explore cues about changes in body image and lifestyle.
8. Make appropriate referrals (e.g., for counseling, vocational rehabilitation, sexuality).
9. Follow up health care referral.
10. Administer heat therapy.

EVALUATION

Outcome Criteria

1. Client can explain the basic nature of the disease.

2. Client demonstrates prescribed program of exercises.
3. Client demonstrates how to apply heat therapy.
4. Client can explain how medications are to be taken, the dosage, the time, and the side effects of medications.
5. Client can describe signs and symptoms that would indicate a need for immediate medical consultation.
6. Client can explain plans for follow-up care.

Complications

1. Significant flexion deformity.
2. Reconstructive surgery to remove a portion of the vertebrae (wedge osteotomy). Total hip replacement may be required to restore hip movement. (Refer to *Osteoarthritis*.)

Reevaluation and Follow-up

Follow up a continuous process, prompted by physical changes in skeletal structures.

RHEUMATOID ARTHRITIS

DESCRIPTION

Rheumatoid arthritis is a major health problem associated with inflammation and has been discussed in Chapter 16. Surgical intervention has helped clients toward well-being and functional independence. Refer to *Osteoarthritis* for nursing care associated with disabling arthritis and surgical intervention.

BURSITIS

DESCRIPTION

Bursitis, an acute or chronic inflammation of a bursa, results from trauma, infection, irritation, or calcareous deposits that form within the bursal walls. The bursae, saclike spaces found between bones, muscles, or tendons, are lined with synovium and contain a small amount of synovial fluid. Usually this fluid cushions joints and permits muscular movements with the least amount of friction. With inflammation, the bursa fills with fluid, causing a joint to become swollen and resulting in restricted joint movement. The most commonly involved joint is the shoulder, although the elbows, knees, and ankles can also be involved. Pain, causing marked disability, is provoked by specific abduction movements and causes a problem commonly referred to as "frozen shoulder." "Tennis elbow" and "housemaid's knee" are common examples of acute bursitis.

PREVENTION

Health Promotion

1. Avoid excessive utilization of joints.
2. Avoid trauma to joints.

Population at Risk

1. Bursitis can occur at any age.
2. Athletes are most affected.

Screening

1. History of pain, swelling, and marked tenderness.
2. Physical examination.

ASSESSMENT

Health History

1. Pain upon movement of joint.
2. Limited movement of joint.
3. History of involvement in athletics: joint trauma.

Physical Assessment

(Refer to *Osteomyelitis*.)

1. Joint pain; swelling; hot, tender area.
2. Restricted joint mobility, especially in abduction.
3. Dependence in activities of daily living.
4. Occupational causation (e.g., jobs involving excessive stress on joints).
5. May be precipated by other problems (e.g., connective tissue disorders) (refer to Chapter 29).
6. May be associated with such physical activities as tennis.

Diagnostic Tests

X-ray film may be ordered to confirm diagnosis; calcification may be seen.

NURSING DIAGNOSES: ACTUAL OR POTENTIAL

1. Alteration in comfort: due to pain and joint swelling.
2. Decreased mobility: pain on movement.

3. Knowledge deficit: regarding the disease process and outcome.

EXPECTED OUTCOMES

1. Joint movement will be increased without pain.
2. Optimal function of joint will be achieved.
3. Client will verbalize knowledge of the disease process and activities that can intensify the problem.

INTERVENTIONS

1. Immobilize affected joint by using pillows, splints, and/or sling.
2. Administer pain medication: analgesics or narcotics (e.g., codeine with or without aspirin).
3. Provide the client with muscle relaxants (e.g., Valium) to prevent muscle spasms.
4. Clients may be given steroids to help reduce inflammation and secondary swelling.
5. Assist with procaine block if indicated, preparing client for procedure. Inject Novocain into joint for temporary relief of pain.
6. Apply moist heat or cold packs to decrease inflammation and swelling.
7. Continue active exercises prescribed by physical therapist, as tolerated (range-of-motion exercises).
8. Teach energy conservation through modifications in activities of daily living.
9. Refer for vocational counseling if bursitis is job-related.
10. Follow up health care referral.
11. Support affected arm, if shoulder is involved, on pillows during sleep to avoid client's rolling over on shoulder.

EVALUATION

Outcome Criteria

1. Client verbalizes awareness that a program of rest should be observed until acute symptoms subside.
2. Client reports modifying the activities of daily living to avoid overuse of the joint associated with the inflamed bursa.
3. Client knows the doses, side effects, and toxic effects of prescribed medication.
4. Client reports increased joint mobility and an absence of pain.

Complications

SUBACROMIAL BURSITIS

This is a condition of inflammation of the supra spinatus tendon.

Assessment

1. Calcification adjacent to tendon.
2. Sudden severe pain.
3. Very painful abduction and external rotation.
4. Increased tenderness over the lateral humeral head.

Revised Outcomes

1. Loss of function will be prevented.
2. Client will rest until pain subsides.

Interventions

1. Phenylbutazone (100 mg tid).
2. Cortisone injections.
3. Rest.
4. Physical therapy after pain subsides.

BICIPITAL TENOSYNOVITIS

This is a condition of inflammation of the synovial sheath of the tendon along the biceps.

Assessment

1. Pain in the bicipital area (radiating to forearm).
2. Pain on abduction.
3. Increased tenderness over biceps.
4. Muscle atrophy, which can occur when problem is chronic.

Revised Outcomes

See *Subacromial Bursitis*, above.

Interventions

See *Subacromial Bursitis*, above.

FROZEN SHOULDER

Frozen shoulder, or adhesive capsulitis, involves pain or decreased use of shoulder as a result of decreased use or impaired function.

Assessment

1. Report of immobilization of joint caused by trauma or fracture.
2. Seen more often in elderly.
3. Reflex sympathetic dystrophy.
4. Reported disuse of joint.
5. Increased inactivity (immobility).
6. Pain on palpation.

Revised Outcomes

1. Optimal joint use will be promoted.
2. Increased joint activity will be achieved through physical therapy.

Interventions
1. Progressive exercise.
2. Nonsteroidal anti-inflammatory drugs.
3. Teaching about the need for exercise and joint use.
4. Support to client and family.
5. Physical therapy.

Reevaluation and Follow-up
1. Reevaluation and follow-up of acute episodes of medical problems are essential.
2. Continued evaluation of joint mobility is important, particularly with the elderly (e.g., after a fractured shoulder).

TUBERCULOSIS OF THE BONES AND JOINTS

DESCRIPTION

Characteristically monarticular in nature, tuberculous arthritis can involve a vertebra, an elbow, a hip, or a knee. During the acute phase of this disease, cold abscesses are produced. Destruction of the joint may occur, resulting in hip deformity or "hunchback." Sinus pathways from a tuberculous joint are known to extend for long distances. In more than half of affected clients there is evidence of pulmonary tuberculosis. The symptoms of pain, wasting of adjacent muscle, weight loss, fever in conjunction with a positive history of tuberculosis, and the monarticular involvement usually suggest the diagnosis. Tuberculous arthritis, as well as tenosynovitis (inflammation of the tendon and tendon sheath) and bursitis, can be caused by *Mycobacterium tuberculosis*. Refer to Chapter 31 for a complete discussion of tuberculosis.

PREVENTION

Health Promotion

Avoidance of unnecessary exposure to individuals with active or quiescent tuberculosis lesions in the lungs.

Population at Risk

1. Skeletal tuberculosis is secondary to foci located elsewhere in the body.
2. Cases with musculoskeletal involvement are seen in children.

Screening

Tuberculin skin sensitivity test.

ASSESSMENT

Health History

1. Slowly developing pain at night; swelling or limp, involving the knee or hip joints.
2. Progressive, more or less painless swelling in tendon sheaths.
3. Vaguely localized unrelenting backaches.
4. Muscle spasm around joint.
5. Weight loss, fatigue, anorexia.
6. Low-grade fever.
7. Night sweats.

Physical Assessment

1. Joint and bone pain.
2. Fever; elevation later in the day.
3. Progressive infectious process.
4. Pulmonary tuberculosis may or may not be present.
5. Weight loss.
6. Dependency, secondary to chronic illness.
7. Muscle atrophy (of adjacent muscles).
8. Increased joint fluid.
9. Deformity in affected joint.

Diagnostic Tests

1. Biopsy of tissue followed by microscopic demonstration of the tubercle bacillus.
2. Culture of bacillus in material aspirated from involved area.
3. Radiographic examination: deterioration and invasion of bone and joint structures.
4. Sedimentation rate: elevated.
5. Radiographic exam and intravenous pyelogram may confirm involvement of the lungs, kidneys, and lymph nodes.

NURSING DIAGNOSES: ACTUAL OR POTENTIAL

1. Decreased activity tolerance: fatigue, muscle wasting.
2. Altered self-concept: secondary to bone and skeletal changes that can accompany the disease process, weight loss.
3. Alteration in comfort: pain, fever.
4. Decreased mobility: secondary to tendon involvement, pain, joint immobility.
5. Knowledge deficit: related to the disease process.

EXPECTED OUTCOMES

(Refer to Chapter 31.)
1. The infectious process will be controlled.

2. Further muscle wasting and skeletal muscular changes will be prevented.
3. Optimal mobility and joint function will be restored.
4. Nutritional status and food intake will improve, as evidenced by weight gain.

INTERVENTIONS

(Refer to Chapter 31.)

1. Maintain client on bed rest for several weeks.
2. Administer pain medication: analgesics.
3. Administer antibiotics and specific chemotherapy for tuberculosis. Usually two of the following are selected (refer to Chapter 31):
   a. Isoniazid (INH).
   b. Rifampin (RM).
   c. Ethambutol (EMB).
4. Observe for toxic effects of medications (e.g., hepatitis).
5. Maintain specific isolation for pulmonary tuberculosis, if present.
6. Implement progressive muscle exercises planned in collaboration with physical therapist.
7. Provide assistive devices for mobility and ambulation (e.g., trapeze, cane, walker).
8. Accept client and his or her behavior and listen for cues of stress.
9. Assist client in working through dependency and encourage self-care.
10. Teach client:
    a. Need for initial bed rest.
    b. Progressive exercises.
    c. Information about medications and their toxic effects.
11. Follow up referrals.
12. Ensure adequate nutrition.
13. Maintain care of casts, body jackets, braces, or splints used to immobilize involved joints.

EVALUATION

Outcome Criteria

1. Client verbalizes knowledge of disease process and related therapeutic plan.
2. Client complies with therapeutic plan and verbalizes the need for continuous use of antituberculosis drugs (refer to discussion in Chapter 31).
3. Client verbalizes concerns and fears associated with a chronic long-term illness.
4. Nutritional patterns are improved, as evidenced by client's log as well as weight gain.
5. Client's overall mobility is improving with continued physical therapy.

Complications

(See Chapter 31.)

Reevaluation and Follow-up

1. Continuous follow-up is essential due to the long-term use of medication and the chronicity of the problem.
2. Follow-up is important to determine compliance and prevent complications.

TRAUMA

FRACTURES

DESCRIPTION

A fracture is a traumatic injury resulting in partial or complete disruption in the continuity of a bone. Fractures can occur in any bone and are defined according to the type and extent of break (refer to Chapter 48 for an illustration of the most common fractures and emergency care). Table 27-2 contains a list of additional fractures along with the descriptions of the type of bone changes that result.

As the bone begins to heal, it progresses through a stage of hematoma formation, beginning regrowth of new tissue, bone and callus formation, and ossification and bone remolding (Brunner and Suddarth, 1980). Refer to Figure 27-1.

PREVENTION

Health Promotion

1. Avoid fatigue of muscles.
2. Maintain adequate nutrition.
3. Use good body mechanics.
4. Employ safety measures in the home and in the hospital.

Population at Risk

1. Individuals who are fatigued with tired, overworked muscles that are unable to support bones adequately.

TABLE 27-2 COMMON BONE FRACTURES

Fracture	Bone Changes
Capillary	Hairline fracture, very thin.
Complete (transverse)	Bone is broken across, with disruption of both sides of the periosteum.
Complex	Closed, with soft tissue damage.
Complicated	Fracture with injury to adjacent organ (e.g., fractured rib with punctured lung.
Compound	Wound communicates from the bone to the surface owing to trauma to both the soft tissue and the bone, or the bone tears through the soft tissues as it fractures.
Linear	Occurs parallel to bone.
Pathological (spontaneous)	Occurs in the presence of a problem or tumor in the bone.
Simple	Clean break in the bone; skin is not disrupted.
Trophic	Due to weakening of the bone from metabolic imbalance.

SOURCE: Adapted from Jones, D. A., et al.: *Medical-Surgical Nursing: A Conceptual Approach*, 2d ed., McGraw-Hill, New York, 1982, p. 1516.

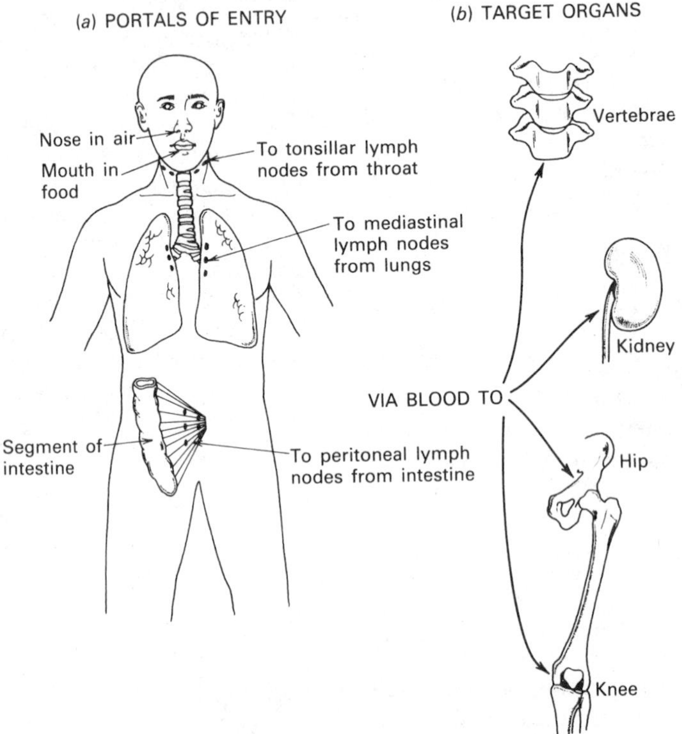

Figure 27-1 Spreading pattern of tuberculosis in the body. (Roaf, R., and Hodkinson, L. J.: *Textbook of Orthopedic Nursing*, 3d ed., Blackwell, Oxford, 1980.)

2. Individuals who have neoplasms and metabolic disorders.
3. Individuals who are malnourished.
4. Individuals whose muscles are atrophied and weakened due to prolonged rest.
5. Individuals whose lifestyles predispose bones to unusual stress, such as athletes, especially those engaged in contact sports.
6. Elderly individuals (refer to *Osteoporosis*).

Screening

1. Observation of injured area.
2. X-ray film (severe break and location of the injury).

ASSESSMENT

Refer to Chapter 48, which discusses early assessment of acute fractures. Additional problems following the acute phase include:

1. Fear of long-term immobility.
2. Potential signs of dehydration.
3. Disruption in skin integrity, especially in compound fracture.
4. Pain.
5. Complaints of changes in bowel and bladder elimination patterns.
6. Abrupt disruption in lifestyle and its consequences.
7. Changes in self-perception; expressed concerns over long-term effects (e.g., scars).

NURSING DIAGNOSES: ACTUAL OR POTENTIAL

1. Alteration in comfort: pain.
2. Anxiety, mild, moderate, severe: secondary to pain, dependence.
3. Alteration in bowel elimination: constipation due to immobility, fluid loss.
4. Impairment of mobility: bed rest, cast, and so forth.
5. Alteration in ability to perform self-care activities: deficit due to immobility, cast.
6. Disruption in skin integrity: due to surgery or injury.
7. Alteration in nutrition (potential): fluid volume deficit, nutritional defect.
8. Respiratory and circulatory dysfunction (potential): secondary to fracture.
9. Fear: regarding long term of fracture.
10. Home maintenance management impaired: potential.

EXPECTED OUTCOMES

1. Respiratory and circulatory functioning will be stabilized.
2. Bone will be immobilized to facilitate healing and proper alignment.
3. Circulatory and/or nerve impairment will be prevented.
4. Pain will be relieved.
5. Cast care will be provided to prevent complications.
6. Constipation will be prevented; fluid intake will be improved.
7. Cast integrity will be maintained.
8. Client self-care will be promoted.
9. Adequate nutrition and fluid intake will be maintained.
10. Complications of immobility will be prevented.
11. Client will be prepared for ambulation.
12. Recurrence of fracture will be prevented.

INTERVENTIONS

Refer to Figure 27-2 for physiology of bone healing.

1. Types of interventions.
   a. *Closed reduction* is the procedure whereby bone fragments are brought into apposition by manipulation and manual traction. A cast is usually applied to immobilize the fracture fragments and to support the injured parts (see below).
   b. *Open reduction* involves surgery on the injured area in order to remove debris, remove bone fragments, or place bones in proper alignment (see *Hip Fractures* for complete discussion).
   c. *Casts* can be applied to the extremities, the complete torso, and the upper torso to include the head and neck. Spica casts are applied to immobilize extremities and are used with shoulder and hip fractures; spica casts can be bilateral, depending on the areas involved. Casting usually includes the joints above and below the fracture.
      (1) Types of cast materials.
         (a) Plaster of Paris.
         (b) Rigid plastic material, such as Lightcase cast.
      (2) Specific nursing interventions for clients with casts.
         (a) Support wet cast with pillows and

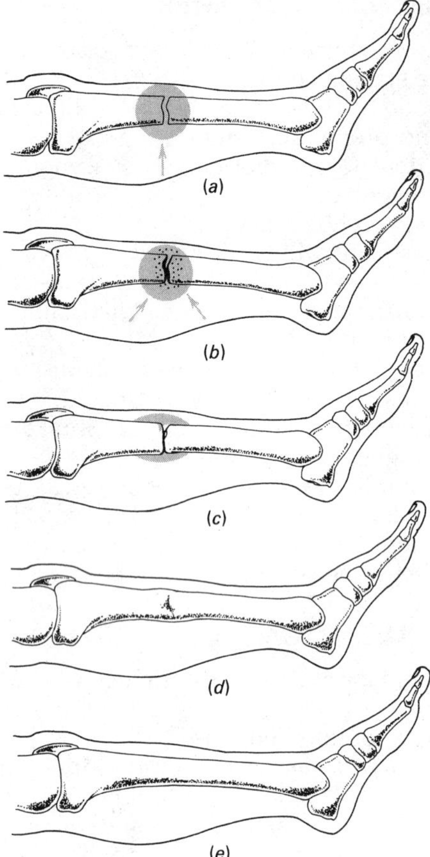

Figure 27-2 Physiology of bone healing. (*a*) Hematoma stage. The local clot serves as a fibrin network for subsequent cellular invasion. (*b*) Cellular proliferation stage. Fibroblastic and endothelial cells invade and colonize the fibrin scaffolding of the cast. (*c*) Callus formation stage. Osteoblasts are derived from mesenchymal cells to produce an osteoid matrix. (*d*) Callus ossification or union stage. Ossification of callus occurs. (*e*) Consolidation and remodeling.

expose cast to air for at least 24–48 h to facilitate drying.

(b) Manipulate cast with palms of hands, rather than fingers, to prevent cracking of cast.

(c) Use fan to increase circulation of air to cast. If the weather is damp, drying may take a longer period of time.

(d) Remove plaster crumbs with moist cloth and petal cast with adhesive tape if edges are rough or unfinished, to prevent skin breakdown.

(e) Use plastic wrap to line edge near genital portion of cast to prevent the cast from becoming damp following excretion and/or urination.

(f) Inspect cast for drainage and inspect under cast edges for lesions.

(g) Assess odors emitted from cast and observe for "hot spots" (hot areas over a particular point of the cast that may indicate infection).

(h) Assess the skin of the exposed distal extremity for pallor, blanch ing, tingling, numbness, temperature differences, cyanosis, edema, and pain.

(3) Teaching plan.

(a) Explain need for elevation of extremity in cast.

(b) Stress that nothing should be placed inside cast.

(c) Instruct client in use of crutches or other assistive devices. Provide instruction on gaits to be used when walking with the assistance of crutches (refer to Figure 27-3).

(d) Inform client of cast removal procedures, need for support to unstable limb after cast removal, and skin care of affected limb.

d. *Traction* is the maintenance of a steady pull on a body part by means of a force to keep two bone fragments in alignment, just touching each other. With traction, there is a forward force produced by weights; counterbalance or countertraction is produced by the backward force of the muscles and the frictional force between the client's body and the bed. Counterbalance is also achieved by elevating the body part placed in traction and by raising the bed on wooden blocks or by traction pull against a fixed body part (e.g., with the use of a Thomas splint, see Figure 27-6, the proximal ring presses against the ischial tuberosity). The most effective traction will have an equal amount of traction and counterbalance.

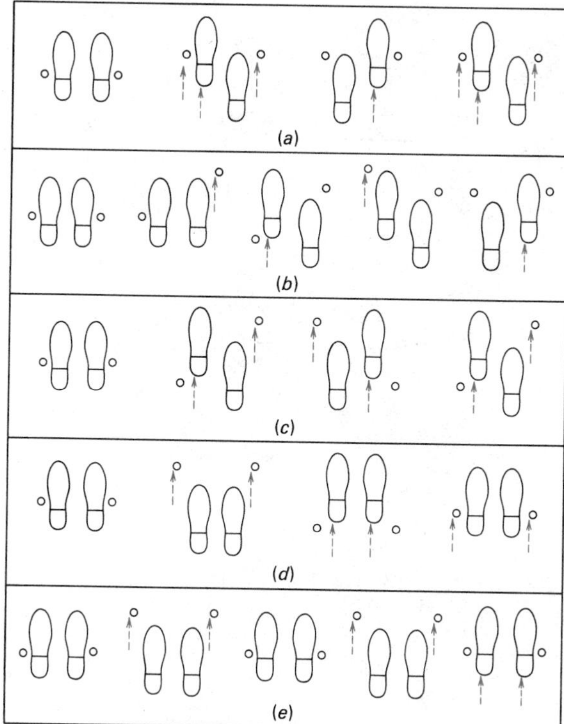

Figure 27-3 Crutch walking. (*a*) Three-point gait with little or no weight bearing on affected limb. (*b*) Four-point gait with partial weight bearing on each limb and support needed for balance. (*c*) Two-point gait used after proficiency with four-point gait is achieved. (*d*) Swing-through gait with weight bearing on both limbs and support needed for balance. (*e*) Swing-to gait with weight bearing on both limbs and support needed for balance.

When this occurs, the traction is considered balanced.

(1) The purposes of traction are:
   (a) To immobilize a reduced fracture.
   (b) To alleviate or eliminate muscle spasm and pain.
   (c) To prevent or correct deformities.
   (d) To permit and/or promote healing of an inflamed joint or extremity by means of immobilization.
(2) Types of traction.
   (a) *Skin traction.* The pulling force is exerted directly on the skin and indirectly on the bone:
      (i) Buck's extension (Figure 27-4).
      (ii) Russell's traction (Figure 27-5).
      (iii) Pelvic or cervical traction.
   (b) *Skeletal traction.* The force is applied directly to the bone by means of a metal pin or wire that is inserted directly into or through the bone.
      (i) Kirschner wire.
      (ii) Steinmann pin.
      (iii) Crutchfield tongs.
      (iv) Thomas splint and Pearson attachment: usually used in conjunction with skeletal traction for fractures of the femur (refer to Figure 27-6).
(3) Specific nursing interventions for clients in traction.
   (a) Monitor attachment of traction frame with the bed in low position, then raise bed (before transfer to unit).
   (b) Use firm mattress with bed board and trapeze before transfer to unit to facilitate movement.
   (c) Position client in recumbent supine position throughout traction unless specified otherwise.
   (d) Assess respiratory functioning to prevent pneumonia secondary to immobility.
   (e) Assist with insertion of Kirschner wire (refer to Chapter 25) and care for wires using sterile technique.
   (f) Examine traction apparatus daily.
      (i) Maintain ropes and pulleys in straight alignment.
      (ii) Keep weights hanging free.
      (iii) Ensure that ropes are unobstructed and not touching client.
      (iv) Keep the heel of affected limb off bed and hip flexion at 20 degrees.
      (v) Use adhesive materials that will not slip out of place.
   (g) Administer medication to relieve pain.
   (h) Maintain the client on a well-balanced diet and provide adequate fluid intake to aid in tissue healing and to prevent problems of elimination.

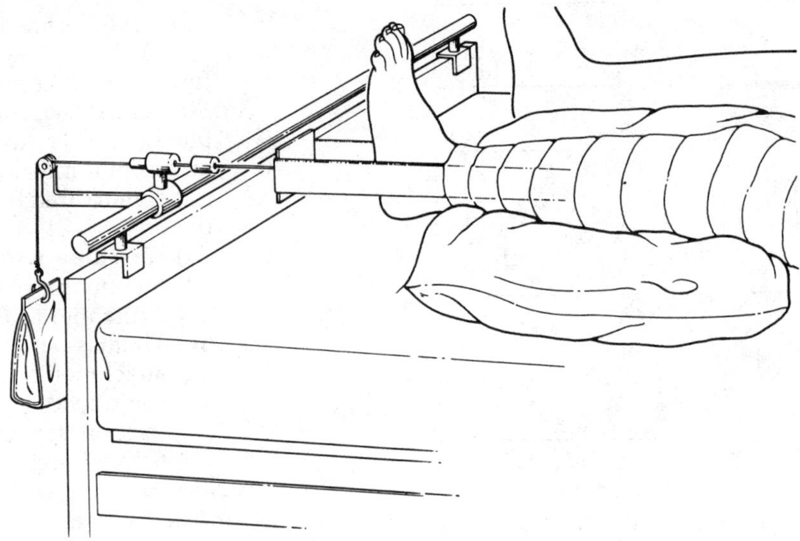

Figure 27-4 Buck's extension. (Adapted from Schwartz, S. I., *Principles of Surgery*, 2d ed., McGraw-Hill, New York, 1974.)

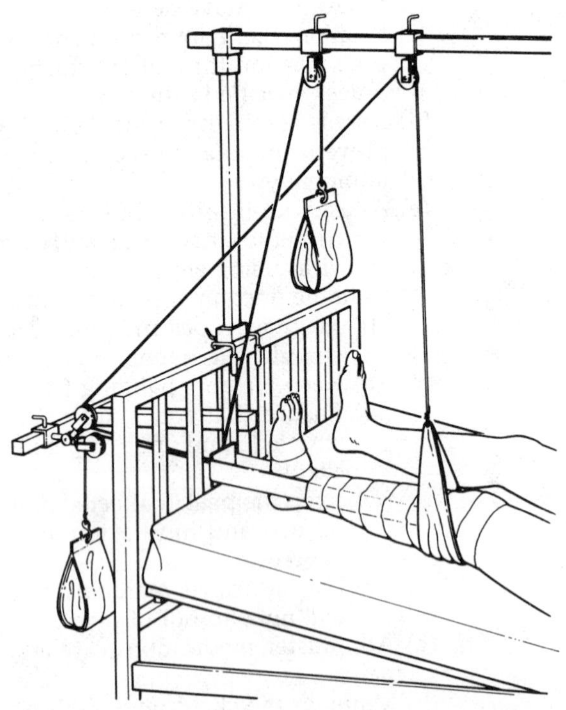

Figure 27-5 Russell's traction. (Adapted from Schwartz, S. I., *Principles of Surgery*, 2d ed., McGraw-Hill, New York, 1974.)

(i) Assess for pressure at popliteal space of the affected limb.
(j) Assess for positive Homan's sign on both legs to evaluate potential of phlebitis (refer to Chapter 29).
(k) Assess for foot drop in affected limb; use footboard to prevent changes.
(l) Assess for circulatory and nerve impairment.
(m) Maintain active exercises to unaffected body parts and muscle strengthening exercises for ambulation. Use isometric exercises for affected limb.
(n) Inspect skin integrity.
  (i) Give skin care to back, coccyx, scapulae.
  (ii) Massage bony prominence every 2–3 h.
  (iii) Examine skin adjacent to traction apparatus.
(o) Rewrap elastic bandages daily to prevent potential embolus formation and reapply elastic stocking twice each day.
(p) Encourage visitors to distract client, provide social interest, and

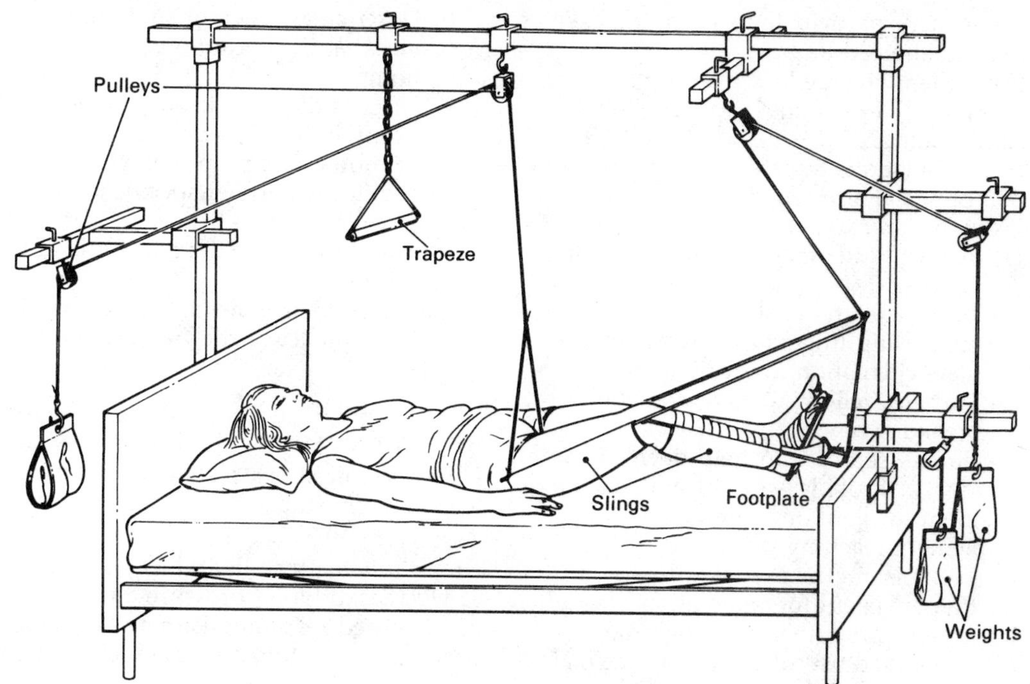

Figure 27-6 Balanced, suspended traction with a Thomas splint and Pearson attachment. (Adapted from Jones, D. A., et al.: *Medical-Surgical Nursing: A Conceptual Approach*, 2d ed., McGraw-Hill, New York, 1982.)

decrease boredom and social isolation.

(q) Explore verbal and nonverbal cues of anxiety. Encourage the client to discuss freely the impact of immobility and explore diversions.

(r) Implement teaching plan. Include:
   (i) Use of trapeze.
   (ii) Limitation of movement to that tolerated.
   (iii) Exercise program.

(s) Allocate time for diversional activities and therapeutic communication.

(t) Plan for discharge and make referrals for follow-up.

2. General nursing intervention for clients with fractures.
   a. Monitor vital signs frequently to assess early signs of infection.
   b. Encourage deep breathing and coughing q2h to prevent respiratory problems.
   c. Elevate injured part with pillows to level of heart or above.
   d. Administer medication for pain as needed (e.g., analgesia, narcotics).
   e. Apply ice bags to injured region to help reduce swelling for the first 24 h after injury.
   f. Massage red areas around bony prominences to prevent tissue breakdown.
   g. Palpate peripheral pulses that are accessible, and evaluate frequently.
   h. Provide well-balanced diet—high in protein, caloric content, and vitamins D and C—to aid in wound healing.
   i. Maintain adequate fluid intake to prevent dehydration and maintain urinary output.
   j. Use fracture bedpan for elimination and schedule elimination similar to patterns before hospitalization.

k. Have client participate in isometric exercises to affected limb.
l. Have client engage in active exercises for unaffected extremities for ambulation conditioning.
m. For ambulation, transfer client to side of bed opposite affected side.
n. Provide skin care.
   (1) Inspect and massage bony prominences.
   (2) Apply cream to skin directly under cast, using fingers or swabs, to stimulate circulation to the area.
   (3) Turn the client q2h to prevent skin breakdown.
o. Encourage self-care to help decrease dependence. Provide support and encouragement to client and family.
p. Implement teaching plan.
   (1) Teach isometric exercises.
   (2) Prepare client for ambulation through muscle strengthening program.
   (3) Encourage use of trapeze to facilitate movement (refer to Figure 27-6).
q. Discharge planning and evaluation of teaching should include:
   (1) Written directions for client regarding such things as exercises, diet, cast care, and medication.
   (2) Return demonstration of teaching, reactivity, exercise, and crutch walking.
r. Follow up on referrals.

EVALUATION

Outcome Criteria

1. The client can describe fracture and care of cast if discharged with applied cast.
2. The client returns to usual state of mobility and self-care; circulatory-respiratory status is stabilized.
3. The client states indication for health care services, safety devices, and knowledge of community resources.
4. The client can explain the limitation of activity to be observed and for what length of time.
5. The client can explain the nature and rationale for prescribed weight-bearing restriction and limitation of joint movement.
6. The client is able to:
   a. Demonstrate safe performance of activities of daily living (ADL) within the prescribed limitations or restriction of activity, weight bearing, or joint movement.
   b. Describe and demonstrate how safety devices and precautions will be used at home.
   c. Discuss diet and keep a log reflecting appropriate food sources.
   d. Demonstrate proper posture, body mechanics, and other specific joint protection techniques.
7. Wound healing occurs and signs of infection are absent.
8. Client verbalizes fears and concerns regarding the impact of the fracture on one's lifestyle.

Complications

HYPOVOLEMIC SHOCK

Hypovolemic shock secondary to fluid or blood loss may develop.

Assessment

(Refer to Chapters 48 and 49.)

1. Decreased blood pressure and pulse.
2. Increased respirations; may be shallow.
3. Restlessness that can be associated with blood loss.
4. Acute anxiety; fear of injury.
5. Complaints of severe pain.
6. Alteration in level of consciousness.

Revised Outcomes

1. Cardiorespiratory status will be stabilized.
2. Bleeding will be terminated.
3. There will be absence of discomfort and return of consciousness.

Interventions

1. Keep client warm; conserve heat.
2. Monitor vital signs.
3. Provide oxygen, if necessary.
4. Check hemoglobin and hematocrit to evaluate blood loss. Evaluate serum sodium, chloride, and potassium levels.
5. Replace or maintain blood volume by transfusion or intravenous fluids. Assess blood reactions.
6. Relieve pain, as it may contribute to hypovolemia.
7. Splint injury to avoid fluid loss and shock.

THROMBOEMBOLISM

(Refer to Chapter 30.)

FAT EMBOLISM

This condition usually occurs in the first few days after injury. It often follows fractures of long bones as a result of release of fatty substances into bone matrix.

Assessment

1. Presence of petechiae in buccal membrane, conjunctival sacs, neck, shoulder, and chest.
2. Tachycardia and chest pain (e.g., precordial) may be assessed.
3. Fever.
4. Increased respiratory rate, especially if embolus lodges in the lung; cyanosis and dyspnea may accompany the problem. A productive, blood-tinged cough may be experienced, and the presence of basal rales or rhonchi may suggest the beginning of pulmonary edema.
5. Altered state of consciousness.

Revised Outcomes

1. Cardiorespiratory status will be stabilized.
2. Consciousness will be returned.
3. Pain and fever will be decreased.

Interventions

1. Reduce shock.
2. Position client for maximum respiration; provide oxygen therapy.
3. Use heparin to prevent additional clot formation.
4. Measure arterial blood gases to assess oxygen and carbon dioxide exchange and perfusion.
5. Give intravenous fluids and glucose to prevent hypovolemia. Dextran may be given as a volume expander.
6. Administer antibiotics, as needed.
7. Monitor urinary output, assess renal perfusion, and evaluate cardiovascular status.
8. Assess neurological signs, especially level of consciousness.
9. Provide a quiet environment to promote rest.
10. Do not turn client; keep client stable to prevent dislodgment of emboli.
11. Administer intravenous corticosteroids to decrease vascular inflammation.
12. Allay apprehension: provide client with information about tests, answer client's questions, and create an atmosphere for open discussion. Support is essential.

CIRCULATORY IMPAIRMENT

This involves arterial and venous impairment.

Assessment

1. Pallor or blanching of toes.
2. Numbness and tingling.
3. Coldness to touch.
4. Pain not relieved by narcotics; the pain intensifies with motion of toes.
5. Peripheral pulses unequal.
6. Venous impairment that may be manifested by cyanosis and edema.

Revised Outcomes

1. Pain will be relieved; peripheral sensation will increase.
2. Color, temperature, and pulse will return to the extremities.

Interventions

1. Assess for tightness of cast.
2. Monitor vital signs.
3. Assess peripheral pulses.
4. Report changes to physician.
5. Open bivalve cast and reapply.
6. Elevate limb (venous impairment).

NERVE IMPAIRMENT

Assessment

1. Tingling or numbness in the affected limb (e.g., the elbow).
2. Decreased ability or inability to move previously functioning toes.
3. Decreased feeling or lack of feeling in toes (paresthesia).
4. When the perineal nerve is involved, the foot and lateral aspect of the ankle are affected.

Revised Outcomes

1. Sensation to the limb will increase.
2. Control over limb movement will increase.
3. Edema will be decreased.

Interventions

1. Assess for edema; monitor peripheral pulses.
2. Assess for cast tightness and release cast (bivalve).
3. Monitor vital signs.
4. Change traction, if necessary.

INFECTION

Assessment

1. An open, contaminated wound (usually a compound fracture) may be present.
2. If infection is deep, gas gangrene or tetanus may develop.
3. Drainage from cast: note color, odor, and amount.
4. Pain may be localized or diffuse.
5. So-called hot spots may be palpated over an affected area of the cast.
6. If gas gangrene is present, cellulitis, fever, tachycardia, discoloration of tissue, and alteration in hemoglobin will be noted.

Revised Outcomes

1. The wound will heal, as evidenced by skin growth, decreased temperature, and decreased edema.
2. Blood and wound cultures will be negative.

Interventions

1. Culture the drainage from wound and note the amount.
2. Inspect skin under cast and remove cast if necessary.
3. Note drainage, encircle drainage area on the cast, and monitor frequently.
4. If gangrene is present, open wound to air, facilitate drainage, irrigate, and apply dressing changes using sterile technique.
5. Give oral antibiotics (e.g., penicillin or tetracycline); check drug allergies.
6. Monitor vital signs.
7. Cast reapplication may be necessary.
8. Administer analgesics and/or narcotics to reduce pain.
9. Cut window in cast to assess site of infection.

DELAYED UNION OR NONUNION

Assessment

1. Radiography: nonunion, lack of callus formation.
2. False motion (pseudoarthrosis).
3. Refer to Assessment under *Fractures*.

Revised Outcomes

Refer to discussion of *Fractures*.

Interventions

1. Surgery (open reduction).
2. Postoperative cast care.
3. Braces.

ORTHOSTATIC HYPOTENSION

(Refer to Chapter 30.)

Assessment

1. Weakness, diaphoresis, and dizziness upon elevation.
2. Syncope upon elevation.
3. Hypotension.

Revised Outcomes

See Chapter 30.

Interventions

1. Place client in dorsal recumbent position.
2. Gradually increase elevation over a period of days.
3. Apply elastic compression bandages and abdominal binder before elevation and ambulation.
4. Engage client in active exercises.
5. Monitor vital signs in supine and Fowler's positions and while affected extremity is dangling.

Reevaluation and Follow-up

1. Evaluate compliance and monitor the healing process.
2. Report any untoward signs.

HIP FRACTURES

DESCRIPTION

The proximal end of the femur that engages with the acetabulum in the innominate bone forms the hip joint. Hip fractures are caused primarily by (1) degenerative and osteoporotic changes and (2) a decreased resistance to normal stresses. Concomitantly there may be normal physiological changes in balance and perception that may occur with senescence. Hip fractures may be *intracapsular,* involving the head and neck of the femur, or *extracapsular,* in which the trochanteric portion of the femur is involved. The characteristic position of a suspected hip fracture is hip abduction and external rotation accompanied by shortening of the affected leg. Also present are muscle spasm and pain. Intracapsular fracture of the femur can easily disrupt the blood supply to the area, and nonunion of the fracture may occur, despite the fact that perfect reduction may have been achieved. Management of the client with a hip fracture is further complicated if there is a history of chronic disease.

PREVENTION

Health Promotion

1. Practice safety measures in the home.
2. See *Fractures*.

Population at Risk

1. Elderly women with degenerative changes.
2. Individuals with osteoporosis.

Screening

1. Observation of affected leg, shortened and externally rotated.
2. X-ray film (reveals break and location of injury).

ASSESSMENT

Health History

(Refer to *Bone Tumors* and *Fractures*.)

1. Age: tendency for this problem to occur in the elderly. Common in women.

2. Occupation may predispose the individual to injuries.
3. Dietary habits: depressed calcium, especially in early development.
4. History of falling, previous fractures, "accident-proneness."
5. Presence of associated diseases (e.g., malignancy, pathological fracture).

Physical Assessment

(Refer to Chapter 48 and *Fractures* in this chapter.)

1. Affected hip in abduction and external rotation.
2. Affected leg is shorter than unaffected leg.
3. Pain aggravated by movement.
4. Muscle spasm intensified by movement.
5. Localized or peripheral edema.
6. Limitation of movement.
7. Temperature inference: affected extremity and toes may be cold.

Diagnostic Tests

(Refer to *Fractures*.)

1. Radiograph of affected hip.
2. Chest plate.
3. ECG to assess cardiac changes.
4. CBC: decreased hemoglobin and sedimentation rate.
5. Others: specifically related to any accompanying illness.

NURSING DIAGNOSES: ACTUAL OR POTENTIAL

Refer to *Fractures*.

EXPECTED OUTCOMES

(Refer to *Fractures*.)

1. Adequate health status will be stabilized and maintained before and after surgery.
2. Extension of affected hip will be maintained.
3. Client will be prepared for surgery.
4. Complications will be prevented.
5. Client's psychosocial needs will be met.
6. Health will be restored.
7. Client will regain independence in activities of daily living and self-care.
8. Client will be prepared for mobilization.
9. Client will be taught how to achieve maximum functional stability of affected hip.
10. Client will be assisted in transition to home care.

INTERVENTIONS

(Refer to *Fractures*.)

1. Use a flotation mattress and trapeze on bed before transfer from emergency room.
2. Transfer client to bed with one person assigned to support affected leg. Apply manual traction, if indicated.
3. Monitor vital signs (e.g., pulse, temperature); evaluate changes.
4. Initiate coughing, deep-breathing exercises.
5. Assess need for pain medication and muscle relaxants; administer as necessary.
6. Assist with application of Buck's extension (Figure 27-4), and explain its purpose.
7. Elevate affected leg on pillow; elevate bed 25 degrees.
8. Check alignment of traction q2h; use trochanter rolls or sandbags if needed to maintain internal rotation.
9. Initiate range-of-motion exercises to unaffected limbs.
10. Inspect toes for circulatory and nerve impairment.
11. Initiate muscle-strengthening exercises to upper extremities, abdomen, and unaffected leg.
12. If client is not placed in traction before surgery, the following turning and positioning techniques can be utilized. Turn q2h, using turning sheets.
    a. Supine position.
        (1) Keep pillow under affected limb from knee to heel.
        (2) Use trochanter roll or sandbag to maintain internal rotation and extension.
        (3) Keep head of bed elevated only if necessary.
    b. Side-lying position.
        (1) Position pillow between client's legs from groin to ankle.
        (2) Bring client close to side of bed.
        (3) Turn client to side with one person always assigned to support affected leg.
        (4) Partial turn to 45 degrees may or may not be tolerated on affected hip.
        (5) Use pillows.
            (a) To back.
            (b) Additional pillow may be necessary to keep hip joint in alignment.
13. Surgical interventions.

a. Preoperative nursing interventions: routine.
b. Open reduction or internal fixation may be performed to expose, realign, and immobilize the hip and related structures in place by means of a metallic device. A metal device, usually vitallium or stainless stell, is nontoxic, inert, nonporous, nonpyrogenic, and nondegradable in the body. Surgical intervention with hip fractures permits early weight bearing and mobility. Bone union usually occurs 4 to 6 months postoperatively.
c. Postoperative nursing interventions.
   (1) Prevent complications (refer to *Osteoarthritis* and see the discussion of complications under *Fractures*).
   (2) Support involved limb; handle gently and carefully.
   (3) Maintain body alignment while client is in bed; maintain hip extension.
   (4) Encourage self-care in activities of daily living; encourage client to move on his or her own.
   (5) Continue range-of-motion and active exercises and begin active assistive exercise in collaboration with physical therapist.
   (6) Ambulate client as soon as possible. When ambulating:
      (a) Apply elastic bandages to both lower extremities.
      (b) Have client get out of bed on unaffected side.
      (c) Assist client in moving slowly, in attaining sitting position, and in maintaining dangling position until balance is attained (monitor vital signs).
      (d) Weight bearing on affected leg may be limited.
      (e) Use of crutches or walker is important to provide assisted ambulation.
   (7) Discharge planning.
      (a) Prepare client and family for home care or for transfer to rehabilitation center.
      (b) Teaching plan should include:
         (i) Adaptation of activities of daily living.
         (ii) Removal of potential hazards at home.
         (iii) Adequate lighting in darkened areas and at night.
         (iv) Slow, purposeful movements and achievement of balance before getting out of bed or up from a chair.
         (v) Need for continuity of care.
   (8) Refer for follow-up care (e.g., visiting nurse). Encourage consideration of an extended care facility.

EVALUATION

Expected Outcomes

1. Client will be walking with a cane or walker at discharge.
2. Client will exercise unaffected leg and both arms.
3. Client will maintain adequate nutrition, especially fluid intake.
4. Client will demonstrate how to perform or modify activities of daily living within the limitations of activity and motion that must be observed.
5. Client understands the limitation of motion and restrictions of activity to be observed and for how long.

Complications

There may be complications of surgery (see Complications under *Fractures* for appropriate intervention).

1. Delayed union or nonunion.
2. Disuse phenomena from immobility.
3. Nerve and circulatory impairment.
4. Respiratory complications.
5. Cardiovascular complications.
6. Wound infection.
7. Alterations in mental acuity.

Reevaluation and Follow-up

Because recovery from a hip fracture involves long-term care, follow-up reevaluation of the client's return to optimal functioning will probably occur for many months after the fracture. This is particularly true of the elderly, in whom the incidence of hip fractures is most significant.

LOWER BACK PAIN

DESCRIPTION

Lower back pain is one of the most common health problems in our society today. It results in great discomfort, disability, and loss of time from work. Among the causes are muscle strains, tension, lack of physical exercise, poor posture, structural abnormalities, and certain systemic diseases. As people grow older, lower back pain becomes more chronic in nature and results from the degenerative processes occurring in the discs and vertebral joints. The therapeutic course is treatment of symptoms.

PREVENTION

Health Promotion

1. Maintain muscle tone of abdomen and back.
2. Wear suitable supporting garments.
3. Maintain good posture.
4. Maintain appropriate weight for skeletal frame.

Population at Risk

1. In children, infection can cause pain in the lower back.
2. In adolescents, a developing bone defect may result in lower back pain.
3. Mechanical strain on the ligaments or discs is the most likely cause in young and middle adults.
4. Back pain in the elderly is the result of some form of bone disease such as osteoporosis or metastatic disease.

Screening

X-ray films (may reveal site and changes at the place of injury).

ASSESSMENT

Health History

1. Pain, severe at times; may radiate down leg.
2. Muscle spasm that may intensify pain.
3. Immobility due to pain.
4. Muscle weakness, unsteady gait.
5. Associated health problem (e.g., fracture, chronic illness).

Physical Assessment

1. Localized tender and painful spot in lumbar region upon palpation.
2. Slight lateral curvature of spine may be present if muscle spasm is asymmetric.
3. Increased back and leg pain on elevation of leg.

Diagnostic Tests

(Refer to *Osteoporosis*.)

1. Serum calcium, phosphorus.
2. Serum alkaline phosphatase.
3. CBC.
4. Sedimentation rate.
5. Urinalysis.
6. X-ray of thoracic and lumbar spine.
7. X-ray film of pelvis and view of sacroiliac joints and hips helpful.

NURSING DIAGNOSES: ACTUAL OR POTENTIAL

1. Alteration in comfort: due to pain, immobility, and muscle spasm.
2. Impaired mobility: due to muscle weakness, numbness, unsteady gait.
3. Potential self-care deficit: due to impaired mobility.
4. Potential for injury (increased): due to paresthesias and unsteady gait.
5. Fear: related to the progressive physical changes caused by the health problem.
6. Knowledge deficit: related to the disease process and its long-term effects.

EXPECTED OUTCOMES

1. Muscle spasm will be relieved.
2. Normal elasticity of affected muscles will be regained.
3. The joint will return to normal function.
4. Any underlying condition will be corrected.
5. A weight-loss program will be planned, if needed.
6. The client will know the immediate and long-term effects of the problem and how to prevent them when possible.
7. The client will verbalize fears and concerns associated with a chronic illness.

INTERVENTIONS

1. Use a firm mattress and bed board; the floor may be used.
2. Apply warm heat (heating pad or hot moist packs).
3. Rest client in Fowler's position. When client

is lying on side, place pillows between client's flexed legs.
4. Administer medication for pain (e.g., Darvon, Tylenol, codeine) and for muscle relaxation (e.g., Valium).
5. Continue exercises initiated in physical therapy, for example:
   a. Abdominal muscle-strengthening exercises.
   b. Exercises to attain mobility of spine.
6. Implement teaching plan. Instruct client to:
   a. Perform daily physical exercise (but avoid strenuous exercises).
   b. Maintain correct posture; make good use of effective body mechanics.
   c. Use a firm mattress and hard plywood board under mattress at home.
   d. Avoid straining or lifting heavy objects.
   e. Avoid sleeping in prone position.
   f. Avoid prolonged sitting, standing, walking, and driving.
   g. Make use of referral for follow-up care.
7. Apply strapping, back brace, or corset for support.
8. Use traction, if necessary (refer to *Fractures*).
9. Provide psychological support to help client deal with anxiety.

EVALUATION

Outcome Criteria

The client:
1. Understands the principles of correct body mechanics.
2. Uses correct methods of stooping, lifting, carrying objects, and sitting.
3. Verbalizes fears and concerns regarding this problem.
4. Optimizes mobility and prevents further injury.
5. Is able to complete activities of daily living without limitations.

Complications

1. Chronic lower back pain syndrome.
2. Nerve blocks and other surgical intervention (refer to Chapter 25).
3. Fracture of spine (refer to Chapter 25).
4. Sprains, strains, dislocations (refer to Chapter 48).

Reevaluation and Follow-up

Long-term follow-up is important because of the course of the disease.

OBSTRUCTIONS

PERIPHERAL VASCULAR DISEASE

DESCRIPTION

Peripheral vascular disease occurs when local cells cannot receive their nutritional requirements because blood supply to the leg is greatly diminished. This may result from peripheral vascular insufficiency caused by atherogenesis and arteriosclerotic changes. A reduction in blood supply to a lower extremity can result in infection, ischemia, and gangrene. All measures to restore circulation are usually attempted before amputation is decided upon (refer to Chapter 30).

PREVENTION

Health Promotion

Refer to Chapter 30.

Population at Risk

Refer to Chapter 30.

Screening

Refer to Chapter 30.

ASSESSMENT

Health History

Refer to Chapter 30.

Physical Assessment

Refer to Chapter 30.

Diagnostic Tests

Refer to Chapter 30. Also:
1. Exercise stress tests: the greater the arterial involvement, the shorter the time to induce claudication.
2. Oscillometry.
3. Serum cholesterol and lipids: increased.
4. Peripheral arteriography.
5. Skin temperature studies.

NURSING DIAGNOSES: ACTUAL OR POTENTIAL

1. Alteration in comfort: pain.
2. Anxiety: mild to severe.

3. Grieving: anticipatory, secondary to a lost limb.
4. Alteration in ability to move effectively: state of dependence.
5. Self-concept: alteration in body image, secondary to amputation.
6. Impairment of skin integrity: secondary to immobility.
7. Alteration in elimination: potential.
8. Alteration in sensory perception: motor loss.
9. Impairment of significant others' adjustment to loss of limb.
10. Disruption in skin integrity.
11. Knowledge deficit.

EXPECTED OUTCOMES

1. Infection will be prevented.
2. Client will verbalize fears and concerns regarding the problem.
3. Client will attain full ambulation to optimal level of function with prosthesis.
4. Pain and discomfort will be eliminated.
5. Client will regain independence at the level before obstruction.
6. Open, honest communication with client and family will be achieved.

INTERVENTIONS

(Refer to Chapter 30 for nonsurgical Interventions.)

1. *Amputation*: the surgical removal of a portion of or an entire limb.
   a. Major reasons for amputation.
      (1) Ischemia due to vascular disease.
      (2) Trauma.
      (3) Revision of congenital anomaly.
      (4) Malignant bone tumors.
      (5) Uncontrolled infection.
   b. Types of amputation.
      (1) Closed or flap amputation.
      (2) Open or guillotine amputation in which the surface of the wound is not covered, usually in presence of actual or potential infection.
   c. Levels of amputation is determined by:
      (1) Type and requirement of prosthesis.
      (2) Function of the limb.
      (3) Adequacy of circulation.
      (4) Muscle balance.
   d. Site of amputation (refer to Figure 27-7).
      (1) Disarticulation: removal by resection of an extremity through a joint, hip, or ankle.
      (2) Partial: amputation through the hand or foot (carpal and metatarsal).
      (3) Above or below a joint.
2. Preoperative interventions.
   a. Place footboard or cradle on bed; elevate head of bed with wooden blocks.
   b. Relieve pain with specified narcotics and/or analgesics.
   c. Prepare the client for surgery; discuss feelings of loss openly. (Refer to Chapter 48 for discussion.)
   d. Maintain upper extremity strength through exercises, especially to muscles of the affected limb.
3. Postoperative interventions.
   a. Apply either a soft dressing to the stump or a rigid dressing, which is a cast to which a pylon and foot piece are attached. This immediate postoperative "prosthesis" reduces edema, shapes the stump, and permits early weight-bearing ambulation.
   b. Prevent stump edema, elevate stump (e.g., with pillows), and prevent contractures.
   c. Stump bandaging (refer to Figure 27-8).
      (1) Use two or three elastic bandages sewn together (4 in total length for amputation below the knee; 6 in total length for amputation above the knee).
      (2) Hip should be flexed about 24 degrees.
      (3) Clean bandage every day.
      (4) Rewrap four times a day.
      (5) Apply before client gets out of bed.
   d. Stump conditioning after healing.
      (1) Wash stump and dry carefully each day.
      (2) Inspect for irritation and pressure.
      (3) Massage stump.
      (4) Push stump into soft pillow, progressing to firm pillow, and finally to hard surface.
      (5) Rub small amount of powder over stump (not incisional site).
      (6) Apply stump sock.
      (7) Apply heat, and change position for muscle spasm.
   e. Facilitate movement as tolerated; use trapeze over bed and foot cradle (for unaffected leg).
   f. Monitor vital signs: prevent shock (hypovolemia); assess and measure drainage from dressings; use Hemovac.
   g. Help the client and family members deal with loss of the limb. Accept behavior

demonstrated, be supportive, and offer the individual and family an opportunity to share feelings. Explore feelings of grief and dependence and perception of body image.

h. Teaching plan for client and family.
   (1) Procedure for alleviating muscle spasm (e.g., warmth, applications).
   (2) Diet to avoid obesity.
   (3) Physical care of remaining extremity, including inspection, hygiene, and nail care.
   (4) Stump care, conditioning, and bandaging (refer to Figure 27-8).
   (5) Modifications of self-care activities if client is confined to wheelchair.
   (6) Crutch walking or other ambulatory adaptations.
   (7) Phantom pain sensations, an annoying phenomenon, decrease with activity. Provide analgesia and/or distraction.

EVALUATION

Outcome Criteria

1. Wound healing is observed.
2. There is an absence of signs of infection at the site of disturbance.
3. Client is attaining full ambulation to optimal level of functioning.
4. There is a decrease to absence of pain.
5. Client verbalizes feelings related to changes in physical appearance.
6. Client reports recognition of those signs of grief and identifies coping strategies to deal with the loss.
7. Client knows the reason for the surgery and the expected outcome and is knowledgeable about those self-care activities that will promote optimal healing.
8. Normal elimination pattern is restored.
9. Client verbalizes increased independence along with increased mobility.

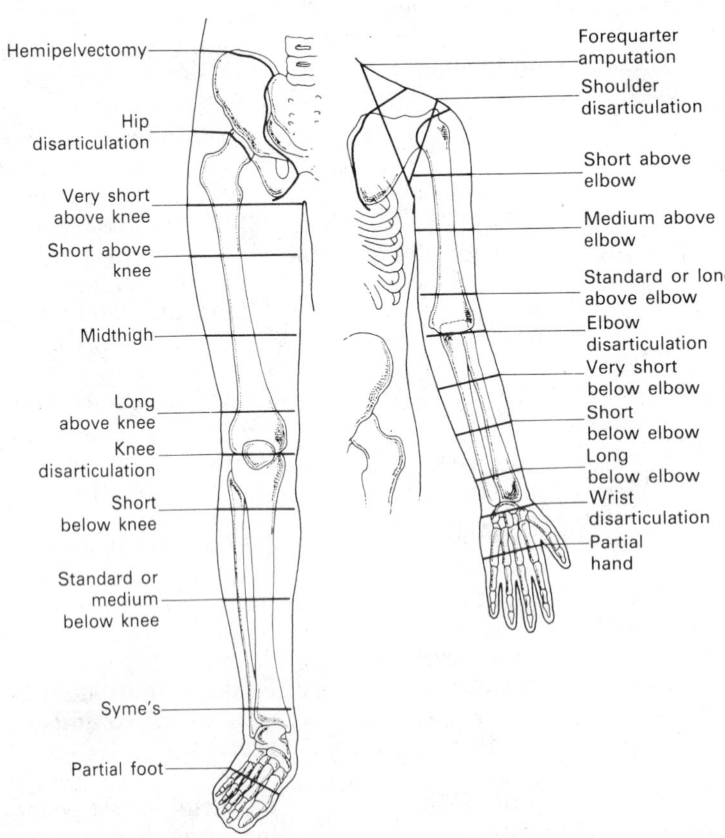

Figure 27-7 Amputation sites.

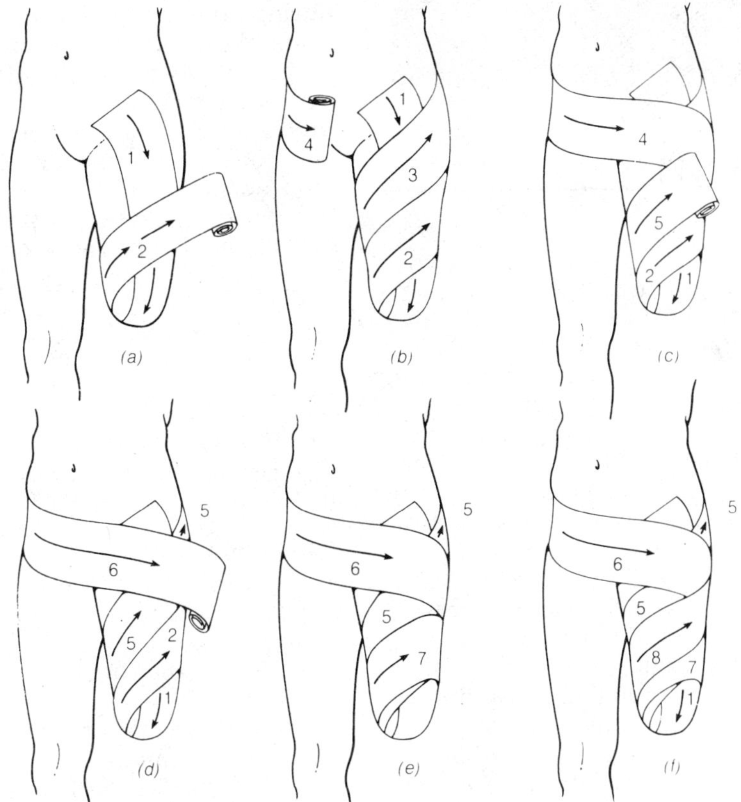

Figure 27-8 Applying a stump bandage. (Jones, D. A., et al.: *Medical-Surgical Nursing: A Conceptual Approach,* 2d ed., McGraw-Hill, New York, 1982.)

Complications

1. Hemorrhage from surgical site; hematoma (refer to Chapter 48).
2. Infection of wound; skin breakdown; wound separation (refer to complications under *Fractures*).
3. Contracture formation (joint) (see Complications under *Fractures*).
4. Phantom limb pain.
5. Delayed grieving (refer to Chapter 45).
6. Stump edema.

Revised Outcomes

1. Client will develop strategies to cope with loss.
2. Infection will be eliminated and healing will be promoted.
3. Pain and edema will be reduced.
4. Contracture will be relieved.
5. Hemorrhage will be terminated.

Interventions

1. Hemorrhage: see Chapter 48.
2. Infection: refer to discussion under *Fractures*.
3. Phantom limb pain: stronger analgesics may be used; counseling; support groups; hypnosis, distraction, and other measures to reduce pain may be used.
4. Stump edema: may be relieved by elevation of the amputated limb; medication may be used to assist the process.
5. Delayed grieving: see Chapter 45.

Reevaluation and Follow-up

1. Recovery from surgical intervention, as evidenced by freedom from pain, healing of tissue, improved circulation.
2. Adjustment to change of lifestyle as result of amputation.
3. Optimal level of functioning at optimal level of independence.

DEGENERATIVE DISEASES

OSTEOARTHRITIS

DESCRIPTION

Osteoarthritis, also known as degenerative joint disease, is a noninflammatory disease affecting the joints. Deterioration and abrasion occur in the articulating cartilage, as well as in the new bone at the articular surface. Osteoarthritis may be idiopathic, occurring with normal use and aging. Structural damage to the joints at an earlier, developmental stage of life can provoke osteoarthritis as one approaches middle age or early senescence.

Osteoarthritis is a localized process found most commonly in the weight-bearing joints of the lower extremities, in the lumbar vertebrae, and in the hands. With aging, the cartilage loses water content and elastic abilities, resulting in softening, separation, and fraying of cartilage. As the cartilage thins and erodes, new bone is stimulated to grow on the articular surface, producing bony spurs that interfere with the mechanical function of the joint. As osteoarthritis progresses, bones, with their eroded cartilage surfaces, come in direct contact with each other, producing pain and restricted motion. As a result, muscle spasms and contractures are common outcomes. Heberden's nodes, bony nodules occurring on the dorsolateral aspects of the distal finger joints, are chronic manifestations of osteoarthritis in the fingers. Table 27-3 gives the differential characteristics between rheumatoid arthritis and osteoarthritis.

PREVENTION

Health Promotion

The cause of this disease is unknown, although there is usually a family history of the condition.

Population at Risk

1. Osteoarthritis is associated with the aging process and is common in middle and old age.
2. Elderly women are more affected than elderly men.
3. Predisposing factors include obesity, trauma, chronic inflammation, faulty body posture and mechanics, and stress.

TABLE 27-3 DIFFERENTIAL CHARACTERISTICS BETWEEN RHEUMATOID ARTHRITIS AND OSTEOARTHRITIS

Rheumatoid Arthritis	Osteoarthritis
Systemic disease; people are sick with malaise, fever, fatigue.	Local joint disease; people have no systemic symptoms.
Signs of inflammation present locally in joints and systemically as pain, fever, soreness, malaise.	Inflammatory signs are less prominent and are local (not systemic) when present.
Fingers and proximal interphalangeal joints are more commonly involved.	Distal interphalangeal nodes are involved more commonly.
Subcutaneous, extra-articular (rheumatoid) nodules are present in tissues around (not in) the joints in 20% of clients.	No periarticular or subcutaneous nodes are present; Heberden's nodes are bony enlargements within the joints.
Bony ankylosis and osteoporosis are common.	Ankylosis and osteoporosis are uncommon.
Elevated sedimentation rate; elevated serum rheumatoid factors.	Normal sedimentation rate and blood chemistries.
Young adults to older adults are affected (25–50 years of age).	Adults are affected during later years (from 45 years of age on).

SOURCE: Mourad, L.: *Nursing Care of Adults with Orthopedic Conditions*, Wiley, New York, 1980.

Screening

X-ray films.

ASSESSMENT

Health History

1. Cultural background.
2. Information regarding client's environment, occupation, finances, education, recreation, and spiritual life relating to habits and social and work roles.
3. Aching pain on weight bearing relieved by rest.
4. Increased pain and stiffness in cold, damp weather.
5. Fatigue with exertion.
6. Stiffness relieved by motion.
7. Associated health problems, current and past.
8. Nutritional history and dietary habits.
9. Relevant family history (e.g., arthritis associated with aging).
10. History of trauma (e.g., fall on affected joint).

Physical Assessment

1. Assess range-of-motion limitations.
2. Position and appearance of extremities: note deformities in affected joints.
3. Joints: tenderness on palpation and pain on motion; some edema may be present.
4. Sensory perception and circulation may not be affected; may be secondary to this problem.
5. Muscle strength: palpation grip test limited.
6. Appearance of affected joints should be normal except for bony enlargement, pain, stiffness, restricted motion, Heberden's nodes.
7. Presence of crepitus on motion: note in affected joints.
8. Vertebral column involvement: motor weakness and paresthesia may be present.
9. Gait unsteady and guarded.
10. Fatigue may be noted, and tolerance (muscle, etc.) may be diminished.
11. Assess general physical health status, including cardiopulmonary status, weight, mental activity.

Diagnostic Tests

1. Arthroscopy.
2. Synovial fluid analysis: normal.
3. Seriology: negative.
4. Arthrography and radiographs of affected joints.
   a. Narrowing of joint space.
   b. Bony sclerosis.
   c. Bony spur formation.
5. Radiographs of vertebral column reveal narrowed spaces between vertebrae.
6. Sedimentation rate: normal.

NURSING DIAGNOSES: ACTUAL OR POTENTIAL

1. Alteration in comfort: discomfort, pain.
2. Immobility: secondary to restricted joint mobility.
3. Alteration in nutrition: more or less than required.
4. Alteration in ability to move effectively; dependence.
5. Alteration in ability to perform self-care activities.
6. Alteration in sensory and motor perception.
7. Associated health problems: potential.
8. Anxiety: mild to severe.

EXPECTED OUTCOMES

1. Pain will be reduced or alleviated.
2. Joint mobility will be maintained or improved.
3. Stresses on affected joints will be reduced.
4. Cause of joint pain will be identified and eliminated.
5. Source of stress on joint will be removed (e.g., weight reduction).
6. Mobility will be maintained or improved, and client will return to optimal level of functioning.
7. Pain will be prevented or controlled.
8. Trauma to weight-bearing joints will be prevented.
9. Maximum joint functioning will be restored.
10. Client will be prepared for surgery, if needed.
11. Client will adjust lifestyle and activities to a level that the involved joint can tolerate.
12. Disability and further disease progression will be prevented.

INTERVENTIONS

1. Apply heat to affected joint for edema.
2. Administer medications to reduce pain.
   a. Corticosteroids to reduce joint inflammation.

   b. Analgesics and/or salicylates to reduce pain and joint inflammation.
   c. Muscle relaxants to reduce muscle spasm.
3. Explain local intra-articular injections (e.g., cortisone) to client and support during injections.
4. Assist in diet selection, considering client's likes and dislikes; control weight and plan diet accordingly.
5. Encourage self-care and other physical activities.
6. Continue exercise regimen and use of ambulatory aid (walker, crutches) initiated in physical and occupational therapy.
7. Refer client to counseling for vocational rehabilitation, if applicable.
8. Provide a back brace or corset if spine is involved.
9. Encourage use of properly fitting shoes to avoid pronated feet.
10. Review principles of good body mechanics and posture.
11. Provide emotional support regarding progressive loss or limitation of motion.
12. Implement teaching plan.
    a. Understanding and cooperation in weight reduction.
    b. Reduction of joint strain.
    c. Rationale and side effects of medication (e.g., steroids, salicylates).
    d. Modification of activities to perform within physical limits and stress on joints; plan physical activity as tolerated.
    e. Rest periods twice per day in recumbent position; periods of sitting.
    f. Proper body mechanics; exercise program to be continued at home.
13. Ensure continuity of health care and follow-up referral.

EVALUATION

Outcome Criteria

1. A balance of rest and activity to maintain optimal health is achieved.
2. ADL are altered to avoid excess use of affected joints.
3. Proper weight is reduced and/or retained via proper nutrition.
4. Client safely uses ambulatory devices.
5. Client takes medications as prescribed and can state their use, dosage, time, route, side effects.
6. Client can safely perform ADL.
7. Client displays knowledge of plans for managing and preventing pain (medication, rest, heat application).
8. Client can describe plans for maintaining mobility (exercises, splints, self-care activities).
9. Client can state limits of activity.
10. Client can describe plans for health maintenance (rest, adequate diet, weight control, adequate urinary and bowel elimination).
11. Client can demonstrate prescribed exercise program.
12. Client makes use of community resources.

Complications

SIDE EFFECTS OF MEDICATION

Assessment

1. Hemorrhagic tendency from salicylates (refer to discussion in Chapter 29).
2. Stress ulcer from corticosteroids (refer to discussion in Chapter 33).
3. Allergies (refer to discussion in Chapter 28).

Revised Outcomes

1. Pain will be alleviated and maximum joint mobility will be attained.
2. Hemorrhage: refer to Chapter 48.
3. Stress ulcer: refer to Chapter 33.
4. Allergies: refer to Chapter 28.

Interventions

1. Institute trial of other medications and combination thereof.
2. Alter exercise program.

PROGRESSION OF DISEASE

Assessment

1. Joint deformity/contraction.
2. Immobility of joint with increased muscle spasm.
3. Continual pain.

Revised Outcomes

1. Motion and stability to the joint will be restored.
2. Deformity will be corrected.
3. Pain will be relieved.

Interventions

1. Surgery.
   a. Synovectomy: removal of the synovial membrane within a joint.
   b. Arthrodesis: fusion of a joint to reduce motion and pain.
   c. Osteotomy: surgical section of a bone (e.g., subtrochanteric).

d. Arthroplasty (total joint replacement): surgical procedure by which the joint is repaired by removal of degenerative or traumatized tissues. Arthroplasties are available for shoulder, elbow, knee, and hip. The hip is a commonly replaced joint and the discussion here is limited to the surgical procedure for total hip replacement (refer to Figure 27-9).

2. Preoperative intervention.
   a. Implement teaching plan.
      (1) Client and family participation in mobility regimen.

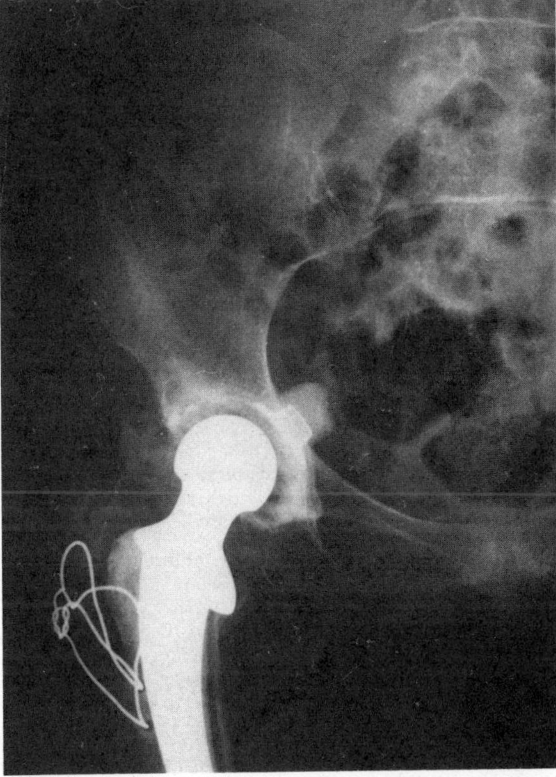

Figure 27-9 Total hip replacement arthroplasty. The acetabulum is replaced with a polyethylene prosthetic part. A metallic prosthesis replaces the femoral head and neck. The wires visible are used to reattach and hold the greater trochanter to the femur for healing. Wires are needed because the muscles attached to the greater trochanter would pull it away, leading to nonunion. Methyl methacrylate is used to cement both the femoral and acetabular parts in place. (Mourad, L.: *Nursing Care of Adults with Orthopedic Conditions,* Wiley, New York, 1980.)

      (2) Postoperative exercise program.
      (3) Techniques in hip abduction.
      (4) Use of urinal and bedpan in recumbent position.
      (5) Postoperative respiratory exercises.
   b. Demonstrate balanced suspension traction apparatus and use of trapeze (see Figure 27-6).
   c. Administer systemic antibiotic and anticoagulant therapy.
   d. Perform bacteriostatic skin scrub preparation: usually pHisoHex and/or Betadine is used.
   e. Explore verbal and nonverbal cues of emotional stress.
   f. Explain and perform routine preoperative procedures.

3. Postoperative intervention.
   a. Use flotation mattress, traction apparatus, and trapeze on bed.
   b. Monitor vital signs.
   c. Provide for adequate respiratory functioning.
   d. Maintain integrity of hip prosthesis.
      (1) Maintain hip in abduction at all times; use wedge-shaped abduction pillow between legs.
      (2) Turn q2h, supine, to unaffected side, keeping hip in abduction.
      (3) Elevate affected extremity on pillows.
      (4) Limit elevation of head of bed to 45 degrees.
   e. Assess circulatory and nerve functioning of affected leg every hour.
   f. Initiate exercise program early, in collaboration with physical therapist.
      (1) Affected leg: isometric exercises.
      (2) Active exercises to unaffected extremities, using footboard.
      (3) Discourage sitting for prolonged periods.
   g. Monitor alignment of traction three to four times per day.
   h. Observe incisional dressing for drainage, bleeding; Hemovac may be present.
   i. Assess for signs of infection in operative site.
   j. Assess for thrombophlebitis and possible emboli.
      (1) Antiemboli stockings, Ace bandages.
      (2) Leg exercises.
      (3) Frequent turning.
   k. Assess for dislocation (subluxation) of hip prosthesis.

(1) Severe pain.
(2) External rotation of hip with noticeable shortening of leg.
(3) Bulge can be palpated over head of femur.

l. Assess bony prominences for skin breakdown.
(1) Air mattress.
(2) Artificial sheepskin.
(3) Skin care q2h.

m. Discharge planning.
(1) Progressive exercise program.
(2) Follow-up care in ambulatory health care setting.

Reevaluation and Follow-up

Evaluation is continuous. Provide information for modification of plans as the client's status changes with increasing or decreasing mobility.

REFERENCES

Brunner, L. S., and Suddarth D. S.: *Textbook of Medical-Surgical Nursing*, 4th ed., Lippincott, Philadelphia, 1980, p. 1294.

Hilt, N. E., and Cogburn, S. B.: *Manual of Orthopedics*, Mosby, St. Louis, 1980, p. 86.

Jones, D. A., Dunbar, C. F., and Jirovec, M. M.: *Medical-Surgical Nursing: A Conceptual Approach*, 2d ed., McGraw-Hill, New York, 1982, p. 1540.

Powell, M.: *Orthopaedic Nursing and Rehabilitation*, 8th ed., Churchill Livingstone, Edinburgh, 1982, p. 562.

Roaf, R., and Hodkinson, L. J.: *Textbook of Orthopedic Nursing*, 3d ed., Blackwell, Oxford, 1980, p. 236.

BIBLIOGRAPHY

Buckwalter, K. C., and Buckwalter, J. A.: "Pain Assessment and Management in the Patient With a Fracture," *Journal of Nursing Care*, **14**:17–20, July 1981. A discussion of causes, symptoms, and appropriate nursing actions to be initiated to relieve pain following reduction and immobilization of a fracture.

Derscheid, G.: "Rehabilitation of Common Orthopedic Problems," *Nursing Clinics of North America*, **16**:709–720, December 1981. Offers a discussion of the general principles of physical therapy that can be initiated by the nurse when physical therapy is not available or acceptable to the client with ankle injuries, knee injuries, arthroplasty of the hips, and knee and shoulder injuries.

Dunnery, E.: "Fractured Hip: How to Position and Mobilize Patients—Without Undoing Their Surgery," *R.N.*, **42**:45–57, June 1979. Preoperative and postoperative nursing care, assessment, and teaching of a client with a fractured hip is presented. A narrative and pictorial description of transfer from stretcher to bed, turning, and chair transfer is included.

Farrell, J.: *Illustrated Guide to Orthopedic Nursing*, 2d ed., Lippincott, Philadelphia, 1982. This book focuses on the nursing care of adult orthopedic clients in the hospital environment—on those factors that influence the client's adjustment, behavior, and recovery. Practical suggestions for assisting the client to readjust to the home environment are presented. Basic information on conditions and disorders is also presented.

Hay, B. K., and Karas, C. B.: "External Fixation: Option for Fractures," *AORN Journal*, **34**:417–423, September 1981. The increasingly popular procedure for external fixation of a grade III open fracture is described in case method format.

Hay, B. K., and Karas, C. B.: "A Teaching Plan for External Fixation," *AORN Journal*, **34**:424–426. An external fixation teaching plan is presented including the instructional content, the teaching activity, and evaluation.

Kerr, A.: *Orthopedic Nursing Procedures*, 3d ed., Springer, New York, 1980. This book deals with initial and emergency care of orthopedic injuries. In addition, the book addresses trauma in general, giving very practical ideas.

Kryschyshen, P. L., and Fisher, D. A.: "External Fixation for Complicated Fractures," *American Journal of Nursing*, **80**:256–259, February 1980. External fixation, its devices, indication for use, application, postoperative nursing care, and advantages are discussed.

Lentz, M.: "Selected Aspects of Deconditioning Secondary to Immobilization," *Nursing Clinics of North America*, **16**:729–737, December 1981. This article explores the possible nursing interventions and their rationales for use with the identified deconditioning changes in the cardiovascular system and the musculoskeletal system resulting from immobilization due to orthopedic conditions.

Levitt, D. Z.: "Multiple Myeloma," *American Journal of Nursing*, **81**:1345–1347, July 1981. A discussion of the pathophysiology, diagnosis, treatment, and complications of a client with multiple myeloma. A chart of client care guidelines related to complications and nursing interventions is included.

Love-Mignogna, S.: "Taping and Splinting: Seven Common Problems and How to Avoid Them," *Nursing 80*, **10**:88–92, October 1980. This article presents solutions, both narrative and pictorial, for common problems, including interdigital maceration, chafing, faulty joint stabilization, "tourniquet" effect, edema, improper positioning, and postprocedural complications.

McWilliams, N.: *Manual of Orthopedic Surgery for Nurses*, Robert J. Brady, Bowie, Md., 1982. This book is intended to be an aid to experienced nurses who wish to practice in the specialty of orthopedic surgery. It is arranged as a self-instructional tool to teach the many principles and skills specific to preoperative and postoperative care.

Miller, L. B.: "Orthopedic Patients in an Ambulatory Surgery Facility," *Nursing Clinics of North America*, **16**:749–758, December 1981. This article describes the advantages and concept of ambulatory surgery, the orthopedic conditions treated by ambulatory therapy and surgery, and the major nursing focus on adequate preparation of the client.

Ritchey, J.: "Traction Review," *The ONA Journal*, **6**:335–340, August 1979. Diagrams of the most common types of skin and skeletal traction (Buck's, Bryant's, split Russell's, side arm, Dunlap's, cervical, pelvic), showing positioning of extremity and weights. Indications for each type of traction are included.

Rodriguez, R. C.: "A Classification System for the Orthopedic Patient," *The ONA Journal*, **6**:398–405, October 1979. A system of classifying orthopedic clients according to their need for care in terms of time, physical condition, and skill of practitioner is presented along with a Kardix/Care Plan that identifies nursing diagnoses and nursing approach.

Walters, J.: "Coping With a Leg Amputation," *American Journal of Nursing*, **81**:1349–1352, July 1981. This article discusses the four phases of adjustment to an amputation: impact, retreat, acknowledgment, and reconstruction. An illustration of lower extremity prostheses is presented.

Wassel, A.: "Nursing Assessment of Injuries to the Lower Extremity," *Nursing Clinics of North America*, **16**:739–748, December 1981. Lower extremity injuries are divided into two groups: (1) vehicular or crushing injuries and (2) nonvehicular, torsion, or overuse injuries. Initial assessment, treatment, and nursing functions are discussed.

28

The Endocrine System

Virginia L. Cassmeyer and Betty L. Hopping

The endocrine system is composed of a variety of specialized tissues spread throughout the body that function to regulate physiological processes in numerous target organs via the secretion of hormones that act as chemical messengers. The regulatory functions are varied and diffuse and affect most of the major organ systems of the body. It is now evident that the hypothalamus controls many of the endocrine functions via stimulation of pituitary secretion. Many of the more common endocrine diseases involve abnormal cellular growth, hypoactivity, or hyperactivity that result in decreased or increased function in the target organs. Therefore, nursing interventions related to endocrine disorders require knowledge of the functioning and pathophysiology of most of the organ systems of the body.

PHYSICAL ASSESSMENT SPECIFIC TO IDENTIFICATION OF ENDOCRINE PROBLEMS

1. General body growth and developmental status.
   a. Height.
   b. Weight.
   c. Depressed body growth may be indicative of thyroid or pituitary problems.
   d. Increased body growth may be indicative of pituitary problems.
   e. Change in weight may be indicative of diabetes mellitus, adrenal cortical excess, or thyroid problems.
   f. Abnormal secondary sex characteristics may be indicative of adrenal, pituitary, or gonadal problems.
2. Total body muscle mass and fat distribution.
   a. Decreased muscle mass may be seen in pituitary, adrenal, or pancreatic endocrine problems.
   b. Changes in fat distribution (buffalo hump, thickened girdle, moon face) are seen in adrenal cortical excess.
3. Integumentary system.
   a. Pigmentation changes may be seen in adrenal cortical problems.
   b. Increased body hair in females may be indicative of increased adrenal androgens.
   c. Lesions (boils, infections, ulcers, yeast, fungus, or monilial infections) are frequently found in uncontrolled diabetics.
   d. Skin over the lower extremities may show changes characteristic of arterial insufficiency (loss of hair, color changes, temperature change, pigmentation changes).
   e. Skin turgor changes may be the result of diabetes mellitus, adrenal cortical insufficiency, hypoaldosteronism, diabetes insipidus.
4. Head, neck, and face.
   a. Eyes.
      (1) Prominent eyes with infrequent blinking.
      (2) Fixed stare with sclera showing both above and below the iris.
      (3) Exopthalmos.

Recognition is given to Jacqueline Sicard Baran, R.N., M.S., who was the original author of this chapter in the previous edition of this book.

b. Face.
   (1) Moon facies.
   (2) Increased facial hair.
c. Neck.
   (1) Noticeable swelling of masses.
   (2) Thyroid.
      (a) In normal clients frequently not palpable.
      (b) Diffuse enlargement of total gland is indicative of goiter due to iodine deficiency or hyperthyroidism.
      (c) Toxic adenomas may cause diffuse enlargement of one lobe.
      (d) Hard nodules may be indicative of cancer.

5. Central nervous system.
   a. Sensory systems.
      (1) Responses to temperature, proprioception, vibration, pain, touch may be decreased due to vascular insufficiency.
      (2) Vision.
         (a) Acuity may be decreased as a result of diabetes or pituitary problems.
         (b) Visual field defect (particularly of peripheral visual field) may occur with pituitary tumors.
   b. Motor functions.
      (1) Reflexes may be hyperactive in hyperthyroidism or hypoactive in diabetes mellitus.
      (2) Generalized weakness, decreased ambulatory ability; tremor may be present in multiple endocrine diseases.
6. Cardiovascular-respiratory system.
   a. Check vital signs (blood pressure, pulse, respiration); check BP and pulse for orthostatic changes.
   b. Monitor for arrhythmias.
   c. Check all peripheral pulses; note presence, strength, and bilateral equality.
   d. Check skin temperature and color of the extremities.
   e. Check for presence of edema, particularly in lower extremities and sacrum in bedridden clients. Fluid overload from abnormal retention or congestive heart failure may be present in many endocrine problems.
   f. Note respiratory pattern, depth, Kussmaul breathing, hypo/hyperventilation.
   g. Listen for breath sounds.
7. Breast.
   a. Examine for change in size in males.
   b. Check for presence of galactorrhea.

ABNORMAL CELLULAR GROWTH

PITUITARY TUMORS

DESCRIPTION

Pituitary tumors result from abnormal growth of one of the cells of the pituitary gland. Pituitary tumors account for 10 percent of all symptomatic intracranial tumors and may arise from the anterior or posterior lobe. Posterior lobe tumors are rare. Anterior lobe tumors have been commonly classified according to the staining qualities of the cells of the tumor, namely, *chromophobic, acidophilic,* or *basophilic.* Approximately three-fourths of the pituitary tumors are chromophobes. Chromophobes in the past were considered to be clinically "nonfunctioning," that is, unable to secrete any pituitary hormones. With the development of finer diagnostic tests it has been found that these tumors do secrete hormones. Chromophobes most frequently are associated with the secretion of prolactin, although they may secrete other hormones. The next most frequently occurring pituitary tumor is acidophilic-staining. These tumors secrete prolactin, growth hormone, or both. Basophilic-staining tumors are associated with the secretion of adrenocorticotropic hormone (ACTH) and rarely thyroid stimulating hormone (TSH). Because classifying by staining quality does not automatically tell the type of endocrine abnormality associated with the tumor, tumors are sometimes classified instead by type of hormone secreted, for example, prolactin-secreting tumor or growth hormone–secreting tumor.

Other intracranial tumors arising from Rathke's pouch (craniopharyngiomas), the hypothalamus, and so on may extend into the pituitary. These tumors are nonsecreting but may cause endocrine problems because they suppress normal hypothalamic-pituitary function.

Depending on the size, location, and secreting capacity of the tumor, three clinical problems may occur: (1) *hypersecretion* of one or more pituitary hormones, most commonly prolactin (PRL), somatotropin (GH), or corticotropin (ACTH); (2) *hyposecretion* of one or more pituitary hormones as a result of compression of normal pituitary tissue; or (3) *neurological symptoms* due to alteration of surrounding tissue by the tumor. (Figure 28-1 illustrates the relationship of the pituitary gland to surrounding structures.)

The cause of pituitary tumors is unknown. Evidence of secreting tumors is often given by their hormonal effects before they cause neurological symptoms. Nonsecreting tumors are frequently asymptomatic until they cause neurological changes.

Table 28-1 lists the hormones secreted by the hypothalamus and anterior pituitary. Of the hypothalamic hormones (factors) listed, only thyroid-releasing hormone (TRH/TRF), luteinizing hormone–releasing hormone (LHRH/LHRF), and somatostatin (GHIH/GHIF) have been fully characterized. The others listed are believed to exist based on research but have not been characterized. There are probably other hypothalamic inhibiting factors, but as yet this is unknown. The hypothalamus also produces two other hormones, antidiuretic hormone (ADH) and oxytocin, which are stored and released from the posterior pituitary.

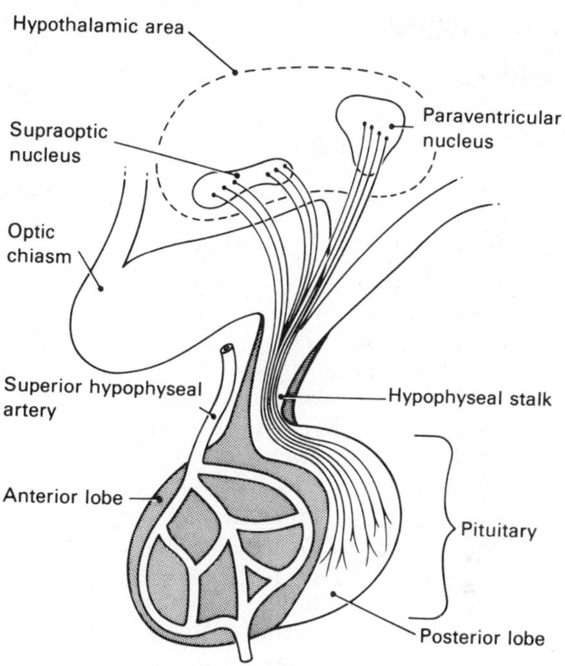

Figure 28-1 Hypothalamic-pituitary relationship.

PREVENTION

Health Promotion

As the cause of pituitary tumors is unknown, there is no known way to prevent the problem. Early detection and treatment is the key to preventing complications.

Population at Risk

There is no known population at risk.

Screening

There are no known screening tests or tools that can be used for mass screening.

TABLE 28-1 HORMONES SECRETED BY THE HYPOTHALAMUS AND ANTERIOR PITUITARY

Hypothalamus	Anterior Pituitary
Growth hormone–releasing factor (GHRF)	Growth hormone (GH)
Growth hormone–inhibiting factor (GHIF, somatostatin)	
Prolactin-releasing factor (PRF)	Prolactin (PRL)
Prolactin-inhibiting factor (PIF)	
Melanocyte-releasing factor (MRF)	Melanocyte-stimulating hormone (MSH)
Melanocyte-inhibiting factor (MIF)	
Corticotropin-releasing factor (CRF)	Adrenocorticotropic hormone (ACTH)
Thyrotropin-releasing factor (TRF)	Thyroid-stimulating hormone (TSH)
Luteinizing hormone–releasing factor (LHRF)	Luteinizing hormone (LH)
Follicle-stimulating hormone–releasing factor (FSH-RF)	Follicle-stimulating hormone (FSH)
Antidiuretic hormone (ADH)	
Oxytocin	

ASSESSMENT

Health History

1. Pituitary tumors in general.
   a. Perceived changes in visual acuity, occurrence of diplopia, and defects in visual field because of compression on the optic pathway.
   b. History of CNS symptoms.
      (1) Seizures.
      (2) Confusion.
      (3) Dizziness.
      (4) Headaches.
2. Growth hormone–secreting tumors.
   a. Perceived changes in the acral parts.
      (1) Increase in ring size.
      (2) Increase in hand span.
      (3) Increase in shoe size.
      (4) Broadening of the mandible, maxilla, and forehead.
   b. Increased sweating.
   c. Mood swings, mental changes, and drowsiness.
   d. Joint and back pain due to osteoarthritis of the joints from overgrowth of the periosteum.
   e. Disturbance in menstrual cycle.
   f. Weight gain.
   g. Change in voice.
   h. Glucose intolerance.
   i. History of items listed under number 1 above.
3. Prolactin-secreting tumors.
   a. Change in menstrual cycle, amenorrhea.
   b. Intermittent lactation.
   c. Increase in breast tissue in males.
   d. Infertility.
   e. History of items listed under number 1 above.
4. ACTH-secreting tumors (see *Adrenocortical Hyperfunction: Hypercortisolism* in this chapter).
5. TSH-secreting tumors (see *Hyperthyroidism* in this chapter).

Physical Assessment

1. Pituitary tumors in general.
   a. Very frequently there will be no changes.
   b. Confrontation examination might reveal visual field defects if tumor is large.
   c. Diplopia, papillary edema.
   d. If the tumor is very large, other CNS changes such as confusion or emotional changes might be seen.

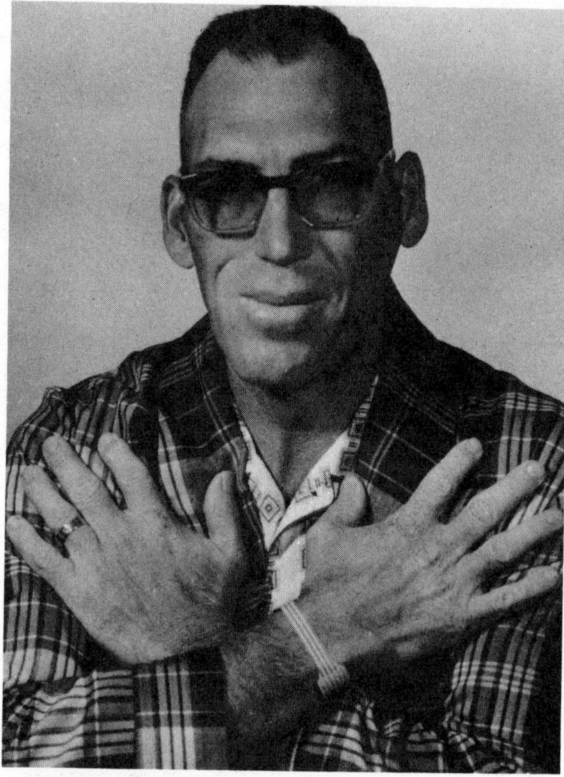

Figure 28-2 Acromegaly. [Hume, D. M., and Harrison, T. S., in S. I. Schwartz et al. (eds.): *Principles of Surgery*, 2d ed., McGraw-Hill, New York, 1974.]

2. Growth hormone–secreting tumors.
   a. All the assessment items listed above under number 1 for tumors in general plus the following.
   b. Musculoskeletal system (see Figure 28-2).
      (1) Acral bone growth.
         (a) Broad spadelike hands.
         (b) Widened fingers.
         (c) Broadening of the feet.
      (2) Broad face, mandibular teeth extending beyond maxillary.
      (3) Widely separated teeth.
      (4) Coarse facial features (broad nose, enlarged lips, prominent forehead).
      (5) Enlarged tongue.
      (6) Enlarged bulk of frame.
      (7) Decreased range of motion in joints and back due to osteoporosis.
      (8) Muscle weakness, atrophy.
   c. Integumentary system.
      (1) Coarsening, thickening of the skin.

(2) Oily skin.
(3) Coarse body hair on face, abdomen, and extremities, particularly in females.
(4) Increased pigmentation.

d. Central nervous system.
(1) Hypoactivity.
(2) Slowing of mental functions.
(3) Emotional liability.
(4) Paresthesia.

e. Other physical manifestations.
(1) Enlarged liver, spleen due to generalized increase in visceral growth.
(2) Husky voice.
(3) Symptoms of other endocrine problems such as diabetes mellitus and thyroid problems.

3. Prolactin-secreting tumors.
a. May have physical assessment changes listed under number 2a through d above.
b. Galactorrhea.
c. Amenorrhea in females.
d. Increased breast tissue in males.

Other Sources of Information

1. Photographs of family members and of the client over time can be helpful in the diagnosis of excessive growth hormone.
2. History information should be validated by family members or other significant others.

Diagnostic Tests

1. Measurement of serum levels of GH, TSH, ACTH, FSH, and LH to identify the secreting capacity of the tumor and to assess the function of the pituitary.
2. Measurement of serum levels of glucocorticoids, T_3 and T_4, estrogen, progesterone, and testosterone to assess functioning of target glands.
3. To identify the presence of tumor:
a. X-ray films of sella turcica, skull.
b. Computerized axial tomography (CAT scan).
c. In some instances pneumoencephalograms or cerebral arteriograms are necessary to define the extent of the tumor.
4. Tangent screen perimetry to assess visual field defects.
5. Special tests for suspected growth hormone–secreting tumors.
a. Radiographic examinations of feet, hands, skull (see Figure 28-3).
b. Suppression test. Glucose tolerance test. Normally 100 g of glucose should suppress growth hormone secretion within 30–90 min. This does not occur in acromegaly (growth hormone excess).
6. Special tests for PRL-secreting tumors.
a. Suppression test. Client is given L-dopa (L-dopa suppresses PRL levels).

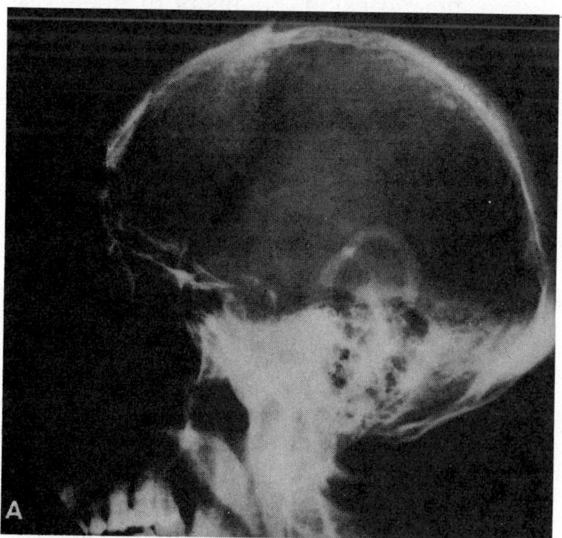

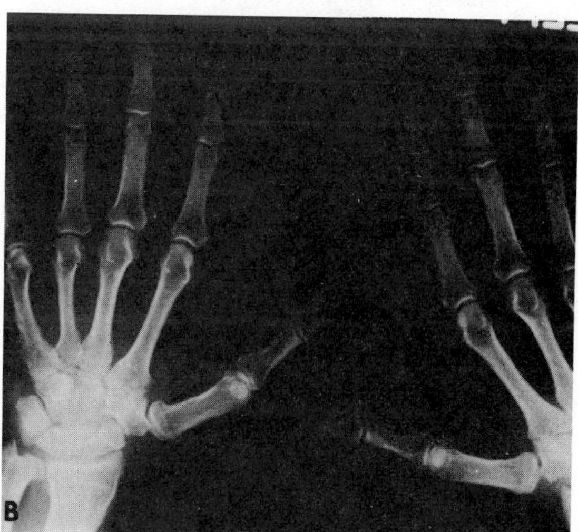

Figure 28-3 X-ray films of lateral skull and hands of client with acromegaly. [Hume, D. M., and Harrison, T. S., in S. I. Schwartz et al. (eds.): *Principles of Surgery*, 2d ed., McGraw-Hill, New York, 1974.]

b. Stimulating test. In normal persons, TRF or chlorpromazine cause an increase in prolactin. In clients with PRL-secreting tumors this response is blunted.

NURSING DIAGNOSES: ACTUAL OR POTENTIAL

1. Pituitary tumors in general.
   a. Permanent or temporary visual loss: related to compression of optic pathway by tumor.
   b. Headache: related to expanding tumor mass in cranium.
   c. Potential for injury: related to seizures, syncope, dizziness, confusion resulting from increased tumor mass.
   d. Fear: related to the seriousness of the disease.
   e. Potential lack of knowledge: regarding diagnostic tests, pathophysiology, and treatment.
2. Growth hormone excess (acromegaly).
   a. Muscle weaknesses: due to changes in muscle growth and metabolism.
   b. Pain: related to osteoporosis in joints and back.
   c. Potential for injury: related to changes in CNS, vision, and mobility.
   d. Alterations of self-concept: related to body changes.
   e. Potential alterations in sexual functions: related to GH excess.
   f. Potential alterations in homeostasis: related to glucose intolerance.
   g. Also diagnoses as listed for pituitary tumors under 1 above.
3. Prolactin excess.
   a. Alteration in sexual functioning: related to PRL excess and fear of sterility.
   b. Alterations in self-concept: related to galactorrhea, amenorrhea, or change in breast tissue mass.
   c. Also diagnoses as listed for pituitary tumors under 1 above.

EXPECTED OUTCOMES

1. Immediate.
   a. Headaches will decrease initially because of appropriate use of pain medications and other therapeutic measures. (Later, headaches will be relieved because of treatment.)
   b. Client will be free of injuries that could result from decreased vision, weakness, changes in mental status. (Later, client will be free of injuries because he or she will have learned how to compensate for visual changes.)
   c. Client will express minimal complaints of discomfort from joint and back pain because of adequate use of therapeutic measures.
   d. Client will demonstrate adequate knowledge of diagnostic tests, as evidenced by the ability to explain tests, purpose of procedures, and special preparation.
   e. Client will demonstrate adequate knowledge of potential treatment (surgery or radiation therapy) by describing:
      (1) Treatment planned.
      (2) Expected effects of the treatment (decrease in hormone excess, no alterations in normal pituitary function, return of normal sexual function, minimal or no changes in body features due to acromegalia, improvement of glucose tolerance, unknown improvement of vision, decrease in headaches).
      (3) Potential complications (loss of normal pituitary function, CNS damage, and infection).
      (4) Expectations after transsphenoidal removal of pituitary tumors (temporary nose packing, no ability to smell, use of oxygen by facial mask, nasal drainage, headaches, frequent monitoring of intake and output, vital signs, and nasal drainage).
      (5) Expectations after radiation therapy (slow decrease in excess hormone secretion, headaches, lethargy, nausea and vomiting after treatments).
      (6) Expectations with removal of tumor by frontal craniotomy (see Chapter 25).
   f. Client will not develop any unrecognized changes in homeostasis that can result from other hormonal imbalance.
   g. Client will demonstrate improved self-concept, as evidenced by talking about self in positive terms, accentuating positive attributes (hairstyle, dressing to minimize body changes), identifying plans to increase social contacts if these were decreased, and setting goals for the future.
   h. Client will demonstrate improvement in

sexual functioning, as evidenced by recognizing that sexual function changes are probably temporary, identifying alternatives available if sterility is permanent, and maximizing secondary sexual characteristics.

i. Client will not develop any complications from treatment that go unrecognized, such as CSF leak, CNS infection, diabetes insipidius, or other hormonal deficits.

2. Long-term.
   a. Client will state need for continual follow-up and specify time and date of first appointment.
   b. Client will understand how to deal with any residual hormonal deficits present, as evidenced by identifying deficits and signs and symptoms of deficits, stating type of hormonal replacement necessary, stating time and amount of therapy, stating signs and symptoms of excess and insufficient therapy, and stating times when more replacement therapy might be necessary.

INTERVENTIONS

1. General.
   a. Determine if headaches are present and institute measures to decrease them (e.g., darkened room, head of bed elevated, quiet environment).
   b. Identify any CNS changes that could result in injury, such as vision changes, seizures, syncope, and confusion.
      (1) Structure environment to prevent injury.
      (2) Structure environment to allow client as much independence as possible.
   c. Give pain medications as soon as possible.
   d. Ensure safety and accuracy of diagnostic tests by:
      (1) Administering diagnostic medications as appropriate and ensuring appropriate collection of specimens.
      (2) Monitoring client for side effects of diagnostic medications.
   e. Instruct client and family regarding diagnostic tests.
      (1) Purpose of tests.
      (2) Routine of tests (medicines to be given, blood to be drawn, length of time test takes, where test is performed, and care after test).
   f. Instruct client and family regarding diagnoses.
      (1) Anatomy and physiology of the pituitary and hypothalamus.
      (2) Functions of hormones.
      (3) How increases or decreases of hormones caused the signs and symptoms client is experiencing.
   g. If appropriate, teach client and family about transsphenoidal removal of pituitary tumors. Teaching plan should include:
      (1) Surgical approach.
      (2) Care needs after surgery (nasal packing and drainage, frequent checking of vital signs, monitoring of intake and output, daily weights, oxygen by facial mask, and mouth care.
      (3) Physical changes after surgery (temporary loss of smell and temporary headaches).
   h. If appropriate, instruct client and family regarding frontal craniotomy (see Chapter 25).
   i. If appropriate, teach client and family about radiation therapy. Teaching plan should include:
      (1) Where and when treatment is done.
      (2) The fact that there will be a gradual relief of symptoms.
      (3) The fact that there might be a gradual onset of signs and symptoms of hormonal deficiency.
      (4) The signs and symptoms that client must monitor for.
      (5) The possibility of nausea, vomiting, and lethargy after treatments.
   j. Allow for discussion of feelings.
      (1) Plan time to be with the client in privacy.
      (2) Allow the client to set the pace in what he or she wants to discuss but be sure client is aware you are available.
      (3) Direct your attention to the client's major concern.
      (4) Be honest with the client about expected outcomes.
   k. Specific postoperative care for transsphenoidal removal of pituitary tumors (Jubiz, 1979).
      (1) Institute assessment regimen. Check:
         (a) Vital signs q4h.
         (b) Intake and output and specific gravity at least q4h; daily weight at

same time, with same clothes, on same scale.

(c) Nasal drainage every 2–4 h. Record amount and color of drainage. Cerebrospinal fluid (CSF) will be clear and will cause a "halo" ring around serous fluid. CSF and nasal drainage appear similar. CSF drainage contains glucose, so drainage can be tested with dipstick for the presence of glucose. If glucose is present in a clear fluid, collect specimen for laboratory analysis and consult with the physician.

(2) Mouth care: Use mouthwash and swabs to clean the mouth. Do not use a toothbrush.

(3) Maintain oxygen by facial mask. Make sure the client is getting enough humidity. This will prevent drying of the mucous membranes.

(4) Administer pain medications for headache. Monitor effectiveness.

(5) Ambulate client the first day after surgery. Do not let client bend over or position head lower than trunk.

(6) Prevent sneezing and coughing. These activities will increase intracranial pressure.

(7) Warn client not to blow nose. This can disrupt the suture line.

(8) Provide soft foods and liquids as tolerated and allowed.

l. In preparation for discharge institute teaching regarding:

(1) Sequence for follow-up after discharge.

(2) Activities allowed.

(3) Rest schedule.

(4) Oral hygiene allowed.

(5) Signs and symptoms of ACTH deficit. It is not usually necessary to teach signs and symptoms of hormonal insufficiency to client, but if pituitary is totally removed, client must know signs and symptoms of deficiency states: adrenocortical insufficiency (see *Adrenocortical Hypofunction* in this chapter): thyroid hormone deficiency (see *Hypothyroidism* in this chapter), diabetes insipidus (see *Diabetes Insipidus* in this chapter), and gonadotropin deficiency (see *Gonadotropin Deficiency* in this chapter).

(6) Medications: Hormonal replacement therapy is not usually necessary, as the normal function of the pituitary is not usually disrupted; but if it is necessary, teaching should include:

(a) Purpose.

(b) Dosage.

(c) Time to take medication.

(d) Signs and symptoms of excess therapy or insufficient therapy.

(7) Follow-up visits: Plan with client to return to the clinic usually 1 month after discharge and then every 6 to 12 months.

(8) Follow-up evaluation: During return visit the client will be observed for signs and symptoms of hormonal deficiency or continual hormonal excess. Serum levels of GH, PRL, ACTH, TSH, glucocorticoids, FSH, LH, estrogen, progesterone, testosterone, and T_3 and T_4 may be measured.

2. Additional interventions if client has a growth hormone–secreting tumor.

a. Identify amount of discomfort from joint and back pain.

b. Institute comfort measures that will decrease pain (e.g., hard mattress, extra support for joints, warmth applied to joints).

c. Identify client's limitations due to fatigue, muscle weakness, or pain.

d. Structure an environment that allows independence within client's limitations (e.g., placing personal belongings and equipment within reach, providing a shower if client cannot get into a tub, providing appropriate type of chair).

e. Assist with activities of daily living as necessary.

f. Plan activities to allow for rest between bath, treatments, tests, meals, and visiting.

g. Institute monitoring schedule to identify other hormonal imbalances.

(1) Perform urine test for sugar and acetone qid.

(2) Monitor for signs of hypo- and hyperglycemia (see *Diabetes Mellitus* in this chapter).

3. Additional interventions if client has a prolactin-secreting tumor.

a. The client may be treated with bromocriptine, an ergot derivative, which is known to inhibit prolactin secretion.

b. Bromocriptine controls symptoms only; it does not decrease size of tumor.
c. Amenorrhea, galactorrhea, and the patient should become fertile.

EVALUATION

Outcome Criteria

1. Headaches are controlled and then completely relieved.
2. Client suffers no injuries.
3. Client's activities are not limited by joint and back pain or weakness.
4. Client is able to perform activities of daily living safely.
5. Client and family can recall with complete accuracy the information presented in teaching session on diagnostic tests.
6. Client and significant others can recall with complete accuracy the information presented regarding the disease and treatment.
7. Client is not developing any complications that were not immediately identified.
8. Client is talking about self in positive terms, dressing to maximize positive characteristics, and discussing planned social contacts.
9. Client is taking medications appropriately, as evidenced by chart he or she is keeping (only if on medications).
10. Client is self-monitoring for signs and symptoms of deficiencies, as evidenced by diary with record of:
    a. Feelings of well-being.
    b. Activity level.
    c. Daily weight.
    d. Presence or absence of nausea, vomiting, headache, dizziness, and fatigue.

Complications

1. Panhypopituitarism. This is a deficiency of all anterior pituitary hormones and at times ADH. Assessment, outcomes, and interventions would be those listed for adrenocortical insufficiency (see *Adrenocortical Hypofunction, Hypothyroidism,* and *Gonadotropic Deficiency,* all in this chapter).
2. Diabetes insipidus (see discussion this chapter).
3. CNS infection (see Chapter 25).

THYROID TUMORS

DESCRIPTION

Tumors of the thyroid gland may be benign or malignant. *Benign tumors,* or *adenomas,* are well encapsulated, noninvading tumors that do not respond to normal physiological controls on growth or synthesis and secretion of hormones, resulting in atrophy of normal thyroid tissue and in some cases hyperthyroidism (toxic adenoma). *Malignant tumors* of the thyroid are uncommon, slow growing, and rarely fatal (accounting for only 0.4 percent of all cancer deaths).

The prognosis associated with thyroid tumors is determined by many factors, namely, the histological features and stage of the tumor and the age and sex of the client. Histologically, tumors can be classified as *papillary* (accounting for 50 percent of all adult and 70 percent of all childhood malignant tumors), *follicular* (30 percent of cases, the incidence of which peaks in adults between the ages of 30 to 50 years), *medullary* (which secrete calcitonin rather than thyroxine and/or triiodothyronine, are frequently associated with other endocrine disorders such as pheochromocytoma, hyperparathyroidism, and Cushing's disease, and may be inherited as an autosomal dominant characteristic), and *anaplastic* tumors, which grow rapidly and invade surrounding tissue extensively and metastasize widely. There are impressive data linking the occurrence of tumors, usually slow-growing papillary or follicular cancer, in children and young adults to therapeutic head and neck or thymus radiation treatment as infants; the tumor may appear 5 to 30 years following the treatment. Thyroid cancers are staged from grade I to grade III, which range from encapsulated, circumscribed cancer with minimal invasion of adjacent tissue and favorable prognosis to extensive local invasion, undifferentiated cells, and possible metastases with poor prognosis. These cancers are at least four times as frequent in women as in men but carry a less favorable prognosis for men. Increasing age, especially after age 40, signifies less favorable prognosis because of the greater possibility of metastases.

PREVENTION

Health Promotion

1. Early diagnosis and treatment.
2. Protection of thyroid gland if x-ray irradiation of head, neck, thymus is essential.

Population at Risk

1. Persons who received x-ray irradiation of head, neck, thymus during infancy.

2. Persons who have a family history of multiple endocrine tumors such as pheochromocytoma, hyperparathyroidism, Cushing's disease.
3. Adults over age 40, especially women.

Screening

Physical examination of thyroid gland.

ASSESSMENT

Health History

1. Family history of endocrine tumors, especially of thyroid, parathyroid, adrenal gland.
2. Nodule in thyroid area with history of increasing size; painless if adenoma or noninvasive tumor, painful if invasive tumor.
3. Complaint of difficulty swallowing (if tumor is large).
4. Complaint of frequent watery diarrhea (if medullary tumor secreting calcitonin).
5. Possible history of hyperthyroidism.

Physical Assessment

1. Palpation of thyroid area for possible nodule.
2. Palpation of supraclavicular area for possible metastases to lymph nodes draining thyroid area.
3. Observation of skin for excessive perspiration and velvety softness associated with hyperthyroidism.
4. Observation for lack of forehead wrinkling on upward gaze, tremors of eyelids upon closing, tremors of hands and tongue on extension—all associated with hyperthyroidism.
5. Examination of rectal/perineal area for excoriation associated with diarrhea.

Diagnostic Tests

1. Radioisotope thyroid scanning.
2. Needle biopsy of nodule.
3. X-ray films of neck.
   a. Barium swallow showing displacement and fixation of the trachea, tracheal stenosis.
   b. Calcifications on one or both sides of the trachea and involved lymph nodes with medullary carcinoma of the thyroid.

NURSING DIAGNOSES: ACTUAL OR POTENTIAL

1. Pain: related to thyroid tumor, surgery.
2. Hyperirritability: related to hyperthyroidism.
3. Discomfort: related to excessive perspiration (if hyperthyroid).
4. Fatigue: related to inadequate oxygenation due to compression of trachea by tumor mass.
5. Inadequate nutrition: related to decreased food intake due to tumor constricting esophagus; fatigue.
6. Psychological distress: related to unknown outcome of tests and lack of definitive treatment.
7. Potential anxiety: related to unfamiliarity with hospital environment, expectations, tests, and treatment modalities.
8. Risk of infection: related to inadequate nutrition. (Negative nitrogen balance is associated with depressed immune function.)
9. Potential for suffocation (following thyroidectomy): related to damage/edema of recurrent laryngeal nerve or inadvertant total parathyroidectomy (either may result in closure of vocal cords obstructing airflow to lungs).

EXPECTED OUTCOMES

1. Pain will be relieved within 30 min of treatment, as evidenced by client's statement to that effect.
2. Hyperirritability will be reduced during hyperthyroid state, as evidenced by decreased activity by client, slowing of speech, ability to rest and sleep.
3. Excessive perspiration will not result in discomfort, as evidenced by statement to that effect by client.
4. Fatigue will be minimized as evidenced by completion of activities of daily living without complaint of fatigue.
5. Nutritional status will be adequate before surgery, as evidenced by no weight loss within 48 h of admission.
6. Psychological distress will be reduced during hospitalization, as evidenced by reduced questioning, trusting relationships with health care personnel, and client's statement to that effect.
7. Anxiety will be reduced during the first 24-h period of hospitalization, as evidenced by client's expectations of self and others congruent with reality, demonstration of knowledge about hospital environment and policies, and ability to describe diagnostic tests and their expected outcomes before tests.
8. There will be no evidence of infections during

hospitalization. Respiratory difficulty will be assessed (following surgery) and treatment instituted before suffocation occurs.

INTERVENTIONS

1. Assess pain to determine its origin.
2. Relieve pain by using prescribed analgesics at intervals appropriate to client's wishes and need.
3. Assess effectiveness of pain treatment 30 min following drug administration.
4. Decrease environmental stimuli (inappropriate ambient room temperature, repeated interruptions of rest periods, excessive visitors, and so forth) to decrease hyperirritability.
5. Approach client in a calm, self-assured manner.
6. Change bedding, client's clothing (or assist client) before saturation by diaphoresis.
7. Maintain a high-calorie, high-protein diet in the consistency appropriate to client's ability to swallow (if client is in negative nitrogen balance).
8. Space activities of daily living with 30-min rest periods and assist as appropriate to prevent undue fatigue.
9. Encourage and allow client to express fears and expectations about disease process and its treatment. Correct with factual information if incorrect. Listen nonjudgmentally.
10. Orient client to hospital surroundings, policies, and expectations within 24 h of admission.
11. Assess client's knowledge of each test to be done; explain test procedure and purpose if unknown by client, answer all questions; acquaint with transporter to test area.
12. Practice good handwashing technique and encourage patient to do the same; use clean or sterile technique, as appropriate for procedures (e.g., catheterization, catheter care; IV insertion and daily care).
13. Assess preoperative teaching needs and formulate teaching plan appropriate to the individual.
14. Keep tracheostomy tray at client's bedside following thyroidectomy.
15. Keep calcium gluconate/calcium chloride at bedside for emergency use.
16. Monitor respirations hourly during first 24 h after surgery

EVALUATION

Outcome Criteria

1. Client states pain is decreased or absent within 30 min of treatment.
2. Client does not exhibit signs and symptoms of hyperirritability, as evidenced by sleeping through the night, being able to rest and relax during rest periods, not responding with irritation to others, not complaining of feeling tense and irritable.
3. Client does not complain of discomfort due to saturated clothing, bedding.
4. Client states that her or his fatigue is absent or minimal following completion of activities of daily living.
5. Client's nutritional status is adequate before surgery, as evidenced by no weight loss during 48 h before operation.
6. Client experiences minimal psychological distress during hospitalization, as evidenced by the client's statement to that effect and effective, trusting relationships with health care personnel.
7. Client does not experience anxiety after the first 24 h of hospitalization, as evidenced by her or his statement to that effect and a calm, relaxed demeanor when moving about the health care facility.
8. Client possesses sufficient knowledge about tests and definitive treatment, as evidenced by ability to describe tests, expectations, and treatment in his or her own words.
9. Client does not have signs of infection, as evidenced by normal vital signs; a clean, dry, surgical incision with no redness or excess pain; lung sounds present and clear in all lung areas; and no pain, burning, or urgency on urination.
10. There is no sign of hypoxia following surgery, as evidenced by respirations of 16 to 22 and no complaints of dyspnea.

Complication

HYPOTHYROIDISM

Assessment

See *Hypothyroidism* in this chapter.

Revised Outcomes

See *Hypothyroidism*.

Interventions

See *Hypothyroidism*.

Reevaluation and Follow-up

1. Clinic visits for evaluation of thyroid function and/or:

2. Monitoring for possible metastases (if tumor was malignant).

ADRENAL MEDULLARY TUMORS

DESCRIPTION

The function of the adrenal medulla is to produce catecholamines (epinephrine and norepinephrine) and secrete them into the circulation. The adrenal medulla is not essential for life because its functions can be carried out by the sympathetic nervous system; therefore, there are no problems associated with adrenal medullary insufficiency. Excess of adrenal medulla secretions results from medullary tumors. These tumors are classified as pheochromocytomas, neuroblastomas, and ganglioneuromas.

Pheochromocytomas, the most common type of tumor, are rare lesions. They occur in all age groups but are most common in adults in the fourth and fifth decade of life. Ninety percent are benign. These tumors as well as the others can arise anywhere along the sympathetic trunk ganglia, but most frequently are found in the abdomen (especially the adrenal medulla). The cause of most pheochromocytomas is unknown, but approximately 10 percent are a familial manifestation of an autosomal dominant defect. Familial pheochromocytomas may occur alone or may be associated with multiple endocrine adenomatosis, neurofibromastosis, or von Hippel-Lindau disease.

Neuroblastomas are usually large, highly malignant tumors. They occur most often in children under 5 years of age and rarely in adults. The most common clinical features are diarrhea, weakness, malaise, and abdominal pain and often are the result of the spread of the tumor.

Ganglioneuromas are rare tumors that can develop during youth but occur more frequently in adulthood. They can be benign or malignant.

In the subsequent outline, the most prominent tumor, pheochomocytoma, will serve as a model for the application of the nursing process.

PREVENTION

Health Promotion

As the cause of pheochromocytoma is unknown, there are no measures to prevent the health problems described below.

Population at Risk

Although there is no way to prevent the problem, screening as described below should be done yearly in the small group of persons with a family history of the disease.

Screening

1. Mass screening is not done.
2. Any client with essential hypertension that is poorly controlled should be screened with the tests described below.

ASSESSMENT

The client may present with a variety of signs and symptoms and thus may give varied information in the history and various signs on the physical examination. All signs and symptoms result from the accentuation of the normal effects of epinephrine and norepinephrine. The effects of epinephrine and norepinephrine on various organs and metabolic functions are listed in Table 28-2.

Health History

1. Cardiovascular.
   a. History of hypertension is the most common symptom if the tumor secretes predominately norepinephrine. The hypertension may be sustained but labile (approximately 50 percent of clients) or paroxysmal (approximately 50 percent of clients).
   b. History of hypotension with syncope may be elicited if the tumor secrets predominately epinephrine.
   c. History of tachycardia and palpatations are common with epinephrine-secreting tumors.
   d. Dilated pupils
2. Neurological.
   a. Pain.
      (1) Headache: abrupt onset, short duration; generalized, throbbing.
      (2) Angina due to increased cardiac oxygen needs.
   b. Paresthesia, tremors.
   c. Nervousness, anxiety.
3. History of precipitating events.
   a. Sneezing.
   b. Postural changes that involve flexion or bending of the body.
   c. Pressure on the abdomen.
   d. Sexual activities.

TABLE 28-2 EFFECTS OF NOREPINEPHRINE AND EPINEPHRINE ON VARIOUS ORGANS OR METABOLIC EVENTS

Organs/Events	Norepinephrine	Epinephrine
Heart rate	No effect	Increased
Cardiac contraction	No effect	Increased
Vascular bed	Vasoconstriction	Vasodilation
Intestinal smooth muscles	Relaxed	Relaxed
Bronchial smooth muscles	No effect	Relaxed
Eyes	Dilated	Dilated
Sweat glands	Increased activity	Increased activity
Piloerection	Yes	Yes
Blood glucose	No effect	Increased

e. Micturation.
f. Valsalva maneuvers.
g. Smoking.
h. Eating.
i. Change in environmental and body temperature.
j. Emotional stressors.

4. Others.
   a. Excess sweating.
   b. Pallor or flushing.

Physical Assessment

1. Loss of weight even though food intake has been normal.
2. Any signs listed above (hypertension, hypotension, tachycardia, dilated pupils, tremors, sweating) occurring continuously or paroxysmally.
3. Retinal changes if sustained hypertension is present.

Diagnostic Tests

1. Tests to rule out other diseases.
   a. Pheochromocytoma can mimic diabetes mellitus because increased catecholamines cause hyperglycemia, ketone formation, and weight loss. Thus the client will have blood glucose and urinary glucose measurements done.
   b. Thyrotoxicosis may also cause some of the same signs and symptoms, thus the client may have thyroid hormone levels measured.
2. Tests to identify abnormal levels of catecholamines.
   a. 12- or 24-h urine collections for catecholamines or their metabolites, vanillylmandelic acid (VMA) and metanephrine.
   b. Spot urines for these same products at time of attacks.
   c. Measurement of plasma catecholamines (but these tests are difficult and expensive).
   d. Pharmacological testing.
      (1) Histamine, glucagon, and tyramine can be given. These drugs stimulate the release of catecholamines.
         (a) May cause severe hypertension.
         (b) Should be used only in client for whom all other tests are inconclusive and yet the person has life-threatening hypertension.
         (c) Client is frequently tested with administration of phenoxybenzamine (Dibenzyline) pretesting to prevent hypertension.
         (d) Urine for catecholamines and their metabolites is used to measure release of catecholamines.
      (2) Phentolamine can be given and the blood pressure measured to see the depressor response. Usually occurs in 2–10 min. Positive results are indicated by a blood pressure fall greater than 35/25. Test frequently gives false positive and false negative results. Severe hypotension can occur.
3. Tests to locate tumor. CAT scan, nephrotomography, arteriograms and venograms. (Before arteriograms and venograms the client is given an autonomic blocker to prevent hypertension.)

NURSING DIAGNOSES: ACTUAL OR POTENTIAL

1. Cardiovascular instability (hypertension, hypotension, arrhythmias): due to abnormal catecholamine levels.
2. Episodic periods of anxiety, nervousness: related to increased catecholamines.
3. Alteration in comfort (headache): related to vasodilation.
4. Alteration in comfort (angina): related to increased cardiac oxygen needs.
5. Potential metabolic imbalance: related to hyperglycemia and ketosis.
6. Sweating: related to increased catecholamines.
7. Paresthesia/tremors: related to increased catecholamines.
8. Lack of knowledge: regarding diagnostic tests.
9. Lack of knowledge: regarding treatment and long-term needs.

EXPECTED OUTCOMES

1. Immediate.
   a. Client will not experience any episodic crises that go undetected.
   b. Discomfort (headache/angina) will be controlled.
   c. Client will have adequate time for rest during the day and periods of uninterrupted sleep during the night.
   d. Client will not experience any discomfort due to sweating.
   e. Client will have controlled homeostasis (glucose and ketone levels).
   f. Client and family will accurately explain diagnostic tests (purpose, procedure, and follow-up care).
   g. Client and family will accurately explain the disease (anatomy and physiology of adrenal medulla, pathophysiology), expected outcomes of the treatment, and potential complications.
2. Long-term.
   a. Client and family will explain the need for continual follow-up and specify date and time of appointment.
   b. Client on chronic medical treatment and family will be able to explain drugs used, purpose of therapy, dosage and time schedule, and side effects of therapy.
   c. Client who has undergone bilateral adrenalectomy and client's family will be able to explain the postoperative hormonal replacement therapy needed and other discharge needs due to adrenocortical insufficiency (See *Adrenocortical Hypofunction* in this chapter).

INTERVENTIONS

1. Immediate.
   a. Minimize stressors that can precipitate attacks (e.g., physical activities such as bending and flexion, pressure on the abdomen, Valsalva maneuvers, changes in environmental temperature, carotid sinus massage, smoking, wearing tight clothing, pain, and emotional upset).
   b. Monitor client for cardiac stability and signs and symptoms of paroxysmal attacks every 1–2 h. Vital signs: orthostatic changes, rate and rhythm of pulse, presence of sweating, pallor, paraesthesia, and headache.
   c. Monitor and record blood sugar status.
      (1) Daily blood sugar levels, if unstable.
      (2) Urine sugar and ketone levels qid.
   d. Plan daily activity schedule with the client and include adequate rest periods.
   e. Administer medications (analgesics, antihypertensives, and agents to control blood sugar) and record results. If not effective, consult with physician.
   f. Provide diet to control hyperglycemia, if necessary, and to maintain or increase weight.
   g. Explore ways to help client cope with periods of anxiety and nervousness and institute these.
   h. Encourage frequent showers or baths to prevent discomfort from sweating.
   i. Instruct client and family regarding diagnostic tests.
      (1) Purpose of the test.
      (2) Procedure.
      (3) Monitoring and care during and after the test.
   j. Instruct client and family regarding disease and treatment.
      (1) Anatomy and physiology of illness.
      (2) Stressors that precipitate attacks and ways to avoid them.
      (3) Type of treatment.
      (4) Expected effects of treatment.
         (a) Unilateral adrenalectomy.

(i) Curative.
(ii) No hormonal therapy necessary.
(b) Bilateral adrenalectomy.
(i) Curative.
(ii) Adrenocortical insufficiency (primary) results.
(c) Medical treatment, if inoperable.
(i) Drugs used.
(ii) Noncurative; controls symptoms.

2. Hypertensive crisis.
   a. Place client on cardiac monitor.
   b. Monitor blood pressure, pulse, respiration every 15 min.
   c. Monitor neurological status every 30 min to 1 h.
   d. Ensure adequate bed rest with head of bed elevated.
   e. Maintain strict intake and output.
   f. Establish intravenous line at keep-open rate for medications.
   g. Administer medications and fluids as ordered and monitor for effectiveness. If not effective, report to physician.
3. After adrenalectomy.
   a. See discussion on abdominal laparotomy in Chapter 33.
   b. If bilateral adrenalectomy, interventions are similar to those described for adrenalectomy in this chapter under *Adrenocortical Hyperfunction: Hypercortisolism.*
   c. If unilateral adrenalectomy, long-term hormonal deficiency is not a problem, but immediately after surgery client may show temporary insufficiency of cortisol and aldosterone.
   d. Monitor vital signs frequently. Hypertension may occur because of the release of excess catecholamines during manipulation of tumor in surgery.
   e. Attend client when ambulating. Postural hypotension may occur due to alpha receptor blockade or inability of sympathetic nervous system to compensate immediately.
      (1) If hypotension occurs, place client in bed, monitor vital signs every 15 min until they return to normal, initiate intravenous therapy, and administer fluids and drugs as necessary.
      (2) Teach client to change position slowly, to flex ankles as soon as she or he stands, and not to stand in one position.
4. Discharge.
   a. Teach client and family about hormonal replacement therapy, if necessary. (See *Adrenocortical Hypofunction* in this chapter.)
   b. Instruct client and significant others regarding follow-up.

EVALUATION

Outcome Criteria

1. Client is developing no undetected paroxysmal crisis.
2. Hypertension is being controlled.
3. Headache, angina are controlled.
4. Sweating does not cause any discomfort.
5. Hyperglycemia and ketosis are not uncontrolled.
6. Client and family can accurately explain the diagnostic tests, the disease process, and the planned treatment and results.
7. Client and family can accurately explain the follow-up planned.
8. Client and family can accurately explain the appropriate information about drug therapy or hormonal replacement therapy (if appropriate).

Complications

1. Hypertensive crisis. See interventions 2a through g above.
2. Hypotensive crisis. See intervention 3e above.
3. Adrenocortical insufficiency. See *Adrenocortical Hypofunction* in this chapter.

Reevaluation and Follow-up

1. Establish plan as necessary for any complications and evaluate until controlled. Then proceed with long-term goals.
2. Client will return to clinic in 1 week after discharge and will be assessed for the same data listed under Health History and Physical Assessment above. If client has been placed on hormonal replacement therapy, refer him or her to a visiting nurses service.

INSULINOMAS

DESCRIPTION

Insulinomas are functioning beta cell tumors of the pancreas. Like most endocrine tumors, they synthesize and secrete their hormone, insulin, without responding to normal feedback mechanisms, resulting in episodic and spontaneous hypoglycemia secondary to excess insulin secretion. Serum glucose levels frequently drop gradually rather than abruptly, resulting in signs and symptoms of central nervous system dysfunction such as headache, blurred vision, diplopia, mental confusion, and incoherent speech, rather than the sweating, nervousness, weakness, hunger, tremor, and tachycardia seen with rapid falls in serum glucose levels. Fasting and exercise precipitate hypoglycemia, thus many persons with this disorder learn to avoid hypoglycemia by frequent feedings throughout their waking hours. Weight gain may occur as a result of increased food intake. Approximately 90 percent of these tumors are benign, and multiple insulinomas are found in approximately 12 percent of cases.

PREVENTION

Health Promotion

Early diagnosis of the disorder.

Population at Risk

1. Those with a family history of diabetes mellitus (25 to 30 percent of persons with this disorder).
2. The majority of cases occur between the ages of 30 to 60 years.

Screening

There are currently no reliable screening tests or maneuvers.

ASSESSMENT

Health History

1. Family history of endocrine disorders, especially diabetes mellitus.
2. Other medical and endocrine problems, especially peptic ulcer associated with tumors or hyperplasia of the pancreatic islets, parathyroids, and pituitary (multiple endocrine adenomatosis, type 1).
3. Increased food intake and/or increased frequency of food intake during waking hours and possible weight gain.
4. Episodes of hypoglycemia precipitated by exercise (exercise increases serum glucose levels in reactive hypoglycemia but increases insulin secretion in insulinoma).
5. Episodes of awakening with headache, blurred vision, night sweats, and mental confusion (all symptoms of night-time hypoglycemia).

Physical Assessment

1. Nervous system.
   a. Sensory: visual disturbances.
   b. Motor weakness.
   c. Light-headedness.
   d. Fatigue.
2. Integumentary system.
   Excessive sweating (sympthetic nervous system manifestation of hypoglycemia).
3. Central nervous system (manifestations of hypoglycemia).
   a. Drowsiness.
   b. Stupor.
   c. Confusion.
   d. Loss of consciousness.
   e. Coma.
4. Mental status (manifestations of hypoglycemia).
   a. Amnesia.
   b. Personality change.
   c. Noisy behavior.

Diagnostic Tests

1. Fasting blood sugar and insulin levels.
2. Prolonged fasting (48–72 h) blood sugar and insulin levels.
3. Glucose tolerance test (limited value).
4. Provocative tests (play secondary role to prolonged fast).
   a. Intravenous tolbutamide.
   b. Intravenous glucagon.
5. Angiography. (Most tumors are highly vascular and can thus be identified with this procedure; however, endocrine tissue is also highly vascular and angiography may fail to demonstrate the tumor if it is small.)

NURSING DIAGNOSES: ACTUAL OR POTENTIAL

1. Potential for injury: related to episodes of weakness, fatigability, and altered mental status.
2. Episodes of hypoglycemia: related to exercise and fasting (fasting necessary to do tests).
3. Potential antisocial behavior: related to hypoglycemia.
4. Potential anxiety: related to lack of knowledge about disease, tests, and treatment.

5. Postoperative pain: related to surgical intervention (if done).

EXPECTED OUTCOMES

1. Client will remain free of injury during episodes of weakness, fatigue, and altered mental status during hospitalization.
2. Exercise- and/or fasting-induced hypoglycemia will be assessed before the occurrence of profound mental changes (e.g., coma) and appropriate treatment will be instituted.
3. Client exhibiting antisocial behavior will be prevented from injuring self or others with the least possible restraint.
4. Client will exhibit decreased anxiety during hospitalization, as evidenced by decreased questioning, relaxed facies and body posture, vital signs within normal range, and client's own statement that he or she feels less anxious.
5. Client will experience postoperative relief of pain within 30 min of treatment (e.g., relaxation, distraction, analgesic administration).

INTERVENTIONS

1. During episodes of weakness, fatigability, and/or altered mental status, protect client from injury.
   a. Use bed rails if client is in bed.
   b. Assist client during ambulation.
   c. Reorient client to time, place, person if disoriented.
   d. Stay with client or encourage family member to sit with client until episode has passed.
2. Assess for signs and symptoms of hypoglycemia during exercise and fasting (e.g., diaphoresis, tremor, tachycardia, change in mental status).
3. Institute treatment for hypoglycemia upon its assessment (quick-acting carbohydrate).
4. Isolate the client exhibiting antisocial behavior and treat for hypoglycemia.
5. Explain all diagnostic procedures and expected outcomes.
6. Assess client knowledge of the disease process and potential treatment. Prepare teaching plan that covers areas of knowledge deficit. (When appropriate include family member or significant other who will act as backup in self-care.) Teaching plan should include: anatomy and physiology of insulinoma; signs and symptoms of hypoglycemia; medical treatment plan/surgical treatment plan, and expected outcomes and consequences. Identify environmental stressors contributing to hypoglycemic attacks.
7. Implement teaching plan with teaching sessions and content appropriate for client's learning ability and style.
8. If partial or total pancreatectomy is done:
   a. Relieve pain as desired by client and as appropriate.
   b. Administer analgesic as ordered.
   c. Help client to realign body to relax tensed muscles.
   d. Distract client's attention from pain (e.g., use of music, television, conversation).
   e. Assess for signs and symptoms of hyperglycemia and hypoglycemia (see *Diabetes Mellitus* in this chapter).
   f. Provide routine postoperative care.
   g. Implement client and family teaching (see number 6 above and/or *Diabetes Mellitus* as appropriate).

EVALUATION

Outcome Criteria

1. Client experiences no injury during hospitalization.
2. Client does not experience profound mental changes during episodes of hypoglycemia.
3. By discharge, client has verbalized no unanswered questions concerning disease process, treatment, expected outcomes of treatment, or self-care activities.
4. By discharge, client has verbalized no feelings of anxiety and has exhibited a relaxed facies and body posture and normal vital signs.
5. Postoperative pain is relieved within 30 min of treatment.

Complications

DIABETES MELLITUS

Overt, following partial or total pancreatectomy.

Assessment/Revised Outcomes/Interventions

See *Diabetes Mellitus* in this chapter.

Reevaluation and Follow-up

1. Clinic visits.
2. Referral to visiting nurses service when self-care is complicated and/or self-care learning is less than optimal.

HYPERACTIVITY AND HYPOACTIVITY

SYNDROME OF INAPPROPRIATE ADH SECRETION

DESCRIPTION

The syndrome of inappropriate ADH (antidiuretic hormone) secretion (SIADH) or excess secretion of ADH results in secretion of concentrated urine with water retention and low plasma tonicity and the risk of severe water intoxication. Figure 28-4 shows the normal mechanisms of ADH regulation.

The stimulus for release of ADH by the posterior pituitary (which stores ADH) is believed to be regulated by osmoreceptors in the hypothalamus, namely, paraventricular and supraoptic nuclei. Changes in the plasma osmolar concentration (amount of solute in body water) are detected by the osmoreceptors, and ADH secretion is either enhanced or decreased. Pressoreceptors (carotid body) in the vascular system also control ADH secretion by sending impulses to the hypothalamus in response to pressure changes in the blood vessels. After being released into the circulation, ADH exerts its water-conserving effect by altering the permeability of the distal convoluted tubules and collecting ducts of the kidneys. Stimulators of ADH secretion include shock, hemorrhage, hyperosmolality, and trauma. Pain and other emotional stressors can stimulate increased ADH. Drugs such as nicotine, morphine, acetylcholine, some tranquilizers, and also some anesthetics can stimulate ADH secretion.

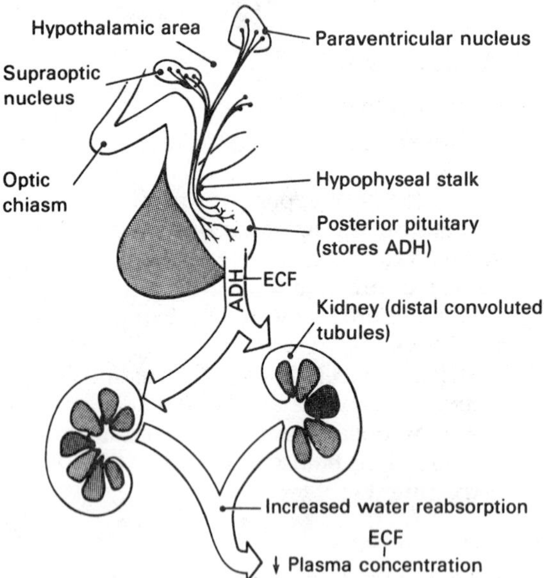

Figure 28-4 ADH regulation. Stimuli → hypothalamic receptors → ↑ ADH by hypothalamus → plus, neural message sent to posterior pituitary to ↑ ADH release → ↑ plasma ADH → altered membrane permeability of the distal convoluted tubules → ↑ water reabsorption by ECF → ↓ plasma concentration, and urine output.

SIADH may occur from ectopic vasopressin secretion. The most common cause of ectopic secretion is bronchogenic cancer. But lung tissue affected by tuberculosis, abscesses, or pneumonia can also secrete ectopic ADH. Clinical disorders of the central nervous system (trauma, neurosurgery on the midbrain, infection, cerebral hemorrhage), emotional stress, and use of certain drugs (chlorpropamide, narcotics, barbiturates, vincristine), can cause SIADH. In some clients no underlying disorder can be found.

PREVENTION

Health promotion

There is no known way to prevent the disease entity.

Population at Risk

1. Clients with bronchogenic cancer.
2. Clients immediately postoperative, especially if they have been experiencing major emotional stressors, have extensive pain, and are receiving large quantities of narcotics.
3. Clients with head injuries.

Screening

1. There are no mass screening techniques available.
2. Clients at risk should be on strict input and output and have serum albumin, BUN, and sodium monitored regularly.

ASSESSMENT

Health History

1. History of weight gain without increased food intake.
2. History of neurological complications.
   a. Weakness.
   b. Lethargy.
3. Rarely does the client complain of edema.

Physical Assessment

1. Weight gain.
2. Decreased output.
3. Mental confusion, convulsions, coma.
4. Rarely does client have edema, congestive heart failure (CHF), or hypertension.

Diagnostic Tests

1. Blood.
   a. Serum albumin low due to hemodilution.
   b. BUN low due to hemodilution.
   c. Serum osmolality less than 275 mosmol/L.
   d. Serum sodium usually less than 130 mEq/L.
2. Urine.
   a. Increased osmolality.
   b. Sodium more than 20 mEq/L.

NURSING DIAGNOSES: ACTUAL OR POTENTIAL

1. Weight gain: related to increased ADH secretion.
2. Altered fluid and sodium balance: related to ADH.
3. Thirst: related to fluid restrictions.
4. Lethargy/weakness: related to altered fluid and sodium balance.
5. Potential for injury: related to convlusions and coma.
6. Knowledge deficit: regarding tests and treatment.

EXPECTED OUTCOMES

1. Weight gain will stop and client's weight will return to normal.
2. Fluid intake will equal output, serum sodium will be more than 130 mEq/L.
3. Client will not complain of thirst.
4. Lethargy and weakness will decrease.
5. Client will suffer no injuries should convulsions occur.
6. Client and family will be able to explain purpose of blood and urine collection.
7. Client and family will be able to explain treatment regimen.

INTERVENTIONS

1. Observe and record:
   a. Intake and output q8h.
   b. Blood pressure, pulse, respiration, and temperature q4h.
   c. Weight daily.
   d. Urine specific gravity every shift.
   e. Mental status every 2–4 h.
   f. Serum albumin, BUN, osmolality, sodium every 1 to 2 days.
2. Institute safety measures if client is confused, restless, or convulsing.
   a. Keep side rails up.
   b. Use padded bed rails.
   c. Keep bed low to floor.
   d. Get client up only with assistance.
   e. Keep airway and suction equipment available.
3. Institute care for coma client (see Chapter 25).
4. Maintain strict adherence to fluid restrictions.
5. Ensure intake of a lot of fluid over 24 h in a manner the client finds satisfactory. Use ice cubes in place of water if client desires.

EVALUATION

Outcome Criteria

1. Client's weight gain stops and client loses weight.
2. Output equals intake.
3. Client's mental status is normal, and lethargy and weakness decrease.
4. Client suffers no injury.
5. Client and family can accurately explain the purpose of urine and blood tests.
6. Client and family can accurately explain the purpose of fluid restrictions.

Complications

CONVULSIONS AND COMA

See Interventions in Chapter 25 and intervention 2a through e above.

WATER INTOXICATION

Assessment

1. Weight gain.
2. Serum sodium less than 120 mEq/L.
3. Deteriorating mental status.

Interventions
1. Maintain client's safety.
2. Administer hypertonic saline and diuretics as ordered.
3. Follow other interventions as listed above.

Revised Outcomes
1. Serum sodium will be elevated to at least 130 mEq/l.
2. Other outcomes will be as originally stated above.

Reevaluation and Follow-up
Institute specific plan to ensure that complications are overcome. Client will return for periodic checks. At that time client's weight and serum sodium, osmolality, BUN, and albumin will be checked for effectiveness of therapy. Monitor client's ability to comply with fluid restrictions if need is still present.

DIABETES INSIPIDUS

DESCRIPTION

The term diabetes insipidus refers to a deficiency of antidiuretic hormone (ADH, or vasopressin). ADH exerts control of urinary water excretion, thereby controlling the concentration of body fluids. A deficiency of ADH results in the excretion of excessive amounts of dilute urine and secondary polydipsia.

Diabetes insipidus can be permanent or transient. Permanent diabetes insipidus results from structural damage to the supraoptic and paraventricular nuclei of the hypothalamus, to the division of the supraopticohypophysial tract above the median eminence, or to the kidneys, causing renal unresponsiveness to ADH (nephrogenic diabetes insipidus). Diabetes insipidus can be caused by idiopathic or familial factors or it may result from head trauma (accidental or neurosurgical), neoplasm, or infections.

PREVENTION

Health Promotion

There is no effective way to prevent diabetes insipidus.

Population at Risk

1. Clients who have just undergone neurosurgery, hypophysectomy.
2. Clients who have had head trauma.

Screening

1. Mass screening is not done.
2. Clients at risk:
   a. Input and output.
   b. Daily weight.
   c. Vital signs.
   d. Serum sodium, osmolality, albumin, BUN, hemoglobin to identify fluid loss.

ASSESSMENT

Health History

1. Most frequently seen after surgery, trauma.
2. Complaints of thirst, polyuria.
3. History of fatigue, lack of sleep may be elicited but this is rare, as most clients drink adequate amounts of fluid to retain normal vascular volume if alert (not comatose).

Physical Assessment

1. Hypotension-postural changes if client does not get fluid replacement.
2. Mucous membranes may be dry.
3. Skin turgor is decreased or feels doughy.
4. Weakness.

Diagnostic Tests

1. Skull x-ray film, CAT scan with view of sella turcica.
2. 24-h urine: volumes of 5–10 L or more.
3. Urine osmolalities: 50–200 mosmol/L.
4. Plasma osmolality: more than 300 mosmol.
5. Specific gravities: 1.000 to 1.005.
6. Water deprivation test (8 h):
   a. Urine volume: remains greater than 30 mL/min.
   b. Urine concentration: less than 200 mosmol/L (280–300 mosmol is normal).
   c. Urine specific gravity: 1.001 to 1.005 (1.020 or above is normal).

NURSING DIAGNOSES: ACTUAL OR POTENTIAL

1. Excessive thirst: related to polyuria.
2. Polyuria: related to diabetes insipidius.
3. Potential for volume depletion: related to inability to concentrate.
4. Fatigue: related to lack of sleep.
5. Potential for injury: related to fatigue and volume depletion.
6. Constipation: related to decreased body water.

EXPECTED OUTCOMES

1. Immediate.
   a. Client's vascular volume will remain normal.
   b. Client's thirst needs will be met.
   c. Client will have rest periods during the day.
   d. Client will be able to explain the purpose of various urine and blood tests and the purpose of procedures for and monitoring during the water deprivation test.
2. Long-term. Client will be able to explain hormonal replacement therapy or other therapy prescribed, list signs and symptoms of successful therapy and insufficient treatment, and be able to administer drugs appropriately.

INTERVENTIONS

1. Monitor:
   a. Intake and output every shift.
   b. Specific gravity every shift.
   c. Weight daily.
   d. Blood pressure and pulse with orthostatic changes q4h.
2. Monitor bowel pattern and administer laxatives and stool softeners as ordered and needed.
3. Provide adequate fluids, ice water, if client prefers.
4. Provide safe environment as needed, such as:
   a. Getting client up only with attendance.
   b. Having client use walker or cane for support if weak.
5. Assist with activities of daily living as needed to lessen fatigue.
6. Provide rest periods during the day.
7. Instruct client and family regarding diagnostic tests.
8. Carefully monitor client during water restriction test.
   a. Weight before test and frequently during test. Loss of 3 to 5 percent of body weight warrants immediate reporting.
   b. Intake and output.
   c. Urine specific gravity: will not change if client has diabetes insipidus.
   d. Mental status.
9. Instruct client and family regarding disease and treatment.
   a. Pathophysiology of diabetes insipidus.
   b. Treatment.
      (1) Pituitary diabetes insipidus.
         (a) DDAVP (desmopressin) spray or snuff every 12–24 h.
         (b) Vasopressin tannate in oil, IM, every 24–72 h.
         (c) Chlorpropamide (oral hypoglycemic agent), clofibrate (Atromid-S), or carbamazepine (Tegretol) for incomplete diabetus insipidus.
      (2) Nephrogenic diabetes insipidus.
         (a) Only treatment is use of diuretics, particularily the thiazides. They decrease sodium and thus decrease glomerular filtration rate, thus enhancing tubular reabsorption of water.
         (b) Sodium intake must also be restricted.
   c. Expected response from treatment.
      (1) Decreased thirst, urination, constipation.
      (2) Less weakness, fatigue.
   d. Signs and symptoms of ineffective therapy.
      (1) Volume of urine large.
      (2) Continued thirst.
      (3) Weakness.
      (4) Fatigue.
      (5) Constipation.
10. Demonstrate and have client return demonstration of:
    a. Use of nasal spray.
    b. Injection technique: mixing ADH (e.g., Pitressin) in oil, withdrawing medicine into syringe, care of syringes.
11. Instruct client to obtain a medic-alert bracelet.

EVALUATION

Outcome Criteria

1. Client's vascular volume remains normal.
2. Thirst needs are being met.
3. Fatigue is decreased.
4. Client can accurately explain tests.
5. Client can accurately explain pathophysiology, dose, time, expected effects of therapy, and signs and symptoms of ineffective therapy.
6. Client can demonstrate skills taught, use of nasal spray, injection technique (preparation of drug, injection, and care of equipment).
7. Client wears medic-alert bracelet or necklace.

Complications

Vascular collapse (shock) if hypodypsia or impairment of consciousness occurs.

Assessment/Revised Outcomes/Interventions

See *Shock* in Chapter 48.

Reevaluation and Follow-up

If complications occur establish plan to meet client needs until outcome is achieved. Client will be followed as necessary in outpatient settings. Refer to a visiting nurse's service if client is placed on injections. On return visits assess client as described under Assessment above.

GONADOTROPIN DEFICIENCY

DESCRIPTION

Absence or deficiency of the gonadotropins (FSH and LH) results in a lack of normal gonadal hormone production in the human being and gives rise to a syndrome called *hypogonadotropic hypogonadism*. The signs and symptoms demonstrated vary depending on when the syndrome occurs. If it occurs before puberty, impaired sexual development occurs. This is described in Chapter 17. Gonadotropin deficiency is the most common hypothalamic pituitary deficiency in adults with either pituitary tumors or craniopharyngiomas. It can also occur from pituitary damage resulting from infectious and granulomatous lesions, physical injury, or vascular disorders.

PREVENTION

Health Promotion

There is no known prevention. Early detection and treatment is the key to preventing complications.

Population at Risk

There is no known population at risk.

Screening

No mass screening tools are available.

ASSESSMENT

Health History

1. *Female*: History of secondary amenorrhea, breast atrophy and, if associated with panhypopituitarism, signs and symptoms of multiple endocrine deficits (ACTH, TSH, and possible ADH deficits). See discussion under *Adrenocortical Hypofunction, Hypothyroidism,* and *Diabetes Insipidus* in this chapter. If condition is associated with pituitary tumors, client will have symptoms as listed under *Pituitary Tumors,* Assessment, Health History, number 1a and b.
2. *Male*: History of decreased libido, decreased potency, weakness, and change in beard growth. If condition is associated with panhypopituitarism, the client will have signs and symptoms of other endocrine deficits as described above; if associated with pituitary tumors, client will have symptoms as listed under *Pituitary Tumors,* Assessment, Health History number 1a and b.

Physical Assessment

1. *Female*: Breast and uterine atrophy may be noted. If condition is associated with panhypopituitarism, other signs might be present; if associated with pituitary tumors, client will have signs as listed under *Pituitary Tumors,* Assessment, Physical Assessment number 1a through d.
2. *Male*: Change in beard growth and decrease in size of testes might be noted. If condition is associated with panhyopopituitarism, other signs might be present; if associated with pituitary tumors, client will have signs listed under *Pituitary Tumors,* Assessment, Physical Assessment number 1a through d.

Diagnostic Tests

1. Serum levels of FSH and LH will be measured. Hormones are pulsatile in nature; several measurements must be taken.
2. Serum levels of testosterone (male) and estrogen and progesterone (female) will be measured. If signs and symptoms of other hormonal imbalances are present, serum levels of other hormones as described under *Pituitary Tumors* will be measured.
3. Sperm count will be done on males.
4. LHRH test to assess the pituitary reserve of gonadotropins.
5. If pituitary tumor is suspected, skull x-ray films with views of the sella turcica, CAT scan, pneumoencephalograms, and arteriograms may be done.

NURSING DIAGNOSES: ACTUAL OR POTENTIAL

1. See diagnoses as listed under Nursing Diagnoses, *Pituitary Tumors.*

2. Embarrassment: due to uncomfortableness with discussing sexuality.
3. Altered body image: due to change in secondary sexual characteristics.

EXPECTED OUTCOMES

1. If condition is associated with pituitary tumor, outcomes are the same as those listed under Expected Outcomes for *Pituitary Tumors.*
2. Client will be free of embarrassment and able to ask questions he or she needs to, as evidenced by: client's statement of not having any unanswered questions, the client's talking comfortably about his or her problem, and the client's being able to explain his or her disease and treatment.
3. Client will demonstrate an improvement in body image, as evidenced by: stating that the changes are reversable with treatment, dressing to minimize the change in body image, talking about future plans, and interacting appropriately with staff and family and friends.

INTERVENTIONS

1. If condition is associated with pituitary tumor, interventions are as listed under *Pituitary Tumors.*
2. If condition is not associated with tumor, teach client and family about hormonal therapy.
   a. If fertility is not desired, males are given long-acting testosterone preparations and females are treated with cyclic estrogen and progesterone products.
   b. If the adult client desires children, the client is treated with gonadotropins.
3. Allow time for the client to share concerns.
   a. Spend time privately with the client.
   b. Talk about the client's problem in a factual way.
   c. Direct your attention to the client's major concern.
   d. Clarify for the client any information given by others.
4. Help the client develop an improved body image.
   a. Make it clear that the body changes are reversible.
   b. Help the client see that many attributes make up an individual.
   c. Make sure the family's concerns and questions are answered so that they can give support to the client.

EVALUATION

Outcome Criteria

Outcomes are as listed under Evaluation, *Pituitary Tumors.*

Complications

Complications are the same as those listed under *Pituitary Tumors.*

Reevaluation and Follow-up

Reevaluation and follow-up is the same as that listed under *Pituitary Tumors.*

DIABETES MELLITUS

DESCRIPTION

Diabetes mellitus is a chronic systemic disease manifesting both metabolic and vascular changes that affect virtually every organ of the body. It is characterized by alterations of carbohydrate, protein, and fat metabolism, vascular changes (thickening of basement membranes, microaneurysms, peripheral vascular disease, early and widespread atherosclerosis), and both transient and permanent neuropathies. Although diabetes is a common disease, no distinct pathogenesis, causes, invariable set of clinical findings, specific tests, or curative therapy exist. The client and family must learn to "manage" the disease within the lifestyle of the client.

Etiological factors associated with diabetes include heredity, viruses, obesity, membrane receptor defects, insulin antibodies, and drugs. Although there is not sufficient evidence that stress per se can produce a permanent diabetic state in genetically normal individuals, a variety of severe stress states (psychological and physical) have been associated with glucose intolerance (e.g., pregnancy, physical and emotional trauma, and acute illnesses). For the population at risk for developing diabetes, stress may be the factor responsible for the overt expression of the disease and may subsequently hinder the individual's response to treatment.

There are two major types of diabetes mellitus, *insulin-dependent* (formerly juvenile onset) and *non-insulin dependent* (formerly adult onset). Insulin-dependent diabetes is frequently manifested by the rapid onset of acute symptoms such as polyuria, polydipsia, polyphagia, weight loss, or frank ketoacidosis before the client's fifteenth birthday, but it is not unknown in adults. Non-insulin dependent diabetes is most frequently found in obese adults between their fortieth and sixtieth birthdays and is manifested by minimal symptoms such as moderate weight gain or loss, nocturia, vulvar pruritus, and other recurrent skin lesions. This type of diabetes may also be manifested first by vascular complications such as blurred or decreased vision associated with diabetic retinopathy or diabetic neuropathies such as paresthesias, impotence, or nocturnal diarrhea. Insulin-independent diabetics rarely develop ketoacidosis; however, they are prone to nonketotic hyperosmolar coma precipitated by carbohydrate loads, infection, exogenous glucocorticoids, thiazide diuretics, Dilantin, or extreme stress.

Diabetes has previously been classified into stages (prediabetes, latent, chemical, and overt); however, the usefulness of this strategy is presently in question. Another term used in reference to diabetes is "brittle." The term refers to an unstable, labile diabetic stage that is difficult to control. The individual fluctuates between ketosis and hypoglycemia with minor changes in insulin dose.

PREVENTION

Health Promotion

1. Encourage maintenance of ideal body weight.
2. Counsel population at risk regarding diet, exercise, use of diabetogenic drugs.
3. Encourage regular medical supervision during pregnancy (maternal population at risk).
4. Provide support and/or refer client to appropriate medical/mental health agency during periods of stress.
5. Suggest genetic counseling to parents contemplating a family if they are at risk for diabetes.

Population at Risk

1. Obese individuals.
2. Family history of diabetes, especially parents, siblings.
3. Females with history of giving birth to large babies, stillbirths, toxemia.
4. Individuals over the age of 40 years.
5. Individuals experiencing physical and/or psychological stress who are categorized as prediabetic or latent/chemical diabetic.
6. Individuals with other endocrine diseases such as Cushing's, acromegaly (secondary diabetes).
7. Individuals using drugs capable of producing glucose intolerance (estrogen-containing drugs, thiazide diuretics, glucocorticoids).

Screening

1. Capillary blood glucose sampling for mass screening.
2. Postprandial blood sugar measurement (2 h).

ASSESSMENT

Health History

1. Recent unexpected weight gain or loss.
2. Polyuria, polydipsia, polyphagia.
3. Complaints of "flulike" symptoms.
4. Nocturia.
5. Persistent and recurrent monilial or fungal vaginitis or skin fold infections.
6. Unexplained fatigue.
7. Sexual dysfunction (impotency, retrograde ejaculation, failure to achieve orgasm).
8. Change in mental status (decreased ability to concentrate, anxiety, nervousness, impaired relationships with others).
9. Recent physical or emotional stress (infection, trauma, divorce, death of significant other, period of rapid growth, pregnancy).
10. Use of diabetogenic drugs (oral contraceptives or other estrogens, glucocorticoids, thiazide diuretics, Dilantin).
11. Family history of diabetes mellitus or other endocrine disorders.

Physical Assessment

1. Findings associated with hyperglycemia.
   a. Hypotension: dry inelastic skin, dull mucous membranes with thick, stringy secretions, flat neck veins while lying flat (associated with dehydration related to solute diuresis).
   b. Blurred vision (associated with osmotic swelling of the lens of the eye).
   c. Headache, drowsiness, stupor, possibly coma (associated with dehydration of brain cells).
   d. Depressed muscle tone and reflexes: possible numbness, tingling, and diminished sensory responses to stimuli of lower ex-

tremities (may be associated with osmotic swelling of nerves and are thus transient).
   e. In early stages nocturia, polyuria (associated with osmotic diuresis), oliguria to anuria in later stages (associated with dehydration). Urine positive for sugar; also positive for acetone if individual is insulin-dependent.
   f. Kussmaul's respirations (physiological compensatory response to metabolic acidosis).
   g. Acetone or fruity odor of breath (acetone, one of the ketoacids, is being blown off).
2. Other findings.
   a. Monilial or fungal infections in skin folds, vagina, perineal areas.
   b. Infected ulcers, diminished or absent pulses, hair loss on lower extremities (associated with diminished arterial blood supply).
   c. Various neuropathies affecting:
      (1) The bladder, resulting in residual urine and increased incidence of urinary tract infections.
      (2) The bowel, resulting in nocturnal diarrhea.
      (3) The lower extremities, resulting in sensory deficits.
      (4) Postural hypotension.

Diagnostic Tests

1. Fasting blood sugar.
2. Postprandial blood sugar (2 h).
3. Glucose tolerance test, either oral or intravenous (oral test most frequently used).

NURSING DIAGNOSES: ACTUAL OR POTENTIAL

1. Acute hyperglycemia.
   a. Fatigue: related to increased metabolic rate, negative nitrogen balance, and inadequate available nutrition.
   b. Dehydration: related to solute diuresis.
   c. At risk for injury: related to altered mental status, hypotension, and decreased visual acuity.
   d. Abdominal pain and muscle aches: related to ketoacidosis or nonketotic hyperosmolar syndrome (may be associated with lactic acidosis in latter syndrome).
   e. Anxiety, fear: related to serious illness, hospital admission, unknown expectations of health care personnel, policies and regulations of health care facility.
2. Maintenance.
   a. Potential hyperglycemia: related to inadequate available insulin in relation to caloric intake and gluconeogenesis.
   b. Potential hypoglycemia: related to administration of too much insulin in relation to blood sugar level.
   c. Potential inability to manage disease process: secondary to lack of knowledge about diabetes, calculating prescribed diet, monitoring self for signs and symptoms of inadequate control of disease, administering prescribed insulin/medication, and making necessary lifestyle changes.
   d. At risk for infection: secondary to glycogen deposits in skin and mucous membranes.
   e. Potential unnoticed injuries to lower extremities: secondary to diminished motor and/or sensory responses in lower extremities, visual deficits.
   f. Potential changes in body image: secondary to diagnosis of chronic disease and possible lifestyle changes necessitated by diabetes and its management.
   g. Potential sexual dysfunction: secondary to neuropathies.
   h. Obesity: secondary to intake of more calories than expended in daily activities (80 percent of non-insulindependent diabetics are overweight at the time of diagnosis).

EXPECTED OUTCOMES

1. Acute hyperglycemia.
   a. Activities of daily living will be completed without fatigue during hospitalization.
   b. Adequate hydration will be present within 24 h of admission and maintained during hospital stay.
   c. Client will not show evidence of injury during hospitalization.
   d. Pain will be relieved within 30 min of treatment (if client desires treatment).
   e. The client will not exhibit signs or symptoms of anxiety or fear during hospitalization.
2. Maintenance.
   a. Hyperglycemia will be assessed and treatment initiated before overt ketoacidosis or nonketotic hyperosmolar syndrome appear.

b. Hypoglycemia will be assessed before profound mental changes occur and treatment is instituted.
c. By discharge, the client and family will describe, in their own words, knowledge of the pathology of diabetes necessary for self-care, will calculate 2 days' menus with 90 percent accuracy of caloric intake and food groups, will draw up and inject insulin with 100 percent accuracy for 2 days, will test and interpret urine for sugar and acetone with 100 percent accuracy for 2 days, will be able to describe signs and symptoms of hyperglycemia and hypoglycemia accurately and without confusion, and will be able to take appropriate action.
d. Client will not exhibit any infection at discharge.
e. Client can both describe and demonstrate her or his daily routine of care of lower extremities and inspection for injury.
f. Body image changes will be identified and discussed (if the client desires) before discharge.
g. Sexual dysfunction will be identified and treatment modalities discussed before discharge.
h. The client (if obese) will lose 1–2 lb/week until prescribed weight loss is accomplished.

INTERVENTIONS

1. Acute hyperglycemia.
   a. Assist client with activities of daily living to avoid fatigue. Space activities with 30-min rest periods.
   b. Monitor intake and output qh until urine output stabilizes at greater than 30 mL/h, then q4h.
   c. Monitor daily weight (weigh before breakfast, after voiding, and before bowel movement).
   d. Assess oral mucosa for signs of adequate hydration (glistening membranes with thin watery secretions) every shift.
   e. Monitor temperature, pulse, respiration, and blood pressure every hour until stable, then every shift.
   f. Monitor for signs and symptoms of hyperkalemia (during potassium replacement therapy).
   g. Help client to avoid injury.
      (1) Keep bed rails up while client is in bed.
      (2) Stay with client or request that family member sit with client during periods of decreased or altered mental function.
      (3) Assist client in and out of bed, to bathroom, to chair, and so forth when client is experiencing fatigue or weakness.
      (4) Remove from immediate environment small objects client could stumble over.
      (5) Ensure that client has unwrinkled stockings, shoes or slippers on when out of bed (to avoid foot injury and blisters).

2. Pain relief measures.
   a. Reposition client; do not allow extremities to remain in dependent position.
   b. Administer analgesics as prescribed for client.
   c. Assess effectiveness of pain relief treatment 30 min after institution of treatment.
   d. Orient client to her or his surroundings; explain all treatments and procedures and your expectation of client's behavior when appropriate.
   e. Encourage client to verbalize fears and expectations.
   f. Listen nonjudgmentally, answer all questions, and correct unrealistic expectations.

3. Maintenance.
   a. Assess for signs and symptoms of hyperglycemia each shift (complaints of weakness or fatigue, increased respirations, abdominal pain, nausea, sugar in urine).
   b. If hyperglycemia is assessed, institute prescribed treatment; if unprescribed, consult with physician.
   c. Assess for signs and symptoms of hypoglycemia during periods of insulin peak activity (regular insulin, 2–4 h; intermediate insulin, 8–12 h; long-acting insulin, 12–24 h), when caloric intake is inadequate for amount of administered insulin (perspiration, headache, tremor, tachycardia, nervousness, hunger).
   d. If hypoglycemia is assessed, institute prescribed treatment and notify physician (so that adjustments in insulin dosage and

diet can be made if necessary). Treatment may be 10 g of quick-acting carbohydrate.

e. Assess client's knowledge of the disease's process and its management. Assess client's ability for self-care. Together with client identify significant other who is willing to serve as back-up caregiver.
f. Prepare a teaching plan that includes:
   (1) Pathophysiology of diabetes mellitus, its chronic nature, necessity of treatment to maintain blood sugar within normal range, and consequences of abnormal blood sugar.
   (2) Diet planning, its relationship to insulin (medication) and exercise, and the necessity for regularity of food consumption.
   (3) Medication administration, expected actions, rotation of injection sites, and care of insulin and syringes or care of insulin pump if insulin is prescribed, timing of medication administration, peak action time of prescribed insulin.
   (4) Exercise routine, its benefits, and its consequences when not correlated with medication and diet.
   (5) Monitoring urine for sugar and/or acetone, and/or home glucose monitoring.
   (6) Signs and symptoms of hyperglycemia and hypoglycemia.
   (7) Stressors that alter body's need for insulin.
   (8) Monitoring and care of lower extremities.
   (9) Common sites of infection, signs and symptoms.
   (10) Guidelines for when to contact physician or nurse clinician for consultation.
g. Implement teaching plan for both client and agreed upon backup person.
h. Assess skin fold areas daily for fungal or yeast infections.
i. Assess lower extremities daily for injuries, blisters, ulcerations, temperature changes, changes in sensory perceptions.
j. Cleanse skin fold areas and lower extremities daily with mild soap and water, dry thoroughly.
k. Assess for signs and symptoms of urinary tract infection (pain and burning on urination, foul smelling urine), upper respiratory infection (cough, elevated temperature, adventitious lung sounds), infection of wound or ulcer (exudate other than serosanguineous, pain increase, redness of surrounding tissue).
l. Practice good handwashing technique and teach client to do the same.
m. Encourage client to discuss her or his expectations regarding changes in lifestyle, job, daily activities, and so forth. Listen nonjudgmentally, correct misconceptions with factual information, and encourage client to think of alternatives.
n. Be open and nonjudgmental of client's discussion of sexual dysfunction. Seek consultation if you are unable to deal constructively with subject.
o. Encourage expression of client's expectation concerning prescribed weight loss, past efforts (successes and failures).
p. Mutually agree on a plan of action for weight loss if client is obese; implement plan.

EVALUATION

Outcome Criteria

1. Client experiences no increase of fatigue during hospitalization, as evidenced by no complaints of fatigue during performance of daily activities.
2. Client is adequately hydrated, as evidenced by glistening mucous membranes with thin, watery secretions, no daily weight loss of greater than 1 lb, no hypotension.
3. Client presents no evidence of injury at discharge. Pain is relieved within 30 min of treatment, as evidenced by patient's statement to that effect.
4. Client exhibits few signs and symptoms of anxiety by the end of 48 h of hospitalization, as evidenced by fewer questions, increased trust of health care personnel, verbalization of decreased anxiety.
5. At discharge, the client verbalizes little anxiety.
6. Client does not experience ketoacidosis or nonketotic hyperosmolar syndrome during hospitalization, as evidenced by no signs or symptoms of the disorders.
7. Client experiences hypoglycemia during hospitalization (so she or he could experience it and know how it feels under controlled situation) but treatment is instituted before profound mental changes occur.

8. By discharge, the client is capable of self-care (or care giver is capable of caring for client), as evidenced by ability to:
   a. Describe in her or his own words pertinent pathology of diabetes and the goals of treatment.
   b. Plan two daily menus with 90 percent accuracy in caloric count or food groups.
   c. Draw up and inject insulin (if prescribed), observing all safety procedures, for 2 days before discharge.
   d. Collect, test, and interpret urine sample for sugar and acetone without error for 2 days before discharge.
   e. Verbally recite, without error, the signs and symptoms of both hyperglycemia and hypoglycemia, differentiate between them, and describe appropriate action to take for each problem.
   f. Demonstrate foot and leg care while reciting procedure and assessment areas without error.
   g. Describe daily routine of exercise accurately.
   h. Explain in own words the relation between diet, exercise, insulin/medication without error.
   i. Describe situations for which consultation with physician or nurse clinician is required.
9. The client has no signs or symptoms of infection at discharge.
10. The client has no evidence of injury at discharge.
11. By discharge, the client verbalizes changes that must be made in lifestyle, job, activities of daily living, her or his reaction to the changes, and accurate expectations regarding meaning and implications of the changes.
12. By discharge, the client describes concrete plans to accomplish necessary lifestyle changes.
13. Sexual dysfunction is described and alternatives for treatment/adjustment are known by client.
14. Prescribed weight loss will be completed by (date), as evidenced by 1–2 lb lost per week.

Complications

DIMINISHED VISION

Related to cataract formation, retinopathy, temporary osmotic swelling of lens due to hyperglycemia:

Assessment
1. Distorted and/or diminished vision.
2. Halos around lights.
3. Corrective lenses no longer adequate.

Interventions
Consultation with physician.

NEPHROPATHY

Related to glomerulosclerosis (Kimmelstiel-Wilson's syndrome), atherosclerosis, hypertension:

Assessment
1. Proteinuria.
2. Increased BP.
3. Signs and symptoms of renal failure.

Interventions
Consultation with physician.

PERIPHERAL VASCULAR DISEASE

Related to atherosclerosis:

Assessment
1. Decreased temperature in lower extremities.
2. Loss of hair.
3. Pain in lower extremities.
4. Ulcer formation.
5. Infection.

Revised Outcomes
1. Circulation will increase.
2. Need for oxygen and nutrients in lower extremities will decrease.

CORONARY ARTERY DISEASE

Related to atherosclerosis:

Assessment
Angina on exertion.

Interventions
Consultation with physician.

Reevaluation and Follow-up
1. For the four complications listed: periodic telephone calls to assess client's self-care competence and knowledge base.
2. Regular clinic visits.
3. Referral to visiting nurse if client agrees.

HYPERTHYROIDISM

DESCRIPTION

The terms *thyrotoxicosis* and *hyperthyroidism* are used interchangeably to describe diseases associated with excess thyroid hormone. Figure 28-5 reviews the normal mechanisms for plasma thyroid hormone regulation.

Overactivity of the thyroid gland itself is the most common cause of hyperthyroidism. An in-

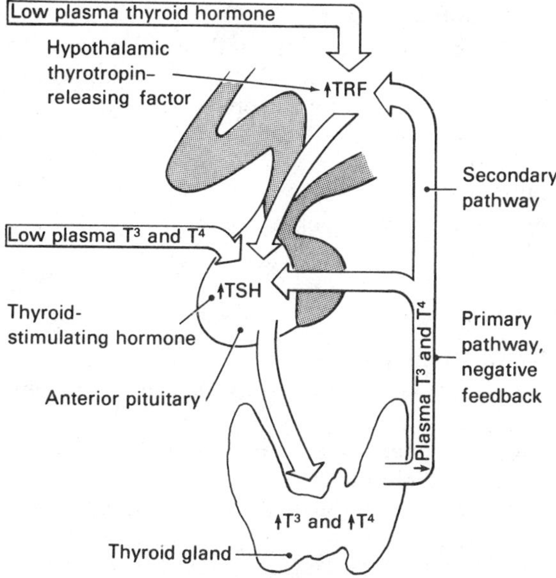

Figure 28-5 Normal mechanism for plasma thyroid hormone regulation. Low plasma T_3 (triiodothyronine) and T_4 (thyroxine) → anterior pituitary ↑ gland T_3 and T_4 ↑→↑ plasma T_3 and T_4 → feedback to anterior pituitary, pituitary, and hypothalamus. More research is needed to clarify the exact role of the hypothalamus in regulating thyroid hormone synthesis. Present evidence suggests a secondary role in which the hypothalamus determines the set point of the feedback threshold. For example, when T_3 and T_4 levels become very elevated, TRF levels drop, producing a fall in TSH levels.

crease in serum thyroxine (T_4) is the mark of hyperthyroidism and is usually accompanied by an increase in triiodothyronine (T_3). *Graves' disease* is the most common form of hyperthyroidism and consists of an enlarged and uniformly affected thyroid gland (diffuse goiter). Other forms include *Plummer's disease* (multinodular goiter) and *toxic adenoma* (uninodular goiter). Hyperthyroidism can also be caused by excessive pituitary TSH (thyroid-stimulating hormone) secretion or by the ectopic production of TSH-like material by neoplasms. The latter situations occur rarely. Pregnancy and excessive ingestion of thyroid hormones are also associated with an increase in circulating thyroid hormones.

The functions of thyroid hormones are to increase the synthesis rate of intracellular proteins (mostly enzymes) and to increase energy production, resulting in an increased rate of consumption of carbohydrates, fats, and oxygen and increased heat production as the metabolic rate of the body is increased. Thyroid hormones also appear to potentiate the effects of catecholamines on body tissues. The signs and symptoms usually associated with hyperthyroidism, therefore, are weight loss despite increased appetite, fatigue, weakness, heat intolerance and diaphoresis, tachycardia, nervousness, tremor of hands, tongue, and closed eyelids, prominent eyes with infrequent blinking, and a steady stare.

Toxic multinodular goiter is a disorder in which hyperthyroidism arises from a nontoxic multinodular goiter of long standing. The mechanism by which the nontoxic goiter escapes from homeostatic control is unknown. The clinical manifestations of the disease are relatively mild in comparison with those of Graves' disease, and the disease is almost never accompanied by infiltrative opthalmopathy.

GRAVES' DISEASE

DESCRIPTION

Graves' disease, a particular type of hyperthyroidism, is a multisystemic disorder characterized by diffuse goiter (see Figure 28-6), infiltrative opthalmopathy, and pretibial myxedema. The exact pathogenesis is unknown; however, the clinical manifestations and course of the disease are modified by factors such as heredity, sex, and possibly emotions. The tendency of Graves' disease to occur in several members of the same family is well documented. The hereditary factor may be associated with an autoimmune response, as suggested by the increased family incidence of other autoimmune disorders such as pernicious anemia and Hashimoto's thyroiditis. Females are seven times more likely to have the disease than males. Graves' disease frequently is precipitated by severe emotional stress such as loss of a significant person or an acute fright such as an automobile accident.

Usual treatment of the disorder is symptom control facilitated by blocking thyroid hormone synthesis and secretion until spontaneous remission occurs. Antithyroid medication (e.g., propylthiouracil) is given to maintain a euthy-

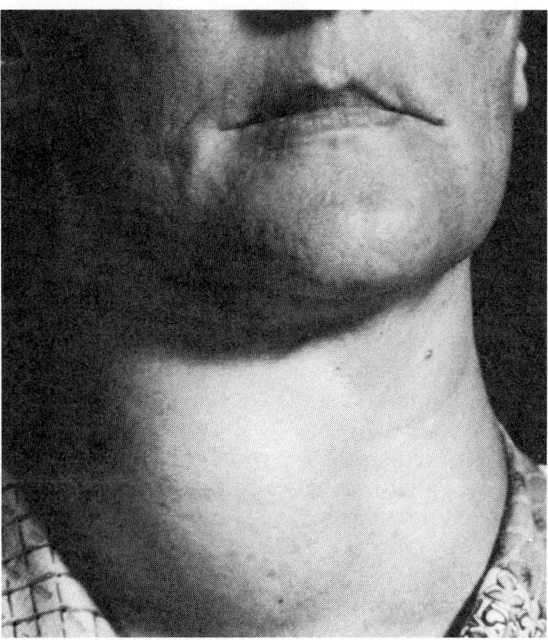

Figure 28-6 Diffuse goiter of hyperthyroidism. (Courtesy of Dr. Louis Avioli.)

roid state for 1 to 3 years, then discontinued to see if remission has occurred. If remission does not occur in 3 to 5 years with such drug therapy, or if the gland is large and unsightly, the majority of the gland is surgically removed, leaving a portion of functioning thyroid tissue to ensure, it is hoped, a euthyroid state. Two weeks before surgery, iodine may be added to the drug therapy to decrease vascularity of the gland and thus reduce the risk of hemorrhage during surgery.

The typical client with Graves' disease is a female between the ages of 30 to 40 years who has had symptoms of hyperthyroidism for at least 6 months before seeking medical assistance. Her eyes appear prominent because of lid retraction, infrequent blinking, and a steady stare; this may or may not be associated with exophthalmos, an infiltration of the orbit, extraocular muscles and eyelids with inflammatory cells, mucopolysaccharide, and edema resulting in some degree of globe protrusion.

PREVENTION

Health Promotion

Early detection and treatment.

Population at Risk

Women between the ages of 30 to 40 years with a family history of Hashimoto's thyroiditis, hypothyroidism, and pernicious anemia and/or recent history of severe stress.

Screening

Serum thyroxine level.

ASSESSMENT

Health History

1. Family history of thyroid disorders and pernicious anemia.
2. Recent severe stress, anxiety, behavior problems, psychotic episode.
3. Onset of heat intolerance, diaphoresis, nervousness, weight loss in spite of increased food intake, decreased or absent menses (if female), decreased libido and impotence (if male), and heart palpitations within the past 6 months.
4. Complaints of angina and possibly diarrhea.

Physical Assessment

1. Prominent eyes with infrequent blinking; fixed stare with sclera showing both above and below the iris; possible frank exophthalmos.
2. Skin texture soft and velvety, warm and damp.
3. Silky hair.
4. Loosening or detachment of the nail from its nailbed.
5. Absence of forehead wrinkling on upward gaze.
6. Fine tremor of outstretched hands, tongue, and closed eyelids.
7. Hyperreflexia.
8. Rapid speech and body movements.
9. Emotional lability.
10. Tachycardia, hypertension, arrhythmias, especially atrial fibrillation.
11. Visably enlarged thyroid gland with right lobe possibly larger than left lobe.
12. Bruit may be heard over thyroid gland.
13. Muscle weakness.

Diagnostic Tests

1. Serum thyroxine (T_4) and triiodothyronine (T_3) levels.
2. Radioactive iodine uptake.

NURSING DIAGNOSES: ACTUAL OR POTENTIAL

1. Fatigue: secondary to muscle weakness, weight loss, and hyperactivity.
2. Inadequate nutritional intake: secondary to increased metabolic rate.
3. Potential change in body image: secondary to large goiter, exophthalmos (if present), altered or absent menses (female), decreased libido or impotence (male).
4. Potential corneal ulceration: secondary to decreased blinking or inability to close eyes due to globe protrusion (exophthalmos).
5. Discomfort: secondary to clothing or bedding saturated with perspiration, too warm ambient room temperature.
6. Potential lack of knowledge necessary for self-care after discharge from hospital.
7. Potential cardiac decomposition: related to tachycardia, increased cardiac output.
8. Potential anxiety, fear: related to hospitalization, not knowing personnel's expectations, or policies and procedures of the institution.

EXPECTED OUTCOMES

1. Fatigue will be decreased within 24 h of hospital admission and absent by discharge, as evidenced by client's sleeping through the night, ability to relax during rest periods, and statement to that effect.
2. Client will not lose weight during hospitalization, as evidenced by monitoring of daily weight.
3. Client will discuss perceived body image changes and integrate them into body image perception if likely to be permanent, or discard them if transient, as evidenced by an accurate assessment of own body image and apparent comfort with that body image.
4. There will be no evidence of corneal ulceration during hospitalization.
5. Client will not complain of discomfort due to perspiration-soaked clothing or bedding during hospitalization.
6. By discharge, client will be capable of self-care, as evidenced by demonstration of knowledge of name, dosage, expected action, and side effects of prescribed drugs and ability to describe accurately the disease process, treatment, and expected outcomes.
7. Cardiac decomposition will be assessed before there are acute manifestations.
8. Anxiety/fear will be slight to absent during hospitalization, as evidenced by client's familiarity with surroundings, willingness to go or be transported to various areas, decreased questioning, trusting relationships with health care personnel, statement that anxiety/fear is decreased or absent.

INTERVENTIONS

1. Assist with activities of daily living and space with 30-min rest periods to avoid fatigue.
2. Reduce environmental stimuli (bright light, noise, interruption of rest periods).
3. Approach client in a calm, unhurried manner.
4. Increase caloric intake to 2,500–3,000 cal/day, using between-meal snacks to avoid weight loss.
5. Weigh client daily in the morning before breakfast and stool and after emptying bladder.
6. Encourage client to verbalize his or her concerns regarding permanence of perceived body image changes. Listen nonjudgmentally. Correct misperceptions with factual information.
7. Accept client without making value judgments regarding physical appearance, behavior.
8. Assess client's ability to completely close eyes and the frequency of blinking. If inadequate, administer prescribed eyedrops.
9. Assess dampness of clothing and bedding at least once each shift; change or assist client to change before there are feelings of discomfort.
10. Assess client's knowledge of treatment regimen, disease process; prepare teaching plan and implement it.
11. Assess cardiac function each shift; notify physician if signs of failure are found. (See *Congestive Heart Failure*, Chapter 30).
12. Orient client to surroundsings within 24 h of admission; introduce to caregivers, roommate (if any).
13. Explain all tests and procedures, their purpose, and client's expected behavior during them.
14. Answer all questions.
15. Include client in care planning and timing.

16. Allow client as much control over his or her activities as is consistent with optimal care.
17. Monitor intake and output.

EVALUATION

Outcome Criteria

1. Client will state that he or she is not experiencing fatigue.
2. Client's body weight will be equal to or greater than admission weight upon discharge.
3. Client's assessment of body image will be accurate and he or she will express comfort with that body image.
4. At discharge, client will exhibit no signs or symptoms of corneal ulceration.
5. At discharge, client will not have experienced discomfort due to perspiration-soaked clothing or bedding.
6. At discharge, client will describe accurately disease process, expected outcomes, and treatment regimen and will be able to name all prescribed drugs and their dosage(s) and schedule without error.
7. Cardiac decomposition will be assessed and treatment instituted before acute manifestations.
8. Client will state that he or she has experienced only slight or no anxiety/fear after the first 24 h of hospitalization.

Complications

PSYCHOTIC EPISODE

Assessment

1. Inappropriate reality testing.
2. Combativeness.

Revised Outcomes

Client will be protected from self-injury and/or injury to others.

Interventions

See Chapter 38, especially *The Threat of Violence.*

Reevaluation and Follow-up

1. Clinic visits to evaluate effectiveness of medication/treatment.
2. Preparation for surgery (if it becomes necessary).

HYPOTHYROIDISM

DESCRIPTION

Hypothyroidism is a disorder that affects every system of the body as a result of the deficiency of thyroid hormones thyroxine (T_4) and triiodothyronine (T_3). Severe hypothyroidism, beginning in infancy, is termed *cretinism. Myxedema coma* is the term used to denote severe hypothyroidism accompanied by neurological involvement leading to impairment of consciousness or frank coma, often precipitated by exposure to cold, infection, trauma, and/or ingestion of CNS depressants.

Hypothyroidism is classified as primary, secondary, or tertiary, depending upon the origin of thyroid hormone deficiency. *Primary hypothyroidism* refers to decreased thyroid hormone production by the thyroid gland itself as a result of destruction by surgery, radiation, idiopathic disease, or defects in thyroid hormone synthesis due to antithyroid drugs (propylthiouracil, lithium carbonate, oral hypoglycemic agents) or iodine deficiency. *Secondary hypothyroidism* results from decreased release of thyroid-stimulating hormone (TSH) from the anterior pituitary gland. *Tertiary hypothyroidism* results from decreased synthesis and/or secretion of thyroid-releasing hormone (TRH) by the hypothalamus. Regardless of the cause, the consequences of decreased thyroid hormones in blood and tissues is the same; the severity of clinical manifestations is dependent on the degree of hormone deficiency.

Hormone replacement therapy will reverse the clinical manifestations of the disorder with the exception of cretinism. Because of the clinical manifestations of the disorder, slowed cognitive and motor function, forgetfulness, and depressed affect, the diagnosis of hypothyroidism may escape detection in the elderly because of its similarity with expected aging changes. As a consequence of this oversight, the elderly individual may be institutionalized for custodial care rather than with hypothyroidism treated.

PREVENTION

Health Promotion

1. Adequate intake of iodine in diet.
2. Early assessment of antithyroid effects of drugs that inhibit the synthesis and secretion of thyroid hormones.

Population at Risk

Either sex, at any age, can become hypothyroid; however, the majority of cases occur in women between the ages of 30 to 40 years.

Screening

Serum thyroxine level.

ASSESSMENT

Health History

1. Family history of goiter or hypothyroidism.
2. History of antithyroid drug ingestion, previous thyroidectomy or radioactive iodine therapy.
3. Insidious onset of weight gain of 10–20 lb, tingling and numbness of hands and feet, constipation, anorexia, impotence/decreased libido (males), heavy and prolonged menstrual periods, exertional dyspnea.
4. Complaints of anorexia, chest pain.

Physical Assessment

1. Deafness (found in one-third of clients).
2. Mental impairment (i.e., forgetfulness, slowed cognitive ability, poor memory, depressed affect).
3. Facial (especially periorbital) and peripheral edema ("hard edema" secondary to mucopolysaccharide deposits).
4. Thinning of lateral aspects of eyebrows.
5. Hair coarse, dry, brittle.
6. Skin pale, coarse, dry, cold with a yellow tinge but normal sclerae (due to block in hepatic conversion of carotene to vitamin A).
7. Hyperkeratosis of elbows and knees.
8. Thyroid gland may be diffusely enlarged (familial goiter secondary to enzymatic defect in hormone synthesis); enlarged, irregular, and firm (suggests chronic thyroiditis); thyromegaly (due to drug-induced hypothyroidism).
9. Thyroid gland not palpable (ablation by surgery or radioactive iodine, atrophy secondary to lack of TSH or TRH, or idiopathic process).
10. Delay in the relaxation phase of deep tendon reflexes.
11. Bradycardia, cardiomegaly.
12. Mild diastolic hypertension.
13. Frank psychosis (dementia, depression) (see Chapters 36 and 45).

Diagnostic Tests

1. Serum T_3 and T_4 and TSH (to distinguish between primary and secondary hypothyroidism).
2. Serum TSH following intravenous injection of TRH (to distinguish between secondary and tertiary hypothyroidism).
3. Metyrapone test to rule out possibility of multiple primary endocrine failure.
4. Laboratory test abnormalities associated with hypothyroidism include anemia, elevated SGOT, LDH, cholesterol, triglycerides, uric acid, and carotene (due to decreased clearance from blood).

NURSING DIAGNOSES: ACTUAL OR POTENTIAL

1. Weakness, fatigue: related to decreased metabolic rate.
2. Dyspnea: related to exertion.
3. Potential constipation: related to decreased bowel motility.
4. Discomfort: related to cold intolerance.
5. Potential lack of knowledge: regarding disease process and treatment regimen.
6. Potential learning dysfunction: related to slowed cognitive function and poor memory.
7. Potential injury: related to weakness, fatigue, slowed mental processes.
8. Potential skin breakdown: related to dry skin.

EXPECTED OUTCOMES

1. Activities of daily living will be completed without excess fatigue, as evidenced by client's statement to that effect.
2. During hospitalization client will complete activities as prescribed.
3. Dyspnea will be slight or absent during hospitalization, as evidenced by client's statement to that effect.
4. Client will have at least one soft-formed stool every other day during hospitalization.
5. Client will not complain of being cold during hospitalization.
6. Client or significant other will have the knowledge necessary for self-care by time of discharge, as eivdenced by correct description of the disease process and treatment regimen.
7. Client will not exhibit evidence of injury during hospitalization.
8. There will be no evidence of skin breakdown during hospitalization.

INTERVENTIONS

1. Assist with activities of daily living as necessary to avoid fatigue.
2. Space activities with 30-min rest periods.
3. Do not rush client in self-care activities.

4. Remind client, as necessary, what the goal of the present activity is in a gentle but firm manner. Coach as appropriate.
5. Assess bowel function and usual medication/treatment for constipation.
6. If there is no bowel movement (or stool is hard/dry) for 48 h, administer prescribed treatment.
7. Provide blankets as necessary to keep client warm.
8. Assess clothing needs to maintain warmth; if clothes are not available within health care facility, ask family member or significant other to provide them.
9. Assess knowledge of client regarding disease process and treatment regimen.
10. Assess client's learning ability and memory function.
11. If client does not have the ability to learn and remember, locate a significant other who will take responsiblity for carrying out the treatment regimen.
12. Formulate a teaching plan that incorporates findings from above assessments; include necessary pathophysiology of disease process, names of drugs used, their effects and side effects, dosage and administration schedule, expected outcome of treatment, and the chronic nature of the disease process necessitating continued treatment throughout life.
13. To avoid injury to client:
    a. Have side rails up when client is in bed.
    b. Assist client, as appropriate, in getting in and out of bed and chair and in ambulation.
    c. Reorient client as necessary.
    d. Do not allow client to get lost.
14. Apply lotion or cream to dry skin areas and pressure areas.
15. Use soap sparingly and rinse well after its use.

EVALUATION

Expected Outcomes

1. Client will not experience excess fatigue during hospitalization, as evidenced by no complaints to that effect.
2. Client will complete all prescribed activities during hospitalization.
3. Client will not complain of dyspnea during activities while hospitalized.
4. Client will have at least one soft-formed stool every other day during hospitalization.
5. Client will not experience discomfort due to being cold during hospitalization, as evidenced by a statement to that effect.
6. Client, or a significant other, will be capable of performing self-care activities at discharge, as evidenced by the ability to:
    a. Accurately describe pertinent pathophysiology of hypothyroidism.
    b. List signs and symptoms of both hypothyroidism and hyperthyroidism and not confuse the two syndromes.
    c. Name the medication(s) prescribed, the expected effects, possible side effects, prescribed dosage, and administration times.
7. Client will exhibit no signs or symptoms of injury at discharge.
8. There will be no evidence of skin breakdown during hospitalization.

Complications

MYXEDEMA COMA

Fifty percent or more of clients lapse into coma after hospitalization (Jubiz, 1979).

Assessment

May be precipitated by exposure to cold, infection, trauma, and/or CNS depressants. Clinical manifestations include:

1. Hypothermia.
2. Hypotension.
3. Ileus, fecal impaction, or urinary retention.
4. Seizures.
5. Respiratory failure.
6. Congestive heart failure.

Revised Outcomes

Potential myxedema coma will be assessed and physician notified before loss of consciousness.

Interventions

1. Assess respiratory and cardiac status at least once each shift.
2. Monitor vital signs q8h.
3. Assess and record bowel function.
4. Notify physician if signs and symptoms of impending coma are present.
5. Take precautions against seizure.

Reevaluation and Follow-up

1. Routine clinic visits to monitor treatment effectiveness.
2. Referral to visiting nurse if self-care competence is questionable or if client is anxious about ability for self-care.

ADRENOCORTICAL HYPERFUNCTION: HYPERCORTISOLISM

DESCRIPTION

Hypercortisolism results in chronically elevated levels of cortisol. *Cushing's syndrome* is the name given to the clinical and chemical abnormalities associated with hypercortisolism. Cushing's syndrome can result from (1) excessive secretion of ACTH by the pituitary (also called *Cushing's disease*), (2) adenoma or carcinoma of the adrenal cortex, and (3) exogenous secretion of ACTH by nonpituitary tumors (malignant neoplasms, particularly lung cancer). Figure 28-7 shows normal cortisol regulation.

PREVENTION

Health Promotion

At this time there is no means to prevent Cushing's syndrome except Cushing's syndrome secondary to exogenous steroid usage. In this instance the steroid therapy is kept as low as possible to prevent side effects. Early detection and treatment is the key to preventing complications.

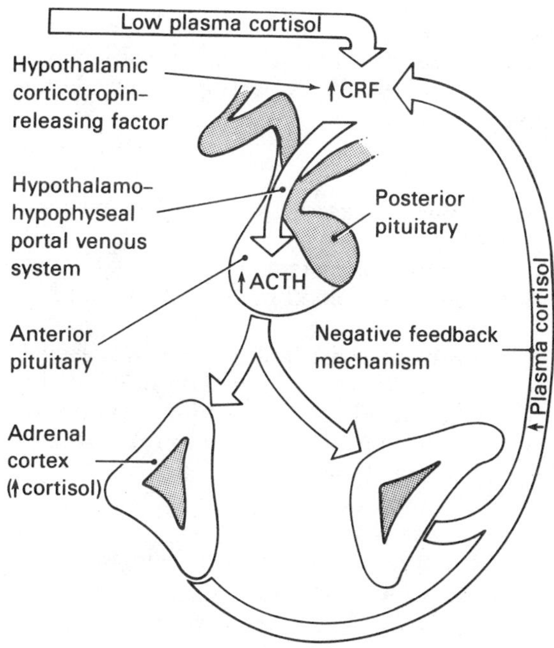

Figure 28-7 Normal mechanism for plasma cortisol regulation. Low plasma cortisol → hypothalamus ↑ CRF → anterior pituitary ↑ ACTH → adrenal cortex ↑ cortisol → ↑ plasma cortisol → hypothalamus.

TABLE 28-3 NORMAL FUNCTIONS OF GLUCOCORTICOIDS

Mobilize amino acids.
Increase breakdown of proteins and promote negative nitrogen balance.
Promote gluconeogenesis.
Increase total body fat.
Prevent inflammatory response.
Decrease movements of white blood cells to area of inflammation and effectiveness of immune response.
Cause some water and sodium retention.

Population at Risk

1. Clients with lung cancer.
2. Clients on exogenous steroids for anti-inflammatory properties.

Screening

1. Mass screening is not done.
2. Any client on steroids should be monitored for Cushing's syndrome.

ASSESSMENT

Because of the numerous functions of glucocorticoids the signs and symptoms of excess are varied and multiple. Also, the client may have varied degrees of excess from only a small increase to major abnormal levels. Signs and symptoms are due to accentuation of normal functions of the glucocorticoids. Table 28-3 lists normal functions of glucocorticoids.

Health History

1. Increased weight and change in body proportions.
2. Hirsutism.
3. Menstrual changes.
4. Weakness, fatigue.
5. Pain in back, joints.
6. Easy bruising, petechia formation.
7. Edema.
8. Hypertension.
9. Mood swings.
10. Gastrointestinal complaints.

Physical Assessment

Refer to Figure 28-8.

1. Nervous system.
   a. Motor.
      (1) Weakness.
      (2) Poor coordination.
   b. Emotional.
      (1) Mood changes.
      (2) Irritability, depression, psychosis.
   c. Pain, back and joints.
2. Integumentary system.
   a. Fragile, thin skin.
   b. Facial plethora due to abnormal dilation of blood vessels.
   c. Bruising on arms, legs.
   d. Purple striae on arms, trunk, thighs, and abdomen.
   e. Petechial hemorrhage.
   f. Poor wound healing.
   g. Hirsutism due to increased androgens.
3. Cardiovascular system.
   a. Hypertension.

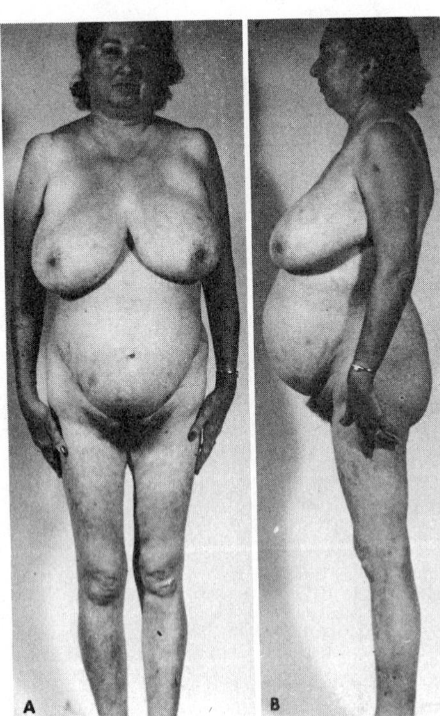

Figure 28-8 Cushing's syndrome. [Hume, D. M., and Harrison, T. S., in S. I. Schwartz et al. (eds.): *Principles of Surgery*, 2d ed., McGraw-Hill, New York, 1974.]

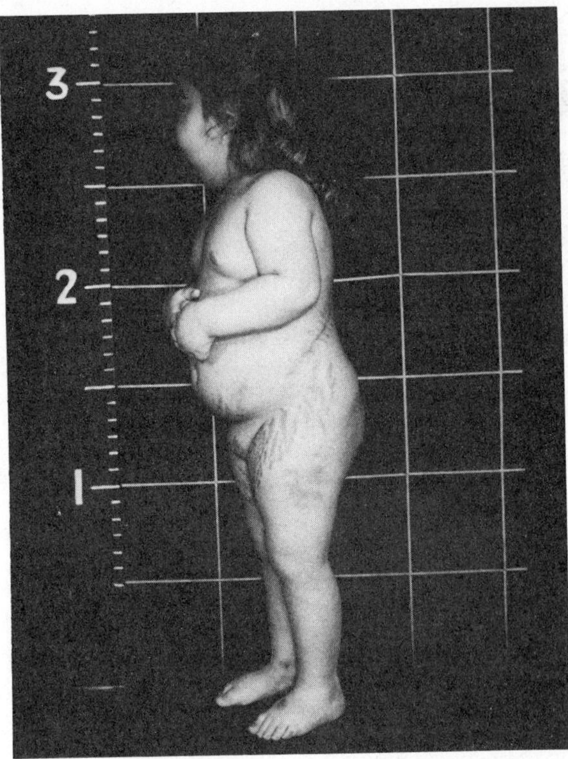

Figure 28-9 Client with Cushing's syndrome. Note proximal distribution of fat and striae over abdomen and thigh. (Courtesy of Dr. Louis Avioli.)

   b. Edema, increased risk of congestive heart failure.
4. Gastrointestinal system.
   a. GI bleeding (blood in stool, vomitus).
   b. Obesity.
      (1) Proximal distribution (see Figures 28-9 and 28-10 for comparison of the distribution of fat in Cushing's syndrome with that in normal obesity).
      (2) Supraclavicular.
      (3) Truncal obesity.
      (4) Buffalo humps.
      (5) Moon face (see Figure 28-11).
5. Musculoskeletal system.
   a. Muscle wasting.
   b. Weakness.
   c. Pain due to osteoporosis.
6. Other manifestations.
   a. Gynecomastia.
   b. Change in secondary sex characteristics.
   c. Enlargement of clitoris.

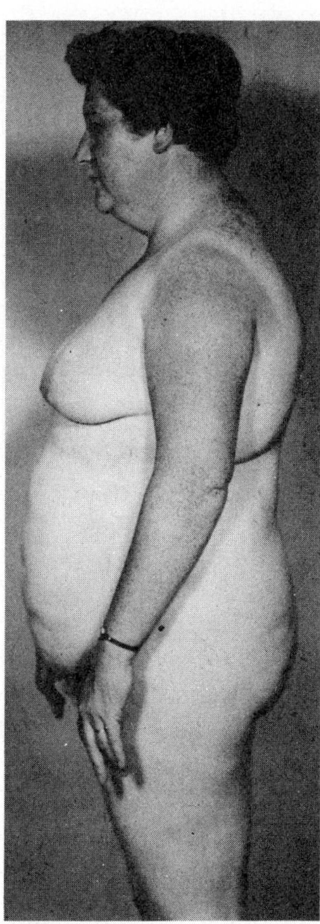

Figure 28-10 Simple obesity, in contrast to Cushing's syndrome. [Hume, D. M., and Harrison, T. S., in S. I. Schwartz et al. (eds.): *Principles of Surgery*, 2d ed., McGraw-Hill, New York, 1974.]

Diagnostic Tests

1. Plasma ACTH levels.
2. Plasma cortisol (at 8 A.M. and 4 P.M.).
3. 24-h urine for 17-OH steroids.
4. Dexamethasone suppression test, both low and high dose test.
5. Metyrapone testing.
6. Blood glucose levels and glucose tolerance test.
7. Serum electrolytes (sodium, potassium, chloride).
8. Skull x-ray films and CAT scan of head to view pituitary.
9. Chest x-ray films for ectopic sites of r duction.
10. CAT scan of abdomen.

NURSING DIAGNOSES: ACTUAL OR POTENTIAL

1. Immediate.
   a. Fluid and electrolyte imbalance (increased sodium and water and decreased potassium): related to increased cortisol.
   b. Hypercalciuria: related to increased osteoporosis.
   c. Obesity: related to increased appetite.
   d. Weakness/fatigue: related to poor muscle strength and electrolyte imbalance.
   e. Potential for injury: related to weakness, fatigue, behavior changes.
   f. Potential abnormal blood sugar: related to hypercortisolism.
   g. Increased risk of infection: related to depressed inflammatory response.
   h. Hypertension: related to fluid retention.
   i. Inability to tolerate stressors: related to emotional lability.
   j. Change in self-image: related to change in appearance (truncal obesity, increase in body hair, etc.).

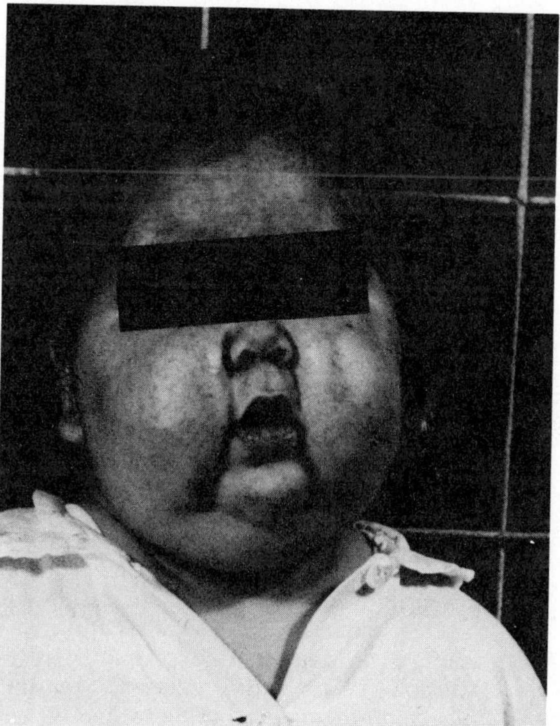

Figure 28-11 Moon face of Cushing's syndrome. (Courtesy of Dr. Louis Avioli.)

k. Midepigastric pain: related to ulcer.
l. Lack of knowledge about diagnostic tests.
m. Lack of knowledge about disease and treatment.

2. After adrenalectomy.
   a. Incisional pain: related to surgery.
   b. Hypotension: related to decreased hormonal level.
   c. Fluid and electrolyte imbalance (decreased sodium and water and increased potassium): related to hypocortisolism.
   d. Poor wound healing: related to depressed inflammatory response.
   e. Lack of knowledge about long-term self-care needs.
3. After transsphenoidal removal of pituitary tumor or radiation therapy to pituitary. Potential inability to maintain homeostasis due to panhypopituitarism (see *Pituitary Tumors* in this chapter).

EXPECTED OUTCOMES

1. Immediate.
   a. Fluid and electrolyte balance will be maintained (input equals output).
   b. Weight gain will stop and weight loss will occur at rate of 1 lb/week.
   c. Weakness and fatigue will decrease.
   d. Client will be free of injuries.
   e. Blood glucose will be kept within normal limits.
   f. Client will not develop any infections.
   g. Psychological stressors (abrupt change in schedule, family crisis, lack of information) will be decreased.
   h. Client will state that midepigastric pain is controlled.
   i. Client will demonstrate improved self-image, as evidenced by talking about self in positive terms, dressing to accentuate positive attributes, talking about future plans, and so forth.
   j. Client and family will demonstrate accurate knowledge of diagnostic test, as evidenced by description of purpose, procedure, monitoring during test and after.
   k. Client and family will demonstrate accurate knowledge about diagnosis and treatment, as evidenced by explaining pathophysiology, type of treatment, reason, expected outcomes, complications.
2. After adrenalectomy.
   a. Client will state pain is controlled.
   b. Client will not develop any symptoms of hypocortisolism or other postoperative complications that go undetected.
   c. Client will not develop a wound or respiratory or genitourinary infection.
   d. Client and family will be able to describe long-term self-care needs, such as:
      (1) If hormonal therapy is necessary, the client will be able to state how to take replacement therapy, the signs and symptoms of excess or deficiency, and when extra hormonal therapy will be needed.
      (2) If on other medications for chronic health problems such as diabetes mellitus and hypertension, the client will know why he or she is on therapy, how to take medication, the side effects of therapy, and the signs and symptoms of effectiveness.
      (3) Follow-up care.
      (4) When the client can return to work.
      (5) Planned activity/rest schedule.
      (6) How to deal with identified stressors and effect of stressors on glucocorticoids.

INTERVENTIONS

1. All clients need orientation to the hospital environment and schedule of activities, but clients with adrenocortical problems particularily need it as they cannot tolerate unexpected changes in activities.
2. Monitor and record:
   a. Intake and output every shift.
   b. Vital signs q4h.
   c. Presence or absence of edema every shift.
   d. Daily weight with the same scale, at the same time, and with the same clothes.
   e. Laboratory results daily.
   f. Urinary glucose/ketones qid.
   g. Check every stool for occult blood.
3. Plan diet to keep glucose and sodium levels within normal limits, to restrict calories to prevent abnormal weight gain, and to provide adequate proteins.
4. Assist with activities of daily living and plan rest periods between activities.
5. Use sterile technique with all invasive procedures.
6. Assess for occurrence of infections: skin lesions, change in respiratory status, and presence of urinary tract infections.

7. Isolate client from other clients with infections.
8. Allow time for client to express fears and anxieties.
   a. Spend time with client.
   b. Do not force client to talk; just let him or her know you are available.
9. Medicate client as appropriate for midepigastric pain.
10. Discuss client's feelings about changes in appearance. Explain reversibility of changes. Discuss ways to maximize positive attributes.
11. Instruct client and family regarding diagnostic test.
   a. Why done.
   b. Procedure.
   c. Monitoring during and after test.
12. Instruct client and family regarding disease and treatment.
   a. Pathophysiology.
   b. Relation of adrenal problem to pituitary ACTH, ectopic ACTH, or adrenal tumor, whichever is appropriate.
   c. Treatment planned.
      (1) Hypercortisolism secondary to increased pituitary ACTH (see teaching plan under Interventions, *Pituitary Tumors* in this chapter).
      (2) Hypercortisolism secondary to ectopic ACTH secretion. Treatment of disease process that causes ectopic secretion (e.g., treatment of lung cancer, as described in Chapter 31).
      (3) Hypercortisolism due to adrenal adenoma or carcinoma.
         (a) Bilateral or unilateral adrenalectomy.
         (b) Resultant adrenal insufficiency with bilateral adrenalectomy.
13. Provide postoperative care after surgical removal of pituitary tumor or radiation therapy for pituitary tumors (see section on *Pituitary Tumors* in this chapter).
14. Provide postoperative care after removal of adrenal gland(s).
   a. Relieve pain with medication, diversion, relaxation techniques, and good body positioning.
   b. Monitor for signs of complication and prevent complications.
      (1) Adrenal crisis (see *Adrenocortical Hypofunction*).
         (a) Definitely will occur if client had bilateral adrenalectomy and is not on replacement therapy.
         (b) May occur in the immediate postoperative period in client having unilateral adrenalectomy because the one gland may not be sufficient to meet needs of the body immediately.
      (2) Shock (hemorrhagic or adrenal insufficiency).
         (a) Check vital signs q1h until stable, then q2h.
         (b) Check operative site for excess bleeding q1h.
         (c) Monitor intake and output.
         (d) Check weight daily.
      (3) Infection.
         (a) Check temperature q4h.
         (b) Check wound for drainage, redness, foul odor. Report to physician.
         (c) Use aseptic technique with all invasive procedures, dressing changes.
         (d) Check coughing and deep breathing q2h.
         (e) Change client's position q2h.
         (f) Auscultate chest q4h. Report signs of increased congestions, poor air exchange, change in sputum.
      (4) Gastrointestinal distress.
         (a) Monitor patency of nasal gastric tube, return of bowel sounds, flatulence, and occurrence of nausea and vomiting.
         (b) Administer antiemetics as necessary and as ordered.
         (c) Ambulate client as soon as possible.
         (d) Irrigate nasogastric tube as ordered. If there is no order and client is vomiting, consult with physician.
         (e) Promote high-protein diet as soon as it can be tolerated. Other dietary restrictions will vary. Client may need low-calorie, increased-potassium, low-sodium diet.
15. Instruct client and family in self-care needs after discharge.
   a. Follow-up appointment.

b. Hormonal replacement therapy (see *Adrenocortical Hypofunction*) if client had a bilateral adrenalectomy.
c. Time period for reversal of body image changes.
d. Signs and symptoms of continual adrenocortical excess.
e. When client can return to work.
f. Self-care needs for residual chronic problems that resulted from adrenocortical excess (hypertension, see Chapter 30; congestive heart failure, see Chapter 30; diabetes mellitus, see this chapter).
g. Effects of physical and emotional stress on steroid needs.
h. Diet that is high in protein with restricted calories. Diet may need to be adjusted for glucose intolerance and hypertension in some cases.

EVALUATION

Outcome Criteria

1. Fluid and electrolyte balance is maintained.
2. Weight loss is occurring at the rate of 1 lb/week.
3. Client states satisfaction with diet.
4. Weakness and fatigue are decreasing.
5. Client has suffered no injuries.
6. Blood glucose is within normal limits.
7. Client has developed no infections.
8. Client states that stressors have been kept to a minimum and appears free of anxiety, as seen by relaxed facial expression, lack of restlessness, interacting appropriately with staff and significant others.
9. Midepigastric pain is controlled; stool for occult blood is negative.
10. Client discusses self in positive terms, is attentive to his or her appearance, talks of future plans, and discusses reversibility of body changes.
11. Client can explain purpose, procedure, and monitoring necessary during and after tests with 100 percent accuracy.
12. Client and family can accurately explain information on diagnostic tests.
13. Client and family can accurately explain diagnosis and treatment information.
14. Client's postoperative pain has been controlled; there are no signs and symptoms of complications (adrenal insufficiency, shock, infection, GI distress).
15. Client and family can accurately explain self-care needs and can demonstrate accurate self-medication routine, as seen by chart the client is keeping.

Complications

1. Adrenal insufficiency.
2. Infection.
3. Gastrointestinal distress.

Assessment/Revised Outcomes/Interventions

For these complications, see Assessment, Expected Outcomes, and Interventions for adrenocortical hyperfunction, above.

Reevaluation and Follow-up

If any of these complications occurs, institute an individualized plan until complications are controlled. Client will return for follow-up care frequently. At these times client should be assessed for signs and symptoms of both continual signs of adrenalcortical excess and insufficiency. Client should be assessed for ability to meet self-care needs.

HYPERALDOSTERONISM

DESCRIPTION

Hyperaldosteronism is a clinical syndrome involving excess secretion of aldosterone. Aldosterone is the primary mineralocorticoid secreted by the adrenal cortex. Excess secretion of the hormone leads to sodium retention, loss of potassium, and hypertension from extracellular volume expansion.

PREVENTION

Health Promotion

There is no known way to prevent the problem. Early detection and treatment is the key to prevention of complications.

Population at Risk

Persons with dehydration, sodium depletion, renal artery stenosis, and cardiac failure are candidates to develop secondary hyperaldosteronism.

Screening

There are no tools for mass screening.

ASSESSMENT

Health History

1. Complaints of hypertension.
2. Complaints of weakness, muscle cramps, headaches, paresthesia, and lethargy.
3. Complaints of excessive thirst and frequent voiding.

Physical Assessment

1. Weakness and lethargy.
2. Hypertension.
3. Cardiac enlargement.

Diagnostic Tests

1. Plasma aldosterone after hypokalemia is corrected.
   a. Supine and upright.
   b. After sodium challenge.
2. 24-h urine aldosterone.
3. Serum electrolytes: sodium and potassium.
4. 24-h urine potassium.
5. Peripheral plasma renin levels.
6. Plasma renin activity (PRA).
   a. After volume depletion.
   b. With postural changes.
   c. After salt loading.
7. Test to locate tumor.
   a. Intravenous pyelogram (IVP).
   b. Renal arteriograms secondary to IVP.
   c. Adrenal vein catheterization with aldosterone levels.

NURSING DIAGNOSES: ACTUAL OR POTENTIAL

1. Pain: related to muscle cramps and paresthesia and headaches.
2. Potential for injury: related to weakness and lethargy.
3. Altered fluid and electrolytes: related to increased aldosterone.
4. Cardiac instability, hypertension/arrhythmias: due to low potassium and high sodium.
5. Thirst: related to polyuria.
6. Lack of interest in activities, hobbies, projects: related to lethargy and weakness.
7. Knowledge deficit: regarding diagnostic tests, disease, treatment, and self-care needs.

EXPECTED OUTCOMES

1. Client will be free of pain as a result of effective use of therapeutic interventions.
2. Client will experience no injuries.
3. Fluid and electrolyte levels will return to normal.
4. Client will state that thirst is not a problem.
5. Client will not develop any undetected cardiac instability.
6. Client will take interest in activities, hobbies, and projects.
7. Client will be able to explain accurately the diagnostic tests planned (purpose, procedure, where test is done, posttest care).
8. Client will be able to explain accurately the anatomy and physiology of the adrenal cortex, the pathophysiology of the disease, and how the disease causes the symptoms.
9. Client will be able to explain accurately the planned treatment (adrenalectomy, expected effect, potential complications, other therapy if surgery is not possible).

INTERVENTIONS

1. General—promote comfort.
   a. Administer pain medications as indicated.
   b. Make use of exercises, warm soaks, muscle relaxants to decrease muscle cramps.
   c. Assess client's potential for injury and structure environment to protect client.
      (1) Get client up only with assistance.
      (2) Use side rails if client is lethargic.
      (3) Avoid chance for burns (e.g., test bath water, etc.).
      (4) Assess and record data with regard to fluid and electrolyte status.
         (a) Vital signs q4h more frequently if client is hypertensive.
         (b) Intake and output every shift.
         (c) Daily weight at the same time, with the same scale, and with the same clothes.
         (d) Lab values particularily of potassium and signs of increasing weakness.
         (e) Presence of edema (rare).
         (f) Cardiac monitor if there is presence of arrhythmias or if client has low potassium.
   d. Provide frequent rest periods between activities, tests, visiting, meals, and so on.
   e. Provide diet that is appropriate and satisfying to the client (usually low-sodium diet).
   f. Spread liquids throughout the day to pre-

vent thirst. Provide liquids that the client finds most satisfying and that are within dietary restrictions.

g. Institute client and family teaching about diagnostic test.
   (1) Purpose.
   (2) Procedure.
   (3) What to expect during the test.
   (4) Care needs after test.
h. Ensure that test is carried out appropriately by seeing that client is prepared appropriately and that specimens are collected appropriately.
i. Institute client and family teaching regarding the disease and treatment.
   (1) Anatomy and physiology of the illness.
   (2) How the hormonal imbalance causes the problems.
   (3) Treatment measures and expected responses. Primary aldosteronism:
      (a) Preferred treatment is the removal of the tumor.
      (b) If no tumor is found, the surgery consists of a left-sided adrenalectomy with removal of 50 percent of right adrenal.
      (c) Surgery should relieve the symptoms.
      (d) Potential for adrenal insufficiency after the surgery (see section on *Adrenocortical Hypofunction* in this chapter).
      (e) If surgery is not possible, the client may be treated with sodium-restricted diet and spironolactone (Aldactone). This treatment is also used for clients who show recurrent signs and symptoms after surgery.
j. Institute client and family teaching for discharge needs.
   (1) Signs and symptoms of hypokalemia.
   (2) Signs and symptoms of adrenal insufficiency.
   (3) Dietary restrictions.
   (4) Rest and activity schedule so that client has time and energy to do the things he or she enjoys.
k. Work with client to help him or her take part in activities that were previously enjoyed. This will mostly include helping the client schedule activities so that the client has the energy to do the activities.

2. Postoperative care of adrenalectomy. See *Adrenocortical Hyperfunction: Hypercortisolism.*

EVALUATION

Outcome Criteria

1. Client states that pain is controlled.
2. Client did not suffer any injuries.
3. Fluid and electrolytes return to normal.
4. Client said that thirst was not a problem.
5. No instability of the cardiac system occurs.
6. Client discusses activities that he or she has planned to take part in.
7. Client can accurately explain the anatomy and physiology of the adrenal cortex and the pathophysiology of the disease.
8. Client and family can accurately describe the diagnostic procedures.
9. Client can accurately explain the planned treatment and the expected effects.

Complications

HYPOKALEMIA

Assessment

Lab values for serum less than 3 mEq/L.

1. Increasing weakness of muscles.
2. Cardiac arrhythmias.

Expected Outcomes

Potassium level will return to normal.

Interventions

1. Place on cardiac monitor.
2. Administer potassium as ordered.
3. Encourage high potassium foods.

Reevaluation and Follow-up

1. If complications should occur, expected outcomes and interventions are instituted as outlined.
2. On return visits, client is checked for compliance to medication regimen, signs and symptoms of hyperaldosteronism, signs and symptoms of hypokalemia, and signs and symptoms of adrenal insufficiency (if surgery was performed).
3. Lab measurements of potassium and sodium are done.
4. Other diagnostic tests as outlined are done if necessary.
5. Client is referred to a visiting nurses service in the event of adrenocortical insufficiency or if lethargy makes it difficult for the client to understand instructions.

ADRENAL INSUFFICIENCY

See *Adrenocortical Hypofunction* in this chapter.

HYPERSECRETION OF ADRENAL ANDROGENS

DESCRIPTION

Impaired production of adrenal androgens can result from enzyme deficits (congenital adrenalhyperplasia) or from development of an adenoma or carcinoma. In children, excess of adrenal androgen leads to adrenogenital syndrome. (See Chapter 17 for a discussion of this problem in children.) In the adult female, excess of adrenal androgen causes virilization and symptoms such as hirsutism, acne, increased sebum production, temporal baldness, deepening of voice, amenorrhea, atrophy of the uterus, decreased breast size, and development of male habitus. This condition is most common in children and thus will not be discussed in this section in detail. If it does occur in adult females, the treatment is adrenalectomy. The problems, expected outcomes, and interventions are the same as for adrenalectomy for Cushing's syndrome (see *Adrenocortical Hyperfunction: Hypercortisolism* in this chapter). The change in sexual characteristics should change with treatment.

ADRENOCORTICAL HYPOFUNCTION

DESCRIPTION

Adrenocortical insufficiency can be primary or secondary. *Primary adrenal insufficiency*, or *Addison's disease*, is the result of destruction of the adrenal cortex, thus impairing the capacity of the gland to secrete cortisol and aldosterone. Most often the cause of primary insufficiency is idiopathic, possibly an autoimmune response. Other known causes of primary adrenal insufficiency included adrenalectomy, infection (tuberculosis, histoplasmosis), adrenal hemorrhage (trauma), amyloidosis, and metastatic disease.

In most instances the destruction of the gland is a gradual process, and for a time the client is able to meet the normal physiological needs of the body in the absence of physiological and psychological stressors. When more than 90 percent of the adrenal cortex is destroyed, internal homeostasis is lost. This causes a clinical picture characterized by an insidious onset of slowly progressing fatigue, weakness, anorexia, nausea and vomiting, weight loss, hypotension, increased pigmentation, and occasionally hypoglycemia. But the symptoms can vary greatly from a complaint of mild fatigue to shock.

The symptoms result from a deficiency in both glucocorticoids and mineralocorticoids (see Table 28-3). The loss of mineralocorticoids causes volume contraction and hyperkalemia. The loss of glucocorticoids causes impaired tolerance to stress, weakness, decreased vigor, and hypoglycemia. The hyperpigmentation is due to the fact that melanocyte-stimulating hormone (MSH) is increased in primary adrenal insufficiency. Some clients with primary adrenal insufficiency will have decreased libido due to decrease in adrenal androgens.

Glucocorticoid deficiency occurring as a consequence of pituitary ACTH deficiency is termed *secondary adrenal insufficiency*. ACTH deficiency may be due to pituitary or hypothalamic disease. Unlike primary adrenal insufficiency, secondary adrenal insufficiency is seldom associated with a deficiency in aldosterone secretion and/or an increase in MSH. Some of the more commonly encountered causes of ACTH deficiency are pituitary tumors or cysts and chronic suppression of ACTH glucocorticoid from an adrenal neoplasm or by exogenous glucocorticoids.

PREVENTION

Health Promotion

There is no known way to prevent primary adrenal insufficiency. Clients on chronic glucocorticoid therapy should be carefully monitored upon withdrawal of therapy to prevent secondary adrenal insufficiency. These clients may need extra adrenal glucocorticoids for up to 1 year after withdrawal in times of major stress. Early diagnosis and treatment is the key to preventing complications.

Population at Risk

1. Clients on chronic glucocorticoid therapy.
2. Addison's disease has been seen with increased frequency in clients with Hashimo-

to's disease, idiopathic hyperparathyroidism, diabetes mellitus, ovarian failure, and pernicious anemia.

Screening

No mass screening tools are available. For clients with a high index of suspicion, diagnostic tests as described below are used.

ASSESSMENT

Health History

1. Complaints of fatigue, weakness. Fatigue at first may be sporadic and may occur only at times of increased stress, but eventually the client may be continually fatigued and require bed rest.
2. GI complaints.
   a. First symptoms noted by the client are frequently gastrointestinal.
   b. Complaints may vary from anorexia to fulminating nausea and vomiting and diarrhea with weight loss.
   c. Ill-defined abdominal pain is often present.
   d. History of drugs used, particularly steroids.
   e. History of known precipitating stressors or events such as trauma, infection, shock.
   f. History of infertility, impotence, irregular menstrual cycle.

Physical Assessment

1. Weight loss.
2. Hypotension; in severe cases may be as low as 80/50. Postural vital sign changes often present, syncope.
3. Weakness and poor coordination.
4. Wasting of fat deposits and muscles.
5. Hyperpigmentation of skin and mucous membranes (seen in primary adrenal insufficiency only), vitiligo, dry skin, loss of skin tone, and loss of body hair.
6. Apathy, lethargy, irritability, confusion, psychosis.

Diagnostic Tests

1. Plasma cortisol (8 A.M. and 4 P.M.).
2. Plasma ACTH: helps to differentiate primary from secondary adrenal insufficiency.
3. 24-h urine for 17-hydroxycorticosteroids and 17-ketosteroids.
4. ACTH stimulation test.
5. Serum electrolytes.

NURSING DIAGNOSES: ACTUAL OR POTENTIAL

1. Fluid and electrolyte imbalance: related to adrenal insufficiency.
2. Fatigue and weakness: related to decreased adrenocortical steroids.
3. Weight loss: related to nausea, vomiting, decreased appetite, abdominal pain, and altered metabolism.
4. Change in self-concept: related to decreased energy and change in sexual characteristics.
5. Alteration in comfort: related to abdominal pain.
6. Altered ability to tolerate stressors (physical and emotional): related to insufficiency of steroids to maintain homeostasis.
7. Knowledge deficit: regarding disease, diagnostic tests, and treatment.
8. Lack of knowledge about self-care needs after discharge.
9. Addisonian crisis.
   a. Severe alteration in homeostasis (shock/arrhythmias): related to abnormal hormonal levels and the inability to secrete more hormones in time of stress.
   b. Impaired CNS function (confusion/stupor/coma): related to hormonal deficit.
   c. Absolute inability to tolerate any stressors.

EXPECTED OUTCOMES

1. Fluid and electrolyte balance will return to normal and will be maintained.
2. Fatigue and weakness will be controlled and will then decrease as therapy is instituted.
3. Weight loss will stop and weight gain as needed will occur.
4. Client will demonstrate improved self-concept, as evidenced by: talking about self in positive terms, talking about future plans, and stating that problem can be controlled and will not interfere with future.
5. Client will not be exposed to any unnecessary stressors.
6. Client will not demonstrate any undetected changes in homeostasis that could result from worsening of adrenal insufficiency or could result from increased stressors requiring more adrenocorticol hormone.
7. Client and family will demonstrate accurate knowledge of diagnostic tests (purpose, procedure, monitoring done during and after test).

8. Client and family will demonstrate accurate knowledge of disease and treatment (anatomy and physiology of the adrenal gland, pathophysiology of the disease, replacement therapy).
9. Client and family will demonstrate accurate knowledge for self-care, as demonstrated by the ability to explain:
   a. Needed replacement therapy.
   b. Dosage and time schedule of therapy.
   c. Times when more therapy is necessary.
   d. Signs and symptoms of adrenocortical excess. (See *Adrenocortical Hyperfunction: Hypercortisolism* and *Hyperaldosteronism* in this chapter.)
   e. Signs and symptoms of insufficient therapy.
   f. The necessity of therapy for life.
   g. The need to wear a medic-alert bracelet or necklace so therapy is always given.
   h. Stressors in their lives and ways to handle them.
   i. Follow-up care.
   j. Daily activity plan that incorporates activities of daily living and working.

INTERVENTIONS

1. Monitor:
   a. Fluid and electrolyte balance.
   b. Intake and output every shift and every hour if client is in addisonian crisis.
   c. Daily weight at the same time, on the same scale, and with the same clothes.
   d. Serum lab values every day.
   e. Vital signs with orthostatic changes q4h; client in addisonian crisis will require vital sign checks every 15 min until stable and then q1h.
2. Administer fluids and drugs as necessary and as ordered until homeostasis is returned.
3. Assist with activities of daily living; if client is in addisonian crisis, some activities such as complete bath will be eliminated.
4. Schedule activities to allow for rest periods between activities.
5. Ambulate client with assistance; maintain on bed rest if in crisis.
6. Provide adequate oral intake.
   a. Medications for nausea and vomiting.
   b. Frequent oral hygiene.
   c. Small, frequent feedings.
   d. Rest before and after meals.
   e. If in crisis, client will be NPO and may have a nasogastric tube.
7. Eliminate environmental stressors and monitor for presence of stressors.
   a. Infection.
      (1) Isolate client from persons with active infection.
      (2) Monitor and record temperature, change in WBC count, respiratory status (breath sounds, productive cough, dyspnea), urinary system (complaints of frequency or dysuria).
      (3) Use aseptic technique with all procedures.
   b. Emotional stressors.
      (1) Make plans with client and avoid changing the schedule.
      (2) Monitor the response of the client to visitors and help the family to assist in decreasing the client's stress.
      (3) Discuss with the client his or her ability to resume preillness activities.
8. Instruct client and family regarding diagnostic tests.
   a. Need for and frequency of blood and urine tests.
   b. Purpose and procedure for ACTH stimulation test.
9. Instruct client and family regarding the disease.
   a. Anatomy and physiology of the adrenal gland.
   b. Pathophysiology.
10. Instruct client and family regarding hormonal replacement.
    a. Primary adrenocortical insufficiency.
       (1) Glucocorticoids.
       (2) Mineralocorticoids.
       (3) Sometimes adrenal androgens.
    b. Secondary adrenal insufficiency.
       (1) Glucocorticoids.
       (2) Mineralocorticoids usually not required.
    c. Necessity of taking medications for remainder of his or her life.
    d. Times when additional therapy is necessary.
11. Instruct client and family regarding self-care needs.
    a. Hormonal therapy as stated above.
    b. As the client must never miss medica-

tions, he or she should wear a medic-alert bracelet or necklace.

c. Client must realize that he or she cannot tolerate irregular schedules. Client should develop a plan of activities that incorporates work, activities of daily living, hobbies, social activities, and rest.
d. Client should be able to identify stressors in his or her life and discuss ways to deal with them.
e. Client must know signs and symptoms of adrenal insufficiency that would signify inadequate therapy. (See Description in this section.)
f. Client must know signs and symptoms of Cushing's disease that would signify excess therapy (See *Adrenocortical Hyperfunction: Hypercortsolism* in this chapter.)
g. Client should be able to describe discharge diet.
h. Client should be able to describe follow-up planned.

EVALUATION

Outcome Criteria

1. Fluids and electrolytes are returning to normal.
2. Weakness and fatigue is decreasing.
3. Weight loss has stopped and client is gaining weight as appropriate.
4. Client states he or she is not experiencing any unnecessary stressors and appears relaxed, as evidenced by relaxed facial expression, comfortable interactions with staff and visitors, and lack of signs of restlessness.
5. Client is not experiencing any worsening in homeostasis.
6. Client and family can accurately explain diagnostic tests.
7. Client and family can accurately explain the disease process.
8. Client and family can accurately explain the hormonal replacement therapy planned.
9. Client and family can accurately explain self-care requirements.

Complications

1. Addisonian crisis. See Expected Outcomes, Interventions, and Evaluation in this section.
2. Vascular volume insufficiency. This occurs as part of addisonian crisis. See *Shock* in Chapter 48.

Reevaluation and Follow-up

If client develops complications, institute goals and interventions as appropriate. Then focus on long-term needs when client's condition stabilizes. Client will return to clinic for follow-up care. At this time client should be checked for signs and symptoms of insufficiency and excess. Client's compliance with discharge teaching should be assessed. Client should be referred to a visiting nurses service for assistance in making necessary adjustments in lifestyle.

HYPERGONADOTROPIC HYPOGONADAL SYNDROMES

DESCRIPTION

The secretion of testosterone, estrogen, and progesterone by the testes and ovaries is necessary for normal sexual development and reproduction. Synthesis of these hormones by the gonads is regulated by the anterior pituitary gonadotropins (LH and FSH). The hypothalamus in turn controls the secretion of pituitary gonadotropins.

Several disorders affecting normal sexual development and reproduction can occur. The most common disorders of abnormal sexual development and function fall into the category of hypergonadotrophic hypogonadal syndromes. These syndromes are characterized by decreased testosterone or estrogen and progesterone. With the decreased levels of gonadal secretions, there is no negative feedback to the pituitary and thus the levels of gonadotropins increase (hypergonadotropic).

Klinefelter's syndrome represents the most common example of male hypergonadism (elevated LH, FSH, and decreased testosterone). The primary etiological factor is an extra X chromosome (47,XXY). The presence of an extra X chromosome in testicular tissue is the factor responsible for failure of the seminiferous tubule (site of spermatogenesis) and the Leydig cell (site of testosterone production). Variant forms of Klinefelter's syndrome occur infrequently. The clinical features of these variant forms are determined by the number of X chromosomes.

Turner's syndrome (ovarian dysgenesis) represents the most common clinical entity of female hypergonadotropic hypogonadism (elevated LH and FSH and decreased estrogen and progesterone). The majority of these clients have a 45,XO sex chromosome constitution. Some isolated cases of male Turner's syndrome have been identified. These disorders usually demonstrate themselves in infancy, childhood, or adolescence.

PREVENTION

Health Promotion

There is no known way to prevent these problems. Early detection and treatment is the primary key to preventing the problems described.

Population at Risk

There is no known population at risk.

Screening

No tools are available for mass screening.

ASSESSMENT

Health History

1. Klinefelter's syndrome: puberty.
   a. History of absence of sexual development.
   b. Decreased libido.
   c. Slowed mental development.
2. Turner's syndrome: puberty.
   a. History of absence of sexual development.
   b. History of amenorrhea.

Physical Assessment

1. Klinefelter's syndrome: puberty.
   a. Lack of secondary sexual characteristics.
   b. Small, firm testes.
   c. Gynecomastia: breast enlargement.
   d. Excessive long bone growth in the extremities.
   e. Possible subnormal intelligence.
   f. Possible emotional problems.
2. Turner's syndrome: puberty.
   a. Short, webbed neck.
   b. Shieldlike chest.
   c. Low-set or deformed ears.
   d. Puffiness over dorsum of the fingers.
   e. Cubitus valgus (deviation of extended forearm).
   f. Sparse pubic hair.
   g. Widely separated nipples.
   h. Short stature.

Diagnostic Tests

1. Klinefelter's syndrome.
   a. Serum FSH and LH.
   b. Serum testosterone.
   c. Buccal smear (Barr body present). Barr bodies appear whenever a double X chromosome is present. This would tell the health team that this client has an extra X chromosome.
   d. Occasionally, testicular biopsy.
   e. Sperm count.
2. Turner's syndrome: puberty.
   a. Serum FSH, LH, and prolactin.
   b. Serum estrogen and progesterone.
   c. Buccal smear (Barr body absent). This would tell the health team members that the client is missing an X chromosome.

NURSING DIAGNOSES: ACTUAL OR POTENTIAL

1. Decreased self-concept: related to inadequate sexual development.
2. Potential social isolation: related to embarrassment and feelings of inferiority.
3. Dependence: related to mental retardation (Klinefelter's syndrome) or immature appearance.

EXPECTED OUTCOMES

1. Client will show an improvement in self-concept, as evidenced by talking about self in positive terms, talking about the future, and making appropriate plans for the future.
2. Client will show an increase in social interactions, as evidenced by talking on the phone with family and friends, talking with staff and other clients, and making plans for future activities.
3. Client will become more independent, as evidenced by taking part in making decisions and being assertive in taking part in planning care.
4. Client and family will demonstrate accurate knowledge about diagnostic tests, the disease, and the treatment.

INTERVENTIONS

1. Assess client's and family's knowledge about disease and treatment.
   a. Develop appropriate teaching plan. Include information regarding:
      (1) Anatomy and physiology of the gonads.
      (2) Pathophysiology.
      (3) Hormonal replacement therapy.

(4) Expected outcomes. (Therapy will restore secondary sexual characteristics but not fertility.)
   b. Institute teaching as necessary.
2. Teach client and family about diagnostic tests.
   a. Purpose of the tests.
   b. Procedures.
3. Identify client's feeling about self.
   a. Spend time alone with the client.
   b. Talk matter-of-factly about sexuality.
   c. Do not force the client to talk but let him or her know you are available.
4. Identify family's feelings about the client.
   a. Spend time with family alone and in private.
   b. Encourage them to share their feelings.
   c. Correct misconceptions about the cause of the disease.
   d. Emphasize the positive effects of treatment.
5. Increase client's independence.
   a. Include client in planning activities.
   b. Allow client some independent decision making.
   c. Seek educational evaluation for the child with mental retardation in order that realistic plans for education can be made so that the client will be allowed to develop to his or her fullest.
6. Increase client's social interactions.
   a. Explore client's interests and help him or her identify ways to become involved in these activities.
   b. Help client minimize the effects of disease by dressing in ways that maximize positive attributes.
7. Refer for family counseling if necessary.
8. Institute discharge teaching (medications, follow-up).

EVALUATION

Outcome Criteria

1. Client shows improvement in self-concept.
2. Client has increased social contacts and is discussing activities he or she plans to become involved in.
3. Client shows increasing independence, as evidenced by making decisions about care and discussing plans for the future.
4. Client and family can accurately recall the information given about diagnostic tests, the disease, the treatment, and self-care management.

Complications

None.

Reevaluation and Follow-up

Client will be followed in clinic after discharge. On return visits, the client should be evaluated for the effectiveness of therapy and for adjustment to the disease.

METABOLIC DISORDERS

HYPERPARATHYROIDISM

DESCRIPTION

Hyperparathyroidism is characterized by excess synthesis and secretion of parathyroid hormone (PTH) and results in hypercalcemia and possibly some degree of bony demineralization over time. (See Figure 28-12 for review of parathyroid hormone functions.)

PTH is responsible for regulating calcium and phosphate metabolism. PTH exerts its effect on three primary sites—bone, kidney, and gastrointestinal tract—stimulating resorption of calcium and phosphate from bone; calcium reabsorption, phosphate excretion, and vitamin D metabolism by the kidneys; and directly and indirectly, absorption of calcium and phosphate from the gastrointestinal tract (presence of vitamin D in the gastrointestinal tract primarily responsible for calcium absorption). PTH activity is regulated by serum calcium levels. A fall in serum calcium stimulates PTH secretion and a rise suppresses PTH secretion (negative feedback mechanism). The effects of PTH are opposed by calcitonin, a hormone produced by the thyroid gland, which acts to lower serum calcium levels.

Hyperparathyroidism can be primary or secondary. *Primary hyperparathyroidism* is the result of a defect in the normal feedback control of PTH secretion. The exact cause is unknown; however, the most common findings are an autonomously functioning adenoma of the parathyroid gland or hyperplasia of the gland. *Secondary*

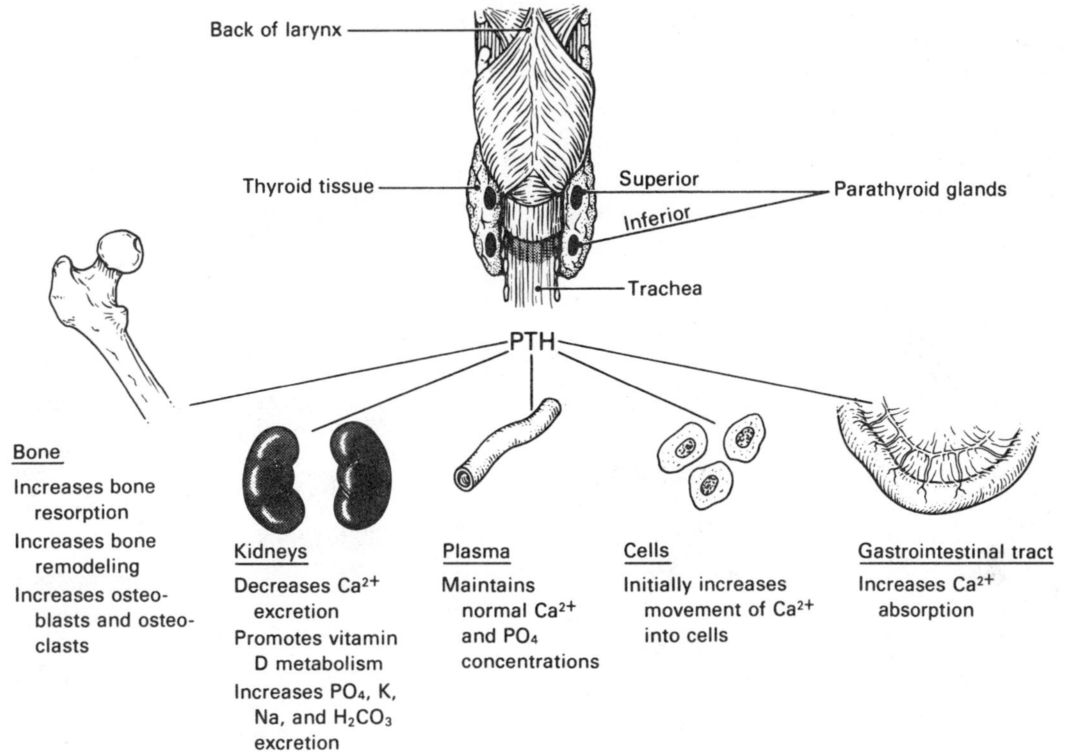

Figure 28-12 Major actions of parathyroid hormone (PTH).

hyperparathyroidism is characterized by a disruption of mineral homeostasis, producing a compensatory increase in PTH secretion such as occurs due to the hypocalcemia of chronic renal failure, rickets, VDRR (vitamin D–resistant rickets), or malnutrition.

The possibility of a multiple endocrine neoplasia syndrome (MEA) should be considered when hyperparathyroidism is present. Two types of MEA exist. *MEA type I* includes (1) pituitary tumors that hypersecrete growth hormone, prolactin, or both, (2) primary hyperparathyroidism, and (3) islet cell tumors of the pancreas, which often secrete gastrin or insulin. *MEA type II* includes (1) medullary carcinoma of the thyroid with hypersecretion of calcitonin, (2) primary hyperparathyroidism, and (3) pheochromocytoma.

The usual treatment of primary hyperparathyroidism includes surgical removal of the hypertrophied or tumor-containing gland following the resolution of hypercalcemia. The treatment of renal osteodystrophy (secondary hyperparathyroidism) includes phosphate-binding in the gut by ingestion of aluminum hydroxide, which corrects hyperphosphatemia and thus decreases PTH secretion.

PREVENTION

Health Promotion

Early detection and treatment.

Population at Risk

1. Persons with chronic renal failure (renal osteodystrophy).
2. Persons subject to genetic transmission of multiple endocrine neoplasia.
3. Persons with vitamin D–resistant rickets.

Screening

Hypercalcemia in concert with hypophosphatemia.

ASSESSMENT

Health History

1. History of anorexia, nausea, constipation, weight loss, urinary tract infection.

2. Family history of multiple endocrine neoplasia.
3. Client may be asymptomatic.

Physical Assessment

1. Dehydration related to solute (calcium) diuresis.
2. Muscular weakness, decreased muscle tone.
3. Lethargy.
4. Cardiac irregularities.
5. Altered mental status: confusion, delusions, stupor, or coma (if hypercalcemia is severe).

Diagnostic Tests

1. Determination of serum calcium, phosphate, chloride, PTH.
2. Chloride-to-phosphate ratio greater than 30.
3. Elevated PTH level.

NURSING DIAGNOSES: ACTUAL OR POTENTIAL

1. Dehydration: realted to solute diuresis.
2. Bone pain: related to bony demineralization/compression fracture.
3. Malnutrition: related to anorexia, nausea, vomiting.
4. Constipation: related to hypercalcemia and dehydration.
5. Injury: related to weakness and fatigue.
6. Changes in mental status: related to hypercalcemia.
7. Skin breakdown contractures: related to immobility (especially if comatose).
8. Anxiety: related to lack of knowledge about disease process and treatment regimen.

EXPECTED OUTCOMES

1. Client will remain adequately hydrated during hospitalization, as evidenced by glistening mucous membranes and thin, watery secretions in oral cavity.
2. Urinary output will be greater than 1,000 mL/24 h.
3. There will be no weight loss greater than 1 lb/24 h.
4. Bone pain will be relieved within 30 min of treatment, as evidenced by client's statement to that effect.
5. Nutritional status will be within normal limits by discharge, as evidenced by no unplanned weight loss compared with admission weight or weight gain if client was underweight.
6. Client will have at least one soft-formed stool every other day during hospitalization.
7. By discharge, the client will not exhibit contractures of extremities or areas of skin breakdown as a result of immobility.
8. Client will exhibit no evidence of injury at discharge.
9. Changes in mental status will be assessed and treatment instituted before frank coma occurs.
10. Client wil exhibit little or no anxiety regarding disease process and its treatment by discharge, as evidenced by client's statement to that effect.

INTERVENTIONS

1. Assess hydration status q 8h by checking mucous membranes of mouth and intake and output.
2. Check daily weight before breakfast and stool, after voiding.
3. Administer pain medication as ordered and assess effectiveness 30 min after administration.
4. Reposition client q2h if client cannot accomplish this alone.
5. Administer antinausea medication as ordered/needed and assess effectiveness 30 min after administration.
6. Offer small, attractive meals six times daily.
7. Assess client's food likes and dislikes and routine intake regimen, including religious and philosophical restrictions. Adhere to these as much as possible.
8. Increase mobility as much as possible to increase hunger, to prevent contractures and pressure areas as well as to retard bony demineralization (e.g., sit client up in chair, ambulate).
9. Assess frequency and consistency of stools and record.
10. Administer laxative or stool softener as desired by client and ordered by physician to ensure one soft-formed stool every other day.
11. Have client perform range-of-motion exercises q8h (if immobilized).
12. Massage bony prominances q8h (if immobilized).

13. Prevent client injury.
    a. Have bed rails up when client is in bed.
    b. Assist client in and out of bed when appropriate.
    c. Assist with ambulation when appropriate.
    d. Have client wear slippers or shoes when out of bed.
    e. Reorient client as necessary.
14. Assess mental status at least q8h; notify physician when deterioration is assessed.
15. Assess knowledge level of client regarding disease process and treatment regimen.
16. Formulate teaching plan appropriate for client, including pathophysiology of disease process, treatment plan, tests, and expected outcomes.
17. Answer all questions and evaluate client's understanding.

EVALUATION

Outcome Criteria

1. Client is adequately hydrated throughout hospitalization, as evidenced by:
    a. Glistening oral mucous membranes with thin, watery saliva.
    b. Urinary output of greater than 1,000 mL/24 h.
    c. Weight loss less than 1 lb/24 h.
2. Client states that pain is relieved no later than 30 min following treatment.
3. By discharge, the client's nutritional status is within normal limits, as evidenced by no unplanned weight loss when discharge weight is compared with admission weight.
4. Client is having at least one soft-formed stool every other day during hospitalization.
5. At discharge, the client shows no evidence of contractures of any extremity.
6. At discharge, the client shows no evidence of injury.
7. Client's mental status is not deteriorating to coma during hospitalization.
8. At discharge, the client states he or she is experiencing no anxiety in relation to lack of knowledge of disease process or treatment regimen.

Complications

COMA

The condition is secondary to hypercalcemia/dehydration.

Assessment

Deterioration of mental status; response to stimuli degenerates from A (alert), to V (voice), to P (pain), to U (unresponsive.)

Revised Outcomes

Client will not experience injury; aspiration of vomitus, fluid, saliva; or skin breakdown during coma.

Interventions

1. Position client on side.
2. Do not feed or administer fluids orally.
3. Keep side rails up.
4. Turn client q2h from side to side.
5. Massage bony prominences.
6. Support arms and legs with pillows or rolled blankets to prevent dependent edema.
7. Maintain oral hygiene each shift with half strength hydrogen peroxide; use padded tongue blade or cotton swab. Have suction machine available if choking occurs.

Reevaluation and Follow-up

1. Home visits by visiting nurse.
2. Clinic visits.

HYPOPARATHYROIDISM

DESCRIPTION

Hypoparathyroidism is a disorder characterized by decreased or absent synthesis and secretion of parathyroid hormone (PTH), most commonly as a result of removal of all four or a significant portion of the parathyroid glands. Surgical removal of the glands may be done as treatment of hyperparathyroidism or inadvertantly during thyroidectomy because of their usual location on the posterior thyroid. Other causes of hypoparathyroidism include idiopathic loss of parathyroid function or loss of functional tissue due to hemorrhage, infection, or thyroid gland irradiation.

Unless there is an acute loss of PTH, hypoparathyroidism may present with few signs and symptoms other than hypocalcemia. An acute loss of PTH, however, perhaps following inadvertant removal of the parathyroid glands during thyroidectomy, may present with laryngeal spasm, stridor, and labored respirations secondary to acute hypocalcemia. Tetany and positive Trousseau's and Chvostek's signs are also manifestations of the disorder.

Hypoparathyroidism is usually treated with large doses of vitamin D and calcium rather than PTH replacement.

PREVENTION

Health Promotion

1. Leaving parathyroid glands in place during thyroidectomy.
2. Early diagnosis and treatment of the disorder.

Population at Risk

1. Persons who have had a thyroidectomy.
2. Persons who have had a total parathyroidectomy.
3. Persons who have had a hemorrhage or infection in region of parathyroid glands.

Screening

Serum calcium and phosphate levels.

ASSESSMENT

Health History

1. Development of tetany during pregnancy.
2. Numbness and tingling of perioral area, hands and feet.
3. Painful muscle contractions, especially in the hands.
4. Complaints of weakness and lack of energy.

Physical Assessment

1. Positive Chvostek's and Trousseau's signs.
2. Hyperactive deep tendon reflexes.
3. Tetany.
4. Laryngeal stridor (if calcium level falls rapidly).

Diagnostic Tests

1. Low serum calcium and elevated serum phosphorus in presence of normal renal function.
2. PTH radioimmunoassay.

NURSING DIAGNOSES: ACTUAL OR POTENTIAL

1. Potential respiratory difficulty: related to laryngeal spasm.
2. Potential knowledge deficit: regarding disease process, treatment regimen.
3. Potential discomfort: related to muscle cramps in hands.

EXPECTED OUTCOMES

1. Respiratory distress will be assessed and treatment instituted before respiratory arrest occurs.
2. By discharge, the client will describe the pathophysiology of hypoparathyroidism essential for self-care, name each medication prescribed, its dosage and schedule, and expected effects as well as untoward side effects.
3. Discomfort will be relieved within 30 min following treatment, as evidenced by the client's statement to that effect.

INTERVENTIONS

1. Assess respiratory status q8h.
2. Consult with physician immediately if respiratory stridor and/or labored respirations are assessed.
3. Assess client's level of knowledge about disease process and treatment regimen.
4. Prepare teaching plan and timetable for teaching. Include essential pathology of the disease, treatment regimen, expected outcome.
5. Answer all questions, explain all tests.
6. Administer pain treatment as prescribed and when appropriately requested by client.
7. Assess effectiveness of pain treatment 30 min following its administration.

EVALUATION

Outcome Criteria

1. Respiratory arrest does not occur during hospitalization, as evidenced by no cessation of respirations.
2. At discharge, the client can describe the pathophysiology of hypoparathyroidism in her or his own words and can give the names of prescribed drugs, correct dosages, schedules, and expected effects as well as untoward side effects without error.
3. Discomfort related to muscle cramps in the client's hands is relieved within 30 min after institution of treatment, as evidenced by client's statement to that effect.

Complications

None.

Reevaluation and Follow-up

Regular clinic visits to assess effectiveness of treatment. (Hypercalcemia may occur secondary to vitamin D intoxication, and nephrolithiasis may result from excessive urinary calcium excretion secondary to lack of PTH.)

INFLAMMATIONS

THYROIDITIS

DESCRIPTION

Inflammatory reactions of the thyroid gland are termed *thyroidits*. Depending upon the stage of infection, hypothyroid or hyperthyroid states may occur, although the latter is uncommon. *Acute thyroiditis* is very rare. Subacute and chronic (Hashimoto's) thyroiditis are the most common inflammatory diseases of the thyroid gland.

Subacute (granulomatous or de Quervain's) thyroiditis is believed to be caused by a viral infection. It often follows an upper respiratory infection, mumps, or some other viral infection such as influenza or Coxsackie virus. The disease usually subsides within a few months, leaving no deficiency in thyroid function. However, repeated infections over many months can produce hypothyroidism.

Hashimoto's thyroiditis is thought to be caused by an autoimmune response which interferes with the normal biosynthesis of thyroid hormones, such as organic binding of thyroid iodide. There is often a family history of Hashimoto's disease, goiter, primary hypothyroidism, or Graves' disease. About 20 percent of the patients are hypothyroid when first examined. If seen during the early phase of the disease, symptoms of mild hyperthyroidism may be present. Clinical hypothyroidism commonly develops in patients who are euthyroid (normal thyroid function) when first seen. The progression to hypothyroidism develops over several years.

Riedel's thyroiditis is a rare disorder with no known cause. The thyroid gland is enlarged, with marked fibrosis. Clinical symptoms are related to compression of adjacent structures, namely, the trachea, esophagus, and recurrent laryngeal nerves. Hypothyroidism occurs occasionally.

PREVENTION

Health Promotion

Early diagnosis and treatment.

Population at Risk

1. Women between the ages of 30 to 50 years.
2. Most common cause of sporadic goiter in children.

Screening

None known.

ASSESSMENT

Health History

1. History of viral infection (subacute thyroiditis).
2. Family history of chronic thyroiditis, goiter, primary hypothyroidism, or Graves' disease.
3. Gradual or sudden pain in thyroid region that may radiate to ears (subacute thyroiditis).
4. Painless enlargement of thyroid gland (chronic thyroiditis).

Physical Assessment

1. Subacute: enlarged, tender thyroid gland.
2. Chronic: painless, firm, enlarged thyroid gland. May have manifestations of either hyperthyroidism or hypothyroidism. (See those sections in this chapter for details.)

Diagnostic Tests

1. Thyroid function tests; T_4 elevated in subacute, variable in chronic thyroiditis.
2. ^{131}I uptake very low in subacute thyroiditis, increased in early chronic thyroiditis.
3. Erythrocyte sedimentation rate elevated in subacute thyroiditis.

NURSING DIAGNOSES: ACTUAL OR POTENTIAL

1. Subacute: discomfort related to pain in anterior neck, ears.
2. Chronic: see *Hypothyroidism*.

EXPECTED OUTCOMES

1. Subacute: the client will experience pain relief within 30 min following treatment administration, as evidenced by the client's statement to that effect.
2. Chronic: see *Hypothyroidism*

INTERVENTIONS

1. Subacute: administration of aspirin or other analgesic prescribed/effective.
2. Assess treatment effectiveness 60 min following administration, if medication is used.

EVALUATION

Outcome Criteria

Client states pain relief is effective within 60 min of administration of treatment.

Complications

See sections on *Graves' Disease* and *Hypothyroidism* in this chapter.

Reevaluation and Follow-up
Clinic visits.

REFERENCES

Jubiz, W.: *Endocrinology; A Logical Approach for Clinicians*, McGraw-Hill, New York, 1979, p. 70.

BIBLIOGRAPHY

Bacchus, H.: *Metabolic and Endocrine Emergencies*, University Park Press, Baltimore, 1977. The author presents a comprehensive review detailing the recognition and management of endocrine emergencies.

Camuñas, C.: "Transsphenoidal Hypophysectomy," *Critical Care Update*,**8**(6):22–27, 1981. An easy-to-read article that briefly describes normal physiology of the pituitary, reasons for hypophysectomy, client assessment, and preoperative and postoperative care needs of client having a transsphenoidal hypophysectomy.

Chaney, P.: *Managing Diabetics Properly*, Intermed Communications, Horsham, Pa., 1977. The physiological and psychosocial aspects of the clinical management of diabetes are discussed in this publication.

Cooperman, D., and Malarkey, W.: "Pituitary Apoplexy," *Heart and Lung*, **7**:450–454, 1978. A comprehensive discussion of pituitary apoplexy. Nursing assessment and care are very well explained.

Cryer, P. E.: *Diagnostic Endocrinology*, Oxford University Press, New York, 1976. This book provides a basic understanding of endocrine diagnostic tests that can be utilized in planning client teaching.

Cuff, M. (consultant): "Controlling Diabetes Mellitus," *American Journal of Nursing*, **80**(10):1827–1850, 1980. A programmed instruction unit on adult-onset diabetes (insulin-independent diabetes).

Fredholm, N. Z.: "The Insulin Pump: New Method of Insulin Delivery," *American Journal of Nursing*, **81**(11):2024–2026, 1981. An overview of the purpose, use, advantages, and disadvantages of the insulin pump by persons who have insulin-dependent diabetes mellitus.

Gotch, P.M.: "Incorporating Activity Into Diabetic Self-Care," *Occupational Health Nursing*, February 1982, pp. 16–19. An overview of physical exercise as it relates to the person with diabetes. Includes descriptions of the activities that some diabetics should not participate in, as well as categories of exercise and caloric expenditure.

Gotch, P. M.: "Teaching Patients About Adrenal Corticosteroids," *American Journal of Nursing*, **81**(1):78–82, 1981. A well-written article that stresses important points clients on chronic steroid therapy must be taught.

Hallal, J.: "Thyroid Disorders," *American Journal of Nursing*, **77**:418–432, 1977. A programmed unit that gives a comprehensive review of all thyroid disorders.

Hamburger, S. (ed.): "Endocrine Metabolic Crises," *Critical Care Quarterly*, **3**(2):1–143, 1980. This is a multiauthored journal with 14 articles. Each article gives a current, up-to-date discussion of the etiology, pathophysiology, and management of a selected endocrine emergency. Nursing care is not detailed but can be extrapolated from the content.

Hite, A. M.: "Clinical Estimation of the Renal Threshold for Glucose in Persons with Diabetes Mellitus," *Nursing Research*, **31**(3):153–158, 1982. Report of a study of the relation between the renal threshold for glucose in diabetics and age, sex, type, and duration of diabetes. Results of the study suggest that urine glucose test results should not be used as a basis for insulin adjustment because they frequently do not correlate with blood glucose levels.

Honigman, R. E.: "Thyroid Function Tests," *Nursing 82*, **12**(4):68–71, 1982. Description of thyroid function tests, their purposes, client preparation, procedures, implications of results, and interfering factors.

Isselbacher, K., Adams, R., Braunwald, E., Petersdorf, R., and Wilson, J.: *Harrison's Principles of Internal Medicine*, 9th ed., McGraw-Hill, New York, 1980. This book gives a clear review of endocrine disorders, manifestations, treatment, and complications.

Jubiz, W.: *Endocrinology: A Logical Approach for Clinicians*, McGraw-Hill, New York, 1979. This book provides a good overview of the physiology and pathology of the endocrine system as well as medical management of these disorders.

Krueger, J. A., and Ray, J. C.: *Endocrine Problems in Nursing*, Mosby, St. Louis, 1976. This book provides a comprehensive summary of the nursing problems frequently encountered in the care of clients with endocrine disorders.

McConnell, E.: "Meeting the Special Needs of Diabetics Facing Surgery," *Nursing*, **766**:30–37, June 1976. A general review of the physiological and psychosocial needs of diabetic clients that is useful for understanding the body's reaction to stress and associated insulin needs is provided in this article. The reader is encouraged to utilize supplemental source(s) for drug management.

Plasse, N. J.: "Monitoring Blood Glucose at Home: A Comparison of Three Products," *American Journal of Nursing*, **81**(11):2028–2029, 1981. Report of a study in which a group of nurses and a group of clients with diabetes each utilized three different products to determine blood glucose levels. Each product used by both the nurses and the clients is discussed in relation to ease of use and accuracy of glucose measurement.

Solomon, B. L.: "Symposium on Endocrine Disorders," *Nursing Clinics of North America*, **15**(3):433–534, 1980. This is a multiauthored journal with eight articles on selected endocrine topics. The articles provide up-to-date information on the physiological alterations of the selected endocrine topic. Clinical nursing implications are presented.

Stevens, A. D.: "Monitoring Blood Glucose at Home: Who Should Do It," *American Journal of Nursing*, **81**(11):2026–2027, 1981. This article discusses the categories of diabetics who can benefit most from home blood glucose monitoring.

Tucker, S.: *Patient Care Standards*, Mosby, St. Louis, 1975. The author presents a comprehensive review of nursing implications.

Williams, R.: *Textbook of Endocrinology*, Saunders, Philadelphia, 1974. This is an in-depth reference for understanding the physiological and psychosocial manifestations of endocrine disorders.

Winters, B.: "Promoting Wound Healing In The Diabetic Patient," *AORN Journal*, **35**(6):1083–1087, 1982. An overview of the complications of diabetes mellitus, especially as they relate to the client undergoing surgery. Gives rationale for why these complications may arise as well as goals of nursing management preoperatively, intraoperatively, and postoperatively.

29

The Hematologic System

Mary Bigelow Huntoon

Blood is a substance composed of many cells: erythrocytes, leukocytes, and so on (refer to Figure 29-1). It circulates continuously throughout the body, transporting oxygen and nutrients, removing carbon dioxide and body wastes, protecting the body from infection, transporting hormones, and helping to regulate body temperature. When a disruption in blood formation or blood composition occurs, the result can be a multiplicity of physical and emotional changes. Gastrointestinal problems, decreased resistance to infection, enlargement of body structures (e.g., the liver and spleen), and bone pain are but a few of the changes observed.

This chapter discusses alterations that occur as a result of disruptions in blood formation, disturbances in blood coagulation, destruction of blood cells, and abnormalities of blood cell growth.

ABNORMAL CELLULAR GROWTH

LEUKEMIA

DESCRIPTION

Leukemia is a neoplastic disease that involves the blood-forming tissues in the lymph nodes, spleen, and bone marrow. Several types of leukemia are recognized, but all are characterized by abnormal and uncontrolled growth of immature leukocytes present in the tissue producing that cell and in the blood. The most common white cells involved are the granulocytes, lymphocytes, and monocytes.

Leukemia is also classified by the course and duration of the disease. *Acute leukemia* (more common in children and young adults) is more serious than chronic leukemia, has a rapid onset, and progresses quickly into the blood-forming organs with immature leukocytes. *Chronic leukemia* (more common in older adults) has a gradual onset and a slower course, as the leukocytes in an adult are more mature and better able to defend the body against infection (refer to Table 29-1). The incidence of leukemia is on the increase, with a 50 percent rise in mortality noted over the last quarter of a century.

The exact cause of leukemia is unknown. Several factors are associated with the disease and may contribute to its development. Viruses have caused leukemia in laboratory animals, and thus it is possible they may also cause leukemia in human beings. Increased exposure to radiation (above "safe" levels) is also linked with development of leukemia. Studies have shown that absorption of certain chemicals and also genetic disorders may be influential in the development of this problem.

The course of development in leukemia is (1) proliferation of abnormal immature leukocytes that arise from the bone marrow; (2) infiltration of the cells into the blood-forming tissue (e.g., lymph nodes), and (3) the eventual infiltration into all the body tissues. Death may result due to primary and secondary causes.

Of all leukemias, both acute and chronic, 90

TABLE 29-1 CLASSIFICATION OF COMMON TYPES OF ACUTE AND CHRONIC LEUKEMIA

Major Category	Subcategory	Synonyms	Characteristic Cells and Clinical Manifestations
		Acute	
Myelogenous	Granulocytic	Myelocytic, AML, AGL (includes congenital leukemia)	Myeloblasts Most common in adults and infants Response to therapy 50%; median prognosis 10–12 months
	Myelomonocytic	Naegli, AMML	Myeloblasts with some monocytic characteristics Prognosis 1–2 years
	Erythroleukemia	DiGuglielmo, EL	Proerythroblasts
	Promyelocytic	Progranulocytic, AProL	Promyelocytes Usually in adults Risk of disseminated intravascular coagulation (DIC)
	Oligoblastic	Smoldering, preleukemia	Slow progression Poor response to therapy
Monocytic	Monocytic, acute	Monoblastic, Schilling, AMonoL	Immature monocytes Usually in children or young adults Response to drugs; prognosis 6 weeks to 3 months Risk of DIC Inflamed gums common sign
Lymphocytic	Lymphocytic, acute	Lymphocytic, ALL	Immature lymphoblast Common in 95% of children; rare in adults Response to therapy; median prognosis 2.5 years Lymphadenopathy
	Undifferentiated	Stem cell, acute, AUL	Stem cell Prognosis very poor
		Chronic	
Myelogenous	Granulocytic	Myelocytic, CML, CGL	Abnormal proliferation of granulocytes Most common in adolescents and young adults Splenomegaly Presence of Philadelphia chromosome in 90% Median prognosis 3 years
Monocytic	Monocytic, chronic		Immature monocytes
Lymphocytic	Lymphocytic, chronic	CLL	Abnormal proliferation of mature lymphoblasts Most common in older adults Enlarged lymph nodes and spleen Median prognosis 5 years

SOURCE: Adapted from Williams, W. J., et al.: *Hematology*, 2d ed., McGraw-Hill, New York, 1977, pp. 810, 820.

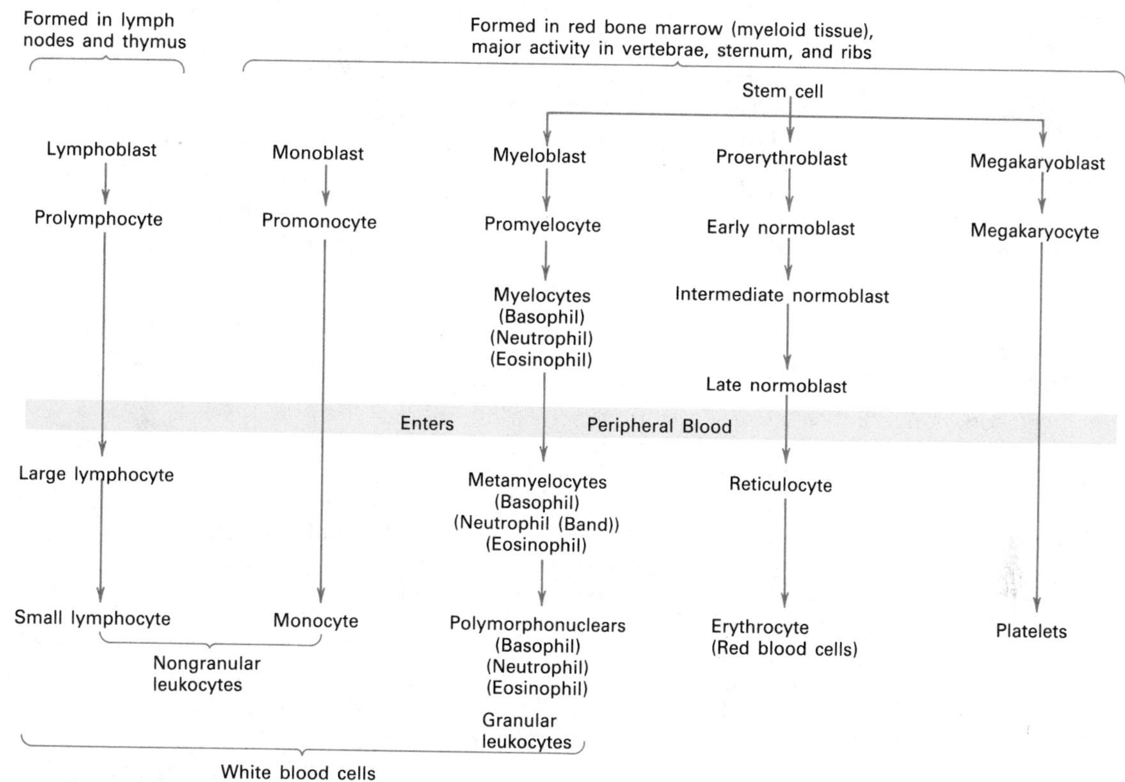

Figure 29-1 Development of the various formed blood elements in the adult. It is now known that all blood cells originate from a single precursor. Among the earliest cells in the differentiation process are the lymphoid stem cells and the progenitor stem cells of the myeloid line. These two precursor cells eventually result in the B and T lymphocytes and in the array of erythrocytes, granulocytes, and thrombocytes. (Tilkian, S. M., Conover, M. B., and Tilkian, A. G.: *Clinical Implications of Laboratory Tests*, 3d ed., Mosby, St. Louis, 1983, p. 28.)

percent are lymphocytic (characterized by hyperplasia of the lymphoid tissues), whereas only 10 percent are monocytic and myelocytic (characterized by hyperplasia of the spleen and bone marrow). Acute granulocytic, chronic granulocytic, and chronic lymphocytic leukemia will be discussed here. (Refer to Chapter 18 for a discussion of acute lymphocytic leukemia.)

ACUTE GRANULOCYTIC LEUKEMIA

A subcategory of *acute myelogenous leukemia*, acute granulocytic leukemia (AGL) is a malignant disease of the *myeloid* stem cells of the bone marrow. Its course is infiltration of bone marrow and organs with myeloblasts, an immature granulocytic precursor. AGL represents over 80 percent of acute leukemias in adulthood and increases in incidence from middle age onward. It is more common in males than in females, but there seems to be no difference in frequency among races.

CHRONIC GRANULOCYTIC LEUKEMIA

The first type of leukemia to be discovered, chronic granulocytic leukemia (CGL) is characterized by abnormal, immature granulocytes (myeloblasts). The disease usually presents itself in the *chronic phase*, in which the myeloid ratio is increased and other organs, besides the bone marrow, are involved in production of granulocytes. After a period of 2 to 3 years, the *blastic phase* occurs, with a rise in the number of myeloblasts. The Philadelphia chromosome

(Ph[1]), discovered in 1960 by Lowell and Hungerford of Philadelphia, is present in 90 percent of the clients and is believed an acquired (inherited) chromosomal defect (Johnson and Hubbard, 1978). Onset of CGL is most common from the age of 25 through 40, and the disease is seen more often in men than in women. Of all cases of leukemia, 20 percent are accounted for by CGL.

CHRONIC LYMPHOCYTIC LEUKEMIA

The most common type of leukemia, chronic lymphocytic leukemia (CLL) affects older adults (it is unusual in persons younger than 30), and the frequency increases with age. It is, again, more common in males. CLL has few symptoms and develops slowly. It is usually the easiest leukemia to diagnose and treat. It is characterized by proliferative and abnormal lymphoid tissues, and it mainly affects the B lymphocytes, thus impairing immunocompetence. Inherited or acquired immunological defects may be significant in this disease.

PREVENTION

Health Promotion

1. Avoidance of exposure to toxic chemicals (e.g., benzol, phenylbutazone) or radiation.
2. Maintenance of good health habits (e.g., rest, nutrition, exercise).

Population at Risk

1. Males and middle-aged adults have a higher incidence of the disease.
2. Persons with exposure to chemicals or radiation or those taking cytotoxic drugs.
3. Persons with frequent viral illnesses.
4. Persons with a familial history of leukemia or those in whom the Philadelphia chromosome is present.
5. Persons who have some genetic syndromes with inherent chromosomal defects (e.g., Down's syndrome) are not at increased risk.

Screening

1. Blood studies to identify abnormal and immature leukocytes or to identify an elevated cell count.
2. Testing to determine the presence of the Philadelphia chromosome.

ASSESSMENT: ACUTE GRANULOCYTIC LEUKEMIA (AGL)

Health History

1. Client complains of fatigue or malaise, usually of several months' duration. Exercise intolerance may be noted, along with dizziness or lightheadedness.
2. Fever may be present with or without a documented infection.
3. Client may also complain of easy bruising, nosebleeds, bleeding gums, or petechiae; menstrual periods may increase in length and in volume.
4. Chronic infections of the skin and respiratory tract are often noted.
5. Client may complain of satiety after meals and of abdominal fullness, due to splenomegaly (Johnson and Hubbard, 1978).
6. Documentation regarding previous treatment of any similar symptoms or a family history of leukemia is necessary, along with any known exposure to chemicals or radiation.
7. Transformation of a chronic myelocytic leukemia into acute leukemia is possible. The change is accompanied by weight loss and progressive anemia.

Physical Assessment

1. A complete assessment of all systems and a full evaluation of general health are necessary for all clients (refer to Table 29-2).
2. Marked pallor of the skin and mucous membranes is usually noted, due to anemia, with petechial hemorrhages and various-sized ecchymoses present. Careful documentation of bruised sites should be noted and evaluated.
3. Malaise and diaphoresis may be present.
4. Tachycardia and cardiac murmurs may be heard.
5. Splenomegaly, hepatomegaly, and lymphadenopathy may be present.
6. Sternal tenderness is often demonstrated in these clients. When firm pressure is applied from the top to the bottom of the sternum, a small area, most commonly in the midportion, is found to be quite tender under pressure. The client will complain of pain at the pressure point but will have been previously unaware of its existence.

Diagnostic Tests

1. Blood studies are done to identify cell changes. The findings reveal:

TABLE 29-2 GENERAL PHYSICAL ASSESSMENT APPLICABLE TO HEMATOLOGIC DISORDERS

1. General appearance.
   a. Lassitude can be noted.
   b. The client may appear thin and pale.
2. Vital signs.
   Fever may be noted in clients with infectious mononucleosis, leukemia, or multiple myeloma.
3. Skin.
   a. Paleness and brittleness of the skin and spoon-shaped nails (koilonychia) are noted in iron deficiency anemia.
   b. Jaundice may be seen in clients with hemolytic anemia; pale yellow skin is often found in vitamin B_{12} deficiency.
   c. Petechiae are commonly seen in aplastic anemia, idiopathic thrombocytopenic purpura, and disseminated intravascular coagulation.
   d. Ecchymoses are seen in leukemia, hypoprothrombinemia, vascular purpura (especially on the extremities, face, groin), and hemophilia.
   e. Plethora (dusky red, ruddy skin color) is present in polycythemia vera.
   f. Skin is easily bruised.
4. Eyes, ears, head, neck, and throat.
   a. Pale conjunctiva are noted in iron deficiency anemia.
   b. Glossitis and hypertrophy of the tongue are seen in vitamin B_{12} and folate deficiency.
   c. Jaundiced sclerae are found in hemolytic anemia.
   d. Mouth, throat, and gum bleeding and ulceration are found, along with frequent sore throat, dysphagia.
   e. Nosebleeds and bleeding gums are common in clients with leukemia.
   f. Blurred vision may accompany the disease of multiple myeloma.
   g. Sore throat is associated with agranulocytosis and infectious mononucleosis.
   h. Tinnitis may interfere with hearing potential.
5. Thorax, heart, breasts, and axillae.
   a. Enlargement of the lymph nodes is seen in leukemia and infectious mononucleosis (especially cervical, axillary, and inguinal).
   b. Tachycardia and palpitations can be present in iron deficiency anemia.
6. Abdomen, rectum.
   a. Hepatomegaly and splenomegaly are common in clients with leukemia and idiopathic thrombocytopenic purpura.
   b. Splenomegaly is also found in polycythemia vera and in vitamin B_{12} deficiency.
   c. Constipation/diarrhea, rectal bleeding, tarry stools, and abdominal fullness are noted.
7. Musculoskeletal system.
   a. Sternal tenderness is often demonstrated in clients with leukemia.
   b. Deformities or asymmetry in the skeleton, a decrease in height, and pain over lesions or pathological fractures are seen in clients with multiple myeloma.
   c. Swollen joints and phlebitis are found in polycythemia vera, along with joint stiffness, gout, and backache.
   d. Peripheral vascular intermittent claudication, thrombophlebitis are noted.
8. Genitoreproductive system.
   Changes in menstrual flow, menorrhagia, postmenopausal or abnormal bleeding are common.
9. Neurological system.
   a. Numbness, tingling, paresthesias are common.
   b. Mood changes and confusion may be noted.

a. A marked increase in the immature leukocytes in the peripheral blood, associated with anemia and thrombocytopenia.
b. An elevated white blood count, with abnormal and immature cells.
c. In approximately one-half of the clients, serum uric acid levels are elevated.

2. Bone marrow biopsy may be done to confirm the diagnosis by examining the cells and platelets for number, size, and shape. It is unnecessary if numerous blasts are found in the blood.
   a. The biopsy is usually done using the sternum as the site, although the iliac crest may be used (refer to Figure 29-2).
   b. For a sternal puncture, the client is placed on his or her back with a pillow under the thoracic spine. For an iliac crest puncture, the client is placed in a side-lying position.
   c. The site is prepared and anesthetized.
   d. A sternal needle is inserted, and a small amount of marrow is aspirated.
   e. Following the removal of the needle, the puncture site is covered with a sterile dressing. Bleeding may occur. Pressure is applied to the site. Ice packs will help control the bleeding.
   f. A slight soreness may be present for several days.

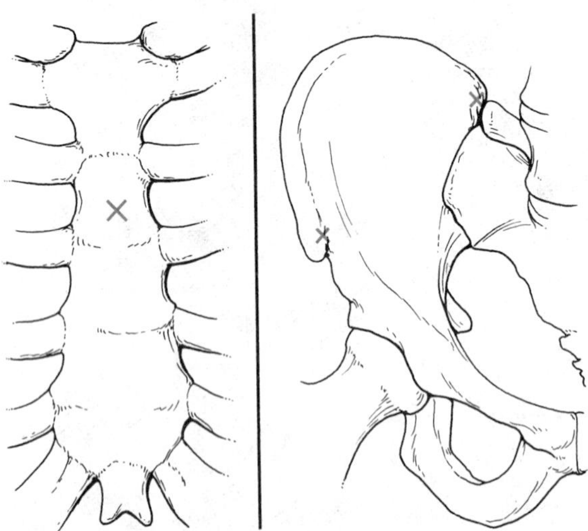

Figure 29-2 The two most commonly used sites for bone marrow aspirations are the sternum, at left, and the anterior or posterior iliac crests, at right. (Adapted from Schwartz, S. O., Hartz, W. H., Jr.,and Robbins, J. H.: *Hematology in Practice*, McGraw-Hill, New York, 1961.)

ASSESSMENT: CHRONIC GRANULOCYTIC LEUKEMIA (CGL)

Health History

1. Complaints of the client are similar to those of clients with acute granulocytic leukemia.
2. The onset is usually gradual and insidious.
3. Complaints of aching and pain in the long bones and discomfort in the upper left abdomen are common.
4. Headaches and confusion or other central nervous system symptoms may be present.

Physical Assessment

(Refer to Table 29-2.)

1. Findings coincide with acute granulocytic leukemia.
2. Sternal tenderness is usually present.
3. Splenomegaly is present; hepatomegaly may be present, but the lymph nodes are usually not palpable.

Diagnostic Tests

1. Blood studies reveal:
   a. A high leukocyte count (100,000–300,000 cells per cubic millimeter, with granulocytes in all stages of development. (In the *chronic phase*, most of the leukocytes are mature; in *blastic crisis*, immature myeloblasts are present.)
   b. Mild anemia.
   c. An elevated platelet count, as opposed to the low count found in acute granulocytic leukemia.
   d. A genetic defect, the Philadelphia chromosome, present in the white cells of 90 percent of all clients.
   e. A decreased leukocyte alkaline phosphatase determination.
   f. An elevated uric acid and serum vitamin B_{12}.
2. X-ray films may reveal osseous lesions in the skeleton.

ASSESSMENT: CHRONIC LYMPHOCYTIC LEUKEMIA (CLL)

Health History

1. Complaints similar to those of clients with AGL and CGL as previously discussed are found.

2. Fatigue and chronic infection are the most outstanding complaints.
3. Documentation of a family history of leukemia is necessary.

Physical Assessment

(Refer to Table 29-2.)

1. Enlargement of superficial lymph nodes is noted. The cervical nodes are most often involved; however, the axillary and mesenteric nodes may also be involved (refer to Figure 29-3).
2. Splenomegaly is usually present.
3. Skin lesions may be apparent. These lesions, the result of actual infiltration of the skin by leukemic cells, are generalized, discrete, and bright red or purple in color. The client may relate a long-standing history of these lesions.

Diagnostic Tests

1. Blood studies reveal:
   a. Elevated, lymphocyte count, abnormal and immature cells (refer to Figure 29-4).
   b. Mild anemia.
   c. Decreased immunoglobulin levels.
   d. Normal uric acid levels.
2. Bone marrow biopsy is of little value in diagnosis.
3. Chest x-ray films can be done to check lymph node involvement.

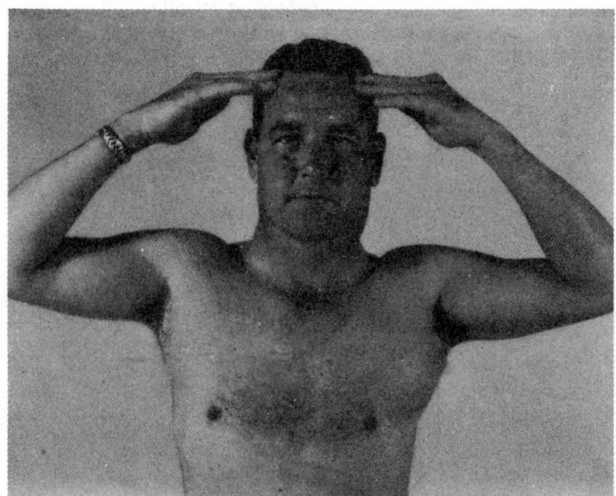

Figure 29-3 Axillary and cervical lymph node enlargements in a client with chronic lymphocytic leukemia (CLL). (Williams, W. J., et al.: *Hematology* 2d ed., McGraw-Hill, New York, 1977, plate 8-1.)

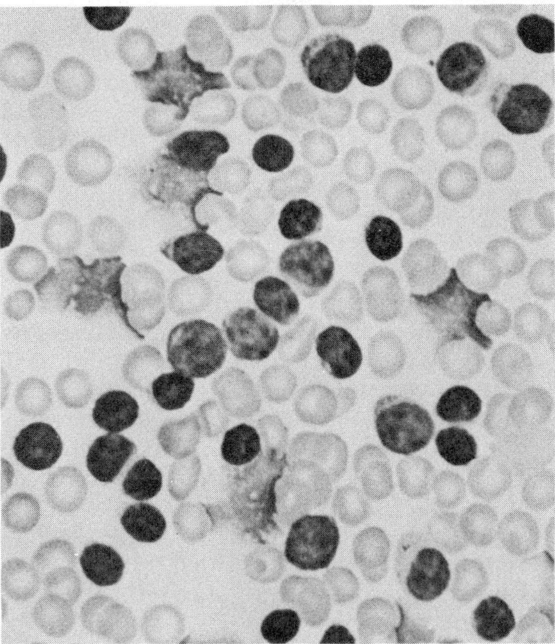

Figure 29-4 Peripheral blood in chronic lymphocytic leukemia. All cells are lymphocytes, showing immaturity. (Hayhoe, F. G. R., and Flemans, R. J.: *Color Atlas of Hematological Cytology*, 2d ed., Wiley, New York, 1982.)

NURSING DIAGNOSES: ACTUAL OR POTENTIAL

1. Increased potential for skin breakdown: due to increased vulnerability to hemorrhage secondary to thrombocytopenia.
2. Increased potential for infection: due to the leukocytes, which are present in large numbers but are immature or abnormal and are unable to fight microorganisms.
3. Alterations in comfort (pain and discomfort): due to fatigue, as a result of anemia, to pain and pressure from enlarged organs on adjacent structures, to tachycardia, and to mouth ulcerations.
4. Nutritional deficit: due to fever, anorexia, and mouth ulcerations that may result from chemotherapy.
5. Alteration in fluid volume: due to fever and anorexia; could result in an impairment in urinary elimination and in fluid and electrolyte imbalance.
6. Alterations in self-concept: due to the disease

process and prognosis and related effects of chemotherapy.

7. Decreased activity tolerance: due to fatigue, anemia.
8. Fear: due to inability to cope with a life-threatening disease, fear of death.

EXPECTED OUTCOMES*

1. Proliferation of leukocytes will decrease or halt, thus inducing a remission, if possible, as evidenced by a decrease of myeloblasts in the bone marrow and an increase in normal marrow elements.
2. Bleeding and hemorrhaging will decrease, due to altered blood values. Client will demonstrate a decrease in bruising, blood in stools and urine, pallor, and fatigue within a specified period of time (for example, within 6 weeks of beginning treatment).
3. Client will give evidence of compliance with plan of care by:
   a. Adhering to medication and therapy regimens, as evidenced by medical and client and family records.
   b. Promoting adequate food and fluid intake in order to meet bodily needs, as evidenced by physical appearance, weight gain, and urine output.
   c. Maintaining optimal functioning and comfort in activities of daily living, as reported by client and family.
4. Client will understand the ways to avoid infection by:
   a. Avoiding persons who are ill, especially those with airborne illnesses.
   b. Washing hands, checking for lesions, and avoiding trauma.
   c. Getting adequate rest, including frequent naps.
   d. Indicating, by recall, early indications of infection that require immediate interventions, such as fever, sore throat, and sores.
5. Client and family will be involved in the client's adjustment to the disease process and possible complications, to psychological needs, and to changes in lifestyle, as evidenced by client–family–health team interactions.
6. Client will verbalize fears and concerns associated with a life-threatening disease.

* Although there are several varieties of leukemia; most of the principles of care are similar (Goldstein, 1980).

INTERVENTIONS

1. Observe client closely for signs of bleeding or hemorrhage.
   a. Check urine, feces, and vomitus for blood, along with frequent checks of the skin surfaces.
   b. Protect client from falls and handle client gently to prevent injury from trauma.
   c. Apply pressure to injection sites or any cuts for several minutes to decrease hematoma formation.
   d. Administer stool softeners if necessary to prevent constipation and rectal trauma.
2. Anemia (or hemoglobin levels less than 8 g/100 mL) will be treated with transfusions of whole blood.
   a. Check blood work frequently to monitor anemic state.
   b. Thrombocytopenia may be managed with platelet transfusions (see discussion under *Idiopathic Thrombocytopenic Purpura* later in this chapter and refer to Chapter 18).
3. Ensure that client receives adequate rest to prevent fatigue and an increased susceptibility to infection.
   a. Encourage client to get 8 h of sleep at night and to take short naps during the day.
   b. Administer sedatives at night if necessary to aid sleeping because of increased bone pain and resulting discomfort.
4. Many types of pain or discomfort accompany leukemia. Bone pain, discomfort due to the enlarged organs and lymph nodes, nerve pain, and throat pain from ulcerations are common. Many interventions are prescribed, including the following:
   a. Repositioning, cooling baths, and mouth care, in addition to medication, are useful.
   b. Acetaminophen (e.g., Tylenol) or propoxyphene hydrochloride (Darvon) with sedatives (if needed) are used.
   c. Stronger analgesics, such as codeine or meperidine hydrochloride (Demerol), in conjunction with promethazine hydrochloride (Phenergan) and chlorpromazine hydrochloride (Thorazine) can be administered in the event of more severe pain.
   d. Oral medications are preferred if thrombocytopenia is present.

5. Increase the comfort of the client by controlling fever.
   a. Antipyretic drugs such as aspirin or acetaminophen in the presence of hemorrhage) may decrease temperature and control mild pain.
   b. Cooling sponge baths in tepid water can help reduce fever.
6. Administer frequent mouth care.
   a. To ease painful ulcerations in the mouth and throat, provide mouth care before meals and at least every 2–3 h. Use viscous lidocaine hydrochloride (Xylocaine) to anesthetize the throat and increase comfort. Ensure that the gag reflex is intact before offering the client food or liquids.
   b. Prevent cracking and crust formation around the lips by lubricating with petroleum jelly.
7. Adrenocortical steroids such as prednisone may decrease lymph node enlargement and increase the client's level of comfort. (For a complete discussion of steroids, refer to Chapter 27.)
8. See that client receives small servings of soft, bland food to improve dietary intake and decrease throat irritation. Also try anesthetic gargles along with cold or frozen foods such as ice cream, sherbet, milk shakes, and high-protein fruit drinks.
   a. Allow the client to choose foods that are most appealing, and consult the dietitian if necessary.
   b. Ensure that the client's diet is high in protein, vitamins, and calories, as these are the most effective nutrition sources for leukemic clients.
9. Anorexia is often present as a result of painful mouth ulcerations, discomfort resulting from enlarged organs (especially the spleen and liver), and possibly chemotherapy or radiation.
   a. Administer antiemetics $\frac{1}{2}$ h before meals to try to control nausea.
   b. If severe vomiting is a problem, check blood electrolytes. Check emesis for occult blood.
   c. If the client has any gastrointestinal bleeding, old blood may accumulate, making the client nauseous.
      (1) Use diluted hydrogen peroxide or lemon and glycerin to cleanse the mouth, remove crusted blood, and decrease halitosis.
      (2) Use soft-bristled toothbrushes or cotton applicators to remove excess debris from the teeth and gums.
10. Ensure that the client with leukemia receives an intake of 3–4 L of fluid per day to prevent dehydration and to dilute the high levels of uric acid that result from the abnormal leukocyte destruction by the antileukemic drugs.
    a. Administer sodium bicarbonate q6h to achieve alkalinization of the urine.
    b. Administer allopurinol (100 mg, tid or qid) to inhibit uric acid crystal formation.
    c. If client is unable to eat and drink, intravenous therapy or hyperalimentation may be required (refer to Chapter 33 for discussion on hyperalimentation).
11. Prevention of infection is a major nursing problem, as immature white cells and the effects of anticancer drugs limit the client's resistance to infection.
    a. Monitor the client continuously for sore throats, temperature elevations, and chills. If infection is suspected, immediately institute treatment with antibiotics, based on blood culture and sensitivity tests, as ordered.
    b. Check blood studies frequently. If there is evidence of pancytopenia (a reduction in all the cellular blood components), place the client in a single room for protection. Reverse isolation precautions may be used. A laminar airflow room with a sterile client environment, established with topical and oral antibiotics, may be used.
    c. Give platelet and WBC transfusions, if ordered, to increase resistance and to decrease bleeding. (Donor matching increases the success rate.)
    d. Treat recurrent infections due to low immunoglobulin levels with prophylactic doses of gamma globulin as ordered.
12. Management and care of the client with leukemia should be structured to allow the client to pursue as many activities and as full a life as possible.
    a. When feasible, the client should live at home, continue work or school, and participate in social activities.
    b. It is important for the client to have the

support of significant others to help in carrying out the activities of daily living.

c. The family, close friends, and employers, in addition to the client, will need information (and teaching) about leukemia, including the symptoms, treatment, complications, and prognosis.

d. Client should be encouraged to verbalize his or her fear of death.

13. Despair and depression.
   a. These are common emotional responses when clients deal with the problem of a chronic, life-threatening illness and the eventual body image changes that may result. Hope for remission may be crucial to the client and family; however, realistic assessment and evaluation of the type of leukemia and its response to therapy are necessary in order to provide support for clients and their families.
   b. The client's psychological responses should be evaluated. Social workers can help the client and family deal with financial problems. (Information about the Visiting Nurse Association, long-term care, special equipment that might be needed, and available in-home nursing and housekeeping care can be obtained from the American Cancer Society.)
   c. Measures to involve a minister or priest, psychiatrist, and occupational or physical therapist may be appropriate to provide the physical and/or emotional support or activities needed to help the client handle the illness. The fear of death is always present and should be discussed, as appropriate.

14. *Medical intervention*. In leukemia medical intervention usually consists of chemotherapy alone or in conjunction with radiation or x-ray therapy. (For a complete discussion of chemotherapy, refer to diseases listed under *Abnormal Cellular Growth* throughout the text.)
   a. *Acute granulocytic leukemia*. In AGL chemotherapeutic agents may be used alone, sequentially, or in combination. The two most commonly used are mercaptopurine (6-MP, Purinethol), a purine antimetabolic given in doses of 2.5 mg/kg per day orally, or a folic acid antimetabolite, methotrexate (Amethopterin), 2.5–5.0 mg/day orally.
   b. *Chronic granulocytic leukemia*.
      (1) In CGL the drug of choice is busulfan (Myleran), an alkylating agent. The dose is usually 2 mg, two to four times daily.
         (a) Once the WBC count falls to normal limits, the drug is given intermittently.
         (b) Platelet counts should be checked daily, as the major toxic effect of busulfan is irreversible thrombocytopenia, a decrease in the number of blasts and promyelocytes in the peripheral blood to below normal.
         (c) Chlorambucil or mercaptopurine may also be used.
      (2) Irradiation of the spleen and administration of radioactive phosphorus may also be used in treating chronic granulocytic leukemia.
   c. *Chronic lymphocytic leukemia*. The chemotherapeutic agent most often selected in CLL is chlorambucil (Leukeran), 0.01–0.2 mg/kg daily in divided doses. This is usually given after meals to decrease gastric irritation. Triethylenemelamine (TEM), 2.5–5 mg daily, is also used with sodium bicarbonate before meals.
   d. Bone marrow transplants in suitable clients with matched donors are now being performed. The results vary.

EVALUATION

Outcome Criteria

1. Client is complying with therapy as evidenced by:
   a. Remission and extended length of survival. (Chronic lymphocytic leukemia has the best prognosis of the three types of leukemia.)
   b. Bleeding and hemorrhage have decreased, based on history and physical examination. Monthly chemotherapy and physical evaluations will be continued.
   c. The chosen medication and therapy regimens are being followed.
   d. Client and family members know side effects of therapy and are aware of the need for compliance (Herbert, 1980). The client has not had to modify activities of daily living and reports no difficulties with food

or fluid intake. Weight gain is noted where weight loss was significant.

2. The client demonstrates no evidence of infection.
3. Family members are providing sensitive support to the client in regard to body image changes and are aware of any alteration in daily living patterns.
   a. Counselors, such as marital or sexual counselors, along with the nurse, are providing additional help.
   b. The client is aware that a decrease in libido, as well as sterility, impotence, and menopausal symptoms, are common side effects of chemotherapy.

Complications

1. The most common complications in leukemia and usually the eventual causes of death are infections, hemorrhage, and renal failure. (Refer to Chapters 32 and 48.)
2. Iatrogenic disorders, resulting from radiation and chemotherapy.

Assessment

Radiation sicknesses, such as nausea, platelet depression, and alopecia (baldness) may be seen.

Revised Outcomes

1. Radiation and chemotherapy will be evaluated. Signs and symptoms will decrease or be eliminated.
2. Other outcomes are as originally stated above under Expected Outcomes.

Interventions

1. Nausea (see previous interventions).
2. Platelet counts must be done frequently to monitor level of depression.
3. For the client's sense of well-being, he or she should be encouraged to wear a wig until alopecia resolves.
4. Client should be allowed to express feelings regarding therapy and the subsequent problems resulting from therapy.

Reevaluation and Follow-up

Long-term monitoring is needed.

MULTIPLE MYELOMA

DESCRIPTION

Multiple myeloma (plasma cell myeloma) is produced by malignant proliferation of plasma cells, which may result in diffuse invasion and overgrowth of the bone marrow and the formation of single or multiple plasma cell tumors at various sites. This causes bone destruction throughout the body due to plasma cell rather than red cell replacement, overproduction of myeloma proteins, and later involvement of the lymph nodes, liver, spleen, and kidneys. By the time of diagnosis, the disease is usually widely spread. (Common sites are the spine, ribs, and pelvis.) The cause is unknown but may be related to genetic composition. The condition occurs most commonly in the 50- to 60-age range and is seen twice as often in men as in women. The prognosis is generally poor, with the median survival rate less than 2 years. The incidence of multiple myeloma has increased over recent years (refer to the brief discussion in Chapter 22). Remissions can occur with a median duration of 21 months; however, the disease progresses and eventually becomes resistant to therapy. Some clients develop acute leukemia. The most common cause of death, accounting for 50 percent of cases, is nonhypertensive renal failure.

PREVENTION

Health Promotion

Early medical help for symptoms of bone pain and fatigue.

Population at Risk

Males and middle-aged adults have a higher incidence of the disease.

Screening

1. Skeletal x-ray films to detect bone lesions or osteoporosis.
2. Urine testing for Bence Jones protein.

ASSESSMENT

Health History

1. The onset of multiple myeloma is slow, and clients may have a long period without symptoms; however, during this period they may suffer from recurring attacks of fever, cough, and bacterial infections, especially pneumonia. Once symptoms appear, they are varied.
2. The client's most common complaint is usually pain. Progressive back or rib pain is usually increased with movements and varies in

intensity. It may correlate with incidence of pathological fractures. Increased pain may be associated with increased neoplastic involvement.
3. The client may complain of weight loss and fatigue.
4. Tingling and numbness in the lower extremities may be experienced.
5. Changes associated with hypercalcemia may be observed (e.g., renal nocturia, anorexia, and confusion, or subtle personality changes).
6. If anemia is present, it may correspond to the loss of weight and general pallor. The client's overall appearance must be considered; however, these complaints may indicate only that something is wrong.

Physical Assessment

(Refer to Table 29-2.)

1. Pressure or gentle palpation over osteolytic or "punched-out" lesions of the skeleton may elicit tenderness or pain (see Figure 29-5.) Pathological fractures may be present due to osteoporosis.
2. The client may demonstrate deformities or asymmetry in the skeleton. A change in height is often detected, due to decreased bone mass.
3. Neurological disorders may be manifest due to spinal cord involvement and compression fractures of the vertebrae.
4. The liver and lymph nodes may be enlarged.
5. Blurred vision and dizziness may be present due to hyperviscosity syndrome.

Diagnostic Tests

1. X-ray studies of the skeleton (e.g., metastatic series and bone scan) indicate osteoporosis, multiple lesions of the bone, and demineralization.
2. A bone marrow biopsy reveals large numbers of atypical or immature plasma cells.
3. Blood studies.
   a. There is an increased concentration of serum globulin, particularly an abnormal M-type globulin. The albumin/globulin ratio is reversed, with a low albumin and an elevated globulin, suggestive of myeloproliferative diseases with hypergammaglobulinemia. Serum electrophoresis will determine the exact type of immunoglobulin.
   b. Anemia is usually present.

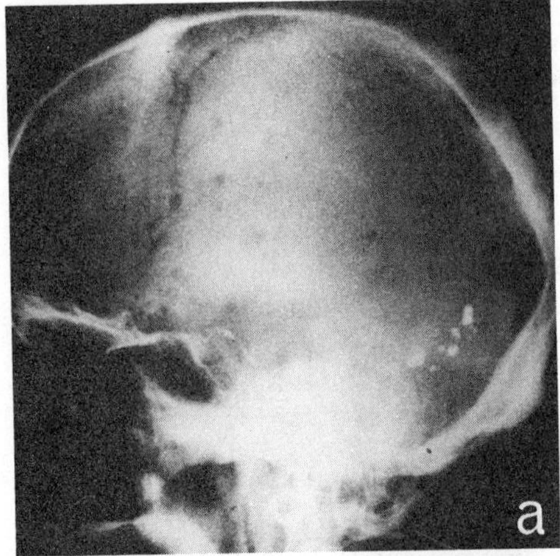

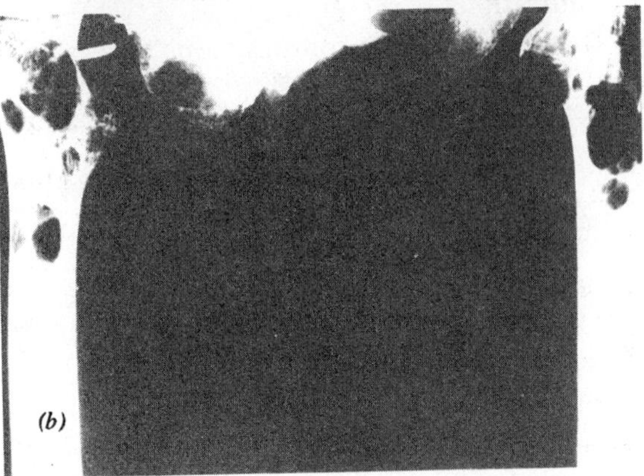

Figure 29-5 X-ray studies of a client with multiple myeloma. (*a*) Small punched-out lesions in the skull. (Williams, W. J., et al.: *Hematology*, 2d ed., McGraw-Hill, New York, 1977, p. 1103.) (*b*) Multiple myeloma (punched-out lesions). (Donahoo, C. A., and Dimon, J. H.: *Orthopedic Nursing*, Little, Brown, Boston, 1977, p. 123.)

4. An abnormal globulin, Bence Jones protein, appears in the urine, the final and most definitive sign of multiple myeloma.
5. Renal function tests (e.g., calcium level tests, uric acid level tests, protein tests, BUN, and creatinine) will give data concerning renal function. (Refer to Chapter 32 for a discussion of tests.)

NURSING DIAGNOSES: ACTUAL OR POTENTIAL

1. Alterations in comfort (pain): may be experienced in the area of skeletal lesions or nerve compression.

2. Vulnerability to infection: due to disturbances in antibody formation.
3. Impairment of mobility: due to pain, pathological fractures, ossification, loss of calcium from the bones, and fear.
4. Decreased activity tolerence: due to fatigue.
5. Potential impairment of urinary elimination: due to hypercalcemia, renal stones, and inadequate hydration.
6. Anxiety (mild to severe): due to the prognosis, the overall effects of the disease, and/or concern regarding the pain and the effects of the illness on family and work responsibilities.
7. Vulnerability to hemorrhage and bleeding: may result from circulatory and hemorrhagic disturbances due to increased blood viscosity.

EXPECTED OUTCOMES

1. Pain will decrease over a specified period of time, as evidenced by client response, by medication intake, and by an increase in activities of daily living. (For example, the client will take medication four times a day for 2 weeks and will maintain activities without complaint or discomfort.)
2. Client will give evidence of compliance with plan of care by:
   a. Adhering to medication and therapy regimens, as indicated by medical and client and family records.
   b. Allowing adequate fluid intake in order to maintain renal function, as evidenced by an intake of 3,000–4,000 mL of fluid a day and by urine output.
   c. Establishing and maintaining an ambulation program in order to increase the effects of chemotherapy and to decrease the complications of immobility.
   d. Indicating, by recall, knowledge of signs and symptoms of the disease.
3. Bone tumor size and growth will be slowed, as evidenced by x-ray studies and by a decrease in abnormal serum and urine globulins.
4. Client will understand the ways to avoid infection in order to prevent a further decrease in resistance. (Refer to the discussion of infection under *Leukemia* in this chapter.)
5. Client and family will be involved in adjustment to illness and in development of supportive roles for family members, as evidenced by client–family interactions.

INTERVENTIONS

1. Pain can generally be controlled with medication.
   a. Give aspirin (acetaminophen in the presence of hemorrhage) and codeine to provide relief in the earlier stages.
   b. If necessary, administer stronger analgesics, such as meperidine hydrochloride (Demerol), as ordered, as the disease progresses.
2. In order to promote bone remineralization, activity, physical therapy, adrenocortical steroids, and vitamin D may be used.
3. Ambulation and maintenance of mobility are necessary to sustain a client and permit remission through chemotherapy.
   a. Encourage ambulation and mobility, as osteoporosis and calcium loss increase with immobility.
   b. Pain or fear of falling may be a major obstacle. Ensure that client is always accompanied when walking, in view of increased vulnerability to falls and accidents.
   c. Use orthopedic supports or braces for the spine, ribs, or extremities to stabilize the client and to prevent further damage, such as fractures and spasms.
   d. Use supports only for a short time because of atrophy and immobilization and usually only until pain is decreased or relieved by radiotherapy or chemotherapy.
   e. Fractures of the long bones may be pinned surgically.
4. If bacterial infection is present, administer antibiotics as prescribed.
   a. Isolate client from sources of infection; teach client and family members about the need for adequate rest, good nutrition, and avoidance of persons with colds or sore throats.
   b. All infections must be cultured and treated promptly.
   c. Frequent blood work to assess the degree of leukopenia is necessary.
5. Clients with multiple myeloma require between 3,000 and 4,000 mL of fluid per day to counteract the calcium overload and to prevent protein precipitation in the renal tubules.
   a. Counteract hyperuricemia by administering allopurinol.
   b. Use saline infusions, thiazides, and steroids, if they are not contraindicated.

c. Nausea and vomiting are often seen in these clients, especially with chemotherapy; therefore, along with forcing fluids, administer antiemetics as ordered.

6. Clients with multiple myeloma have a grave prognosis. Provide support and encouragement to promote client's mobility and receptiveness to chemotherapy.
   a. Give client ample opportunity to express fears and ask questions.
   b. Support family members and encourage them to participate in care and to interact with client.
   c. Answer client's and family's questions honestly and realistically.
   d. As necessary, involve additional support systems via referrals to counselors, social workers, and other significant persons the client and family may want to involve.
   e. Adjustments in lifestyle will have to be made, because fear, anger, and grieving are client reactions that will often be seen.
7. *Medical intervention*. The most common medical treatment for multiple myeloma is chemotherapy.
   a. Alkylating agents such as L-phenylalanine mustard (L-PAM, melphalan) and cyclophosphamide (Cytoxan) are used with an approximately 35 percent chance of survival for 2 years.
   b. Prednisone has also been combined with intermittent doses of L-PAM or other agents; this is believed to enhance the effects of the alkylating agent and to increase the remission rate to greater than 60 percent. The choice of chemotherapy, agents, and dose schedule varies greatly and depends on many factors such as age, degree of debility, state of disease, and hematologic status.
   c. Radiotherapy may prove effective for localized bone lesions.

EVALUATION

Outcome Criteria

1. Pain is controlled by current medication regimen. Client is able to maintain activities of daily living.
2. Medical therapy is evaluated as effective at this time. Continual follow-up will be done with assessment of the client's health status, measurement of serum and/or urine protein concentrations, and evaluation of complications.
3. Client has an intake of an average of 3,500 mL of fluid per day.
4. Client has established a daily ambulation plan and is progressing through the first phase of the plan.
5. Client is able to recall major signs and symptoms of the disease.
6. No apparent infection is noted.
7. The client's adjustment to physical changes and level of mobility is being evaluated. The client and family members are seeing a psychologist regarding adjustment to the illness and prognosis.

Complications

1. Neurological complications may cause spinal cord compression. If they do, a surgical laminectomy is indicated. Paraplegia may result (refer to Chapter 25).
2. Pathological fractures may occur. (See discussion of treatment under Interventions above.)
3. Anemia is treated with androgens and transfusions of whole blood or red blood cell concentrations.
4. Complications of chemotherapy are many and may be varied, depending on the agent used.
5. Hemorrhagic complications may be responsive to fresh blood or platelet transfusions. If they are due to hyperviscosity, plasmapheresis is necessary to remove enough plasma containing the monoclonal protein to reduce plasma volume. Prednisone or other steroids may aggravate these symptoms.
6. Hyperviscosity syndrome, indicating increased intravascular resistance.

Assessment

1. Hyperviscosity of blood, due to excessive amounts of abnormal proteins, is present.
2. It is accompanied by heart failure, visual disturbances, and renal failure.

Revised Outcomes

1. Plasma load will be reduced within normal limits.
2. Other outcomes are as originally stated under Expected Outcomes above.

Interventions

Plasmapheresis, a method by which hyperviscous blood is removed in an effort to lower total plasma volume, is done when necessary.

Reevaluation and Follow-up

1. A plan to monitor viscosity and resultant symptoms should be established.
2. Revision in teaching or instituting counseling may be necessary, based on assessment of adjustments.

POLYCYTHEMIA VERA

DESCRIPTION

Polycythemia vera (primary polycythemia) is a disease of unknown cause. It is classified as a myeloproliferative disorder caused by neoplastic overproduction of one or more of the bone marrow cells related to differentiation of the stem cell. The problem is characterized by a marked increase in erythrocytes, reflected by an elevated hematocrit and usually an increase in the leukocytes and thrombocytes. This results in an increase in blood viscosity, resulting in a slowing of blood flow, an increase in the total blood volume (as much as two to three times normal), and a severe congestion of all tissues and organs with blood.

PREVENTION

Health Promotion

As the cause of the disease is unknown, there are no known preventive measures.

Population at Risk

1. Clients are usually 50 to 60 years of age or older.
2. Clients are often white males of Jewish extraction.

Screening

There are no known effective screening measures.

ASSESSMENT

Health History

1. Headaches.
2. Dizziness and tinnitus.
3. Dyspnea.
4. Visual disturbances.
5. Weakness of long duration.
6. Possible gastrointestinal complaints of nausea, vomiting, and abdominal pain.
7. Often, an increase in bruising with nosebleeds and gingival bleeding.

Physical Assessment

1. Classic sign of dusky red and ruddy skin color (plethora), due to blood volume and viscosity is noted, especially on the face, ears, nose, lips, and distal parts of the extremities.
2. The spleen is usually palpable.
3. Portal congestion may lead to liver enlargement.
4. If early pump failure is present, tachycardia and lung congestion may be noted.
5. Hypertension is often present.
6. Painful, swollen joints, related to uric acid deposits, are found.
7. Phlebitis, due to thrombi, is common.

Diagnostic Tests

1. Blood tests demonstrate, by chromium tagging, an increase in red cell mass; also a decreased erythropoietin level and increased uric acid level are often seen. Leukocytosis and microcythemia are present in approximately 50 percent of clients.
2. Examination of bone marrow shows hyperplasia with a noted proliferation of red blood cells.

NURSING DIAGNOSES: ACTUAL OR POTENTIAL

1. Nutritional deficit due to fullness.
2. Decreased activity tolerance due to immobility: fatigue.
3. Altered comfort due to joint swelling.
4. Knowledge deficit: lack of information regarding the health problem.

EXPECTED OUTCOMES

1. Client will report compliance with therapeutic plan.
2. Joint pain will diminish gradually.
3. Nutritional balance will be restored; feelings of fullness will diminish.
4. Activity tolerence will improve; fatigue will decrease.

INTERVENTIONS

As the cause of polycythemia vera is unknown, interventions and treatment are administered on a symptomatic basis. Nursing interventions focus on promoting client comfort, preventing complications, and encouraging client independence.

1. Increased bleeding can be a problem. The client must be taught to guard against injury and to use caution in personal activities.
2. Gastrointestinal bleeding, plus the increased number of red cells in the body, calls for dietary planning to avoid foods high in iron content (liver, legumes) and to have small, bland meals.
3. Hyperuricemia may lead to gouty arthritis and renal calculi.
   a. A large fluid intake, causing a decrease in blood viscosity, and dietary modifications in purine intake may be needed.
   b. Treatment of acute gouty arthritis is treated in a manner similar to primary gout (refer to Chapter 27).
   c. Uricosuric agents, such as allopurinol, may be given.
   d. Clients should be taught to test their own urine for alkalinity.
5. Fatigue may occur, due to anemia, therapy, and/or treatments. Rest periods and adequate nutrition may be helpful in alleviating the fatigue.
6. Pruritis, believed to be due to an increase in histamine, may be disabling to some clients. Relief may be obtained from antihistamines (e.g., Benadryl), medicated baths, and/or antipruritic lotions.
7. Alteration in mobility and maintenance of activities of daily living may be a problem. Clients should be encouraged to ambulate or, if bedridden, should be turned frequently with passive range-of-motion exercises, in order to prevent development of urine stasis and thrombi.
8. Discomfort related to joint swelling can be treated with heat, elevation and/or analgesics.
9. *Medical intervention*. Prompt treatment will help reverse the more acute changes.
   a. The most common medical treatment is a *phlebotomy*. The number of 500-mL phlebotomies needed varies from individual to individual, but it is desirable to keep the hematocrit around 40 to 45. Phlebotomy can be used as a sole means of treatment for a period of time in approximately two-thirds of the clients.
   b. Irradiation with a myelosuppressant agent, such as radioactive phosphorus, can be used to control proliferating cells.
   c. Intravenous use of alkylating agents and chemotherapy is often preferred over irradiation.

EVALUATION

The survival rate for clients with polycythemia vera is approximately 13 years.

Complications

1. Many clients develop leukemia-like symptoms and eventually die.
2. Common complications are decreased blood flow and venous stasis; venous thrombosis; infection secondary to the disease or therapy chosen; and congestive heart failure (refer to Chapter 30 for discussion of changes to be assessed).

HYPERACTIVITY AND HYPOACTIVITY

APLASTIC ANEMIA

DESCRIPTION

Aplastic ("having deficient or arrested development") anemia is a disorder associated with hypoproliferation of the precursor red blood cells in the bone marrow, resulting in a decrease in circulating erythrocytes. It is characterized by erythrocyte cellular depletion and fatty replacement of the bone marrow. It is accompanied by thrombocytopenia and pancytopenia (or a reduction in all the cellular blood components), and it affects all age groups and both sexes. The cause of approximately 50 percent of the cases of aplastic anemia seen is unknown, as clients have nonsignificant histories; however, the source of the injury to the stem cells that causes their decreased proliferation is theorized to be acquired by environmental factors (such as exposure to pollutants) or idiopathic genetic factors (such as the lack of a necessary humoral or poietic factor or the presence of some suppressor).

The diagnosis of aplastic anemia comes largely from exclusion of other diseases; however, the most common *known* causes of aplastic anemia are chemical and physical agents such as drugs (chloramphenicol is most often identified), radiation, and infections, both viral (hepatitis) and bacterial (tuberculosis) (refer to Table 29-3).

Death usually occurs within a few months. The overall mortality in adults is 70 percent, with a mean survival rate of 3 months. Recent changes in choices of therapy may change these results.

PREVENTION

Health Promotion

1. Reduced exposure to pollution and occupational toxins.
2. Avoidance of unnecessary drug ingestion.
3. Public education regarding the hazards of certain drugs and chemicals.

Population at Risk

1. Persons with exposure to toxic substances or drug ingestion.
2. Persons with a known predisposition to bone marrow failure.
3. A history of tuberculosis, hepatitis, or infection may increase the risk of aplastic anemia.
4. Persons with a known history of drug sensitivity; familial tendencies should also be noted.
5. Glue sniffing, improper use of insecticides, and overuse of Kwell shampoo have caused the disease.

TABLE 29-3 AGENTS ASSOCIATED WITH APLASTIC ANEMIA

Consistently associated (at a sufficient dose)
Benzene, its derivatives (trinitrotoluene) and related agents
Ionizing radiation (x-rays, radioactive isotopes, etc.)
Sulfur or nitrogen mustard and congeners (busulfan, melphalan, cyclophosphamide, etc.)
Antimetabolites (antifolic compounds and purine or pyrimidine analogues, such as 6-mercaptopurine, thioguanine, cytosine arabinoside)
Antimitotic agents (e.g., colchicine, periwinkle alkaloids)
Certain antibiotics (e.g., daunorubicin, doxorubicin hydrochloride)
Other toxic agents (e.g., inorganic arsenic, dichlorovinylcysteine, estrogens)
Occasionally associated
Antimicrobial agents (chloramphenicol, organic arsenicals, quinacrine)
Anticonvulsants (methylphenylethylhydantoin, trimethadione)
Analgesics (phenylbutazone)
Gold compounds
Rarely associated (single or very few reports)
Antimicrobial agents (streptomycin, penicillin, methicillin, oxytetracycline, chlortetracycline, sulfonamides, sulfisoxazole, sulfamethoxypyridazine, amphotericin B)
Anticonvulsants (methylphenylhydantoin, phenacemide, ethosuximide, phenytoin)
Antithyroid drugs (carbethoxythiomethylglyoxaline, methylmercaptoimidazole, potassium perchlorate, propylthiouracil)
Antidiabetic agents (tolbutamide, chlorpropamide, carbutamide)
Antihistamines (tripelennamine)
Analgesics (acetylsalicyclic acid, indomethacin, carbamazepine)
Sedatives and tranquilizers (meprobamate, chlorpromazine, promazine, chlordiazepoxide, mepazine)
Insecticides (chlorophenothane, parathion, chlordane, pentachlorophenol, lindane)
Miscellaneous (acetazolamide, hair dyes, dinitrophenol, thiocyanate, bismuth, mercury, colloidal silver, carbon tetrachloride, solvents)

SOURCE: Goldstein, M.: "The Aplastic Anemias," *Hospital Practice*, **15**(5):86, May *1980*.

Screening

Blood studies to document the decrease of red blood cells.

ASSESSMENT

Health History

1. The client usually complains of a slow onset of fatigue and weakness in conjunction with nosebleeds, fever, or infection.
2. A careful documentation of recent infections is needed (e.g., in granulocytopenia there is a decreased resistance to disease).
3. A suspected history of drug ingestion or exposure to other toxic substances should be noted. (Studies have shown that reactions can occur up to 1½ years after exposure.) Occupation may be a source of toxin (e.g., carbon tetrachloride or DDT).
4. Bleeding episodes should be clearly explained and documented.

Physical Assessment

1. The examination may show nothing remarkable except a slight pallor.
2. Small petechiae (purpura) might be seen upon skin inspection, especially around the shoulders and ankles, along with hemorrhages in the mucous membranes, especially around the gums (thrombocytopenia).
3. Upon eye examination, retinal hemorrhages are usually noted.
4. Enlargement of the spleen may be noted.

Diagnostic Tests

1. Blood studies reveal RBC, WBC, and platelet counts all below normal. Reticulocyte count is depressed (refer to Table 29-4).
2. Bone marrow aspiration will reveal thin, bloody material showing a decrease in bone marrow elements and an increase in fatty deposits. A biopsy may be done at the same time to avoid delay in diagnosis and to allow determination of the severity of the disease, which may influence the choice of therapy.

NURSING DIAGNOSES: ACTUAL OR POTENTIAL

1. Potential for infection (increased): due to decreased WBC count.
2. Fluid volume deficit: due to hemorrhage secondary to decreased platelet blood cell count.
3. Alterations in activities of daily living (decreased): due to fatigue and anemia.
4. Anxiety (mild to moderate): due to disease process and diagnosis.

EXPECTED OUTCOMES

1. If identified, the offending agent or drug will be withdrawn *immediately* to prevent further damage.
2. A spontaneous remission will be obtained within a specified period based on initial evaluation of the client (e.g., the client will demonstrate signs of a remission within a month's time).
3. The client and family will demonstrate adjustment to the disease process, as evidenced by their interactions, allowing the client to be as comfortable as possible while "buying time" until a remission occurs.
4. Activity tolerence will increase, as evidenced by client's verbal report of participation in activities of daily living.
5. No evidence of infection will be present.

INTERVENTIONS

1. The chemical or infectious agent must be identified and removed or treated.
2. Restrictions and safeguards for the client are needed in order to protect and support the client. They include the following focus.
   a. Provide the client and family with frank and realistic information about the seriousness of the disease and the goals of intervention.
   b. Make referrals to resource persons, such as a psychologist, as necessary, to allow the client to ventilate fears and anxieties and to provide information needed to make adjustments in lifestyle.
3. Anemia may be treated with blood transfusions of platelets, whole blood, or granulocytes. The transfusions are stopped when bone marrow function resumes.
4. Infections are common and are also the usual cause of death; however, unless it is absolutely necessary not to, encourage the client to continue his or her accustomed lifestyle.
   a. Reverse isolation may be necessary. Reduce the client's exposure to numbers of people, wash hands with an antiseptic before contact with clients, and wear a mask. A laminar airflow room may be used.

   b. Observe closely for signs and symptoms of infection.
   c. Use antiseptic soap to reduce skin infection.
   d. Administer antibiotics as ordered to treat known infections.
5. Excessive bleeding is also a common problem. Teach the client to take care to prevent injury.
   a. Stress the importance of avoiding skin injuries and of having any noted bleeding or bruising examined for causes and then treated.
      (1) Avoid intramuscular injections and venipunctures. Hold site of injection until bleeding stops.
      (2) Suggest that an electric razor be used.
   b. Stress the need for care in oral hygiene. Instruct the client in proper technique, if necessary, and to use a soft toothbrush and to avoid trauma to the gum tissue.
   c. Suggest the use of a stool softener to avoid straining at defecation and rectal bleeding.
   d. Excessive menstrual flow is treated with suppressive hormonal therapy.
   e. Corticosteroids may decrease capillary bleeding.
   f. Encourage client to follow a diet high in vitamins and protein.
   g. Platelet transfusions can be given.
6. *Medical intervention.* To stimulate bone marrow function, the following medical courses of action may be considered.
   a. Androgens (e.g., fluoxymesterone, oxymesterone, testosterone) may be given in small doses and over a short time of several months. Drugs used may be varied. The result is at least partial restoration of function. Transfusions are given concurrently.
   b. Bone marrow transplants can be done, but compatible donors are hard to find and results have been varied. They are more successful early in the disease before sensitization to antigens by transfusion occurs. Rejection and infection are problems.
   c. Pilot studies using antithymocyte globulin suggest the results of this therapy may be as good as transplants. Antithymocyte globulin suppresses T cell-dependent autoimmune responses that cause stem cell death and/or prevent cellular differentiation (Goldstein, 1980).
   d. A splenectomy may be performed if the organ is enlarged and/or interfering with the development of normal cells. It can increase the effective life span of available circulating blood cells, but it is not common because of the risks and variable results. (For pre- and postoperative preparation similar to that of general surgery, refer to Chapter 18.)

EVALUATION

Outcome Criteria

1. The offending agent is or is not identified; however, all possibilities have been carefully evaluated. Reassessment is continuous. Blood studies are followed closely.
2. Remission has occurred.
3. Supportive therapy continues, and complications are treated symptomatically. Client and family are demonstrating appropriate adjustment and coping mechanisms to the disease process.
4. There are no signs of infection.

Complications

Hemorrhage and infection are the most common complications. The client with a history of recent exposure to bone marrow toxins seems to do the best; the client with a history of hepatitis does poorly.

Complete remissions are rare, but approximately one-third of patients with remissions seen are cured. If severe pancytopenia is present, death may occur from hemorrhage or overwhelming infection.

AGRANULOCYTOSIS

Agranulocytosis is a rare disorder manifested by a decrease in granulocytes leading to lowered resistance and possible bacterial invasion. It is caused by a suppression of bone marrow activity with a resulting decrease in production. It can occur at any age but is seen most often in adult women. The exact cause is not known, but it appears to be an immunological or leukocytic antibody reaction (to drug administration) by an inherently sensitive individual. This idiosyncratic drug reaction is most often seen with phenothiazines, promethazine hydrochloride (Thorazine), sulfonamides, and penicillin, but

TABLE 29-4 COMPARATIVE BLOOD PICTURE[a]

Test	Abbreviation	Normal Values	Variance	Clinical Implications	Subsequent Laboratory Studies, Comments, and/or Conclusive Symptoms
Complete Blood Count					
Hematocrit	Hct	Male: 40–54% Female: 38–47%			
Hemoglobin	Hgb	Male: 13.5–18.0 g/dL Female: 12.0–16.0 g/dL	↓[b]	Anemia	
			↓ (borderline) with ↓ (borderline) hematocrit and normal RBC count	Hypochromic microcytic anemia: iron deficiency, thalassemia major and minor, sickle cell anemia, and hemoglobin C disease	Bone marrow biopsy, decreased serum iron level, hemoglobin electrophoresis
			↓	Normochromic normocytic anemia	History, reticulocyte count
			↓ with ↑ MCV and ↑ MCHC	Macrocytic anemia, folic acid deficiency, vitamin B_{12} deficiency (pernicious anemia)	
Red blood cell count	RBC	Male: 4.6–6.2 × 10^6/μL Female: 4.2–5.4 × 10^6/μL	↑ (primary)	Polycythemia vera (leukemia)	↓ erythropoietin level
White blood cell count	WBC	4,500–11,000/μL	↑ (mild to moderate)	Infectious disease, mainly bacterial and moderate	History, physical, and differential
Erythrocyte Indices					
Mean corpuscular volume (ratio of hematocrit: packed cell volume to RBC count)	MCV	82–98 μm³ (fl)	↓	Hypochromic microcytic anemia, iron deficiency, thalassemia	
			Normal	Normocytic, normochromic anemia, aplastic anemia, congenital hemolytic anemia, anemia of leukemia	
			↑	Macrocytic, normochromic anemia, folic acid deficiency, vitamin B_{12} deficiency (pernicious anemia)	
Mean corpuscular hemoglobin (weight of Hgb in average RBC, related to MCV)	MCH	27–31 pg	↓	Same as above	
			Normal	Same as above	
			↑	Same as above	
Mean corpuscular hemo-	MCHC	32–36%	↓	Same as above	
			Normal	Same as above	

	(140,000–440,000) Brecher-Cronkite method		cytopenia (various causes)	
Additional findings		↑	Polycythemia	
		Spherocytosis, polychromatophilia, and erythrocyte agglutination	Compensated, acquired hemolytic anemia	
		Spherocytosis with polychromatophilia	Hereditary spherocytosis	Fragility test
		Macrocytosis and hypersegmental neutrophils	Vitamin B_{12} and/or folic acid deficiency	Serum folate, RBC folate
		Rouleaux formation	Multiple myeloma	Bone marrow biopsy, serum protein electrophoresis
		Atypical lymphocytes	Infectious mononucleosis	
		↓ Neutrophils and increased lymphocytes	Agranulocytosis	
		Blast (primitive) forms	Acute leukemia	
Reticulocyte count	25,000–75,000 cells/μL	↓	Vitamin B_{12} anemia (pernicious anemia), aplastic anemia	
		↑	Hemolytic anemia	
WBC Differential (Adult)				
Lymphocytes	Mean %: 34% Range of absolute counts: 1,000–4,800/μL	↑ 80–90% ↑ (marked) leukocytes	Chronic lymphocytic leukemia	
		↑ (marked with ↑ moderate leukocytes)	Infectious diseases: infectious mononucleosis	Bone marrow biopsy, peripheral smear
Basophils	Mean %: 3%	↑	Myeloproliferative disease	Bone marrow biopsy, serum protein electrophoresis, serum albumin/globulin ratio

SOURCE: Adapted from Tilkian, S. M., Conover, M. B., and Tilkian, A. G.: *Clinical Implications of Laboratory Tests*, 3d ed., Mosby, St. Louis, 1983, pp. 53–56.

[a] Only significant hematology studies are presented; not all tests are included.

[b] ↑ = elevated; ↓ = depressed.

may also be seen after large doses of antimetabolite drugs and after radiation and radioisotope therapy over a long period of time.

A thorough *health history* of recent exposure to drugs or chemical agents is needed.

1. Any family history of increased drug or chemical sensitivity should be noted.
2. Early symptoms include fatigue, weakness, headache, and restlessness.

Physical assessment reveals:

1. The majority of individuals complain of a sore throat, which progresses rapidly into chills, high fever, and dysphagia.
2. Necrotic areas are often seen in the oral mucosa.

Blood tests show:

1. White blood cell count is less than 5,000 per cubic millimeter.
2. Cultures are positive for bacteria, usually gram positive.
3. Bone marrow examination reveals hypoplasia.

Interventions focus on treatment for removal of the offending agent.

1. Teach the client to avoid any further contact with drugs, chemicals, or physical agents that may affect bone marrow.
2. Provide general supportive care, including:
   a. Elimination of infection with antibiotics.
   b. Prevention of future infections (including reverse isolation, if necessary).
   c. Adequate rest periods and increased fluid intake.
3. Encourage good oral hygiene and adequate nutrition with a diet high in protein, vitamins, and calories. Instruct the client to avoid foods and beverages that may irritate the throat.
4. Institute hot saline gargles, an ice collar, and administering analgesics to provide comfort.
5. Administer antipyretics and suggest tepid baths to reduce fever.

Recovery results vary depending on the promptness of treatment, the granulocyte count, bone marrow production, and whether the disease is acute or chronic; however, the recovery is usually fairly rapid if infection is prevented and sepsis is avoided. In chronic agranulocytosis, leukocyte transfusion or splenectomy may eventually be necessary.

ACQUIRED IMMUNE DEFICIENCY SYNDROME*

Acquired immune deficiency syndrome (AIDS) is a present-day health problem of unknown cause. Recently, the Centers for Disease Control (CDC) defined AIDS as a disease of at least a moderately predictive defect in cell-mediated immunity, occurring in a person with no known cause for diminished resistance to diseases. These diseases have included atypical mycobacteriosis, candidiasis, toxoplasmosis, Karposi's sarcoma, and others of fungal, viral, bacterial, and protozoal origin.

The first cases of AIDS were reported in 1979 in the Los Angeles area. Other literature, however, suggests that a similar syndrome was observed in tropical countries such as Africa, Haiti, and Barbados years earlier. To date there have been over 1,600 reported cases of AIDS throughout the United States. New York, California, New Jersey, and Florida report high incidences of this syndrome. Although several hundred persons have died from AIDS, it is not considered to be a problem of epidemic proportions within the general population.

The exact cause of AIDS is unknown, but several hypotheses have been postulated as to its origin. Some researchers suggest that AIDS is caused by *Herpes virus*, including the simplex, cytomegalovirus, and Epstein-Barr virus. Other researchers, such as those at the National Cancer Institute, have demonstrated that a human T-cell leukemia virus (HTLV) may be responsible for AIDS. This virus, they believe, causes a rare cancer in human beings and has been shown to attack specific T cells within the immune system of the AIDS victim.

Although much research is being conducted to isolate and define the problem, further study continues to be essential. Evidence to date indicates that AIDS is most probably transmitted by blood and blood products, semen, and saliva. Additional reports support the belief that AIDS

* This section contributed by Dorothy A. Jones, R.N., C., M.S.N., FAAN.

appears to have an epidemic pattern similar to that of hepatitis B. Because AIDS presents with such a wide variety of signs and symptoms, isolation of the cause of AIDS is, at best, difficult. Based upon this, researchers also believe that the AIDS victim is usually subjected to repeated infections that weaken the immune system, decrease resistance to further infections and, if allowed to continue, will result in death due to "burnout" of the immune system.

The incubation period of AIDS can be as short as 1 month or as long as 24 months. The mean time frame ranges between 8 to 18 months. As the cause of AIDS is unknown, efforts of health providers center on health promotion activities and early treatment of infectious processes.

Proposed *health promotion activities* include:

1. Maintaining a healthy lifestyle (i.e., effective nutritional pattern, adequate sleep, and regular exercise).
2. Conserving energy.
3. Decreasing exposure to high-risk AIDS groups and persons.
4. Limiting the number of anonymous sexual partners.
5. Avoiding sexual contact with AIDS victims.
6. Encouraging all health care workers to use extra caution when handling all secretions, particularly from suspected AIDS victims (e.g., wearing gloves and masks and using special procedures when handling specimens).
7. Seeking immediate health care for specific changes in health status. These changes include:
   a. Enlarged single or multiple lymph glands (especially in the groin, neck, and armpit).
   b. Unexplained weight loss of 10 or more pounds over a 2-month period.
   c. Night sweats without shaking chills and unrelated to a specific viral infection.
   d. Persistent unexplained diarrhea.
   e. Purple spots or lumps that do not heal.
   f. Persistent fatigue in the presence of good health habits.
   g. Unexplained shortness of breath upon exertion.
   h. Other symptoms related to an infectious process.

There are several specific *populations at risk* for AIDS. They include homosexuals, intravenous drug users, Haitian people, hemophiliacs, and persons receiving blood transfusions. Of the more than 1,600 reported cases of AIDS, 6 percent have been women. Children have also been included in these statistics, particularly children of AIDS victims. Continued health promotion and public education among these and other groups may help diminish the spread of AIDS.

To date, there are also no specific *screening tests* avilable to detect AIDS. Because each victim presents with a different cluster of symptoms, laboratory tests often validate only a specific organism. Although there is no specific serologic indicator for AIDS, there is speculation that certain antibody titers may be AIDS precursors. Cell mediated immunity (T cells) and humoral immunity (B cells) may play a role in AIDS, but data are inconclusive.

When clients enter the health care system they will require much attention and support. At times, victims of AIDS may be forced to disclose lifestyle events to family, friends, or other health care providers, resulting in fear and anxiety. Counseling and support will be needed along with increased emphasis on health teaching activities to improve the person's health status.

Depending upon the nature of the presenting symptoms and related infectious processes, medical treatments will vary. If hospitalized, the client will be placed on isolation precautions. Frequently, less ill clients are treated at home with supportive interventions. In the more severe cases, broad-spectrum antibiotics and intravenous replacement therapies are used. Currently research is being focused on the use of interferon as the drug of choice. The results are now under investigation and are inconclusive at this time.

Throughout the United States considerable funding is being devoted to AIDS research. This action is in response to citizen and health providers' concerns and fears related to the potential spread of AIDS. In time, there will be more facts available that will describe AIDS, define its cause and presenting signs and symptoms, and propose a cure. Until that time, the public is encouraged to seek medical attention for any alteration in health (particularly among high-risk populations), to report all suspected cases of AIDS to appropriate health personnel and, most importantly, to engage in health promotion activities that support optimal health.

METABOLIC DISORDERS

PERNICIOUS ANEMIA

DESCRIPTION

Pernicious anemia, the most common manifestation of vitamin B_{12} deficiency, is a chronic, progressive, megaloblastic anemia characterized by a deficiency of the intrinsic factor. Vitamin B_{12} is necessary for normal red blood cell maturation and for normal nervous system functioning. Vitamin B_{12} is obtained from foods (or the extrinsic factor) and cannot be absorbed in the small intestine unless the intrinsic factor, believed to be a glycoprotein secretion of the gastric mucosa, is present in sufficient quantities. Vitamin B_{12} deficiency, thought to be an autoimmune disorder, impedes deoxyribonucleic acid (DNA) synthesis, resulting in the appearance of megoblasts (large, primitive erythrocytes) in the blood and bone marrow and also resulting in thrombocytopenia and leukopenia.

Pernicious anemia affects approximately 0.1 percent of the population. The highest incidence is found mainly in men and women over age 50. It is seen fairly often in fair-skinned, blue-eyed Scandinavians and may be due to a genetic predisposition in that nationality.

Other vitamin B_{12} deficiencies that may be seen are due to inadequate dietary intake, increased vitamin B_{12} requirements, such as in hyperthyroidism, defective absorption caused by a total gastrectomy, and failure of absorption in the small intestine. The most common causes of lack of small intestine absorption are malabsorption syndromes, such as celiac disease, blind loop, and tapeworm infestation (refer to Table 29-5). Vitamin B_{12} deficiency can result in degeneration of the lateral and dorsal columns of the spinal cord, peripheral nerve damage and parasthesia, and altered food digestion; however, symptoms vary with the severity of the disease (refer to Table 29-6).

PREVENTION

Health Promotion

1. Public education regarding the causes and signs and symptoms of vitamin B_{12} deficiency.
2. Increased public awareness of the need for good nutrition.

Population at Risk

1. People over 50, both males and females.
2. Persons of Scandinavian heritage.
3. People with type A blood.
4. Vegetarians.
5. Persons with a history of peptic ulcer or pancreatic disease, bowel resection or gastrectomy, ileal conditions, gastritis, or gastric atrophy.
6. Alcoholics.
7. Persons with a familial history of vitamin B_{12} deficiency.
8. Persons with a history of long-term use of neomycin, colchicine, para-aminosalicylic acid (PAS), megadoses of vitamin C, and/or slow-release potassium chloride (Herbert, 1980).
9. Persons with diseases with a high rate of hemopoiesis (e.g., sickle cell anemia or thalassemia) or a history of iron deficiency that causes atrophy of the gastric mucosa.

Screening

1. Blood studies to show a decreased serum vitamin B_{12} level.
2. Screening test to measure the absorption of radioactive vitamin B_{12}.

ASSESSMENT

Health History

1. The client usually complains of a slow, steady onset of weakness, anorexia, indigestion, and numbness and tingling in the extremities.
2. A weight loss may have been noted. Diarrhea is commonly seen.
3. Early graying of the hair may have been noted.
4. Complaints of tinnitus may be described if auditory nerve involvement is present.
5. Irritability and mood swings may be noted.
6. The dietary history (although not often seen) may indicate a poor dietary intake, such as a "strict vegetarian" diet or alcoholism.
7. In older clients, shortness of breath, dizziness, palpitations, and the development of angina after exertion may be the most common complaints.
8. The deficiency may develop slowly because the bodily requirement of vitamin B_{12} is low; therefore, symptoms may appear gradually.

TABLE 29-5 ETIOLOGICAL MECHANISMS OF MEGALOBLASTIC ANEMIAS

Vitamin B_{12} Deficiency	Folic Acid Deficiency
Decreased intake: Poor diet Impaired absorption and/or utilization: Intrinsic factor (IF) deficiency: Pernicious anemia Gastrectomy (total and partial) Destruction of gastric mucosa by ingested caustics Anti-IF antibody in gastric juice Abnormal intrinsic factor molecule Intrinsic intestinal disease Familial selective malabsorption (Imerslund syndrome) Ileal resection, ileitis Sprue, celiac disease Infiltrative intestinal disease (lymphoma, scleroderma, etc.) Drug-induced malabsorption Competitive parasites: Fish tapeworm infestation Bacteria in diverticula of bowel Bacteria in blind loops and pouches Chronic pancreatic disease Increased requirement, excretion, or destruction: Pregnancy Neoplastic disease Hyperthyroidism	Decreased intake: Poor diet: Alcoholism Infancy Hemodialysis Impaired absorption and/or utilization: Intestinal absorption, due to inhibition of conjugase enzyme Steatorrhea Sprue, celiac disease Intrinsic intestinal disease Anticonvulsants, oral contraceptives Increased requirement, excretion, or destruction: Pregnancy Infancy Hyperactive hemopoiesis Neoplastic disease Skin disease Blocked activation by folic acid antagonists

SOURCE: Williams, W. J., et al.: *Hematology*, 2d ed., McGraw-Hill, New York, 1977, p. 304.

Physical Assessment

(Refer to Table 29-2.)

1. The client appears pale, wasted.
2. A pale yellow or lemon-yellow tinge to the skin or sclera may be noted due to increased destruction of malformed red blood cells.
3. The mucous membranes may be inflamed, and the tongue is smooth and beefy red.
4. Bleeding of the gingivae may be noted.
5. The spleen is usually enlarged and palpable.
6. The most significant findings are those made upon neurological examination. Signs of posterior and lateral column disease may be symmetrical paresthesias in the feet and fingers. Incoordination, impairment of position (apragnosia) and vibratory sense, and an absence of reflexes may be noted. Alteration in balance and proprioception may be noted.
7. Bowel sounds may be increased if diarrhea is present.
8. Dyspnea may be present, increasing upon changes in position. Slowed capillary refill will also be noted.
9. Tachycardia and premature ventricular beats may be heard. In advanced stages, signs of pump failure may be noted.

Diagnostic Tests

1. Blood studies will show a decreased erythrocyte count and a decreased serum vitamin B_{12} level.
2. Bone marrow biopsy reveals an increased number of megaloblasts.

TABLE 29-6 PROBABLE BIOCHEMICAL AND HEMATOLOGIC SEQUENCE OF EVENTS IN INADEQUATE VITAMIN B_{12} AND FOLATE DEFICIENCY

Vitamin B_{12} Deficiency	Folate Deficiency
Day 1: Inadequate absorption of food B_{12} and reabsorption of bile B_{12}; serum B_{12}-binding capacity 40% ± 10% saturated; serum B_{12} normal (>200 pg/ml)	3 weeks: Low serum folate; slight increase in size of average bone marrow normoblast
1 to 2 years: Serum B_{12} below 150 pg/ml; B_{12} in reproducing cells approximately one-half normal; early bone marrow and peripheral blood changes; hypersegmentation; MCV elevated	5 weeks: Hypersegmentation in neutrophils in bone marrow
1½ to 2 years: Early damage to myelin	7 weeks: Hypersegmentation in peripheral blood; bone marrow shows increased and abnormal mitoses and basophilic intermediate megaloblasts
2 to 3 years: Serum B_{12} below 100 pg/ml; serum B_{12}-binding capacity less than 10% saturated; B_{12} in reproducing cells approximately 10% of normal; bone marrow unequivocally megaloblastic; low red cell folate; serum folate normal or elevated	10 weeks: Bone marrow shows same large myelocytes and a number of polychromatophilic intermediate megaloblasts
2½ to 3 years: Severe damage to myelin	14 weeks: Orthochromatic intermediate megaloblasts in bone marrow
	17 weeks: Low RBC folate
	18 weeks: Macrocytosis; many large myelocytes in bone marrow
	19 weeks: Overtly megaloblastic marrow
	20 weeks: Anemia

SOURCE: Herbert, V.: "The Nutritional Anemias," *Hospital Practice,* **15**(3):67, 68, March 1980.

3. A definitive test for pernicious anemia is the Schilling test, which consists of a measurement of the absorption of radioactive vitamin B_{12} both before and after parenteral administration of the intrinsic factor.
4. Gastric juice analysis for the presence of free hydrochloric acid is another important test. Analysis follows histamine administration, which usually stimulates gastric juice production. A low-volume, high-pH gastric juice with no free hydrochloric acid is seen in pernicious anemia.
5. A biopsy can be done to determine the presence of the intrinsic factor.
6. A therapeutic trial of B_{12} can be given.

NURSING DIAGNOSES: ACTUAL OR POTENTIAL

1. Potential noncompliance with vitamin B_{12} therapy: due to neurological involvement.
2. Knowledge deficit: due to a lack of understanding regarding medical treatment.
3. Nutritional deficit: stemming from gastrointestinal disturbances due to the decrease in hydrochloric acid that affects chemical digestion of food, decreased absorption of vitamin B_{12}.
4. Decreased activity tolerance: due to fatigue, shortness of breath.
5. Potential for injury: related to paresthesia,

mental confusion, and ataxia, which are the results of vitamin B_{12} deficiency.
6. Sensory deficit (hearing deficit): due to tinnitis.
7. Ineffective coping: due to increased irritability, mood swings.

EXPECTED OUTCOMES

1. There will be a decrease in symptoms after a 10-day trial period of vitamin B_{12} therapy.
2. Client will give evidence of compliance with plan of care by:
   a. Allowing adequate nutritional intake, as measured by 24-h dietary recall.
   b. Indicating understanding of the need for protection because of neurological symptoms.
   c. Establishing frequent rest periods to promote maximum functioning.
   d. Demonstrating knowledge, by recall, of disease process and the need for maintenance of vitamin B_{12} therapy for the client's lifetime.
   e. Allowing family involvement as a support system.

INTERVENTIONS

1. Nursing interventions are in conjunction with medical therapy. Immediate vitamin B_{12} therapy is initiated with administration of cyanocobalamin, 100 μg IM daily for 10 doses.
   a. Folic acid is sometimes given in conjunction with vitamin B_{12}. Caution should be used with folic acid administration, as neurological symptoms may be intensified.
   b. Iron supplements of ferrous sulfate, 0.2 g, or ferrous gluconate, 0.3 g, tid after meals, may be given.
   c. In extreme cases, blood transfusions may be needed.
   d. In the presence of peripheral edema, diuretics and decreased sodium intake will be prescribed.
2. Vitamin B_{12} therapy must be continued for the rest of the client's life. Involve the client in a teaching plan that includes information about:
   a. Injections of cyanocobalamin: 100 μg may be given twice monthly or oral vitamin B_{12} may be given in daily 500- to 1,000-μg doses.
   b. The importance of continued medical observation and treatment.
   c. The risks of interrupted therapy.
   d. The importance of being well informed regarding pernicious anemia and having a basic grasp of the need for continued medication in order to increase chances of a good prognosis.
3. Treat gastrointestinal symptoms when observed.
   a. Perform mouth care carefully in the client with severe glossitis. Provide frequent oral hygiene before and after meals to ease discomfort and cleanse the mouth.
   b. Instruct the client to avoid highly seasoned, coarse, or irritating foods and also foods that may be difficult to digest.
   c. Administer hydrochloric acid (HCl) after meals if dysphagia is present. Because HCl stains the teeth, be sure it is well diluted in water and administer it through a straw.
   d. Administer appropriate medication in case of constipation or diarrhea.
4. Emphasize the importance of a nutritious diet to the client with pernicious anemia. Encourage client to eat foods high in protein, iron, and vitamins such as vitamin B_{12}; these include meat, poultry, liver, fish, eggs, and dairy products.
5. Ensure that client receives adequate bed rest if severe anemia is present.
   a. Encourage client to exercise as tolerated. Unless contraindicated, permit client bathroom privileges and short periods out of bed in a chair.
   b. If the client is bedridden, turn frequently, encourage range-of-motion exercises, and see that client receives physical therapy.
6. If neurological disturbances are present:
   a. Keep side rails up and use restraints.
   b. Protect the client from falls, especially if a gait disturbance has been noted.
   c. Accompany the client at night, as perception disturbances cause great difficulty in maneuvering in the dark.
   d. Use heating pads and hot compresses with care, as reduced sensations to heat and pain are often present.
   e. Provide extra blankets for comfort, as increased sensation to cold is also a problem.
   f. Employ foot cradles to take the undue pressure of blankets off the feet.
   g. Observe bladder for rectal sphincter in-

volvement due to advanced disease process, as it may complicate nursing care and be a source of infection.
7. Use restraints, mild sedation, and counseling if the behavioral changes that accompany pernicious anemia necessitate.
   a. Provide a quiet environment to soothe the client.
   b. Provide the support and reassurance that are most critical in facilitating relaxation.

EVALUATION

Outcome Criteria

1. Client has an immediate reversal of symptoms manifested by absence of neurological involvement, improved appetite, increased physical activity, and sense of well-being.
2. Client is demonstrating compliance with therapeutic regimen, as evidenced by verbal reports of dietary intake, freedom from injury, increased activity tolerance, planned rest periods, and family involvement in care of the client.

Complications

1. Follow-up is necessary, as relapses may indicate infection, renal insufficiency (refer to Chapter 32), gastric carcinoma, benign polyps, or gastrointestinal bleeding (refer to Chapter 33).
2. With neurological complications, the prognosis is related to the extent and duration of involvement. Vigorous therapy and treatment can reverse some of the neurological problems.
3. Vitamin B_{12} deficiency can result in folic acid and/or iron deficiency.

FOLIC ACID ANEMIA

DESCRIPTION

Folic acid anemia is relatively common, especially in adults. The causes of this condition vary and are very similar to the causes of vitamin B_{12} deficiency (refer to Table 29-6). Folic acid is necessary for normal red blood cell maturation, and its deficiency affects the synthesis of DNA. This megaloblastic anemia, like vitamin B_{12} deficiency, is characterized by the appearance of megaloblasts in the blood and bone marrow.

The incidence of folic acid anemia is higher in countries with poor nutritional sources. Although in the United States dietary intake of folic acid is high, the bodily reserves are low, and the symptoms of folic acid anemia can appear rapidly in 12 to 16 weeks with depletion of the total body stores (refer to Table 29-6).

PREVENTION

Health Promotion

1. Public education regarding the causes and signs and symptoms of folate deficiency.
2. Increased public awareness of nutrition.

Population at Risk

1. Persons with poor dietary habits, especially those who overcook food; alcoholics and narcotic addicts.
2. Persons with a history of liver disease or gastrointestinal malabsorption.
3. Elderly persons.
4. Pregnant women.
5. Persons who use certain oral contraceptives, anticonvulsants, and antimetabolites.

Screening

1. Blood studies to show a decreased serum folate level.

ASSESSMENT

Health History

1. The client's complaints are very similar to those of pernicious anemia or vitamin B_{12} deficiency (see previous section in this chapter).
2. Fatigue and shortness of breath may be the major complaints.
3. An extensive dietary history is very important. A poor intake of green vegetables or fresh fruits along with excessive cooking of food may result in folic acid anemia.
4. Chronic alcoholics are especially susceptible, partially due to diet but also due to increased alcohol levels that block bone marrow response to folic acid.
5. A history of liver disease or gastrointestinal malabsorption, such as sprue (intolerance of wheat, protein, or gluten ingestion) or regional enteritis, may be found.
6. A history of any previous anemia should be noted, along with any treatment given.
7. Drug ingestion of certain anticonvulsants (Dilantin, phenobarbital), oral contraceptives,

and antimetabolites (such as methotrexate, a folic acid antagonist) must be determined.

8. Folic acid requirements are increased during growth, pregnancy (especially during the last trimester), and in certain disease states, such as cancer and leukemia.
9. Care must be taken to be sure the client has folic acid anemia and not vitamin B_{12} deficiency.

Physical Assessment

(Refer to Table 29-2.)

1. The appearance of the client is similar to that in pernicious anemia.
2. The client is pale and emaciated.
3. Glossitis is usually present.
4. The neurological changes present in pernicious anemia are *not* seen in folic acid anemia, unless they are linked to chronic alcoholism.
5. Other disorders, such as protein and iron deficiency and electrolyte imbalances, may be seen in conjunction with folic acid anemia.

Diagnostic Tests

1. Blood studies reveal macrocytic, megaloblastic blood cells, with decreased erythrocytes, leukocytes, and platelets.
   a. A decrease is seen in the serum and red cell and folate levels.
   b. The Schilling test and serum vitamin B_{12} level are normal.
2. Hydrochloric acid is present in the gastric juice.
3. Bone marrow examination reveals an increased number of megaloblasts.
4. A favorable response to a therapeutic trial of folic acid, 0.5–1 mg IM daily for 10 days, is indicative of folic acid anemia.

NURSING DIAGNOSES: ACTUAL OR POTENTIAL

1. Noncompliance: due to inability to alter dietary habits or lack of understanding of disease.
2. Nutritional deficit: due to an intake of less than minimal daily requirements.
3. Alterations in comfort: due to irritations of the oral mucosa.

EXPECTED OUTCOMES

1. There will be a decrease in symptoms after a 10-day period of folate therapy.
2. Client will demonstrate understanding of adequate nutrition to supplement and increase folic acid intake, as evidenced by a dietary log and by discussion with the dietitian.
3. Client will understand information regarding prevention of future folic acid deficiency taught in teaching sessions, as evidenced by 85 percent accuracy on a written test.

INTERVENTIONS

1. Oral doses of folic acid, 0.25–1 mg daily, are given until the blood studies improve or the cause of intestinal malabsorption is corrected. If malabsorption is a problem, parenteral doses are given initially. (Usually folate, 1 mg, is given for approximately 10 days.)
2. Vitamin C is sometimes also prescribed, in addition, because it augments folic acid in promoting erythropoiesis. One-half to one cup of orange juice per day can maintain folic acid stores.
3. Dietary habits and food intake must be considered.
   a. A dietitian working closely with the client may be able to suggest foods high in folic acid and plan meals that are attainable to the client.
   b. Consideration must be given to cost and availability.
   c. Fruits and dark leafy green vegetables, including such choices as lemons, bananas, melons, liver, kidney, cauliflower, spinach, broccoli, lettuce, and lima beans, are necessary to provide adequate folic acid intake. Brewer's yeast is also high in folic acid.
4. Refer to *Pernicious Anemia* for care of the mouth.

EVALUATION

Outcome Criteria

1. Client demonstrates a decrease in symptoms. Periodic blood determinations to evaluate the client's response to drug therapy are continuing.
2. Client and family can verbalize their understanding of the disease and related dietary therapy.
3. Client can recall accurately, both in writing and verbally, the content presented in teaching sessions.
4. Client reports increased activity tolerance.

Complications

If folic acid anemia is misdiagnosed and is in reality vitamin B_{12} deficiency, neurological symptoms will develop.

IRON DEFICIENCY ANEMIA

DESCRIPTION

Iron deficiency anemia is one of the most common anemias, and it affects 10 to 30 percent of the world population. It is characterized by decreased or absent iron stores in the bone marrow, spleen, and liver; a low serum iron and a low hemoglobin level, which means decreased oxygen-carrying capacities; and the presence of microcytic, hypochromic (small and devoid of pigment) red blood cells (refer to Figure 29-6). It is caused by inadequate intake or absorption of dietary iron to compensate for iron requirements, by increased loss of iron due to bleeding, whether physiological or pathological, or by increased requirements, such as pregnancy. The distribution of this anemia is related to geographic location, economic and social class, age, and sex. Iron deficiency is common in underdeveloped areas where nutrition is poor and in tropical areas where parasites such as hookworm are prevalent. Menstruating and pregnant women and young children are the most common victims. One study has concluded that in the United States, 25 percent of infants, approximately 6 percent of children, 15 percent of menstruating women, and 30 percent of pregnant women are iron deficient (Herbert, 1980). If pathological bleeding is involved, the chronic blood loss is usually from the gastrointestinal tract. Symptoms will increase and intensify unless replacement therapy begins (refer to Table 29-7).

PREVENTION

Health Promotion

1. Public education regarding the causes and signs and symptoms of iron deficiency.
2. Increased public awareness of positive nutrition.

Populations at Risk

1. Persons in areas of poor nutrition and in tropical areas where hookworm is prevalent.
2. Women, especially teen-agers and menstruating and pregnant women.
3. Elderly persons who have poor eating habits (e.g., only tea and toast for a meal).
4. Alcoholics.
5. Persons with a history of gastrointestinal bleeding.
6. Black male adolescents (Ten-State Nutrition Survey, 1972).

Screening

Blood studies to show decreased iron stores and serum iron.

ASSESSMENT

Health History

1. Fatigue, irritability, and headaches are common complaints. Numbness in hands and feet may be present.

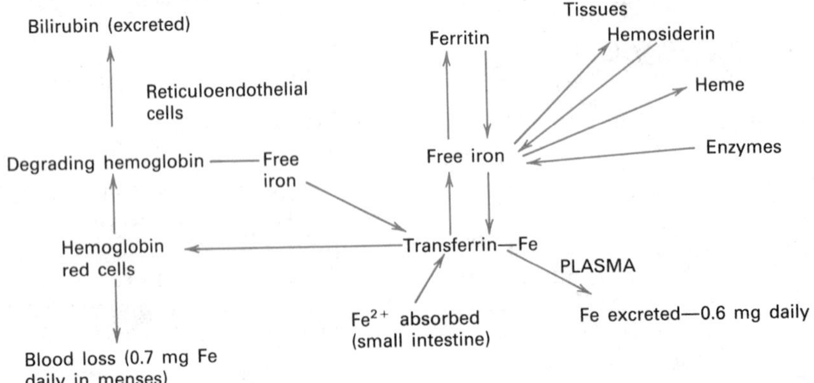

Figure 29-6 Iron transport and metabolism. (Guyton, A. C.: *Textbook of Medical Physiology*, Saunders, Philadelphia, 1976, p. 62.)

TABLE 29-7 ESTIMATED DIETARY IRON REQUIREMENTS

	mg/day[a]
Normal men and non-menstruating women	5–10
Menstruating women	7–20
Pregnant women	20–48[b]
Adolescents	10–20
Children	4–10
Infants	1.5 mg/kg[c]

SOURCE: Herbert, V.: "The Nutritional Anemias," *Hospital Practice,* **15**(3):66, March 1980.

[a] Assuming 10% absorption.
[b] More than can be derived from diet: mandates iron supplementation in latter half of pregnancy.
[c] To maximum of 15 mg.

2. In severe anemia, shortness of breath upon exertion and tachycardia may be noted.
3. A complete dietary history should be obtained. If a small amount of animal protein is eaten or if clay (pica) and starch are ingested, these may be the source of the deficiency. Often clients have low levels of income or do not feel like properly preparing meals.
4. Any history of previous anemias should be checked in both the client and the family members.
5. Menstrual histories are important. Recent pregnancies and any difficulties with pregnancies should be noted.
6. Chronic bleeding, diarrhea, malabsorption syndromes, or gastric surgery should be investigated, as any recent problem may be related to the cause of this anemia.
7. Clients may have a history of a recent infection or nonbacterial inflammation, such as rheumatoid arthritis.
8. Regular blood donation can result in iron loss.
9. Iron deficiency anemia may be observed more frequently in young adults and teen-agers due to poor dietary intake.

Physical Assessment

(Refer to Table 29-2.)

1. The client will appear pale.
2. The mucous membranes and conjunctiva are pale, and the normal redness in the palms of the hands is missing.
3. Inflammation of the mucosa of the mouth (stomatitis), cracks in the corner of the mouth, and glossitis (atrophy of the papillae of the tongue) are often seen.
4. The skin is dry.
5. Flattening or concavity of the nails (koilonychia) may be noted, along with brittleness of the hair and nails (see Figure 29-7).
6. There may be a slight enlargement of the liver noted upon palpation.
7. Because another health problem (e.g., carcinoma, vascular occlusions, rectal bleeding) may be the primary cause of the anemia, a complete physical is essential.

Diagnostic Tests

1. Blood studies reveal:
   a. Red blood cells are microcytic and hypochromic.
   b. Blood hemoglobin is reduced.
   c. A decrease in the serum iron level may be found.
   d. Any one of these tests (a) iron stores, (b) iron binding capacities, or (c) serum ferritin level, which determines the serum saturation of transferrin, can be used to determine iron deficiency anemia (refer to Figure 29-8).
2. On bone marrow examination, hemosiderin (an insoluble form of storage iron) is absent.
3. Stool may demonstrate the presence of occult blood.
4. Once diagnosed, additional studies may be necessary to determine the cause of the ane-

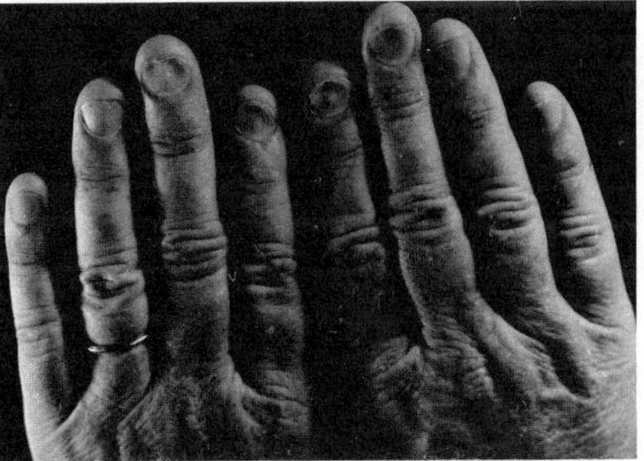

Figure 29-7 Spoonlike concavity of the fingernails seen in iron deficiency anemia (koilonychia). (Courtesy of Dr. Wayne Rundles.)

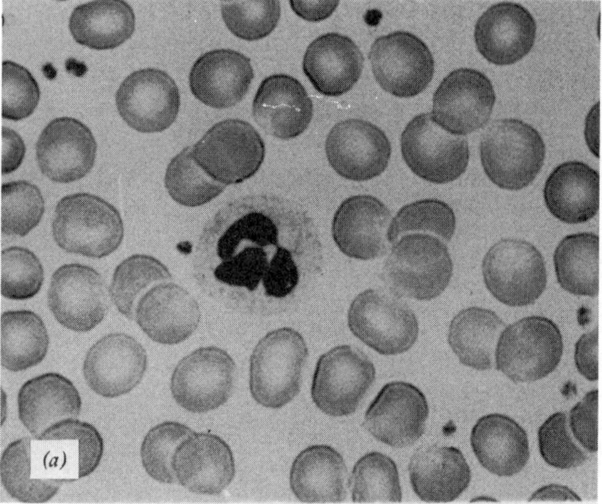

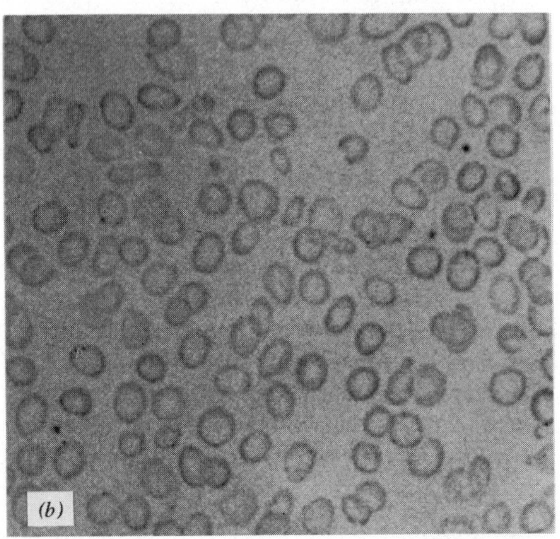

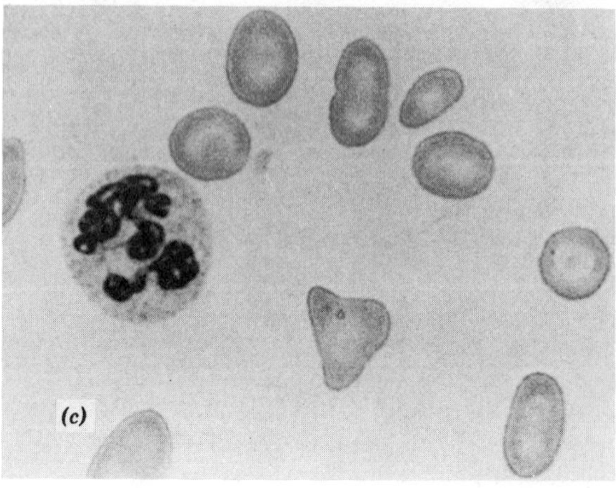

mia, for example, gastrointestinal. If gastrointestinal bleeding is suspected, numerous diagnostic tests must be performed. X-ray studies of the gastrointestinal tract, stool examinations for occult blood, and gastroscopy and sigmoidoscopy examinations may be done.

NURSING DIAGNOSES: ACTUAL OR POTENTIAL

1. Potential alterations in comfort: due to glossitis, headaches, and possible gastrointestinal disturbances from iron therapy.
2. Nutritional alteration deficit: due to inadequate intake of foods high in iron.
3. Knowledge deficit: regarding the need to find the source of the deficiency.
4. Decreased activity tolerance: due to fatigue and dyspnea.
5. Potential for infection: increased.
6. Noncompliance: due to knowledge deficit.

EXPECTED OUTCOMES

1. The underlying cause of the anemia will be determined and corrected within a specified amount of time (e.g., client will have a decrease in symptoms of iron deficiency within 1 month, as indicated by client interview, physical assessment, and evaluation of response to therapy).
2. Client will give evidence of compliance with plan of care by:
   a. Adhering to medication and therapy regimens, as evidenced by medical and client and family records.
   b. Demonstrating understanding of adequate nutrition to supplement and increase food iron intake, as evidenced by a dietary log and by discussion with the dietitian.

Figure 29-8 Blood smears of normal peripheral blood, iron deficiency anemia, and folate deficiency. In contrast to the normal peripheral blood smear (*a*) with normochromic, normocytic red cells, that of iron deficiency anemia (*b*) reveals hypochromic, microcytic cells. Seen in the smear from a client with megaloblastic anemia (*c*) are the macroovalocytes and a hypersegmented polymorphonuclear leukocyte, characteristic of B_{12} or folate deficiency. (Herbert, V.: "The Nutritional Anemias," *Hospital Practice*, **15**(3):82, 83, March 1980.)

c. Indicating, using recall, early symptoms of recurrence.

INTERVENTIONS

1. Teach the client about test procedures; provide support and comfort during and after tests. Encourage the client and family to ask any questions they might have regarding diagnostic tests or the disorder.
2. Administer iron orally or parenterally.
   a. Oral medications, such as ferrous sulfate, 0.2 g, or ferrous gluconate, 0.3 g, tid after meals, are preferred. Enteric-coated preparations reduce gastric irritability.
   b. Give iron salts following food as they are gastric irritants. Some dyspepsia may result anyway; however, do not give salts with milk, as absorption will not take place.
   c. Because liquid iron preparations stain the teeth, dilute them and administer through a straw.
   d. Inform the client that iron will make stools appear tarry or dark green and that this is a harmless side effect.
   e. Ascorbic acid will help to promote iron absorption; give vitamin C or orange juice with the iron preparations.
   f. Instruct the client regarding the importance of following a diet high in iron. Foods high in iron include red meat (e.g., liver, kidney), egg yolk, leafy green vegetables like spinach, dried fruits, and iron-fortified cereals.
   g. Administer parenteral iron therapy only when it is necessary because of oral intolerance or continual blood loss. Give iron dextran (Imferon) in doses of 100–250 mg daily or every other day on demand.
      (1) Take care to prevent the medication's leaking into the tissues. To accomplish this, use a double-needle technique, using 0.5 mL of an air bubble to follow injection while skin surface is moved to the side and maintained in that position.
      (2) The Z-tract injection technique is usually used.
         (a) Insert needle at a 90-degree angle; inject material; hold needle in place for 5–10 s following injection of medication; withdraw.
         (b) Movement increases absorption. Warn client to avoid excessive exercise or constricting garments. Do not massage the skin surrounding an injection site.
         (c) Check previous sites for complications (e.g., hemorrhage, skin staining) throughout the course of therapy.
   h. Inform client that iron therapy will be necessary for 2 to 3 months after the hemoglobin returns to normal because the iron stores replenish at a slower rate.
      (a) Instruct the client especially regarding iron overload (hemosiderin). Warn the client that additional iron preparations (e.g., vitamins) may cause iron overload and heart failure.
      (b) Treatment of hemosiderin includes administration of deferoxamine, which chelates with iron, and a phlebotomy.
3. Refer to the other anemias for further interventions.

EVALUATION

Outcome Criteria

1. The cause of the anemia has been determined and is being treated. Signs and symptoms of the deficiency have resolved.
2. Compliance to therapeutic plan can be measured by return of normal blood values (hemoglobin level), verbal reports of dietary change, increased activity tolerance, absence of glossitis.
3. Client is taking ferrous sulfate daily, has improved dietary iron intake, and knows the signs and symptoms of recurrence.
4. There is an absence of infection.

Complications

1. Complications are rare.
2. Recurrence of anemia is often seen in cases where iron deficiency was treated, but the underlying cause was not.
3. Persons at risk should be followed because they may be in the early stages and may develop the deficiency later.
4. Iron deficiency may cause folic acid deficiency due to increased red blood cell hemolysis, thus increasing the amount of folate needed to regenerate the cells. The deficiency may also appear in conjunction with vitamin B_{12} deficiency.

HYPOPROTHROMBINEMIA

Hypoprothrombinemia is a disorder characterized by a deficient amount of circulating prothrombin. Prothrombin is produced in the liver, and the presence of vitamin K is necessary for prothrombin synthesis to take place. If a person is vitamin K deficient, it may be due to improper diet, gastrointestinal tract disorders that interfere with vitamin K absorption, extensive liver damage, or antibiotic therapy that sterilizes the bowel and thus prevents vitamin K production. Dicumarol, an anticoagulant, can cause hypoprothrombinemia in toxic doses by interfering with the conversion of vitamin K to prothrombin.

The health history may be vague, with the client complaining of minor bleeding episodes or ecchymosis following minimal trauma. On examination, ecchymosis may be present and blood studies reveal an elevated prothrombin time. Hematuria and gastrointestinal bleeding may be overt symptoms. Treatment includes administration of a vitamin K supplement, such as menadiol sodium diphosphate (Synkayvite), 5 mg IM, or phytonadione (Mephyton), 5 mg PO, for minor bleeding. For more severe bleeding, larger doses of phytonadione (as Aquamephyton), 10–15 mg, can be given IV. Prothrombin can be replaced directly by transfusion.

INFLAMMATIONS

INFECTIOUS MONONUCLEOSIS

Infectious mononucleosis (also known as *glandular fever*) is a common, benign condition seen most often in young adults from 17 to 25 years of age. It is very prevalent among college students. The cause is believed to be a herpeslike virus, known as the Epstein-Barr virus (EBV), and transmission is probably due to oral contact with saliva exchange. Although infectious mononucleosis is an acute, but self-limiting disease, its symptoms are varied and its effects are seen throughout the body. The incubation period is approximately 30 to 50 days, and the onset of symptoms may be gradual.

The *health history* of a person affected with mononucleosis reveals:

1. Decreased rest, poor eating habits, increasing fatigue, and exposure to an individual having similar symptoms are not uncommon.
2. Early complaints include chills, headache, and malaise.
3. There may also be nausea, loss of appetite, and distaste for cigarettes.
4. In 80 percent of reported cases, the classic triad is fever, sore throat, and swollen lymph nodes.

The diagnosis of infectious mononucleosis is based on both the clinical picture and blood test results. Upon *physical assessment*, the following conditions are commonly present.

1. The pharynx is usually reddened, with infected mucous membranes near the tonsils.
2. Exudate, petechiae, and white patches may be noted on the palates.
3. Cervical lymph nodes are enlarged and palpable bilaterally. This may be in conjunction with enlarged axillary and inguinal nodes.
4. In severe cases, the liver and spleen are palpable.

Characteristic findings of the *diagnostic blood tests* (most often seen within 10 days) are:

1. Leukocytosis, with a white blood cell count of 12,000 to 18,000 per cubic millimeter, of which 60 percent are large, atypical lymphocytes (Down cells).
2. A positive heterophil agglutination test.
3. The presence of EBV antibodies.

Interventions should focus on relieving the problems and preventing complications. The prognosis for infectious mononucleosis is usually excellent. However, no specific interventions hasten the process. Therefore, providing comfort and symptomatic intervention are of primary concern, as convalescence varies.

1. Strongly encourage the client to get plenty of bed rest until the fever, headache, and fatigue decrease.
2. Warn the client not to engage in any strenuous activity, as this may result in a decrease in resistance to infection or may cause a splenic rupture.
3. Admonish the client to avoid blows to the abdomen, lifting, and straining.

4. Decrease the fever and discomfort of the sore throat and swollen glands in order to improve client's appetite and relieve dysphagia. Aspirin or other analgesics and warm saline gargles, along with cool sponge baths and a large fluid intake, will help.
5. Encourage intake of nutritious foods with a high-protein and high-vitamin content. These foods should be nonirritating to the throat and might include soup, milk shakes, fruit juices, and soft cheeses.
6. Adrenocortical steroid treatment, such as prednisone, and intravenous therapy may be indicated if the throat swelling is severe.
7. Isolate the client from possible sources of infection, as a secondary streptococcal infection of the throat is not uncommon. Note any increase in throat pain or fever so that antibiotic therapy may be started.

Although infectious mononucleosis is a benign condition, serious *complications* can occur.

1. Splenic rupture is always of concern in the acute phase of infectious mononucleosis. The two major indicators are abdominal pain, left-sided and radiating, and shock.
2. Tachycardia is often present. If this occurs, an emergency splenectomy is necessary.
3. Acute airway obstruction can occur with extreme hyperplasia of the pharyngeal tissue.
4. Neurological manifestations with central nervous system involvement can be seen in the presence of these severe changes.

OBSTRUCTIONS

PURPURA (VASCULAR)

Purpura is the name given to a group of disorders characterized by the appearance of ecchymoses or small hemorrhages (petechiae) in various places on the body or mucous membranes. The causes are unknown or poorly understood. Often the platelet count and function are normal, so the hemorrhages are believed to be associated with the inability of the blood vessels, usually capillaries, to maintain integrity. Thus, the blood is permitted to seep into the subcutaneous tissue. This postulated abnormality in the vascular factors involved in hemostasis may be in conjunction with increases in fragility and permeability. The causes are varied: an autoimmune reaction, due to allergy or specific drugs (iodine, belladonna); bacterial or viral infection (subacute bacterial endocarditis, Rocky Mountain spotted fever); hereditary or acquired structural disorders (Cushing's disease, scurvy); or a result of various disease processes, such as certain skin or chronic diseases (refer to Table 29-8).

Diagnosis of purpura is usually made by exclusion. The client may have a *health history* of:

1. Bleeding, either acute or chronic, (a familial history may be indicated).
2. Hepatic, splenic, or renal disease.
3. Anticoagulant therapy, which is known to interfere with platelet or bone marrow marrow function.
4. Bruising or spontaneous bleeding into the tissues.

TABLE 29-8 PURPURAS

1. Vascular
   a. Nonthrombocytopenic purpura.
      (1) Purpura simplex.
      (2) Mechanical purpura.
      (3) Orthostatic purpura.
      (4) Senile purpura.
      (5) Adrenocortical hyperfunction.
      (6) Hereditary disorders of connective tissue.
      (7) Scurvy.
      (8) Purpura associated with dysproteinemia.
      (9) Purpura associated with infections.
   b. Autoerythrocyte sensitivity.
   c. DNA sensitivity.
   d. Allergic purpura.
2. Hereditary hemorrhagic telangiectasia.
3. Thrombocytopenic purpura.
   a. Idiopathic thrombocytopenic purpura.
   b. Secondary thrombocytopenic purpura.

SOURCE: Williams, W. J., et al.: *Hematology*, 2d ed., McGraw-Hill, New York, 1977, p. 1313.

5. Other associated findings, such as pain and gastrointestinal bleeding; however, the incidence varies widely depending on the process involved. Upon *physical assessment*, hemorrhages are usually seen on the extremities, face, or groin area or at the site of noted trauma. *Blood studies* usually are not definitive.

Interventions should include the following.

1. Continuous observation of the client for signs of bleeding is imperative. Teach the client and family to:
   a. Watch for signs of internal hemorrhage, including weakness, dizziness, tachycardia, abdominal pain, and confusion.
   b. Treat nosebleeds and cuts immediately.
   c. Check urine and stools for frank blood.
   d. Examine the skin and mucous membranes for petechiae or ecchymoses.
2. Instruct the client always to carry an identification card that states the type of blood disorder, blood type, and his or her physician's name.
3. Warn the client to prevent trauma by avoiding extreme heat and dehydration, straining, and lifting heavy objects.
4. Instruct the client to maintain meticulous skin care.
5. Teach the client to apply pressure to the site of a cut for several minutes and to check the site often. A pressure dressing may be needed.
6. Stools should be kept soft to prevent trauma of the rectal mucosa; advise use of laxatives or stool softeners as needed.
7. Instruct the client to use only electric razors and soft-bristled toothbrushes.
8. Advise the client that dietary modification, to prevent mucous membrane and gastrointestinal urinary irritation, may be needed.
9. Instruct the client's family regarding purpura, its complications, and how they can help and support the client in maintaining as normal a lifestyle as possible.

IDIOPATHIC THROMBOCYTOPENIC PURPURA

The cause of idiopathic thrombocytopenic purpura (ITP) is unknown, but the major theory is that autoantibodies sensitize platelets, making them vulnerable to premature destruction by the spleen, or that the autoantibodies interfere with the production of platelets. Chronic ITP affects all ages and more women than men; acute ITP is most common in children (refer to Chapter 18).

The *health history* is usually not indicative of any obvious sources; however, it often reveals:

1. Clients with leukemia, aplastic anemia, or a history of infections, of taking certain types of drugs (e.g., myelosuppressive or estrogens), or of radiation exposure are known to have an increased risk of developing ITP.
2. Certain nutritional deficiencies, such as folic acid or pernicious anemia, may also increase the risk (McFarlane, 1982).
3. The most common physical manifestations are petechiae, especially on the distal parts of extremities, and minor bleeding episodes. The bleeding may have been noted for years (e.g., spontaneous nosebleeds, gingival bleeding, epistaxis, or menorrhagia).
4. Fatigue may be present.
5. In more advanced cases, dyspnea, decreased joint movement, and pain are added complaints.

Upon *physical assessment*, in addition to the petechiae and ecchymosis, the liver and spleen may be palpable.

Blood studies (see Table 29-9) reveal:

1. A decreased platelet count, below 200,000 per cubic millimeter.
2. A prolonged bleeding time (clot retraction test).
3. An increased capillary fragility.
4. A normal prothrombin time.

Interventions include control of the bleeding and rest.

1. Adrenocortical steroids, such as prednisone, 10–20 mg qid, increase the platelet count, thus reducing the bleeding tendency. Platelet transfusions have been used (refer to Chapter 17) for care of the client who is receiving steroids.
2. If steroids are not effective or if large doses are necessary, a splenectomy is done. After a splenectomy, 80 percent of the clients improve or go into a remission.
3. Immunosuppression has been used with

TABLE 29-9 LABORATORY TESTS USED IN THE DIAGNOSIS OF HEMATOLOGIC DISORDERS

Name of Test	Purpose	Normal Values	Interpretation of Findings
Bleeding time (Bl time)	Measures rate of platelet clot formation after small puncture wound.	3–8 min in adults	Bleeding over 10 min is abnormal; prolonged bleeding occurs in vascular maladies, thrombocytopenia, and after aspirin ingestion.
Platelet count	Measures number of circulating platelets in venous or arterial blood.	250,000–450,000/ mm^3	Low count results in prolonged bleeding time and impaired clot retraction; diagnostic of thrombocytopenia.
Partial thromboplastin time (PTT)	Complex method for testing normalcy of coagulation process; employed to identify deficiencies of coagulation factors, prothrombin, and fibrinogen.	39–53 s	Prolongation of time indicates coagulation disorder due to deficiency of a coagulation factor; not diagnostic for platelet disorders.
Prothrombin time (Pro time)	Determines activity and interaction of factors V, VII, X, prothrombin, and fibrinogen; used to determine dosages of anticoagulant drugs.	12–15 s (one-stage method)	Prolongation of time indicates client is receiving anticoagulants; abnormally low fibrinogen concentration; deficiencies of factors II, VII, V, and X; presence of circulating anticoagulants as seen in lupus erythematosus; impaired prothrombin activity.
Coagulation (clotting time)	Crude measure of coagulation process in venous blood; used to control heparin therapy.	9–12 min (Lee-White method)	Prolonged time occurs in severe coagulation problems; therapeutic administration of heparin.
Thromboplastin generation test (TGT)	Measures generation of thromboplastin; if result is abnormal, second stage is done to identify missing coagulation factor.	12 s or less (100%)	Abnormal values are found in hemophilia.
Clot retraction	Indicates function and number of platelets; measures time needed for contraction of an undisturbed clot.	Clot retraction begins within 2 h and is finished within 24 h.	Clot retraction is retarded in thrombocytopenia; clot is small and soft in thromobocythenia (functional disturbance of platelets).
Tourniquet test (Rumpel-Leede test; capillary fragility test)	Crude test of vascular resistance and platelet number and function; done by placing blood pressure cuff on arm for 5 min and then counting petechiae.	No petechiae	Petechiae appear in thrombocytopenia and vascular purpura.

SOURCE: Adapted from Luckmann, J., and Sorensen, K. C.: *Medical-Surgical Nursing, A Psychophysiologic Approach*, 2d ed., Saunders, Philadelphia, 1980, p. 1076.

some success in clients who did not respond well to the splenectomy (Williams et al., 1977).

Complications include hemorrhages, especially cerebral. Rest and prevention of undue stress through excess activity, sneezing, or straining are necessary.

DISSEMINATED INTRAVASCULAR COAGULATION

Disseminated intravascular coagulation (DIC) is an acute disorder that is characterized by widespread fibrin deposits in capillaries and arterioles and hemolysis of platelets, thrombin, and other clotting factors that results in bleeding. The excessive clotting to retard the bleeding activates the fibrinolytic mechanism to produce fibrin split end products, thus further inhibiting platelet clotting and ultimately leading to more bleeding. The result is decreased blood flow and increased tissue damage due to microcirculatory obstruction and hypoperfusion of organs. The cause of DIC is not understood, but it is related to thromboplastic substances that are released into the blood. This may be due to certain chronic disease states, obstetric complications (e.g., abruptio placentae), surgical trauma, gram-negative sepsis, or shock, or may be seen after rapid transfusion of a large amount of blood. DIC may last for several hours or days. Unless this process can be reversed, death will ensue due to severe renal problems and/or hemorrhage.

The *health history* may not be indicative of the onset of disseminated intravascular coagulation. Nevertheless:

1. Questioning regarding specific predisposing factors (e.g., infections, malignant diseases, heat stroke, burns, and obstetrical complications) should be included.
2. Bleeding, if noted, should be carefully assessed as to the type, severity, location, and mode of onset.

Physical assessment will reveal:

1. Petechiae or ecchymotic areas on the skin and mucous membranes.
2. Hemorrhaging may be overt.
3. Signs of shock, including oliguria and seizures, may be present and confuse the diagnosis.

Blood studies indicate:

1. A prolonged prothrombin time.
2. A low platelet count.
3. The lack of blood coagulation.

Interventions focus on immediate treatment of the underlying condition that initiated DIC.

1. Heparin is administered to block coagulation.
2. The consumed clotting components are replaced after heparin is started. Platelet concentrates, fresh or fresh-frozen plasma, and fibrinogen are used.
3. Bleeding and shock, if present, are treated.

Complications of organ injuries resulting from DIC are often seen.

DEGENERATIVE DISORDERS

HEMOPHILIA

The hemophilias are relatively rare disorders characterized by a defective mechanism in the coagulation process. The most common is *hemophilia A*, or *classic hemophilia*, which is a deficiency or nonfunction of factor VIII. This represents approximately 80 percent of the inherited coagulation disorders. The other type of hemophilia seen is *hemophilia B*, which is a factor IX, or "Christmas" factor, deficiency (refer to Figure 29-9). Hemophilia is a sex-linked recessive trait seen almost exclusively in males, although females are carriers. However, approximately one-third of the people with hemophilia have no family history of the disease. The severity of the clotting defect can range from mild to severe and is manifested by prolonged bleeding from trauma to the tissues and joints. Hemophilias are classified as childhood disorders, but because of new developments in treatment this disease now extends into adulthood.

A thorough *health history* is extremely important for clients with suspected hemophilia.

1. A family history of "bleeders" maybe is indicative of hemophilia, as the genetic defect is hereditary.
2. Any association of bleeding episodes with other illnesses, procedures, drugs, and diet should be noted, along with age of onset.
3. A detailed description of all past operations (dental extractions or surgery) and traumas and the duration of bleeding in relation to the above are significant.

The client may exhibit a variety of signs and symptoms, as this disorder varies in severity from family to family. The *physical assessment*, however, usually confirms the health history.

1. The client exhibits signs of current or past hemorrhage.
2. Characteristics of chronic joint deformities,

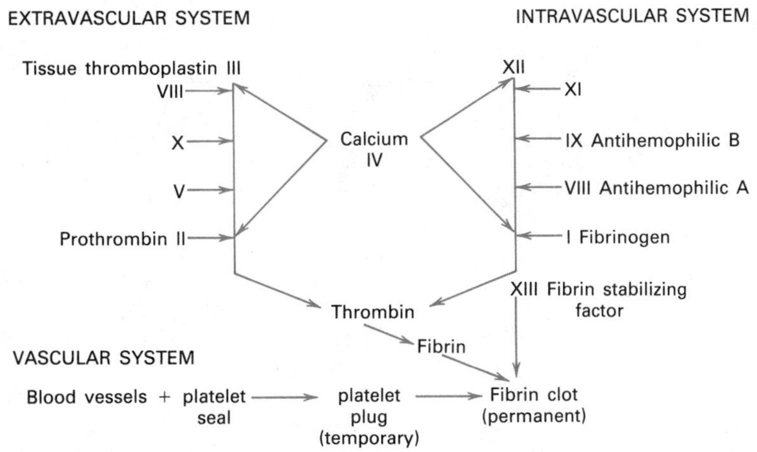

EXTRAVASCULAR SYSTEM

INTRAVASCULAR SYSTEM

Tissue thromboplastin III
VIII
X
V
Prothrombin II
Calcium IV
XII
XI
IX Antihemophilic B
VIII Antihemophilic A
I Fibrinogen
XIII Fibrin stabilizing factor
Thrombin
Fibrin

VASCULAR SYSTEM

Blood vessels + platelet seal → platelet plug (temporary) → Fibrin clot (permanent)

Figure 29-9 Sequence of coagulation. Factor VIII, known as the antihemophilic factor A of antihemophilic globulin (AHG), is a plasma globulin derivation necessary for thromboplastin formation and the change of prothrombin to thrombin. Factor IX, known as the Christmas factor, antihemophilic factor B, or plasma thromboplastin component, has its source in the liver and influences production of thromboplastin. Both factors will demonstrate a normal prothrombin time and an abnormal partial thromboplastin time. (Jones, D. A., et al.: *Medical-Surgical Nursing: A Conceptual Approach*, McGraw-Hill, New York, 1978, p. 807.)

due to hemarthrosis, or bleeding into the joint may be noted.

3. Contractures or muscle atrophy may be present, along with hematuria, epistaxis, hematemesis, and melena.
4. Severe abdominal pain and bruising are common.

Diagnostic tests include:

1. Screening tests for coagulation factors to determine the type of bleeding disorder and to distinguish between factor VIII and factor IX deficiencies.
2. Blood studies to show a prolonged partial thromboplastin (PTT) and prothrombin time (PT).
3. X-ray studies of the joints.

Interventions include:

1. The missing factor is replaced by transfusions of fresh or fresh-frozen whole blood or plasma.
2. Antihemophilic factor (AHF) levels can be raised by administration of commercial AHF concentrates such as cryoprecipitate and Hemophil (self-infusion is possible in some states).
3. Prophylactic treatment of the missing factors before surgery or dental extractions is necessary.
4. Trauma must be avoided and the client educated to prevent bleeding episodes.
5. Bleeding can be delayed for periods of time in hemophilia, and the manifestations of that bleeding are not seen until much later, so continual observation for internal bleeding is important.
6. Topical bleeding can be controlled by pressure, using Gelfoam or hemostatics such as thrombin.
7. Clients must identify the fact that they have hemophilia to doctors, teachers, dentists, and employers. An identification card should be carried.
8. Hemarthrosis is treated with AHF or whole blood administration, rest, protection (sometimes in a cast), and ice.
9. Adrenocortical steroids may reduce joint inflammation.

The major *complication* associated with hemophilia is that repeated transfusion and AHF therapy will cause the client to become sensitized to AHF and to develop autoimmune anticoagulants (anti-AHF factor). This client will not respond to further therapy and consequently dies as a result of hemorrhaging.

HEMOLYTIC ANEMIAS

DESCRIPTION

Hemolytic anemia is a broad descriptive name given to numerous diseases characterized by a shortened erythrocyte life span. It is caused by increased destruction by the reticuloendothelial elements and failure of the bone marrow to produce sufficient erythrocytes to compensate for the vast numbers of red cells destroyed. Much about these diseases is yet unknown; however, they are most often classified as either hereditary, or intracorpuscular, or acquired, or extracorpuscular, defects.

A *hereditary,* or *intracorpuscular, defect* takes place within the erythrocyte. The genetic result is usually due to (1) defects in the red cell membrane, (2) defects of the glycolysis and related metabolic system enzymes, (3) defects of the hemoglobin molecule and its synthesis, and (4) defects in the immune response to the erythrocyte. An *acquired,* or *extracorpuscular, defect* is due to factors or mechanisms external to the erythrocyte, such as drugs, plasma components, infections, chemical or physical agents (refer to Table 29-10).

Hemolytic anemias are found in all age groups and both sexes. The anemia may be acute or chronic, mild or severe, depending on the rate of hemolysis. Racial and geographic factors are noted in many of the diseases.

In adults, *hereditary spherocytosis,* or congenital hemolytic jaundice, is one type of hemolytic anemia seen, characterized by spherocytes (spherically shaped erythrocytes) in the blood smear and increased osmotic fragility. *Glucose 6-phosphate dehydrogenase* (G6PD) deficiency is rare and appears to be an enzymatic sex-linked defect that is manifested in response to certain chemical oxidants, such as food and drugs. The problem maybe observed in greater numbers in th population carrying the sickle cell trait (see Chapter 18). *Thalassemia* is a biochemical defect in hemoglobin synthesis characterized by target cells and an insufficient number of polypeptide chains. *Autoimmune hemolytic anemia* is an acquired defect, the exact mechanism of which is not known. It is theorized to result from an alteration in the red cell antigen, to be a cross-reaction of that antigen, or to be induced by the lymphoid cells that produce antibodies against normal red cells.

Hemolytic "crisis" is often characterized by fever, abdominal discomfort, nausea, and vomiting. Comfort measures are referred to under the other anemias; other care for anemia is discussed under the other anemias (refer to *Metabolic Disorders* in this chapter).

PREVENTION

Health Promotion

1. Education of persons with certain cultural and ethnic backgrounds as to the signs and symptoms of the disease.
2. Avoidance of exposure to infection and radiation.

Population at Risk

1. Certain factors of race, sex, age, and geography increase the risk of disease.
   a. Glucose 6-phosphate dehydrogenase is believed to be sex linked and is manifested in blacks and persons of Mediterranean extraction.
   b. Thalassemia major and sickle cell anemia are first seen in children. Thalassemia is common in blacks and those of Mediterranean, southern Chinese, or central African heritage (refer to Chapter 18).
2. Persons with certain infections and those exposed to certain chemicals and drugs have a higher incidence of hemolytic anemia.

Screening

Disease-specific blood studies could be done (refer to Figure 29-10).

ASSESSMENT

Health History

1. The major complaints of clients with hemolytic anemia are those common to most anemias: weakness and fatigue. Dypsnea of exertion may also be noticed.
2. If the client is in hemolytic crisis (which may be precipitated by an acute infection), ma-

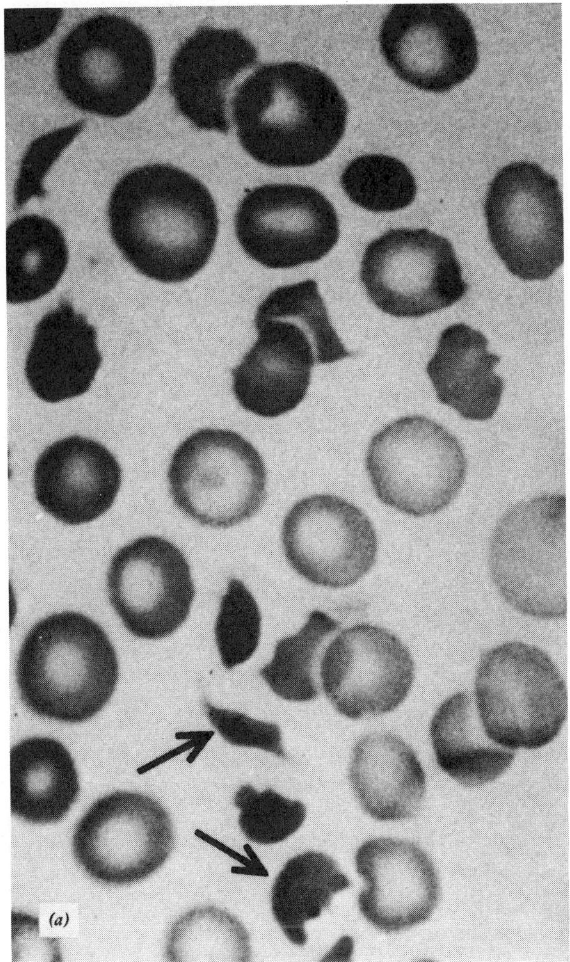

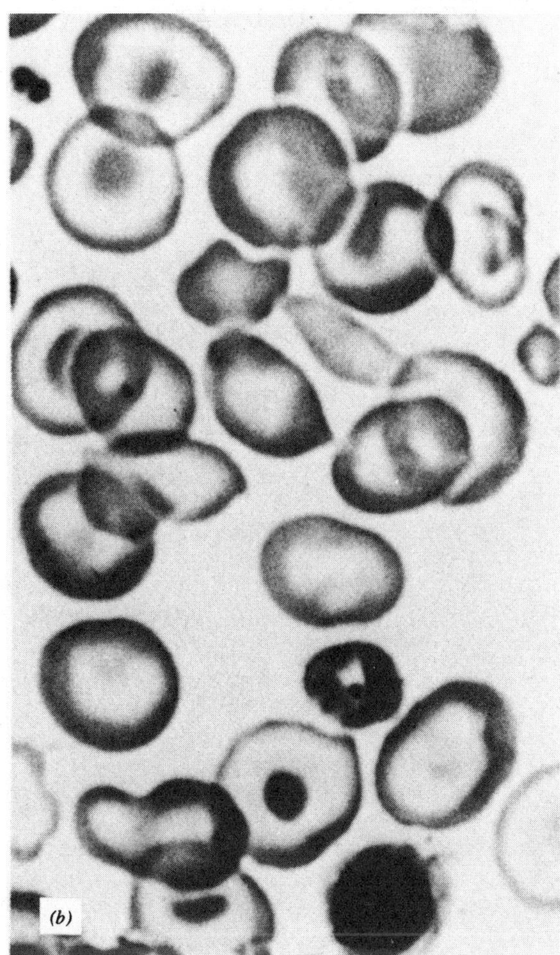

Figure 29-10 Blood smears of hemolytic anemia. (*a*) Microangiopathic hemolytic anemia is a result of mechanical trauma to red cells. Intravascular hemolysis is associated with the presence of strikingly abnormal RBCs, for example, schistocytes, or helmet cells (arrows). (*b*) Characteristic blood smear of thalassemia shows marked hypochromia, target cells (upper left), poikilocytes (abnormally shaped red cells), and nucleated red cells. (Forget, B. G.: "Hemolytic Anemias: Congenital and Acquired," *Hospital Practice*, **15**(4):76–77, April 1980.)

laise, chills, fever, aches, and pains in the back and abdomen may accompany the complaint of fatigue.

3. A strong family history of certain kinds of hemolytic anemias or signs and symptoms in other family members may be noted, including a history of jaundice, gallstones, or anemia. Some hemolytic anemias are genetic and sex linked.
4. Any bleeding episodes should be noted.

Physical Assessment

(Refer to Table 29-2.)

1. Pallor may be noted, along with jaundice. A slight scleral icterus may be the only observable sign.
2. Splenomegaly is present in inherited hemolytic anemias, except for sickle cell anemia.
3. Cholelithiasis is common, especially in hereditary spherocytosis.
4. Leg ulcers may be noted, especially around

TABLE 29-10 CLASSIFICATION OF COMMON HEMOLYTIC DISEASES

1. Hereditary or intracorpuscular hemolytic disorders.
   a. Erythrocyte membrane defects.
      (1) Hereditary spherocytosis.
      (2) Hereditary elliptocytosis.
      (3) Stomatocytosis.
   b. Enzyme deficiencies in the metabolic pathways.
      (1) Glucose 6-phosphate dehydrogenase (G6PD).
      (2) Pyruvate kinase.
   c. Defects in globin structure and synthesis.
      (1) Sickle cell anemia.
      (2) Thalassemia major.
2. Acquired or extracorpuscular hemolytic disorders.
   a. Immunohemolytic anemias.
      (1) Transfusion of incompatible blood.
      (2) Erythroblastosis fetalis.
      (3) Autoimmune hemolytic anemia due to warm-reactive antibodies.
         (a) Idiopathic.
         (b) "Secondary."
            (i) Virus and *Mycoplasma* infections.
            (ii) Lymphosarcoma, chronic lymphocytic leukemia.
            (iii) Other malignant diseases (e.g., hypertension).
            (iv) Systemic lupus erythematosus.
         (c) Drug-induced.
            (i) Quinidine.
            (ii) Penicillin.
            (iii) Methyldopa.
      (4) Autoimmune hemolytic anemia due to cold-reactive antibodies.
   b. Traumatic and microangiopathic hemolytic anemias.
      (1) Prosthetic valve replacement and cardiac abnormalities.
      (2) Thrombotic thrombocytopenic purpura.
      (3) Disseminated intravascular coagulation.
   c. Infections.
      (1) Malaria.
      (2) Bacteria.
      (3) Virus.
   d. Chemicals, drugs, and venoms.
      (1) Antimalarials.
      (2) Sulfonamides.
      (3) Antipyretics and analgesics.
      (4) Mothballs.
      (5) Fava beans.
      (6) Certain snake and spider venoms.
      (7) Mushrooms.
      (8) Lead poisoning.
   e. Physical agents.
      (1) Thermal injury.
      (2) Ionizing irradiation (questionable).
   f. Hypersplenism.

SOURCE: Adapted from Wintrobe, M. W., et al.: *Clinical Hematology*, 7th ed., Lea & Febiger, Philadelphia, 1975, p. 721.

the ankles. They are usually bilateral and are often seen in hereditary spherocytosis and sickle cell anemia.

5. Skeletal abnormalities of the skull and of the frontal and parietal bones are often observed in severe thalassemia major.
6. Clients having acquired hemolytic anemia may exhibit only pallor and a slight jaundice.

Diagnostic Tests

1. Blood studies reveal:
   a. Normocytic, normochromic anemia (an exception is thalassemia).
   b. Increased reticulocytes due to the efforts of the bone marrow to compensate for excessive erythrocyte destruction.
   c. Increased red cell fragility.
   d. Shortened erythrocyte life span.
   e. An increased serum lactate dehydrogenase (LDH) (often noted).
   f. Increased serum bilirubin.
2. The direct Coombs test can detect certain antigen-antibody reactions and can determine varieties of hemolytic anemia.
3. As a variety of disorders are found in the hemolytic anemias, further diagnostic tests

and exhaustive health histories must be obtained to diagnose causative factors (see Table 29-11).

4. Hyperplasma in the bone marrow is found upon examination.
5. Hemoglobinuria results from the excretion of hemoglobin into the urine. The urine appears pink to red to almost black. This can be distinguished from hematuria microscopically. Intravascular hemolysis is the major cause of hemoglobinuria.
6. Fecal and urine urobilinogen reflect the increased catabolism of cells with the resulting breakdown of hemoglobin.

NURSING DIAGNOSES: ACTUAL OR POTENTIAL

1. Potential impairment of urinary elimination: due to severe hemolysis, resulting in renal failure.
2. Self-care deficit: interrupted activities of daily living due to sickle cell crisis and anemia.

TABLE 29-11 DIAGNOSIS AND TREATMENT OF HEMOLYTIC ANEMIAS

Type of Anemia	Diagnosis	Therapy or Prevention
Hemolytic anemia in general	Complete blood count; reticulocytosis (5%); erythroid hyperplasia of bone marrow; unconjugated hyperbilirubinemia; increased urobilinogen in urine (and feces); decreased serum haptoglobulin level; possibly elevated LDH; shortened ^{51}Cr red cell survival.	See therapy for specific anemias, below
Intravascular hemolysis	Elevated free plasma hemoglobin; absent serum haptoglobin; decreased serum hemopexin; methemalbuminemia; hemoglobinuria; hemosiderin in urine	
Hereditary spherocytosis, elliptocytosis, stomatocytosis	Incubating osmotic fragility test	Splenectomy with prior antipneumococcal vaccination
Sickle cell syndromes	Screening tests (sickle cell prep. and solubility tests); hemoglobin electrophoresis	Treatment of complications; supportive therapy for anemia
Thalassemias	Hemoglobin electrophoresis; examination of cells from blood and bone marrow aspirate for inclusion bodies by supravital staining; inclusion bodies induced with the dye BCB in Hb H disease	Lifelong transfusions in beta-thalessemia major; folic acid replacement; splenectomy in some cases
G6PD enzyme deficiency	RBCs screened for ability to reduce dyes; quantitative assays, methemoglobulin elution slide test; cyanide ascorbate test of Jacob and Jandl	No specific therapy; avoidance of oxidant substances
Immune hemolytic anemias	Coombs test with broad and specific antisera	Treatment of any primary disease; corticosteroids; splenectomy; immunosuppressive drugs; avoidance of exposure to cold (in cold agglutinin disease)
Traumatic hemolytic anemias	Striking morphologic abnormalities in red cells and evidence of intravascular hemolysis (see above).	Primary disorder is treated to remove cause of trauma if possible; transfusions; splenectomy in cases of severe hypersplenism
Unstable hemoglobins	Supravital staining of blood preparation for Heinz bodies; heat-instability test; isopropanol stability test	Avoidance of oxidant chemicals and drugs; supportive therapy for anemia
Paroxysmal nocturnal hemoglobinuria (PNH)	Sucrose-water hemolysis test; Ham acid serum lysis test	No satisfactory therapy; repeated transfusions in severe cases; iron replacement
Pyruvate	Specific enzyme assays	No specific therapy

SOURCE: Forget, B. G.: "Hemolytic Anemias," *Hospital Practice,* **15**(4):73, April 1980.

3. Alterations in comfort: secondary to pain.
4. Decreased activity tolerence: due to fatigue and dyspnea.
5. Knowledge deficit: due to lack of understanding of the disease process.

EXPECTED OUTCOMES

1. Causative factors that may precipitate hemolysis, such as certain drugs and infections, will be eliminated.
2. Renal tubule necrosis will be prevented, as indicated by renal function and urine output, and anemia will be treated, as indicated by normalization of hemoglobin level and a decrease in fatigue.
3. Client will understand information regarding causative factors leading to disease process taught in teaching sessions, as indicated by recall.
4. Client will comply with the therapeutic plan and will verbalize increased knowledge of disease process.
5. There will be an increase in client's self-care ability.
6. Client will experience increased comfort and an absence of pain.

INTERVENTIONS

1. Once the diagnosis is made, elimination of the causative factor and client education as to the source are necessary.
2. Renal function and fluid and electrolyte balance must be maintained.
   a. Ensure that client takes in large amounts of water to dilute the effects of the red cells.
   b. Monitor input and output carefully and check electrolytes, as renal tubule absorption may be impaired.
   c. Administer intravenous therapy if necessary.
   d. Administer infusions of sodium bicarbonate or sodium lactate to alkalize the urine.
3. Treat anemia with blood transfusions as ordered. Caution must be used, as the transfused cells will rapidly be destroyed in clients with an autoimmune hemolytic disease.
   a. Administer adrenocortical steroids, such as prednisolone, as ordered, in 10- to 20-mg doses qid until normal hemoglobin levels return.
   b. Instruct clients to avoid infection while taking adrenocortical steroids.
4. A splenectomy is often the treatment of choice in hemolytic anemias. A measure of the severity of the disease can be determined by radioisotope infusion. This will help predict the success of a splenectomy.
5. Administer immunosuppressive drugs as ordered if adrenocortical steroids and/or a splenectomy are not successful.

EVALUATION

Outcome Criteria

1. Causative factors have been eliminated. Continual follow-up is necessary to prevent recurrence. The prognosis of the disease varies, but in certain disorders, such as thalassemia minor and hereditary spherocytosis, the prognosis is very good.
2. The signs and symptoms of the disease process have decreased. Renal function studies, hemoglobin level, and urine output are within normal limits.
3. Client and family education regarding the disorder has been completed.

REFERENCES

Goldstein, M.: "The Aplastic Anemias," *Hospital Practice*, **15**(5):85, 86, May 1980.

Herbert, V.: "The Nutritional Anemias," *Hospital Practice*, **15**(3):66, 73, March 1980.

Johnson, B. L. and Hubbard, S. M.: "The Leukemias and Lymphomas," in D. A. Jones, et al. (eds.): *Medical-Surgical Nursing: A Conceptual Approach*, McGraw-Hill, New York, 1978, pp. 243–246.

McFarlane, J. M.: "Disturbances in the Oxygen Carrying Mechanism," in D. A. Jones, et al. (eds.): *Medical-Surgical Nursing: A Conceptual Approach*, 2d ed., McGraw-Hill, New York, 1982, p. 804.

Ten-State Nutrition Survey, 1968–1970, DHEW Publication No. (HSM) 72-8134. Health Services and Mental Health Administration, Washington, D.C., 1972.

Williams, W. J., et al.: *Hematology*, 2d ed., McGraw-Hill, New York, 1977, p. 1055.

BIBLIOGRAPHY

Brain, M. C.: "Hemolytic Anemia: A Systematic Approach to Management," *Postgraduate Medicine*, **64**:127–136, October 1978. This article discusses treatment for the intrinsic and extrinsic causes of hemolytic anemia.

Centers for Disease Control: "Update on Acquired Immune Deficiency Syndrome" *MMWR*, **31**(37):507–508, 513–514, 1982.

———: "Acquired Immune Deficiency Syndrome (AIDS): Precautions for Clinical and Laboratory Staffs," *MMWR*, **31**(43):577–580, 1982.

———: "Prevention of Acquired Immune Deficiency Syndrome (AIDS): Report of Inter-Agency Recommendations," *MMWR* **32**(8):101–103, 1983.

The above reports provide current information available at the CDC, where active research on AIDS continues.

Flynn, K. T.: "Iron Deficiency Anemia Among the Elderly," *Nurse Practitioner: The American Journal of Primary Health Care*, **3**(6):20–24, November–December 1978. A logical presentation of diagnosis and interventions for iron deficiency anemia in the elderly.

Forget, B. G.: "Hemolytic Anemias: Congenital and Acquired," *Hospital Practice*, **15**(4):67–78, April 1980. A discussion of the wide variety of causative factors and therapy in hemolytic anemia.

Goldstein, M.: "The Aplastic Anemias," *Hospital Practices*, **15**(5):85–96, May 1980. This article discusses the alternative treatments of bone marrow transplantation, androgen administration, and antithymocyte globulin administration.

Herbert, V.: "The Nutritional Anemias," *Hospital Practice*, **15**(3):65–89, March 1980. An excellent presentation of folate, iron, and vitamin B_{12} anemias with a major focus on iron deficiency.

Jacob, H. S.: "Severe Bone Marrow Failure: Possible Pathophysiologic Mechanisms," *Postgraduate Medicine*, **64**:97–99, October 1978. A discussion of pathophysiological mechanisms, such as damage to microenvironment stem cells, viral damage, marrow infarction, and marrow replacement with inflammatory tissue.

Keating, M. J., et al.: "Acute Leukemia," *CA: A Cancer Journal for Clinicians*, **27**:2, February 1977. An excellent discussion of acute lymphocytic and myelocytic leukemia, including diagnosis, treatment, and supportive care.

McCredie, K. B.: "Current Concepts in Acute Leukemia," *Postgraduate Medicine*, **61**:221, January 1977. An interesting discussion of maintenance of remission using combinations of chemotherapy.

Najean, Y., et al.: "Prognostic Factors in Acquired Aplastic Anemia: A Study of 352 Cases," *American Journal of Medicine*, **67**:564–571, 1979. A study looking at all grades of severity and at high-dose androgen therapy. A prognostic index with 73 percent accuracy was developed.

O'Brian, B. S., and Woods, S.: "The Paradox of DIC," *American Journal of Nursing*, **78**:1878, November 1978. A concise presentation of symptoms, pathophysiology, and treatment of disseminated intravascular coagulation.

Scarlato, M.: "Blood Transfusions Today: What You Should Know and Do," *Nursing 78*, **8**(2):72, February 1978. This article clarifies component transfusions and provides an overview of care.

Viera, F., and Frank, E.: "Acquired Immune Deficiency in Haitians," *The New England Journal of Medicine*, **308**(3):125–129, 1983. This article describes the incidence and characteristics of AIDS in the Haitian population.

West, S.: "One Step Behind a Killer," *Science*, March 1983, pp. 36–45.

Williams, W. J., Beutler, E., Ersler, A. J., and Wayne, R. R.: *Hematology*, 2d ed., McGraw-Hill, New York, 1977. An excellent and thorough presentation of all hematologic disorders.

Wood, C.: "Macrocytic Megaloblastic Anemias," *Nurse Practitioner*, **2**:24, 25, 29, July 1977. A concise summary of the physiology of vitamin B_{12} and folic acid anemia.

30

The Cardiovascular System

Rose Pinneo

Cardiovascular nursing is the care of individuals with an alteration in cardiovascular physiological functioning. It encompasses both cardiac and peripheral circulatory disturbances. In caring for persons with these disturbances, the nurse needs an understanding of the pathophysiology of related conditions as a basis for collecting meaningful data, formulating nursing diagnoses, establishing expected outcomes of care, planning interventions, and evaluating outcomes. In performing these various aspects of the nursing process, the nurse works collaboratively with the physician and other members of the health team so that high-quality care is delivered to the client.

This chapter provides the practicing nurse with a quick reference relating to the care of clients with selected cardiovascular disorders. Because the scope of content is broad, it is not possible to provide in-depth information about each disorder; therefore, the reader is referred to the bibliography and other sources for further information. It is hoped that the information provided in this chapter will motivate the nurse to seek other resources to increase her or his knowledge.

The cardiovascular system is a remarkable, integrated network of blood vessels and a pump. When there are alterations in one part of the system, compensatory mechanisms are brought into operation to maintain homeostasis so that tissues receive oxygen and nutrients and eliminate waste products.

When caring for clients with cardiovascular disorders, the nurse has a responsibility not only to care for the immediate needs but to prevent further cardiovascular problems. This is achieved by educating the client and the client's family about risk factors and encouraging them to change the client's lifestyle in such a way that cardiac problems are less likely to occur. This preventive aspect is more effective in decreasing cardiovascular disease than caring for people after damage is done; however, as complete eradication of cardiovascular diseases is impossible at the present time, the nurse needs to provide care in such a way that clients are rehabilitated to their optimal level.

ASSESSMENT SPECIFIC TO THE CLIENT WITH CARDIOVASCULAR PROBLEMS

Past Medical History

1. Childhood diseases, such as rheumatic fever, mumps, and chickenpox.
2. Medications that the client has been taking, such as digitalis, quinidine, diuretics, and tranquilizers.
3. Thrombophlebitis or any clotting disorder that can precede pulmonary embolism.
4. History of diabetes or gout. (Such metabolic disorders are related to the development of atherosclerosis.)
5. Weight gain or loss in recent months.

Family History

1. Occurrence of congenital heart disease, cardiac disease, hypertension, heart murmurs, cerebrovascular disease, diabetes, gout, rheumatic fever, and renal disease.
2. Premature death from coronary heart disease.

Client Profile

1. Occupational history to determine physical work load, degree of stress, emotional involvement, and financial status.
2. Marital history to determine the number of marriages, number of years married, age of spouse, and sexual relationships.
3. Number of children and ages.
4. Educational background, in order to assess at what level teaching can start.
5. Habits and life patterns, such as physical exercise, relaxation, vacations, diet, recent stressful life changes, and the use of alcohol, drugs, coffee, tea, and cigarettes.

Symptoms of Cardiovascular Problems

1. *Chest discomfort.* Determine:
   a. Onset and duration.
   b. Location and radiation.
   c. Quality and intensity.
   d. Associated symptoms.
   e. Precipitating and relieving factors.
2. *Dyspnea.* This is defined as labored or difficult breathing. Types of dyspnea include:
   a. *Exertional dyspnea,* which occurs when the client exercises and disappears at rest.
   b. *Orthopnea,* which occurs when the client has dyspnea while lying flat in bed but is relieved in an upright position.
   c. *Paroxysmal nocturnal dyspnea,* which occurs suddenly at night when a client awakens gasping for air. It is usually relieved when a window is opened and the patient sits in an upright position.
   d. *Acute pulmonary edema,* which is a severe form of dyspnea that occurs during day or night when fluid accumulates in the pulmonary alveoli, preventing exchange of gases across alveoli membranes. The client experiences acute dyspnea, cyanosis, tachycardia, acute anxiety, diaphoresis, and frequently blood-tinged sputum.
3. *Fatigue.* The client complains of easy fatigability after mild exertion. It is due to the inability of the heart to pump sufficient blood to meet demands of cells and tissues for oxygen and nutrients.
4. *Palpitations.* The client is aware that the heart is beating rapidly, especially after mild exertion. The rhythm may be regular or irregular, depending on the arrhythmia causing it.
5. *Syncope.* This is fainting or loss of consciousness due to sudden decreased cerebral perfusion.
6. *Edema.* This is an abnormal accumulation of fluid in interstitial spaces in dependent portions of the body or throughout the body, if severe (*anasarca*). Assess edema by weight gain, puffiness of ankles in ambulatory clients or sacrum and buttocks in bedridden clients.
7. *Cyanosis.* This is a bluish discoloration of the skin resulting from increased amounts of reduced hemoglobin in the blood. When looking for the presence of cyanosis, observe color of ear lobes, lips, fingernail beds, and mucous membranes of the eyes. Look for clubbing of toenails or fingernails, especially in prolonged cyanosis.
8. *Neck vein distension.* Increased enlargement of the jugular veins indicates a high central venous pressure, a common finding in right-heart failure. Observe jugular veins while the client is sitting at a 45-degree angle, comparing the level of distension with the sternal angle.

New York Heart Association Functional Classification of Cardiac Client

Developed in 1964, the following classification is useful in communicating the client's ongoing status among all disciplines involved in the client's care:

Class I. No limitation of physical activity. Ordinary physical activity does not cause undue fatigue, palpitation, dyspnea, or angina.

Class II. Slight limitation of physical activity. No symptoms at rest, but ordinary activity results in fatigue, palpitations, dyspnea, or angina.

Class III. More severe limitations. Usually comfortable at rest. Less than ordinary activity causes fatigue, palpitation, dyspnea, or angina.

Class IV. Inability to carry on any physical activity without discomfort. Symptoms of cardiac insufficiency or of angina may be present even at rest. If any physical activity is undertaken, discomfort is increased.

Physical Assessment

The four main methods for examining the heart are:

1. *Inspection.* Examine for precordial pulsations at the end of a normal or forced expiration. The apical impulse is normally at the

fifth intercostal space, midclavicular line, 7–9 cm left of the midsternal line. The location of the apical impulse is called the *point of maximum impulse* (*PMI*).

2. *Palpation.* Palpate by placing the hand over the anterior precordium and shifting the second and third fingers until the apical impulse is felt at the mitral area (PMI).

   Continue palpating for other pulsations and thrills, using the flat portions of three fingers, at the second intercostal space to the right and left of the sternum (aortic and pulmonic areas) and at the left lower sternal border (tricuspid area) for a right ventricular lift, indicating a possible right ventricular hypertrophy (see Figure 30-1).

3. *Percussion.* Percussion is not done often, as the chest x-ray study is more reliable for cardiac size.

   By placing the middle finger on the skin, percuss by tapping it with the middle finger of the other hand over the left third, fourth, and fifth interspaces. Begin laterally and proceed medially while listening for a change of sound from resonance to dullness. At this point, the lateral border of the heart is outlined and normally should be 4, 7 and 10 cm left of the sternum for the three intercostal spaces, respectively.

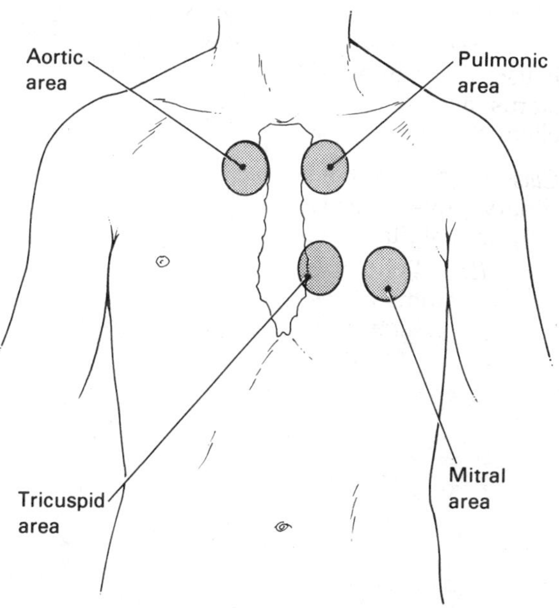

Figure 30-1 Areas on the chest where vibrations are palpated and heart sounds are heard. Aortic area: second intercostal space right of sternum; pulmonic area: second intercostal space left of sternum; tricuspid area: fifth intercostal space left of sternum; and mitral area: fifth intercostal space left of midclavicular line.

4. *Auscultation.*
   a. *Cardiac cycle.* A review of the cardiac cycle helps to understand the meaning of heart sounds. In response to electrical stimulation, the following mechanical events take place:
      (1) Atria contract (atrial systole) to empty blood into ventricles through the opened atrioventricular valves (mitral and tricuspid).
      (2) As the atria relax (atrial diastole), the ventricles contract (ventricular systole) to force blood into the pulmonary artery from the right ventricle through the pulmonic valve and into the aorta from the left ventricle through the aortic valve.
      (3) As the ventricles relax, the pulmonic and aortic valves close (see Figure 30-2).
   b. *Heart sounds.* The sounds heard on the skin with the stethoscope are produced by vibrations caused by the movement of blood and valvular closing. Following is a description of the four heart sounds:
      (1) First heart sound (S_1), "lubb," results from the closure of the tricuspid and mitral valves at the beginning of ventricular systole.
      (2) Second heart sound (S_2), "dup," results from the closure of the aortic and pulmonic valves at the end of ventricular systole.
      (3) Third heart sound (S_3) results from the inrush of blood from the atria to the ventricles in the first third of diastole. When combined with S_1 and S_2, it sounds like the gallop of a horse and is called a *ventricular gallop*. This sound is normal in children and young adults but is diagnostic of cardiac disease if heard in adults.
      (4) Fourth heart sound (S_4) results from ventricular filling in response to atrial contraction late in diastole before S, of the next cardiac cycle. When combined with S, and S_2, it gives the sound of a gallop and is called an *atrial gallop*. It is uncommon to hear this sound in adults

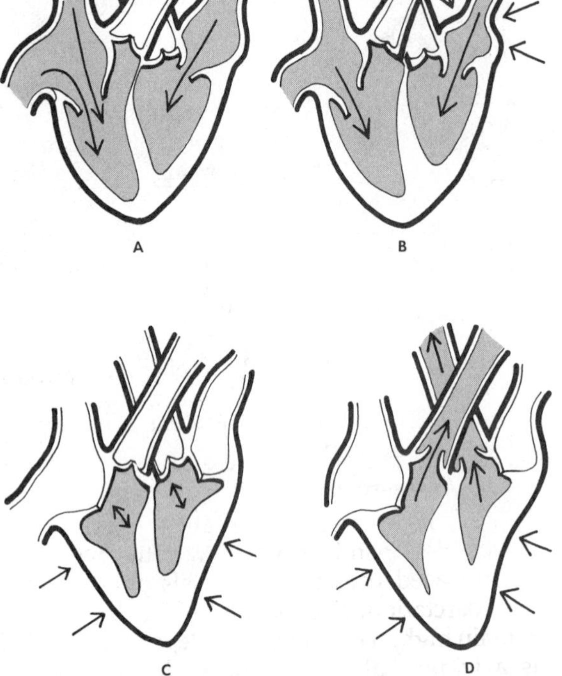

Figure 30-2 (*a*) Diastole (atrial and ventricular): early passive filling phase; (*b*) atrial systole: late active filling phase; (*c*) beginning of ventricular systole (isovolumic contraction); (*d*) ventricular systolic ejection. (Tilkian, A., and Conover, M.: *Understanding Heart Sounds and Murmurs*, Saunders, Philadelphia, 1979, p. 6. Used by permission of the publisher.)

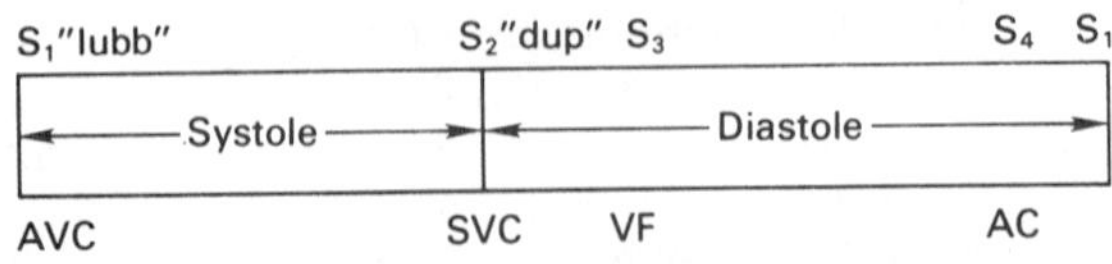

Figure 30-3 Relation of heart sounds to systole and diastole of one cardiac cycle. AVC = atrioventricular valvular closure (mitral and tricuspid valves); SVC = semilunar valvular closure (aortic and pulmonic valves); VF = ventricular filling; AC = atrial contraction, causing further ventricular filling.

and may indicate cardiac disease (see Figure 30-3).

c. *Heart murmurs.* Heart murmurs are produced by vibrations from turbulent blood flow during systole or diastole and are named according to their position in the cardiac cycle. When recording heart sounds and murmurs by phonocardiography, the vibrations causing them are shown as rapid vertical lines (see Figure 30-4).

d. *Technique for listening to heart sounds.*
   (1) Put the client in a comfortable supine position.
   (2) Be sure the room is warm and quiet.
   (3) Provide appropriate draping for female clients.
   (4) Warm the stethoscope before applying it to the skin.
   (5) Systematically inch the stethoscope, using the diaphragm and the bell from one area to another—aortic, pulmonic, tricuspid, and mitral—listening to S_1 and S_2, obtaining the heart rate and

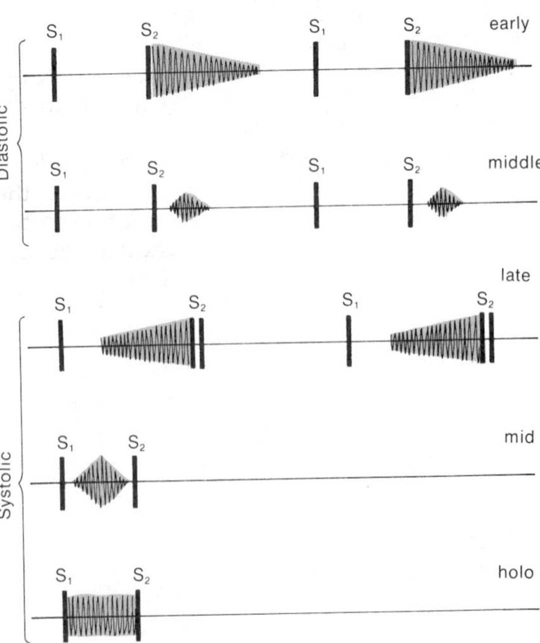

Figure 30-4 Phonocardiogram: a recording of heart sounds and murmurs. (Tilkian, A., and Conover, M: *Understanding Heart Sounds and Murmurs*, Saunders, Philadelphia, 1979, p. 54. Used by permission of the publisher.)

rhythm, and then listening for extra sounds and murmurs.

ABNORMAL CELLULAR GROWTH

CONGENITAL HEART DISEASE: COARCTATION OF THE AORTA

DESCRIPTION

Coarctation of the aorta is a constriction of the aorta, usually occurring distal to the left subclavian artery. The severity of the problem depends on the number of other congential defects that occur at the same time, such as patent ductus arteriosus and ventricular septal defects.

If the constriction occurs alone and does not completely occlude the aorta, a person can live to adulthood before symptoms are obvious. This is because blood is pumped through the narrow stricture and through collateral vessels that bypass the stricture to provide circulation to the rest of the body.

However, when symptoms become evident, surgical treatment is needed to correct the anomaly and allow improved circulation to the body; otherwise, this condition induces degenerative changes.

PREVENTION

Health Promotion

Prevention of congential cardiac anomalies in utero by preventing rubella in the mother during the first trimester of pregnancy.

Population at Risk

Persons with other congenital anomalies often have coarctation as well.

Screening

Blood pressure screening of the population at risk. Blood pressures of upper extremities are compared with blood pressures of lower extremities.

ASSESSMENT

Health History

1. Age: Coarctation is usually diagnosed when the client is an adult because increasing symptoms bring the person to medical attention or because routine physical examinations identify signs of the condition.
2. Occupation: Client may be restricted in activities associated with occupation because of restricted cardiac output and the accompanying cardiac insufficiency.
3. Sex: The condition appears twice as frequently in males as in females.
4. Symptoms described by the client: These include headache, dizziness, epistaxis, dyspnea on exertion, and occasionally chest pain.
5. Claudication in lower extremities: This is an infrequent finding.

Physical Assessment

1. Systolic blood pressure is higher in the upper extremities than in lower extremities because of increased pressure in vessels proximal to the coarctation. The diastolic blood pressures remain high in both arms and legs; thus, there is a wider pulse pressure in the upper extremities than in the lower extremities.
2. Pulses in the lower extremities may be diminished or absent.
3. There may be muscle cramps in lower extremities, especially after exercise.
4. There are forceful arterial pulsations in the suprasternal notch or in the neck.
5. The arm and shoulder muscles may be extensively developed.
6. A soft systolic ejection murmur may be heard along the left sternal border.
7. An S_4 may be present, caused by left ventricular failure.
8. Headaches and epistaxis may occur from the hypertension due to the coarctation.
9. Dyspnea is due to left ventricular failure.

Diagnostic Tests

1. Electrocardiogram shows left ventricular hypertrophy or strain.
2. Chest x-ray studies reveal a dilated left subclavian artery high on the left mediastinal border, an enlarged aorta, and left ventricular hypertrophy. They also reveal bilateral rib notching due to intercostal arterial dilation and extensive collateral circulation.

3. Cardiac catheterization and aortography are indicated when other cardiac anomalies are suspected.
4. Echocardiography may show increased left ventricular muscle thickness and, possibly, aortic valve abnormalities and the site of the coarctation.

NURSING DIAGNOSES: ACTUAL OR POTENTIAL

1. Anxiety of client and family: associated with the increasing severity of the situation.
2. Discomfort: due to symptoms (and later surgical intervention).
3. Potential of infection: bacterial endocarditis.
4. Knowledge deficit: regarding treatment plan.

EXPECTED OUTCOMES

1. Headaches will decrease, as evidenced by the client's verbal report.
2. Anxiety of the client and family will be lessened, as evidenced by verbalization of fears and concerns and by nonverbal behaviors.
3. Dyspnea will subside.
4. Infections will be prevented.
5. Client will identify the treatment plan and its rationale.

INTERVENTIONS

1. Give analgesics for the accompanying headaches.
2. Provide a restful, quiet environment to prevent excessive stimulation.
3. Explain diagnostic tests to client and family to allay anxiety. Allow client to express concerns.
4. Teach the client and the family the nature of the disorder, what the surgery entails, what drugs will be given, and what to expect following surgery.
5. Surgical intervention: surgical resection with end-to-end anastomosis of the aorta or insertion of a prosthetic graft at the site of the constriction (see Figure 30-5).
6. After corrective surgery:
   a. Monitor blood pressure carefully, using an intraarterial line. Compare blood pressure in all extremities.
   b. Monitor intake and output.
   c. If hypertension develops and nitroprusside is required, administer it by using an infusion pump. Watch for hypotension and regulate the dose carefully.
   d. Provide pain relief.
   e. Encourage a gradual increase in activity. Note the difference between resting and recovery pulse and blood pressure.
   f. Promote adequate respiratory functioning by turning, coughing, and deep breathing.
   g. Monitor chest tubes for patency, correct functioning, and quantity of drainage.
   h. Teach the client about medications, dosages, and side effects. Stress the need for compliance with therapy, especially if antihypertensives are used.

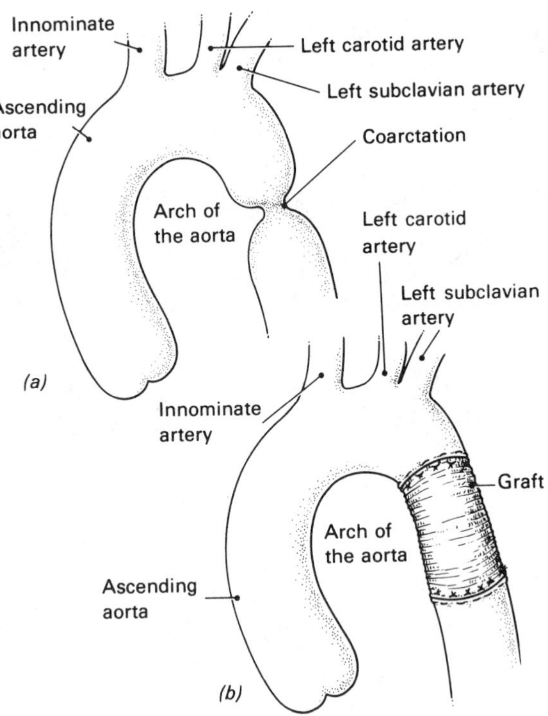

Figure 30-5 (*a*) Coarctation of the aorta. (*b*) Repair of coarctation of the aorta with a graft.

EVALUATION

Outcome Criteria

Dyspnea is subsiding.

Complications

1. Congestive heart failure (see discussion in this chapter).
2. Bacterial endocarditis (see discussion in this chapter).
3. Cerebrovascular accident (see Chapter 25).

Reevaluation and Follow-up

1. Assess blood pressures in upper and lower extremities during periodic clinic visits.
2. Repeated electrocardiograms and chest x-rays will detect the presence of arrhythmias and cardiac enlargement.
3. Assess presence of headaches or episodes of epistaxis.
4. Assess problems with circulation in lower extremities, such as claudication or muscle cramps, and relationship to activities.
5. Assess the client's knowledge of drug therapy in controlling hypertension and in preventing heart failure or bacterial endocarditis.

RHEUMATIC HEART DISEASE

DESCRIPTION

Rheumatic heart disease occurs as a sequela in 50 percent of the clients with an earlier episode of acute rheumatic fever, a hypersensitive reaction to group A beta-hemolytic streptococcal infection. As a result of the inflammatory process, there may be damage to the endocardium, myocardium, or pericardium.

1. *Endocardial involvement.* Ulcerations of valve tissue cause valve leaflet swelling and scarring. Beadlike vegetations, consisting of blood, platelet, and fibrin, are deposited on the leaflets. The mitral valve is most often affected. The aortic valve is also affected frequently. Occasionally, the tricuspid is affected and the pulmonic valve only rarely. In addition, the chordae tendineae are also inflamed, resulting in fibrosis with shortening, thickening, and fusion.
2. *Myocardial involvement.* Characteristic lesions, called *Aschoff bodies,* cause cellular swelling and fragmentation of interstitial collagen, leading to formation of fibrotic nodules and interstitial scars. Contractility of myocardial tissue is affected by this process, resulting in weakness of the myocardium.
3. *Pericardial involvement.* Adhesions form between the two layers, visceral and parietal pericardium, resulting in constrictive pericarditis and adhesions to surrounding tissues. The pericardium can become thickened, thus restricting the relaxation and filling of the heart during diastole.

The development of rheumatic heart disease in adult life depends on the severity of the damage at the time of the earlier episode of acute rheumatic fever, especially if there were repeated episodes.

PREVENTION

Health Promotion

1. Maintenance of good health habits: adequate rest and nutrition.
2. Prevention of exposure to cool, damp environment.
3. Avoidance of contact with persons with streptococcal infections.
4. Seeking medical assistance for symptoms of recurrent streptococcal infections: sudden sore throat, redness of the throat, pain on swallowing, and elevated temperature.
5. Promotion of good dental hygiene to prevent gingival infection.
6. An understanding on the part of individuals of the need for antibiotic therapy for any streptococcal infections or for any possible infections from dental work.

Population at Risk

1. Persons with previous attacks of acute rheumatic fever.
2. Persons with inadequate nutrition. (These people are prone to have repeated attacks of rheumatic fever.)
3. Persons who develop recurrent upper respiratory infections and streptococcal sore throats.
4. Persons living in substandard, poor, or crowded environments.

Screening

1. Persons with histories of acute rheumatic fever should be frequently screened for abnormal heart sounds, abnormal electrocardiographic changes, and any signs of an infectious process.
2. For the general population, abnormal heart sounds and electrocardiographic changes on routine physical examinations may indicate a previous episode of acute rheumatic fever without having obvious symptoms.

ASSESSMENT

Health History

1. History of acute rheumatic fever (although there are some cases without this history) during childhood or teenage years.

2. Easy fatigability, especially on exertion.
3. Repeated respiratory infections and sore throat.
4. Dyspnea, especially on exertion.
5. Anxiety when symptoms occur with normal activity levels.
6. Angina with overexertion.

Physical Assessment

1. Cardiac murmurs during systole or diastole, depending on which valve is affected and whether there is stenosis or regurgitation.
2. Increased intensity of the first heart sound (S_1).
3. Pericardial friction rub if pericarditis is present.
4. Dyspnea, rapid respirations, and basilar rales due to increased left atrial pressure.
5. Diaphoresis.
6. Hemoptysis may be present.
7. Giant *a* wave in the jugular veins if tricuspid stenosis is present.

Diagnostic Tests

There are, unfortunately, no specific laboratory tests, but the following can be helpful in establishing the medical diagnosis:

1. Confirmation of the organism by throat culture.
2. Electrocardiographic tracings show a prolonged PR interval and possible atrial fibrillation.
3. Echocardiography demonstrates any abnormal valve function.
4. Chest x-ray study may show evidence of left atrial enlargement, especially if mitral stenosis is present. Enlarged left ventricle may also be present.
5. Cardiac catheterization will determine the specific valve or valves involved.

NURSING DIAGNOSES: ACTUAL OR POTENTIAL

1. Activity intolerance: due to decrease in cardiac output.
2. Potential for increased risk of respiratory infections.
3. Noncompliance: due to knowledge deficit.

EXPECTED OUTCOMES

1. Client will be able to state the activities that can safely be performed without producing symptoms.
2. Dyspnea will be reduced during usual activities.
3. Fatigability will lessen during usual activities.
4. Client will reduce respiratory or other infections and receive antibiotic therapy for any that occur.
5. Client will show compliance with antibiotic therapy, when ordered, by showing evidence the medications are used.
6. Client will understand the reasons for cardiac surgery and what to expect before and after surgery.

INTERVENTIONS

1. Teach the client the relation of activities to cardiac work by providing an activity list with related expenditure of energy.
2. Emphasize the importance of avoiding contact with persons with respiratory or other infections and of reporting such contact when it does occur so that additional antibiotic therapy can be given.
3. When giving antibiotic therapy, check for hypersensitivity and teach the client the reason for the use of the drug.
4. Prepare the client both psychologically and physically for diagnostic tests.
5. Prepare the client for cardiac catheterization and provide care after catheterization (see discussion under *Valvular Heart Disease* in this chapter).
6. Teach the client and family about the disease and its treatment.
7. Teach the client about what surgery involves and the postoperative expectations (see discussion on surgery under *Valvular Heart Disease* in this chapter).

EVALUATION

Outcome Criteria

1. Client participates in activities that do not cause symptoms of dyspnea and fatigue.
2. Client complies with therapeutic regimen, as evidenced by absence of infections or other complications.
3. If surgical intervention was needed: (1) The client shows an understanding of expectations following valvular surgery by answering questions; (2) postoperative care reduces complications after surgery.

Complications

CONGESTIVE HEART FAILURE

See *Congestive Heart Failure* in this chapter.

HEMORRHAGE FROM CARDIAC CATHETERIZATION SITE

Assessment
1. Fresh blood appears suddenly on dressings over catheterization site.
2. Blood pressure decreases and pulse increases in a few minutes.

Revised Outcomes
Bleeding will be controlled immediately.

Interventions
1. Call the physician.
2. Apply pressure with a sterile gauze pad over the site.
3. Apply pressure over arterial pressure points proximal to the site (if an arterial site).

THROMBOSIS AT CATHETERIZATION SITE

Assessment
1. There is a lack of palpable pulse distal to the catheterization site.
2. The skin appears mottled and the temperature of the extremity is cold.

Revised Outcomes
Thrombi will be removed so that normal circulation to the extremity can be resumed.

Interventions
1. Call the physician.
2. Elevate the involved extremity.
3. Keep the client from moving.

Reevaluation and Follow-up

Every 6 months, evaluate:
1. Presence of congestive heart failure.
2. Changes in heart sounds.
3. Physical endurance.
4. Presence of streptococcal infections.

VALVULAR HEART DISEASES

DESCRIPTION

Valvular diseases of the heart may develop from inflammations or infections, such as acute rheumatic fever, bacterial endocarditis, or syphilis. They may also develop from congenital malformation of the valves or from rupture of the chordae tendineae. The damage results in stenosis (narrowing) or regurgitation (insufficiency). These changes cause a disturbance in blood flow and increased work load on the heart. If stenosis is present, an increased force is needed for blood to move forward through the valve, thus adding stress to the pumping mechanism and eventually leading to a decreased cardiac output. When regurgitation occurs, the valve leaflets shorten and do not close completely after contraction. The blood, therefore, goes in a reverse direction from normal flow and returns to an area from which it was ejected. This puts a burden on the heart, for an increased amount of blood is pumped by the heart to meet the demands of the body.

The valves most often affected are those in the left heart (mitral and aortic) because of the higher pressure load as compared with that of the right heart. The tricuspid valve between the right atrium and right ventricle is less often affected.

PREVENTION

Health Promotion

1. Persons with histories of acute rheumatic fever should avoid exposure to individuals with upper respiratory infections.
2. Persons of low socioeconomic status should be counseled regarding selecting essential nutrients within their budget and getting sufficient rest.
3. Persons with a history of acute rheumatic fever should inform their dentists so penicillin will be given.

Population at Risk

1. Persons living in crowded, damp environments, as their resistance to infections is low.
2. Persons with prior history of acute rheumatic fever.
3. Individuals with a family history of rheumatic fever.
4. Individuals with cardiac problems or those who have elevated cholesterol levels, hyperlipidemia, and hypertension due to atherogenic changes of the valves.

Screening

1. Chest x-ray study for heart size.
2. Echocardiogram for function of valves.
3. Electrocardiogram for hypertrophy and arrhythmias.

ASSESSMENT

Health History

1. Dyspnea on exertion or a history of progression with less and less exertion.
2. Previous history of streptococcal infections or other infections.
3. Angina on exertion.
4. History of cardiovascular and related pathologies in client and family members.
5. Fatigue (possibly incapacitating).

Physical Assessment

1. *Mitral stenosis.* The mitral valve narrows because of scar formation at its commissures, which prevents adequate opening during diastole. This impedes blood flow from the left atrium to the left ventricle. Symptoms are:
   a. Atrial fibrillation develops because of left atrial enlargement. Its likely consequence is thrombus formation from stasis of blood leading to embolization to cerebral arteries.
   b. On auscultation, three significant findings are apical diastolic murmur, increased intensity of the first heart sound (S_1), and an opening snap.
   c. Dyspnea, the most important symptom, appears when atrial pressure produces transudation of fluid into alveoli. It first appears with extreme exertion but later occurs even at rest. It may also appear with emotional excitement or stress, which increases cardiac output.
   d. Excessive fatigue.
   e. Cough and hemoptysis.
   f. Peripheral edema, jugular venous distention, ascites, hepatomegaly from right-heart failure.
   g. Client may appear thin and frail with signs of muscular wasting.
2. *Mitral insufficiency.* There is scarring, thickening, shortening, and deformity of the cusps of the mitral valve with restriction at the free margins. As a result, there is incomplete closure of the mitral valve during systole, allowing for regurgitation of blood. Symptoms are:
   a. Fatigue.
   b. Dyspnea on exertion, orthopnea, and paroxysmal nocturnal dyspnea.
   c. On auscultation, a pansystolic murmur is heard best at the apex (due to reflux of blood and increased force of the apical impulse).
   d. Peripheral edema, jugular venous distention, hepatomegaly (from right-heart failure.)
   e. Atrial fibrillation is frequent with chronic disease.
3. *Aortic stenosis.* Valve cusps of the aortic valve become stiff and calcified with fusion of the commissures. This closure causes impedence to left ventricular emptying. Symptoms are:
   a. Angina pectoris is usually the most common symptom. It is due to the disparity between oxygen need and supply because of the increased work load caused by aortic stenosis.
   b. Syncope develops after effort. It is commonly associated with angina.
   c. Left ventricular failure is a grave development and demands immediate therapy.
   d. Diminished carotid pulses.
   e. Auscultation reveals a midsystolic murmur that begins after S_1, increases in frequency, and then decreases before S_2. This finding reflects the increased left ventricular ejection velocity through the stenosed valve. it is loudest at the aortic area with radiation to carotids.
   f. Narrowed pulse pressure in advanced cases (less than 30 mmHg pressure).
   g. Dyspnea with exertion.
4. *Aortic insufficiency.* This condition results from scarring, restriction, and stiffening of the free borders of aortic valve leaflets. If the valve is very deformed and rigid, varying degrees of stenosis may be present also. Symptoms are:
   a. There is palpitation or throbbing in the chest, particularly when lying on the left side.
   b. Exertional dyspnea and easy fatigability occur as the disease worsens. It may progress to orthopnea, paroxysmal nocturnal dyspnea, and pulmonary edema.
   c. Angina pectoris has a different pattern from that of aortic stenosis. It usually occurs after evidence of left ventricular failure. This symptom is thought to be due to a reduced coronary blood flow secondary to a low diastolic aortic pressure coupled with an increased requirement for blood by the hypertrophied left ventricle.
   d. Neck pain is usually acute in onset and persists from hours to as long as 5 to 6 days. It is ascribed to the stretching of the carotid sheaths.

e. Abdominal pain may be present. It is a pounding or aching sensation in the epigastric region and is possibly due to constant stretching of the abdominal aorta.
f. Dizziness is due to temporary cerebral ischemia caused by rapid, marked pressure changes in cerebral vessels subject to a wide pulse pressure.
g. Wide pulse pressure reflects the high systolic and low diastolic pressures. The range is between 80 to 100 mmHg.
h. The pulse wave in peripheral arteries reveals a rapidly rising and collapsing pulse due to the rapid ejection from the left ventricle and the loss of blood volume across the incompetent aortic valve. This characteristic feature of the pulse is called *Corrigan's pulse,* or *water-hammer pulse.*
i. On auscultation, a soft, blowing decrescendo diastolic murmur, starting with S_2 and decreasing in intensity, may be heard. It is heard best over the aortic area and at the third interspace to the left of the sternum with the client leaning forward.

5. *Tricuspid stenosis.* Organic disease of the tricuspid valve is almost always due to rheumatic fever and is always seen in association with disease of the mitral valve. There is fusion of the commissure, thus leaving a small central opening for passage of blood. In order to maintain blood flow across the stenosed tricuspid valve, the right atrium must increase its pressure. This increased right atrial pressure is reflected in peripheral edema. Symptoms are:
   a. The a wave of jugular venous pulsations may be large because of resistance to right atrial emptying. If atrial fibrillation is present, this a wave is lost because of ineffective atrial contractions.
   b. On palpation, a diastolic thrill, accentuated during inspiration, may be felt along the left sternal border.
   c. Auscultation reveals a split S_1, from the delay in tricuspid closure, heard best at the lower left sternal border. This split S_1 increases in intensity during inspiration.

      There is usually no normal physiological splitting of S_2 in tricuspid stenosis because the normal increase in right ventricular and diastolic volume during inspiration is inhibited.

      A middiastolic low-pitched murmur is heard at the left sternal border in the fourth or fifth intercostal space. It increases in intensity with inspiration. This is the most valuable auscultatory assessment of tricuspid stenosis.
   d. Symptoms of right-sided heart failure may occur, such as dependent edema, ascites, and extreme fatigue.
6. *Tricuspid insufficiency.* There are thickening, curling, and retraction of valve leaflets. In addition, there is shortening and fusion of the chordae tendineae. Moderate degrees of tricuspid insufficiency are tolerated well because the regurgitated blood is dissipated well into the venous system with little adverse influence on the circulation. Symptoms are:
   a. Atrial fibrillation is a common finding, probably due to the regurgitant blood from the right ventricle.
   b. Prominent systolic venous pulsations are observed in the jugular veins.
   c. On auscultation, a holosystolic murmur is usually found at the 4th intercostal space to the left of the sternum. It is augmented on inspiration, thus indicating a tricuspid valvular origin. This is related to increased filling of the right ventricle due to lower intrathoracic pressures during inspiration.
7. Pulmonic valvular disease is extremely rare and is usually congenital rather than rheumatic in origin.

Diagnostic Tests

1. Electrocardiogram may be normal in mild cases. In severe cases, it will show hypertrophy of heart chambers, depending on which valve is involved. Atrial fibrillation is a common arrhythmia found in many valvular disorders.
2. Chest x-ray study will show cardiac enlargement when left-heart failure is present.
3. Echocardiogram is the use of ultrasound to record a reflected sound wave, or "echo," from an interface between varying tissue densities. Thus, valvular disorders can be detected. The technique is noninvasive. A transducer is positioned at various sites on the chest to send and receive ultrasound waves. The wave forms seen on a screen show normal or abnormal valvular functions.
4. Cardiac catheterization is a definitive means of visualizing specific chambers and determining pressures and oxygen content and direction of blood flow through the heart. Cath-

eters are inserted via the right or left brachial vein or a femoral artery to the heart. Thus, data on structural damage to the heart valves, the cardiac output, and any congenital anomalies are obtained.

NURSING DIAGNOSES: ACTUAL OR POTENTIAL

1. Activity intolerance: due to hemodynamic changes.
2. Alteration in comfort: secondary to episodes of angina pectoris.
3. Lack of compliance with therapeutic regimen: due to knowledge deficit.
4. Anxiety: due to fears of possible surgery.

EXPECTED OUTCOMES

1. There will be increased activity tolerance resulting in decreased fatigue and angina.
2. Client will give evidence of compliance with therapy by:
   a. Adhering to medical regimen, as indicated by a record kept by the client.
   b. Avoiding contact with persons with respiratory infections.
   c. Establishing a routine of activity and rest periods.
3. Client will understand information taught in teaching sessions, as evidenced by 85 percent accuracy in answering questions.
4. Client will live within the limitations of valvular damage if surgical intervention is not feasible.

INTERVENTIONS

1. Promote a rest and activity program by assessing the client's knowledge and teaching according to the client's needs.
2. Teach the client about:
   a. Prevention of infections.
   b. Reasons for diagnostic tests and expectations of the client during the tests.
   c. Surgical procedures that are needed, including preoperative preparation and postoperative care.
   d. Medications, such as nitroglycerin for chest pain, digitalis preparations, and diuretics if heart failure is present.
3. Medical therapy.
   a. Treat congestive heart failure, if present, with digitalis, sodium and fluid restriction, diuretics, and limitation of activity.
   b. Administer antibiotic therapy to prevent recurrences of infection.
4. Provide psychological support as the client experiences diagnostic tests and interventions.
5. Surgical interventions. Valvular defects can lead to pump failure if cardiac output is decreased and medical therapy (e.g., a combination of diuretics, digitalis, low-sodium diet, oxygen, and rest) is inadequate to prevent or treat it. Clients progress to a point where surgical intervention is necessary to correct the defect or replace a defective valve. Surgical intervention may be by means of:
   a. Closed heart surgery.
      (1) A closed commissurotomy for mitral stenosis is used for younger clients without a history of emboli or signs of extensive valvular calcification.
      (2) Through this technique, commissures of the valve are opened by direct digital pressure of the surgeon's finger or a dilator inserted through the left atrial appendage. It does not require the use of the heart-lung machine (cardiopulmonary bypass) (Fitzmaurice, 1980).
   b. Open heart surgery. Through the use of the heart-lung (cardiopulmonary bypass) machine, which diverts blood from the heart and lungs during surgery and maintains oxygen and carbon dioxide exchange functions throughout the body, the heart can be incised and defective valves replaced by direct visibility. Pacemaker wires are implanted prophylactically in case of need during postsurgery (see Figure 30-6).
6. Nursing care for clients having cardiac surgery.
   a. Preoperative nursing care.
      (1) Encourage the client to share fears and concerns; prepare client for psychological changes after surgery.
      (2) Instruct the client and family regarding:
         (a) Reason for surgery.
         (b) Type of incision to expect.
         (c) Probable length of hospitalization.
         (d) Anatomy of the heart.

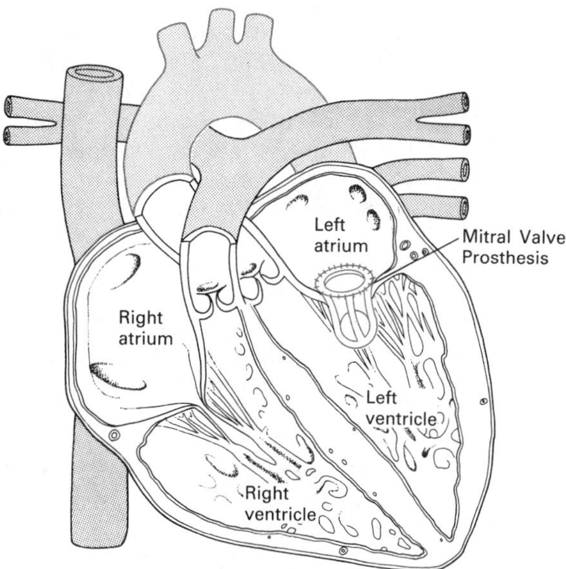

Figure 30-6 Position of mitral valve prosthesis in the heart.

(e) Expectations for client after the operation, such as inability to speak (because of an endotracheal tube), the use of a respirator, chest tubes, venous and arterial lines, and the amount of pain.

(3) Orient the client and family to the recovery room, the intensive care unit, and the equipment to be used and discuss the continuous care given in these settings.

(4) Demonstrate and have the client practice deep breathing, coughing, and range-of-motion exercises.

(5) Explain reasons for the numerous laboratory tests such as urinalysis, blood gases, electrolytes, enzymes, electrocardiogram, echocardiogram, cardiac catheterization, and pulmonary function tests.

(6) Give preoperative skin preparation with a bacteriostatic soap for several days before the surgery. Shave the incisional site.

(7) Provide a low-sodium diet and explain its purpose.

(8) Weigh the client daily to provide baseline measurements to be used later for fluid replacement and drug dosage calculation.

(9) Monitor vital signs, including apical-radial pulse, arrhythmias, variations in quality of the pulse, any respiratory difficulty and abnormalities in body temperature.

b. Postoperative nursing care.

(1) Assess vital signs frequently to detect any changes in:

(a) Arterial blood pressure, via catheters in arteries connected to a monitor.

(b) Calcium blockers (e.g., verapamil).

(c) Heart rate and rhythm (arrhythmias), by using a cardiac monitor. This continuous assessment of arrhythmias provides important information about the cardiac output and cardiac status. When the rate is extremely high, antiarrhythmic drugs may be indicated; if extremely low, pacing may be needed.

(d) Rate and quality of peripheral pulses in order to determine adequacy of perfusion to the area. Palpate the radial, dorsalis pedis, and popliteal arteries, comparing the left and right extremities with each other. In addition, monitor the apical-radial pulse.

(e) Pulmonary artery wedge pressure readings if a Swan-Ganz catheter (which provides information about left atrial and ventricular function) is in place.

(2) Control respirations by using a respirator attached to an endotracheal tube and the concentration of oxygen according to individual needs.

(3) Connect drainage tubing and pumps to the nasogastric tube; measure and record quantity of drainage.

(4) Connect chest tubes to water seal drainage or pleurevac equipment. Frequently strip or milk the drainage tubes to prevent the formation of clots in the tubes. Carefully measure, observe, and record the amount and character of drainage in the collecting bottle. Report drainage in excess of 30 mL/h.

(5) Check the surgical dressings for ex-

cessive drainage and bleeding. If there is a lateral incision, check for drainage posteriorly.

(6) Monitor urinary output carefully by measuring and recording urinary drainage through the indwelling urinary catheter every hour. Less than 20 mL/h indicates hypovolemia or low cardiac output.

(7) Assist the client with deep breathing and coughing by splinting the chest. Turn the client from side to side for improved lung expansion.

(8) Give parenteral fluids and blood transfusions carefully to avoid overloading the client.

(9) Assist with drawing blood specimens for various laboratory studies that include electrolytes, arterial blood gases via the arterial line already in place or an arterial puncture, and hematocrit, hemoglobin, prothrombin time, and serum fibrinogen.

(10) Weigh the client daily to assess fluid loss or retention. Compare the weights with previous recordings.

(11) Give pain medication in small doses. This prevents overmedicating and thus does not hinder the cough reflex and deep breathing.

(12) Give the usual medications, which include antibiotics to prevent endocarditis, anticoagulants to prevent thromboembolism on prosthetic valves, and digitalis preparations to increase contractility of the myocardium.

(13) Ambulate the client the evening of surgery by assisting the client to dangle. On the following day, help the client will get out of bed to a chair for a short time; increase ambulation thereafter.

(14) Monitor activity tolerance by measuring pulse and blood pressure response to progressive activity.

(15) Provide psychological support to the client and family by explaining the procedures, reassuring them about the normal expectations and progress, and allowing them to express concerns and fears. Continuously reorient the client to time and place. Help the client regain some control over the situation by allowing him or her to communicate feelings and to make some choices in resting, eating, or ambulating whenever possible.

(16) As the client improves and goes through rehabilitation, teach the client about:
  (a) Exercise in relation to energy costs with signs of stress.
  (b) Medications: Purposes and side effects of digitalis, antiarrhythmics, diuretics, anticoagulants.
  (c) Low-sodium diet: List foods to avoid that are rich in sodium.
  (d) Taking pulse daily, if feasible, and reporting significant changes in pulse rate and rhythms.
  (e) Taking temperature and reporting a fever, as this might indicate endocarditis.

EVALUATION

Outcome Criteria

1. Dyspnea subsides within 1 week of surgery.
2. Activity tolerance levels increase within 2 weeks of surgery, resulting in decreased fatigue.
3. Angina pectoris episodes cease.
4. Client shows compliance with therapy by the time of discharge.
5. Client understands information about the heart and therapy, as evidenced by answering questions with 85 percent accuracy.
6. Client lives within limitations of valvular damage if surgical intervention is not feasible.

Complications

CARDIAC TAMPONADE

This is a serious complication and is due to bleeding into the pericardial sac surrounding the heart. Consequently, the myocardium is compressed, thus preventing adequate filling during diastole.

Assessment

1. Low arterial blood pressure.
2. Pulsus paradoxus.
3. Narrow pulse pressure.
4. Elevated central venous pressure.
5. Weak, thready pulses.
6. Dyspnea, which causes extreme anxiety to the client.

Revised Outcomes

1. Cardiac output will return to a normal range.
2. Blood will be removed from pericardium so that it will not put external pressure on the heart.
3. The source of bleeding into the pericardial sac will be found and bleeding will cease.

Interventions

1. Prepare for and assist with a pericardial tap.
2. If assessment indicates no change, surgery will be necessary to locate and treat the source of bleeding into the pericardium.
3. Monitor vital signs to evaluate effectiveness of intervention.
4. Provide psychological support for the client, as fear is extreme at this time.

ARRHYTHMIAS

Atrial fibrillation often occurs following valvular surgery. It may be associated with the hypothermia produced during surgery or with the presence of the prosthetic valve. The danger is decreased cardiac output to as much as 40 percent of normal when atrial fibrillation occurs. Other arrhythmias may also occur. (See *Arrhythmias*.)

Assessment

1. Identify atrial fibrillation and other arrhythmias on the cardiac monitor.
2. Note the frequency of ventricular response; if extremely rapid (above 100/min) or slow (below 50/min), symptoms of low cardiac output are usually evident. If within a normal range, symptoms are usually absent.

Revised Outcomes

1. The ventricular response to atrial fibrillation or other arrhythmias will be within normal limits (60–100/min).
2. Normal sinus rhythm will be restored.

Interventions

1. Administer antiarrhythmic drugs (quinidine, procainamide, or lidocaine) to suppress irritable foci.
2. Prepare client for electrical countershock (synchronized cardioversion) that will be used if the ventricular rate does not decrease with drug therapy.

THROMBOSIS AND EMBOLIZATION

Mural thrombi form within the heart near the site of the prosthetic valve or in the atria when stasis of blood results from atrial fibrillation. These thrombi can be released and can migrate to other areas, such as coronary arteries (producing coronary ischemia), cerebral circulation (producing a cerebrovascular accident), or to extremities (causing occlusion of arterial circulation). Thrombi can also arise from veins in legs. These can migrate to the lungs, causing pulmonary emboli.

Assessment

1. Symptoms of a myocardial infarction (see discussion under *Coronary Heart Disease* in this chapter).
2. Mental confusion or irritability, weakness of one side of the body if cerebral circulation is affected.
3. Increased respiratory rate, shallow respirations, acute chest pain aggravated by respiratory movements, and dyspnea. Po_2 is 80 mm Hg or below.
4. A cold, numb extremity with lack of peripheral pulses and changes in skin color, indicative of occlusion of a peripheral artery.

Revised Outcomes

1. See Expected Outcomes for myocardial infarction under *Coronary Heart Disease* in this chapter.
2. See Expected Outcomes for clients with cerebrovascular accidents in Chapter 25.
3. See Expected Outcomes for clients with pulmonary embolism or infarction in Chapter 31.
4. Occlusion of an artery in an extremity will be relieved.

Interventions

1. See Interventions for myocardial infarction under *Coronary Heart Disease* in this chapter.
2. See Chapter 25 for interventions for cerebrovascular accidents.
3. For a suspected peripheral arterial occlusion, an angiogram is done to make a definitive diagnosis. Give analgesics for the pain, place the affected extremity in a dependent position, and wrap the extremity loosely with cotton to preserve body heat. If there is no relief within a few hours, an endarterectomy may be needed.
4. For pulmonary embolism or infarction, heparin is used, or fibrinolytic therapy with urokinase or streptokinase, if massive, to enhance fibrinolysis of the emboli. Vasopressor drug therapy may be needed. Possibly, surgery will be needed for clients unable to take anticoagulants or those who have recurrent emboli in spite of anticoagulant therapy. Surgery consists of vena caval ligation plication

or insertion of a device ("umbrella" filter) to filter blood returning to the heart and lungs (Nurses Reference Library, 1981).

SHOCK

Shock can be caused by a failing heart (cardiogenic) or by hypovolemia (from loss of fluid and/or blood). The result of shock is decreased tissue perfusion, decreased venous return, and low cardiac output.

Reevaluation and Follow-up

1. The client is discharged home by about the tenth day. By this time, the client will have had discharge planning regarding activity schedule, medications, diet and may have had a referral to a public health agency for further follow-up care.
2. Reevaluation includes assessment of:
   a. Cardiac status: palpation of pulses for rhythm and quality, blood pressure determination, and auscultation for abnormal heart sounds.
   b. Respiratory status: respiratory rate and depth of respiration, presence of dyspnea and its association with emotional status and activity.
   c. Client's compliance with the regimen:
      (1) Medications (anticoagulant therapy).
      (2) Diet.
      (3) Activity.
   d. Client's and family's knowledge of therapy and side effects that need to be reported.

HYPERTROPHIC OBSTRUCTIVE CARDIOMYOPATHY

DESCRIPTION

Hypertrophic obstructive cardiomyopathy (HOCM) is characterized by hypertrophy of the left ventricle, involving the interventricular septum and sometimes the right ventricle as well. There is a genetic basis to the disease in that it can occur in many members of the same family. This abnormality affects the outflow tract from the left ventricle, resulting in obstruction to left ventricular systolic ejection. This condition is called by various names: hypertrophic obstructive cardiomyopathy, idiopathic hypertrophic subaortic stenosis (IHSS), or muscular subaortic stenosis (MSS).

Most commonly, the condition occurs in young adults, predominantly in the third and fourth decades. The prognosis depends on the extent of obstruction to left ventricular ejection, although the course is extremely variable and death can occur suddenly without warning. The development of atrial fibrillation is a poor prognostic sign because cardiac output decreases with this arrhythmia.

PREVENTION

Health Promotion

Because of the risk of sudden death in clients with this disease, strenuous exercise is inadvisable.

Population at Risk

Adults with familial history of the disease.

Screening

1. Electrocardiogram for cardiac hypertrophy.
2. Echocardiogram for valvular movement.
3. Chest x-ray study for cardiac size.

ASSESSMENT

Health History

1. Although the age of clients ranges from birth to 85 years, the majority are in the third and fourth decades.
2. Clients give a history of exertional dyspnea and angina pectoris. In addition, dizziness and fainting spells are common, especially when they suddenly assume an erect posture.

Physical Assessment

1. A jerky arterial pulse with a sharp upstroke is typical. A bifid pulse may be palpated, especially over the carotid artery. The initial peak results from an early unobstructed rapid ventricular ejection and the later peak from relief of dynamic outflow obstruction.
2. Many clients have a thrill along the lower precordium and/or at the apex.
3. A systolic murmur, usually grade III over VI or louder, commences after a brief pause following S_1. It is heard along the left sternal border and at the apex and is not transmitted to the neck.
4. A prominent S_4 is frequently evident.

5. Client's symptoms include:
   a. Exertional dyspnea.
   b. Angina pectoris.
   c. Dizziness and syncope.
   d. Palpitations if arrhythmias are present.

Diagnostic Tests

1. An electrocardiogram shows signs of left ventricular hypertrophy, abnormal broad Q waves in leads II, III, aVF (due probably to septal hypertrophy). It also shows features of Wolff-Parkinson-White (W-P-W) syndrome, left anterior hemiblock, bundle branch block, and atrial and ventricular arrhythmias.
2. An echocardiogram is the most useful diagnostic tool for this disease for detecting the presence of the abnormality as well as following the progression in clients. It shows increased thickness of the interventricular septum and the left ventricular posterior wall and their movements during systole. The motion of the mitral valve is analyzed during systole also. Abnormal systolic anterior motion of the anterior mitral leaflet with its opposition against the septum localizes the outflow obstruction of HOCM.
3. A chest x-ray study may not be helpful and may even be normal. Evidence of left ventricular enlargement may be subtle, as the cavity size is not increased.
4. Cardiac catheterization with angiography. One of the most important features of the disease is the variability in the severity of obstruction. For instance, large variations in the systolic pressure gradient occur in the course of a single study. This increased pressure gradient can be demonstrated by exercise, elevation of legs, Valsalva maneuver, or by giving certain drugs such as isoproterenol. The angiogram characteristically reveals marked thickening of the left ventricular wall. The left ventricular cavity tends to be unusually small and may almost be obliterated at the end of ejection.

NURSING DIAGNOSES: ACTUAL OR POTENTIAL

1. Activity intolerance: secondary to cardiac dysfunction.
2. Fear: associated with dizziness or syncope.
3. Knowledge deficit: regarding reportable signs and symptoms.

EXPECTED OUTCOMES

1. There will be a gradual improvement in exercise tolerance.
2. Fear of attacks of dizziness and syncope will be reduced.
3. Client will identify reportable signs and symptoms.

Interventions

1. Teach the client to increase exercise gradually and to avoid strenuous exercise.
2. If syncope occurs, elevate client's legs to augment venous return to the heart.
3. Medical therapy.
   a. Give oxygen therapy for dyspnea.
   b. Beta-adrenergic blockers, to diminish anginal attacks and arrhythmias by slowing the heart rate. Teach the client the purpose of the drug.
   c. Avoid giving digitalis preparations except for rapid atrial fibrillation when other drugs are unsuccessful.
   d. Do not administer nitrates, as they are contraindicated.
   e. Use diuretics carefully in order to avoid hypovolemia.
   f. Use anticoagulants if atrial fibrillation is present to prevent thrombi.
4. Surgical therapy involves an incision of the muscular ridge at the left ventricular outflow tract. (See the discussion of pre- and postsurgical cardiac care in this chapter.)

EVALUATION

Outcome Criteria

1. Anginal attacks and the heart rate are decreased.
2. Exercise tolerance improves within 3 months of therapy.
3. Arrhythmias causing palpitations are reduced by the time of discharge.

Complications

1. Heart failure (see the discussion under *Congestive Heart Failure* in this chapter).
2. Following surgery (see the discussion of cardiac surgery in this chapter).

Reevaluation and Follow-up

1. Assess the presence of systolic murmurs and the quality of the pulse.
2. Assess the presence of arrhythmias causing

the discomfort of palpitations and activity intolerance.
3. Relate the frequency of anginal, dizziness, and syncopal attacks to the time of medication administration.
4. Reevaluate the client's knowledge of medications and exercise tolerance.

HYPERACTIVITY AND HYPOACTIVITY

CONGESTIVE HEART FAILURE

DESCRIPTION

Congestive heart failure is a syndrome in which the heart is unable to pump an adequate supply of blood to meet the oxygen and nutritional needs of the body.

The causes are factors that:

1. Increase the work of the heart, such as:
   a. Systemic or pulmonary hypertension.
   b. Fast-rate arrhythmias.
   c. Demands for increased cardiac output (high output failure) such as hyperthyroidism, high fever from infectious diseases, and anemia.
2. Decrease cardiac contractility, such as:
   a. Myocardial infarction.
   b. Arrhythmias of all types related to disturbances to impulse initiation or conduction.
   c. Pericarditis or cardiac tamponade.
3. Hinder or deter the flow of blood within the heart, such as:
   a. Valvular defects.
   b. Congenital cardiac anomalies.

Cardiac reserve is the ability of the heart to compensate for increased demands placed upon it. *Cardiac output* is the amount of blood ejected by the heart per minute. It is determined by:

1. Heart rate, which is governed by the balance between the sympathetic (increases) and the parasympathetic (decreases) nervous systems.
2. Stroke volume, which is regulated by the Frank-Starling law of the heart. This law states that by increasing the filling volume and stretching the myofibrils, there will be a proportionate increase in contractility. This process continues to a point. After this, further stretch no longer produces increased contractility (see Figure 30-7).

There are three main *compensatory mechanisms* by which the heart is able to compensate for beginning failure. When limits for these mechanisms are exceeded, decompensation is said to exist and symptoms become evident. These mechanisms are:

1. Increased sympathetic nervous system activity via the transmitter, norepinephrine, which is stored in vesicles in the myocardium and secreted by the adrenal medulla. The result is increased heart rate, increased contractility, and vasoconstriction to increase return of blood to the heart.
2. Increased retention of sodium by the kidneys. This is accomplished through increased renin, which then increases angiotensin, which then increases aldosterone. Finally, al-

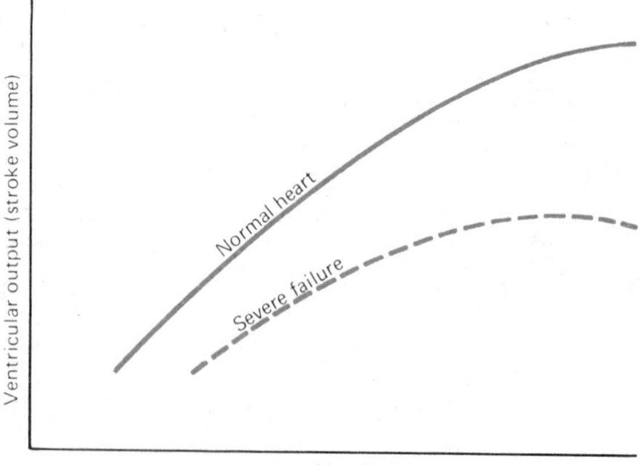

Figure 30-7 Graph of ventricular function curves. In the normal heart, increased myofibril length increases stroke volume. In the failing heart, a point is reached when increased lengthening no longer increases the stroke volume. (Pinneo, R.: *Congestive Heart Failure*, Appleton-Century-Crofts, East Norwalk, Ct., 1978, p. 17. Used by permission of the publisher.)

dosterone causes retention of sodium. The posterior pituitary gland senses this increased sodium and secretes antidiuretic hormone to further increase the retention of fluid.

3. Hypertrophy and dilatation of the heart. Hypertrophy is the thickening of the muscle walls to increase contractility. Dilatation is the stretching of myofibrils to increase size of chambers. Both of these have limitations in effectiveness in increasing cardiac output.

There are several forms of heart failure. The heart consists of two separate but related pumping systems: the left heart, which is the pump for the systemic circuit and the right heart, which is the pump for the pulmonary circuit. Heart failure may involve the left heart, the right heart, or both.

1. *Left-sided heart failure* always results from damage to the myocardium of the left ventricle. This damage causes a decrease in the pumping ability of the left ventricle, which results in its failure to eject its full quota of blood when the heart contracts. As more blood enters the left ventricle, it meets resistance from this remaining blood. This causes the left atrium to increase its pressure to overcome this resistance. In turn, this increased pressure is reflected in the pulmonary veins and capillaries. These congested pulmonary vessels impede the exchange of oxygen and carbon dioxide across the walls of the aveoli of the lungs and the capillaries. As the situation continues, fluid from the capillaries is forced by the increased pressure into the alveoli of the lungs.
2. *Right-sided heart failure* is often a sequela to left-sided heart failure, for the increased pressure in the pulmonary vascular system causes the right ventricle to dilate and hypertrophy to meet the increased work load. Right-sided heart failure may also occur when pulmonary diseases are present, which puts an added burden on the right ventricle. When the right ventricle fails, it no longer ejects its normal quota of blood volume and some remains after contraction. The residual volume now impedes blood flow from the right atrium, which has to increase its pressure to exceed the pressure in the right ventricle in order to empty blood into it. This then creates a backward pressure throughout the entire peripheral venous system.

PREVENTION

Health Promotion

1. Early detection and treatment of predisposing factors of heart failure, such as hyperthyroidism, infectious diseases, anemia, valvular defects, congenital heart defects, or coronary artery disease.
2. Follow-up care of persons with any cardiovascular disease for the first symptoms of heart failure.
3. Instruction of persons with cardiovascular problems to:
   a. Maintain good health habits.
   b. Maintain a regular exercise program according to individual tolerance levels.
   c. Report symptoms of heart failure immediately.
   d. Avoid high altitudes or unpressurized airplanes.
   e. Avoid extremes of environmental temperatures or increases in humidity that increase cardiac work; use air conditioners or dehumidifiers to help control the environment.
4. Avoidance of stressful situations that increase anxiety and the work of the heart.
5. Monitoring the rate of intravenous fluids of hospitalized clients to avoid overloading the circulatory volume.

Population at Risk

1. Persons who have had an acute myocardial infarction.
2. Persons with elevated cholesterol levels.
3. Persons with history of rheumatic heart disease, infections, hypertension, alcoholism, and structural heart defects.
4. Persons who are obese, anemic, or have a vitamin deficiency.
5. Pregnant women with a history of cardiac problems.

Screening

1. Electrocardiogram.
2. Chest x-ray study.
3. Auscultation of the heart for a ventricular gallop (S_3).

ASSESSMENT

Health History

1. Client complains of fatigue that increases throughout the day.
2. Complaints of restlessness and insomnia are common and may be due to beginning dyspnea.
3. If dyspnea is a complaint, find out what activities precipitate it, what time of day or night it occurs, and whether its occurrence causes a change in normal routine activities. Also, find out whether pillows are needed at night.
4. Inquire about any subtle behavior change such as confusion or decreased memory span, as these may indicate cardiac decompensation.
5. An increase in cough with expectoration should be inquired about to determine whether it occurs after exertion or at night, when it may interfere with sleep.
6. Client may have experienced a recent weight gain and swelling of the ankles.

Physical Assessment

1. Left-sided heart failure. The following symptoms develop because of congestion in the lungs due to the back pressure from the left side of the heart.
   a. Dyspnea (shortness of breath). This may be the earliest symptom of left-sided failure. At first it may occur only on exertion. Later, it occurs with normal activities or at rest.
   b. Orthopnea. If dyspnea occurs when the client is recumbent and is relieved when the client sits upright, this condition is called orthopnea.
   c. Paroxysmal nocturnal dyspnea. Sudden dyspnea occurs when the client is asleep. Client awakens, feels suffocated, and usually coughs and wheezes. The client often finds relief by sitting upright in bed or opening the window.
   d. Acute pulmonary edema. This is the most extreme form of left-sided heart failure. Massive accumulation of fluid occurs in the alveoli of the lungs, which greatly interferes with gaseous exchange and results in hypoxia. Unless it is corrected immediately, this leads to death from severe hypoxia and arrhythmias.
   e. As cardiac output from the left ventricle falls. arterial pressure in the kidneys decreases. The body compensates for what it senses as low blood volume by increasing enzymes that retain sodium and water. This serves to increase venous return to the heart and increases the work load of the heart.
   f. Cerebral anoxia. When the left ventricle fails and cardiac output is decreased, the amount of oxygen going to the brain is decreased. This causes irritability, restlessness, and confusion. For some reason, this seems to happen at night more than during the daytime, possibly because fluid is transferred from interstitial spaces to the circulatory system and the heart cannot accept this increased volume.
   g. Fatigue and muscular weakness. Another effect of a low cardiac output is profound exhaustion. Oxygen to the tissues is diminished and removal of metabolic wastes is delayed.
   h. Physical signs to watch for are:
      (1) Rales. On auscultation of the bases of the lungs, one can detect abnormal breath sounds that reflect the presence of fluid in the alveoli. As the situation worsens, rales are heard higher in the lung fields. Therefore, the height of where rales are heard in the chest is indicative of the extent of heart failure.
      (2) Gallop rhythm. By auscultation of heart sounds, a triple rhythm can be heard that consists of S_1, S_2, and S_3. The third heart sound is abnormal in the adult and indicates dilatation of the left ventricle with an increase of fluid volume entering it.
      (3) Pulsus alternans. A strong heart beat alternates with a weak heart beat because of variation in the stroke volume.
      (4) Tachycardia is often present to compensate for a decreased cardiac output.
2. Right-sided heart failure. When the right side of the heart fails, the symptoms relate to the retention of sodium and water within the body, which causes edema and venous congestion within the organs.
   a. Distended neck veins. These are due to increased venous pressure. Normally, neck veins do not remain distended when a client is sitting at an angle of 45 degrees. In the client with right-sided heart failure,

however, the neck veins remain distended at this angle because of the increased back pressure from the right atrium. This may be one of the earliest signs of right-sided heart failure and should be observed by turning the client's neck slightly and using tangential lighting.

b. Peripheral edema. This is caused by the increased pressure in the venous circulation that forces fluid from the capillaries into interstitial spaces. It is necessary to look for edema in dependent parts of the body, such as the ankles, if the client is sitting in a chair, or in the sacrum, if the client remains in bed. If edema is generalized and found throughout the body, the term *anasarca* is used.
c. Weight gain. A gain in weight corresponds to the fluid retention mentioned above. Weighing the client is a far more precise measurement of fluid retention than observing for edema, for a person can accumulate up to 10 lb of fluid before edema is obvious.
d. Liver enlargement and abdominal pain. As the liver becomes congested with fluid, it enlarges and thus stretches the capsule surrounding it. This causes tenderness in the abdomen and is often accompanied by anorexia and nausea. When pressure is applied over an engorged liver, neck veins distend. This phenomenon is called *hepatojugular reflux.*
e. Coolness of the extremities. This is due to the reduction of peripheral blood flow.
f. Anxiety and fear. The client realizes that his or her heart is diseased and knows the significance of this. The client may have sleep disturbances, become very depressed, or withdraw from reality and use denial as a coping mechanism.

Diagnostic Tests

1. Electrocardiogram shows an enlarged heart and tachycardia.
2. Chest x-ray study shows an enlarged heart and pulmonary involvement if there is pulmonary edema.
3. Although not done routinely, an arm-to-tongue circulation time may be done to determine if circulation is prolonged. Normal range is 9–16 s. In heart failure, this time is increased.

NURSING DIAGNOSES: ACTUAL OR POTENTIAL

1. Alteration in comfort: due to dyspnea.
2. Anxiety: due to the disease process.
3. Noncompliance: due to knowledge deficit.
4. Alteration in mentation: due to decreased cerebral perfusion.
5. Fatigue: due to decreased oxygenation of tissues.

EXPECTED OUTCOMES

1. Immediate.
   a. Fluid volume will be decreased.
   b. Fatigue and dyspnea on exertion will decrease.
   c. Pulse rate will decrease.
   d. Anxiety will decrease.
2. Long-range.
   a. Client will adapt a lifestyle compatible with the cardiac status.
   b. Client will know, with 85 percent accuracy the reasons for therapy and the symptoms to be reported.
   c. Client will know the energy costs of activities and their relationship to cardiac endurance.

INTERVENTIONS

1. To increase contractility of the myocardium, digitalis preparations will be used. When giving these drugs, the nurse should understand:
   a. The effects of digitalis preparations.
      (1) They enhance the force of myocardial contraction, thus increasing the cardiac output.
      (2) They slow the heart by vagal stimulation, thus decreasing fast-rate arrhythmias and allowing increased filling time for better contraction.
   b. The toxic effects of digitalis preparations.
      (1) On the cardiovascular system:
         (a) Arrhythmias: ventricular bigeminy, paroxysmal atrial tachycardia with block and atrioventricular block. These may be due to potassium depletion, especially when diuretics are given concurrently.
         (b) Changes in heart rate, particularly rates below 60 (may be due to an atrioventricular block).

(c) Pulse deficit between the radial pulse rate and the apical rate, indicating a variation in stroke volume as in atrial fibrillation.

(2) On gastrointestinal system:
 (a) Early symptoms: nausea and vomiting, and then anorexia.
 (b) Later symptoms: diarrhea and abdominal pain.

(3) On the central nervous system:
 (a) Visual disturbances, particularly yellow vision.
 (b) Confusion, lethargy, headache.

(4) If there are symptoms of digitalis toxicity, inform the physician before giving further digitalis preparations (see Table 30-1).

2. Oxygen therapy and rest will help to reestablish the balance between myocardial oxygen supply and demand.
 a. Use oxygen therapy by means of nasal cannulas or masks. Be sure to maintain humidification of the oxygen.
 b. Provide mental and physical rest so that the work of the heart will decrease and oxygen needs are met. Avoid complete client immobility because of its complications. Encourage client to use a bedside commode and to perform self-care activities to some extent, such as feeding and bathing.
 c. Provide supportive help for client's anxiety after identifying its cause. Include the family in counseling when appropriate.

3. To decrease the work of the heart by reducing blood volume returning to the heart:
 a. Use diuretics, which interfere with the reabsorption of sodium by the kidneys, thus, aiding in excreting fluid from the body. Diuretics used in heart failure include:
 (1) Thiazides. Used for moderate heart failure.
 (a) Chlorothiazide (Diuril).
 (b) Hydrochlorothiazide (Hydrodiuril).
 (2) Furosemide (Lasix). Rapid acting when given intravenously and, therefore, may cause electrolyte imbalance. May also be given orally.
 (3) Ethacrynic acid (Edecrin). Rapid-acting when given intravenously and, therefore, may cause electrolyte imbalance. May also be given orally.
 (4) Aldosterone antagonists: spironolactone (Aldactone). Used in mild heart failure. Blocks action of aldosterone, thus increasing urinary excretion of fluid.
 b. Be on the alert for symptoms of hypokalemia (low potassium) when using diuretics. These include weakness, gastrointes-

TABLE 30-1 COMMON CARDIAC GLYCOSIDES USED IN PUMP FAILURE

	Total Digitalizing Dose (usually given in divided dosages over a period of time)	Maintenance Dose (daily)	Onset of Action[a]	Peak Effect[a]	Gastro-intestinal Absorption	Means of Elimination
Digoxin	2.9–3.0 mg PO 0.75–1.5 mg IV	0.25–0.75 mg PO	15–30 min	1–5 h	60–85%	Renal
Digitoxin	1.2–1.6 mg PO 1.2–1.6 mg IV	0.05–0.2 mg PO	½–2 h	4–12 h	90–100%	Hepatic-renal
Deslanoside	1.2–1.6 mg IV or IM		10–30 min	1–2 h	Erratic	Renal
Ouabain	0.25–0.5 mg IV		5–10 min	½–2 h	Erratic	Renal

SOURCE: Jones, D., Dunbar, C., and Jirovec, M.: *Medical-Surgical Nursing: A Conceptual Approach*, McGraw-Hill, New York, 1978, p. 825. Used by permission of the publisher.

[a] The onset of action and peak effect are based on the initial IV administration of the digitalizing dose.

tinal complaints, and arrhythmias. Clients on digitalis preparations and diuretic therapy are particularly prone to develop hypokalemia; therefore, potassium supplements in the forms of medications or an increase in potassium-rich foods are used.

c. Use a sodium-restricted diet to prevent, control, and eliminate fluid by lowering the amount of sodium in the body. To make this measure effective, also restrict the client's fluid intake. Make this diet more palatable by suggesting seasoning, such as lemon juice, vinegar, lime juice, or mint. Salt substitutes can be suggested if the physician agrees to them.

d. Give morphine sulfate to relieve anxiety, especially when dyspnea is present. It also causes some venous dilatation, thus relieving the heart of some fluid load.

4. To help the client adopt a lifestyle compatible with the heart condition:
   a. Teach the client and family the need for a balance between rest and activity and how to know the caloric expenditure of energy associated with various activities.
   b. Assist the client and family in achieving a low-salt diet by reading labels on food products to determine their ingredients and by providing a list of foods with their related sodium content.
   c. Weigh the client the same time each day in the hospital and teach its importance after discharge. Weight comparisons can then be made and weight gain due to fluid accumulation can be confirmed and interventions adjusted.
5. To help the client understand the reasons for interventions and symptoms of problems:
   a. Teach the client the necessity for digitalis therapy according to the physician's prescription but to report side effects if they occur. Teach the client and family to take the pulse and report changes.
   b. Teach the client the reason for diuretic therapy and to avoid taking the medication near bed time to avoid its diuretic effect at night. Also teach the client the possible side effects, especially hypokalemia, and what foods to supplement that are high in potassium unless the physician has ordered potassium replacements as drug therapy.
   c. Emphasize routine follow-up care, which includes an electrocardiogram and serum electrolytes. In addition, teach the client symptoms indicating worsening of the heart failure, such as severe dyspnea, increased peripheral edema, cough, weakness, and lethargy.

EVALUATION

Outcome Critiera

1. Cardiac work load resumes more normal function, as evidenced by:
   a. Decrease in dyspnea, edema, weight, and fatigue.
   b. Pulse rate decreases and is stronger.
2. Anxiety is lessened.
3. Client adopts a lifestyle compatible with cardiac status.
4. Client understands reasons for therapy.
5. Client understands the effect of activities on the work of the heart.

Complications

ACUTE PULMONARY EDEMA

This condition is an extreme form of left-sided heart failure. Because of increased capillary pressure within the pulmonary capillaries, fluid with some blood cells from the blood seeps across the interstitial spaces into the alveoli of the lungs.

Assessment

1. Acute respiratory distress with severe dyspnea, noisy moist respirations, frothy red-tinged sputum, cough, and cyanosis.
2. Intense fear and a sense of doom.
3. Coarse rales or rhonchi heard in lower parts of the lungs.
4. Tachycardia as a compensatory mechanism to increase cardiac output.
5. Diaphoresis.

Revised Outcomes

1. Circulatory volume of fluid to the heart and lungs will decrease.
2. Oxygen supply to tissues will be increased.
3. Myocardial contractility will improve.
4. Respirations will improve.
5. Fear and anxiety will decrease.

Interventions

1. Decrease the volume of fluids to the heart and lungs:
   a. Use rapid-acting diuretics, such as furosemide (Lasix) 40–80 mg IV push, or ethacrynic acid (Edecrin) 50 mg IV push. When giving these drugs, watch for po-

tassium depletion. Potassium replacement is usually needed. Be sure to dilute the potassium in IV fluids; *never* give potassium as an IV push in a concentrated form.

b. Use rotating tourniquets (Figure 30-8). These are applied high on the four extremities, except where intravenous fluids are administered. Three of the four are tightened to trap blood in the extremities and thus reduce venous return to the heart. Although not used frequently today because of improved rapid-acting diuretics, the nurse may have occasion to know the correct use of them in some situations.
   (1) Tighten only enough to occlude venous circulation and not arterial circulation. Take the pulse distal to the tightened tourniquet to make sure of this. Put an X mark at the locations of pulses to save time for later checks.
   (2) Prepare a diagram and a chart to make sure that the clockwise rotation will continue every 15 min.
   (3) Use a small towel under each tourniquet to prevent skin irritation.
   (4) When terminating, loosen only one tourniquet at a time every 15 min to prevent a sudden increase in circulating blood to the heart.

c. A phlebotomy or venesection is done to remove approximately 500 mL of blood. Be sure to check the blood pressure before this procedure is done. If there is hypotension, the phlebotomy would make it worse.

2. Increase oxygen supply to tissues by giving oxygen in high concentrations, initially by an intermittent positive pressure breathing machine and a tight-fitting mask. Alcohol (20 to 50 percent) is sometimes used in the nebulizer of the equipment for its antifoaming action in reducing pulmonary secretions.
3. Increase myocardial contractility by giving a rapid-acting digitalis preparation intravenously.
4. Improve respirations by the above measures and by:
   a. Giving aminophylline intravenously or

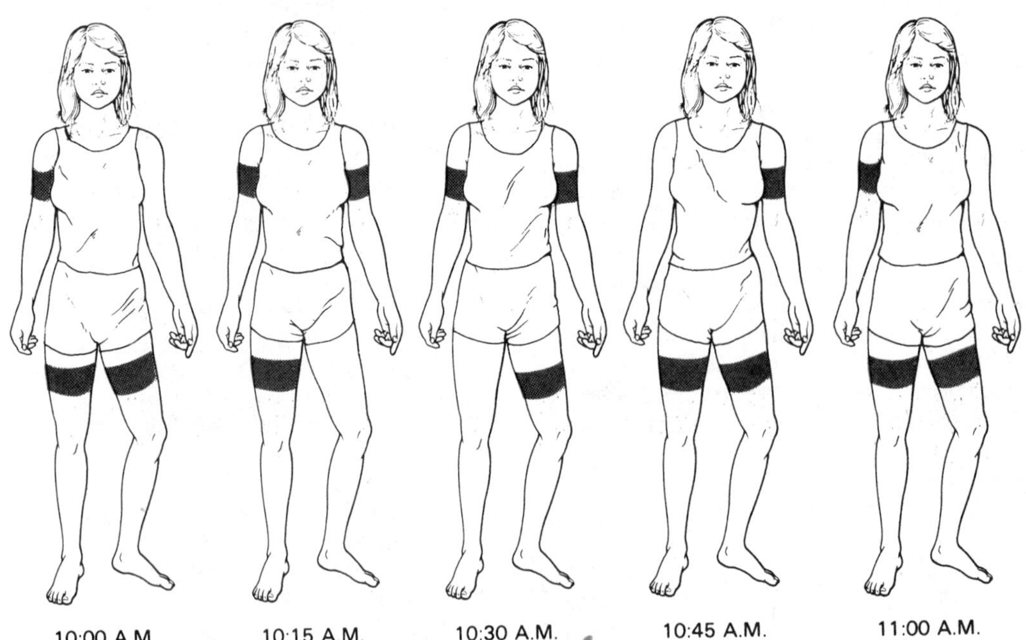

Figure 30-8 Rotating tourniquets. (Luckmann, J., and Sorensen, K., *Medical-Surgical Nursing: A Psychophysiologic Approach*, 2d ed., Saunders, Philadelphia, 1980, p. 812. Used by permission of the publisher.)

via suppository to relieve bronchospasm, which interferes with respirations. It is given in a dosage of 250–500 mg diluted in 50 mL fluid over a 15-min period. Monitor the client for the development of tachycardia and increased arrhythmias.
   b. Placing the client in a high Fowler's position allows the lungs to expand by depressing the diaphragm. This assists breathing by gravitational forces that allow fluid to accumulate in the lower lungs.
5. Decrease fear and anxiety by:
   a. Giving morphine, 10–15 mg intravenously. This also slows the rapid respiratory rate and creates some peripheral vasodilatation.
   b. Explaining to the client and family diagnostic tests and interventions.
   c. Having a nurse remain with the client until the acute phase has subsided.
6. If intervention for heart failure is unsuccessful, the client may proceed to develop *cardiogenic shock*, an extreme form of pump failure (see the discussion of this complication under *Cardiogenic Shock* in this chapter).

Reevaluation and Follow-up

Clients with congestive heart failure need to have continued follow-up care as, in most cases, the precipitating cause of the heart failure cannot be removed. This follow-up care should include an appraisal of:

1. The client's knowledge of the cardiac condition and the importance of continuing with the interventions.
2. The client's change in lifestyle in restriction of activities, planned rest, and awareness of the effect of stress on the heart.
3. The avoidance of activities that cause dyspnea, fatigue, weakness, and palpitations.

PULMONARY HEART DISEASE

DESCRIPTION

Pulmonary heart disease (cor pulmonale) is hypertrophy of the right ventricle resulting from diseases affecting the function and/or the structure of the lungs, such as chronic obstructive pulmonary disease (COPD). The common factor preceding right ventricular hypertrophy is pulmonary hypertension, which causes an increased pressure work load on the right ventricle.

The pathophysiological changes associated with pulmonary heart disease include:

1. Pulmonary capillary destruction and pulmonary vasoconstriction (usually secondary to hypoxia) reduce the cross-sectional area of the pulmonary vascular bed.
2. To compensate for the extra work needed to force blood through the lungs, the right ventricle dilates and hypertrophies.
3. In response to low oxygen content, the bone marrow produces more red blood cells, causing erythrocytosis. When the hemotocrit exceeds 55 percent, blood viscosity increases. This further aggravates pulmonary hypertension and increases the hemodynamic load on the right ventricle.
4. Right ventricular failure results (Nurses Reference Library, 1981).

PREVENTION

Health Promotion

1. Avoidance of cigarette smoking.
2. Avoidance of exposure to individuals with upper respiratory infections.
3. Reduced exposure to air pollution (as in industrialized communities).
4. Avoidance of exposure to occupational pollution (asbestos, dust, cotton, silica) by using protective devices such as masks.

Population at Risk

1. Persons with genetic predisposition, such as alpha-antitrypsin deficiency (Jones, 1978). (Alpha-antitrypsin is an enzyme that normally protects lung tissue during inflammation.)
2. Persons having chronic bronchitis or frequent respiratory infections.
3. Cigarette smokers.
4. Persons living in densely populated industrial cities.
5. Elderly men more often than women.

Screening

1. Ventilatory screening with the use of a spirometer. If abnormal results are found, further pulmonary function tests should be done.
2. Chest x-ray study. This is helpful only for advanced pulmonary disease.

ASSESSMENT

Health History

1. Progressive exertional dyspnea and gradual restriction of activities over a period of time.
2. If cough is a complaint, inquire about its characteristics: frequency, whether it is productive or nonproductive, and time of day.
3. Cigarette smoking history and onset, number of cigarettes per day, number of years. If smoking has stopped, determine reasons for quitting.

Physical Assessment

1. General appearance: thin individual with a barrel chest.
2. Increased respiration rate with a prolonged expiratory time.
3. Anteroposterior diameter of the chest increases and accessory muscles of respirations are used.
4. Dyspnea is progressive and worsens with exertion.
5. Clubbing of fingers and toes may be present, due to chronic hypoxia to extremities.
6. Decreased expansion of the chest because of hyperinflation.
7. On percussion, hyperresonance is noted over the chest wall.
8. On auscultation of breath sounds, sonorous rhonchi are produced by secretions in the airway and may clear after productive coughing. Wheezes, high-pitched musical sounds, are produced by airflow through narrowed airways and are more pronounced on expiration.
9. Pansystolic murmur at left lower sternal border due to tricuspid insufficiency. Its intensity increases on inspiration.

Diagnostic Tests

1. Spirometry is used to measure lung volumes, capacities, and flow rates.
2. Chest x-ray study shows large central pulmonary arteries and an enlarged right heart.
3. Echocardiography indicates right ventricular enlargement.
4. Arterial blood gases show decreased Po_2 (often less than 70 mmHg and never more than 90 mmHg).
5. Electrocardiogram shows arrhythmias during severe hypoxia; may also show right bundle branch block, right axis deviation, and right ventricular hypertrophy.
6. Complete blood count reveals an elevated hemoglobin and hemotocrit with secondary polycythemia associated with chronic hypoxia.
7. Pulmonary artery pressure measurements (by pulmonary artery catheter) show increased right ventricular and pulmonary artery pressure. Right ventricular systolic and pulmonary artery systolic pressures will be more than 30 mmHg.

NURSING DIAGNOSES: ACTUAL OR POTENTIAL

1. Lack of compliance: secondary to knowledge deficit.
2. Ineffective airway clearance: secondary to increased accumulation of bronchial secretions.
3. Anxiety: due to limitation of activities and accompanying symptoms.
4. Potential for respiratory infections.
5. Activity intolerance: secondary to respiratory dysfunction.

EXPECTED OUTCOMES

1. Client will give evidence of compliance with the plan of care by:
   a. Reducing the number of cigarettes by one-half or eliminating smoking within 1 month.
   b. Avoiding environmental and industrial irritants and pollutants.
   c. Adhering to the drug regimen, as indicated by recordkeeping.
   d. Establishing an effective exercise and rest regimen in the lifestyle.
   e. Adhering to a low-salt diet.
2. Client will decrease bronchial secretions within 2 weeks of therapy, as evidenced by clear lung sounds.
3. Client will demonstrate effective deep breathing and postural drainage techniques.
4. Anxiety will be lessened within 1 month as exercise tolerance increases.
5. Client will learn how to avoid respiratory infections.
6. Client will pace activities, as evidenced by decreased fatigue and dyspnea after activities.

INTERVENTIONS

1. Make sure the client understands:
   a. The effect of cigarette smoking and environmental polutants on the respiratory system.

   b. The importance of maintaining a low-salt diet.
   c. How to detect dependent edema. Teach the client to press the skin over the shin and observe for finger impression after release.
   d. How to avoid respiratory infections and to report early symptoms of infection (sputum production, cough or wheeze, fever).
   e. How to establish an exercise and rest regimen.
   f. Postural drainage techniques.
   g. The procedure for breathing and exhaling through pursed lips and then taking another breath and cough on expiration.
2. Administer prescribed bronchodilators (ephedrine or aminophylline) and prophylactic antibiotics to reduce inflammation and promote liquefaction and removal of excess secretions.
3. Give carefully controlled low concentrations (24 to 40 percent) of oxygen, depending on the arterial Po_2.
4. Give low-salt nutritious diet, restricted fluid intake, and diuretics to reduce edema.

EVALUATION

Outcome Criteria

1. Client shows compliance by:
   a. Decreasing number of cigarettes by one-half within 1 month.
   b. Avoiding pollutants.
   c. Maintaining a record of medications.
   d. Showing evidence of a balanced exercise-rest regimen.
   e. Keeping on a low-salt diet.
2. Lung sounds show no evidence of rales or rhonchi within 2 weeks.
3. Anxiety about being ill has diminished, and client is coping more effectively with ADL.
4. Exercises and activities have been increased to optimum levels for the client.

Complications

RIGHT-HEART FAILURE

Assessment

1. Ankle edema.
2. Distended neck veins.
3. Abdominal pain resulting from liver distention.
4. On auscultation, a ventricular gallop (S_3) heard over the left sternal border at fifth intercostal space.
5. Tachycardia of 90 to 110 heart rate per minute.
6. Rapid respiratory rate.

Revised Outcomes

See those on right-heart failure under *Congestive Heart Failure* in this chapter.

Interventions

See those on heart failure under *Congestive Heart Failure* in this chapter.

Reevaluation and Follow-up

1. At 6-month intervals, evaluate the client's level of activities as it relates to symptoms. If none occur, increase activities slowly.
2. Evaluate the client's compliance with decreasing in smoking, avoiding pollutants, and avoiding respiratory infection.
3. Assess the client's emotional responses to the disease and provide psychological support.
4. Evaluate the presence of complications.

CARDIOGENIC SHOCK

DESCRIPTION

Cardiogenic shock is defined as inadequate tissue perfusion in the body as the result of decreased efficiency of the left ventricle to function as a pump. Acute myocardial infarction is frequently the cause because of tissue destruction and the subsequent loss of contractility.

As the result of the severe damage to the myocardium, the stroke volume and cardiac output are greatly reduced. This marked decrease in cardiac output causes the arterial blood pressure to fall. Finally, decreased tissue perfusion results. This means that body tissues are deprived of essential nutrients and oxygen.

The body has a wonderful ability to use compensatory mechanisms to restore adequate cardiac output and tissue perfusion. Following is a sequence of events by which cardiac output may be maintained for a time:

1. Baroreceptors sense changes in arterial pressure.
2. The sympathetic nervous system is stimulated by the vasomotor center in the medulla.
3. Release of catecholamines causes peripheral vasoconstriction and an increased heart rate.
4. As renal vasoconstriction occurs, renin is released. This stimulates angiotensin, which causes further vasoconstriction and stimu-

lates increased aldosterone from the adrenal cortex. Aldosterone retains sodium in the kidney to increase blood volume by retaining fluid.

5. Osmoreceptors in the hypothalamus sense the increased sodium levels and stimulate the posterior pituitary gland to secrete antidiuretic hormone (ADH). This results in further fluid retention (see Table 30-2).

Physical Assessment

1. Hypotension: Systolic blood pressure falls below 90 mmHg, causing a narrowed pulse pressure, as systolic pressure falls more quickly than diastolic pressure. Hypotension alone does not constitute shock; unless the hypotension is accompanied by other clinical findings of inadequate tissue perfusion, the diagnosis of shock is not justified.
2. Mental apathy, disorientation, confusion, and restlessness indicate cerebral ischemia from low cardiac output.
3. The pulse rate is fast and quality of pulse is weak. There may be a pulse deficit, identified by comparing the apical and radial pulse rates.
4. Respirations are rapid and shallow resulting from an accumulation of carbon dioxide, which stimulates the respiratory center. On auscultation of breath sounds, rales are heard in lung bases.
5. There is oliguria or anuria from diminished renal blood flow and the failure of the kidneys to function adequately. Normally, at least 60 mL/h of urine is excreted; in shock, urinary output is less than 30 mL/h.
6. The skin is cold and moist because of peripheral vasoconstriction.
7. Pallor or cyanosis is present because of decreased cardiac output.
8. Arrhythmias may be due to the lactic acidosis from anaerobic metabolism, which occurs in the absence of adequate oxygen.
9. Anxiety of client and family is extreme due to fear of outcomes.

Diagnostic Tests

1. Intraarterial pressure measurements provide accurate systolic, diastolic, and mean pressure readings on a continuous basis.
2. Arterial blood gases show low P_{O_2} and low pH (because of metabolic acidosis).
3. Electrocardiogram indicates an acute myocardial infarction and/or the presence of arrhythmias.
4. Central venous pressure measurements assess vascular volume and efficiency of the right ventricle (normal value is 5–8 cm H_2O).
5. Pulmonary artery pressure monitoring: increased pulmonary artery pressure (PAP) and increased pulmonary capillary wedge pressure (PCWP) via a Swan-Ganz catheter threaded into the pulmonary artery (see Figure 30-9).
6. Hemoglobin and hematocrit are usually decreased.
7. Blood urea nitrogen and creatinine levels are increased due to decreased kidney function.

TABLE 30-2 MECHANISM OF CARDIOGENIC SHOCK

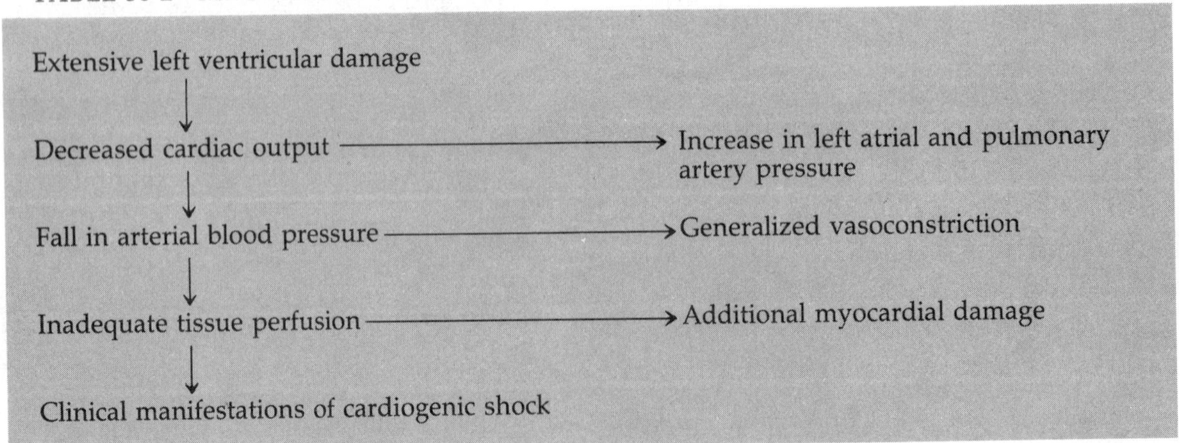

SOURCE: Meltzer, L., Pinneo, R., and Kitchell, J. R.: *Intensive Coronary Care*, 3d ed., Robert J. Brady, Co., Bowie, Md., 1977, p. 91. Used by permission of the publisher.

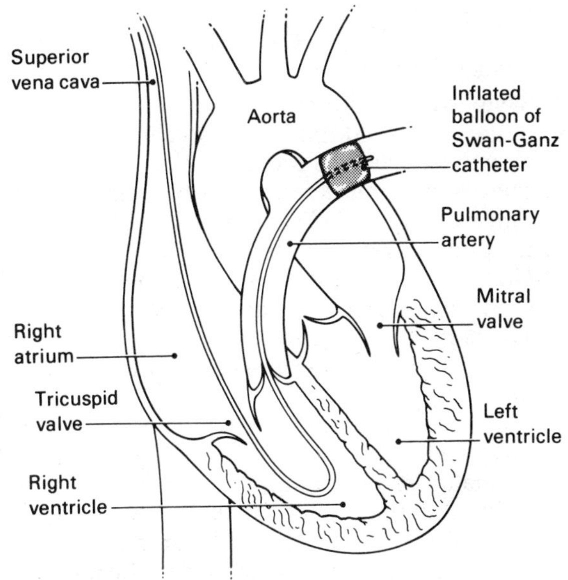

Figure 30-9 Insertion of a Swan-Ganz catheter through the right side of the heart to the pulmonary artery. Note the inflated balloon at the tip of the catheter for obtaining pulmonary capillary wedge pressure measurements.

NURSING DIAGNOSES: ACTUAL OR POTENTIAL

1. Discomfort: related to peripheral vasoconstriction.
2. Alteration in levels of consciousness: secondary to cerebral hypoperfusion.
3. Anxiety (client and family): due to fear of death.
4. Immobility: secondary to fatigue, invasive monitoring, and therapeutic devices.

EXPECTED OUTCOMES

1. Skin will be warm and dry.
2. Client will be oriented to time, person, and place.
3. Anxiety of client and family will be lessened.
4. Effects of immobility will be lessened.
5. Client will be comfortable without signs of extreme dyspnea.

INTERVENTIONS

1. Circulatory assistance.
   a. An intraarterial catheter is inserted for accurate assessments of blood pressure measurements, as cuff pressures are unreliable from the peripheral vasoconstriction. Observe the monitor connected to the catheter to assess blood pressure values and report abnormal values to the physician.
   b. Monitor cardiac rate and rhythm continuously using a cardiac monitor. Use drug therapy to slow the fast rates (antiarrhythmic drugs or sedatives) or increase slow rates (atropine).
2. Administration of drugs.
   a. Give plasma volume expanders, such as low molecular weight dextran or albumin. Watch for fluid overload by monitoring the central venous and pulmonary artery pressures. If whole blood is used, check for blood transfusion reactions.
   b. Use inotropic drugs (dopamine or dobutamine) to raise the blood pressure through selective vasoconstriction and to improve the cardiac output by improving ventricular contractility. Watch for arrhythmias and for tissue infiltration at infusion sites.
   c. Another measure to improve cardiac output is through the use of vasodilator drugs, such as sodium nitroprusside and phentolamine. These reduce the resistance in the arteries against which the left ventricle must pump, thus reducing the work of the heart. Because nitroprusside is light-sensitive, keep the infusion bottle containing it covered to protect it from light.
   d. Catheterize the client with an indwelling catheter and connect it to a collecting bottle. Measure urine output hourly and record the amount. Urea and mannitol may be given to prevent acute renal tubular damage.
3. General measures.
   a. Give oxygen therapy by using a tight-fitting mask or assisted respiratory devices. It is possible that endotracheal intubation or a tracheostomy might be needed if respiratory distress is severe.
   b. Because of client's mental confusion and altered levels of consciousness, stay with the client or have another nurse relieve you in order to provide reassurance to the client.
   c. Keep the client comfortably warm to restore normal body temperature.

d. Inform the client, if oriented, and a family member about the progress being made and plans for therapy to relieve anxiety. Allow time for them to share concerns.
e. Turn the client frequently and ask the client to deep breathe and cough at periodic intervals. Do passive range-of-motion exercises of extremities not being used for intravenous fluids or invasive monitoring.

4. Mechanical assistance. When clients do not respond to drug therapy, mechanical circulatory assistance may be used. A balloon catheter is threaded through a femoral artery to an area distal to the left subclavian artery and attached to a gas-pumping machine that uses helium or carbon dioxide to inflate the balloon around the catheter. Through synchrony with the ECG, the machine inflates the balloon during diastole and deflates it during systole. This method assists the left ventricle by lowering resistance against which it pumps during systole and enhances coronary artery filling during diastole. As the client improves, the machine can be changed in the ratio to heart beats so that, instead of inflating for each heart beat, it can be regulated to inflate for every second, every fourth, or every eighth beat (see Figure 30-10).

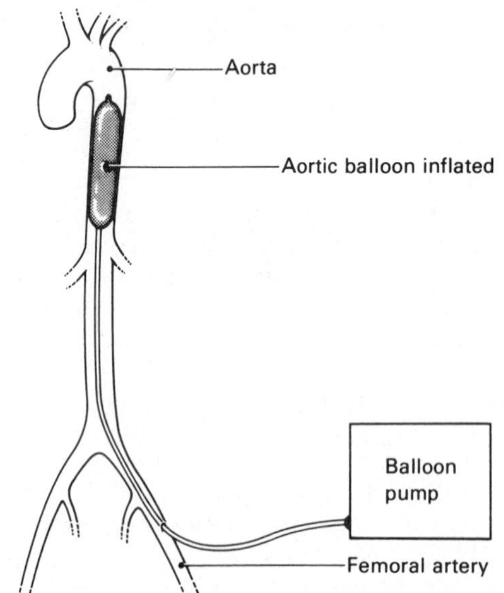

Figure 30-10 Intra-aortic balloon threaded into descending aorta via the femoral artery. By inflation and deflation in synchrony with the heartbeat, the left ventricle is assisted in its cardiac output.

EVALUATION

Outcome Criteria

1. Systolic blood pressure improves to at least a range of 90–100 mmHg, as evaluated by intraarterial pressure monitoring.
2. The client's heart rate is within the normal range of 60 to 100 beats per minute.
3. Respiratory rate is within normal range.
4. Urinary output is at least 60 mL/h.
5. Client is oriented to time and place.
6. The skin is warm and dry.

The nurse's role in the use of this device is to:

a. Frequently and carefully check the involved extremity for any changes in color, quality of pulsation, and temperature.
b. Instruct the client to avoid flexing the legs, for this movement could displace the balloon catheter that is inserted in the femoral artery.
c. Closely monitor for appropriate timing of balloon inflation and deflation.

7. The anxiety of the client and family is decreased.
8. There are no complications from immobility.

Complications

INFECTION

The infection may be caused by invasive monitoring techniques or therapy.

Assessment

1. Body temperature increases above normal values.
2. Pulse rate increases.
3. Respiratory rate increases.
4. Redness occurs on the skin at the site of infection.

Revised Outcomes

Signs of infection will cease.

Interventions

Administer antibiotic therapy specific for the organism causing the infection.

ARRHYTHMIAS

See discussion under *Arrhythmias* in this chapter.

THROMBOPHLEBITIS

See *Thrombophlebitis* in this chapter.

CARDIAC ARREST

Refer to the discussion in Chapter 49.

HEMORRHAGE AT THE SITES OF INTRAARTERIAL CATHETERS

Assessment

1. The dressings over the site of the catheter show bright red blood.
2. Blood pressure decreases.
3. All symptoms of shock become exaggerated.

Revised Outcomes

Hemorrhage will cease.

Interventions

1. Apply pressure over the area.
2. Call physician. Prepare equipment for suturing the artery.
3. If possible, elevate the involved extremity.

INFILTRATION OF INOTROPIC DRUGS AT INFUSION SITES

Assessment

1. Area around the infusion site becomes puffy.
2. Skin around the infusion site becomes blanched.

Revised outcomes

1. Tissue infiltration will cease.
2. Tissue damage will not occur.

Interventions

1. Remove intravenous fluids with the inotropic drugs.
2. Have phentolamine (Regitine) available for direct injection into tissues.

THROMBUS FORMATION WHEN CATHETERS ARE IN ARTERIES

Assessment

1. Color of extremity distal to the thrombus will be pale.
2. The pulse distal to the thrombus will be absent.
3. Temperature of the skin distal to the thrombus will be decreased.

Revised Outcomes

There will be no further formation of thrombi.

Interventions

1. Use heparin to prevent thrombi.
2. Instruct the client to avoid flexing the legs.

Reevaluation and Follow-up

1. Assess blood pressure, pulse, and repirations frequently to detect problems. (See Complications above.)
2. Assess the client daily for changes in physical and emotional state that may indicate future problems.
3. Teach the client the principles of energy expenditure related to various activities and indicate which activities are safe within the limits of his or her capabilities.
4. Evaluate progress toward rehabilitation; encourage the client on the basis of small progress.

METABOLIC, NUTRITIONAL, AND TOXIC DISORDERS

HYPERTENSION

DESCRIPTION

Hypertension is a persistent elevation of the systolic blood pressure above 140 mmHg and of the diastolic pressure above 90 mmHg. A sustained elevation of blood pressure is clinically significant because it can lead to such conditions as cerebrovascular accidents (strokes), hypertensive heart disease, nephrosclerosis, and retinal abnormalities.

There are two general ways to classify hypertension, (1) *systolic* or *diastolic* hypertension or (2) *primary* or *secondary* hypertension.

1. Systolic and diastolic hypertension.
   a. Systolic hypertension is most commonly related to arteriosclerotic changes in arterial blood vessels with advancing years in which there is a decrease in elasticity. It may also be seen in thyrotoxicosis, severe anemia, fever, and aortic valvular insufficiency as a result of an elevated cardiac output.
   b. Diastolic hypertension is a true disease phenomenon resulting from atherosclerosis of arteries. It is a reflection of the pressure exerted against the walls of small arteries, exclusive of the pressure exerted by contraction of the left ventricle.
2. Primary and secondary hypertension.
   a. Primary hypertension, also known as *essential hypertension,* constitutes 90 percent of all cases of hypertension. Its cause is unknown. Types include:
      (1) *Benign hypertension*: gradual onset and prolonged course.
      (2) *Malignant hypertension*: abrupt onset

and a short, dramatic course that is rapidly fatal unless treatment is successful.

b. Secondary hypertension develops as a result of other primary diseases of the cardiovascular system, renal system, adrenal glands, or neurological system.

Although there may be no obvious pathological changes in the blood vessels and organs early in the course of hypertension, in time there are widespread pathological changes in both the small and large blood vessels and in organs supplied by these blood vessels, namely the heart, kidney, and brain. Small vessel damage includes intimal damage, which causes accumulation of fibrin, local edema, and intravascular clotting. Large vessels become sclerosed and tortuous; their lumina narrow and may become completely occluded, resulting in diminished blood flow or hemorrhage. Death due to hypertensive cardiovascular disease results either from irreparable damage to kidneys, brain, and myocardium as a result of small vessel damage or from occlusion or hemorrhage of a large vessel.

PREVENTION

Health Promotion

1. Education regarding the significance of high blood pressure.
2. Having blood pressure checked at least yearly, especially those persons with any family history of hypertension.
3. Identifying and eliminating (as much as possible) potential stressors, including psychosocial factors or occupational stressors.
4. Awareness of the effects of obesity, smoking, and oral contraceptives on hypertension.
5. A well-balanced, low-cholesterol, salt-restricted diet.

Population at Risk

1. Men develop hypertension more frequently than women.
2. After menopause, the rate in women rapidly approaches that in men and becomes higher in old age.
3. Blacks in the United States develop hypertension twice as often as the white population.
4. Persons with familial history of hypertension.
5. Persons subjected to emotional stress.
6. Persons using quantities of salt on food.
7. Persons taking oral contraceptives.
8. Persons who have smoking habits.

Screening

1. Hypertension screening at public places and for children in schools.
2. Referral to a physician for individuals who have had two or more elevated blood pressure readings.
3. Routine blood pressure measurement for all individuals seeking health care in all specialties and settings, such as preemployment and insurance physical examinations.

ASSESSMENT

Health History

1. Identify factors in the client's lifestyle that might be related to hypertension (smoking, oral contraceptives, salt in the diet, and psychosocial stress).
2. Determine at what age the client's blood pressure first became elevated.
3. Identify any renal or cardiovascular diseases in the client's history.
4. Identify any family history of hypertension.
5. Determine whether the client has suddenly lost weight (sign of pheochromocytoma) or gained weight (edema).
6. Client often complains initially of a headache upon rising in the morning that gradually lessens as the day progresses.
7. Dizziness and fatigue are often reported in the history.
8. Palpitations and dyspnea on exertion may be described.
9. There may be complaints of blurring of vision.
10. Epistaxis (nosebleeds) may be reported.

Physical Assessment

1. The blood pressure is consistently higher than 140 mmHg systolic and 90 mmHg diastolic.
2. Eye signs: by an ophthalmoscopic examination, the retina shows blood vessels that are tortuous, thin, and shiny with exudates and hemorrhage.
3. Severe headaches associated with nausea and vomiting are present, especially in the morning hours.
4. Palpation of peripheral pulses reveals a delayed or weak femoral pulse as compared with carotid or radial pulse taken simulta-

neously (may suggest coarctation as the cause).
5. Peripheral edema may be present if there is right-heart failure as a consequence of hypertension.
6. There may be polyuria and nocturia due to the kidney's decreased ability to concentrate the urine; thus, there is an increased urinary excretion.
7. Epistaxis (nosebleeds) may occur from ruptured nasal capillaries from increased vascular pressure.

Diagnostic Tests

1. Blood pressure readings are taken on both arms while the client is supine and then when the client is erect and the findings are compared. For accuracy, readings are taken repeatedly over a period of 1–2 h.
2. Ophthalmoscopic examination may demonstrate vascular changes in the retina. If hemorrhage, exudate, or papilledema are present, there is definite vascular change.
3. The electrocardiogram shows evidence of left ventricular hypertrophy or other cardiac abnormalities.
4. Chest x-ray study suggests cardiac enlargement.
5. Urinalysis shows proteinuria, hematuria, or pus cells, indicating kidney disease and low specific gravity.
6. An intravenous pyelogram is helpful in revealing parenchymal disease of the kidney by visualizing the size, shape, position, and filling of the kidneys and the ureters.
7. Blood tests show evidence of elevated blood urea nitrogen and serum creatinine.
8. Serum potassium levels are determined to assess the possibility of primary aldosteronism in mild or moderate hypertension.

NURSING DIAGNOSES: ACTUAL OR POTENTIAL

1. Anxiety: due to fear related to symptoms.
2. Lack of compliance with therapy: due to knowledge deficit.
3. Dizziness and fatigue: secondary to alterations in decreased cardiac output.

EXPECTED OUTCOMES

1. Anxiety will be lessened.
2. Client will show compliance with the care plan by:
   a. Eliminating smoking, if a smoker.
   b. Losing weight, if obese.
   c. Returning for check-ups as ordered.
3. Client will identify adverse symptoms and side effects and methods of management.

INTERVENTIONS

1. General measures.
   a. Help the obese client to lose weight.
   b. Teach the client the content and purposes of a sodium-restricted diet (about 2 g sodium a day).
   c. Help the client to stop smoking, if a smoker.
   d. Encourage regular physical exercise.
   e. Give sedatives or tranquilizers for anxiety or headaches.
   f. Provide a quiet environment.
   g. Assist the client in coping with stress and anxiety.
   h. Teach the client and the family about hypertension, the need for a change in lifestyle, and the need for continued therapy.
   i. Use ice packs over the bridge of the nose or back of the neck for nosebleeds.
2. Drug therapy. Antihypertensive drug therapy will be ordered to reduce the blood pressure and thus relieve secondary health problems. As no two clients are alike in their response to drug therapy, observe each client carefully for expected and side effects. Generally, two categories of drugs are available: *diuretics* and *vasodilators*.
   a. Diuretics: for mild to moderate benign hypertension.
      (1) Thiazides: chlorothiazide (Diuril), hydrochlorothiazide (Hydrodiuril).
         (a) Block tubular reabsorption of sodium and potassium.
         (b) Potassium may need replacement through food or medication if thiazides and a digitalis drug are used together.
      (2) Spironolactone (Aldactone).
         (a) Antagonizes the action of aldosterone, thus promoting diuresis by inhibiting sodium reabsorption.
         (b) Spares potassium excretion; therefore, do *not* use potassium supplements for clients on this drug.
   b. Vasodilators.

(1) Reserpine (Serpasil).
 (a) Depletes stores of norepinephrine, thus producing vasodilatation.
 (b) Can cause emotional depression; therefore, observe client for despondency.
 (c) Can also cause nasal stuffiness that causes discomfort to the client.

(2) Guanethidine (Ismelin).
 (a) Produces postganglionic blockade of norepinephrine.
 (b) Can cause orthostatic hypotension (low blood pressure with change of body position); therefore, warn clients to change body positions slowly.
 (c) Can also cause an inability to ejaculate, thus causing impotence.

(3) Hydralazine (Apresoline).
 (a) Dilates peripheral vessels directly.
 (b) Increases cardiac output and renal blood flow.
 (c) Can cause tachycardia, palpitations, and angina pectoris.

(4) Methyldopa (Aldomet).
 (a) Displaces norepinephrine in the sympathetic nerve endings with alpha norepinephrine, called a "false transmitter."
 (b) Dilates peripheral arterioles, usually increasing glomerular filtration and cardiac output.
 (c) May cause drowsiness and dryness of the mouth.
 (d) May also cause orthostatic hypotension.
 (e) Toxic effects: hepatitis and hemolytic anemia.

(5) Propranolol (Inderal).
 (a) Blocks beta-adrenergic receptor sites, thus lowering heart rate and myocardial contractility. This action decreases cardiac output and plasma renin.
 (b) May cause depression, aggravation of bronchial asthma, and gastrointestinal symptoms.
 (c) Should be used with caution for clients with pump failure or bradycardia, for it intensifies them.

3. Surgical intervention.
 Sympathectomy: This procedure results in the blockage of stimuli from the sympathetic nerve fibers to the blood vessels. This surgery is done on those few clients who cannot tolerate drug therapy. This used to be the method of choice, but it has its side effects, especially orthostatic hypotension, neuritis, loss of ejaculation in the male, and loss of perspiration in areas innervated by the sympathetic nerves.

4. Teaching and rehabilitation:
 a. Teach the client that hypertension is controllable, not curable.
 b. Inform the client that rehabilitation will be adjusted to the particular needs of each client so that there will be maximum compliance with the regimen.
 c. The following points should be included in the teaching plan:
  (1) Teach the client how to take his or her own blood pressure so that this can be done at home.
  (2) Instruct the client to continue with the medications as ordered. Admonish the client to take the drugs on time, not to skip doses, not to take more than ordered, and to report side effects to the physician.
  (3) Dietary restrictions: Instruct the client to avoid large, heavy meals. Teach the reasons for the sodium-restricted diet and what foods can be included or excluded. Teach the client not to drink large amounts of fluid, as increased fluid will increase blood volume, which in turn causes increased blood pressure.
  (4) Emphasize a planned, moderate exercise program, including activities such as daily walks, gardening, and golf. Warn the client to avoid strenuous exercise.
  (5) Encourage the client to develop interesting hobbies.

EVALUATION

Outcome Criteria

1. Headaches become less frequent within 2 weeks of therapy.
2. Nosebleeds are controlled and decreased in frequency within 1 month of therapy.
3. As symptoms decrease, anxiety decreases.
4. Client shows compliance by taking medications as directed, adhering to the prescribed

diet, and ceasing to smoke cigarettes within 6 months of therapy.
5. Fatigue has decreased, as evidenced by client's increased ability to tolerate activity and stress.

Complications

VISUAL CHANGES

Assessment
Assess the fundus for papilledema or hemorrhage in macular area.
Revised Outcomes
Prevent further visual problems and protect client from injury.
Interventions
1. Encourage the client to wear eyeglasses and have yearly eye exams.
2. Protect the elderly client from falls.
3. Teach the client and family to observe safety precautions.

CEREBROVASCULAR ACCIDENT

This is caused by intracerebral hemorrhage or ruptured blood vessel (see Chapter 25).

RENAL FAILURE

See discussion in Chapter 32.

CONGESTIVE HEART FAILURE

Refer to the discussion under *Congestive Heart Failure* in this chapter.

CORONARY HEART DISESAE

See the discussion under *Coronary Heart Disease* in this chapter.

HYPERTENSIVE EMERGENCIES

These occur in an acute crisis when the diastolic level exceeds 140 mmHg. Such a situation is a threat to life and must be treated immediately.
Assessment
1. Sudden, abrupt elevation of diastolic pressure above 140 mmHg.
2. Paralysis.
3. Coma.
4. Convulsions.
5. Severe headaches.
6. Vomiting.
7. Blindness.

Revised Outcomes
Blood pressure will be reduced quickly without producing side effects.
Interventions
1. Drug therapy will be parenteral vasodilators, such as sodium nitroprusside (Nipride), reserpine, diazoxide, methyldopa, or hydralizine (Apresoline)
2. Monitor blood pressure constantly to observe for hypotension and shock.

Reevaluation and Follow-up

Clients should be seen and reevaluated at periodic intervals, depending on the severity of their hypertension. During these visits:
1. Evaluate compliance with medications, diet, and changes in lifestyle, such as ceasing to smoke and doing regular exercises.
2. Check blood pressure at least twice over a period of several minutes.
3. Examine the retina for vascular changes.
4. Do a physical examination of the heart. When auscultating, listen for an S_3 gallop.
5. Do a laboratory examination of the urine for protein and blood.
6. Obtain blood specimens for serum creatinine and BUN.
7. Evaluate loss of weight (if obesity had been a problem).

ANEMIA AND HEART DISEASE

DESCRIPTION

Anemia is defined as a condition in which the oxygen transport capacity is below normal due to a decreased number or quality of erythrocytes or a reduction of hemoglobin. *Tissue hypoxia* results from these reductions and is the underlying cause of all symptoms that accompany anemia. The anemic state may result from (1) inadequate production of erythrocytes because of abnormal function of the bone marrow, (2) insufficient quantity of erythrocytes because of acute or chronic blood loss, (3) inadequate maturation of erythrocytes because of absence of the essential factor (as in pernicious anemia), and (4) increased destruction of erythrocytes resulting from acquired or hereditary factors (Beland and Passos, 1981).

Compensation for the anemia and the resultant hypoxia include tachycardia and an increased stroke volume to produce an increased cardiac output. If this compensation is ineffective in increasing the cardiac output sufficiently, myocardial ischemia may develop because of insufficient oxygenation of the myocardium, thus causing angina or myocardial infarction or congestive heart failure from the overworked myocardium.

Therapy for the anemia is given according to the type of anemia that is present and its underlying cause, such as iron deficiency, factors related to bone marrow inadequacy, hemolysis, or blood loss. When the anemia is associated with repeated incidences of anginal pain or congestive heart failure, the correction of the anemia is a necessary part of the treatment of the heart condition. If packed cells or whole blood transfusions are given, they should be given slowly so that pulmonary edema does not result, especially in any client with congestive heart failure (for details of the anemias, see Chapter 29).

ARRHYTHMIAS

DESCRIPTION

Arrhythmias are disorders of the heartbeat. They are due to exercise, pharmacological causes, emotions, anemia, myocardial ischemia or infarction and to systemic causes such as fever, hormonal imbalances, and hyperthyroidism. Arrhythmias are especially important because of their effect on cardiac output. Factors associated with arrhythmias that affect the cardiac output are (1) extremes in heart rate (slow or fast); (2) irregularity; (3) lack of effective atrial contraction, called *atrial boost*; (4) lack of synchrony between atrial and ventricular contractions; and (5) ventricular ectopy (abnormal initiation of an impulse). Arrhythmias are related to disorders of the initiation of the impulse or to the transmission of the impulse through the heart.

Basic electrocardiography. Arrhythmias can be definitely identified only by means of devices that record the electrocardiographic wave forms. Therefore, it is essential that a usable knowledge of electrocardiography be attained in order to develop skills in arrhythmia detection.

Impulse formation. Each normal heartbeat results from an electrical impulse that originates in a special node, called the *sinoatrial (SA) node*, located in the right atrial wall near the entrance of the superior vena cava. For this reason, the SA node is considered the normal pacemaker of the heart. If the SA node is depressed, other inherent pacemakers throughout the heart can assume pacemaking function. In addition, ectopic pacemakers assume pacemaking function when the myocardium is irritable from various causes or when the rate of SA node is extremely slow.

Impulse conduction. The impulse initiated in the sinoatrial (SA) node is transmitted through the heart along a specialized network of fibers called the *conduction system* (see Figure 30-11). The myocardium is stimulated to contract in response to the electrical impulse. The impulse is conducted along the conduction system as follows:

1. The impulse originates in the SA node.
2. It spreads through the atrial myocardium along three bands of tissue known as the *internodal tracts*. This causes atrial contraction.
3. It reaches the atrioventricular node (AV), where it is momentarily delayed before its transmission.
4. The impulse then is transmitted to the common bundle of His and to its branches, the right bundle branch and the left bundle branch.
5. Finally, the impulse reaches the terminal Purkinje fibers and from here it crosses the Purkinje-myocardial junction.

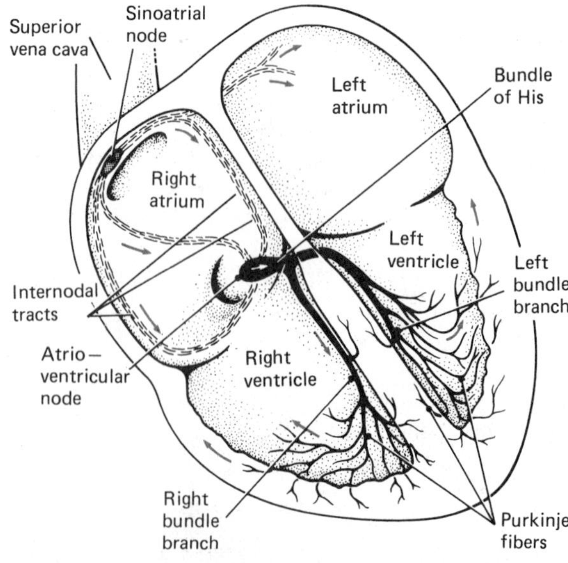

Figure 30-11 Conduction system of the heart.

6. As a result of the impulse's reaching the ventricular myocardium, ventricular contraction occurs (see Figure 30-11).

Electrocardiogram. The electrical activity associated with the impulse conduction through the heart can be detected by specialized equipment such as an electrocardiograph machine, the electrodes of which are applied to skin surfaces. Varying the location of these electrodes on skin surfaces or turning a lead selector dial will produce a variation in the resultant electrocardiogram configuration on an oscilloscope or on electrocardiogram paper.

The electrical activity as shown on the electrocardiogram during a cardiac cycle is designated as five separate waves or deflections from the baseline as P, Q, R, S, and T (see Figure 30-12). The meaning and significance of the waves and time intervals must be thoroughly understood in order to interpret an electrocardiogram.

1. *P wave.* This wave represents the conduction of the impulse from its initiation in the SA node through the atria via the internodal tracts.
2. *PR interval.* This represents the time for the impulse to go from the SA mode through the atria, AV node, bundle of His, to the ventricles. This interval is measured from the beginning of the P wave to the beginning of the QRS complex. Its normal time is between 0.12 s (three small squares on ECG paper) to 0.20 s (fivesmall squares on the ECG paper).
3. *QRS complex.* This represents the time for the impulse to depolarize the ventricles. It consists of a Q wave (small downward deflection), the R wave (tall upward deflection), and the S wave (a second downward deflection). These three deflections constituting the QRS complex vary in size depending upon the lead being recorded; in some, there may be absence of one or two of these deflections.

   The QRS complex is measured from the beginning of the Q wave to the end of the S wave (if any deflections are absent, measurement is from the beginning to the end of the observed waves). The normal duration of the QRS complex is between 0.06–0.10 s.
4. *ST segment.* This interval represents the period of time between the completion of ventricular depolarization and the beginning of repolarization (recovery) of the ventricular myocardium. Normally, this segment is isoelectric, meaning it is neither elevated nor depressed. Elevation or depression of the ST segment indicates abnormal recovery of the ventricles from depolarization, usually from an ischemic process.
5. *T wave.* This wave represents the electrical recovery (repolarization) of the ventricles. Ischemia of the myocardium may cause the T waves to invert.

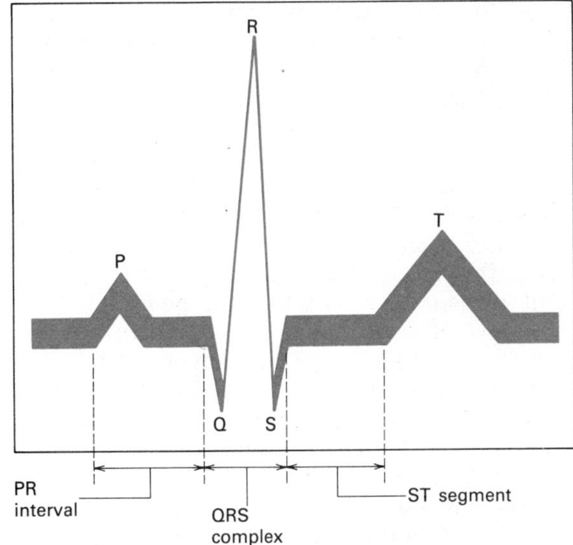

Figure 30-12 Electrocardiographic configurations of one cardiac cycle.

CARDIAC MONITORING

As the electrical impuse is conducted through the heart, as described above, it also spreads outward from the heart to the skin, where it can be detected on a cardiac monitor attached to the client via cables and electrodes. Although cardiac monitoring does give valuable information to help in the care of clients with cardiac problems, it should never be construed as a replacement for direct nursing observations of the client.

Although cardiac monitors vary, the basic cardiac monitor consists of the following components:

1. Electrodes, which are attached to the skin to transmit electrical impulses initiated in the heart to the cable of the cardiac monitor.
2. An oscilloscope, which displays the client's

continuous electrocardiogram. As the heart beats, the tracing moves across the screen.

3. A pulse rate indicator, which displays the heart rate per minute as a digital display or on a rate scale indicator. The monitor counts the number of R waves and displays a light and sounds an audible beep for each heart beat (the beeper is often turned off if the sound is annoying).
4. Alarm system, which alerts the staff by audio and visual alarms when the heart rate falls below or exceeds the preset pulse rate settings. Because of the dependence of the staff on the alarm system, the pulse rate settings should be individualized for each client and rechecked regularly to be sure the system is operative.
5. Additional components:
   a. Direct write-out mechanism, which provides a printed record of the electrocardiogram seen on the oscilloscope. This rhythm strip permits documentation of an arrhythmia and is valuable for comparing tracings over a period of time. This write-out mechanism can be triggered automatically when pulse-rate alarms occur or on demand when a recording is desired.
   b. "Freeze" or "hold" device, which stops the movement of the electrocardiogram across the oscilloscope, thus keeping a particular pattern in place for observation.
   c. Memory systems, which are designed to store and play back the electrocardiogram of the preceeding 15–60 s (or more).
   d. Computers, which are incorporated into monitors and are capable of displaying the name of arrhythmias and retreiving trends of information for the previous hours.
   e. Mutichannel records, which monitor respiratory rates and central venous, pulmonary artery, pulmonary wedge, and arterial pressures, which may be displayed on a continuous basis. In some systems, these measurements are stored in computers from which data can be retrieved when needed.

The basic operation of a cardiac monitor is described below:

1. Prepare the client before starting cardiac monitoring. Explain the purpose, how the system works, and the possibility of false alarms. Encourage the client to express concerns and anxieties.
2. Turn on the cardiac monitor.
3. Use the following steps in applying electrodes to the chest:
   a. Choose the sites for the electrodes on the chest for the cardiac monitor being used in your unit. The two most common electrode positions are those shown in Figure 30-13.
   b. Prepare the skin for the sites by shaving hair (on male client) in 4-in areas around the intended electrode sites and cleaning the area with alcohol; allow time for the skin to dry.
   c. Peel the protective cover from each pregelled electrode as it is to be applied.
   d. Apply the electrode to the prepared site and press firmly on the adhesive tape around the electrode.
   e. Connect the electrode to the receptacle of the client cable, matching the electrode placement with the correct openings in the receptacle.
   f. Pin the cable to the client's gown to allow for movement.
4. Cardiac monitor adjustments.
   a. Adjust the client's tracing on the oscilloscope by using the centering and amplitude knobs.
   b. Set the low and high pulse rate alarm settings. Generally, it is customary to set the low rate at 50 and the high rate at 140 for normal heart rates. If, however, the rate

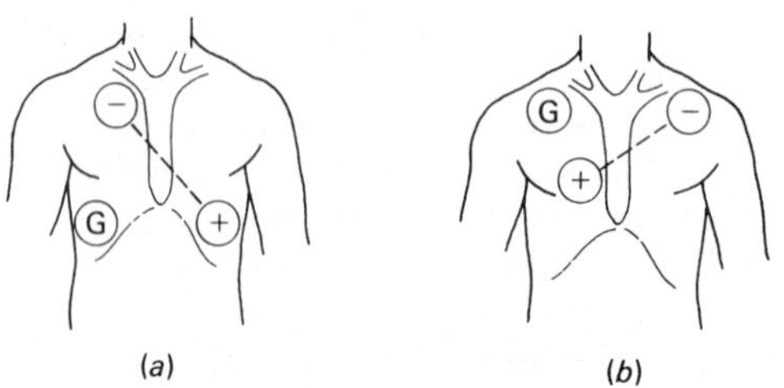

Figure 30-13 Two electrode positions: (*a*) conventional monitoring (lead II), (*b*) modified chest lead (lead V_1 or MCL). (Modified from Meltzer, L., Pinneo, R., and Kitchell, J. R.: *Intensive Coronary Care*, 3d ed. Robert J. Brady Co., Bowie, Md., 1977, p. 127. Used by permission of the publisher.)

is very slow or very fast, the pulse rate alarm settings should be narrowed so that the staff will be alerted for deviations beyond these settings.

INTERPRETATION OF ARRHYTHMIAS

In identifying and interpreting arrhythmias, the nurse plays an essential role. To fulfill this role, the nurse needs a clear understanding of which arrhythmias are innocuous and require no therapy, which arrhythmias are forewarnings of catastrophic events and require aggressive therapy, and finally, which arrhythmias are life-threatening and require immediate resuscitative management. In addition, the nurse needs to know the anticipated drug therapy and, in some cases, must proceed to give it according to written protocols; the nurse must also know the anticipated emergency resuscitation measures, as she or he must often initiate them while other personnel are on the way to assume their roles.

A logical approach to identifying an arrhythmia is to classify arrhythmias as due to disturbances in impulse initiation or to disturbances in impulse transmission. By following a series of five basic steps and comparing the findings with characteristics of the various arrhythmias, identification is achieved, as follows:

1. Calculate the heart rate. Count the number of R waves in a 6-in strip of ECG tracing (which equals 6 s). Multiply the number obtained by 10 to get the average number per minute.
2. Measure the regularity (rhythm) of the R waves by comparing the distances between R waves.
3. Examine the P waves to determine whether they precede each QRS complex and whether they are of normal shape.
4. Measure the PR interval to determine if it is 0.12–0.20 s in time.
5. Measure the width of the QRS complex. It should be less than 0.10 s.

Normal sinus rhythm (NSR) is said to exist when the SA node generates impulses between 60 and 100 times a minute and each impulse is conducted normally. The ECG characteristics of NSR are: (1) R wave rate is 60 to 100 times a minute; (2) R wave rhythm is regular; (3) P waves of normal shape precede each QRS complex; and (4) the QRS complex width is within normal limits (see Table 30-3). An arrhythmia exists when these criteria are not met.

Table 30-4 gives a summary of the most frequent arrhythmias and their abnormal characteristics. Note that the rhythm strips shown in the table reduced in size; therefore, use the 3-s markings on the strips to count the rate. Also note that only the abnormal characteristics of the representative arrhythmias are stated. The other characteristics are normal. These arrhythmias are organized as to whether they are due to disturbances in impulse initiation or to impulse transmission.

PREVENTION

Health Promotion

Persons prone to develop arrhythmias should:
1. Avoid stimulants such as coffee.

TABLE 30-3 NORMAL SINUS RHYTHM AND ITS CHARACTERISTICS

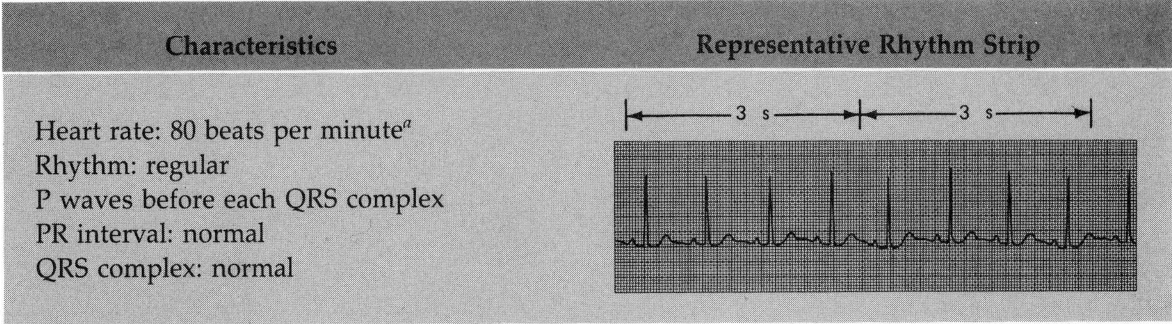

Characteristics	Representative Rhythm Strip
Heart rate: 80 beats per minute[a] Rhythm: regular P waves before each QRS complex PR interval: normal QRS complex: normal	3 s — 3 s

[a] Note the "3 s" markings at the top of the tracing. Count the R waves within 6 s and multiply by 10 to obtain the heart rate per minute.

TABLE 30-4 ARRHYTHMIAS AND THEIR ABNORMAL CHARCTERISTICS[a]

Arrhythmias and Characteristics	Representative Rhythm Strip
Arrythmias Due to Disturbances in Impulse Formation	
1. Sinoatrial (SA) node arrhythmias: impulses originate in the SA node.	
a. *Sinus tachycardia*. Heart rate: 100–150 beats per minute. Here the rate is 110 per minute.	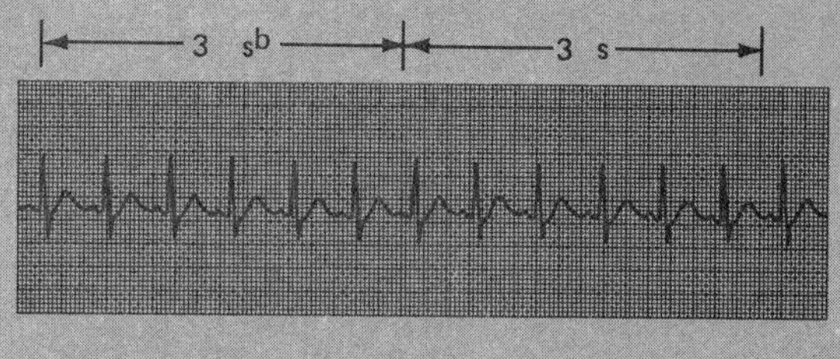
b. *Sinus bradycardia*. Heart rate: 40–60 beats per minute. Here the rate is 40 per minute.	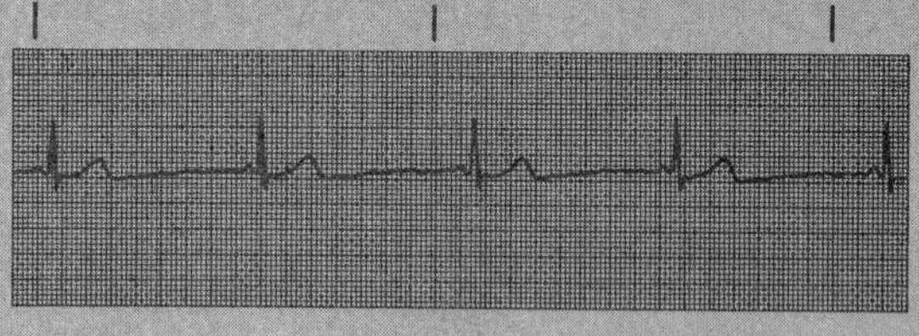
c. *Sinus arrhythmia*. Irregular rhythm of QRS complex: fast rate alternating with slow rate. Increased rate is related to respiratory inspiration; decreased rate is related to respiratory expiration.	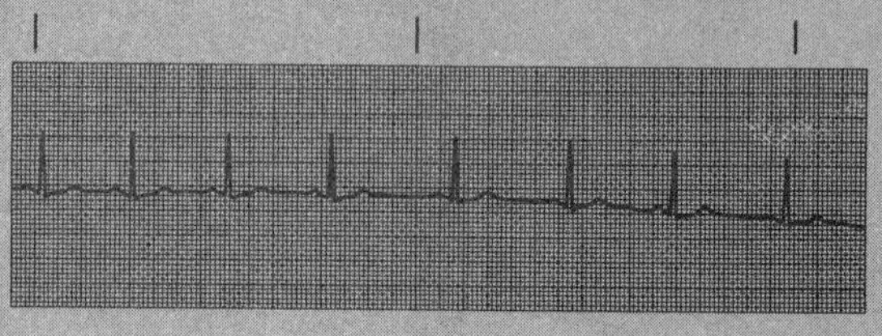
2. Atrial arrhythmias: impulses originate in the atria.	
a. *Premature atrial complexes* (PAC). A premature beat preceded by an abnormally shaped P wave. Note the PACs shown by arrows.	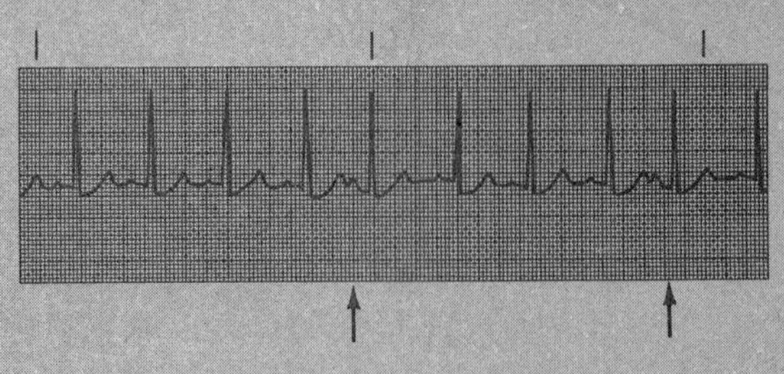
b. *Paroxysmal atrial tachycardia*. Heart rate: 150–250 beats per minute. P waves, if seen, are abnormal in shape and may be combined with T waves. Here the rate is 200 per minute.	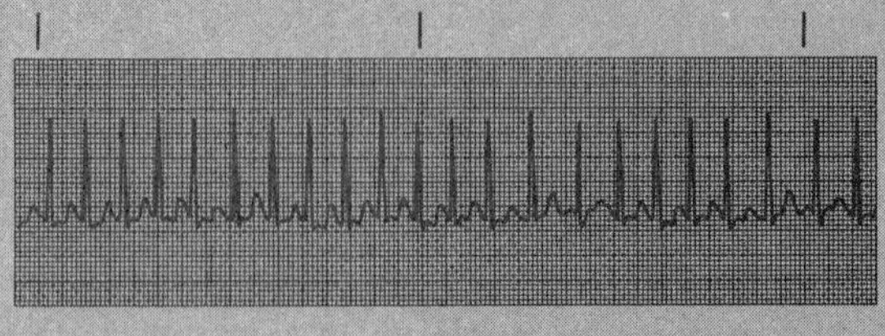
c. *Atrial flutter*. Sawtooth-appearing flutter waves instead of P waves. There is usually a ratio of these flutter waves to QRS complexes, as only a proportion are conducted to the ventricles. Ratio is expressed as 2:1, 3:1, or 4:1 atrial flutter. Note that P waves are superimposed on T waves.	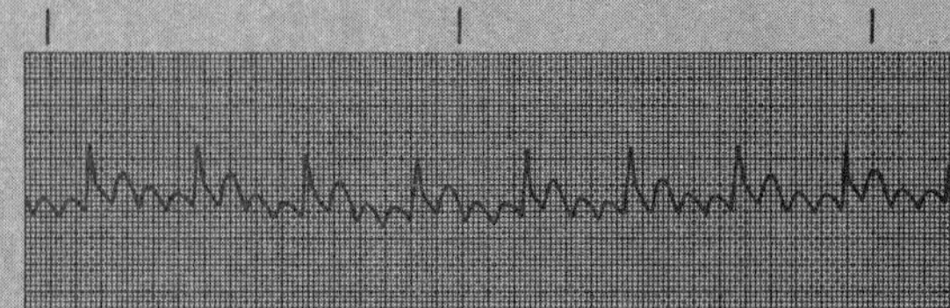

TABLE 30-4 *(continued)*

Arrhythmias and Characteristics	Representative Rhythm Strip
Arrythmias Due to Disturbances in Impulse Formation	
d. *Atrial fibrillation.* Irregular ventricular rhythm. P waves are not present; instead there are small irregular fibrillation waves and irregular rhythm of QRS complexes.	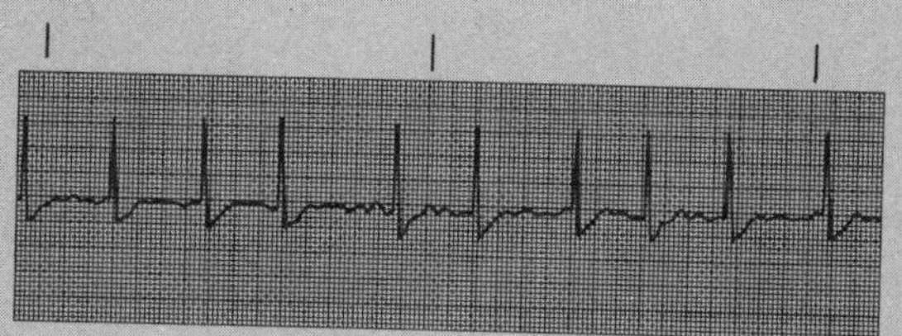
3. Junctional arrhythmias: impulses originate near the atrioventricular (AV) node.	
a. *Premature junctional complex.* Shape and position of P waves may vary. There may be inverted preceding or following QRS complexes or may be hidden in the QRS complexes. The cardiac cycle comes earlier than expected. Here the arrow indicate two premature junctional complexes.	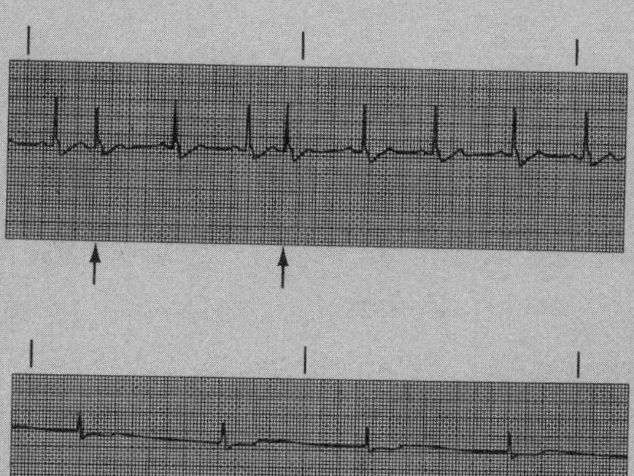
b. *Junctional rhythm.* Slow rate: 40–60 beats per minute. P waves have the same characteristics as in premature junctional complex (above). All the beats have the characteristics stated above. (There are no identifiable P waves in the rhythm strip to the right.) Here the rate is 40 per minute.	
4. Ventricular arrhythmias: impulses originate in the ventricles.	
a. *Premature ventricular complex* (PVC). Premature beat having no P wave. Widened, distorted QRS complexes. T wave oppositely directed from the QRS complex. Full pause follows the premature beat. Various patterns include ventricular bigeminy, multifocal PVC, frequent PVCs, R-on-T pattern. Note the one PVC shown by arrow.	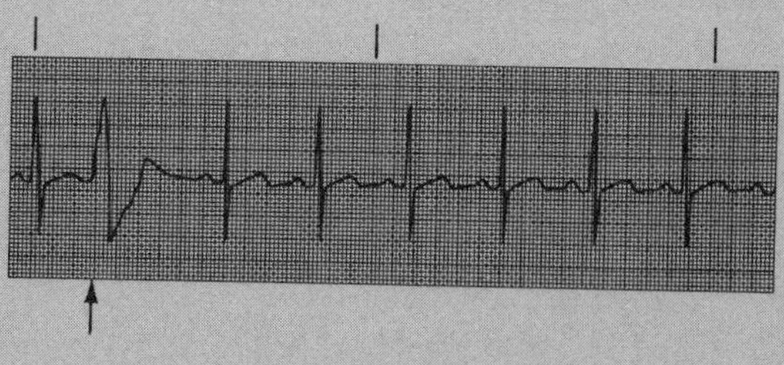
b. *Ventricular tachycardia.* Heart rate: 140–220 beats per minute. Slightly irregular rhythm. No identifiable P waves. Widened, distorted QRS complexes. T wave oppositely directed from QRS complexes. Here the rate is 150 per minute.	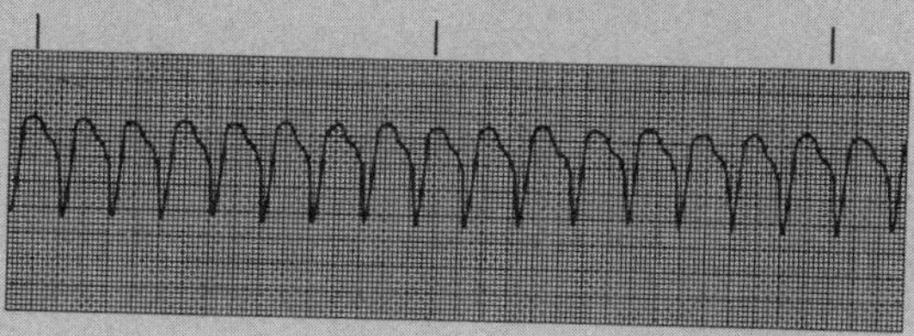

TABLE 30-4 *(continued)*

Arrhythmias and Characteristics	Representative Rhythm Strip
Arrythmias Due to Disturbances in Impulse Formation	
c. *Ventricular fibrillation.* Chaotic waves of varying height and width. No pattern. Client soon became unconscious because of no cardiac output. Death results unless the arrhythmia is treated immediately. No heart rate or rhythm can be determined because the chaotic waves are not QRS complexes.	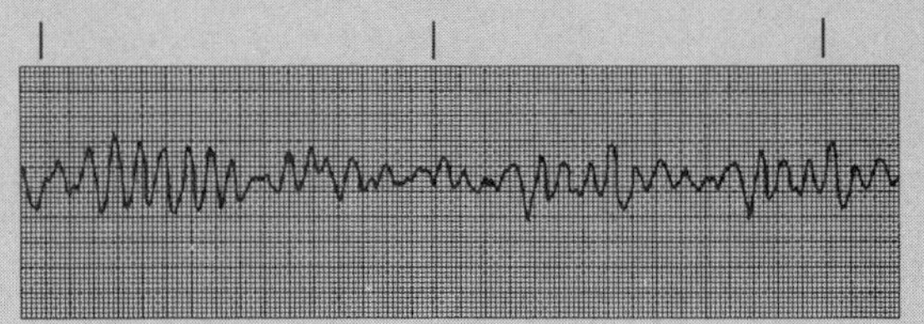
Arrhythmias Due to Disturbances in Impulse Transmission	
1. Atrioventricular node heart blocks.	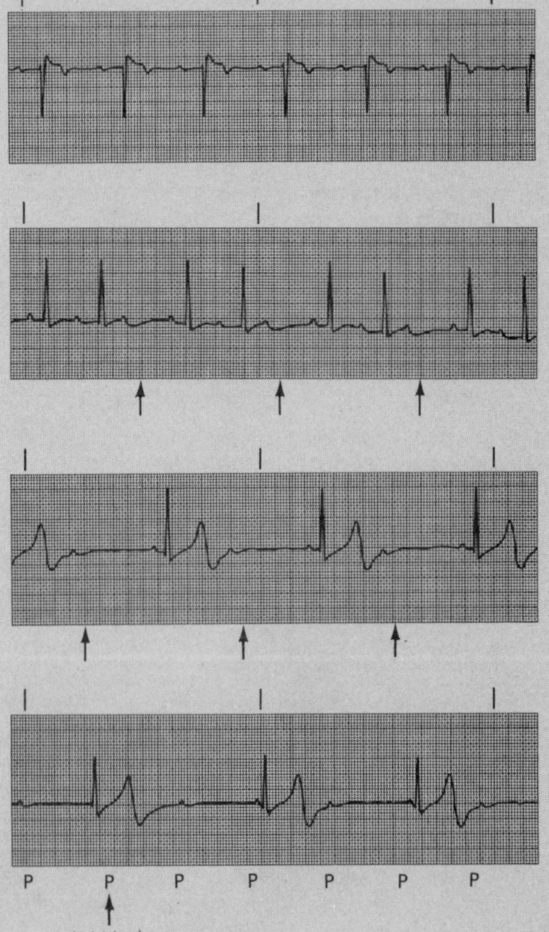
a. *First-degree AV heart block.* PR interval prolonged beyond 0.20 s (five small squares on ECG paper). Here the PR interval is 0.28 s.	
b. *Second-degree AV heart block.*	
(1) *Wenckebach type.* Progressive lengthening of PR interval from beat to beat until a P wave is not followed by a QRS complex (arrows); then the sequence is repeated.	
(2) *2:1 AV heart block.* A ratio of P waves to QRS complexes of 2:1 (as in rhythm strip on right), 3:1, or 4:1. Beats are dropped in this ratio (arrows indicate where P waves are not conducted).	
c. *Third-degree AV heart block (complete).* Slow ventricular rate: 30–40 beats per minute. P waves independent of QRS complexes. QRS complexes are regular in rhythm. Here the heart rate is 30 per minute. Note the regular sequence of P waves and the varying PR interval, indicated lack of relationship between P waves and QRS complexes.	

TABLE 30-4 *(continued)*

Arrhythmias and Characteristics	Representative Rhythm Strip
Arrythmias Due to Disturbances in Impulse Transmission	
2. Intraventricular blocks. *Bundle branch block.* P waves precede wide, distorted QRS complexes. QRS complexes exceed 0.12 s (three small squares on ECG paper).	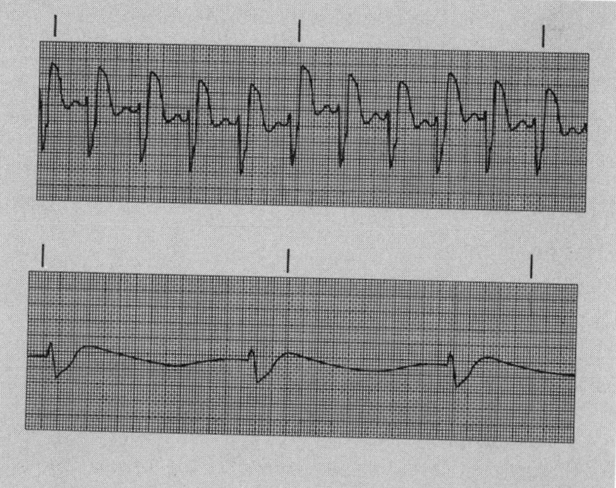
3. Ventricular standstill. P waves may be seen with sudden cessation of QRS complexes, or P waves are absent and QRS complexes are very slow in rate, 10–25 beats per minute, and are widened. They may be absent and only a straight line is seen. Client is unconscious. Death results unless resuscitation is immediate.	

[a] Only the abnormal characteristics are stated; others are normal.
[b] Note the markings at the top of each rhythm strip for counting the heart rate. The space between one mark to the next indicates 3 s.

2. Avoid cigarette smoking.
3. Avoid strenuous exercises.

Population at Risk

1. Persons with an acute myocardial infarction.
2. Persons with congestive heart failure.
3. Persons with Wolff-Parkinson-White syndrome (having an accessory conduction system between atrium and ventricle).
4. Persons with fever, hyperthyroidism, or an electrolyte imbalance.
5. Persons on digitalis drugs.
6. Persons with hypertension.
7. Persons with high anxiety levels.

Screening

1. A full electrocardiogram annually during routine physical examinations for persons age 40 or above.
2. Cardiac monitor for clients admitted with acute myocardial infarction, angina pectoris, congestive heart failure, or other cardiac problems.
3. Holter tape recorder to relate activity levels to the occurrence of arrhythmias.

ASSESSMENT

Health History

1. Previous episodes of acute myocardial infarction, angina pectoris, congestive heart failure, or arrhythmias.
2. Information about all the drugs the client has been taking, especially digitalis drugs, diuretics, and antiphypertensive drugs.
3. Lifestyle: regarding amount of coffee the client drinks, the number of cigarettes smoked per day, and the amount and kind of physical activity usually engaged in.
4. Client's coping ability when faced with stress and the level of anxiety the client exhibits.

Physical Assessment

1. Apical-radial pulse: presence of a pulse deficit occurs when there is a variation in the stroke volume (giving a higher rate at the apex than at the radial artery).
2. Venous distention of the great veins in the neck.
3. Anxiety.

4. Palpitations (sensation of heart beating rapidly) caused by a fast-rate arrhythmia.
5. Dyspnea due to fast-rate arrhythmias.
6. Blood pressure: if it falls, it might be due to low cardiac output caused by an arrhythmia.
7. In ventricular fibrillation and ventricular standstill, the client will be unconscious.
8. Syncope or dizziness due to temporary loss of cerebral perfusion from decreased cardiac output.
9. Pulse: irregularity, premature beats and the rate.
10. Sensation of "skipped beats."

Diagnostic Tests

1. Electrocardiogram.
2. Cardiac monitor.
3. Holter tape recorder.
4. Telemetric cardiac monitor.
5. Exercise testing to define the severity of the arrhythmia.
6. Bundle of His recordings via an electrode-tipped catheter threaded into the right side of the heart near the tricuspid valve. As this involves a cardiac catheterization, it is done selectively for clients with conduction deficits.

NURSING DIAGNOSES: ACTUAL OR POTENTIAL

1. Anxiety: due to the arrhythmias and being on a cardiac monitor.
2. Knowledge deficit: regarding reportable signs and symptoms.
3. Alteration in the level of consciousness: due to decreased cardiac output.

EXPECTED OUTCOMES

1. Anxiety will decrease.
2. Palpitations will subside.
3. Dyspnea will decrease.
4. Blood pressure will be within normal levels.
5. Consciousness will be restored.

INTERVENTIONS

Medical and nursing care focuses on (1) reducing or eliminating the factors causing the arrhythmias, such as drugs, fever, hyperthyroidism, or anxiety; and (2) using a therapeutic approach for the arrhythmias: drug therapy, precordial shock, and cardiac pacing. It is important for the nurse to assess the emotional needs of clients with arrhythmias and to meet these needs through direct nursing care.

A summary of medical and nursing interventions follows:

Slow-Rate Arrhythmias (Bradyarrhythmias)

1. *Drug therapy.*
   a. Atropine 0.6–1.0 mg to block vagal stimulation of the heart, resulting in an increase in rate. Avoid its use if glaucoma or prostatic hypertrophy is present.
   b. Isoproterenol (Isuprel) 2–4 mg/1000 mL IV fluids. Always dilute this drug; never give as a bolus dose. Isoproterenol stimulates conduction and contraction, thus increasing the rate. Watch for ventricular arrhythmias caused by irritability.
2. *Cardiac pacemaker.* An artificial cardiac pacemaker is an electrical device that is used to inititate the heartbeat when the client's rate is slow from a variety of causes, such as AV heart block and bundle branch blocks. The pacemaker consists of a battery pack taht may be placed outside the body (external) or embedded under the skin (internal). The battery pack is attached to electrodes through which the electrical stimulation reaches the tissues of the heart.
   a. The methods of pacing are:
      (1) Fixed rate, which stimulates at a preset rate, regardless of the client's heart rate. Although not used much at present, there may be occasions to use it if the client's rate is regular.
      (2) Demand pacing, which stimulates when the client's heart rate falls below the rate set on the pacemaker.
   b. Types of pacemakers are:
      (1) Temporary pacemakers, which are used for temporary heart block, as in acute myocardial infarction. A pacemaker catheter with electrodes near its tip is threaded through the great veins into the right side of the heart until it touches the endocardium of the right ventricle. The pacemaker battery is outside the body and is attached to the end of the pacemaker catheter. Its rate, voltage, and sensitivity are controlled by knobs on the pacemaker battery. To avoid electrical hazards as well as the

chance of the client's changing the controls, the pacemaker battery should be enclosed in a plastic cover or in a rubber glove. Pay careful attention to the site on the skin where the catheter penetrates to avoid infection through sterile technique during dressing change and the topical application of an antibiotic.

(2) Permanent pacemakers.

(a) Epicardial pacemaker electrodes are inserted on the epicardium (outside layer) of the heart via a surgical incision through the chest wall. The pacemaker is then embedded under the skin of the chest or the abdomen.

(b) Transvenous endocardial pacemaker electrodes are at the tips of the pacemaker catheter, which is threaded into the right side of the heart until it touches the endocardium of the right ventricle. Its position is evaluated with the use of fluoroscopy. The end of the catheter is attached to a pacemaker that is embedded in a surgically made pocket under the skin of the chest wall (see Figure 30-14).

(c) Nursing role: preoperative care.

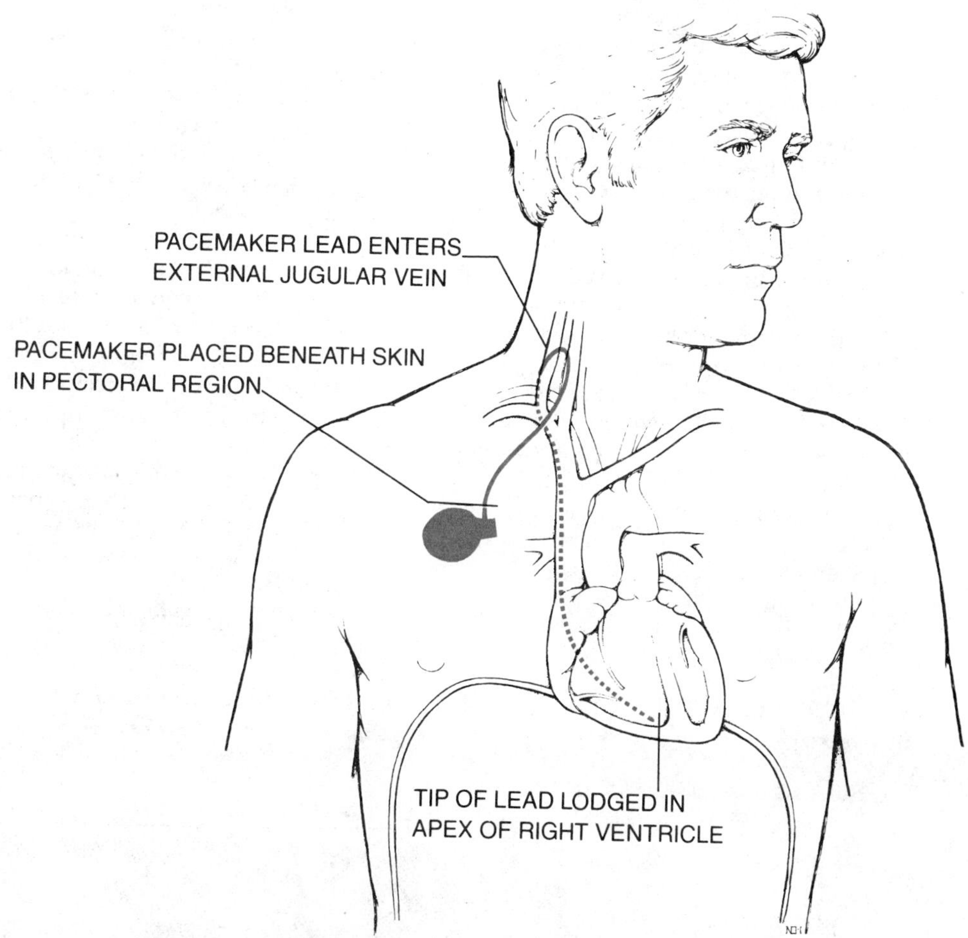

Figure 30-14 Placement of pacemaker and pacemaker catheter. (Brunner, L., and Suddarth, D.: *Textbook of Medical-Surgical Nursing*, 4th ed., Lippincott, Philadelphia, 1980, p. 589. Used by permission of the publisher.)

(i) Prepare the client and family for the procedure and for what to expect following it, such as bulging of the pacemaker embedded under the chest wall (although this problem has lessened with the advent of newer, smaller pacemakers), soreness, and discoloration of the area where it is embedded.

(ii) Provide psychological support by listening to the client's concerns.

(iii) Assess the client's understanding of the pacemaker and how it will help the heartbeat and help the client feel better.

(iv) Ask the client to do range-of-motion exercises postoperatively to prevent a "frozen shoulder" from developing.

(d) Nursing role: postoperative care.

(i) Prevent infection by using sterile dressings over the operative site and giving antibiotics for several days (if ordered).

(ii) Monitor the cardiac rhythm. Verify the correct functioning of the pacemaker by observing the rhythm strip from the monitor. When the pulse rate of the client drops below the rate set on the pacemaker (if a demand mode), there should be a pacemaker spike seen on the electrocardiogram. Following this pacemaker spike, a QRS complex should occur if the pacemaker is capturing the heartbeat. If there is a pacemaker spike not followed by QRS complexes, or if the client's heart rate falls very low and there are no pacemaker spikes, the pacemaker is not functioning correctly and the physician should be so notified (see Table 30-5).

(iii) Assist the client in moving his or her shoulder by passive range-of-motion exercises to prevent the development of a frozen shoulder.

(iv) Provide psychological support by allowing the client to express feelings about having a pacemaker. Help the client deal with any fears and anxieties

(e) Nursing role: rehabilitation and long-term care.

(i) Assess the client's understanding of the pacemaker and its purpose.

(ii) Include in client instruction: normal function of the heart, the pacemaker function, how to take one's pulse, the importance of follow-up visits to the clinic or physician's office, how to recognize symptoms of malfunctioning of the pacemaker (dizziness, syncope), and warnings about being near electrical equipment with high-frequency signals (e.g., microwave ovens).

(iii) Emphasize the positive aspects

TABLE 30-5 PACEMAKER-INDUCED RHYTHM AND ITS CHARACTERISTICS

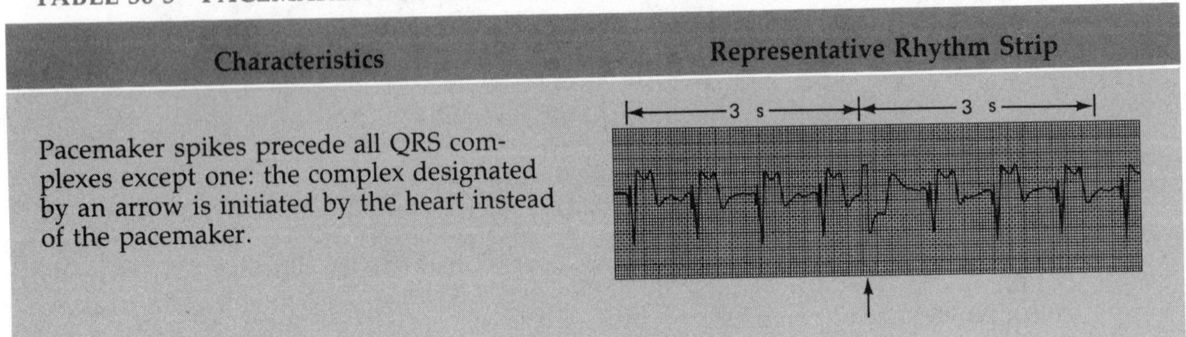

Characteristics	Representative Rhythm Strip
Pacemaker spikes precede all QRS complexes except one: the complex designated by an arrow is initiated by the heart instead of the pacemaker.	

following insertion of a pacemaker and stress that normal activities can be pursued.

(iv) Many medical centers can follow up on the function of pacemakers by using a telephone network. A rhythm strip can thus be produced with the client's leaving home.

3. *Cardiopulmonary resuscitation* for ventricular standstill (see Chapter 49).

Fast-Rate Arrhythmias (Tachyarrhythmias)

1. *Drug therapy.*
   a. Digoxin may be used for atrial fibrillation with a rapid ventricular rate or to terminate other fast-rate arrhythmias originating above the ventricles. Its action is on the vagus nerve to slow impulses going through the AV node, thus reducing the number of impulses conducted to the ventricles.
   b. Quinidine is usually given orally to depress ectopic foci in the atria; therefore, it is helpful in controlling the atrial arrhythmias.
   c. Procainamide (Pronestyl) is used to depress ventricular ectopic foci primarily, but it also has been used for atrial arrhythmias. When given intravenously, it has a tendency to cause hypotension.
   d. Lidocaine is used to suppress ventricular ectopic activity and, therefore, is effective for premature ventricular complexes and ventricular tachycardia. It has an advantage over procainamide in that it does not cause hypotension.
   e. Propronolol (Inderal) reduces sympathetic stimulation of the heart by blocking beta-receptor cells of the heart. It decreases the strength of ventricular contraction and, therefore, should not be used if heart failure is present.
2. *Electric countershock.* By delivering a high voltage of electric current of brief duration through the heart, depolarization of the entire heart is accomplished. This allows the SA node to regain its pacemaking function. Its use is:
   a. For ventricular fibrillation. The machine is set at its highest voltage and the synchronizer switch is turned off. The current will flow through the heart as soon as the button for the electric discharge is pushed. This is called *defibrillation.*
   b. For tachyarrhythmias (other than ventricular fibrillation). The machine is set at low voltage levels (depending on the physician's preference) and the synchronizer switch is turned on. The current will flow through the heart when the machine senses an R wave. This procedure is called *elective cardioversion* (see Figure 30-15).
3. *Carotid sinus pressure.* This is vagal stimulation applied by using slight pressure over the carotid sinus in a carotid artery where baroreceptors are located. It is most effective for paroxysmal atrial tachycardia and is used by the physician. Be sure the client is lying down, for this maneuver can cause a very slow heart rate and possibly syncope.

EVALUATION

Outcome Criteria

1. Anxiety lessens as arrhythmias are controlled.
2. Palpitations are no longer sensed.
3. Dyspnea is relieved.
4. Normal blood pressure is maintained.
5. Client is fully conscious and aware of surroundings.

Complications

1. Congestive heart failure can be caused by fast-rate arrhythmias (see the discussion under *Congestive Heart Failure* in this chapter).
2. Cerebrovascular accident may occur in clients with atrial fibrillation. This increases the likelihood of thrombus foundation. The thrombus can break loose and travel in the blood stream to cerebral arterials (see the discussion in Chapter 25).

Reevaluation and Follow-up

1. On follow-up visits, do an electrocardiogram to assess arrhythmias.
2. Assess effectiveness of therapy in controlling arrhythmias.
3. If the client has a pacemaker, assess correct functioning of the pacemaker in a pacemaker clinic or via special telephone communication. In addition, evaluate the client's knowledge of the pacemaker and problems the client is having in the adjustment to a pacemaker.
4. Assess client's compliance with therapy.

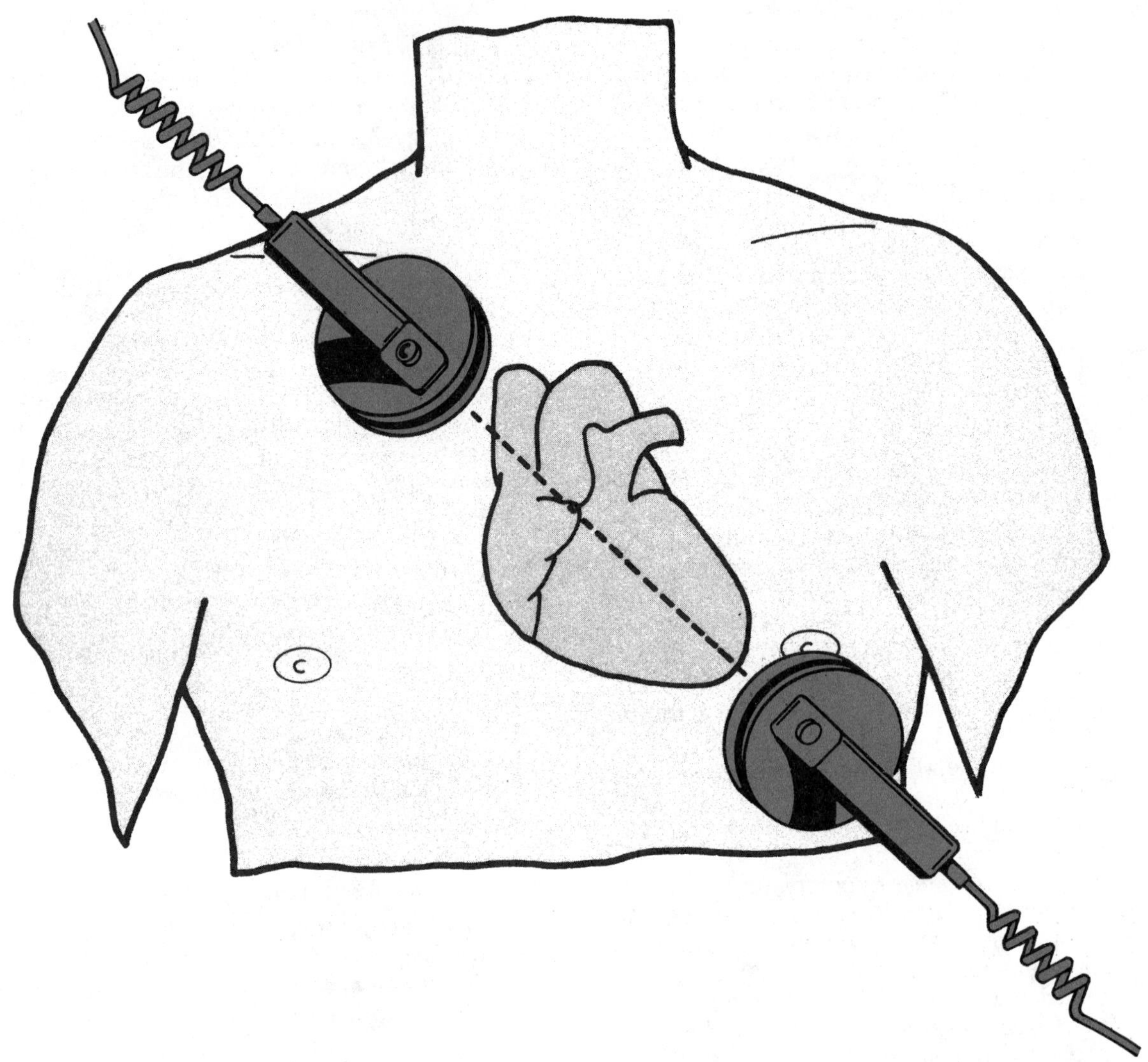

Figure 30-15 Placement of paddles for precordial shock (defibrillation or cardioversion). One paddle is to the right of the chest and the other is over the apex of the heart. (Meltzer, L., Pinneo, R., Kitchell, J. R.: *Intensive Coronary Care*, 3d ed., Robert J. Brady Co., Bowie, Md., 1977, p. 232. Used by permission of the publisher.)

SCLERODERMA

DESCRIPTION

Scleroderma (systemic sclerosis) is a chronic collagen disease of unknown cause characterized by sclerosis of the skin and subcutaneous tissues as well as internal organs. Cardiac involvement may appear late in the disease. Although all three layers of the heart are affected singly or in combination, the myocardium is affected more frequently and more seriously than the others. The myocardium is replaced by connective tissue in various degrees: (1) patchy scarred areas, (2) overgrowth of vascular connective tissue that separates muscle bundles, and (3) massive replacement of cardiac muscle by nonvascular connective tissue (Hurst et al., 1978).

PREVENTION

Health Promotion

1. Wearing of warm clothing, socks, and gloves and avoidance of cold temperatures to extremities.
2. Avoidance of fatigue by pacing activities and organizing work schedules to include rest periods.
3. Performance of range-of-motion exercises to prevent muscle contractures.

Population at Risk

1. Women are affected twice as frequently as men.
2. Onset is usually between 30 to 50 years of age. The disease rarely affects children.

Screening

There are no screening tests.

ASSESSMENT

Health History

1. Complaints of dyspnea on exertion or at rest.
2. Swelling and stiffness of fingers or toes.
3. Dysphagia from dysfunction of neuromusculature of the esophagus.
4. Weight loss.

Physical Assessment

1. The disease begins with Raynaud's pnenomenon: blanching, cyanosis, erythema of fingers and toes in response to exposure to cold.
2. The fingers swell, giving a sausagelike appearance. The skin then thickens and becomes taut and shiny.
3. Ulcerations may appear at fingertips.
4. Facial skin also becomes tight and unelastic, causing a masklike appearance.
5. Gastrointestinal dysfunction causes dysphagia, leading to weight loss.
6. Cardiac and pulmonary involvement may produce arrhythmias, dyspnea, and chest pain.
7. Renal involvement is manifested by hypertension that leads to renal failure.

Diagnostic Tests

1. Elevated erythrocyte sedimentation rate.
2. Proteinuria, hematuria, and casts with renal involvement.
3. X-ray studies of hand show subcutaneous calcification.
4. Chest x-ray studies show an enlarged heart with cardiac involvement.
5. Pulmonary function tests show decreased diffusion and vital capacity.
6. Electrocardiogram indicates possible nonspecific abnormalities.
7. Skin biopsy indicates marked thickening of the dermis.

NURSING DIAGNOSES: ACTUAL OR POTENTIAL

1. Body image disturbances: due to skin changes.
2. Potential for aspiration: due to dysphagia.
3. Nutritional deficit: due to dysphagia.
4. Skin breakdown: due to underlying disease process.
5. Anxiety and fear: secondary to the progress of the disease.

EXPECTED OUTCOMES

1. Client will adjust to changes in body image.
2. Client will show compliance with care plan by:
   a. Avoiding fatigue and planning rest periods.
   b. Participating in skin care of fingers and toes.
   c. Preventing exposure of extremities to cold temperature and wearing proper clothing.
   d. Taking medications as prescribed.
3. Dysphagia will subside and the weight will increase.
4. Skin will remain intact.
5. Anxiety and fears will decrease as the client and family learn to cope with the problems.

INTERVENTIONS

1. Encourage the client to express feelings regarding the appearance of the face and extremities. Help the client adjust to the changes in body image.
2. Teach the client:
   a. To avoid fatigue by organizing work schedules to include necessary rest.
   b. Information about the disease.
   c. To wear warm socks and gloves and to avoid exposure of hands and feet to cold temperatures.
   d. To eat small, frequent meals, to chew food

slowly, and to drink liquids with meals to minimize dysphagia.
3. Medical treatment may involve vasodilators for the Raynaud's phenomenon.
4. Chemotherapy and immunosuppressives may also be ordered as palliative treatment.

EVALUATION

Outcome Criteria

1. Client and family understand reasons for the changes in body image.
2. Client shows compliance with the plan of care.
3. Dysphagia subsides and weight increases.
4. Chest pain, arrhythmias, and dyspnea cease.
5. Anxiety and fears lessen.

Complications

1. Arthralgias and arthritis (see Chapter 27).
2. Renal involvement (see Chapter 32).
3. Congestive heart failure (see the discussion in this chapter under *Congestive Heart Failure*).

Reevaluation and Follow-up

As scleroderma is progressive, complete cessation of the symptoms is unrealistic. When doing follow-up evaluation:

1. Evaluate the client's compliance with the plan of care.
2. Evaluate the condition of the skin of the fingers and toes.
3. Evaluate any new complications and provide interventions for them.

LUPUS ERYTHEMATOSUS

DESCRIPTION

Lupus erythematosus (LE), the most common of the collagen diseases, is characterized by inflammatory lesions involving many body systems: the skin, joints, kidneys, cardiopulmonary system, and central nervous system. In about one-half of clients the heart is involved. When it is involved, the endocardium, myocardium, and pericardium are affected singly or in combination. The lesions in the endocardium are Libman-Sacks lesions, which are wartlike in appearance and are commonly found under the mitral valve leaflets. The myocardial lesions are due to deposition of fibrinoid material in the septa between the myocardial cells. The pericardium shows fibrinoid degeneration and necrosis of connective tissue.

The onset is insidious and the course is variable and unpredictable. Generally, there are two types: *acute*, which is severe in nature, and *subacute*, which is milder and accounts for the majority of cases. The present therapy and prognosis are still far from satisfactory.

PREVENTION

Health Promotion

As the cause of this disease is unknown, there is no way to prevent it.

Population at Risk

1. Found predominantly in females during child-bearing ages.
2. Occurs more frequently in black Americans and Asians than in Caucasians.

Screening

There is no effective screening tool for LE.

ASSESSMENT

Health History

1. Client describes an insidious onset of general symptoms: chills, low grade fever in the afternoon, aching, weakness, fatigue, malaise, loss of appetite, and decreased weight.
2. Women give a history of irregular menstrual periods or cessation.
3. Client reports painful erythematous, or scaly, rashes on face, neck, and upper extremities that may be induced by exposure to the sun.
4. Some clients are sensitive to cold temperatures. After exposure to the cold, the skin on hands and feet show color changes.
5. Some clients bruise easily and experience pinpoint bleeding into the skin.
6. Painful ulceration of the mouth, pharynx, and vagina occurs in early disease.
7. Sometimes clients state a problem of forgetfulness or transient states of depression, hyperirritability, and anxiety due to central nervous system involvement.

Physical Assessment

This is a multisystem disease with many problems and many possible physical manifestations including:

1. Skin and mucous membranes.
   a. Erythematous rash over the bridge of the

nose (butterfly lesion), on the neck, extremities, or trunk. This rash is aggravated by exposure to the sun.
   b. Bruises or petechiae of the skin or mucous membranes.
   c. Hair loss (alopecia) in some clients.
   d. Ulcerations of the mouth, pharynx, and vagina.
   e. Raynaud's phenomenon: if severe, can cause gangrene of digits.
2. Cardiopulmonary system.
   a. Sinus tachycardia.
   b. Murmurs and gallop rhythm.
   c. Friction rub due to pericarditis.
   d. Dyspnea and chest pain due to pleurisy.
3. Musculoskeletal system.
   a. Arthritis (differs from rheumatoid arthritis in that it is nondeforming).
   b. Arthralgia: joints are red and swollen, causing decreased mobility.
4. Gastrointestinal system.
   a. Abdominal pain.
   b. Nausea and vomiting.
   c. Anorexia.
   d. Bloody stools.
   e. Hepatomegaly.
5. Kidneys.
   a. Hematuria.
   b. Proteinuria.
6. Central nervous system.
   a. Seizures.
   b. Forgetfulness.
   c. Hyperirritability.
   d. Psychosis.
7. General symptoms.
   a. Aching.
   b. Weakness.
   c. Fatigue.
   d. Low-grade fever.
   e. Chills.
   f. Weight loss.

Diagnostic Tests

1. Erythrocyte sedimentation rate is elevated.
2. Urea clearance test evaluates renal function.
3. Proteinuria is the best indicator of disease activity in the kidney.
4. Skin biopsy of skin lesions.
5. Synovial fluid analysis of involved joints.
6. Electrocardiogram may show conduction defects and cardiac enlargement.
7. Chest x-ray study shows size of heart and pulmonary involvement.
8. Antinuclear antibody test is positive (but is not specific for lupus).
9. LE factor is strongly suggestive if positive.
10. Anti-DNA test is the most specific; correlates well with disease activity.

NURSING DIAGNOSES: ACTUAL OR POTENTIAL

1. Potential for physical injury: due to neurological changes.
2. Impaired mobility: due to joint pain.
3. Knowledge deficit: regarding skin care.
4. Decreased activity tolerance: due to generalized weakness.
5. Discomfort: related to the disease process.
6. Disturbance in self-concept: related to perception of disease as chronic.

EXPECTED OUTCOMES

1. Dermal symptoms will subside.
2. Mobility will improve so that falls are prevented.
3. Normal digestion will be restored.
4. Client will demonstrate proper skin care.
5. Client will verbalize a sense of well-being as the general systemic problems are solved.
6. Client will know:
   a. The value of rest.
   b. The reasons for diagnostic tests.
   c. How to do range-of-motion exercises.
   d. The rationale for medications.

INTERVENTIONS

1. Skin treatment:
   a. Teach client to avoid direct sunlight and cold temperatures on hands and feet; advise client to wear protective clothing.
   b. Give antimalarial drugs (chloroquine or Plaquenil), as ordered. An ophthalmological examination should be done every 6 months to observe for retinal damage.
   c. Advise client to eliminate cigarette smoking.
   d. Use corticosteroid ointments for skin care.
2. Medications:
   a. Place client on diuretics, digitalis, and low-sodium diet if heart failure is present.
   b. Administer morphine for chest pain.
   c. Use prednisone in high doses initially, followed by gradual decrease; warn the client about side effects.

d. Use antihypertensive drugs for hypertension.
   (1) Weigh client daily.
   (2) Evaluate intake and output.
   (3) Observe characteristics of urine.

3. Mobility:
   a. Give aspirin for joint pain and inflammation.
   b. Help the client develop an activity-rest schedule unless client is acutely ill.
   c. Apply heat packs to relieve joint pain and stiffness.
   d. Encourage full range-of-motion exercises to prevent contractures.
4. Nutrition: assist the client in the selection of a well-balanced diet.
5. Safety measures::
   a. Use seizure precautions. Maintain a safe environment.
   b. Orient the client to time and place.
6. Teaching and counseling:
   a. Teach the client:
      (1) How to cope with stress.
      (2) To avoid exposure to infections.
      (3) To maintain regularity in the lifestyle.
   b. Provide psychological support.

EVALUATION

Outcome Criteria

1. Dyspnea, chest pain, and tachycardia subside.
2. Skin lesions diminish.
3. Mobility is increased as joint pain decreases.
4. Client maintains a well-balanced diet.
5. Urinary output is normal and laboratory values for kidney function are within normal limits.
6. The psychological effects of the disease are diminished and cerebral functioning is normal.
7. Client has a sense of well-being.

Reevaluation and Follow-up

A community health nurse referral should include the following:

1. Observe client for exacerbation of the disease.
2. Evaluate client's compliance regarding:
   a. Avoidance of direct sunlight.
   b. Protection of hands and feet from cold temperatures.
   c. Regular exercise.
   d. Drugs: corticosteroids.
3. Evaluate client's functional ability to perform activities of daily living.
4. Evaluate vocational ability to tolerate pace and activities in a work situation.
5. Assess the client's emotional status and the ability to cope with the disease.

INFLAMMATIONS

BACTERIAL ENDOCARDITIS

DESCRIPTION

Bacterial endocarditis is a severe bacterial infection of the endocardium. The basic lesion is a friable vegetation on the heart valves, the endocardial lining of a heart chamber, or the endothelium of a blood vessel. The vegetation is made up of platelets, fibrin, white blood cells, red blood cells, some bacteria, and varying amounts of necrosis. As healing takes place, the exposed area of the vegetation becomes covered with fibrous tissue and phagocytosis of the bacteria occurs. Previous rheumatic endocarditis is the most common cause of bacterial endocarditis. The mitral valve is the site most often involved. Because of the location of these vegetations and their friable characteristic, peripheral arterial embolism is common in this disease. As the result of the embolization to other parts of the body, septic infarction and abscess formation occur, most commonly in the kidney, brain, and spleen.

There are two forms of bacterial endocarditis:

1. *Acute bacterial endocarditis:* This is a severe infection, characterized by high fever, heart murmurs, embolic phenomena, and an enlarged spleen. It follows a rapid course. The endocardium is damaged early in the disease.
2. *Subacute bacterial endocarditis:* This is a less severe infection, characterized by a continuous fever, weight loss, fatigue, joint pains, and an enlarged spleen. Its onset is insidious, and the course is prolonged. With adequate therapy, there is little or no damage to the endocardium.

Infection may originate from:

1. Preexisting disease or injury of the heart valve, which predisposes the endocardium to infection.
2. Acute infection elsewhere in the body (tonsils, teeth, kidneys).
3. Heart surgery when poor technique is used.
4. Contaminated needles and careless technique in parenteral administration of drugs or IV therapy (drug addicts are prone to develop infection).

PREVENTION

Health Promotion

1. Avoidance of exposure to infections, especially if rheumatic fever is in the person's history.
2. Use of excellent sterile technique for all procedures (parenteral drug or IV) administration, catheterization, cardiac surgery.
3. Education of teachers and parents regarding the association between sore throat and rheumatic fever.

Population at Risk

1. Persons with preexisting disease or injury to heart valves, especially from rheumatic fever.
2. Drug addicts who use contaminated needles and careless techniques.
3. Individuals with a family history of rheumatic fever.
4. Persons with frequent infections.

Screening

1. Throat cultures for a suspected person with streptococcal sore throat.
2. Throat cultures for family members when "strep throats" appear frequently in a family.

ASSESSMENT

Health History

1. History of rheumatic fever.
2. Recent dental work.
3. Previous acute infection of tonsils, kidneys, gums, teeth, lungs.
4. Previous surgery or invasive techniques, such as cardiac catheterization, parenteral fluids or medications.
5. Repeated sore throats.
6. Complaints of fatigue, anorexia, angina, and dyspnea on exertion.

Physical Assessment

1. Intermittent fevers, chills, diaphoresis.
2. Weight loss.
3. Tachycardia.
4. Clubbing of fingers and toes late in disease.
5. Pallor.
6. Loud, regurgitant murmur.

Diagnostic Tests

1. Blood culture, repeated over several days, to identify specific organism. Blood is drawn before antibiotic therapy is begun.
2. Elevated sedimentation rate.
3. Low hematocrit.
4. Increased white cell count (leucocytosis).
5. Hematuria, proteinuria, and casts.
6. Electrocardiogram may show atrial fibrillation that accompanies valvular damage.
7. Echocardiography may identify valvular damage.

NURSING DIAGNOSES: ACTUAL OR POTENTIAL

1. Fatigue: due to increased cardiac work.
2. Anxiety: secondary to symptoms.
3. Nutritional deficit: related to anorexia.
4. Lack of compliance: due to knowledge deficit.

EXPECTED OUTCOMES

1. Client will increase activity tolerance level without fatigue.
2. Anxiety will subside.
3. Appetite will improve and weight will increase.
4. Client will show compliance with the plan of care.

INTERVENTIONS

1. Provide supportive care.
   a. Relieve anxiety.
   b. Give aspirin and provide cooling measures for fever.
   c. Maintain adequate fluid intake.
2. After the causative organism has been identified through diagnostic blood cultures, administer antibiotic therapy. (Find out if client is allergic before giving.)
   a. Penicillin is the backbone of therapy, for it penetrates the fibrin of the vegetation to reach the bacteria.
      (1) It is given over 4 to 6 weeks.
      (2) It is given by slow, continuous IV drip.

   b. If the client has an allergic reaction to penicillin, diphenhydramine (Benadryl) may be administered intravenously.
   c. Alternative antibiotic therapy such as cephalosporins are prescribed in the event of allergies to penicillin.
3. Provide bed rest to decrease work of the heart for signs of heart failure or fever.
4. Teach the client and family:
   a. About the disease.
   b. The need for prolonged treatment.
   c. Symptoms to watch for (fever and anorexia).
   d. Activity level compatible with client's progress.
5. Surgery of the involved valve may be necessary after the infectious process is controlled if heart failure continues.

EVALUATION

Outcome Critiera

1. Symptoms of infection subside within 1 week.
2. Activity tolerance improves with decreased fatigue and/or chest pain.
3. Anxiety decreases.
4. Appetite improves and weight increases.
5. Client is compliant with the plan of care.

Complications

EMBOLIZATION

Embolization from the heart to other tissues often occurs within 3 months.

Assessment

1. Tenderness and enlargement of the spleen (if emboli travel to spleen).
2. Hematuria and flank pain if kidneys are involved.
3. Sudden visual problems, inability to speak, and paralysis if cerebral embolization has occurred.
4. Circulatory problems such as gangrene in extremities if emboli have lodged in arteries of the extremities.
5. Severe dyspnea, hemoptysis, cough, and pleuritic pain in pulmonary embolism.
6. Petechiae (pinpoint hemorrhages) under the skin.

Interventions

See the discussion on emboli in this chapter under *Acute Arterial Occlusion by Arterial Embolism.*

Revised Outcomes

Further embolization will be prevented.

HEART FAILURE

Refer to *Congestive Heart Failure* in this chapter. Replacement of the injured valve may be necessary in refractory heart failure (see the discussion of valvular cardiac surgery in this chapter).

Reevaluation and Follow-up

1. Be aware that effective control of bacterial endocarditis is determined by the following criteria:
   a. Fever, sweats, and tachycardia disappear.
   b. Weight increases.
   c. There are negative blood cultures.
   d. Urinary function improves.
2. Watch for complications.
   a. Heart failure.
   b. Embolization to other organs.
3. Assist the client in rehabilitation for activities of daily living according to progress of the disease.

MYOCARDITIS

DESCRIPTION

Myocarditis is an inflammatory process involving the myocardium caused by viral, bacterial, parasitic, or rickettsial infections. It is frequently associated with acute pericarditis. When this problem is present, the heart is unable to contract properly because the inflammatory process interferes with contractile function of the myocardial cells.

PREVENTION

Health Promotion

1. Effective treatment of infectious diseases.
2. Avoidance of contact with persons with infectious diseases.

Population at Risk

1. Persons experiencing any infectious process are at risk.

Screening

Throat cultures of susceptible persons.

ASSESSMENT

Health History

1. History of previous infections, such as rheumatic fever, diphtheria, or tuberculosis.
2. Family history of infections.
3. Complaints of fatigue, dyspnea, palpitations, and mild, continuous pressure or soreness in the chest.
4. Gastrointestinal complaints: nausea, vomiting, and anorexia.

Physical Assessment

1. The disease begins like influenza and is followed by clinical features associated with cardiac enlargement and failure.
2. Persistent fever with tachycardia that is disproportionate to the degree of fever.
3. Pericardial friction rub if pericarditis is present.
4. Gallop rhythms: S_3 and S_4.
5. Pulsus alternans.
6. Arrhythmias: supraventricular and ventricular.

Diagnostic Tests

1. Cardiac enzymes: elevated creatine phosphokinase (CPK), isoenzyme (CPK_2), SGOT, LDH.
2. Increased white blood cell count.
3. Increased sedimentation rate.
4. Elevated antibody titers, such as antistreptolysis O (ASO titer) in rheumatic fever.
5. Electrocardiographic changes are the most reliable diagnostic aid: ST-segment and T-wave abnormalities. In addition, prolonged PR intervals are found.
6. Stool and throat cultures may identify the bacteria or isolate the virus.
7. Chest x-ray study may show an enlarged heart.

NURSING DIAGNOSES: ACTUAL OR POTENTIAL

1. Activity intolerance: related to cardiac dysfunction.
2. Alteration in comfort due to palpitations from arrhythmias.
3. Nutritional deficit: due to gastrointestinal symptoms: nausea, vomiting, anorexia.

EXPECTED OUTCOMES

1. Body temperature will be within normal range.
2. Activity tolerance will improve.
3. Appetite will return as nausea, vomiting, and anorexia decrease.
4. Chest discomfort will cease.

INTERVENTIONS

1. Give antibiotics for bacterial infection.
2. Provide bed rest to decrease work load of the heart. Assist with bathing as necessary; provide a bedside commode.
3. Give reassurance that activity limitations are temporary. Offer diversional activities that are not physically demanding.
4. Give antiarrhythmic drugs for arrhythmias as ordered (quinidine or procainamide).
5. Assess cardiovascular status frequently to watch for complications of heart failure. If digitalis is used, watch for toxicity, for clients are hypersensitive to even small doses because of the inflammatory process.
6. Provide nutrition in small amounts and in appropriate consistency.
7. Give analgesics for chest discomfort.

EVALUATION

Outcome Criteria

1. Fever disappears and body temperature is normal within 2 days of therapy.
2. Palpitations decrease.
3. Appetite returns as nausea, vomiting, and anorexia decrease.
4. Chest discomfort ceases.

Complications

1. Heart Failure (see the discussion under *Congestive Heart Failure* in this chapter).
2. Thromboembolism (see the discussion under *Acute Arterial Occlusion by Arterial Embolism* in this chapter).

Reevaluation and Follow-up

1. Effective control of myocarditis can be determined by:
   a. Relief of symptoms related to heart failure.
   b. Normal body temperature.
   c. Decrease in cardiac symptoms.
   d. Decrease in the heart size as determined by chest x-ray study.
   e. No ST-segment and T-wave abnormalities on electrocardiogram.
2. Increase in the client's sense of well-being is due to:

   a. Decrease in fatigue, nausea, vomiting, and anorexia.
   b. Increase in activity level.
3. During recovery, the client should resume normal activities slowly and avoid competitive sports.

PERICARDITIS

DESCRIPTION

Acute pericarditis is an inflammatory process involving the pericardium. It may occur as a primary process but is usually secondary to other diseases. Pericarditis may occur with or without an exudate. When there is an exudate, it accumulates between the two layers of pericardium (parietal and visceral) and impairs the heart function because of its constrictive action. Occasionally, the acute process heals with fibrosis, which constricts the heart action also. Pericarditis is classified as acute or chronic:

1. *Acute pericarditis* may be fibrinous or exudative.
   a. *Acute fibrinous*: Delicate adhesions form around the pericardiac sac. There is a pericardial friction rub, described as scratchy.
   b. *Acute exudative*: A fluid accumulates in the pericardial sac, it prevents the heart from filling during diastole. If it occurs rapidly, tamponade results.
2. *Chronic constrictive pericarditis*: The pericardium becomes a thick, fibrous, calcified band of tissue around the heart. It eventually causes cardiac failure.

PREVENTION

Health Promotion

Prevention of infectious diseases (bacterial, fungal, or viral) and myocardial infarction.

Population at Risk

1. Persons with hypersensitivity to autoimmune diseases.
2. Persons with infectious diseases.
3. Persons who have had coronary artery disease.

Screening

1. Electrocardiograms on susceptible persons.
2. Assessment of pericardial friction rub in susceptible persons.

ASSESSMENT

Health History

1. Previous infectious diseases.
2. Previous myocardial infarction.
3. Previous radiation to the chest.

Physical Assessment

1. Sharp and sudden chest pain that radiates to the neck, shoulders, back, and arms. Unlike myocardial infarction pain, it is pleuritic and increases with deep inspiration and decreases when sitting up or leaning forward.
2. Pericardial friction rub occurs as the heart moves during systole and diastole. It has a scratchy, grating sound, heard best during forced exhalation.
3. Dyspnea.
4. Tachycardia.
5. Fever.
6. In constrictive pericarditis, pulsus paradoxus occurs. This is an abnormal (more than 10 mmHg) inspiratory fall in systolic blood pressure during normal breathing.

Diagnostic Tests

1. Electrocardiogram: elevated ST segment the first few days; T wave inverts as the subacute phase starts. Pathological Q waves, seen in acute myocardial infarction, do not occur. Atrial arrhythmias are observed.
2. White blood cell count may be elevated to 10,000 to 20,000 per centimeter.
3. Echocardiography shows a widened space between the pericardial layers when pericardial effusion is present.
4. Erythrocyte sedimentation rate is elevated.
5. Culture of pericardial fluid may identify the causative organism.

NURSING DIAGNOSES: ACTUAL OR POTENTIAL

1. Discomfort: related to pericardial friction.
2. Discomfort: due to fever, sharp chest pain, or dyspnea.
3. Anxiety: due to the disease process.

EXPECTED OUTCOMES

1. Chest pain will be reduced.
2. Client will be free of dyspnea.
3. Anxiety will lessen.

INTERVENTIONS

1. To relieve dyspnea and chest pain, place the client in an upright position. Provide analgesics and oxygen as needed.
2. Stress the importance of bed rest.
3. Reassure the client having acute pericarditis that the condition is usually temporary and that it responds well to therapy.
4. Explain all diagnostic procedures.
5. Give aspirin for the inflammation and fever.
6. Give antibiotics as ordered for identified infections.
7. Administer steroids if ordered if aspirin is ineffective when the diagnosis is clearly not tuberculosis.
8. Pericardiectomy (excision of the fibrinous pericardium) for constrictive pericarditis is performed for chronic cases. If this is to be done, explain the procedure to the client and what to expect after surgery.

EVALUATION

Outcome Criteria

1. Chest pain ceases within 3 days of treatment.
2. Dyspnea is relieved.
3. Body temperature is normal.
4. Anxiety lessens.

Complications

1. Congestive heart failure (see the discussion in this chapter).
2. Cardiac tamponade (accumulation of fluid in pericardium) (see complications under *Valvular Heart Diseases*).

THROMBOPHLEBITIS

DESCRIPTION

Thrombophlebitis is the inflammation of a vein with clot formation. *Phlebothrombosis* is clot formation in the vein without or followed secondarily by inflammation. It is difficult to tell in some clients which condition came first, for after several days inflammation and thrombi coexist.

Many factors are associated with thrombophlebitis. Venous stasis damage to the endothelium and hypercoagulability of the blood are contributory causative mechanisms. The use of oral contraceptives is correlated with increased intravascular clotting, although the exact mechanism for this association is unknown.

PREVENTION

Health Promotion

1. Persons working in jobs requiring continuous standing should wear support hose.
2. Persons working in sedentary jobs should increase physical activity.
3. Tight, constricting clothing involving the lower extremities, such as round garters or girdles, should be avoided.
4. Women taking oral contraceptive drugs should be taught about the danger of thrombosis.
5. Pressure on the back of the knee, such as in crossing the legs, should be avoided.
6. If obesity is present, the person should lose weight.

Population at Risk

1. Persons experiencing long periods of immobility or prolonged periods without positional changes.
2. Persons taking oral contraceptive drugs.
3. Persons with injuries to extremities.
4. Persons with existent vascular problems creating disturbance in blood flow, such as varicosities or Buerger's disease.

Screening

No screening test is available.

ASSESSMENT

Health History

1. Previous history of thrombus formation.
2. History of an injury to an extremity.
3. Presence of a coexisting vascular disease.
4. Complaints of mild or severe pain and tenderness localized to a specific area. Activity may or may not aggravate the pain.
5. Sedentary lifestyle.

Physical Assessment

1. Mild calf pain aggravated by walking.
2. Swelling of the extremity. Compare circumference of the involved extremity with the normal extremity. A difference of 5 mm is significant.
3. Redness along the course of the involved vein.
4. Calf of the involved leg is warm.
5. Homan's sign (pain in the calf with forced dorsiflexion) in about one-half of the clients.
6. Body temperature may be elevated to 38.3°C (101°F).
7. Anxiety.

Diagnostic Tests

1. Phlebography is done by injecting a radiopaque medium and using fluoroscopy to determine how well the vein fills with blood and the location of the thrombi.
2. Venous pressure measurements: In the affected leg, the venous pressure is higher than in the other. This is due to back pressure of the blood. When collateral circulation is established, venous pressure in the involved leg may no longer be elevated.
3. Radioactive isotopes, such as fibrinogen labeled with radioactive iodine, are injected into the involved vein. A counter determines how concentrated the iostopes are in the areas of thrombi.
4. An ultrasonic flow detector is used as a diagnostic tool to study blood flow. Failure to detect normal flow constitutes a positive test. Usefulness is limited to the acute period.

NURSING DIAGNOSES: ACTUAL OR POTENTIAL

1. Pain: due to inflammation in the affected extremity.
2. Knowledge deficit: regarding treatment plan.

EXPECTED OUTCOMES

1. The pain in the extremity will cease.
2. Client and family will learn preventive measures.
3. Client will identify medications in terms of name, dose, action, frequency, and side effects.

INTERVENTIONS

1. Relieve calf pain.
   a. Apply warm, moist compresses to the affected area.
   b. Use analgesics (codeine or Darvon).
   c. Put the client on bed rest with elevation of the involved extremity until symptoms of inflammation subside.
   d. Teach client not to massage the affected leg.
2. Prevent further thrombosis and possibly embolism.
   a. Administer anticoagulants (if there is deep vein thrombosis).
   b. Use streptokinase and urokinase (fibrinolytic drugs) to disolve thrombi.
3. Counsel the client to wear elastic stockings.
4. Teach the client about medications and what side effects to report.

EVALUATION

Outcome Criteria

1. Calf pain is decreased.
2. Anxiety lessens.
3. Embolism is not present.
4. Client and family can recall with 85 percent accuracy measures that will prevent another episode of thrombophlebitis.

Complications

Pulmonary embolism due to displacement of thrombus to the lungs (see Chapter 31).

Reevaluation and Follow-up

1. Evaluate client's compliance with preventive measures.
   a. Physical activity and specific exercises.
   b. Avoidance of constrictive clothing.
   c. Loss of weight, if obese.
   d. Avoidance of oral contraceptives.
   e. Use of elastic stockings.
2. Evaluate compliance with medications, such as anticoagulants, and knowledge of side effects to report (bleeding).
3. Evaluate client's knowledge of recurrent symptoms of thrombophlebitis.

TRAUMA

CARDIAC AND GREAT VESSEL TRAUMA

DESCRIPTION

There are two categories for injuries to the heart and great vessels: *injuries due to external forces* and *injuries due to diagnostic, medical, or therapeutic procedures*.

1. Injuries due to external forces.
   a. *Cardiac tamponade.* This is usually caused by gunshot and stab wounds. Tamponade is the result of as little as 50–100 mL of blood in the pericardium. Wounds of the atria are likely to heal spontaneously be-

cause of the low pressure; wounds of the ventricles, however, will bleed and result in death unless treatment abates the process.

b. *Shunts.* These are abnormal communications between parts caused by trauma, such as ventricular septal defect, fistula between the left ventricle and the coronary sinus, and a fistula between the aorta and the right ventricle. Congestive heart failure occurs if the shunt is large.
c. *Valvular insufficiency.* This condition results from injury to the valves of the heart. Usually, the injury is a blunt trauma, such as a sharp blow to the chest wall.
d. *Myocardial contusion.* Myocardial contusion follows blunt trauma. Hemorrhage occurs in the contused area and is followed by infarction. Tachycardia and arrhythmias occur frequently. The contused area can rupture.
e. *Coronary arterial insufficiency.* Coronary arterial injury is rare as a result of blunt trauma. Usually, if the coronary artery is injured, the injury has caused additional serious injuries to other areas of the heart. The result of coronary arterial injury is *hemopericardium.*
f. *Rupture or aneurysm (or both) of the aorta.* Penetrating trauma of the aorta usually has fatal results. Clients will be in severe shock or near death by the time they reach the emergency department.
g. *Arterial involvement.* Major arterial injuries may result from either penetrating trauma or from blunt trauma. Either a complete or partial laceration of the artery may take place. By the time the client is seen there may be a pulsating hematoma and formation of a false aneurysm.
h. *Embolization.* A penetrating object can cause clot formation on its surface. Such clots are likely to move as emboli to other parts of the body.

2. Injuries due to medical or therapeutic procedures.
   a. *Cardiac surgery.* Various accidental events can happen following surgery, such as a prosthetic aortic valve impinging on the right coronary ostium, embolization of calcified material following the removal of a calcified valve, and creation of a dissecting aneurysm.
   b. *Cardiac catheterization.* There may be laceration of the left ventricle, hemorrhage into a ventricular wall following injection of contrast material during angiocardiography, and perforation of the right atrium by a catheter that had migrated there after prolonged intravenous therapy.

See Chapter 48, Traumatic Injuries, for further details on emergency care. Subsequent care following the transfer of the client to an intensive care unit from the emergency department or operating room will depend upon the type of injury that occurred. Generally, the care initiated in the emergency department continues in the intensive care unit.

OBSTRUCTIONS

CORONARY HEART DISEASE

DESCRIPTION

The ability of the heart to function as a pump to meet the many demands placed upon it is dependent on an adequate blood supply to the myocardium via coronary arteries. If these coronary arteries are occluded or narrowed, blood is hindered from reaching myocardial tissues supplied by these vessels. Ischemia develops from this occlusive process and may progress to infarction, depending on the extent of hypoxia of the tissue.

The primary cause of this occlusive process is *atherosclerosis,* a progressive development of fatty deposits called *plaques* along the intimal lining of the blood vessels. A combination of several factors, such as cigarette smoking, high cholesterol intake, and hypertension is highly correlated with the development of atherosclerosis. The two most common manifestations of coronary heart disease are:

1. *Angina pectoris,* which is temporary ischemia of the myocardium without tissue damage.
2. *Myocardial infarction,* which is extreme ischemia with tissue damage.

Both forms result from atherosclerosis but differ from each other in extent of ischemia.

PREVENTION

Health Promotion

1. Control of coronary heart disease risk factors:
   a. Cessation of cigarette smoking.
   b. Lowering of cholesterol intake.
   c. Identification and control of hypertension.
   d. Maintenance of optimum weight.
   e. Physical exercise.
   f. Reduction of stress.
2. Correction or control of health problems, such as anemia, diabetes, hyperthyroidism, congenital cardiac anomalies.
3. Attention to the development of risk in persons with a family history of coronary heart disease.

Population at Risk

1. Males more than females until age 50; then incidence is equal in both sexes.
2. Persons with family history of premature coronary heart disease.
3. Persons with previous episodes of coronary heart disease.
4. Persons with a combination of risk factors.

Screening

1. Electrocardiogram to detect changes in ST segment and T wave at the time of an anginal attack and large Q waves in a myocardial infarction.
2. Exercise testing to determine the effect of physical exercise on the electrocardiogram, pulse, and blood pressure.

ASSESSMENT

Health History

1. Family history of premature coronary disease, sudden death, or other cardiac problems.
2. Excessive intake of saturated fats.
3. Sedentary lifestyle.
4. Cigarette smoking.
5. History of diabetes mellitus.
6. Hypertension.
7. Previous episodes of chest pain.
8. Amount of stress associated with occupation.
9. Type A personality (ambitious, competitive).
10. Precipitating factors preceding the present episode.

Physical Assessment

1. Angina pectoris.
   a. Anxiety: during an anginal attack.
   b. Description of pain: crushing, squeezing burning sensation under the sternum; usually radiates to the neck and arms (most often the left arm).
   c. Precipitating causes: physical exercise, overeating, emotional excitement, or exposure to cold weather.
   d. Onset and duration: gradual or sudden onset: usually lasts less than 15 min.
   e. Relief of pain: cessation of precipitating cause or administration of nitroglycerine sublinqually.
   f. Additional assessments: once pain is relieved, the client is usually free of symptoms.
2. Myocardial infarction.
   a. Anxiety: severe, from fear of impending doom.
   b. Description of pain: persistent, severe squeezing, burning sensation under the sternum; usually radiates as in angina pectoris; more severe than in angina pectoris.
   c. Precipitating causes: pain occurring following similar precipitating causes, as for angina pectoris, or pain unrelated to such causes.
   d. Onset and duration: sudden onset; lasts 30 min to 2 h.
   e. Relief of pain: unrelieved by rest or nitroglycerine; analgesics such as morphine as needed.
   f. Additional assessments: dyspnea and increased respiratory rate; nausea and vomiting; pallor; diaphoresis; elevated BP at first, then possibly decreased; extreme weakness; tachycardia.

Diagnostic Tests

1. Angina pectoris.
   a. Electrocardiogram shows ST segment and T wave changes if taken during the anginal attack; otherwise, it may be normal.
   b. Coronary angiogram (necessitating a cardiac catheterization, a dye injection into coronary arteries, and x-ray films) shows the sites of the occlusive process. Decision for coronary bypass surgery is made according to findings.
2. Myocardial infarction.
   a. Electrocardiogram will show ST-segment

and T-wave changes initially and Q-wave changes after 24 h. These changes are observed in those leads nearest the injured part of the myocardium.

b. Serum enzymes increase from ischemic cells.
   (1) Creatine phosphokinase (CPK) rises within 6 h and returns to normal in 2 to 3 days. The presence of the myocardial band (MB), an isoenzyme of CPK, is specific for ischemia of cardiac cells.
   (2) Serum glutamic oxaloacetic transaminase (SGOT) rises within 6–8 h and returns to normal in 4 to 8 days. It is nonspecific and may rise from other causes; therefore, it is not used much.
   (3) Lactic dehydrogenase (LDH) rises on the second or third day and returns to normal after 5 to 7 days. LDH_1, and LDH_2, isoenzymes, are specific for myocardial infarction.

c. Leukocytosis may appear several days after the infarction. The ratios of LDH_1 to LDH_2 reverse after a myocardial infarction because of rapid increase in LDH_1.

d. Elevated sedimentation rate occurs in response to inflammation after a few days.

NURSING DIAGNOSES: ACTUAL OR POTENTIAL

1. Anxiety: due to fear of outcomes.
2. Alteration in comfort: secondary to chest pain.
3. Decreased activity: due to imbalance between myocardial oxygen supply and demand.
4. Lack of compliance: secondary to knowledge deficit.

EXPECTED OUTCOMES

1. Anxiety will lessen.
2. Chest pain will be relieved.
3. Fatigue will lessen.
4. Dyspnea will cease.
5. Client's compliance will be evidenced by:
   a. Avoidance of controllable risk factors.
   b. Adherence to instructions regarding medications, diet, and exercise.

INTERVENTIONS

1. Angina pectoris.
   a. During attacks of chest pain:
      (1) Have client stop physical activity and remain quiet.
      (2) Give nitroglycerin sublingually when the pain starts. Repeat every 5–10 min up to three times, if needed. If pain or discomfort continues, the client should immediately be evaluated in the nearest emergency room. (Remember to teach the client to keep the medication in a dark bottle because it is light-sensitive, to expect a stinging sensation under the tongue, and possibly a headache when using it, and to renew the prescription within 6 months.)
      (3) Monitor blood pressure and heart rate.
      (4) Take an electrocardiogram during the attack.
      (5) Provide psychological support.
      (6) Record duration of pain, medication required to relieve it, and any accompanying symptoms.
   b. Prevent attacks of chest pain:
      (1) Give long-acting nitrates such as isosorbide dinitrate (Isordil) orally or topical ointment on the skin ($\frac{1}{2}$ in, 1 in, or 1 $\frac{1}{2}$ in on measured paper, according to physician's orders).
      (2) Give propranolol (Inderal) orally to reduce oxygen requirements of the myocardium.
      (3) Teach the client:
         (a) To use follow a low-salt, low-cholesterol diet.
         (b) To maintain regular exercise.
         (c) To abstain from cigarette smoking.
      (4) If necessary, prepare the client for cardiac catheterization and angiography by explaining the purpose and the method of how the procedure is done. If an angioplasty is to be done with the catheterization, explain that its purpose is to relieve the coronary obstruction. Following the procedure, monitor the catheter site for bleeding, check distal pulses, and assess vital signs.
      (5) Coronary artery bypass surgery.
         (a) After identification, by coronary angiography, of which coronary arteries are occluded, coronary by-

pass surgery is performed to increase blood supply. A saphenous vein is used as the graft and is attached at one end to the aorta and the other end to a coronary artery distal to the occlusion. Open heart surgery with the use of the heart-lung machine is the technique employed (see Figure 30-16).

(b) Before surgery, explain the procedure to the client and family and answer questions. Take them on a tour of the intensive care unit.

(c) After surgery, provide meticulous care for IV, pulmonary artery catheter, endotracheal tube, and chest tubes. Monitor blood pressure, intake and output, breath sounds, and cardiac rhythm.

(d) Near time of discharge, provide instructions on medications, diet, and activity.

2. Myocardial infarction.
   a. Acute care in a coronary care unit (CCU).
      (1) Relieve the client's anxiety by:
         (a) Orienting client and family to CCU.
         (b) Encouraging expression of fears.
         (c) Reducing potential stressors.

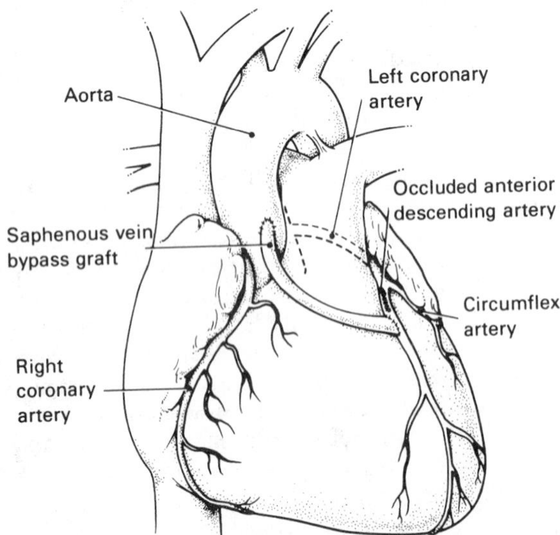

Figure 30-16 Saphenous vein graft for an occluded coronary artery.

         (d) Reassuring and supporting by commending any small progress.
         (e) Giving sedatives or mild tranquilizers as needed.
      (2) Relieve chest pain with morphine sulfate or meperidine (Demerol) intravenously as ordered.
      (3) Lessen fatigue by providing bed rest, a liquid diet, and stool softeners (to avoid straining at stool).
      (4) Relieve dyspnea by:
         (a) Elevating the head of the bed.
         (b) Giving oxygen via nasal cannulae.
      (5) Increase the client's compliance by teaching the client and family:
         (a) The meaning of a heart attack.
         (b) The need for reducing the work of the heart.
      (6) Assess beginning complications by:
         (a) Monitoring for arrhythmias on a cardiac monitor.
         (b) Reporting significant arrhythmias and giving ordered medications.
         (c) Monitoring vital signs.
   b. Subacute care (after transfer from CCU).
      (1) Relieve anxiety by:
         (a) Encouraging client's expression of concerns about work, home, sex.
         (b) Reassuring and supporting the client about progress and future outcomes.
      (2) Prevent fatigue by alternating rest periods with gradually increasing activities. Assess physiological response to activities (BP and pulse rate).
      (3) Increase client's compliance and reinforce education by asking the client to:
         (a) State names of drugs being taken.
         (b) State foods allowed and not allowed on the prescribed diet.
         (c) Follow instructions regarding activity level.
   c. Convalescent care.
      (1) Continue to relieve anxiety of the client and family regarding needed adjustments following discharge.
      (2) Reinforce client education regarding control of risk factors.
      (3) Increase activity level according to the client's tolerance and teach the client symptoms to observe for when the tolerance has been exceeded (angina, dyspnea, palpitations, dizziness).

EVALUATION

Outcome Criteria

1. Angina pectoris.
   a. Chest pain decreases in frequency within 1 month of therapy.
   b. Anxiety decreases as chest pain decreases.
2. Myocardial infarction.
   a. Chest pain ceases within 3 days.
   b. Anxiety gradually decreases.
   c. Dyspnea decreases within 12 h of admission.
   d. Arrhythmias subside by the fourth day and cease by the seventh day.
   e. Compliance is shown by client's:
      (1) Avoiding risk factors, as expressed by the client.
      (2) Taking medications as ordered.
      (3) Eating the diet as ordered.
      (4) Performing activities within tolerance level.

Complications

1. Angina pectoris
   When there are repeated and increased frequency of attacks, an increased risk of myocardial infarction exists.
2. Myocardial infarction.
   a. Congestive heart failure.
   b. Cardiogenic shock.
   c. Arrhythmias.
   d. Myocardial rupture.

Assessment

1. BP suddenly drops.
2. Pulse is fast and feeble, then becomes imperceptible.
3. Cardiac monitor reveals ventricular fibrillation or standstill.

Revised Outcomes

Cardiac output will be restored.

Interventions

See Chapter 49, Medical Emergencies.

Reevaluation and Follow-up

1. Angina pectoris.
   a. Evaluate frequency of anginal attacks. Drug therapy may need to be changed.
   b. Evaluate the client's knowledge of drug therapy.
   c. Evaluate client's compliance with controlling risk factors (cigarette smoking).
2. Myocardial infarction.
   a. Exercise testing is often done to determine a prescription for activities according to the client's tolerance. The amount of energy required for various activities is expressed in METs (1 MET is the metabolic equivalent or metabolic equivalents of energy required at rest).
   b. Evaluate client's compliance with controlling risk factors and with following instructions (e.g., drug therapy, exercise).
   c. Provide psychological support by encouraging the client to express concerns and assisting the client to solve problems.
   d. Evaluate the level of client's knowledge regarding the nature of the cardiac problem.
   e. An electrocardiogram is done to compare the status of the heart with previous tracings.
   f. Planned sessions, such as in "coronary clubs" or "sharing and caring" groups are useful in providing social support for the client and family. In these sessions, concerns and problems are shared with others who have similar experiences.

PERIPHERAL ARTERIAL DISEASES

ARTERIOSCLEROSIS AND ATHEROSCLEROSIS

DESCRIPTION

Arteriosclerosis is the loss of elasticity and the hardening of the media (middle layer) of the blood vessel wall by the deposition of calcium. The cerebral arteries and arteries of the lower extremities are the most commonly affected. It is referred to as hardening of the arteries or "pipe-stem" arteries associated with the aging process.

Atherosclerosis is a type of arteriosclerosis in which plaques containing cholesterol, fatty acids, and other substances develop along the intima (inner layer) of the vessel wall. Causative factors are elevated serum cholesterol, hypertension (by producing mechanical stress), and diabetes.

PREVENTION

Health Promotion

1. Control of hypertension by following prescribed medications.
2. Cessation of cigarette smoking.
3. Reduction of weight if obesity is a problem.
4. Reduction of cholesterol intake.
5. Education regarding prevention throughout formal education from elementary school through college (nutritional counseling, cholesterol screening, hypertension screening, weight reduction).
6. Control of emotional stress.

Population at Risk

1. Males between 25 and 64 years of age (more than females).
2. Cigarette smokers.
3. Diabetic persons.
4. Hypertensive persons.
5. Persons with a family history of arteriosclerosis or atherosclerosis.

Screening

1. Blood pressure measurements: if hypertension is present, therapy is needed to control it.
2. Blood sugar measurements to detect presence of diabetes.
3. Weight: if the person is overweight, counsel weight reduction.

ASSESSMENT

Health History

1. Smoking habits.
2. High cholesterol content of foods.
3. Familial history.
4. Diabetes mellitus.
5. Complaints of pain in lower extremities brought on by exercise and terminating when exercise ceases (intermittent claudication).
6. Identification of other risk factors such as lack of exercise, obesity, and stress.

Physical Assessment

1. Analysis of the pain includes:
   a. Location: in the calf of the leg.
   b. Factors that initiate or eliminate pain: for example exercise, external temperature, or humidity.
   c. Numbness and coldness of the extremity is noted.
2. Skin color of the affected extremity may be pale or cyanotic. When the limb is raised above the level of the heart, blanching is noted.
3. Upon palpation of peripheral pulses, dorsalis pedis and posterior tibial may be absent or difficult to identify.
4. Upon auscultation over an affected peripheral artery, a bruit is heard, indicating a narrowed blood vessel.
5. There may be limited joint mobility due to decreased joint use and increased pain on movement. Muscle atrophy may also result.
6. Leg ulcerations may be present as a result of ischemia.
7. The skin appears smooth and taut with dryness. There may be loss of hair, thickening of nails, and muscle wasting from the lack of nutrition to the tissue.

Diagnostic Tests

There are seven commonly used tests.

1. Oscillometry: through applying a blood pressure cuff around the extremity at various levels and attaching it to an oscillometer (manometer), pressure readings are recorded; abnormal findings indicate the level of arterial occlusion.
2. Skin temperature studies: skin warmth and coolness of the extremities are compared by varying methods. If the client is anxious, skin temperature may be altered, thus making these studies unreliable when anxiety is present.
3. Arteriography: by injecting contrast media into the arteries and taking x-rays films, abnormalities of blood flow can be detected.
4. Exercise tests: client exercises and a record is made of the time from the onset of exercise to the onset of pain.
5. Lumbar sympathetic block: this is done by injecting a local anesthetic into the sympathetic ganglia; if there is decrease in limb pain and increased skin temperature as a result, it means that a sympathectomy would be indicated to improve circulation.
6. Doppler ultrasound velocity detector: this involves using a stethoscope to obtain qualitative and quantitative data about blood flow.
7. Plethysomography: this records pulse changes with each heart beat.

NURSING DIAGNOSES: ACTUAL OR POTENTIAL

1. Discomfort in lower extremities: secondary to decreased blood supply.
2. Impaired mobility: due to pain on movement.
3. Alteration of body image: due to skin breakdown.
4. Noncompliance: due to knowledge deficit.

EXPECTED OUTCOMES

1. Pain in lower extremity will decrease.
2. Mobility will improve within 2 months.
3. Thrombus formation will not occur.
4. Client will comply with therapy, as evidenced by:
   a. Ceasing cigarette smoking by the time of discharge.
   b. Taking medications as ordered and stating their purposes with 80 percent accuracy.
   c. Reducing cholesterol content of diet within 3 months.
   d. If hypertensive, taking antihypertensive medications as ordered by the time of discharge.
   e. Taking mediculous care of the skin.

INTERVENTIONS

1. Give analgesics or narcotics, as ordered, for pain in the extremity. Vasodilating drugs may be used to dilate constricted arteries.
2. Prevent skin breakdown by using mild soaps and lotions to prevent drying of the skin. Avoid extremes in temperature of bath water. Promote circulation in the extremities by graduated increases in walking on a flat surface. Teach client to avoid round garters or crossing legs, which constrict arterial blood supply.
3. Administer mild tranquilizers if the client is anxious. Counsel the client and family about the part stress plays in the progress of the disease.
4. Administer anticoagulants, if ordered, to prevent thrombus formation.
   a. Heparin interferes with platelets releasing thromboplastin and prothrombin-forming thrombin. Antidote: protamine sulfate.
   b. Coumadin depresses prothrombin. Antidote: vitamin K.
5. Teach the client to:
   a. Reduce cholesterol in the diet.
   b. Stop cigarette smoking.
   c. Lose weight, if obese.
   d. Control other problems, such as diabetes and hypertension.
   e. Check peripheral pulses.
   f. Give skin meticulous care.
   g. Avoid cold temperatures to extremities.

EVALUATION

Outcome Criteria

1. Mobility improves without accompanying pain.
2. Body image is restored as extremity skin appears more normal.
3. Thrombosis is prevented.
4. Client compliance with diet, medications, avoidance of risk factors, and care of the extremities is achieved.

Complications

Acute arterial occlusion by arterial embolism. See the discussion following in the next section of this chapter.

Reevaluation and Follow-up

1. Observe for improved symptoms.
   a. Intermittent claudication is decreased.
   b. Skin color and temperature are normal.
   c. Client is increasing exercise without experiencing pain.
2. Evaluate client's long-term compliance with avoiding risk factors and maintaining drug therapy as ordered.
3. Provide counseling regarding adjustments to changed lifestyle and occupation. Be alert for concerns of the client and family and provide the support they need.

ACUTE ARTERIAL OCCLUSION BY ARTERIAL EMBOLISM

DESCRIPTION

Arterial embolism is frequently the cause of acute arterial occlusion. It occurs as a sudden catastrophic event appearing without warning and threatening the loss of a limb or a life. In most cases, arterial emboli originate in the heart and, therefore, should be regarded primarily as a symptom of serious underlying heart disease. The three main causes are (1) mitral stenosis, (2) atrial fibrillation, and (3) myocardial infarction. Most of the emboli originating in the heart lodge in the arteries of the extremities. They tend to lodge at the bifurcation of a major artery, such as the site where the abdominal aorta divides into the two iliac arteries to the legs. When this happens, the tissues perfused by such arteries are deprived of oxygen.

One of the greatest threats from an embolus is that it may lodge in the cerebral circulation, resulting in stroke. Most often, these affected vessels are intracranial and cannot be reached by surgery for the removal of the embolus.

The physiological consequences of an arterial embolus are the immediate onset of ischemia with resulting anoxia of tissues distal to the occlusion. Within a few hours after the lodging of an embolus, thrombi form in the artery distal to it where the flow of blood has become stagnant. Necrosis develops in the ischemic tissues several hours after the embolus has obstructed the artery. The rate of necrosis varies according to the collateral circulation.

The survival of the client as well as of the involved limb depends upon prompt recognition and intelligent management.

PREVENTION

Health Promotion

Anticoagulant therapy for cardiac conditions that are likely to cause thrombi. (These thrombi can break loose and travel to peripheral or cerebral arteries.)

Population at Risk

1. Persons with mitral valve disease and enlargement of the left atrium.
2. Persons who have had an acute myocardial infarction.
3. Persons with congestive heart failure from any cause.
4. Persons with atrial fibrillation.
5. Persons with peripheral arterial diseases.

Screening

None.

ASSESSMENT

Health History

1. History of cardiac diseases.
2. History of peripheral arterial diseases.
3. Sudden onset of burning or aching in areas distal to the site of occlusion with increasing intensity (although occasionally it may be painless).
4. Coldness, numbness, and muscle weakness in the affected limb.
5. Aggravation of pain by motion of the limb.
6. Complaint of pain at rest by client with advanced peripheral arterial occlusion.

Physical Assessment

1. There are five *P*'s included in the assessment of clients with acute arterial occlusion.
   a. Pain in the involved extremity is the most distinctive symptom. As the disease progresses, the pain occurs with less and less exertion until in advanced peripheral arterial occlusion the pain occurs even at rest. This often occurs at night. The person finds some relief when sitting in a chair or dangling the legs over the side of the bed. The pain is characterized as burning, throbbing, sharp, and shooting.
   b. Paresthesia (tingling or numbing sensations) is due to ischemia of the peripheral nerves.
   c. Pallor in the affected extremity can be seen upon elevation of the extremity above the level of the heart and slowly changes to normal color upon lowering of the extremity.
   d. Pulselessness in the affected extremity gives information about the site of occlusion. This is the most significant finding of arterial occlusion. Pulses should be compared bilaterally.
   e. Paralysis is a late symptom. It indicates a severe ischemic insult and probable necrosis (Rutherford, 1977).
2. Leg ulcerations that drain and fail to heal may be present.
3. Client may complain of a sense of heaviness and fullness in the involved extremity due to edema. This edema may be pitting or nonpitting in character, depending on the extent of venous and/or lymph involvement.
4. Because of decreased blood supply to the involved extremity, muscle size may be less than the uninvolved extremity due to muscle wasting. To determine this, the relative sizes of the two extremities should be compared by measuring their circumferences.
5. The skin is cold to the touch. Skin tempera-

ture should be assessed when the client is at rest and the extremities compared bilaterally.
6. Tissue necrosis and gangrene may be present. If this occurs, the area is hard, dry, and black in appearance.
7. On auscultation, a bruit over the constricted artery may be heard.
8. Acute anxiety occurs as the client realizes the significance of the situation.

Diagnostic Tests

1. An electrocardiogram is done to rule out myocardial infarction, atrial fibrillation, or ventricular hypertrophy as possible causes.
2. An arteriogram is done if there is uncertainty about the location of an embolus. It is a technique in which contrast dye is injected into an artery followed by x-rays or fluoroscopy to visualize the course of the dye in the arteries.
3. Oscillometry may be of value in recording pulsations or absent pulsations in the involved extremity. By using a blood pressure cuff, pressure readings are obtained that provide information about the site of the occlusion.

NURSING DIAGNOSES: ACTUAL OR POTENTIAL

1. Discomfort: due to circulatory changes.
2. Impaired mobility: due to pain in the extremity.
3. Impairment in skin integrity: due to decreased tissue perfusion.
4. Anxiety: due to possible loss of limb.

EXPECTED OUTCOMES

1. Discomfort will be reduced.
2. Mobility will be resumed.
3. Further skin breakdown of the extremity will be prevented.
4. Anxiety will be lessened as the status of the limb improves.
5. If amputation is necessary, client will demonstrate the ability to cope with decision making.

INTERVENTIONS

Immediate action within a few hours is necessary if complete arterial occlusion is diagnosed.

1. Relieve the pain with analgesics.
2. Give tranquilizers and emotional support to reduce anxiety provoked by the pain.
3. Administer vasodilators as ordered to help increase the blood supply to the area and reduce the pain.
4. A heparin infusion is given to prevent further clot formation.
5. Place the head of the bed on 6- to 8-in blocks to put the lower extremities in a dependent position. This position promotes increased blood supply to the extremities by gravity.
6. Instruct the client to avoid crossing the legs and feet (at ankles) so that stasis of blood in the lower extremities is prevented.
7. Provide a warm environment and dress the client warmly to prevent vasoconstriction; however, do not apply direct heat to any extremity with poor circulation.
8. Instruct the client on ways to decrease emotional stress and to stop cigarette smoking.
9. To prevent skin ulceration, provide good skin care that includes: preventing pressure areas, using lamb's wool on the involved extremity, using lotions and skin creams to prevent dryness, and changing the client's position frequently.
10. Surgery. There are several operative procedures that can be done.
    a. Preoperative nursing interventions.
        (1) Explain to the client and family why the surgery is needed and what the surgery entails.
        (2) Allow sufficient time for expressions of anxieties and concerns.
    b. Surgical procedures.
        (1) *Embolectomy.* An arteriotomy is made over the involved artery. A balloon-tipped catheter is then introduced into the artery and pushed through the embolus. The balloon is then inflated and the catheter is gently pulled, removing the embolus with the inflated balloon.
        (2) *Endarterectomy.* This procedure increases arterial blood flow by the removal of the arterial obstruction and the intima and media of the involved area of the artery.
        (3) *Combined endarterectomy and bypass grafts.* After an endarterectomy is done, a bypass graft made of the client's own saphenous vein or a dacron graft is anastomosed above and

below the obstructed artery. The saphenous vein bypass graft is usually used for the femoropoliteal obstruction, in which case the vein is turned the opposite way, and the dacron graft is used for the aortoiliac obstruction.

(4) *Amputation*. This procedure is needed when irrerversible gangrenous changes occur. (See Chapter 27, The Musculoskeletal System.)

c. Postoperative interventions for the above procedures (except amputations).
   (1) Palpate peripheral pulses.
   (2) Check for changes in skin color and temperature and for any signs of further occlusion (thrombosis at the area of anastomosis).
   (3) Check the vital signs.
   (4) Assess urine output, as the blood flow along the renal arteries may have been interrupted during aortic clamping.
   (5) Report if hypotension develops, for its presence enhances thrombus formation from the stasis of blood.
   (6) Check for hemorrhage at the sites of anastomosis. Instruct the client to avoid flexing the extremity with the bypass graft.
   (7) Use heparin intravenously to prevent clot formation.
   (8) Use antibiotics and carefully handle surgical dressings and wounds to prevent infections.

EVALUATION

Outcome Criteria

1. Pain in extremity ceases.
2. Anxiety decreases as condition improves.
3. Client can move extremities without experiencing pain.
4. Skin breakdown is healed, if ulcerations were present.
5. Extremity is normal in color, sensation, and temperature.
6. Amputation is not necessary.

Complications

Marked necrosis or gangrene necessitating an amputation (see Chapter 27, The Musculoskeletal System).

Reevaluation and Follow-up

1. Check pulses in extremities to evaluate status of circulation.
2. Correct sources of emboli, such as valvular heart disease with surgery, atrial fibrillation with drug therapy or cardioversion, and congestive heart failure with drug therapy.
3. Evaluate the client's tolerance for physical activity.
4. Provide counsel on preventive measures, such as stopping cigarette smoking and avoiding other risk factors.
5. Evaluate client's compliance with changes in lifestyle. Reinforce educational program.

THROMBOANGIITIS OBLITERANS (BUERGER'S DISEASE)

DESCRIPTION

This is a disease characterized by inflammation of the walls of blood vessels with thrombus formation, fibrous thickening and scarring, and eventual occlusion. Although superficial veins may be involved early in the disease, small- and medium-sized arteries are primarily involved. The feet are usually affected most often, but vascular changes may also occur in the hands and eventually throughout the body. The outcome of acute attacks depends on the extent of area deprived of normal blood supply and the available collateral circulation.

PREVENTION

Health Promotion

1. Avoidance of cigarette smoking.
2. Prevention of exposure of extremities to cold temperatures by using warm clothing or by moving to a warm climate.
3. Avoidance of constricting garments.
4. Prevention of mechanical, chemical, or thermal injuries to the feet.
5. Prevention of infection by proper care of the feet (e.g., cutting nails).

Population at Risk

1. Men between 20 and 40 years of age.
2. Cigarette smokers.
3. Incidence is highest among those with Jewish ancestry.

Screening

There are no available screening tests.

ASSESSMENT

Health History

1. Intermittent claudication of the instep may be the first symptom noticed by the client. This is pain that is aggravated by exercise and relieved by rest. This pain pattern is increased by emotional disturbances, smoking, or cold temperature.
2. The feet initially become cold, cyanotic, and numb when exposed to low temperatures; later, they become hot and produce a tingling sensation.

Physical Assessment

1. Extremities are pale when elevated above the heart level and red when dependent.
2. Arterial pulses in the involved extremities diminish as the disease progresses.
3. Ulceration and gangrene are frequent complications.
4. Edema is common in advanced cases.

Diagnostic Tests

1. Doppler ultrasonography shows diminished circulation in the peripheral vessels.
2. Arteriography (injection of a dye followed by x-rays) locates lesions.

NURSING DIAGNOSES: ACTUAL OR POTENTIAL

1. Discomfort: due to circulatory changes.
2. Knowledge deficit: regarding risk factors and methods of management.
3. Anxiety: due to fears of outcomes.
4. Impaired skin integrity: secondary to decreased blood circulation.

EXPECTED OUTCOMES

1. Circulation to the extremity will improve, as evidenced by:
   a. Decreased pain, numbness, tingling.
   b. Improved skin color of the extremity.
   c. Palpation of peripheral pulses.
2. Client will cease cigarette smoking.
3. Compliance will be evidenced by the client's demonstrating proper care of the feet.
4. Anxiety will lessen.
5. Skin ulceration and gangrene will be prevented.

INTERVENTIONS

1. Teach the client to stop cigarette smoking in any form, for it causes constriction of blood vessels.
2. Teach client to take proper care of feet by using warm clothing, by having properly fitting shoes, avoiding cold or overheating from appliances, and by avoiding constricting clothing (garters).
3. Provide psychological support for anxieties and concerns over lifestyle changes and their effect on the client and family.
4. Give vasodilator drug therapy as ordered.
5. Counsel the client concerning reduction of stress.
6. Teach the client to do Buerger-Allen exercises to alternately fill and empty blood vessels to promote circulation.
   a. Client lies flat.
   b. Legs are raised above level of the heart for $1\frac{1}{2}$–3 min until blanching occurs.
   c. Legs are lowered below the level of the heart. Feet are exercised for 3 min until skin color is pink.
   d. Client lies flat for 5 min with legs covered.
   e. Client repeats five times. Entire set is done three times a day.

EVALUATION

Outcome Criteria

1. Pain in the extremity decreases.
2. Skin color of extremity is normal.
3. Peripheral pulses are palpable.
4. Cigarette smoking ceases.
5. Client takes proper care of the feet.
6. Anxiety lessens.

Complications

ULCERATION AND GANGRENE OF THE LEG

Assessment

1. Ulceration and gangrene usually first occur at terminal digits in one extremity at a time. They may occur spontaneously or from trauma.
2. Edema of the legs usually accompanies these skin changes.

Revised Outcomes

1. Circulation will increase by vasodilation of extremity blood vessels.
2. Ulcerated and gangrenous areas will be removed if necessary.

Interventions

1. Sympathetic block or lumbar sympathectomy to produce vasodilation.
2. Amputation if necessary. (See Chapter 27, The Musculoskeletal System, for preoperative and postoperative care.)

Reevaluation and Follow-up

1. Check that smoking has ceased completely.
2. Evaluate the client's compliance with the care of the feet.
3. Evaluate the effect of Buerger's exercises on circulation of the leg.
4. Assess the symptoms: pain, numbness, tingling, burning sensations in leg.
5. Reevaluate the drug therapy (vasodilators).
6. Reevaluate client's lifestyle and suggest adaptations where necessary.
7. Reinforce the education of the client and family.

RAYNAUD'S DISEASE

DESCRIPTION

Raynaud's disease is a peripheral vascular disorder of the extremities, usually the hands, of unknown cause. It is characterized by paroxysmal spasm of the arteries brought on by exposure to cold temperatures or by emotional stress. Pallor and cyanosis occur during the spasm followed by rubor from vasodilation. It is thought that there is abnormal sympathetic innervation or hypersusceptibility to certain stimuli as possible causes. Vasospasms in the arterial wall lead to occlusion of the circulation, atrophy, and possibly gangrene of the tips of the digits.

PREVENTION

Health Promotion

1. Avoidance of exposure to cold temperatures.
2. Avoidance of smoking.
3. Wearing warm clothing.

Population at Risk

1. Women between 16 and 40 years of age.
2. Persons who smoke cigarettes.
3. Persons who live in cold climates.

Screening

There are no screening tests. Symptoms are the main reason for seeking help.

ASSESSMENT

Health History

1. The client may have an early age of onset when only the distal portion of one or more digits are involved. Later, all digits become involved.
2. Cold temperature or emotional factors trigger episodes of arterial spasm.
3. Other family members may have a peripheral vascular disease.

Physical Assessment

1. During a severe spasm of a few minutes, the color of the skin appears white (pale), then blue (cyanotic), then hyperemic (red).
2. Both hands are involved (bilateral involvement).
3. Radial and ulnar pulses are palpable and normal.
4. Skin of the hands appears white, smooth, taut, shiny; nail deformity and loss of hair may eventually occur.
5. Later in the course of the disease, scars from healed ulcerations are noted along with absence of radial or ulnar pulses.
6. Repeated attacks of vasospasm may progress to ulceration and gangrene in only 1 percent of persons with the disease.
7. Anxiety of the client increases as the spasms increase.

Diagnostic Tests

There are no specific diagnostic tests. Diagnosis is made according to clinical criteria of:

1. Skin color changes induced by cold or stress.
2. Bilateral involvement.
3. Absence of gangrene or, if present, minimal cutaneous gangrene.
4. Normal arterial pulses.
5. History of symptoms for longer than 2 years.

NURSING DIAGNOSES: ACTUAL OR POTENTIAL

1. Discomfort: due to impaired circulation to both hands.
2. Anxiety: secondary to the symptoms.
3. Alteration in lifestyle: due to limitations caused by the disease.

EXPECTED OUTCOMES

1. Episodes of vasospasm will decrease.
2. Anxiety will lessen.

3. Client will adapt to changes in lifestyle required by treatment.

INTERVENTIONS

1. Instruct the client to:
   a. Avoid exposure to cold temperatures.
   b. Wear warm clothing and warm gloves when going out in cold weather.
   c. Avoid defrosting refrigerator and use gloves when handling frozen food from freezer.
   d. Avoid exposure of hands to water and to detergents, which lead to drying and fissuring of the skin. Use an emollient to the hands.
   e. Avoid injury of the fingers by careful handling of sharp objects.
   f. Avoid smoking in any form.
   g. Consider moving from cold to warm climate.
2. Reassure the client that the disease is benign and will not lead to amputation. Allow the client to express anxieties and concerns.
3. Vasodilator drugs may be helpful: phenoxybenzamine hydrochloride (Dibenzyline), cyclandelate (Cyclospasmol), or reserpine.
4. Surgery. A sympathectomy is helpful for the client who has progressed to having trophic changes in the fingers.
5. Assist the client in controlling emotional factors that bring on episodes of vasospasm.

EVALUATION

Outcome Criteria

1. Frequency of episodes of vasospasms has decreased.
2. Anxiety is lessened.
3. Client shows compliance by changing lifestyle, including:
   a. Protecting hands from cold temperatures by wearing gloves and avoiding handling cold objects.
   b. Ceasing smoking in any form.
   c. Taking prescribed vasodilators.
   d. Controlling emotions.

Complications

TROPHIC ULCERATIONS OF DIGITS OF THE HANDS

Assessment

Open sores at the tips of digits.

Revised Outcomes

Infection will be prevented.

Interventions

Continue with above interventions with special emphasis on keeping the involved digits clean in order to avoid infections.

Reevaluation and Follow-up

1. Provide continuous reassurance.
2. Evaluate condition of tips of fingers for ulcerations.
3. Evaluate the relation of episodes to precipitating factors. Reinforce education regarding the effect of cold temperatures on the arteries in the hands and controlling emotional factors.
4. Reinforce instruction regarding avoidance of trauma to the hands by careful handling of sharp objects.

DEGENERATIVE DISORDERS

VARICOSE VEINS

DESCRIPTION

Varicose veins are dilated, tortuous, elongated, superficial veins caused by incompetent valves. The greater and lesser saphenous veins and their branches are most commonly affected.

Because of the incompetent valves, there is incomplete emptying of the veins because of backward pressure on these veins from the effect of gravity when a person is in an upright position. As the blood becomes stagnant in these veins, thrombosis results. As the back pressure further increases in the veins, there is extravasation of red blood cells through the capillary walls into surrounding tissues. When these red blood cells disintegrate, they produce a characteristic brown pigmentation (hemosiderin) to the skin. In addition, chronic edema of the subcutaneous tissue leads to inflammation, fibrosis, and atrophy. Finally, the cells die and ulceration of the skin occurs (see Figure 30-17).

PREVENTION

Health Promotion

1. Avoidance of prolonged standing or sitting.
2. Avoidance of crossing legs at the thigh.

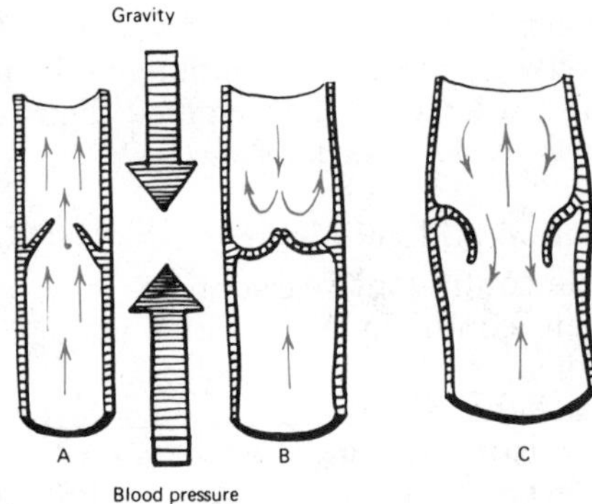

Figure 30-17 Competent and incompetent valves in lower extremity veins. (*a*) Competent valve in open position; (*b*) competent valve in closed position, preventing backflow of blood; (*c*) incompetent valve allowing backflow of blood from the effect of gravity. (Brunner, L., and Suddarth, D.: *Textbook of Medical-Surgical Nursing*, 4th ed., Lippincott, Philadelphia, 1980, p. 645. Used by permission of the publisher.)

3. Avoidance of elevating the bed under the knees.
4. Avoidance of wearing constricting clothes such as round garters.
5. Use of elastic support hose.
6. Elevation of lower extremities to promote venous return.

Population at Risk

1. Persons, generally over 30, with family history of varicosities.
2. Persons in occupations requiring prolonged standing.
3. Persons who are obese.
4. Persons with thrombophlebitis.
5. Pregnant women with a family history of varicosities.

Screening

Trendelenburg test (see Diagnostic Tests below).

ASSESSMENT

Health History

1. Aching in the legs usually occurs after a period of standing and is relieved by elevation of the legs.
2. Edema of the lower leg appears during the course of the day and becomes aggravated by prolonged standing. Because of this edema, the person senses a heaviness due to fluid accumulation.
3. There may be complaints of night cramps in the calves of the legs and the feet due to contractions of muscles in the leg.
4. Varicose veins may be secondary to thrombophlebitis of the deep veins.
5. Familial history of venous diseases may be present.
6. Complaints of diffuse dull aches, muscle cramps, and fatigability of muscles in lower extremities that are relieved by elevating the legs.

Physical Assessment

1. Dilated, tortuous veins while legs are dependent. The sclerosed valves may appear as nodular protrusions.
2. Brownish pigmentation of the lower leg (from extravasation of RBCs into tissues), dryness, scaling, and some pruritis over prominent varices, particularly at the ankle.
3. Skin infections over the varices are likely to occur.
4. Ulcerations occur with long-standing varicose veins. They are usually shallow but can possibly erode veins or even arteries causing hemorrhage.
5. Varicosities usually occur in both legs, unless they are secondary to other disease mechanisms.
6. Discomfort in the legs is increased in hot weather or when there is a change from low to a high altitude.

Diagnostic Tests

1. Venous pressure changes during walking. Normally, there is a marked decrease in the saphenous vein pressure with exercise, for muscular action increases the flow of blood. Those clients with varicose veins have less of a decrease in venous pressure during exercise because of the reflux of blood down the veins from loss of elasticity and valvular function.
2. Trendelenburg's test will demonstrate the backward flow of blood through the incompetent valves into the saphenous veins. The client lies down and elevates the involved leg until the superficial veins collapse. Then a tourniquet is applied high on the leg to occlude the superficial veins. The client then stands and the tourniquet is taken off. If the

valves are incompetent, the veins distend quickly because of the backflow of blood.

3. Phlebography: angiographic contrast medium is injected into the saphenous veins followed by x-rays before and after the client stands. This permits visualization of the valves.

NURSING DIAGNOSES: ACTUAL OR POTENTIAL

1. Alteration in body image: secondary to altered appearance of legs.
2. Discomfort: due to circulatory changes.
3. Potential skin breakdown.

EXPECTED OUTCOMES

1. Circulation of blood in veins of lower leg will be promoted within 2 weeks, as evidenced by:
   a. Improved appearance of the legs.
   b. Increased comfort.
   c. Increased ability to stand.
   d. Absence of skin breakdown and infection.
2. Client will learn proper care of the legs and feet.

INTERVENTIONS

1. Educate the client about:
   a. Proper use of elastic support hose to decrease venous pooling in veins. Support hose should be individually prescribed for proper fit.
   b. Avoidance of restricting clothing to the legs.
   c. Proper care of the legs and feet (avoidance of trauma).
   d. Using bland, oily lotions to prevent scaling and dryness.
2. Use antigravity measures to increase blood flow from the veins in lower legs to the heart.
   a. Teach the client to elevate the legs at regular 2- to 3-h intervals throughout the day.
   b. Have client sleep with the foot of the bed elevated 6 in by placing blocks under the foot of the bed. If pillows are used for elevating the leg, place them so that they support the entire length of the extremity to prevent compression under the knee.
   c. Instruct client to avoid periods of prolonged standing.
   d. Encourage an obese client to reduce weight.
   e. Advise walking, which promotes circulation by muscle contraction of leg muscles around the veins.
3. Measure and record the circumference of the affected leg daily and compare with the normal leg if the problem is unilateral.
4. Surgical intervention. *Ligation* and *stripping of veins*. The great saphenous vein is ligated at the groin and is stripped from groin to ankle by threading a wire into the vein and pulling the vein with the wire.

   Postoperative interventions:
   a. Elevate the affected leg.
   b. Relieve pain with an analgesic.
   c. Frequently check circulation in toes (color and temperature) and observe for bleeding.
   d. Rewrap elastic bandages at least once a shift, wrapping from toe to thigh with leg elevated.
   e. Watch for signs of complications: sensory loss (which could indicate nerve damage), calf pain (thrombophlebitis), and fever (infection).

EVALUATION

Outcome Criteria

1. Appearance of the legs has improved.
2. Comfort in legs has increased and the client can stand for longer periods.
3. There is no further skin breakdown or infection.

Complications

VARICOSE ULCERS

Assessment

1. Skin becomes pigmented and edematous.
2. Pruritis and discomfort at the area are noted.
3. Ulcers develop spontaneously or from small bruises.

Revised Outcomes

1. The ulcer will heal.
2. Circulation will be adequate.

Interventions

1. Put client on bed rest with the feet elevated above the level of the heart.
2. Apply warm compresses to eliminate infection, stimulate granulation of tissue, and relieve discomfort.
3. Protect the area from trauma and infection.

4. Administer antibiotics for specific organisms.
5. After a few days, apply an Elastoplast or Unna's paste boot to allow ambulation.
6. If arterial supply is adequate and grannulation has started, skin grafts applied to the ulcer help healing.

Reevaluation and Follow-up

1. Assess the legs for edema, pigmentation of skin, skin breakdown, and pruritis.
2. Evaluate how quickly the veins fill and empty by using the retrograde filling test.
3. Relieve anxiety if progress seems slow to client.
4. Evaluate client's compliance with care of legs and feet.

ANEURYSMS

DESCRIPTION

An aneurysm is dilatation of an artery, most often caused by arteriosclerosis. Other causes are syphilis, trauma, or local infection. The main problem is weakness of the arterial wall, causing distention at the weakened point. A wall of scar tissue develops around the aneurysm, but it is never sufficient or rapid enough to prevent a slowly growing, pulsating tumor filled with blood, which has a propensity to thrombose and become emboli if broken loose.

The various types and most common locations of aneurysms are:

1. *Fusiform* (spindle-shaped dilatation of a segment of an artery). This type is found most often in the aorta, especially the abdominal aorta, and in the iliac arteries.
2. *Saccular* (outpouching from one side of an artery due to thinning of the media). Saccular aneurysms are found most often in the abdominal aorta and popliteal arteries; they may also occur in the femoral artery.
3. *Dissecting* (splitting the arterial wall by blood that is forced between the layers because of a tear or weakness in the intima). This type is found most often in the thoracic aorta with other arteries being involved by its extension into their walls. As dissection progresses, branch vessels become obliterated, thus cutting off arterial circulation to tissues normally supplied by them (see Figure 30-18).

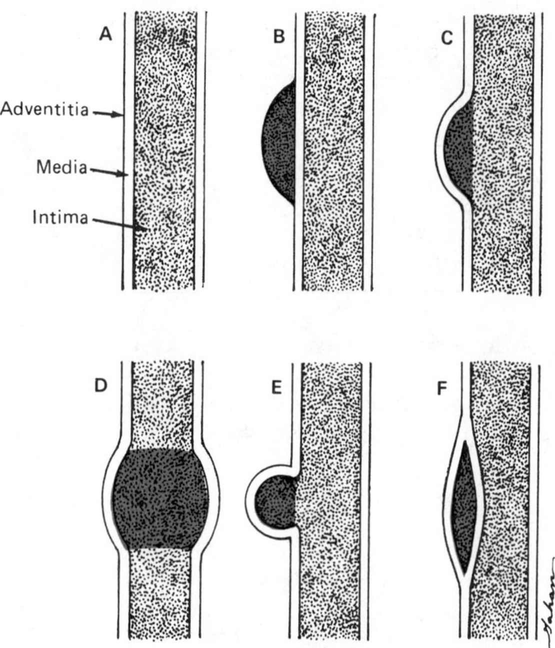

Figure 30-18 Arterial aneurysms. (*a*) Normal artery. (*b*) False aneurysm, actually a pulsating hematoma. The clot and connective tissue are outside the arterial wall. (*c*) True aneurysm. One, two, or all three layers may be involved. (*d*) Fusiform aneurysm, a symmetrical spindle-shaped expansion of entire circumference of involved vessel. (*e*) Saccular aneurysm, a bulbous protrusion of one side of the arterial wall. (*f*) Dissecting aneurysm, usually a hematoma that splits the layers of the arterial wall. (Brunner, L., and Suddarth, D.: *Textbook of Medical-Surgical Nursing*, 4th ed. Lippincott, Philadelphia, 1980, p. 623. Used by permission of the publisher.)

PREVENTION

Health Promotion

1. Control of hypertension, if it exists, for the increased pressure within arteries increases the chance of rupture.
2. Prevention of the development of arteriosclerosis by dietary control and ceasing cigarette smoking.

Population at Risk

1. Males over age 50.
2. Persons with hypertension, because of increased pressure against the arterial wall.

Screening

1. Compare blood pressure of upper and lower extremities.

ASSESSMENT

Health History

1. Hypertension.
2. Trauma.
3. Syphilis.
4. Cigarette smoking.
5. Other cardiovascular diseases.

Physical Assessment

1. Aneurysm of the thoracic aorta.
   a. May be asymptomatic unless large in size.
   b. Pain is the most prominent pressure symptom. It is characterized as being constant and boring due to erosion of a vertebra or rib by pressure of the pulsating sac. If the aneurysm is dissecting, there is a sudden onset of severe, persistent pain described as "tearing" or "ripping." This pain begins in the anterior thorax, usually, but may be between or below the scapulae. If sudden collapse or syncope occurs, pain may be absent.
   c. Dyspnea as the result of the pressure of the sac against the trachea, bronchus, or lung tissue.
   d. Paroxysmal cough that has a brassy quality.
   e. Hoarseness or complete aphonia due to pressure of the aneurysm against the left recurrent laryngeal nerve.
   f. Dyspnea, due to pressure on the esophagus.
   g. Anxiety.
2. Aneurysm of the abdominal aorta.
   a. Abdominal pain is the most common symptom. This pain may be persistent or intermittent and is sensed in the middle or lower abdomen to the left of the midline.
   b. Low back pain, usually due to rupture, is felt.
   c. Abdominal pulsating mass is palpated.
   d. Systolic blood pressure in the legs is abnormally low in comparison with the arms in most clients (opposite from normal).
   e. On auscultation, a systolic bruit is heard over the aneurysm.
   f. Anxiety.

Diagnostic Tests

1. Chest x-ray study for thoracic aneurysms.
2. ECG helps differentiate aneurysm from myocardial infarction.
3. Echocardiography may help identify dissecting aneurysm of the aortic root.
4. Aortography, the most definite test, shows the location of the aneurysm by injecting a dye and visualizing the x-rays.

NURSING DIAGNOSES: ACTUAL OR POTENTIAL

1. Pain: due to circulatory changes.
2. Anxiety: due to progress of disease.

EXPECTED OUTCOMES

1. Pain will cease.
2. Anxiety will lessen.
3. Symptoms related to pressure of the aneurysm will subside.

INTERVENTIONS

1. Surgery is indicated. Resection of the aneurysm and replacement of the segment with a prosthetic graft or an antogenous saphenous vein graft, doing end-to-end anastomosis. Extracorporeal circulation with a pump oxygenator is used when the aneurysm is in the ascending aorta.
2. Postoperative interventions.
   a. Monitor blood pressure, pulse rate, pulmonary capillary wedge pressure, central venous pressure, and level of consciousness.
   b. Assess pain, respirations, and carotid, radial, and femoral pulses.
   c. Observe and record type and amount of chest tube drainage.
   d. Assess heart and lung sounds.
   e. Monitor IV therapy.
   f. Watch for signs of infection.
   g. Give antibiotics to prevent infection, if ordered.
   h. Observe for hemorrhage on dressing.
   i. Assist with range-of-motion exercises of legs to prevent venous stasis during prolonged bed rest.
   j. After stabilization, encourage and assist the client in turning, coughing, and deep breathing.

k. Before client's discharge, ensure compliance with therapy by explaining the need to continue drug therapy (antihypertensive drugs) and the expected side effects. Teach the client how to monitor blood pressure.
l. Throughout client's hospitalization, offer psychological support to the client and family. Answer questions honestly and provide reassurance.

EVALUATION

Outcome Criteria

1. Pain ceases.
2. Symptoms due to pressure of aneurysm on other organs cease (dyspnea, cough, hoarseness).
3. Anxiety lessens.
4. Rupture does not occur.

Complications

RUPTURE OF THE ANEURYSM

Assessment

1. Sudden, severe pain with a tearing or ripping sensation in thorax or anterior chest.
2. Symptoms of shock from blood loss: low BP, weak thready pulse, increased respiratory rate.
3. Melena if rupture is into the retroperitoneal duodenum.

Revised Outcomes

1. Bleeding will cease.
2. Pain will cease.
3. Caridac output will be restored and symptoms of shock will cease.

Interventions

Immediate surgery.

Reevaluation and Follow-up

1. After discharge blood pressure measurements should be done by the client or a member of the family regularly and reported to physician.
2. Follow-up visits to evaluate the presence of pain, the status of peripheral pulses, and the presence of murmurs in the aortic area.
3. Comparison of follow-up x-ray studies with previous studies.
4. Check that cigarette smoking has ceased.
5. Provide psychological support to the client and family.

REFERENCES

Beland, I., and Passos, J.: *Clinical Nursing: Pathophysiological and Psychosocial Approaches*, Macmillan, New York, 1981, p. 783.

Fitzmaurice, J.: *Rheumatic Heart Disease and Mitral Valve Disease*, Appleton-Century-Crofts, New York, 1980, p. 47.

Hurst, J. W., Logue, R. B., Schlant, R., and Wenger, N. (eds.): *The Heart*, 4th ed., McGraw-Hill, New York, 1978, p. 1694.

Jones, D. A., Dunbar, C. F., Jirovec, M. M.: *Medical-Surgical Nursing: A Conceptual Approach*, McGraw-Hill, New York, 1978, p. 1015.

Luckmann, J., and Sorensen, K.: *Medical-Surgical Nursing: A Psychophysiologic Approach*, 2d ed., Saunders, Philadelphia, 1980, pp. 1110–1111.

Nurses Reference Library: *Diseases*, Nursing '81 Books, Intermed Communications, Inc., Horsham, Pa., 1981, p. 480.

Rutherford, R. (ed): *Vascular Surgery*, Saunders, 1977, p. 426.

BIBLIOGRAPHY

The American Heart Association Heartbook, Dutton, New York, 1980. An up-to-date reference on the advances in diagnosis and treatment of cardiovascular disease designed for educating the public and professionals.

Beland, I. L., and Passos, J. Y.: *Clinical Nursing: Pathophysiological and Psychosocial Approaches*, 4th ed., Macmillan, New York, 1981. A comprehensive text on clinical nursing designed for the nursing student. It uses a conceptual approach to the care of clients with a wide variety of disorders.

"Cardiac Arrhythmias—The Indiana University School of Medicine Symposium—Part II," *Heart and Lung*, **10**:629–650, July–August 1981. This is a series of excellent articles on atrioventricular dissociation, supraventricular arrhythmias, and arrhythmias during exercise. Each article includes the hemodynamic effects and treatment of arrhythmias.

Comoss, P. E., Burke, A., and Swails, S.: *Cardiac Rehabilitation: A Comprehensive Nursing Approach*, Lippincott, Philadelphia, 1979. A comprehensive text on the professional nurse's role in cardiac rehabilitation. Each unit of the text covers a phase of cardiac rehabilitation.

Cromwell, R., Butterford, E., Brayfield, F., and Curry, J.: *Acute Myocardial Infarction: Reaction and Recovery*, Mosby, St. Louis, 1977. A book written for health professionals about the findings of a study on stress, personality, and nursing care factors involved in the recovery from acute myocardial infarction.

Czerwinski, B.: *Manual of Patient Education for Cardiopulmonary Dysfunctions*, Mosby, St. Louis, 1980. A practical approach to client education through the use of diagrams and teaching tools.

Dawber, T.: *The Framingham Study*, Harvard University Press, Cambridge, Mass. 1980. The report of the findings from the Framingham Study encompassing 24 years and adding significant information regarding data about cardiac risk factors.

Fardy, P., et al.: *Cardiac Rehabilitation: Implications for the Nurse and other Allied Health Professionals*, Mosby, St. Louis, 1980. A practical, multidisciplinary look at cardiac rehabilitation programs. Included are the roles of nurses and other health professionals, concepts in exercise programming, psychosocial management of the client and family, and administrative aspects.

Finnerty, F.: "Treatment of Hypertensive Emergencies," *Heart and Lung*, **10**:275–284, March–April 1981. A comparison of rapid-acting antihypertensive drugs used in hypertensive crisis and a description of therapies for malignant hypertension, toxemia of pregnancy, acute pulmonary edema, dissecting aortic aneurysm, and stroke.

Goldberger, E., and Wheat, M.,: *Treatment of Cardiac Emergencies*, Mosby, St. Louis, 1977. A helpful reference on cardiac emergencies, divided into three sections: description of cardiac emergency syndromes, discussion of equipment and apparatus used in cardiac emergencies, and description of drug therapy.

Hurst, J. W., Schlant, R., and Wenger, N.: *The Heart*, 4th ed., McGraw-Hill, New York, 1978. A complete, thorough text on medical aspects of the disorders of the heart, arteries, and veins. An excellent resource for etiology, symptoms, and treatment.

Jackle, M., and Halligan, M.: *Cardiovascular Problems: A Critical Care Nursing Focus*, Robert J. Brady Co., Bowie, Md., 1980. An excellent teaching guide for nurses in making appropriate decisions in the care of acutely ill clients with cardiovascular problems. It contains clear diagrams and questions and answers to reinforce learning.

Jones, D. A., Dunbar, C. F., Jirovec, M. M.: *Medical-Surgical Nursing: A Conceptual Approach*, 2d ed., McGraw-Hill, New York, 1982. An excellent resource for nursing, using a conceptual approach for a wide range of diseases. The nursing care is described at four levels with emphasis on the nursing assessment and intervention for each.

Luckmann, J., and Sorensen, K.: *Medical-Surgical Nursing: A Psychophysiologic Approach.*, 2d ed., Saunders, Philadelphia, 1980. This general nursing text devotes nine chapters to the cardiovascular system. It is an excellent resource for nurses at all levels.

McGurn, W.: *People with Cardiac Problems: Nursing Concepts*, Lippincott, Philadelphia, 1981. This book presents a synthesis of concepts drawn from nursing and other sciences related to the care of people with cardiac problems. It is an excellent resource for nurses caring for the acutely or chronically ill cardiac client.

Meltzer, L., Pinneo, R., and Kitchell, J. R.: *Intensive Coronary Care*, 3d ed., Robert J. Brady Co., Bowie, Md., 1977. A basic text for nurses working in coronary care units or with coronary clients on general medical divisions. Its focus is the nursing care related to acute myocardial infarction and its complications.

Nurses Reference Library: *Diseases*, Nursing '81 Books, Intermed Communications, Inc., Horsham, Pa., 1981. A handy reference covering a broad range of disorders. The section on cardiovascular diseases gives a succinct description of the conditions and implications for nursing care.

Pinneo, R.: *Congestive Heart Failure*, Unit I of Series 1: *Myocardial Infarction*, Appleton-Century-Crofts, East Norwalk, Ct., 1978. A practical book that briefly describes the pathogenesis, compensatory mechanisms, clinical assessments, and treatments of congestive heart failure.

Tilkian, A., and Conover, M.: *Understanding Heart Sounds and Murmurs*, Saunders, Philadelphia, 1979. A good reference for understanding heart sounds and murmurs through a discussion of their hemodynamic aspects. Each heart sound is illustrated with a phonocardiogram correlated with the electrocardiogram.

Wenger, N., Hurst, J. W., and McIntyre, M.: *Cardiology for Nurses*, McGraw-Hill, New York, 1980. A text written for nurses working primarily with cardiac clients. The focus is on the nurse's role in obtaining a data base, preparing clients for diagnostic tests, assessing clients and planning and implementing interventions.

31

The Respiratory System

Dorothy L. Sexton and Mary E. Eddy

Adequate and effective oxygenation is contingent upon an intact respiratory system. When physiological changes occur, the actions of the respiratory structures are diminished. Such problems as inflammation, infection, obstruction, cellular proliferation, and trauma can interfere with gas exchange and affect the body as a whole.

This chapter discusses common health problems that can affect respiration and oxygen–carbon dioxide exchange. Each problem is explored in terms of its overall impact on the persons so afflicted. Client care is discussed using the vehicle of the standards of practice in order to develop a realistic plan of care.

ABNORMAL CELLULAR GROWTH

CANCER OF THE LUNG

DESCRIPTION

A *malignant neoplasm* is an abnormal growth of new tissue that does not serve a useful purpose to the body and may metastasize to other tissues. Pulmonary neoplasms may be primary or metastatic lesions. The primary neoplasms include (1) *squamous cell* (*epidermoid*) *carcinoma*, which occurs predominantly in males and is almost always associated with cigarette smoking; (2) *undifferentiated* (*anaplastic*) *carcinoma* (includes oat cell, round cell, large cell), which is more common in males and younger age groups and tends to metastasize early; (3) *adenocarcinoma*, which is associated with peripheral lesions and tends to remain clinically silent until distant metastases have occurred; and (4) *bronchioalveolar cell* (*alveolar cell*) *carcinoma*, which is a less common tumor type characterized by a diffuse lesion and thought by some to be a variety of adenocarcinoma.

Secondary pulmonary neoplasms metastasize from other malignant tumors in body sites such as the breast, prostate, kidney, gastrointestinal tract, and bone. (Refer to Table 31-1.)

While the exact cause is not known, data from epidemiological and animal exposure studies provide evidence that carcinogenic substances inhaled over a long period of time are a major causative factor. Agents associated with the development of primary lung carcinoma are cigarette smoke, asbestos, and uranium.

The incidence of lung cancer is reflected in several epidemiological studies that have confirmed that a relationship exists between heavy cigarette smoking and lung cancer. In fact, statistical analyses have demonstrated a direct correlation between the number of cigarettes a person smokes and risk of that person's developing lung cancer. Other factors such as exposure to asbestos, iron oxide, ionizing radiation, and air pollution have been implicated in the development of primary lung cancer. Statistical analyses point out that if a person is exposed to an in-

TABLE 31-1 DEFINITIONS FOR STAGING BRONCHOGENIC CARCINOMA

TO	No evidence of primary tumor.
TX	Tumor proven by the presence of malignant cells in bronchopulmonary secretions but not visualized roentgenographically or bronchoscopically, or any tumor that cannot be assessed.
TIS	Carcinoma in situ.
T1	A tumor that is 3.0 cm or less in greatest diameter, surrounded by lung or visceral pleura, and without evidence of invasion proximal to a lobar bronchus at bronchoscopy.
T2	A tumor more than 3.0 cm in greatest diameter, or a tumor of any size that either invades the visceral pleura or which has associated atelectasis or obstructive pneumonitis extending to the hilar region. At bronchoscopy, the proximal extent of demonstrable tumor must be within a lobar bronchus or at least 2.0 cm distal to the carina. Any associated atelectasis or obstructive pneumonitis must involve less than an entire lung, and there must be no pleural effusion.
T3	A tumor of any size with direct extension into an adjacent structure such as the parietal pleura, the chest wall, the diaphragm, or the mediastinum and its contents; or a tumor demonstrable bronchoscopically to involve a main bronchus less than 2.0 cm distal to the carina; or any tumor associated with atelectasis or obstructive pneumonitis of an entire lung or pleural effusion.
NO	No demonstrable metastasis to regional lymph nodes.
N1	Metastasis to lymph nodes in the peribronchial or the ipsilateral hilar region, or both, including direct extension.
N2	Metastasis to lymph nodes in the mediastinum.
MO	No distant metastasis.
M1	Distant metastasis such as in scalene, cervical, or contralateral hilar lymph nodes, brain, bones, liver, or contralateral lung.

Occult Carcinoma	Stage 1	Stage 2	Stage 3
TX NO MO	TIS NO MO T1 NO MO T1 N1 MO T2 NO MO	T2 N1 MO	T3 any N or M N2 any T or M M1 any T or N

SOURCE: Carr, D. T., and Rosenow, E. C.: "Bronchogenic Carcinoma," *Basics of R D*, **5**(5):5, May 1977.

dustrial carcinogen and is a cigarette smoker, his or her chances of developing lung cancer are increased. It is estimated that there will be 117,000 new cases (85,000 in men, 32,000 in women) of lung cancer in 1980 (American Cancer Society).

The prognosis of primary lung cancer is directly related to the specific cell type and the status of the lesion (extension or nonextension) at the time of diagnosis. Primary cancer of the lung is the most common cause of deaths due to cancer in men, and the death rate from primary cancer of the lung in women is increasing steadily. Deaths attributed to lung cancer are projected to be 101,300 (74,800 in men, 26,500 in women) for 1980 (American Cancer Society).

PREVENTION

Health Promotion

1. Abstinence from cigarette smoking.
2. Decreased exposure to side-stream smoke.
3. Decreased exposure to industrial carcinogens and air pollution.
4. Use of respiratory mask and protective cloth-

ing when exposure to agents such as asbestos cannot be prevented.
5. Health assessment for persistent cough or a change in a smoker's cough.

Population at Risk

1. Cigarette smokers (moderate or heavy).
2. Persons who are exposed to agents such as asbestos and uranium over long periods.
3. Persons who have extensive inflammatory or fibrotic lung tissue changes.

Screening

1. Sputum specimen for cytology.
2. Chest x-ray study.

ASSESSMENT

Health History

1. Age: usually occurs during the middle years or later.
2. Sex: the incidence in males is greater (especially for squamous cell and undifferentiated cell types). Recent studies indicate a startling increase in females who smoke.
3. Occupation: description of job activities, for example if there is exposure to agents such as asbestos or uranium.
4. Smoking habits: statistics reveal a high correlation (80 to 90 percent) of lung cancer with cigarette smoking. Data should include:
   a. Number of years individual has smoked.
   b. Number of cigarettes smoked per day.
   c. Whether person inhales smoke.
5. History of cough: duration of cough; time of cough (morning or evening); the amount and frequency of sputum production; and a description of the sputum (e.g., blood-tinged).
6. Lifestyle: areas of potential stress; whether individual lives alone; occupational investment; person's involvement in family; support system.
7. Family history of cancer, especially lung cancer.
8. Present condition of teeth: cancer may cause ulceration and bleeding of gums.
9. Client may complain of chest pain, which may be localized or affected by breathing. It can be mild to severe and referred to other body areas.
10. Client may express fear of cancer or a general sense of anxiety, especially in the presence of such changes as hemoptysis or dyspnea.

Physical Assessment

1. Examination of the chest may be normal or there may be changes, such as dullness on percussion (unilateral or bilateral), increased breath sounds, increased tactile fremitus, and bronchial breath sounds.
2. If there is chest pain, the person may guard the affected side and decrease chest excursion (bilateral). Dyspnea, aggravated by exertion, may be present.
3. Person may have a mild cough or may report a change in smoker's cough.
4. Complaints of hoarseness may be made, associated with involvement of the recurrent laryngeal nerve.
5. Examination of the lower extremities should be made for evidence of thrombophlebitis, which is sometimes associated with an early lung carcinoma.
6. The client's general appearance may reveal significant weight loss and apprehension at initial encounter. A complete physical examination will be required in order to assess the total effects of this problem.
7. Careful palpation of lymph nodes should be done and notation made of other physiological changes that may indicate metastatic spread of the disease.

Diagnostic Tests

1. Chest x-ray films: indicate the presence of a lesion, a mass in the hilar region, or changes such as atelectasis, pneumonitis, pleural effusion, or erosion of the ribs or vertebrae.
2. Sputum for cytology: may reveal malignant cells, depending upon the stage of the lung cancer. Client is asked to cough deeply in order to extract mucus from the lungs. Nebulization is used to facilitate the raising and expectoration of sputum.
3. Fiberoptic bronchoscopy: insertion of a fiberscope through the oral cavity to visualize the bronchus. The flexible nature of the scope allows the examiner to visualize the bronchi. The scope also permits biopsy, regional lung washings, and cytologic brushing of lesions (see Figure 31-1).
4. Scalene node biopsy: excision of node for examination (scalene node located in supraclavicular area).

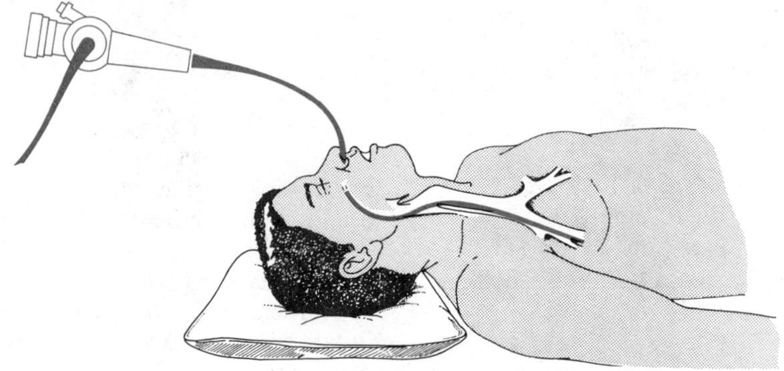

Figure 31-1 The fiberoptic bronchoscope.

5. Mediastinoscopy: insertion of a mediastinoscope (through a skin incision) to view the right and left hilar lymph nodes (the latter are accessible for biopsy). Mediastinoscopy is used routinely to establish a tissue diagnosis. (In most institutions mediastinoscopy has replaced scalene node biopsy.)
6. Pleural biopsy: thoracentesis and needle biopsy of the pleura are frequently performed when pleural effusion is present.
7. When the physical assessment or initial diagnostic procedures suggest that metastases may be present, the following procedures are usually performed:
   a. X-ray films of the skull, EEG, brain scan.
   b. Liver scan, liver biopsy.
   c. Radioisotope bone scan.

NURSING DIAGNOSES: ACTUAL OR POTENTIAL

1. Respiratory dysfunction (tumor within lung tissue): reduction in oxygenation due to obstruction.
2. Alteration in comfort: discomfort secondary to unilateral chest pain.
3. Nutritional alteration deficit: secondary to fatigue/weakness and metabolic changes.
4. Anxiety (moderate to high): secondary to diagnosis, diagnostic procedures, treatment (surgery, radiation, chemotherapy).
5. Alteration in self-concept: due to physical changes that accompany cancer.
6. Alteration in activity level: decreased tolerance secondary to fatigue/weakness.
7. Knowledge deficit: due to current health state and related problems.

EXPECTED OUTCOMES

1. Anxiety level will be reduced, as evidenced by client's ability to cooperate during diagnostic tests and his or her understanding of proposed treatment plan.
2. Client will meet nutritional needs, as evidenced by gradual weight gain (or no further weight loss).
3. Client's activity tolerance will be increased, as demonstrated by the ability to walk about the room and in corridor.
4. Client's self-concept will show improvement, as evidenced by participation in future goal setting.
5. Client will give evidence of compliance in care plan by:
   a. Abstaining from cigarette smoking.
   b. Eating prescribed diet and nutritional supplements.
   c. Performing prescribed exercises.

INTERVENTIONS

1. Help client and family deal with the psychological trauma of cancer diagnosis. Provide support and counseling as needed. Answer questions honestly.
2. Prepare client for diagnostic tests (e.g., sputum for cytology, bronchoscopy, mediastinoscopy).
3. Prepare client for treatment program selected by the health team (e.g., surgery, radiation, chemotherapy).
4. Monitor vital signs; identify changes.
5. Provide oral hygiene frequently, especially if there is an increase in secretions. Half-

strength hydrogen peroxide or sodium bicarbonate with water may be used.

6. Observe for signs of dehydration. Offer fluids on a regular basis in order to maintain hydration.
7. Counsel client regarding the need to abstain from smoking. Help client develop a plan to stop smoking (this may include a smoking clinic or hypnosis).
8. Promote adequate nutrition through diet counseling.
9. Reduce pain by administering analgesia (e.g., narcotic).
10. Help client develop methods to reduce pain. (This may include relaxation exercises and visual imagery.)
11. Alert client and family to additional symptoms that may develop as well as the need for medical evaluation.
12. Teach about:
    a. Coughing and deep-breathing regimen.
    b. Medications: dose and side effects.
    c. Need for proper rest and activity to help maintain natural resistance.
    d. Diet: to maintain nutritional status and weight.
    e. Follow-up schedule and additional symptoms that may develop.

EVALUATION

Outcome Criteria

1. Pain is diminishing, as evidenced by client's increased activity and increased rest/sleep time.
2. Client is taking medications at appropriate times and in correct amounts, as indicated by chart the client is keeping.
3. Client is gaining weight (or is not losing additional weight).
4. Client has abstained from smoking during the past 2 weeks.
5. Client can recall with 85 percent accuracy either verbally or in writing the content presented in teaching sessions.

Complications

1. Respiratory insufficiency (see Complications under *Chronic Bronchitis* later in this chapter).
2. Bronchopneumonia (see the discussion under pneumonia).

LARYNGEAL CANCER

DESCRIPTION

Laryngeal neoplasms may involve the true vocal cords (*intrinsic lesion*) or may extend to the supraglottic or infraglottic areas (*extrinsic lesion*). *Carcinoma in situ* is characteristically confined to the true vocal cord. *Verrucous cancer* (sessile appearance) is a laryngeal lesion that is considered to be histologically benign but is treated as malignant. Approximately 95 percent of laryngeal neoplasms are squamous cell, and the remainder are classified as sarcoma or adenocarcinoma. Metastases to the larynx from other organs rarely occur (refer to Table 31-2).

Although no specific causative agent has been identified, an association has been noted between laryngeal lesions and several factors: heavy cigarette smoking, alcohol consumption, excessive use of voice, exposure to fumes and pollution, and familial history.

Cancer of the larynx typically develops in white males over age 60; however, an increasing number of persons in the 20 to 30 age group are being diagnosed (LeJeune, 1951).

When the lesion develops only on the true vocal cord and proper treatment is instituted, an 85 to 90 percent 5-year survival rate may be expected. This is in part due to the presence of few lymph vessels. If the lesion extends to the extrinsic larynx, the anticipated 5-year survival rate drops to about 70 percent. The prognosis is less favorable when neck metastases are present (DeWeese and Saunders, 1977).

PREVENTION

Health Promotion

1. Abstinence from cigarette smoking.
2. Decreased alcohol intake.
3. Decreased exposure to irritants and noxious fumes.
4. Avoidance of voice abuse.
5. Health assessment for persistent hoarseness of laryngitis.
6. Medical follow-up of clients with leukoplakia and laryngeal polyps.

Population at Risk

1. Cigarette smokers (heavy use).
2. Persons who consume excessive amounts of alcohol.

TABLE 31-2 TNM CATEGORIES FOR CANCER OF THE LARYNX

T	Primary tumor.
TIS	Carcinoma in situ.
Supraglottis	
Both anterior and posterior surfaces of epiglottis (including the tip), aryepiglottic fold, arytenoid, ventricular bands (false cords), ventricular cavities (right and left).	
TIS	Carcinoma in situ.
T1	Tumor confined to site of origin with normal mobility.
T2	Tumor involves adjacent supraglottic site(s) or glottis without fixation.
T3	Tumor limited to larynx with fixation and/or extension to involve postcricoid area, medial wall of pyriform sinus, or pre-epiglottic space.
T4	Massive tumor extending beyond larynx to involve oropharynx, or soft tissues of neck, or destruction of thyroid cartilage.
Glottis	
True vocal cords (right and left), anterior glottic commissure.	
TIS	Carcinoma in situ.
T1	Tumor confined to vocal cord(s) with normal mobility (includes involvement of anterior or posterior commissures).
T2	Supraglottic and/or subglottic extension of tumor with normal or impaired cord mobility.
T3	Tumor confined to larynx with cord fixation.
T4	Massive tumor with thyroid cartilage destruction and/or extension beyond confines of larynx.
Subglottis	
Subglottic region, exclusive of the under surface of true cords.	
TIS	Carcinoma in situ.
T1	Tumor confined to subglottic region.
T2	Tumor extension to vocal cords with normal or impaired cord mobility.
T3	Tumor confined to larynx with cord fixation.
T4	Massive tumor with cartilage destruction or extension beyond confines of larynx.

SOURCE: *Manual for Staging of Cancer, 1978.* American Joint Committee, 55 East Erie St., Chicago.

3. Persons whose jobs involve excessive use of their voice.
4. Persons who have persistent exposure to pollutants and noxious fumes.

Screening

Laryngeal mirror exam.

ASSESSMENT

Health History

1. Health patterns: smoking cigarettes, alcohol intake.
2. Age: tends to occur more in persons in late middle years (age 60) and older.
3. Males (white) are more apt to develop laryngeal cancer.
4. Prolonged period of hoarseness (chronic laryngitis) that does not improve over time (due to the presence of abnormal tissue around the vocal cords). Client should be asked to describe date of onset and accompanying factors, if any.
5. Cough (productive or nonproductive) should be investigated. Duration of cough as well as type and amount of sputum should be evaluated.
6. Sensation of an obstruction (lump) in the throat is commonly described.
7. Pain upon swallowing may be evident in later stages. (Because of the tendency for ulcerations to occur in extrinsic lesions, pain and burning upon drinking hot fluids or orange juice may occur even in early stages.)
8. Metastases may be present and associated with complaints of weight loss, difficulty swallowing, dyspnea, and an odor to the breath.
9. Nutrition: maintenance of adequate nutrition may be a problem and weight loss is not uncommon.

Physical Assessment

1. Head and neck examination may reveal a painless lump.
2. Lymph nodes should be palpated. They may be enlarged, especially if metastases are present.
3. Examination of the larynx will usually reveal the initial lesion.
4. The person is often apprehensive and may fear the diagnosis.
5. If the tumor has interfered with the person's eating habits, weight loss may be apparent.

Diagnostic Tests

1. Indirect laryngoscopy: use of a mirror to examine the larynx.
2. Direct laryngoscopy: visualization of the larynx through a laryngoscope. Many laryngologists routinely use the Zeiss operating microscope with a suspension laryngoscope.
3. Biopsy of lesion in order to analyze the tumor tissue.
4. Laryngogram to define the limits of the neoplasm.
5. Barium esophagogram to define the neoplasm's borders. The person swallows a barium preparation and is then x-rayed.

NURSING DIAGNOSES: ACTUAL OR POTENTIAL

1. Alteration in comfort: secondary to hoarseness, throat pain, cough, dysphagia.
2. Respiratory dysfunction: decreased oxygenation due to obstruction.
3. Impaired communication process: ineffective communication secondary to the lesion on vocal cords.
4. Potential nutritional alteration (decrease): secondary to dysphagia and/or decreased food and fluid intake.
5. Alteration in self-concept: changes in body image secondary to physical changes from surgery.
6. Anxiety: secondary to anticipation of loss of voice and the disfigurement caused by surgery.

EXPECTED OUTCOMES

1. Client and family will be able to deal with the psychological impact of the diagnosis of cancer.
2. Discomfort localized at lesion will be alleviated.
3. Support will be provided before and during diagnostic procedures.
4. Client will be prepared for the prescribed treatment (e.g., radiation therapy, surgery).
5. Infection will be prevented. Client and family will maintain medical asepsis at all times.
6. Client will meet hydration and nutritional needs by demonstrating gradual weight gain (or no further weight loss).
7. Client and family will understand information taught in teaching sessions, as evidenced by 85 percent accuracy during performance

of procedures:
   a. Suctioning and cleaning laryngectomy tube.
   b. Changing bib.
   c. Administering tube feeding (if ordered).
8. Client will understand information taught in teaching sessions concerning prevention and rehabilitation, as evidenced by 85 percent accuracy in writing.
9. Client will give evidence of compliance with recommendations by:
   a. Beginning to learn altered mode of communication as soon as healing has occurred.
   b. Decreasing exposure to irritants and pollutants.
   c. Abstaining from smoking.
   d. Decreasing intake of alcoholic beverages.
   e. Participating in self-help group such as New Voices (if needed).
   f. Obtaining and using a Medic Alert bracelet and vial of life (placed in refrigerator at home).

INTERVENTIONS

1. Preoperative.
   a. Decrease anxiety. Promote an environment in which the client and family feel free to discuss planned diagnostic tests and impending surgery.
   b. Administer oral hygiene to relieve halitosis and prevent infection. Hydrogen peroxide diluted with saline or water may be used.
   c. Provide fluids and soft foods that are easy to swallow (e.g., oatmeal, custard, mashed potatoes, cottage cheese, scrambled eggs). Avoid hot or acidic foods and fluids (e.g., orange juice).
   d. Provide support before and during diagnostic tests.
   e. Decrease anxiety by allowing client to verbalize fear of surgery.
   f. Provide reassurance and support during the period preceding surgery.
   g. Interpret surgeon's information (as needed) for client and family in order to reduce misconceptions and clarify surgery (see Table 31-3).
   h. Arrange for spiritual counseling if desired.
   i. Teach about:
      (1) Use of magic slate or notepaper for communication.
      (2) Breathing and coughing through laryngectomy tube.
      (3) Need for suctioning through laryngectomy tube.
      (4) Need for nasogastric tube or pharyngostomy tube.
      (5) Initial dressing and use of Hemovac.
      (6) Fluid administered via IVs and then tube feedings, until able to swallow.
      (7) Use of oxygen and mist collar (if needed).

TABLE 31-3 TYPES OF SURGICAL INTERVENTION FOR LARYNGEAL TUMORS

Procedure	Description
Excision using suspension laryngoscopy	The technique of suspension laryngoscopy (and magnification with the operating microscope), which facilitates the excision of carcinoma in situ and other minimally invasive lesions.
Laryngofissure with partial laryngectomy	An incision into the thyroid cartilage in order to excise the neoplasm. Usually only one true cord is excised.
Supraglottic laryngectomy	A horizontal incision above the true cords, which permits only the diseased tissue to be removed.
Total laryngectomy	Removal of the thyroid cartilage, the hyoid bone, the cricoid cartilage, and two or three tracheal rings.
Radical neck resection	Removal of an extensive amount of facial tissue, nerves, bone, and lymph glands surrounding the lesion.

SOURCE: Modified from DeWeese, D. D., and Saunders, W. H.: *Textbook of Otolaryngology*, 6th ed., Mosby, St. Louis, 1982, pp. 123–128.

j. Evaluate client's overall response to teaching.

2. Postoperative.
   a. Elevate head of bed to 30 degrees to facilitate drainage and preserve the airway (in particular after total laryngectomy).
   b. Administer oral hygiene to lubricate mucosa, prevent infection, and reduce odor.
   c. Assess vital signs. Note changes and report as appropriate.
   d. Provide humidified oxygen as needed.
   e. Medicate with analgesic or narcotic for pain as needed. Monitor the client's response to the drug. (Usually little pain is experienced because nerves are severed during the surgery.)
   f. Observe operative site for bleeding, subcutaneous emphysema, signs of wound infection.
   g. Provide laryngectomy tube (or tracheostomy) care: clean skin around tube, clean tube, suction as needed.
   h. Monitor IV or tube feeding.
   i. Monitor nasogastric tube (or pharyngostomy tube) for patency.
   j. Assist client in initial attempts to establish alternate means of communication.
   k. Reassure client that cough will lessen when the ability to swallow improves.
   l. When client can tolerate them, give soft foods, such as custard, oatmeal, scrambled eggs, cottage cheese, mashed potatoes.
   m. Teach client to care for laryngectomy tube (remove, clean, suction, replace) and to administer tube feedings (if needed).
   n. Counsel about abstaining from smoking and decreasing intake of alcohol.
   o. Counsel about use of Medic Alert bracelet, vial of life, and the benefits of participating in a self-help group such as New Voices.

EVALUATION

Outcome Criteria

1. Client is free of preventable complications such as wound infection.
2. Client provides needed care for laryngectomy tube: removing, suctioning, cleaning skin, replacing tube (if needed).
3. Client describes symptoms/signs (which may signal a complication) about which he or she should notify physician or nurse practitioner.
4. Client selects a bib or scarf (or other porous material) to wear over stoma and can explain the reason for doing so.
5. Client eats soft foods and has improved in ability to swallow foods.
6. Client recalls with 85 percent accuracy, either verbally or in writing, the content presented in teaching sessions.
7. Client takes medications at appropriate times and in correct amounts, as evidenced by chart the client keeps.
8. Client has gained 2 lb during the past 2 weeks.
9. Client has given up cigarette smoking and has decreased intake of alcohol.
10. Client wears Medic Alert bracelet and has placed vial of life in home refrigerator.
11. Client is learning an alternate manner for speech.
12. Client participates in a self-help group.

Complications

FISTULA FORMATION

Fistula formation may occur between reconstructed hypopharynx and the skin.

Assessment

1. Increased secretions in localized area.
2. Appearance of vegetable dye on skin surface and/or dressing, when drops of dye have been instilled into hypopharynx.

Revised Outcomes

1. Fistula will heal and continuity of skin will be restored.
2. Other outcomes are as originally stated above under Expected Outcomes.

Interventions

1. Assist with debridement of fistula tract (if needed).
2. Maintain strict septic technique when cleansing area near suture line and tracheostomy.
3. Explain to client that there can be no food or fluid by mouth for several days.
4. Provide nutrition via total parenteral nutrition.

RUPTURE (OR BLOWOUT) OF CAROTID ARTERY

Rupture of the carotid artery is associated with radical neck resection. Clients who have received preoperative irradiation therapy for head–neck tumor are vulnerable.

Assessment
1. Extensive amount of bright red blood spurting through side of neck.
2. Apprehension.
3. Tachycardia.
4. Hypotension/hypovolemia.

Revised Outcomes
1. Circulating blood volume will be restored.
2. Ruptured blood vessel will be repaired.
3. Other outcomes are as originally stated above.

Interventions
1. Apply pressure over site of rupture to curb the outpouring of blood.
2. Assist with the administration of plasma expanders and then whole blood.
3. Position client as flat as can be tolerated.
4. Administer humidified oxygen via nasal prongs.
5. Monitor arterial blood gases and vital signs.
6. Monitor neurological signs every hour.
7. Monitor urine output every hour.
8. Prepare client for immediate surgery: carotid repair and/or ligation.

STENOSIS OF TRACHEOSTOMY

Assessment
1. Shortness of breath (continually).
2. Altered nutrition.

Revised Outcomes
1. Patency of airway will be restored.
2. Other outcomes are as originally stated above.

Interventions
1. Teach client to insert progressively larger tracheostomy tubes or plastic tracheostomy buttons.
2. Prepare client for surgery: surgical revision of tracheostomy.

Reevaluation and Follow-up

Establish a specific individualized plan to ensure that the complication is overcome (short-term) and that long-term surveillance and necessary interventions are provided.

SARCOIDOSIS

DESCRIPTION

Sarcoidosis is an idiopathic disorder that is characterized by a granulomatous reaction in multiple body systems. The most common sites for the granulomas to develop include lungs, lymph nodes, eyes, skin (especially scars), liver, spleen, and heart. The characteristic granulomatous inflammatory changes are those of sarcoidosis and may be found in almost any organ. Typically the inflammatory tissue reaction is minimal. The histological picture of sarcoidosis is not specific; therefore, other disorders need to be excluded. For example, similar histological changes may be noted in lymphomas, tuberculosis, fungus infections, foreign body reaction, and "farmer's lung." The symptoms are usually mild or absent, whereas the specific clinical manifestations depend upon the site of involvement and the activity level of the sarcoid process.

The exact cause of sarcoidosis is unknown. It has been suggested that sarcoidosis is an autoimmune disorder. Most investigators speculate that the sarcoid reaction develops when a genetically predisposed person is exposed to a stimulus that may be one or more infectious agents (e.g., viruses, fungi, tuberculosis); that is, sarcoidosis may develop more because of the host response than the particular agent. Although family cases have been reported, one consistent mode of inheritance has not been noted.

The clinical course of sarcoidosis is variable. The acute process has a high incidence of complete and spontaneous remission in less than 2 years. The chronic disorder may involve the skin exclusively or may take the form of a multisystem debilitating entity. Morbidity can be severe in that pulmonary involvement causes dyspnea and fatigue, ocular disease may lead to blindness, and renal granulomas may cause renal failure. Although sarcoidosis is seldom the cause of death (mortality rate is 3 to 6 percent), cardiac sarcoidosis may lead to sudden death.

PREVENTION

Health Promotion

1. Good health habits (rest, nutrition, exercise, etc.).
2. Avoidance of upper respiratory infections (URI); prompt treatment of colds and flu.
3. Reduced exposure to pollution and environmental dusts.
4. Use of protective devices (e.g., masks) to avoid potential occupational and environmental hazards.

5. Avoidance of exposure to individuals with upper respiratory infections.
6. No smoking.

Population at Risk

1. Young adults (often noted in adults aged 25 to 34 years).
2. Blacks (especially those living in the developed countries).
3. Women (occurs 10 times more frequently in women).
4. Persons who have exposure to harmful substances (e.g., fungi, beryllium, viruses).
5. Persons whose family members have sarcoidosis.
6. Persons who have scars or areas of skin that have had recurrent damage by infection, radiation, or mechanical trauma.

Screening

1. Chest x-ray study.
2. Skin biopsy.

ASSESSMENT

Health History

1. Family history: familial tendency observed.
2. Ethnic background: seen more frequently and more severely in blacks.
3. Exposure to agents that are associated with the sarcoid reaction (e.g., fungi, tubercule bacillus, beryllium) are often described.
4. Increasing complaints of fatigue, dyspnea, and cough are common. (Some persons experience chest pain.)
5. Weight loss may be reported.
6. Arthralgia or arthritis may occur initially or as the disorder progresses.

Physical Assessment

1. Auscultation of the chest may indicate fine respiratory rales. Shortness of breath (dyspnea) may be noted with varying degrees of activity.
2. The skin may be warm to the touch, especially if fever is present. Plaques or papules may be present. Erythematous nodules (erythema nodosum) are often noted along the anterior tibia.
3. Areas of skin may reveal repeated damage and scarring because of infection, radiation, or mechanical trauma.
4. Joint swelling and decreased movement may be observed (wrists, knees, ankles are commonly affected).
5. Generalized lymphadenopathy may be noted.
6. The person often appears tired and pale and may report fatigue and weight loss.
7. A complete physical examination is needed to fully assess the extent of the process (e.g., secondary cardiopulmonary changes, hepatic and splenic enlargement, visual changes, and renal involvement).
8. Clubbing of the digits may be present.

Diagnostic Tests

1. Chest x-ray study reveals bilateral hilar adenopathy. Diffuse symmetrical pulmonary infiltrates may also be noted.
2. Pulmonary function tests permit assessment of the movement of gases in the airways. Typical findings include reduced vital capacity, decreased compliance, and impaired diffusion of oxygen and carbon dioxide. In later stages the arterial blood gases (Pa_{O_2} and Pa_{CO_2}) should be assessed.
3. Transbronchial lung biopsy with a fiberoptic bronchoscope usually yields tissue with characteristic changes.
4. The Kveim-Siltzbach test will yield local, papulonodular lesions in 4 to 6 weeks that should then be biopsied. (This test is often used to confirm the diagnosis; however, a high rate of false-positive and false-negative sarcoid reactions is reported.)
5. Lymph node biopsy should be performed on palpable lymph nodes.
6. Lesions (nodules, papules, plaques) in scars should be biopsied.
7. Biopsy of the lower lip has usually revealed characteristic tissue changes.
8. Liver biopsy is usually performed only if other areas (lung, muscle, lower lip) do not yield tissue with characteristic changes.
9. Laboratory blood tests will demonstrate:
   a. Hypercalcemia.
   b. Hyperglobulinemia.
   c. Elevated urine calcium.
   d. Elevated erythrocyte sedimentation rate (ESR).
   e. Elevated serum angiotensin-converting enzyme (not diagnostic in itself, but supportive of the diagnosis). Serum levels have been observed to parallel the disease activity (Hanno and Callen, 1980).

f. Elevated alpha-globulin levels.
g. Presence of circulating immune complexes.
h. Abnormal complement levels.
i. Evidence of depressed cellular immunity.

10. Refer to *Renal Tumors* in Chapter 32 for additional diagnostic tests.

NURSING DIAGNOSES: ACTUAL OR POTENTIAL

1. Respiratory dysfunction (mild to severe): dyspnea secondary to adenopathy and pulmonary parenchymal changes.
2. Alteration in comfort (discomfort): fatigue secondary to dyspnea and impaired cardiopulmonary status.
3. Alteration in food intake: weight loss secondary to fatigue, dyspnea, and cough.
4. Altered activity/exercise pattern: secondary to fatigue, dyspnea, cough, and arthralgia.
5. Alteration in rest/sleep pattern (potential): secondary to cough, dyspnea, and arthralgia.
6. Alteration in fluid volume (potential for depletion): secondary to fever and lowered intake due to cough.

EXPECTED OUTCOMES

1. Client will feel less fatigued within 7 to 10 days of regimen initiation.
2. Arthralgia will be relieved within 3 to 5 days of regimen initiation.
3. Cough and dyspnea diminish within 3 to 5 days of regimen initiation.
4. Body temperature will return to normal within 3 to 5 days of regimen initiation.
5. Client will gain 4 lb within the next 2 weeks and will gain 10 lb during the 2 months after discharge.
6. Client will understand information taught in teaching sessions, as evidenced by 85 percent accuracy on written tests.
7. Client will give evidence of compliance with care plan by:
   a. Adhering to medication regimen, as indicated by chart maintained by client.
   b. Establishing and maintaining an effective rest and activity regimen.
   c. Adhering to fluid and diet intake plan, as indicated by chart maintained by client.
   d. Gaining weight as recommended.
   e. Eliminating smoking.
   f. Avoiding environmental irritants and pollutants.
   g. Adhering to follow-up schedule and being aware of symptoms of complications.

INTERVENTIONS

1. Provide a quiet, nonstimulating environment.
2. Provide an environment free of irritants and pollutants (no smoking, damp dusting, use of electrostatic filter or air purifier).
3. Promote a rest and activity program.
4. Give frequent mouth care to increase the appeal of food and liquids.
5. Provide a high-protein, moderate-carbohydrate, low-calcium diet. Plan menu with client.
6. Administer indomethecin (25 mg orally, tid to qid) to provide relief for erythema nodosum or arthralgia.
7. Administer corticosteroid eye drops if acute uveitis (inflammation of the iris and ciliary body) is present.
8. Administer methotrexate (25 mg/week) if chronic cutaneous sarcoid lesions are present. (Skin lesions are treated aggressively because they can cause scarring. Topical steroids are seldom effective, perhaps due to lack of penetration.)
9. Provide lozenges to soothe membranes irritated by coughing.
10. Administer systemic corticosteroids when disorder has progressed. (Administer antacids to decrease gastritis.)
11. Counsel about nonsmoking.
12. Teach about:
    a. Medications: dose, side effects.
    b. Diet (high-protein, low-calcium) to maintain health and promote weight gain.
    c. Rest and activity to help maintain resistance to infections and to increase stamina.
    d. Elevating lower extremities to decrease edema and decrease discomfort in knees and ankles.
    e. Avoidance of pollution and other irritants.
13. Plan activity program with gradual increments.

EVALUATION

Outcome Criteria

1. Breath sounds are clearing or are clear; adventitious sounds are absent.

2. Cough decreases in frequency and then ceases.
3. Client is able to walk up to six steps without dyspnea, fatigue, or joint discomfort.
4. Fever decreases and body temperature returns to normal.
5. Client has gained 4 lb during the past 2 weeks.
6. Client stops smoking.
7. Client recalls with 85 percent accuracy, either verbally or in writing, the content presented in teaching sessions.
8. Client takes medications at appropriate times and in correct amounts, as indicated by chart or log.
9. Client adheres to the daily rest and activity program, as evidenced by self-monitored chart.
10. Client reduces exposure to irritants and pollutants in ambient air; uses air purifier.

Complications

1. Blindness can result from untreated ocular disease (see discussion of blindness in Chapter 26).
2. Renal failure can result from granulomatous involvement and nephrocalcinosis (see discussion under *Acute Renal Failure* and *Chronic Renal Failure* in Chapter 32).
3. Lung cancer: a three-fold increase is seen, perhaps because of changes in immunological parameters (see *Cancer of the Lung* in this chapter).
4. Malignant lymphoma: an 11-fold increase is seen, also perhaps influenced by aberrations in immunological parameters (see the discussion in Chapter 29).
5. Respiratory failure (see Complications under *Chronic Bronchitis* later in this chapter).
6. Cor pulmonale (refer to Chapter 30 for a complete discussion).

Assessment

1. Dyspnea: increased.
2. Cough: more productive.
3. Wheezing: increased amount of rales noted upon inspiration.
4. Cyanosis: due to cardiovascular compromise.
5. Loud pulmonic second sound.
6. Hypoxemia: decreased Pa_{O_2} (refer to Table 31-14).
7. Hypercapnia: increased Pa_{CO_2} (refer to Table 31-15).

Revised Outcomes

1. Oxygenation will be restored within normal limits; respiratory embarrassment will cease.
2. Other goals are as originally stated (also see Expected Outcomes under *Cor Pulmonale* in Chapter 30).

Interventions

1. Administer humidified oxygen (as needed).
2. Provide for longer rest periods, but be cautious about hazards of immobility.
3. Provide diet and liquids that are low in sodium.
4. Administer diuretics (refer to Chapter 30 under *Coronary Heart Disease* for a complete discussion).
5. Administer digitalis (refer to Chapter 30 for a complete discussion).
6. Obtain ECG to monitor cardiac changes.
7. Monitor arterial blood gases to evaluate effectiveness of treatment.

Reevaluation and Follow-up

Establish a specific individualized plan to ensure that the complication is overcome (short-term) and that long-term surveillance and necessary interventions are provided.

POLYPS

DESCRIPTION

A polyp is a benign, epithelial pseudotumor with a pedicle. Polyps appear as gray or gray-blue grapelike lesions and are sometimes translucent. Usually nasal polyps are multiple. The pseudotumor must be differentiated from a variety of benign or malignant neoplasms.

Most polyps develop from an outpouching of the mucosa that covers the maxillary or ethmoid sinuses. Nasal polyps develop over time. Initially the polyp is small; however, as the submucosal edema increases, the polyp becomes larger until it resembles a tumor. Polyps cause symptoms because they protrude into the airway.

Allergic rhinitis ("hay fever") is the most common predisposing factor. Polyps tend to recur when the underlying allergic disorder is not well controlled.

PREVENTION

Health Promotion

1. Avoidance of upper respiratory infections (URI). Prompt treatment of colds.
2. Prompt treatment of episodes of sinusitis.
3. Control of underlying allergic disorder.

4. Prompt treatment of episodes of asthma (if present).

Population at Risk

1. Persons who have allergic rhinitis (hay fever).
2. Persons who have sinusitis.
3. Persons who have asthma.

Screening

Nares exam.

ASSESSMENT

Health History

1. Health patterns: smoking, nutrition, use of medications.
2. Preceding URI.
3. Season: may be seasonal if associated with allergic rhinitis.
4. Age: occurs in children but is most often noted in adults.
5. History of allergies (e.g., rhinitis, aspirin hypersensitivity), sinusitis, asthma.
6. Impaired sense of smell.

Physical Assessment

Nasal exam with speculum or mirror reveals:

1. Thickened mucous membrane.
2. Smooth, mobile, gray or gray-blue grapelike lesion in middle meatus.

Diagnostic Tests

"Differentiation and identification is made easier by using a decongestant spray in the nose such as 1% ephedrine or 0.25% Neo-Synephrine solution. . . . A nasal suction tip may then be utilized not only to aspirate secretions for easier inspection but to palpate the soft tissue lesion" (Adams, et al., 1978).

NURSING DIAGNOSES: ACTUAL OR POTENTIAL

1. Alteration in comfort: discomfort secondary to headache, nasal discharge.
2. Respiratory dysfunction: nasal congestion, swelling.
3. Sensory or perceptual alteration: diminished smell.
4. Alteration in sleep–rest pattern: secondary to respiratory discomfort.

EXPECTED OUTCOMES

1. Client will experience reduced nasal obstruction and discharge, as evidenced by breathing sounds and less mouth breathing.
2. Client will have fewer episodes of headaches, as evidenced by reduced intake of aspirin substitutes.
3. Client will understand information taught, as evidenced by 85 percent accuracy in verbal report.
4. Client will give evidence of compliance with care plan by:
   a. Adhering to medication regimen, as indicated by chart maintained by client.
   b. Avoiding exposure to irritants and pollutants.
   c. Reducing the number of cigarettes (smoked per day) by one-half within 2 weeks of last visit.

INTERVENTIONS

1. Administer antihistamines and decongestants to reduce secretions from the nasal passage. (Persons who have hypertension or who are taking monoamine oxidase inhibitors should not be given any drug containing ephedrine.)
2. Provide moist inhalations to lubricate mucosa and prevent drying.
3. Provide oral hygiene frequently, especially if there is an increase in secretions. Half-strength hydrogen peroxide or sodium bicarbonate with water may be used.
4. Administer analgesics (aspirin substitutes) to reduce inflammation of surrounding mucosa and relieve headache.
5. Injection of steroid solution into polyp to reduce inflammation is done by the physician.
6. Surgery: polypectomy, a surgical procedure to remove polyp obstructing the airway. "In patients in whom the condition is severe, a more extensive operation, such as intranasal ethmoidectomy and sphenoidectomy and the Caldwell-Luc procedure will be needed to prevent recurrence" (DeWeese and Saunders, 1977).
7. Lubricate nares entry to prevent skin breakdown.
8. Serve foods that are colorful and appetizing to improve oral intake when client is unable to smell.
9. Teach about:
   a. Control of underlying allergic disorder.
   b. Avoiding irritants.
   c. Medications: dose, side effects.
10. Counsel about nonsmoking.

EVALUATION

Outcome Criteria

1. Nasal obstruction and discharge gradually diminish.
2. Episodes of headaches gradually become fewer.
3. Client is taking medications at appropriate times and in correct amounts, as indicated by chart the client keeps.
4. Client can recall with 85 percent accuracy, either verbally or in writing, the content presented in teaching sessions.
5. Client has reduced the number of cigarettes being smoked.

Complications

1. Hemorrhage (see *Epistaxis* later in this chapter).
2. Infection:

Assessment

1. Increased temperature and pulse.
2. Headache.
3. Nasal obstruction; mouth breathing occurs.

Revised Outcomes

1. Temperature, pulse will be reduced to normal range within 3 days.
2. Headache will be reduced within 3 days.
3. Nasal obstruction will be relieved within 3 days and mouth breathing will diminish.

Interventions

1. Assess vital signs.
2. Administer antibiotics.

Reevaluation and Follow-up

Establish a specific individualized plan to ensure that the complication is overcome (short-term) and that long-term surveillance and necessary interventions are provided.

METABOLIC DISORDERS

RESPIRATORY FAILURE

See Complications under *Chronic Bronchitis* later in this chapter.

CYSTIC FIBROSIS

Refer to the discussion in Chapter 20.

INFLAMMATIONS

PNEUMONIA

DESCRIPTION

Pneumonia is an inflammation in the lung parenchyma involving the respiratory bronchioles, alveolar ducts, alveolar sacs, and alveoli. The inflammation causes consolidation of lung tissue as the alveoli fill with exudate. Four stages of the disease that may appear in a single lesion include (1) edema, (2) red hepatization, (3) gray hepatization (many leukocytes), and (4) resolution (Wittner, 1974). Inflammation may result from different causes and may manifest a variety of symptoms. Pneumonia may occur in healthy people but is usually associated with conditions that alter the body's defense mechanisms. The term *pneumonia* most commonly refers to acute infections. The acute pneumonias have been classified etiologically into the five broad categories presented in Table 31-4.

The causative agent gains access to the lungs by (1) inhalation of microbes present in the air; (2) aspiration of organisms from naso-/oropharynx, the most common cause of bacterial penumonia; (3) hematogenous spread from a distant focus of infection; or rarely, (4) direct spread from a contiguous site of infection (Isselbacher et al., 1980).

Pneumococcal pneumonia caused by gram-positive pneumococci is outlined in detail below because it is the most common type of bacterial pneumonia and generally typifies pneumonia caused by an infectious agent (Brunner and Suddarth, 1982).

PREVENTION

Health Promotion

1. Maintenance of natural resistance (rest, nutrition, exercise, etc.).
2. Avoidance of upper respiratory infections (URI) and exposure to cold and dampness; prompt treatment of colds and flu.
3. Avoidance obliteration of cough reflex and aspiration of secretions; maintenance of gag reflex.
4. Adequate bronchial hygiene by turning, coughing, and deep breathing frequently;

TABLE 31-4 ETIOLOGICAL CLASSIFICATION OF THE PNEUMONIAS

I. Bacteria

- Pneumococci, 83 capsular types
- Hemolytic streptococci, mostly group A; other aerobic streptococci
- *Staphylococcus aureus*
- *Hemophilus influenzae*, type b; other capsular types; rough, noncapsulated
- *Bordetella pertussis*
- *Pasteurella tularensis; P. pestis*
- *Legionella pneumophila*
- *Neisseria meningitidis*
- *Klebsiella pneumoniae* (Friedländer's bacillus) types 1, 2, 4, 5, and others
- Gram-negative rods; *Escherichia coli, Proteus* spp., *Enterobacter* spp., *Pseudomonas aeruginosa*, others
- *Pseudomonas pseudomallei*
- *Salmonella* spp.; *S. typhi*, and others
- *Bacillus anthracis*
- *Bacillus* spp., *B. cereus*
- Anaerobic bacteria: *Bacteroides* spp.; *Fusobacterium* spp.; various streptococci; *Clostridium perfringens*
- *Mycobacterium tuberculosis*
- Atypical mycobacteria
- *Actinomycetes*
  - Aerobic: *Nocardia asteroides; N. brasiliensis*
  - Anaerobic: *Actinomyces israeli; A. bovis*

II. Fungi and Yeasts

- *Cryptococcus neoformans*
- *Blastomyces dermatiditis*
- *Histoplasma capsulatum*
- *Coccidioides immitis*
- *Candida albicans; C. stellatoides*
- *Aspergillus fumigatus*
- *Phycomycetes; Rhizobium* sp.; *Mucor* sp.

III. Filter-Passing Agents

- Influenza virus A, B, C (?)
- Parainfluenza types 1, 2, 3, 4
- Adenoviruses
- Respiratory syncytial virus
- Coxsackie: A21; others
- Measles
- Varicella (chickenpox)
- Variola (smallpox)
- Reovirus
- Herpes simplex
- Cytomegalovirus
- Rhinoviruses
- Rickettsias: Typhus, Rocky Mountain spotted fever; Q fever
- *Chlamydia psittaci; C. trachomatis*
- *Mycoplasma pneumoniae*

IV. Parasites

- Amebiasis
- Schistosomiasis
- Trichinosis
- Paragonamiasis
- Filariasis
- Toxoplasmosis
- *Pneumocystis carinii*
- Flagellates (?)
- Tropical eosinophilia (?)
- Malaria

V. Miscellaneous

- Rheumatic pneumonia
- Allergic (Löffler's eosinophilia)
- Chemical; inhalation; aspiration
- Thermal burns
- Drug reactions: nitrofurantoin; others?
- Physical: radiation

SOURCE: Finland, M.: "Pneumonia and Pneumococcal Infections, with Special Reference to Pneumococcal Pneumonia," *American Review of Respiratory Diseases*, **120**:483, 1979.

ambulating; suctioning when necessary during the postoperative period.

5. Sitting upright when possible or side-lying (Sim's position).
6. Awareness that the actions and side effects of medications and alcohol suppress bronchopulmonary defense mechanisms.
7. Frequent oral hygiene.

8. Prevention spread of infection by using appropriate medical asepsis.
9. Avoidance of smoking.

Population at Risk

1. Immobilized persons (elderly, postoperative clients).
2. Smokers (mild or heavy); excessive alcohol consumers; drug users.
3. Persons who have poor health habits (regarding rest, nutrition, exercise, etc.).
4. Persons exposed to intense cold, damp weather.
5. Persons sustaining upper respiratory infections.
6. Persons living in overcrowded areas with hot, dry air or exposure to air pollution.
7. Persons debilitated by cardiac failure, CNS disorders (seizures, CVA, head injury, neuromuscular disease), chronic obstructive lung disease (COLD), cancer, lymph disorders, pain, trauma, abdominal-thoracic surgery.

Screening

1. Sputum cultures.
2. Chest x-ray studies.

ASSESSMENT

Health History

1. Health patterns: smoking, rest, nutrition, exercise, use of drugs and alcohol.
2. Preceding URI: exposure to cold and dampness.
3. Season: increased susceptibility in winter although problem can also occur in the other seasons.
4. Age: prognosis adversely affected in old age and infancy.
5. Males suffer three times more than females from pneumonia.
6. Presence of other debilitating disorders.
7. History of recent surgery should be noted along with length of time spent under anesthesia.
8. Decreased mobility due to disease process or treatment.
9. Cough and chest pain.
10. Shortness of breath, especially after coughing.
11. Production of sputum, purulent, often bloody.
12. Anxiety, confusion, and disorientation may be present.
13. Nausea and vomiting.

Physical Assessment

1. Skin will appear pale, flushed, warm, and dry. Skin turgor may be affected. The appearance of herpes simplex is not uncommon.
2. Flaring nostrils may be seen and cyanosis of the nailbeds noted.
3. Client will often be lying on the affected side and will guard the affected side when coughing.
4. Severe chest pain is aggravated by chest excursion; chest movement may be limited.
5. Deviation of the trachea away from the affected lung may be noted if empyema or pleural effusion develop.
6. Abdominal distention may be noted.
7. Respirations may be rapid, shallow, and dyspneic. Tachycardia may be present.
8. Client usually has a fever, as high as 40°C to 41°C (104°–106°F); 80 percent have shaking chills.
9. Tactile fremitus is decreased initially and then will increase with consolidation.
10. Upon percussion, dullness will be noted from consolidation or accompanying pleural effusion.
11. Auscultatory findings at first are high-pitched with end-inspiration crackles. Secretions in airway may cause low-pitched early or midinspiration crackles. Consolidated lung surrounding a patent bronchus often gives rise to bronchial breath sounds.

Diagnostic Tests

1. Sputum culture and sensitivity to evaluate pathogen.
2. Blood work may reveal:
   a. Leukocytosis (20,000 to 35,000 white blood cells per cubic milliliter).
   b. Decreased sodium and increased bilirubin.
   c. Decreased chloride and increased sedimentation rate.
   d. Thrombocytopenia.
   e. Leukopenia (an overwhelming infection in the aged or in alcoholics).
3. Blood culture is positive for pneumococci in 25 percent of untreated cases.
4. Blood gases may be altered, depending on extent of problem.
5. Chest x-ray study will demonstrate lung infiltration; areas of consolidation may be vague.

NURSING DIAGNOSES: ACTUAL OR POTENTIAL

1. Respiratory dysfunction: due to impairment of lung tissue.
2. Alteration in cardiac output: decreased/increased.
3. Depletion of body fluid: secondary to increased body temperature.
4. Alteration in comfort: discomfort secondary to pleuritic pain, fever, and respiratory dysfunction.
5. Disturbance in nutrition and fluid intake: secondary to nausea and vomiting, fever, and respiratory dysfunction.
6. Altered levels of consciousness: due to decreased oxygenation.
7. Impairment of skin integrity (potential): due to decreased position changes.
8. Anxiety (mild to moderate): secondary to dyspnea and elevated body temperature.

EXPECTED OUTCOMES

1. Productivity of cough will increase to remove secretions from lungs (initial). Client will have diminished coughing and sputum production, as evidenced by clearing breath sounds within days of initiation of treatment.
2. Body temperature, pulse, and respirations will return to normal within days after treatment is begun.
3. Ability to rest and be comfortable will increase, as evidenced by relief of pain, coughing, fever, and anxiety and diminished disorientation.
4. Spread of infection will be prevented. Client will maintain medical asepsis at all times.
5. Client will meet hydration and nutritional needs by demonstrating gradual weight gain (or weight loss, depending upon the client).
6. Client will understand information taught in teaching sessions, as evidenced by 85 percent accuracy, verbally or in writing.
7. Client will give evidence of compliance with care plan by:
   a. Performing coughing and deep breathing regimen.
   b. Maintaining natural resistance (rest, nutrition, exercise, etc.).
   c. Adhering to medication regimen, as indicated by chart maintained by client.
   d. Maintaining medical asepsis.
   e. Reducing the number of cigarettes by one-half within 2 weeks after discharge.
   f. Avoiding chilling, overcrowded areas with hot, dry air and environmental pollution.
   g. Adhering to follow-up schedule and being aware of signs of complications.

INTERVENTIONS

1. Administer prescribed antibiotics, cough suppressants, expectorants, and analgesics to reduce infection and increase removal of secretions.
2. Promote a safe, quiet environment conducive to rest.
3. Assess level of consciousness.
4. Collect and evaluate results of sputum and blood specimens.
5. Assess vital signs and breath sounds frequently to evaluate client's progress.
6. Administer humidified oxygen, if necessary, to assist respiration. Mechanical ventilation may be needed if respiratory malfunction is severe.
7. Assist with frequent coughing and deep breathing. Chest splinting is important.
8. Perform chest physiotherapy to assist with removal of secretions from lungs. Suctioning may be needed.
9. Offer comfort and support.
10. Assist with normal activities of daily living (ADL).
11. Perform range-of-motion (ROM) exercises; help decrease side effects of immobility.
12. Offer skin care; keep the client warm and dry. Lubricate lips if dry and cracked.
13. Provide oral hygiene; increase the amount of fluids and use good mouth care to prevent infection.
14. Encourage a well-balanced diet with good hydration; record intake and output of fluids.
15. Assist with intercostal block, if necessary.
16. Teach about:
    a. Coughing and deep-breathing regimen.
    b. Medications: dose, side effects.
    c. Medical asepsis to prevent spread of infection.
    d. Proper rest and exercise to help maintain natural resistance.
    e. Diet: as needed to maintain health and modify weight as indicated.

f. Avoidance of chills, overcrowded areas with hot, dry air, and environmental pollution.
g. Follow-up schedule and signs of complications.

17. Counsel about nonsmoking.

EVALUATION

Outcome Criteria

1. Cough becomes more productive initially; then secretions and coughing decrease.
2. Breath sounds are clearing to clear.
3. Temperature, pulse, and respirations are nearing normal to normal.
4. Pain has diminished, as evidenced by increased activity, diminished anxiety, relief of coughing.
5. Client is taking medications at appropriate times and in correct amounts, as indicated by chart client is keeping.
6. Client is adhering to medical asepsis techniques.
7. Client is gaining or losing weight.
8. Client can recall with 85 percent accuracy, either verbally or in writing, the content presented in teaching sessions.
9. Client is reducing the number of cigarettes smoked.

Complications

1. Pleurisy (see the discussion later in this chapter).
2. Pleural effusion (see Complications under *Pleurisy*).
3. Pulmonary edema (see the discussion under *Congestive Heart Failure* in Chapter 30).
4. Lung abscess (see the discussion later in this chapter).
5. Superinfection.
   a. Pericarditis (see discussion in Chapter 30).
   b. Bacteremia (see discussion in Chapter 48).
   c. Meningitis (see discussion in Chapter 25).

ATELECTASIS

Area of lung that is collapsed, airless, and shrunken.

Assessment

1. Pleuritic pain: increased over the affected area.
2. Rapid respirations.
3. Increased dyspnea.
4. Weakness: generalized malaise.
5. Anxiety.
6. Cyanosis.
7. Increased temperature, pulse, and blood pressure.
8. Breath sounds absent over the affected area.
9. Percussion: flat.
10. Mediastinal shift toward affected side noted.

Revised Outcomes

1. Aeration of lung and exchange of gases will be restored when lung is reexpanded; dyspnea and cyanosis will cease.
2. Other goals are as originally stated above under Expected Outcomes.

Interventions

1. Assist with bronchoscopy.
2. Assist with thoracentesis (the insertion of a tube into the chest cavity to remove fluid and to help reinflate the lung).
3. Monitor condition after thoracentesis.
4. Assess vital signs, breath sounds.
5. Encourage coughing, deep breathing.
6. Suction when necessary to help remove secretions.
7. Position on unaffected side.
8. Increase activity gradually.
9. Perform chest physiotherapy.
10. Administer antibiotics.

EMPYEMA

Accumulation of purulent exudate in the pleural cavity.

Assessment

1. Orthopnea.
2. Localized chest pain: constant or on inspiration.
3. Unequal chest expansion.
4. Diminished or absent breath sounds over affected area.
5. Percussion: dull over involved area.
6. Productive cough.

Revised Outcomes

1. Oxygenation will be restored when exudate is removed; pain, respiratory dysfunction, and cough will diminish.
2. Other goals are as originally stated above under Expected Outcomes.

Interventions

1. Administer oxygen (humidified).
2. Place client in semi-Fowler's position.
3. Assess vital signs, breath sounds, and chest expansion.
4. Encourage coughing and deep breathing.

5. Perform chest physiotherapy.
6. Assist with thoracentesis.
7. Monitor chest tubes (see discussion under *Trauma*).

Reevaluation and Follow-up
Establish a specific individualized plan to ensure that the complication is overcome (short-term) and that long-term surveillance and necessary interventions are provided.

TUBERCULOSIS

DESCRIPTION

Tuberculosis is a reportable, communicable, infectious, inflammatory, chronic disease. The tubercle bacillus, *Mycobacterium tuberculosis*, is disseminated by droplets and enters the body by inhalation. The droplet nuclei become implanted on alveolar tissue, generally in the best-ventilated portions of the lungs where the highest oxygen tension exists. After several weeks an allergy to the bacilli develops, thus producing an inflammatory reaction. Soon leukocytes arrive, which are replaced by macrophages that form a loose focus of infiltrated tissue (tubercle). Eventually the cells become compact, and necrosis of the control portion of the lesion occurs. If the necrotic tissue fails to liquefy, it persists as a yellowish cheesy mass called *caseous material*. The healing of tuberculosis lesions may involve resolution, fibrosis (scarring), or calcification.

A primary infection is usually well controlled by the body's defense systems so that generally no illness develops. When the primary lesion heals, spots of calcium are left that appear on x-ray films. It is the *hematogenous seeding* of bacilli that accompanies the primary infection that sets the stage for chronic tuberculosis at a later date. Persons who have been infected previously are generally protected from reinfection by specific immunity that is medicated by T lymphocytes.

Chronic adult tuberculosis is the awakening of bacilli in dormant lesions when resistance is low. This stage of the disease is the most serious and contagious. Vigorous treatment is necessary to interfere with the multiplications of organisms. The American Lung Association has developed a table of basic classification of tuberculosis (see Table 31-5).

Adult tuberculosis is generally located in the upper regions of the lungs in the apical posterior segments of the upper lobes, involving the lung parenchyma. The disease spreads to other regions by the bronchogenic routes. Tuberculosis develops most often in the lungs, but lesions do arise in the kidneys, bones, and lymph nodes.

In 1976 in the United States about 32,000 new cases of clinical tuberculosis developed, an incidence of 15 per 100,000, down from 24 in 1966 and 53 in 1953 (Hall and Colman, 1975).

PREVENTION

Health Promotion

1. Avoidance of contact with an infectious case of tuberculosis.
2. Maintenance of natural resistance (rest, nutrition, exercise, etc.).
3. Reduced exposure to overcrowded, inadequately ventilated, poorly sanitized areas.
4. Avoidance of smoking.
5. Chemoprophylaxis.
   a. Isoniazid (INH) is given (dosage and frequency vary) to high-risk persons in order to prevent the development of active clinical disease. Such therapy is highly recommended for:
      (1) Household contacts.
      (2) Recent converters of any age (persons whose skin tests for tuberculosis were originally negative but later became positive).
      (3) Persons under 20 years of age with inactive tuberculosis and positive reactions.
      (4) Individuals in special clinical situations who are highly susceptible.
      (5) Newly infected persons.
      (6) Significant tuberculin skin test reactors with abnormal results of chest x-ray study.
      (7) Significant tuberculin skin test reactors up to and over 35 years of age.
   b. Bacillus Calmette-Guérin (BCG) vaccine, which contains antigens, may be used to treat tuberculin-negative persons, in an attempt to produce increased resistance to clinical tuberculosis. It has limited use in the United States due to low infection rate here. It offers limited protection but is not completely prophylactic. Because BCG changes tuberculin skin tests from a neg-

TABLE 31-5 CLASSIFICATION OF TUBERCULOSIS

0. *No tuberculosis exposure, not infected* (no history of exposure, reaction to tuberculin skin test not significant).
1. *Tuberculosis exposure, no evidence of infection* (history of exposure, reaction to tuberculin skin test not significant).
2. *Tuberculous infection, no disease* (significant reaction to tuberculin skin test, negative bacteriologic studies, if done, no clinical and/or roentgenographic evidence of tuberculosis).
   Chemotherapy status (preventive):
   - None
   - On chemotherapy since (date)
   - Chemotherapy terminated (date):
     - Complete (prescribed course of therapy)
     - Incomplete
3. *Tuberculosis: current disease* (*M. tuberculosis* cultured, if done; otherwise, *both* a significant reaction to tuberculin skin test *and* clinical and/or roentgenographic evidence of current disease).
   Location of disease:
   - Pulmonary
   - Pleural
   - Lymphatic
   - Bone and/or joint
   - Genitourinary
   - Disseminated (miliary)
   - Meningeal
   - Peritoneal
   - Other

   The predominant site shall be listed. Other sites may also be listed. Anatomic sites may be specified more precisely.

   Bacteriologic status:
   - Positive by:
     - Microscopy only (date)
     - Culture only (date)
     - Microscopy and culture (date)
   - Negative (date)
   - Not done

   Chemotherapy status:
   - On chemotherapy since (date)
   - Chemotherapy terminated, incomplete (date)

   The following data are necessary in certain circumstances:

   Roentgenogram findings:
   - Normal
   - Abnormal:
     - Cavitary or noncavitary
     - Stable or worsening or improving

   Tuberculin skin test reaction:
   - Significant
   - Not significant
4. *Tuberculosis: no current disease* (history of previous episodes of tuberculosis, or abnormal stable roentgenographic findings in a person with a significant reaction to tuberculin skin test, negative bacteriologic studies, if done, no clinical and/or roentgenographic evidence of current disease).
   Chemotherapy status:
   - None
   - On chemotherapy since (date)
   - Chemotherapy terminated (date):
     - Complete
     - Incomplete
5. *Tuberculosis suspect* (diagnosis pending).
   Chemotherapy status:
   - None
   - On chemotherapy since (date)

SOURCE: *Diagnostic Standards and Classification of Tuberculosis and Other Mycobacterial Diseases*, American Thoracic Society, New York, 1981.

ative to a positive reaction, it interferes with case-finding programs. It is recommended for persons with nonsignificant tuberculin skin test results.

Population at Risk

1. Persons with general physical debilitation and lowered resistance.
2. Persons in contact with an infectious case of tuberculosis in the family or occupation (hospital or nursing home personnel especially).
3. Persons living in crowded conditions with poor sanitation and ventilation (slums, migrant work areas, large cities).
4. Persons reacting positively to tuberculin skin tests; those who have converted within the

past year from negative to positive; those having reaction of 10 mm or more of induration.
5. Persons with previous history of pleural effusion, pneumonia, chronic malignancy, diabetes, gastric resection, chronic alcoholism, recent pregnancy; those receiving prolonged steroid treatment or anti-inflammatory drugs.

Screening

1. Tuberculin skin tests (see Table 31-6 for interpretation of results).
   a. Mantoux test (skin test), purified protein derivative (more specific product), or old tuberculin extract injected into forearm.
   b. Tine test, multiple puncture test (screening purposes).
   c. Jet injection used for screening purposes.
2. Chest x-ray study.
3. Sputum cultures.

ASSESSMENT

Health History

1. Exposure to an infectious case of tuberculosis.
2. Health maintenence patterns (rest, nutrition, exercise, smoking).
3. Living conditions: crowded with poor sanitation and ventilation.
4. Positive reaction to tuberculin skin tests.
5. Previous illness: pleural effusion, pneumonia, diabetes, gastric resection, chronic alcoholism; recent pregnancy; receiving corticosteroid treatment.
6. Disease affects males two times more than females; individuals over age 45.
7. Tuberculosis is four times more common in nonwhites than in whites (North American Indians and African blacks have high incidence and increased susceptibility).
8. Persistent cough may be present. Can become more frequent with production of mucoid or mucopurulent sputum.
9. Sputum production is contingent upon the progression of the disease; when present, sputum usually is odorless, green or yellow, and generally raised in the morning; streaking with small amounts of blood may accompany the cough.
10. Lassitude, fatigue, irritability, anxiety, and depression.
11. Persistent loss of weight.
12. Indigestion with accompanying anorexia, nausea, and vomiting may be present.
13. Headaches in evening may occasionally be noted.
14. Night sweats.
15. Resistance may be lowered by diabetes and immunosuppressive drugs or in the postpartum period.

Physical Assessment

1. Pallor may be noted.
2. Rales over affected lung after forced expiration. This is followed by a short cough and a quick, deep inspiration. In long-standing tuberculosis, there is an inadequate apical dullness, course rales, a deviation of the trachea, and a diminished mobility in one hemithorax.
3. Dyspnea and persistent cough with sputum may be present.
4. Temperature elevation (late afternoon).
5. Shortness of breath, palpitations upon exertion.

Diagnostic Tests

Refer to Table 31-6.

1. Mantoux (skin test): Tuberculin unit dose of purified protein derivative (PPD); record induration. A reaction of 10 mm or more of induration is significant; 5 mm or more is significant in persons at risk of exposure.
2. Negative response to PPD does not rule out diagnosis of tuberculosis.
3. Chest x-ray study is done to detect lesions.
4. Algorithm for diagnosis and treatment of tuberculosis (see Figure 31-2).
5. Sputum culture for acid-fast bacillus (AFB): positive for tuberculosis. Often three or more specimens are examined to confirm diagnosis.
6. Blood work (routine) will reveal:
   a. Increased sedimentation rate.
   b. WBC usually normal.
   c. Hemoglobin and hematocrit usually normal.

NURSING DIAGNOSES: ACTUAL OR POTENTIAL

1. Respiratory dysfunction: secondary to cough, dyspnea.
2. Impairment of alveolar integrity (potential).
3. Anxiety (mild to moderate).
4. Grief: secondary to diagnosis of long-term illness.
5. Impairment of significant other's adjustment to illness.

TABLE 31-6 RECOMMENDED INTERPRETATION OF SKIN TEST REACTIONS

1. *Intracutaneous Mantoux and jet injection tests* (with standard test dose).
   a. *10 mm or more of induration = positive reaction.* This is interpreted as positive for past or present infection with *Mycobacterium tuberculosis* because reactions this large most likely represent specific sensitivity. The test does not need to be repeated for confirmation in ordinary circumstances, unless there is reason to question the validity of the test.
   b. *5 to 9 mm of induration = doubtful reaction.* Reactions in this size range reflect sensitivity that can result from infection with either atypical mycobacteria or *M. tuberculosis;* hence they are classed as doubtful. However, a person with a doubful reaction who is known to have been in close contact with an infectious person, i.e., a subject with infectious sputum, or a person having radiographic or clinical evidence of disease compatible with tuberculosis, should be regarded as probably infected with *M. tuberculosis.* For all other persons, if an appropriate antigen for atypical mycobacteria is available, an intracutaneous test with such an antigen may be applied at the same time as a repeat tuberculin test.
   c. *0 to 4 mm of induration = negative reaction.* This reflects either a lack of tuberculin sensitivity, or a low-grade sensitivity that most likely is not caused by *M. tuberculosis* infection. No repeat test is necessary unless there is also suggestive clinical evidence of tuberculosis. If the person is in contact with a tuberculosis subject, he or she should be followed up according to the established routine for contacts.
2. *Multiple-puncture tests.* In determining the size of induration, measure the diameter of the largest single reaction. If the reaction consists of discrete papules, the diameters of separate areas of induration should not be added. For screening tests, the following interpretation is suggested.
   a. *Vesiculation = positive reaction.* If vesiculation is present, the test may be interpreted as positive, in which case the management of the subject is the same as that for one classified as positive to the Mantoux text.
   b. *2 mm or more of induration = doubtful reaction.* Even though such reactions may be due to *M. tuberculosis,* a significant proportion of them may not be confirmed by a positive standard Mantoux test. This is particularly true of smaller reactions. Therefore, a standard Mantoux test should be done on all subjects in this group, and management should be based on the reaction to the Mantoux test or on the results of dual testing using PPD-tuberculin and PPD-B.
   c. *Less than 2 mm of induration = negative reaction.* There is no need for retesting unless the individual is in contact with a case of tuberculosis or there is clinical evidence suggestive of the disease.

SOURCE: *Diagnostic Standards and Classification of Tuberculosis and Other Mycobacterial Diseases,* American Lung Association, New York, 1974, pp. 18–19.

6. Alteration in nutrition: secondary to indigestion, vomiting, cough.
7. Alteration in comfort: discomfort and fatigue.
8. Depletion of body fluids (potential): secondary to vomiting, diaphoresis, and fever.

EXPECTED OUTCOMES

1. Sputum will be negative in a few weeks following initiation of chemotherapy.
2. Productivity of cough will increase to remove secretions from lungs (initial). Client will have diminished cough secretions, as evidenced by alteration in breath sounds.
3. Body temperature and respirations will return to normal after treatment initiation.
4. Ability to rest will increase, as evidenced by acceptance of illness, diminished anxiety and irritability, and relief of discomfort and respiratory dysfunction.
5. Spread of infection will be prevented. Client will maintain medical asepsis at all times. A

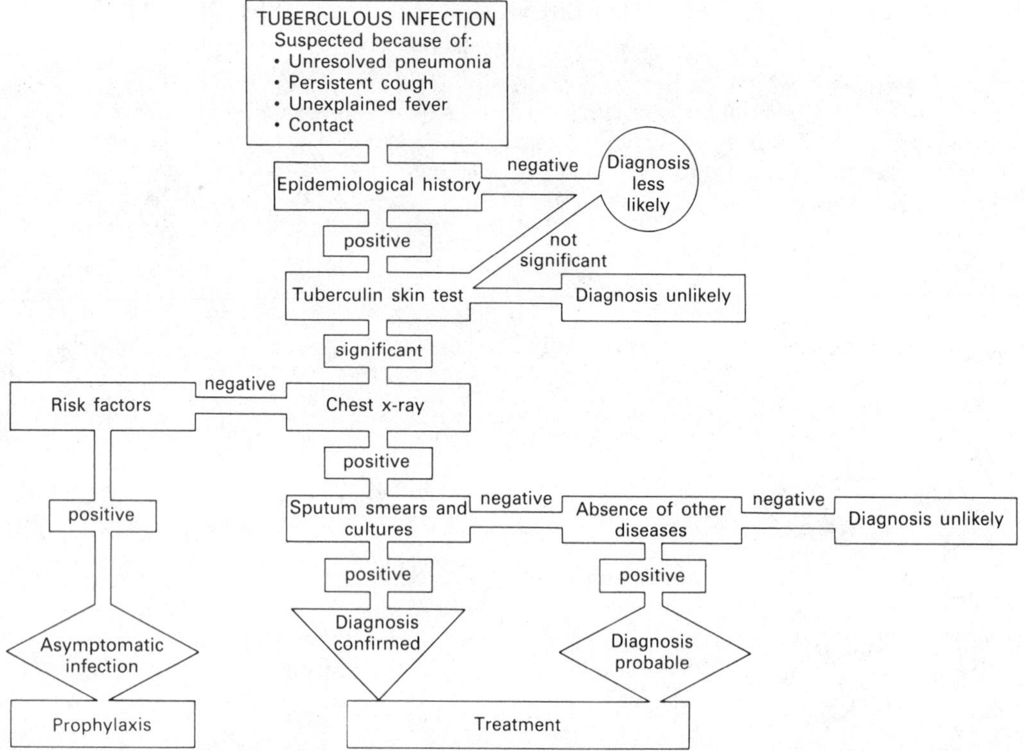

Figure 31-2 Algorithm for the diagnosis and management of tuberculosis: a logical progression. (*Tuberculosis: What Every Physician Should Know,* American Lung Association, New York, 1982, adapted from Daniel, T. M.: "Tuberculosis," *Journal of Infectious Disease,* **134**:419, 1976.)

noninfectious state will be achieved soon after therapy is initiated.

6. Client will meet hydration and nutritional needs, as demonstrated by increase in appetite and gradual weight gain (or weight loss, depending upon the client).
7. Client will understand information taught in teaching sessions, as evidenced by 85 percent accuracy, verbally or in writing.
8. Client will give evidence of compliance with care plan by:
   a. Adhering to medication regimen, as indicated by chart maintained by client.
   b. Gaining (or losing) weight as recommended.
   c. Avoiding overcrowded areas with poor ventilation or sanitation.
   d. Reducing number of cigarettes.
   e. Establishing and maintaining a plan for coughing and deep breathing exercises, rest, recreational activities.
   f. Maintaining medical asepsis.
   g. Adhering to follow-up schedule and being aware of signs of complications.

INTERVENTIONS

1. Provide a quiet, restful environment.
2. Administer prescribed chemotherapy. Teach the client about purpose, dosage, and side effects. Frequently treatment is begun even though positive bacteriological results are not yet avoidable. The principles that guide the selection of drug therapy are found in Table 31-7 and Figure 31-2. Chemotherapy consists of (a) rapid reduction of tubercle bacilli and (b) continuous treatment to eliminate persisting organism. Constant uninterrupted therapy is the key to success. Multiple drug therapy is generally used to treat active tuberculosis (see Table 31-8).
3. Maintain asepsis technique (consult protocol of facility).

TABLE 31-7 PRINCIPLES OF CHEMOTHERAPY IN TUBERCULOSIS

To be effective in therapy, a drug must interfere with a vital function of the tubercle bacillas without harming the host. The choice of therapy should be guided by several well-established principles:

1. Drugs should be chosen to which the bacilli are likely to be susceptible. Fortunately, in the United States this presents little difficulty in most newly discovered cases because most strains are susceptible to the major drugs. If a patient has been treated previously or contracted the infection in an area where drug resistance is common (e.g., Southeast Asia, Philippines, Mexico), it must be assumed that the bacilli will be resistant to isoniazid (INH) and the regimen should include at least two other drugs until the results of susceptibility studies are known.
2. Even in a generally susceptible population of bacilli, a naturally resistant mutant occurs about once in 10^5 to 10^6 organisms. For this reason at least two effective drugs should always be given to patients with clinical tuberculosis to avoid multiplication of drug-resistant mutants.
3. Bactericidal drugs are always preferred. Both rifampin and isoniazid are bactericidal for both extra- and intracellular bacilli. For this reason these two drugs are effective both for immediate reduction in the large extracellular population of bacilli and for ultimate eradication of the smaller intracellular population.
4. When treatment appears to be failing (bacteriology fails to become negative within 3 to 4 months), the addition of a single drug is an invitation to disaster. Therapy should always be changed to an entirely new regimen of at least two new drugs, and great care should be taken to ensure that the patient takes the medication regularly.
5. Therapy must be continued long enough to eradicate the bacilli from the body. When two bactericidal drugs are used, this can be accomplished in 9 months, but when one of the drugs is bacteriostatic, a treatment period of 18 to 24 months is required.
6. All medications should be given before breakfast and in a single dose, if possible, in order to achieve a single combined peak concentration for maximum effect on the bacilli.

SOURCE: Isselbacher, K., et al.: *Harrison's Principles of International Medicine*, 9th ed, vol. 1, McGraw-Hill, New York, 1980, p. 708.

4. Ensure adequate air ventilation; decontamination of air is achieved by noncirculating air conditioning or ultraviolet lighting.
5. Collect and evaluate sputum specimens.
6. Provide oral hygiene.
7. Assess vital signs and breath sounds.
8. Manage cough and pain if present.
9. Encourage coughing, deep breathing.
10. Perform chest physiotherapy.
11. Offer support and encouragement.
12. Provide diversion (e.g., occupational therapy).
13. Teach client about:
    a. Clinical condition; brief hospitalization if condition requires it; follow-up and signs of complications.
    b. Medications: dose, side effects.
    c. Rest and diversion to maintain resistance against other infections.
    d. Diet: as needed to maintain health and modify weight.
    e. Avoidance of overcrowded areas with poor ventilation and sanitation.
    f. Prevention of the spread of infection.
    g. Planning a program for coughing and deep breathing.
14. Counsel about nonsmoking.

EVALUATION

Outcome Criteria

1. Sputum cultures are negative.
2. Cough becomes productive; then sputum production and cough diminish.

TABLE 31-8 TREATMENT OF TUBERCULOSIS IN ADULTS AND CHILDREN

	Dosage[a]		Most Common Side Effects[a]	Tests for Side Effects[a]	Remarks[a]
	Daily	Twice Weekly			
Commonly Used Drugs					
Isoniazid	10–20 mg/kg up to 300 mg PO or IM	15 mg/kg PO or IM	Peripheral neuritis, hepatitis, hypersensitivity	SGOT/SGPT (not as a routine)	Bactericidal, pyridoxine 10 mg as prophylaxis for neuritis; 50–100 mg as treatment
Ethambutol	15–25 mg/kg PO	50 mg/kg PO	Optic neuritis (reversible with discontinuation of drug; very rare at 15 mg/kg), skin rash	Red-green color discrimination and visual acuity[b]	Use with caution with renal disease or when eye testing is not feasible
Rifampin	10–20 mg/kg up to 600 mg PO	600 mg PO	Hepatitis, febrile reaction, purpura (rare)	SGOT/SGPT (not as a routine)	Bactericidal, orange urine color; affects action of other drugs
Streptomycin	15–20 mg/kg up to 1 g IM	15–30 mg/kg	8th nerve damage, nephrotoxicity	Vestibular function, audiograms;[b] BUN and creatinine	Use with caution in older patients or those with renal diseases
Pyrazinamide	20–40 mg/kg up to 2 g PO		Hyperuricemia, hepatotoxicity	Uric acid, SGOT/SGPT	Under study as first-line drug in short-course regimens
Less Commonly Used Drugs					
Capreomycin	15 mg/kg up to 1 g IM		8th nerve damage, nephrotoxicity	Vestibular function, audiograms;[b] BUN and creatinine	Use with caution in older patients; rarely used with renal disease
Kanamycin	15 mg/kg up to 1 g IM		Auditory toxicity, nephrotoxicity, vestibular toxicity (rare)	Vestibular function, audiograms;[b] BUN and creatinine	Use with caution in older patients; rarely used with renal disease
Ethionamide	15–30 mg/kg up to 1 g PO		GI disturbance, hepatotoxicity, hypersensitivity	SGOT/SGPT	Divided dose may help GI side effects
Para-amino-salicylic acid (aminosalicylic acid)	200–300 mg/kg up to 12 g PO		GI disturbance, hypersensitivity, hepatotoxicity, sodium load	SGOT/SGPT	GI side effects very frequent, making cooperation difficult
Cycloserine	10-20 mg/kg up to 1 g PO		Psychosis, personality changes, convulsions, rash	Psychologic testing	Very difficult drug to use; side effects may be blocked by pyridoxine, ataractic agents, or anticonvulsant drugs

SOURCE: *Tuberculosis: What Every Physician Should Know*, American Lung Association, New York, 1982.

[a] Check product labeling for detailed information on dose, contraindications, drug interaction, adverse reactions, and monitoring.

[b] Initial levels should be determined at start of treatment.

3. Breath sounds are clearing to clear.
4. Body temperature and respirations are returning to normal.
5. Client adheres to aseptic technique.
6. Client takes medications at appropriate times and in correct amounts, as indicated by the charts he or she keeps.
7. Client rests and participates in recreational activities with lessening fatigue, diminished discomfort, and anxiety.
8. Client is gaining (or losing) weight.
9. Client has reduced the number of cigarettes smoked.
10. Client recalls with 85 percent accuracy, either verbally or in writing, the content presented in teaching sessions.

Complications

1. Relapse of tuberculosis: The relapse rate of clients with documented pulmonary tuberculosis who completed an adequate course (18 to 24 months) of combined therapy with isoniazid as one of the drugs is less than 1 percent per year for the first 3 years and less than 0.5 percent thereafter. Relapse rate may be as high as 15 to 25 percent for abbreviated courses of therapy or irregular treatment (Hinshaw, 1979).
2. Pleurisy (see the discussion in this chapter).
3. Hemoptysis (see the discussion under *Pneumonia* and also Evaluation, complication 3, under *Bronchiectasis*).
4. Atelectasis (see Evaluation, complication 6, under *Pneumonia*).
5. Spontaneous pneumothorax (see the discussion under *Pneumothorax*).
6. Bronchopleural fistula: persistent communication between the pleural cavity and the broncheal tree; surgical intervention may be necessary if chemotherapy fails:

Interventions

1. Preoperative intervention (see Interventions under *Cancer of the Lung*).
2. Types of surgical intervention.
   a. *Lung resection*: removal of the diseased lobe(s) of the lung, or the lung itself, in order to terminate the disease process and secondary effects.
   b. *Decortication*: removal of the lung covering (external).
3. Postoperative intervention (see Interventions under *Cancer of the Lung*).

Reevaluation and Follow-up

Establish a specific individualized plan to ensure that complications are overcome (short-term) and that long-term surveillance and necessary interventions are provided.

LUNG ABSCESS

DESCRIPTION

A lung abscess is a localized collection of pus within a cavity that has been formed by the necrosis of inflammatory tissue and lung tissue. Abscess formation is an attempt to wall off an infection. For a while the abscess remains somewhat isolated, but eventually it erodes and ruptures into a bronchus.

Location of the abscess is in those segments of the lungs that are most dependent at the time of aspiration: the posterior segment of the upper or superior segment of the lower lobes, especially on the right lung when the client is supine, or the basilar segments of the lower lobes when upright.

Several different types of disorders are associated with abscess formation (see Table 31-9). The onset and duration of the disease symptoms vary greatly.

The incidence of lung abscesses has decreased due to early and effective antimicrobial treatment and skillful surgical management (Luckman and Sorensen, 1980).

PREVENTION

Health Promotion

1. Maintenance of good oral hygiene, dental health.
2. Functioning swallow reflex. Lack of this reflex would allow entrance of aspiration, which is associated with loss of consciousness, drug overdose, or central nervous system diseases.
3. Avoidance of chemical injury to airway that would impair clearance of microorganisms.

Population at Risk

1. Persons with poor oral hygiene.
2. Persons who could aspirate foreign bodies, infectious materials, or dental deposits: alcoholics, drug users, epileptics, or persons with central nervous system disorders.
3. Persons suffering from bacteremia, septic em-

TABLE 31-9 CLASSIFICATION OF LUNG ABSCESSES ACCORDING TO CAUSE

1. Necrotizing infections.
   a. Pyogenic bacteria (*Staphylococcus aureus, Klebsiella*, group A streptococcus, *Bacteroides, Fusobacterium*, anaerobic and microaerophilic cocci and streptococci, other anaerobes, *Nocardia*).
   b. Mycobacteria (*Mycobacterium tuberculosis, M. kansasii, M. intracellularis*).
   c. Fungi (*Histoplasma, Coccidioides*).
   d. Parasites (amebas, lung flukes).
2. Cavity infarction.
   a. Bland embolism.
   b. Septic embolism (various anaerobes, *Staphylococcus, Candida*).
   c. Vasculitis (Wegener's granulomatosis, periarteritis).
3. Cavitary malignancy.
   a. Primary bronchogenic carcinoma.
   b. Metastatic malignancies (very common).
4. Other.
   a. Infected cysts.
   b. Necrotic conglomerate lesions (silicosis, coal miner's pneumoconiosis).

SOURCE: Murray, J. F., in Isselbacher, K., et al.: *Harrison's Principles of Internal Medicine*, 9th ed., McGraw-Hill, New York, 1980, p. 1228.

boli, right-sided endocarditis, or septic thrombophlebitis or from infections in extremeties or abdominal cavity.

4. Persons exposed to occupational pollution (e.g., coal miners).

Screening

Chest x-ray study of those persons with predisposing illness.

ASSESSMENT

Health History

1. Health maintenance patterns: poor oral hygiene, alcoholism, drug use, smoking, nutritional practices.
2. Exposure to URI.
3. Occupational exposure (e.g., pneumoconiosis).
4. History of pneumonia, central nervous system disorders, recent unconsciousness.
5. Three times more males are affected by disease than females.

Physical Assessment

1. Malodorous breath.
2. Sputum will be prevalent, often fetid, and bloody with dyspnea.
3. Clubbing of fingers and toes may be noted in chronic cases.
4. Anxiety and lack of understanding of disease process may be present.
5. Increased production of foul-smelling sputum with a cough and dyspnea.
6. Fever may be present.
7. Oral exam usually discloses poor dentition with caries, gingivitis, and periodontal infection.
8. Chest percussion may reveal a dull area of consolidation and pleural thickening associated with empyema.
9. Pain: pleuritic or dull.
10. Breath sounds: normal or cavernous sounds with rales may be heard over the involved area.
11. Weight loss, anorexia, and weakness.

Diagnostic Tests

1. Chest x-ray study shows wall around lucent area must be present.
2. Sputum culture and sensitivity help isolate pathogen. Specimen should be obtained by transtracheal or transthoracic aspiration.
3. Bronchogram isolates the abscess and surrounding cavity.
4. Blood work will reveal:
   a. Leukocytosis.
   b. Anemia and hypoalbuminemia.
5. Needle aspiration is performed to remove liquid strainage and to isolate the organism.

NURSING DIAGNOSES: ACTUAL OR POTENTIAL

1. Respiratory dysfunction: dyspnea secondary to cough, pain, and sputum production.
2. Impaired integrity of lung membrane.
3. Alteration in comfort: pleuritic pain, cough, fever.
4. Depletion of body fluids: secondary to inflammatory response, fever.
5. Knowledge deficit: due to lack of understanding of disease and oral hygiene.

6. Anxiety (mild to moderate): due to disease process.
7. Difficulty in coping: secondary to the diagnosis of a potentially chronic problem.
8. Alteration in nutrition (deficit): secondary to malaise, anorexia.

EXPECTED OUTCOMES

1. Productivity of cough will increase and secretions will be removed, followed by diminished cough and sputum production, as evidenced by clearing breath sounds.
2. Body temperature and respirations will return to normal following treatment initiation.
3. Client will demonstrate gradual weight gain over a specified period of time.
4. Client will understand information taught in teaching sessions, as evidenced by 85 percent accuracy, verbally or in writing.
5. Client will give evidence of compliance with care plan by:
   a. Adhering to medication regimen, as indicated by chart maintained by client.
   b. Establishing and maintaining an effective oral-dental hygiene program.
   c. Performing a coughing and deep breathing regimen.
   d. Avoiding environmental irritants.
   e. Being able to rest with decreased anxiety, pain, fever, and coughing.
   f. Maintaining nutrition-hydration pattern necessary to modify weight and increase natural resistance.
   g. Reducing smoking, alcohol intake, or drug use.
   h. Adhering to follow-up schedule (it may take a long time for x-ray film to clear) and being aware of signs of infection.

INTERVENTIONS

1. Administer prescribed antibiotics for about 6 weeks, aerosolized bronchodilators or vasoconstrictors (drugs must be able to reach involved portion of lungs).
2. Instruct client how to cough effectively (refer to Table 31-10).
3. Perform chest physiotherapy; suction if necessary.
4. Assist with bronchoscopy. Prepare the client. Instruct the client not to eat or drink after this test, because of the anesthetic effect. (Refer to Bronchoscopy.)

TABLE 31-10 EFFECTIVE COUGHING

Effective coughing requires a forward flexion motion and cannot be done while lying flat in bed.

1. The patient is first instructed to assume the "cough friendly" sitting position (head flexed, shoulders relaxed and slightly rolled forward, feet supported). A pillow may be placed on the patient's lap to assist in elevating the diaphragm.
2. Then the head drops, the chest sinks, and the patient slowly bends forward while blowing out through slightly parted or pursed lips with an expiratory airflow just below that which will cause collapse of the airways. Facial plethora or venous distention of the head or neck veins is an obvious sign of increased intrathoracic pressure and indicates the need to breathe out more slowly.
3. Sitting up, the patient is now told to sniff slowly, increasing aeration of the lung bases. Fast, gasping breaths do not aerate mucus-filled areas of the lung but are preferentially directed to the upper thorax and low-resistance areas of the lower thorax. A sufficient column of air behind the mucous plugs is necessary to propel them out of the airways.
4. After three or four repetitions (bending forward and sitting up), the patient may feel the mucus that has mobilized from the distal branches but is told to refrain from coughing until several additional repetitions have escalated even more secretions to the major bronchi. When the patient is ready to cough, she or he must first take a comfortably deep abdominal breath (feeling the abdomen push out against the pillow) and then bend forward to produce a soft, staged, staccato cough, generating an expiratory force sufficient to maintain maximum possible expiratory flow without airway collapse.

SOURCE: Lagerson, J.: "Nursing Care of Patients with Chronic Pulmonary Insufficiency," *Nursing Clinics of North America*, **9**:165–179, March 1974.

5. Measure and record amount and color of sputum.
6. Encourage well-balanced diet with adequate hydration to avoid reinfection.
7. Encourage rest and offer support and encouragement.
8. Have client perform range-of-motion exercises.
9. Provide oral hygiene to help relieve malodorous breath. Use diluted hydrogen peroxide, lemon, glycerin, or other substances.
10. Teach self-care.
    a. Medications: dose, side effects.
    b. Diet: as needed to maintain health and modify weight as indicated.
    c. Coughing and deep-breathing exercises.
    d. Oral and dental hygiene.
    e. Avoidance of environmental irritants.
    f. Follow-up schedule and signs of complications.
11. Counsel about nonsmoking or decreasing alcohol or drug use.

EVALUATION

Outcome Criteria

1. Cough becomes more productive initially; secretions and cough are decreased.
2. Breath sounds are clearing to clear.
3. Temperature and respirations have returned to normal.
4. Client maintains oral and dental hygiene program and coughing and deep breathing regimen.
5. Client is maintaining nutritional plan and is gaining weight.
6. Client is taking medications at appropriate times and in correct amounts, as indicated by chart client is keeping.
7. Client can recall with 85 percent accuracy, either verbally or in writing, the content presented in teaching sessions.
8. Client has reduced number of cigarettes or use of alcohol or drugs.
9. Client can rest and experiences decreased to absent pain, dyspnea, and diminished anxiety.

Complications

1. Chronic pulmonary abscess: development of abscess that is continuously present.
2. Empyema pus in the pleural cavity, due to a lung infection.
3. Shock (see discussion in Chapter 48).
4. Bronchopleural fistula (see Evaluation, complication 6, under *Tuberculosis* in this chapter).
5. Hemorrhage (see discussion in Chapter 48).
6. Brain abscess (see discussion in Chapter 25).

Reevaluation and Follow-up

Establish a specific individualized plan to ensure that complications are overcome (short-term) and that long-term surveillance and necessary interventions are provided.

PLEURISY

DESCRIPTION

Pleurisy is an acute or chronic inflammation of a small part of or the entire surface of the pleura. This condition may occur at the onset or during the course of many pulmonary diseases. The inflammation usually resolves itself with subsidence of the primary disease. Pain develops when the two inflamed pleural walls rub together. *Fibrinous (dry) pleurisy* deposits a fibrinous exudate on the pleural surface. *Serofibrinous (wet) pleurisy* is due to an increase in nonpurulent pleural fluid and may result in pleural effusion.

PREVENTION

Health Promotion

1. Avoidance of exposure to respiratory infection.
2. Maintenance of good health habits (diet, rest, exercise, etc.).
3. Avoidance of trauma.

Population at Risk

Clients with pneumonia, tuberculosis, pulmonary infarction, neoplasm, chest trauma, thoracotomy, pericarditis, or lung abscess.

Screening

Chest x-ray study.

ASSESSMENT

Health History

1. History of pneumonia, tuberculosis, pulmonary infarction, neoplasm, chest trauma, thoracotomy, pericarditis, or lung abscess.
2. Health maintenence patterns: smoking, diet, activity, etc.

Physical Assessment

1. General appearance: pallor and anxiety.
2. Chest motion limited on affected side: decreased chest excursion.
3. Lying on affected side: splinting; cough present.
4. Shallow, rapid breathing.
5. Occasional hemoptysis with coughing.
6. Pleuritic pain may be present.
7. Pain: varies from intercostal tenderness to severe, sharp knifelike chest pain, usually near the lower half of the thorax, especially on inspiration. The pain is augmented by coughing or sneezing and is minimal or absent when breath is held. It may be referred to upper abdomen and along costal margins. Neck and shoulder pain may be present with diaphragmatic pleurisy.
8. Temperature: high fever usually present.
9. Percussion: dullness due to the presence of increased fluid.
10. Breath sounds: diminished; pleural friction rub is heard 28–48 h after the onset of pleurisy. Auscultated on inspiration and expiration.
11. Heart sounds: pleural-pericordial rub auscultated.

Diagnostic Tests

1. Chest x-ray films reveal areas of consolidation.
2. Sputum examination identifies pathogen.
3. Pleural biopsy rules out metastases.
4. Increased WBC (leukocytosis).
5. Thoracentesis with removal of pleural fluid for examination.

NURSING DIAGNOSES: ACTUAL OR POTENTIAL

1. Alteration in comfort: pain secondary to pleurisy.
2. Respiratory dysfunction; dyspnea, diminished respiratory excursion.
3. Anxiety (mild to moderate): intensified by pain and dyspnea.
4. Decreased activity tolerence: due to dyspnea, fatigue.
5. Depletion of body fluids: secondary to inflammatory response, fever.
6. Knowledge deficit: due to lack of information about disease process.

EXPECTED OUTCOMES

1. Client will be able to rest when anxiety has diminished and pain has decreased.
2. Respirations and temperature will return to normal.
3. Client will have an increase in nutritional and fluid intake as exercise and malaise decrease.
4. Client will understand information taught in teaching sessions, as evidenced by 85 percent accuracy, verbally or in writing, on tests.
5. Client will give evidence of compliance with care plan by:
   a. Adhering to medication regimen, as indicated by chart maintained by client.
   b. Establishing and maintaining proper nutritional, hydration, rest, and exercise patterns.
   c. Maintaining follow-up schedule, being aware of long healing process, and observing for signs of complication.
   d. Reducing number of cigarettes smoked.
   e. Other outcomes will relate to primary disease.

INTERVENTIONS

1. Administer analgesics that reduce pain.
2. Assess vital signs.
3. Apply heat or cold over area of pain to reduce inflammation and to relieve discomfort.
4. Provide chest physiotherapy.
5. Splint rib cage when client coughs.
6. Encourage client to cough and breathe deeply to rid the body of secretions.
7. Provide restful environment; prevent stressful situations that may increase energy consumption.
8. Instruct client to lie on affected side to prevent organisms from traveling to the unaffected side.
9. Assist with procaine intercostal block (used to relieve pain).
10. Offer fluids for hydration and a well-balanced diet to maintain body weight and to help liquefy secretions.
11. Provide reassurance; be supportive to relieve anxiety.
12. Teach about:
    a. Medications: dose, side effects.
    b. Diet and hydration: as needed to maintain health.

c. Rest and activity to help maintain resistance.
d. Follow-up schedule and signs of complications.
13. Counsel about nonsmoking.

EVALUATION

Outcome Criteria

1. Client is able to rest and partake in activities as pain and anxiety decrease.
2. Breath sounds are clearing to clear.
3. Client maintains nutritional, fluid, rest, and exercise patterns.
4. Client takes medications at appropriate times and in correct amounts, as indicated by chart he or she keeps.
5. Client recalls with 85 percent accuracy, either verbally or in writing, the content presented in teaching sessions.
6. Client has reduced number of cigarettes smoked.

Complications

PLEURAL EFFUSION

Assessment

1. Shortness of breath.
2. Localized chest pain.
3. Decreased local expansion of chest wall.
4. Dull percussion; absence of breath sounds; pleural friction rub.
5. Increased pulse.
6. Pallor.
7. Prostration.
8. High fever.
9. Dry cough.

Revised Outcomes

1. Oxygenation will be restored; dyspnea and discomfort will decrease.
2. Other outcomes are as originally stated under Expected Outcomes above.

Interventions

1. Assist with thoracentesis and insertion of intercostal drainage tube (Figures 31-3 and 31-4).
2. Monitor chest drainage.
3. Check vital signs and breath sounds.
4. Provide chest physiotherapy and splint chest when client is coughing.
5. Offer frequent oral hygiene.
6. Provide range-of-motion exercises.
7. Provide skin care.

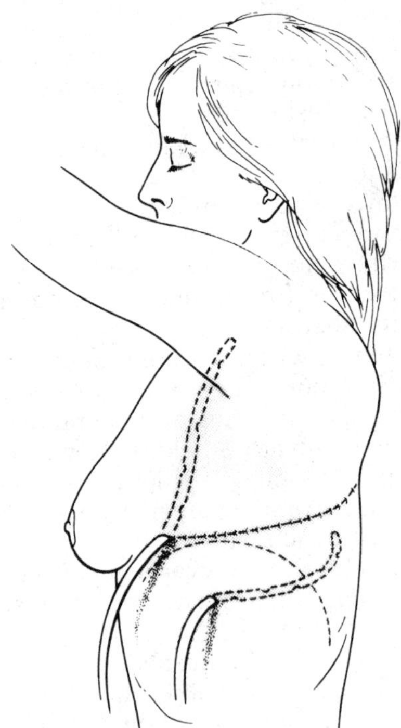

Figure 31-3 Chest tube. (Jones, D. A., Dunbar, C. F., and Jirovec, M. M.: *Medical-Surgical Nursing: A Conceptual Approach,* McGraw-Hill, New York, 1978.)

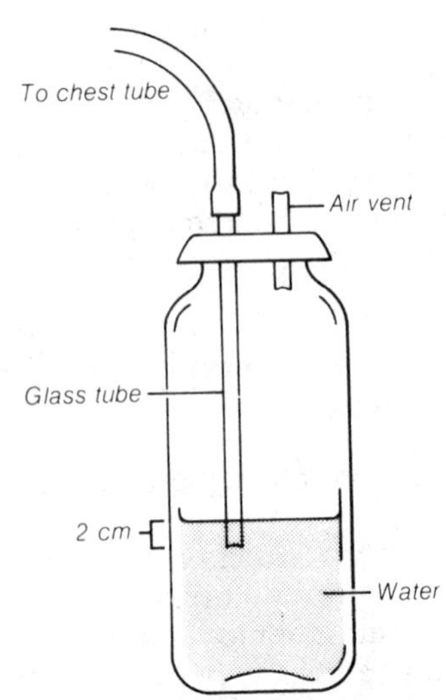

Figure 31-4 Single-bottle, closed, water seal drainage system. (Jones, D. A., Dunbar, C. F., and Jirovec, M. M.: *Medical-Surgical Nursing: A Conceptual Approach,* McGraw-Hill, New York, 1978.)

8. Encourage well-balanced diet with adequate hydration.

CHRONIC ADHESIVE PLEURITIS

Assessment
Marked pleural thickening.
Revised Outcomes
Oxygenation will be restored when thickened pleura is removed.
Interventions
Surgical: *decortication*—removal of thickened pleura.
Reevaluation and Follow-up
Long-term surveillance is necessary and follow-up should be instituted as necessary.

RHINITIS

DESCRIPTION

Rhinitis is an acute or chronic inflammation of the mucous membrane of the nose. Common causes of rhinitis include infection, allergic reaction, or nonallergic reaction.

1. Viral infection is common and is a manifestation of the common cold, influenzal infections of the upper respiratory tract, or a bacterial infection, elsewhere in the body, that invaded the nasal mucosa. At first there is transient vasoconstriction followed by dilation, edema, and increased activity of the seromucinous glands and goblet cells.
2. Allergic reaction.
3. Nonallergic reaction is chronic, intermittent nasal obstruction or nasal stuffiness resulting from nervous tension, repeated respiratory infections, exposure to noxious materials, deviated septum, or polyps.

PREVENTION

Health Promotion

1. Avoidance of dusty, crowded rooms and environmental irritants.
2. Avoidance of abrupt changes in temperature, humidity, and ventilation.
3. Maintenance of natural resistance (diet, rest, exercise, etc.).
4. Avoidance of persons with upper respiratory infection (URI).
5. Avoidance of smoking.
6. Prevention of spread of infection by using medical asepsis.

Population at Risk

1. Persons with nasal obstruction (deviated septum, enlarged adenoids, polyps).
2. Persons with decreased natural resistance due to fatigue, lack of exercise, or poor nutritional intake.
3. Persons with exposure to environmental irritants and climate changes.
4. Persons suffering from renal, hepatic, or blood disorders; diabetes; or endocrine diseases.
5. Children are most frequently affected while their immunity is gradually being acquired.

ASSESSMENT

Health History

1. Peak incidence: late October, early January, and March.
2. Exposure to climate changes or environmental irritants.
3. Complaints of burning and irritation with discharge and obstruction of nasal passage.
4. General malaise, chills, slight fever, headache, sneezing, and watery eyes.
5. Complaints of disturbance in voice patterns and sense of smells.
6. Health maintenance patterns: smoking, rest, nutrition, exercise altered.

Physical Assessment

1. Headache and general malaise may be present.
2. Tearing of the eyes may be present.
3. Catarrh, crusting of membrane with fetid odor (ozena), hoarseness, and disturbed sense of smell.
4. Frequent sneezing; drainage from the nose is usually clear.
5. If fever is present, the client may be pale and warm to the touch.
6. Disturbances of sense of smell may be reported.
7. Inspection of nasal chamber reveals:
   a. Edematous mucous membranes: complaints of congestion.
   b. Nasopharynx smooth and glistening.
   c. Posterior turbinates enlarged and possibly intruding into nasopharynx.
   d. Abnormal amount of connective tissue,

hypertrophy of nasal septum, atrophy of membrane and cartilage (chronic rhinitis).
e. Caseosa: accumulation of offensive cheeselike masses with serous purulent discharge.

Diagnostic Tests

1. Rhinoscopic exam: examination of the nasal chamber. This test will reveal reddened, swollen membranes.
2. Blood work when infection is present may include:
   a. Leukocytosis.
   b. Slight rise in sedimentation rate.

NURSING DIAGNOSES: ACTUAL OR POTENTIAL

1. Respiratory dysfunction. Impairment of mucous membrane of nose.
2. Alteration in comfort: discomfort secondary to congestion.
3. Alteration in sense of smell and voice pattern.
4. Depletion of body fluids (potential).

EXPECTED OUTCOMES

1. Client will be able to breathe through clear nasal passages with decreased swelling and congestion in 3 to 7 days.
2. Client will be able to rest with minimal discomfort from congested, irritated mucous membranes.
3. Body temperature will return to normal in 5 to 10 days.
4. Voice pattern and sense of smell will return to normal.
5. Client will meet hydration and nutritional needs.
6. Spread of infection will be prevented. Client will maintain medical asepsis at all times.
7. Client will understand information taught in teaching sessions.
8. Client will give evidence of compliance with care plan by:
   a. Adhering to medication regimen, as indicated by chart maintained by client.
   b. Avoiding persons with URI, environmental irritants.
   c. Maintaining natrual resistance by rest, nutrition, exercise, and so on.
   d. Blowing nose with correct technique.
   e. Maintaining medical asepsis.
   f. Reducing the number of cigarettes smoked.
   g. Being aware of signs of complications.

INTERVENTIONS

1. Provide restful environment with increased humidity.
2. Offer adequate fluids and well-balanced diet.
3. Administer prescribed antipyretics, antihistamines, analgesics, and aspirin to help relieve inflammation, congestion, and discomfort.
4. Teach about:
   a. Blowing nose with mouth slightly open, through both nostrils at the same time, not too frequently or too hard.
   b. Medications: dose, side effects.
   c. Medical asepsis to prevent spread of infection.
   d. Proper rest, nutrition, hydration, and exercise to help maintain natural resistance.
   e. Avoidance of persons with URI, environmental irritants, and climate changes.
   f. Signs of complications.
5. Counsel about nonsmoking.

EVALUATION

Outcome Criteria

1. Nasal congestion and swelling decrease.
2. Temperature is normal.
3. Discomfort is diminished, as evidenced by relief of congestion, discharge, fever, and malaise.
4. Hoarseness and disturbed sense of smell have disappeared.
5. Client reports taking medications at appropriate times and in correct amounts.
6. Client recalls with 85 percent accuracy, either verbally or in writing, the content presented in teaching sessions.
7. Client has reduced the number of cigarettes smoked.
8. Client is adhering to medical asepsis techniques.

Complications

1. Sinusitis (see the following discussion).
2. Otitis media (see the discussion in Chapter 26).
3. Bronchitis (see the discussion later in this chapter).

4. Pneumonia (see the discussion in this chapter).

Reevaluation and Follow-up
Long-term follow-up and necessary appointments made as needed.

SINUSITIS

DESCRIPTION

Sinusitis is an inflammatory reaction of the sinus mucosa to the retention of secretions or the presence of allergens or pathogens. The disorder is referred to as *ethmoid, frontal, maxillary,* or *sphenoid* sinusitis or, if they all are involved, *pansinusitis.* Because the nasal and sinus mucous membranes are continuous, infections spread rapidly from the nasal passages to the sinuses (Figure 31-5).

Typical causes of sinusitis include viral infections, dental infections, allergic rhinitis, and inadequate drainage due to obstructions (polyps, deviated septum, enlarged turbinates), as well as changes in intranasal pressures. Sinusitis (especially chronic sinusitis) occurs more commonly in cold, wet climates. Persons who have dental conditions, facial fractures, deviated septum, or nasal polyps are more apt to develop sinusitis. Persons who swim and dive are prone to develop sinusitis.

Acute sinusitis is usually resolved within 10 to 14 days with treatment. Complications such as abscess and osteomyelitis rarely occur because of the use of antibiotics.

When the ostium (sinus opening) is obstructed (nasal polyps, deviated septum, swollen mucous membrane), the air (oxygen) in the sinuses is absorbed. The negative pressure that results causes pain over the sinus region. In the presence of the negative pressure, transudate from the mucous membrane fills the sinus and serves as a medium for bacterial growth. Subsequently there is an outpouring of leukocytes, and the mucous membranes evidence hyperemia and edema changing pressure.

PREVENTION

Health Promotion

1. Maintenance of natural resistance (rest, nutrition, exercise, etc.).
2. Avoidance of upper respiratory infections (URI) and exposure to cold and dampness; prompt treatment of colds and flu.
3. Abstinence from smoking.
4. Yearly dental exams to detect periodontal conditions and apical abscesses.
5. Daily oral hygiene to prevent dental infections and periodontal disease.
6. Treatment of underlying allergic disorders.
7. Control of exposure to allergens.
8. Correction of conditions such as nasal polyps and deviated septum.

Population at Risk

1. Persons who have nasal polyps and/or deviated septum.
2. Persons who have dental conditions (molar

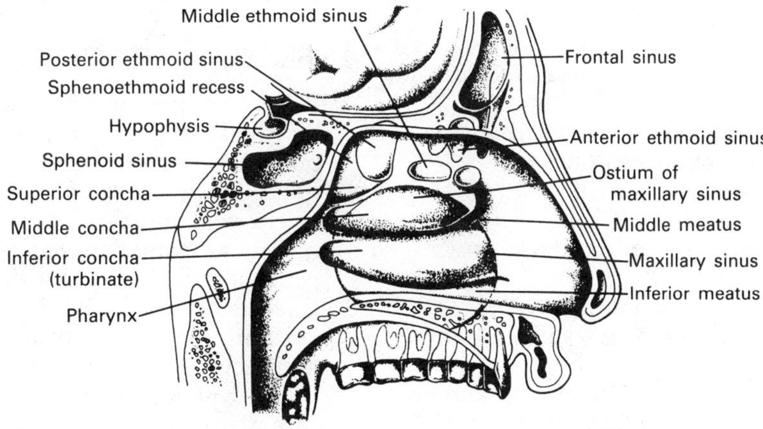

Figure 31-5 Sagittal section of the nasal cavity showing anatomy of the sinuses.

extraction, apical abscess, peridontal disease).
3. Persons who have facial fractures or maxillofacial deformities.
4. Persons who swim and dive in contaminated water.
5. Persons who are exposed to changes in atmospheric conditions (cold, dampness, humidity, dryness).
6. Smokers and those who are exposed to smoke.

Screening

1. Nares exam with speculum.
2. Transillumination of sinuses.

ASSESSMENT

Health History

1. Health patterns: rest, nutrition, exercise.
2. Habits: smoking, snuff, drugs (e.g., cocaine).
3. Preceding URI; exposure to cold and dampness.
4. Season: often associated with allergic rhinitis.
5. Presence of other conditions: nasal polyps, deviated septum, facial fractures, maxillofacila deformities.
6. History of dental conditions: recent molar extraction; apical abscess, periodontal disease.
7. Residence: more common in cold, damp climate.
8. Recent air travel.

Physical Assessment

1. Nasal chamber exam may reveal:
   a. Blood-tinged, purulent mucous.
   b. Enlarged turbinates.
   c. Mucosa that is hyperemic and edematous (a vasoconstrictor may be used to shrink turbinates).
   d. Deviated septum (not always present).
   e. Nasal polyps (not always present).
2. Nasopharynx exam may reveal:
   a. Inflamed mucosa.
   b. Purulent secretions, often thick, green-yellow.
3. Paranasal sinus examination may reveal:
   a. Tenderness over involved sinus (a constant finding).
   b. Swelling over involved sinus: right and/or left nasal cavity or orbital area.
4. Person's temperature is usually only slightly elevated 37.22°–37.50°C (99°–99.5°F).

Diagnostic Tests

1. Transillumination of the sinuses: decreased light transmission may indicate mucosal thickening or the presence of fluid in the cavity.
2. Culture and sensitivity of secretions to identify involved organisms: common organisms include *Streptococcus pneumoniae, Streptococcus, Staphylococcus, Hemophilus influenzae, Klebsiella*.
3. X-ray exam reveals:
   a. Cloudy appearance.
   b. Air–fluid level (not always seen).
4. A-mode ultrasound examination: used to confirm the presence of fluid within the maxillary sinus (also used in differentiating solid tumors from fluid-filled sinuses that often present similar radiographic appearances) (Isaacson and Edell, 1978).
5. White blood count is usually within normal limits; leukopenia (5,000 to 6,000) is common.

NURSING DIAGNOSES: ACTUAL OR POTENTIAL

1. Respiratory dysfunction: secondary to inflammatory and increased accumulation of secretions in sinuses.
2. Alteration in comfort: pain/discomfort secondary to changes in upper respiratory system.
3. Nutritional alteration: (potential) weight loss secondary to anorexia, malaise, and purulent secretions.
4. Disturbed sleep pattern: difficulty sleeping at night secondary to changes in upper respiratory system.

EXPECTED OUTCOMES

1. Pain/discomfort will be relieved, as indicated by client's ability to rest and sleep.
2. Sinus congestion will be decreased, as evidenced by increased flow of mucus via nares.
3. Client will meet hydration and nutritional needs, as demonstrated by gradual weight gain (or no additional weight loss).
4. Client will understand information taught in teaching sessions, as evidenced by 85 percent accuracy verbally or in writing.
5. Client will give evidence of compliance with care plan by:
   a. Maintaining natural resistance (rest, nutrition, exercise, etc.).

b. Adhering to medication regimen, as indicated by chart maintained by client.
c. Reducing the number of cigarettes smoked by one-half within 2 weeks after discharge.
d. Avoiding cold, damp areas, overcrowded areas, and environmental pollution.
e. Seeking consultation for management (surgery: removal of nasal polyps, repair of deviated septum or desensitization).
f. Blowing nose with caution (not too often and not too vigorously).
g. Using steam inhalations and hydration to relieve edema and congestion.
h. Adhering to follow-up schedule and being aware of signs of complications.

INTERVENTIONS

1. Administer prescribed analgesics to reduce pain/discomfort.
2. Administer prescribed antihistamines, vasoconstrictors (nose drops/nasal spray, 2 percent ephedrine, 0.25 percent phenylephrine, and antibiotics to relieve congestion, promote removal of secretions, and prevent infection.
3. Provide a quiet environment for rest; use Fowler's position to promote drainage and relieve edema.
4. Provide soothing steam inhalations and warm, moist packs.
5. Provide oral hygiene and warm gargles; increase the amount of fluids and use good mouth care to prevent infection.
6. Provide a nutritious, appealing diet that is easy to chew and swallow.
7. Teach about:
   a. Medications: dose and side effects.
   b. Administering nose drops and nose sprays.
   c. Proper rest, diet, and exercise to help maintain natural resistance.
   d. Avoidance of damp, cold areas, overcrowded areas, areas of high humidity and environmental pollution (including tobacco smoke).
   e. Follow-up schedule and signs of complications.
9. Counsel about not smoking.

EVALUATION

Outcome Criteria

1. Pain/discomfort diminishes, as indicated by ability to rest and sleep.
2. Sinus congestion decreases, as evidenced by increased mucus drainage.
3. Client has gained 2 lb during the past week.
4. Client is taking medications at appropriate times and in correct amounts, as indicated by chart he or she keeps.
5. Client recalls with 85 percent accuracy, either verbally or in writing, the content presented in teaching sessions.
6. Client has reduced the number of cigarettes smoked to one-half pack per day.
7. Client uses steam inhalations and hydration at recommended times, as indicated by chart the client is keeping.
8. Client has secured consultation regarding management, as evidenced by consultant's report.

CHRONIC SINUSITIS

Chronic sinusitis is a sinus infection that extends over months or years (see Figure 31-6).

Assessment

1. Pain, tenderness over the involved sinus.
2. Headaches: pattern usually determined by sinus involved.
3. Purulent nasal discharge.
4. Fever (low grade) and malaise.
5. Foul breath.

Revised Outcomes

1. Sinus congestion and pressure will be reduced when sinus cavity is surgically drained.
2. Other goals are as originally stated under Expected Outcomes above.

Interventions

Refer to Table 31-11.

1. Administer antibiotics intravenously.
2. Assist with surgical drainage of involved sinus.
3. Monitor condition after drainage procedure.

Reevaluation and Follow-up

As needed.

ORBITAL CELLULITIS

This is a condition of diffuse inflammation of periorbital tissues that occurs when the infectious process extends through the lateral ethmoid sinus wall.

Assessment

1. Edema, inflammation of eyelids and inner canthus.
2. Chills.
3. Elevated temperature.

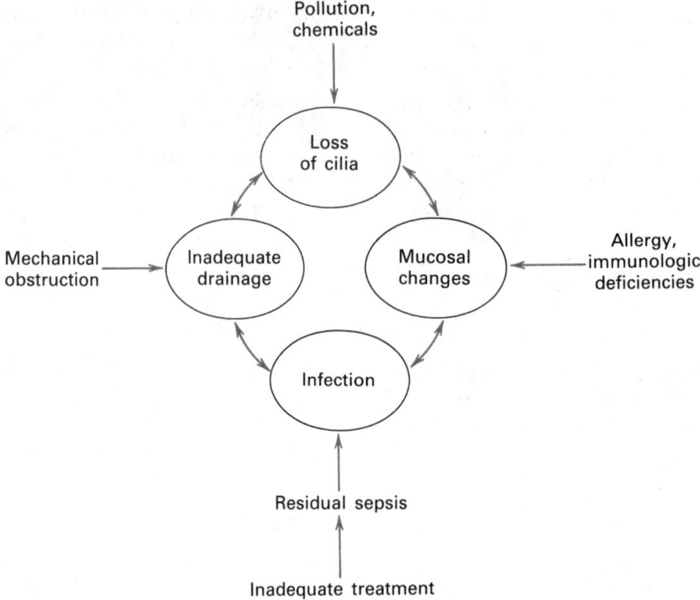

Figure 31-6 Cycle of events leading to chronic sinusitis. (Adams, G. L., Boies, L. R., and Paparella, M. M.: *Boies' Fundamentals of Otolaryngology,* 5th ed., Saunders, Philadelphia, 1978, p. 400.)

4. Painful eye movements.
5. Chemosis (red, edematous, thickened conjunctiva).

Revised Outcomes

1. Chills and elevated temperature will cease.
2. Edema of eyelids, painful eye movements, and chemosis will diminish.
3. Other outcomes are as originally stated above.

Interventions

1. Administer intravenous antibiotics.
2. Administer analgesics as needed.
3. Apply warm, moist compresses.

Reevaluation and Follow-up

As needed.

ORBITAL ABSCESS

This is the extention of the infectious process into orbital tissues.

Assessment

1. Orbital pain.
2. Exophthalmos.
3. Limited movement of eye globe.
4. Edema of eyelids and inner canthus.
5. Elevated temperature.
6. Elevated WBC (10,000 to 20,000).
7. Culture of nasal secretions, conjunctiva, blood.
8. Nasal exam.
9. Ultrasonic exam to assess medial orbit.
10. CT scan to determine extent of abscess in posterior orbit and to ascertain overall dimension of abscess.

Revised Outcomes

1. Orbital pain will cease.
2. Edema of eye tissues, exophthalmos, and limited eye movements will be resolved.
3. Other outcomes are as originally stated above.

Interventions

1. Administer intravenous antibiotics (ampicillin, penicillin, cephalothin).
2. Administer analgesics as needed.
3. Assist with incision and drainage.
4. Monitor temperature, WBC.
5. Monitor visual acuity.

Reevaluation and Follow-up

As needed.

TABLE 31-11 PROCEDURES USED IN THE MANAGEMENT OF CHRONIC SUPPURATIVE SINUSITIS

Sinus	Procedure
Maxillary	*Antral irrigation:* the wall of the maxillary sinus is punctured and the cavity is irrigated with normal saline. *Antral window:* a window is made through the lateral wall of the nose under the inferior turbinate. This window allows retained pus to drain into the nose by gravity. *Caldwell-Luc operation:* through an antral window, all of the diseased mucosa and periosteum is removed.
Ethmoid	*Ethmoidectomy* (intranasal or external): removal of ethmoid air cells, all infected tissue, and the medial wall of the orbit, *or* the lateral wall of the nose medial to the ethmoid area.
Frontal	*Frontoethmoidectomy:* the floor of the frontal sinus is excised to remove *all* of the lining mucosa of the frontal sinus. (The ethmoid air cells are always removed when the frontal sinus is exenterated in order to provide adequate drainage.)

SOURCE: DeWeese, D. D., and Saunders, W. H.: *Textbook of Otolaryngology*, 6th ed., Mosby, St. Louis, 1982, pp. 241–249.

TONSILLITIS (ACUTE)

Tonsillitis is an inflammation of the tonsils or lymphatic tissue mass located on the lateral walls of the oropharynx. It is the most common form of streptococcal infection in human beings. Its incubation period is 3 to 5 days. As the process develops, a general inflammation and swelling of the tonsil tissue is noted. There is also an accumulation of leukocytes, dead epithelial cells, and pathogenic bacteria in the tonsillar crypts. The tonsils are usually spotted and may be covered with a gray-yellow exudate.

Often group A beta-hemolytic streptococci are the cause; however, pneumococci, staphylococci, and hemolytic influenza can also be involved. Acute tonsillitis is endemic in most areas; however, it occurs more commonly during the colder months, especially in children and young adults. Acute tonsillitis may be epidemic in military recruits.

Although discomfort and malaise may be noted for 48–72 h, acute tonsillitis usually subsides in 7 to 10 days if the person rests and follows the prescription.

Refer to Chapter 20 for a discussion of tonsillitis in children.

ACUTE TRACHEOBRONCHITIS

DESCRIPTION

Acute tracheobronchitis is an acute inflammation of the mucous membranes of the trachea and the bronchial tree. Tracheobronchitis may be caused by extension of an upper respiratory tract infection (URI) or exposure to pollution (dust, fumes, smoke). This precipitating factor causes temporary impairment of the cilia, thus permitting bacterial invasion and the subsequent accumulation of mucopurulent exudate and cellular debris.

The disorder occurs most often in the winter months and in persons who are cigarette smokers and/or who have chronic pulmonary disease. Usually the disorder is self-limiting, with eventual complete healing and return of function. Although tracheobronchitis may be a minor disorder for most persons, it can be life-threatening to persons who have chronic pulmonary or cardiac disease.

PREVENTION

Health Promotion

1. Avoidance of exposure to individuals who have URI.

2. Reduced exposure to pollution and occupational dusts.
3. Use of masks (or other protection devices) when exposed to dust, smoke, or fumes.
4. Avoidance of smoking.

Population at Risk

1. Persons who have URI.
2. Persons who have continual exposure to pollutants (e.g., dust, smoke, fumes).
3. Smokers (mild to heavy).

Screening

Not applicable.

ASSESSMENT

Health History

1. Presence of URI.
2. Exposure to pollutants or other irritants that may stimulate an inflammatory response.
3. Chest tightness may be present.

Physical Assessment

1. Erythema of pharynx: dryness and laryngitis may be present.
2. Anterior cervical lymphadenopathy is usually present.
3. Rhonchi are usually heard. Cough may be productive. Sputum may be thick.
4. Wheezing may be heard upon auscultation. Moist rales are usually heard at the lung base.
5. Fever and general malaise are present.

Diagnostic Tests

1. Chest x-ray study to rule out bronchopneumonia.
2. Sputum culture to determine whether infection is present and, if so, to identify the pathogen.
3. Increased leukocytes.

NURSING DIAGNOSES: ACTUAL OR POTENTIAL

1. Respiratory dysfunction (mild to severe).
2. Alteration in comfort: discomfort secondary to substernal tightness and pleuritic pain.
3. Alteration in body fluids: decrease secondary to potential decreased intake and fever 38.33–38.89°C (101°–102°F).

EXPECTED OUTCOMES

1. Body temperature will return to normal within 2 to 3 days of initiation of regimen.
2. Ability to rest and be comfortable will increase, as evidenced by relief of pain and fever and control of coughing.
3. Extension of infection will be prevented.
4. Client will meet hydration and nutritional needs by demonstrating adequate urine output and no weight loss.
5. Productivity of cough will increase to remove secretions from lungs (initial). Client will have diminished coughing and sputum production, as evidenced by clearing breath sounds within 3 to 4 days of initiation of treatment.
6. Client will understand information taught in teaching sessions, as evidenced by 85 percent accuracy, verbally or in writing.
7. Client will give evidence of adherence to care plan by:
   a. Adhering to medication regimen, as indicated by chart maintained by client.
   b. Reducing the number of cigarettes by one-half within 2 weeks of illness episode.
   c. Using cold steam inhalations.
   d. Adhering to fluid intake schedule as recommended.
   e. Adhering to follow-up schedule and being aware of signs of complications.

INTERVENTIONS

1. Administer prescribed antibiotics, expectorants, and analgesics to reduce infection, promote removal of secretions, and control discomfort.
2. Provide a quiet, nonstimulating environment conducive to rest.
3. Provide frequent mouth care to prevent halitosis and mucosal dryness. These measures increase the appeal of fluids and food.
4. Assess vital signs and breath sounds frequently to evaluate client's progress.
5. Provide fluids and diet as tolerated.
6. Give soothing inhalations (humidify inspired air).
7. Teach about:
   a. Medications: dose, side effects.
   b. Diet: as needed to maintain health and modify weight.
   c. Rest and activity to help maintain resistance to other infections and increase stamina.
8. Counsel about not smoking.

EVALUATION

Outcome Criteria

1. Cough becomes more productive initially; then secretions and coughing decrease.
2. Breath sounds are clearing to clear; wheezing is diminished.
3. Temperature, pulse, and respirations are within normal range, as indicated on chart kept by client.
4. Pain has diminished, as evidenced by increased activity and decreased need for analgesics.
5. Client takes medications at appropriate times and in correct amounts, as indicated by chart client is keeping.
6. Client recalls with 85 percent accuracy, either verbally or in writing, the content presented in teaching sessions.
7. Client has reduced the number of cigarettes smoked to one-half pack per day.

Complications

1. Bronchopneumonia (see the discussion in this chapter).
2. Respiratory insufficiency (see Complications under *Chronic Bronchitis*).

Reevaluation and Follow-up

Short-term surveillance and necessary interventions should be provided as needed.

PHARYNGITIS (ACUTE)

DESCRIPTION

Acute pharyngitis is a common inflammation of the pharyngeal wall. Initially the walls of the pharynx show evidence of hyperemia and edema, then secretions are noted. The secretions change from serous to thicker mucoid and often become dry and adhere to the wall. The adjacent lymphoid tissue, the tonsils, or the lymphoid follicles (on the posterior pharyngeal wall) become inflamed and swollen.

Acute pharyngitis may be viral in origin or may be caused by organisms such as streptococci, staphylococci, pneumococci, or the influenza bacillus. The problem occurs in all age groups. It may arise by extension from tonsils, nose, or sinuses, or from common cold, infected teeth, or other disorders involving the oral cavity. Unless there is a secondary infection, the symptoms usually remain mild and resolve within 4 to 6 days.

PREVENTION

Health Promotion

1. Maintenance of natural resistance (rest, nutrition, etc.).
2. Avoidance of upper respiratory infections (URI) and exposure to cold and dampness.
3. Avoidance of smoking.

Population at Risk

1. Persons who have poor health habits (rest, nutrition, exercise, etc.).
2. Smokers (mild or heavy).
3. Persons with exposure to cold, damp weather.
4. Persons living in overcrowded areas.

Screening

Examination of throat.

ASSESSMENT

Health History

1. Health patterns: smoking, rest, nutrition, and so on.
2. Exposure to cold and dampness.
3. Season: increased susceptibility in winter.
4. History of mild sore throat with some difficulty in swallowing.
5. History of referred pain to ear.

Physical Assessment

1. An examination of the throat will reveal:
   a. Hyperemic, edematous mucosa (vesicle formation, herpes, strongly suggests a viral cause).
   b. Exudate usually present.
2. Anterior an posterior lymphadenopathy.
3. Temperature elevation.

Diagnostic Tests

1. Examination of the throat.
2. Throat culture and sensitivity to identify causative organisms.
   a. Streptococcal (group A beta hemolytic) is common.
   b. Staphylococcal tends to occur in debilitated persons.

NURSING DIAGNOSES: ACTUAL OR POTENTIAL

1. Alteration in comfort: pain due to sore throat, fever, headache.
2. Body fluid loss (potential): due to fever.

3. Nutritional alteration (potential): secondary to dysphagia.
4. Respiratory dysfunction: cough.
5. Decreased activity tolerence: fatigue.
6. Altered communication: secondary to throat discomfort.
7. Knowledge deficit: regarding pharyngitis.

EXPECTED OUTCOMES

1. Pharyngeal mucosal congestion and discomfort will diminish within a few days of treatment, as evidenced by ability to swallow with ease.
2. Headache and muscle and joint discomfort will be reduced within a few days of treatment, as evidenced by reduced need for analgesics.
3. Temperature will return to normal within a few days of treatment.
4. Client will meet hydration needs, as demonstrated by absence of tenting and an adequate urine output.
5. Client will meet nutritional needs, as evidenced by no weight loss.
6. Client will understand information taught in teaching sessions, as evidenced by 85 percent accuracy, verbally or in writing.
7. Client will give evidence of compliance with therapeutic plan by achieving an improved health state.

INTERVENTIONS

1. Administer nasal decongestants to relieve edema and congestion (e.g., Actifed, dimetapp, Chlortrimeton).
2. Administer analgesics to reduce headache and muscle and joint pain.
3. Administer antibiotics (e.g., penicillin) in the presence of group A beta streptococcus.
4. Apply lubricant to lips to prevent cracking and potential herpes.
5. Provide a warm, nonstimulating environment for rest and sleep.
6. Provide fluids and soft foods that are thermally, chemically, and mechanically nonirritating.
7. Provide steam inhalation to help loosen secretions and prevent dryness of the pharynx.
8. Use/teach oral hygiene to lubricate the mucosa and prevent halitosis; encourage saline gargles.
9. Provide lozenges with topical anesthetic.
10. Counsel not to smoke.
11. Arrange for follow-up.
12. Counsel regarding potential need for tonsillectomy and/or adenoidectomy, depending upon the number of streptococcal infections and whether client still has tonsils.

EVALUATION

Outcome Criteria

1. Pharyngeal mucosal congestion and discomfort are alleviated.
2. Hoarseness is alleviated, as evidenced by ability to communicate in normal tone of voice.
3. Throat discomfort has diminished, as demonstrated by ability to swallow liquids and soft foods.
4. Body temperature returns to normal.
5. Client is taking medications at appropriate times and in correct amounts, as indicated by chart client is keeping.
6. Client has a normal amount of urine output.
7. Client has not lost weight; normal weight is maintained.
8. Client's lips and oral mucosa are moist and lubricated.
9. Client reports reduction in the number of cigarettes being smoked.
10. Client can recall with 85 percent accuracy, either verbally or in writing, the content presented in teaching sessions.

Complications

1. Otitis media (see the discussion in Chapter 26).
2. Sinusitis (see *Sinusitis*).
3. Rheumatic fever (see *Rheumatic Heart Disease* in Chapter 30).
4. Acute glomerulonephritis (see Chapter 32).

Reevaluation and Follow-up

Establish a specific individualized plan to ensure that any complications are overcome. Follow-up assessment scheduled.

LARYNGITIS

Laryngitis is an inflammation of the larynx. Common causes of laryngitis include (1) an infection involving the vocal cords, (2) an upper respiratory infection, and (3) straining the voice. Laryngitis may also be associated with infections such as measles, diphtheria, bronchitis, pneumonia, and influenza. The inhalation of irritation substances or toxic fumes is also known to cause laryngitis.

Laryngitis is common in all age groups. It is often associated with paninfection involving the sinus, ear, larynx, and bronchial tubes. When acute laryngitis occurs in conjunction with another disorder, it usually resolves with the primary disorder.

Individuals should avoid upper respiratory infections as well as smoking and inhalation of irritants.

For a complete discussion of nursing care, refer to *Pharyngitis* in this chapter. (Refer to Chapter 20 for additional information.)

HERPES SIMPLEX

Herpes simplex is a vesicular eruption, or "cold sore," that develops on the lips, on the skin around the mouth, and/or on the oral mucosa. Initially the lesion appears as small, clear vesicles that rupture and form shallow ulcers. An area of inflammation surrounds the weeping ulcer, which gradually forms a crust.

Cold sores are associated with the herpes simplex virus (*Herpesvirus hominis*, HVH). It is estimated that 70 to 90 percent of the population have experienced a primary episode by the age of 14. It is thought that the virus remains dormant in the skin or nerve ganglia. The herpes virus tends to be activated when the person's resistance is lowered. Approximately 50 percent of the adult population may be vulnerable. In many instances the triggering agent is unknown; however, common precipitants include sunlight, fever, colds, food allergies, abrasion of the lips, and dental trauma. Lesions generally last for 7 to 10 days. Secondary infection is a threat.

TRAUMA

Chest trauma refers to those injuries sustained in major traffic or industrial accidents or in attempted suicide or homicide. Trauma may damage the chest walls, lungs, heart, great vessels, and other mediastinal structures and may be penetrating or nonpenetrating. Trauma to the lung reduces oxygen and carbon dioxide exchange due to destruction of the parenchyma and respiratory units. This can lead to hypoxia and hypercapnia.

PNEUMOTHORAX

DESCRIPTION

Pneumothorax refers to the collapse of a lung due to collection of air in the thorax, When air collects within the intrapleural space, it is called a *closed pneumothorax*. *Spontaneous pneumothorax* results when there is a rupture of an emphysematous bleb on the pleural surface. *Tension pneumothorax* occurs because of an open chest wound with a flap that acts as a one-way valve; air entering on inspiration is unable to escape on expiration, and the lung collapses as intrathoracic tension increases. *Hemothorax* results from pulmonary laceration or torn intercostal blood vessels. This causes blood to accumulate in the chest cavity, thus compressing the lung. A flail chest will result from multiple fractures of one or more ribs in different places (see Figure 31-7).

Pneumothorax can result from penetrating chest wounds caused by stabbing, bullets, or any missile moving at a high speed. Nonpenetrating injuries to the chest wall include fractured ribs, electric shock, drowning, blast injuries, or alteration in barometric pressure (see Figure 31-8). Such injuries are potentially life-threatening because multiple organs may be affected and the cardiopulmonary processes may be disturbed. Because the trauma results in pressure change, the expansion of the unaffected lung is affected and there may be shifting back and forth of the collapsed lung and mediastinum. This shifting interferes with the filling of the right side of the heart, which lessens cardiac output. Figure 31-9 illustrates the physiological events that may be caused by chest injuries.

PREVENTION

Health Promotion

Avoidance of occupational trauma, recreational hazards, and driving accidents.

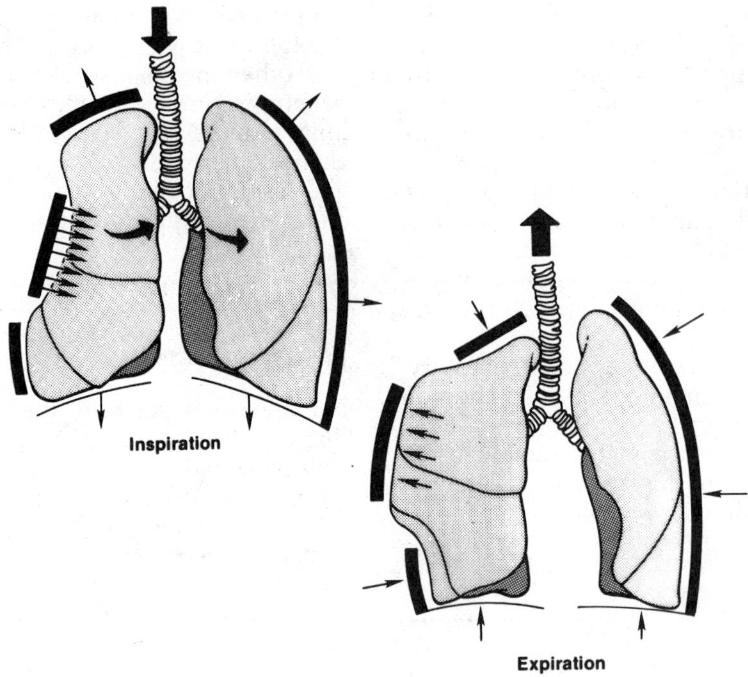

Figure 31-7 Flail chest. (Jones, D. A., Dunbar, C. F., and Jirovec, M. M.: *Medical-Surgical Nursing: A Conceptual Approach,* McGraw-Hill, New York, 1978.)

Population at Risk

1. Persons with another related health problem, (e.g., malignancy, head injuries).
2. Clients receiving mechanical ventilation.

Screening

Not applicable.

ASSESSMENT

Health History

1. History of accident or occupational injury.
2. Health patterns: alcohol, drugs, smoking.
3. Age: problem can occur at any time.
4. Chest pain may be present.
5. Cough (with or without hemoptysis).
6. Complaints of vertigo are not uncommon.
7. Anxiety may be present.

Physical Assessment

Refer to Chapter 48.

1. Paleness and cyanosis of mucosa and nail beds may be present.
2. Level of consciousness may be affected.
3. Dyspnea may be present. Use of accessory muscles may be evident. Rapid shallow breathing.
4. Asymmetrical chest movement related to mediastinal shift may be observed, also crepitus (fluid and air in intrapleural cavity).
5. Diaphoresis with elevated temperature may be present.
6. Tachycardia with weak pulse may be found.
7. Hypotension may be present.
8. Determine whether injury is closed or contused and search for wounds of entrance and exit.
9. Palpation and percussion.
   a. Determine equality and amplitude of all pulses.
   b. Determine cardiac size and point of maximal impulse (PMI).
   c. Evaluate chest expansion (excursion) and check for areas of hyperresonance or dullness.
   d. Determine areas of tenderness or pain, abnormal mobility of ribs or sternum, tracheal shift, or crepitation.

10. Breath sounds may be absent on affected side, or rhonchi may be heard on expiration but clear with coughing.

Diagnostic Tests

1. Chest x-ray study will reveal collapsed lung.
2. Blood gases indicate the adequacy of oxygen–carbon dioxide exchange.
3. Blood work: electrolytes to assess fluid and electrolyte balance; hemoglobin and hematocrit to assess blood loss.
4. ECG to identify cardiac changes.
5. Lung biopsy to assess lung tissue.
6. Mediastinoscopy to visualize the mediastinal pleural surfaces and the diaphragm.

NURSING DIAGNOSES: ACTUAL OR POTENTIAL

1. Respiratory dysfunction: dyspnea secondary to thoracic trauma.
2. Alterations of cardiac output: secondary to thoracic trauma.
3. Anxiety (mild to severe): secondary to injury.
4. Depletion of body fluids: dehydration, diaphoresis, blood loss.
5. Impaired lung tissue, destruction of respiratory units.
6. Alteration in comfort: pain (thoracic), cough.
7. Knowledge deficit: regarding diagnosis.

EXPECTED OUTCOMES

1. Gas exchange will return to normal as breath sounds clear.
2. Client will be able to rest and to partake in an effective coughing and deep breathing regimen.
3. Body temperature, pulse, and respiration will return to normal.
4. Client will meet nutritional and hydration needs.

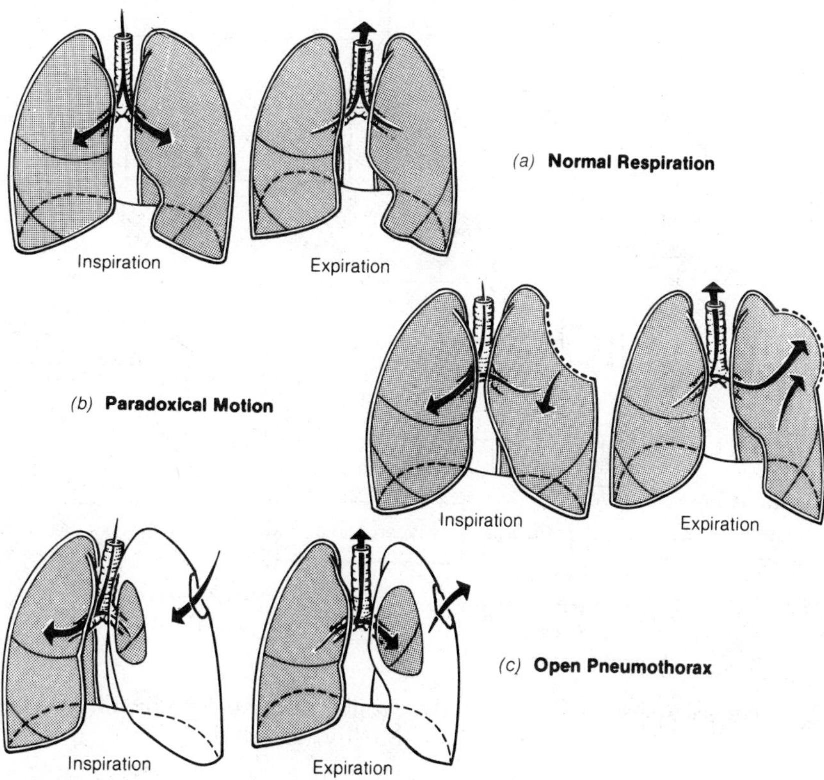

Figure 31-8 Pathogenesis of pneumothorax. (Jones, D. A., Dunbar, C. F., and Jirovec, M. M.: *Medical-Surgical Nursing: A Conceptual Approach*, McGraw-Hill, New York, 1978.)

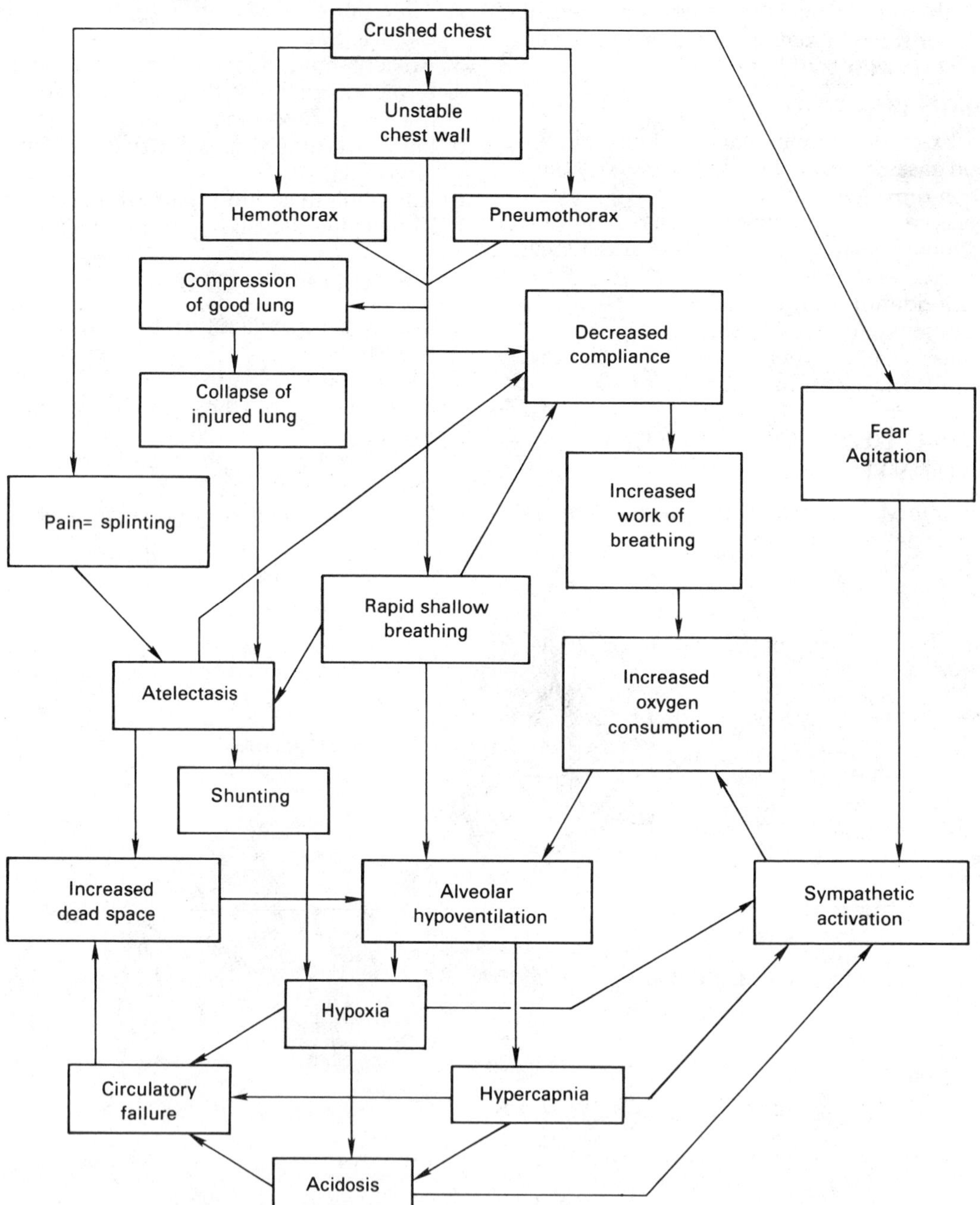

Figure 31-9 Factors causing respiratory failure following crushed chest injuries. (Adapted from Bendixin, H. H., et al.: *Respiratory Care,* Mosby, St. Louis, 1965.)

5. Client will understand information taught in teaching sessions, as evidenced by 85 percent accuracy either verbally or in writing.
6. Client will give evidence of compliance with care plan by:
   a. Adhering to medication regimen, as indicated by chart maintained by client.
   b. Performing coughing and deep-breathing regimen.
   c. Caring for puncture area with proper technique.
   d. Maintaining a well-balanced diet with adequate fluid intake.
   e. Avoiding URI and environmental and recreational hazards.
   f. Adhering to follow-up schedule and being aware of signs of complications.
   g. Reducing the number of cigarettes smoked.

INTERVENTIONS

1. Administer prescribed antibiotics and analgesics to reduce pain and to prevent infection from developing.
2. Continuously assess vital signs, breath sounds, chest expansion, and blood gases.
3. Administer humidified oxygen therapy.
4. Place client in semi-Fowler's position to facilitate drainage and ease breathing.
5. Provide restful environment; keep dry and warm. Allow the client to increase activity as tolerated.
6. Perform range-of-motion exercises and include chest physiotherapy to help decrease the hazards of immobility.
7. Instruct client to avoid stretching or sudden movements, as they could cause recurrence of the problems.
8. Maintain diet and fluid intake as ordered or as tolerated; measure intake and output (Guenter, 1977).
9. Assist with insertion of closed chest drainage in order to remove air and fluid from the thoracic cavity and facilitate lung reexpansion. Explain procedure carefully to client to help reduce anxiety.
   a. A thoracotomy is done, and one or more chest tubes are inserted (refer to Figure 31-3) above the area of the second or third rib.
   b. Each tube is connected to a closed drainage system, for example, water seal drainage (refer to Figure 31-4) or Pleur-evac.
   c. Carefully observe the drainage system to ensure its proper function. Take care to avoid interruption in the airtight system via dislodgement of the tubing or bottle breakage.
10. Provide tracheostomy care and suctioning as needed (see Table 31-12 and Figure 31-10).
11. Intermittent positive pressure can be used to facilitate removal of secretions and aid in lung reexpansion.
12. Teach about:
    a. Coughing and deep-breathing regimen.
    b. Medications: dose, side effects.
    c. Proper rest, activity, and nutritional intake to maintain natural resistance.

TABLE 31-12 TRACHEOSTOMY CARE

1. Before care be sure the client is well oxygenated.
2. Suction as needed to remove secretions (the use of humidified O_2 will help liquefy secretions).
3. Rest between suctionings.
4. Perform care at least every 6–8 h, more frequently, if needed.
5. Change dressing by sterile technique.
6. Utilize prepackaged tracheostomy kits, if available.
7. Be sure to secure new neck tapes before beginning the procedure.
8. Use a 3% hydrogen peroxide solution to clean the cannula.
9. Emergency tracheostomy set should be kept at bedside in case the cannula slips out or is coughed out by the patient.
10. If emergency opening is necessary, a Kelly clamp, kept at the bedside at all times, may be used to keep the tracheostomy open until help arrives.
11. Cuffed tracheostomy tubes as well as endotracheal tubes need to be deflated frequently to prevent tissue necrosis at the tracheal site. Before deflating the cuff, the nurse should be certain that the patient has been adequately suctioned.

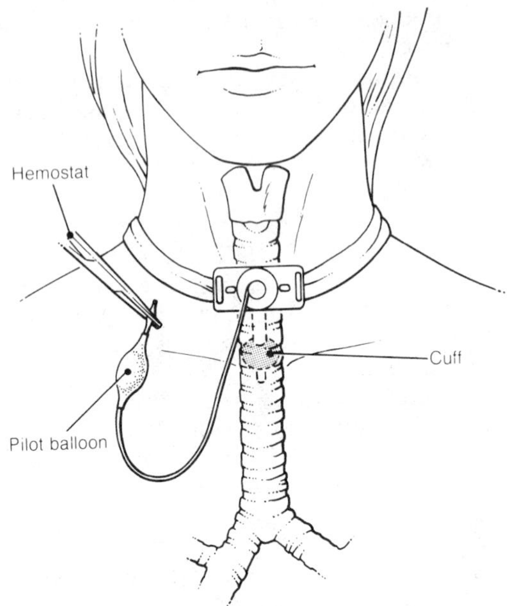

Figure 31-10 Tracheostomy tube. (Jones, D. A., Dunbar, C. F., and Jirovec, M. M.: *Medical-Surgical Nursing: A Conceptual Approach*, McGraw-Hill, New York, 1978.)

   d. Avoidance of accidents and environmental hazards.
   e. Follow-up schedule and signs of complications.
13. Counsel about nonsmoking.

EVALUATION

Outcome Criteria

1. Ventilations are returning to normal, as evidenced by clear to clearing breath sounds.
2. Temperature, pulse, and respiration are returning to normal.
3. Pain is diminishing. Relief of anxiety and cough is evident.
4. Client reports taking medications at appropriate times and in correct amounts.
5. Client performs coughing and deep breathing regimen.
6. Client has reduced the number of cigarettes being smoked.

Complications

WET LUNG SYNDROME

This is the presence of fluid in the lungs (mucus, blood, serum) as the result of severe chest injury and contusion of pulmonary tissue. Results are an inability to cough, airway obstruction, and atelectasis.

Assessment

1. Constant loose cough, wheezing.
2. Dyspnea.
3. Noisy respirations, rales upon auscultation.
4. Tachycardia.
5. Cyanosis.

Revised Outcomes

1. Cardiopulmonary function will be restored by improving tracheobronchial breathing.
2. Other outcomes are as originally stated under Expected Outcomes above.

Interventions

1. Encourage client to cough; support chest.
2. Perform chest physiotherapy.
3. Administer bronchodilators and analgesics.
4. Assist with intercostal nerve block.
5. Aspirate secretions, if necessary.
6. Provide pre- and post-thoracentesis care.
7. Assist with tracheostomy and perform follow-up.
8. Assess and maintain ventilatory support systems.

ADULT RESPIRATORY DISTRESS SYNDROME (ARDS) (SHOCK LUNG)

This is a descriptive term that has been applied to many acute diffuse infiltrative lung lesions of diverse causes (see Table 31-13). These conditions are often present in combination and may be obvious at different times, but the clinical characteristics of ARDS are quite similar regardless of the cause.

Assessment

1. Dyspnea.
2. Tachypnea.
3. Diffuse bronchial breath sounds.
4. Cyanosis.
5. Altered cardiac output.
6. Decreased tidal volume.
7. Blood gases: decreased Po_2 and Pco_2.
8. X-ray study reveals patchy infiltrates progressing to opacity.

Revised Outcomes

Gas exchange will improve when cause is treated; cyanosis and dyspnea will cease.

Interventions

1. Provide oxygen therapy.
2. Assess and maintain mechanical support of respirations, utilize positive end-expiratory pressure (PEEP) and intermittent positive-

TABLE 31-13 CONDITIONS THAT MAY LEAD TO THE ADULT RESPIRATORY DISTRESS SYNDROME

1. Diffuse pulmonary infections (e.g., viral, bacterial, fungal, pneumocystic)
2. Aspiration (e.g., gastric contents with Mendelson's syndrome, water with near-drowning)
3. Inhalation of toxins and irritants (e.g., chlorine gas, NO_2, smoke, ozone, high concentrations of oxygen)
4. Narcotic overdose pulmonary edema (e.g., heroin, methadone, morphine, dextropropoxyphene)
5. Nonnarcotic drug effects (e.g., nitrofurantoin)
6. Immunologic response to host antigens (e.g., Goodpasture's syndrome, systemic lupus erythematosus)
7. Effects of nonthoracic trauma with hypotension ("shock lung")
8. In association with systemic reactions to processes initiated outside the lung (e.g., gram-negative septicemia, hemorrhagic pancreatitis, amniotic fluid embolism, fat embolism)
9. Postcardiopulmonary bypass ("pump lung," "postperfusion lung")

SOURCE: Ingram, R., in Isselbacher, K., et al.: *Harrison's Principles of Internal Medicine,* 9th ed., McGraw-Hill, New York, 1980, p. 1276.

pressure breathing (IPPB) so as to increase lung volume.
3. Restrict fluids.
4. Administer diuretics, steroids, and human serum albumin.
5. Monitor pulmonary arterial pressure and pulmonary arterial wedge pressure.
6. Assess sputum culture; observe for secondary bacterial infection.

FRACTURED NOSE

A fractured (broken) nose, with or without displacement, results from direct injury. Such trauma may cause bilateral nosebleeds, pain, and later, swelling and hematoma of the nose and both lower eyelids. Generally, serious consequences do not arise, but a deformity could lead to nasal obstruction, facial disfigurement, and chronic rhinitis (Ballantyne and Graves, 1979).

EPISTAXIS

Ninety-five percent of epistaxes, or nosebleeds, arise from the anterior plexus of the blood vessels located in the mucosa of the nasal septum. Typically, bleeding is from only one naris and is only from one area. Bleeding from the posterior portion, involving the large vessels, is frequently profuse. Causes of epistaxis are numerous: trauma, the aftereffects of surgery, deviated septum, picking of nasal crusts, blowing the nose too hard, sclerotic blood vessels, straining, pregnancy, vicarious menstruation, bleeding diatheses, hypertension, acute sinusitis, high altitudes, and foreign bodies.

OBSTRUCTIONS

PULMONARY EMBOLI

DESCRIPTION

Pulmonary emboli are generally fragments of a thrombus that originated somewhere in the venous system, most often in the veins of the lower extremities, pelvic area, or in the right side of the heart. As the embolus travels, one or more of the pulmonary arteries may be partially or completely obstructed. Other materials, such as tumors, amniotic fluid, air, bone marrow, fat, and a variety of foreign bodies, may also obstruct the arteries.

The three factors involved in thrombogenesis are (1) stasis, (2) abnormalities in the vessel wall, and (3) alteration in the blood coagulation system. Respiratory and hemodynamic events result. The obstruction produces a zone of lung that is ventilated, not perfused. Arterial hypoxemia is common but not a universal occurrence. The primary hemodynamic consequence is a reduction of the available cross-sectional area of the pulmonary-arterial bed. Pressure increases in the pulmonary artery, which in turn causes an increase in the volume and pressure in the great veins. The blood volume in the left atrium is decreased, thus decreasing the stroke volume and leading to shock. Serotonin may be released from the platelets, causing pulmonary hypertension.

The yearly incidence of pulmonary emboli in the United States probably exceeds 500,000. Available data suggest that less than 10 percent of all pulmonary emboli result in death (Bushnell, 1973).

PREVENTION

Health Promotion

1. Avoidance of immobilization; early ambulation after surgery.
2. Performance of range-of-motion and regular exercises for clients on complete bed rest.
3. Avoidance of letting legs dangle without support, crossing legs, and prolonged sitting and standing.
4. Avoidance of constricting clothing (e.g., garters, girdles).
5. Awareness by females of the potential clotting effect of oral contraceptives.
6. Anticoagulant prophylaxis for susceptible clients.
7. Monitoring of length of time IV lines are in place; assessment of surrounding tissue; IV change every 24 h.
8. Avoidance of smoking.

Population at Risk

1. Postoperative clients, especially following pelvic surgery.
2. Persons on long-term immobilization with paralysis; elderly.
3. Pregnant women; particularly during the postpartum period.
4. Users of estrogen-containing contraceptives combined with smoking.
5. Persons with congestive heart failure, chronic pulmonary disease, deep venous insufficiency, carcinoma, obesity, myocardial infarction, previous venous thromboembolism, or cerebrovascular accident.
6. Persons with fractures or injuries to lower extremities.
7. Persons whose employment requires continuous sitting.

Screening

Methods for early detection of deep venous thrombosis:
1. Ultrasound (Doppler-flow technique).
2. Radiolabeled fibrinogen method.
3. Impedance plethysmography.

ASSESSMENT

Health History

1. Recent surgery; immobilization.
2. History of emboli, pregnancy, obesity, or varicose veins.
3. Health maintenance patterns: smoking, limited activity, use of alcohol, drugs, or caffeine.
4. Job: requiring continuous sitting with little position change.
5. Presence of congestive heart failure, chronic pulmonary disease, deep venous insufficiency, carcinoma, myocardial infarction, cerebrovascular accident.
6. Incidence increases with age.
7. Breathlessness, sudden onset of dyspnea.
8. Cough and hemoptysis, occasionally.
9. Complaints of pleuritic chest pain when infarction has occurred; substernal oppressive discomfort may be present with extensive emboli.
10. Syncope.
11. Apprehension and fear.

Physical Assessment

1. General appearance will be pale; cyanosis and diaphoresis may be present.
2. Signs of neck vein engorgement may be present.
3. Chest expansion may be limited due to chest pain.
4. Overt signs of peripheral phlebitis may be present in extremities.
5. Possible alteration in consciousness and thought process due to cerebral anoxia.
6. Anxious and apprehensive.
7. Respirations rapid and gasping.
8. Tachycardia; arrhythmias may be present.
9. Hypotension may be present.
10. Breath sounds: disclose a few atelectatic rales; localized wheezing is rare; pleural friction rub or evidence of pleural effusion may be present if infarction has occurred.
11. Heart sounds: scratchy systolic ejection-type murmur may be heard in the pulmonic area;

systolic or continuous murmur, accentuated by inspiration, may be audible over the lung fields; wide, often fixed, splitting of the second heart sound may be present (Isselbacher et al., 1980).

TABLE 31-14 OBSERVABLE SIGNS INDICATING CHANGE IN Po_2[a] VALUE

Approximate Po_2 Value, mmHg	Observable Signs
85–100	Normal.
80–95	Breathes with mouth open. Respiratory rate 25 breaths/min. (May be ambulatory but short of breath.)
75–80	Increased use of facial muscles (frontalis, nostrils). Creases in forehead with each breath. Telegraphic speech—short broken sentences, two to three words at a time. Tachycardia—pulse rate increased.
70	Mild duskiness. Respiratory rate 30–35 breaths/min.
60 and lower	Restless. Combative—may fight restraints, pull out tubes, etc. No response to morphine—patient cyanotic and more combative. Sweating, starting at forehead. Tugs on throat, trouble getting air in, coughs on respiration. Respirations more than 40 breaths/min.
	Gray cyanosis. Blood pressure decreases. Patient is within minutes of cardiac arrest.

SOURCE: Murphy, E. R.: "Intensive Nursing Care in a Respiratory Unit," *Nursing Clinics of North America*, **3**:423–436, September 1968.

[a] Partial pressure of oxygen in artery.

TABLE 31-15 OBSERVABLE SIGNS INDICATING CHANGE IN Pco_2[a] VALUE

Approximate Pco_2 Value, mmHg	Observable Signs
20	Tetany, cerebral deterioration.
35–45	Normal.
53	Headache, dizziness.
76	Dizziness, muscle twitching, unconsciousness.
110	Convulsions, coma.
200	Deep coma.

SOURCE: Murphy, E. R.: "Intensive Nursing Care in a Respiratory Unit," *Nursing Clinics of North America*, **3**:423–426, September 1968.

[a] Partial pressure of carbon dioxide in artery.

Diagnostic Tests

1. Chest x-ray study may show a parenchymal infiltrate and evidence of a pleural effusion if infarction has occurred.
2. Pulmonary perfusion photoscans show abnormalities of distribution of blood flow. Ventilation scan with emboli demonstrates normal wash in and normal wash out from embolized lung zones.
3. Angiography provides anatomical information.
4. ECG is normal in most clients; with extensive embolization there may be evidence of acute pulmonary hypertension; rightward shift of QRS axis; a tall, peaked P wave; and ST-T changes may be indicative of right ventricular "strain" and ischemia. These changes are often transient, lasting minutes to hours, or persist with pulmonary vascular obstruction.
5. Fluoroscopy is done to discover a nonpulsatile vessel.
6. Arterial blood gases: see Tables 31-14 and 31-15. Findings with massive embolism reveal:
   a. Arterial hypoxemia.
   b. Hypocapnia.
   c. Respiratory alkalosis.

7. Blood work: findings may be as follows but have limited value:
   a. Normal or increased SGOT.
   b. Increased LDH.
   c. Increased serum bilirubin.
   d. Increased creatinine.
   e. Decreased phosphokinase.

NURSING DIAGNOSES: ACTUAL OR POTENTIAL*

1. Alteration in comfort: pleuritic pain, cough.
2. Alteration in cardiac output: decreased circulation; hypotension.
3. Anxiety (moderate to severe): due to fear of death.
4. Respiratory dysfunction: secondary to obstruction of pulmonary vessels.
5. Depletion of body fluids: secondary to diaphoresis, hemoptysis.
6. Altered perception/levels of consciousness: due to decreased cerebral circulation.
7. Knowledge deficit: due to disease.
8. Decreased activity tolerence: fatigue and dyspnea.

EXPECTED OUTCOMES†

1. Cardiopulmonary functions will be restored. Pulse, respirations, and blood pressure will return to normal.
2. Client will be able to rest with less discomfort and diminished apprehension and anxiety. Bed rest is generally required for 5 to 7 days.
3. Client will be free from cough, hemoptysis, and diaphoresis.
4. Client will understand information taught in teaching sessions.
5. Client will give evidence of compliance with care plan.

INTERVENTIONS

1. Acute phase.
   a. Main IV line for administration of medications.
      (1) Anticoagulants: heparin inhibits thrombus growth and inhibits platelet aggregation.
      (2) Analgesics, sedatives to decrease anxiety.
      (3) Cardiotonics (see Chapter 30 under *Coronary Heart Disease*).
      (4) Diuretics (see Chapter 30 under *Hypertension*).
      (5) Prothrombinopenic drugs for protection for prolonged periods.
      (6) Thrombolytic agents for treatment of clients with massive embolism.
   b. Place client on bed rest in semi-Fowler's position to facilitate breathing.
   c. Administer humidified oxygen therapy. Mechanical ventilation may be necessary.
   d. Monitor vital signs, blood gases, blood work, ECG, and breath sounds.
   e. Provide emotional support to help relieve anxiety. Provide reassurance and clarification of situation.
2. Subacute phase.
   a. Provide elastic stockings.
   b. Encourage liberal intake of fluid; measure intake and output of fluids.
   c. Maintain rest, increasing activities gradually.
   d. Encourage range-of-motion exercises.
   e. Administer skin care.
   f. Check the color, amount, and consistency of sputum.
   g. Provide oral hygiene.
   h. Avoid constipation.
   i. Administer anticoagulants to keep coagulation within therapeutic limits.
      (1) Check coagulation, bleeding time, prothrombin time.
      (2) Have appropriate antidote available (e.g., vitamin K or protamine sulfate).
      (3) Assess for untoward bleeding following shaving, bleeding of gums, nosebleeds, bruises, and blood in stool or urine.
   j. Teach about:
      (1) Medications: dose and side effects.
      (2) Rest and activities with a regular exercise regimen.
      (3) Follow-up schedule and signs of complications.
      (4) Proper clothing to wear and the need not to cross or dangle legs and to avoid sitting or standing.

* The effects of a pulmonary embolus are extremely variable and depend on the size and location of the embolus.

† Medical goals include (1) immediate inhibition of thrombus growth, (2) promotion of thrombus resolution, and (3) prevention of emboli recurrence.

(5) Informing dentist about medications currently being taken.

k. Counsel about nonsmoking.

EVALUATION

Outcome Criteria

1. Cardiopulmonary functions are restored, as evidenced by laboratory values, decreased cough. Vital signs and breath and heart sounds are normal.
2. Client is able to rest and perform activities with diminished discomfort.
3. Client reports reduction in the number of cigarettes smoked.
4. Client adheres to medications regimen, taking medications at appropriate times and in correct amounts, as indicated by chart being kept by client.
5. Client is performing the daily exercise plan and tolerating it well.
6. Client can recall with 85 percent accuracy, either verbally or in writing, the content presented in teaching sessions.

Complications

1. Shock (see discussion in Chapter 48).
2. Recurrence of embolism. If anticoagulant therapy is deemed inadequate or impractical, surgical treatment may be employed to prevent immediate recurrence (refer to Chapter 30 under discussion of *Coronary Heart Disease*).

Intervention

Venous interruption and pulmonary embolectomy.

Reevaluation and Follow-up

1. Establish a specific individualized plan to ensure that any complications are overcome.
2. Long-term surveillance and necessary interventions are provided.

BRONCHIECTASIS

DESCRIPTION

Bronchiectasis is a congenital or acquired disorder characterized by chronic dilatation of the medium-size airways and destruction of bronchial elastic and muscular structures. Bronchiectasis occurs after repeated and prolonged respiratory tract infections and prolonged bronchial obstruction. It may also occur as a sequela to some other process that has caused an alteration in normal bronchial structure.

The *infectious process*, which is the major factor in the development of bronchiectasis, destroys segments of bronchial mucosa that are then replaced by fibrous tissue. These resulting deformed and dilated airways contribute to the retention of secretions that become infected. The affected lung segments then harbor a chronic necrotizing infection.

The disorder typically developed in childhood and young adulthood during the preantibiotic years. The actual prevalence of chronic childhood bronchiectasis is decreasing; however, the number of individuals with late-onset bronchiectasis is increasing. This population includes those who have cystic fibrosis, atopic asthma, or an immune deficiency disorder.

Bronchiectasis is not a reversible disorder. Exacerbations may be precipitated by exposure to inflammatory agents (smoking, particulates, infections). Pulmonary hypertension and cor pulmonale typically develop in the late stages.

PREVENTION

Health Promotion

1. Immunization against childhood diseases and influenza.
2. Prevention of severe respiratory infections.
3. Immediate removal of aspirated foreign bodies.
4. Prompt and complete treatment of severe respiratory infections.
5. Evaluation of the cause of all chronic coughs.
6. Avoidance of smoking.
7. Avoidance of exposure to individuals with upper respiratory infections (e.g., influenza).
8. Reduced exposure to particulates and fumes.

Population at Risk

1. Persons who have repeated and prolonged respiratory tract infections.
2. Persons who have a chronic disorder (e.g., cystic fibrosis, bronchitis, asthma) associated with severe respiratory infections.
3. Persons who have an occluded airway because of an aspirated foreign body.

Screening

1. Chest x-ray study.
2. Sputum culture.

ASSESSMENT

Health History

1. History of childhood diseases (especially measles or pertussis complicated by respiratory infections).
2. History of chronic bronchitis.
3. Chronic cough that may occur in paroxysms.
4. Expectoration of yellow or green sputum that may be blood streaked (hemoptysis is not uncommon).
5. Recurrent respiratory tract infections (especially in the winter) that progress to pneumonia.
6. Health maintenance patterns: smoking, exposure to infection, nutritional practices (decreased appetite).
7. Sleep habits: number of pillows used, amount of rest needed.
8. Shortness of breath, especially on exertion.
9. Exposure to pollutants (e.g., particulates, fumes).

Physical Assessment

1. Limited chest expansion is noted.
2. Inspiratory rales and rhonchi may be auscultated over affected areas (rhonchi tend to diminish after productive coughing).
3. Cough may be in paroxysms; dyspnea is usually present.
4. Clubbing of the fingers is usually present.
5. The client is likely to be thin, weak, and pale.

Diagnostic Tests

1. X-ray films of the chest may appear normal. In moderate or advanced cases increased markings are noted, as well as inflammatory changes at the lung bases. Large dilated bronchi may be reflected in a honeycombed pattern.
2. Pulmonary function tests (PFTs) reflect the degree of lung involvement. If the disease process is localized, the PFT values may be within normal limits. When diffuse disease is present, the PFT values are similar to those found in chronic bronchitis.
   a. Decreased VC (vital capacity).
   b. Decreased FEV (forced expiratory volume).
   c. Decreased MVV (maximum voluntary ventilation).
   d. Increased RV (residual volume).
3. Bronchoscopy allows identification of sites of endobronchial disease.
4. Bronchogram permits radiographic visualization of the bronchial tree by introduction of a radiopaque dye. The distorted and tortuous bronchi in bronchiectasis are only confirmed by bronchography. (Beacuse of its untoward effects, bronchography is usually indicated only when surgical resection is planned.)
5. Sputum culture is done to identify the pathogen.
6. Arterial blood gases are done to estimate the progression of the disorder. Even when the structural changes are limited, a decreased Pa_{O_2} is usually present because of ventilation/perfusion aberrations.

NURSING DIAGNOSES: ACTUAL OR POTENTIAL

1. Respiratory dysfunction (mild to severe): dyspnea secondary to retained bronchial secretions.
2. Alteration in comfort: discomfort secondary to respiratory changes.
3. Alteration in food intake: weight loss secondary to respiratory dysfunction.
4. Altered/decreased activity tolerence: secondary to respiratory dysfunction (dyspnea, cough, hypoxia).
5. Lack of compliance with therapeutic plan (potential): due to knowledge deficit.

EXPECTED OUTCOMES

1. There will be regular drainage of secretions from lungs.
2. Client will have no evidence of superimposed infection.
3. Client will understand information taught in teaching sessions, as evidenced by 85 percent accuracy when tested.
4. Client will demonstrate gradual weight gain over a 2-month period following discharge. (Client will gain 2 lb within 3 weeks and 6 lb within 2 months after discharge.)
5. Client will give evidence of compliance with care plan by:
   a. Reducing number of cigarettes by one-half within 3 weeks of discharge, or
   b. Eliminating smoking.
   c. Gaining weight as recommended.
   d. Avoiding environmental pollutants and irritants.
   e. Adhering to medication regimen, as indicated by chart maintained by client.

f. Adhering to postural drainage regimen, as indicated by chart maintained by client.
g. Adhering to oral hygiene regimen, as demonstrated by chart maintained by client and also by absence of fetid breath.
h. Establishing and maintaining an effective activity regimen.

INTERVENTIONS

1. Promote a rest and activity program.
2. Administer prescribed mucolytics and antibiotics to reduce inflammation and promote liquefaction and removal of secretions.
3. Give frequent mouth care to cleanse the mucosa and facilitate the appeal of food and fluids.
4. Provide diet and fluids as tolerated.
5. Teach about:
   a. Medications: dose, side effects.
   b. Postural drainage (see Figure 31-11).
   c. Diet: as needed to maintain health and modify weight as indicated.
   d. Rest and activity to help maintain resistance to other infections.
   e. Avoidance of pollution and other irritants.
6. Counsel about nonsmoking.
7. Plan activity program with gradual increments.

EVALUATION

Outcome Criteria

1. Cough continues to be productive and secretions drain regularly.
2. Breath sounds consist of fewer rales and rhonchi.
3. Client is able to walk up eight steps without fatigue or dyspnea.
4. Client recalls with 85 percent accuracy, either verbally or in writing, the content presented in teaching sessions.

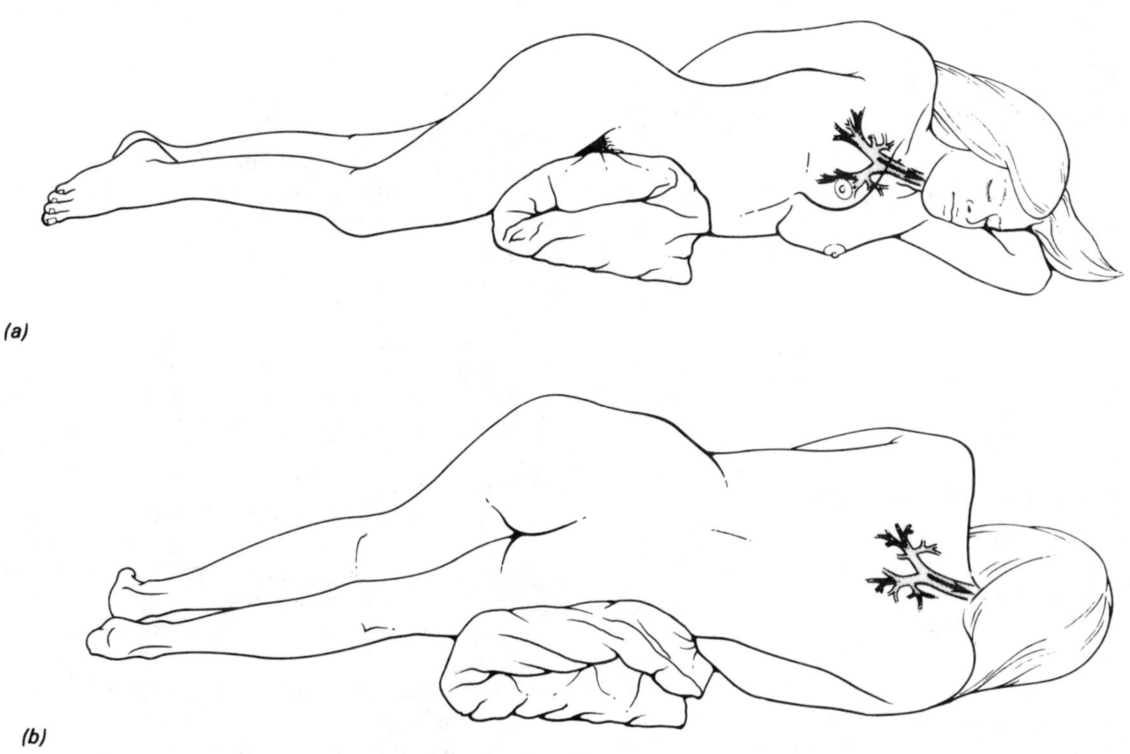

Figure 31-11 Postural drainage. (*a*) Left lateral decubitus position. (*b*) Right lateral decubitus position. (Jones, D. A., Dunbar, C. F., and Jirovec, M. M.: *Medical-Surgical Nursing: A Conceptual Approach*, McGraw-Hill, New York, 1978.)

5. Client has gained 2 lb during the past 3 weeks.
6. Client reports a reduction in the number of cigarettes smoked to six per day.
7. Client takes medications at appropriate times and in correct amounts, as indicated by chart he or she is keeping.
8. Client adheres to daily activity program and is progressing through phase 1 of the program.

Complications

1. Bronchopneumonia (see the discussion in this chapter under Pneumonia).
2. Cor pulmonale (see the discussion in Chapter 30).
3. Hemoptysis:

Assessment

1. Expectoration: bright red, frothy blood.
2. Apprehension.
3. Discomfort in chest: burning or bubbling.
4. Salty taste in mouth.
5. Sensation in throat: tickling.
6. Restlessness.

Revised Outcomes

1. Oxygenation will be restored within normal limits; apprehension and restlessness will cease.
2. Bleeding will be controlled; expectoration of bright red, frothy blood will diminish; chest discomfort will cease.
3. Other outcomes are as originally stated above.

Interventions

1. Provide suctioning as needed.
2. Administer humidified oxygen as needed.
3. Provide reassurance.
4. Monitor vital signs.
5. Place ice bag on thorax.
6. Monitor arterial blood gases.

Reevaluation and Follow-up

1. Establish a specific individualized plan to assess complication.
2. Long-term surveillance and necessary interventions should be provided.

DEVIATED SEPTUM

DESCRIPTION

A deviated septum is a cartilaginous and bony septum containing rounded lumps or sharp projections that deflect from the midline of the nose. It may be bent or inclined to one side or may encroach on the nasal chamber and sinus ostia. Deviations could be either in the vertical or horizontal plane, usually involving both the cartilage and the bone.

PREVENTION

Health Promotion

Avoidance of traumatic injury to nose.

Population at Risk

1. Some infants who had abnormal intrauterine posture. The nose was further exposed to torsion forces during parturition.
2. Persons who have sustained a traumatic injury to the nose.
3. Persons with a family history, often congenital.

Screening

Not applicable.

ASSESSMENT

Health History

1. Age: children and older adults.
2. Persons with a family history or those who had a difficult parturition.
3. History of recent traumatic injury.
4. Difficulty in breathing; postnasal drip may be present.
5. Headaches may develop.
6. Anxiety may be associated with dyspnea.
7. Severe deviation affects nasal functions with obstruction, drying, and pain.

Physical Assessment

1. Dyspnea, mild; postnasal drip may be present.
2. Inflamed nasopharynx, with occasional nasopharyngitis, may be evident.
3. Physical examination of nasal chamber reveals:
   a. Visible alteration in the shape of the nasal chamber.
   b. Dry, crusting mucosa.
   c. On occasion, evidence of bleeding.

Diagnostic Tests

Routine preoperative tests are required.

NURSING DIAGNOSES: ACTUAL OR POTENTIAL

1. Respiratory dysfunction (mild): dyspnea secondary to nasal obstruction.
2. Alteration in sensory perception: gustatory and olfactory senses altered.
3. Anxiety (mild): secondary to dyspnea and results of surgery.
4. Alteration in comfort: discomfort secondary to respiratory dysfunction, obstructions, postnasal drip, crusty mucosa, headaches, and occasional inflammation.
5. Disruption in skin integrity: due to surgical wound.

EXPECTED OUTCOMES

1. Following surgery, the client will be able to breathe with less difficulty and discomfort as anxiety and obstruction decrease.
2. Healing of surgical wound will be complete. Client will mouth breathe and avoid straining.
3. Function of senses will return to normal.
4. Client will understand information taught in teaching sessions, as evidenced by 85 percent accuracy, verbally or in writing.
5. Client will give evidence of compliance with care plan postoperatively by:
   a. Breathing through mouth.
   b. Not coughing vigorously, not swallowing blood or blowing nose.
   c. Avoiding straining, heavy lifting, and pressure.
   d. Adhering to follow-up schedule and being aware of signs of complications.

INTERVENTIONS

1. Preoperative interventions.
   Teach about:
   a. Purpose of treatment, surgical procedure, and anesthesia administration.
   b. Mouth-breathing technique.
   c. Purpose of packing; full feeling in nose is normal with packing; packing will be checked periodically.
   d. Discoloration and swelling around eyes may follow; discomfort may be present; final cosmetic result is not immediately evident.
2. Surgical procedures.
   a. Submucous resection.
   b. Nasal septum reconstruction.
3. Postoperative interventions.
   a. Assess vital signs (rectal temperature); slight temperature elevation is normal with packing.
   b. Check position of string attached to nasal packing; check mustache dressing.
   c. Check position of splint; observe underlying skin for evidence of pressure.
   d. Place client in semi-Fowler's position.
   e. Provide oral hygiene.
   f. Foster appetite; provide liquids and food as tolerated. Explain why it is difficult to swallow.
   g. Assess discomfort; offer sedatives, analgesics.
   h. Apply ice compress over the nose.
   i. Offer comfort and support.
   j. Teach about:
      (1) Not lifting heavy weights for 2 weeks.
      (2) Avoiding pressure on nose from eyeglasses.
      (3) Consulting doctor about wearing contact lenses.
      (4) Presence of tarry stools (normal).
      (5) Utilizing stool softener to avoid straining.

EVALUATION

Outcome Criteria

1. Client is able to breathe with less difficulty and discomfort from obstruction and anxiety.
2. Surgical wound has healed completely.
3. Sense of taste and smell have returned to normal.
4. Client can recall with 85 percent accuracy, either verbally or in writing, the content presented in teaching sessions.

Complications

HEMORRHAGE

Assessment

1. Bright red blood on external dressing.
2. Expectorating or vomiting bright red blood.
3. Swallowing repeatedly followed by belching.
4. Altered vital signs.
5. Restlessness.

Revised Outcomes

1. Patent airway will be maintained.
2. Gas exchange will be restored as bleeding ceases and vital signs return to normal.

Interventions

1. Raise upper body.

2. Reinforce dressing.
3. Prepare to observe site and repack.

Reevaluation and Follow-up
Evaluate a specific individualized plan to ensure recovery from complications.

ENVIRONMENTAL DISORDERS

ASTHMA

DESCRIPTION

Asthma is a disorder "characterized by an increased responsiveness of the airways to various stimuli and manifested by slowing of forced expiration which changes in severity either spontaneously or as a result of therapy" (American College of Chest Physicians, 1975). Evidence suggests that persons with asthma are hypersensitive to extrinsic allergens or to intrinsic infectious agents of the respiratory tract. It is posited that an allergen–antibody mechanism may cause the release of chemical mediators, such as acetylcholine, histamine, or SRS-A (slow-reacting substance of anaphylaxis), which generate an inflammatory response. Chemical mediators cause bronchial constriction and excess mucus production. In addition, there is enlargement of the mucous glands, edema of the bronchial wall, and infiltration by eosinophils. The abnormal mucus (thick, tenacious, slow-moving) forms plugs, which occlude the airways and are later coughed up in the sputum (see Figure 31-12).

No one factor has been identified as the causative agent of asthma. An episode of asthma may be associated with allergy or infection as well as environmental, occupational, and psychological factors. Approximately 8 million individuals in this country are affected by asthma. Asthma may develop at any age; however, close to one-third of the cases occur before age 10 and another one-third develop before age 40. During the past 10 years an increased morbidity from asthma has been noted.

Asthma attacks are episodic and usually reversible. Typically they are short-lived and tend to last from a few minutes to a few hours. Status asthmaticus may evolve if an asthmatic attack does not respond to treatment.

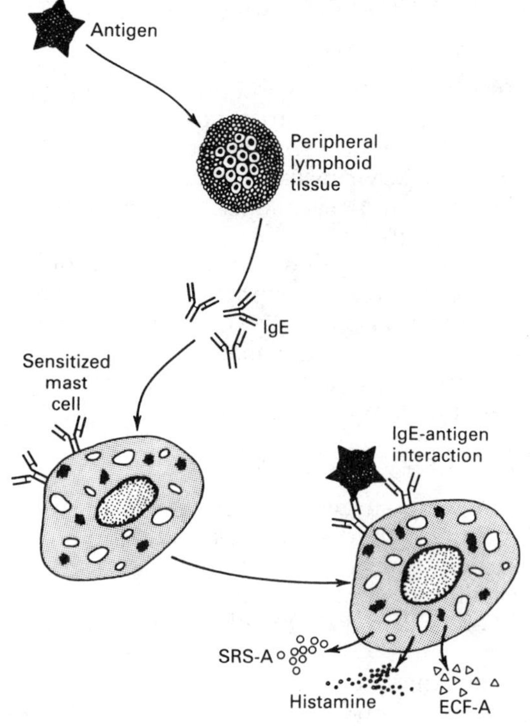

Figure 31-12 Molecular mechanisms of mediator release in asthma. Antigen exposure stimulates peripheral lymphoid tissues in atopic individuals to synthesize IgE. The IgE antibody becomes fixed by its Fc fragment to certain cells (e.g., basophils circulating in the blood or mast cells in the tissues). On repeated exposure, the same antigen reacts with antigen receptors on the Fab fragment of two IgE molecules. The IgE–antigen interaction activates enzyme systems within the cell that cause the release of mediators of anaphylaxis. In lung tissues, at least three mediators may be released, including histamine (bronchospasm), SRS-A, and ECF-A. (Gold, W: "Cholinergic Pharmacology in Asthma," in K. F. Austen and L. M. Lichtenstein, eds.: *Asthma: Physiology, Immunopharmacology, and Treatment*, Academic, New York, 1972, p. 170.)

PREVENTION

Refer to Chapter 20 under *Bronchial Asthma* for Health Promotion, Population at Risk, and Screening.

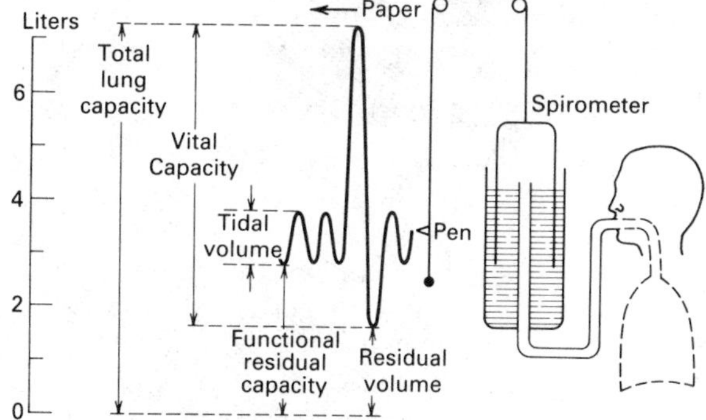

Figure 31-13 Lung volumes. Note that the functional residual capacity and residual volume cannot be measured with the spirometer. (West, J. B.: *Respiratory Physiology: The Essentials*, 2d ed., Williams & Wilkins, Baltimore, 1979, p. 13.)

ASSESSMENT

Refer to Chapter 20 under *Bronchial Asthma* for Health History and Physical Assessment.

Diagnostic Tests

1. Chest x-ray study allows visualization of the lungs and identifies areas of infiltration and demonstrates the presence of atelectasis, pneumothorax, or pneumonitis.
2. Pulmonary function tests permit an assessment of the movement of air in the airways and demonstrate decreased VC (vital capacity); decreased FEV_1 (forced expiratory volume in 1 s) increased RV (residual volume) (see Figures 31-13 and 31-14).
3. Sputum examination (Wright's or Hansel's stain) determines the presence of eosinophils.
4. Arterial blood gases estimate the progression of the asthma attack: Pa_{O_2} is decreased due to airway obstruction; Pa_{CO_2} is lowered or normal because the diffusing capacity remains normal. A rising Pa_{CO_2} in an asthmatic is indicative of severe airway obstruction and impending respiratory failure.
5. Determine serum levels of immunoglobulin IgE (see Table 31-16).
6. A base line of blood values should be ob-

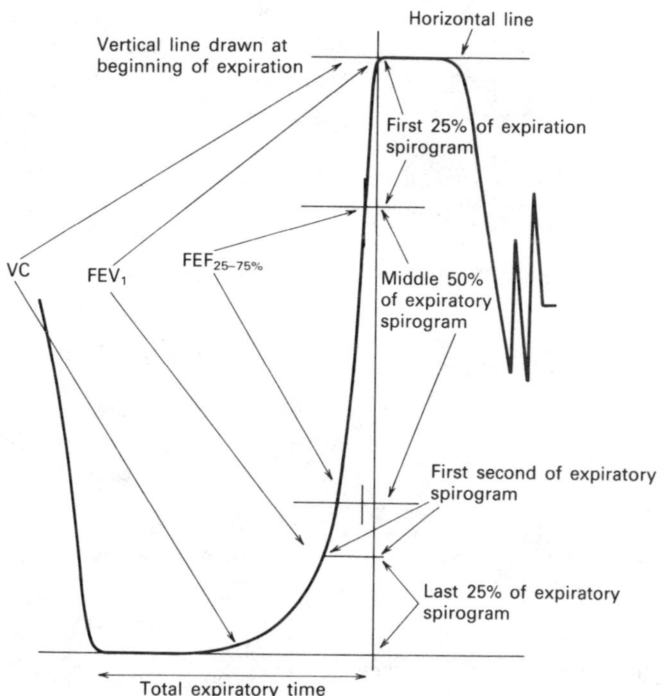

Figure 31-14 Reproduction of normal spirogram (lines are added to facilitate analysis of C, FEV_1, and $FEF_{25-75\%}$). (Petty, T. L.: *Pulmonary Diagnostic Techniques*, Lea & Febiger, Philadelphia, 1975, p. 5.)

TABLE 31-16 CLASSIFICATION OF IMMUNOGLOBULINS

Class	Quantity	Location	Function
IgG	About 75% of total immunoglobulins	Plasma and interstitial fluid	Produces antibodies against bacteria, viruses, and toxins; largely responsible for secondary immune response reactions; activates the complement system
IgA	About 15% of total	Large quantities in tears, saliva, milk, and other exocrine secretions, small quantities in serum	Functions in mucous membrane protection and defense of exposed body surfaces, particularly from infectious agents
IgM	About 10% of total	Serum	In combination with IgG, has specific antitoxin action; provides the "natural" antibodies that include the rheumatoid factor and the ABO isoantibodies; largely responsible for the primary immune response reaction; activates the complement system
IgD	Less than 1% of total	Serum	Unknown
IgE	Less than 1% of total	Serum and interstitial fluid; present also in exocrine secretions	Allergic reactions: atopy and anaphylaxis

SOURCE: Jones, D. A., Dunbar, C. F., and Jirovec, M. M.: *Medical-Surgical Nursing: A Conceptual Approach*, McGraw-Hill, New York, 1978, p. 287.

tained: white blood count, hemoglobin, hematocrit, eosinophils, serum electrolytes.

NURSING DIAGNOSES: ACTUAL OR POTENTIAL

Refer to Nursing Diagnoses under *Bronchial Asthma* in Chapter 20.

EXPECTED OUTCOMES

Refer to Expected Outcomes under *Bronchial Asthma* in Chapter 20.

INTERVENTIONS

Refer to Interventions under *Bronchial Asthma* in Chapter 20.

EVALUATION

Outcome Criteria

Refer to Outcome Criteria under *Bronchial Asthma* in Chapter 20.

Complications

STATUS ASTHMATICUS

Assessment

1. Hypoxemia: decreased Pa_{O_2} (refer to Table 31-14).
2. Hypercapnia: increased Pa_{CO_2} (refer to Table 31-15).
3. pH: respiratory acidosis.
4. Anxiety.
5. Restlessness.
6. Breathless, pale, exhausted.

7. Tachycardia, signs of dehydration evident (dry skin, elevated temperature, concentrated urine).
8. Audible wheezing or a "silent chest" (indicates mucus plugs occluding airways).

Revised Outcomes
1. Oxygenation will be restored within normal limits.
2. Anxiety, restlessness, and breathlessness will cease.
3. Other outcomes are as originally stated under Expected Outcomes for *Bronchial Asthma* in Chapter 20.

Interventions
1. Administer aminophylline by continuous infusion (dosage is based on client's age, weight, and previous response).
2. Administer corticosteroid (Solu-Cortef) by intravenous infusion.
3. Administer sodium bicarbonate by intravenous infusion, if the pH drops to 7.2 or lower (adrenergic drugs are thought not to be effective when the pH falls below 7.2).
4. Administer a broad-spectrum antibiotic by intravenous infusion (infections often precipitate status asthmaticus).
5. Monitor arterial blood gases and pH.
6. Monitor theophylline levels.
7. Administer oxygen by nasal prongs or by Venturi mask.
8. Assist with fiberoptic bronchoscopy to remove mucus plugs (if needed).

Reevaluation and Follow-up
1. Reassess client's health.
2. Continue follow-up as needed.

CHRONIC BRONCHITIS

DESCRIPTION

Chronic bronchitis is "a condition associated with prolonged exposure to nonspecific irritants and accompanied by mucus hypersecretion and certain structured alterations in the bronchi" (American College of Chest Physicians, 1975). Long-term exposure to chemical irritants and dusts impairs the function of cilia and causes mucosal edema and mucous gland hypertrophy with excessive secretion of viscid mucus. These factors along with mucus plugging contribute to diminished airflow and create an environment conducive to bronchopneumonia. During the healing process, fibrosis of tissues contributes to dilation or distortion of bronchioles.

Chronic bronchitis is an environmental disorder associated with cigarette smoking and exposure to pollutants and industrial irritants such as dusts and fumes. It is considered to be more common in men than in women and more common among cigarette smokers than in nonsmokers. The disorder has been reported to occur more often in urban dwellers and in those who are socioeconomically disadvantaged. Chronic bronchitis evolves into a year-round disability that is characterized by acute exacerbations.

PREVENTION

Health Promotion
1. Avoidance of smoking.
2. Reduced exposure to pollution and occupational dusts.
3. Avoidance of exposure to persons with upper respiratory infections.
4. Use of protective devices (e.g., masks) to avoid potential environmental and occupational hazards.
5. Maintenance of good health habits (rest, nutrition, etc.).
6. Regulations enforcing environmental health.

Population at Risk
1. Smokers (mild to heavy).
2. Persons living in densely populated areas.
3. Persons with continual exposure to harmful irritants (e.g., cotton hemp, asbestos, dust).

Screening
1. Chest x-ray study.
2. Spirometry: FEV_1 (forced expiratory volume in 1 s).

ASSESSMENT

Health History
1. Exposure to pollutants or other irritants that may stimulate an inflammatory response.
2. Repeated or chronic respiratory infections.
3. Recurrent cough that becomes increasingly persistent over many years.
4. Increased production of sputum, particularly upon arising, which may be tiring to the client.
5. Shortness of breath, especially upon exertion.

6. Sleep habits: number of pillows used, amount of rest needed, adequacy of rest and sleep.
7. Health maintenance patterns: smoking, exposure to infection, nutritional practices.

Physical Assessment

1. Chest excursion is diminished.
2. Scattered, moist rales are noted upon auscultation over the affected areas.
3. Wheezing may be auscultated. Wheezing intensifies with inspiration of cold air.
4. Musical rhonchi may also be heard, especially if respiratory infection is present.
5. Dyspnea is frequently present. Cough is persistent. Sputum is not initially present, but as bronchitis becomes more chronic, sputum becomes thicker and more copious.
6. Clubbing of the fingers may be present.
7. Client is likely to be pale and may tire easily. Cyanosis may be observable around lips and nail beds.
8. Pedal edema may be noted. Jugular vein distention may be present.
9. Dry mucous membranes and poor skin turgor may be present, especially if the client is febrile.

Diagnostic Tests

1. Chest x-ray films allow visualization of the lungs and identification of areas of increased markings.
2. Reid index (a measure of mucous gland enlargement in relation to the thickness of the bronchial wall) indicates gradual enlargement of mucous glands.
3. Sputum culture is done to determine whether infection is present and, if so, to identify the pathogen.
4. Sputum cytological examination: presence of eosinophils indicates an underlying allergic disorder.
5. Arterial blood gases estimate the progression of the disease: as pulmonary obstruction worsens, blood gases become increasingly altered (low Pa_{O_2}, elevated Pa_{CO_2}).
6. Pulmonary function tests show:
   a. Decreased FEV_1 (forced expiratory volume in 1 s).
   b. Decreased $FEF_{25-75\%}$ (the forced expiratory flow during the middle half of the forced vital capacity).
   c. Decreased MVV (maximum voluntary ventilation).
   d. Increased residual volume.

NURSING DIAGNOSES: ACTUAL OR POTENTIAL

1. Respiratory dysfunction (mild to severe): dyspnea secondary to increased accumulation of bronchial secretions.
2. Alteration in comfort: discomfort secondary to respiratory changes.
3. Lack of compliance with therapeutic regimen (potential): due to knowledge deficit.
4. Alteration in food intake: weight loss secondary to respiratory dysfunction.
5. Altered activity/tolerance: secondary to respiratory dysfunction (dyspnea, cough).
6. Loss of body fluids: secondary to fever.
7. Alteration in elimination patterns: constipation.
8. Alteration in patterns of sexuality: secondary to dyspnea and fatigability.
9. Social isolation (potential): secondary to dyspnea, cough, sputum expectoration, and fatigability.
10. Fear (potential): secondary to fear of suffocation.
11. Impaired grieving processes (potential): depression; anxiety.

EXPECTED OUTCOMES

1. Productivity of cough will increase to remove secretions from lungs (initial). Client will be free from cough and excessive secretions in lung, as evidenced by the return of clearing lung sounds within 2 to 5 days after treatment is started.
2. Sputum will be less sticky and will change from yellow-green to mucoid within 3 to 5 days after treatment is begun.
3. Body temperature will return to normal within 2 to 5 days of treatment initiation.
4. Ventilatory capacity will increase weekly, as evidenced by decreased fatigue after a selected activity.
5. Client will understand information taught in teaching sessions, as evidenced by 85 percent accuracy, verbally or in writing.
6. Client will lose 4 lb during the next 4 weeks and 6 lb during the second month after discharge.
7. Client will give evidence of compliance with care plan by:
   a. Reducing number of cigarettes by one-half within 2 weeks of discharge, or
   b. Eliminating smoking.

c. Losing weight as recommended.
d. Avoiding environmental pollutants and irritants.
e. Adhering to medication regimen, as indicated by chart maintained by client.
f. Establishing and maintaining an effective activity regimen.

INTERVENTIONS

1. Provide a quiet, nonstimulating environment.
2. Promote a rest and activity program.
3. Provide humidified oxygen therapy (if needed).
4. Administer prescribed bronchodilators, mucolytics, and prophylactic antibiotics to reduce inflammation and promote liquefaction and removal of excess secretions.
5. Give frequent mouth care to increase the appeal of food and fluids; these measures help to keep the client hydrated and to liquefy secretions and diminish fever.
6. Administer Colace or Metamucil to facilitate motility of intestional contents.
7. Give soothing inhalations (humidify inspired air).
8. Provide fluids and diet as tolerated.
9. Monitor vital signs as needed.
10. Monitor arterial blood gases and spirometry as needed.
11. Monitor theophylline levels as needed.
12. Teach about:
    a. Medications: dose, side effects.
    b. Diet: as needed to maintain health and control weight.
    c. Rest and activity to help maintain resistance to other infections and to increase stamina.
    d. Avoidance of pollution and other irritants.
    e. Monitoring changes in sputum.
    f. Preventing respiratory infections.
    g. Effective coughing technique (see Table 31-10).
    h. Postural drainage and percussion (see Figure 31-11).
    i. Breathing control.
    j. Relaxation techniques.
13. Counsel client about nonsmoking and weight control and maintenance.
14. Plant activity/exercise program with gradual increments.
15. Counsel about participation in Better Breathing Club, American Lung Association education series, or a community support group.
16. Counsel about influenza vaccine and pneumovax (pneumonia vaccine).

EVALUATION

Outcome Criteria

1. Cough becomes more productive initially; then secretions and coughing decrease.
2. Breath sounds are clearing; adventitious sounds are diminished.
3. Client walks up five stairs without fatigue or dyspnea.
4. Client recalls with 85 percent accuracy, either verbally or in writing, the content presented in teaching sessions.
5. Client has lost 2 lb during the last 2 weeks.
6. Client has reduced the number of cigarettes smoked to one-half pack per day.
7. Client reports taking medications at appropriate times and in correct amounts, as indicated by chart client is keeping.
8. Client follows the daily exercise plan and is progressing through the plan.

Complications

BRONCHOPNEUMONIA

See the discussion in this chapter (see discussion under *Pneumonia*).

COR PULMONALE

Refer to the discussion in Chapter 30.

RESPIRATORY INSUFFICIENCY

Assessment

1. Hypoxemia: decreased Pa_{O_2} (refer to Table 31-14).
2. Hypercapnia: increased Pa_{CO_2} (refer to Table 31-15).
3. pH: respiratory acidosis or normal.
4. Restlessness.
5. Headache.
6. Shallow, rapid respirations.

Revised Outcomes

1. Oxygenation will be restored within normal limits.
2. Headache, restlessness, and respiratory embarrassment will cease.
3. Other outcomes are as originally stated under Expected Outcomes above.

Interventions

1. Provide suctioning as needed.
2. Administer a nebulized bronchodilator, aminophylline, and mucolytics to reduce bronchospasm and decrease bronchial constriction.
3. Administer humidified oxygen via nasal prongs or Venturi mask (as needed).
4. Assist ventilation as needed.
5. Obtain ECG to determine cardiac status.
6. Monitor arterial blood gases to evaluate effectiveness of treatment.
7. Monitor electrolytes.

RESPIRATORY FAILURE

This is a state in which the alveolar ventilation is inadequate for the body's needs, even at rest. (It is commonly accepted that respiratory failure exists when the Pa_{O_2} is below 60 mmHg and the Pa_{CO_2} is above 50 mmHg.)

Assessment

1. Hypoxemia: Pa_{O_2} less than 60 mmHg (see Table 31-14).
2. Hypercapnia: Pa_{CO_2} more than 50 mmHg (see Table 31-15).
3. pH: respiratory acidosis (pH = 7.30 or lower).
4. Apprehensive.
5. Restlessness.
6. Tachycardia.
7. Shallow, rapid respirations.
8. Increased use of accessory muscles.
9. Confusion.
10. Headache.
11. Cyanosis, especially lips, beneath fingernails, ear lobes.
12. Chest x-ray study will show atelectatic areas and increased heart size. Areas of pneumonia may be noted.
13. ECG will show evidence of right-heart strain.
14. Sputum culture is done to determine if infection is present and, if so, to identify the pathogen.

Revised Outcomes

1. Oxygenation will be restored within normal limits.
2. Headache, restlessness, and respiratory embarrassment will cease.
3. Underlying respiratory infection will be cured.
4. Other outcomes are as originally stated under Expected Outcomes above.

Interventions

1. Provide suctioning as needed.
2. Administer humidified oxygen via nasal prongs or Venturi mask to maintain Pa_{O_2} at 60–70 mmHg. (If Pa_{O_2} is not maintained at 60 mmHg and pH falls below 7.30, ventilatory assistance is indicated. A nasal endotracheal tube with a volume-cycled ventilator with assist control is commonly used.)
3. Administer theophylline by intravenous infusion.
4. Monitor theophylline levels (the therapeutic range is 10–20 μg/mL serum).
5. Monitor arterial blood gases and pH.
6. Monitor electrolytes.
7. Administer prescribed antibiotics to eliminate underlying respiratory infection.
8. Assist with insertion of Swan-Ganz catheter.
9. Monitor pulmonary wedge pressure.
10. Assist with fiberoptic bronchoscopy (at bedside) to aspirate secretions and remove mucus plugs.

Reevaluation and Follow-up

1. Evaluate a specific individualized plan.
2. Follow up and reassess as necessary.

PULMONARY EMPHYSEMA

DESCRIPTION

Pulmonary emphysema is a disease characterized by "an abnormal enlargement of the air spaces distal to the terminal nonrespiratory bronchiole, accompanied by destructive changes of the alveolar walls" (American College of Chest Physicians, 1975). Inflammation, infection, retained secretions, and endoproteases from macrophages contribute to the destructive changes that are thought to begin in the smaller bronchioles. The loss of elastic recoil in the narrowed, tortuous airways causes premature airway collapse and air trapping. The destruction of the alveolar walls and the vascular bed decreases airway support and limits the amount of oxygen–carbon dioxide exchange.

The tissue changes characteristic of pulmonary emphysema are thought to be initiated and aggravated by factors such as cigarette smoking, recurrent infection, and inhaled irritants. A familial form of primary emphysema has been associated with a deficiency in α-antitrypsin (a glycoprotein that has an inhibitory effect on several proteases).

Pulmonary emphysema is diagnosed more often in men, in cigarette smokers, and in those who live in urban settings. Emphysema is usually diagnosed by age 50 or 60; however, those who have an α_1-antitrypsin deficiency usually have manifestations before age 40.

Pulmonary emphysema is an irreversible disorder that is punctuated by episodes of respiratory infections, bronchopneumonia, and respiratory insufficiency. As the pulmonary destructive process continues, the individual becomes more hypoxic and more hypercapnic and succumbs to bronchopneumonia and respiratory failure.

PREVENTION

Health Promotion

1. Avoidance of smoking.
2. Reduced exposure to pollution and occupational dusts.
3. Use of protective devices (e.g., masks) to avoid potential occupational hazards.
4. Avoidance of exposure to individuals with upper respiratory infections.
5. Prompt treatment of respiratory infections.
6. Maintenance of good health habits (rest, nutrition, etc.).
7. Regulations enforcing environmental health.

Population at Risk

1. Smokers (mild to heavy).
2. Persons with α_1-antitrypsin deficiency.
3. Persons who have had recurrent upper respiratory infections.
4. Persons continually exposed to harmful irritants (e.g., dusts, fumes, fibers).
5. Persons living in densely populated areas (e.g., large industrial cities).

Screening

1. Chest x-ray films.
2. Spirometry: FEV_1 (forced expiratory volume in 1 s).

ASSESSMENT

Health History

1. Shortness of breath, especially upon exertion.
2. Cough, sometimes productive of mucoid sputum.
3. Persistent weight loss.
4. Repeated or chronic respiratory infections.
5. Family history of α_1-antitrypsin deficiency.
6. Repeated exposure to pollution or other irritants that may stimulate the inflammatory response.
7. Sleep habits: number of pillows used, amount of rest needed, adequacy of rest and sleep.
8. Health maintenance patterns: smoking, exposure to infection, nutritional practices.

Physical Assessment

1. Breath sounds are faint, and adventitious sounds are usually absent.
2. Wheezing may be heard during expiration.
3. The chest is hyperinflated with hyperresonance.
4. There are shallow respirations with prolonged expiration.
5. There is evidence of increased use of accessory muscles with retraction of supraclavicular fossae.
6. Heart sounds are faint but may be heard over the epigastrum or at the apex.
7. Increased anterior diameter of the chest gives it a barrel-shaped appearance.
8. Clubbing of the fingers may be present.
9. Face may be ruddy to cyanotic (does not always occur).
10. Client is likely to be thin and pale and easily fatigued.
11. Client is air hungry and is usually found sitting and leaning forward with arms on chair arm or thighs.

Diagnostic Tests

1. Chest x-ray study allows visualization of the lungs and identification of the following changes (in relatively advanced cases):
   a. Overaeration of lungs and increase in the retrosternal space.
   b. Decreased vascular markings at lung peripheries.
   c. Increased anterior-posterior chest diameter.
   d. Low, flat diaphragm images.
   e. Widening of the intercostal spaces.
2. Pulmonary function tests will show:
   a. Reduced FEV_1.
   b. Reduced $FEF_{25-75\%}$ (forced expiratory flow during the middle half of the forced vital capacity).
   c. Reduced VC (vital capacity).
   d. Reduced MVV (maximum voluntary ventilation).

e. Increased TLV (total lung volume).
f. Increased RV (residual volume).

3. Arterial blood gases estimate the progression of the disease (refer to Tables 31-14 and 31-15) and show:
   a. Pa_{O_2} is decreased.
   b. Pa_{CO_2} is increased.
4. pH is normal or decreased.
5. α_1-antitrypsin is done to verify deficiency and a diagnosis of primary emphysema. A flat alpha globulin curve is demonstrated in the presence of a deficiency.
6. Sputum culture is done to determine whether infection is present and, if so, to identify the pathogen.

NURSING DIAGNOSES: ACTUAL OR POTENTIAL

1. Respiratory dysfunction (mild to severe): dyspnea secondary to air trapping and alveolar wall destruction.
2. Alteration in comfort: discomfort secondary to respiratory changes.
3. Anxiety (potential): secondary to fear of suffocation.
4. Depression (potential): secondary to loss of ability to perform activities of daily living.
5. Alteration in food intake: weight loss secondary to respiratory dysfunction and fatigue.
6. Alteration in bowel elimination: constipation secondary to dyspnea and fatigue.
7. Altered activity/exercise pattern: secondary to respiratory dysfunction.
8. Lack of adherence to therapeutic regimen (potential): due to knowledge deficit.
9. Impaired thought processes: secondary to elevated Pa_{CO_2}.
10. Social isolation: secondary to dyspnea, cough, fatigue.
11. Alteration in patterns of sexuality (decreased): secondary to dyspnea and fatigue.

EXPECTED OUTCOMES

1. Productivity of cough will increase to remove secretions from lungs (initial). Cough will lessen within 2 to 4 days after treatment is started.
2. Ventilatory capacity will improve weekly, as evidenced by decreased fatigue when walking about room.
3. Client gains 2 lb within the next 3 weeks and 6 lb within 2 months after discharge.
4. Client understands information taught in teaching sessions, as evidenced by 85 percent accuracy, either verbally or in writing.
5. Client complies with care plan as evidenced by:
   a. Reducing number of cigarettes by one-half within 2 weeks of discharge, or
   b. Eliminating smoking.
   c. Gaining weight as recommended.
   d. Avoiding environmental irritants and pollutants.
   e. Adhering to medication regimen, as indicated by chart maintained by client.
   f. Practicing relaxation techniques as recommended.
   g. Establishing and maintaining an effective activity/exercise regimen.

INTERVENTIONS

1. Provide a quiet, nonstimulating environment.
2. Promote a rest and activity program.
3. Provide humidified oxygen at 2–3 L by nasal prongs (if needed).
4. Administer prescribed bronchodilators and prophylactic antibiotics to decrease bronchoconstriction and prevent infection.
5. Provide fluids (2–3 L/day) to help liquefy secretions and replace body fluid.
6. Provide a diet of soft foods and fluid in small amounts 4 to 5 times a day.
7. Give frequent mouth care to increase appeal of foods and fluids; these measures help to keep the client hydrated and to liquefy secretions.
8. Administer stool softeners (Colace, Metamucil) and increase hydration to relieve constipation.
9. Monitor vital signs and arterial blood gases (as needed).
10. Provide program of activity and exercise to assess tolerance levels.
11. Teach about:
    a. Medications: dose, side effects.
    b. Diet: as needed to maintain health and promote weight gain.
    c. Hydration to liquefy secretions, relieve constipation, and replace body fluids.
    d. Postural drainage and percussion: as needed to facilitate mobilization of secretions.

e. Avoidance of pollution and other irritants.
f. Effective coughing and controlled breathing techniques.
g. Coordination of breathing and activity.
h. Rest and activity to help maintain resistance to other infections and to increase stamina.

12. Counsel about nonsmoking.
13. Counsel about participation in American Lung Association client education programs and support groups.

EVALUATION

Outcome Criteria

1. Cough becomes more productive initially; then secretions and coughing decrease.
2. Client walks across room without fatigue or dyspnea.
3. Client recalls with 85 percent accuracy, either verbally or in writing, the content presented in teaching sessions.
4. Client has gained 2 lb during past 3 weeks.
5. Client has reduced the number of cigarettes smoked to one-half pack per day.
6. Client takes medications at appropriate times and in correct amounts, as indicated by chart the client is keeping.
7. Client performs postural drainage as needed, as indicated by absence of pulmonary congestion and chart maintained by client.
8. Client follows daily exercise plan and is progressing through phase 1 of the plan.

Complications

1. Bronchopneumonia (see the discussion in this chapter under *Pneumonia*).
2. Cor pulmonale (see the discussion in Chapter 30).
3. Respiratory insufficiency (see Complications under *Chronic Bronchitis* in this chapter).
4. Respiratory acidosis: an excessive retention of carbon dioxide occurring in the presence of bronchiolar obstruction and diminished alveolar surface area:

Assessment

1. Hypoxemia: decreased Pa_{O_2}.
2. Hypercapnia: increased Pa_{CO_2}.
3. pH: decreased.
4. Cardiac arrhythmias may occur.
5. Drowsiness.
6. Decreased shallow respirations.

Revised Outcomes

1. Pa_{CO_2} will be decreased to within normal range; respiratory embarrassment will cease.
2. Oxygenation will be restored within normal limits; respiratory embarrassment will cease.
3. Other outcomes are as originally stated under Expected Outcomes above.

Interventions

1. Administer humidified oxygen, 2–3 L via nasal prongs or Venturi mask (as needed).
2. Assist ventilation as needed.
3. Administer intravenous bronchodilator to diminish bronchoconstriction.
4. Administer percussion to mobilize secretions.
5. Obtain ECG to determine cardiac changes.
6. Monitor arterial blood gases and pH to evaluate effectiveness of treatment.
7. Monitor vital signs as needed.
8. Monitor electrolytes.

Reevaluation and Follow-up

Establish a specific individualized plan to ensure that the complication is overcome (short-term) and that long-term surveillance and necessary interventions are provided.

PNEUMOCONIOSIS

DESCRIPTION

Pneumoconiosis refers to a parenchymal lung disease that is caused by the lung's reaction to dusts and fibers that are inhaled and retained. The dusts or fibers (5–10 μm) that are inhaled and retained in the lungs elicit an inflammatory response and an outpouring of macrophages. Enzymes from the destroyed macrophages cause the fibrosis, or scarring, of the lung tissue. The distorted lung architecture is reflected in the loss of elasticity (compliance) and the decreased diffusion of gases.

The inhaled particulates exert harmful effects by various mechanisms. Organic materials (moldy hay) cause a hypersensitivity reaction and produce granulomas. Fiber dust (cotton) may elicit allergic responses. Particulate matter such as silica and asbestos may cause pulmonary fibrosis.

Pneumoconiosis is found among workers who are employed in quarries, foundries, the pottery industry, textile factories, and tunneling projects. Family members are exposed to the particulates when they handle workers' contaminated garments. Pneumoconiosis is an irreversible disease that is characterized by hypoxia and recurrent respiratory infections. As the disorder worsens, the individual succumbs to bronchopneumonia and respiratory failure.

PREVENTION

Health Promotion

1. Avoidance of smoking.
2. Reduced exposure to pollution and occupational dusts (use of protective devices such as masks).
3. Avoidance of exposure to garments contaminated with harmful dust and fibers.
4. Avoidance of exposure to persons with upper respiratory infections.
5. Maintenance of good health habits (rest, nutrition, etc.).
6. Regulations enforcing environmental health.

Population at Risk

1. Persons who work with harmful dusts and fibers in textile mills, foundries, mines, quarries, and the pottery industry.
2. Persons who handle garments/equipment contaminated with harmful dusts.
3. Smokers, especially cigarette smokers.
4. Persons who have repeated upper respiratory infections.

Screening

1. Chest x-ray study.
2. Spirometry (e.g., FEV_1 = forced expiratory volume in 1 s).

ASSESSMENT

Health History

1. Residence: all places of residence.
2. Occupation: all types of employment.
3. Exposure to occupational vapors, dusts, fibers (e.g., silica cotton, uranium, aluminum, coal, asbestos, talc).
4. Exposure to environmental pollutants (e.g, carbon monoxide, sulfur dioxide, ozone).
5. Smoking, especially cigarettes.
6. Repeated or chronic respiratory infections.
7. Health maintenance patterns: exercise, nutritional practices, exposure to infection, exposure to tuberculosis.
8. Hobbies: use of glues, sealants, paints, sanding.
9. Sleep habits: number of pillows used, amount of rest needed, adequacy of rest and sleep.
10. Recurrent cough that becomes increasingly persistent over many years.
11. Production of sputum, especially upon rising.
12. Shortness of breath, which is aggravated by exertion.

Physical Assessment

1. Chest expansion is diminished.
2. Diaphragm excursion is decreased.
3. Breath sounds are diminished in intensity.
4. Areas of hypo- and hyperresonance are noted.
5. Wheezing may be auscultated, especially during exertion.
6. Dyspnea and cough are present. These are associated with the accompanying chronic bronchitis or emphysema.
7. Sputum may be dark gray to black.
8. Clubbing of the fingers may be present.
9. Chest pain may be present.
10. A loud second pulmonic heart sound may be noted.
11. Tachycardia is often present.

Diagnostic Tests

1. Chest x-ray study permits visualization of the lungs and identification of shadows and opacities, as well as patterns of nodules and calcifications.
2. Lung function tests show:
   a. Reduced VC (vital capacity).
   b. FEV_1 may be normal or greater than normal.
   c. Reduced MVV (maximum voluntary ventilation).
   d. Decreased diffusion capacity (movement of oxygen and carbon dioxide across the alveolar-capillary membrane).
3. Fiberoptic-transbronchial lung biopsy.
4. Arterial blood gases estimate progression of disease: as pulmonary fibrosis worsens, blood gases become increasingly altered (low Pa_{O_2}, elevated Pa_{CO_2}).
5. PPD to determine reaction to purified protein derivative.

NURSING DIAGNOSES: ACTUAL OR POTENTIAL

1. Respiratory dysfunction (moderate to severe): dyspnea secondary to pulmonary fibrosis.

2. Alteration in comfort: discomfort secondary to respiratory changes.
3. Altered activity/exercise pattern: secondary to respiratory dysfunction (dyspnea, cough).
4. Lack of compliance with therapeutic regimen (potential): due to knowledge deficit.

EXPECTED OUTCOMES

1. Productivity of cough will increase to remove secretions from lung (initial). Cough will diminish and excessive secretions will cease within 2 to 4 days after treatment is begun.
2. Ventilatory capacity will show some improvement, as evidenced by less fatigue when walking about room.
3. Client will understand information taught in teaching sessions, as evidenced by 85 percent accuracy verbally or in writing.
4. Client will give evidence of compliance with care plan by:
   a. Reducing number of cigarettes by one-half within 2 weeks of discharge, or
   b. Eliminating smoking.
   c. Avoiding environmental pollution and irritants.
   d. Adhering to medication regimen, as indicated by chart maintained by client.
   e. Establishing and maintaining an effective exercise regimen.

INTERVENTIONS

1. Provide a quiet, nonstimulating environment.
2. Promote a rest and activity program.
3. Provide oxygen therapy if needed.
4. Administer prescribed bronchodilators to reduce bronchoconstriction and promote removal of secretions.
5. Administer PPD (purified protein derivative). (Persons with silicosis are more vulnerable to pulmonary tuberculosis.)
6. Give frequent mouth care to increase the appeal of food and fluids; these measures help keep the client hydrated.
7. Provide diet and fluids as tolerated.
8. Monitor vital signs and arterial blood gases as needed.
9. Teach about:
   a. Medications: dose, side effects.
   b. Diet: as needed to maintain health and keep weight within normal range.
   c. Rest and activity to help maintain resistance to respiratory infections, increase stamina, and promote muscle strength.
   d. Prevention of respiratory infections.
   e. Avoidance of pollution and other irritants.
10. Plan activity/exercise program with gradual increments.
11. Counsel regarding NIOSH (National Institute for Occupational Safety and Health) standards and safety measures in occupational setting.
12. Counsel regarding possible need to change occupations or to retire; nonsmoking; and participation in American Lung Association client education groups or support groups.

EVALUATION

Outcome Criteria

1. Cough becomes more productive initially; then secretions and cough decrease.
2. Breath sounds are clearing to clear; adventitious sounds are absent.
3. Client walks up six steps without dyspnea or fatigue.
4. Client recalls with 85 percent accuracy, either verbally or in writing, the content presented in teaching sessions.
5. Client reaction to PPD is not positive.
6. Client has reduced the number of cigarettes smoked to one-half pack per day.
7. Client takes medications at appropriate times and in correct amounts, as indicated by chart maintained by client.
8. Client follows the daily exercise plan and is progressing through phase 1 of the plan.

Complications

1. Bronchopneumonia (see the discussion in this chapter).
2. Cor pulmonale (see the discussion in Chapter 30).
3. Pulmonary tuberculosis (see the discussion under *Tuberculosis* in this chapter).
4. Cancer of the lung (see the discussion in this chapter).
5. Bronchiectasis (see the discussion in this chapter).
6. Pulmonary emphysema (see the discussion in this chapter).
7. Respiratory failure (see Complications under *Chronic Bronchitis*).

REFERENCES

Adams, G. L., Boies, L. R., and Paparella, M. M.: *Boies' Fundamentals of Otolaryngology*, 5th ed., Saunders, Philadelphia, 1978, p. 347.

American Cancer Society: *Cancer Facts and Figures—1980*, American Cancer Society, New York, 1979, p. 9.

American College of Chest Physicans, American Thoracic Society: "Pulmonary Terms and Symbols," *Chest*, **67**(5):583–593, May 1975.

Ballantyne, J., and Graves, J.: *Scott Brown's Diseases of Ear, Nose, and Throat*, 4th ed., vol. 3, "The Nose and Sinuses," Butterworth, London, 1979.

Brunner, L., and Suddarth, D.: *The Lippincott Manual of Nursing Practice*, Lippincott, Philadelphia, 1982.

Bushnell, S.: *Respiratory Intensive Care Nursing*, Little, Brown, Boston, 1973.

Guenter, C. A., and Welch, M. H., eds.: *Pulmonary Medicine*, Harper & Row, Hagerstown, Md., 1977.

DeWeese, D. D., and Saunders, W. H.: *Textbook of Otolaryngology*, 5th ed, Mosby, St. Louis, 1977, p. 123.

Hall, I., and Colman, B.: *Diseases of the Nose, Throat and Ear*, Churchill Livingstone, New York, 1975.

Hanno, R., and Callen, J. R.: "Sarcoidosis," *Medical Clinics of North America*, **64**(5):847–866, September 1980.

Hinshaw, H.: *Diseases of the Chest*, 4th ed., Saunders, Philadelphia, 1979.

Isaacson, S., and Edell, S. L.: "A-mode Ultrasound Evaluation of Macillary Sinusitis," *Otolaryngology*, **86:**ORL-231–235, March-April 1978.

Isselbacher, K., et al.: *Harrison's Principles of Internal Medicine*, 9th ed., vols. 1 and 2, McGraw-Hill, New York, 1980.

LeJeune, F. E.: "Symposium: Carcinoma of Larynx; Surgical Treatment of Early Carcinoma of Larynx," *Laryngoscope*, **61**(6):488–495, June 1951.

Luckmann, J., and Sorensen, K.: *Medical-Surgical Nursing*, Saunders, Philadelphia, 1980.

Sexton, D. L.: "The Place of Cromolyn Sodium in the Management of Asthma," *Nurses' Drug Alert*, **III**(12):117–120, 1979.

Wittner, M.: *Pneumococcal Pneumonia*, Abbot Laboratories, Ill., 1974.

BIBLIOGRAPHY

DeWeese, D. D., and Saunders, W. H.: *Textbook of Otolaryngology*, 5th ed., Mosby, St. Louis, 1977. Reviews anatomy, physiology, diagnosis, treatment, and rehabilitation of otolaryngological disorders. Contains excellent figures and photographs.

Dudley, D. L., Glaser, E. M., Jorgenson, B. N., and Logan, D. L.: "Psychological Concomitants to Rehabilitation in Chronic Obstructive Pulmonary Disease," *Chest*, **77**(3):413–420 (part 1 of 3), 1980. Discusses psychosocial concomitants of COPD, such as isolation, denial, and repression in relation to dyspnea, anxiety, and depression. The article also focuses on guidelines for treating the psychosocial aspects, including breathing retraining, meditation, behavior modification, and the experimental use of biofeedback.

Fishman, A.: *Pulmonary Diseases and Disorders*, vols. 1 and 2, McGraw-Hill, New York, 1980. Presents a comprehensive discussion of the manifestations of lung disease, assessment and diagnostic tests, and treatment regimens.

Fitzmaurice, J., and Sasahara, A.: "Current Concepts of Pulmonary Embolism: Implications for Nursing Practice," *Heart and Lung* **5:**209–218, March-April 1974. Signs and symptoms, diagnosis and treatment, and implications for nursing care for pulmonary embolism are outlined.

Karus, C.: "Tuberculosis: An Overview of Pathogenesis and Prevention," *The Nurse Practioner*, **8**(2):23, February 1983. An excellent article providing recent facts about the disease, preventive methods for persons at risk, and diagnostic tests and treatment.

Maurer, J. M.: "Providing Optimal Oral Health," *Nursing Clinics of North America*, **12**(4):671–685, December 1977. This article discusses the factors causing alterations in oral physiology and includes guidelines for assessing oral health and the choice of agents to be used in oral care.

Mechner, F.: "Patient Assessment: Examination of the Chest and Lungs, Part I," *American Journal of Nursing*, **76:**1–23, September 1976. This article is a programmed instruction of assessment techniques for examining the adult chest.

Owens, J.: "Respiratory Failure after Injury: A Review and Plea for Accuracy," *Heart and Lung*, **6:**303–307, March-April 1977. Reviews clinical presentation, pathophysiology, and management of the adult respiratory syndrome.

Reichman, L. B. (ed.): "International Conference on Tuberculosis," *Chest*, **76:**737–817, December 1979 (supplement). This issue is devoted to a report of a continuing education conference about tuberculosis. Aspects such as diagnosis, chemotherapy, and adherence to treatment program are emphasized.

Rosenow, E. C., and Carr, D. T.: "Bronchogenic Carcinoma," *CA—A Cancer Journal for Clinicians*, **29:**233–245, July-August 1979. This article outlines the histology, manifestations, staging, treatment, and prognosis of bronchogenic cancer.

Sexton, D. L.: *Chronic Obstructive Pulmonary Disease: Care of the Child and Adult*, Mosby, St. Louis, 1981. Includes the pathophysiology, assessment, and management of asthma, chronic bronchitis, emphysema, and bronchiectasis. Final chapters focus on psychosocial aspects and coping with chronic obstructive pulmonary disease.

Sovik, C.: "The Nursing Care of Lung Cancer Patients," *Nursing Clinics of North America*, **13:**301–318, June 1978. This article provides an overview of the treatment for lung cancer and reviews the nursing implications.

Sweetwood, H. M.: *Nursing in the Respiratory Care Unit*, Springer, New York, 1979. Outlines respiratory diseases; good illustrations and references.

32

The Urinary System

Margaret Allen Murphy

Optimal functioning of the genitourinary system depends on the regulatory mechanisms and integrated functioning of the cardiovascular, nervous, and endocrine systems. A disturbance in excretory, regulatory, or secretory functioning of the kidney may result in a disturbance in other parts of the genitourinary system or other parts of the body. Conversely, an obstruction of the free flow of urine or a disturbance in performance below the pelvis of the kidney may eventually result in destruction of nephrons.

In this chapter, each phase of the nursing process is discussed. When applying this format to an actual client situation, the nurse must assess the client's needs and delineate specific, appropriate expected outcomes in terms of the individual client. The health history of the client and sound professional judgment on the part of the nurse will indicate essential areas of investigation, diagnosis, intervention, and evaluation (see Table 32-1).

ABNORMAL CELLULAR GROWTH

RENAL TUMORS

DESCRIPTION

Masses in the kidney may be caused by fluid-filled cavities, by cysts, or by solid tumors. Tumors of the kidney are rarely benign. Neoplasms of the kidney can be divided into three major categories:

1. Tumors developing from embryonic tissues.
2. Tumors originating in the renal parenchyma of the adult kidney.
3. Tumors developing in the renal pelvises or calyces of adults.

Nephroblastomas, or Wilms' tumors, the most common renal malignancies occurring in children, originate from embryonic tissues and contain epithelial and mesodermal elements. Rarely occurring bilaterally, this neoplasm appears in infancy or early childhood, usually before age 7.

Tumors of the renal parenchyma, often called hypernephromas or adenocarcinomas, are the most commonly seen neoplasms in the adult kidney and rarely occur before age 30. These tumors are usually unilateral and are encapsulated. Men are more frequently affected than women. Growth of this renal neoplasm compresses surrounding renal tissue and displaces and distorts the renal pelvis, calyces, and blood vessels. Invasion of the renal vein and metastasis to the liver, lungs, and long bones are characteristic of adenocarcinomas.

Squamous cell tumors of the renal pelvis or calyces are far less common. Believed to be caused by carcinogens in the urine, these tumors arise from the epithelium of the renal pelvis. The neoplasms are often associated with bladder and ureteral tumors. Involvement of regional lymph nodes and the renal vein occurs, but metastases to distant organs are uncommon.

Regardless of the origin of the renal neoplasm, obstruction of urinary drainage or de-

TABLE 32-1 ASSESSMENT FINDINGS ASSOCIATED WITH URINARY SYSTEM PROBLEMS

1. General appearance.
   The client presenting for assistance with a concern related to the urinary tract will usually appear acutely ill, whether resulting from inadequate kidney clearance, obstruction, or infection. Even minor alterations in function will cause:
   a. Dramatic changes in the skin, such as pruritus, petechiae, crystal formation, excess perspiration, and skin color change.
   b. Abdominal or flank pain.
   c. Fever.
   d. Obvious edema, such as periorbital edema or facial edema.
   e. Recent weight loss or gain.
   f. Expressions of pain and distress.
   g. Signs of dehydration may appear throughout the body.
2. Family history (specific).
   Determine whether family members have had:
   a. Tuberculosis: TB of kidney can occur as result of TB at another site.
   b. High blood pressure: can cause end-organ damage in kidney.
   c. Heart failure: accumulation of fluid.
   d. Diabetes mellitus: neurogenic bladder and renal or vascular disease, UTI, and pyelonephritis.
   e. Diabetes insipidus: affects ability to concentrate urine.
   f. Beta hemolytic streptococcal sore throat: foci of infection in kidney can occur.
   g. Rheumatic fever: foci of infection in kidney can occur.
   h. Scarlet fever: foci of infection in kidney can occur.
   i. Gout or gouty arthritis: deposit of sodium urate crystals from excess uric acid in blood.
3. Nutritional assessment.
   a. General dietary assessment to verify fluid intake, protein intake, and intake of calcium, sodium, potassium, and phosphorus.
   b. Complaints of metallic taste may occur in the presence of toxic materials in the system.
   c. Complaints of nausea, vomiting, and loss of appetite are not uncommon.
4. Concurring complaints.
   a. Headaches: associated with renal artery stenosis, excess renin excretion, and hypertension.
   b. Fatigue, lethargy, decreased muscle tone, peripheral neuropathy.
   c. Changes in sleep patterns.
   d. Alterations in sexual patterns.
5. Urinary pattern assessment.
   To determine changes in pattern of micturation (urination). Assessment should focus on:
   a. The frequency of involuntary or unexpected voiding.
   b. The amount of urine in 24 h: usually equal to normal intake (1,500–3,000 cc).
   c. The amount of urine per voiding: 400–500 ml in normal adult.
   d. The number of voidings q 24h; increase in the number of voidings per night.
   e. The color, odor, and dilution of urine: accumulation of waste products can cause discoloration.
   f. The presence of dysuria, pain or burning in urethra on urination occurring as result of:
      (1) Central nervous system involvement: tabes, multiple sclerosis.
      (2) Peripheral nervous system involvement: diabetic neuropathy.
      (3) Inflammation in urinary tract or bladder.
      (4) Obstruction in urinary tract or bladder.
   g. Urgency: inflammation, stones, or tumor.
   h. Frequency: inflammation, tumor.

TABLE 32-1 *(continued)*

i. Hesitancy: tumor or other obstruction.
j. Burning: inflammation.
k. Strangury: slow, painful emission of urine.
l. Tenesmus: obstruction, painful spasms of the bladder after voiding.
m. Hematuria or change in color of urine.
n. Urethral discharge.

6. Physical assessment.
Includes:
a. Inspection: observe urinary stream.
b. Palpation: differentiate meatal stenosis, urethral caruncle, urethral prolapse (caruncle is painful, prolapse is not).
c. Transillumination of contents of scrotum (edema fluid transilluminates, blood or bowel does not).
7. Abdominal changes.
Can include:
a. Suprapubic bulge of distended bladder.
b. Easily palpable kidneys may indicate severe renal damage.
c. Costovertebral angle tenderness may alert the examiner to potential inflammation and renal damage.
d. Edema of the abdomen (fluid waves, puddles sign) are indicative of fluid accumulation that may be observed in the presence of severe renal damage.
8. Cardiovascular alterations.
a. Arrhythmias related to accumulation of electrolytes in serum (K, Ca).
b. Pulmonary changes, including lung rales, may be suggestive of congestive failure or pulmonary edema.
c. Increase in blood pressure.
d. Tacchycardia: presence of S_3 (gallop rhythm) may be found in the presence of fluid volume overload.
9. Neurologic changes.
Can include:
a. Drowsiness or disorientation due to accumulation of toxic products.
b. Superficial reflexes: cremasteric reflex tests L_1, L_2, L_3; gluteal reflex texts L_4, L_5.
c. Deep tendon reflexes: patella reflex tests segmental level L_3, L_4; Achilles reflex tests segmental level S_2.
d. Parasympathetic nerves: S_1, S_2, S_3, S_4 control bladder.
e. Sympathetic nerves: L_1, L_2 control trigone and urethra.

SOURCE: Malasanos, L., et al.: *Health Assessment*, Mosby, St. Louis, 1981, p. 555.

struction of renal tissue may eventually result. Most renal neoplasms grow insidiously and relatively quickly. Many fail to produce distinctive symptoms early in the course of the disease, since symptoms often do not occur until 80 to 90 percent of the nephrons are damaged.

PREVENTION

Health Promotion

1. Avoid smoking and other exposure to known carcinogens.
2. Insist local water supplies be tested periodically, especially if known industrial waste sites are nearby.
3. Support public interest in environmental issues.

Population at Risk

1. Smokers.
2. Persons living near industrial waste sites.
3. Persons exposed to industrial chemicals.
4. Men over age 30.

Screening

1. Industrial surveys (cytology reports).
2. Occupational history of exposure to toxins.
3. Gross or microscopic intermittent hematuria (> 2 RBCs, or red blood cells, per high power field, or hpf).

ASSESSMENT

Health History

Refer to Table 32-1.

1. Age: hypernephromas rarely occur before age 30.
2. Sex: tumors occur more often in men.
3. Occupation: possible exposure to carcinogens.
4. Home environment: proximity to waste disposal sites.
5. Weight (usual and present): weight loss or gain.
6. Nutritional assessment to verify intake.
7. Past health history: previous physical examinations, hospitalizations, and/or surgery.
8. History of allergies (particularly to iodine) and blood type.
9. History of drug use (particularly nephrotoxic agents and drugs, and anticoagulants). Include information about:
   a. Type of drug used.
   b. Whether drug is medically prescribed or self-prescribed.
   c. The reason for taking the drug.
   d. Length of time used.
   e. Method and frequency of administration.
   f. Response to drug.
10. Perception of the client and family regarding expectations of hospitalization, future decision-making structure, and available support systems and resources.
11. Health perception, motivation for self-care, and adaptability to disruptions in health.
12. Nonurologic complaints that may be indicative of metastasis to surrounding or distant organs.
13. Presence, location, intensity, quality, and precipitating or aggravating factors of pain (present in advanced cases, especially "dragging" flank pain).
14. Agents or factors that aid in pain relief.
15. Voiding patterns and characteristics of urination, particularly intermittent or continuous painless hematuria, gross or microscopic.

Physical Assessment

1. Palpable or visible mass in affected flank (not always present).
2. Depending on the extent of tumor invasion and/or metastasis, the following may be present:
   a. Elevated temperature.
   b. If bleeding is present and anemia is noted, the client will appear pale, with poor capillary refill noted.
   c. Muscular weakness, malaise, and lethargy.
   d. Dyspnea and/or cough.
   e. Edema in lower extremities.
   f. Distention of abdominal veins.

Diagnostic Tests

Many tests are used to diagnose renal tumors. The following discussion focuses on some of the major ones. As with all diagnostic tests, the client requires a complete explanation of each procedure. Tests provide information on structural integrity, functional capability, and renovascularity.

1. The following tests are concerned with structural integrity.
   a. X-ray flat plate of ureters, kidneys, and bladder.
   b. Cystoscopy: inspection of the bladder with a cystoscope via the urethra for defects, malformations, and abnormal cellular growth in the bladder.
      (1) The procedure is usually performed under general anesthesia, although local anesthesia may be used.
      (2) Client receives nothing by mouth (NPO) before procedure; intravenous fluids are given to allow for collection of specimens.
   c. Cystoureterogram: introduction of radiopaque dye into bladder and urethra.
   d. Intravenous pyelogram (IVP): a radiopaque substance is used to visualize the size and shape of the kidney and the urinary tract; it is administered IV.
      (1) A screening of creatinine level precedes the test.
      (2) Client usually receives NPO from the midnight before the test.
      (3) Client receives a cathartic and/or enema before the x-ray so that a better view of the urinary structures can be achieved.
      (4) Client should be observed for an

allergic response to the dye (redness, blotching, itching, and signs of respiratory distress should be noted/reported immediately).

(5) A test dose is usually given to detect possible serious side effects of the radiopaque substance.

(6) Following the test, fluids are forced to flush out excess dye and prevent dehydration.

(7) Emergency epinephrine should be available in case of anaphylactic reaction.

e. Retrograde pyelogram: visualization of ureters and renal pelvis by use of radiopaque contrast medium, introduced via ureteral catheter.

f. Retroperitoneal pneumography: carbon dioxide or oxygen is used as a contrast gas to outline adrenal tumors or retroperitoneal tumors.

g. Ultrasonogram: high-frequency sound waves projected into the body are reflected back onto an oscilloscope screen that shows computerized images of soft tissue; effectively assesses size of organs and identifies masses, obstructions, and malformations in the urinary tract.

h. Nephrotomogram: computerized axial tomography of the kidneys that detects small tumors in paranchyma of kidney; may be done with contrast material (IV).

i. Metastatic series (x-ray) to evaluate progression of the tumor and metastasis to other areas.

2. The following tests give information on the physiologic functional capacity of the kidneys and involve blood chemistries or urinalysis.

a. Single-voiding urinalysis.

(1) Gross and microscopic evaluation of sugar, acetone, protein, hemoglobin, red blood cells, or gross blood in the urine.

(2) Urine for culture and sensitivity to detect the number of bacteria per high power field and sensitivity to antibacterial agents (clean catch or catheterized urine specimen).

(3) Urine for cytology or Papanicolaou examination to detect atypical cells of malignancy.

b. Urine specimens q24h for chemical content culture for tubercle bacillus or proteinuria.

c. Glomerular filtration rate: tests actual function of kidneys by comparing timed samples of blood and urine and calculating the rate at which creatinine is cleared from the plasma (110–113 mL/min corrected for body surface area).

d. Urine concentration tests.

(1) Specific gravity 1.010–1.026; as nephron function falls, specific gravity falls.

(2) Fishberg concentration test: withholding fluids; tests the ability of the kidney to conserve fluid.

e. Blood chemistry tests.

(1) Blood urea nitrogen (BUN) 10–20 mg/100 mL; measures kidney's ability to excrete nitrogenous products of protein breakdown.

(2) Serum creatinine 0.9–1.5 mg/100 mL, as above.

f. Concentration of serum electrolytes: ability of kidneys to clear or resorb electrolytes; gives information on kidney function.

(1) Sodium (Na) 138–148 mEq/L.

(2) Potassium (K) 3.5–5.0 mEq/L.

(3) Calcium (Ca) 9–11 mg/100mL.

(4) Chloride (Cl) 100–106 mEq/L.

(5) Phosphorus (Ph) 3–4.5 mg/100 mL.

3. The following tests give information on the renal vascular lymph supply and drainage.

a. Renogram: isotopic evaluation of renal vascularity and glomerulofiltration; probe registers isotope count over each kidney.

b. Renal scan: radioactive mercury injected intravenously is detected and printed out by probe and photography; not effective for areas of disease less than 1 inch.

c. Renal angiogram: venogram contrast medium introduced via femoral artery outlines arterial or venous circulation.

(1) Observe for bleeding over catheter site.

(2) Palpate for intact pedal pulses.

(3) Observe for reaction to dye used.

d. Retroperitoneal lymphangiogram: outlines by contrast medium lymphatic drainage to detect metastasis; observe for lipoid pneumonia.

NURSING DIAGNOSES: ACTUAL OR POTENTIAL

1. Fear due to impending diagnostic studies, surgery, radiation, or chemotherapy.
2. Lowered self-esteem due to body changes.
3. Alteration in urinary elimination pattern due to fluid volume deficit or excess.

4. Nutritional alteration due to altered body requirements secondary to nausea, vomiting, diminished food ingestion.
5. Alteration in bowel pattern due to retention of feces, or constipation.
6. Knowledge deficit regarding effects of surgery, chemotherapy, radiation, course of alteration, and discharge plans.
7. Alteration in skin integrity due to accumulation of toxins, calcium, and fluid.
8. Alteration in comfort due to pressure of abdominal mass diagnostic tests, surgery, radiation, or chemotherapy.
9. Decreased activity tolerance due to fatigue, muscle weakness, immobility, or cardiovascular deficit.
10. Nonproductive coping patterns due to increased need for assistance and lack of environmental resources.
11. Alteration in cardiac function due to renovascular deficit.
12. Alteration in sexual pattern due to hypotensive agents, impotence, decreased libido, or changes in body image.
13. Impaired reasoning ability due to accumulation of toxic products in central nervous system.

EXPECTED OUTCOMES

1. Client will cope with discomfort and inconvenience of diagnostic and therapeutic procedures with minimum distress.
2. Body functions will be maintained as close to normal as possible.
3. Client and significant others will use information sources and other support systems to maintain desired lifestyle throughout course of illness.
4. Client will achieve optimal wellness in view of a life-threatening illness.

INTERVENTIONS

1. Review with client the processes and outcomes associated with diagnostic procedures, surgery, radiation, and chemotherapy, including sensations to be expected, time frame, positions assumed, and dietary and bowel preparation.
2. Establish rapport with client and family. Actively attend to client's concerns, both verbal and nonverbal. Answer questions honestly. Assess level of coping.
3. Determine client's usual pattern of bladder elimination from nursing history and attempt to restore pattern.
   a. Identify aids used in initiating and maintaining usual patterns of urine elimination.
   b. Assist client in forcing or restricting fluid intake according to physician's prescription.
   c. Measure specific gravity and test urine for blood at every voiding and observe for presence of clots (if client can do so, teach procedures).
   d. Prepare client for diagnostic tests, nephrectomy, radiation, chemotherapy, hemodialysis, and peritoneal dialysis (see *Acute Renal Failure* and *Chronic Renal Failure*).
   e. If indwelling catheter is ordered, insert prescribed indwelling bladder catheter. Initiate measures to maintain a sterile, closed system (Begg, 1981).
      (1) Insert urinary catheter using proper sterile technique and the following sterile equipment: gloves, a fenestrated drape, sponges and an iodophor solution for periurethral cleansing, a lubricant jelly, and an appropriate-size urinary catheter. Following insertion, secure catheter properly to prevent movement and urethral traction.
      (2) Always use a closed, sterile drainage system. Do not disconnect distal urinary catheter and proximal drainage tube, thus opening the closed system (see Figure 32-1).
      (3) Do not disconnect catheter tubing for ambulating or transporting the client. Do not use catheter plugs.
      (4) If catheter irrigations are necessary, use needle and syringe method for irrigation. Use and then discard a large-volume sterile syringe, 21-gauge needle, and sterile irrigant. If frequent irrigations are necessary, a triple lumen catheter permitting continuous irrigation within a closed system is preferable.
      (5) Aspirate small volumes of urine for culture and/or urinalysis from distal catheter using a sterile syringe and 21-gauge needle; prepare catheter with

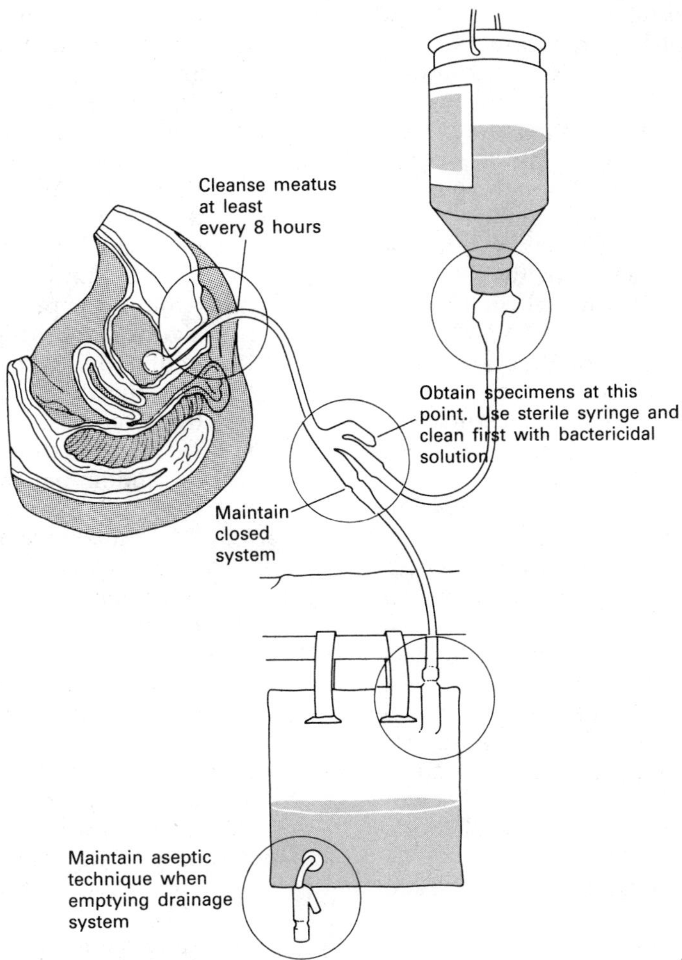

Figure 32-1 Major points to consider when an indwelling catheter is present.

tincture of iodine and/or alcohol. Urine for chemical determinations (i.e., glucose, electrolytes, or osmolarity) can be obtained from the drainage bag by sterile means.

(6) Maintain unobstructed "downhill" flow at all times; this requires emptying the collection bag regularly, replacing poorly functioning or obstructed catheters, and ensuring that collection bags remain below the level of the bladder.

(7) Immediately replace all closed collecting systems contaminated by inappropriate technique, accidental disconnection, leaks, or other means.

(8) In clients with chronic indwelling catheters, replace when concretions can be palpated in catheter or when malfunction or obstruction occurs. In clients with urinary catheterization of less than two weeks' duration, routine catheter change is not necessary except when obstruction, contamination, or other malfunction occurs (Horsley, 1981).

(9) Inspect skin carefully around catheter and assess urinary drainage.

(10) Measure accurately and record intake and output of all fluids.

4. Assist client undergoing surgical excision of kidney.

a. Types of surgical intervention.
   (1) Lumbar nephrectomy: formation of a fistula in the pelvis of the kidney made through flank incision.
   (2) Transperitoneal nephrectomy: formation of a fistula within the pelvis of the kidney made through an opening through the peritoneum.
   (3) Transthoracic nephrectomy: formation of a fistula within the pelvis of the kidney made through an incision.

b. Preoperative interventions.
   (1) Decrease fear through reassurance and well-established nurse–client relationship (see Nursing Diagnoses).
   (2) Encourage support from family and significant others.
   (3) Provide pastoral care and counseling if appropriate.
   (4) Provide teaching regarding physical and psychological preparation for surgery.
   (5) Offer information about immediate and long-term postoperative expectations and activities, including the intensive care unit, coughing and deep breathing exercises, intravenous fluids, and Foley catheter drainage.
   (6) Introduce need to establish long-range rehabilitaton goals.
   (7) Type and crossmatch blood to be kept on call.

c. Postoperative interventions.
   In general, the nursing care of a client following a nephrectomy is similar to the care of a client after major abdominal surgery.
   (1) Assess for alterations in vital signs.
   (2) Use meticulous measurement and correlate intake and output every hour.
   (3) Assess dressings for serosanguineous drainage or urinary drainage in immediate postoperative period.
   (4) Maintain fluid and electrolyte balance. Administer prescribed intravenous fluids.
   (5) Assess for bladder distension.
   (6) Provide meticulous indwelling bladder catheter care with prescribed continuous irrigation.
   (7) Assess function of each drainage tube and area being drained.
   (8) Assess urine for clots. Maintain adequate and safe outflow of urine through drainage system (see Figure 32-1).
   (9) In the case of transthoracic nephrectomy, assess placement and drainage of catheter in pleural cavity.
   (10) Provide respiratory care, including deep breathing, coughing, and turning every hour. Splint operative area. Use caution if drains are present.
   (11) Administer pain relief measures: analgesics, massage, relaxation, therapeutic touch, and/or moist heat.
   (12) Administer NPO until peristaltic activity returns.
      (a) Assess return of bowel sounds via abdominal auscultation.
      (b) Gradually increase food according to tolerance as prescribed.
      (c) Provide rigorous oral hygiene when oral fluids are limited.
   (13) Encourage early mobility and ambulation as prescribed operatively. Use elastic knee-length stockings. Discourage sitting in a chair for long periods.
   (14) Provide reassurance and assistance in dealing with possible altered body image and loss of body part. If signs of grieving are apparent, the nurse should provide support (see Chapter 45).
   (15) Assess for signs and symptoms of infection. Examine the drainage and operative site for poor healing and signs of inflammation.
   (16) Administer prescribed antibiotics. Change dressing as ordered.
   (17) Initiate teaching-learning transaction (include family and/or significant others) regarding the following:
      (a) Medications, especially name, dosage, rationale, expected action, side effects, and signs of toxicity.
      (b) Nutritional counseling.
      (c) Signs and symptoms of urinary tract infections and appropriate responses.
      (d) Importance of health care follow-up.

d. Follow-up interventions.
   (1) (a) Measure intake and output q8h.

(b) Help client to force or restrict fluids as necessary.
(c) Stress attractive meals that follow dietary prescription (restricted protein decreases nitrogenous waste products and conserves kidney function).
(d) Develop teaching plan regarding importance of nutrition in maintaining kidney function, energy level, and general well-being.
(e) Assess factors that may contribute to inadequate nutrition, anorexia, vomiting, nausea, noncompliance, altered taste, and lack of resources for shopping and food preparation.
(f) Refer for dental problems.
(g) Monitor weight each morning before food or fluids to evaluate fluid retention (1 kg body weight = 1 L fluid).
(h) Restrict sodium as prescribed.
(i) Assess skin daily (see Table 32-1).

(2) (a) Determine client's usual pattern of bowel elimination from nursing history.
(b) Identify aids used in maintenance of usual bowel pattern.
(c) Consult physician for stool softener or bulk-forming laxatives if necessary (avoid those containing magnesium).
(d) If phosphate binders are used to decrease serum calcium, they can cause constipation.

(3) Develop individualized teaching plan at every stage of tumor growth and related management. Consider client's educational level, emotional factors, and style of learning.

(4) Provide pain relief measures.
(a) Administer prescribed analgesics before pain is established.
(b) Provide distractors as appropriate.
(c) Use therapeutic touch, massage, visual imagery, counterstimulation, music therapy, and relaxation response in management of discomfort.

(5) Plan daily activity–rest schedule with client, considering role activities, renal function, energy level, and muscle strength.
(a) Check vital signs.
(b) Assess energy level (by report).
(c) Test for deep tendon reflexes, decreased sensation, position sense, two-point discrimination, and restless leg syndrome.
(d) Consult with physician and physical therapist regarding muscle cramps or alteration in electrolyte level.
(e) Assess for acidosis, since potassium and hydrogen may be retained by poor renal functions.

(6) Include specific plans for:
(a) Teaching client the relationships among medications, diet, fluid intake, stress, rest, and activity.
(b) Acting as resource person for client, providing referral to local and national organizations or client self-help groups.
(c) Advising client regarding resources available for future care.
(d) Providing atmosphere that fosters self-care and maximal independence.

(7) Monitor the client's health state.
(a) Assess vital signs (can be taught to client or primary care provider).
(b) Check serum electrolytes as available.
(c) Check hemoglobin and hematocrit as available.
(d) Weigh client each day before food or fluids (can be taught to client or primary care provider).

(8) Support the client's relationship with spouse.
(a) Assist client and partner in planning personal lives to maximize sexual potency.
(b) Refer client to sexual counselor.

(9) Help client maintain ADL.
(a) Assist client in maximizing renal function by adherence to therapeutic regimen, including diet, exercise, medications, treatments, and self-care.
(b) Assess neuromuscular integrity, including muscle strength, sensation, muscle cramps, footdrop.

(c) Provide safe, comfortable environment for compromised function.
(d) Assess need for assistive devices.
(e) Initiate seizure precautions in the presence of elevated BUN levels.
(f) Provide physiologic body alignment with adequate pillow support to prevent pathological fractures.

EVALUATION

Outcome Criteria

1. Client tolerates diagnostic procedures with minimal discomfort and stress, as evidenced by self-rating of less than 4 on distress scale of 1–10 (8 h postprocedure).
2. Client and family maintain open communication with each other and staff concerning effectiveness of coping mechanisms as evaluated by primary care provider/self.
3. Clear urine output is equal to intake each 24 h (+400–600 cc for other modes of fluid excretion); specific gravity in normal range (1.010–1.026).
4. Client reports no nausea or vomiting and maintains optimal weight within 5 lb of predetermined baseline on each follow-up visit.
5. Client and primary home care provider achieve 80-percent mastery on quizzes of 10 items related to diet, medications, elimination, and symptoms of renal decompensation or metastatic spread.
6. Client verifies bowel elimination of soft brown stool every 1–2 days.
7. Skin is intact, smooth, elastic, and nonpruritic on daily or weekly assessment.
8. Client is following daily exercise plan with safety and comfort as evaluated according to schedule by primary care provider or self.
9. Hemoglobin 13.5–18 g/100 mL in men, 12–16 g/100 mL in women.
10. Dyastolic blood pressure below 90 mmHg.
11. Client and partner report mutually satisfactory sexual relationship on each follow-up visit.
12. Neuromuscular exam is within normal limits daily while in hospital and on each follow-up visit after discharge.

Complications

1. Complications related to personal social status.
   a. Situational depression.
   b. Social isolation.
2. Complications related to surgery, tumor growth, or medical management.

INTERNAL HEMORRHAGE

Assessment

1. Tachycardia, hypotension, and shortness of breath.
2. Increased restlessness and changes in mental status.
3. Pallor, skin clamminess, and apprehension.
4. Excessive drainage on dressing. Bleeding may be frank or mixed with urine.
5. Abdominal distension.

Revised Outcomes

1. Bleeding will terminate.
2. Physiologic balance will be restored.

Interventions

1. Monitor and assess vital signs every 15 min; administer oxygen as needed.
2. Administer blood replacements as prescribed; observe for volume overload.
3. Institute measures to prevent hypovolemic shock (refer to Chapter 48).
4. Assess hematocrit and hemoglobin; evaluate arterial blood gases.
5. If bleeding is external, apply a pressure dressing over the incision while awaiting physician.
6. Measure fluid intake and output accurately.

Evaluation

Outcome criteria:

1. Hemoglobin is maintained at 13.5–18 g/100 mL in men, 12–16 g/100 mL in women.
2. Hematocrit is maintained.
3. Fluid volume is maintained as evidenced by stable blood pressure, pulse, and central venous pressure every 4 h.
4. Acute renal failure does not occur; output will be maintained at more than 400 cc in 24 h.

OBSTRUCTION IN LOWER URINARY TRACT (BLADDER AND/OR URETHRA) DUE TO BLOOD CLOTS OR SLOUGHED TUMOR TISSUE

Assessment

1. Blood clots, mucous threads, or particles of tumor tissue in the urine.
2. Oliguria with accompanying bladder distension (less than 400 cc urine output in 24 h).
3. Increased pain.
4. Altered vital signs, especially increased blood pressure.

5. Moderate to severe anxiety, restlessness, and diaphoresis.

Revised Outcomes
1. Clots will be eliminated.
2. Tissue will be sloughed.
3. Urinary output will be restored.

Interventions
1. Insert prescribed indwelling bladder catheter with continuous irrigation (see intervention 3e, item 4, on page 1122 and Figure 32-1).
2. Increase oral fluid intake for internal irrigation. Monitor and correlate intake and output.
3. Administer prescribed antispasmodics and analgesics.
4. Maintain blood volume; administer prescribed transfusions. Monitor and assess vital signs frequently.
5. Offer reassurance and support.

Evaluation
Outcome criteria:
1. Urine output is maintained clear; check q4h.
2. Volume follows intake each day.

OBSTRUCTION IN THE UPPER URINARY TRACT (URETER AND/OR KIDNEY PELVIS) DUE TO ABNORMAL CELLULAR PROLIFERATION AND/OR BLOOD CLOTS

Refer to *Obstructions*.

HEMORRHAGE DUE TO INVASION OF INTRARENAL CIRCULATION

Assessment
1. Pallor, skin clamminess, and diaphoresis.
2. Hypotension and rapid, thready pulse.
3. Continuous gross, frank hematuria.
4. Increased pain in affected flank.
5. Severe apprehension and restlessness.

Revised Outcomes
1. Hemorrhage will be terminated.
2. Physiologic balance will be restored.

Interventions
1. Insert prescribed indwelling bladder catheter with continuous irrigation. Be sure to include irrigation fluids in the intake and output recordings.
2. Monitor and assess vital signs every 15 min. Observe for signs of increasing hypovolemia.
3. Maintain blood volume. Administer transfusions as prescribed.
4. Maintain fluid and electrolyte balance; administer prescribed intravenous fluids.
5. Institute measures to prevent hypovolemic shock (refer to Chapter 48).
6. Monitor and assess hematocrit and hemoglobin.
7. If hemorrhage cannot be controlled, a nephrectomy may be performed regardless of the presence of metastasis. Begin preoperative preparation.

Evaluation
Outcome criteria:
1. Blood pressure is maintained ±10 mmHg of baseline every 30 min.
2. Pulse is maintained strong and equal bilaterally every 30 min.
3. Absence of gross blood on dressing or in urine (check every 30 min).
4. Client appears relaxed when checked every hour around the clock (more often if blood pressure and pulse are unstable or bleeding continues).

RENAL FAILURE

Refer to *Acute Renal Failure* and *Chronic Renal Failure*.

PNEUMONIA

See discussion in Chapter 31.

EFFECTS OF RADIATION AND/OR CHEMOTHERAPY

Assessment and Revised Outcomes
See *Tumors of the Urinary Bladder*.

Interventions
1. Since radiation and chemotherapy do not appear to be very effective, support client, family, and /or significant others in dealing with the poor prognosis.
2. Assist client in developing realistic and attainable goals.
3. Initiate teaching regarding untoward effects of treatment regimen. Assist client and family in dealing with side effects of radiation and chemotherapy.
4. Initiate referral for follow-up home care.

Evaluation
Outcome criteria (follow-up visits every 3–6 weeks):
1. Client maintains regimen at home per evaluation criteria.
2. Client reports positive feelings despite life-style constraints.

BOWEL OBSTRUCTION

See Chapter 33.

PRURITIS AND JAUNDICE

See Chapter 33.

CARDIAC FAILURE

See Chapter 30.

AZOTEMIA AND RENAL FAILURE

See *Acute Renal Failure* and *Chronic Renal Failure*.

METASTATIC DISEASE

Discussed throughout the text under *Abnormal Cellular Growth*.

DEATH AND GRIEVING

See Chapter 45.

Reevaluation and Follow-up

Renal tumors follow a progressive downhill course. Metastasis complicates the picture, as does renal failure (see *Acute Renal Failure* and *Chronic Renal Failure*).

TUMORS OF THE URINARY BLADDER

DESCRIPTION

Tumors of the bladder occur more frequently in men than in women, and the incidence seems to increase with age. The etiology of the pathogenesis of tumors of the urinary bladder is obscure; however, the ingestion, inhalation, or cutaneous application of certain chemical compounds is believed to cause bladder tumors.

Bladder tumors arising in the mucous membrane layer of the bladder wall constitute the majority of these genitourinary tumors. These tumors are papillary in nature.

Benign tumors protrude from the mucosal surface of the bladder wall as small outgrowths. They may undergo malignant degeneration with successive recurrences. *Nonepithelial infiltrating tumors* usually do not invade beyond the muscular layer of the bladder wall. They are malignant but occur less frequently than papillary tumors. *Adenocarcinomas* and *sarcomas*, though rare, tend to penetrate deeply into the bladder wall and beyond.

Tumors of the urinary bladder generally originate near the bladder floor. Consequently, ureteral and urethral orifices are often obstructed by abnormal cellular proliferation.

PREVENTION

Health Promotion

1. Monitor maintenance of clean, fresh water supply for those at home, at work, or in public places.
2. Maintain level of fluid intake at 4,000 cc per day to dilute unknown toxins or carcinogens in the environment.

Population at Risk

1. Workers in the following categories:
   a. Asphalt workers.
   b. Coal tar and pitch workers.
   c. Gas stokers.
   d. Still cleaners.
   e. Dyestuffs users.
   f. Rubber workers.
   g. Textile dyers.
   h. Paint manufacturers.
   i. Leather and shoe workers.
2. Persons exposed to cigarette smoke; excessive use of sodium, saccharin, and coffee may incur high risk for bladder cancer, but a cause-effect relationship has not been proven.

Screening

1. Implementation of cytodiagnostic programs in rubber and chemical industries should be undertaken.
2. Since potential carcinogens have only recently begun to be identified, all health-promotion and illness-related assessments should include complete occupational histories, with chemical exposures noted.

ASSESSMENT

Health History

The health history, as well as the physical examination, should focus on those changes that have occurred before and during hospitalization (refer to *Renal Tumors* and Table 32-1).

1. History of recurrent urinary tract infections (particularly cystitis). Indicate the frequency with which they occur.
2. History of intermittent or continuous gross painless hematuria (present in 60–80 percent of clients).
3. Voiding patterns and characteristics of urine, particularly frequency, urgency, nocturia, and dysuria.
4. Presence, location, intensity, quality, and precipitating or aggravating factors of pain. Investigate factors that aid in analgesia. Pain is not always present. Pain in bladder, rectum, pelvis, flank, back, or legs is usually present in advanced disease process.

Physical Assessment

1. Palpable suprapubic or pelvic mass (rare). A pelvic mass may be palpable through the abdominal wall or on bimanual examination of a woman.
2. Edema in lower extremities may be noted. This often indicates venous obstruction caused by invasive tumor.
3. Fever and severe flank pain may be observed. This may indicate renal infection. Elevation of white blood counts in serum and urinalysis may be present.
4. Uremic symptoms may be present secondary to impaired renal function (see *Acute Renal Failure* and *Chronic Renal Failure*).

Diagnostic Tests

1. Cystoscopy (see *Renal Tumors*). Ultraviolet cystoscopy.
2. Biopsy of bladder wall, with bimanual examination under anesthesia.
3. IVP-filling defect may indicate presence of bladder tumor (for a complete discussion, see *Renal Tumors*).
4. Excretory urogram: radiological viewing of the urinary tract showing excretion of intravenous fluids or opaque dye.
5. Urinary cytologic examination to study cell composition of the urine.
6. Microscopic urinalysis, specifically for hematuria. A clean catch urinalysis or sterile urine collection is often used.
7. Renal function studies: usually normal unless obstruction has resulted in damage to renal parenchyma (refer to *Renal Tumors*).
8. Hematocrit and hemoglobin to evaluate blood loss.
9. Coagulation studies to rule out predisposition to bleeding.
10. Blood typing and crossmatching.
11. Metastatic series, including bone scan to assess metastases.

NURSING DIAGNOSES: ACTUAL OR POTENTIAL

1. Altered urinary elimination patterns: incontinence, retention, or dysuria due to infection or anatomical obstruction related to tumor growth.
2. Fear due to impending diagnostic studies and unconfirmed medical diagnosis.
3. Altered bowel elimination patterns: constipation due to palpable mass in abdomen.
4. Decreased activity tolerance due to fatigue associated with anemia.
5. Reactive (situational) depression due to poor prognosis, spiritual distress, need for career change, or role change.
6. Perceived powerlessness due to poor prognosis and invasive nature of the medical regimen.
7. Altered body image due to surgical interventions (see Interventions, below).
8. Sexual dysfunction due to depression or decreased libido.
9. Alteration in comfort or pain due to dysuria (as above), constipation, or tumor growth.

EXPECTED OUTCOMES

See *Renal Tumors*.

INTERVENTIONS

1. Immediate interventions.
   a. Monitor gross and occult blood in urine.
   b. Monitor urinary output q24h (quantity and quality). Weigh client daily to assess fluid retention.
   c. Administer medications as ordered (antibiotics if infection is present).
   d. Monitor catheter irrigation or instillation if present. Follow clinical protocol for catheter care (see interventions under *Renal Tumors*). Repeated local instillation of triethylenethiophosphoramide is sometimes effective in the treatment of multiple lesions and in the prevention of recurrences.
2. Develop a teaching plan.
   a. Prepare client for diagnostic studies by describing the procedural and sensory components of each test. Arrange for client to talk with another person who has undergone procedure.
   b. Provide preoperative teaching, assure informed consent, and monitor postoperative course if urinary diversion and/or total cystectomy is the treatment of choice.
   c. Prepare client for effects of supervoltage radiation if that is the treatment of choice.
3. Develop plan for support of client's own bowel elimination pattern. Consult physician for stool softeners if necessary.
4. Develop plan for activity around energy level and expressed desired role functions.
5. Assist client in dealing with possible altered body image.

a. Offer information on physical changes as appropriate and as tolerated.
b. Assist client in discussing effect of altered body image on values, beliefs, roles, and relationships.

6. Maintain environment that fosters maximal self-care.
   a. Guide transition from total dependency to self-care using feedback from client and family and problem-solving approach.
   b. Assist client and family in developing realistic rehabilitative goals.
   c. Refer to American Cancer Society or Ostomy Association for group support.
   d. Refer to any necessary assistance with home care.
7. See *Renal Tumors* for additional nursing interventions.
8. Response to surgical interventions.
   a. Transurethral resection and fulguration: transurethral resection involves the resection of small tumors not involving the muscle tissue using a resectoscope, which enters the area via the urethra; fulguration is the process of destroying tissue thought to be malignant by use of electric current.
      (1) Preoperative interventions (refer to *Renal Tumors*).
      (2) Postoperative interventions.
         (a) Measure and correlate intake and output q4h for first 24 h, progressing to q8h when appropriate.
         (b) Test urine for blood at each voiding if no indwelling catheter is present; if catheter is present, test urine at least q2h. (Urine may be pink-tinged, and gross bleeding may be intermittent.) Hemoglobin and hematocrit levels should be checked to assess suspected blood loss.
         (c) Observe urine for clots. Maintain free, unobstructed flow of urine.
         (d) Provide meticulous and safe indwelling bladder catheter care. (Refer to discussion under *Renal Tumors*.)
         (e) Maintain oral fluid intake at 2,500–3,000 mL/24 h.
         (f) Administer prescribed blood replacements: transfusions, intravenous fluids, and electrolytes.
         (g) Administer prescribed analgesics and antispasmodics for pain and complaints of spasm. Administer a sitz bath or moist heat to provide relief from bladder spasms.
         (h) Observe for signs of infection. Administer prescribed prophylactic antibiotics, and assess temperature frequently.
         (i) Initiate teaching-learning transaction (include family and/or significant others) regarding:
            (i) Medications, especially name, dosage, rationale, expected action, side effects, and signs of toxicity.
            (ii) Nutritional counseling (e.g., counseling is needed concerning decreased bladder capacity following the removal of the urethral catheter).
            (iii) Continued intake of approximately 3,000 ml per 24-h period. (Tell client to space oral intake.)
            (iv) Need for follow-up and cystoscopic examination every 3 months for 1 year, and every 6 months thereafter.
   b. Segmental resection of the bladder.
      (1) Preoperative interventions (refer to *Renal Tumors*).
      (2) Postoperative interventions (see 8a, item 2, under Interventions above).
         (a) Monitor and assess drainage from cystostomy tube and indwelling bladder catheter. Include cystostomy drainage in total urinary output.
         (b) Offer reassurance that bladder capacity will gradually increase. Immediate postoperative bladder capacity may not be more than 60 ml. This should increase from 200 to 400 ml postoperatively.
         (c) Instruct client on how to time ingestion of fluids to prevent frequent urination due to decreased bladder capacity.
            (i) Consume large amounts of fluids at one time.
            (ii) Limit fluids at least 2 h before going out.
            (iii) Consume no fluids after 6 P.M.
   c. Cystectomy: the complete removal of the

bladder. This type of surgical procedure is usually performed after assessing the size of the lesion, the depth of tissue involvement, the client's general health status, and whether the cellular growth is curable. The type of surgery will result in permanent urinary diversion. There are several procedures that can be performed, and each requires special management following surgery.

(1) Types of urinary diversion.
   (a) Rectal bladder: formation of a sigmoid colostomy with implantation of the ureters into the rectum (Figure 32-2a).
   (b) Ureterosigmoidostomy: transplantation of the ureters into the intact colon (Figure 32-2b).
   (c) Ureterileostomy (ileal conduit): transplantation of ureters into an isolated section of ileum, which is sutured closed at one end; the open end is brought to the skin (Figure 32-2c).

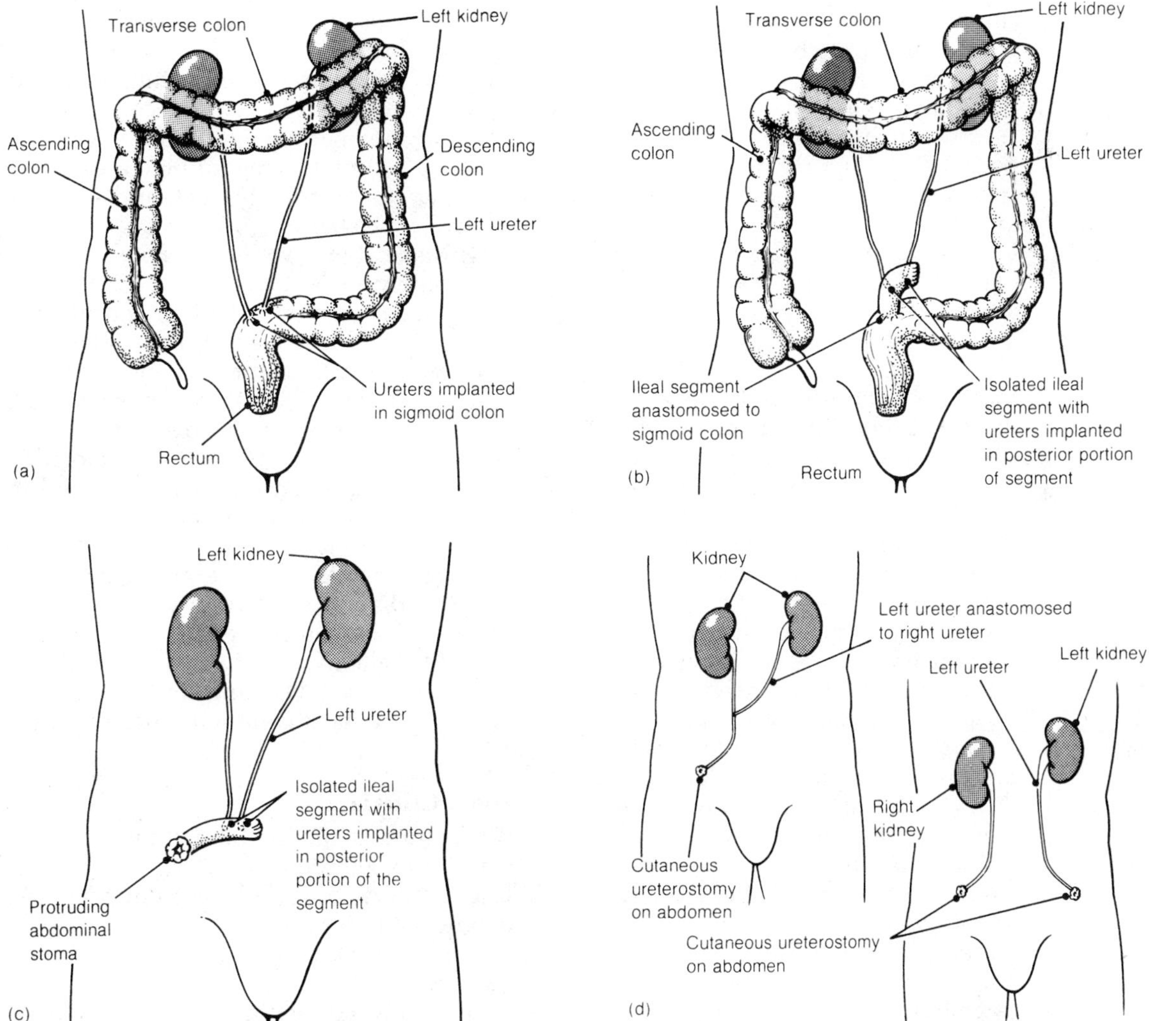

Figure 32-2 Urinary diversion. (From Jones, D.A., et al., eds: *Medical-Surgical Nursing: A Conceptual Approach*, 2d ed., McGraw-Hill, New York, 1982.)

(d) Cutaneous ureterostomy: implantation of the ureters directly onto abdominal skin (Figure 32-2d).

(2) Preoperative interventions (see *Renal Tumors*).

(a) Prepare the client psychologically for urinary diversion. This is vital, since changes in body image may be of much concern to the client. Offer reassurance, encouragement, and support.

(b) Create an atmosphere that fosters open discussion to relieve anxiety.

(c) Perform a bowel preparation, usually several days before surgery, including a cathartic, an enema, and a sulfonamide such as neomycin.

(d) Give the client a clear liquid diet (for 3 days). Give vitamins B and K as ordered if a deficiency is suspected (fluid supplements via intravenous therapy may be used).

(3) Postoperative interventions.

(a) Label catheters and maintain their patency. Irrigations may be prescribed as frequently as q2h. Measure, assess, and correlate fluid intake and output hourly.

(b) Maintain unobstructed flow of urine. Observe for edema around stoma. If a collection bag is attached, empty it frequently to prevent backflow.

(c) Observe for signs of infection. Measure temperature at least q2h. Peritonitis can occur through escape of feces into peritoneal cavity.

(d) Administer pain relief measures. Initiate measures to prevent postoperative complications.

(e) Observe for distension of lower abdomen, particularly with ileal conduit, since distension can cause tension on the suture line and can result in rupture. Frequently, a nasogastric tube is used after surgery to reduce bowel distension.

(f) Observe for electrolyte disturbances, especially following ureterosigmoidoscopy, because of reabsorptive powers of the sigmoid.

(g) Provide meticulous skin care around stoma. Consult enterostomal clinical nurse specialist. Use protective devices and preparations. Assess response to interventions. Measure the stoma carefully and determine the size of the opening accurately. Use a bag that fits firmly and does not exert pressure on the stoma.

(h) Depending on the type of urinary diversion performed, initiate early teaching regarding use of ostomy equipment, only if appropriate. This intervention may be inappropriate, depending on the client. Assess anxiety level and readiness to learn.

(i) Begin discharge teaching and planning early. Instruct client, family member, or significant other, if appropriate, regarding care of the stoma, activity, diet, and so on. Be specific.

(4) Medical interventions.
Support client's response to:

(a) Intracavity radiation: introduction of radioactive isotopes contained in the balloon of a Foley catheter is rarely used, since external radiation is more effective.

(b) Supervoltage external radiation: used when tumor is large and invasive or if client's condition will not tolerate surgery.

(c) Combination therapy: external radiation and surgery may be used for maximum effect.

(d) Palliative chemotherapy: 5 fluorouracil (5FU) and andriomycin are the most commonly used agents.

EVALUATION

Outcome Criteria

1. Clear urine is eliminated daily without discomfort (3,000 cc).
2. Client reports comfort level 1 day after each diagnostic procedure.
3. Client has soft brown stool according to basic pattern.
4. Activity prescription is followed as documented in daily log and tolerated without undue fatigue.

5. Client reports positive contacts with family and friends or pleasurable solo activities on two of every three visits.
6. Client reports positive relationship with spouse.
7. Vital signs and weight are within normal range of baseline.
8. Hemoglobin 13.5–18 g/100 mL in men, 12–16 g/100 mL in women. Hematocrit 45–50 vol/100 mL in men, 40–45 vol/100 mL in women.
9. Medication and diet prescriptions are followed exactly on follow-up visit every 7 days.
10. Serum electrolytes are maintained in normal range.
11. Client demonstrates knowledge of therapeutic regimen by making two appropriate adjustments in lifestyle during the first month at home.
12. Client returns for evaluative cystoscopy every 3 months as prescribed.

Complications

1. Complications of transurethral resection and fulguration.
   a. Hemorrhage: if hemorrhage cannot be controlled, surgical reintervention may be necessary.
   b. Obstruction in lower urinary tract (refer to *Obstructions*): radical cystectomy with pelvic lymph node dissection and urinary diversion; for men, this involves radical prostatoseminal vesiculectomy, resulting in impotence.
2. Complications of urinary diversion.
   a. Peritonitis (see Chapter 33).
   b. Urethritis and pyelonephritis (see *Urethritis* and *Pyelonephritis*).
   c. Obstruction of urinary outlet (see *Obstructions*).
   d. Renal failure (see *Acute Renal Failure* and *Chronic Renal Failure*).

Reevaluation and Follow-up

1. Evaluate outcomes met and not met at 1-month follow-up.
2. Reassess (see Assessment under *Tumors of the Urinary Bladder*).
3. Revise interventions depending on level of self-care ability and progression of tumor (exacerbation or remission).

CARCINOMA OF THE PROSTATE

DESCRIPTION

Carcinoma of the prostate is the most common type of malignant tumor of the genitourinary tract. Men over age 40 are most frequently affected; the incidence of this condition rises with advancing age. Prostatic carcinoma arises in the periurethral and posterior portions of the prostate, which is adjacent to the rectum. Most prostatic carcinomas are classified as adenocarcinomas. Clients with prostatic cancer usually remain asymptomatic until late in the course of the disease when bladder obstruction or symptoms of pelvic or distant metastases occur.

PREVENTION

Health Promotion

Cleaner air may be associated with lower incidence in rural areas.

Population at Risk

1. Sex: male.
2. Age: 40 or over.
3. Race: incidence among blacks is almost double that among whites.
4. Environment: urban dwellers have a higher incidence than rural residents.

Screening

Yearly or biannual.

1. Digital rectal examination in all men over age 40 is the best means of detecting early and operable tumors.
2. Radioimmunoassay (RIA) is a newly developed but expensive screening tool used to detect prostatic carcinoma.
3. Counterimmunoelectrophoresis determination of prostatic acid phosphatase is currently under investigation for detection of early intracapsular carcinoma of the prostate.

ASSESSMENT

Health History

Refer to *Renal Tumors* (see Table 32-1).

1. Race.
2. Family history of cancer.
3. Time of last voiding.

4. Difficulty in starting and maintaining urinary stream.
5. Diminished caliber and force of stream and "dribbling" of urine after micturition completed.
6. Frequency, urgency, nocturia, and burning on urination.
7. Hematuria (late manifestation).
8. Presence, location, intensity, quality, and precipitating or aggravating factors of pain. (Pain in body structures may indicate metastasis.)

Physical Assessment

1. Palpation of solitary firm nodule confined to the posterior or lateral portion of the prostate gland on rectal examination may be an early operable tumor.
2. Bladder distension present in acute or chronic urinary retention.
3. Limited range of motion of lower back from tumor extension.

Diagnostic Tests

1. Prostatic biopsy necessary to confirm diagnosis.
2. Cystoscopy and IVP to rule out associated renal pathology (refer to discussion under *Renal Tumors*).
3. Excretory urogram.
4. Metastatic series: x-ray examination of skeletal structures, especially pelvis, spine, ribs, and skull.
5. Lymphangiography to demonstrate metastatic lymphatic spread.
6. Renal function studies.
7. Serum acid phosphatase elevated when prostatic carcinoma has penetrated the prostatic capsule.
8. Serum alkaline phosphatase elevated when body metastasis is present.
9. CBC and electrolyte determinations.
10. Microscopic urinanalysis, urine cultures, and antibiotic sensitivities.

NURSING DIAGNOSES: ACTUAL OR POTENTIAL

1. See nursing diagnoses listed under *Tumors of the Urinary Bladder*.
2. Body image altered due to castration, impotence, or ineffective sphincter control.

EXPECTED OUTCOMES

See *Renal Tumors*.

INTERVENTIONS

1. See *Tumors of the Urinary Bladder*.
2. Assist client with response to surgical intervention, such as radical resection of prostate gland and removal of entire prostate gland, prostatic capsule, seminal vesicles, and adjacent tissue.
   a. Preoperative intervention (refer to *Renal Tumors*).
   b. Postoperative interventions.
      (1) Observe dressing for drainage.
      (2) Avoid dislodging urethral catheter, since it serves as a splint for urethral anastomosis.
      (3) Encourage use of perineal exercises.
      (4) Assist client in rebuilding self-esteem and positive body image.
      (5) Initiate sexual counseling, since impotence is usual.
3. Assist client with response to other types of surgical intervention.
   a. Huggins treatment: the elimination of androgens by orchidectomy (see Chapter 21).
   b. Bilateral adrenalectomy (see Chapter 28).
   c. Hypophysectomy (see Chapter 28).
   d. Cryosurgery reduces size of obstructive lesion by freezing of prostatic tissue.
   e. Transurethral resection to relieve obstruction.
   f. Supapubic cystosomy provides for drainage if transurethral resection cannot be done.
4. Assist client with response to medical management of inoperable neoplasm.
   a. Radiation therapy to decrease tumor size.
   b. Administration of estrogenic hormones, usually diethylstilbestrol.
5. Use support group and/or significant others in helping client regain positive self-perception.
   a. Talk with client concerning mind–body interaction, wellness concepts, role of imagery, and relaxation.
   b. Assist client in normalizing diet, sleep patterns, and exercise and activity and to adjust medical regimen and lifestyle interaction.

6. Answer client's questions honestly and consult with physician, social worker, and family concerning plans for terminal or continuing care as necessary.

EVALUATION

Outcome Criteria

1. See outcomes listed under *Tumors of the Urinary Bladder*.
2. Client reports at each follow-up visit positive feelings about effects of therapy in spite of altered body image and limitation of life goals.

Complications

ACUTE RETENTION OF URINE

Assessment

1. Suprapubic pain.
2. Distended bladder.
3. Frequent, urgent urination with small amounts of urine.

Interventions

1. Validate intake and output.
2. Use voiding measures.
3. Catheterize as ordered.
4. Assist and teach client technique of catheterization if able and willing.

Reevaluation and Follow-up

1. Arrange for home visits as needed.
2. Evaluate success of home care for client and care provider.
3. Discuss hospice care with client and family.
4. Reassess on each visit and by phone as needed.

HYPERACTIVITY AND HYPOACTIVITY

ACUTE RENAL FAILURE

DESCRIPTION

Renal failure may be classified as acute or chronic according to the length of time associated with the development of the condition and whether it is short-lived or prolonged. Acute renal failure (ARF) is a sudden, severe reduction of renal functioning resulting in the accumulation of metabolic waste products in the blood and a disturbance in fluid and electrolyte concentrations. *Acute renal failure* and *acute tubular insufficiency* are synonymous. *Acute tubular necrosis*, although sometimes used interchangeably with *acute renal failure*, represents a different histological pattern and is characterized by abnormal handling of sodium in the proximal tubule. This causes an increase in plasma renin levels and a decrease in blood flow to the kidney. When the kidneys are unable to eliminate body wastes and maintain fluid and electrolyte balance, the client develops azotomia.

Acute renal failure has been classified on the basis of etiology as prerenal, or functional renal insufficiency due to extrarenal causes; renal, an internal failure of the kidney to function properly; and postrenal, involving the distal portion of the urinary tract and usually associated with obstruction (Walters, 1982, p. 507). The prognosis of ARF varies, depending on the length of the oliguric phase, the severity of the underlying causative disease process, and the rate of urea production. If ARF continues unabated, chronic uremia, a clinical syndrome, develops.

PREVENTION

Health Promotion

1. Health teaching concerning behavioral correlates or urinary tract infection: fluid intake, hygiene.
2. Health teaching concerning careful labeling and storing of toxins, poisons.
3. Safety in the workplace, specifically concerning exposure to hazardous materials.
4. Comprehensive prenatal care.

Population at Risk

1. Surgical clients who may experience hypotension, shock, or renal ischemia.
2. Persons with frequent urinary tract infections or obstructions.
3. Workers exposed to hazardous materials or toxins.
4. Pregnant women, especially eclamptics and those undergoing abortion.
5. Persons taking antibiotics or analgesics.

Screening

1. Inclusion of occupational history in routine examinations.

2. Careful follow-up of urinary tract infections.
3. Early pregnancy detection.
4. Identification of self-medication.

ASSESSMENT

Health History

Since renal failure, both acute and chronic, is an extremely complex condition, all body systems must be assessed. The following areas should be investigated in detail with each client. This is not intended to be an exhaustive list of items to include in a nursing health history. Each client is an individual; therefore, the nurse must individualize the health history by expanding or deleting certain areas (refer to Table 32-1).

1. Age.
2. Sex.
3. Marital status.
4. Occupation.
5. Socioeconomic status and educational background.
6. Family structure and significant others, lifestyle, religion, ethnic background, description of home environment (explore family resources).
7. Level of consciousness and mental and emotional status.
8. Height and usual weight; present weight.
9. Family history of renal disease.
10. Previous medical history.
    a. Discuss previous health problems that may be of significance (e.g., diabetes mellitus, systemic lupus erythematosus, streptococcal pharyngitis, gout, etc.).
    b. Investigate previous hospitalizations, surgery, radiation, and medical and nursing care.
    c. Investigate for congenital malformation of the ear, spinal cord anomalies, imperforate anus, or genital anomalies (congenital renal anomalies and these defects frequently occur in the same client).
11. Complete and detailed nutritional assessment (include history of anorexia, diarrhea, nausea and vomiting; food preferences and dislikes; dietary restrictions, self- or medically imposed).
12. History of allergies and drug use (e.g., nephrotoxic drugs).
13. Activity, rest, and sleep patterns; activities of daily living.
14. Voiding patterns and characteristics of urine, including decreased volume.
    a. Oliguria: 24-h total of approximately 500 mL.
    b. Anuria: 24-h total of approximately 250 mL.
15. Sexual history and contraceptive practices.
    a. Development of secondary sexual characteristics.
    b. Actual or perceived alterations in sexual drive and/or functioning.
    c. History of menstrual cycle for women.
16. Alteration in body image and/or self-esteem. Assess response to illness, motivation for self-care, body image disturbances, role disturbances, and coping mechanisms.

Physical Assessment

1. Enlarged kidney(s) palpable.
2. Elevated blood pressure: renin-angiotensin system may be involved.
3. Weight gain due to edema and decreased removal of body fluids.
4. Skin: pallor due to anemia, urate crystals, pruritis, dry and cracked mucous membranes; assess skin turgor.
5. Eye changes: retinal hemorrhages, papilledema (not always present; usually associated with markedly elevated blood pressure).
6. Mouth: halitosis due to acidosis, urinous breath, ammonia odor from breakdown of urea secreted into saliva.
7. Edema in face, abdomen, and extremities. Pitting edema may be palpated in presence of decreased urinary output.
8. Muscular twitching may be present.
9. Elevated body temperature may be present.
10. Deviations from the norm in any body system.

Diagnostic Tests

1. IVP (see *Renal Tumors*).
2. Chest x-ray examination.
3. Electrocardiogram (refer to Chapter 30).
4. Renal arteriography.
5. Renal biopsy, renal scan, radioactive renogram.
6. Blood studies.
    a. Nonprotein nitrogen.
    b. Plasma alkaline phosphatase.
    c. BUN usually elevated.
    d. Serum creatinine usually elevated.

  e. Serum magnesium.
  f. Serum uric acid.
  g. Serum chloride.
  h. Serum potassium may be elevated to dangerous levels in cardiac arrest.
  i. Serum calcium usually decreased.
  j. Serum sodium.
  k. CO_2 content usually low.
  l. Inorganic serum sulfates.
  m. Arterial blood gases (refer to Chapter 30).
7. Blood coagulation studies to rule out predisposition to bleeding.
8. Hematocrit and hemoglobin: anemia almost always present.
9. White blood cell differential count: leukocytosis usually present.
10. Blood typing and crossmatching.
11. Urine culture and antibiotic sensitivities.
12. Microscopic urinalysis usually indicates low fixed specific gravity, some proteinuria, casts, hematuria, and cellular debris. Urine osmolarity tends to be maintained at 1.010 despite variations in fluid intake; this is called isosthenuria.

NURSING DIAGNOSES: ACTUAL OR POTENTIAL

1. Impaired urinary elimination.
2. Nutritional alteration due to fluid volume excess and diminished food ingestion.
3. High risk of infection due to increased stress and decreased physiologic balance.
4. Decreased activity tolerance secondary to immobility and altered elimination of toxins.
5. Alteration in skin integrity secondary to edema.
6. Alteration in comfort or discomfort.
7. Alteration in bowel/bladder elimination due to alteration in fluid volume.
8. Impaired thought process secondary to increased toxins and increased fluid retention.
9. Knowledge deficit.
10. Situational independence–dependence conflict.
11. Reactive (situational) depression.
12. Inadequate support system.

EXPECTED OUTCOMES

1. Initial cause of renal failure will be identified and removed if possible.
2. As normal a fluid and electrolyte balance as possible will be maintained.
3. Infection will be prevented.
4. Overhydration will be prevented.
5. Workload of the kidneys will be decreased; level of serum toxic materials will be reduced.
6. Acidosis will be prevented, and protein catabolism will be minimized.
7. Further renal damage and decrease in function will be prevented.
8. Adequate nutritional status will be maintained while metabolic demands are decreased.
9. Hypertension will be controlled.
10. Renal function will be restored.
11. Client will comply with treatment regimen.

INTERVENTIONS

1. Assist in determining and eliminating the cause of ARF.
2. Dietary restrictions.
   a. Administer prescribed diet, usually nonprotein, low in potassium and sodium, and high in carbohydrates (at least 100 g/day) and fat. This diet reduces endogenous protein catabolism and helps prevent ketosis.
   b. Enforce fluid restrictions. (Rule of thumb: fluid intake should be 400 mL plus amount of total output on previous day.)
   c. Serve food at the proper temperature.
   d. Allow client choice in food whenever possible. Allow client to choose from exchange list.
   e. Allow client to choose distribution of fluid restriction.
   f. Give wet cloth or ice chips to suck to help allay thirst (include in total oral intake).
   g. Measure fluid intake and output meticulously and accurately every hour.
   h. Weigh client daily on same scale (preferably a bed scale), with the same amount of clothing, at the same time of day, preferably before breakfast.
   i. Refer to nutritionist.
   j. Teach client, family, and food preparer regarding the reading of labels on processed foods and avoiding the use of salt substitutes (most are low in sodium but high in potassium).

k. Administer intravenous hypertonic carbohydrate solution if oral intake impossible.

3. Prevention of infection.
   a. Give meticulous attention to all sterile procedures.
   b. Promote environmental asepsis. (Client should be in private room.)
   c. Avoid exposing client to any kind of infection.
   d. Recognize and report signs of infection. (Client may have hypothermia even in presence of infection; client may have leukocytosis without infection.)
   e. Administer prescribed antibiotics if infection occurs. Continue to protect from infection. Avoid use of potassium penicillin, to prevent potassium overload.
   f. Avoid chilling, but maintain carefully ventilated room.
   g. Avoid unnecessary instrumentation of any kind. If indwelling bladder catheter used, seek order for continuous irrigation with antibiotic solution.
   h. Turn frequently. Administer pulmonary care to prevent pneumonia.
   i. Use reverse isolation precautions when necessary.
   j. Instruct client about personal hygiene and avoiding contact with individuals who have an upper respiratory infection.
4. Activity restrictions to decrease metabolic rate.
   a. Encourage strict bed rest in acute phase.
   b. Provide diversional activity if appropriate. Consult the client to enlist aid of family and/or significant others.
   c. Encourage passive and active exercises to prevent muscle atrophy.
   d. During diuretic phase, assist and encourage progressive ambulation.
5. Electrolyte imbalance and fluid disturbance.
   a. Monitor ECGs for arrhythmias and/or heart block. Client should be on cardiac monitor (see Chapter 30).
   b. Monitor and assess central venous pressure every hour until condition stabilizes.
   c. Monitor and assess vital signs every hour. Assess radial and apical pulses.
   d. Observe for signs of sudden or severe hypotension. Measure postural signs.
   e. Assess heart sounds. Listen for friction rub and tachycardia. Watch for signs of developing effusion and cardiac tamponade. Be prepared for emergency pericardiocentesis.
   f. Assess pulmonary status (lung sounds). Assess for Kussmaul's respirations, which are present in acidotic state.
   g. Observe for congestive heart failure, chest pains, pericarditis, and pulmonary edema (see Chapter 30).
   h. Observe for signs of hyperkalemia (flaccid paralysis, slow respirations, anxiety, convulsions, and cardiac arrest).
   i. Initiate measures to reduce hyperkalemia. Administer prescribed medications:
      (1) Cation exchange resins increase potassium excretion from the bowel. Acidosis may result as a side effect.
      (2) Insulin and glucose intravenously promote removal of potassium from extracellular fluid.
      (3) Intravenous calcium gluconate or calcium chloride protects the heart from the effects of hyperkalemia but does not reduce serum potassium.
      (4) Intravenous sodium bicarbonate assists in combating acidosis.
      (5) Observe for signs of hypokalemia.
   j. Administer prescribed aluminum hydroxide gel with meals to reduce absorption of phosphorus, thus causing an increase in serum calcium (avoid gels with magnesium because of danger of magnesium toxicity).
   k. Observe for signs of hypernatremia during oliguric phase and hyponatremia during diuretic phase.
      (1) Hypernatremia: characterized by fluid retention, weight gain, and systemic edema. Restrict sodium intake.
      (2) Hyponatremia: characterized by dry mouth, loss of skin turgor, and hypotension. Administer prescribed sodium supplements.
   l. Administer prescribed diuretics during early acute renal failure (mannitol is frequently used).
   m. Observe for signs of developing or increasing acidosis. Administer prescribed medications. Watch for development of side effects.

n. Observe for signs of hypocalemic tetany and convulsions if acidosis is corrected. Administer prescribed medications.

6. Skin care and oral hygiene.
   a. Perform oral hygiene before each meal. Give sour balls to help alleviate metallic ammonium halitosis. Vinegar (0.25 percent acetic acid) neutralizes ammonium.
   b. Keep nasogastric tube free of encrustations.
   c. Use bland soaps that do not contain perfume.
   d. If uremic frost present, bathe client frequently to remove crystals. It is not necessary to use soap because the skin is dry enough.
   e. Systematically examine bony prominences q4h.
   f. Turn the client q2h. Use nondrying agents to massage bony prominences. Prevent decubitus ulcers.
7. Environmental conditions.
   a. Keep noise to a minimum. Maintain calm, quiet atmosphere. Plan rest periods.
   b. Allow for self-care and maintain independence as much as possible. Assist with hygiene as needed.
   c. Institute seizure precautions. Use padded tongue blade, airway, suction, oxygen, and padded side rails.
   d. Promote environmental safety.
8. Combat anemia and bleeding tendency.
   a. Avoid unnecessary trauma. Keep client's fingernails trimmed.
   b. Instruct client on safety. Use soft toothbrush, avoid constipation, avoid vigorous nose blowing, rough contact sports, and so on.
   c. Observe for evidences of bleeding.
   d. If blood administered, observe for signs of reaction (washed packed red cells frequently used because transfusions may add to potassium level).
9. Psychological status.
   a. Explain to the client and family that periods of confusion are expected outcomes of the disease process. Reorient the confused client. Responses may be slowed. Allow time for client response; avoid requiring that complex choices be made.
   b. Offer reassurance, support, and encouragement.
   c. Reassess level of consciousness and mental status q4h.
   d. Keep bed in low position and side rails elevated.
10. General nursing considerations.
    a. Observe for drug toxicity.
    b. Monitor and assess all blood values.
    c. Initiate referral for sexual and vocational counseling.
    d. Keep avenues open to allow client to discuss anxieties, fears, concerns, and apprehensions regarding alteration in sexual patterns. Include spouse in conferences.
    e. Initiate social service and nutritional consultation.
    f. Initiate teaching-learning transaction (include family and/or significant others) regarding:
       (1) Nature of the disease process.
       (2) Dietary allowances and restrictions.
       (3) Medications, specifically name, dosage, rationale, expected action, side effects, and signs of toxicity.
       (4) Symptoms that require medical attention.
       (5) Symptoms of infection, fluid retention, and hypertension.
       (6) General health care practices.
       (7) Importance of health care follow-up.

EVALUATION

Outcome Criteria

1. Urinary output increases to 2–6 L within 6 weeks.
2. Electrolytes stabilize within early diuretic period.
   a. Serum creatinine .9–1.5 mg/100 mL.
   b. BUN 10–20 mg/100 mL.
   c. Serum calcium 9–11 mg/100 mL.
   d. Serum potassium 3.5–5 mg/100 mL.
   e. Serum phosphate 3.0–4.5 mg/100 mL.
3. Temperature 98.6°F. Blood pressure within 5 mmHg of baseline.
4. Activity and exercise plan is carried out each day.
5. Low-sodium (10–40 g/day), low-protein, high-carbohydrate, high-fat, low-potassium

diet is maintained as ordered. Client's log reflects adherence on early follow-up visit.
6. Body weight is maintained ± 1 kg.
7. Cardiovascular, gastrointestinal, neuromuscular, and integument assessment are within normal limits.
8. Hematocrit, hemoglobin, and coagulation studies within normal limits.
9. Client's behavior exhibits decreased role conflict and depression.
10. Before discharge, the client:
    a. Explains relationship between ARF and three randomly selected prescribed therapies.
    b. Identifies all medications and dosages according to regimen.
    c. Describes signs and symptoms of chronic renal dysfunction.

Complications

CARDIAC FAILURE

See Chapter 30.

PULMONARY EDEMA

See Chapter 31.

SEPTIC SHOCK

See Chapter 48.

CHRONIC RENAL FAILURE

Assessment
See *Chronic Renal Failure.*

Interventions
1. Peritoneal dialysis (see Interventions under *Chronic Renal Failure*).
2. Hemodialysis (see Interventions under *Chronic Renal Failure*).
3. Kidney transplant (see Interventions under *Chronic Renal Failure*).

Evaluation
See *Chronic Renal Failure.*

Reevaluation and Follow-up
Reassess on follow-up each 2–4 weeks for 6 months, each 6 months for 2 years.

CHRONIC RENAL FAILURE

DESCRIPTION

Chronic renal failure is progressive irreversible deterioration of renal functioning that may develop insidiously over a period of years or following an unresolved bout of acute renal failure. The nephrons are gradually destroyed until uremia develops, resulting in death if dialysis and/or kidney transplantation is not part of the treatment plan.

Uremia is a complex clinical syndrome associated with the end stages of renal disease. Uremia results from acute or chronic renal failure. The uremic syndrome is characterized by markedly elevated blood urea nitrogen, elevated serum creatinine (which is less affected by external variables than is BUN), and increased serum sodium, serum potassium, serum magnesium, serum phosphate, and serum sulfate. Serum calcium and serum chloride levels may be decreased (Walters, 1982, p. 579).

PREVENTION

Health Promotion

1. Assure availability of pure, fresh water supply.
2. Encourage consumption of 8 glasses of water a day.
3. Introduce coping and stress reduction programs in school-age populations to decrease hypertension.
4. Offer nutritional counseling to public.
5. Encourage early prenatal care.

Population at Risk

1. Persons living or working in area whose water supply is contaminated by bacteria.
2. Persons working with hazardous industrial materials.
3. Hypertensives.
4. Diabetics.

Screening

1. Regular and complete physical examination including blood pressure reading and urinalysis.
2. Pregnancy testing in population at risk.

ASSESSMENT

Health History

See *Acute Renal Failure.*

Physical Assessment

1. Pallor or sallow or brown skin discoloration due to retained urinary chromogen.
2. Periorbital edema and edematous extremities due to fluid retention.

3. Arterial hypertension.
4. Halitosis (ammonia odor).
5. Frothy urine.
6. Muscle twitching, numbness, pericarditis, and pleuritis may occur as a result of accumulation of toxins in blood and at cellular level.
7. Pruritis due to increased phosphate crystals.

Diagnostic Tests

1. Blood urea nitrogen is increased.
2. Serum creatinine is increased and creatinine clearance time is increased.
3. Normochromic, normocytic anemia is present due to decreased production and increased destruction by diseased kidney or erythropoietin of RBCs.
4. Acidosis is present as a result of potassium and hydrogen ion retention.

NURSING DIAGNOSES: ACTUAL OR POTENTIAL

1. Nutritional excess and/or deficit intake due to excess body fluids secondary to or depleted body fluid due to altered renal output.
2. Decreased activity tolerance due to anemia, electrolyte imbalance, lack of protein in diet, and increased fatigue.
3. Alteration in self-care activities and potential self-care deficit.
4. Impaired thought process due to retained toxins.
5. Alteration in comfort or discomfort due to pruritis, muscle spasm, or cramps.
6. Disturbance of sleep and rest activity due to alteration in comfort.
7. Ineffective family coping secondary to dealing with chronic illness.
8. Independence-dependence conflict.
9. Potential for physical injury due to decreased sensory perception.
10. Altered pattern of sexuality due to decreased hormonal activity.

EXPECTED OUTCOMES

1. Renal functioning will be restored and preserved.
2. Fluid and body chemistry balance will be improved.
3. Alterations in other body organs will be reversed.
4. The need for dialysis and transplantation will be minimized.
5. The quality of life and comfort level will be improved.

INTERVENTIONS

See *Acute Renal Failure.*

1. Provide for nourishment according to blood electrolyte and chemistry levels and clinical status of client.
   a. Provide appropriate motivation for staying on prescribed diet. Offer praise for a job well done. Assist client in using behavior modification techniques (e.g., goal setting, contacting). Refer client and family to organized groups with similar dietary restrictions.
   b. Restrict salt in the oliguric or anuric client to 400–2,000 mg/day.
   c. Restrict potassium, usually to 1,000–2,000 mg/day.
   d. Assess need for vitamin supplements.
   e. Keep caloric intake at 2,000–2,500 cal/day. The ratio of nonprotein to protein kilocalories should be 5:1.
   f. Enforce fluid restriction during advanced stages to avoid overhydration, but avoid dehydration.
   g. Administer prescribed alkaline salts to combat acidosis. (Caution: clients with far-advanced renal disease cannot tolerate sodium bicarbonate because of possibility of hypernatremia.)
   h. Administer prescribed diuretics to decrease circulating fluid volume and decrease hypertension. Reinforce measures to control hypertension to prevent further renal damage.
2. Assist client and family in psychosocial adaptation.
   a. Allow client time to mourn loss of important bodily function (see Chapter 45).
   b. Assist client, family, and significant others in accepting and dealing with this chronic illness and in accepting responsibility for own health care.
   c. Assist in planning future in realizing implication of decisions.
   d. Initiate early discussion of use of dialysis and/or transplantation.
   e. Allow client and family to consider changes in occupation, residence, and finances to enhance family coping.

f. Provide an atmosphere for open discussion of problems with family and client (assist with problem-solving skills). Emotional response to illness will require multiple repetitions and repeated reinforcements of material taught.

3. Initiate teaching-learning transaction (include client, family, and/or significant others) regarding:
   a. Positive aspects of client's condition. Encourage family to avoid overprotectiveness.
   b. Medication and dietary information. Give in written form as well as orally.
   c. Avoidance of any medication without the consent of a physician.
   d. Self-care practices.
   e. Development of self-observational skills: client should note daily weight, note development of edema, and measure fluid intake and output.
4. During period of conservative management, assess client's ability and willingness to cooperate in chronic hemodialysis and/or transplantation.
5. Initiate referral for vocational and sexual counseling.
6. Seek dietary and social service consultations if necessary.
7. Peritoneal dialysis: the term *dialysis* denotes the physical movement of solutes from an area of greater concentration through a semipermeable membrane into an area of lesser concentration until the concentration of solutes in both areas is equal; such differential diffusion for the removal of endogenous or exogenous toxins and other substances can be achieved intracorporeally by peritoneal dialysis or extracorporeally by hemodialysis. Either treatment can be used in acute and chronic renal failure to sustain life until the damaged kidney can repair itself and regain function, to overcome uremia, and/or to physically maintain a client for transplantation. The goals of dialysis therapy include removal of toxic substances and metabolic wastes (end products of protein metabolism), regulation of fluid balance through removal of excessive body fluid, maintenance of serum electrolyte balances, and correction of acid-base imbalances.

   Intermittent or continuous ambulatory peritoneal dialysis (CAPD) uses the principles of osmosis, diffusion, and filtration to move low-molecular-weight substances such as urea, glucose, and electrolytes through the peritoneum, which acts as an inert semipermeable membrane. These substances move between the dialyzing solution, which is introduced into the peritoneal cavity, and the blood vessels of the abdominal cavity. When the concentrations of solutes in the dialyzing solution and the blood are equal, the dialyzing solution, dialysate, is drained from the peritoneal cavity by the use of gravity. Additional dialysate may be used to remove excess nitrogenous products and to restore normal fluid and electrolyte balance (see Figure 32-3).

   Peritoneal dialysis may be utilized in both acute and chronic renal failure. Frequently, clients with chronic renal failure are maintained on peritoneal dialysis while being evaluated for chronic hemodialysis or transplantation. Greater emphasis within the health professions on the benefits of self-care is reflected by the increased use of continuous ambulatory peritoneal dialysis by clients in their homes. The decreased need for expensive, complicated equipment and the decreased restrictions on lifestyle are balanced by an increased need for careful and complete teaching and follow-up by the nurse. Special protocols have been developed for clients with varied physical restrictions. CAPD utilizes the continuous presence of dialysate fluid in the peritoneum, 24 h per day, 7 days a week. Dialysate is drained and replaced with fresh solution 3 to 5 times per day. Daytime exchanges last 4 to 6 hours; nighttime, 8 to 12 hours, depending on client's sleeping schedule and lifestyle (Prowant and Fruto, 1980).

   The following protocol is for peritoneal dialysis carried out in a health facility. Specific prescriptions are given for infusion rate, dialysate strength, time for equilibrium to be reached, and number of treatments per day or week.
   a. Interventions before dialysis.
      (1) The nurse should explain:
         (a) The purpose of the procedure.
         (b) Insertion of the catheter.
         (c) Cycling of fluid.
         (d) Allowed activity during dialysis.
         (e) Expected length of procedure

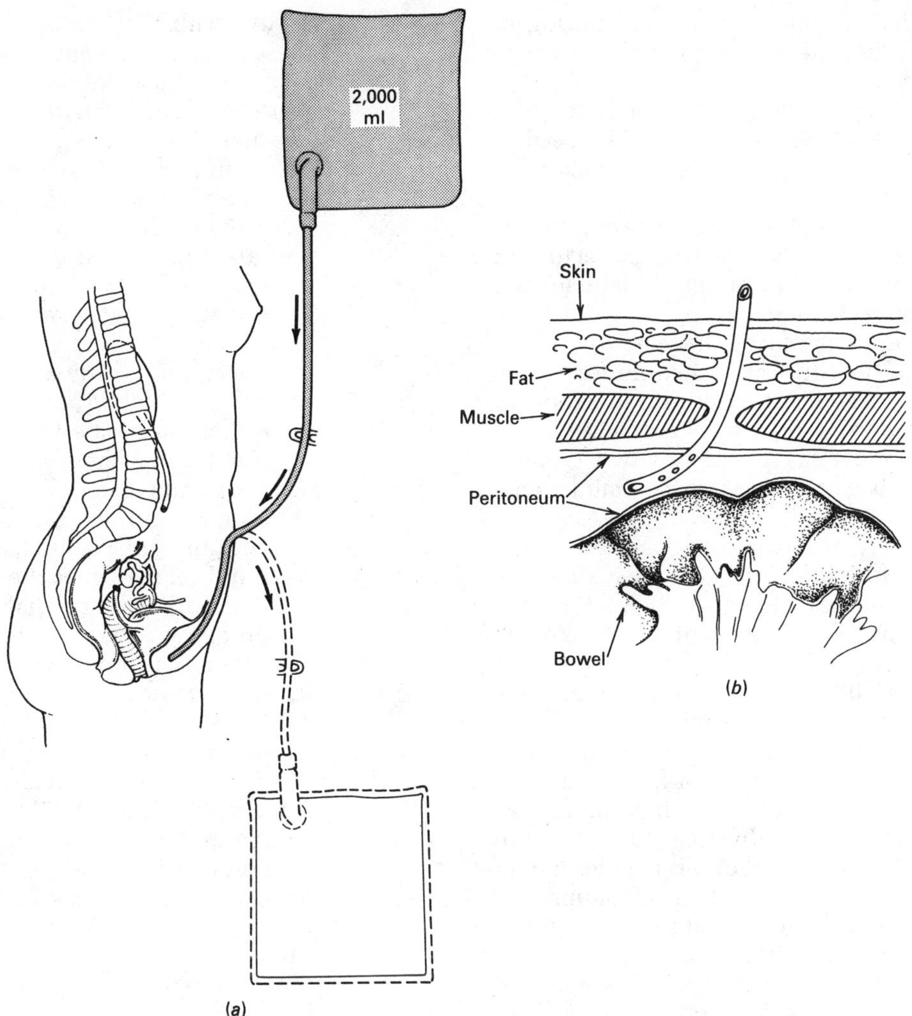

Figure 32-3 (*a*) Diagram illustrating peritoneal dialysis. Note that 2 L of dialysate are connected at one time to reduce risk of infection. Direction of arrows indicates direction of the flow of dialysate. Inflow clamps are open during instillation, while outflow clamps are closed. The reverse is true during outflow. (*b*) Placement of dialysis tubes in the abdomen.

(usually 36–72 h, longer if BUN levels are high; CAPD involves continuous maintenance of 2 L of dialysate exchanged through a permanent catheter 4 or 5 times per day).

(2) Provide a reassuring, supportive attitude. Assess client's anxiety level and intervene appropriately. (Some clients desire and need only minimal information, while others desire and benefit from exact and detailed information.)

(3) Allow client avenue for expressing fears and anxieties. Offer reassurance. Allow time for questions. Informed written consent is necessary for CAPD.

(4) Ask client to void. If client cannot void, a urethral catheter may be inserted to ensure that the bladder is empty. This decreases the likelihood

that it will be perforated during insertion of the trocar into the peritoneum.

(5) Measure weight for baseline information. Bed scale should be used.

(6) Measure vital signs for baseline information.

(7) Assist in physically preparing the trocar insertion site and the actual insertion of the catheter. Maintain sterile technique.

b. Interventions during dialysis.

(1) Adhere to time schedule for cycling as prescribed by physician. Common dialyzing flow rates are 2–2½ L/h.

(2) Connect as prescribed two L-bottles or bag of dialysate to Y-administration tubing.

(3) Dialysate should be warmed to 38°C before infusion. (This helps increase peritoneal clearance, helps the client maintain a constant body temperature, and appears to be more comfortable.) Overheating the dialysate can damage abdominal organs.

(4) Heparin may be added to dialysate to prevent formation of fibrin plugs. Infuse dialysate according to time specifications of physician (usually 10–15 min). Do not allow air to enter tubing, as this can result in abdominal discomfort and drainage difficulties. Clamp administration tubing.

(5) Wait for equilibration to occur according to physician's orders (usually 30–45 min).

(6) Allow fluid to drain from peritoneal cavity and close outflow valve. Time is specified by physician (usually 20 min).

(7) Observe color of outflow fluid. Normally it is clear, pale yellow, and may be blood-tinged during first few cycles because of traumatic insertion of catheter. If it is blood-tinged after first few cycles, suspect abdominal bleeding.

(8) If drainage of dialysate is difficult, check for kinks in tubing, "milk" the tubing, have the client change positions, apply firm pressure using both hands, and/or irrigate the peritoneal cavity with heparinized saline. If these measures do not increase drainage, notify the physician. A new catheter may need to be inserted.

c. Interventions after dialysis.

(1) Maintain dialysis flow sheet.

(a) Record type of dialysate, medications added, amount of dialysate infused and drained, precise timing of inflow and outflow, observations regarding outflow dialysate, net fluid balance of each cycle, and cumulative net fluid balance. Notify physician of fluid balance at least every 8 h. Report significant changes in fluid balance immediately.

(b) Monitor and assess all other forms and amounts of intake and output. Diet may be higher in protein than diet before dialysis, since protein is lost in the dialysate.

(2) Monitor and compare vital signs with baseline readings.

(a) Measure vital signs every 15 min during the first exchange and every 1 to 4 h thereafter.

(b) Client should be on a cardiac monitor. Evaluate apical pulse and observe for arrhythmias.

(3) Measure weight every 24 h after beginning dialysis. Weigh client at the same point in the dialysis cycle each time (1 L of dialysate weighs approximately 1 kg).

(4) Monitor and assess blood electrolyte determinations every 12 h or more frequently if necessary.

(5) Test urine for glucose, ketones, specific gravity, protein, blood, pH, and so forth at each voiding.

(6) Observe for hyperglycemia, hypotension, hypovolemia, infection, overhydration, hyponatremia, and hypoproteinemia (about 0.2–0.8 g/L of protein is lost).

(7) Provide necessary comfort measures.

(a) Provide diversional activity, since the procedure is very time-consuming.

(b) Encourage self-care as much as possible.

(c) Obtain physician's order before allowing client out of bed for short periods of time.

(8) Observe physiologic and psychological effects of treatment.

(a) Observe for signs of peritonitis (abdominal pain, tenderness, abdominal rigidity, fever, leukocytosis, and cloudy drained dialysate). If suspected, send dialysate overflow for culture and sensitivity. Peritonitis is the major problem associated with CAPD.

(b) Observe for signs of perforated bowel (pain and fecal material in outflow dialysate).

(c) Stop dialysate and notify physician.

(d) Observe for signs of pulmonary edema (rapid respiratory rate, rales, tachycardia, markedly reduced respiration depth due to fluid in the peritoneal cavity pushing the diaphragm upward). If suspected, stop inflow phase, elevate the head of the bed, and notify the physician.

(e) Observe for signs of leakage of dialysate into abdominal tissues, chest cavity, and scrotum. If this occurs, change the dressing around the catheter site and notify the physician.

(f) Provide constant reassurance and support. Maintain therapeutic nurse–client relationship. Provide avenue for expression of frustrations and anxieties. Assist client in maintaining self-esteem and body image.

(g) Observe for behavioral changes that may accompany dialysis disequilibrium.

(h) Provide for safety needs.

(9) Assist client undertaking CAPD.

(a) Develop teaching plan for client and dialysate partner. Emphasize importance of aseptic technique, since the major problem associated with CAPD is peritonitis. Teaching may be on an inpatient or outpatient basis, takes 5 to 10 days, and is reimbursable under third-party health care provider guidelines.

(b) Self-monitoring by the client or dialysate partner must be supplemented by nurse follow-up, when criteria for goal achievement are evaluated (Bruce et al., 1980).

8. Hemodialysis, or extracorporeal dialysis, is a complex mode of therapy that is extremely expensive and psychologically and physically demanding. Hemodialysis uses the same physical principles as peritoneal dialysis. In hemodialysis, blood is removed from the client's radial or brachial artery and pumped through a semipermeable cellophane membrane while the dialysate flows on the outside of the membrane. The waste products of metabolism, water, and electrolytes flow freely across the semipermeable membrane from the blood into the dialysate. Since end-stage renal disease has both reversible and irreversible biochemical components, long-term dialysis can only partially serve as a substitute for normal renal function (see Figure 32-4) (Sampson, 1980).

Hemodialysis is indicated for use in clients with acute or chronic renal failure when very rapid or frequent dialysis is necessary or when peritoneal dialysis is contraindicated, such as in cases of poisoning or severe uremia. Since the facilities for hemodialysis are limited and the cost is prohibitive, the selection of candidates for hemodialysis is often complex. The nurse frequently brings valuable information to a multidisciplinary conference for evaluating the feasibility and value of long-term hemodialysis.

a. Interventions related to lifestyle adaptations.

(1) Support client in identification of strengths and use of adaptive mechanisms.

(2) Assist client in mourning the loss of health, independence, financial stability, and possibly employment. Assist in developing and exploring interests and hobbies.

(3) Observe for signs of severe depression.

(a) Noncompliance such as improper cannula care, ingesting foods high

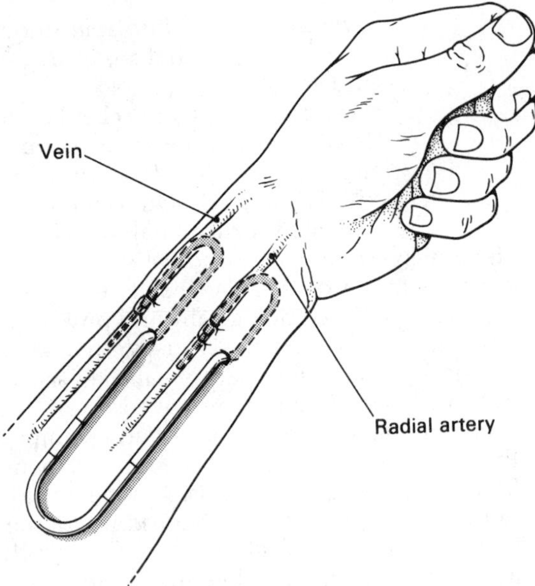

Figure 32-4 Schematic representation of a silastic shunt. This cannula allows easy access to both the artery and the vein without repeated venipuncture. (Adapted from Fellows, B.J.: "The Role of the Nurse in a Chronic Dialysis Unit," *Nursing Clinics of North America*, **1**(4):259, 1966.)

in potassium, and the like may be a manifestation of depression.

(b) Insomnia, a physical response to dialysis, can contribute to depression.

(4) Help client and family to develop realistic expectations and to avoid overprotectiveness.

(a) Maintain and encourage independence.

(b) Encourage responsibility for maintenance of therapy regimen within the realistic limitations of the client's condition.

(5) Counsel client and spouse regarding decreased libido and impotence.

(6) Advise that marital stability before dialysis carries through the stresses of dialysis and that role reversal is common.

(7) Assist the family in supporting the client. Use of denial by the family may be destructive; the family should be allowed avenues for expressing anxiety, hostility, and guilt. Be supportive, nonjudgmental, and objective in achieving this goal.

(8) Support development of and participation in family–client dialysis groups to help combat social isolation and provide avenues for teaching and sharing common experiences.

(9) Recognize and deal with staff reactions through staff conferences with a psychologist or psychiatrist to aid in dealing with personal reactions to dialysis. Health team attitudes are communicated to clients, and consistency of a multidisciplinary team is vital.

(10) Assist client in dealing with financial difficulties.

(a) Refer to appropriate agencies.

(b) Initiate appropriate referrals for vocational rehabilitation, social services, and follow-up home care.

(11) Evaluate feasibility of home dialysis.

b. Interventions related to physiological adaptation.

(1) Discontinue use of antihypertensive medications several hours before dialysis is begun.

(2) Identify history of bleeding and past dietary compliance.

(3) Maintain aseptic technique throughout the hemodialysis.

(4) Observe client's general condition and mood during hemodialysis. Measure and record weight, blood pressure (standing and lying down), temperature, pulse, respiration, and clotting time.

(5) Prepare client for blood sample for baseline electrolytes.

(6) Monitor condition of fistula or cannula access using only a mature, patent, fistula (2–4 weeks). Avoid taking blood pressure or drawing blood from canulated arm.

(7) Monitor the position, intactness, patency of tubing, and security of insertion site. Tape and position as necessary, avoiding air or kinking in tubing.

(8) Identify individualized dialysate so-

lution, blood flow rate, dialysate flow rate, length and frequency of dialysis, degree of ultrafiltration.

(9) Initiate dialysis by slowly increasing flow rates while noting vessel spasm, pain, needle position, pump speed, and bleeding from needle puncture site.

(10) Be familiar with information from monitor and alarm systems, including the blood leak detector, air bubble detector, flow rate indicator, and indices of changes in dialysate concentration and temperature.

(11) Monitor for signs of disequilibrium syndrome, duct cerebral edema (hypertension, headache, confusion, nausea, and vomiting).

(12) Monitor for signs of hypovolemia, hypervolemia, electrolyte imbalance, shock, and hemorrhage.

c. Interventions related to comfort and safety.

(1) Carefully observe for bleeding and equipment failure.

(2) Position client with legs elevated slightly to prevent vascular pooling.

(3) Provide recreation, diversion, position change, special meals, back rubs, and assistance with hygiene.

(4) Supervise cleaning and sterilization of equipment for reuse.

9. Renal transplantation involves the surgical transfer of a human kidney from one person to another. Organs may be obtained from a living donor or a cadaver. Regardless of the source, the donor kidney is placed in the iliac fossa, the donor renal artery is anastomosed end to end to the recipient's hypogastric artery, and the donor renal vein is anastomosed to the recipient's internal iliac vein. The donor ureter is implanted into the bladder wall in such a way as to prevent reflux (Phipps et al., 1980). Before transplantation, a bilateral nephrectomy may be performed.

a. Preoperative interventions: recipient.

(1) Answer questions honestly regarding the surgery, immediate postoperative period, and discharge plans.

(2) Encourage maintenance of self-care and maximal independence. Allow client to express fears.

(3) Refer for psychotherapy if necessary to prevent development of severe emotional disturbances.

(4) Include interventions listed under *Chronic Renal Failure.*

(5) Identify and support medical treatment of all infectious processes. Prepare client for postoperative reverse isolation.

(6) Assist in the collection of specimens to ascertain tissue compatibility.

b. Preoperative interventions: donor.

(1) Perform physical preparation similar to that for a client undergoing abdominal surgery. Assist in collection of specimens to ascertain tissue compatibility.

(2) Promote psychological preparation by:

(a) Identifying motivation for donating kidney.

(b) Assisting with psychiatric and physical evaluations of donor.

(c) Answering questions openly and honestly. Clarifying misconceptions for donor.

(d) Allowing donor to refuse being a donor; letting donor know that it is all right to say no.

c. Postoperative interventions: recipient.

(1) Implement immediate reverse isolation procedures (usually recipient does not go to the recovery room, because few recovery rooms are equipped to manage reverse precautions). Provide care similar to that for a client recovering from general anesthesia.

(2) Maintain fluid balance and renal functioning.

(a) Measure urine output every hour. Inspect and monitor composition of urine.

(b) Monitor and assess serum electrolyte and renal function values q24h, progressing to three times a week as condition stabilizes.

(c) Monitor vital signs, including central venous pressure (CVP), every hour.

(d) With a return to normal function in 48–72 h, urine output may ex-

ceed 2,000 mL/h. Bladder spasms resulting from use of previously underused urinary tract are common.
(e) Collect 24-h urine specimen for creatinine clearance and sodium, potassium, and protein excretion.
(f) After 24 h, monitor vital signs q4h and fluid intake and output q8h.
(g) Daily weights essential.
(3) Early mobility to maintain optimal pulmonary functioning.
(a) Begin ambulation 24 h after surgery. Client may lie on operative side in bed. Elevate head of bed 30–45 degrees.
(b) Instruct client to avoid sitting for extended periods (may cause kinking of ureter, tension on anastomosis, or rotation of the graft).
(4) Prevent infection.
(a) Administer prescribed immunosuppressive drugs (usually azathioprine) and corticosteroids. Administer prescribed antacids with corticosteroids.
(b) Monitor white blood counts every day.
(c) Maintain strict aseptic precautions. Careful handwashing is vital. Avoid exposure to anyone with infections.
(d) Observe meticulous catheter care.
(e) Obtain routine cultures of likely signs of infection.
(5) Initiate teaching-learning transaction (include family and/or significant others) regarding:
(a) Self-assessment and self-care: measuring fluid intake and output, recording weight, taking blood pressure, collecting urine specimens, and so on.
(b) General health habits and activity levels: oral and personal hygiene essential.
(c) Dietary counseling.
(d) Signs and symptoms of infection and/or rejection.
(e) Importance of follow-up care.
(6) Assist client in dealing with new body image and emotional feelings of obligation to the donor. Allow client opportunities to express fears of rejection and other feelings. Emphasize positive aspects of client's life.

d. Postoperative interventions: donor.
(1) Physical care similar to that for a client following major abdominal surgery.
(2) Assist donor in working through depression and feelings of not being adequately regarded for personal sacrifice.
(3) In cases of rejection reactions, assist donor in working through feelings of guilt.

e. Initiate referral for follow-up and reevaluation.

f. Deal with pre- and posttransplantation reactions by staff and family.

EVALUATION

Outcome Criteria

1. Client complies with prescribed diet; weight reflects established baseline ± 1 kg.
2. Absence of edema: periorbital, extremities, sacral, pulmonary (lungs clear of fluid excess upon examination).
3. Client is able to explain relationship between fluid sodium intake and weight gain.
4. Calcium, phosphorus, potassium levels are maintained.
   a. Calcium 9–11 mg/100 mL.
   b. Phosphorus 3.5–5.5 mg/100 mL.
   c. Potassium 3.5–5.0 mg/100 mL.
5. Temperature 98.6°F. Blood pressure within 5 mmHg of baseline.
6. Absence of pruritus, muscle spasm, and cramps.
7. Sensory and perceptual functions are intact.
   a. Extremities respond to light touch and sensations of sharp, dull, hot, and cold.
   b. Client has position sense.
   c. Romberg test is within normal limits.
8. Memory is intact: client is able to recall recent and remote facts.
9. Client can describe self-care activities, an exercise and activity schedule, and a sleep and rest plan that are compatible with age, stage, and progress of disease.
10. Client reports maintenance of positive family relationships and established, desired pattern of sexuality.

11. Client can describe signs and symptoms of chronic renal dysfunction.
12. Client can describe cannula and/or fistula care and precautions if applicable.

Complications

1. Complications of peritoneal dialysis.
   a. Loss of the catheter into the abdomen; removed by laparoscopy.
   b. Perforation of the bowel (refer to Chapter 33).
   c. Perforation of the bladder (refer to *Trauma to the Urinary Bladder*).
   d. Peritonitis, especially in CAPD.
   e. Wound infection.
   f. Arrhythmia due to removal of potassium (refer to Chapter 30).
   g. Hyperglycemia (refer to Chapter 28).
   h. Hypernatremia.
   i. Hyperosmolarity.
   j. Reactive hypoglycemia sometimes occurs 24–48 h after dialysis, most often in diabetics.
2. Complications of hemodialysis.
   a. Hyper- or hypovolemia.
   b. Hemolysis.
   c. Dialysis disequilibrium syndrome.
   d. Transfusion hazards.
   e. Psychological dysfunction.
   f. Continuation of uremic problems despite dialysis.
      (1) Anemia.
      (2) Hypertension.
      (3) Peripheral neuropathy.
      (4) Renal osteodystrophy.
      (5) Reproductive system abnormalities such as gynecomastia and menorrhagia.
      (6) Pruritis: use of porcine rather than bovine heparin may reduce itching; sometimes responds to lidocaine infusions or antihistamines (Miller and Sayers, 1981).

Reevaluation and Follow-up

1. Changes in protocols must be made as client's health status, age, and energy level change.
2. Maintaining support systems through counseling and use of homemaker and respite care is key to maintaining a satisfactory lifestyle for these clients and their families.
3. Clients need assistance in dealing with transplant rejection and resumption of dialysis. When these modes of treatment have been exhausted or the client grows weary of the struggle, terminal care is indicated.

INFLAMMATIONS

URETHRITIS

DESCRIPTION

Urethritis, inflammation of the urethra, may be acute or chronic. In either case, the inflammation is generally limited to the epithelial and subepithelial layers of the urethra. Urethritis may be nonspecific, in that no organism can be identified as the causative agent. Exposure to chemicals in some bubble baths and spermicidal jellies has been identified as an etiological factor, as has catheterization. However, in the majority of cases, urethritis is caused by bacteria, particularly *Neisseria gonorrhoeae*, which is transmitted by direct sexual contact. Exposure to other organisms, such as viruses, fungi, and protozoa from the vagina and/or rectum, may also be a cause. Repeated infection may cause stricture and obstruction of the urinary tract.

PREVENTION

Health Promotion

1. Support the teaching of sexual and urinary hygiene in school health classes.
2. Drink 4–6 glasses of fluid per day if not contraindicated.
3. Void completely at specific times (e.g., every 4–6 h) during the day.

Population at Risk

1. Sexually active men and women.
2. Persons experiencing trauma of urethra.
3. Persons with obstructions of urinary meatus.

Screening

1. Preemployment, school history, and physical and functional pattern assessment.
2. Culture of midstream urine specimen in symptomatic persons.
3. Hematuria and pyuria on routine urinalysis.
   a. Hematuria $>$ 2 RBCs/hpf.

b. Marked pyuria > 20 WBCs/hpf (Kamaroff and Winickoff, 1977).

ASSESSMENT

Health History

Refer to Table 32-1.

1. Past history of urinary tract infections, location, frequency of recurrence, severity, duration, and mode of treatment.
2. History of hygienic self-care practices (particularly use of bubble baths, perfumed soaps, and/or feminine hygiene deodorant sprays).
3. Identification of possible causative factors (e.g., catheterization or other traumas).
4. Sexual history and contraceptive practices (particularly use of spermicidal jellies).
5. Voiding patterns and characteristics of urination (particularly frequency, nocturia, urgency, burning upon initiating micturition).
6. Irregular voiding patterns.

Physical Assessment

1. Elevated body temperature.
2. Edema and erythremia around urinary meatus.
3. Discharge from urethra (usually present in males but not always in females).
4. Pain in urethra upon movement.

Diagnostic Tests

1. Culture and antibiotic sensitivities of urethral discharge.
2. Urine culture and antibiotic sensitivities; midstream urine specimen.
3. Microscopic urinalysis.
4. Visual inspection of several urine specimens in glass receptacles to identify site of infection (multiple-glass test).
5. White blood cell differential count.
6. Serologic test for syphilis.

NURSING DIAGNOSES: ACTUAL OR POTENTIAL

1. Altered urinary elimination pattern due to inflammatory process.
2. Health management deficit related to poor personal hygiene or other poor health habits.
3. Alteration in comfort or pain due to urethritis.
4. Sleep pattern disturbance due to nocturia or dysuria.
5. Mild to moderate anxiety due to pain, frequency, or sexual dysfunction.
6. Sexual dysfunction related to alteration in comfort.

EXPECTED OUTCOMES

1. Transmission of causative organism will be prevented, if urethritis is of infectious origin.
2. Existing inflammatory or infectious process will be eradicated.
3. Urinary stasis will be prevented.
4. Pain, discomfort, and anxiety will be reduced.
5. Causative factors will be identified and removed.
6. Extension of inflammatory or infectious process will be prevented.
7. Recurrence will be prevented through client education.

INTERVENTIONS

1. Initiate precautionary isolation measures (linen, towels, clothing, etc. should be treated as contaminated items; be particularly careful when discarding contaminated urine).
2. Administer prescribed antibiotics (usually broad-spectrum). Penicillin used if urethritis is from gonorrhea. Tetracycline antibiotics used if client allergic to penicillin.
   a. Assess urethral discharge for response to antibiotics.
   b. Monitor culture and antibiotic sensitivities of urethral discharge during first week of therapy to determine effect.
3. Increase fluid intake to 3,000 mL per 24-h period (unless contraindicated by other coexisting physical condition).
4. Monitor and assess correlation between intake and output.
5. Administer prescribed analgesics and other appropriate pain relief measures.
6. Examine urethra for patency, observe voiding, and palpate bladder for possible distention.
7. Monitor and assess temperature q4h (more frequently if indicated by marked deviation from the norm).
8. Provide environment that promotes improvement of general physical and psychological health.
9. Offer reassurance that voiding patterns will return to state before urethritis (barring complications).
10. Decrease anxiety regarding sexual concerns by presenting a supportive atmosphere.

11. Initiate teaching-learning transaction (include family and/or significant others) regarding:
    a. Home care of linen, towels, clothing, and so on until infectious process has been successfully treated.
    b. Avoidance of sexual intercourse to prevent transmission of the infection before antibiotics act.
    c. Hygienic practices, particularly proper cleansing after urination and defecation and avoidance of bubble baths (see *Cystitis* for more information).
    d. Medications, desired effects, and side effects.
        (1) Alert client that some medications cause discoloration of urine.
        (2) Advise continuation of full course of medications despite cessation of symptoms.
    e. Signs of recurrence or reinfection and appropriate responses to these signs.
    f. Avoidance of other identified cause.
12. Refer for evaluation of alternative means of contraception if spermicidal jelly or diaphragm is used (Lach et al., 1980).
13. Counsel and refer sexual partner(s) for investigation and treatment of causative organism.
14. Follow-up and reevaluation.

EVALUATION

Outcome Criteria

1. Temperature returns to normal within 48 h after start of antibiotic.
2. Pain diminishes sufficiently to allow client to sleep at night within 48 h start of antibiotic.
3. Urinary output increases until equal to input q24h (3,000 cc recommended).
4. Client reports hygiene practices compatible with guidelines.
    a. Women.
        (1) Client cleans perineal region carefully, wipes front to back, and washes hands with soap and water after bowel movement.
        (2) Client empties bladder before and immediately after intercourse (Lach et al., 1980).
        (3) Client showers with antibacterial soap and avoids tub baths.
        (4) Client wears cotton underpants.
    b. Men. Client reports avoiding prolonged bladder distension and empties bladder every 4–6 hours.
5. Client reports adhering to medication schedule; client reports side effects of medication.
6. Client can list indications for contact with health care provider (see *Assessment* under *Urethritis* and *Cystitis*).

Complications

RECURRENCE OR REINFECTION

Assessment

Symptoms of fever, frequency, and urgency do not resolve, and the following symptoms develop:

1. Bladder spasms, increased cramps, and suprapubic pain.
2. Low back pain and rectal pain in perineal area.
3. Hematuria.
4. Enlarged, tender prostate, which to avoid bacterial spread, should not be massaged.
5. Noncompliance with therapeutic plan.

Revised Outcomes

See expected outcomes under *Cystitis*.

Interventions

See *Cystitis*.

Evaluation

See outcome criteria under *Cystitis*.

ASCENDING INFECTION: CYSTITIS AND ACUTE PROSTITIS

Assessment

1. Symptoms and signs of urethritis reappear 7–10 days to 6 months after one sterile midstream microscopic urinalysis.
2. Elicit history of infection from personal hygiene lapse or sexual exposure.

Revised Outcomes

See expected outcomes under *Cystitis*.

Interventions

1. Refer to physician for reevaluation because of treatment failure.
2. Reinforce client teachings listed above with primary interventions for urethritis.

Evaluation

Outcome criteria:

1. Clean catch urine specimen and culture of discharge indicate no recurrence or reinfection when evaluated against initial specimens in weekly follow-up.

2. Client compliance with revised outcomes are met.

URETHRAL STRICTURE

Assessment
1. Physical assessment of patency by inspection.
2. Reported inability to urinate.

Revised Outcomes
See expected outcomes under *Cystitis*.

Interventions
Assist client undergoing urethral dilation.

Evaluation
Outcome criteria:
1. Client forces fluids to 3,000 cc/24 h.
2. Client seeks health care if symptoms recur.

HEMORRHAGIC CYSTITIS

Assessment
1. Increased number of RBCs in urine (0–2/hpf is normal).
2. No response to antimicrobial therapy.
3. Symptoms persist 5–7 days and subside spontaneously.

Revised Outcomes
See expected outcomes under *Cystitis*.

Interventions
1. Monitor RBCs in urine.
2. Consult physician.
3. Reassure client.
4. Force fluids.

Evaluation
Revised outcome criteria: complete resolution of symptoms in 5–7 days.

Reevaluation and Follow-up
Refer for urologic evaluation after three episodes of infection in 6 months in women and after the first occurrence in men.

CYSTITIS

DESCRIPTION

Cystitis, inflammation of the wall of the urinary bladder, may occur as a primary condition; however, it is more frequently associated with an infectious process elsewhere in the urinary tract. Cystitis may also be related to the obstruction of the free flow of urine (urethral obstruction). Women are more frequently affected than men. Contamination of the urethra from the rectum and vagina may be causative. Cystitis in males is usually associated with urinary retention caused by an enlarged or infected prostate gland.

Chronic cystitis may develop when the underlying cause or predisposing factors are not eliminated. Urine cultures may reveal no growth of organisms in the chronic state, and clients may be asymptomatic in the presence of increased bacterial counts.

Interstitial cystitis, also known as Hunner's ulcer, most frequently affects middle-aged women. This condition is characterized by decreased bladder capacity and actual splitting of the epithelium in the presence of bladder distention. The etiology remains obscure, and treatment is extremely difficult; however, fulguration of the bleeding ulcer under general anesthesia has been successful.

PREVENTION

Health Promotion

1. Drink 2,500–3,000 mL fluids per day.
2. Empty the bladder completely or nearly completely every 4–5 h.
3. Avoid urinary tract trauma.
4. Teach public importance of urinary hygiene.
5. Promote excretion of acid urine by acid-ash diet.

Population at Risk

1. Sexually active women.
2. Persons with neurogenic bladder and/or immobility, especially if catheterized.
3. Diabetics.
4. Pregnant women.
5. Persons with obstructions of the urinary tract.

Screening
1. Careful preemployment history, physical, and functional health pattern assessment.
2. Elevated WBCs and RBCs on routine urinalysis.
   a. Marked pyuria > 20 WBCs/hpf.
   b. Hematuria > 2 RBCs/hpf.

ASSESSMENT

Health History

Health history is important, since recurring bladder infections should be carefully documented for further follow-up (see Table 32-1).

1. Voiding patterns and characteristics of micturition (particularly frequency, nocturia, ur-

gency, tenesmus, and burning throughout voiding or at the end of micturition).
2. Description and characteristics of urine (particularly pyuria, hematuria, and/or malodor).
3. Frank hematuria with pyuria (pus in urine) and sterile urine cultures may indicate tuberculosis of the urinary tract.

Physical Assessment

1. Elevated body temperature.
2. Suprapubic pain or flank pain.
3. Cloudy, malodorous urine.
4. Abdominal discomfort on palpation and fullness in abdominal cavity.

Diagnostic Tests

1. Microscopic urinalysis: specimens will show alkaline pH, albuminuria (common in chronic cases), and hematuria (WBCs > 20/hpf).
2. Urine culture and antibiotic sensitivities.
3. Visual inspection of several urine specimens in glass receptacles (random specimens will contain sediment).
4. White blood cell differential count.

NURSING DIAGNOSES: ACTUAL OR POTENTIAL

See *Urethritis*.

EXPECTED OUTCOMES

See *Urethritis*.

INTERVENTIONS

1. Assess urine cultures and antibiotic sensitivities to determine response to chemotherapy.
2. Encourage fluid intake (oral and parenteral) of at least 3,000 mL per 24-h period to reduce residual urine (unless contraindicated by medications, coexisting disease conditions, and/or complete obstruction of urine flow).
3. Encourage mild to moderate activity to prevent urinary stasis (some restrictions are imposed during the acute phase).
4. Administer prescribed antispasmodics to reduce tenesmus.
5. Administer prescribed analgesics and/or other measures to relieve pain.
6. Establish nurse–client relationship that encourages discussion of anxieties regarding sexual activity, sexual hygiene, and choice of contraceptives.
7. Personalize a plan for education including principles of hygiene, medications, fluids, and symptoms of reinfection or recurrence.
8. If urinary stasis, obstruction, or neurogenic bladder is a problem, teach strict aseptic technique, self-catheterization, or the use of external catheter.

EVALUATION

Outcome Criteria

1. Temperature returns to normal.
2. Urinary output reflects increased fluid intake (3,000 cc recommended).
3. Client reports continued adherence to medication schedule.
4. Pain diminishes sufficiently to allow client to sleep within 48 hours and totally subsides within 5 days.
5. Client reports return to desired sexual activity within 10 days.
6. Urinary bacterial count returns to normal (10,000/hpf) in 5 days.
7. Client reports understanding of and adherence to hygiene program (see expected outcomes for *Urethritis*).

Complications

CHRONIC CYSTITIS

Assessment

1. History of three or more episodes of acute cystitis in 6 months in women; history of one other episode in men.
2. Thorough abdominal, genitourinary, and neurological assessment to determine any structural and functional abnormalities of the urinary tract, obstruction to flow of urine, or impaired bladder innervation, which may cause stasis.
3. Thorough history of sexual and reproductive patterns, including developmental aspects and use of contraceptives.
4. In-depth review of client's health and hygiene habits, elimination pattern, activity and exercise pattern, and coping stress tolerance pattern to determine behavioral aspects of health deficit.
5. Assess catheter care or self-catheterization technique by client or care provider.

Revised Outcomes

1. Client will remain symptom free and maintain bacterial count of 10,000/hpf.

2. Repeat urinalysis following completion of antibiotic course to determine bacterial count.

Interventions
1. Refer to physician for further workup.
2. Establish cause of repeated infections if possible.
3. Develop management plan with client considering life goals, lifestyle.
4. Assist client with behavior modification if behavioral aspects are identified.

Complications
1. Pyelonephritis (refer to *Pyelonephritis*).
2. Septicemia (see Chapter 49).

Reevaluation and Follow-up
Follow up with client every 3 months for 2 years (can be done by phone).

PYELONEPHRITIS

DESCRIPTION

Acute pyelonephritis is an inflammation of one or both kidney pelvises caused by a bacterial infection. Gram-negative enteric bacilli are the most commonly encountered organisms that enter the urinary system. *Escherichia coli* is frequently the causative organism. In addition to developing from an ascending infection in the lower urinary tract, acute pyelonephritis may be caused by a blood-borne infection such as streptococcus.

Females, particularly girls under the age of 10 and women in their early childbearing years, are more frequently affected than males. Persons with diabetes mellitus and women in the first trimester of pregnancy appear to have a particular predisposition to pyelonephritis.

Of prime concern in dealing with acute pyelonephritis is the possible cessation of symptoms with the persistence of an asymptomatic infection that eventually develops into destruction of the kidneys.

PREVENTION

Health Promotion

Careful teaching of those clients with urinary tract infection concerning hygiene practices.

Population at Risk

1. Pregnant women.
2. Persons experiencing trauma or obstruction of urinary tract.
3. Hypertensives, diabetics, and persons with polycystic kidneys.
4. Persons exposed to renal toxins (e.g., from analgesic abuse).

Screening

1. Preemployment and school physicals and family and functional pattern area assessments.
2. Early pregnancy testing and prenatal care.

ASSESSMENT

Health History

Because of the nature of the predisposing factors associated with acute pyelonephritis, the nurse should review the nursing health history outlines related to the obstruction of the free flow of urine due to any cause and/or infection in any part of the urinary tract. (Refer to Table 32-1.) In addition, the nurse should investigate:

1. Onset of symptoms and treatment to date (onset is usually manifested by violent chills).
2. Presence, location, intensity, quality, and precipitating or aggravating factors of pain. Determine agents and/or factors that aid in analgesia.
3. Voiding patterns and characteristics of urination, particularly frequency, urgency, nocturia, and burning on urination.
4. Description and characteristics of urine, particularly malodorous, cloudy, or bloody urine.
5. Description of other contributing factors, such as pregnancy, diabetes, or advanced age.

Physical Assessment

1. Elevated body temperature.
2. Tenderness in affected costovertebral angle (may be bilateral).
3. Enlarged kidney may be palpable (possibly bilaterally).
4. Slightly rigid abdominal flank pain and lower abdominal pain.
5. Lethargy and malaise.

Diagnostic Tests

1. Review of diagnostic studies to rule out obstruction of urine due to any cause and infections of the urinary tract distal to the kidney pelvis.
2. IVP to detect dilatations of urinary pelvis.
3. Cystoscopy to view the bladder and related structures.

4. Renal biopsy.
5. Microscopic urinalysis to isolate organisms involved; may show pyuria, bacteriuria, proteinuria, and cysts.
6. WBCs elevated with increase in band cells.
7. Urine specific gravity usually less than 1.010.

NURSING DIAGNOSES: ACTUAL OR POTENTIAL

1. Health management deficit due to activity intolerance.
2. Urinary elimination pattern altered.
3. Decreased activity tolerance (level III) related to toxicity.
4. Alteration in comfort or pain due to flank pain.
5. Sleep pattern disturbance due to pain.
6. Fear related to toxic state, hospitalization, and potential effects on pregnancy.
7. Sexual dysfunction due to pain or bacteremia.
8. Ineffective or compromised family coping related to health status and/or hospitalization.

EXPECTED OUTCOMES

1. Pain, discomfort, and fever will be reduced.
2. Existing infection will be permanently eradicated.
3. Transmission of causative organism will be prevented.
4. Urinary stasis will be prevented.
5. Urinary output will be maintained at least 1,500 mL per 24-h period.
6. Anxiety and fear related to illness, hospitalization, and effect on pregnancy, job, and lifestyle will be reduced.
7. Permanent renal damage will be prevented.
8. Recurrence will be prevented through client education.

INTERVENTIONS

1. Administer prescribed analgesics, back massages, and/or other measures to relieve pain.
   a. Assess response to pain relief measures.
   b. Determine whether more vigorous nursing or medical measures are needed.
2. Administer prescribed broad-spectrum antibiotics (determined by urine cultures and antibiotic sensitivities).
3. Assess urine cultures and antibiotic sensitivities to determine response to chemotherapy. Reculture urine after antibiotics are discontinued and periodically for 1 year after infection.
4. Encourage fluid intake (oral and parenteral) of at least 3,000 mL per 24-h period to reduce residual urine and prevent stasis (unless contraindicated).
5. Monitor and assess correlation of intake and output q4h (more frequently if indicated). Urinary output should be maintained at no less than 30–40 mL/h.
6. Test urine for specific gravity, protein, pH, and hematuria q2h.
7. Observe for signs of obstruction; drainage of urine proximal to obstruction may be necessary. Nephrostomy, ureterostomy, cystostomy, urethral catheterization, or surgery to repair congenital anomalies and defects may be necessary.
   a. Ensure unobstructed urine flow through urinary drainage system to prevent reflux and/or stasis.
   b. Provide meticulous catheter care (refer to *Renal Tumors*).
8. Monitor and assess vital signs, especially temperature, q4h or more frequently as indicated by marked deviation from norm.
   a. Carry out comfort measures during periods of hyperpyrexia (tepid sponge baths; fresh, dry linen and bed clothes, etc.).
   b. Administer prescribed medications to reduce temperature.
   c. Assess response to interventions.
9. Encourage strict bed rest during acute phase, but avoid total immobility to prevent stasis of urine.
10. Weigh client daily (on the same scale, with the same amount of clothes, at the same time of day, preferably before breakfast and after voiding).
11. Monitor and assess renal function studies and electrolyte determinations, especially blood urea nitrogen, sodium, and chloride and serum creatinine.
12. Assist client in determining possible causative factors.
13. Establish therapeutic nurse–client relationship that encourages discussion of anxieties and concerns regarding diagnostic testing, treatment regimen, and future implications of illness.
14. Provide environment that fosters maximal self-esteem and self-care activities despite initial restrictions.

15. Initiate teaching-learning transaction (include family and/or significant others). (Refer to *Renal Tumors*.)
16. Refer to social service for financial and homemaker assistance.

EVALUATION

Outcome Criteria

1. Client is hospitalized or has necessary home assistance from others for initial period of illness (3–5 days).
2. Urinary elimination is maintained at rate of 40 cc/h.
3. Client reports decrease in pain within 24 h of antibiotic therapy. Pain is controlled (below 5 on intensity scale of 1–10) by analgesics, massage therapy, position change, relaxation response, and therapeutic touch during initial 24 h.
4. Client reports at least 6 h of uninterrupted sleep each night.
5. Client freely discusses fears related to health status, family coping, and sexuality by third hospital day or on first follow-up visit if treated in ambulatory setting.
6. Temperature, white blood cell count, and urine culture return to normal within 72 h.
7. Client can list all medications, actions, effects, side effects, and frequency of dosage before discharge or on follow-up visit if ambulatory.
8. Client can list symptoms of recurrence or reinfection (see Assessment).
9. Client can list hygienic measures listed under *Urethritis* and *Cystitis*.
10. Client engages in self-care activities and reports gradually increasing activity tolerance.

Complications

Chronic pyelonephritis is believed to be related to multiple episodes of acute pyelonephritis, which cause healing with the formation of large scars, fibrosis, and tubular dilatation characteristic of chronic disease. Generally, the glomeruli are spared injury except in advanced cases.

Assessment

1. Most clients offer a history of repeated attacks of acute pyelonephritis or chronic bacteriuria.
2. Client may complain of dull flank pain (unilateral or bilateral), low-grade fever, fatigue, headache, and anorexia often accompanied by weight loss and lethargy.
3. Decreased specific gravity of urine (indicative of kidney failure to adequately concentrate urine), polyuria, and excessive thirst may also be noted.
4. IVP, cystoscopy, and renal biopsy may be ordered.

Revised Outcomes

Kidney function will be maintained at current level with diet, fluid, and activity control.

Interventions

1. Refer to discussion under *Chronic Renal Failure* for nursing interventions that promote psychological adjustment to chronic condition.
2. Chronic suppressive therapy may be instituted in an attempt to prevent acute flare-ups (e.g., sulfamethoxazole, trimethoprim, and nitrofurantoin).

Complications

1. Bacteremic shock (refer to Chapter 48).
2. Renal failure (refer to *Acute Renal Failure* and *Chronic Renal Failure*).

Reevaluation and Follow-up

Continuous nursing and medical management every 3 months is indicated.

ACUTE GLOMERULONEPHRITIS

DESCRIPTION

Acute glomerulonephritis is a disease in which the glomeruli of both kidneys are seriously damaged and partially destroyed by an inflammatory process that originates as an allergic or autoimmune response. This allergic or autoimmune response may be stimulated by a beta-hemolytic streptococcus infection that precedes the glomerulonephritis by 2 or 3 weeks or by lupus erythematosis. The exact mechanism of this response is not known. Hypertension, diabetes, and disseminated intravascular coagulation are other causes. The pathology is characterized by diffuse inflammatory changes in glomeruli and an increase in permeability of the systemic capillary bed. All renal tissues are affected to varying degrees, and nephrotic changes result in the formation of increasing amounts of scar tissue, resulting in atrophy and complete destruction of the nephrons.

This disease most often affects children and young adults. Males are more frequently affected than females. Ninety percent of children and 50 percent of adults have a complete recovery (Isselbache et al., 1980).

PREVENTION

Health Promotion

1. Drink 2,500–3,000 mL of clear, fresh water every day.
2. Health teaching at middle school, high school, and college level of importance of urinary hygiene.
3. Careful explanation of the importance of throat cultures and of completion of antimicrobial therapy is important, but there is no evidence that it is preventive.

Population at Risk

1. Persons with history of beta-hemolytic streptococcal infections (especially of the throat).
2. Persons with recurrent cystitis.

Screening

Careful preemployment and school health functional pattern assessments should identify those people at high risk.

ASSESSMENT

Health History

See *Acute Renal Failure* (refer to Table 32-1).

1. History of beta-hemolytic streptococcal infections (particularly of the throat).
2. Visual disturbances due to retinal edema, weakness, nausea, anorexia, headaches, and dizziness.

Physical Assessment

1. Enlarged kidneys may be palpable.
2. Periorbital edema and dependent edema.
3. Papilledema and/or retinal hemorrhage (not always present).
4. Elevated temperature and elevated arterial blood pressure (renin-angiotensin system may be involved).
5. Tenderness in costovertebral angles.

Diagnostic Tests

1. IVP or retrograde pyelograms.
2. Appropriate cardiovascular and pulmonary function tests.
3. Antistreptolysin (ASO) titer and C-reactive protein (CRP): both elevated during the course of acute glomerulonephritis.
4. Blood chemistry determinations (e.g., serum electrolytes).
5. Renal function studies: elevated BUN and serum creatinine; decreased plasma protein; phenolsulfonphthalein and creatinine clearance test may show decreased excretion in urine specimens.
6. Hematocrit and hemoglobin: anemia may be present because of hematuria and disturbance of the hemopoietic mechanism initiated by release of erythropoietin from the kidney.
7. Microscopic urinalysis: oliguria or anuria; hematuria almost always present; color is smoky brown or mahogany; low specific gravity (1.020–1.025); leukocytosis; many casts; large amounts of albumin; pH usually acid.

NURSING DIAGNOSES: ACTUAL OR POTENTIAL

1. Altered urinary elimination pattern due to glomerular destruction.
2. Total self-care deficit related to complete bed rest, lassitude, fatigue, and fever.
3. Potential for infection or reinfection.
4. Alteration in nutritional requirements related to high-carbohydrate, low-sodium, fluid-restricted diet.
5. Potential fluid volume deficit associated with retained sodium: inability of kidney to concentrate urine.
6. Temporarily impaired home maintenance management due to bed rest (full recovery can take up to 2 years).
7. Noncompliance with therapeutic regimen because client does not feel ill and bed rest may be protracted.

EXPECTED OUTCOMES

1. Nephron destruction will be limited.
2. Metabolic demands on compromised kidney will decrease.
3. Hypertension and infection will be controlled.
4. Complications will be recognized and treated early.
5. Renal functioning will be restored.
6. Anxiety and apprehension will be reduced.
7. Recurrence will be prevented.

INTERVENTIONS

See *Acute Renal Failure*.

1. Administer prescribed antibiotics.
2. Provide safe environment. Initiate seizure precautions (uremic seizures may develop).

3. Provide and encourage total physical and psychological rest. Bed rest essential during acute phase. Activity may be increased as renal function improves. Provide reassurance, encouragement, and support. Provide avenue for expression of anxieties.
4. Measure and assess vital signs q4h.
5. Measure weight and assess water retention every day.
6. Massage skin and change position every hour. Encourage and carry out passive and active range-of-motion exercises. Assess condition of skin and surface membranes.
7. Maintain oral hygiene.
8. Provide prescribed diet. Foods high in carbohydrates and fats allowed. Carbohydrates provide energy and reduce catabolism of protein. Diet is usually low in protein (depending on BUN levels) and limited in sodium and potassium. Fluid restriction usually 1,200 mL per 24-h period.
9. Meticulously measure and assess intake and output.
   a. Measure total amount and frequency of voided urine.
   b. Test specific gravity, hematuria, and albumin at each voiding or q2h if catheter present.
10. Maintain strict aseptic technique.
11. Initiate teaching-learning transaction (include family and/or significant others) regarding:
    a. Avoiding overexertion.
    b. Avoiding exposure to all acute and chronic infections. If infectious process develops, prompt attention and treatment necessary.
    c. Prophylactic immunizations to prevent secondary infections.
    d. Early prenatal care (if appropriate).
    e. General health care practices.
12. Initiate social service consultation (necessary because of prolonged convalescence). Economic problems frequently develop.
13. Initiate referral for follow-up home care.

EVALUATION

Outcome Criteria

1. BUN and creatinine level remain compatible with:
   a. BUN 8–28 mg/100 mL.
   b. Serum creatinine 0.5–1.2 mg/100 mL.
2. Urine specific gravity 1.010–1.025.
3. Blood pressure, proteinuria, and edema do not increase with prescribed activity.
4. Client has care provider for self-care and home-care needs during acute phase (up to 2 months).
5. Client remains free of infection as exhibited by normal temperature and no signs of upper respiratory infection (URI).
6. Client can describe rationale for rest and medication even though symptoms may be absent.
7. Client reports adherence to diet and has 2-kg or less weight gain per month.
8. Client freely discusses feelings about illness, restrictions, and lifestyle changes and maintains interest in recovery process at each follow-up visit.

Complications

REINFECTION

Assessment
1. Chills, elevated temperature, sore throat.
2. Reported exposure to streptococcal infection.

Revised Outcomes
Client will remain infection free.

Interventions
1. Refer to physician for possible prescription of prophylactic antibiotic.
2. Advise to avoid crowds and fatigue.

FLUID OVERLOAD OR PULMONARY EDEMA

Assessment
1. Edema: periorbital, sacral, or of the ankles.
2. Paroxysmal nocturnal dyspnea or rales in lung bases.
3. Hypertension.
4. History of dietary noncompliance.

Revised Outcomes
Client will exhibit no signs of fluid overload (as listed above).

Interventions
1. Refer to physician for possible prescription of diuretics.
2. Revise dietary teaching plan and consult dietitian.

NONCOMPLIANCE

Assessment
1. History of noncompliance.
2. Signs of reinfection or fluid overload.
3. Verbal report of noncompliance with therapeutic plan.

Revised Outcomes
1. Client will exhibit no fluid overload.
2. Client will avoid depression (see Chapter 36).

Interventions
1. Instruct client in keeping diet and activity log.
2. Consult dietitian on development of diet guidelines that include client's ethnic and/or favorite foods.
3. Encourage support group for client and family.
4. Assist client in use of contracting to achieve goals.

Reevaluation and Follow-up
Recovery, though common, is protracted and frustrating. Follow-up over a 5-year period is advisable, frequently during the first 2 years, half-yearly thereafter.

TUBERCULOSIS OF THE URINARY TRACT

DESCRIPTION

Mycobacterium tuberculosis is the causative organism of tuberculosis (TB) of the urinary tract. This disease process, unilateral or bilateral, originates from a pulmonary or gastrointestinal lesion and reaches the kidney via the bloodstream.

Lesions in the renal parenchyma gradually erode into the renal pelvis, and eventually large cavities develop, with complete destruction of the kidney. The infection usually descends via the ureters into the bladder, causing symptoms similar to cystitis and urethritis. Development of fibrous tissue and urethral strictures is not uncommon.

Complaints of gross hematuria, frequency, burning on urination, and dull flank pain accompanied by fatigue and gradual weight loss should alert the nurse to suspect tuberculosis. In addition to urine cultures and skin testing to confirm the diagnosis, identification of the primary sources of the disease is vital.

PREVENTION

Health Promotion

1. Employee health policies that include tuberculosis control.
2. Careful following of post-TB clients and those with positive tuberculin tests.

Population at Risk

1. Active TB clients.
2. Post-TB clients.
3. Families and others exposed to persons with TB.

Screening

Culture of first morning voiding in persons with symptoms of hemorrhagic cystitis and history of positive tuberculin test. Pus in urine and sterile urine culture is suggestive of TB.

ASSESSMENT

Refer to *Cystitis* and to the discussion of tuberculosis in Chapter 31.

NURSING DIAGNOSES: ACTUAL OR POTENTIAL

1. Altered urinary elimination pattern due to destruction of renal calices.
2. Alteration in nutritional requirements related to decreased renal function.
3. Decreased activity tolerance related to fatigue and need for rest.
4. Potential noncompliance related to fact that client may feel well but medication must be taken for at least 1 year.
5. Self-esteem disturbance related to chronic communicable disease state.
6. Knowledge deficit related to need for isolation, sexual transmissibility, genital involvement, and affect on fertility.
7. Home maintenance management deficit due to need for rest and long convalescence.

EXPECTED OUTCOMES

1. Destruction of functional kidney will be reduced.
2. Demand on kidney will be decreased through diet and activity control.
3. Active pulmonary tuberculosis will be ruled out.
4. Client will adapt to contagious, chronic disease with implications for sexuality and fertility.

INTERVENTIONS

1. Administer antituberculosis medications, specifically isoniazid, sodium para-aminosalicylate, and cycloserine. Streptomycin, kanamycin, ethionamide, rifampin, and viomy-

cin sulfate may be used if drug resistance or intolerance to previously mentioned medications develops.
2. Initiate precautions to prevent transmission of the organism. Initiate teaching regarding use of protective devices (condom) during sexual intercourse to prevent transfer of organism. Continue all precautions until urine cultures negative.
3. Assist client in dealing with actual, perceived, or self-imposed social isolation.
4. Initiate teaching-learning transaction (include family and/or significant others) regarding:
   a. Disease process and treatment regimen.
   b. General health care measures (adequate rest and avoidance of overexertion).
   c. Medications.
   d. Importance of routine health care follow-up.
5. Support medical management of primary lesion.
6. Initiate referral for occupational therapy, social service, and follow-up home care.
7. Initiate referral for screening of family members, contacts, and so on.

EVALUATION

Outcome Criteria

1. Kidney function and demand compatible with:
   a. BUN 8–28 mg/100 mL whole blood.
   b. Serum creatinine 0.5–1.5 mg/100 mL adjusted for age and sex.
2. Client reports compliance with dietary regimen, as evidenced by elimination of symptoms, and compliance with medication regimen on each follow-up.
3. Client explains need for isolation, sexual precautions, and activity prescription.
4. Client's lifestyle, roles, and relationships are adapted to need for special health management routines.

Complications

GENITAL INVOLVEMENT

Assessment
Men: scrotal pain or tenderness and swelling in the vas, seminal vesicles, and/or prostate gland. Women: abdominal pain, white vaginal discharge, sterility, or ectopic pregnancy.

Revised Outcomes
1. Infectious process will be resolved.
2. Spread of infection will be prevented.

Interventions
See interventions under *Tuberculosis of the Urinary Tract*.

INFECTION OF SEX PARTNER

Assessment
Periodic screening.

Revised Outcomes
1. Infectious process will be resolved.
2. Spread of infection will be prevented.

Interventions
See interventions under *Tuberculosis of the Urinary Tract*.

Reevaluation and Follow-up
Lifelong follow-up and family supervision are required.

OBSTRUCTIONS

URETHRAL STRICTURE

See complications under *Urethritis*.

BENIGN PROSTATIC HYPERTROPHY

DESCRIPTION

Benign prostatic hypertrophy is an enlargement of the prostate gland that occurs in the majority of men over age 50. Because the prostate gland surrounds the proximal portion of the urethra, enlargement leads to obstruction of the bladder outlet and urinary stasis.

PREVENTION

Health Promotion

Since the cause remains obscure, health promotion activities are not known; their determination depends on the determination of physiological and behavioral etiology.

Population at Risk

1. Men over age 50.
2. Men who are exposed to cold and/or ingest alcohol may be at risk of obstruction.

Screening

Rectal examination for palpable enlarged prostate gland (unless hyperplasia is confined to the median lobe, in which case it may not be felt).

ASSESSMENT

Health History

Refer to Table 32-1.

1. Recent exposure to cold or ingestion of alcohol may be noted.
2. Voiding patterns and characteristics of urination: difficulty in starting and maintaining urinary stream, diminished caliber and force of stream and "dribbling" of urine after urination, frequency, urgency, nocturia, hematuria, and burning on urination.

Physical Assessment

1. Enlarged prostate on rectal examination (may not always be felt).
2. Bladder distension due to acute/chronic urinary retention (only in marked obstruction).
3. Examination may be entirely normal.

Diagnostic Tests

1. Intravenous pyelogram is usually done to determine renal effects of obstruction and/or stasis.
2. Voiding cystourograms indicate degree of obstruction.

NURSING DIAGNOSIS: ACTUAL OR POTENTIAL

1. Altered urinary elimination pattern due to obstruction of bladder neck.
2. Potential for infection due to prolonged incomplete bladder emptying.
3. Sleep pattern disturbance due to nocturia.
4. Body-image disturbance due to frequency or dribbling.

EXPECTED OUTCOMES

1. Urinary complications secondary to prolonged incomplete bladder emptying will be prevented.
2. Client will maintain positive body image and self-esteem.
3. Urinary obstruction and bladder rupture will be prevented.

INTERVENTION

1. Teach client effects of exposure to cold and ingestion of alcohol.
2. Avoid use of anticholinergic drugs, which decrease sphincter control.
3. Teach client signs of bladder obstruction.
   a. Increased difficulty starting stream.
   b. Enlarged bladder and suprapubic pain.
4. Assist client in use of relaxation technique to assist bladder emptying.
5. Assist client in fluid regulation to minimize nocturia.
6. Assess bladder distension at each visit or every hour during hospitalization.
7. Consult physician for periodic evaluation of status.
8. Catheterize client as ordered.
   a. Maintain aseptic technique and meticulous catheter care.
   b. Teach client self-catheterization as necessary.

EVALUATION

Outcome Criteria

1. Urinary output is maintained, with no bladder distension on physical examination.
2. Client reports less than 2 sleep interruptions per night due to nocturia.
3. Client reports no episodes of cystitis on follow-up visits.

Complications

CYSTISIS

See *Cystitis*.

SIGNIFICANT OR COMPLETE URETHRAL OBSTRUCTION

Assessment

1. Marked bladder distension is present.
2. Severe suprapubic pain is present.
3. Increased blood pressure pulse and inspiration may be present.
4. Diaphoresis and marked apprehension are usually present.
5. If obstruction is complete, catheter cannot be passed.

Revised Outcomes

1. Client will report no urinary incontinence 3 weeks after surgery.
2. Client will report no difficulty initiating urinary stream and no nocturia 3 weeks after surgery.
3. Client will report appropriate sexual adjustment 6 weeks after surgery.
4. Client will list symptoms of cystitis and obstruction and describe mechanism for initiating contact with health care system.

Interventions

1. Assist client with response to medical management.
   a. Offer reassurance and support to client, family, and/or significant others.
   b. Monitor and assess vital signs frequently.
   c. Administer antispasmodics, urinary antiseptics, and analgesics as prescribed.
   d. Prepare client for prostatic massage if anticipated.
   e. Teach client self-catheterization if no corrective surgery is planned.
2. Assist client with response to surgical management.
   a. Suprapubic cystostomy: surgical incision through the abdominal wall into the bladder is done to drain urine. A suprapubic catheter is usually left in place to prevent another episode of acute retention.
      (1) When prescribed, clamp catheter for 4 h and unclamp for 15–30 min.
      (2) Assess client's ability to void while catheter is clamped.
      (3) Catheter is removed according to physician's direction after patient is able to void while suprapubic catheter clamped.
      (4) Once removed, place sterile dressing over suprapubic catheter site.
   b. Transurethral resection: removal of the prostate with instruments introduced transurethrally. No incision is needed.
   c. Suprapubic prostatectomy: removal of the hypertrophied prostate gland through an abdominal incision that extends into the bladder.
   d. Perineal prostatectomy: removal of the prostate through a perineal resection. Postoperative wound contamination, incontinence, and impotence are likely sequelae.
   e. Retropubic prostatectomy: removal of the prostate gland through an incision between the pubic arch and the bladder. No incision is made into the bladder.
3. Preoperative interventions.
   a. Initiate teaching-learning interaction regarding postoperative activities and expectations.
      (1) Avoid attempting to void around catheter.
      (2) Avoid straining when having a bowel movement (may cause prostatic hemorrhage).
      (3) Do perineal exercises to decrease incontinence.
   b. Encourage client to discuss possibility of impotence with wife and nurse in case of perineal prostatectomy.
   c. Carry out prescribed bowel preparations.
4. Postoperative interventions.
   a. Administer prescribed analgesics and antispasmodics. Wean client from antispasmodics 24 h before removal of urethral catheter.
   b. Maintain free, unobstructed flow of urine. Inspect catheter(s) for signs of obstruction from blood clots or, occasionally, pieces of tissue. Continuous irrigation frequently ordered. Monitor and assess drainage from wounds and catheter sites.
   c. Observe closely for signs of hemorrhage. Some hematuria expected. Test urine for blood. Measure specific gravity. Monitor and assess vital signs, particularly blood pressure and oral temperature.
   d. Maintain strict aseptic technique at all times; consult physician if temperature is elevated or drainage is purulent.
   e. Maintain fluid intake (oral and parenteral) at 2,500–3,500 mL per 24-h period (unless contraindicated by coexisting condition).
   f. Monitor and correlate intake and output q2h immediately postoperatively, progressing to q8h as condition stabilizes.
   g. Avoid taking rectal temperatures, using rectal tubes, or administering enemas (particularly following perineal resection).
   h. Initiate measures to prevent postoperative complications: turning q2h, passive and active range-of-motion exercises, early ambulation, and antiembolism stockings. Encourage nonvigorous coughing.

i. Review preoperative teaching plan, particularly perineal exercises and instructions not to attempt to void around catheter. Perineal exercises should be started 2–3 days postoperatively.
j. Seek order for laxative or stool softener 3–4 days postoperatively.
k. Provide nutritional information to avoid constipation postdischarge.
l. Instruct client to avoid vigorous exercises and heavy lifting for at least 3 weeks postoperatively. Instruct client:
   (1) That any sign of bleeding should be reported to member of health care team (physician or nurse) immediately.
   (2) About signs of developing urethral strictures and infection.
   (3) That abstinence from sexual activity for at least 4 weeks is essential.
   (4) That high oral fluid intake is to be continued following discharge.
m. Initiate referral for sexual counseling in case of perineal prostatectomy (postoperative incontinence may be a problem; impotence may create marital discord).
n. Reassure, encourage, and support client, family, and/or significant others. Depression is common because of inability to regain bladder control immediately. Encourage diversional activity. Elicit assistance from family.
o. Observe client for signs of water intoxication due to salt wasting from large amounts of irrigating fluid and characterized by irritability, hypertension, polyuria, and decreased serum sodium.

Reevaluation and Follow-up

See client every 2–3 weeks for 2 months and/or until expected or revised outcomes are achieved.

NEPHROLITHIASIS

DESCRIPTION

Urinary calculi may develop in the kidney, ureter, bladder, or urethra and may be multiple and bilateral. Ninety percent of urinary calculi are composed of calcium salts, while nearly all the rest are urate stones. Cystine stones develop in clients with a rare hereditary metabolic disorder. Like uric acid stones, they develop in an acidic environment. Infection, urinary stasis, and high urinary concentration predispose to precipitation of urinary salts. Middle-aged persons and men have a higher incidence than the rest of the population.

Calcium stone formation can be caused by hyperparathyroidism (which causes excretion of calcium), excessive ingestion of vitamin D, Cushing's syndrome, acute osteoporosis due to immobilization, or acute renal tubular acidosis. Alkaline urine causes calcium to come out of solution and crystallize.

Uric acid stones are formed only in an acidic urine (pH less than 5.5). Increased excretion of uric acid due to gout or a persistently acidic urine result in the formation of uric acid stones.

The size of calculi varies from small sandy particles (gravel) to large staghorn stones that may occupy the entire renal pelvis. Silent calculi are large stones that remain in the renal pelvis and produce no symptoms (see Figure 32-5). These stones (usually the large ones) may remain in the kidney pelvis, or they may pass down through the ureters into the bladder and eventually be excreted through the urethra. Renal colic may develop if calculi are unable to pass through the narrow lumen of the ureters.

PREVENTION

Health Promotion

1. Maintain high urine output, especially if there is history of renal stones (4,000 mL/24 h) (Metheny, 1982).
2. Maintain level of activity and exercise to avoid excessive release of calcium from bones, especially in clients with bone fractures.
3. Void frequently to avoid urinary stasis.
4. Control symptoms of gout to decrease excretion of uric acid.
5. Reinforce need for reporting signs of urinary infections and seeking early treatment.

Population at Risk

1. Persons with family history of cystine stones (congenital cystinuria).
2. Clients immobilized by bone fractures.
3. Persons with hyperparathyroidism or gout.
4. Persons with history of renal stones or from families of stone formers: risk is 10 times greater than for rest of population.
5. Persons with urinary stasis related to obstruction: urethral stricture or benign prostatic hypertrophy.

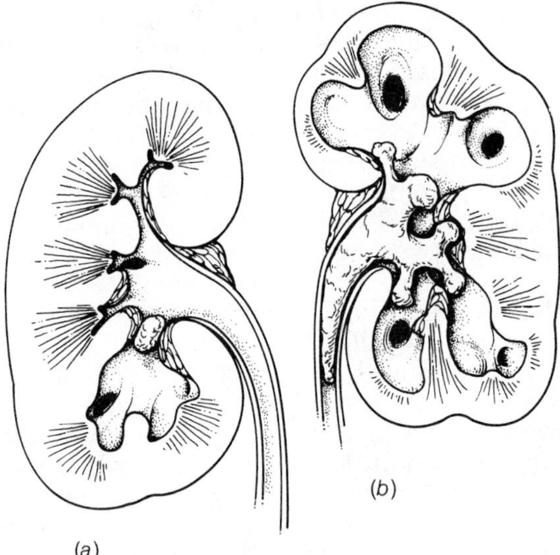

Figure 32-5 (*a*) Single calculus obstructing and dilating the lower renal calyx. (*b*) "Staghorn" calculus obstructing and dilating all the renal calyces. (Adapted from Flocks, R.H.: "Urology," in Liechty, R.D., and Soper, R.T., eds.: *Synopsis of Surgery*, 2d ed., Mosby, St. Louis, 1972.)

6. Chronically dehydrated persons with inadequate fluid intake or chronic diarrhea.
7. Persons undergoing treatment for neoplastic disease, causing rapid cell distinction.
8. Persons from the southeastern, southwestern, and Great Lakes regions of the United States.

Screening

Persons with health history of frequent urinary tract infection, previous renal calculi, immobility due to fracture, hyperparathyroidism, and gout are in high-risk category.

ASSESSMENT

Health History

See Table 32-1.

1. Past history of any condition predisposing to stasis of urine (extended periods of immobilization, infections, etc.).
2. Comprehensive nutritional assessment.
3. Past history of urinary calculi (method of treatment, etc.).
4. Voiding patterns and characteristics of urination (particularly frequency, urgency, hematuria, and intermittent stream).
5. Pain: presence, location, frequency, intensity, quality, precipitating or aggravating factors, and factors that aid in relief.
6. Health perception and identification of response patterns to crisis situation.

Physical Assessment

1. Sharp, excruciating pain radiating from affected flank toward groin and testes or labia.
2. Tenderness over involved kidney and ureter on palpation.

Diagnostic Tests

1. Microscopic urinalysis, particularly for albuminuria, pH, and hematuria.
   a. Alkaline urine associated with stones of calcium salts.
   b. Acidic urine associated with uric acid and cystine stones.
2. Urine culture and antibiotic sensitivity to determine coexisting infection.
3. Sulkowitch test to determine calcium content of urine from a single specimen.
4. Twenty-four-hour urine specimen for calcium and uric acid.
5. Blood studies: serum calcium, serum phosphorus, and serum uric acid.
6. Renal function tests: BUN, creatinine, and creatinine clearance.
7. Radiologic studies: IVP, cystogram, cystoscopy with retrograde pyelography (uric acid stones not radiopaque), and various radiologic imaging techniques.

NURSING DIAGNOSES: ACTUAL OR POTENTIAL

1. Alteration in comfort or pain due to renal colic.
2. Severe anxiety (panic) related to uncontrolled pain.
3. Sleep pattern disturbance related to alteration in comfort.
4. Impairment of urinary elimination related to retention due to urinary obstruction.
5. Potential for infection related to urinary stasis.

EXPECTED OUTCOMES

1. Obstruction of urinary flow will be relieved.
2. Pain will be relieved and anxiety reduced.
3. Symptoms of urinary colic will be relieved.
4. Urinary tract infection will be controlled (prevented if possible).

5. Renal functioning will be preserved.
6. Client will regain positive body image and self-esteem.
7. Cause of stone formation will be identified.
8. Further stone formation will be prevented.

INTERVENTIONS

1. Reassure and support client, family, and/or significant others.
2. Provide avenue for client to verbalize concerns and anxieties regarding his or her reaction to severe pain.
3. Assist client in dealing with altered body image and self-esteem.
4. Observe for spontaneous passage of stone. Teach client to strain all urine at each voiding.
5. Observe urine for hematuria. Measure specific gravity at each voiding to assess renal functioning.
6. Monitor and assess vital signs (particularly temperature) q4h.
7. Observe for signs and symptoms of urinary complications resulting from retention and/or stasis.
8. Initiate pain relief measures (e.g., analgesics, antispasmodics, moist heat, sitz bath, visual imagery, relaxation technique).
9. Insert prescribed indwelling bladder catheter; maintain aseptic technique.
10. Increase fluid intake to 4,500 mL per 24-h period (unless contraindicated by coexisting condition). Calculi re-formers should have fluid intake around the clock.
11. Monitor and assess intake and output q8h (more frequently if necessary).
12. Encourage moderate activity to prevent stasis of urine.
13. Monitor and assess studies of renal functioning.
14. Provide nutritional counseling (see Table 32-2 for specific information).
15. Refer client with recurrent calcium stones to physician for possible prescription of a mixture of neutral phosphates of sodium and potassium, which may prevent growth of new calculi.
16. Refer client with recurrent calcium stones to physician for possible prescription of thiazide diuretics, which reduce urinary calcium by half.
17. Refer client with uric acid stones to physician for possible prescription of allopurinol, the treatment of choice; it is sometimes used with antineoplastic drugs to reduce uric acid residue from rapid cell destruction.
18. Refer client with struvite stones to physician for possible treatment, including surgical removal, long-term antibiotic therapy, and use of acidifying agents (note that commercial cranberry juice is only 26 percent juice and

TABLE 32-2 DIETARY MANAGEMENT OF NEPHROLITHIASIS

Type of Stone	Dietary Management	pH Maintenance
Calcium oxalate stones	Curtail intake of asparagus, cabbage, celery, chocolate, lamb, rhubarb, spinach, tomatoes, chard, beets, parsley, nuts, cocoa, tea, vitamin C supplements	Form in any urine pH
Calcium phosphate stones	Same as above; also avoid poultry, fish, whole-grain cereals	Are soluble in acid urine
Uric acid stones	Limit meat, spinach, dried beans, peas, tea, coffee, chocolate, alcohol	Maintain alkaline urine (pH > 6.5)
Cystine stones		Maintain alkaline urine (pH = 7.6–8.0)
Struvite stones		Maintain acid urine (pH < 6.5)

may not be practical for acidifying urine) (Kinney and Blount, 1979).

EVALUATION

Outcome Criteria

1. Client reports pain reaction of 4 or less on pain scale of 1–10.
2. Client sleeps 6 h or more q24h.
3. Urinary output equals intake ± 300–500 ml in 24 h (4,000 mL recommended).
4. Temperature 98.6°F (37°C). Pulse and respiration equal to baseline.
5. Client exhibits no symptoms of cystitis (see *Cystitis*).
6. Client experiences no recurrence of symptoms (see Assessment).
7. Client communicates dietary prescription before discharge.

Complications

CLIENT UNABLE TO PASS STONE

Assessment

1. Continued severe pain.
2. Renal colic.
3. Complete obstruction.
4. Infection uncontrolled by antimicrobial agents.
5. Hydronephrosis (see *Hydronephrosis*).
6. Renal failure (see *Acute Renal Failure* and *Chronic Renal Failure*).

Revised Outcomes

1. Client will report pain reaction of 4 or less on a scale of 1–10 within 48 h after surgery.
2. Urinary elimination pattern will be reestablished in baseline range within 72 h after surgery.
3. Client will report fluid intake of 5,000 ml/24 h.
4. Nurse or client will log diet and activity compatible with that prescribed every 24 h for 1 week.
5. Diet and medication prescriptions will be revised depending on analysis of stones removed.

Interventions

If client is unable to spontaneously pass stone through medical interventions, one of the following surgical interventions may be employed. Treatment depends on the position, location, and size of the stone and the client's general condition. Coexisting conditions must also be considered.

1. Types of surgical intervention.
   a. Insert ureteral catheter into renal pelvis by cystoscopy.
   b. Cystolithectomy: removal of stone from the bladder.
   c. Ureterolithotomy: removal of a stone that is lodged in the ureter.
   d. Pyelolithotomy: removal of a stone lodged in the kidney pelvis.
   e. Nephrolithotomy: removal of a stone from the kidney through an incision into the kidney.
   f. Litholapaxy: crushing of a stone in the bladder followed by immediate washing out of the crushed fragments through a catheter (see Figure 32-6).
   g. Nephrectomy may be necessary if kidney is functionless (see *Renal Tumors* for preoperative and postoperative intervention).
   h. New modes of interventional radiology utilizing fiberoptics and radiologic imaging are minimally invasive techniques of fragmenting and removing stones.
2. Preoperative interventions (see *Renal Tumors*).
3. Postoperative interventions following ureteral surgery should include the following nursing measures:
   a. Offer reassurance, support, and understanding. The abdominal incision will drain urine for approximately 3 weeks.
   b. Prevent dressing from being constantly wet with urinary drainage. Initiate appropriate measures.
   c. Initiate meticulous care of skin, using protective powders, ointments, and so on (see discussion of urinary diversion under *Tumors of the Urinary Bladder*).
   d. Encourage free fluid intake to decrease urine concentration.
   e. Maintain odorless environment.
   f. Observe incision for signs of infection.
   g. Maintain patency of ureteral catheter for adequate drainage. Intermittent irrigation may be necessary. Check physician's orders. (NOTE: since the kidney pelvis normally holds 3–5 mL of fluid, exercise extreme care in irrigating ureteral catheters).
4. Postoperative interventions following flank (kidney) incision. The following nursing measures should be considered:
   a. Assess for alterations in vital signs.

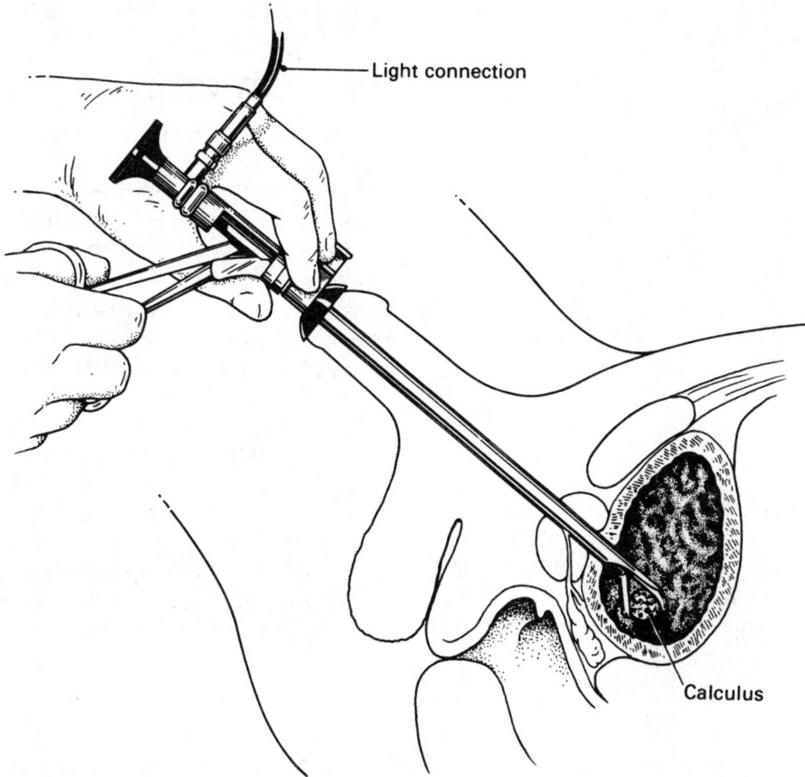

Figure 32-6 Litholapaxy: removal of stone by crushing forceps. (Adapted from Liechty, R.D., and Soper, R.T., eds.: *Synopsis of Surgery*, 2d ed., Mosby, St. Louis, 1972.)

b. Meticulously measure and correlate fluid intake and output q2h. Assess color of urine. Observe for clots. Meticulous catheter care. Monitor intake (4,500 mL/24 h recommended).
c. Assess dressing for serosanguineous drainage.
d. Maintain fluid and electrolyte balance.
   (1) Administer prescribed intravenous fluids.
   (2) Monitor and assess blood electrolytes.
e. Provide vigorous respiratory care, including deep breathing, coughing, and turning q2h. Splint the operative area (incision is directly below diaphragm). Provide oral hygiene as needed.
f. Assess response to interventions. Respiratory therapy consultation may be necessary.
g. Administer prescribed narcotic analgesics; utilize back massage as pain relief measure. Assess response to interventions.
h. Encourage early mobility. Teach passive and active range-of-motion exercises. Start ambulation 24 h postoperatively. Use elastic knee-length stockings.
i. Discourage sitting in chair for long periods.
j. Assess for signs of infection and administer prescribed antibiotics to prevent infection.
k. Provide nephrostomy tube care (see Figure 32-7).
   (1) Maintain adequate drainage of urine.
   (2) Ensure patency of nephrostomy tube.
   (3) When positioning client, support nephrostomy tube with pillows and the like to prevent kinking of tubing.
l. Initiate teaching-learning transaction (include client, family, and/or significant oth-

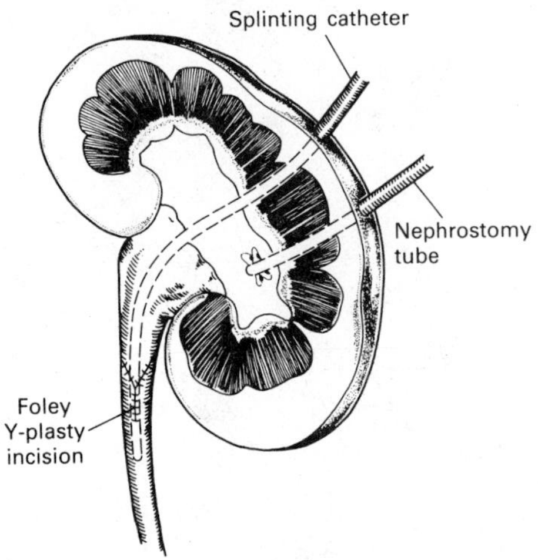

Figure 32-7 Schematic representation showing the placement of a nephrostomy tube. The nephrostomy tube is used to drain urine while the splinting catheter is used to support the Y incision. (Adapted from Shafter, K.N., Sawyer, J.B., McCluskey, A.M., Beck, E.L., and Phipps W.J.: *Medical-Surgical Nursing*, 6th ed., Mosby, St. Louis, 1975.)

ers) regarding:
(1) Medications: name, dosage, rationale, desired effects, side effects, and signs of toxicity.
(2) Nutritional counseling: adjust to client's culture and food preferences and according to chemical analysis of stone.
(3) Continued intake of large amounts of fluids (4,500–5,000 mL/24 h) unless contraindicated by coexisting condition.
(4) Prevention of urinary tract infection, detection of signs of urinary tract infection, and appropriate responses.
(5) Avoidance of long periods of immobilization.
(6) Possible vocational counseling if present occupation predisposes client to dehydration through excessive perspiration.
(7) Teach client to test pH with test tape.

Reevaluation and Follow-up
Diet, activity, fluid, and medication prescriptions are reviewed with client. Signs or symptoms of recurrence dictate follow-up.

HYDRONEPHROSIS

DESCRIPTION

Hydronephrosis is the distension of the kidney pelvis (may be bilateral) and its calyces beyond their normal capacity of 3–10 mL. Hydronephrosis is caused by a gradual, partial, or intermittent obstruction of the free flow of urine. As discussed earlier, any interference with the flow of urine (stasis) can result in infection that may produce narrowing and further obstruction. If obstruction is intermittent but frequent, there may be an increase in pressure and the renal parenchyma begin to atrophy in a retrograde manner. The collecting tubules dilate and atrophy. Fibrous tissue replaces the dilated, muscular wall of the kidney pelvis. If the obstruction is located in the bladder or urethra, hydronephrosis may develop bilaterally; however, if the obstruction is in the ureter, hydronephrosis may develop in the related kidney.

PREVENTION

Health Promotion

Health teaching referral and follow-up of clients with recurrent inflammation of the urinary tract.

Population at Risk

Clients who have repeated urinary tract infections should be referred for renal workup.

Screening

Careful history of urinary elimination patterns (including developmental patterns) from all preemployment, school, and health maintenance assessments.

ASSESSMENT

Health History

See *Inflammatory Disorders* and *Obstructions* (see Table 32-1).

Physical Assessment

1. Costovertebral angle tenderness is usually present.
2. Abdominal pain radiating to genitals or thigh due to dilated kidney may be present.
3. Nausea and vomiting due to ureteral spasm may be present.
4. Symptoms of urinary stasis or cystitis may be present.

Diagnostic Tests

See *Cystitis, Pyelonephritis,* and *Benign Prostatic Hypertrophy.*

NURSING DIAGNOSES: ACTUAL OR POTENTIAL

1. Altered urinary elimination pattern due to urinary statis or destruction of kidney pelvis.
2. Altered nutritional requirements due to kidney failure.
3. Alteration in comfort or pain due to abdominal mass.
4. Potential for infection related to urinary statis.
5. Self-management deficit due to pain.
6. Body-image disturbance related to kidney malfunction.

EXPECTED OUTCOMES

1. Kidney functioning will be maintained and danger due to obstruction or inflammation will be limited.
2. Client will maintain positive self-image and health perception.
3. Self-care–health-provider balance will be encouraged through health teaching.

INTERVENTIONS

1. Support medical interventions to identify and relieve underlying cause of urinary stasis.
   a. Initiate care of nephrostomy tube: may be inserted to drain the kidney pelvis when high ureteral obstruction present (only a temporary measure) (see Figure 32-7).
      (1) Assess for bleeding or drainage from cutaneous nephrostomy site.
      (2) Because of limited fluid capacity of kidney pelvis, do not clamp the nephrostomy tube.
      (3) Exercise extreme caution when performing prescribed irrigations. (Must be done gently. Follow policies of individual institution. May be considered a medical intervention.)
   b. Initiate care for ureteral catheter: inserted if nephrostomy tube insertion contraindicated. Exercise extreme caution to prevent dislodging. Label the catheter *ureteral.* (Catheter will exit the body through the urinary meatus.) Tape catheter to the shaved thigh. (NOTE: irrigation of ureteral catheter is not considered a nursing function.)
2. Refer to interventions under *Obstructions.*
3. See *Pyelonephritis* (pyelonephritis may develop as a result of obstruction and the subsequent stasis of urine).
4. Initiate preoperative interventions. (Surgery may be indicated if conservative management cannot relieve the underlying cause of obstruction.)
5. See *Acute Renal Failure* (acute renal failure may develop if obstruction is of acute onset with sudden cessation of renal functioning).

EVALUATION

Outcome Criteria

1. Kidney function tests are compatible with optimum kidney function:
   a. Urinary elimination equals intake ± 250 mL unless there is heavy water loss from exposure or manual labor.
   b. Client documents no pain or signs of infection q24h (may use log or telephone report).
   c. Client maintains desired role and family relationships and reports satisfaction with these on each follow-up visit.

Complications

RENAL FAILURE

See *Acute Renal Failure* and *Chronic Renal Failure.*

COMPLETE IRREVERSIBLE URETERAL OBSTRUCTION

Assessment

Diagnostic tests indicate blocked ureter(s) (see diagnostic tests under *Renal Tumors*).

1. Retrograde pyelogram and ultrasonogram.
2. Buret test: calibrated buret at kidney level is attached to nephrostomy tube. The supine client at rest will not experience increased manometer readings over 24-h period if ureter is patent (medical procedure).

Revised Outcomes

Client exhibits ureteral patency: no infection or obstruction postsurgery.

Interventions

1. For plastic repair of resection of ureter in which a segment of ilium is grafted onto the ureter at point of stricture, leave a splinting catheter that may or may not drain urine in place 2–3 weeks to assure patency (consult with surgeon).

2. See interventions under *Acute Renal Failure* and *Chronic Renal Failure.*

Reevaluation and Follow-up

Client should be assessed at least every 6 months if no symptoms occur, more often if symptoms of infection, obstruction, or renal failure are present. Since nephrostomy tube may be left in place 3–4 months, frequent (weekly) follow-up may be necessary postsurgery.

DEGENERATIVE DISEASES

CHRONIC GLOMERULONEPHRITIS

DESCRIPTION

Chronic glomerulonephritis is an inflammation of the glomeruli that usually does not follow poststreptococcal glomerulonephritis, although it can. Occurrence is gradual and often idiopathic. Mild proteinuria and moderate hypertension are often discovered incidentally or on routine physical examination. The course of the disease is slowly or rapidly progressive, depending on etiology. There is no known cure, and management is directed toward retarding progressive renal failure by control of fluid and electrolyte balance.

PREVENTION

See *Acute Glomerulonephritis, Acute Renal Failure,* and *Chronic Renal Failure.*

ASSESSMENT

Health History

1. Diabetes.
2. Lupus erythematosus.
3. Acute glomerulonephritis.
4. Exposure to known nephrotoxins (antibiotics, analgesics, poisons, solvents, and insecticides) may or may not be contributory.

Physical Assessment

1. Moderate hypertension.
2. May be normal.
3. Mild proteinuria.
4. See *Acute Renal Failure* and *Chronic Renal Failure.*
5. Problems: since there is no cure, treatment is symptomatic until renal insufficiency becomes apparent (see *Acute Renal Failure* and *Chronic Renal Failure*).

EXPECTED OUTCOMES

Adequate kidney functioning will be maintained as long as possible.

NURSING DIAGNOSES: ACTUAL OR POTENTIAL

1. Body-image disturbance related to body organ failure.
2. Unresolved independence-dependence conflict related to questionable course of disease.
3. Knowledge deficit related to asymptomatic body-system deficit.
4. See diagnoses under *Acute Renal Failure* and *Chronic Renal Failure.*

INTERVENTIONS

1. Teach client about antihypertensives (prescribed as needed).
2. Individualize sodium-restricted diet as prescribed.
3. See interventions under *Acute Renal Failure* and *Chronic Renal Failure.*
4. Counsel daily if necessary to assist client with lifestyle adjustments and potentially shortened life span.

EVALUATION

Outcome Criteria

See *Acute Renal Failure* and *Chronic Renal Failure.*

Complications

See *Acute Renal Failure* and *Chronic Renal Failure.*

Revised Outcomes

See *Acute Renal Failure* and *Chronic Renal Failure.*

Reevaluation and Follow-up

Follow-up every 4–6 months from diagnosis, with more frequent appointments as change occurs.

NEPHROTIC SYNDROME

DESCRIPTION

Nephrotic syndrome, or nephrosis, is not a disease entity but a group of symptoms that develop with increased permeability of the glomerulus to plasma protein. The nephrotic syndrome is frequently found in association with glomerulonephritis, systemic lupus erythematosus, nephrotoxic reactions, pregnancy, and diabetic glomerulosclerosis. Etiology remains obscure in 80 percent of the cases that develop in children. Although young people are most frequently affected, people of any age may develop this condition (refer to Chapter 21).

PREVENTION

See *Acute Glomerulonephritis*.

ASSESSMENT

Health History

See *Acute Renal Failure* and *Acute Glomerulonephritis*.

Physical Assessment

1. Generalized edema, particularly around the eyes, neck, genitalia, and lower extremities. Ascites frequently develops.
2. Foamy urine; color deeper than usual; oval fat bodies present.
3. Skin: waxy pallor due to edema.
4. Circulatory overload and hypertension.

Diagnostic Tests

1. Plasma albumin levels: concentration < 1 g/100 mL and reversed albumin/globulin (A/G) ratio.
2. Serum cholesterol: hyperlipidemia.
3. Electrolyte determinations, particularly hypernatremia.
4. Renal function studies: elevated BUN, creatinine, and so on, reflecting underlying renal pathology.
5. Renal biopsy to determine potential response to corticosteroids.
6. Electron microscopy.

NURSING DIAGNOSES: ACTUAL OR POTENTIAL

1. Body-image disturbance related to interstitial fluid retention.
2. Potential for infection related to decreased plasma protein.
3. Potential impairment of skin integrity due to infection, decreased protein, tissue repair, and edema.

EXPECTED OUTCOMES

See *Chronic Glomerulonephritis*.

INTERVENTIONS

1. Refer to physician for possible prescription of dietary management: a high-protein diet is indicated because of excessive losses in the urine.
2. Refer to physician for possible prescription of corticosteroids, which are responsible for remission in most cases.
3. See *Chronic Glomerulonephritis*.

EVALUATION

See *Chronic Glomerulonephritis*.

POLYCYSTIC DISEASE OF THE KIDNEY

DESCRIPTION

Multiple cysts replace the renal parenchyma in this familial congenital disorder. In adults, the disease progresses slowly from presentation in the thirties or forties characterized by hematuria, mild hypertension, and flank pain to end-stage renal disease in the fifties or sixties.

PREVENTION

Genetic counseling could be effective in eradicating the disease and should be arranged for clients with a family history of disease.

ASSESSMENT

Health History

Except for family history, health history is often noncontributory. There may be history of flank pain that is relieved by lying down.

Physical Assessment

1. Hypertension is usually present.
2. Bilateral palpable kidneys are usual.
3. Liver and spleen may be palpable.

Diagnostic Tests

1. IVP demonstrates enlarged kidneys with elongation of the pelvis.
2. Specific gravity is low due to inability to concentrate urine.
3. Hematuria may be present.
4. Tests associated with renal insufficiency develop over time (see *Chronic Renal Failure*).

NURSING DIAGNOSES: ACTUAL OR POTENTIAL

1. Potential for infection related to pressure of cysts.
2. Potential fluid volume deficit related to salt wasting.
3. Alteration in nutritional requirement.
4. Decreased activity tolerance.
5. Alteration in comfort due to flank pain.
6. Reactive depression due to chronic illness.

EXPECTED OUTCOMES

1. Flank pain will be controlled.
2. Episodes of hematuria and infection will be minimized.
3. Family concerns regarding genetic counseling will be addressed.
4. Lifestyle issues related to diet, possible limited earning power, dialysis, and kidney transplant must be addressed.

INTERVENTIONS

1. Arrange frequent rest periods to avoid flank pain and abdominal pressure.
2. Personalize diet prescription to provide adequate fluid, protein, carbohydrate, and oral sodium supplements to compensate for sodium wasting.
3. Develop teaching plan to assist client in recognizing signs of pyelonephritis and ways to avoid infection.
4. Use iron supplements and/or tight abdominal binder if hematuria is pronounced.
5. Develop teaching plan related to hypertension.
6. Consult genetic counselor.
7. Observe for signs of depression.
8. Assist client in accepting altered life span and lifestyle.

EVALUATION

Outcome Criteria

1. Client reports adherence to diet, fluid, and medication regimens.
2. No episodes of pyelonephritis occur. Temperature 98.6°F and sterile microscopic urinalysis at each follow-up.
3. Client plans energy output compatible with tolerance, as evidenced by minimal flank pain and frequent rest periods.
4. Client reports satisfactory lifestyle adjustment to illness.

Complications

See *Chronic Renal Failure.*

Revised Outcomes

See *Chronic Renal Failure.*

Reevaluation and Follow-up

Client will need support throughout life, depending on stage of disease process.

TRAUMA

TRAUMA TO THE KIDNEY

DESCRIPTION

The kidneys are afforded a great deal of protection by the rib cage and the heavy muscles that line the back. Trauma to the kidneys may be due to penetrating wounds, crushing injuries, or blunt blows directly to the flank or abdomen. In addition to causing renal damage, trauma usually involves other viscera as well.

Kidney trauma are classified as contusions (minor bruising of parenchyma and capsule or major bruising with rupture of parenchyma and perirenal hematoma formation), lacerations (tears in the renal parenchyma with or without rupture of the drainage system), and ruptures of vascular pedicle. Following injury, the presence of a local mass may be due to extravasation of blood and/or urine. There may be leakage of urine from an open wound.

PREVENTION

Health Promotion

1. Teach the importance of careful driving, wearing seatbelts, and driver education.
2. Teach normal functioning and signs and symptoms of dysfunction in health education classes.

Population at Risk

1. Young adults who participate in contact sports: football, wrestling, boxing.

2. Drivers, especially those who drink and drive.

Screening

Abdominal bleeding or bruising should be investigated in trauma victims.

ASSESSMENT

Health History

Refer to *Renal Tumors*.

1. Identification of circumstances surrounding the injury (what happened and how) and the anatomical location of the traumatic blow.
2. Past history of conditions affecting urinary tract.
3. Voiding patterns and characteristics of urination before and since injury.
4. Health perception and identification of response patterns to crisis situations.

Physical Assessment

1. Tenderness and/or pain in affected costovertebral angle and/or abdominal quadrant.
2. Expanding mass in affected costovertebral angle due to extravasation of blood and/or urine.
3. Hematuria that is often painless and can persist for several days.

Diagnostic Tests

Refer to *Renal Tumors*.

1. Radiologic tests of the kidneys, ureter, and bladder.
2. IVP (absolutely essential), supplemented by retrograde pyelography.
3. Renal arteriogram.
4. Miscroscopic urinalysis, specifically for hematuria: < 2 RBCs/hpf.
5. Urine culture and antibiotic sensitivities.
6. Hematocrit and hemoglobin.
7. Renal function studies.

NURSING DIAGNOSES: ACTUAL OR POTENTIAL

1. Altered urinary elimination pattern.
2. Potential for infection.
3. Alteration in nutritional requirements.
4. Decreased activity tolerance.
5. Self-care deficit.
6. Alteration in comfort due to pain.
7. Mild to severe anxiety.
8. Alterations in socialization.

EXPECTED OUTCOMES

1. Extent of damage at injury site will be recognized early.
2. Unobstructed flow of urine will be maintained.
3. Organisms will not be introduced into traumatized urinary tract.
4. Pain and anxiety will be reduced.
5. Hemorrhagic shock will be prevented.
6. Optimal renal functioning of previous state will be maintained.
7. Client, family, and/or significant others will recognize signs that require medical attention.
8. Client and family will recognize importance of safety.

INTERVENTIONS

1. Insert indwelling bladder catheter. Prevent unnecessary instrumentation.
   a. Exercise meticulous catheter care (refer to *Renal Tumors*).
   b. Provide safe and unobstructed flow of urine.
2. Test specific gravity of urine at least q2h.
3. Test urine for blood at least q2h.
   a. Inspect for presence of clots.
   b. Observe for obstruction of urinary drainage by clots.
4. Administer prescribed intravenous fluids and/or blood transfusions.
5. Administer prescribed diet. (Client is usually on NPO status until condition stabilizes; then feeding gradually increases according to tolerance.)
6. Measure and correlate fluid intake and output q2h. Oral and parenteral intake of fluids should be sufficient to provide internal irrigation but not beyond functional renal capacity.
7. Enforce strict bed rest. Take measures to prevent complications of bed rest. Activity increases as condition stabilizes.
8. Administer prescribed prophylactic antibiotics and analgesics. (Narcotics and analgesics may mask abdominal symptoms.)
9. Monitor and assess vital signs every hour unless otherwise indicated.
10. Monitor hematocrit, hemoglobin, and renal function studies every 24 h (more frequently if indicated).

11. Assess hematoma and/or mass for any increase in size. Check abdominal girths q4h.
12. Provide support and reassurance to client, family, and/or significant others during time of crisis. Assist client in dealing with possible alteration in body image.
13. Initiate teaching-learning transaction (include family and/or significant others) regarding:
    a. Need for follow-up care.
    b. Signs that require attention of the health care team.
    c. Home care activities, medications, diet, and so on.

EVALUATION

Outcome Criteria

1. Gross and microscopic hematuria clear within 3 days (72 h).
2. Intravenous pyelogram shows no anatomic deformity or obstruction.
3. Client communicates pain-free condition in 48 h.
4. Client communicates method of contacting health care provider if flank pain or hematuria result.

Complications

SHOCK

Due to torn pedicle, extensive intraperitoneal hemorrhage and/or retroperitoneal hemorrhage (see Chapter 48). If hemorrhage cannot be controlled, emergency surgery is indicated. Frequently the kidney can be repaired; however, if the laceration is extensive, a nephrectomy may be necessary.

PERIRENAL ABSCESS

Assessment

1. Sudden onset of fever, chills, and pain in affected flank.
2. Palpable tenderness and gradual onset of low-grade fever.
3. Malaise, anorexia, and gradual weight loss.
4. Leukocytosis may be present.

Revised Outcomes

Anatomic deformity leading to obstruction, stone formation, or hypertension will be prevented.

Interventions

1. Surgical interventions.
    a. Drainage of abscess.
    b. Removal of kidney (nephrectomy) if not functioning.
2. Preoperative interventions.
    a. Monitor and assess vital signs (especially temperature) q2h.
    b. Administer prescribed analgesics, antibiotics, and antipyretics.
    c. Maintain fluid and electrolyte balance.
    d. Administer prescribed intravenous fluids.
3. Postoperative interventions: similar to those employed following a lumbar nephrectomy (see *Renal Tumors*).
4. Complications of surgery.
    a. Reflex paralytic ileus due to retroperitoneal hemorrhage.
    b. Traumatic renal failure (see *Acute Renal Failure* and *Chronic Renal Failure*).

Reevaluation and Follow-up

Follow-up IVP should be performed in 3 months if hematuria persists.

TRAUMA TO THE URINARY BLADDER

DESCRIPTION

Trauma to the urinary bladder is most frequently caused by fracture of the symphysis pubis. A distended bladder, especially in the young client, may be easily ruptured by blunt trauma, such as a light kick or blow to the lower abdomen or impact during a motor vehicle or bicycle accident. Accidental injury during surgery or from a penetrating missile may also result in a ruptured bladder.

PREVENTION

Health Promotion

See *Trauma to the Kidney*.

Population at Risk

See *Trauma to the Kidney*.

Screening

See *Trauma to the Kidney*.

1. Evaluate persons with fractured pelvis for ruptured bladder.
2. Determine time of pretrauma urination if possible, and assess voiding patterns.

ASSESSMENT

Health History

1. See *Trauma to the Kidney.*
2. Ascertain time of last voiding before injury to assess past trauma voiding patterns.

Physical Assessment

1. Diffuse abdominal pain or palpation.
2. Urine draining from open wound.
3. Free fluid in peritoneal cavity on palpation.
4. Abdominal distention or abdominal rigidity may indicate intraperitoneal rupture.

Diagnostic Tests

1. Cystogram and execretory urogram.
2. Radiologic tests of the kidneys, ureter, and bladder.
3. IVP (not a definitive diagnostic study).
4. Microscopic urinalysis (particularly for hematuria).
5. Urine culture and antibiotic sensitivities.
6. Hematocrit and hemoglobin.
7. Blood typing and crossmatching.

NURSING DIAGNOSES: ACTUAL OR POTENTIAL

See *Trauma to the Kidney.*

EXPECTED OUTCOMES

See Chapter 48.

INTERVENTIONS

See Chapter 48 for nursing care during the acute emergency phase. Surgical intervention is usually immediate.

EVALUATION

Outcome Criteria

1. Client excretes 2,000–3,000 cc clear urine every 24 h via urinary drainage system: cystostomy and ureteral catheters.
2. Client expresses concern about temporary urinary drainage system within 24 h after initiation.
3. Client can describe daily diet and fluid prescriptions and keeps log of intake and output if able.
4. Client expresses fears associated with reparative surgery 12–24 h before planned repair.
5. Temperature and blood pressure are in range of baseline reading q8h.

Complications

INFECTION

See *Cystitis* and *Pyelonephritis.*

Revised Outcomes

See *Cystitis* and *Pyelonephritis.*

PERITONITIS

Refer to Chapter 33.

HEMORRHAGE AND SHOCK

Refer to Chapter 48.

Reevaluation and Follow-up

Follow-up every 2–3 months for 2 years to assure anatomical integrity and efficient bladder functioning (no obstruction or incontinence).

REFERENCES

Begg Marino, L.: *Cancer Nursing*, Mosby, St. Louis, 1981, p. 587.

Bruce, G. L., et al.: "Implementation of ANA's Quality Assurance Program for Clients with End-Stage Renal Disease," *Advances in Nursing Science*, **2**(2):79–97, January 1980.

Horsley, J., et al.: *Closed Urinary Drainage Systems: CURN Project*, Grune and Stratton, New York, 1981, p. 7, 8.

Isselbache, K. J., et al.: *Harrison's Principles of Internal Medicine*, 9th ed., McGraw-Hill, New York, 1980, p. 982.

Kamaroff, A. L., and Winickoff, R. N.: *Common Acute Illnesses*, Little, Brown, Boston, 1977, p. 45.

Kinney, A. B., and Blount, M.: "Effects of Cranberry Juice on the Urinary pH," *Nursing Research* **28**(287):28, September–October 1979.

Lach, P., et al.: "Sexual Behavior and Urinary Tract Infection," *The Nurse Practitioner*, **5**(1):29, January–February 1980.

Malasanos, L., et al: *Health Assessment*, Mosby, St. Louis, 1981, p. 555.

Metheny, N.: "Renal Stones and Urinary pH," *American Journal of Nursing*, **82**(9):1372–1375, September 1982.

Miller, T., and Sayers, V.: "Porcine Heparin as a Contributing Factor for Pruritis in Hemodialysis Patients," *Nephrology Nurse*, August 1981, p. 35.

Phipps, W., et al.: *Shafer's Medical-Surgical Nursing*, 7th ed., Mosby, St. Louis, 1980, p. 654.

Prowant, B., and Fruto, L. V.: "Continuous Ambulatory Peritoneal Dialysis," *Nephrology Nurse*, January–February 1980, p. 8.

Sampson, N.: "Peritoneal Dialysis as a Treatment Modality," *Nephrology Nurse*, January–February 1980, p. 15.

Walters, J. B.: *Principles of Disease*, Saunders, Philadelphia, 1982, p. 507, 579.

BIBLIOGRAPHY

Bielski, M.: "Preventing Infection in the Catheterized Patient," *Nursing Clinics of North America*, **15**(4):703–715, December 1980. Offers principles as well as preventive techniques that serve to reduce the high incidence of infection in catheterized clients.

Bruce, G. L., et al.: "Implementation of ANA's Quality Assurance Program for Clients with End Stage Renal Disease," *Advances in Nursing Science*, **2**(2):79–91, January 1980. This article reports the application of the ANA's Quality Assurance Program to a particular target population. Of particular importance is a discussion of the process of developing criteria to evaluate patient progress and the effectivenss of nursing interventions.

Brundage, D. J.: *Nursing Management of Renal Problems*, 2d ed., Mosby, St. Louis, 1980. Renal failure is the major problem addressed by this book. Sections are devoted to exploring the causes of acute and chronic renal failure. Psychosocial as well as physiologic needs are discussed, and practical theory-based nursing interventions are suggested in this comprehensive text.

Cain, L., Bigongiare, L. R.: "The Percutaneous Nephrostomy Tube," *American Journal of Nursing*, **82**(2): 296–298, 1982. Recent improvements in technique and tools for this procedure, which is used to relieve ureteral obstruction, are discussed, with case studies and visual representations focusing on nursing care.

Gordon, M.: *Manual of Nursing Diagnosis*, McGraw-Hill, New York, 1982. This compact manual designed for clinical use includes all diagnostic categories accepted by the National Conference Group for Classification of Nursing Diagnosis. For each diagnosis, a definition including characteristics and etiologies is listed, and all diagnoses are organized according to functional health pattern typology.

Gordon, M.: *Nursing Diagnosis: Process and Application*, McGraw-Hill, New York, 1982. A thorough treatment of decision-making processes used by nurses in the implementation of the nursing process is presented, along with the functional pattern area approach to gathering data and organizing the nursing diagnoses approved for testing by the National Conference Group for Classification of Nursing Diagnosis.

Horsley, J., et al.: *Closed Urinary Drainage Systems: CURN Project*, Grune and Stratton, New York, 1981. Part of a series of monographs from the Conduct and Utilization of Research in Nursing Project cosponsored by the Michigan Nurses' Association. It offers research-based clinical protocols designed for implementation and evaluation in clinical units.

Jones, D. A., et al. (eds.): *Medical-Surgical Nursing: A Conceptual Approach*, 2d ed., McGraw-Hill, New York, 1982. Chapters on renal dysfunctions include all phases of the nursing process. Assessment techniques and nursing diagnoses are fully described. Nursing actions are organized according to primary, secondary, and tertiary levels of intervention.

Lancaster, L. E.: *The Patient with End-Stage Renal Disease*, Wiley, New York, 1979. Detailed and comprehensive coverage of the client with end-stage renal failure is the emphasis of this publication. Dialysis, dietary management, and related nursing care are covered in this text.

Metheny, N.: "Renal Stones and Urinary pH," *American Journal of Nursing*, **82**(9):1372–1375, September 1982. Chemical composition and physiologic formation of renal stones are presented as the background for a thorough discussion of dietary and pharmaceutical control of the pH. Specific dietary prescriptions are offered, and medications used to create alkaline or acidic urine are discussed.

Tucker, S. M.: *Patient Care Standards*, Mosby, St. Louis, 1980. Standards for a number of kidney and bladder-related medical and surgical problems are delineated. Rationales are offered for standards, organized by medical diagnosis. Standards for client teaching in areas such as self-catheterization and dialysis are helpful in designing expected outcomes.

Walter, J.B.: *An Introduction to the Principles of Disease*, 2d ed., Saunders, Philadelphia, 1982. Relevant chapters review background material on the pathophysiology and biochemistry of urinary dysfunctions.

33

The Gastrointestinal System

Mary Marmoll Jirovec

Effective functioning of the body's gastrointestinal components is essential for adequate body metabolism. Disruptions in such components as ingestion, digestion, absorption, and elimination can alter gastrointestinal function and contribute to a variety of health problems. This chapter focuses on major and minor health problems that occur in conjunction with gastrointestinal disturbances.

ABNORMAL CELLULAR GROWTH

ORAL CANCER

DESCRIPTION

Of all human cancer, 8 percent occurs in the oral cavity, and 95 percent of this is squamous cell (epidermoid) carcinoma (Rush, 1979). Extraoral cancer usually occurs on the lower lip, while the tongue is the most common site of intraoral cancer. The gingiva, floor of the mouth, buccal mucosa, and soft and hard palates may also be affected. The speed of metastasis varies with the type and location of the lesion. Oral cancers usually spread by direct invasion, with the submaxillary and cervical lymph nodes the first to become involved. Prognosis is good with early detection.

PREVENTION

Health Promotion

Involves public education and direct client teaching.

1. Extraoral cancer. Client should:
   a. Reduce exposure to intense sunlight.
   b. Avoid chronic irritation to the lip by avoiding smoking cigarettes and cigars.
2. Intraoral cancer. Client should:
   a. Minimize use of tobacco and snuff.
   b. Maintain good oral hygiene.
   c. Support programs to prevent the spread of syphilis.
   d. Encourage early treatment of syphilis associated with syphilitic glossitis.
   e. Avoid excessive alcohol ingestion.
   f. Minimize long-term dental trauma.

Population at Risk

1. Tobacco users.
2. Persons exposed to excessive, intense sunlight.
3. Persons who use sunlamps regularly.
4. Persons with a history of leukoplakia.

Screening

Early evaluation of oral lesions.

ASSESSMENT

Health History

1. Area in or around mouth noted to be roughened, ulcerated, or overgrown.
2. Area usually painless, although local tenderness may be present.

3. Swelling, numbness, or loss of feeling in part of the mouth.
4. Color changes in mouth and/or tongue to white, gray, dark brown, or black.
5. Sore not healed after 2 weeks.
6. Unexplained or persistent bleeding.
7. Low-grade pain, constant or intermittent, in face or ear.
8. Cancer of the tongue usually begins with an area of hyperkeratosis that progresses to an ulcerated lesion. When the posterior half of the tongue is involved, client may experience dysphagia and pain on swallowing, as well as halitosis and weight loss. As the cancer invades muscle, pain increases, with soreness when hot or seasoned foods are eaten, and tongue motion is limited. If untreated, neighboring structures become invaded and client will salivate more, speech will become slurred, and the sputum may be blood-tinged. Extensive invasion can result in trismus (tonic contraction of the muscles used for mastication), the inability to swallow, and constant pain in the ears, face, and teeth.
9. Clients with gingival cancer often describe a mass or slight tenderness with loose teeth. With more extensive involvement, the lesion may ulcerate and bleed, mastication may be affected, and the mandibular nerve may become involved.
10. The initial complaints of a client with cancer in the floor of the mouth are minimal. As the lesion spreads, however, clients experience pain, difficulty eating and speaking, and a swollen tongue.
11. Cancer of the buccal mucosa usually begins with an ulcer and spreads locally.
12. When the lesion is in the *hard palate,* the client often notes a painless mass, which becomes tender with time.
13. Soft palate lesions most frequently result in pain and dysphagia.

Physical Assessment

1. All oral surfaces should be examined for roughness, white and patchy areas, abnormally pigmented areas, redness, or ulcerations. Any lesion that has not healed in 3 weeks should be suspect. Lesions may appear as small swellings, ulcerated areas (see Figure 33-1), or overgrowths (see Figure 33-2).
2. Asymmetry may be present. Any swelling in

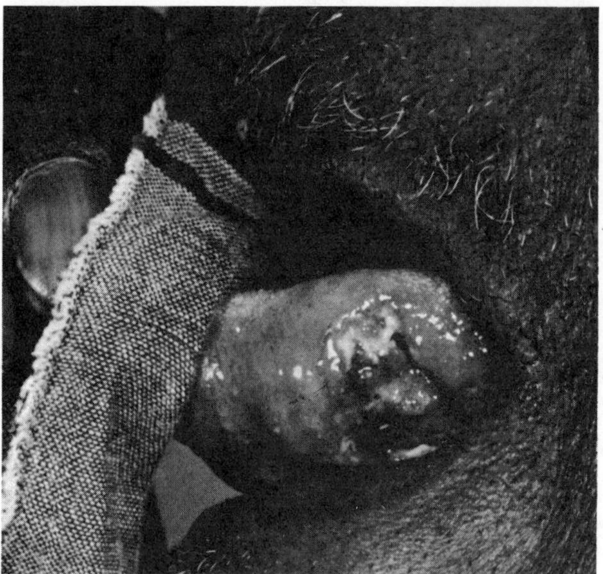

Figure 33-1 Squamous carcinoma of the lateral border of the middle third of the tongue. The lesion is deeply invasive and much larger than the area of ulceration would indicate. The curled, raised border is characteristic. (From Schwartz, S.I., et al., eds.: *Principles of Surgery,* McGraw-Hill, New York, 1974.)

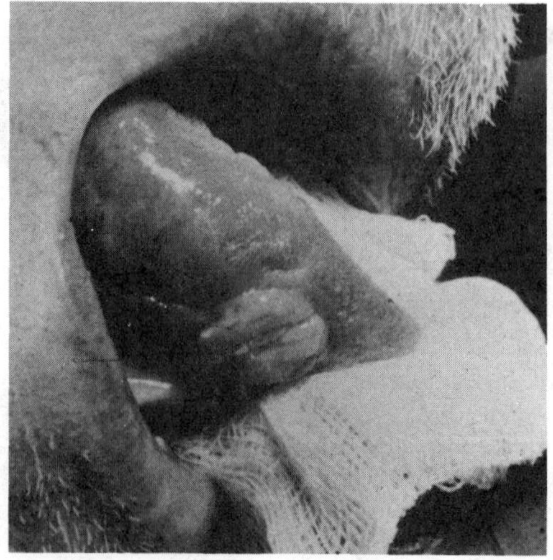

Figure 33-2 Squamous carcinoma of the tip of the tongue. The exophytic, fairly superficial lesion shows a well-differentiated histologic structure. The prognosis for such a lesion is excellent. (From Schwartz, S.I., et al., eds.: *Principles of Surgery,* McGraw-Hill, New York, 1974.)

the oral cavity should be palpated and tenderness noted.
3. Loose teeth may be detected.
4. Difficulty speaking and swallowing may occur due to enlargement caused by the lesion or related structures.
5. There may be loss of sensation over areas in the oral cavity.
6. Metastatic spread may be reflected in enlarged lymph nodes palpated in the head and neck.
7. Client with long-standing oral cancer often appears wasted, with a significant weight loss noted when compared with a previous weight record.

Diagnostic Tests

1. Application of a dye such as toluidine blue to the area enhances visualization of the lesion.
2. Exfoliative cytology allows examination of the cells scraped from the lesion under a microscope.
3. Biopsy is usually done on an outpatient basis. A small piece of tissue is removed using a skin punch and examined for evidence of malignancy.

NURSING DIAGNOSES: ACTUAL OR POTENTIAL

1. Alterations in comfort due to pain in the area of the lesion or surrounding tissue, which will worsen secondarily to extended involvement of the ears, face, or teeth.
2. Alterations in self-concept due to mouth odors noticed by self and others as a result of tissue degeneration, drooling, or speech change.
3. Nutritional deficit due to increased salivation and drooling secondary to difficulty in swallowing and possible increase in saliva or exudate and difficulty chewing foods resulting from lesion or pain.
4. Impairment of verbal communication due to slurring of speech caused by abnormal growth.
5. Grieving due to anxiety and fears related to cancer and changes in body image due to surgery.
6. Role disturbance due to prolonged illness, which can interfere with family and work responsibilities.

EXPECTED OUTCOMES

1. A patent airway will be maintained at all times.
2. Client will ingest nutrients adequate to maintain desired weight.
3. Pain will be controlled so that client is able to perform activities of daily living.
4. Mouth odors will diminish, allowing comfortable interaction with client.
5. Client and family will be able to interact according to previously established patterns.
6. Client will begin to accept changes in self-image and gradually assume previous life activities as far as possible.
7. Client will comply with care plan by:
   a. Reducing tobacco use.
   b. Avoiding excessive exposure to sun.
   c. Maintaining weight.

INTERVENTIONS

1. Surgical interventions: the most common treatment for oral cancer is surgical excision of the cancerous area (often involving wide resection) and radical neck resection, if necessary. Radiation may also be used with some types of cancer, either alone or in combination with surgery. Some head and neck neoplasms also respond to chemotherapy. In its early stages, squamous cancer of the face or lip will respond to topical 5-fluorouracil.
   a. Glossectomy (hemiglossectomy): removal of all or part of the tongue.
   b. Mandibulectomy: removal of part of the mandible.
2. Preoperative interventions.
   a. Administer prescribed medication to control pain.
   b. Give frequent mouthwashes with oxidizing agents such as potassium permanganate (1:10,000) or half-strength hydrogen peroxide to control halitosis. Oral lavages and power sprays aid in cleaning lesions and removing necrotic tissue. If client is a mouth breather, glycerin, mineral oil with lemon juice, or milk of magnesia swabs are helpful. Keep the room well ventilated.
   c. To prevent aspiration, the diet should be bland and in soft or liquid form. A teaspoon or straw may be helpful in taking only small amounts. Suction equipment should be kept at the bedside. Local an-

esthetics should be used with caution to avoid disrupting the function of the gag reflex.

d. Suction frequently for excessive salivation; position to prevent aspiration (refer to Chapter 31 for discussion of suctioning).
e. Allow client to communicate fears, ask questions, and interact with others. Questions should be answered honestly without destroying all hope.
f. Refer for counseling as appropriate.
g. Support the family in interacting with the client.
h. Contact social service agencies to assist with economic difficulties or extended hospitalization.
i. Plan a means of communication with the client after surgery, as speech is often temporarily or permanently affected (e.g., pad and pencil or "magic slate").

3. Postoperative interventions.
   a. Position to prevent aspiration and maintain a patent airway.
      (1) Keep prone, lateral, or supine, with the head turned.
      (2) Perform tracheostomy care to prevent respiratory distress due to postoperative edema, (refer to Chapter 31).
      (3) Suction orally as needed to prevent aspiration; should be done gently to prevent trauma to the suture line.
   b. Administer prescribed analgesics to control pain; mild sedatives may be used to reduce anxiety.
   c. Administer intravenous and nasogastric fluids to meet initial nutritional needs. Depending on the extent of the surgery, a gastrostomy tube may be used. As healing occurs, oral fluids will be reinstituted.
   d. Maintain meticulous and frequent oral hygiene to prevent infection and promote comfort. Gentle lavage with a power spray or mouth irrigations using normal saline, diluted hydrogen peroxide, a weak sodium bicarbonate solution, or an alkaline mouthwash are helpful. Occasionally, an antibiotic solution may be used.
   e. Instruct client in care of prosthetic device to replace some or all of the hard palate (to facilitate chewing and swallowing) if appropriate.
   f. Refer for long-term speech rehabilitation, including speech therapy and/or a prosthesis, if necessary.
   g. Encourage social interaction and help the family adjust to the change. Fear, anger, and grief are normal reactions with which the client should be helped.
   h. Teach client about:
      (1) Nutritional needs.
      (2) Avoidance of infection.
      (3) Avoidance of tobacco, snuff, and alcohol.

EVALUATION

Outcome Criteria

1. Client is able to perform oral hygiene unassisted.
2. Client maintains optimal weight (or gains or loses $2\frac{1}{2}$ lb every 2 weeks, as appropriate).
3. Client is able to communicate with others and continues speech therapy as indicated.
4. Client discusses changes in self-concept and reactions to body image changes realistically.
5. Family discusses fears and concerns with client and assists client in coping with changes in physical appearance.

Complications

HEMORRHAGE

Assessment

1. Frank bleeding during postoperative period. Can occur several days after surgery.
2. Continuous swallowing; vomiting of blood.
3. Signs of hypovolemia present if blood loss is excessive.

Revised Outcomes

Bleeding will stop.

Interventions

1. Apply local pressure initially.
2. Surgical repair.
3. Control volume loss if needed.

Reevaluation and Follow-up

Monitor closely for further blood loss.

RECURRENCE OF CANCER OR METASTASES

Regular follow-up care, especially in the first 2 years, is important to detect recurrence or metastases.

LEUKOPLAKIA

Leukoplakia is the most common precancerous lesion. It can occur anywhere in the mouth or on the lips and is found most frequently in men over age 40. In fair-skinned persons, it often occurs on the lip. It appears to be a reaction to long-term chemical, thermal, or physical irritation and has been associated with heavy smoking, tobacco chewing, and ill-fitting dentures. It consists of a painless, dry, inflamed area that is usually white or blue. The plaque is slightly raised and irregular, with sharp borders. After many years, leukoplakia can hypertrophy or degenerate into fissures or ulcers. The lesion itself can potentially become malignant, and any irritations should be removed.

Because the lesion is premalignant, it should be watched closely and a biopsy taken if any changes are noted. Any initiating factors, such as tobacco use, should be minimized and dentures evaluated for proper fit. Good oral hygiene should be maintained. Vitamin A may also be given. Follow-up care is essential.

SALIVARY TUMORS

Tumors of the salivary glands are most frequently benign. Adenocarcinoma is the most common malignant growth and usually occurs in the sixth decade. It is a slow-growing tumor that spreads widely through both lymph and blood vessels. Mucoepidermoid carcinoma is seen most frequently in the parotid gland. Its degree of malignancy and rate of growth varies. Squamous cell carcinomas are rapidly growing, highly invasive tumors. Malignant tumors initially cause enlargement of the gland involved. As the growth spreads, pressure on sensory and motor nerves results in varying degrees of pain and paralysis.

Clients with salivary tumors are usually in pain and may have to cope with some oral motor impairment that makes chewing, swallowing, or talking difficult. Changes in body image due to surgery are often a major concern. Treatment involves surgical excision of the malignancy. Because of the proximity of the facial nerve during surgery, damage to it can easily result. If possible, the nerve is preserved. During a parotidectomy, the mandibular branch of the facial nerve is most often damaged, causing paralysis. This is, however, often temporary, and the nerve regenerates, with a return of function in 18–24 months. Some salivary malignancies are radiosensitive, and irradiation will be coupled with surgical intervention.

ESOPHAGEAL TUMORS

Benign tumors of the esophagus are rare. Malignant neoplasms are more common and are responsible for 2 percent of all cancer deaths. Squamous cell carcinomas are most common. Cancer of the esophagus is seen more often in men than in women. Its peak incidence is in the sixth and seventh decades. Its cause is unknown, but it has been associated with esophageal damage from lye, achalasia, and the use of alcohol and tobacco. It is thought that genetic differences and chemicals in the diet may also play a role.

The cancer spreads by lymph channels via regional lymph nodes, by blood to the liver and lungs, and through direct invasion, although seldom entering the stomach. Signs and symptoms appear late and spread so quickly that early detection is difficult. Initially, the client experiences only slight dysphagia and transient difficulty passing food through the esophagus. As the dysphagia progresses, the client has trouble swallowing solids, then semisolid food, and finally liquids. As the tumor spreads, there is pain on swallowing and vague, burning, retrosternal pain. As food intake diminishes, weight loss occurs. Halitosis develops, the client has a bad taste in the mouth, and regurgitation occurs. With obstruction of the esophagus, the client may aspirate, and severe coughing episodes often develop.

Interventions focus on relieving the problems and arresting the malignant growth. Whatever the specific treatment selected, the cure rate is low. Surgical excision and irradiation may be used alone or in combination. Some physicians use preoperative irradiation. The type of surgical procedure depends on the cancer and the client's condition. It is often difficult to resect all the cancer. Therefore, the goal of any intervention is to prolong the client's ability to eat normally. This may be accomplished with an esophagectomy and/or implanting an artificial esophagus, using a segment of colon as the esophagus, creating a channel through the tumor, or bringing the stomach into the mediastinum to anastomose the ends of the esophagus. Radiation therapy may also be used as a palliative procedure to reduce the size and slow the growth of the tumor.

Pain may be controlled with analgesic medication. Within the limits of the individual situation, the diet should be made as nutritional as possible. When oral intake is delayed, hyperalimentation may be used. Frequent mouth care will improve the client's appetite and foster nutrition. Because aspiration is a danger, the client should be cautioned to take small bites and chew food thoroughly. Eating alone should be avoided, and a suction machine should be kept at the bedside. Tracheoesophageal fistulas may develop postoperatively and prolong hospitalization.

GASTRIC TUMORS

Of all gastric tumors, 95 percent are malignant. The most common types are adenocarcinoma, lymphoma, and leiomyosarcoma. While the incidence of gastric cancer is decreasing in the United States, it is the fourth leading cause of cancer deaths in men. It is seen in men twice as frequently as in women, has its peak incidence between 50 and 69 years of age, and occurs in blacks and orientals twice as often as in whites. Its cause is unknown, but it has been associated with genetic factors, polyps, changes in the gastric mucosa (i.e., chronic gastritis), and peptic ulcer disease.

Gastric cancer spreads by direct invasion (usually into the pancreas), through lymphatic channels (which occurs early), via the bloodstream to the liver, lungs, and bones, and by growing across the peritoneum. While spread occurs early, symptoms appear late and are often vague. Anorexia often develops, and weight loss is common. The pain can vary in intensity. The client often describes a feeling of rapid filling after eating. Vomiting occurs in about half the clients, and if the cancer is high in the stomach, dysphagia may develop. The client often fatigues easily. Occult bleeding is common, and anemia can develop.

Nursing care should focus on supporting the client and offering reassurance, improving nutrition, relieving pain, and correcting the anemia. The most effective treatment is surgery with complete excision. This usually involves some type of subtotal gastrectomy. Total gastrectomy is seldom indicated. (See *Peptic Ulcers* for a complete discussion of gastric surgery.) Irradiation for gastric cancer has not been tried frequently. Chemotherapy using 5-fluorouracil will occasionally show results if the tumor is inoperable. Follow-up care is essential.

SMALL BOWEL TUMORS

Both benign and malignant tumors are infrequent in the small bowel. Malignant neoplasms account for less than 1 percent of gastrointestinal cancers in the United States. The most common types are adenocarcinomas, lymphomas, and leiomyosarcomas. Small bowel cancer spreads to the liver and local lymph nodes. While its cause is not known, it is associated with chronic small bowel disease (i.e., regional enteritis). Genetic factors have also been implicated.

Clients usually experience malaise, anorexia, weight loss, and abdominal pain. Bleeding is frequent as the lesion ulcerates. Depending on the lesion's location in the small intestine, malabsorption, biliary obstruction, or intestinal obstruction can occur.

Nursing care should focus on promoting adequate nutrition and rest, relieving pain, preventing anemia, and relieving obstructions. Surgical excision is the most effective treatment, although the survival rate remains low. Irradiation, alkalating agents, nitrogen mustard, and corticosteroids may be helpful in treating lymphomas. Follow-up care and continuous evaluation are important.

COLORECTAL TUMORS

Rectocolonic cancer comprises 15 percent of all cancers and accounts for 20 percent of cancer deaths. Carcinoma is the most frequently occurring tumor of the colon or rectum. It usually occurs after age 55. In younger people, it is often associated with ulcerative colitis. Rectal cancer is more common in men, while cancer of the colon is found more frequently in women. Its incidence has been associated with environmental factors, such as diets low in fiber and high in refined carbohydrates, diets high in animal meats and fats, and genetic factors.

Rectocolonic cancer can spread by direct invasion, often into the bladder or vagina, via the regional lymphatics, through the blood to the liver, lungs, kidneys, and bones, and by multiple peritoneal implants. Signs and symptoms usually vary with the location. The usual presenting symptom is a significant change in bowel habits. The client often experiences increasing constipation or constipation alternating with diarrhea and colicky lower abdominal pain. The pain often increases when climbing stairs or bending over. Blood is often present in the stool and may be visible if the tumor is on the left side. Anorexia, nausea, and/or vomiting may be present, and weight loss is common. The client often describes a feeling of fullness in the bowel after defecation.

Interventions focus on arresting tumor growth and relieving obstruction. Nursing care should promote adequate nutrition and rest, alleviate pain, prevent anemia, and help allay fears. Surgical resection is the most effective treatment and may be curative or palliative. It involves large bowel resection with anastomosis of healthy ends or resection and formation of a colostomy. (See *Intestinal Obstructions* for a more complete discussion.)

If the tumor is small, well differentiated, and noninvasive, electrocoagulation, radiation, cryosurgery, and/or local excision may be used. Radiotherapy and chemotherapy (5-fluorouracil used most frequently) are most often used to convert an inoperable tumor into an operable one or to palliate recurrences after surgery. The use of immunotherapy and chemotherapy in conjunction with surgery is being investigated in an effort to improve the host's immunologic response to the tumor (Bland and Garrison, 1979).

TUMORS OF THE LIVER

Both malignant and benign tumors of the liver are rare. Malignant tumors account for only 1–2 percent of all cancers in North and South America and Europe. In Africa and Asia, however, where hepatic carcinogens, expecially aflaxins, are found in the food, hepatic carcinoma accounts for 20–30 percent of all malignancies. In the United States, tumors of the liver are most frequently associated with hepatic cirrhosis. Other etiological factors include genetic factors, malnutrition, iron overload, drugs, parasites, and chemicals. The hepatitis B virus has also been implicated as a possible cause of primary liver cell cancer (Bassendine et al., 1979). Metastatic tumors of the liver are usually from lung, gastrointestinal, or breast carcinomas.

Many of the effects of hepatic carcinoma are similar to those of cirrhosis. For this reason, its development may be overlooked in the severely ill client with cirrhosis. It may be distinguished by the fact that it is painful (usually moderate upper abdominal pain), causes bloody ascitic fluid, and results in a friction rub, or bruit, over the liver. Palpation usually reveals massive hepatomegaly, tenderness, and multiple nodes. Jaundice may occur, depending on the type of cancer. When cancer metastasizes to the liver in the absence of previous liver pathology, the liver becomes enlarged, the abdomen swells and pain and jaundice develop.

Nursing care should focus on relieving the many problems associated with hepatic failure (see *Hepatic Cirrhosis*). Surgery may be tried if the client is young, a good surgical risk, and spread of the cancer is not extensive. The procedure used usually involves a partial hepatectomy. Liver transplantation has been of limited value. Chemotherapy may be used as a palliative measure to relieve pain.

PANCREATIC TUMORS

Pancreatic masses most frequently result from cysts or carcinoma. Pancreatic cysts consist of a collection of fluid that is encapsulated. Retention cysts arise from dilatation of pancreatic ducts within the gland. Pseudocysts are collections of pancreatic juice and cellular debris that can develop 3–4 weeks after an attack of acute pancreatitis. They usually cause aching pain and form a tender, palpable mass. Because of the danger of rupture, surgical drainage is usually employed.

Pancreatic cancer is the fourth leading cause of cancer death in the United States, and its incidence has tripled in the last 40 years (Malagelada, 1979). It affects men twice as frequently as women and is usually seen after age 50. It can affect the head or the body and tail of the pancreas and rapidly spreads by direct invasion into the rest of the pancreas, the liver, the biliary tract, and the duodenum. Quickly adhering to adjacent structures, metastases are carried by lymphatic and blood vessels. Chronic pancreatitis, heavy alcohol use, diabetes mellitus, cigarette smoking, a high-protein and high-fat diet, and industrial carcinogens such as banzidine, betanaphthylamine, and alkylating chemotherapeutics have all been implicated as possible causes.

Physical and behavioral symptoms vary with the location of the tumor. Usually pain is present and may be severe, radiating into the midback if the body or tail of the pancreas is involved. With biliary tract involvement, jaundice develops. Weight loss is common, and digestive disturbances may include anorexia, an aversion to food, nausea, vomiting, gastric fullness, flatulence, constipation, or diarrhea in some clients. When the body or tail is involved, the client often experiences emotional disturbances, with depression and a feeling of doom. Prognosis for pancreatic carcinoma is usually poor, and death is often swift.

With early diagnosis, surgery involving some combination of the following is employed: Whipple operation (removal of pyloric antrum, duodenum, lower common bile duct, head of pancreas, upper jejunum, and regional lymph nodes), total pancreatectomy (*Whipple procedure* plus removal of spleen, tail and body of pancreas, and thorough lymphadenectomy), and regional resection (*total pancreatectomy* plus removal of transpancreatic portion of portal vein, celiac axis, superior mesenteric artery, and middle colic vessels). Because early diagnosis is difficult, fewer than a quarter of cases can be surgically resected. Palliative surgery to relieve obstruction may be the only feasible alternative. Irradiation and chemotherapy have not proven effective but may also be employed for palliation. Testolactose and 5-fluorouracil have been most useful. A sound, nutritionally balanced diet may be coupled with insulin therapy and pancreatic enzyme replacement. Rest should be promoted and narcotics used to relieve pain. Good skin care is essential, particularly in the presence of pruritus. Long-term care is required. Emotional support is needed for family and client. Fears and concerns associated with the disease and consequences should be explored.

HYPERACTIVITY AND HYPOACTIVITY

PEPTIC ULCERS

DESCRIPTION

A peptic ulcer is a clearly defined break in tissue involving the mucosa, submucosa, or musculature of the gastrointestinal track. Of all North Americans, 10 percent have a chronic peptic ulcer at some time. The problem occurs most frequently in the stomach or duodenum but can occur in any area exposed to gastric acid, such as the esophagus, or the jejunum after gastric surgery.

A peptic ulcer develops when the digestive ability of the gastric secretions exceeds the mucosal defenses. This occurs when hydrochloric acid secretion is excessive or when mucosal resistance is decreased by poor circulation, inadequate tissue regeneration, or inadequate mucous production. Gastric ulcers are associated with normal or low levels of acid production. The mechanism involved may be related to acid diffusing back into the gastric mucosa, causing damage. Duodenal ulcers are associated with excess acid production. Stress may be a factor in their development, stimulating the vagus nerve, which increases acid production. The physical stress of a severe burn can result in Curling's ulcer, while a central nervous system lesion can lead to Cushing's ulcer.

PREVENTION

Health Promotion

1. Avoid drugs that increase acid secretion or decrease mucosal resistance (e.g., salicylates, corticosteroids, reserpine, histamine, and indomethacin, or Indocin).
2. Avoid alcohol in excess, caffeine, and cigarettes.
3. Minimize emotional, psychological, and physical stress.

Population at Risk

1. Gastric ulcers generally found in older persons, with men affected twice as frequently as women.
2. Duodenal ulcers found more frequently in young and middle-aged men.
3. Nervous, competitive, compulsive workers in demanding positions often develop duodenal ulcers.
4. Persons with a family history of peptic ulcer.
5. Persons with type O blood.
6. Persons experiencing sustained physical or emotional stress.

Screening

1. Assessment of lifestyle and coping mechanisms.

2. Identification of stressors (physical, psychological, social).
3. Family history.

ASSESSMENT

Health History

1. Previous history of peptic ulcer or chronic indigestion.
2. Blood type O.
3. Medications taken (e.g., Indocin, aspirin, steroids).
4. Occupation and daily habits (executive position; highly stressful, demanding occupation).
5. Complaints of pain described as burning, gnawing, aching, sharp, stabbing, cramplike, a fullness, a sinking feeling, or gas pain. Pain is usually felt in the area of epigastrium and behind the xiphoid cartilage.
6. Nausea, vomiting, or pyrosis (a burning sensation coupled with the regurgitation of acid fluid into the throat) may be present.

Physical Assessment

1. Nervous and anxious appearance.
2. Superficial tenderness in the epigastrium is present on palpation. Occasionally, this discomfort is associated with cutaneous hyperesthesia.
3. With duodenal ulcers, the pain may be experienced over much of the abdomen, with increased intensity in the upper right quadrant. Abdominal pain associated with gastric ulcers is usually left of the midline and localized. Peptic ulcer pain often radiates behind the lower sternum. The pain is often rhythmic and associated with meals. Usually, pain occurs when the stomach is empty and may often wake the client at night. The pain of duodenal ulcers is usually decreased for 1–4 h after eating, while gastric ulcer pain is relieved for $\frac{1}{2}$ to $1\frac{1}{2}$ h.
4. Weight loss may be significant, depending upon the duration of the symptoms.

Diagnostic Tests

1. Barium swallow: used to visualize the ulcer. The client is given barium, a radiopaque substance, orally or through a nasogastric tube, and x-ray films are taken that visualize the ulcer. A laxative or enema may be given subsequently to prevent fecal impaction by the barium.
2. Gastrointestinal endoscopy: used to visualize the ulcer directly. The client should take nothing orally for several hours preceding the test. After applying a local anesthetic to the pharynx, a long, flexible, lighted fiberscope is passed through the mouth into the stomach. The ulcer can be visualized and specimens for cytology taken.
3. Gastric analysis: used to analyze gastric secretions. After an 8-h fast, the gastric secretions are withdrawn via a nasogastric tube and examined for acidity. Subsequently, another analysis may be done, stimulating gastric secretion with histamine. In both analyses, acid secretion is higher than normal with duodenal ulcers.
4. Examination of stools and gastric secretions for occult blood is also performed.

NURSING DIAGNOSES: ACTUAL OR POTENTIAL

1. Alteration in comfort due to discomfort in the epigastric regions that may radiate to the back, secondary to increased production of hydrochloric acid, decreased mucosal resistance, and so on.
2. Nutritional deficit due to alteration in food intake resulting from frequent nausea with vomiting several hours after eating.
3. Mild to severe fear associated with concern about family and work responsibilities and worries about own health.
4. Maladaptive coping patterns secondary to inability to handle daily stress (e.g., occupation, roles, and relationships).

EXPECTED OUTCOMES

1. Nausea and vomiting will stop and pain will be relieved within 1 week.
2. Client will identify stressors in the internal and external environment that precipitate stress responses and reduce them.
3. Client will comply with care plan by:
   a. Avoiding overexertion and taking frequent rests.
   b. Decreasing workload that produces stress.
   c. Avoiding stressful interactions.
   d. Identifying common stressors in life pattern and trying to minimize them.
   e. Working to develop healthy coping strategies to handle stress.

4. Ulcerated area will heal completely in 4–6 weeks.

INTERVENTIONS

1. Provide diet therapy.
   a. Allow client to eat a fairly normal diet while eliminating foods that are not well tolerated, such as foods that may be chemically irritating (e.g., spicy foods), thermally irritating (e.g., very hot foods), or mechanically irritating (e.g., popcorn). (Traditionally, bland foods were used frequently; today more liberal diets have evolved.)
   b. Give client with severe pain milk and antacid on an alternating schedule q½h before diet progresses to three meals a day, with between-meal and bedtime snacks. If the client is experiencing night pain, awaken client once or twice during the night and give milk or antacid (see below).
2. Administer prescribed medications to neutralize acid, decrease gastric secretion and mobility, and reduce anxiety.
   a. Nonsystemic antacids, which are not absorbed, are used to buffer gastric acid. Some tend to be constipating, such as aluminum hydroxide (Amphogel), while those that include magnesium salts (Maalox) may cause diarrhea. Antacids that combine these groups afford fewer complications (Gelusil and Delcid). An alternating schedule of the two types decreases side effects. Observe the contents of antacids, as some are high in sodium (Mylanta) and may affect clients on low-sodium diets.
   b. Anticholinergic drugs are used to decrease gastric motility and secretion but are associated with toxic side effects, including mouth dryness, nausea and vomiting, decreased visual acuity, and urinary retention.
   c. Sedatives may be used to decrease anxiety and restlessness, allowing physical and psychological relaxation.
   d. Synthetic histamine H_2-receptor antagonists that decrease HCl secretion have been investigated. Cimetidine (Tagamet) has been effective in healing duodenal ulcers and preventing recurrence when given for a year's maintenence (Bodemar and Walaw, 1978). It is apparently safe; however, asymptomatic relapses have been known to occur when the drug is discontinued.
3. Teach client about:
   a. Medications: rationale, schedule of administration, likely side effects, and adverse effects that should be reported. Caution client against abuse and overuse of antacids, since they can predispose an individual to acid–base imbalances. Give client a list of drugs known to predispose to ulceration.
   b. Diet: frequency and timing of meals and foods to be avoided. Include the primary food preparer in the teaching and emphasize what is allowed rather than what is not. Coffee, tea, and cola drinks should be avoided because of their stimulating effects. Alcohol intake should be minimized, although alcohol taken with milk or an antacid is not contraindicated.
   c. Reduction or cessation of smoking: the nervous tension associated with this activity must be weighed against the effect of smoking in enhancing gastric secretions.
4. Explore stressful situations with client and family. Stress perceptions vary with each individual. Identify client's perception of particular situations as stressful (e.g., work, family, roles and relationships). Seek ways to decrease stress and help the client develop alternative coping strategies in order to facilitate this process.
5. Refer to physician for irradiation to the stomach to destroy parietal and chief cells, decreasing the secretion of pepsin and hydrochloric acid; used when pain is intractable and recurrent and the client is severely ill with associated disease that makes surgery too great a risk.

EVALUATION

Outcome Criteria

1. Client complies with therapeutic regimen, including taking medication at appropriate times and in correct amounts, as indicated by records he or she keeps.
2. Within 1 week, nausea and vomiting are alleviated and pain is relieved. There is no recurrence of pain after 4–6 weeks.
3. Client follows dietary restrictions, as indicated by lack of pain associated with food.

4. Client reduces stressors in environment by resting more, delegating responsibilities at work, and working with family and/or counselor to develop alternative coping mechanisms.

Complications

HEMORRHAGE

Ulceration penetrates an artery, vein, or capillary bed.

Assessment

1. Hematemesis or melena.
2. Nausea.
3. Pain decreased as lost blood buffers acid.
4. Signs of developing shock (see discussion of shock in Chapters 48 and 49).
5. Hematocrit and hemoglobin to evaluate blood loss.

Revised Outcomes

1. Bleeding will stop and circulatory volume will return to normal. Indications of shock will cease.
2. Other expected outcomes will occur as stated above for *Peptic Ulcers*.

Interventions

1. Expand blood volume with intravenous solutions that often include whole blood and plasma.
2. Sedate to decrease apprehension and anxiety.
3. Insert nasogastric tube (see Figure 33-3) and perform gastric lavage (200 cc instilled for 1–2 min) with iced saline to stop the bleeding. Often, milk and antacids will be administered through the nasogastric tube after the bleeding has subsided. A large-bore Ewald tube may be used to facilitate clot removal.
4. Perform gastric cooling with a gastric balloon after the stomach is emptied of blood and clots. A cooling solution is circulated through the balloon to promote vasoconstriction and temporarily depress secretions. This is often used as an interim measure until surgery can be considered. A Levin tube is used to aspirate stomach contents while the balloon is in place.
5. Monitor vital signs and urinary output closely.
6. Institute appropriate measures to combat shock (see Chapters 48 and 49).

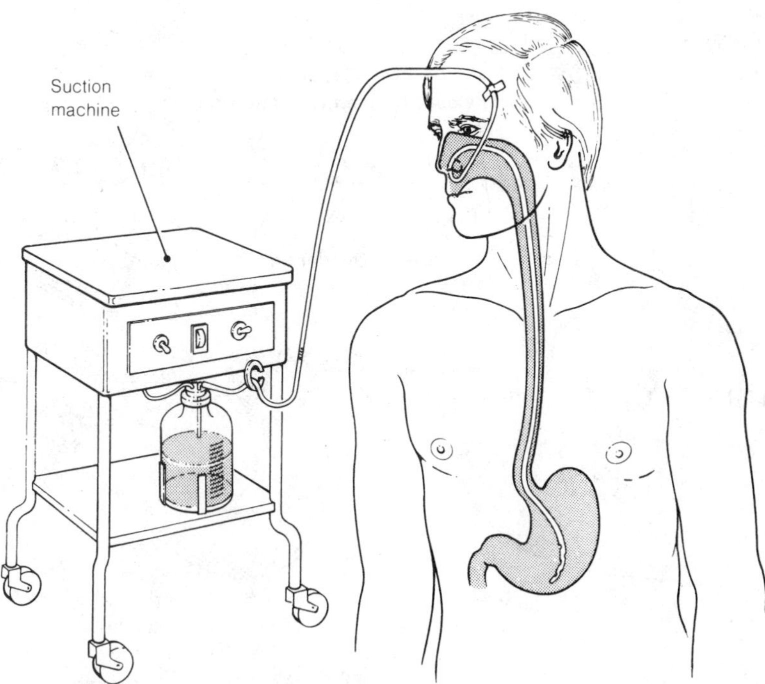

Figure 33-3 Nasogastric tube to suction. (From Jones, D.A., et al., eds.: *Medical-Surgical Nursing: A Conceptual Approach,* 2d ed., McGraw-Hill, New York, 1982.)

7. Surgical intervention: gastric surgery if the bleeding is not countered by blood transfusions after 12 h, if the bleeding persists after 24 h, or if the bleeding recurs while the client is in the hospital. Common surgical procedures include gastric resection (removal of a portion of the stomach), subtotal gastrectomy (removal of 70–80 percent of the stomach; see Figure 33-4a), truncal vagotomy (dividing branches of the vagus nerve), suturing of the ulcer, pyloroplasty (repair of the pylorus), and antrectomy (excision of walls of the antrum; see Figure 33-4b). Because truncal vagotomy often causes diarrhea, sometimes with urgency, and gastric stasis and retention, some surgeons prefer a proximal gastric vagotomy, in which parasympathetic nerves to the corpus and fundus are cut, leaving vagal stimulation to the antrum intact (Kelly, 1980).

Postoperative Interventions

1. Observe for bleeding. Initial drainage from the nasogastric tube will be bright red but should turn dark red after 12 h and greenish yellow in 36 h.
2. Provide prescribed diet. After several days the client will be given clear liquids, and, as tolerated, the nasogastric tube will be removed and the diet progressed.

Reevaluation and Follow-up

Continue to assess progress.

DUMPING SYNDROME

This postoperative complication develops in about 50 percent of clients after gastric surgery. The problem involves the rapid emptying of the gastric contents into the intestines, which draws fluid into the intestinal lumen and causes a decrease in the circulating blood volume. The client experiences a feeling of fullness and nausea with diaphoresis, pallor, dizziness, a feeling of warmth, headache, and palpitations. Because of excess insulin secretion at this time, clients experience weakness, tremors, diaphoresis, and an anxious feeling 2–3 h after eating. A high-protein, high-fat, low-carbohydrate diet con-

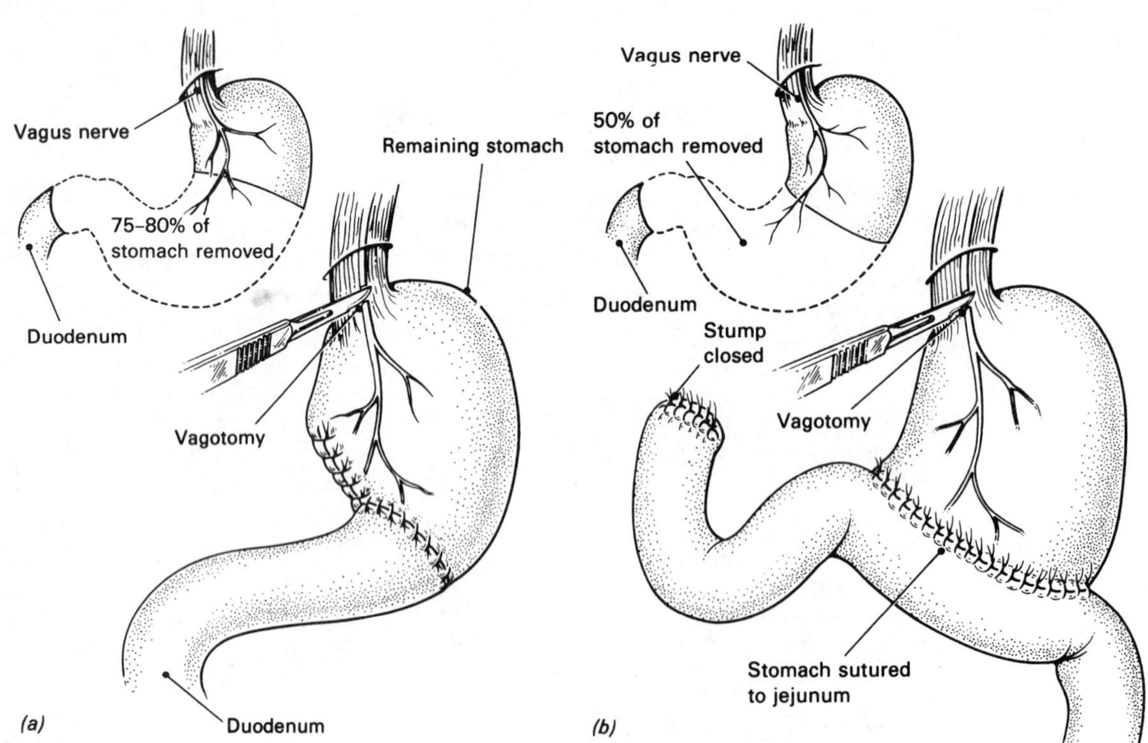

Figure 33-4 (*a*) Billroth I: subtotal gastrectomy. (*b*) Billroth II: antrectomy.

sisting of small, frequent meals is helpful. Fluids should be avoided around mealtimes. Lying down after eating and eating while semirecumbent are also helpful. The problem usually subsides in 6–12 months.

PERFORATION

Ulceration penetrates the stomach wall, spilling the gastric and duodenal contents into peritoneum. Chemical irritation results in peritonitis, an inflammation of the peritoneum.

Assessment

1. Sudden severe epigastric pain that spreads through the abdomen and is worse in the right lower quadrant.
2. Prostration with the knees drawn up.
3. Extremely tender, rigid, boardlike abdomen with rebound tenderness present upon palpation.
4. Nausea and vomiting.
5. Signs of hypovolemia and shock as fluid is lost to peritoneal cavity (see Chapters 48 and 49).
6. Absence of bowel sounds if paralytic ileus develops.
7. Rapid and shallow respiration.
8. Extreme apprehension.

Revised Outcomes

1. Perforation will be closed and leakage of gastrointestinal secretions into peritoneum stopped.
2. Blood volume will be restored.
3. Pain will be relieved and apprehension eased.

Interventions

1. Insert nasogastric tube to empty stomach of secretions.
2. Administer medications to relieve pain.
3. Discuss changes with client and family to allay fears and reduce stress.
4. Combat shock (see Chapters 48 and 49).
5. Surgical intervention: repair to close perforation. Usually a patch of omentum is used. More extensive gastric surgery may be performed (see above under *Hemorrhage*) if client's condition warrants.

Reevaluation and Follow-up

Essential.

PYLORIC OBSTRUCTION

Obstruction results from inflammation and edema around the pylorus. Gastric emptying decreases, resulting in gastric dilatation.

Assessment

1. Classic ulcer pain (refer to discussion under *Peptic Ulcers*).
2. Distension after eating.
3. Anorexia.
4. Weight loss
5. Vomiting of undigested food.
6. Distended abdomen, with visible peristalsis.
7. Succussion splash, evidencing fluid and air in the stomach.

Revised Outcomes

1. The distension will be relieved immediately.
2. The obstruction will subside in 48 hours.
3. Fluid and nutritional requirements will be met.

Interventions

1. Insert nasogastric tube with intermittent suction (see Figure 33-3).
2. Administer intravenous fluids to meet nutritional and fluid needs initially.
3. Give oral fluids after about 48 h when obstruction subsides.
4. Surgical intervention: pyloroplasty, the surgical opening of the pylorus, if the obstruction does not subside or if the pyloric opening is significantly narrowed.
5. Provide support and counseling regarding the complication, and provide interventions to relieve anxiety.

Reevaluation and Follow-up

Essential.

ACHALASIA

DEFINITION

Achalasia (cardiospasm) is a condition characterized by the failure of swallowed food to pass from the esophagus into the stomach. It is thought to result when esophageal peristalsis is feeble or absent and the cardiac sphincter fails to relax after swallowing. As food accumulates in the esophagus, its terminal end dilates (megaesophagus). Impairment of cholinergic innervation may be a factor, but the cause is not known. Occasionally, it is precipitated by emotional stress such as a death of someone close or feelings of guilt after sex. It occurs most frequently in women between the ages of 20 and 40. The course of achalasia is usually chronic and progressive, with remissions and exacerbations.

The client experiences mild dysphagia, which increases with excitement or tension. There is a feeling of fullness that is relieved after a while as the food passes into the stomach. A dull ache or pain radiating to the base of the neck, left shoulder, or scapular area may be experienced. The client is unable to belch, loses weight, and often has a mild esophagitis. Halitosis is usually a problem. With megaesophagus, pressure on the trachea and/or blood vessels can cause difficulty.

Nursing care focuses on promoting nutrition and comfort, minimizing stress, and preventing respiratory difficulties. Medical treatment usually focuses initially on dilating the cardiac sphincter (see Figure 33-5) and, if unsuccessful, surgically cutting it (esophagocardiomyotomy) to promote passage of food into the stomach.

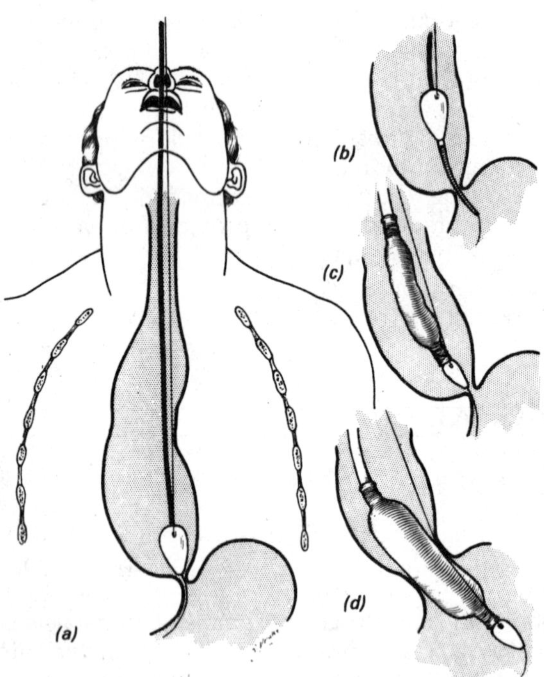

Figure 33-5 Hydrostatic dilatation of the lower esophagus to relieve achalasia. (*a*) An olive-tipped bougie is passed to the stomach. (*b*) A sound is passed through the sphincter, guided by a previously swallowed flexible wire. (*c*) The hydrostatic dilator is then passed through the sphincter and (*d*) distended to dilate the sphincter. (From Schwartz, S.I., et al., eds.: *Principles of Surgery*, McGraw-Hill, New York, 1974.)

The client will often be taught self-dilatation (bougienage) and instructed to do it every 3–7 days.

Food passage can be further facilitated by encouraging a soft diet and teaching the client to eat slowly, chew all food well, take fluids while eating, and arch the back, strain, and flex the chin to the sternum after swallowing. Clients should avoid eating at night or when emotionally stressed and should remain upright after meals. Small doses of sedatives may be given to relieve emotional stress, and smooth muscle relaxants may be tried. The latter are associated with adverse side effects.

CONSTIPATION

Constipation may be defined as a failure of the rectum to evacuate its contents normally. As this occurs, stool accumulates in the rectum, which becomes chronically distended. As water is absorbed from the stool, making it dehydrated, fecal impaction of hard, puttylike stools results. Constipation can result from mechanical obstruction, decreased colonic contractility (i.e., paralytic ileus and megacolon), or, most frequently, when the defecation reflex fails. Dietary changes, inactivity, muscle weakness, overuse of laxatives, chronic suppression of the urge to defecate, and emotional stress can contribute to its development. It often results in anorexia, a bloated feeling, belching, flatus, malaise, weakness, headache, dizziness, and mild abdominal distension. If fecal impaction develops, watery diarrhea occurs as stool passes around the impaction, and crampy lower abdominal pain ensues.

Nursing care focuses on relieving the constipation and preventing its recurrence. To empty the rectum, an enema (water or soapsuds), stool softeners, and mild laxatives are used. Fecal impactions may be softened with an oil retention enema and then removed with a tap water enema or digitally broken and removed. Diet therapy is the most effective way to prevent recurrence. Eating high-fiber foods should be encouraged. Prune juice with breakfast is often helpful, and fresh fruits and vegetables should be eaten liberally. Ingestion of fluids, including water, should be encouraged. The sustained use of laxatives should be discouraged.

METABOLIC DISORDERS

OBESITY

DESCRIPTION

In areas of the world where the food supply is good, obesity is the most common type of metabolic disorder. It is estimated that about 15 percent of the United States population is overweight, with women affected more frequently than men. Approximately 15–30 percent of school-age children are thought to be obese (Hayles and Huse, 1979). Simply defined, obesity involves an excess accumulation of fat that occurs when caloric intake exceeds energy requirements. It can be caused by either endogenous or exogenous factors. Endogenous obesity results when there is a disturbance within the individual, such as a hypothalamic lesion in the ventromedial nucleus or a hormonal imbalance. Exogenous obesity occurs when external factors lead to overeating. These include psychological, sociocultural, economic, and physical influences.

PREVENTION

Health Promotion

1. Avoid caloric intake that exceeds caloric requirements for body size, activity, and lifestyle.
2. Maintain daily exercise program that includes at least moderate exertion.
3. Increase knowledge of good nutrition and its benefits.

Population at Risk

1. Persons with one or both parents overweight.
2. Persons who eat to relieve tension.
3. Persons with sedentary lifestyles.
4. Older persons whose basal metabolic rate and physical activity have decreased without a concomitant decrease in caloric intake.
5. Persons whose work requires eating socially.
6. Persons who have been overweight in the past.

Screening

1. Evaluation of eating habits.
2. Regular height-weight comparisons.

ASSESSMENT

Health History

1. Dietary history of what was eaten in the last 24 h, few days, or week: type and amount of food eaten, when and where it was eaten, activity just before and during eating, and feelings before, during, and after eating.
2. Established eating patterns (e.g., eating alone or with others, use of a shopping list).
3. Onset of obesity: precipitating factors, time of onset, length of time person has been overweight.
4. History of diabetes mellitus, gout, gallbladder disease, atherosclerosis, or coronary artery disease: all associated with obesity.
5. Self-concept (body image) related to being overweight.
6. Previous dieting plans: success versus failure.
7. Ability to identify changes in eating habits related to stress.

Physical Assessment

1. Pattern of fat accumulation will differ. Women tend to develop adiposity below the waist, while men will often carry excess fat on their trunks. Depending on body build, occasionally a person will be obese without obvious visible evidence.
2. Weight, when compared with standard height and weight tables (see Table 33-1), will be excessive.
3. Auscultation through adipose tissue diminishes the sounds, making breath, heart, and bowel sounds difficult to hear. Palpating through fat is also more difficult. Pulses may be difficult to find, and the abdominal examination may be uninformative. Percussion sounds will be duller.
4. Tachycardia, hypoventilation, and/or mild hypertension can be present, particularly following activity. In addition, obese clients may be at risk for changes associated with other health problems (e.g., diabetes mellitus, atherosclerosis.)
5. Excoriation, skin breakdown, and/or infection is often noted in the skin folds.

Diagnostic Tests

1. Calipers to estimate obesity—involves the measurement of the thickness of skin folds in different parts of the body. Comparing the results with normal values presents a fairly accurate estimate of obesity.

TABLE 33-1 STANDARD HEIGHTS AND WEIGHTS[a]

Men					Women				
Height					Height				
Feet	Inches	Small Frame	Medium Frame	Large Frame	Feet	Inches	Small Frame	Medium Frame	Large Frame
5	2	128–134	131–141	148–150	4	10	102–111	109–121	118–131
5	3	130–136	133–143	140–153	4	11	103–113	111–123	120–134
5	4	132–138	135–145	142–156	5	0	104–115	113–126	122–137
5	5	134–140	137–148	144–160	5	1	106–118	115–129	125–140
5	6	136–142	139–151	146–164	5	2	108–121	118–132	128–143
5	7	138–145	142–154	149–168	5	3	111–124	121–135	131–147
5	8	140–148	145–157	152–172	5	4	114–127	124–138	134–151
5	9	142–151	148–160	155–176	5	5	117–130	127–141	137–155
5	10	144–154	151–163	158–180	5	6	120–133	130–144	140–159
5	11	146–157	154–166	161–184	5	7	123–136	133–147	143–163
6	0	149–160	157–170	164–188	5	8	126–139	136–150	146–167
6	1	152–164	160–174	168–192	5	9	129–142	139–153	149–170
6	2	155–168	164–178	172–197	5	10	132–145	142–156	152–173
6	3	158–172	167–182	176–202	5	11	135–148	145–159	155–176
6	4	162–176	171–187	181–207	6	0	138–151	148–162	158–179

SOURCE: 1979 Build Study, Society of Actuaries and Association of Life Insurance Medical Directors of America, 1980. Copyright 1983 Metropolitan Life Insurance Company.

[a] Weights at ages 25–59 based on lowest mortality. Weight in pounds according to frame (indoor clothing weighing 5 lb for men and 3 lb for women; shoes with 1-in. heels).

2. Laboratory tests to detect the development of any of the medical problems commonly associated with obesity (e.g., fasting blood sugar, and tests of glycosuria and ketonuria to detect diabetes; serum cholesterol for atherosclerosis; an electrocardiogram to evaluate cardiac functioning).

NURSING DIAGNOSES: ACTUAL OR POTENTIAL

1. Nutritional alteration due to intake in excess of requirements, often secondary to anxiety, stress, or depression.
2. Respiratory dysfunction due to intolerance of even moderate activity without becoming short of breath (tires quickly with minimal exertion, contributing to inactivity).
3. Impairment of skin integrity due to reddened, raw areas in skin folds.
4. Alteration in self-concept due to increased body size and, possibly, problems with body odor.
5. Social isolation resulting from the use of eating to satisfy psychological needs and from a tendency to isolate self.
6. Ineffective coping resulting from the use of food to handle stress.

EXPECTED OUTCOMES

1. Client will demonstrate gradual weight loss over a specified period of time. For example, client will lose 2½ lb every 2 weeks until ideal weight is reached.
2. Client will gradually increase activity to include moderate exercise without becoming short of breath.
3. Excoriated areas in skin folds will heal.
4. Client will develop a healthy self-concept, as demonstrated by positive comments about self and by interest in weight-reduction program.

5. Client will interact socially to a greater degree by spending less time alone.
6. Client will comply with care plan, as demonstrated by:
   a. Adherence to dietary regimen.
   b. Losing weight as recommended.
   c. Avoiding situations that lead to overeating.
   d. Maintaining an effective exercise regimen.
   e. Developing a healthy body image, as evidenced by positive comments about self.
   f. Demonstrating an understanding that some dietary restriction will be a necessary lifelong activity.

INTERVENTIONS

1. Educate about a diet that includes modest caloric reduction with a low-fat, high-protein content. Protein tends to increase satiety and decrease blood glucose level. Since low fat content may cause constipation, encourage intake of fresh fruit and bulk foods. A stool softener may be needed.
2. Identify behaviors that lead to overeating and develop strategies to modify them.
3. Refer for group therapy with long-term reinforcement to focus on behavior modification. Lay groups such as TOPS (Take Off Pounds Sensibly) and Weight Watchers have also been of value. Diet program should complement client's needs and lifestyle.
4. Do not recommend starvation diets for long-term use, because they are associated with loss of protein tissue. In severely obese clients, fasting may be used initially because the resulting weight loss encourages the client. Such diets should be carried out under physician supervision.
5. Promote an exercise regimen suitable for an overweight client to promote circulation.
6. Discourage drugs (amphetamines) that depress the appetite because any associated weight loss is usually temporary.
7. Teach client to clean and dry skin folds. Inserting cotton in the fold to absorb moisture and taping the fold of tissue up to expose the area to the air are helpful.
8. Encourage daily baths or showers and more frequent cleansing of the armpits and perineum.
9. Surgical interventions.
   a. Surgical bypass of the intestine: an extreme procedure that may be considered in morbid obesity if the client's life is threatened from respiratory or cardiac failure, severe hypertension, or severe peripheral edema with ulceration. Various procedures are used and usually involve a jejunoileal shunt, in which about 6 m of the ileum and jejunum are resected and the remaining jejunum and ileum are anastamosed (see Figure 33-6). In effect, a

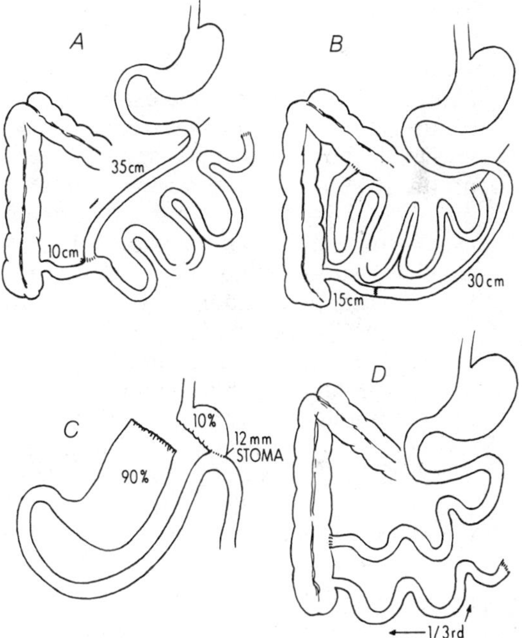

Figure 33-6 Bypass operations. (*a*) Payne-DeWind operation. The proximal 35 cm of jejunum is anastomosed end-to-side to the ileum 10 cm above the ileoceal valve. (*b*) Scott operation. The proximal 30 cm of jejunum is anastomosed end-to-end to the distal 15 cm of ileum; the proximal end of the divided ileum is anastomosed to the transverse colon. (*c*) Mason operation. The distal 90 percent of the stomach is surgically excluded; the proximal pouch is anastomosed by a narrow stoma to the jejunum. (*d*) Buchwald-Vasco operation. The distal one-third of the small intestine is excluded; the proximal intestine is anastomosed end-to-side to the ascending colon. (From Schwartz, S.I., et al., eds.: *Principles of Surgery*, McGraw-Hill, New York, 1974.)

malabsorption syndrome is created, and diarrhea that may last into the second postoperative year is a result.

Complications following intestinal bypass can include electolyte disturbances from persistent diarrhea, vitamin deficiencies, renal calculi, and mild hepatic dysfunction. Cirrhosis of the liver is a rare complication, but alcohol should be avoided. Transient arthritis sometimes occurs, and gallstone formation may also be accelerated.

b. Gastric partitioning: a procedure that involves excluding the lower 90 percent of the stomach from the upper 10 percent by stapling or transecting the stomach (see Figure 33-6c). The rationale for the procedure is that the smaller stomach reservoir will stimulate satiety sooner. Continuity of the gastrointestinal tract is maintained by leaving a small opening along the staples or anastomosing the small intestine to the small upper reservoir. Gastric perforation is the most common complication, making care and patency of the nasogastric tube a primary concern. Intake is initially limited to 30 cc of clear liquids at any given time and progresses to small, frequent feedings after approximately 8 weeks. Before 8 weeks postoperation, no more than 300 cc should be taken at any time.

EVALUATION

Outcome Criteria

1. Client loses $2\frac{1}{2}$ lb every 2 weeks until ideal weight is reached. Client then maintains ideal weight.
2. Client verbalizes reasons for any eating binges and returns to compliance with prescribed therapy.
3. Client tolerates moderate exertion without shortness of breath when ideal weight is reached.
4. Client maintains personal hygiene, as evidenced by lack of body odor and healing of excoriated areas.
5. Client speaks positively about self and avoids activities that foster social isolation.

Complications

1. Diabetes mellitus (see Chapter 28).
2. Atherosclerosis (see Chapter 30).
3. Osteoarthritis (see Chapter 27).
4. Gallbladder disease (see *Cholecystitis*).
5. Pickwickian syndrome: hypoventilation syndrome that results when the weight of the chest wall decreases chest expansion.

Assessment

1. Hypoventilation.
2. Somnolence.
3. Polycythemia.
4. Cyanosis.

Revised Outcomes

1. Oxygenation will be restored within normal limits.
2. Other expected outcomes will occur as stated above for *Obesity*.

Interventions

1. Provide oxygen therapy.
2. Perform other interventions listed above for *Obesity*.

Reevaluation and Follow-up

Continuous and essential.

ANOREXIA NERVOSA

Anorexia nervosa is a chronic, psychoneurotic disorder characterized by self-induced weight loss, amenorrhea, and psychopathology. It occurs most frequently in young girls around the time of puberty and is rare in boys. While the cause is unknown, it is associated with a hypothalamic disorder that causes the menstrual changes. Psychological conflicts regarding puberty and adolescence are common, and a relationship between self-image and culturally determined attitudes about body size have been implicated in its genesis. The client with anorexia nervosa fears becoming fat and avoids food, especially carbohydrate foods. Self-induced vomiting and the abuse of purgatives are not uncommon (see Bulimia below). Weight loss occurs and, if it is severe, emaciation, with apathy, weakness, and marked depression, develops. The client is often impatient and irritable. The decreased body weight leads to susceptibility to cold, and hypokalemia is often present secondary to the vomiting.

Nursing care focuses on improving nutritional intake and providing psychological support. Foster adequate dietary intake. Initially, give a 1,500-cal diet; after 1 week, progress to a 3,000- to 5,000-cal diet. Establish a sound, trusting nurse–client relationship, determine the possible cause of the anorexia, and gently supervise the client at each meal. The use of purgatives should be terminated, and vomiting should be made difficult by supervision and support. As weight is gained, the client should be complimented on his or her appearance. Long-term psychiatric therapy is indicated, as relapses are common.

MALABSORPTION SYNDROMES

Malabsorption syndromes are complexes of conditions characterized by inadequate absorption of one or more substances by the small intestine. A wide variety of conditions can result in a malabsorption syndrome. Their classification usually includes inadequate digestion (e.g., pancreatic insufficiency), inadequate bile salts (e.g., cholestasis), inadequate absorptive surface (e.g., intestinal bypass), lymphatic obstruction (e.g., Whipple's disease), cardiovascular disorders (e.g., congestive heart failure), absorptive defects of the mucosa of inflammatory origin (e.g., tropical sprue), mucosal absorptive defects of biochemical origin (e.g., nontropical sprue), and endocrine or metabolic disorders. Physical symptoms usually consist of severe weight loss, malnutrition, anorexia, abdominal distention, borborygmi, muscle wasting, and diarrhea. Stools are often light yellow to gray and are greasy and soft. As malnutrition becomes severe, various protein, vitamin, and electrolyte disturbances occur. Table 33-2 sum-

TABLE 33-2 PATHOPHYSIOLOGIC BASIS FOR SYMPTOMS AND SIGNS IN MALABSORPTIVE DISORDERS

Symptom or Sign	Pathophysiology
Generalized malnutrition and weight loss	Malabsorption of fat, carbohydrate, and protein → loss of calories
Diarrhea	Impaired absorption or increased intestinal secretion of water and electrolytes; unabsorbed dihydroxy bile acids and fatty acids → lowered absorption of water and electrolytes; excess load of fluid and electrolytes presented to the colon may exceed its absorptive capacity
Nocturia	Delayed absorption of water, hypokalemia
Anemia	Impaired absorption of iron, vitamin B_{12}, and folic acid
Glossitis, cheilosis	Deficiency of iron, vitamin B_{12}, folate, and other vitamins
Peripheral neuritis	Deficiency of vitamin B_{12}
Edema	Impaired absorption of amino acids → protein depletion → hypoproteinemia
Amenorrhea	Protein depletion and "caloric starvation" → secondary hypopituitarism
Bone pain	Protein depletion → impaired bone formation → osteoporosis Calcium malabsorption → demineralization of bone → osteomalacia
Tetany, paresthesias	Calcium malabsorption → hypocalcemia; magnesium malabsorption → hypomagnesemia
Hemorrhagic phenomena	Vitamin K malabsorption → hypoprothrombinemia
Weakness	Anemia, electrolyte depletion (hypokalemia)
Eczema	Cause uncertain

SOURCE: Greenberger, N. J., and Isselbacher, K. J.: "Disorders of Absorption," in Thorn, G. W., et al. (eds.): *Harrison's Principles of Internal Medicine,* 8th ed., McGraw-Hill, New York, 1977, p. 229.

marizes the signs and symptoms observed and their pathophysiologic bases.

Nursing care focuses on improving nutrition and preventing fluid and electolyte imbalances. Specific treatment varies with the type of malabsorption syndrome. For instance, tropical sprue is treated with a broad-spectrum antibiotic, while adult celiac disease (nontropical sprue) responds to a gluten-free diet. Depending on the particular syndrome, clients are often managed with one or more of the following: calcium, magnesium, iron, fat-soluble vitamins, folic acid, vitamin B_{12}, vitamin B complex, pancreatic supplements, broad-spectrum antimicrobials, salt-poor human albumin, immune serum globulin, corticosteroids, antidiarrheal agents, cholestryamine, caloric supplements, and/or antiparasitic agents. Reassessment and long-term care are essential.

BULIMIA

Bulimia is an episodic eating disorder primarily found in adolescents and young adults. The disorder involves the rapid uncontrolled ingestion of large amounts of high-calorie foods within a relatively short period of time (the binge), which terminates with the client's feeling physically uncomfortable due to fullness. Following this period of excess food ingestion, the client feels remorse and guilt and attempts to lose weight through rigid dieting, use of cathartics, and self-induced vomiting. The cause of this problem has not been isolated, and there is no specific treatment for it. Counseling about nutrition and exploration of the client's self-concept may help to diminish the problem.

INFLAMMATIONS

ULCERATIVE COLITIS

DESCRIPTION

Ulcerative colitis is a diffuse inflammation involving the mucosa and submucosa of the rectum and colon. It begins in the rectum, spreading proximally into adjacent bowel, and may involve all or part of the colon. Multiple ulcerations and crypt abscesses develop and are often replaced by scar tissue. When only the rectum is involved, it is called proctitis. If all of the colon is involved, the term used is pancolitis. The course of the disease can be intermittent or continuous, although most frequently it is characterized by remissions and exacerbations. The etiology associated with ulcerative colitis is not known, although several factors have been implicated, including infection, autonomic stimulation, genetic predisposition, immunologic and autoimmune mechanisms, excessive enzymes, basement membrane changes, hypersensitivity reactions, and psychogenic factors. An intolerance to cow's milk is frequently found in these clients. The onset of the disease or an exacerbation is frequently precipitated by a traumatic emotional experience.

PREVENTION

Health Promotion

1. Teach children to express feelings of anger and aggression overtly.
2. Develop coping strategies that foster the outward expression of feelings.

Population at Risk

1. Peak incidence is at ages 20–25 and 50–60.
2. Women are affected more often than men.
3. Non-Jewish whites are affected more often than Jews or blacks.
4. Persons with family history of ulcerative colitis (10–20 percent of families) have multiple cases.

ASSESSMENT

Health History

1. Diarrhea may have a sudden or gradual onset. The occurrence of stools can range from a few semisoft stools a day to several liquid stools every 30 min to 1 h. Feces often contain blood, mucus, and pus. In more severe cases, tenesmus (spasmatic contraction of the anal sphincter accompanied by pain and urgency) may occur.
2. Mild, cramping, lower abdominal pain that is worse before defecation and may be referred to the back.
3. Complaints of malaise and fatigue.
4. Personality structure and coping strategies

may exhibit characteristic feelings of helplessness and hopelessness in coping with stress, difficulty with interpersonal relationships, and an underlying hostility.
5. Emotional stress precipitating the problem may have occurred in the past months and should be isolated.
6. Changes in appetite described (anorexia most common).
7. Family history of ulcerative colitis.

Physical Assessment

1. Appears thin and weak; may be wasted and emaciated.
2. Weight loss, often significant.
3. Abdomen may appear flat, with visible peristalsis. Bowel sounds are often increased. As the inflammation worsens, the abdomen can become distended. There may be guarding and tenderness on palpation, especially along the descending colon and in the left lower quadrant.
4. Anus may be reddened and excoriated. During digital exploration, the rectum is usually found to be empty, anospasm may be felt, and the presence of fissures or abscesses may be noted.
5. Fever is often present.
6. Dehydration may be noted, with severe diarrhea.
7. Skin lesions such as erythema nodosum, which are common in women, and pyoderma gangrenosum, which occur on the legs and ankles, may be noted.
8. The eyes may appear reddened, pupil reactions may be sluggish, and pupil size small.
9. Client often complains of blurred vision. These changes may be due to a variety of ocular inflammations, such as episcleritis, iritis, uveitis, or keratitis (refer to Chapter 26).
10. The liver can become infiltrated with fat, which is evidenced by jaundice.
11. Joint manifestations (e.g., knees, hips) are the most common of these inflammations, occurring in 10–20 percent of ulcerative colitis clients.

Diagnostic Tests

1. Laboratory examinations to evaluate changes:
   a. The red blood cells are usually decreased, depending on the blood loss.
   b. White blood cells may be slightly increased.
   c. The erythrocyte sedimentation rate is usually elevated, and the serum albumin may be depressed.
   d. Serum chemistries may show electrolyte disturbances from the fluid loss.
   e. Stools may evidence blood, pus, or mucus.
2. Barium enema: barium, a radiopaque substance, is instilled into the rectum and visualized with a fluoroscope. The usual bowel preparations are often too rigorous, and the colon is sufficiently cleansed with a high fluid intake (240 ml/h for 8–10 h) and a mild cathartic.
3. Sigmoidoscopy: to visualize directly the rectum and sigmoid colon. The colon is cleansed before the examination. Cathartics and enemas may be used for this purpose. A sigmoidoscope, an inflexible, straight instrument, is then inserted. The client will experience some cramping and discomfort during the procedure.
4. Colonoscopy: direct visualization of the entire colon through the use of a flexible fiberscope. The procedure and preparation are similar to those for sigmoidoscopy. The client is given clear liquids for a few days before the procedure is performed. Biopsies are often taken at the same time. Because these clients are often tense, the nurse must be most supportive when preparing them for each test. Careful, clear explanations may be helpful.

NURSING DIAGNOSES: ACTUAL OR POTENTIAL

1. Alteration in comfort due to cramping pain in lower abdomen that worsens before bowel movements.
2. Alteration in bowel elimination patterns characterized by frequent loose stools, often containing blood, mucus, and pus, possibly secondary to stress or ingestion of an irritating food.
3. Alteration in comfort resulting from moderate temperature elevation due to pain.
4. Impairment of mobility due to fatigue and inability to maintain normal activity level secondary to poor appetite and anemia.
5. Alteration in nutrition characterized by deficit due to malnourishment or anorexia.
6. Alteration in fluid balance due to severe diarrhea, possibly resulting in dehydration.

7. Alteration in tissue integrity characterized by potential for inflammation in the eyes, joints, skin, and/or liver.
8. Maladaptive coping patterns due to feelings of helplessness in stressful situations and lack of strong, supporting, interpersonal relationships.

EXPECTED OUTCOMES

1. Frequency of stools will decrease, and consistency will increase.
2. Fluid balance will be restored, and fluid losses will not exceed fluid intake.
3. Body temperature will return to normal.
4. Pain will be relieved.
5. Client will engage in mild physical activity without fatigue.
6. Extracolonic inflammations will be relieved.
7. Client will gradually gain weight over a specified period of time.
8. Client will adhere to care plan by:
   a. Gaining weight as recommended.
   b. Adhering to medication regimen, as indicated by record kept by client.
   c. Increasing activity tolerance and avoiding overexertion.
   d. Adhering to dietary restrictions, as evidenced by lack of diarrheal attacks associated with diet.
   e. Increasing ability to identify and manage stress.

INTERVENTIONS

1. Administer prescribed anti-inflammatory drugs. Salicylazosulfapyridine (Azulfidine) is used most frequently, although its mode of action is not known. When use of this fails or if diarrhea is severe, corticosteroids may be used.
2. Administer prescribed anticholinergic drugs to decrease spasm and pain. Antidiarrhetics are used to increase the stool consistency.
3. Provide adequate rest, as physical activity increases intestinal motility. A mild tranquilizer may promote general body relaxation.
4. Administer prescribed analgesic drugs to help reduce pain. Opiates should be avoided because of their addicting effect. A hot water bottle to the abdomen may promote comfort. If the anus is sore and excoriated, a cortisone-containing ointment may be used; sitz baths may be soothing.
5. Give blood transfusions if indicated. Observe client for signs of transfusion reaction (e.g., rash, urticaria) (see Chapter 49).
6. Give NPO initially. Supplement calories, electrolytes, and vitamins intravenously. As improvement occurs, fluids and then food are given orally. Serum electrolytes should be monitored and signs of dehydration noted.
7. A preliminary trial with thalidomide employing strict birth control measures has shown marked improvement of colitis (Waters et al., 1979), but more extensive research is needed before its usefulness can be established.
8. Administer total parenteral nutrition (TPN) if protein losses from the bowel are severe. Infusion of a highly concentrated solution of amino acids, dextrose, electrolytes, vitamins, and trace elements into a large vein (e.g., the superior vena cava) is given, usually supplemented with isotonic emulsion solutions through a peripheral vein. The technique of administration varies, but all procedures include:
   a. Maintenance of absolutely sterile technique (including the use of gowns, masks, and gloves).
   b. Changing of all external tubing at least every other day.
   c. Careful observation of the client for signs of inflammation, including redness, pain, swelling at the catheter site, and body temperature elevation because of the danger of infection and/or thromboembolus. If drainage is present, culture the infection site.
   d. Changing dressing daily or as the institution prescribes.
   e. Cleaning skin around catheter site and using an antibiotic ointment (Betadine) as prescribed.
   f. Covering the catheter with a sterile dressing and securing carefully.
   g. Weighing the client daily.
   h. Careful monitoring before, during, and after infusion. Hyperglycemia occurs during infusion and rebound hypoglycemia is frequently seen when TPN is discontinued.
   i. When the dose of TPN approaches the

client's energy requirements, appetite suppression results and persists for a period after TPN is stopped. Appetite is not affected when the dose is 30 percent or less of the client's requirements (DeSomery and Hansen, 1978).

9. Progress and educate about diet after initial period. Explain components and purpose of a high-calorie, high-protein, low-residue diet. Roughage is avoided to minimize mechanical irritation. Chemically irritating foods should be avoided. Clients with a history of milk intolerance should restrict their milk intake. Iron may also be supplemented orally.
10. Reassure client and provide explanations of the disease and modes of treatment during the acute stage. Minimize emotional stress. Psychiatric consultation may be indicated, and individual, group, or family therapy may be beneficial. Occasionally, antidepressant drugs may be given.

EVALUATION

Outcome Criteria

1. Client has 1–3 soft to semisoft formed stools per day.
2. Fluid balance is restored as evidenced by laboratory tests and physical signs (skin turgor, moist mucous membranes, etc.).
3. Client is relatively pain free and does not need analgesic medication. Inflammations from extracolonic manifestations are relieved.
4. Client is able to tolerate moderate activity without fatigue.
5. Client complies with therapeutic plan, as indicated by written record of medications taken at appropriate times and in correct amounts and adherence to dietary restrictions, manifested by a 2½-lb weight gain every 2 weeks.

Complications

CANCER OF THE COLON

Clients with the disease for 10 years or longer are more susceptible. Usually detected through regular sigmoid oscopy (see *Colorectal Tumors*).

RECTAL FISSURES, FISTULAE, AND ABCESSES

A fissure is a cracklike sore, a rectal fistula is a tubelike passage from the rectum to surrounding tissue, and an abscess is a collection of pus.

Assessment

1. Burning associated with defecation.
2. Bright red blood in stool.
3. Drainage of pus.
4. Palpable abscess.

Revised Outcomes

1. Pain associated with defecation will be relieved.
2. Infection will be healed.
3. Other expected outcomes will occur as stated for *Ulcerative Colitis*.

Interventions

1. Surgical incision and drainage of abscess.
2. Surgical excision of associated fistulae.

INTESTINAL OBSTRUCTION

Occurs as lumen of colon narrows from fibrosis, perforation, hemorrhage, toxic megacolon (rapid dilation of transverse colon as motor function becomes paralyzed), and failure of intestines to respond to treatment.

Assessment

1. Obstruction (see *Intestinal Obstructions*).
2. Perforation (see *Peptic Ulcers*).
3. Hemorrhage (see Chapters 48 and 49).
4. Megacolon: marked abdominal distension and weak bowel sounds (see Chapter 22).
5. Failure to respond: unrelieved diarrhea, weight loss, fluid loss, and so on.

Revised Outcomes

1. Acute condition of client will be stabilized.
2. General resistance will be improved.

Interventions

1. Surgical intervention indicated in 15–40 percent of hospitalized clients. The procedure is usually permanent and involves total colectomy and ileostomy. The colon and rectum are removed, and the end of the ileum used to create an opening to the abdomen (see Figure 33-7b). Recently, the continent ileostomy, with an intra-abdominal pouch and an artificial sphincter, has been developed (see Figure 33-7e).
   a. Preoperative care involves increasing the client's resistance with blood, albumin, electrolytes, vitamins, diet, and/or total parenteral nutrition, as needed, and cleansing the bowel. Oral antibiotics may be used to "sterilize" the bowel. Clients should be prepared for the drastic change in elimination. Teaching should include anatomy and physiology, with visualiza-

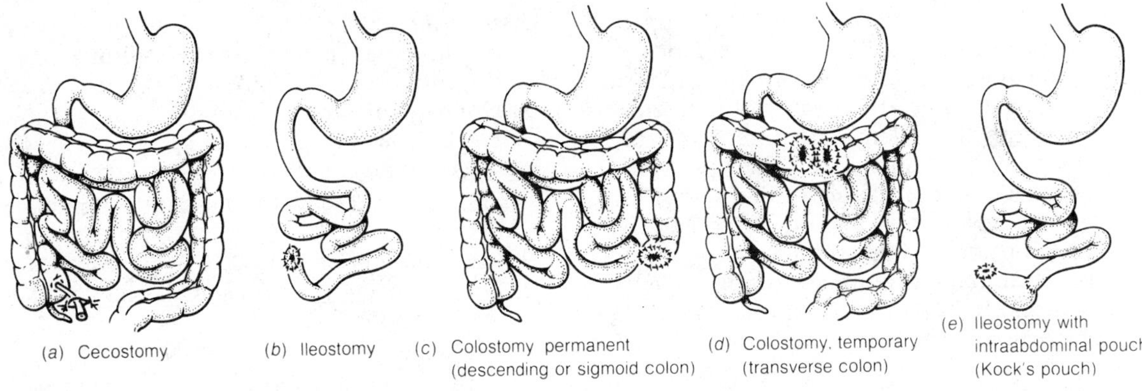

Figure 33-7 Various procedures for fecal diversion. (From Jones, D.A., et al., eds.: *Medical-Surgical Nursing: A Conceptual Approach*, 2d ed., McGraw-Hill, New York, 1982.)

tion of planned changes. Often, a visit from another client with an ileostomy is helpful.

b. Postoperatively the client will have an abdominal wound, the stoma, and a perineal wound. Nothing will be given orally, and a nasogastric tube will be in place until bowel sounds return. Measures to relieve pain should also be implemented.

2. Teach about ileostomy care:
   a. A close-fitting appliance after the stomal edema has subsided. Drainage from an ileostomy is generally semiliquid to soft and continuous, making a permanent appliance necessary.
   b. Care of skin around the stoma will be needed to prevent skin breakdown. It should be cleaned, rinsed, and dried well, and a protective covering (such as *Sterculia* powder or rings) applied.
   c. No specific dietary restrictions. Foods that had a laxative effect prior to surgery should be avoided. It is often best to add foods to the diet one at a time so that intolerance can be pinpointed and eliminated. Clients with a continent ileostomy may find that mushrooms, peanuts, lettuce, and corn tend to plug the ileostomy.
   d. Resumption of normal activities of work, socialization, and sexual relationships.

Outcome Criteria
1. Client is able to manage the ostomy.
2. Client and family adjust to changes.
3. Client is financially able to obtain equipment.
4. Nutritional status is maintained at optimal level.

Reevaluation and Follow-up
Essential.

CHOLECYSTITIS

DESCRIPTION

Cholecystitis is an inflammation of the gallbladder that usually results from the presence of gallstones (cholelithiasis). Most commonly, a stone becomes impacted in the neck of the gallbladder or cystic duct, interfering with gallbladder emptying and resulting in inflammation. Initially, the inflammation is chemical, resulting from the action of bile. The normal bacterial flora soon proliferate, and infection ensues. The associated edema causes vascular congestion, with the development of thromboses and eventual infarction. The presence of the gallstone itself results in ischemia, necrosis, and ulceration.

PREVENTION

Health Promotion
1. Avoid high-fat diet.
2. Maintain proper weight.
3. Avoid lithogenic drugs such as estrogen and clofibrate, which double the risk.

Population at Risk
1. Incidence increases with age.
2. Obese persons.
3. Women twice as susceptible as men.
4. Persons with hemolytic disease or cirrhosis.

Screening

1. Dietary history.
2. Height and weight evaluation.

ASSESSMENT

Health History

1. History of cholelithiasis or cholecystitis.
2. Dietary history and fat content in the diet.
3. Onset of discomfort often related to ingestion of a heavy, fatty meal.
4. Pain called biliary colic: initial episodes are often mild, characterized by a constant epigastric ache or mild indigestion. As the inflammation becomes acute, the pain steadily increases in severity. Complaints of extreme pain (worse in the right upper quadrant and radiating to the shoulder or subscapular area) are common.
5. Anorexia: may have nausea and/or vomiting.
6. Dark urine with common bile duct obstruction and clay-colored stools.
7. Increased weight above normal parameters.

Physical Assessment

1. Palpable gallbladder may be felt as a tender mass.
2. Guarding during abdominal exam secondary to abdominal pain is often present.
3. Discomfort is present with fist percussion over the liver.
4. Abdominal distension and absence of bowel sounds are noted if inflammation is severe enough to cause paralytic ileus.
5. Slight icterus is common; more severe jaundice usually indicates obstruction of the common bile duct by calculi or edema.
6. Temperature is elevated secondary to infection.
7. Mild tachycardia and hypotension present if complications have not developed.
8. Splinting during respirations may result from severe pain.
9. Rales may be hard at the bases of the lungs.

Diagnostic Tests

1. Oral cholecystography to visualize the gallbladder. The client is given an oral radiopaque substance, such as isopanoic acid (Telepaque), sodium ipodate (Oragrafin), or sodium tyropanoate (Bilopaque), which concentrates in the gallbladder, making it visible on x-ray film. Usually, 6 tablets are given, preferably at 5-min intervals, the evening before, although the test must often be repeated for adequate visualization. Some authorities recommend giving 6 tablets the day before over a 6-h period and preceding their administration with a meal containing fat to maximize absorption. Nonvisualization after the second test is indicative of impairment in bile excretion.
2. Intravenous cholangiography visualizes the gallbladder by means of an intravenous dye containing iodine.
3. Percutaneous cholangiography involves injecting the dye directly into a bile duct using a long, spinal-type needle. Fluoroscopy shows ductal filling and localizes obstructions.
4. Endoscopic retrograde cholangiopancreatography (ERCP) involves insertion of a flexible fiberscope into the small intestine and passage of a cannula through the scope to the ampulla of Vater and into the bile duct. Obstructions can be directly visualized.
5. Ultrasonic scanning to detect calculi.
6. Techetium-99m-pyridoxylidine glutamate scanning to visualize gallbladder: cholecystitis confirmed if the isotope is visible in the small bowel but the gallbladder is not seen.
7. Laboratory tests
   a. Leukocyte count elevated secondary to the inflammation.
   b. Slight hyperbilirubinemia.
   c. Serum alkaline phosphatase elevated with bile obstruction.
   d. Serum glutamic-oxaloacetic transaminase (SGOT) and lactic dehydrogenase (LDH) levels elevated.
   e. Serum cholesterol elevated with bile obstruction.
   f. Urine bilirubin levels may be elevated.
   g. Urobilinogen in the feces decreased.

NURSING DIAGNOSES: ACTUAL OR POTENTIAL

1. Alterations in comfort due to pain, often severe, especially in the right upper quadrant and radiating to the shoulder; temperature elevated with occasional chills secondary to inflammatory response.
2. Nutritional deficit due to loss of appetite, fatty foods tolerated poorly, and nausea with occasional vomiting.
3. Respiratory dysfunction characterized by

shallow breathing secondary to abdominal pain and leading to chest congestion.

4. Impairment of skin integrity characterized by slight jaundice, making the skin susceptible to breakdown.
5. Alteration in comfort due to itching secondary to pronounced jaundice.
6. Mild to severe anxiety secondary to worsening pain and fear of possible surgery.

EXPECTED OUTCOMES

1. Pain will be relieved and temperature will return to normal 2–5 days after treatment.
2. Nausea will be relieved, and there will be no further episodes of vomiting.
3. Respirations will increase in depth, and secretions will be removed from lungs with productive coughing.
4. Skin integrity will be maintained.
5. Itching will be relieved (eased), and scratching will be minimized.
6. Client will verbalize fears, especially in relation to surgery, if needed.
7. Client will comply with care plan, as manifested by:
   a. Adhering to dietary restrictions.
   b. Losing weight as recommended.

INTERVENTIONS

1. Administer NPO to minimize gallbladder stimulation.
2. Insert nasogastric tube (see Figure 33-3) to relieve nausea and vomiting and keep the stomach empty.
3. Administer antiemetics as prescribed to relieve nausea and vomiting.
4. Administer parenteral meperidine as prescribed to control pain (morphine is avoided because of its strong spasmogenic effect on the bile duct).
5. Administer anticholinergic drugs as prescribed to decrease secretion and muscle spasm.
6. Administer parenteral fluids to meet nutritional needs and replace fluid losses from the edema, nasogastric tube, diaphoresis, and kidney.
7. Encourage bed rest to promote healing (75 percent of cases will remit in 1–4 days).
8. Gradually increase intake to a high-carbohydrate, high-protein, low-fat diet.
9. Administer replacement therapy with oral bile salts for clients with intolerance to fatty foods; administer fat-soluble vitamin supplements.
10. Administer antibiotics that concentrate well in the biliary tract as prescribed (e.g., ampicillin, tetracycline, or a cephalosporin) to decrease infection.
11. Encourage deep breathing and coughing to clear lungs (splinting the abdomen may help reduce resulting pain). Position should be changed frequently to prevent respiratory congestion and skin breakdown.
12. Discourage itching. Cholestyramine resin may be helpful in lessening pruritus. Frequent skin care will also be helpful.
13. Administer chenodeoxycholic acid, an experimental drug, as prescribed to dissolve cholesterol stones (investigations have combined chenodeoxycholic acid and β-sitosterol and chenodeoxycholic acid and lecithin.
14. Teach about a decrease in fat intake, avoidance of fatty foods, and weight reduction as needed.
15. Surgical intervention considered the immediate treatment of choice by some authorities.
    a. Cholecystectomy (removal of the gallbladder), often accompanied by choledochotomy (exploration and drainage of the common bile duct). Cholecystotomy (removal of stones from the gallbladder) is performed if the client is unable to tolerate a more extensive procedure.
    b. Postoperative care.
       (1) Drains often inserted during surgery to determine whether bile is leaking; they are removed in 4–5 days.
       (2) T tube (see Figure 33-8) often placed in the common bile duct and left in place for 7–10 days to ensure patency of duct.
       (3) Provide skin care to area around the T tube.
       (4) Teach about:
          (a) Avoidance of fatty meals. Following cholecystectomy, bile production continues, discharged into the intestine at a somewhat constant rate.
          (b) Supplementation with fat-soluble

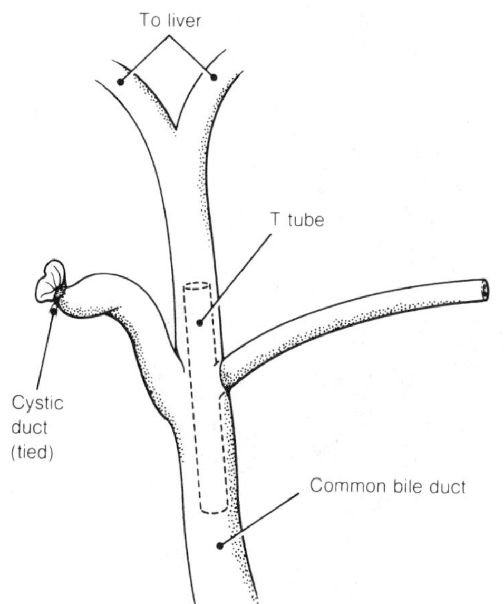

Figure 33-8 The T tube. (From Jones, D.A., et al., eds.: *Medical-Surgical Nursing: A Conceptual Approach*, 2d ed., McGraw-Hill, New York, 1982.)

vitamins because of the decrease in absorption.
(c) Weight reduction if indicated.

EVALUATION

Outcome Criteria

1. Pain is relieved, and client has no further episodes of biliary colic.
2. Client has no further nausea or vomiting.
3. Cough is productive initially as respiratory depth increases; then cough decreases and lungs are clear.
4. Skin integrity is maintained, and client does not scratch in response to itching.
5. Client avoids fatty foods and high-fat meals, as evidenced by lack of episodes of pain and/or indigestion.
6. Client loses $2\frac{1}{2}$ lb every 2 weeks until ideal weight is attained.
7. Surgical wound heals, and drains are removed.

Complications

1. Recurrence of cholecystitis (see discussion above).
2. Acute perforation with peritonitis (see *Peptic Ulcers*).
3. Subacute perforation with abscess formation.
4. Biliary fistula formation.
5. Pancreatitis (see *Acute Pancreatitis*).

ACUTE PANCREATITIS

DESCRIPTION

Acute pancreatitis is a severe, incapacitating illness characterized by inflammation of the pancreas. Its genesis involves the activation of pancreatic proteolytic and lipolytic enzymes within the pancreas, resulting in autodigestion of pancreatic tissue. Initially, the inflammation results in edema, but as venous congestion develops, pancreatic necrosis results. As enzymatic action destroys tissue, vessels can become involved and hemorrhage can occur. Lipases are liberated from the pancreas, and fat necrosis often develops (see Figure 33-9). It usually involves the pancreas and surrounding fatty tissue but can become widespread. As necrotic tissue builds up, infection becomes an increasing danger. The exact mechanism involved in the development of acute pancreatitis is not known, although several etiologic factors have been implicated. These include pancreatic duct obstruction, biliary tract disease, infection, ischemia, drugs, hypersensitivity reactions, autoimmune phenomena, alcoholism, mumps, and trauma. In 10–15 percent of cases, no cause is evident.

PREVENTION

Health Promotion

1. Avoid excess alcohol consumption.
2. Avoid abdominal trauma.

Population at Risk

1. Adults, most frequently over age 40.
2. Alcoholics.
3. Persons with a history of gallbladder disease or mumps.

ASSESSMENT

Health History

1. Intense upper abdominal pain in the area of the epigastrium or in the left or right upper quadrant. The pain is usually steady and may

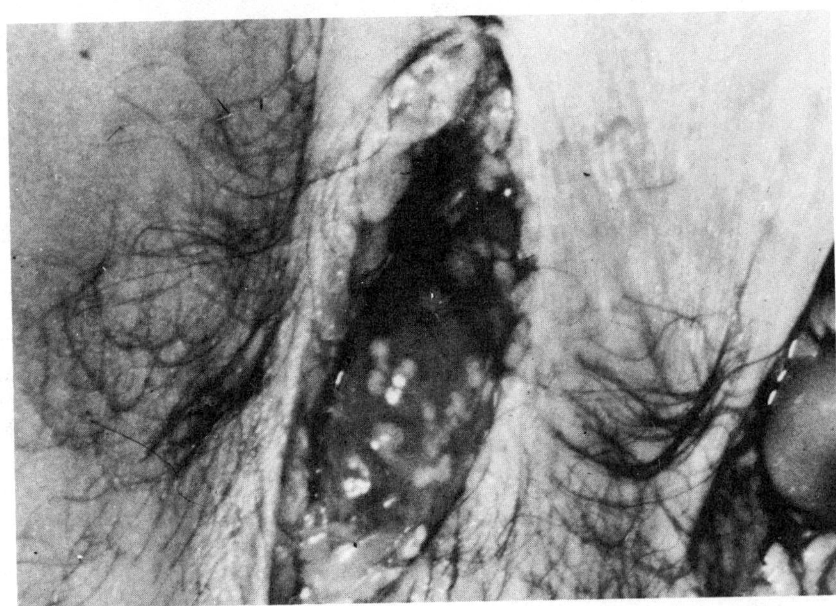

Figure 33-9 Fat necrosis on the external surface of a femoral hernia sac in a client who died of acute pancreatitis. (From Bogoch, A.: *Gastroenterology*, McGraw-Hill, New York, 1973.)

be referred to the area of the twelfth thoracic vertebra. Initially, the pain is localized but after a time may diffuse to the back, chest, or lower abdomen.

2. Client may be too distressed to respond to questions, and the family may have to be questioned regarding onset. The pain often develops after a large meal or significant alcohol intake.
3. Vomiting, often forceful, which continues after the stomach is empty and causes an increase in pain.
4. History of excess alcohol consumption or gallbladder disease may be present.

Physical Assessment

1. Restlessness, distress, and apprehension will be noted.
2. Persons may be curled up with both arms over the abdomen to relieve pain.
3. Guarding in the epigastrium will be evident during the abdominal exam.
4. Abdominal distension and tenderness on deep palpation will be present. Rebound tenderness will also be present.
5. Boardlike rigidity of the abdominal wall will be evident as the inflammation becomes more widespread.
6. Bowel sounds are diminished or, if paralytic ileus has developed, absent.
7. Signs of hypovolemia and shock as fluid losses to edema are marked. Skin often appears mottled and feels cold and moist. Tachycardia is present, and blood pressure falls.
8. Turner's sign, a blue-green-brown discoloration in the flanks from blood accumulation, or Cullen's sign, a similar discoloration around the umbilicus, may be seen 3–6 days after onset and results from hemorrhage.
9. Respirations are often shallow and rapid. Rales may be heard in the lower lobes, and pleural effusion, especially on the left side, may develop.
10. Temperature is usually elevated after a few days.
11. Jaundice may become evident, and urine may darken if edema compresses the common bile duct. Stool specimens are often difficult to examine because constipation is present.

Diagnostic Tests

1. Serum amylase commonly increased above 250 Somogyi units; begins to return to normal after 48 h.

2. Serum lipase elevated.
3. Hypocalcemia, with widespread fat necrosis.
4. Serum calcium may be low.
5. Blood glucose elevation from islet cell damage.
6. Hemoconcentration and an increase in the hematocrit secondary to fluid losses to the edema.
7. White blood cells increased.
8. X-ray examination of the abdomen will reveal gaseous distention, and calcification of the pancreas from previous inflammations may be seen.
9. Chest x-ray film will show an elevation on the left side of the diaphragm, and left pleural effusion may be seen.

NURSING DIAGNOSES: ACTUAL OR POTENTIAL

1. Alteration in comfort due to constant, severe, upper abdominal pain that radiates to the back and elevated temperature.
2. Nutritional deficit due to forceful vomiting, with retching, that increases pain; hyperglycemia from impaired glucose metabolism.
3. Fluid volume deficit due to fluid loss secondary to the edema and vomiting and potential hypovolemia.
4. Alteration in fluid electolyte balance due to tetany secondary to hypocalcemia.
5. Respiratory dysfunction characterized by restricted chest expansion secondary to pain, resulting in shallow respirations and potential congestion.
6. Fear secondary to pain and anxiety and fear of outcome.
7. Decreased activity tolerance due to generalized weakness and pain.

EXPECTED OUTCOMES

1. Pain will be eased during acute stage of pancreatitis and then relieved.
2. Vomiting will be relieved, then eliminated.
3. Fluid and electrolyte balance and blood volume will be restored and/or maintained, as evidenced by vital signs within normal limits and the serum calcium level.
4. Ventilatory capacity will be increased as pain is relieved; breath sounds will remain clear.
5. Body temperature will return to normal.
6. Cellular nutrition will be maintained, as evidenced by blood glucose levels within normal limits.
7. Client will understand various procedures and verbalize feats associated with this altered health state.
8. Evidence of compliance with long-range care plan evidenced by:
   a. Verbalizing adherence to dietary restrictions.
   b. Reports of taking medications as prescribed.
   c. Keeping follow-up appointments.

INTERVENTIONS

1. Give intravenous plasma, human serum albumin, electrolyte solutions and/or whole blood to maintain blood volume.
2. Monitor vital signs, hematocrit, central venous pressure, and urine output to titrate intravenous therapy.
3. Place on a cardiac monitor to observe for changes in cardiac rhythm (see Chapter 30).
4. Administer meperidine to control pain. Opiates are avoided because they cause spasm of the sphincter of Oddi. Pentazocine may also be used. If maximum doses of meperidine are not effective, however, morphine must be considered.
5. Position client on one side, with the knees and back flexed to ease pain. A sedative given in conjunction with the analgesic is often helpful. On rare occasions, a nerve block is used to relieve the pain.
6. Encourage deep breathing and coughing, and change position frequently to avoid pulmonary congestion. Intermittent positive-pressure breathing may be helpful.
7. Insert a nasogastric tube with intermittent suction to keep the stomach empty, relieve distension, and decrease gastric acid stimulation of pancreatic secretions.
8. Give NPO. Antacids may be administered through the nasogastric tube to further decrease gastric acidity.
9. Administer medications to decrease pancreatic secretions. Acetazolamide (Diamox), a carbonic anhydrase inhibitor, decreases the volume and bicarbonate concentration of pancreatic secretions. Anticholinergics may also be used to decrease pancreatic secretion. The use of glucagon is being investigated. It decreases enzyme, protein, and bi-

carbonate secretion from the pancreas, as well as gastric acid production. Aprotinin (Trasylol), an antiproteolytic substance that inhibits kallikrein, chymotrypsin, and trypsin, may also be given, but its use is not fully established (Regan, 1979).

10. Administer antibiotics as prescribed to treat or prevent infection.
11. Monitor serum calcium level and give calcium gluconate as prescribed.
12. Administer intravenous corticosteroids as prescribed if shock does not respond to intravascular volume replacement.
13. Monitor urine and serum glucose levels and give insulin as prescribed to control hyperglycemia.
14. Give sips of water after initial fasting period; progress diet to carbohydrate drinks as tolerated.
15. After pain has subsided for at least 1 week, progress diet to low-fat intake of small, frequent meals.
16. Avoid a high-carbohydrate diet with concentrated sweets and refined sugar. Avoid alcohol and caffeine.
17. Supplement with enteric-coated pancreatic digestive enzymes, if indicated, when pancreatic destruction has been extensive.
18. Teach about:
    a. Dietary restrictions and medication schedule.
    b. The disease process.
    c. Signs and symptoms of diabetes.
19. Surgery is avoided unless the client fails to improve or complications develop. Procedures may involve cleansing the peritoneal cavity, draining the area of the pancreas, or relieving compression in the bilary tract. More extensive procedures include opening the pancreatic duct and anastomosing it to the jejunum or removing part or almost all of the pancreas (pancreatectomy).

EVALUATION

Outcome Criteria

1. Pain is eased initially; then client is pain free.
2. Vomiting terminates initially; eventually a low-fat diet can be tolerated.
3. Client breathes deeply; breath sounds remain clear.
4. Blood volume is maintained, as indicated by stabilization of vital signs.
5. Serum chemistries are maintained within normal limits, as indicated by calcium and glucose levels.
6. Body temperature returns to normal.
7. Anxiety is decreased, as evidenced by cooperation with procedures, questioning, and seeking counseling as needed.
8. Client can list dietary restrictions and adheres to them, as evidenced by no episodes of indigestion or pain.
9. Client takes medications at appropriate times and in correct amounts, as indicated by client's records.
10. Client can list signs and symptoms of diabetes mellitus.

Complications

1. Recurrence and development of chronic pancreatitis.
2. Diabetes mellitus (see Chapter 28).
3. Abscesses from infection 2–4 weeks after attack, manifested by upper abdominal pain, mass or tenderness, fever, and abdominal distention. The goal of care is to relieve the accumulation of pus through surgery and to reverse infection. Follow-up and reevaluation are essential. The mortality rate is 50 percent.
4. Pancreatic pseudocyst: fluid-containing cavity attached to or surrounding the pancreas. The problem is assessed through identification of abdominal pain, usually epigastric, which may also be felt in the back; nausea and vomiting; upper abdominal fullness; anorexia; and weight loss. The problem may resolve spontaneously, but surgical drainage procedures may be necessary to relieve fluid accumulation.
5. Pancreaticocolonic fistula occurs after severe, protracted inflammation and is manifested by diarrhea, fever, hematochezia, disappearing abdominal mass, and rectal bleeding. The goal of care is to prevent hemorrhage and infections and to close the fistula through surgery. There is a high mortality rate if the problem is not diagnosed early. Fulminating sepsis is common.

Reevaluation and Follow-up
Essential.

CHRONIC PANCREATITIS

Chronic pancreatitis is a long-term inflammation of the pancreas. It usually begins after 30 to 40 years of age and is found in men more often than in women. Many factors have been implicated as causative agents. The most common of these is chronic alcohol ingestion; other causes include biliary tract disease and trauma. Symptoms usually develop in two stages. Initially, the inflammation causes an acute episode, with attacks of abdominal pain. As chronicity develops, the pain becomes constant. Significant portions of the pancreas are destroyed, and its production of endocrine (insulin and glucagon) and exocrine hormones (pancreatic enzymes) becomes impaired. Digestion is incomplete, with azotorrhea and steatorrhea, characterized by bulky, frothy, glistening, foul-smelling stools. Weight loss occurs, and complaints of nausea, vomiting, a feeling of fullness, and abdominal distension are common. Diabetes mellitus results from the endocrine disorder.

Nursing care and treatment during an acute attack are similar to those during acute pancreatitis (see above). Care during chronic disease must focus on avoidance of alcohol. A bland, low-fat diet will be given, and pancreatic extracts will be used to improve digestion. Overeating should be avoided, and anticholinergics may relieve pain. Cimetidine, an H_2-receptor antagonist, has been used successfully in conjunction with propantheline to reduce gastric acid and therefore its stimulation of secretin, but its safety is still questioned. Because of the chronic nature of the disease, narcotics are avoided. Vitamin and electrolyte supplements are given as needed. Diabetes mellitus is treated if present (refer to Chapter 28). Follow-up care is essential.

HEPATITIS

DESCRIPTION

Hepatitis may be defined as an inflammation of the liver. When caused by a substance that is toxic to the liver, it is called toxic or drug-induced hepatitis. Some of the offending agents include industrial toxins, such as carbon tetrachloride and yellow phosphorus, the toxin associated with mushroom poisoning, halothane, diphenylhydantoin, α-methyldopa, chlorthiazide, and oxyphenisatin. The more common type of hepatitis involves viral infection. The most common types are hepatitis A and hepatitis B. A third viral type, sometimes referred to as type C or non-A, non-B hepatitis, has also emerged; it appears to be associated with blood transfusions, has a variable incubation period (usually 6–7 weeks), and is less severe than type B hepatitis. The pathologic changes observed in all hepatitis involve inflammation of the liver with hepatic cell necrosis, interference with regenerative activity, Kupffer cell hyperplasia and varying degrees of bile stasis. Symptoms of the infection usually progress through three phases: prodromal phase, icteric stage, and recovery period.

Type A viral hepatitis may be called infectious hepatitis, short-incubation hepatitis, MS-1 hepatitis, or epidemic hepatitis. The type A virus is usually transmitted through the fecal-oral route, although parenteral transmission can occur. After entry into the body, its incubation period is 15–50 days before symptoms begin. Type A occurs throughout the world but is most common in areas with poor sanitation facilities. It occurs most often in the fall and early winter. Type B viral hepatitis has been called serum hepatitis, long-incubation hepatitis, MS-2 hepatitis, and Australia antigen-positive hepatitis. The incubation period for type B is 50–180 days. It is most frequently transmitted when the blood of an infected person comes in contact with the blood or mucous membrane of another person. This can occur with transfusions, needle puncture, skin cut, sexual intercourse, hemodialysis, kissing, and so on. Type B hepatitis can also be transmitted through the fecal–oral route. Types A and B hepatitis differ in onset. With type A, it is often sudden and febrile, while the prodromal phase with type B is usually insidious and fever is seldom evident. Morbidity and mortality are greater with type B.

PREVENTION

Health Promotion

1. Avoid crowded, unsanitary living conditions.
2. Support and stimulate programs that:
   a. Regulate sanitation and housing standards.
   b. Regulate persons who work with food.
   c. Enforce drug laws.
   d. Help drug addicts.
   e. Regulate industrial exposure to toxins.
   f. Solicit blood donations from healthy donors.
3. Support and stimulate research into screening tests for potential blood donors.
4. Give gammaglobulin (human immune serum

globulin, or ISG) to persons exposed to type A hepatitis during the incubation period to stimulate antibody production and provide immunity for 6–8 weeks (usually 0.02–0.05 mL/kg of body weight).
5. Give hyperimmune (anti-HB_s) gammaglobulin within 7 days of needle stick when hepatitis B virus (HBV) is suspected.
6. Research currently being done on a formalin-treated vaccine for HBV (Kiernan and Ramgopal, 1979).

Population at Risk

1. Children and young adults more frequently affected.
2. Drug addicts.
3. Persons living in crowded, unsanitary conditions.
4. Persons exposed to injury by contaminated needles (e.g., health care workers).
5. Institutionalized persons and military personnel living in group shelters.
6. Tourists and foreign service workers. Ingestion of shellfish (e.g., snails) from contaminated water.
7. Persons needing blood transfusions, especially clients with uremia or lymphoma or those taking immunosuppressants.

Screening

1. Test potential transfusion blood for HBV.
2. HB_sAg by radioimmunoassay or enzyme immunoassay to detect HBV.

ASSESSMENT

Health History

1. Possible exposure to hepatitis (onset type A 15–50 days, type B 45–180 days).
   a. Contact with jaundiced persons.
   b. Recent camping trips where there is poor sanitation.
   c. Shellfish ingestion, especially from contaminated waters.
   d. Traveling in areas outside the United States where sanitation is poor.
   e. Seasonal type A: high in winter and fall. Type B: year round.
   f. Blood transfusions in the last 6 months.
   g. Recent ear piercing or tattooing.
   h. Occupational exposure (e.g., nursing entails risk of contact with persons with hepatitis).
   i. Living quarters, large population, unsanitary conditions, poor storage of food, or poor removal of excreta.
   j. Any drugs taken (e.g., heroin) under conditions with potential for needle contamination.
2. Prodromal phase (preicteric phase) usually lasts 3–4 days but may extend to 2 weeks or more.
   a. Anorexia, fatigue, malaise, and lassitude.
   b. Nausea, vomiting, and diarrhea.
   c. Aversion to food and distaste of cigarettes.
   d. Fullness or discomfort in the epigastrium or right upper quadrant late in this phase.
   e. Fever and flulike symptoms, especially with type A.
   f. Skin rash, urticaria, angioneurotic edema, or polyarthritis occasionally occur.
   g. Darkened urine, a lighter stool color, and some itching during last few days of this stage.
3. Icteric phase.
   a. Jaundice, becomes maximum in 1–2 weeks and lasts 6–8 weeks.
   b. Client feels better, with the gastrointestinal symptoms and fever decreasing.
   c. Anicteric hepatitis is infrequent.
4. Recovery period lasts 3–4 months, during which the client finds that he or she fatigues easily.

Physical Assessment

1. Temperature may be mildly elevated during the prodromal phase.
2. Weight loss commonly occurs.
3. Liver is usually tender and palpable 2–3 cm below the costal margin. Liver size begins to decrease 1–2 weeks after the onset of jaundice.
4. Jaundice is present and is best observed in the sclera of the eyes.

Diagnostic Tests

1. Liver function tests (see Table 33-3).
2. Serum hepatitis B antigen (Hb_sAg, Australia antigen) distinguishes type A from type B hepatitis. During the incubation and early acute phase, 80 percent of clients with type B hepatitis have this antigen circulating in their serum.
3. The serum of clients who have had hepatitis A will contain antibody to the hepatitis A antigen (anti-HA). The anti-HA titer increases late in the course of hepatitis A but is not a definitive diagnostic tool.

TABLE 33-3 TESTS OF LIVER FUNCTION

Test	Normal	Comment
Blood Clotting and Blood Cell Count		
Prothrombin time	12–15 s	Prothrombin time is the most important test in assessing liver pathology. In liver disease, blood takes longer to clot due to decreased ability of the liver to synthesize the protein prothrombin. Also, there is decreased absorption of vitamin K, which is essential for prothrombin synthesis. Failure of the liver to return the prothrombin time to normal in presence of vitamin K indicates clinically significant liver cell damage. The degree of liver impairment can fairly accurately be estimated by the degree of prothrombin abnormality.
Hematocrit	35–45%	
WBC	5,000–10,000 cells/mm^3	Count is normal early in cirrhosis and hepatitis. Leukopenia with enlarged, overactive spleen. Leukopenia accompanies fever in hepatitis.
Clearance Studies		
Indocyanine green (ICG) Bromsulphalein (BSP)	Less than 5% remaining in serum 45 min after injection of 5 mg/kg body weight	Procedure: client fasts for 12 h before test. Dose is reduced if clinical symptoms already present. Dye retained in liver cell damage.
Serum Enzyme Studies		
SGPT	5–35 U/mL	Damage to liver cells causes release of these enzymes into blood, but the increased levels in the serum do not directly correlate with the amount of liver impairment. Elevations occur in other diseases. Blood withdrawn from vein.
SGOT	5–40 U/mL	
LDH	400 U/mL (varies with method used)	
Alkaline phosphatase	2–5 Bodansky units (varies with method)	Synthesized in liver, bone, and kidney and excreted in the biliary tract. A measure of biliary obstruction.
γ-Glutamyl transpeptidase		Enzyme found in biliary tract and not in cardiac or skeletal muscle. Elevated in hepatitis. More sensitive in detecting hepatic disease than alkaline phosphatase.

TABLE 33-3 *(continued)*

Special Tests		
Hepatitis B surface antigen (HB_sAg)		HB_sAg is normally absent from the serum and, if present, is diagnostic for viral hepatitis, type B. Tests for HB_sAg include counterelectrophoresis and radioimmunoassay. Not found in serum of clients with type A viral hepatitis.
Liver scan		Through the injection of a radioactive substance, the therapist can visualize the size and shape of the liver. Serves as a guide for liver biopsy.
Liver biopsy		Used to determine microscopic, cellular pathology of liver cells.
Hepatic hemodynamic studies (in clients with suspected cirrhosis)		Splenoportogram is used to determine the adequacy of portal blood flow. Diminished in cirrhosis. Endoscopy to view esophageal varices. Measurement of portal vein pressure.
Metabolic Studies		
Protein metabolism:		Serum proteins are synthesized by the liver. Serum albumin is markedly decreased in liver cellular damage. Gamma globulin is usually elevated in liver disease and markedly elevated in chronic active liver disease.
Serum albumin	3.5–5.5 g/100 mL	
Plasma fibrinogen	10.2–0.4 g/100 mL	
Serum globulin	2.5–3.5 g/100 mL	
Total protein	6.0–8.0 g/100 mL	
Serum protein electrophoresis:	50–65% of total	
Albumin	4–7.5%	
α_1-globulin	4–7.5%	
α_2-globulin	7–12%	
α_2-globulin	7–12%	
β-globulin	10–20%	
γ-globulin		
Ammonia	30–70% µg/100 mL	In liver disease, less ammonia is converted to urea, and thus the serum ammonia concentration increases.
Carbohydrate metabolism:		
Galactose or glucose tolerance tests	Removed from blood in 1–2 h	Injected intravenously. Serial samples are drawn from the vein. If serum galactose remains elevated after 75 min, liver function is impaired. If serum glucose remains elevated after 1–2 h, the liver cells are damaged or utilization of glucose by body tissues is impaired.

TABLE 33-3 *(continued)*

Metabolic Studies *(continued)*		
Fat metabolism: Serum cholesterol Serum phospholipids Triglycerides	 150–250 mg/100 mL 125–300 mg/100 mL 30–135 mg/100 mL	Blood drawn after low-cholesterol diet. Cholesterol esters 70% of total cholesterol. Lipids decreased in liver parenchymal cell damage, elevated in biliary duct obstruction.
Bilirubin metabolism Serum bilirubin Direct (conjugated soluble) Indirect (not conjugated, not water soluble) Total bilirubin	 0.2 mg/100 mL 0.8 mg/100 mL 1.0 mg/100 mL	Venous blood drawn. Bilirubin is a product of RBC hemoglobin breakdown, and elevation may cause jaundice. Total bilirubin measures both direct and indirect bilirubin. Direct bilirubin elevated with obstructed biliary ducts or impaired excretion of conjugated bilirubin. Indirect bilirubin elevated with accelerated erythrocyte hemolyis, absence of glucuronyl transferase, and/or damaged liver cells.
Urine bilirubin Urobilinogen: Urine Feces	None 0–4 mg/24 h 40–280 mg/24 h	A measure of conjugated bilirubin. If bilirubin present in urine, shaking the specimen results in a yellow tint in the foam. Urinary and fecal urobilinogen decrease with bile duct obstruction. Antibiotics reduce the urobilinogen levels. Fecal urobilinogen seldom measured.

SOURCE: Alyn, I. B.: "Disturbances in Hepatic Function," in Jones, D. A., et al. (eds.): *Medical-Surgical Nursing: A Conceptual Approach*, 2d ed., McGraw-Hill, New York, 1982.

4. SGOT and SGPT elevated 7–14 days prior to jaundice.
5. Direct and indirect bilirubin increased.
6. Bromsulphalein retention mildly increased.
7. Serum alkaline phosphatase mildly increased.
8. Hypoalbuminemia mild.
9. Globulin slightly increased.
10. Leukopenia if fever develops.
11. Urine urobilinogen usually normal initially and later increased.
12. Urine bilirubin increased.
13. Stool bilirubin and urobilinogen decreased.

NURSING DIAGNOSES: ACTUAL OR POTENTIAL

1. Nutritional deficit due to poor appetite, dislike of food, and occasional nausea and vomiting, resulting in weight loss over last few weeks secondary to decreased appetite.
2. Diminished activity and exercise tolerance due to tiring easily, resulting in inability to meet work requirements.
3. Alteration in comfort due to epigastric discomfort, aching in muscles or joints, and/or itching.
4. Alteration in temperature regulation due mild fever secondary to infection.
5. Potential impairment of skin integrity due to jaundice, making skin susceptible to breakdown, and itching.
6. Potential for injury to others through spread of infection.
7. Social isolation due to potential for spreading infection.
8. Role disturbance due to inability to fulfill nor-

mal role functions and to occupy self to avoid boredom.
9. Ineffective coping due to anger and stress resulting from social isolation, the effects of long-term illness, and related lifestyle changes.

EXPECTED OUTCOMES

1. Infection will be confined to client. Persons coming in contact with client will remain free of infection.
2. A gradual weight gain (if indicated) over a specified period of time will be observed.
3. A balanced, alternating rest–mild activity regimen will be established according to tolerance level.
4. Pain will be relieved, and itching will be minimized.
5. Temperature will return to normal 3–4 days after treatment initiated.
6. Skin integrity will be maintained, and pruritus will be relieved.
7. Client will understand isolation restrictions and will engage in activities to occupy self.
8. Individual will express fears, concerns, and frustrations associated with role change and a long-term health problem.

INTERVENTIONS

1. Prevent spread of infection.
   a. Follow procedures to prevent spread from the gastrointestinal or parenteral route, including hand washing; isolation of linen; use of separate toilet facilities, separate or disposable dishes, no communal items (e.g., washcloths and toothbrushes), and disposable needles; and avoiding sexual contact.
   b. Teach all visitors about isolation procedures.
2. Provide adequate rest. Bed rest with bathroom privileges is usually recommended. Stress should be minimized.
3. Promote adequate nutrition, which is essential for liver healing and regeneration. Usually a high-calorie (3,000 cal), high-carbohydrate, high-protein diet in small, frequent feedings is recommended. Fat is usually restricted because of intolerance. Alcohol should be avoided for at least 6 months following the onset of hepatitis.
4. Administer medication as prescribed. Corticosteroids may be used to decrease the inflammation in severe cases. Sedatives and analgesics should be used cautiously; those eliminated through the kidney are preferable. If the prothrombin time is prolonged, vitamin K may be given parenterally.
5. Plan time to discuss client's concerns and to explore and develop strategies to deal with this health problem and its impact on lifestyle.

EVALUATION

Outcome Criteria

1. Infection control is effective, as evidenced by no new cases of infections in persons having contact with client.
2. Client can state isolation procedures and the reasons for the restrictions and cooperates with the procedures, as evidenced by explaining procedures to visitors.
3. Client begins to verbalize gradual increase in activity, along with increased activity tolerance.
4. Client is pain free and does not scratch.
5. Client's temperature is within normal limits.
6. Client has gained weight that was lost (if appropriate) by the end of 4 months.
7. Individual verbalizes fears and concerns associated with illness and develops strategies to cope with changes in lifestyle.

Complications

1. Relapse: 5–25 percent have relapse during first 4 months.
2. Recurrence: clients with type A and B hepatitis generally have a lasting immunity to the specific type (however, clients have been known to develop a second case of hepatitis, suggesting that there may be more than one type A virus).
3. Posthepatitis syndrome develops after an episode of hepatitis and lasts 6–12 months. It is characterized by fatigue, weakness and malaise, anorexia, vague upper abdominal discomfort, and poorly defined gastrointestinal symptoms. Expected outcome criteria are similar to those described above. Continued rest and good nutrition are essential. Follow-up and reevaluation are essential to avoid more life-threatening complications.
4. Postnecrotic cirrhosis (see *Hepatic Cirrhosis*).

ORAL AND PERIORAL INFLAMMATIONS

A variety of inflammations can occur in or around the oral cavity. Gingivitis is an inflammation of the gums. It can result from infectious origin because of poor dental hygiene, such as food debris in the mouth, from excessive dryness of the mouth, or as a manifestation of systemic disease. Chronic, desquamative gingivitis occurs in postmenopausal women. Vincent's angina (trench mouth) is an infectious gingivitis thought to be caused by bacteria that are normally found in the mouth. Local trauma, poor oral hygiene, nutritional deficiencies, and debilitation have been implicated as precipitating factors. It is a malodorous infection with painful ulcers found along the margins of the gums. The ulcers have a punched-out appearance. Regional lymph nodes are often enlarged, salivation is increased, and fever is present. Occasionally, the infection will spread to the cheeks, lips, tongue, palate, and/or pharynx.

Periodontitis involves inflammation of the gums and structures in the periodontal pockets that support the teeth. As the inflammation destroys tissue, the teeth loosen.

Stomatitis is an inflammation of the mouth. Its most common causes are mechanical (e.g., jagged teeth), chemical, or infectious (e.g., virus, bacteria, yeast, mold). It is usually associated with a loss of appetite, halitosis, and increased salivation. Stomatitis medicamentosa can develop as a reaction to drugs, such as iodides, barbiturates, antibiotics, sulfonamides, salicylates, and cytotoxic drugs. Stomatitis venenata is a contact stomatitis that can be caused by cosmetics, mouthwashes, toothpaste, drugs, or snuff. Aphthous stomatitis (canker sores) is the most common mouth inflammation and can occur on the lips, gums, inner surface of the cheeks, palate, tongue, or labia. It is associated with small, reddened macules that form vesicles, necrose, and ulcerate, leaving a lesion with a gray-white base and reddened halo. The lesions are usually painful and heal spontaneously in 1–2 weeks. The cause is not known, but it is most common in young women, often recurs rhythmically, and may be preceded by emotional or physical stress.

Herpes simplex is an inflammation of the mouth caused by the herpes simplex virus, usually consisting of cold sore(s) and fever blister(s). It is often preceded by fever, headache, and malaise. Vesicular lesions develop and progress to multiple, small ulcers with red bases. The lesions are painful and may form on the lips, gums, inner cheeks, tongue, and/or oropharynx. The fever and pain last for about 1 week, and the regional lymph nodes are often tender and enlarged. The ulcers usually crust over and heal without scarring in about 2 weeks. Herpes simplex will often recur in the same spot and may be precipitated by fatigue, fever, emotional stress, or an irritant (e.g., sunlight).

Nursing care focuses on symptomatic relief of inflammation, including frequent oral hygiene, use of mouthwashes, and teaching the client the importance of good oral hygiene. All local and systemic factors that predispose to the inflammation should be removed, including local physical irritants. Penicillin and/or antispirochetal agents may be used for infections. Nutrition should be encouraged, with a soft, bland diet and supplemental multivitamins. Topical medications may include steroids, silver nitrate, or local anesthetics. Estrogen supplements may be given in cases where menopausal changes may have contributed to the inflammation. Referral for dental care is critical in cases in which tooth structures are involved.

INFLAMMATION OF THE SALIVARY GLANDS

While any of the salivary glands may become inflamed, parotitis (inflammation of the parotid glands) is the most common. The best known of these is epidemic parotitis (mumps), an acute and highly contagious infection, usually seen in children, that can affect the salivary glands (especially the parotid), testes, pancreas, meninges, and/or central nervous system. It is caused by a virus whose incubation period is 8–28 days. The person is contagious from several days before to 10 days after the onset of symptoms, which include anorexia, malaise, fever, sore throat, and parotid tenderness. Treatment is symptomatic. With the development of a mumps vaccine, incidence has decreased. More frequently seen in adults is an acute suppurative parotitis that is usually caused by *Staphylococcus aureus* and may develop as a complication of severe illness. Debilitation and dehydration are thought to contribute to its development. The parotids become swollen and tender, with local pain, fever, and chills. If the swelling is severe, facial paralysis may develop.

Nursing care focuses on preventing dissemination of the bacteria and promoting healing of the infection. Antibiotics are given to fight the infection, and status must be carefully monitored to prevent dehydration and ensure adequate secretion by the salivary glands. Heat may be applied locally to foster vasodilatation and hasten healing. If the swelling is severe and unrelieved, the gland may be incised and drained.

ESOPHAGITIS

Esophagitis is an inflammation of the esophagus that can result from esophageal trauma (discussed below), gastric reflux, or systemic conditions, such as scleroderma or tuberculosis. Peptic (reflex) esophagitis is the most common and results from the backflow of gastric secretions into the lower esophagus. While it can occur at any age, its incidence increases from ages 40 to 60. Reflux esophagitis has been associated with hiatus hernia, pregnancy, obesity, straining, peptic ulcer disease, gastroesophageal surgery, persistent vomiting, intubation, and severe systemic infection. It causes a generalized inflammation that can erode and ulcerate, eventually healing with fibrosis and scar tissue formation.

Esophagitis causes retrosternal, epigastric pain that may radiate to the throat, jaws, arms, or back. It generally begins a few minutes after eating and persists for a couple of hours. Belching may offer some relief. The client often has difficulty swallowing and complains that food "sticks" in the lower esophagus. The dysphagia is worse when eating solids and at the beginning of a meal. Coughing and choking may be evident, especially at night or in the recumbent position. If bleeding occurs, it is usually mild and chronic.

Nursing focuses on minimizing discomfort, alleviating pain, preventing aspiration, and promoting good nutrition. A bland diet, with four or five small feedings, eaten slowly and chewed well, is recommended. Because dietary indiscretions (e.g., spicy foods) and alcohol are associated with exacerbations, they should be avoided. Keeping the head elevated after eating is also helpful. Obese clients should be encouraged to lose weight. Milk and antacids are often given q1–2h. For severe pain, an anesthetic–antacid preparation may be given. A constant intraesophageal drip of antacid may also be used. Barbiturates are sometimes given to decrease spasm. Anticholinergics should be avoided because they tend to increase reflux. Emotional stress should be minimized, as it can cause painful esophagospasm.

ACUTE GASTRITIS

Acute gastritis, or inflammation of the stomach, can result from a variety of causes, including acute alcoholism; thermal, chemical, or bacterial irritants; infiltrative diseases; food poisoning; various drugs; acute illness; heavy metal poisoning; uremia; and shock. It usually results in anorexia, nausea, and vomiting, with epigastric pain and fever. If severe, hemorrhage can develop. The inflammation can last several hours to days and usually heals spontaneously. Nursing care is usually supportive and often includes administration of antacids to neutralize stomach acid, antispasmodics, and a bland diet. Any offending agent (e.g., alcohol) should be eliminated. If the inflammation causes erosion with hemorrhage, iced saline lavage, gastric cooling, and/or gastric resection may be necessary. Prevention of dehydration is important. Urinary output and fluid intake should be monitored. Intravenous therapy may be required in severe cases of fluid imbalance.

CHRONIC GASTRITIS

Chronic gastritis is found more frequently in older people and may involve inflammatory or atrophic changes. Its cause is unknown, but its occurrence is associated with chronic alcoholism, aspirin use, endocrine disorders, pernicious anemia, carcinoma, polyps, gastric ulcer, and chronic debilitating disease. Often it is asymptomatic but may cause occasional nausea and anorexia. Vomiting occurs after eating, and the client often awakes with a bad taste in the mouth. Dull epigastric discomfort may be felt.

Nursing care focuses on promoting nutrition, with frequent small feedings of a bland diet, and preventing dehydration. Antacids may offer some relief. Any possible precipating factors should be eliminated or treated, and stress should be avoided.

REGIONAL ENTERITIS

Regional enteritis (Crohn's disease) is a chronic inflammatory disease of the small bowel. The terminal ileum is involved in 40 percent of cases, although occasionally the colon and rectum are involved and, in rare cases, the stomach. The problem is seen most frequently in young people, although any age group can be affected. While many factors have been implicated, the cause is not known. The onset is insidious, with slow development of malaise, loss of appetite, mild episodes of diarrhea, intermittent pain, weight loss, and fever. The stool usually contains occult blood, and anemia is common. Pain is felt most frequently around the umbilicus and in the right lower quadrant. Cramping is often increased after eating and lessened with defacation. The formation of rectal fissues, fistulas, and abscesses may occur.

Nursing care is similar to that discussed under *Ulcerative Colitis*. A well-balanced, high-calorie, high-protein diet is encouraged. Problems such as pain, cramps, and diarrhea are treated symptomatically. Surgical intervention is unpopular because recurrence of enteritis after surgery occurs in 50 percent of cases.

DYSENTERY

Dysentery refers to a variety of intestinal disorders characterized by inflammation of the gastrointestinal tract. They can be of bacterial, viral, protozoal, parasitic, or chemical origin. *Salmonella* infections are the most common bacterial cause. Viral infections are often referred to as intestinal flu. Dysentery is associated with some degree of diarrhea, ranging from moderately loose stools to frequent, watery stools that contain blood and pus. Flatulence is often present and colicky, abdominal pain experienced. Fever is usually evident. Bacterial and viral infections are most often associated with gastroenteritis (inflammation of the stomach and intestine) and often result in nausea, vomiting, and malaise as well as diarrhea. Nursing care focuses on symptomatic relief, promoting comfort, and helping to prevent fluid and electrolyte imbalances. Diarrhea is often controlled with antidiarrheal agents, anticholinergic drugs, and/or narcotics. Appropriate antimicrobial agents are employed to eliminate the offending organism. Fluid and electrolyte status should be monitored and losses replaced orally or parenterally.

DIVERTICULITIS

Diverticula are small outpouchings that can occur anywhere in the gastrointestinal tract. They are not common in the esophagus and rarely occur in the stomach. The most common type found in the small intestine is Meckel's diverticulum, which is a developmental anomaly that usually does not cause difficulties. Diverticula are found most often in the colon. The occurrence of multiple diverticula is called diverticulosis. Of all persons over 50 years of age in the United States, 20 percent are thought to have diverticulosis. The cause is not known, but it may be associated with colonic hypermotility. Diets high in fiber tend to decrease its occurrence. It is most often a silent condition that does not cause difficulty. About one-fifth of cases, however, become inflamed (diverticulitis). Inflammation is thought to develop when the pouches do not empty completely and food and bacteria collect. Lower abdominal pain that often lasts 1–10 days results. The pain is worse after eating, and guarding may be evident. Some degree of constipation and abdominal fullness develops, and fever is usually present. Chronic blood loss may also occur. If the diverticulum ruptures, peritonitis, ileus, and shock will quickly develop.

Nursing care focuses on decreasing potential for infection, promoting adequate hydration and comfort, and fostering normal elimination. Bed rest is indicated until the infection is controlled. A broad-spectrum antibiotic is given and liquids are encouraged. Anticholinergic drugs are often used to decrease pain. Initially, a liquid diet and stool softener are given to minimize mechanical stimulation. As the inflammation subsides, diet teaching focuses on a diet high in vegetable and fruit fiber. Supplemental unprocessed bran and/or laxatives may also be indicated. In severe case, in which medical management fails or attacks occur repeatedly in the same area, surgical intervention may be considered (refer to *Intestinal Obstructions*).

TRAUMA

ESOPHAGEAL TRAUMA

DESCRIPTION

The esophagus can be injured in several ways. The most common of these is a burn from the ingestion of corrosive or hot liquid. Foreign bodies can also lodge in the esophagus, traumatizing tissue. In addition, the esophagus can be injured from external trauma such as during an esophagoscopy. This discussion will be limited to chemical burns of the esophagus (acute corrosive esophagitis). The agents involved in chemical burns are usually alkalis (e.g., ammonia, washing soda, bleach, lye, drain cleaners, and dishwashing detergents) or acids (e.g., toilet bowl cleaners, rust removers, iodine, silver nitrate, and sulfuric, nitric, hydrochloric, acetic, or oxalic acid). Both types of agent result in intense inflammation, with mucosal edema and esophagospasm. Areas of necrosis develop and are surrounded by intensely inflamed areas. With sloughing of necrotic tissue, ulcers form. Fibrous healing then occurs, and strictures often develop. Because of the esophagospasm, entrance of the agent into the stomach is limited, decreasing injury to the gastric mucosa. Burns caused by alkalis are usually deeper than acid burns.

PREVENTION

Health Promotion

1. Encourage mental health care to decrease suicide risk.
2. Support and stimulate programs that foster home safety.

Population at Risk

1. Persons susceptible to harming themselves.
2. Children, especially toddlers (refer to Chapters 22 and 48).

ASSESSMENT

Health History

1. Description of the type and amount of substance ingested. Information should be sought from the client or family. Ideally, a sample of the substance should be obtained for analysis, especially if the nature of the substance is in question.
2. Attempts at first aid and the occurrence of any vomiting should be identified.
3. Past history of psychiatric difficulties should be noted to see if the ingestion was intentional.
4. Intense, violent pain behind the sternum and often referred to the back and neck may be present. It may be accompanied by vomiting, which will increase injury to the pharynx, mouth, and lips.
5. Pain and/or difficulty with swallowing.

Physical Assessment

1. The client is acutely ill and severely distressed.
2. Respiratory distress is present secondary to edema in the throat, decreasing patency of the airway. As the throat becomes occluded, stridor becomes evident.
3. Hypovolemia and shock secondary to fluid losses associated with edema (see Chapters 48 and 49).
4. Burns of the lips and mouth are often noted.
5. Salivation is increased.
6. Vomiting may lead to retching, and the vomitus usually contains blood and mucus.
7. Fever is often present.

Diagnostic Tests

Esophagoscopy may be performed to determine the extent of injury after the acute inflammation has subsided.

NURSING DIAGNOSES: ACTUAL OR POTENTIAL

1. Potential for respiratory distress due to airway obstruction secondary to severe laryngeal edema.
2. Alteration in comfort due to severe retrosternal pain that radiates to the neck and back.
3. Alteration in fluid balance characterized by fluid volume deficit due to dehydration, decreased ingestion of fluids, and edema fluid losses.
4. Nutritional deficit due to alteration in food

intake resulting from difficult and painful swallowing.
5. Potential for injury due to large areas of open lesions that can become infected.
6. Ineffective coping patterns; if ingestion was intentional.

EXPECTED OUTCOMES

1. Patent airway will be maintained.
2. Pain will be relieved.
3. Fluid volume will be restored and maintained.
4. Nutritional requirements will be met.
5. Client will remain free of infection.
6. Professional counseling will be sought if ingestion was intentional.

INTERVENTIONS

1. Administer substances to neutralize the chemical ingested. The corrosive chemical should be neutralized within a few minutes with alkaline agents. Acidic chemicals can be diluted with milk, water, sodium bicarbonate, or 1 tablespoon of milk of magnesia in 1 cup of water. Areas that are accessible should be washed with copious amounts of water.
2. Monitor closely for the development of laryngeal edema. Keep a tracheostomy set at the bedside (refer to Chapter 31 for discussion of tracheostomy care).
3. Monitor vital signs and urine output frequently to detect development of hypovolemia.
4. Give parenteral fluids to replace fluid losses.
5. Administer analgesic medication to relieve pain.
6. Administer prescribed corticosteroids for 4–6 weeks to decrease the inflammation and thus subsequent scar tissue formation.
7. Insert nasogastric tube (see Figure 33-3) to maintain patency of the esophagus during the acute inflammation.
8. Give prophylactic antibiotics to prevent secondary infection.
9. Give clear liquids and milk orally after a few days, if the client can swallow, does not have a fever, and there is no danger of perforation.

EVALUATION

Outcome Criteria

1. Patent airway is maintained during the acute stage; client has no difficulties breathing.
2. Client is relatively pain free, and no infection is present.
3. Fluid balance is maintained within normal limits.
4. Client begins ingesting clear liquids and milk after a few days; client gains (if indicated) or maintains weight after healing by ingesting a balanced diet.
5. If appropriate, client can describe plans for regular psychiatric counseling.

Complications

STRICTURE FORMATION WITH ESOPHAGEAL OBSTRUCTION

Can occur in most cases of severe burns. Symptoms include dysphagia, difficulty or inability to pass food and/or liquids, and regurgitation, occasionally into nasal passages. The goals of therapy are to establish or maintain esophageal patency and meet nutritional requirements through oral intake and to establish psychological care.

Interventions

1. Esophageal dilation started about a week after ingestion of the chemical to decrease stricture formation. The procedure involves passing a well-lubricated, small-caliber bougie daily and gradually increasing its size until the lumen of the esophagus is stable. Some physicians use an olive-shaped metal dilator for the same purpose (see Figure 33-5).
2. Retrograde passage used if stricture formation prevents dilating the esophagus through esophageal dilation. A string is passed through the nose and esophagus into the stomach and brought out through a gastrostomy tube. The two ends are joined, making a continuous loop. Dilators can then be attached and pulled through from the stomach.
3. Surgical repair if stricture formation does not respond to bougienage. The procedure usually involves resection of the esophagus or replacement of it with a piece of colon or jejunum.

Reevaluation and Follow-up

1. Nutritional status should be monitored, weights checked periodically, and dietary teaching reviewed.
2. A long-term plan of psychiatric help should be provided.
3. Repeated bougienage is often required, and esophageal lumen size must be periodically reassessed.

OBSTRUCTIONS

INTESTINAL OBSTRUCTIONS

DESCRIPTION

Intestinal obstruction occurs when the intestinal contents fail to progress through the small and/or large intestine. It can be caused by mechanical or nonmechanical factors. Some of the mechanical factors include gallstones, worms, adhesions, hernias, volvulus (a twisting of the bowel upon itself), intussusception (slipping of part of the intestine into the part below it), and tumors. Nonmechanical factors can result in an adynamic (paralytic) ileus or a dynamic (spastic) ileus. Paralytic (adynamic) ileus occurs most frequently in response to trauma (i.e., surgery), peritoneal irritation, hypoxia, or metabolic changes (i.e., hypokalemia), while dynamic ileus is uncommon and is often associated with toxic conditions. Table 33-4 summarizes some of the causes of intestinal obstruction.

Uncomplicated intestinal obstruction has a 15 percent mortality rate, to which 9,000 deaths per year in the United States can be attributed. It causes widespread pathophysiologic changes that make the client severely ill. As obstruction occurs, air and fluid accumulate in the proximal intestine, and distension develops. About 70–80 percent of the gaseous distension is attributed to swallowed air. Fluid accumulates primarily from that produced by the intestines. Normally, about 8 L of fluid is produced and reabsorbed. As obstruction occurs, not only is this production increased, but reabsorption is decreased, increasing further the fluid losses to the intestinal lumen. In the first few hours after obstruction, the intestine attempts to "push past" the obstruction by increasing peristalsis. As the bowel dilates, however, motility decreases, and eventually atony develops.

As distension increases, pressure decreases the venous return to the intestinal wall. Fluid from the intestinal capillaries is lost to the lumen, bowel wall, and peritoneal cavity. As the splanchnic circulation becomes inadequate, intramural hemorrhage and necrosis occur. The bowel wall becomes permeable, and fluid and bacteria are lost to the peritoneal cavity. The fluid losses into the intestinal lumen and peritoneal cavity eventually cause dehydration. If the intraluminal pressure is unrelieved, the bowel will eventually burst. These changes are usually gradual but can develop rapidly if an obstruction strangulates part of the intestine.

PREVENTION

Health Promotion

1. Avoidance of factors contributing to gallbladder disease (see *Cholecystitis*).
2. Proper care of hernias (see *Hernias*).
3. Prevention and early detection of intestinal cancer (see *Small Bowel Tumors* and *Colorectal Tumors*).
4. Health teaching regarding cancer risks.
5. Close monitoring of severely ill clients.

Population at Risk

1. Persons with a history of gallstones, intestinal surgery, hernias, or intestinal tumors.
2. Severely ill clients with peritoneal irritation, hypoxia, metabolic imbalances, or toxic conditions.
3. Persons undergoing abdominal surgery, especially those requiring extensive bowel manipulation.
4. Elderly persons, particularly with an altered health state such as listed above.

Screening

1. Cancer screening.
2. Monitor bowel sounds of acutely ill clients.

ASSESSMENT

Health History

1. History of cancer, polyps, chronic inflammatory conditions such as diverticulitis or ulcerative colitis, and abdominal operations.
2. Increasing constipation, vague and diffuse pain, lower abdominal cramps, and/or occasional abdominal distention.
3. Rhythmical, colicky pain that reaches a peak and then subsides, associated with mechanical obstruction. In small bowel obstruction, the pain is usually in the midabdomen, while the pain associated with large bowel obstruction is frequently located in the lower abdomen and is less severe.
4. No pain experienced with adynamic ileus until the distension becomes severe and the abdomen tight.

TABLE 33-4 CAUSES OF SMALL BOWEL OBSTRUCTION

1. Mechanical occlusion of lumen.
   a. Intrinsic defects of intestine.
      (1) Congenital defects.
         (a) Errors in rotation of intestine.
         (b) Duplications and cysts.
         (c) Meckel's diverticulum.
      (2) Inflammatory lesions.
         (a) Regional enteritis.
         (b) Tuberculosis.
         (c) Diverticulitis.
         (d) Eosinophilic granuloma.
      (3) Tumors.
         (a) Benign.
         (b) Malignant.
      (4) Traumatic lesions.
         (a) Strictures.
         (b) Hematomas.
      (5) Intussusception.
      (6) Radiation strictures.
      (7) Endometriosis.
      (8) Pneumatosis intestinalis.
   b. Obturation obstruction.
      (1) Gallstones.
      (2) Bezoars.
      (3) Foreign bodies.
      (4) Enteroliths.
      (5) Worms.
      (6) Balloons of intestinal tubes.
   c. Volvulus.
      (1) Primary.
      (2) Secondary.
         (a) Associated congenital abnormality.
         (b) Secondary surgical artifact.
         (c) Secondary bands, adhesions, stenosis, or obturation.
   d. Extraintestinal lesions.
      (1) Adhesions and bands.
      (2) Hernia.
         (a) Extra-abdominal: inguinal, femoral, umbilical, ventral, diaphragmatic, lumbar, epigastric, interstitial, prevesical, obturator, sciatic, perineal, Richter's or Littre's.
         (b) Intra-abdominal: paraduodenal, foramen of Winslow, paracecal, intersigmoid, through omental or mesenteric defect, or through broad ligament.
      (3) Compression by extraintestinal mass.
         (a) Carcinomatosis.
         (b) Intraperitoneal abscess.
         (c) Adjacent tumor.
         (d) Pregnancy.
         (e) Foreign body.
         (f) Superior mesenteric artery duodenal obstruction.
         (g) Annular pancreas.
         (h) Wandering spleen.
   e. Obstruction secondary to surgical operation (other than adhesions).
      (1) Intraperitoneal abscess.
      (2) Wound dehiscence.
      (3) Anastomotic obstruction (stricture or edema).
      (4) Anastomotic leak.
      (5) Obstruction at external stoma.
      (6) Hernia through peritoneal defect.
      (7) Volvulus about fixed point.
2. Obstruction with open lumen.
   a. Paralytic ileus.
   b. Spastic ileus.
   c. Mesenteric vascular occlusion.

SOURCE: Bogoch, A.: *Gastroenterolgoy*, McGraw-Hill, New York, 1973.

5. Nausea and vomiting: the higher the obstruction is located, the earlier these symptoms occur and the greater their severity. The client initially will vomit the stomach contents and then the intestinal contents, until the vomitus eventually becomes fecal in character.
6. Absolute constipation (obstipation) after the intestine distal to the obstruction is empty.

Physical Assessment

1. Distended abdomen: the lower the obstruction, the worse the distension. Early in the obstruction, peristalsis may be visible, and as the proximal intestine contracts, high-pitched gurgling and eventually tinkling sounds are head on auscultation. As motility decreases and eventually ceases, so do bowel sounds.

With adynamic ileus, bowel sounds are diminished or absent from the onset. Percussion of the abdomen reveals tympany, and with mechanical obstruction, guarding and abdominal tenderness are present during palpation.
2. Obstructions in the rectum may be felt during rectal examination.
3. Vital signs and fluid status reflect developing dehydration, shock, or sepsis. If the obstruction is strangulated and becomes gangrenous, pain worsens, tachycardia develops, temperature rises, and blood pressure falls. If a strangulated obstruction becomes perforated, sepsis ensues, manifested by pallor, sweating, cold and clammy extremities, tachycardia, hypotension, and disorientation.

Diagnostic Tests

1. Flat film x-ray of the abdomen to show gas-filled intestines.
2. Sigmoidoscopy or proctoscopy to visualize a low obstruction: the procedure is very painful and uncomfortable for clients with obstruction, since it involves the insertion through the rectum of an inflexible tube through which the bowel can be visualized and biopsies taken (see *Ulcerative Colitis*). The client is forced to assume a jackknife-type position for the duration of the test in order to make the visualization of the bowel more accessible.
3. Barium enema may be carefully attempted if colonic obstruction is suspected. This will occasionally correct obstructions caused by volvulus or intussusception. (See *Ulcerative Colitis* for discussion of procedure.)

NURSING DIAGNOSES: ACTUAL OR POTENTIAL

1. Alteration in comfort due to colicky pain that may be centered in the mid- or lower abdomen secondary to distention and obstruction.
2. Respiratory dysfunction characterized by limited respiratory expansion secondary to abdominal distention.
3. Nutritional alteration due to inability to take food orally and vomiting of stomach and intestinal contents.
4. Alteration in fluid volume due to the loss of large amounts of fluid to the abdomen and from vomiting; potential for hypovolemia.
5. Anxiety due to extreme apprehension and difficulty comprehending what is happening.
6. Potential alteration in self-concept due to fear of disruption in body image secondary to radical surgery.

EXPECTED OUTCOMES

1. Pain will be relieved.
2. Ventilatory capacity will be increased, and respiratory expansion will be unhindered.
3. Distension will be relieved and the obstruction reversed.
4. Vomiting will be relieved, and nutritional requirements will be initially met with parenteral fluids. After the obstruction is relieved, client will be able to resume normal diet.
5. Fluid volume will be restored, and blood volume will be maintained within normal limits.
6. Client will become less fearful and will understand the physical and emotional changes resulting from this altered health state.
7. Client will accept change in self-concept if surgery is necessary.

INTERVENTIONS

1. Insert nasogastric tube (see Figure 33-9) attached to intermittent suction for decompression if the obstruction is high in the intestine. Some physicians prefer inserting a tube to the point of obstruction, which is accomplished by inserting a long intestinal tube with a weighted tip through the nose and into the stomach. The weighted tip then allows the tube to be advanced by peristalsis. Once in the intestine, the tube will be advanced by the nurse at regular intervals until it reaches the point of obstruction. The location of the tube should be frequently checked during insertion by x-ray examination or fluoroscopy. It is usually attached to low, continuous suction. When intestinal tubes are used, a nasogastric tube is also necessary to keep the stomach empty.
2. Administer medication for pain to clients with mechanical obstruction. As the intestinal distention is relieved, the pain will lessen.
3. Administer broad-spectrum antibiotics as prescribed if sepsis becomes a threat from strangulation.
4. Provide intravenous fluid to replace fluid losses. The amount is usually determined by the urine output, central venous pressure, and hematocrit. Unless the obstruction is

very high, acidic fluids from the stomach and alkaline fluids from the intestines are both lost, and acid–base imbalances do not develop. Saline intravenous fluids with added potassium chloride will usually meet the client's needs.

5. Give NPO until the obstruction is relieved. Nutritional needs will be met by intravenous glucose solutions with supplemental vitamins.
6. Provide symptomatic care and/or remove the causative factor for clients with paralytic ileus to effect a return of peristalsis. For example, hypoxia should be reversed and hypokalemia corrected. Occasionally, a medication regimen will be tried in which the client is first given a sympathetic blocking agent to decrease the antiperistaltic effect and then given a cholinergic drug to promote the parasympathetic effect of increasing motility.
7. Offer explanations frequently and allow client to ventilate fears.
8. Surgery to relieve most mechanical obstructions.
   a. Surgical decompression: a palliative measure that may be employed when client is too ill to undergo more extensive surgery. It involves the insertion of a cecostomy tube in an opening in the bowel. The tube is then brought out through the abdominal wall (see Figure 33-7).
   b. Bowel resection to remove diseased portion of the bowel and anastomose the ends.
   c. Colostomy to create an avenue for bowel excretion by opening the colon and bringing it to the abdominal wall (see Figure 33-10).
      (1) A temporary colostomy is done when there is hope that the lower (distal) portion of the colon will heal and normal elimination can be restored (e.g., as in trauma, diverticulitis). It is usually kept 3–6 months and involves bringing a loop of bowel to the abdominal surface and creating two holes, one to allow the proximal intestine to empty and the second to communicate with the distal portion of the colon (see Figure 33-7).
      (2) A permanent colostomy is most frequently done when there is cancer close to the anal sphincter. The colon is opened and brought to the surface, while the rectum and distal section are removed (see Figure 33-7).
         (a) Preoperative care focuses on cleaning the intestine and preparing the client psychologically. Continuous support is critical. For all surgeries that involve opening the bowel, special attention is given to cleaning the intestines. Cleansing enemas are given, and often poorly absorbed antibiotics are used in an attempt to "sterilize" the bowel. The nature of the surgery is fully discussed with the client, and time is provided for questions and concerns. When possible, the family is included in the discussions. Often a visit preoperatively from another client with a colostomy helps alleviate some anxiety and provides the client with an additional opportunity to discuss pertinent issues.
         (b) Postoperative care initially focuses on the usual concerns following surgery: hemorrhage, atelectasis,

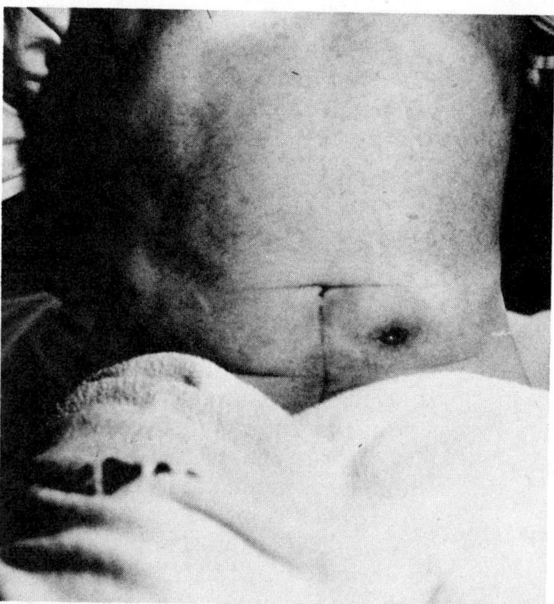

Figure 33-10 Colostomy stoma. (From Jones, D.A., et al., eds.: *Medical-Surgical Nursing: A Conceptual Approach*, 2d ed., McGraw-Hill, New York 1982.)

thrombophlebitis, and infection. When the client is ready physically and psychologically, he or she should be taught to care for the colostomy. Clients with colostomies can often be trained to perform regular evacuation of soft to formed stool with suppositories, irrigations, or finger dilation. Appliances should be properly fitted and community resources made available. Dietary restrictions are minimal and usually dictated by the client's needs. If diarrhea is a problem, residue is decreased. For constipation, clients are taught to increase residue. In general, flatus can be partly controlled by avoiding gas-forming foods. Clients must adjust to a significant change in body image and should be given support in this process.

EVALUATION

Outcome Criteria

1. Client is pain free.
2. Respirations are unhindered, and breath sounds are clear.
3. Abdominal distension is relieved and obstruction reversed, as evidenced by passage of fluid and air through the intestines.
4. Bowel patterns gradually return to normal.
5. Weight is within normal limits without dietary constraints.
6. Fluid volume remains within normal limits.
7. Anxiety is relieved, as evidenced by client's cooperating with procedures and asking questions as appropriate.
8. Client who has undergone colostomy evidences acceptance of the change in bodily appearance:
   a. Initially client is able to look at colostomy.
   b. Client begins to help care for colostomy.
   c. Client assumes total responsibility for colostomy care.
   d. Client develops diet that promotes regular evacuations.

Complications

Mortality rate increases to 35–40 percent if complications develop.

1. *Strangulation* (blood supply to a segment of bowel is cut off) and gangrene.
2. Perforation (see discussion under *Peptic Ulcers*).
3. Hypovolemia and shock (refer to Chapters 48 and 49).
4. Infection (refer to *Inflammatory Disorders*).
5. Pneumonia as the abdominal distension presses on the diaphragm, decreasing lung expansion (refer to Chapter 31).
6. Aspiration pneumonitis (see Chapter 31).

HERNIAS

A hernia is a projection (rupture) of the abdominal contents through a weakness in the muscular wall that encloses the peritoneal cavity. Penetration of the intestines through the opening can be constant or intermittent. If the intestines can be returned into the peritoneal cavity, the hernia is reducible. If this is not possible, it is considered irreducible or incarcerated. When the size of the abdominal opening compromises the blood supply to the protruding intestine, the hernia is strangulated. Hernias result from a defect in the abdominal wall that can be caused by a congenital weakness, trauma, aging, or increased intra-abdominal pressure. The latter can be caused by obesity, pregnancy, heavy lifting, coughing, or trauma. Hernias occur in a variety of sites. Among the more common are indirect inguinal hernias, which pass through the inguinal ring into the canal and can descend into the scrotum; direct inguinal hernias, which pass through a weakness in the abdominal wall; femoral hernias, which pass through the femoral ring; hiatus hernias, which result in the stomach's partially entering the thorax through a weakness in the diaphragm; umbilical hernias, seen most frequently in children; and incisional hernias. Often the client experiences only a lump that disappears when lying down. Vague discomfort and epigastric pain may be felt. If the hernia becomes strangulated, however, the pain increases and the client becomes acutely ill (refer to *Intestinal Obstructions*).

Nursing care focuses on preoperative and postoperative care, as surgical repair is recommended because of the danger of strangulation and intestinal obstruction. If surgery is not a viable alternative, the client should be taught to keep the hernia reduced with a belt, truss, or well-fitting corset. A pad or sponge may be placed over the hernia. The client should be instructed to avoid heavy lifting both before and after surgery.

HEMORRHOIDS

Hemorrhoids are varicosities of the hemorrhoidal venous plexus that occur in the anorectal area. They are considered external if covered by skin and internal if covered by mucous membrane. They have been associated with standing erect for long periods, anorectal sepsis, straining, rectal cancer, pregnancy, portal hypertension, and diarrhea. If uncomplicated, hemorrhoids are usually asymptomatic. Acute episodes can develop, however, if they become thrombosed, causing severe pain. Internal hemorrhoids may bleed and can prolapse through the anus, predisposing to thrombosis.

Nursing care focuses on symptomatic relief until the thrombosis resolves. This may include bed rest with the feet elevated to increase venous return, analgesics, suppositories (Anusol), sedation, good anal hygiene, witch hazel compresses, and a laxative such as milk of magnesia. After the acute attack, sitz baths and a low-residue diet may be considered, with evacuation of the clot in external hemorrhoids or hemorrhoidectomy for internal hemorrhoids.

DEGENERATIVE DISORDERS

HEPATIC CIRRHOSIS

DESCRIPTION

Hepatic cirrhosis is a chronic, diffuse liver disease that involves hepatic cell loss and necrosis with fibrosis, scar tissue formation, and regeneration. The most common type of cirrhosis is that caused by chronic alcoholism (Laennec's cirrhosis, alcoholic cirrhosis, fatty cirrhosis). Laennec's cirrhosis is often preceded by an alcoholic hepatitis and is associated with fatty infiltration of the liver. Malnutrition contributes to its development and may be a major factor in cirrhosis. Laennec's cirrhosis occurs in both sexes and all ages but is found more frequently in men of about 50 years of age after 5–15 years of alcoholic abuse.

While alcoholic abuse is the most frequent cause of cirrhosis, the disorder can result from other factors. Postnecrotic cirrhosis can follow the liver damage caused by viral infections of the liver, chemical intoxications, or hepatic infections. Biliary cirrhosis results from bile duct obstruction or intrahepatic cholestasis of unknown etiology. Hemachromatosis leads to liver damage and cirrhosis as hemosiderin is deposited in hepatic tissue. Congestive heart failure can lead to vena caval hypertension, increasing pressure in hepatic circulation and causing cirrhosis. Hepatic cirrhosis has also been associated with metabolic disorders, infectious diseases, infiltrative diseases, and gastrointestinal disorders.

Hepatic cirrhosis results in widespread disruption of liver function. Metabolic functions such as the conversion of carbohydrates, fats, and proteins into various nutrients and substances; the storage of vitamins A, D, and E and carotene; and the synthesis of albumin are diminished. The liver's ability to detoxify ammonia, estrogen, the antidiuretic hormone, aldosterone, adrenocorticosteroids, and various drugs, poisons, and heavy metals is decreased. Storage of vitamin B_{12} and iron is impaired, as are vitamin K storage and the synthesis of fibrinogen, prothrombin, and factors V, VII, and X. The ability of the liver to remove bilirubin from circulation is also diminished. As cirrhosis in the liver becomes widespread, hepatic microcirculation becomes disrupted, and pressure increases in the portal vein. Fluid retention results from portal hypertension (increasing portal hydrostatic pressure), hypoalbuminemia (decreasing the vascular colloid osmotic pressure), and sodium and water imbalance. With increasing pressure, collateral circulation develops primarily around the anus (causing hemorrhoids), the esophageal gastric junction (causing esophageal varices), and the abdominal wall and periumbilical area. The pressure from portal hypertension is also communicated to the spleen, causing splenomegaly.

The onset of hepatic cirrhosis is insidious, and changes usually appear late because of the liver's ability to maintain function, with loss of up to 75 percent of its mass. After 4–5 years, the pathology becomes evident on examination.

PREVENTION

Health Promotion

1. Avoid excessive alcohol consumption.
2. Support and stimulate programs to reduce alcoholism.
3. Encourage early treatment of hepatitis.
4. Prevent spread of hepatitis.
5. Encourage measures to reduce gallbladder disease.
6. Encourage treatment of congestive heart failure.

Population at Risk

1. Alcoholics.
2. Persons with history of severe hepatitis.
3. Persons with gallbladder disease.
4. Persons with severe congestive heart failure.
5. Persons who use alcohol as a way of handling stress or who engage in excessive social drinking.

ASSESSMENT

Health History

1. Generalized weakness, lassitude, and easy fatigability.
2. Vague upper abdominal discomfort or a dull ache in the upper right quadrant.
3. Anorexia, nausea, and complaints of gagging and retching in the morning.
4. Episodes of slight jaundice, ankle edema, changes in the color of urine or stool, and itching (seldom occurs) noted by the client.
5. Changes in menstrual history and/or sexual function. In men a decreased libido and impotence are common, and women often develop amenorrhea or irregularity.
6. History of alcohol use, including age when drinking began, amount of alcohol ingested daily and related eating habits, and relationship to stress and coping patterns.
7. History of hepatic infections, biliary disease, cardiac disease, metabolic disorders, or gastrointestinal problems.
8. Drugs the client takes or chemicals to which he or she has been exposed (e.g., toxic substances).
9. Identify social interactions, lifestyle, occupation, and so on.

Physical Assessment

1. Weight loss is usually evident, and some clients appear emaciated.
2. The characteristic yellow color of jaundice is usually noted and best observed in the sclera of the eyes.
3. Purpura and bruises may be present, secondary to decreased synthesis of clotting factors.
4. Loss of body hair (alopecia), pubic hair, and auxiliary hair and enlarged breasts (gynecomastia) may be noted in men, secondary to decreased estrogen detoxification.
5. Spider angiomas (spider nevi) are often seen.
6. Mottled redness of the palms (palmar erythema), clubbing of the fingers, and Dupuytren's contracture (flexion of the ring and little fingers into the palm) may be present.
7. Skin is dry, and there is musculoskeletal wasting.
8. Tongue may be swollen and red.
9. Intermittent, low-grade fever without chills is present in 25–50 percent of cases.
10. Abnormal collections of fluid should be noted. Ascites is present initially; peripheral edema develops later. Abdominal girth is increased. Serial measurements usually reveal a gradual increase in size.
11. Abdominal examination reveals:
    a. Spider nevi, distension, and dilated periumbilical veins (caput medusae).
    b. Fluid in the peritoneum, as evidenced by shifting dullness and the puddle examination (see Physical Assessment section at beginning of this chapter).
    c. Vascular bruits over the upper abdomen.
    d. Enlarged liver will be evident, with a round, firm edge.
    e. Palpable spleen.
12. Hemorrhoids are usually noted, and rectal palpation often reveals prostatic atrophy from the estrogenic effect. Testicular atrophy may also be noted.

Diagnostic Tests

1. Clearance studies to evaluate liver function. After a 12-h fast, a dye such as Bromsulphalein (BSP) or indocyanine green (ICG), which is removed from the serum by the liver, is injected intravenously. Any retention of the dye in the blood indicates hepatic dysfunction.
2. Prothrombin time to evaluate liver's ability to store vitamin K and synthesize various clotting factors; prolonged in cirrhosis.

3. Hemoglobin, hematocrit, and red blood cell count reflect anemia, which results from blood loss from esophageal varices, folic acid deficiency, hypersplenism (overactivity of the spleen), and the toxic effect of alcohol on the blood.
4. Leukopenia and thrombocytopenia secondary to folic acid deficiency, hyperinsulinism, and the toxic effect of alcohol.
5. Serum ammonia level increased reflecting liver's inability to convert ammonia to urea.
6. Serum alkaline phosphatase elevated, some of which is synthesized by the liver and is excreted in the biliary tract.
7. Bilirubin elevated, as it is conjugated by the liver and eliminated in the bile. With hepatic dysfunction indirect bilirubin (unconjugated) and total bilirubin will be increased. If biliary excretion is impaired, direct bilirubin (conjugated) will also be elevated.
8. Urine bilirubin and urobilinogen increased.
9. Serum enzymes, such as serum glutamic-oxaloacetic transaminase (SGOT) and serum glutamic-pyruvic transaminase (SGPT), are liberated during hepatic damage and will be elevated but are not specific indicators of hepatic damage alone.
10. Serum cholesterol, serum phospholipids, and triglycerides decreased, reflecting decreased synthesis of fats by the liver.
11. Serum albumin, which is synthesized by the liver, is decreased, and the serum globulins, especially IgG, are elevated.
12. Liver scan infrequently done to visualize the size of the liver. Used as a guide to liver biopsy and involves the injection of a radioactive substance.
13. Photoscan (Scintiscan) to outline the liver.
14. Liver biopsy to evaluate the microscopic cellular hepatic changes. The procedure involves the insertion of a needle intercostally into the liver and the aspiration of hepatic cells through it. Because of the liver's vascularity, bleeding is a problem. Prothrombin time should be checked prior to the test, and vitamin K should be given as needed. Following biopsy, the client's vital signs should be closely monitored until all chance of bleeding has passed. The client should be kept supine or lying on the right side. The latter position causes the abdominal contents to fall against the liver, applying slight pressure.
15. Radiography to evaluate the circulatory changes associated with portal hypertension. The procedures involve the injection of a radiopaque dye into a vessel and subsequent x-ray examination or fluoroscopy to examine the flow of blood. Studies may include splenoportography, hepatoportography, or celiac arteriography.
16. Esophagoscopy to visualize esophageal varices and/or the gastric mucosa directly. The procedure involves the insertion of a flexible tube with a lighted tip and lens into the esophagus and sometimes through to the stomach.

NURSING DIAGNOSES: ACTUAL OR POTENTIAL

1. Alteration in nutrition characterized by nutritional deficit due to loss of appetite, occasional nausea, vomiting in the morning, weight loss (especially noticeable in a decreased muscle mass), and signs of vitamin deficiency, secondary to malnutrition.
2. Decreased activity and exercise tolerance related to fact that client fatigues easily and is unable to maintain normal activity level.
3. Alteration in fluid balance due to fluid excess and retention, noticeable in pitting pedal edema and ascites.
4. Alteration in electrolyte balance due to predisposition to hyponatremia and hypokalemia.
5. Respiratory dysfunction characterized by inability to fully expand chest, resulting in shortness of breath secondary to abdominal distention.
6. Impairment of skin integrity due to jaundice, making skin susceptible to breakdown.
7. Alterations in comfort due to itching over entire body secondary to jaundice or due to abdominal pain.
8. Alteration in level of consciousness related to occasional disorientation and a heightened response to sedatives, hypnotics, barbiturates, and narcotics secondary to decreased liver detoxification capability.
9. Alterations in self-concept due to concern and embarrassment about abdominal distension, enlarged breasts, hair loss, and sexual difficulties.
10. Ineffective, maladaptive coping patterns related to alcoholism.

EXPECTED OUTCOMES

1. Gradual weight gain will occur over a specified period of time.
2. Client will exhibit increased tolerance of activity by increasing exercise without fatigue.
3. Fluid and electrolyte balance will be restored, as evidenced by decreasing ascites and pedal edema and normal laboratory values.
4. Respiratory excursion will be increased, breath sounds will remain clear, and dyspnea on exertion will not occur.
5. Skin integrity will be maintained and pruritus will diminish.
6. Pain will be relieved.
7. Client will understand reasons for physical changes and will be able to verbalize feelings about them.
8. Client will comply with a program of sobriety and learn to manage stress more effectively.
9. Client will be oriented to time, place, and person.

INTERVENTIONS

1. Provide a high-protein (1 g/kg of body weight), high-calorie (2,000–3,000 cal) diet in three to four small feedings, with nutritional supplements between meals (e.g., eggnog or ice cream) if there is no indication of neurologic involvement. Liquid protein supplements may be used initially. Supplemental multivitamins are given, and all alcohol is restricted.
   a. Encourage client to eat and make environment conducive to stimulating the appetite.
   b. Give frequent oral hygiene.
   c. Encourage minimal movement to decrease nausea and vomiting.
   d. Administer antiemetics if necessary.
2. Restrict sodium and water.
3. Administer diuretic therapy as prescribed.
4. Administer salt-poor albumin intravenously.
5. Monitor fluid balance.
   a. Measure intake and output.
   b. Weight client daily.
   c. Measure abdominal girth daily.
6. Elevate edematous extremities to promote fluid return and decrease retention.
7. Provide bed rest to decrease fatigue and improve client's overall condition.
8. Give iron supplements and vitamin B_{12} therapy to treat anemia.
9. Watch closely for possible sites of infection. Cutdown sites and skin breaks should be cleansed regularly. Personal hygiene should be encouraged. Temperature should be monitored and exposure to infections be minimized.
10. Control itching (includes daily assessment of skin).
    a. Give cholestyramine (Cuemid); avoid dry skin.
    b. Decrease anoxia, which increases itching (i.e., correcting anemia).
    c. Minimize perspiration and overexertion.
    d. Decrease anxiety and emotional stress.
11. Avoid drugs eliminated through the liver (e.g., narcotics, sedatives, hypnotics, and barbiturates).
12. Discuss body image changes. Allow client time to ventilate concerns.
13. Paracentesis to relieve abdominal distension if ascites causes respiratory embarrassment or hernia. The procedure involves the insertion of a trocar with an obturator and the removal of fluid from the peritoneal cavity. Because the ascitic fluid is rich in albumin, it is removed slowly, usually no more than 1,000 mL at a time. Vital signs are monitored until stable.
14. Promote ways to stimulate abstinence from alcohol. This is extremely difficult, but all resources should be considered when plans are set. Individual, family, and/or group therapy may be needed. Lay groups such as Alcoholics Anonymous and Al-Anon are often used.
15. LeVeen peritoneal jugular shunt: a recently developed procedure to relieve ascites without depleting body of valuable proteins (LeVeen et al., 1979).
    a. Involves insertion of multilumen catheter into peritoneal cavity, a subcutaneous extraperitoneal valve, and a catheter running from the valve through subcutaneous tissue into the jugular vein (see Figure 33-11).
    b. Abdominal binder and/or blow bottles for maximal inspiration may be used to increase intraperitoneal pressure.
    c. Decreases ascites bý continually reinfusing ascitic fluid.

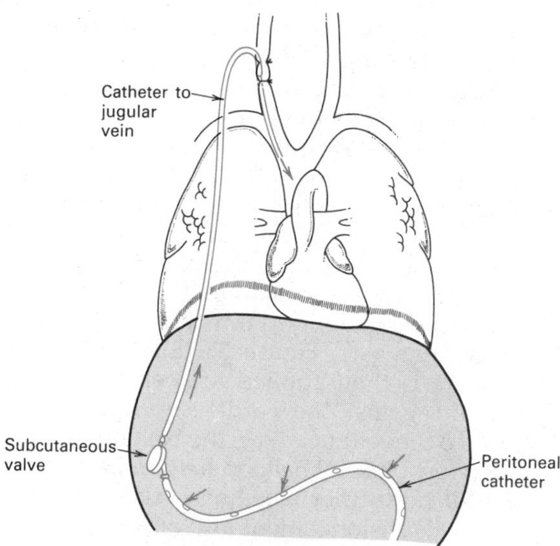

Figure 33-11 As intra-abdominal pressure increases, the subcutaneous valve opens, allowing fluid to pass through catheter into jugular vein. During inspiration, ascitic fluid escapes from the abdomen as abdominal pressure increases and intrathoracic pressure decreases.

   d. Complications including disseminated intravascular coagulopathy, hepatic coma, and sepsis must be carefully observed for.

16. Teach client about:
   a. Diet to ensure adequate nutrition and fluid balance measures.
   b. Medications to be taken.
   c. Drugs to avoid.
   d. Activity tolerance and plan for increasing daily exercise.
   e. The disease process and impact on physical appearances.

EVALUATION

Outcome Criteria

1. Client eats a balanced diet and takes vitamin supplements.
2. Client follows a daily exercise regimen and does not fatigue with moderate exercise.
3. Client has no ascites or pedal edema.
4. Breath sounds are clear, and client has full respiratory excursion.
5. Client is pain free and pruritus is relieved.
6. Skin integrity is maintained.
7. Client is fully aware of surroundings and is able to assume responsibility for self.
8. Client discusses physical changes openly and honestly and recognizes impact of the disease on health status and others (e.g., family).
9. Client does not ingest alcohol and regularly attends sessions that offer support for sobriety.

Complications

HEPATIC COMA

Secondary to ammonia buildup in the blood and interference with normal brain metabolism. Also called hepatocerebral intoxication, ammonia intoxication, and portosystemic encephalopathy.

Assessment

1. Initially, slight apathy and/or euphoria observed, with incoordination that progresses to forgetfulness, confusion, and an inversion of the normal sleep rhythm. Then client becomes restless and untidy and behaves inappropriately, with picking at the bedclothes. Lethargy and stupor ensue, and finally coma develops. Rarely, seizures develop, but rigidity, hyperreflexia, and a characteristic flapping tremor (asterixis) of the hands are usually present.
2. Fetor hepaticus, a musty breath odor.
3. Electroencephalogram changes present.

Revised Outcomes

1. Blood ammonia level will be decreased, and brain functioning will return to normal.
2. Client will not harm self during periods of disorientation and will be able to state name, time, and place.
3. Other expected outcomes will occur as stated for *Hepatic Cirrhosis*.

Interventions

1. Administer low-protein, high-calorie diet to minimize endogenous protein breakdown and ammonia absorption from the gastrointestinal tract. Lactovegetarian diet especially useful. Avoid foods high in ammonia and/or preformed amines such as cheese, salami, and lima beans.
2. Encourage frequent small meals rather than three large meals.
3. Abstain from alcohol.
4. Avoid constipation, which increases ammonia formation in gastrointestinal tract.

5. Avoid drugs with ammonium salts and/or urea.
6. Control gastrointestinal bleeding, as blood is a source of protein. A large-bore Ewald tube is often used so large clots can be removed. Laxatives and/or an enema are used to empty the colon of nitrogenous products.
7. Administer neomycin, a poorly absorbed antibiotic, to decrease intestinal bacteria. Bacterial action on protein produces ammonia.
8. Administer lactulose to acidify the colon and decrease ammonia absorption.
9. Monitor potassium level and administer supplements, as hypokalemia increases ammonia reabsorption by the kidneys.
10. Administer L-dopa as prescribed to control symptoms until ammonia level is decreased.
11. For severe cases, exchange blood transfusions, hemodialysis, plasmaphoresis, cross-circulation with humans or animals, extracorporeal pig liver perfusion, charcoal hemoperfusion, and liver homotransplant are being investigated.

Reevaluation and Follow-up

1. Establish an individualized plan to ensure sobriety.
2. Evaluate compliance with goals established.

HEMORRHAGE

Secondary to esophageal varices becoming overextended and bleeding. Control of this bleeding can be complicated if the liver pathology has resulted in clotting defects.

Assessment

1. Indications of hypovolemia and shock (see Chapters 48 and 49).
2. Black, tarry stools if blood loss is slow. All stools should be tested (guiac) for the presence of blood.
3. Bright red or coffee ground emesis (hematemesis) may be present if blood loss is rapid.

Revised Outcomes

1. Blood loss will be stopped, and blood volume will be maintained.
2. Hepatic coma will be prevented.

Interventions

1. Control bleeding and prevent shock. Replace blood loss intravenously; intravenous vasopressin may also be used to control hypotension and decrease bleeding. Vitamin K is given if the prothrombin time is prolonged (refer to Chapters 48 and 49).
2. Administer gastric lavage with iced saline, to control bleeding initially and remove blood from the stomach. Administer continuously until fluid begins to clear.
3. Insert a Sengstaken-Blakemore tube to compress bleeding varices. It consists of a three-lumen tube, one going to the stomach for suctioning, one ending in a gastric balloon, and one ending in an esophageal balloon. After insertion, correct positioning is determined by x-ray examination, and the two balloons are inflated (see Figure 33-12). Continuous pressure is then applied to keep the gastric balloon against the cardioesophageal junction. To prevent necrosis, the balloons are deflated (esophageal balloon first) in 24 h. After 48 h, if no further bleeding occurs, they are removed. Dislodgement and airway obstruction are constant dangers while using the tube and scissors should be kept at the bedside to deflate balloons in an emergency.

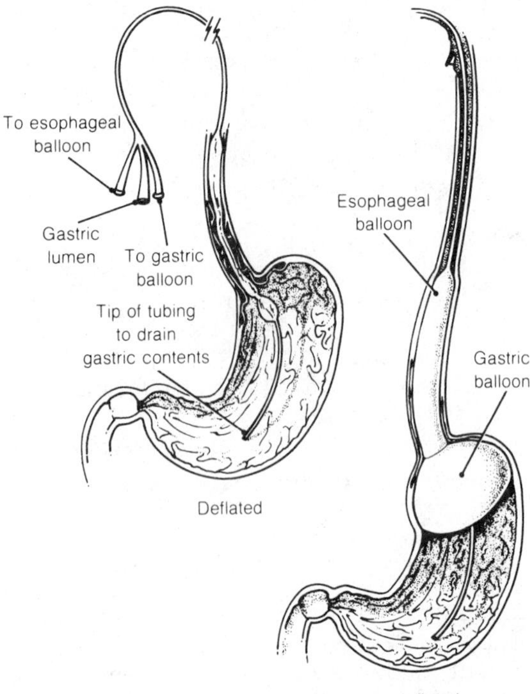

Figure 33-12 Sengstaken-Blakemore tube for bleeding espophageal varices. (From Jones, D.A., et al., eds.: *Medical-Surgical Nursing: A Conceptual Approach*, 2d ed., McGraw-Hill, New York, 1982.)

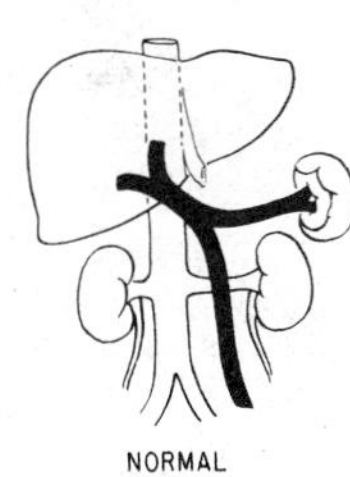

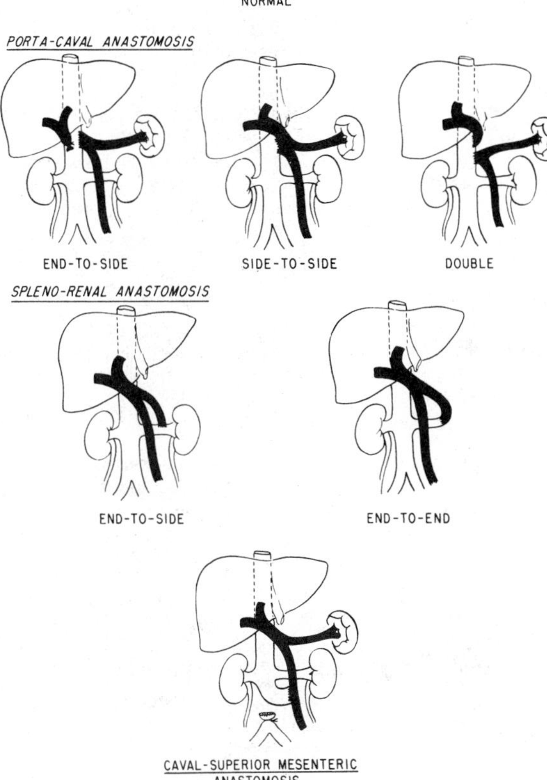

Figure 33-13 Diagrammatic representation of major portosystemic shunts. (From Schwartz, S.I.: *Surgical Diseases of the Liver*, McGraw-Hill, New York, 1964.)

4. Surgical intervention utilizing a portosystemic shunt if medical management does not control the hemorrhage. The procedure involves diverting blood from the portal vein so that pressure is relieved and esophageal varices are drained (see Figure 33-13). Because the procedure diverts splanchnic blood from the liver, the ammonia absorbed from the intestine is not detoxified as readily by the liver, and hepatic encephalopathy can develop.
5. Take measures to reduce blood ammonia levels (see interventions under *Hepatic Coma*).

Reevaluation and Follow-up

1. Establish individualized plan to ensure sobriety.
2. Provide long-term surveillance to evaluate response to and compliance with therapy.

REFERENCES

Bassendine, M. F., Chadwick, R. G., Lyssiotis, T., et al.: "Primary Liver Cell Cancer in Britain: A Viral Aetiology," *British Medical Journal*, **1**(6157):166, January 20, 1979.

Bland, K. I., and Garrison, R. N.: "Colorectal Carcinoma: Overview of Management Techniques," *Postgraduate Medicine*, **66**(3):106–115, September 1979.

Bodemar, G., and Walan, A.: "Maintenance Treatment of Recurrent Peptic Ulcer by Cimetidine," *The Lancet*, **1**(8061):403–407, February 25, 1978.

DeSomery, C. H., and Hansen, B. W.: "Regulation of Appetite During Total Parenteral Nutrition," *Nursing Research*, **27**(1), January–February 1978.

Kelly, K. A.: "Which Operation for Duodenal Ulcer?" *Mayo Clinic Proceedings*, **55**:5–9, January 1980.

Kiernan, T. W., and Ramgopal, M.: "Viral Hepatitis: Progress and Problems," *Medical Clinics of North America*, **63**(2):611–609, May 1979.

Hayles, A. B., and Huse, D. M.: "Obesity—Who Is to Blame?" (Editorial), *Mayo Clinic Proceedings*, **54**:749, November 1979.

LeVeen, H. H., Wapnick, S., Diaz, C., et al.: "Ascites: Its Correction by Peritoneovenous Shunting," *Current Problems in Surgery*, **16**(2):3–56, February 1979.

Malagelada, J. R.: "Pancreatic Cancer," *Mayo Clinic Proceedings*, **54**:459–467, July 1979.

Patek, A.: "Alcohol, Malnutrition, and Alcoholic Cirrhosis," *American Journal of Clinical Nutrition*, **32**:1304–1312, June 1979.

Regan, P. T.: "Medical Treatment of Acute Pancreatitis," *Mayo Clinic Proceedings*, **54**:432–434, July 1979.

Rush, B. F.: "Tumors of the Head and Neck," in Schwartz, S. I., et al. (eds.): *Principles of Surgery*, 3d ed., McGraw-Hill, New York, 1979, p. 602.

Waters, M., Laing, A., Ambikapathy, A., et al.: "Treatment of Ulcerative Colitis with Thalidomide," *British Medical Journal*, **1**(6166):792, March 24, 1979.

BIBLIOGRAPHY

Baranowski, K., Greene, H., and Lamont, J.: "Viral Hepatitis," *Nursing 76*, **6**(5):31–38, May 1976. Excellent discussion of type A and B hepatitis and related nursing care.

Beeson, P.: "The Growth of Knowledge About the Disease: Hepatitis," *American Journal of Medicine*, **67**:366–370, September 1979. Reviews general information regarding hepatitis to date.

Bell, J.: "Just Another Patient with Gallstones? Don't You Believe It," *Nursing 79* **9**(10):26–33, October 1979. Reviews nursing care of client with gallbladder disease, including diagnosis, preoperative care, postoperative care, and discharge.

Borgen, L.: "Total Parenteral Nutrition in Adults," *American Journal of Nursing*, **78**(2):224–228, February 1978. Excellent overview of TPN. Includes table of complications and how to prevent or correct them.

Bromley, B.: "Applying Orem's Self-Care Theory in Enterostomal Therapy," *American Journal of Nursing*, **80**(2):245–249, February 1980. Enterostomal therapist discusses approach to nursing care based on putting theory into practice.

Burkle, W.: "What You Should Know About Tagamet: New Drug Therapy for Peptic Ulcers," *Nursing 80*, **10**(4):86, April 1980.

Daly, K. M.: "Oral Cancer: Everyday Concerns," *American Journal of Nursing*, **79**:1415–1417, August 1979. Excellent discussion of postsurgical problems and ways to cope from client's perspective.

Gruber, M., and Nywer, N.: "Treating Esophageal Varicies with Injection Sclerotherapy," *American Journal of Nursing*, **82**(8):1214, August 1982. Good discussion of alternative endoscopic technique, as opposed to shunting procedure, to control esophageal bleeding.

Jones, D. A., et al. (eds.): *Medical-Surgical Nursing: A Conceptual Approach*, 2d ed., McGraw-Hill, New York, 1982. Excellent general medical-surgical text with pathophysiology, physical assessment, and preventative, ambulatory, and acute care incorporated throughout. Metabolic disorders are covered in depth.

Kosel, K., and Matas, P. G.: "Total Pancreatectomy and Islet Cell Autotransplantation," *American Journal of Nursing*, **82**(4):568, April 1982. Good discussion of new procedure to reduce discomfort of chronic pancreatitis.

Kratzer, J. B., and Rauschenberger, D. S.: "What to Tell Your Patient About His Duodenal Ulcer," *Nursing 78*, **8**(1):54–56, January 1978. Discusses teaching plan and reviews major areas to be covered.

Long, G. D.: "GI Bleeding: What To Do and When," *Nursing 78*, **8**(3):44–50, March 1978. Covers usual emergency care of GI bleeding and ways of differentiating possible causes.

Mahan, L. K.: "A Sensible Approach to the Obese Patient," *Nursing Clinics of North America*, **14**(2):229, June 1979. Excellent discussion. Includes comprehensive table summarizing the many treatments for obesity, with comments of effectiveness of each.

Malagelada, J.: "Medical Versus Surgical Therapy for Duodenal Ulcer," *Mayo Clinic Proceedings*, **55**:25–32, January 1980. Good discussion of drugs used, with their benefits and averse effects.

Samborsky, V.: "Drug Therapy for Peptic Ulcer," *American Journal of Nursing*, **78**(12):2064–2066, December 1978. Discusses use of cimetidine in peptic ulcer. Includes action and side effects.

Seybert, P. L., Gordon, K. M., and Jackson, B. S.: "The LeVeen Shunt: New Hope for Ascites Patients," *Nursing 79*, **9**:24–31, January 1979. Excellent description of new procedure with preoperative and postoperative care. Includes case study to illustrate.

Sherman, D. W., et al.: "Realistic Nursing Goals in Terminal Cirrhosis," *Nursing 78*, **8**(6):43–46, June 1978. Reviews case study of evolving cirrhosis. Includes insert explaining esophageal varices and shunt procedure.

Sweet, K.: "Hiatal Hernia," *Nursing 77*, **7**(8):36–43, August 1977. Excellent discussion of etiology, effects, diagnosis, treatment, and care of hiatal hernia.

Wentworth, A., and Cox, B.: "Nursing the Patient with Continent Ileostomy," *American Journal of Nursing*, **76**(9):1424–1428, September 1976. Very good discussion of postoperative care and management of internal ileostomy pouch.

Wilson, J., and Colley, R.: "Meeting Patients' Nutritional Needs with Hyperalimentation," *Nursing 79*, **9**(8):56–63, August 1979. Photographic study and discussion focusing on teaching clients to administer TPN at home.

34

The Reproductive System

Mary Suzanne Tarmina

Problems common to both the female and male reproductive systems are presented in this chapter with the exception of infertility problems, which can be found in Chapter 14, The Infertile Family, and problems of the male urogenital system, which can be found in Chapter 32, The Urinary System. In addition, a more detailed discussion of sexually transmitted diseases can be found in Chapter 24, Communicable Diseases.

The majority of the problems encountered with the reproductive system are related to abnormal cellular growth and inflammation; therefore, early screening and preventive interventions are of utmost importance in decreasing the morbidity and mortality resulting from diseases of this system. Nursing plays a vital role in teaching clients early signs and symptoms of the major reproductive problems as well as the need for periodic examinations.

Most malignant tumors of the reproductive tract require surgical removal. Irradiation and chemo- or hormone therapy may be alternative or additional choices of treatment. To the client and family undergoing such procedures, the gynecological nurse provides invaluable physical and emotional support as educator, counselor, and mediator. Because of the nature of the disease and its highly specialized treatment regimens, the gynecological nurse may represent an important link in the chain of gynecologist, surgeon, radiologist, medical social worker, and family.

FEMALE REPRODUCTIVE SYSTEM

ABNORMAL CELLULAR GROWTH

CERVICAL CARCINOMA

DESCRIPTION

Cervical carcinoma is a rapid cellular dysplasia that begins at the cervical squamocolumnar junction (transformation zone) and, if unabated, then infiltrates the cervical stroma, vagina, uterus, pelvic cavity, and distant organs in metastasis. The *transformation zone* is that area of the cervix where the single layer of columnar epithelium covering the cervix meets the stratified layers of simple squamous epithelium covering the vagina mucosa (Figure 34-1). The squamocolumnar junction is usually located just inside the external os of the cervix, but in clients with severe dysplasia the junction is often found outside the os because of endocervical eversion or erosion. Approximately 95 percent of cervical cancers arise from the squamous epithelium as a preinvasive carcinoma in situ or invasive carcinoma and 5 percent from the columnar epi-

Recognition is given to Nancy Reame, R.N., PhD., who was the original author of this chapter in the previous edition of this book.

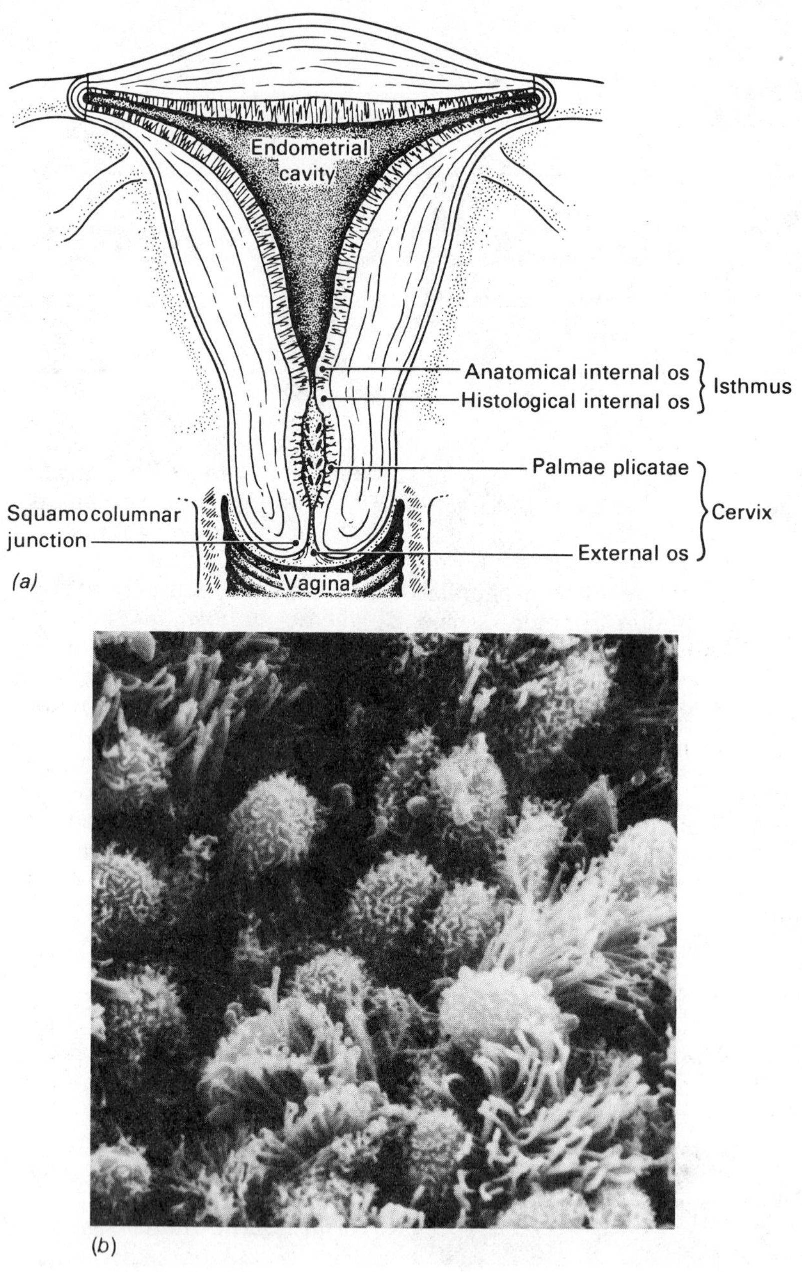

Figure 34-1 The transition zone (squamocolumnar junction) is a common site for cervical cancer. (*a*) Anatomy of the cervix. (*b*) Area above the squamocolumnar junction (endocervix) composed of a single layer of ciliated and secretory cells. (Adapted from Romney, S. L., et al.: *Gynecology and Obstetrics: The Health Care of Women*, McGraw-Hill, New York, 1975.)

thelium as adenocarcinomas (Gusberg and Depper, 1982).

Squamous cell carcinoma of the cervix is divided into two phases. The *preinvasive phase* begins with mild dysplasia and progresses to carcinoma in situ, which moves rapidly through the epithelium but does not penetrate the basement membrane. If treated in this phase, a 100 percent 5-year survival rate is predicted (Beller et al., 1974). The *invasive phase* includes the spread of the tumor into the stroma of the cervix, down the vaginal wall, into the broad ligaments and pelvic wall, and through the lymphatic vessels, involving the paracervical, hypogastric, obturator, and external iliac nodes and possible metastasis of adjacent or distant organs. The clinical stages of invasive carcinoma have been documented by international convention from stage 0, carcinoma in situ, through stage IV, infiltration into the bladder, rectum, and other organs (UICC, 1977). The prognosis for recovery for these stages decreases from 85 percent in stage I to 5–10 percent in stage IV.

Early stages of the preinvasive phase may be removed by biopsy, cautery, or cryosurgery. Radiotherapy and surgery are the treatment modalities for the invasive phase, and chemotherapy is used for recurrent lesions.

PREVENTION

Health Promotion

1. Abstinence from sexual activity and avoidance of pregnancy at an early age.
2. Maintenance of a monogamous sexual relationship.
3. Abstinence or use of a condom if partner has herpes virus type 2 or prostatic or penile cancer or is uncircumcised.
4. Periodic Pap test; prompt report of abnormal bleeding to health care provider.

Population at Risk

1. Women of low socioeconomic status.
2. Women whose first coitus took place at an early age.
3. Women whose first pregnancy took place at an early age.
4. Female prostitutes.
5. Women engaging in coitus with uncircumcised and/or with multiple partners.
6. Women infected with herpes virus type 2.
7. Non-Jewish, black, or Mexican-American women.
8. Women whose partners have prostatic or penile cancer.

Screening

1. Family history of blood relatives with gynecological cancer.
2. Periodic Pap stain of cervical smears.

ASSESSMENT

Health History

1. Age: medium age for preinvasive carcinoma is about 10 years younger than age for invasive cervical cancer.
2. Race: non-Jewish, black, Mexican-American.
3. Nonreversible weight loss.
4. Socioeconomic status.
5. Partner status: years with current partner; stability of relationship.
6. Menstrual history: regularity of cycle, noncyclic bleeding, intermenstrual bleeding, postmenopausal bleeding.
7. Obstetrical history: number of pregnancies, type of delivery, age at first pregnancy.
8. Sexual history: age at first coitus, number of partners, number of uncircumcised partners, contact with herpes virus type 2, penile or prostatic cancer, postcoital spotting, dyspareunia.
9. Personal hygiene habits.
10. Previous cervical problems: symptoms, diagnostic tests, treatment.
11. Previous vaginal, vulval infections: type of discharge, herpes virus type 2, antibiotics used.
12. Abdominal discomfort: asymptomatic, nausea and vomiting, unusual dull cramping, lower quadrant fullness.
13. Rectal problems: bleeding, constipation.
14. Urinary discomfort: burning, hematuria, CVA tenderness.
15. Referred flank or leg pain; persistent leg edema.
16. Level of anxiety; fear of cancer or death.
17. Family history: carcinoma of specific part of reproductive system.

Physical Assessment

1. *Preinvasive phase:* normal external genitalia; cervix and vaginal mucosa pink and clear; bimanual exam unremarkable, possible cervical bleeding after exam (stage 0).

2. *Invasive phase:* enlarged cervix; friable, granular, red and yellow fungating mass centering around external os, possible purulent, sanguineous, or serous exudate; irregular cervical surface; mass and/or vaginal extension on bimanual exam; parametrial infiltration on rectovaginal exam (stages I–IV).

Diagnostic Tests

1. Pap test: mild to severe dysplasia—preinvasive carcinoma in situ; unattainable if massive necrotic lesion present, thus presenting distorted cellular morphology of invasive carcinoma.
2. Schiller test or colposcopy and punch biopsy of squamocolumnar junction: positive—preinvasive carcinoma in situ; diagnostic curretage of endocervical canal positive—invasive phase.
3. Cone biopsy: malignant invasion of stromal tissue (stage I).

NURSING DIAGNOSES: ACTUAL OR POTENTIAL

1. Anxiety (mild to severe): fear of cancer, disfigurement, death.
2. Alteration in self-concept: implications of surgery on body image, sexuality, fertility, maternal role.
3. Alteration in comfort: pain.
4. Grieving: loss of body part.

EXPECTED OUTCOMES

1. Anxiety and fear of surgery or radiation and dying will be reduced.
2. Client will adapt and cope positively with cancer diagnosis.
3. Client will reevaluate self-concept and adapting to surgical or radiation changes.
4. Preventive measures will be taken to reduce risk of recurrence.

INTERVENTIONS

1. Medical-surgical interventions.
   a. Carcinoma confined to cervix: cone biopsy; simple hysterectomy.
   b. Microinvasive stromal carcinoma: radical hysterectomy (removal of uterus, tubes, ovaries, upper third of vagina, parametrium; ureteral, obturator, hypogastric, iliac lymph node dissection), or radiotherapy with intracavity radium therapy (IRT) (radium implant by cervix) and external radiation therapy (SRT) irradiating regional nodes.
   c. Invasive carcinoma of vagina, parametrium: radiotherapy (IRT and ERT) if lesion is receptive; otherwise, radical hysterectomy.
   d. Extension of carcinoma into pelvic wall: radiotherapy; chemotherapy.
   e. Extension of carcinoma into bladder, rectum, and other organs: individualized exploration for exenteration (removal of invaded pelvic reproductive organs, lymph nodes, bladder and distal ureters, rectum and distal sigmoid colon, perineum and pelvic floor, perineum and levator muscles).
2. Preoperative interventions.
   a. Encourage discussion of fears and anxieties about cancer, dying; allow ventilation of feelings; provide information on 5-year survival rates based on extent of regional involvement.
   b. Provide information and demonstration to the client and family, about:
      (1) Type of medical intervention and procedure: hysterectomy, radiotherapy, possible side effects (anorexia, nausea, vomiting, diarrhea, stomatitis, vaginal discharge); extent of surgical procedure and appearance of wound.
      (2) Anesthesia.
      (3) Preoperative procedures, hospital routines: abdominal perineal shave; NPO after midnight; enema, douche; intravenous fluid; Foley catheter.
      (4) Postoperative procedures and routines.
         (a) Vital signs taken at regular intervals; client turns and coughs q2h.
         (b) Inspiratory maneuvers or techniques used to prevent respiratory complications.
         (c) Foley catheter kept in place 1 to 2 weeks (depending on extent of surgery) to prevent wound contamination and measure urinary output accurately.
         (d) Pain and nausea medications given every 3–4 h as needed.
         (e) IV feedings given first 2 days after surgery; diet progressed from liquid to soft to solid foods.

(f) Hemovac used to drain incision.
(g) Antiembolism stockings worn to prevent edema and thrombophlebitis.
(h) Footboard used to encourage leg exercises and prevent circulatory problems.
(i) Air mattress used to provide comfort and prevent pressure sores.
(j) Bed cradle may be used to keep incision free of bed covers.
(k) If radium implant placed, minimal movement in bed required; "log-roll" turning employed.
(l) Activity is increased from feet dangling first day to standing and walking second day.
(m) Scheduled routine of bed bath, bed pan use, sitz baths, showers.
(n) Number of visitors, hours.

(5) Common misinformation (radioactivity of client); use of shield barrier, limited nursing time in room, telephone visitor contact if radium implant in place.
(6) Resumption of intercourse within 3 months depending on extent of surgery and healing process.

c. Offer counseling through therapeutic use of self or referral concerning sexuality, femininity, cancer, dying, spiritual needs (see Chapters 38 and 45).
d. Provide preoperative nursing care: initiate deep breathing exercises; identify baseline vital signs; control foods and fluids; maintain mouth care; monitor GI or catheter tubes; modify temperature, rest, activity; maintain emotional support.

3. Postoperative interventions.
   a. Assess vital signs, pain, input-output (hydration), vaginal drainage, incision drainage.
   b. If present change perineal and groin dressings frequently to keep as dry as possible.
   c. Have client take sitz baths after voiding and bowel movement to decrease risk of contaminating incision.
   d. Debride wound with hydrogen peroxide or antibacterial solutions using asepto bulb syringe; dry wound area after irrigation with heat lamp or hair dryer.
   e. Maintain indwelling catheter for 7 to 14 days (depending on extent of surgery) to prevent urethral stenosis and urinary incontinence; after catheter is removed, have client urinate while standing to decrease strain on sutures.
   f. Promote rest, relaxation, relief of pain: offer pain medication 20 min before client coughs; splint incision while client is deep breathing and coughing.
   g. Decrease leg edema by continued use of elastic stockings.
   h. Promote healing through deep breathing, turning, coughing, exercise, ambulation.
   i. Promote optimal nutritional intake: high protein, low cholesterol, low fat, moderate carbohydrate intake; supplement vitamin and mineral deficiencies; control nausea and vomiting with frequent carbohydrate snacks; allow no fluids at meals; elevate head of bed during and after meals.
   j. Maintain mouth, skin, and tube care.
   k. Reinforce preoperative teaching and support; initiate sexuality, depression counseling.
   l. Assess abdominal surgical complications through hemorrhage, untoward pain, fever, distorted self-concept.
   m. Prepare client for discharge: explain rationale for periodic screening; identify community organizations for cancer and posthysterectomy clients; discuss home activity of no lifting for 6 weeks, stair climbing only after 2 to 3 weeks to avoid undue strain on abdominal muscles; no tub bathing for 6 weeks to prevent infection in cervical stump.

EVALUATION

Outcome Criteria

1. Client was initially dependent on nursing management but is now taking responsibility for deep breathing, coughing, ambulation, and rest.
2. Client openly communicates feelings about surgery and loss of reproductive ability.
3. Client initiates discussion of questions and concerns about prognosis.
4. Client indicates positive beliefs about self-worth.
5. Client actively participates in arranging re-

turn appointment to outpatient clinic; keeps appointment.

Complications

RECURRENT CARCINOMA IN VAGINAL VAULT

Assessment

1. Class III or IV Pap test.
2. Foul-smelling green, yellow, purulent, or sanguineous discharge.
3. Postcoital bleeding, dyspareunia.
4. Rectovaginal exam reveals parametrial infiltration.
5. Punch biopsy of vaginal vault identifies invasive carcinoma.
6. Client moderately to severely anxious and concerned (see discussion of anxiety in Chapter 36).

Revised Outcomes

1. Client will regain hope via new treatment modality.
2. Anxiety and fear of another recurrence will be reduced.
3. Fear of dying will be openly discussed.
4. Preventive measures will be continued to reduce risk of further recurrence.

Interventions

1. Teach client about radiotherapy (IRT and ERT) (implant procedure, restricted nursing contact, use of lead shield), including side effects of anorexia, nausea, vomiting, diarrhea, complete bed rest with restrictive movements, Foley catheter, fracture pan or emesis basin for bowel movements.
2. Evaluate anxiety and offer emotional support (see discussion of anxiety in Chapter 36).
3. Assess nausea, diarrhea, skin reaction, and fatigue; initiate a bland low-fiber diet; keep irradiated skin dry and well aerated.
4. Promote rest and healing by answering client's signal light promptly; position body in good alignment; encourage passive range of motion movements.
5. Give discharge instructions, including resuming sexual intercourse within 7 to 10 days depending on cervical and vaginal reaction to radiotherapy, douching to control vaginal discharge (distilled vinegar water solution), avoiding direct sunlight to areas of radiation exposure, using emollient cream to reduce pruritus.
6. Assess client's support system and need for visiting nursing service after discharge.

Reevaluation and Follow-up

1. Establish a specific individualized plan for assessing the recurrence of complications through periodic return exams, telephone contact, and home health evaluation.
2. Develop a long-term surveillance plan to ensure the provision of appropriate interventions.

RECURRENT CARCINOMA IN BLADDER OR RECTUM

Assessment

1. Backache, abdominal discomfort, urinary and rectal discomfort.
2. Blood in urine and/or feces.
3. CVA tenderness.
4. Palpable suprapubic mass upon abdominal exam; tenderness upon palpation.

Revised Outcomes

See Revised Outcomes for *Recurrent Carcinoma in Vaginal Vault* immediately above.

Interventions

1. Prepare client for further diagnostic tests, for example, intravenous pyelogram, bone scan, liver enzymes, barium enema.
2. Prepare client and family for pelvic exenteration (total, anterior, posterior) by discussing the purpose and alternatives of surgery, preoperative procedures and hospital routines, changes in body image and excretory and sexual function, changes in daily living habits.
3. Evaluate client's emotional stability, family support systems, financial situation, facilities for home care, need for nursing care in home.
4. Prepare bowels for surgery: antibiotics, laxative, enemas, intestinal tube, abdominal preparation.
5. Assist in placement of central venous pressure line.
6. Offer continuous emotional support.
7. Evaluate immediate postoperative condition by assessing cardiac changes, signs of shock, kidney function.
8. Promote return of physiological homeostasis and healing (see postoperative interventions originally stated under Interventions).
9. Reduce anxiety, discomfort (see discussion of anxiety in Chapter 36).
10. Provide postoperative teaching of client and family concerning dressing changes, stoma care, diet (see postoperative interventions under Interventions).

11. Provide postoperative counseling and support concerning grief over bodily mutilation, extent of surgery, change in body functions and lifestyle, fear of sudden death, relapse (see Chapters 38 and 45).
12. Promote continuity of care and support during convalescence by visiting nurse referral and visit in hospital, periodic calls to client at home, continued teaching, counseling at physician's visits concerning sexual function and new problems, referral for sexual counseling for couple if desired.

Reevaluation and Follow-up

See Reevaluation and Follow-up under *Recurrent Carcinoma in Vaginal Vault* above.

METASTASIS TO SPINE

Assessment

1. Backache, pelvic pain.
2. Weight loss, fatigue.
3. Depression, despair (see discussion of depression in Chapter 36).

Revised Outcomes

See Revised Outcomes for *Recurrent Carcinoma in Vaginal Vault* above.

Interventions

1. Prepare client for chemotherapy: maintain nutritional and health status; teach about purpose, procedure, side effects, and treatment of side effects; counsel and provide emotional support.
2. Reduce discomfort of side effects (i.e., pain, nausea, vomiting, mouth bleeding, skin irritation, diarrhea).
3. Reduce risk of infection.
4. Promote family support and environment for expression of feelings.
5. Observe for signs of drug tolerance.
6. Discuss hospice care.

Reevaluation and Follow-up

See Reevaluation and Follow-up under *Recurrent Carcinoma in Vaginal Vault* above.

BREAST CARCINOMA

DESCRIPTION

Breast cancer is a malignant neoplasm that develops from the epithelial lining of the mammary ducts. The carcinoma evolves through hyperplasia of ductal cells, increasing cellular atypia, progressing to intraductal (in situ) carcinoma, and finally stromal invasion. Multiple sites of malignancy are found in 50 percent of breasts removed for a clinically single focus of cancer (Donegan, 1982). Metastasis often occurs in distant lymph nodes, axial skeleton, pleura, lungs, liver, and finally the intracranium. The cause is unknown, but a genetic predisposition has been suggested for some families as well as environmental factors of high fat consumption, obesity, and exposure to carcinogens.

Segmental, modified, and radical mastectomies are still the major treatment modalities with irradiation, chemotherapy, and endocrine-hormone therapy used in disseminated breast cancer. Approximately 78 percent of clients with no axillary node involvement (stage I) will survive 5 years after a mastectomy (Fisher et al., 1975). Invasive mammary carcinoma has been classified into four clinical stages:

1. *Stage I:* breast tumors less than 2 cm in diameter.
2. *Stage II:* breast tumors 2–5 cm or cancers with small mobile axillary lymph node metastases.
3. *Stage III:* breast tumors over 5 cm with lymph node metastases or skin involvement.
4. *Stage IV:* distant metastases.

Noninvasive cancers are classified as stage TIS (tumor-in-situ) (AJC, 1978).

PREVENTION

Health Promotion

1. Avoidance of extended use of oral contraceptives if established fibrocystic disease or strong family history of breast cancer is present.
2. Maintenance of monthly self breast exams (SBE) (70 percent of breast carcinomas are found by clients themselves) (Donegan, 1982).
3. Avoidance of environmental factors of high fat consumption, obesity, and exposure to carcinogens.
4. Avoidance of first full-term pregnancy after age 35.
5. Reduced ingestion of methylxanthine-containing foods that can aggravate development of fibrocystic disease (e.g., tea, coffee, cola drinks, chocolate) (Minton et al., 1979).
6. Avoidance of prolonged, high dose, exogenous estrogen exposure.

7. Annual mammogram for women over age 50 and from 40 to 49 years of age for those with history of breast cancer in mother, sister, or daughter or previous cancer of one breast.

Population at Risk

1. Women 40 years of age and older.
2. Jews and Western Caucasian women.
3. Women with a high fat-consumption diet.
4. Obese women.
5. Women living in an urban and highly industrialized area, Western hemisphere, or cold climate.
6. Women of high socioeconomic status.
7. Daughter, sister, mother of breast cancer client.
8. Women with previous benign breast disease or cancer of one breast.
9. Women with previous endometrial, ovarian, or colon cancer.
10. Women exposed to excessive breast irradiation.
11. Women with Cowden's disease (multiple hamartoma syndrome).
12. Women on high prolonged doses of conjugated estrogens for natural or surgical menopause.
13. Women who experienced menarche before age 12 years and/or menopause after age 50 years.
14. Women with 30 or more years of active menstrual activity.
15. Nulliparas or women who had a first full-term pregnancy after age 35.
16. Women with established fibrocystic breast disease who have made extensive use of oral contraceptives.
17. Men with Klinefelter's syndrome (XXY sex chromosomes).

Screening

1. Annual breast exam by health care provider.
2. Monthly SBE.
3. Mammography.

ASSESSMENT

Health History

1. Age: over 40.
2. Race: Jewish, Caucasian.
3. Residence, socioeconomic status.
4. Stature: obese.
5. Diet: high fat consumption.
6. Reproductive system: menarche; aggregate lifetime menstrual cycle; age of menopause; age of first full-term pregnancy; number of pregnancies; previous cancer of the endometrium, ovary, colon and type of treatment; previous operations, cause; LNMP.
7. Drugs: use and length of time on oral contraceptives; dose, years of use of conjugated estrogens.
8. Skin and mouth: small raised tumors (trichoepitheliomas) on face or hands or in oral cavity.
9. Breast: benign breast disease; previous cancer of one breast; excessive irradiation of breast tissue; persistent erosion or crusting of a nipple; nontender mass sometimes associated with discomfort; dimpling; unilateral nipple discharge; recent nipple retraction, swelling, erythema, ulceration, pain, ecchymoses; enlarged tender lymph nodes (supraclavicular).
10. Family history: mother or sister with breast cancer.

Physical Assessment

1. Skin, month: small circumscribed nodules (trichoepitheliomas) on face or hands or in oral cavity.
2. Breast examination.
   a. Previous mastectomy.
   b. Asymmetry in size or shape.
   c. Localized edema, erythema, pink satellite nodules within the skin, ulceration, ecchymoses, pain on palpation and by history, skin dimpling.
   d. Hard, ill-defined mass; nontender on palpation; usually immobile; blocks transillumination.
   e. Moist ulcerated, crusted lesion on or around nipple; sanguineous nipple discharge; deviated or inverted nipple resisting temporary eversion.
3. Client is restless, agitated, intense.

Diagnostic Tests

1. Fine-needle aspiration: increased resistance to passage of needle; small sanguineous aspirate with mass remaining.
2. Mammogram.
3. Incisional (small specimen from large mass) or excisional (complete removal) biopsy.
4. Estrogen-progresterone receptor protein (ER) analysis of tumor tissue.
5. Ultrasound with automated water-bath scan-

ner to visualize discrete cysts from solid lesions.

NURSING DIAGNOSES: ACTUAL OR POTENTIAL

1. Anxiety (mild to severe): fear of cancer, death, body disfigurement (see discussion of anxiety in Chapters 36, 38, and 45).
2. Grieving: loss of body part, femininity.
3. Impairment of significant others to illness.
4. Alteration in self-concept: body image, self-esteem, role performance, personal identity.
5. Alteration in patterns of sexuality: minimization of breast stimulation in sexual foreplay.

EXPECTED OUTCOME

1. Fear of cancer, death, and body disfigurement will be reduced.
2. Cancer diagnosis will be accepted by positive coping mechanisms.
3. Postoperative healing will occur without complications.
4. Client will regain full range of motion (ROM) and function of arm on affected side.
5. Client and family will adapt to surgical changes of body image by reevaluating self-concept.
6. Preventive measures will be taken to prevent risk of recurrence.

INTERVENTIONS

1. Medical-surgical interventions.
   a. Stage TIS: lumpectomy; total mastectomy (all mammary parenchyma, axillary tail of Spence) and dissection of lower axillary lymph nodes.
   b. Stage I: lumpectomy and irradiation; segmental mastectomy (removal of involved section of breast leaving only skin, nipple intact) or modified radical mastectomy (removal of entire breast and varying amount of axillary tissue only) and irradiation or chemotherapy if ER negative; hormone therapy if ER positive.
   c. Stage II: modified radical mastectomy and irradiation or chemo/hormone therapy.
   d. Stage III: radical mastectomy (removal of skin, entire breast, pectoralis minor and major muscles, deep facia and entire axillary contents) and irradiation or chemo/hormone therapy.
   e. Stage IV: chemo- or hormone therapy based on ER analysis of carcinoma.
2. Preoperative interventions.
   a. Encourage client and family to discuss fears and anxieties about cancer, dying, body disfigurement, and other concerns.
   b. Provide information to client and family about:
      (1) Type of mastectomy, irradiation, chemo/hormone therapy; possible side effects (anorexia, nausea, vomiting, local discomfort, hair loss).
      (2) Anesthesia.
      (3) Preoperative procedures, hospital routines.
      (4) Postoperative procedures: pressure dressings or catheter suction; pain; rest; treatment of affected arm; daily routine; coughing, deep-breathing, ROM exercises; visitors.
   c. Offer counseling through therapeutic use of self or referral concerning femininity, body disfigurement, cancer, dying, spiritual needs (see Chapters 36, 38, and 45).
   d. Provide preoperative care: initiate deep breathing exercises; identify baseline vital signs; control food and fluids; modify rest and activity; maintain emotional support.
3. Postoperative interventions.
   a. Assess vital signs, pain, discomfort, incisional drainage (avoid taking blood pressure, venipuncture, giving injections or vaccinations on affected arm to reduce chance of infection or decreased circulation).
   b. Evaluate wound drainage on pressure dressing or in hemovac; check for swelling in immediate area, amount and color of drainage; assess wound each shift; change dressing using sterile technique.
   c. Maintain support of affected arm by keeping hand higher than elbow, which is higher than shoulders, by using two pillows under hand and one pillow under elbow; keep in good body alignment.
   d. Prevent injury to desensitized area.
   e. Promote rest, relaxation, relief of pain: offer pain medication 20 min before coughing, deep breathing exercise.
   f. Promote healing: deep breathing, turning, coughing, range-of-motion exercises for affected arm, using hand and arm after surgery, squeezing bandage roll or ball 10

times an hour, ambulation, appropriate nutrition.

g. Reinforce preoperative teaching.
h. Maintain emotional support; assist client in accepting pathological report, extent of disease, further treatment.
i. Assess anxiety level, coping mechanisms, grieving process, self-concept, emotional support systems (see Chapters 36, 38, and 45).
j. Promote adjustment and return to activities of daily living; encourage upright posture when ambulating through Reach to Recovery referral, breast prosthesis, sexual counseling.
k. Prepare client for discharge.
   (1) Explain short-lived dependency on family after discharge.
   (2) Review arm exercises and SBE on remaining breast and incision area.
      (a) Hand grips: beginning day after surgery client should squeeze ball (size of lemon) or bandage roll with hand on affected side, beginning 10 times per hour, continuing at home several times per day.
      (b) Hair brushing; sitting by table client should rest affected arm initially on books and brush hair, working around head; as arm strengthens, client will brush without supporting arm.
      (c) Arm lifting: keeping elbow straight, client should raise arm from side to front and back to side, repeating several times a day.
      (d) Walking the wall: facing wall, client should place palms on wall at shoulder level, walk fingers up wall, and slide palms back to shoulder level, repeating several times; client should mark progress on wall with tape, advancing an inch each day arms extend straight above head.
      (e) Pulley: client should place a 6-ft rope over rod (shower curtain) and grasp an end in each hand and pull back and forth.
   (3) Encourage client to protect hand and arm by wearing gloves if injury is possible, wearing mitts to avoid burns while cooking, wearing rubber gloves when in water for prolonged period, pushing not cutting cuticles, avoiding excessive sun exposure to affected side.
   (4) Instruct client to prevent swelling by elevating arm while sitting (rest on back of chair or sofa); keeping jewelry, sleeves, watch band loose on affected arm; not carrying heavy purse or objects on affected arm.
   (5) Encourage scheduled return appointments.
   (6) Maintain open, supportive communication.

EVALUATION

Outcome Criteria

1. Client was initially dependent on nursing care but is now taking responsibility for deep breathing, coughing, arm exercises, ambulation, and rest.
2. Client openly communicates thoughts about loss of breast, fear of cancer, prognosis.
3. Client follows through with Reach to Recovery Program and independently maintains daily activities and wall climbing, pendulum, pulley, broom-raising, and rope-turning exercises.
4. Client wears prosthesis and participates in arranging return appointment.

Complications

RECURRENT CARCINOMA ON AFFECTED SIDE

Assessment

1. Lump in chest wall at site of incision.
2. Enlarged remaining axillary nodes.

Revised Outcomes

1. Recurring fear of cancer and death will be reduced.
2. Client and family will adapt positively to second cancer diagnosis.
3. Client will experience minimal side effects from irradiation, chemo- or hormone therapy.
4. Preventive measures will be taken to prevent risk of recurrence.

Interventions

1. Prepare client for further diagnostic tests (i.e., metastatic series, ER analysis, mammogram of remaining breast).
2. Assist in preparation for irradiation.
   a. Assess client's knowledge level and perceptions of therapy.
   b. Explain principles of radiation, physical

environment encountered, time involvement per day, expected reactions.
c. Discuss portal markings on skin to indicate therapy boundary that must be left on skin until treatment is terminated.
d. Review therapy reactions: lungs (shortness of breath, respiratory distress); skin (reddening or sunburn reaction to severe necrosis); general malaise.
e. Discuss management of therapy reaction: optimal activity/rest schedule; avoiding lotions, creams, oils to irradiated skin—using only mild soap and warm water; using soft, nonconstrictive cotton bra.

3. Prepare client for chemo/hormone therapy.
   (1) Discuss side effects: nausea, vomiting, possible alopecia, hemorrhagic cystitis, stomatitis, fever, diarrhea, constipation.
   (2) Teach preventive measures.
      (a) Using mouthwash and soft toothbrush q4h; inspecting mouth for white or red patches or sores.
      (b) Eating high-protein, high-calorie foods; doubling fluids—2 to 3 L/day; eating six small meals instead of three large ones.
      (c) Preventing constipation or diarrhea by eating a balanced diet, including bran, vegetables, fruits, meats.
      (d) Preventing infection by inspecting skin, hands, feet daily; exercising in fresh air; preventing bleeding; avoiding aspirin, vitamins.

Reevaluation and Follow-up

1. Assist client and family in maintaining strong support system with consultation and referral as needed.
2. Establish an individualized plan to overcome complications, evaluate interventions, and identify potential health problems.

CARCINOMA OF FORMERLY UNAFFECTED BREAST

See Assessment, Expected Outcomes, and Interventions under *Breast Carcinoma* and Reevaluation and Follow-up under *Recurrent Carcinoma on Affected Side* directly above.

METASTASIS OF OTHER ORGANS

Assessment

1. Backache, pain with breathing, right upper quadrant abdominal distension and discomfort, urinary discomfort, bowel changes, mental status change.
2. Weight loss, fatigue.
3. Depression, despair.

Revised Outcomes

1. Fear of dying will be reduced through support, referral, and consultation.
2. Client and family will adapt to metastasis diagnosis.
3. Client will experience minimal side effects from irradiation and/or chemo- or hormone therapy.

Interventions

1. Reduce pain and discomfort by maintaining good body alignment, supporting pressure areas, anticipating prn pain medication.
2. Prevent spine fractures by supporting axial skeleton and attending client when ambulatory.
3. Assist in preparation for irradiation and/or chemo- or hormone therapy (see Interventions under *Recurrent Carcinoma on Affected Side* above).

Reevaluation and Follow-up

See Reevaluation and Follow-up under *Recurrent Carcinoma on Affected Side* above.

VULVAR CARCINOMA

Vulvar carcinoma, which constitutes 3 to 4 percent of all primary malignancies of the genital tract, is classified as carcinoma in situ, Paget's disease, and invasive carcinoma (Woodruff, 1982). Unfortunately there is often a long delay between the appearance of symptoms and the diagnosis of carcinoma because the initial symptom of pruritus is common to many minor vaginal disorders and is often tolerated for an indefinite period of time.

The average age of all clients with vulvar cancer is 60 to 65 years. Carcinoma in situ occurs at any age and is not uncommon during the third and fourth decades of life (Woodruff). Although the most common complaint of all vulvar cancers is pruritus, the lesion may be asymptomatic or may appear as a lump or white hyperkeratic plaque on an erythematous background (Paget's disease). A 5-year survival rate of 85 to 90 percent can be expected if no lymph nodes are involved. Metastases to inguinal and femoral lymph nodes have a 5-year survival rate of 30 to 35 percent (Woodruff).

Treatment is basically surgical with a wide local excision or removal of the entire vulva (vulvectomy) and the superficial and deep inguinal and femoral lymph nodes. Because of cross lymphatic circulation, a bilateral procedure is recommended.

Postoperative nursing procedures generally include dressing changes, sitz baths, catheter irrigations, and preventive care against leg edema. Vulvectomy clients may require special counseling in dealing with body disfigurement and the effects on sexuality.

CARCINOMA OF THE VAGINA

Primary malignancy arising in the vagina represents less than 1 percent of all genital cancers (Woodruff, 1982). In situ epidermoid carcinomas occur with other similar lesions in the genital area, after incomplete surgery for carcinoma in situ of the cervix, or following radiation for invasive carcinoma of the cervix. The lesions are often asymptomatic but can be recognized early with routine cytology.

The most common malignancy of the vagina is an *invasive neoplasma*. Two-thirds of all clients are over age 50 and present with a bloody vaginal discharge. Vaginal prolapse, urgency, and pain on urination and defecation can occur with diagnosis confirmed by biopsy.

Primary adenocarcinoma arising in benign adenosis tissue is developed most commonly in young women (7 to 27 years of age) whose mother received estrogen therapy during pregnancy (diethylstilbesterol). Women exposed in utero to this drug are at risk for developing the proliferation of endocervical granular epithelium in the vaginal wall in place of the normal squamous epithelium. Of this population at risk, only 0.1 percent develop adenocarcinoma (Herbst, 1978). Routine cytologic and thorough biannual exams are preventive. All vaginal malignancies are treated by surgery and/or radiotherapy or chemotherapy.

CARCINOMA OF THE ENDOMETRIUM

Endometrial carcinoma is the third highest malignancy of the reproductive system of women (Beller, 1974). Clinical conditions associated with carcinoma of the endometrium are menopausal women (75 percent of all endometrial cancers), premenopausal women with long periods of amenorrhea or menorrhagia, women with estrogen-secreting ovarian tumors, clients who have taken estrogen therapeutically, and women with endometrial polyps. The phenotype of a woman with endometrial cancer is one of obesity, diabetes or a diabetic glucose-tolerance curve, and hypertension.

Cystic hyperplasia resulting from a static endometrium is one of the earliest carcinoma stages. Over the years the cysts change, forming a complex glandular tissue called *adenomatous hyperplasia*. In time another transformation of dysplasia occurs, ending in carcinoma in situ. The next stage is invasive with neoplastic glands producing a visible tumor projecting into the lumen of the uterine cavity. The tumor extends into the surrounding endometrium and then invades the myometrium and the pelvic lymph nodes. The lymphatic spread results in metastases to the vaginal vault, rectum, and ovaries. Invasion of blood vessels results in metastases to the liver, lungs, and bone marrow.

The most common characteristic of endometrial cancer is dysfunctional uterine bleeding (*metrorrhagia*) presenting as a mucoid, sanguineous vaginal discharge. Cramping, occasional contractions, and an increased sense of pressure may be present. Aspiration curettage or endometrial biopsy is the diagnostic method employed.

Several schemas of treatment exist: total hysterectomy and bilateral salpingo-oophorectomy following several weeks of radium implantation or external radiation following the hysterectomy and oophorectomy. Postoperative x-ray and/or hormonal or cytotoxic chemotherapy is used for disseminated disease beyond the uterus and into the myometrial and aortic lymphatics.

ENDOMETRIOSIS

DESCRIPTION

Endometriosis is characterized by the presence and proliferation outside the uterus of endometrial tissue that responds to hormonal stimulation. Retrograde tubal flow of menstrual fragments leads to implantation and growth of endometrium on ovaries, cul-de-sac, and uterosacral ligaments that then respond to hormonal influence. Other theories address the inflammatory stimulus of specific cells on endometrial tissue or the release of chemical-inducing substances from transported endometrium-activating undifferentiated tissue to form endometrial tissue as the cause. Nutrition, intercourse during menstruation, and the use of tampons have also been suggested as causative factors. Common sites for endometrial cell attachment are the vulva, vaginal vault, urinary bladder, pelvic peritoneum, uterus, fallopian tubes, ovaries, small intestine, large intestine, cul-de-sac, and rectovaginal septum. The incidence of women having endometriosis is about 25 percent. The fertility rate of clients with endometriosis is 66 percent as opposed to 88 percent in the general population (Merrill, 1982).

PREVENTION

Health Promotion

1. Maintenance of a well-balanced diet.
2. Refraining from intercourse during menstruation.
3. Use of pads instead of tampons during menstruation.
4. Avoidance of tubal insufflation, which causes the reflux of endometrial tissue through the fallopian tubes into the peritoneal cavity where implantation occurs.
5. Avoidance of hysterosalpingography, during which endometrial tissue can be inadvertently transplanted.
6. Avoidance of cervidilation during menstrual flow because of the reflux result of forcing endometrial cells out through the tubes.
7. Avoidance of pregnancy at an early age.

Population at Risk

1. Women between the ages of 30 and 48.
2. Women whose mothers, grandmothers, aunts, or sisters have a history of the disease.
3. An initial pregnancy in the late twenties or the thirties or forties.
4. A very unbalanced diet.
5. Women who consistently have intercourse during menstruation or use only tampons.
6. Women who have had a tubal insufflation, hysterosalpingography, or cervidilation during menstruation.

Screening

1. Laparoscopy.
2. Regularly scheduled periodic pelvic examinations.

ASSESSMENT

Health History

1. Age: late twenties, thirties.
2. Family history: occurrence in other women in the maternal blood line.
3. Diet: frank nutritional deficiencies.
4. Reproductive history: age at first pregnancy; past history of tubal insufflation, hysterosalpingography, or cervidilation; infertility.
5. Sexual history: consistent intercourse during menstruation; deep dyspareunia; asymptomatic.
6. Menstrual history: use of only tampons during mensturation; dysmenorrhea; dull, aching, or cramping lower abdominal or sacral pain associated with menstruation and decreasing as flow begins; abnormal flow, duration of cycles; asymptomatic.
7. Abdominal pelvic symptoms: pain with bowel movements; constant or intermittent pain with ovulation continuing as vaginal aching, cramping, or bearing down sensation through to menses; asymptomatic.

Physical Assessment

1. Pelvic exam: multiple, tender nodules palpable along the uterosacral ligaments or above the posterior fornix of the vagina; fixed retrograde (tipped) uterus; thickened nodular adnexa and/or an immobile ovarian cyst.
2. Abdominal exam: right or left lower quadrant mass; bloating or distension; pain on palpation.

Diagnostic Tests

1. Laparoscopy to visualize the lesions.
2. Hematocrit or hemoglobin.

NURSING DIAGNOSES: ACTUAL OR POTENTIAL

1. Anxiety (mild to severe): fear of infertility, loss of reproductive status (see discussion of anxiety in Chapter 36).
2. Alteration in self-concept: implications of surgery on body image, maternal role, personal identity.
3. Alteration in comfort: pain.
4. Grieving: loss of body part.
5. Functional performance: variations in ability to perform activities of daily living, work.
6. Alteration in nutrition: fewer body requirements.

7. Alteration in sexuality patterns.
8. Dysrhythm of sleep or rest activity.

EXPECTED OUTCOMES

1. Anxiety and fear of surgery or loss of reproductive status will be reduced.
2. Client will adapt to body image and role change and cope positively with the treatment modality.
3. Pain and discomfort will be eliminated.
4. Client will be able to perform daily functions and have intercourse or a bowel movement without discomfort.
5. Client will maintain a nutritionally balanced diet and demonstrate a normal hematocrit.
6. Sleep patterns will return to normal.

INTERVENTIONS

1. Medical-surgical interventions: based upon childbearing goals of the client and individualized to alleviate symptoms.
   a. Analgesics to relieve dysmenorrhea and abdominal and pelvic pain.
   b. Hormonal therapy of estrogen, testosterone, oral contraceptives, or antigonadotropins for 6 to 9 months.
   c. Selective surgical removal of the endometriosis tissue or bilateral salpingo-oophorectomy and hysterectomy.
2. Preoperative interventions. See the preoperative interventions under Interventions for *Cervical Carcinoma*.
3. Postoperative interventions. See the postoperative interventions under Interventions for *Cervical Carcinoma*.

EVALUATION

Outcome Criteria

1. Client is compliant with hormonal regimen and makes and keeps return appointments.
2. If surgery was performed, client is transferring to self the dependency formerly placed on nursing management for deep breathing, coughing, ambulation, rest, and dietary intake by third or fourth postoperative day.
3. Open communication occurs about surgery and loss of reproductive function.
4. Client indicates positive beliefs about changed role status and self-worth.
5. Activities of daily living and comfortable intercourse are fully restored by 3 months, asymptomatic bowel movement in 2 to 6 weeks.
6. Client is eating a well-balanced diet and maintains a weight-per-height ratio appropriate for body build and hematocrit within normal range within 2 to 3 months.
7. Normal sleep patterns are resumed by 2 to 6 weeks.

Complications

Infertility: see the discussion in Chapter 14, The Infertile Family.

CHORIOCARCINOMA OF THE UTERUS

This reproductive disease is a malignant neoplasm arising from the trophoblastic epithelium of the embryo. Pregnancies in rapid succession and protein deficiency are believed to be predisposing factors. Clinical symptoms may mimic signs of abortion or dysfunctional bleeding.

Although the disease is rare, choriocarcinoma is the outstanding example of a malignancy that can be successfully treated with chemotherapy. Methotrexate is used in conjunction with total hysterectomy or alone in low-risk clients. It blocks the conversion of folic acid to tetrahydrofolic acid, thus interrupting the life cycle of the malignant cell by inhibiting DNA synthesis (Bloomfield, 1976). The drug's side effects include gastric bleeding, ulcers, and bone marrow depression.

CARCINOMA OF THE FALLOPIAN TUBE

Oviduct carcinoma is rare, constituting less than 1 percent of all reproductive system cancers in women age 17 to 80. The highest incidence occurs in the fifth decade, and malignancy is very difficult to diagnose, with 20 percent of all tubal carcinoma clients asymptomatic. The most common symptoms are a yellow or slightly blood-tinged discharge, abnormal vaginal bleeding, menstrual irregularities, and pain. An adnexal mass is the most common physical finding but occurs in only 50 percent of clients. The disease is often found in association with healed or subacute salpingitis and is spread by direct extension rather than through the lymphatics. Abdominal hysterectomy and bilateral salpingo-oophorectomy with postoperative external beam radiation is the preferred treatment. The 5-year survival rate varies from 0 to 44 percent (Merrill, 1982).

OVARIAN CANCER

Malignant neoplasms of the ovary are the fourth leading cause of death from cancer among American women following cancer of the breast, colon, and lung. Predisposing factors include lower parity (especially with history of infertility), repeated spontaneous abortion, delayed onset of childbearing, and family history of malignancy. Approximately 60 percent of malignant ovarian tumors occur in women aged 40 to 60 and 20 percent under 40 and over 60, respectively. There are many different kinds of malignant ovarian lesions, differing histologically. The silent nature of the lesions until well advanced in a malignant growth pattern is nonsupportive of early diagnosis. A consistent pattern of increased abdominal girth, vague lower abdominal discomfort, dyspepsia, weight gain or loss, and other GI abnormalities usually occur late in the disease. Postmenopausal bleeding occurs in about 30 percent of all malignancies. Any palpable ovarian mass greater than 5 cm should be suspect. Ascites occurs with omentum metastases, and pleural effusions, supraclavicular, axillary, and inguinal nodes are additional sites. Total abdominal hysterectomy, bilateral salpingo-oophorectomy, and omentectomy should be followed by radio- or chemotherapy; involved lymph nodes are also excised (Nelson and Dolan, 1982).

BENIGN LESIONS OF THE REPRODUCTIVE TRACT

With the exception of the oviducts, reproductive organs including the breasts are especially susceptible to the proliferation of normal cells of muscle, glands, and connective tissue. Unlike malignancies, benign lesions have a limited growth potential, remain localized, and are usually not life-threatening. Genital lesions have been classified according to tissue of origin, gross features, cell type, and degree of proliferation. Several types appear to be dependent and responsive to the reproductive hormones that have been used in suppressive therapy.

The signs and symptoms of abnormal growth depend on the size and location of the lesion. Many are found incidentally on gynecological examination or in hysterectomy specimens. *Inappropriate uterine bleeding* is the most common manifestation of both benign and malignant tumors. In women of childbearing age, symptoms of benign growth may sometimes be mistaken for pregnancy. Pain does not generally occur unless the growth is large enough to produce tension on surrounding structures. Treatment usually involves surgical removal. Some of the more common sites of benign lesions are shown in Figure 34-2.

CERVICAL POLYPS

Polyps are the second most common lesion of the cervix and are found in all ages but are more common during the reproductive years. Presenting as soft, velvety red lesions, polyps usually are pedunculated and commonly arise from the lower end of the endocervix. The most common symptom for the client is genital bleeding following contact from coitus, douching, or tampon insertion. Many polyps are asymptomatic. Treatment usually consists of avulsion of the polyp as an office procedure unless a malignancy is suspected (Merrill, 1982).

FIBROID TUMORS

A uterine fibroid (leiomyoma, myoma, fibromyoma, fibroma) is a well-circumscribed, pseudocapsulated, benign tumor composed mainly of smooth muscle and some fibrous connective tissue. The lesion is the most common pelvic tumor in women, frequently found in the fourth and fifth decades of life, and more commonly in a black client. The tumors are usually found in the intramural, subserous or submucous layers of the corpus uterus and can grow into the cavity of the uterus, projecting into the cervical canal or into the pelvis and broad ligament and thus distorting the uterine contour. Fibroids may be asymptomatic and can cause abnormal uterine bleeding; bladder or rectal pressure; pelvic pressure resulting in edema or leg varicosities; gradual, intermittent pain; dull, aching soreness; abdominal distortion; and fertility

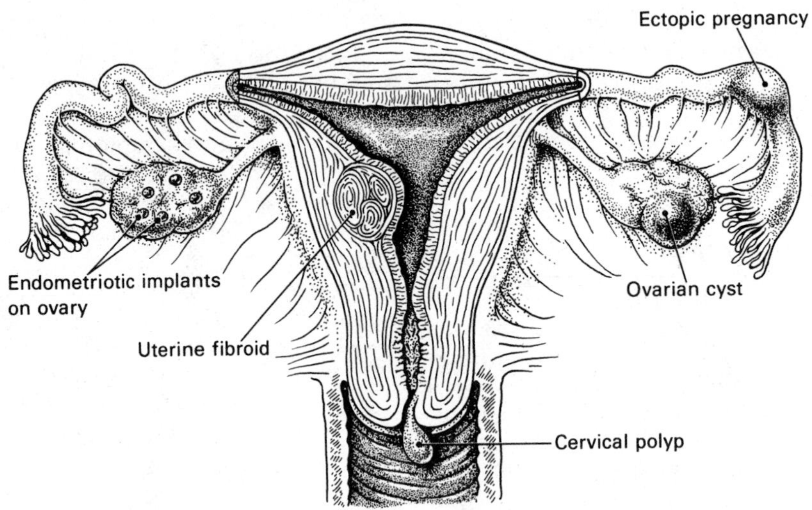

Figure 34-2 Common sites of benign lesions of the female reproductive tract.

impairment. Once menopause occurs the tumor often regresses, sometimes completely supporting a treatment regimen of reevaluative exams every 3 to 6 months for complications.

Myomectomy (removal of tumors) or a total hysterectomy is indicated when a myomatous uterus is larger than a 3-month pregnancy or sudden tumor growth occurs, particularly in a postmenopausal woman. The removal of a single pedunculated tumor has few complications and preserves a childbearing uterus. Adhesions, bowel obstruction, and fibroid recurrence are common after a multiple myomectomy, with a total hysterectomy the procedure of choice for the majority of clients (Merrill, 1982).

FUNCTIONAL OVARIAN CYSTS

Functional ovarian cysts can develop from the continued growth of a follicle when ovulation does not occur, cystic development of the corpus luteum following ovulation, or the cystic enlargement of atretic follicles during pregnancy. Most cysts are asymptomatic and are found incidentally. Symptoms present with larger cysts or the complication of torsion, rupture, or hemorrhage. Ectopic pregnancy can be simulated through amenorrhea and irregular uterine bleeding, and rupture or hemorrhage can produce sharp, aching, or colicky pelvic pain, tenderness, nausea, or vomiting (Merrill et al. 1982).

INFLAMMATIONS

VAGINITIS

DESCRIPTION

Vaginitis is an inflammation or hormonal change of the vaginal mucosa caused by abnormal organisms (*Trichomonas*), an increase in the number of the normal flora (*Candida, Gardnerella vaginalis*, anaerobes), estrogen deprivation, mechanical irritants, or contact allergans (see Figure 34-3). The simple squamous epithelium of the vagina is maintained in an acid pH of 3.5 to 5.0 by the lactic acid secretion of Döderlein's bacillus, a gram-positive nonmotile rod. A change in the vaginal pH, a decrease in Döderlein's bacillus growth, or an increase in vaginal glycogen can result in monilial, trichomonal, or nonspecific vaginitis (*G. vaginalis* plus anaerobic bacteria). A decrease in estrogen, seen in postmenopausal women, can result in atrophic vaginitis. Vaginal infections are the most common gynecological problem, transmittable through sexual contact but treatable once diagnosed (Eschenbach, 1982).

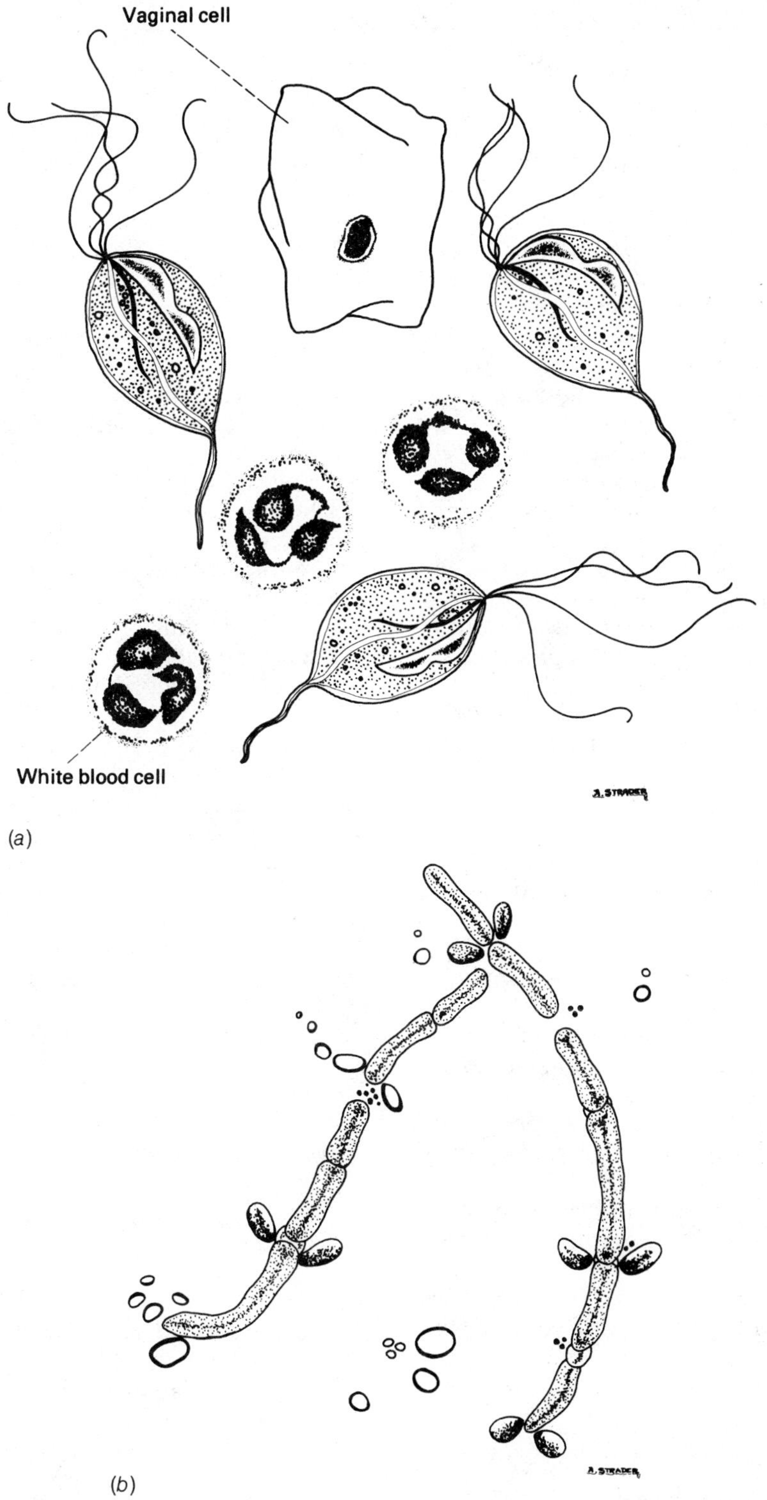

Figure 34-3 Specific findings in diagnosing the causative agent for vaginitis. (*a*) *Trichomonas* as viewed by the light microscope. (*b*) The spores and hyphae of *Candida albicans* as seen microscopically with potassium hydroxide suspension. (Romney, S. L., et al.: *Gynecology and Obstetrics: The Health Care of Women*, McGraw-Hill, New York, 1975.)

PREVENTION

Health Promotion

1. Decreased ingestion of refined sugar products, which are secreted as glycogen in the vagina, thus stimulating *Candida* overgrowth.
2. Avoidance of the use of oral contraceptives or vaginal contraceptive agents if diagnosed as causing repetitive monilial vaginitis.
3. Maintenance of vaginal acidity by avoiding the use of deodorized tampons, feminine hygiene sprays, bubble bath, or vaginal douches (unless prescribed by a physician).
4. Promotion of normal vaginal flora growth when taking broad-spectrum antibiotics.
5. Avoidance of sexual contact with infected partners.
6. Maintenance of normal blood glucose levels.
7. Promotion of vaginal hygiene by wearing cotton-crotch underpants, wiping from front to back, and rinsing well after soaping in bath or shower.
8. Diagnosis of unrecognized diabetes by glucose tolerance test if recurrent vaginal yeast infections occur.
9. Avoidance of emotional stress.

Population at Risk

1. Diabetic women with elevated blood glucose levels.
2. Pregnant women.
3. Women treated with broad-spectrum antibiotics.
4. Vaginal or oral contraceptives users.
5. Women who ingest large amounts of refined carbohydrates.
6. Persistent users of deodorized tampons, bubble baths, feminine hygiene sprays, or vaginal douches.
7. Women who wear occlusive clothing, wipe back to front, and do not rinse well after shower or bath.
8. Women in emotional stress.
9. Women who engage in sexual contact with an infected partner.

Screening

1. Microscopic examination of KOH or NaCl wet mount.
2. Gram stain of suspected fungi.
3. Urinary estrogen excretion; serum FSH and LH.

ASSESSMENT

Health History

1. Medication use: oral contraceptives, recent course of antibiotics, immunosuppressive drugs, IUD.
2. History of diabetes mellitus or other debilitating disease; control of disease.
3. Family history of diabetes.
4. Dietary history: refined carbohydrate intake.
5. Menstrual history: age at menarche; age at menopause; length of cycles, duration, amount of flow; breakthrough bleeding; LNMP.
6. Sexual history: partner status, number of partners, oral or rectal intercourse, dyspareunia, history and presence of urogenital infections of partner.
7. Obstetrical history: possibility of pregnancy.
8. Past medical history: previous vaginal infections, gonorrhea, sexually transmitted diseases (STD).
9. Exercise: type; clothing worn; bath or shower afterwards.
10. Vaginal hygiene: vaginal deodorants, feminine hygiene sprays, douches, bubble bath, deodorized tampons, wiping practices, bath or shower, type of undergarment worn.
11. Urogenital history: internal or external dysuria; vulvar or vaginal pruritis; vulvar pain.
12. Current vaginal discharge: type, amount, odor.
13. Recent emotional stress.
14. Level of anxiety: fear of communicable disease.

Physical Assessment

1. Vulva:
   a. Edematous.
   b. Geographic erythema.
   c. Fissures.
2. Vagina:
   a. *Candida* (*Monilia*): dry vagina; bright red in color, mottled by adherent white, curdy plaques; sometimes no discharge or erythema.
   b. *Trichomonas vaginalis*: profuse, malodorous, sometimes frothy discharge; subepithelial cervical hemorrhages (strawberry spots); often no discharge present.
   c. Nonspecific vaginitis: thin, homogene-

ous, foul-smelling ("fishy"), adherent yellow-gray discharge.
   d. Atrophic vaginitis: disappearance of rugae; thinning mucosa; whitish, viscid discharge.
3. Bimanual pelvic exam: foreign body; possible vaginal-cervical tenderness; no uterine-adnexal tenderness or swelling.

Diagnostic Tests

1. *Candida* (*Monilia*).
   a. Microscopic examination of vaginal plaques, discharge, or vulvar scrapings mixed with 10% KOH on a wet-mount glass slide revealing hyphae, pseudohyphae, or budding.
   b. Gram stain of plaques, discharge, or scrapings demonstrating fungi.
2. *Trichomonas vaginalis*.
   a. Microscopic examination of vaginal discharge mixed with normal saline on wet-mount glass slide revealing motile teardrop-shaped trichomonads and many polymorphonuclear leukocytes.
   b. Pap test revealing nonmotile trichomonads.
   c. Culture of *T. vaginalis* when diagnosis is suspected but organism cannot be identified in wet mount or Pap test.
   d. Gonorrhea culture: 60 percent of women with gonorrhea have trichomoniasis.
3. Nonspecific vaginitis.
   a. Microscopic examination of vaginal discharge mixed with normal saline on wet-mount glass slide revealing vaginal epithelial cells covered with gram-negative *G. vaginalis* bacteria (clue cells).
   b. Absence of polymorphonuclear leukocytes and lactobacilli (Döderlein's).
   c. Vaginal discharge plus 10% KOH demonstrating "fishy" amine odor of anaerobes.
4. Atrophic vaginitis.
   a. Urinary estrogen secretion: low tonic estrogen output.
   b. Serum gonadotropins: elevated FSH and LH.

NURSING DIAGNOSES: ACTUAL OR POTENTIAL

1. Anxiety (mild): due to concern about sexual relationship.
2. Alteration in comfort: pain, pruritis burning.
3. Alteration in patterns of sexuality.
4. Impairment of skin and integrity of mucous membranes.

EXPECTED OUTCOMES

1. Pruritus, edema, vaginal-vulvar tenderness, dysuria, dyspareunia will subside with treatment.
2. Normal vaginal flora and pH 3.5 to 5.0 will be restored.
3. Debilitating diseases will be controlled.
4. Client will maintain a well-balanced diet.
5. Client will practice healthy vaginal hygiene principles.
6. Client will use alternative coping mechanisms to manage emotional stress.
7. A comfortable sexual relationship will be restored.
8. Reinfection or recurrence of vaginitis will be prevented.
9. Anxiety and fear will be dispelled.

INTERVENTIONS

1. Explain mechanism of action, vaginal insertion or oral medication dosage, precautions (avoidance of alcohol intake with metronidazole therapy), and side effects (gastrointestinal irritation from metronidazole therapy) of medication prescribed for vaginitis.
2. Explain rationale for treatment of partner and encourage health evaluation.
3. Provide information about alternative forms of contraception, vaginal and personal hygiene habits, and predisposing factors to vaginitis.
4. Promote a balanced diet through nutritional counseling.
5. Reinforce treatment regimen in controlling any debilitating disease.
6. Instruct client to promote comfortable sexual relationship by resting vaginal mucosa (early stage of vaginitis) and using water soluble lubricants (atrophic vaginitis).
7. Encourage using a condom to prevent cross contamination.
8. Encourage return appointment for treatment evaluation (Fleury, 1981).

EVALUATION

Outcome Criteria

1. Client keeps return appointments.
2. No vaginal-vulvar discomfort, dysuria, or dyspareunia is indicated by the client.
3. A normal, cyclic vaginal discharge is present.
4. Client is eating a well-balanced diet and avoiding refined carbohydrate sugars.
5. Debilitating diseases are in control through client compliance to treatment regimen.
6. Client uses vaginal hygiene principles appropriately.
7. Client exhibits no measurable stress symptoms.
8. Client indicates satisfaction with health status.

Complications

1. Concurrent infectious disease (see *Gonorrhea* and *Syphilis* in Chapter 24, Communicable Diseases).
2. Coexistent vaginal infection (candidiasis and trichomoniasis often occur at the same time, with the predominant symptoms focusing the cure on one agent. Persistent discharge after adequate treatment should be reassessed).
3. Monilial vaginitis after antibiotic treatment of nonspecific vaginitis (see *Vaginitis* in this chapter).

GENITAL HERPES

DESCRIPTION

Herpes simplex virus (HSV) is the most common viral genital infection, characterized by the primary presentation of multiple vesicles that rapidly progress to painful coalescent alterations of the vulva, vagina, or cervix. Incubation period is 3 to 7 days after exposure; lesions can last 3 or more weeks and fever, malaise, headache, or urinary retention last about 1 week. After the primary infection, a latency stage occurs when HSV enters the nervous system at the sacral ganglion or locally in the dermis, where it remains asymptomatic. A secondary infection from the latent virus usually occurs weeks to months after the primary infection. The lesions are less painful, more localized, last 3 to 10 days and systemic reactions rarely occur. The virus returns to the ganglion nearest the original infection site and remains dormant until activated by such factors as vaginal, anal, or oral-genital contact; fever; sun; menstruation; gastrointestinal upsets; psychological stress; corticosteroid use, or immunosuppresant therapy. HSV type 2 causes 75 to 80 percent of the genital infections, and HSV type 1 (primary cause of lip and perioral infections) the remaining 20 to 25 percent.

The highly infectious HSV virus 1 or 2 is transmitted through vesicular or ulcer contact. HSV has been associated with cervical cancer and serious fetal effects during pregnancy (Eschenbach, 1982).

PREVENTION

Health Promotion

1. Primary prevention.
   a. Avoidance of direct contact with vesicular or ulcerative lesions identified as HSV infection.
   b. Avoidance of oral or genital contact with undiagnosed partners.
2. Recurrent prevention.
   a. Avoidance of individual precipitating factor known to activate dormant phase.
   b. Reduced exposure to sunlight through the use of protective clothing and sun-screening preparations.
   c. Maintenance of good health habits (e.g., rest, nutrition).
   d. Development of positive coping mechanisms during psychological stress or gastrointestinal problems.
   e. Minimization of any concurrent stress factors during the presence of a fever or menstruation.
   f. Awareness of the 1 to 10 percent HSV transmission occurring with contact of asymptomatic carriers.

Population at Risk.

1. Primary risk profile.
   a. Any individual in direct contact with an HSV vesicle or ulcer.
   b. One to ten percent of individuals in contact with asymptomatic carriers.
   c. Person of early age at first coitus (see discussion of herpes in adolescents in Chapter 23).
   d. Person who has a multiple number of sex partners.

2. Recurrent risk profile. An HSV carrier in the dormant phase exposed to a precipitating factor such as sunlight, local or systemic trauma, stress, or sexual intercourse.

Screening

1. Tissue culture.
2. Smear test.
3. Antibody titers.

ASSESSMENT

Health History

1. Sexual history: age at first coitus, number of sexual partners, dyspareunia.
2. Urogenital history: dysuria, urinary retention, frequency and urgency, pruritus, burning, tingling, tenderness in affected area, radiating pain, vaginal discharge.
3. Systemic symptoms: fever, malaise, headache.
4. History of past disease.
   a. Precipitating factor (sunlight, sexual contact, fever, menstruation, GI tract disturbance, stress, trauma).
   b. Description of former symptoms: site of onset, location and distribution of lesions, character and radiation of pain.
   c. Number of previous outbreaks.
   d. Success of treatment.
5. Level of anxiety: concern about sexual relationships, future pregnancies, social stigma, fear of cervical cancer.

Physical Assessment

1. External genitalia exam.
   a. Inguinal lymph enlargement and tenderness.
   b. Local erythema and edema of labia or vulva.
   c. Scattered painful vesicles or coalescent mass of fluid-filled lesions; gray-yellow secretion covering some lesions; located on labia major and/or perineal area, vagina, thighs.
   d. Ulcerated lesions over labia, vulva, thighs.
2. Vaginal-cervical exam.
   a. Vagina: vesicular or ulcerated lesions.
   b. Cervix: diffusely erythematous, edematous, and bleeding easily when touched; granulomatous masses covered with gray exudate; large ulcerated areas between masses; profuse thin, white discharge.
3. Temperature greater than 37.8°C (100°F) orally.

Diagnostic Tests

1. Tissue culture: swabbing the affected area, steaking the swab across monolayer live tissue cells; evaluating tissue layer daily for cell destruction (cytopathic effect).
2. Cytological smear test: stained cells from affected area to visualize multinucleated giant cells.
3. Serum antibody level: to determine initial or primary infection, asymptomative client exposed to HSV, and levels of HSV1 and HSV2 (Bettoli, 1982).

NURSING DIAGNOSES: ACTUAL OR POTENTIAL

1. Anxiety (mild to severe): fear of intimate contact with others; fear of cervical cancer; concern about the outcome of future pregnancies and the health of the infant.
2. Alteration in self-concept: implications of disease on future lifestyle, social acceptance, self-esteem.
3. Alteration in sexuality patterns.
4. Potential and actual impairment of skin integrity from eroding ulcers.
5. Alteration in comfort: tingling, burning, pain with active phase.

EXPECTED OUTCOMES

1. Anxiety and the fear of intimate personal contact, outcome of future pregnancies, and cervical cancer will be reduced.
2. Client will adapt positively to herpes diagnosis and will use preventive measures to reduce the spread of disease and recurrences.
3. Client will reevaluate self-concept and adjust to any ulcer scarring or loss of self-esteem.
4. Client will change sexual patterns to promote healthy relationships.
5. Skin integrity will be restored.
6. Tingling, burning, and pain will be reduced through treatment.

INTERVENTIONS

1. Instruct client to:
   a. Keep lesions clean and dry.
   b. Take sitz baths three or four times a day and dry well afterward.

c. Avoid sexual intercourse or sore-to-skin contact during lesion eruptions; avoid touching sores to control spreading to other parts of body.
d. Avoid tight-fitting clothing and wear cotton underwear.
e. Urinate in bath water after bathing or while pouring warm water on vulva if dysuria is present.
f. Establish periodic routine Pap tests for early detection of cervical cancer.

2. Administer prescribed agents for symptomatic relief.
3. Reduce stress by teaching alternative relaxation techniques.
4. Evaluate nutritional intake and adjust nutrients to provide a balanced diet.
5. Teach preventive measures to avoid recurrences.
6. Help client to identify precipitating factors.
7. Encourage discussion of fears and anxieties about cancer, intimate relationships, future pregnancies.
8. Offer information about the education and support provided by the Herpes Resource Center and their publication, *The Helper* (Herpes Resource Center, Box 100, Palo Alto, CA 94302) (Belloli, 1982).

EVALUATION

Outcome Criteria

1. Client openly discusses fears and anxieties and identifies preventive measures.
2. HSV precipitating factors are assessed and appropriate coping methods adopted.
3. Client is compliant with treatment regimen and keeps appointments for periodic scheduled Pap tests and reevaluations.
4. Client uses precautionary measure to prevent recurrent episodes.
5. Skin integrity is restored with minimal scarring.
6. Client is eating a balanced diet, as demonstrated by a 24-h recall evaluation.

Complications

1. Recurrent herpetic disease (see Assessment, Expected Outcomes, and Interventions under *Genital Herpes* above).
2. Cervical cancer (see *Cervical Carcinoma* earlier in this chapter).

VULVITIS

Inflammation of the vulva may be caused by a local manifestation of a dermatological or systemic infectious disease or by a secondary infection of the genital tract. Common symptoms include pruritus, which stimulates prolonged scratching or pain and soreness. The inguinal lymph nodes may be enlarged and tender. Soap, detergent, and antiseptic solutions either applied directly or used in laundering underwear may cause a local allergic reaction. Excretion through the urine of drugs such as antibiotics and sulfonamides may also be responsible.

Genital herpes and condyloma acuminatum (venereal warts) are the most common vulvar infections. The genital wart caused by a DNA virus thrives in the moist genital area and is usually sexually transmitted. After a 3-month incubation period single lesions occur on the labia or posterior fourchette and can become confluent if untreated (see Figure 34-4). Condyloma acuminatum needs to be differentiated from the papular growths of syphilitic condyloma lactum and vulvar carcinoma in situ.

Repetitive topical treatment can control the disease. Nursing interventions should include the relief of local pain and itching and teaching

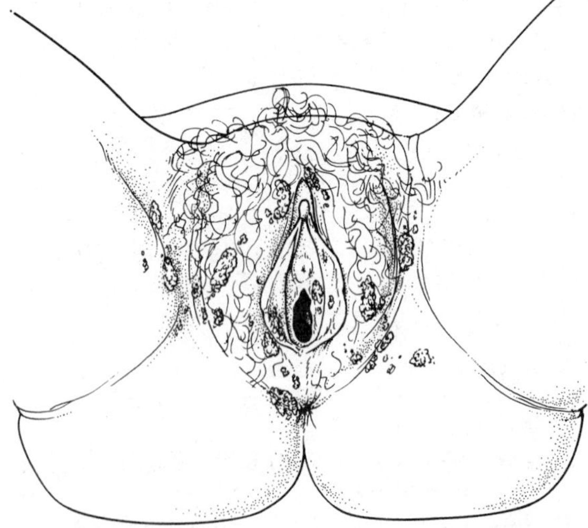

Figure 34-4 Condylomata acuminata. (Adapted from Beller, F. K., et al.: *Gynecology: A Textbook for Students*, Springer-Verlag, New York, 1974.)

appropriate personal hygiene measures to prevent the spread of infection and cross infection (Eschenbach, 1982).

CERVICITIS

The main symptom of inflammation of the cervix is increased cervical discharge, although cervical mucorrhea may be seen under physiological as well as pathological conditions. Secretions of the cervical gland are increased under the influence of estrogen, as at the time of ovulation or in pregnancy. Excess mucous production also occurs normally in the newborn and in adults, as a result of sexual or other emotional stimulation. Oral contraceptives produce cervical mucous properties similar to those seen during the luteal (progestogenic) phase of the menstrual cycle.

Cervicitis is common after vaginal delivery as a result of subsequent infection of cervical lacerations. Gonorrhea and chlamydia produce an acute cervicitis that may become chronic due to secondary infection by streptococci. Other factors in the pathogenesis of cervicitis are poor hygiene, decreased resistance to infection, irritation by foreign bodies, and neoplastic disease of the upper genital tract.

The acute inflammatory reaction of the cervix is characterized by a thick, purulent, whitish discharge with an acrid odor. Dysuria may also be present. The general well-being of the client is unaffected. Chronic infection of the cervix results in hyperactivity of the cervical gland cells, resulting in excess secretions, hypertropy, and hyperplasia. There is a forward growth or displacement of the squamocolumnar junction, producing an eversion and redness about the external os with new cervical glands developing where they do not normally exist. Chronic cervicitis is a major etiological factor in infertility, dyspareunia, and abortion.

As with other inflammatory disorders of the reproductive tract, a complete health history should be obtained to aid in the identification of the source(s) of infection. Specific medical treatment will depend on the infectious agent, age of the client, her desire for pregnancy, and the severity of cervical involvement. Cervical cauterization or electrocoagulation (to destroy diseased gland tissue) is indicated when erosion and infection are extensive (Benson, 1977).

DEGENERATIVE CHANGES

MENOPAUSE

Menopause is defined as the physiological cessation of menses associated with decreased ovarian function and diagnosed retrospectively after 1 year with no menses (between ages 45 and 50). *Climacteric* is defined as the transitional period in a woman's life in which reproductive function gradually diminishes. It is marked by closer menses cycles with notably heavy bleeding early in transition and scanter lighter blood flow later in transition. Physiologically menopause begins with a critical loss of oocytes associated with follicular atresia, decline in estrogen secretion, and irregular uterine bleeding. When the ovary is no longer stimulated to follicule maturation, follicule stimulating hormone (FSH) rises, with luteinizing hormone (LH) following and remaining elevated for life (Jones and Wentz, 1982). Although the estrogen levels are lower than recorded during reproductive years, 40 percent of menopausal women maintain moderate levels of lifetime estrogen activity (McLennan and McLennan, 1971). The postmenopausal ovarian stroma produces androgenic steroids, mainly androstenedione and testosterone, in sufficient quantity for extraglandular conversion to estrogen.

The only physiological symptom documenting this normal developmental phase in women is the "hot flash." It is a vasomotor phenomenon, associated with estrogen deprivation and occurring in the climacteric and menopausal periods. The flash has a variety of preceding events, trigger points, and progression patterns. Most women can predict their own unique flash origin and spread (Voda, 1982).

The acceptance of menopause as a natural phase in a woman's life cycle began deteriorating in the 1960s when menopause was diagnosed as a deficiency disease, analogous to diabetes, requiring hormone replacement (Goodman, 1982). This unfortunate analogy and the focus of the media on the youth concept in our society has hindered women from progressing normally through middlescence. Common psychological symptoms associated with the menopausal syndrome include dizziness, headaches, irritability, anxiety, and depression and are attributed to the woman's loss of the traditional reproductive role in our society supplemented by a fear of sexual inadequacy worthlessness, helplessness, and loneliness. Married women with only a primary education, low income, and completion of childbearing at an early age are more likely to develop these psychological symptoms.

Although all women experience the cessation of menses, the incidence and severity of these symptoms has many variations (Jaszman et al., 1969). Physical changes in the menopausal woman are frequently as much a part of a physiological aging process as of estrogen deficiency. Dyspareunia, leukorrhea, pruritus, mucosal thinning, and disappearance of rugae are atrophic vaginal changes related to estrogen deprivation rarely occurring until 10 years after cessation of menses. The occasional narrowing and shortening of the vagina is related to disuse and deposition of fibrous tissue in the submucosa (Jones and Wentz, 1982).

Because estrogen replacement therapy (ERT) for women in the postmenopausal years is controversial, the care of each client should be individualized. The beneficial effect on the cardiovascular and skeletal symptoms is still being evaluated, while the elimination of hot flashes and prevention of genitourinary mucosal atrophy has been well documented. The long-term carcinogenic side effects of estrogen treatment remain to be explored (Friederich, 1982).

Nurses need to be aware of the possible psychological implications associated with the loss of reproductive capacity for a client with menopausal symptoms. If the client's purpose in life has centered around her childbearing functions, she may need support in developing a new role and lifestyle.

Although pregnancy is unlikely, contraceptive measures should be continued until 4 years after the last menstrual period; however, oral contraceptives are not advised for women over 40 because of the suspected association with heart disease. In addition, women taking birth control pills may not recognize the onset of menopause, as regular bleeding usually continues while estrogen and progesterone are taken cyclically.

THE MALE REPRODUCTIVE SYSTEM

ABNORMAL CELLULAR GROWTH

BENIGN PROSTATIC HYPERPLASIA OR HYPERTROPHY

Prostatic enlargement is believed to be caused by either hyperplasia of the periurethral glands, compressing the prostatic tissue, or hyperplasia of the prostatic tissue in the two lateral and subcervical lobes infiltrated by the periurethral glands, developing a glandular component. Enlargement begins in most men by age 50, with the majority presenting a palpable change in the prostate by age 60. The cause is unclear; an androgen-estrogen imbalance has been suggested as a causative factor, having implications as one of the results of male menopause.

For a detailed discussion of benign prostatic hyperplasia, see Chapter 32.

PROSTATIC CANCER

Cancer of the prostate is rare before age 60. It increases in frequency with age and afflicts 25 to 50 percent of men over age 80. The disease is rare in Orientals, more common in blacks, Maoris, white New Zealanders, and Scandinavians. Familial incidence is documented, and multiple cancers are common in these clients. The cause is unknown, but the neoplastic growth is strikingly influenced by sex hormones: Androgens usually increase tumor growth rate, whereas estrogens slow growth. A correlation between a previous gonorrhea infection and the development of prostatic cancer has been found.

For a detailed discussion of prostatic cancer, see Chapter 32.

TESTICULAR NEOPLASMS

Carcinoma of the testicle accounts for less than 1 percent of all neoplastic deaths in men but is the third most frequently found tumor in men between the ages of 20 and 34. Incidence is higher in men with undescended testicles, even when the retained testicle is removed. The tumor usually is a hard, heavy, firm, nontender mass that does not transilluminate but is occasionally smooth and resilient, thus complicating the diagnostic findings. Metastasis usually occurs in the left supraclavicular or preaortic lymph nodes or lungs. Surgical removal of the involved testicles and lymph nodes combined with radio- and chemotherapy are the treatment modalities. Fear of death, disfigurement, sexual rejection, anxiety, and an altered self-concept focus nursing interventions on education, counseling, and the development of a support system network (Smith, 1981).

CARCINOMA OF THE PENIS

The most common cause of cancer of the penis is a chronic inflammation from an infection of the foreskin and glans of an uncircumsized male. Penal neoplasms are epithelial in origin and often malignant. If the tumor is localized to the foreskin or glans with no metastasis, the 5-year survival rate is 70 to 90 percent. Lymph node involvement has a cure rate of 30 percent.

The lesion may first appear as a raised red, firm plaque; an enlarging warty growth; or a spreading ulcer, all of which are painless but require biopsy to rule out syphilis and other venereal diseases. Edema from the infection can cause the foreskin to be nonretractable. A bloody, foul-smelling discharge often emanates from the prepuce pouch while a solid, hard lump is palpated on the glans. Treatment involves local incision of contained lesions, amputation of more extensive lesions, radiotherapy of involved nodes, and chemotherapy of metastases. The devastating disfigurement and life-threatening prognosis should require continual support and extensive counseling (see discussion of loss and death in Chapter 45).

HYDROCELE

A hydrocele is a cystic mass that occasionally is so full of clear, straw-colored fluid that a solid mass is simulated. As an extratesticular mass it usually surrounds the testis completely, can be transilluminated, and should be aspirated to allow palpation of underlying structures if another primary cause is suspected, such as epididymitis, trauma, or a testicular tumor.

SPERMATOCELE

A spermatocele is an intrascrotal cystic mass separate from but on the upper pole region of the testis. Aspiration reveals a typical thin, milky fluid containing sperm.

VARICOCELE

The dilatation of scrotal veins is caused by an increased pressure on the valves of the internal venous system, resulting in a retrograde flow from the renal vein into the scrotal circulation. Although 90 percent of the varicoceles occur in the left scrotum because of the venous anatomy, cross-venous circulation in the testes causes both sides to be affected. Varicoceles have a "bag of worms" appearance on physical exam, are usually nontender, and decrease in size when the client is recumbent. Varicocelectomy is a very successful surgical procedure by which all varicosities are removed so that retrograde flow is completely arrested.

INFLAMMATIONS

EPIDIDYMITIS

Epididymitis is the most common of all intrascrotal infections and occurs mainly in adults. Organisms enter the epididymis from the bladder, posterior urethra, prostate, or seminal vesicles where the initial infection occurred. Three classifications have been developed to identify the pathogens. (1) *Nonspecific epididymitis* is caused by common pyogenic organisms (staphylococci, various colon bacilli, and streptococci) usually forced into the vas deferens by straining. (2) *Traumatic epididymitis* is caused by a direct or indirect incident activating a dormant infection. A traumatic strain is believed to force urine into the epididymis or lessen the resistance of the tissue to an infection in another reproductive tract organ. (3) *Specific epididymitis* includes infections caused by gonorrhea, syphilis, tuberculosis, brucellosis, and other identifiable contagious agents.

The disease may be subacute, acute, chronic, or recurrent. Infection can remain localized or may develop into an abscess and extend into the testicle or scrotal wall. The client usually complains of a tender, swollen posterior testicle, and physical exam verifies the symptoms. An accompanying hydrocele is often present.

Rest, scrotal support, and observation for abscess formation are the general treatment modalities. When the causative agent has been identified, the appropriate antibiotic is given. In severe cases, broad-spectrum antibiotics and chemotherapy are recommended. If the disease remains refractory to all antibiotics and develops an abscess and invades adjacent structures, epididymectomy under local anesthetic is advised. Instrumentation or surgery on the reproductive system can be the traumatic incident initiating an epididymitis infection. If procreation is not a goal of the client, a preoperative vasectomy reduces the incidence of epididymitis (Nickel and Plumb, 1978). Nursing measures should address preventive education, rest, scrotal support, modified activities of daily living, and good hygiene and health habits.

ORCHITIS

An acute infection involving solely the testis is rare in clinical urology. The rich blood and lymphatic supply provides a high resistance threshold, and metastatic infection rarely occurs. Orchitis is usually secondary to a primary disease located elsewhere in the body. The most frequent orchitis is seen accompanying mumps in 18 percent of the outbreaks. Orchitis usually appears 4 to 6 days after clinical parotitis but can occur without any symptoms. Unilateral involvement is seen in 70 percent of all orchitis infections, and 50 percent of the involved testes develop some atrophy. Impotence and sterility are concerning complications. Nausea, vomiting, chills, and testicular swelling (hydrocele) after the first 48 h are symptoms of the disease. After 7 to 10 days the orchitis subsides. Bed rest, scrotal support, hot and cold applications, and diethylstilbesterol diminish the degree of pain, swelling, and fever. Plasma, gamma globulin, ACTH, cortisone, and prednisone injections are believed to lower the incidence of orchitis. Aspirating the hydrocele to reduce the pressure is also recommended (Smith, 1981).

REFERENCES

Beller, F. K., Knorr, K., Lauritzen, C., and Wynn, R.: "Benign and Malignant Neoplasms," in *Gynecology: A Textbook for Students*, Springer-Verlag, New York, 1974, p. 315.

Benson, R. C.: *Handbook of Obstetrics and Gynecology*, Lange Medical Publications, Los Altos, Calif. 1977, pp. 513–519.

Bettoli, E. J.: "Herpes: Facts and Fallacies," *American Journal of Nursing*, June 1982, pp. 924–926.

Bloomfield, R. D.: "Current Cancer Chemotherapy in Obstetrics and Gynecology," *American Journal of Obstetrics and Gynecology*, **109**:487–528, 1976.

Donegan, W. L.: "Diseases of the Breast," in D. N. Danforth

(ed.), *Obstetrics and Gynecology,* 4th ed., Harper & Row, Philadelphia, 1982, p. 1193.

Eschenbach, D. A.: "Pelvic Infections," in D. N. Danforth (ed.), *Obstetrics and Gynecology,* 4th ed., Harper & Row, Philadelphia, 1982, pp. 993–996.

Fisher, B., Slack, N., Katryck, D., and Wolmark, N.: "Ten-Year Follow-up Results of Patients with Carcinoma of the Breast in a Cooperative Clinical Trial Evaluating Surgical Adjuvant Chemotherapy," *Surgical Gynecology and Obstetrics,* **140:**528, 1975.

Fleury, F. J.: "Adult Vaginitis," *Clinical Obstetrics and Gynecology,* **24**(2):407–438, 1981.

Friederich, M. A.: "Aging, Menopause, and Estrogens: The Clinician's Dilemma," in A. M. Voda (ed.), *Changing Perspectives on Menopause,* University of Texas Press, Austin, 1982, pp. 333–345.

Goodman, M. J.: "A Critique of Menopause Research," in A. M. Voda (ed.), *Changing Perspectives on Menopause,* University of Texas Press, Austin, 1982, pp. 272–287.

Gusberg, S. B., and Depper, G.: "Malignant Lesions of the Cervix and Corpus Uteri," in D. N. Danforth (ed.), *Obstetrics and Gynecology,* 4th ed., Harper & Row, Philadelphia, 1982, pp. 1054, 1056.

Herbst, A. I.: *Intrauterine Exposure to Diethylstilbesterol in the Human,* American College of Obstetricians and Gynecologists, Chicago, 1978, pp. 24–27.

Jaszman, L., van Lith, N. D., and Zaat, J. C. A.: "The Perimenopausal Symptoms: The Statistical Analysis of a Survey," *Medical Gynecological Society,* **4:**268–275, 1969.

Jones, G. S., and Wentz, A. C.: "Adolescence, Menstruation, and the Climacteric," in D. N. Danforth (ed.), *Obstetrics and Gynecology,* 4th ed., Harper & Row, Philadelphia, 1982, pp. 172–174.

McLennan, M. T., and McLennan, C. E.: "Estrogenic Status of Menstruating and Menopausal Women Assessed by Cervical Vascular Smears," *Obstetrics and Gynecology,* **37:**325, 1971.

Merrill, J. A.: "Lesions of the Fallopian Tube, Benign Lesions of the Cervic Uteri, Endometriosis," in D. N. Danforth (ed.), *Obstetrics and Gynecology,* 4th ed., Harper & Row, Philadelphia, 1982, pp. 1105–1112.

Merrill, J. A., Gusberg, S. B., and Depper, G.: "Lesions of the Corpus Uteri," in D. N. Danforth (ed.), *Obstetrics and Gynecology,* 4th ed., Harper & Row, Philadelphia, 1982, pp. 1081–1088.

Merrill, J. A., Nelson, J. H., Jr., and Dolan, T. E.: "Lesions of the Ovary," in D. N. Danforth (ed.), *Obstetrics and Gynecology,* 4th ed., Harper & Row, Philadelphia, 1982, pp. 1114–1139.

Minton, J. P., Foeching, M. K., Webster, D. J. T., and Matthews, R. H.: "Caffeine, Cyclic Nucleotides, and Breast Disease," *Surgery,* **1:**105, 1979.

Nelson, J. H., Jr., and Dolan, T. E.: "Malignant Lesions of the Ovary," in D. N. Danforth (ed.), *Obstetrics and Gynecology,* 4th ed., Harper & Row, Philadelphia, 1982, pp. 1139–1164.

Nickel, W. R., and Plumb, R. T.: "Other Infections and Inflammations of the External Genitalia," in *Campbell's Urology,* Saunders, Philadelphia, 1978, pp. 682–684.

Smith, D. R.: *General Urology,* 10th ed., Lange Medical Publications, Los Altos, Calif. 1981, pp. 296–302.

UICC American Joint Committee for Cancer Staging, "Classification and Staging of Malignant Tumors in the Female Pelvis," ACOG Technical Bulletin, No. 47, June 1977.

Voda, A. M.: "Menopausal Hot Flash," in A. M. Voda (ed.), *Changing Perspectives on Menopause,* University of Texas Press, Austin, 1982, pp. 136–159.

Woodruff, J. D.: "Lesions of the Vulva and Vagina," in D. N. Danforth (ed.), *Obstetrics and Gynecology,* 4th ed., Harper & Row, Philadelphia, 1982, p. 1035.

BIBLIOGRAPHY

Benton, B. D. A.: "Stillbestrol and Vaginal Cancer," *American Journal of Nursing,* **74:**900–901, 1974. This article presents a concise review of the etiology of this disorder and focuses on nursing management of the adolescent client with vaginal cancer.

Britt, S. S.: "Fertility Awareness: Four Methods of Natural Family Planning," *Journal of Obstetrical, Gynecological, and Neonatal Nursing,* **6:**9–18, 1977. This article provides the physiological rationale and a clear description of each method of natural family planning.

Dan, A. J., Graham, E. A., and Beecher, C. P. (eds.): *The Menstrual Cycle,* Vol. 1, Springer, New York, 1980. The text offers a synthesis of the current interdisciplinary research on the menstrual characteristics in women's health care including theoretical, methodological, developmental, physiological, and psychological aspects.

Dyche, M. E.: "Pelvic Exenteration: A Nursing Challenge," *Journal of Obstetrical, Gynecological, and Neonatal Nursing,* **4:**11–19, 1975. This article focuses on the problems and nursing management of the cancer client undergoing pelvic exenteration.

Einhorn, L. H. (ed.): *Testicular Tumors: Management and Treatment,* Masson New York, 1980. A thorough presentation of the pathophysiology, diagnosis, and care of benign and malignant tumors in the testicles is presented.

Fleury, F. J.: "Adult Vaginitis," *Clinical Obstetrics and Gynecology,* **24**(2):407–438, 1981. The diagnosis and management of bacterial, fungal, and abnormal organisms in the vagina are discussed.

Fogel, C. I., and Woods, N. F.: *Health Care of Women, A Nursing Perspective,* Mosby, St. Louis, 1981. A complete text of the diagnosis, medical treatment, and nursing management of multiple problems affecting women.

Foreman, J. R.: "Vasectomy Clinic," *American Journal of Nursing*, **73**:819–821, 1973. This article explains the procedure and describes nursing management of the postvasectomy couple.

Ginsberg, S. J.: "Timely Detection: Key to Opitmal Management of Breast Cancer," *Geriatrics*, **37**(1):97–99, 103, 105–106, 1982. The author stresses the value of early detection and management of carcinoma of the breast.

Girtanner, R.: "Ovarian Cancer: Diagnosis and Treatment," *Comprehensive Therapy*, **6**(5):30–38, 1980. The detection and management of ovarian cancer is well delineated.

Glassburn, J. R.: "Carcinoma of the Endometrium," *Cancer*, **48**(2, supplement):575–581, 1981. This article reviews the diagnostic process in evaluating endometrial carcinoma.

Gribbons, C. A., and Aliapoulios, M. A.: "Treatment for Advanced Breast Carcinoma," *American Journal of Nursing*, **72**:678–682, 1972. This article presents medical and nursing problems related to the client with recurrent breast cancer.

Griffiths, B. L.: "Genital Infection with Herpes Simplex Virus," *Nursing Times*, **78**(13):545–548, 1982. The author discusses the pathology and nursing care of genital herpes.

Herbert, P., Welch, I., and Jackson, E.: "Colposcopy—What Is It?" *Journal of Obstetrical, Gynecological, and Neonatal Nursing*, **5**:29–32, 1976. This article presents a review of the procedure, its indications, and role of the nurse in preparing the client for colposcopy.

Katzman, E. M.: "Common Disorders of Female Genitalia from Birth to Older Years: Implications for Nursing Interventions," *Journal of Obstetrical, Gynecological, and Neonatal Nursing*, **6**:19–21, 1977. The author discusses common disorders in children, adult women, and older women. Principles for prevention and nursing intervention are offered.

Kommenich, P., McSweeney, M., Noack, J. A., and Elder, N. (eds.): *The Menstrual Cycle*, Vol. 2, *Research and Implications for Women's Health*, Springer, New York, 1981. This book evaluates some of the behavioral and physiological aspects of the menstrual cycle, research (past, present, and future), the rights and responsibilities for women under hormone therapy, and the implications for women's health care.

McNall, L. K. (ed.): *Contemporary Obstetric and Gynecologic Nursing*, Mosby, St. Louis, 1980. The book discusses the effects of the women's movement on women's health care, antepartum, postpartum, and neonatal care, assault and battery, and the preventive management of various gynecological problems.

Minkin, S.: "Depo-Provera: A Critical Analysis," *Women's Health*, **5**(2):49–69, 1980. The author evaluates the use, risks, and benefits of the drug Depo-Provera.

Morley, G. W.: "Cancer of the Vulva: A Review," *Cancer*, **48**(2, supplement):597–601, 1981. The current medical management of cancer of the vulva with implications for nursing.

Piver, M. S.: "Early Diagnosis of Ovarian Cancer," *Hospital Medicine*, **18**(1):43–47, 50–52, 1982. This article addresses the insidious development of ovarian cancer, emphasizing the initial cues that have implication for client teaching.

Quirk, B.: Part I, "This Is VD Too? Moniliasis, Trichomoniasis, Vaginalis, Herpes Simplex, Condylomata Acuminata," *Journal of Obstetrical, Gynecological, and Neonatal Nursing*, **4**:13–15, 1975. This article reviews the less commonly considered types of venereal disease and discusses the nursing role in their management.

Sulewski, J. M.: "Endometriosis: What to Do and When to Refer," *Consultant*, **20**(7):160–161, 163, 165–166, 169, 1980. This article discusses the management of limited to extensive endometriosis.

UICC Committee on Professional Education: *Clinical Oncology*, Springer-Verlag, New York, 1973. This manual for clinicians presents a concise description of neoplasia, organized by organ systems and classified according to stage, survival rate, and treatment.

"Vaginalis, Herpes Simplex, Condylomata Accuminata," *Journal of Obstetrical, Gynecological, and Neonatal Nursing*, **4**:13–15, 1975. This article reviews the less commonly considered types of venereal disease and discusses the nursing role in their management.

Voda, A. M., Dinnerstein, M., and O'Donnell, S. R. (eds.): *Changing Perspectives on Menopause*, University of Texas Press, Austin, 1982. This book explores the anthropological, biological, physiological, and psychological parameters of menopause, various research models, and facts and falacies.

Wahl, T. P., and Blythe, J. G.: "Chemotherapy in Gynecological Malignancies—and Its Nursing Aspects," *Journal of Obstetrical, Gynecological, and Neonatal Nursing*, **5**:9–14, 1976. This article describes the indications, applications, and complications of cancer chemotherapy and the role of the gynecological nurse as an educator, listener, and friend.

Woods, N. F.: "Influences on Sexual Adaptation to Mastectomy," *Journal of Obstetrical, Gynecological, and Neonatal Nursing*, **4**:33–37, 1975. This nursing article focuses on the problems in sexuality faced by the postmastectomy client.

35

The Integumentary System

Meredith Censullo

An intact integumentary system is vital in maintaining body temperature, protecting the body against infectious pathogens, preserving body fluids, and contributing to personal appearance. Disruptions of the integument can be precipitated by such things as trauma, abnormal cellular growth, and inflammation. When these disturbances occur, they result in a variety of behavioral and pathophysiological changes. This chapter discusses common health problems which alter the integumentary system, identifies related psychosocial and physiological effects, and discusses the nursing care that can be applied to each health problem.

ABNORMAL CELLULAR GROWTH

SKIN TUMORS

DESCRIPTION

Skin tumors include all benign, precancerous, and cancerous lesions of the skin. The depth of cutaneous layers involved and pattern of growth can be indicative of potential for malignancy. Prompt reporting and treatment of any suspicious lesions are strongly encouraged. Most pigmented lesions have a characteristic appearance and predictable clinical course.

Basal cell epithelioma is found in the epithelial layer of the skin in locations of greatest sebaceous gland concentration. It is the most common skin cancer, but it rarely metastasizes. It can slowly invade underlying tissues, specifically if found around the nose, eyes, mouth, or ears. The initial lesion is a papule, which enlarges laterally. Over a period of several months it will progress to an ulcer, with a shiny, translucent border and telangiectasis. The lesion bleeds easily. The majority are found on the face between the hairline and upper lip. After excision, other lesions may occur.

Squamous cell cancer or epidermoid carcinoma develops from the prickle cells of the epidermis. It begins as a yellowish pink papule or plaque. It grows peripherally and inwardly. The tumor spreads rapidly if located at the mucocutaneous junction. The original lesion may ulcerate, leaving a crusted ulcer with a hard, firm base. Frequently the lesions are found on the mucous membranes as well as the skin of sites exposed to chronic irritation, e.g., the mouth of a pipe smoker and the glans penis in an uncircumcised male.

Nevi or moles are circumscribed, pigmented papules or macules composed of nevus cells, specialized epithelial cells containing melanin. Intradermal or common moles are benign lesions. The melanocyte is located in the corium rather than the epidermal layer of the skin. Hairy moles are usually intradermal. Functional nevi can be benign or precancerous. The melanocyte is contained at the junction of the dermal and epidermal layers of the skin. The lesion is flat or slightly elevated, dark brown or black (see Chapter 23 for an in-depth discussion).

Melanoma is the most common fatal illness seen by the dermatologist. There has been a significant increase in the incidence of melanoma in the past decade, and it now accounts for 1 percent of all cancer deaths. The disease progresses from a period in which the lesion is invasive, but not metastasized (growing superficially and laterally through the epdermis and upper dermis) to a period of deep penetration and metastasis. Survival is based on the level of invasion, and early detection is essential. The disease is divided into four types: superficial spreading, nodular, lentigo maligna, and acrolentiginous. The problem commonly occurs during the reproductive years, ages 20 to 60. Lentigo maligna melanoma is seen predominately in the elderly. In men the most common sites are head, neck, back, and upper extremities; for women the sites are the same in addition to the lower leg. In Oriental and black ethnic groups common sites are palms, nail beds, soles of the feet, and mucous membranes. The most significant clinical characteristics of the lesion are the mixture of colors, (blues, reds, blacks, browns, and white) and the irregularity of the borders. Superficial spreading melanoma begins as a raised lesion, spreads laterally for one to seven years, then develops nodules, notching margins, and variegated colors. Nodular melanoma develops as an invasive nodule with a lateral spread. It is an elevated, dark, blueberry-like lesion with scattered black nodules on the surface.

Lentigo maligna melanoma occurs on exposed surfaces in the elderly. It has a flat, variegated color (tan, brown, black), and grows slowly. *Acrolentiginous melanoma* appears similar to lentigo maligna, but the clinical course is more aggressive.

PREVENTION

Health Promotion

1. Avoid excessive exposure to sunlight.
2. Avoid exposure to chemical carcinogens: industrial, mechanical, and environmental.
3. Encourage use of protective devices: clothing and medication, PABA sunscreens.
4. Support and stimulate regulations enforcing occupational safety, environmental health, and consumer product safety.

Population at Risk

1. Skin type: people with lightly pigmented skin.
2. Environment, geography: higher incidence in areas closer to the equator because of the increased exposure to ultraviolet rays.
3. Occupation: fishermen, housepainters, industrial exposure to chemical irritants in factories, farmers using insecticides.

Screening

1. Controversy regarding the significance of precursor lesions (congenital nevi) with melanoma.
2. Watch all lesions closely; report changes promptly.
3. Melanoma during the period of lateral growth can be diagnosed and cured by surgical excision before metastasis occurs.

ASSESSMENT

Health History

1. Age at time of onset (varies): young adult through elderly.
2. Occupation pertinent if establishes history of chronic irritant.
3. Establish history of irritant: sun, specialized clothing, boots, pipe, helicopter pilots in World War II exposed to constant wind on side of face.
4. Data regarding knowledge of the problem needed; important in planning care for the chronically or terminally ill person.
5. Clients will often complain of a suspicious lesion which does not heal over time but changes its characteristics, begins to grow rapidly, gets darker, becomes painful, ulcerates or bleeds.

Physical Assessment

Refer to definition above. Additional information should include the following:

1. Evaluation of the direction and rate of cellular growth.
2. Observation and description of the lesion with a hand lens in bright light, including details, onset, location, size, shape, margins, growth rate, color and changes in color, and presence or absence of pain.
3. Palpation of the lesion for hardness, softness, flatness, or elevation.
4. Identification of telangiectasis, crusting, ulceration, bleeding, or irritation.

DIAGNOSTIC TESTS

Biopsy of tissue (lesion) to evaluate composition, selecting tissue from multiple sites, including nodule, border, and pigmented area. Observe for halo around tumor.

NURSING DIAGNOSIS: ACTUAL OR POTENTIAL

1. Impaired skin integrity secondary to lesion.
2. Anxiety: mild to moderate; fear of metastasis and death.
3. Alteration in comfort: pain.
4. Self-concept: alteration in body images secondary to diagnosis and surgery.

EXPECTED OUTCOMES

1. Skin integrity will be restored.
2. In cases of metastasis the client will achieve maximum functioning, depending upon the limitations imposed by the treatment and the amount of tissue removed.
3. Anxiety will be managed, evidenced by the client's ability to maintain usual activities of daily living and personal social relationships.
4. Comfort will be restored, evidenced by the decrease in pruritus and pain.
5. Self-concept will be maintained.
6. Client will actively participate in activities of daily living.

INTERVENTIONS

1. Supportive counseling throughout diagnostic period and long-term follow-up. Reassurance and careful explanation of each problem essential.
2. Basal cell epithelioma:
   a. Preparation of client and supportive counseling throughout treatment and biopsy.
   b. Tumor excised by electrodesiccation, curettage, x-ray therapy, surgery, or cryosurgery.
3. Squamous cell epithelioma:
   a. Preparation of client and support throughout treatment and biopsy.
   b. Irradiation by superficial or deep x-ray, surgical excision.
   c. Identify external irritant and remove when possible.
4. Suspicious nevi:
   a. Preparation and support throughout procedure.
   b. Lesion excised with wide margins and biopsy performed.
5. Malignant melanoma:
   a. Definitive treatment is surgical excision.
   b. Prognosis is related to the level of invasion, thickness of the primary tumor, and extent of regional lymph node involvement.
   c. Based on the assessment of the risk factors, some clients are then placed on immunotherapy (BCG) combined with chemotherapy (CCNU, DTIC).
   d. In cases where the prognosis is poor, the client is supported through the grieving process and is helped to cope with a terminal illness.
   e. Emphasis must be placed in teaching clients to seek early diagnosis and treatment of any suspicious lesion.

EVALUATION

Outcome Criteria

1. Skin (biopsy or surgical site) is healed.
2. Client is receiving treatments or has completed course of treatment.
3. Client has been able to continue normal lifestyle.
4. Pain and pruritus are resolved; comfort is increased.
5. In cases of malignancy the client is compliant with the treatment as evidenced by keeping appointments for chemotherapy and immunotherapy.
6. There is an absence of infection or contractures.
7. Clients nutrition is maintained as evidenced by maintenance of optimal weight.
8. Exposure to chronic irritant is terminated.

Complications

1. Secondary infection.
2. Metastasis.

WARTS (VERRUCAE)

DESCRIPTION

A wart is a benign contagious epithelial tumor caused by the papilloma virus. It is spread by autoinoculation. The course of infection is erratic and over half the infections spontaneously clear. Warts are classified as common, plantar, flat, and venereal. *Common warts* (Figure 35-1) appear as yellowish flesh-colored papules that grow over several weeks, increasing in discoloration. They are found most often on the

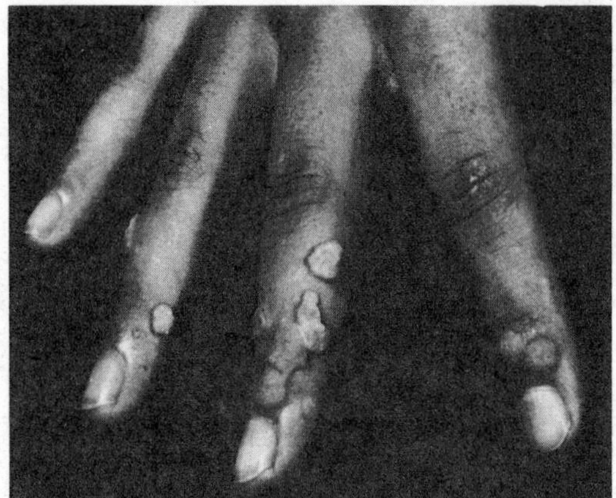

Figure 35-1 Common warts. (From Fitzpatrick, T.B., et al., eds.: *Dermatology in General Medicine*, 2d ed., McGraw-Hill, New York, 1975. Reproduced with permission.)

hands. *Plantar warts* (Figure 35-2) are firm, elevated, or flat lesions that interrupt natural skin folds. Red or black capillary dots are seen. They can form a mosaic, a group of multiple warts in one large, flat lesion. *Flat warts* are yellowish pink or tan, soft papules found on the face, neck, or extensor surfaces of forearms and hands. *Venereal warts* (*Condylomata acuminata*) occur in clusters in warm, moist, intertriginous areas, usually in the anogenital region. They are sexually transmitted and may appear up to 6 months following exposure. Therefore, the client under treatment should be followed for 6 months to be checked for previously undetected lesions.

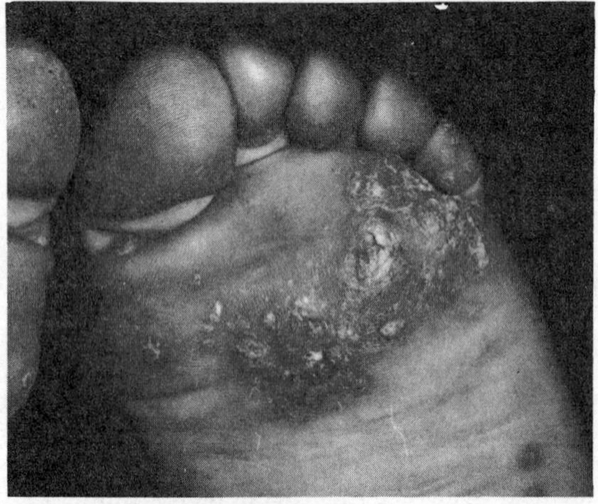

Figure 35-2 Plantar warts. (From Fitzpatrick, T.B., et al., eds.: *Dermatology in General Medicine*, 2d ed., McGraw-Hill, New York, 1975. Reproduced with permission.)

PREVENTION

Health Promotion

1. Maintain good health habits.
2. Wear correct footware (warts found in areas of calluses or pressure).

Population at Risk

1. Clients who have immunological suppression or have defect in cell-mediated immunity.
2. School population, ages 12–20.

NURSING DIAGNOSIS: ACTUAL OR POTENTIAL

1. Disruption in skin integrity: lesions disrupt skin.
2. Alteration in comfort: pain secondary to skin lesion.
3. Anxiety: mild to severe secondary to stress of chronic health problem.

EXPECTED OUTCOMES

1. Skin integrity will be restored by the disappearance of the warts.
2. Pain will be reduced as lesions resolve in pressure sites, palmar surface of the feet and genitalia.
3. Client will participate in the long course of therapy if needed.
4. Client will demonstrate medication application correctly as evidenced by no irritation from overtreatment or signs of secondary infection.

INTERVENTION

1. General
   a. Prepare and support client by explaining the application of the medication.
   b. Stress the importance of keeping follow-up appointments.
2. Common warts: Treatment includes:
   a. Removal of warts through electrodesiccation process causes superficial destruction by dehydrating cells.
   b. Curretage and cryosurgery (freezing with liquid nitrogen) may also be used.
   c. Explain all procedures indicating that electrodesiccation and curretage may be uncomfortable but not painful.

d. When cryosurgery is used, the client usually develops a blister at the site which will slough with some inflammation.
e. Administer keratolytic agents, 5–20 percent salicylic acid or 5–20 percent lactic acid.
f. Instruct the client to apply medication by washing the area for five minutes. Roughen the surface with a nail file and apply the medication with a wooden match tip, dry to the air. Seal bottle carefully. Apply only once a night. Expect 12 weeks for results. Do not use after cryosurgery until the inflammation has resolved.
g. Administration of podophyllin resin (25 percent in compound tincture of benzoin) is accomplished by applying the medication over night and removing it carefully in the morning. This medication is very irritating, and contact with surrounding tissue should be avoided. Effectiveness may be increased by occluding area with adhesive tape.

3. Flat warts:
   a. Assist with cryosurgery.
   b. Instruct the clients in the home use of keratolytic agents.
4. Plantar warts:
   a. Flatten lesion with a pumice stone to relieve the pressure. Usually left untreated, they will eventually resolve.
   b. Active treatment can cause these warts to spread by autoinoculation. If treatment is necessary because the warts are painful and spreading rapidly, apply keratolytic agent as above. Concurrently the warts are debrided twice a month by curretaging. If liquid nitrogen is used, it may cause discomfort in walking for several days due to the blister formation and inflammation.
5. Condylomata acuminata: Weekly painting of the lesion with 25 percent podophyllin resin in compound tincture of benzoin. Very irritating to healthy tissue. Do not allow agent to touch uninvolved area. Allow site to dry thoroughly, then powder before the client dresses. At the beginning of the treatment remove the medication in an hour, progress to 4–6 hours. Client should be aware that the treated lesions may be painful. Topical anesthetics may be prescribed. For large lesions only a portion may be treated at a time.

EVALUATION

Outcome Criteria

1. Skin integrity will be restored.
2. Comfort level will be restored. Itching will be eliminated. Pain will decrease.
3. Client will verbalize compliance with therapy.

Complications

1. Excoriation of healthy tissue: discontinue plaster.
2. Secondary infection: antiobiotics may be needed along with continued follow-up care.

Reevaluation and Follow-up

1. Prepare client for a long course of treatment, as removal of warts may require several follow-up visits.
2. Caution client against overzealous self-treatment, as it may be harmful to surrounding tissue and could affect healing.
3. Emphasize follow-up. Compliance is necessary for successful treatment. However, since warts may return even with compliance, the client may become frustrated easily. Reassurance and encouragement will be needed.

HYPERACTIVITY AND HYPOACTIVITY

PSORIASIS

DESCRIPTION

Psoriasis is a classic example of hyperactivity. It is a chronic, recurrent epidermal disease which begins usually in early adult life. Hormonal influence has also been associated with psoriasis. The problem is characterized by rapid cell proliferation of the epidermis (which is replaced in 4 days, compared to 28 days in normal skin). The epidermal cells of psoriatic lesions synthesize DNA and divide more rapidly, producing a thick, dry, silvery, scaly epidermis. The course is prolonged and unpredictable. For most clients the disease is localized. In severe cases it can cover the whole body. Spontaneous clearing is rare, although it has been reported temporarily to clear with pregnancy. This is a lifelong disease. Unexplained exacerbations are common. Topical treatment temporarily clears up most lesions. Since psoriasis is not life-threatening, systemic treatment with the related risk of side effects is reserved for severe cases that are resistant to topical therapy. A small percentage of psoriatic clients develop arthritis of the distal, interphalangeal joints. Cosmetic and psychological effects for some clients can be socially disabling. Unaesthetic lesions can be wrongly associated with disfigurement, contagion, or uncleanliness, leading to social isolation. This disease dictates the occupational, social, and sexual life of the client. These restrictions, combined with additional stress and anxiety, frequently precede exacerbations.

PREVENTION

Health Promotion

Maintain good health habits, adequate rest, activity and nutrition.

Population at Risk

1. Family history, inherited polygenic trait.
2. Environmental insults influence the first clinical appearance; trauma, burns, lacerations, chemical injuries.
3. Clients on certain systemic drugs, especially steroids and chloroquine, are more susceptible.
4. Since the problem is associated with low humidity, it should be avoided in a population at risk.

ASSESSMENT

Health History

1. Onset slow but continuous.
2. Scaling plaques pruritus; in severe cases the client may shiver while warm.
3. Psoriastic arthritis presents with tenderness, morning stiffness, and pain in small joints of hands and feet in early stages.
4. Later, intense pain in large joints, cervical and lumbar spine.
5. Anxiety associated with physical appearance.
6. History of psoriasis in family members (inherited autosomal traits).
7. Age: psoriasis usually appears late in childhood, in adolescence, and in middle-aged adults.
8. Occupation. Assess presence of mechanical injury. Identify environmental problems, e.g., dryness.
9. Identify stress factors within the client's environment, as this may aggravate the condition.
10. History of streptococcal infection.

Physical Assessment

1. Lesion is erythematous, consisting of sharply circumscribed plaques and papules, covered by silvery white scales. Localized to elbows, scalp, knees, sacrum, and behind the ears (see Figure 35-3) with profuse scaling.
2. Lesions are dry, and pruritus may be present.
3. Pitting, plating, ridging, or total destruction of fingernails and toenails.
4. Bilateral symmetry of the lesion observed.
5. Lesions can appear at sites of injury, scratches, surgical scars, sunburn, or occur following systemic illness, drug reaction, use of antimalarial drugs, or steroid withdrawal.
6. Acute psoriatic arthritis: distal phalanges have sausagelike appearance, with swollen, erythematous, painful joints.
7. Depending upon the extent of the lesion or the multiplicity of lesions, the client's general appearance may be changed. The client may appear withdrawn.

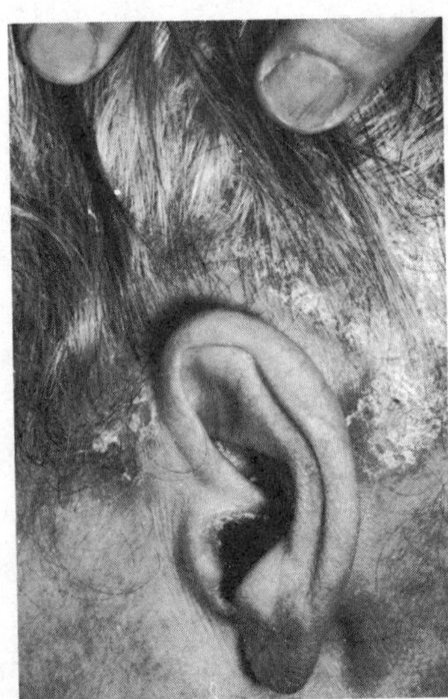

Figure 35-3 Psoriasis (hairline). (From Fitzpatrick, T.B., et al., eds.: *Dermatology in General Medicine*, 2d ed., McGraw-Hill, New York, 1975. Reproduced with permission.)

Diagnostic Tests

1. Sedimentation rate: elevated.
2. Rheumatoid factor: negative.

NURSING DIAGNOSIS: ACTUAL OR POTENTIAL

1. Impaired skin integrity; potential infection.
2. Altered self-concept and altered body image secondary to lesions.
3. Social isolation secondary to skin lesion.
4. Alterations in comfort: pain and pruritus due to erythema.
5. Anxiety: mild to moderate, secondary to physical appearance.

EXPECTED OUTCOMES

1. Number of erythematous, scaling lesions will be reduced.
2. Pruritus and pain will lessen varying with the degree of skin involvement and the individual course of the disease.
3. Social isolation will be alleviated because of the decrease in the lesions and amount of scaling.
4. Anxiety will diminish with a decrease in symptoms.
5. Positive self-image will be fostered with restored skin integrity.
6. Client will adhere to the medical regimen, as noted by verbal report of skin healing, avoiding trauma, and taking medications.

INTERVENTIONS

1. The choice of treatments of outpatient or inpatient depends on the extent, location, and degree of discomfort. Clients are hospitalized until condition is under control.
2. The choice of medication depends on the client's response to previous therapy, location of lesions, and the extent of the body surface involved.
3. Administer and teach the use of medications.
   a. Coal tar ointment (Psori-Gel, Estar). Used at night and rubbed into lesions. Apply thin film in intertriginous areas to avoid irritation. Enhances effectiveness of ultraviolet light (B wavelength) therapy.
   b. Fluorinated corticosteroids (Valisone, Synalar, Halog, Lidex, Hydrocortisone). These medications are used in varying strengths and preparations, and the method of application depends on the stage of treatment. Creams in a water base are used first because they alleviate dryness, remove scales, and allow the medication to penetrate the skin. Ointments have a petrolatum base, are greasy, and also remove scales, enhancing absorption. Long-term use of topical steroids can lead to irreversible skin changes and systemic absorption. Topically, skin thins, atrophies, forms striae, and becomes hypopigmented. Systemically, steroids can cause atrophy of the adrenal cortex, resulting in a decreased response to stress. Preoperatively, clients may be given supplemental medications. The nurse should be alert to side effects of topical steroids used to treat chronic dermatologic problems and should document their use.
4. Application of medication.
   a. The medications are applied three times a day to local lesions, with occlusive dressings at night.
      (1) Teach the application of airtight dressings at home.
      (2) Wash area well while skin is moist; rub medication thoroughly into the lesion.
      (3) Cover area with plastic wrap.
      (4) Seal edges with airtight paper tape.
      (5) Corticosteroids can be used in combination with coal tar. Because of the required nightly use, treatment is very costly. The dressings are awkward, and clients need encouragement for continued use. Occlusive dressings with ointment can cause folliculitis. As lesions subside use dressings less, while adding use of a bland emollient to medical regimen.
      (6) Psoralen and ultraviolet light (A wavelength), PUVA. Drug taken in pill form with excellent results, still being tested.
      (7) Coal tar therapy (Estar Gel) at night in combination with corticosteroids during the day, preceded by a bath to remove coal tar, plaques, and scaling and followed by ultraviolet light treatment (regimen used for hospitalized clients).
   b. Administration of ultraviolet light (B wavelength). This intervention is used alone and in conjunction with topical med-

ications. It should be used for restricted time periods, with a timer and eye protection. Usually exposure is desired until minimal erythema is attained. The dose is gradually increased. Use caution and time carefully.

c. The client should be taught good scalp care. The scalp can be washed with a mild shampoo, with vigorous scrubbing to remove scales. The hair is parted and a kerolytic agent (phenol and sodium chloride solution or Kerolytic Gel) can be applied. The client should be instructed to remove all medication before reapplication. Sometimes the medication may remain on overnight with showercap. Thoroughly wash hands after application of medication (very irritating to healthy skin). May be followed by steroid solution (Synalar, Valisone).
d. The client will require constant encouragement. The disease is treatable. The nightly, somewhat messy dressing and expensive medication are a constant source of discouragement. In addition, the physical changes in personal appearance can be frustrating. The nurse should emphasize that the disease can be controlled with consistent care. Support and encouragement will be needed throughout the course of treatment.
e. Teach, evaluate, and reteach home care as needed. The importance of appropriate use of medications and application of dressings cannot be overemphasized.
f. Family members should be included in all stages of treatment. Encourage the client and family to touch the skin without fear.
g. Provide an opportunity for clients to express their feelings regarding self-image, verbalize discouragements, and ask questions regarding the treatment and expectations of improvement.
h. Explore stress factors within the client's environment, and select possible solutions to decrease them.
i. Refer to counseling if client is socially disabled by illness and the alterations of physical appearance.
j. Support the client during quiescent periods to continue skin care nightly and apply emollients faithfully (Eucerin, Alpha Keri, bath oil without perfumes).
k. In more severe cases treatment of thick plaques requires the administration of anthralin paste on an inpatient or outpatient basis. This method stains, is irritating, and is difficult to apply. At night, bathe the client in coal tar, scrub off the scales, apply the paste with a glove, cover it with powder, then a gauze dressing, or old pajamas. In the morning the client bathes in mineral oil and applies low-strength corticosterods during the day. The anthralin paste can be very irritating to intertriginous areas (these areas can be protected by strips of soft cloth during the night). Salacylic Acid Cream 3–6% will remove the stain of the paste from the skin and is used to rim the lesions to limit the paste margins during application.
l. Clients require strong support due to chronic course of illness and the continual demand for constant care and attention. Psoriasis clients have formed mutual support groups in various parts of the country. Write the National Psoriasis Foundation for further information.

EVALUATION

Outcome Criteria

1. Lesions decrease in size and the amount of scaling is reduced.
2. Client is able to maintain normal lifestyle and social activity.
3. Pruritus and joint pain are absent; comfort level is improved.
4. Client verbalizes and develops strategies for handling stressors. Sources of stress and anxiety are reduced, as evidenced by continuation of normal sleeping habits, nutrition, and relationships.

Complications

1. Continued skin breakdown.
2. Secondary infection.

Assessment
Presence of pruritus, vesicles, and pustules.

Diagnostic Tests
Culture and sensitivities for causative organism and appropriate antibiotic.

Revised Outcomes
1. Infection will be cured.
2. Previous goals as stated will be achieved.

Interventions
Administration of antibiotic with instructions.
Reevaluation and Follow-up
1. Infection resolved.
2. Psoriasis clearing.

SYSTEMIC LUPUS ERYTHEMATOSUS

DESCRIPTION

Systemic lupus erythematosus (SLE) is a chronic inflammatory disease with occasional exacerbation of connective tissues associated with lesions in the vascular system, dermis, and serous and synovial membranes. It is characterized by multiple autoantibodies which participate in immunologically medicated tissue injury. The etiology is unknown. It affects individuals of all races, most often those between ages 15 to 25 years. Incidence of genetic factors and viral etiology are areas of recent ongoing investigation.

PREVENTION

Health Promotion

Protection from over exposure to sunlight.

Population at Risk

1. Persons taking certain drugs, i.e., hydralazine, procainide.
2. Continuous exposure to sunlight (e.g., frequent sunbathing).

ASSESSMENT

Health History

Include family history.
1. Tends to occur in certain ethnic groups and among immediate relatives, especially an identical twin.
2. General malaise and weakness.
3. Present medications: SLE can be drug-induced.
4. Chills.

Physical Assessment

1. May complain first of constitutional symptoms:
   a. Generalized aching.
   b. Low-grade fever.
   c. Weight loss.
2. Skin.
   a. Butterfly rash.
   b. Discord lesion.
   c. Any skin reaction to sun.
3. Musculoskeletal system.
   a. Nonerosive arthritis.
   b. Arthralgias.
4. Central nervous system.
   a. Seizures.
   b. Psychosis.
   c. Cranial nerve involvement.
5. Cardiopulmonary system.
   a. Chest pain on breathing: pleurisy.
   b. Substernal or precordial pain aggravated by movement may indicate pericardial involvement.
6. Renal system.
   a. Blood cells and protein in urine.
   b. Elevated blood pressure on several different readings.

Diagnostic Tests

1. Lupus erythematosus cell preparation.
2. Antinuclear antibody.
3. Complement testing.
4. False-positive serology for syphilis.

NURSING DIAGNOSES: ACTUAL OR POTENTIAL

1. Alteration in comfort: generalized aching; elevated temperature, thoracic pain.
2. Altered self-concept: changes in body due to rash; lesion.
3. Altered level of consciousness in response to seizure activity.
4. Nutritional deficit: weight loss due to decreased appetite.
5. Diminished activity tolerance: fatigue, malaise, joint pain.
6. Ineffective coping: secondary to mood changes, anxiety; depression due to diagnosis.
7. Altered elimination pattern: constipation.
8. Alteration in fluid balance secondary to retention of fluids.
9. Potential alteration in skin integrity: increased bleeding tendency.

EXPECTED OUTCOMES

1. Prevent exacerbations.
2. Maintain lifestyle and activity.

3. Promote adequate nutrition.
4. Relieve discomfort.
5. Promote adequate rest.
6. Promote effective coping. Decrease anxiety.
7. Increase self-concept and overall body image.

INTERVENTIONS

1. Teach client, family, and significant others about:
   a. Pathology of disease.
   b. Possible course of disease.
   c. Medications and side effects.
   d. Warning signs which indicate flare-up, i.e., constitutional symptoms.
2. Explain emotional involvement and mood swings to client and family.
3. Plan activity and rest schedule; promote gradual activity as symptoms diminish.
4. Discuss possible effects of stress and different ways to cope.
5. Explain to employer the disease process and patient's need to continue to be productive.
6. Administer antiinflammatory medications: aspirin, nonsteroids (Indocin). Skin lesions: use antiinflammatory creams; skin care; avoid trauma, sunburn, antimalarial medications.
7. Reduce joint inflammation: salicylates, exercise regularly.
8. Relieve nutritional deficit through use of bland diet, medication (e.g., malox or enteric-coated aspirin may be used to avoid the side effects of antiinflammatory medications).
9. Cardiopulmonary dysfunction: regulate exercise, monitor vital signs, observe for signs of pneumonia and other secondary lung infections.
10. Vascular involvement: observe for tarry stools, abdominal pain and distension, abnormal bowel sounds.
11. Renal problems: monitor blood pressure and temperature, observe for edema in lower extremities, weigh daily (indications of fluid retention).
12. Central nervous system involvement: observe for ptosis, diplopia, seizures, alterations in consciousness.
13. Vascular spasms: observe for signs of Raynaud's syndrome (sensitive, ulcerative, or gangrenous digits).
14. Hematologic problems: observe for malaise, chills, and fever; check urine for hematuria; check for back and abdomen pain.
15. Bruising and petechiae: observe for blood in stools and gastric secretions, nosebleeds, or any other bleeding.
16. Corticosteroid therapy:
    a. Observe for toxic effects: diabetes, peptic ulcers, secondary infections, necrosis.
    b. Provide for adequate rest and nutrition: control inflammation.
17. Provide support in handling stress: reduce susceptibility to secondary infections.
18. Immunosuppressant therapy: uncertain action: observe for possible toxic effects. Relief of constipation facilitated by diet and laxatives.

EVALUATION

Outcome Criteria

1. Remission of symptoms, no bleeding, decreased pain, normal cardiovascular function.
2. Follows drug regimen manifested by symptom remission.
3. Gradual increase in mobility and activity tolerance.
4. Continues previous lifestyle as nearly as possible.
5. Return to normal laboratory values.
6. No indication of further systemic involvement.
7. Gradual improvement of nutrition manifested by weight gain.
8. Improvement of coping strategies; decreased anxiety, diminished depression.
9. Absence of CNS involvement (e.g., no seizure activity).
10. Return of fluid balance; absence of peripheral edema; normal levels of urinary output maintained.

Reevaluation and Follow-up

1. Acute phase
   Clinic visits should be determined on individual basis depending on severity of symptoms; needed support and adjustment of client to this health problem.
2. Chronic phase
   a. The client must be followed by health team for remainder of life.

b. Consistency of health team members of utmost importance.
c. Group therapy with other clients or involvement in Lupus Club may be beneficial.

CHRONIC DISCOID LUPUS ERYTHEMATOSUS

DESCRIPTION

Chronic discoid lupus erythematosus (CDLE) is a rare, benign, self-limiting, sometimes disfiguring disease. Lesions are characterized by well-defined erythematous papules which spread with an irregular outline, while the center of the lesion heals with scarring, atrophy, loss of pigmentation, and scaling. Lesions are located mostly on the butterfly areas of the face (scalp, forehead, and ears). In widespread CDLE, lesions extend to the neck, back, shoulders, forearms, and legs. Exacerbations are aggravated by physical trauma, emotional stress, and exposure to cold and sunlight. Adults between the ages of 25 and 45 years are at highest risk, with women being effected twice as often as men. There are no abnormal laboratory values. The diagnosis is made by biopsy. Nursing interventions include support during the diagnostic evaluation and prevention of exacerbations by teaching the client to reduce exposure to sunlight through the use of clothing and sunscreens.

The treatment of choice for isolated lesions is intralesional infiltration of corticosteroids. The effect lasts several weeks to months. For widespread lesions corticosteroid creams or ointments with occlusive dressings are used. On occasion systemic therapy using 4-aminoguinoline group of antimalarial drugs are administered in doses higher than used to treat malaria. Clients are treated until the lesions resolve, then the drugs are maintained on the lowest dose possible. Treatment is stopped during quiescent periods. The drug is contraindicated in clients with psoriasis. There are numerous side effects, including gastrointestinal distress, nausea, dizziness, headache, tinitus, drug eruption, decreased auditory acuity, and retinal damage (not reversible).

INFLAMMATIONS

ACNE VULGARIS

DESCRIPTION

Acne vulgaris is a chronic inflammatory condition of the pilosebaceous structures (sebaceous follicles), usually involving the face, shoulders, back, chest, and upper arms. The problem results when excessive sebum is secreted into the follicle. Bacteria (e.g., *Corynebacterium* acnes) then break up the fatty acid of the sebum and keratin increases. This substance is irritating to the skin and its presence results in the formation of comedones (blackheads), formed by increased compaction of keratin, or milia (whiteheads), which result from closure of the follicular opening and trapping of oil in the skin.

These lesions may be cystic, papular, or pustular. They usually affect people from the age of puberty to middle years (age 40). There may be periods of remission, or the problem can be aggravated by a particular season of the year, menstrual problems, gastrointestinal disturbances, hormonal changes (e.g., ACTH), or stress.

There are a variety of lesions that characterize acne. These can be noninflammatory and/or chronic (see Figure 35-4), or an acute inflammatory response which results in pitting and facial scarring (see Figure 35-5). These physical changes in appearance may lead to social withdrawal and isolation. (Refer to Chapter 23 for a discussion of acne in children and adolescents.)

PREVENTION

Health Promotion

1. Avoid repeated pressure, leaning, touching, or scrubbing to acne prone areas.
2. Avoid oil in face creams, moisturizers, makeup, pomade.
3. Maintain good hygiene, clean hair.
4. Inform medical provider when taking systemic drugs (acne can be aggravated by use of INH, Dilantin, steroids, lithium, hyperalimentation, oral contraceptives, cobalt irradiation).

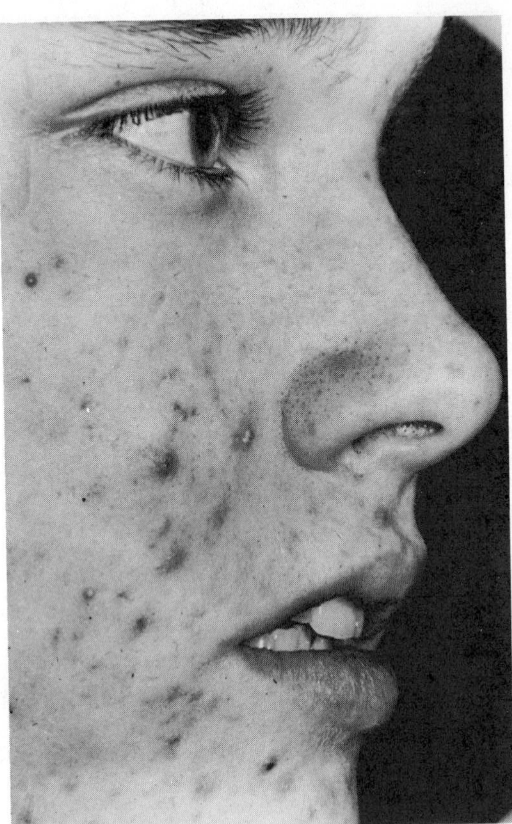

Figure 35-4 Milk acne. (From Fitzpatrick, T.B., et al., eds.: *Dermatology in General Medicine,* 2d ed., McGraw-Hill, New York, 1975. Reproduced with permission.)

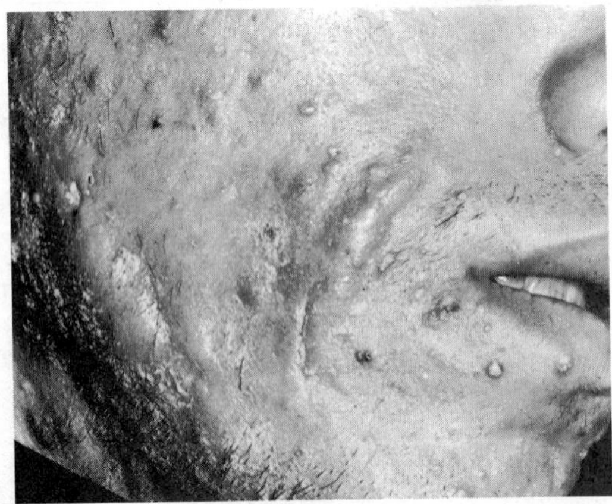

Figure 35-5 Cystic acne. (From Fitzpatrick, T.B., et al., eds.: *Dermatology in General Medicine,* 2d ed., McGraw-Hill, New York, 1975. Reproduced with permission.)

5. When possible avoid humid environments and excessive sweating.

Population at Risk

1. Preadolescents.
2. Adolescents
3. Adults.

ASSESSMENT

Health History

1. Complaints of chronic eruptions on face, back, shoulders, arms, chest.
2. Previous history of skin lesion (familial, self).
3. Age: onset of problem common around puberty to middle years.
4. History of menstrual, gastrointestinal, or hormonal health problems.
5. History of systemic medication (e.g., cortisone).
6. Stress response: identify issues within the environment that may be stress-producing; identify coping patterns.
7. Elicit socialization pattern and interactions with age group.
8. Evaluate occupation in terms of continued exposure to dirt, and review hygiene habits.
9. Medical treatment utilized at home or in the past.

Physical Assessment

1. Examine scalp, skin, and hair for oily appearance.
2. Examine lesions for drainage and note color and odor of discharge.
3. Examine face, back, arms, chest, and shoulders for the presence of comedones.
4. Closed follicles (comedones) will appear white or pale and slightly elevated; upon stretching the skin they are more easily observed.
5. Open comedone will be slightly raised with a central black or brown appearance due to the collection of keratin.
6. Pruritus and complaints of itching may be present.
7. Upon palpation the lesion may feel cystic, papular, or pustular (see Figure 33-5).

Diagnostic Tests

1. Occasionally there will be a positive culture for *Staphylococcus*.
2. X-ray films may demonstrate local calcium deposits.

NURSING DIAGNOSIS: ACTUAL OR POTENTIAL

1. Impaired skin integrity, potential for infection.
2. Self-concept: altered self-image secondary to lesions, scar formation.
3. Alteration in comfort: pruritus and/or pain.
4. Alterations in roles and relationships: withdrawal secondary to physical appearance.

EXPECTED OUTCOMES

1. Pruritus and pain will be relieved. Time frame will depend on the number and frequency of lesions.
2. Number and size of lesions will diminish within 8–10 weeks of the start of therapy.
3. Positive self-image will be maintained with the disappearance of lesions.
4. Factors that precipitate the problem will be reduced, preventing scarring.

INTERVENTIONS

1. Encourage client conscientiously to follow instruction for treatment throughout exacerbations and remissions. Client's perception of severity of problem is a guide to selecting treatment.
2. Teach self-care; purpose is to decrease oil accumulation on the skin.
   a. Cleanse face with abrasive soaps or lotions (Pernox, microsyn). Caution against overtreatment to avoid further irritation.
   b. Apply drying preparations both day and night (e.g., Benoxyl and Desquamx). The purpose of these medications is to achieve mild drying and erythema without discomfort.
   c. For more severe sores with pustules, cysts, and abscesses, systemic antibiotics are used to reach the sites of inflammation. Tetracycline, 250 mg, is the drug most commonly used. Tetracycline prevents new lesions from forming but does not affect those already present. It is the least expensive antibiotic. Clients should be told not to expect results until 4 to 6 weeks after treatment begins. When the client is receiving tetracycline, he or she should be taught to take the drug 1 hour before or after meals because it is irritating to GI tract without milk or milk products. Infection from *Candida (Monilia vaginitis)* can occur as a side effect of tetracycline therapy. Medication is not used during pregnancy; also, there may be an increased sensitivity to sunlight. Clients should be protected accordingly.
   d. Topical application of benzoylperoxide and vitamin A acid may be used to prevent formation of milia and comedones.
   e. Ultraviolet light may be used to dry lesions. Midday sun is also good. When a sun lamp is used at home, the client should be encouraged to protect eyes always, never use when sleepy, and use a timer to prevent facial burns.
   f. Encourage good hygiene, keep face and hair clean and free of oil, shampoo as often as necessary.
   g. Encourage person to verbalize feelings toward acne, self-image, and treatment. The nurse should be supportive and create an atmosphere in which this problem can be discussed.
   h. Diet counseling: research has not isolated a specific dietary pattern to use in the presence of acne other than a well-balanced diet. Avoid irritating foods.
3. Surgery.
   a. Acne surgery relieves pressure and prevents the progression of the lesion. The procedures are removal with comedone extractor, incision and drainage of cysts, intralesional injection of steroids, and cryosurgery, causing desquamation and involution of lesions.
   b. Plastic surgery.

EVALUATION

Outcome Criteria

1. Lesions decrease in size and amount.
2. Inflammation resolved in 8–10 weeks of treatment.
3. Scarring prevented.
4. Continued compliance measured by few new lesions, no exacerbations.
5. Client maintains personal hygiene by keeping body and hair clean and avoiding oily creams and make-up.
6. Self-image fostered, evidenced by positive relationships with peers.
7. Good response to necessary surgery.

Complications

1. Infection.
2. Permanent scarring.

DERMATOPHYTOSIS

DESCRIPTION

Dermatophytosis infections are contagious, superficial, fungal infections classified as *Tinea corporis* (ringworm of body), *Tinea capitis* (ringworm of the scalp; see Figure 35-6), *Tinea cruris* (ringworm of the area, or jock itch), and *Tinea pedis* (ringworm of the feet or athlete's foot). These diseases are highly transmissable by direct contact or contact with fomites (hairbrush, hats, shoes, floors, socks, towels). With specific antifungal treatment along with prevention the problem can be totally eliminated.

PREVENTION

Health Promotion

1. Protection: keep skin dry, change clothing and towels frequently.
2. Avoid contact with fomites.
3. Avoid use of personal articles of infected persons.

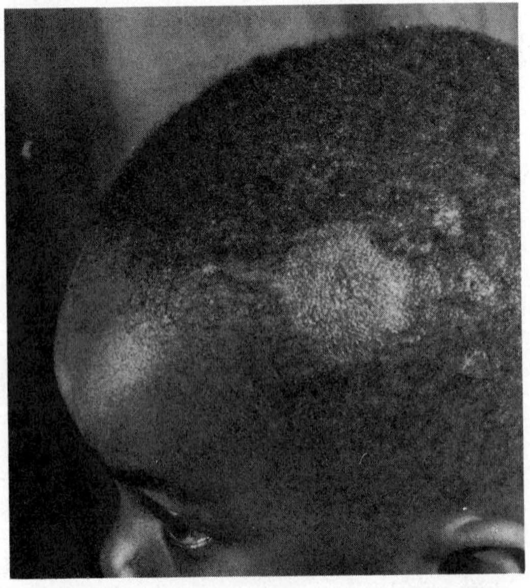

Figure 35-6 Tinea capitis. (From Fitzpatrick, T.B., et al., eds.: *Dermatology in General Medicine*, 2d ed., McGraw-Hill, New York, 1975. Reproduced with permission.)

Population at Risk

1. Persons with poor hygiene and nutrition.
2. Persons living in hot humid climates.
3. Persons in frequent contact with infected persons or fomites; i.e., swimmers using public pools.
4. Person with debilitating diseases.

ASSESSMENT

Health History

1. Assess recent exposure to pools, woods, pets, or locker rooms.
2. Determine recent exposure to fungus (e.g., *Tinea capitis*), in a school population; in a day-care center, from other family members, etc.
3. Client complains of pruritic, spreading lesions.
4. Loss of hair may be a response to fungus (*Tinea capitis*).
5. Poor hygiene and lack of foot care often noted in history.
6. Age: this problem can occur in any age group (*Tinea capitis* is more often observed in children).
7. Heredity may be involved in the development of this problem (particularly, *Tinea pedis*), e.g., sweating and immunological reactions.
8. Men may be more affected than women (*Tinea pedis*).

Physical Assessment

1. *Tinea pedis*.
   a. Acute inflammatory response involving one or both feet. A red rash is often observed in the interdigital spaces and on soles of feet.
   b. Lesions are vesicular in nature with scaling.
   c. Toenails may be involved in the inflammatory reaction. When this occurs, the nails become brittle and break easily, and brownish discoloration may be observed.
   d. Itching is not uncommon, and this can contribute to generalized swelling. If there are breaks in the skin, cellulitis may occur.
   e. Another form of tinea pedis may lead to fissures developing between the toes. Laceration of the skin may be observed.
2. Tinea corporis.
   a. Lesions are usually vesivular, with redness and scaling found on nonhairy skin.
   b. Lesion can begin as a red papule and spread peripherally with central healing.

c. The outer borders of the lesion are sharply defined and may appear in clusters.
d. Lesions are often observed on the scalp, hair, nails.

3. Tinea capitis.
   a. Most commonly found in the scalp, hair.
   b. Granulomatous lesions on scalp, inflammation, scaling, red macules (raised lesions, crusting may be noted) (see Figure 35-6).
   c. Hair loss may be observed. Hair becomes brittle (temporarily).
   d. Seen in children most often.
4. Tinea cruris.
   a. Aggravated by obesity, increased sweating, friction, seen more frequently in men.
   b. Sharp, symmetric eruptions observed in groin and thigh, and may spread to buttocks.
   c. Pustules are present at margin of lesions. Scaling and brownish discoloration observed.

Diagnostic Tests

1. Microscopic examination of scraping of lesion reveals hyphae of fungi.
2. Culture for fungi (scraping on a slide for direct visualization).
3. Wood's lamp in tinea capitis: affected hairs fluoresce.

NURSING DIAGNOSIS: ACTUAL OR POTENTIAL

1. Impaired skin integrity, secondary to lesion; break in skin.
2. Alteration in comfort: pruritus.
3. Potential risk of spreading infection.

EXPECTED OUTCOMES

1. Prevent transmission.
2. Relieve pruritus.
3. Restore skin integrity.
4. Prevent reinfection or secondary infection.

INTERVENTIONS

1. Instruct client on self-care, proper use of medication, course of illness, cause.
2. Administration of antifungal medications used topically, such as Lotrimin, Tinactin, and Halotex. Tinea capitus systemic treatment: grisiofulvin should be taken orally with meals (the presence of fat enhances absorption). Side effects include epigastric pain, nausea, and leukopernia. Contraindicated in clients with Psophyria. Effects of grisofulvin decreased with use of phenobarbital.
3. Teach client to decrease moisture in affected areas, as this will facilitate treatment and reduce chance of reinfection. Encourage the person to wear cotton next to skin and to change clothing and socks whenever wet to avoid accumulation of moisture. Restrictive shoes and tight clothing should also be avoided.
4. Intradigital spaces dried thoroughly and talcum applied if needed.
5. The nurse should teach the client and family members to protect themselves and others by wearing shoes in public showers, not sharing personal articles, i.e., towels, combs, in order to reduce transmission of these problems. Pets should be checked and treated if fur has moth-eaten appearance, as they may be the source of the problem.
6. All contacts should be screened and referred for treatment if symptomatic.
7. Follow the client and family members until infection has cleared.
8. Use drying powder (Lotrimin) after infection has cleared to prevent reinfection.

EVALUATION

Outcome Criteria

1. Itching decreased.
2. Healing of infection contained and spread of infection limited.
3. Skin integrity restored.

Complications

Secondary infection, e.g., cellulitis and lymphadermatitis; administer appropriate antibiotic after cultures.

Reevaluation and Follow-up

Should continue until the problem is eliminated.

DERMATOSIS: ATOPIC DERMATITIS

DESCRIPTION

Atopic dermatitis, or eczema, is a superficial inflammation of the skin. Although the etiology is unknown, it is thought to be due to sensitization to a particular substance. Usually there is a familial history of some type of allergy. The lesion often results in itching and scratching, and leads to secondary infection and lichenification, triggering the "itch-scratch cycle." Typical lesions are found in local areas of the body, usually flexor surfaces, around the eyes, and the hands, but there may be total body involvement. The course of the disease is periodic, unpredictable, and discouraging with exacerbations and partial remissions. Exacerbations occur often during periods of psychological or physical stress. Certain factors trigger the itch. This condition is often worse in the winter, intensified by extremes in temperature and irritated by sweating and substances such as wool or silk, occlusive clothing, oil, soaps, detergents, and environmental allergens.

PREVENTION

Health Promotion

1. Avoid dry skin. Disease is common in the winter and fall; utilization of a humidifier or open containers of water in the home may be helpful.
2. Reduce excessive moisture and sweating because it aggravates itchy skin. Exercise should not be restricted but overheating should be avoided.
3. Avoid soap because it is an irritant (contains lye). Soap also removes natural oils causing further drying and itching.
4. Avoid wools, furry fibers, and synthetic materials because they are irritating to the skin and stimulate the itch-scratch cycle.
5. Do not use lotions and creams. Their water content causes dryness through evaporation.
6. Emotional factors; anger, excitement, and distress can trigger itching.

Population at Risk

1. May occur at any age: the most common is infantile eczema.
2. Affects 1 percent of school children.
3. Usually family history of allergies; hay fever, eczema, or asthma.

ASSESSMENT

Health History

1. Intense pruritic scaling, erythematous patches described.
2. Obtain a personal or family history of past allergies. Determine if home treatment has been initiated.
3. May occur at any age.
4. Environmental and psychological factors which precipitate the problem should be determined (e.g., season, clothing, stress).

Physical Assessment

1. Erythema and scaling progressing to excoriations secondary to itching.
2. Lesions may appear anywhere on the body. Often noted (in adults) on face, neck, upper chest, and flexures of the arms and legs.
3. Scratching leads to dry, lichenified, hyperpigmented, or hypopigmented plaques.

NURSING DIAGNOSIS: ACTUAL OR POTENTIAL

1. Impaired skin integrity, potential infection.
2. Alteration in comfort: discomfort secondary to pruritus.
3. Disturbed sleep-rest pattern secondary to presence of "itch-scratch" cycle.
4. Ineffective coping: increased anxiety (mild to moderate) or stress.

EXPECTED OUTCOMES

1. Pruritus will be relieved, "itch-scratch" cycle stopped (length of time varies with the extent of involvement).
2. Erythematous, scaling lesions will be reduced in number, further excoriations with oozing and crusting will be avoided.
3. Client will be able to sleep at night without itching.
4. External stresses will be identified, reduced, and eliminated when possible.
5. Bacterial skin infection will be prevented.

INTERVENTIONS

1. Support client through long, discouraging course of treatment by consistent, positive approach throughout the interaction.
2. Prepare for treatment by explaining that the rationale for interventions is to identify the trigger mechanism and then prevent the pruritus from occurring.
3. Suppress the itch-scratch cycle.
   a. Keep skin moist and supple.
   b. Bathing with antipruritus additives (Aveeno) rather than soap.

c. After bathing pat the skin dry, leaving some moisture. Seal in the moisture with an emollient (petroleum jelly, Crisco, Eucerin, Alpha Keri bath oil).
d. Administer topical corticosteroids, Valisone, Synalar, Lidex, Aristocort (see *Psoriasis* for use of cortisone cream).

4. Caution client against excessive bathing and high humidity; these may aggravate symptoms. Avoid contact with wool, silk, and other trigger factors.
5. Promote rest by providing a quiet environment, well ventilated. Antihistamines are used for the pruritus. Itching is usually worse at night, so sleepiness is induced with the administration of antihistamines.
6. Identify stresses causing exacerbations (job, family, or situational crisis) and select strategies to cope more effectively.
7. Explain to the client that initially useful medications may become ineffective for periods of time and will be changed accordingly.
8. Alert the client to avoid exposure to chicken pox and the vaccination. Also avoid persons with a herpes infection and persons recently vaccinated.
9. Remind client to have yearly eye exam, because of an increased incidence of cataracts.
10. Urge consistency in treatment and keeping follow-up appointments.

EVALUATION

Outcome Criteria

1. Pruritus relieved within 48 hours of instituting treatment. Varies with the severity of involvement.
2. Lesions healing, erythema resolved with the pruritus.
3. Client can sleep without interruptions caused by itching.
4. Exacerbations kept to a minimum by avoiding excessive sweating, and termination of the "itch-scratch cycle."

Complications

SECONDARY INFECTION

Intervention

Stop topical steroids and emollients. Administer antibiotics; compress with Burow's solution. Alumin acetate diluted 1:20, as wet dressings to promote drying, soothing, and cleaning of the infected area. Use until oozing and crusting resolved.

DERMATOSIS: CONTACT DERMATITIS

DESCRIPTION

Contact dermatitis is a superficial inflammation which results from a sensitization of the skin due to skin contact with natural or synthetic substances (nonallergic). Reactions may be immediate or delayed, with symptoms occurring within hours or weeks. Allergic contact dermatitis is delayed hypersensitivity to exposure to contact allergens by sensitized people, e.g., poison ivy, poison oak. Primary irritants in contact dermatitis are plants, trees, chemicals, therapeutic agents, cosmetics, fabrics, and metals (nickel). Successful intervention and removal of the precipitating irritant should relieve the symptoms.

Erythema, vesicles, ulcers, edema, and oozing are observed. Chronic exposure may lead to fissuring of the skin with dryness and thickness. Burning and pain may be noted. Distribution of contact dermatitis is significant. Usually the area has sharp, straight borders, due to direct contact with primary irritant. Skin thickness is noted in prolonged cases. Hemorrhagic bullae may develop in more severe cases.

Treatment of contact dermatitis depends on stage of the problem and related symptoms. Acute (mild to moderate) contact dermatitis: apply compresses of Burow's solution directly to vesicles. These can be followed by applying a soothing, drying solution (e.g., calamine). In severe cases of bullae and edema, steroids may be used. After vesiculation decreases, topical corticosteroids may be applied.

During the chronic stage use tar compounds in combination with steroids and occlusive dressings. Antihistamines can be used to decrease pruritus. Prevention of reoccurrence essential. Therefore, the source of irritation is most important. Use of rubber gloves, skin testing, and avoiding the source of the problem should eliminate symptoms. Follow-up is critical.

SEBORRHEIC DERMATITIS

DESCRIPTION

An acute, inflammatory dermatosis of oily skin, seborrheic dermatitis is usually found in those parts of the body containing large sebaceous glands. The lesions are pruritic and characterized by dry, moist, or greasy scales and crusted yellowish plaques; when located in the scalp, it is known as dandruff.

Fine, dry scaling on scalp, eyebrows, postauricular folds, and beard is noted. In distinct borders, greasy yellow scales can form. Irritation may occur in men in hairy areas of the chest.

Interventions include promoting skin healing by teaching administration of topical cortiosteroids to control skin inflammation. Valisone lotion or Synalar on the scalp may help relieve the problem. Scrub the scalp with mild shampoo; remove crusts and previous medications before reapplication of a shampoo. Sebulex, Selson, Zincon are available in drugstores and may be used for this purpose. Follow-up is necessary until the condition improves, as this problem may become chronic. Threat of secondary infection is always present. Therefore, good hygiene is essential.

SCABIES

DESCRIPTION

Scabies is a parasitic skin infection, characterized by fine, superficial burrows and intense pruritus. The disease is caused by the burrowing itch mite, *Sarcoptes scabiei*. Scabies is readily transmissible by intimate contact. The burrows are a result of female mites entering the superficial layers of skin and depositing eggs. Symptoms appear when larvae hatch, up to 3 weeks after exposure. Lesions are generally found on the interdigital webs of the hands, wrists, intertriginous spaces, lower abdomen, around nipples, genitalia, and ankles, and usually not on the scalp or back (see Figure 35-7).

PREVENTION

Health Promotion

1. Avoid exposure to the mite; i.e., intimate physical contact with a person who has scabies, and with fomites (organism is found to live 48 hours away from the host), bedding, sleeping bags, shag rugs. Small animals can also be hosts.
2. Good hygiene.

Population at Risk

Highly communicable; most of the population is at risk.

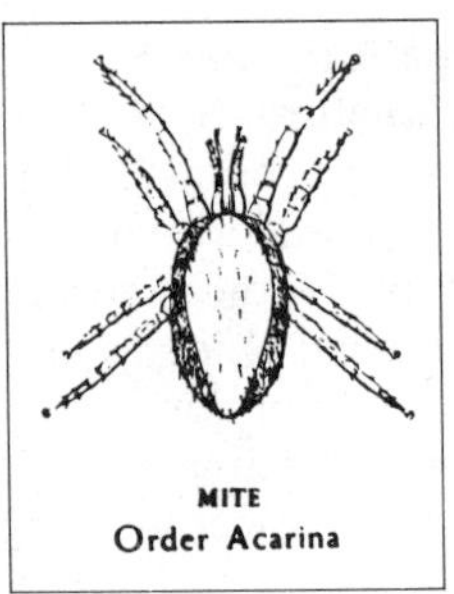

Figure 35-7 Mite (scabies). (From Fitzpatrick, T.B., et al., eds.: *Dermatology in General Medicine*, 2d ed., McGraw-Hill, New York, 1975. Reproduced with permission.)

ASSESSMENT

Health History

1. Environmental exposure: increased incidence in areas with substandard hygienic conditions.
2. Contacts, e.g., dogs, cats, small animals, sexual contacts, fomites (bedclothes).
3. Intense itching, worse at night. Obtain history of the medication or treatment already started at home.
4. Age of client important; pregnant women should also be identified.

Physical Assessment

1. Upper skin layer involved; fingers, interdigital spaces, flexor surfaces, wrists, elbows, axilla, genitalia.
2. Erythema and papules present. May appear at the end of fine wavy lines, grayish in appearance. May be visualized better by holding a flashlight to taut skin.
3. Generalized excoriation can occur at sites of scratching.
4. Urticarial and papular rash may be observed.

Diagnostic Tests

Scraping of lesions and microscopic confirmation. Observe mite, larvae, or brown-black fecal material.

NURSING DIAGNOSIS: ACTUAL OR POTENTIAL

1. Impaired skin integrity; potential infection, secondary to excoriation.
2. Alteration in comfort: discomfort secondary to pruritus.

3. Fear (mild to severe): anxious about the presence of parasite under skin; change in body image.

EXPECTED OUTCOMES

1. Pruritus will be reduced within 24 hours.
2. Rest will be promoted within 12 hours.
3. Contacts will be referred for treatment immediately.
4. Skin integrity will be restored within two weeks.
5. Recurrence will be prevented by removing original source.

INTERVENTIONS

1. Explain course of the disease, its highly contagious nature, its cause and treatment to client and family.
2. Teach client application of medication:
   a. 1 percent Kwell Lotion (Gamma Benzene Hexachloride, GBH), cream and shampoo. Caution with use, since 10% of the topically applied drug may be absorbed systemically. It is not recommended for infants, young children, and pregnant women. Instruct client to apply to the entire body, from the neck to the lower extremities for 24 hours, following a soap and water bath. Reapply to areas where lotion is removed during that 24 hours, i.e., hands and genitalia. The medication is used in laundering clothing, bed linen combined with detergent and hot water. Nonwashables should be dry cleaned.
   b. Alternative medications: Crotamiton (10% N-ethyl-o-crotonotoluide) and Eurax are effective medications applied twice in 48-hour period. They will relieve pruritus. Clients are warned to expect stinging. These drugs are a second choice of therapy.
3. Client is strongly urged to follow all of the instructions. Caution against overzealous treatment, which can lead to contact dermatitis and irritation, must be stressed.
4. Teach client to expect the pruritus to persist after treatment is completed. Utilization of topical emollients or antipruritics (Aveeno) will provide relief. Antihistamines may be prescribed orally. Reinstitution of the use of the medication should not begin without consulting with their primary provider.
5. Promote rest by the proper use of medication. Explain the itch-scratch cycle. Encourage client to utilize distractions to interrupt the cycle; i.e., physical exercise or a walk before retiring.
6. Contacts should be treated prophylactically and simultaneously, because of the contagious nature of this problem.
7. Reduce anxiety by reassuring the client that the proper use of the medication will stop the process. Prepare them to expect the pruritus to resolve more slowly.

EVALUATION

Outcome Criteria

1. Pruritus will decrease in intensity to eventually full elimination of discomfort.
2. Erythema and burrows no longer visible within a week of initial treatment.
3. Excoriation resolved; no new lesions or infection present.
4. Sleep restored in 24 hours.
5. Good hygiene, clean skin is reported by the client and observed on assessment of skin integrity.

Complications

SECONDARY INFECTION

See *Dermatosis: Atopic Dermatitis*.

CONTACT DERMATITIS

From overtreatment.

PERSISTENT ITCHING

Assessment
Resistance to GBH.
Intervention
Change to another medication.

HYPERSENSITIVITY

Assessment
Pruritic nodules. Neurodermatitis.
Intervention
Interlesional corticosteroids injection, topical corticosteroids, or a short course of oral corticosteroids.

ALTERED SLEEP PATTERNS

TRANSMISSIBLE VIA CONTACT: POTENTIAL

ERYTHEMA MULTIFORME

DESCRIPTION

Erythema multiforme is an inflammatory hypersensitivity reaction. Onset begins similar to a viral illness. Symptoms usually begin a few days after a fever. The course of the problem generally lasts 2 to 3 weeks in mild cases and 6 to 8 weeks in a more severe form. (Stevens-Johnson syndrome). Many factors, e.g., drugs, barbiturates, penicillin, malignancy, endocrine changes, viral illness, and most often herpes simplex, can precipitate the occurrence of this illness. This disease responds to treatment but may reoccur. In severe forms the problem may be life-threatening due to infection. Secondary blindness may develop if eyelids are involved. Leakage of fluid into the dermis (caused by blistering) can lead to tissue necrosis.

PREVENTION

Etiology unknown.

ASSESSMENT

Health History

1. Complaints associated with an upper respiratory infection. Fever is not uncommon.
2. Initial eruption may be symptomless. Some clients complain of stinging and burning.
3. Dietary changes may be noted if oral mucosa is involved.
4. History of herpes simplex is not uncommon.
5. Identification of the precipitating cause is critical. (Screen for history of recent vaccination. Use oral contraceptives, radio therapy, and pregnancy.)
6. The problem is rarely observed before the age of 2 or after age 50.
7. It is often precipitated by the cold weather, increasing in incidence in December, January, and February.

Physical Assessment

1. Lesions are red blotches which erupt suddenly (see Figure 35-8). They are symmetrically distributed.
2. The face, neck, legs, dorsal surface of the hands, forearms, feet, and oral mucosa may be affected.
3. The iris or target lesion often appears as a white central vesicle, surrounded by alternating pale concentric rings of erythema.
4. In severe forms the client will have generalized lesions that blister, with bullae and hemorrhage involving mucous membranes of eyes and mouth.
5. The skin becomes dusky as the lesions progress (age). As fluids leak into the dermis (e.g., from blisters), they can cause tissue necrosis.
6. Oral mucous membranes may be involved, with purulent drainage.
7. Body temperature may be increased.

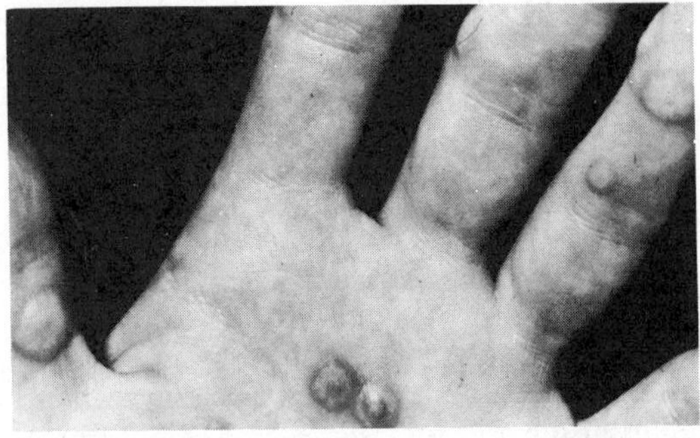

(a)

(b)

Figure 35-8 Erythema multiforme: (a) target lesions; (b) major lesions. (From Fitzpatrick, T.B., et al., eds.: *Dermatology in General Medicine,* 2d ed., McGraw-Hill, New York, 1975. Reproduced with permission.)

Diagnostic Tests

1. CBC: anemia may be present.
2. Leukocytosis may be observed.

3. Serology tests.
4. Chest x-rays to rule out pneumonia and malignancy (mycoplasma).
5. Liver function tests to rule out hepatitis, mononucleosis, and Australia antigen.
6. Skin tests for TB and fungal infection.
7. Rule out mycoplasmic infections and histoplasmosis.
8. Culture for streptococcus, mycoplasma, coccidomycosis.
9. Biopsy: assess histologic picture.

NURSING DIAGNOSIS: ACTUAL OR POTENTIAL

1. Impairment of skin integrity; potential necrosis and infection.
2. Alteration in nutrition, secondary to oral mucosa involvement.
3. Potentially life-threatening problem.
4. Alteration in comfort: pain.
5. Anxiety: mild to moderate.
6. Self-concept: alteration in body image, secondary to lesions.

EXPECTED OUTCOMES

1. Adequate fluid balance and nutrition will be maintained.
2. Attempts will be made to identify the precipating cause.
3. Pain will be relieved.
4. Anxiety will be reduced with the onset of treatment.
5. Skin integrity will be restored and serious complications avoided.

INTERVENTIONS

1. Reassure client, explain treatment, provide physical and emotional comfort, and offer support to client and family.
2. Administer steroids orally to reduce inflammation; antibiotics are used when infection is present or suspected.
3. Apply open wet compresses to bullae and erosive lesions to help reduce inflammation and promote comfort. Cover only one-third of the body at a time to avoid hypothermia.
4. Oral hygiene: mouthwash for cleanliness (3% hydrogen peroxide), Dyclone solution, viscous Xylocaine for pain (used topically) in order to reduce halitosis and to limit infection.
5. Provide bland diet to make oral intake possible and to promote comfort while eating.
6. Administer analgesics: aminosalicylic acid (ASA), 600 mg as circumstances require and antihistamines.
7. With severe cases (client is hospitalized) monitor IV fluids, mouth care, and eye care. Administer prednisone (systemically) to help reduce inflammation. Compresses continued.
8. Create an environment in which client can discuss fears and apprehension, especially if the cause of the problem is unknown.
9. Observe closely, record changes.
10. Encourage follow-up of diagnostic tests.

EVALUATION

Outcome Criteria

1. Nutritional and metabolic balance restored as evidenced by fluid and electrolyte balance and maintenance of body weight.
2. Verbal comprehension of the disease process evidenced by decrease in fear of lesion; changes in self-concept.
3. Restoration of body image as lesion begins to respond to treatment.
4. Restoration of skin integrity evidenced by healing; increased comfort, and decreased skin irritation and pain.

Complications

1. Secondary infection.
2. Blindness (refer to Chapter 26).
3. Toxic reaction to tissue necrosis.
4. Kidney damage (refer to Chapter 32).
5. Malignancy: suspected when lesions appear after the age of 50.

TRAUMA

The most common wounds or injuries to the skin are burns. Therefore, most of the following section will focus on nursing care of the burn patient. The reader is referred to Chapter 48 for a complete discussion of the immediate care of the client with mild to severe burns.

BURNS

DESCRIPTION

Burns are a profound trauma to the skin that interrupt the normal skin function. As a result there is an ineffective barrier against infection, loss of body fluids, disruption in temperature control, destruction of sweat and sebaceous glands, and an alteration in sensory receptors. The causes of burns include prolonged exposure to flames, hot liquids, chemicals, electricity, and radiation. Burns are classified as first, second, and third degree, depending on depth of skin traumatized. First-degree burns are superficial injuries of the epidermis resulting in localized erythema and edema. Second-degree burns are partial thickness injuries involving the epidermis and part of the dermis. Erythema, edema, and bullae appear. Sebaceous glands, sweat glands, and hair follicles remain intact. Pain is often severe. Third-degree burns are full thickness injuries that destroy all layers, leaving necrotic tissue. No regeneration can occur. These burns destroy the skin appendages, nerve endings, fascia, and blood supply. Skin grafting is required for healing since no new epithelialization can occur. The area is painless because of nerve destruction.

1. When an individual sustains a burn there is initial fear, pain, and anxiety (neurogenic shock). (See Chapter 48.)
2. Physiologically, vasodilatation and increased capillary permeability occur.
3. Extracellular fluid shifts to the site of injury accompanied by sodium and protein. The escape of these substances into the wound causes edema and blister formation, or loss through the open wound.
4. Fluid is also depleted from the circulating blood as fluid extravasates into deeper tissues. Half of the extracellular fluid can shift from the interstitial spaces and the bloodstream to the site of a severe burn.
5. Plasma also seeps into the tissue.
6. Hypovolemic shock (refer to Chapter 48) results, accompanied by a fall in blood pressure and inadequate kidney perfusion (leading to anuria). Pump failure, hormonal disturbances, and cerebral anorexia result.
7. The shock stage is accompanied by dehydration, hyperproteinemia, electrolyte imbalance, and increased stress on the kidney due to decreased blood volume and increased by-products of hemolyzed cells being excreted.
8. Blood potassium elevates due to decreased urinary output, and cardiac arrhythmias may be seen.
9. Anemia develops because red blood cells are trapped in the burn site and destroyed.
10. Heat is lost through open wounds by evaporation, increasing the metabolic rate and leading to weight loss.
11. Adrenocortical activity increases in response to the generalized stress.
12. Respiratory distress is a problem for head and neck injuries or when a substance (e.g., smoke) is inhaled.
13. After the first 24 to 36 h, fluid shifts from the extravascular space and returns to the vascular system. Caution at this stage to avoid fluid overload by carefully monitoring cardiac output, renal output, and intravenous intake cannot be overemphasized.
14. The next stage of physiologic change is the period of burn slough and infection. The burned necrotic tissue or eschar separated from underlying viable tissues leaves an open wound with a high risk for infection. Before repair can begin, the eschar must be removed. If some of the original layer of skin remains, the skin will regenerate. If all the layers are destroyed, only granulation tissue remains to form unsightly scars. Therefore, skin grafting is utilized to prevent scarring and promote early healing.

The homeostatic mechanisms of the severely burned client are disturbed. Most victims of second-degree burns and all victims of third-degree burns, inhalation burns, and burns of the face and neck require hospitalization. The psychological toll on the client is devastating. Physiologically, death may occur during any period of treatment; therefore, care becomes most demanding. Depending upon the severity of the injury, rehabilitation may require many months or even years of nursing and medical care. Long-term nursing interventions are needed for clients with chronic health problems, and referral to a variety of health resources will be required, again depending upon the depth of the burn and the extent of tissue involvement. Permanent alteration in body image may necessitate counseling.

PREVENTION

Health Promotion

1. Care to turn pot handles in, so that they are not overhanging the edge of the stove.
2. Avoid use of appliances with frayed electrical cords.
3. Be careful when cooking with long hair, long sleeves, or full garments.
4. Caution when handling hot liquids, place in from the edge of the table.
5. Avoid dangling electrical cords from irons, coffeemakers, and electric frypans.
6. Caution when using combustible liquids, gasoline, charcoal lighter.
7. Attention not to touch electrical items when not properly grounded.
8. Store combustibles in a well ventilated place out of reach of children.
9. Use proper protection when working with volatile materials.

Population at Risk

1. General public.
2. Children.
3. Elderly.

ASSESSMENT

Health History

May be obtained from family or friend if client is unable to talk.

1. Age: Developmentally significant, especially if disfigurement is anticipated. Age is also significant in determining treatment (e.g., fluid replacement).
2. Occupation: Was the injury job-related? If so, was there an explosion? Identify the materials that were burning and the source of the fire.
3. Complete medical history: Screen for cardiac or renal diseases, diabetes, ulcers, allergies, and factors that may complicate treating the burn, e.g., emotional illness, alcoholism, or epilepsy.
4. History of the injury.
   a. Identify the material that directly burned the individual materials that were inhaled, and length of time patient was exposed to burning substance.
   b. Identify when and where first aid was given, the treatment given, and whether or not tetanus toxoid was given prophylactically.
   c. Identify the amount and type of fluid replacement instituted, if any.
   d. Question if other losses were involved in the fire, e.g., home or family members.
5. Personal history: Identify the client's relationships, previous coping patterns, personal needs, needs of family and significant others, life-style, sleep patterns, nutritional habits, and educational background.
6. Socioeconomic factors: Assess financial status and insurance benefits, as long-term care may be costly.
7. Assess current health status (prior to injury). Evaluate past health perceptions.

Physical Assessment

For initial assessment, refer to Chapter 48.

1. A complete physical examination is necessary in order to assess whether there are other injuries (e.g., fractures and internal trauma).
2. General appearance: Observe for alertness, anxiety, vital signs, blood pressure, signs of impending shock.
3. Neurological: Note changes in consciousness, e.g., fear, hysteria. Neurological evaluation is important.
4. Skin: Temperature changes (cold), peripheral circulation other than burn site (refer to Table 35-1).
5. Cardiorespiratory:
   a. Lung changes indicative of inhalation injury: rales or cough (if productive, note color and amount of sputum), cyanosis, labored breathing (dyspnea), stridor, singed nasal hairs. Tracheostomy or endotracheal tube may be inserted (refer to Chapter 31).
   b. Cardiac status: blood pressure, pulse (arrhythmias, signs of failure), alterations in circulation due to shifting fluid, cyanosis, capillary refill.
6. Musculoskeletal: Decreased mobility, check for fractures. Observe for deformity secondary to immobility, observe for exposure of muscle tissue and bone structure.
7. Urogenital: Urinary output decreased in fluid-shock phase, increases as fluid shifts after the first 24 to 36 h. Hematuria indicates renal stress.
8. Gastrointestinal: Head and mouth injuries, check for edema, nausea, and vomiting.
9. Observe stomach contents for blood, indic-

ative of stress ulcer. Assess bowel sounds and abdominal distension. Client usually has a nasogastric tube placed while in the emergency room. Observe for paralytic ileus and bleeding of the internal organs. (Refer to Chapter 33.)

10. Observe for signs of infection, including prevalent drainage, increased body temperature.
11. Complete assessment of pain or lack of it. Accurate reporting of pain duration, intensity, quality, location, etc., important throughout the care of each client.
12. Behavioral assessment, including verbal and nonverbal responses, assessment of memory, judgment, level of consciousness, and orientation to time and place, are important parameters.

Diagnostic Tests

1. Serum electrolyte to evaluate fluid loss: potassium increases, sodium chloride decreases.
2. Blood gases: assess arterial oxygen level (refer to Chapter 30).
3. Hematocrit, hemoglobin: assess blood loss.
4. Blood urea nitrogen, creatinine: assess renal function.
5. Hourly urine for amount, pH, protein, sugar, acetone, specific gravity, blood.
6. Leukocyte and sedimentation rate: evaluate inflammation.

NURSING DIAGNOSIS: ACTUAL OR POTENTIAL

1. Body fluids: depletion, secondary to impaired skin function and fluid shift.
2. Impaired mobility, secondary to immobilization after injury; contractures.
3. Nutritional deficit alteration: less than required, due to decreased appetite, impaired ingestion.
4. Self-concept: altered body image secondary to tissue destruction.
5. Alteration in comfort: pain, moderate to severe.
6. Fear: moderate to severe, life-threatening situation.
7. Sleep-rest pattern disturbance: due to pain; discomfort; disturbance caused by frequent monitoring.
8. Loss of privacy, invasion of territorial space; secondary to immobility and dependency.
9. Altered ability to perform self-care activity.
10. Grieving: acute, delayed; secondary to physical loss, dependency.
11. Impairment of significant others' adjustment to illness.
12. Sensory perception: altered due to disruption in normal body rhythms and sensory stimulation.
13. Thought process impaired: potential due to altered level of consciousness.
14. Cardiac output: depleted potential.
15. Alteration in socialization: potential secondary to physical appearance.

EXPECTED OUTCOMES

1. Physiologic balance will be restored and health state stabilized.
2. Shock will be prevented.
3. Stress and fear will be managed, gradually improving with skin healing, restoration of physical health, and knowledge gained through questioning and information sharing.
4. Pain will be relieved, comfort level improved.
5. Skin integrity will be restored and healing promoted.
6. Self-esteem will be maintained and self-concept will be improved with healing.
7. Contractures will be prevented.
8. Body integrity will be preserved.
9. Client will be helped to develop coping strategies with the physical changes, treatments, and rehabilitation resulting from injury.
10. Normal sleep patterns will be restored.
11. Client will be helped through the grieving process.
12. Family will be helped through support and education to cope with the burn victim.
13. Cognitive processes and level of conscious awareness will be gradually restored.
14. There will be gradual improvement in socialization with others, usually congruent with physical health.

INTERVENTIONS

1. Monitor fluid replacement to counteract the fluid loss of intravascular and extravascular fluid into the burn wound. Various formulas are utilized for the initial replacement therapy. See Table 35-2 for the description of the

TABLE 35-1 ASSESSMENT OF BURNS

Degree	Skin Involvement[a]	Health History	Assessment
First degree	Epidermis	Complaints of tingling, throbbing, hyperesthesia, pain	Skin red; area blanches with pressure Slight edema may be present Scabbing may appear as wound heals; peeling may be seen
Second degree (superficial)	Tissue destruction occurs up to dermis	Often result of burn from boiling/hot water	Blistering, edema and redness may occur
Second degree (deep)	Dermis affected	Complaints of pain, hyperesthesia Clothing burns may be the causative agent	Blistering, edema, and redness may occur Skin may be broken and may weep liquid (usually clear) Recovery in 2–3 weeks; scarring may be present Infection may occur
Third degree	Complete tissue destruction, including subcutaneous tissue	Painless Symptoms of shock, depending upon severity and extent of damage Exposure of tissue may be noted	Dry, pale, or brownish leathery appearance Edema, with skin broken; fat tissue may be observed Hematuria Loss of shape and function of a limb
Fourth degree	Full thickness, tissue destroyed, plus underlying structures	Exposure of tissue may be prolonged	Deep electrical burns may result in charring (black) of skin; may produce harmful toxins Signs of hypovolemic shock may accompany this problem

SOURCE: Adapted from Crews, E.R.: *A Practical Manual for Treatment of Burns*, 1964, courtesy of Charles C Thomas, Publisher, Springfield, Ill.

[a] Depends on depth of burn, intensity, and duration.

Brooke, Parkland, and Evans Formula. Selection and implementation of the formulas vary with medical providers and the institutional setting. With each formula it is important to start calculations from the time that the burn occurs.

2. Urinary output maintained at 30 to 50 mL/h in order to prevent congestion in the renal tubules. Oliguria may be present at first after burns. After the first 36 h, fluid shifts from the extravascular spac back to the vascular systems.
3. As urinary output increases, intravenous intake should decrease.
4. Central venous pressure catheter should be inserted in order to monitor the effects of

fluid replacement. Readings should be taken frequently (e.g., every 1 to 2 h) to assure adequate blood volume without causing fluid overload. A pulmonary wedge catheter may also be used. See discussion of shock in Chapter 48.

5. Routine indwelling catheter care needed for continuous recording of urinary output (see Chapter 32 for discussion of catheter care).
6. Oral hygiene, care of nasogastric tube important. Intake of oral fluids as tolerated. Administration of prophylactic penicillin to prevent group A betahemolytic Streptococcus, especially where there are multiple skin breaks.
7. Administration of multivitamins to facilitate tissue growth.
8. Provide physical comfort and emotional support. Observe client's reaction to condition. Discuss changes, fears, and anxiety openly.
9. Administer pain medication, e.g., morphine sulfate. Observe responses to medication. Prevent drug dependency.
10. Establish open communication with client and family. Help prevent social isolation, especially if reverse isolation is being used.
11. Wound care begins once antishock treatment is established, with the client in isolation. Most fresh burns require aseptic care. After 48 to 72 h, gram-negative and gram-positive organisms begin to grow. *Staphylococcus aureus* and *Pseudomonas aeruginosa* are the most common types of infections. Necrotic tissue is a source of infection and therefore must be debrided (removed) before topical medication is applied. Initiate treatment as prescribed; bactericidal and bacteriostatic ointments are used. The type depends on the extent of the injury and the organism cultured from the wound.
    a. Silver sulfadiazine ointment, 1% (water-soluble base), is smeared over the burn area. The use of this drug is still under investigation. It does not appear to cause acid-base imbalances and is not painful to apply. Cutaneous sensitivity can occur. Drug of choice; not absorbed systemically, nonallergenic, available and affordable.
    b. Sulfamylon cream, 10% (mafenide acetate) penetrates eschar and requires exposure to the air. No dressing is used. Client needs turning to prevent maceration. Not drug of choice; causes pain and electrolyte imbalance.
    c. Gentamicin sulfate (Garamycin Creme, 0.1%) is an antibiotic specifically effective against gram-negative bacteria, including many strains of Pseudomonas. The ointment spreads easily and is painless to apply. There is a tendency for the organism to develop resistance, so the medication is reserved for life-threatening situations. Does not stain, used on face (2 times a day).
    d. Silver nitrate solution, 0.5% (nonallergenic), increases sodium loss through the burn. Large supplements of sodium are required in the diet to replace this loss. The drug is applied with wet dressings. The area is covered with circular gauze bandages, moisture-retaining stockinets, and Ace bandages. A stockinet alone is used in the first 36 h due to edema. Client must be covered with dry blankets to assure a warm environment around the wet dressings and to minimize heat loss by evaporation. This drug stains anything it

TABLE 35-2 FLUID RESUSCITATION OF BURNED CLIENTS: PARKLAND FORMULA

First 24 h:

Electrolyte solution (lactated Ringer's): 4 mL/kg body weight per percent of second- and third-degree burn

Administration rate: $\frac{1}{2}$ first 8 hr, $\frac{1}{4}$ second 8 h, $\frac{1}{4}$ third 8 h

Urine output: 30–70 mL/h

Second 24 h:

Glucose in water (D_5W): To replace evaporative water loss, maintaining serum sodium concentration of 140 mEq/L

Colloid solution (plasma): To maintain plasma volume in clients with more than 40% second- and third-degree burns

Urine output: 30–100 mL/h

SOURCE: Schwartz, S. I., et al., *Principles of Surgery*, © 1979 by McGraw-Hill Book Company. Used with permission of McGraw-Hill Book Company.

comes in contact with, and care should be used during administration. The injured parts should be covered by sterile sheets. Difficult to ambulate client; can damage healthy tissue.

12. Reduce anxiety. Distinguish irritability, restlessness, and discomfort due to pain from hypoxia due to hypovolemia. Listen and explain procedures carefully. Administer pain medication before painful procedures. Encourage client to verbalize positive and negative feelings. Answer questions, explain clinical course, guide client's expectations. (Use of other interventions to reduce pain, e.g., distraction, white noise, etc., may be used.)
13. Reduce social isolation. Teach family the rationale for medications and procedures.
14. Encourage visitors as allowed, and encourage continuation of outside interests.
15. Encourage touching to decrease sensory deprivation and physical isolation.
16. Promote self-esteem by providing opportunities for the client to make choices and participate in self-care.
17. Encourage client and family, pointing out progressive stages of healing.
18. Refer both client and family for counseling as necessary.
19. Provide therapeutic diet. After removal of nasogastric tube, diet gradually increased from clear liquid to high protein. Administer oral fluids slowly so tolerance can be observed. Be alert for signs of Curling's ulcer (refer to Chapter 33); incidence is in proportion to extent of burn. Appetite needs to be encouraged. Avoid painful procedures around meal times. When appropriate, select those foods which are nutritious and enjoyed by the patient.
20. Provide environment that helps person stay oriented to counteract sensory deprivation and disturbed body rhythms. Use clocks, pictures, television, radio, and visitors.
21. Control edema and prevent decubiti by positioning in supine semi-Fowler's position. Change position often.
22. Lower extremities should be extended and elevated with slight abduction and external rotation of the hips and heels off the bed. Upper extremities are elevated and abducted, with supination of the hands and external rotation of the humerus. This positioning facilitates respiration and decreases risk of contracture but limits the mobility.
23. Further prevention of contractures is obtained by a footboard; have the individual feed self; splint hands at night only.
24. Constant observation and reassessment of physical and psychological needs as client progresses from the acute stage.

EVALUATION

Outcome Criteria

1. Health state stabilized, as evidenced by normal blood gases, fluid intake and output within normal limits for the stage of the burn injury; cardio-respiratory status stable.
2. Identify cause early (ideally at the time of emergency).
3. Shock (hypovolemic, cardiogenic, neurogenic) prevented.
4. Pain relieved, may become more intense as healing progresses and nerves regenerate. Use of pain medication decreases in accordance with increased comfort.
5. Fears gradually decreasing. Effective intervention instituted and continually reevaluated.
6. Self-esteem will be maintained as evidenced in the persons' self-care behavior, affected areas are healing without signs of infection. Healthy granulation tissue is observed.
7. Optimal and full range of motion of extremities maintained.
8. The client is oriented and involved in treatment, as evidenced by questions and compliance with therapeutic plan; orientation to time, place, etc.
9. Person maintains relationships and communicates with family members, peers, and medical providers.
10. Evidence of appropriate grieving response and development of coping strategies to deal with physical and other losses.
11. Return of nutritional intake as evidenced by decreased use of IVs and increase in body fat (not fluid).

Complications

INFECTION

Assessment

1. Culture the wound.
2. Note any change in symptoms.

3. Note increased restlessness.
4. Check vital signs.
5. Watch for fever.

Intervention
Administration of medication (antibiotic) specific to organism.

STRESS ULCER OR CURLING'S ULCER

Refer to Chapter 33.

Assessment
1. Distension.
2. Bleeding.
3. Abdominal pain.
4. Hemoptosis.
5. Guaiac-positive stools.
6. Change in vital signs.

Intervention
See discussion of ulcers in Chapter 33.

RESPIRATORY CHANGES

Pneumonia or respiratory distress (see Chapter 31).

Assessment
1. Rate.
2. Sound.
3. Quality of respirations:
   a. Dullness on palpation.
   b. Decreased chest excursion.
   c. Rales and ronchi.
4. Stridor.
5. Labored breathing.
6. Cough.
7. Hoarseness.
8. Increased temperature.
9. Cyanosis.

Intervention
Refer to Chapter 31.
1. Observe for change.
2. Have a tracheostomy set ready.
3. Have oxygen equipment easily accessible.

SHOCK

Refer to Chapter 48.

DEPRESSION

Assessment
1. Change in sleep.
2. Activity.
3. Alteration in appetite.
4. Changes in affect.

Intervention
Refer to discussion of depression in Chapter 36.

CONTRACTURES

Assessment
Limitation of mobility.

Intervention
1. Range-of-motion exercises: first passive, then active.
2. Whirlpool.
3. Footboard.

Intervention
Surgery.
1. Skin grafting: use of hemografts, heterografts over burn area to facilitate tissue regrowth.
2. Eschar removal: incisions made into burn to release tissue and facilitate movement, e.g., chest.
3. Bone reconstruction following formation of contractures.
4. Additional care (refer to Chapter 27).

DEGENERATIVE DISORDERS

SYPHILIS

Refer to *Syphilis* in Chapter 24 and *Neurosyphilis* in Chapter 25 for further discussion.

DESCRIPTION

Syphilis is a serious, contagious, venereal disease caused by the motile spirochete *Treponema pallidum*. The course of illness can be fatal without adequate treatment. Syphilis is spread primarily by sexual contact but can also be the result of congenital transmission and accidental inoculation. The incubation period of syphilis is anywhere from 9 to 90 days, with an average incubation of 3 to 4 weeks. Generally syphilis is classified according to stages. Treatment and transmission of the disease depend upon the stage being observed.

1. *Primary stage*. During this stage a painless chancre (indurated) appears with a roughly circular shape. It may appear as papule, vesicle, or ulcer. Usually it is observed at the point of entry of the spirochete, 9 to 90 days after sexual contact (see Figure 35-9). In the

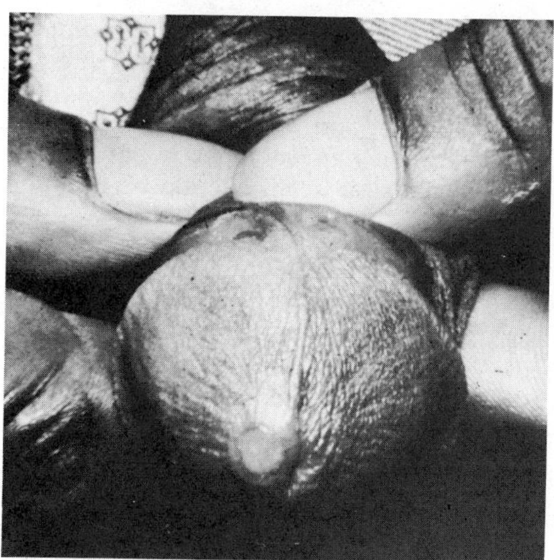

Figure 35-9 Primary chancre. (From Fitzpatrick, T.B., et al., eds.: *Dermatology in General Medicine,* 2d ed., McGraw-Hill, New York, 1975. Reproduced with permission.)

female, the chancre can go unnoticed if it is located on the cervix or vaginal wall. In homosexual males the chancre is often located in the rectum or the mouth. A chancre can appear at any site of sexual contact, including penis, lips, labia, oral cavity, or anus. Lymphadenopathy may be found in the node that drains the affected site. Without treatment, the chancre heals by itself in 1 to 5 weeks. However, the disease continues to develop and remains transmissible.

2. *Secondary stage.* During this stage a generalized skin rash appears along with flulike symptoms. This is often noted within 6 months following the date of exposure. The description of rash varies, and can be visualized as erythematous papules on face, shoulders, upper arms, chest, back, abdomen, palms of the hands, and soles of the feet. These papules turn coppery brown and gradually fade away. The rash is generally nonpruritic (see Figure 35-10). A rash on the palms and the soles of the feet is significant, since few rashes manifest at these sites. *Condylomata lata* form in warm, moist areas. These are moist papules, pink or greyish, which contain serous fluid and are highly infectious. Mucous patches are greyish white with dull red borders that can appear in mucous membranes of mouth or tonsils, perhaps resulting in a sore throat. Rash may be accompanied by a feeling of malaise, headache, nausea, constipation, anorexia, pain in long bones, alopecia, and low-grade fever. Without treatment symptoms usually disappear in 2 to 8 weeks, but secondary relapse can occur during latent stage.
3. *Latent stage.* Syphilis is asymptomatic, but gives a positive serology and negative spinal tap. The client may experience a relapse of secondary symptoms during the first 2 years of latent syphilis. Within 2 to 4 years client is no longer infectious to sexual partners.
4. *Tertiary stage.* There are three types. Not all untreated cases of syphilis progress to tertiary stage of immunologic reactions.

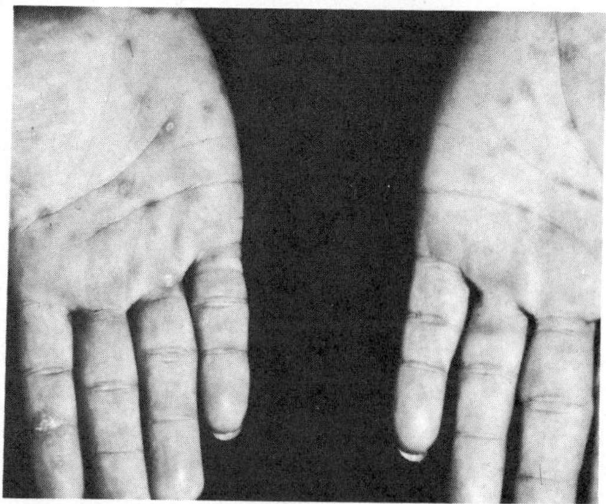

(*a*)

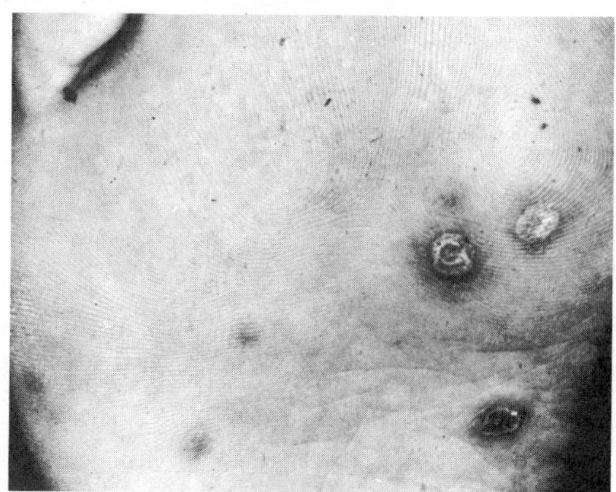

(*b*)

Figure 35-10 Secondary syphilis. (From Fitzpatrick, T.B., et al., eds.: *Dermatology in General Medicine,* 2d ed., McGraw-Hill, New York, 1975. Reproduced with permission.)

a. Benign late, which affects skin, muscles, digestive organs, liver, lungs, eyes, and endocrine glands. The characteristic lesion is a gumma, which occurs in any tissue and results in necrosis.
b. Cardiovascular effects: blood vessels and heart. The characteristic lesion is an aortic aneurysm.
c. Neurosyphilis involves the meninges, brain, and spinal cord. Today, symptoms of tertiary syphilis are rarely seen, since screening and treatment methods currently in use pick up the disease much sooner. Clients suspected of having syphilis are often found in a local clinic or emergency room. Cases are reported to local health department. Contacts should be treated.

PREVENTION

Health Promotion

1. Maintaining good personal hygiene, particularly before and/or after sexual relations.
2. Know sexual partners.
3. Use protective devices during sexual relations (e.g., condoms, foam, and jelly).
4. Routine screening blood test with physical examinations (optional).
5. Encouraging reporting of sexual partners.

Population at Risk

1. Sexually active persons.
2. Persons coming in contact with blood or lesions of infected persons (i.e., laboratory personnel).
3. Rape victims.

Screening

1. Premarital blood tests. VDRL may be required.
2. Blood test in the first and third trimester of pregnancy.
3. Screening blood test is usually required with routine physicals or when entering school or the armed services.
4. Following a rape.
5. Blood test when documented case of gonorrhea.

ASSESSMENT

Health History

1. Age: highest incidence is 20 to 40 years; next highest, 15 to 19 years.
2. Sexual preference: recent sexual contacts.
3. History of a painless chancre or symptoms of secondary syphilis and the dates they occurred.
4. History of last and previous contact, sites of exposure, and names of steady partners.
5. General physical health should be explored.
6. Lifestyle.
7. History of allergies.

Physical Assessment

Observable signs discussed under Definition. Client should have complete physical examination and thorough medical history should be taken.

Diagnostic Tests

1. Dark-field microscopic examination visualizes spirochete.
2. Serology test for screening a blood test (reagin antigen tests) designed to detect reagin in the blood. Less expensive than treponemal tests. If client shows a positive reaction on initial screening, treponemal test and qualitative titer are done to determine extent of the reaction and may be negative up to 8 weeks after becoming infected. False positives may occur with clients who have mononucleosis, malaria, hepatitis, vaccinia, and collagen diseases (lupus erythematosus, rheumatoid arthritis) and in heroin users. Biologic false positives ordinarily have positive APR but negative FTA-ABS.
3. Commonly used blood tests are:
   a. Venereal disease research lab (VDRL).
   b. Blood serology (RPR). If the RPR screening test is returned positive or reactive, then automatically, quantitative RPR and the fluorescent treponemal antibody absorption test (FTA-ABS) should be done.
4. Treponemal test for diagnosis. FTA-ABS. Blood test to detect specific syphilis antibodies. Done following all positive RPRs.
5. Spinal tap: fluid sent for RPR (refer to *Neurosyphilis* in Chapter 25).

NURSING DIAGNOSIS: ACTUAL OR POTENTIAL

1. Impaired skin integrity: potential.
2. High risk to infection to self and others: transmissible disease.
3. Fear (mild to moderate) regarding the disease and related complications.
4. Alterations in self-concept, secondary to social stigma of syphilis.

5. Neurological deficit: secondary to the prognosis.

EXPECTED OUTCOMES

1. Treatment will be instituted immediately to limit side effects of the health problem.
2. Contacts will be identified and referred for treatment immediately.
3. Required follow-up blood tests will be explained and schedule instituted.
4. Progression of stages will be halted and resolution of symptoms noted.
5. Protective health care measures will be incorporated into lifestyle.

INTERVENTION

1. Explain illness, course, rationale for treatment, importance of follow-up of client and contacts. Be supportive to the client, as discussion of the problem is often difficult and embarrassing.
2. Administration of penicillin. Check carefully for a history of allergy:
   a. *Early, primary, secondary, and latent* (*less than a year's duration*). Administer benzathine penicillin 2.4 million units, intramuscularly, times one, or procaine penicillin 600,000 units intramuscularly, daily for ten days. Benemid may be given PO to enhance the effectiveness of the antibiotic. Oral treatment with an antibiotic is not recommended. In cases of penicillin allergy, tetracycline or erythromycin are prescribed.
   b. *Syphilis of more than a year's duration.* Administer benzathine penicillin 2.4 million units intramuscularly once a week for three weeks. Procaine penicillin 600,000 units intramuscularly daily, for 15 days.
3. Encourage follow-up. Serology (RPR) should be repeated monthly for a year, then every 3 months until negative. In cases of primary syphilis, if RPR is not negative within a year, reevaluate and retreat. In cases of secondary syphilis and latent syphilis, allow 2 years.
4. Identify and refer clients to public health associate at the state level who will gather information regarding contacts. Primary contacts are those within the past 3 months plus the duration of the chancre. Secondary contacts are those within 6 months plus the duration of the secondary symptoms.
5. Discuss prevention. Encourage washing areas of sexual contact with soap and water following sexual activity. Routine serological, physical, and gynecological examinations are important.
6. Supportive counseling. Sexually transmitted disease carries moral implications for some clients. Be objective and informative; encourage clients to ask questions and verbalize positive and negative feelings toward the problem.
7. Reportable disease. For the procedure in your local area, contact the state health department. Usually requires a phone referral and written report.
8. Instruct client to abstain from sexual contact until treatment completed.
9. Use caution when handling specimen for laboratory. Also, if chancre is present, culture may be necessary.
10. NOTE: Penicillin treatment for gonorrhea is curative for incubating syphilis.

EVALUATION

Outcome Criteria

1. Quantitative titer measured every three months should decrease at least fourfold within a year.
2. Contacts treated, as evidenced by records of the state epidemiologist.
3. Client reports improved health care habits regarding sexual hygiene.

Complications

CLINICAL DISEASE CONTINUES OR RECURS

As indicated by a diagnostic quantitative titer increasing fourfold.

ANAPHYLAXIS REACTION

Assessment

1. Subjective.
   a. Fear of impending death.
   b. Apprehension.
   c. Chest constriction.
   d. Immobility.
   e. Paresthesia.
2. Objective.
   a. Syncope.
   b. Seizure.
   c. Decreased blood pressure.
   d. Urticaria.
   e. Wheezing.
   f. Cyanosis.
   g. Thready pulse.

Intervention
1. Administer epinephrine.
2. Maintain patent airway.
3. Assist with fluid replacement for shock.
4. Administer antihistamines, steroids, oxygen.

PROCAINE REACTION

Assessment
1. Subjective.
   a. Fear of impending death.
   b. Apprehension.
   c. Auditory and visual hallucinations.
   d. Restlessness.
   e. Faintness.
2. Objective.
   a. Syncope.
   b. Seizure.
   c. Increased blood pressure.
   d. Cyanosis.
   e. Strong pulse.

Intervention
1. Reassure client.
2. Restrain if necessary.
3. Symptoms transitory; stay with client.
4. Administer phenobarbital, observe.

NEUROLOGICAL

Paresthesia, tabes dorsalis, dementia, meningitis, Charcot's joint (refer to Chapter 25).

OPTIC ATROPHY

Result of late syphilis.

CARDIOVASCULAR

Aortitis, scarring of vessel lining (e.g., intima), aneurysm, or aortic heart block (see Chapter 30).

CONGENITAL SYPHILIS

Refer to Chapter 24.

BIBLIOGRAPHY

Amann, L. P.: "Psoriasis, Looking for a Cure," *Nursing Times* **75**:407, March 1979. Pictorial discussion of psoriasis.

Arnold, V. et al.: "Phototherapy for Psoriasis," *American Journal of Nursing*, **79**:466, March 1979. Pictorial explanation of treatment.

Arndt, K.: *Manual of Dermatologic Therapeutics*, Little, Brown, Boston, 1971. Excellent, concise reference manual of dermatologic problems seen in an ambulatory setting.

Baker, M., Eppeson, C., Vandergnff, J.: "Safe or Sorry Exposure to Radiation" *Pediatric Nursing* **8**(4):237, 1982.

Bielan, B.: "What a Rash Really Means," *RN* **43**:58, February 1979. Pictorial explanation of rashes.

Bhantooa, D.: "Fluid Replacement with Special Reference to Burned Patients Management During Infusion," *Nursing Times* **73**:337, March 1977. Good reference, discussion of nursing care.

Fears, T., Scotto, J., and Schneiderion, M.: "Skin Cancer, Melanoma and Sunlight," *American Journal of Nursing* **66**:461, May 1976. A good discussion of skin cancer and the part sunlight plays in the incidence.

Fitzpatrich, T. B. et al., eds.: *Dermatology in General Medicine*, 2d edition, McGraw-Hill, New York, 1979. Current, thorough medical description of most dermatology disorders, with copious photographs.

Friberg, T.: "Assessment: Could That Itching Be Scabies?" *Nursing Update* **7**:1, August 1979. Discussion and assessment of scabies.

Grant, M.: "Kidney and Fluid and Electrolyte Imbalances," in Jones, D., Dunbar, C., Jirovec, M., eds., *Medical-Surgical Nursing: A Conceptual Approach*, 2d ed., McGraw-Hill, New York, 1982. Excellent resource for complete nursing care of burns. Photographs of burn injuries inside the back cover help provide the reader with a complete in-depth picture of all the parameters involved when caring for a client who sustains a burn injury.

Quan, R. N., Strack, R., Rodney, W.: "Treatment of Acne Vulgaris," *Journal of Family Practitioner*, **11**:1041, 1980.

Roach, L.: "Color Changes in Dark Skin," *Nursing '77*, **7**:48, January 1977. Photographic description depicting skin lesions and related color changes as observed in dark-skinned individuals.

Robinson, L.: "Sun Exposure and Sun Protection," *Pediatric Nursing* **8**(4):272, 1982. Discusses need for protection and resources to be used when exposed to sunlight.

Wolfe, L., Weitzel, M., Feurst, E.: *Fundamentals of Nursing*, 6th Edition, Lippincott, New York, Toronto, 1979. General discussion of basic nursing interaction; care of the skin, promoting comfort, sleep, healing, maintaining fluid balance, administration of therapeutic agents and compresses.

THE NURSING CARE OF ADULTS AND CHILDREN WITH MENTAL HEALTH PROBLEMS

PART V

PART V CONTENTS

CHAPTER 36 ANXIETY AND THE AFFECTIVE DISORDERS 1297

Anxiety **1297**
Description 1297
Prevention 1298
Assessment 1299
Nursing diagnoses: actual or potential 1301
Expected outcomes 1301
Interventions 1302
Evaluation 1306

Depression **1306**
Severe depression 1306
Description 1306
Prevention 1307
Assessment 1308
Nursing diagnoses: actual or potential 1308
Expected outcomes 1309
Interventions 1309
Evaluation 1312
Mild to moderate depression 1313
Description 1313
Prevention 1313
Assessment 1313
Nursing diagnoses: actual or potential 1313
Expected outcomes 1313
Interventions 1314
Evaluation 1314

Elation **1314**
Description 1314
Assessment 1314
Nursing diagnoses: actual or potential 1314
Expected outcomes 1314
Interventions 1315
Evaluation 1316

CHAPTER 37 INTERPERSONAL PROBLEMS OF ADULTS 1319

Alterations in Self-Care Activities **1319**
Description 1319
Prevention 1320
Assessment 1320
Nursing diagnoses: actual or potential 1320
Expected outcomes 1320
Interventions 1321
Evaluation 1321

Self-Imposed Social Isolation **1321**
Description 1321
Prevention 1322
Assessment 1322
Nursing diagnoses: actual or potential 1322
Expected outcomes 1322
Interventions 1323
Evaluation 1323

Sensory-Perceptual Alteration **1324**
Description 1324
Prevention 1324
Assessment 1324
Nursing diagnoses: actual or potential 1324
Expected outcomes 1324
Interventions 1325
Evaluation 1325

Manipulation **1325**
Description 1325
Prevention 1326
Assessment 1326
Nursing diagnoses: actual or potential 1326
Expected outcomes 1326
Interventions 1327
Evaluation 1328

Alterations in Self-Concept **1328**
Dependent behavior 1328
Description 1328
Prevention 1329
Assessment 1329
Nursing diagnoses: actual or potential 1330
Expected outcomes 1330
Interventions 1330
Evaluation 1332

Maladaptive Coping Patterns **1332**
Demanding behavior 1332
Description 1332

PART V CONTENTS *(continued)*

Prevention 1332
Assessment 1333
Nursing diagnoses: actual or potential 1333
Expected outcomes 1333
Interventions 1333
Evaluation 1333
Compulsive-ritualistic behavior 1334
Description 1334
Prevention 1334
Assessment 1334
Nursing diagnoses: actual or potential 1334
Expected outcomes 1335
Interventions 1335
Evaluation 1335

Compromised Decision Making **1336**
Description 1336
Prevention 1336
Assessment 1336
Nursing diagnoses: actual or potential 1336
Expected outcomes 1336
Interventions 1337
Evaluation 1337

CHAPTER 38
THREATS TO SURVIVAL 1339

The Threat of Suicide **1339**
Description 1339
Prevention 1340
Assessment 1340
Nursing diagnoses: actual or potential 1342
Expected outcomes 1342
Interventions 1342
Evaluation 1344

The Threat of Violence **1344**
Description 1344
Prevention 1344
Assessment 1345
Nursing diagnoses: actual or potential 1345
Expected outcomes 1345
Interventions 1345
Evaluation 1347

CHAPTER 39
DISRUPTIONS OF PERCEPTUAL AND COGNITIVE FUNCTIONS **1351**

Hallucinations **1351**
Description 1351
Prevention 1352
Assessment 1352
Nursing diagnoses: actual or potential 1352
Expected outcomes 1352
Interventions 1352
Evaluation 1353

Delusions **1354**
Description 1354
Prevention 1354
Assessment 1354
Nursing diagnoses: actual or potential 1355
Expected outcomes 1355
Interventions 1355
Evaluation 1355

CHAPTER 40
MENTAL HEALTH PROBLEMS OF CHILDREN 1357

Impulsivity in Children **1357**
Description 1357
Prevention 1357
Assessment 1358
Nursing diagnoses: actual or potential 1359
Expected outcomes 1359
Interventions 1360
Evaluation 1361

Depression in Children **1362**
Description 1362
Prevention 1362
Assessment 1364
Nursing diagnoses: actual or potential 1365
Expected outcomes 1365
Interventions 1365
Evaluation 1366

PART V CONTENTS (*continued*)

CHAPTER 41
PERSON ABUSE 1369

Spouse Abuse 1369
Description 1369
Prevention 1369
Assessment 1370
Nursing diagnoses: actual or potential 1371
Expected outcomes 1372
Interventions 1372
Evaluation 1374

Child Abuse 1375
Description 1375
Prevention 1375
Assessment 1377
Nursing diagnoses: actual or potential 1379
Expected outcomes 1379
Interventions 1380
Evaluation 1381

Sexual Abuse 1382
Description 1382
Prevention 1382
Assessment 1382
Nursing diagnoses: actual or potential 1383
Expected outcomes 1383
Interventions 1383
Evaluation 1384

Elder Abuse 1385
Description 1385
Prevention 1385
Assessment 1386
Nursing diagnoses: actual or potential 1386
Expected outcomes 1386
Interventions 1386
Evaluation 1387

CHAPTER 42
GROUP WORK IN INPATIENT SETTINGS 1391

Description 1391
Assessment 1391
Nursing diagnoses: actual or potential 1396
Expected outcomes 1396
Interventions 1399
Evaluation 1400

CHAPTER 43
FAMILY WORK IN INPATIENT SETTINGS 1405

Description 1405
Prevention 1411
  Population at risk 1411
Assessment 1411
  Family history 1411
  Physical assessment 1412
  Family diagram 1412
Nursing diagnoses: actual or potential 1413
Expected outcomes 1413
Interventions 1413
Evaluation 1414
  Outcome criteria 1414
Case example 1414
Specific interventions directed at emotional isolation or depression 1415

36

Anxiety and the Affective Disorders

Ruth Dailey Knowles

The purpose of this chapter is to describe the implementation of the nursing process for clients with dysfunctional affective states (i.e., anxiety, depression, and elation). These affective states (particularly anxiety and depression) are associated, in varying degrees, with all illnesses and are experienced by most clients regardless of medical diagnosis.

The nurse can be the key health professional to use appropriate interventions in anxiety or mild to moderate depression; nurses can often be catalysts in helping clients to avoid serious depressive or high-anxiety states through knowledgeable intervention at early stages of illness or other stress.

Nursing goals, interventions, and evaluations in this chapter are oriented toward all clients whether hospitalized or at home and should expand the repertoire of meaningful nursing interventions of all nurses in dealing with the most common affective disorders. Nurses caring for clients in any clinical area can utilize selected principles reflected in this chapter. Useful behavioral techniques are described fully in the text.

ANXIETY

DESCRIPTION

Definition

1. Anxiety is a feeling of apprehension evoked by a threat to some value that the individual holds essential to his or her existence as a personality; it includes feelings of impending doom, dread, and uneasiness.
2. Some anxiety is necessary for normal functioning.
   a. Low anxiety motivates us to action.
   b. Moderate anxiety may interfere with thinking, learning, perceptions, and general functioning.
   c. High anxiety incapacitates the individual, as perceptions are so narrowed that judgment may be impaired, and aberrant behavior and immobility may result.

Cause

1. Anxiety underlies all other emotions and accompanies them, whether the emotion is anger, love, or depression.
2. Any threat can precipitate anxiety.

Incidence

1. Everyone has anxiety every day in varying amounts.
2. High anxiety occurs more frequently in tense individuals (who turn their anxiety into body tension), in phobic individuals, or in those who internalize strong emotions, keeping them locked within the self.

Prognosis

1. Excessive anxiety is learned, and it can be unlearned.
2. Anxiety is useful in real situations as a self-protective mechanism (e.g., fight or flight).
3. Irrational anxiety can be identified and lowered through learning on the part of the individual.

4. Behavioral and cognitive techniques can help the individual be aware of, lower, and control anxiety.

Pathophysiology

1. Anxiety can be somatized (that is, turned into physical symptoms and conditions) or can exacerbate existing conditions:
   a. Cardiovascular system: symptoms.
      (1) Increased pulse rate.
      (2) Palpitations that are transient and not relieved by rest or cessation of exercise.
      (3) Chest pain.
      (4) Vasomotor flushing.
   b. Cardiovascular system: conditions, diseases.
      (1) Coronary artery disease.
      (2) Myocardial infarction.
      (3) Raynaud's disease.
      (4) Buerger's disease.
      (5) Stroke due to hypertension related to stress.
      (6) Migraines.
   c. Respiratory system: symptoms.
      (1) Increased respiratory rate.
      (2) Hyperventilation.
      (3) Transient respiratory distress (i.e., wheezing or inability to take a deep breath).
      (4) Sighing.
   d. Respiratory system: conditions, diseases.
      (1) Asthma.
      (2) Emphysema.
      (3) Allergies.
   e. Gastrointestinal (GI) system: symptoms.
      (1) Diarrhea or constipation.
      (2) Nausea.
      (3) "Butterflies" in stomach.
      (4) Spasm of cardiac or pyloric sphincters.
      (5) Intestinal irritability, abdominal cramps.
      (6) Anorexia or excessive eating, bulimia.
      (7) Indigestion.
      (8) Dry mouth.
      (9) Dysphagia.
   f. Gastrointestinal system: conditions, diseases.
      (1) Ulcers (epigastric, duodenal, stomatitis, etc.).
      (2) Ulcerative colitis.
      (3) Hyperchlorhydria.
   g. Musculoskeletal system: symptoms.
      (1) Weakness and tremors.
      (2) Tense posture.
      (3) Muscle soreness.
      (4) Posture-related problems.
   h. Integumentary system: symptoms.
      (1) Sweating.
      (2) Pallor.
      (3) Itching and hives.
      (4) Allergies.
      (5) Ecxema.
   i. Other physical symptoms.
      (1) Vertigo and/or syncope.
      (2) Dilated pupils.
      (3) Urinary frequency.
      (4) Wavering voice.
      (5) Sleeplessness.
      (6) Fidgety movements.

PREVENTION

Health Promotion

1. Teach relationship between stress/anxiety and psychological distress and physical symptoms.
2. Assist client to learn to "level" anxiety.
3. Teach breathing exercises.
4. Teach progressive relaxation exercises to use prophylactically, to become a more tranquil, in-control person.
5. Teach thought-stopping procedure.
6. Encourage self-esteem-enhancing activities, thoughts, and experiences.
7. Teach specific means for handling anxiety, anger, jealousy, and fear as a means of directly dealing with anxiety rather than internalizing it into depression or somatic complaints.

Population at Risk

1. Everyone has anxiety and copes with it in varying ways. Low anxiety spurs us to action; high anxiety can be immobilizing.
2. Adults in competitive jobs who are overly time-conscious, tense, have few physical-energy outlets, are heavy smokers, heavy eaters, have high-pressure lifestyles, and who live "to accomplish," are at highest risk for coronary artery disease. These behaviors are known as "type A behaviors" or "coronary prone behaviors."
3. Fearful individuals who *avoid* the feared object or situation, thereby slowly, but progressively, limiting their activities until they are moderately to severely restricted in their existence.

4. Individuals from families where somatic complaints have been a way to get and maintain attention by significant others; consequently, anxiety is transformed into physical symptoms that are transient *or* life-threatening conditions and diseases.

Screening

1. Identify *where* an individual first feels anxiety.
   a. This is usually in the body system most vulnerable to damage.
   b. This sensation is a consistent physical cue that anxiety is rising and may be used to alert the individual to the need for early intervention.
   c. Life changes can be made to promote longevity when the individual identifies his/her unique individual first sensation of anxiety. For example, individuals who "feel" their anxiety first in their heart region usually come from families with a history of heart disease. Consequently, the informed individual should recognize the propensity to convert anxiety into coronary-related symptoms and/or conditions; realizing this vulnerability, one could decide to reduce the risk level by stopping smoking, increasing exercise, reducing weight, limiting saturated fats in the diet, and decreasing stress-related/coronary prone activities and behaviors in his or her life. In addition, this individual might decide to engage in relaxation exercises two to three times every day or take up jogging/brisk walking as a means of reducing his or her stress level. Nursing psychotherapy could be a useful adjunct to the individual's increased control over the potentially harmful coronary prone behavior that had been a part of his or her life.
2. Identify level of anxiety. To practice this efficiently, set a kitchen timer to a random number of minutes. When it rings, "level" anxiety; if it is high, lower it through relaxation or breathing exercises. Reset timer, and continue throughout the day.
3. The nurse's knowledge of psychosomatic influence is a potent screening tool, as he or she may interpret and then validate with the client anxiety-related symptoms/conditions, as the preliminary step toward teaching the client control over various symptoms and the situations that exacerbate the symptoms.
4. Identify somatic outcomes of the client's internalization of anxiety, discussing with the client ways in which strong emotions might be more effectively and appropriately discharged.
5. Determine life changes within the past 1 year. If many changes have taken place (e.g., the client has lost job, gotten married, gotten pregnant, and moved to a new city), the individual is at much higher risk of developing serious physical illness within the next 2 years.

ASSESSMENT

Health History

1. Chief complaint.
2. Medical diagnoses (if applicable).
3. History of current illness or symptoms, and relevant past history.
   a. Duration of symptoms.
   b. Date of onset of symptoms.
   c. Manner of onset and predisposing factors.
      (1) What happened immediately before the onset?
      (2) What does the client think is causing the situation?
      (3) How often do the symptoms occur?
      (4) When, in the past, have similar symptoms/situations occurred?
      (5) What did the client do to treat or help alleviate the symptoms in the past?
4. Other symptoms, difficulties, and so on that might be significant in the assessment and intervention of anxiety (see Table 36-1).
5. Treatment.
   a. Has client sought treatment before?
   b. How is the client's health in general?
   c. Prescribed medications used.
   d. Nonprescribed medications used.
   e. Effectiveness of prior, or ongoing, treatment.
6. Review of systems for anxiety-related symptoms. (See Description, above, for symptoms/conditions to identify.)
   a. Respiratory.
   b. Cardiovascular.
   c. Gastrointestinal.
   d. Neurological.
   e. Musculoskeletal.
   f. Integumentary.
   g. Genitourinary.
   h. Eyes and ears.

TABLE 36-1 CHECKLIST FOR CLIENT TO IDENTIFY SYMPTOMS/BEHAVIORS/SITUATIONS THAT MIGHT CLARIFY OR EXPAND HEALTH HISTORY

Directions: Underline any of the following that apply to you:

Addicted to drugs
Arthritis
Asthma
Avoid people
Bad home situation
Blackouts
Breathing disturbances
Can't keep a job
Chest pains
Chills/warmth all over
Compulsions
Conflict in the family
Constipation
Convulsions
Depressed
Dizziness
Difficulty with
- Concentration
- Making decisions
- Memory

Don't like weekends or vacations
Drinking excessively
Edema/swelling
Excited/jittery
Fainting
Family problems
Fatigue
Fear of going crazy
Fear of losing control
Fear of being alone
Feel different from others
Financial problems
Flushing
Hallucinations
Headaches
Heart problems
Homosexual fantasies or fears
Hopeless outlook
Indigestion
Insomnia
Job dissatisfaction
Leg cramps
Lonely
Loss of appetite
Loss of sleep
Loss of temper
Lump in throat
Marriage conflict
Migraines
Nausea
Nightmares
No friends
Numbness of feet or hands
Obsessions
Overambitious
Overeating
Pallor
Palpitations
Panic attacks
Phobias
Recent weight gain
Recent weight loss
Severe anxiety
Sexual problems
Shaking of hands/feet
Shy
Shortness of breath
Speech problems
Stomach trouble
Suicidal thoughts
Sweating excessively
Take drugs frequently
Tensions
Tics
Tire easily
Tremors
Trouble communicating
Ulcers
Unable to have a good time
Unable to relax
Upset easily
Urinary problems
Use painkillers often
Use sedatives often
Use street drugs
Use over-the-counter remedies
Weakness in legs/knees
Worries

Now, go back and circle any word or phrase that is of major importance in describing you.

7. Past history.
   a. Allergies.
      (1) Drugs.
      (2) Food.
      (3) Respiratory (seasonal or perennial).
   b. Major illnesses and dates.
   c. Major operations and dates.
   d. Hospitalizations and dates.
8. Habits.
   a. Smoking (include amount).
   b. Drinking alcoholic beverages (include type/amount).
   c. Hard drugs (include type/amount).
   d. Soft drugs (include names/amount).
9. Psychosocial history.
   a. Current feelings, about chief complaint and predisposing factors.
   b. Worries.

   c. Recent life-change events within the family.
   d. Recent changes in mental status (e.g., confusion, irritability, mental fatigue, depression, etc.).
10. Previous coping skills used with similar problems.
   a. How is stress handled at home?
   b. How is stress handled at work?
   c. How does this differ from manner of handling stress before presenting symptoms?
   d. What does the client do when angry, sad, frustrated, anxious?
11. Thoughts.
   a. Are there thoughts that are disturbing to the client?
   b. What are some of the "not helpful thoughts" experienced?
   c. What thoughts are prohibiting the client from becoming the person he or she wants to be?
12. Support systems.
   a. Does the client have close friends/family with whom to talk honestly?
   b. Can this person(s) provide the support the client needs?
   c. What is the client's relationship with co-workers?
   d. How does the client respond in social situations?
   e. How does the client feel about self in social and/or work situations?
   f. What problems are there in the family that inhibit support?
   g. What are sources of support within the family?
   h. What organizations, groups, clubs does the client belong to, and how significant are they to the client?
   i. Are there other people, pets, activities on which the client relies for support?
   j. To whom is the client closest?
13. Motivations for treatment at this time.
   a. What does the client see as the goal of treatment?
   b. What are some of the client's expectations for treatment?
   c. What current behaviors does the client wish to change?
   d. What behaviors does the client wish to increase or decrease, in order to live a better life?
   e. What, specifically, caused the client to seek treatment at this particular time?

Physical Assessment

For anxiety, the nurse would not necessarily conduct a physical assessment. Most necessary information can be elicited from the health history.

Diagnostic Tests

See Screening.

NURSING DIAGNOSES: ACTUAL OR POTENTIAL

1. Anxiety due to a perceived threat to any aspect of the self.
2. Maladaptive coping patterns.
   a. Due to learned somatization as an unconscious defense against anxiety.
   b. Due to internalization of anxiety, causing free-floating anxiety and/or depression.
3. Alteration in patterns of sexuality.
   a. Due to concern over sexual performance after transient sexual difficulty (e.g., erectile difficulty or preorgasmic state).
   b. Due to gender-identity anxieties.
4. Sleep-rest activity.
   a. Dysrhythm due to anticipation of inability to sleep.
5. Ineffective family relationships.
   a. Demonstrated in open family conflict.
   b. Demonstrated in pathology in one or more children.
   c. Demonstrated in somatic complaints in one or more family members.
   d. Family disruption.

EXPECTED OUTCOMES

1. The client will be able to, at his or her own rate
   a. Level anxiety and report measurement level.
   b. Lower anxiety through use of breathing exercises and relaxation training.
   c. State situations that precipitate high levels of anxiety.
   d. Prepare for and rehearse interactions before these high-anxiety situations.
   e. Consciously lower anxiety repeatedly during the day.
   f. Demonstrate the relaxation response.
   g. Demonstrate thought stopping and report decreased frequency of occurrence of the anxiety-producing thought.
   h. Substitute adaptive behaviors and coping patterns for maladaptive ones.

i. Use fewer tranquilizers and other psychotropic drugs as self-control methods of decreasing anxiety are learned, practiced, and mastered.
j. Decrease somatic complaints.
k. Control high levels of anxiety by intervening at lower levels through habitual use of relaxation and other cognitive-behavioral approaches.
l. Select additional coping mechanisms to use in intervening with anxiety.
m. Expand relationships with significant others.
n. Reduce the frequency of "not helpful thoughts," self-depreciation, and decreased hope and faith in the self.
o. Be functional in sexual situations.
p. Sleep regularly and deeply.
q. View family relationships realistically and not necessarily be reactive to upsetting family situations.
r. Make assertive requests and responses.
s. Express hostility and anger appropriately.
t. Be a happier, more productive, and functional person.

INTERVENTIONS

1. Teach client to level his or her anxiety. Most of the time, individuals are not aware of their level of anxiety. They can recall relaxed times, and they can recall panic times. The nurse can teach clients to become more aware of their level of anxiety. This leads not only to increased identification of rising anxiety, but also to documentation, in the minds of clients, that they can reduce anxiety levels.

   Have clients identify on a scale of 0 to 10 their anxiety levels (0 = asleep, 10 = absolute panic). During interviews the nurse may periodically ask clients to identify or "level" their anxiety and to report it to the nurse. Before teaching any relaxation or thought-stopping techniques, the nurse should ask the client to level the anxiety. Immediately after participating in behavioral exercises, clients should be asked again to identify the level of anxiety. In most cases, clients will identify a lowered level; hence this is an indication to them that they can affect anxiety levels and exert control, to some degree, over this discomfort. Encourage clients to level their anxiety frequently. Whenever their anxiety reaches the level of 5 or 6 they should engage in an anxiety-reducing behavior. This reporting of the level of anxiety is also helpful to the nurse in identifying content areas that produce tension in the client, since frequently anxiety may be disguised. When clients report a level of increased anxiety, both they and the nurse are objectively able to incorporate this information for therapeutic purposes.
2. Teach client breathing techniques.
   a. Breath-holding technique. Instruct the client about leveling anxiety procedure; then have him or her put a number on their present level of anxiety; then instruct as follows: "Take a deep breath, hold it for a count of three, then as you let it out slowly, let your body sag slightly, and say in your mind: *relax*. Take another deep breath, hold it, hold it, hold it, and as it flows out, let your body go limp and loose." Immediately after the client has let out all the breath, ask, "What is your level of anxiety now?" Usually individuals report a drop of one or two levels of anxiety. One can reinforce this, such as, "Two whole points!! And you *did* something about your anxiety, *all by yourself*. What a powerful tool to have when you find yourself anxious."
   b. Quiet breathing technique. Breathe normally for 1 to 2 minutes, and with each expiration, mentally say "one" or "calm" or "peace." In your mind, "watch" the air entering your nostrils, going down your throat, into the trachea, bronchi, bronchioles and filling each of the alveoli, exchanging oxygen for CO_2, and leaving the body. Listen to what your breathing sounds like as you normally breathe in and out. Fill yourself with the sensations of breathing, as you continue to say your word with each expiration.

      To say words on expiration, as well as giving the individual a picture, sound or feeling to attend to, fills the mind, distracts it, and gives it something to think about that can interfere with other thoughts (usually anxiety-provoking thoughts). One might continue, ". . . and as you pay attention to your breathing, you may notice that a quiet feeling comes over you. Experience that feeling, focus on slowing down your mind and body, and enjoy remaining in this state for a few minutes. Before you return to the activities of your day, you might wish to tell yourself that you will be able to bring the comfortable feeling of relaxation with you to your activities, and that you will feel alert, rested, and energetic." When the body is relaxed, the mind is open to self-suggestion, and clients can be encouraged to utilize this phenomenon in a way that will feel good to them.

3. Teach client progressive relaxation techniques. Relaxation is a normal and natural activity of the body, but under most circumstances we are not usually very relaxed. Anxiety and tensions promote the nonrelaxed state, but excess anxiety and tension can be reduced through conscious relaxation of body parts. Since tension and relaxation are incompatible, relaxation can be used to overcome tension.

   The nurse may wish to practice relaxation for the purpose of learning how to relax by lowering his or her own anxiety or tension level. Only after the nurse has become adept at self-relaxation and has become knowledgeable of the ramifications of relaxation from the literature should the nurse teach relaxation to others (see the Bibliography at the end of this chapter for references related to progressive relaxation training). Practice on friends and family will help the nurse to refine relaxation-teaching techniques before these are taught to clients.

   To teach relaxation, the nurse will have the client assume a comfortable position with shoes off, contact lenses out, tight clothing loosened, bladder emptied, eyes closed, and all body parts supported. A quiet, private, slightly darkened room will facilitate relaxation.

   Relaxation can be achieved by either of two methods: the tension-relaxation method or the relaxation-alone method. For the tension-relaxation method, the nurse will direct the client to try to get in a comfortable position, concentrate on her or his toes, tightly contract the muscles in the toes (to about three-fourths of maximum strength), hold the tension to the count of three, and then when the nurse says "Relax," to let go instantly of the tension. The discrepancy between the tensed and relaxed states heightens the client's awareness of the feeling of relaxation. This tension-relaxation method is best used with individuals who have difficulty in relaxing.

   Regardless of which method is used, the nurse will continue, using a soft, slow, somewhat monotonous voice, instructing the client to concentrate next on the ball of the foot, then the instep, the heel, and the ankle and move up the leg (paying particular attention to relaxing the muscles in the front of the leg) to the knee, upper leg, pelvic area (including sphincters), buttocks, waist, and chest and around to the back, upper chest, and shoulders. Have the client pay particular attention to relaxing the shoulders, which are usually in a perennial state of tension and need to be "pulled down" to relax. Encourage the client to move at any time to facilitate relaxation of a body part.

   Continue with relaxing the upper arms, elbows, lower arms, wrists, hands, and each finger. Statements can be made such as "Notice the difference between the feeling of your body in the relaxed state from the way it felt a few minutes ago," or "You may notice that there is some tingling in your fingers, signifying that even your blood vessels are becoming opened and relaxed."

   Return to the shoulders and neck, first the front and then the back, smoothing out the large neck muscles, and then have the client extend the relaxed state over the scalp and top of the head and "flow" down over the forehead into the eyebrows, eyes, cheeks and nose, mouth, tongue, and jaw muscles.

   When the client is completely relaxed, have her or him experience what it feels like to be relaxed all over. Allow the client to remain relaxed at least 1 minute before announcing that you will count backward from five to one. Add that, when you get to one, the relaxation will end but, having found relaxation so comfortable, she or he will probably wish to return to the relaxed state on her or his own soon. Then count slowly from five to one. When the client's eyes are open, ask how she or he feels. Additionally, you may request that the level of anxiety be reascertained. Usually, the client will report that anxiety is lower after relaxing than it was before. This is additional "objective evidence" to the client that one can control to some degree her or his own anxiety level. This control on the part of the client should be reinforced by the nurse, as it leads to independence, increased self-esteem, and acceptance by the client that feelings and behavior are not beyond self-control.

After skill has been gained in relaxing according to one of the methods described, the client will probably find shortcuts to the procedures (e.g., the entire legs can be relaxed at once, then the torso, arms, head, and neck). After practice, the client should be able to relax in a matter of minutes or seconds.

Relaxation can be used in a variety of ways to decrease anxiety, overcome specific tensions, and to obtain an overall increased sense of calm and control. Relaxation may be used as a tool to lower feelings of tension in an anxiety-provoking situation, by the client's consciously and inconspiciously relaxing legs, torso, and shoulders. If the client feels anxiety rising to uncomfortable heights, she or he may retire to a private area to relax completely for a few minutes.

A third way to relax is to set aside one or two 10- to 15-minute periods in the day to relax the body privately, gently sweeping all thoughts from the mind and attempting to concentrate only on the feeling of relaxation. While in this relaxed state, the mind is more open to suggestion, and the client may wish to attempt, through autosuggestion, to make her- or himself feel refreshed, less irritable, less depressed, and more alert upon "awakening" from the relaxed state, almost as one would feel if one had taken a short nap.

For optimum safety and success, plus control on the part of the client, relaxation should be taught as something that the patient does for her- or himself and not as an activity imposed by another. Encourage the client to practice relaxing until it is an easy activity and until parts of the body can easily be relaxed on command.

In public situations, clients may wish to use a variation of the relaxation technique. They should take a moderately deep breath, hold it for a count of three or four, and then as they slowly exhale tell themselves subvocally to relax. This may be repeated only twice, as more than a total of three times may lead to hyperventilation and subsequent reinstitution of the anxiety state.

For clients who frequently find themselves in very high states of anxiety, to the degree that they cannot think of what to do, the nurse may suggest that they carry with them a card that lists, in order of helpfulness to them, all the things they can do to reduce their anxiety, for example, take deep breath and hold, then relax; tell self that the anxiety has always gone away and it will go away this time; find a place to do progressive relaxation; call a friend who is a calming individual; engage in physical activity; knead some clay (kept handy for the occasion); do thought stopping, and so on.

All anxiety and tension cannot be alleviated on each occasion by the use of behavioral techniques, but clients should discover that use of the techniques usually decreases the anxiety or makes it manageable. Since these techniques are taught to clients to prescribe for themselves *and use*, they should eventually come to believe that they have increased control over their anxiety and tensions.

4. Teach the client thought-stopping techniques. Many individuals, healthy or not, have repeated thoughts that might be classified as "not helpful" thoughts, that is, worries, thoughts of low self-worth, obsessions, and ruminations. It is possible to control to some degree the thoughts that one has by utilizing the thought-stopping technique. To teach this to the client, the nurse should first instruct the client to identify in his or her mind two or three situations or remembrances that bring pleasurable thoughts. When the client has sufficiently identified these remembrances to him- or herself (they need not be shared with the nurse), the nurse should instruct the client to list, in written form, all not helpful thoughts and then to reorder these thoughts in priority of how disturbing they are and how frequently they occur.

The nurse should select one not helpful thought that occurs the most frequently or is the most disturbing to the client. The nurse will ask the client to begin to think this thought and to visualize it vividly. When the client signals that he or she is strongly aware of the not helpful thought, the nurse should shout, "*Stop*." Of course, the client will be startled but should be immediately asked, "Are you still thinking the not helpful thought?" The client will invariably report no, whereupon the nurse should point out that the client has evidence of being able to stop not helpful thoughts, having just done so. The client should be instructed to use this behavioral technique every time he or she is aware of thinking a not helpful thought, by either shouting stop verbally or shouting it only in his or her head (particularly useful in public). To further reinforce this ability to stop a thought, the client should be instructed to immediately think of the pleasurable situation identified earlier as soon as stop has been said. If the not helpful thought returns, it should be stopped again. Many individuals find that after stopping a thought repeatedly, the frequency of the occurrence of the thought decreases.

5. Teach the client to use self-statements that lower anxiety and enhance self-esteem and confidence in the self. Although many individuals think that feelings and thoughts are separate, it does take a thought to initiate a feeling. Our personalities and self-concepts are formed by the "self-statements" we give ourselves. If our parents told us that we were bad, we incorporated this as a self-statement and experienced a subjective feeling of distress associated with this thought. Over time, perception of negative statements about the self are telescoped into an almost instantaneous feeling, usually resulting in feelings of lowered self-esteem. We bypass the statement, for example, "I am ugly; therefore no one likes me; therefore I am worthless," and we have feelings of depression and anxiety when we identify ourselves as ugly.

   The nurse can help the client to identify methodically the self-statements given to the self in an attempt to replace negative statements with positive ones. This may be done as:

   Thought: I am ugly.
   Replaced thought: My face has character and is different.
   or
   Thought: I am ugly.
   Replaced thought: Although I am ugly, I have a fantastic personality.

   Have clients list the negative thoughts they have that affect their self-esteem, and then have them write beside these negative thoughts the correlative positive thoughts to insert into their consciousness whenever the negative thoughts appear.

   A second self-enhancing technique to use is to instruct the client to purchase one hundred 3- by 5-inch index cards, number them, and then write one statement on each card that represents something they like about themselves, for example, "I am smart," "I am kind to others," "I have good posture," "I can play the violin," "I am interested in improving myself." These cards should be placed in a frequently visited location (such as near the telephone, in the bathroom, or in the glove compartment of the car) and should be reviewed several times per day. Frequent review of these positive self-statements will help replace or partially negate negative self-statements.

6. Teach the client to monitor thoughts that are precursors of anxious feelings.
7. Teach the client to identify irrational, as opposed rational thoughts, to determine the consequences of each, and to consciously dispute the irrational thoughts that are disturbing.
8. Teach the client to use appropriately assertive behaviors.
   a. Use role model of the assertive nurse.
   b. Practice rehearsals of assertive behavior to be used first with strangers, and then later with friends/family.
   c. Before a "big" assertion, rehearse either before a mirror, on a tape-recorder, or with a comfortable other.
   d. Learn how to make "I-statements," rather than "you-statements." An "I-statement" includes
      (1) Good, warm eye-contact.
      (2) A (affect/feeling)
         "I feel. . ."

B (behavior)
"... when you..."
C (consequences)
"... the outcome is..."
D (desire)
"... I would prefer..."

e. Teach self-reinforcement (self-congratulations) to enhance further assertive behaviors.
f. Teach how to evaluate the assertive outcomes.

9. Teach the use of imagery, to imagine self being successful in an anxiety-provoking situation.

   In the relaxed state, have the client imagine the situation, first seeing the events, then hearing the probable sounds, then feeling the customary response, but this time with the relaxed state he or she is experiencing. If anxiety level rises, have the client return to a "peaceful scene," then with anxiety reduced, once again face the anxiety situation until it can be thought about clearly without associated anxiety. This is practice for real life situations, and facility at handling a situation in imagery increases its appropriate handling in real life.
10. Have client keep a diary of all activities. Each activity should be rated concerning the client's degree of feelings of accomplishment, mastery, or pleasure.
11. Encourage client to complete tasks related to anxiety for the purpose of gaining feelings of accomplishment.
12. Encourage client to use behaviors (according to a hierarchy from lowest anxiety producer to highest) that engender anxiety, in conjunction with progressive relaxation exercises.
13. Direct client to postpone large decisions until in a less anxious state.
14. Have client make a list of positive self-statements to use when anxious, for example
    a. "I have been anxious before and I got over it."
    b. "This feeling is temporary."
    c. "Nothing actually happens to me when I get anxious."
    d. "What is the worst thing that can happen to me in this situation?"
15. Have client list strengths and talents, and encourage client to find opportunities to use them.
16. Assist client in identifying threats or stresses in personal environment that might be removed.
17. Teach appropriate assertive behavior.
18. Provide a role model of assertive behavior.
19. Do role playing with client related to situations calling for assertive behavior.
20. Be available to client or advise client whom to contact during periods of high anxiety.
21. Provide anticipatory guidance for future anxiety situations.

EVALUATION

Outcome Criteria

Effective use of the aforementioned techniques will help the client to meet each of the expected outcomes listed above. Each of the outcomes, when met, will be observable by the nurse and client except outcomes m-t, which will be measurable by the client through self-report.

Reevaluation and Follow-up

1. Reevaluation can be implemented at any time after treatment. Clients return for one or two "booster sessions" when severe life stress arises. Either the client is reinforced and reminded of coping skills within his/her ability, or new goals are identified for further psychotherapeutic work.
2. Referral to a nurse psychotherapist for ongoing psychotherapy is appropriate.

DEPRESSION

SEVERE DEPRESSION

DESCRIPTION

Definition

1. Depression is characterized by a feeling of sadness, lowered self-esteem, and a mood stage of melancholy inactivity, and self-depreciation.
2. Depression can vary in intensity, ranging from "Monday morning blues" to psychotic depression in which the client is out of touch with reality and may require hospitalization.

Etiology

1. Dynamic theory: the turning inward of anger.
2. Behavioral theory: absence of reinforcement.
3. Learning theory: learned helplessness from family and/or life experiences. Depressive lifestyle.
4. Physical theory: hormonal imbalances, chemical imbalances, illness.
5. Loss theory: depression is the manifestation of great or cumulative losses.
6. Combination theory: depression is caused in varying degrees by the combination of one or more of the above.

Incidence

1. Most common psychiatric condition.
2. Increases with age.
3. Found to some degree in most psychiatric disorders.
4. Associated with most physical illnesses.
5. Expected side effect of certain chemical, hormonal, or medication-induced imbalances.

Prognosis

1. Depends on the cause.
   a. Client's motivation to eradicate the depression.
   b. Lifelong learning patterns.
   c. Ability to incorporate new modes of behavior.
   d. Course of physical illness and rehabilitation.
   e. Coping style and mechanisms of the individual.
   f. Reversal of chemical and hormonal imbalances.
2. If suicidal (see also Chapter 38), lethality rises if also present are
   a. Devastating loss, that is, recently widowed or divorced.
   b. Elderly, living alone.
   c. Near important anniversaries, holidays.
   d. Sleep disturbances.
   e. Giving away prized possessions.
   f. Suicide note.
   g. Previous suicide attempt.
   h. Accessible agents.
   i. Views death as a release.
   j. Parents or close friend committed suicide.
   k. Psychotic, injurious, or threatening hallucinations, impulsivity.
   l. Intoxication.
   m. Coming out of a depression.
   n. Euphoria suddenly after depression.
   o. Tidying up life.
   p. Extreme hopelessness.

Pathophysiology

1. Anxiety usually accompanies depression, and any of the signs of anxiety may be present (see Pathophysiology section of *Anxiety*, above).
2. Physical observations or complaints reported by the patient can include
   a. Crying.
   b. Neglect of grooming.
   c. Bowed posture when sitting or walking.
   d. Limited verbal communication.
   e. Anorexia.
   f. Loss of weight.
   g. Decreased movements and/or slow, deliberate movements.
   h. Sad facies.
   i. Disturbed sleep patterns (e.g., goes to sleep early, awakens early, and is unable to go back to sleep).
   j. Sleeplessness.
   k. Constipation.
   l. Abdominal pain.
   m. Nausea.
   n. Headaches; pressure band around the head.
   o. Poor concentration; slowed thoughts.
   p. Fatigue; tired and unrefreshed after period of sleep.
   q. Gastrointestinal upsets.
   r. Back pain (may be related to stooped posture).
   s. Palpitations unrelated to exercise, caffeine intake.
   t. Dizziness.
   u. Flushing.
   v. Withdrawal.

PREVENTION

Health Promotion

1. Teach relationship between depression and life-change events that revolve around loss.
2. Teach client to identify situations in life that result in angry feelings.
3. Teach relationship between stress and physical symptoms.
4. Encourage use of specific appropriate means for handling anxiety, anger, frustration, and fear as a means of directly dealing with the

anger rather than internalizing it into depression or somatic complaints.
5. Encourage self-esteem-enhancing activities, thoughts, and experiences.
6. Teach client to "level anxiety."
7. Teach client progressive relaxation exercises to use prophylactically.
8. Teach client thought-stopping procedures.
9. Teach client breathing exercises for stress management.
10. Teach client imagery exercises.

Population at Risk

1. Those who have learned in their families that anger is a "not-OK" emotion.
2. Those who have learned in their families that it is alright, even desirable, to occasionally be depressed and sad.
3. Those who have strong feelings of needing to be perfect, to always excel, to compete directly or indirectly with others.
4. Individuals who are physically ill.
5. Individuals who are temporarily or permanently disabled.
6. Individuals who have few outlets for the expression of actual or imagined anger, for strenuous physical exercise, or for anxiety.

Screening

1. Individuals who convert anger into depression. "When something unfortunate happens to you, what is your first reaction?"
   a. If anxiety symptoms, teach stress management techniques.
   b. If somatic illness, teach interrelationship between emotions and illness.
   c. If depression, encourage client to find more appropriate and less personally damaging ways to deal with anger/frustration.
2. Individuals from "learned helplessness" families.
   a. "Do you rationally wish to live your life the way your family has?"
   b. "There are ways to convert learned helplessness to productive behavior."
3. See Screening section under *Anxiety*, above.

ASSESSMENT

Health History

See Health History section under *Anxiety*.

Physical and Behavioral Assessment

See Pathophysiology section under *Anxiety*.

1. General feelings reported or implied by client may include
   a. Sad and miserable.
   b. Pessimistic.
   c. Self-blaming, filled with guilt.
   d. No interest in sexual or other activities.
   e. Depersonalization.
   f. Worthlessness.
   g. Unloved and unlovable.
2. Other behavior related to severe depression and reported by, or observed in, client. For example
   a. Awakens at 4 A.M. every morning and is unable to return to sleep.
   b. Cries approximately one-half of each therapeutic session.
   c. Complains of nausea at mealtimes.
   d. Refuses to eat, stating that he or she is not worthy of eating.

Diagnostic Tests

See Screening sections above and under *Anxiety*.

NURSING DIAGNOSES: ACTUAL OR POTENTIAL

1. See also Nursing Diagnoses section under *Anxiety*.
2. Maladaptive coping patterns.
   a. Due to internalization of anxiety and frustration, causing depression.
   b. Due to depressive lifestyle.
3. Ineffective family coping.
   a. Due to learned helplessness from family.
   b. Due to habitual behavior in which depression is reinforced by friends, family, and/or employment situation.
4. Grieving.
   a. Anger over perceived loss is turned inward onto the self and is being converted into depression.
   b. Client may be fixated in anger/depression stage of grieving at overwhelming loss.
5. Alterations in self-concept.
   a. Negative feelings about self.
   b. Hopelessness about self, the world, and the future.
   c. Unrealistic attending to negative detail, with inattention to positive ideation.
6. Sleep-rest activity (dysrhythm).
   a. Early morning awakening.

   b. Concern over not getting enough sleep.
   c. Napping occasionally throughout the day.
   d. Escaping painful, depressed thoughts by excessive sleeping.
7. Social isolation.
   a. Self-imposed isolation.
   b. Absence of reinforcing social relationships.
   c. Increased negative ideation when alone.
   d. Paranoid or suspicious that others will not want to see them depressed.

EXPECTED OUTCOMES

1. Immediate goals. The client will
   a. Be protected from carrying out destructive acts toward self.
   b. Begin to eat small quantities of food and increase nutritional status.
   c. Implement medication regimen.
   d. Increase verbalization with nurse.
   e. Decrease self-deprecating statements.
   f. Report suicidal thoughts.
   g. Stay in room no more than a total of 1 hour during daytime hours.
   h. Talk briefly with other clients.
   i. Engage in simple tasks assigned by the nurse.
   j. Engage in occupational therapy that involves nonverbal release of tension and energy.
   k. Dress self in morning.
   l. Drink at least 1,500 mL of fluids per day.
   m. Walk at least every 2 hours.
   n. Improve grooming.
2. Long-range goals. The client will
   a. Seek out staff members and other clients with whom to talk.
   b. Show congruence between words and affect.
   c. Identify situations in life that seem to precipitate depression.
   d. Identify previous patterns in family or in self in which depression was the lifestyle.
   e. Identify alternative behaviors to achieve the secondary gains formerly satisfied by depression.
   f. Demonstrate increased use of coping skills.
   g. Identify individuals who can be most supportive to self.
   h. Gain insight into precursors of depression in self.
   i. Recognize when he or she is starting to become depressed.
   j. Identify when he or she is feeling sad, angry, frustrated, or anxious.
   k. Begin to express hostility appropriately.
   l. Begin to make assertive requests and responses.
   m. Relate appropriately to staff, other clients, and family.
   n. Identify ways of relieving stress and tension.
   o. Be able to think about and work on painful aspects of self.
   p. Accomplish tasks assigned.
   q. Engage in recreational activities within the hospital unit.
   r. Engage in recreational activities and hobbies enjoyed previously.
   s. Remain reality oriented.
   t. Make positive statements about self and others.
   u. Decrease use of antidepressant medications.
   v. Accomplish activities of daily living without assistance from others. The client will
      (1) Eat a nutritionally balanced diet.
      (2) Eliminate regularly.
      (3) Dress appropriately.
      (4) Stand erectly.
      (5) Sleep throughout the night.
   w. Report decrease in all physical symptoms.

INTERVENTIONS

1. General interventions. See Interventions section under *Anxiety*.
2. Specific interventions. The following interventions are to be used with the severely depressed client hospitalized in a psychiatric unit.
   a. Use short, declarative sentences when talking with client.
   b. Allow client time to respond.
   c. Talk about neutral topics initially.
   d. Avoid undue cheerfulness with client.
   e. Encourage client to stay out of bed and out of bedroom.
   f. Encourage others to talk with client.
   g. Give brief explanation of treatments and procedures.
   h. Encourage client to postpone major decisions (e.g., divorce, separation, quitting

job, selling house) until after depression lifts.

i. Encourage client to engage in small tasks that can be accomplished.

j. Encourage use of strengths. Have client list strengths and assets.

k. Encourage replacement of negative thoughts with positive ones (see Intervention 5 under *Anxiety*).

l. Environment should be made conducive to decreasing depression.

m. Have client room with another client who is verbal but not intrusive toward others.

n. Provide sparse furniture, softly colored walls and furnishings; avoid bright colors in room if possible.

o. Assign room near enough to the nurses' station that client can be observed frequently.

p. As client becomes less depressed, suicidal potential increases. Observe and listen for signs of suicidal ideation or planning (see Chapter 38).

q. Remove all objects from environment that could potentially be used by client to injure self.

r. Inquire of any suicidal thoughts when interviewing client.

s. Do not leave client alone in bath or shower.

t. Foods and fluids.
   (1) Food intake should be kept nutritionally adequate.
   (2) Help client find place to eat among others.
   (3) Eat with client to assist and encourage intake.
   (4) Assist client in preparing tray.
   (5) Suggest first bite and first drink.
   (6) Assume client will eat, and convey this expectation.
   (7) Record accurate intake.
   (8) Provide soft, easily chewed, but nutritious foods.
   (9) Provide small amounts of food frequently during the client's waking hours.
   (10) Ascertain and provide client's food preferences.
   (11) Provide hand foods if use of utensils is too difficult for the client.
   (12) Use feeding tube or intravenous (IV) fluids as a last resort.
   (13) Provide at least six glasses of fluids per day.

u. Elimination.
   (1) Record accurate output.
   (2) Force fluids if urine output is low.
   (3) If there is no bowel movement for 2 days
      (a) Increase passive and active exercise.
      (b) Increase raw and bulky foods in diet.
      (c) Add bran to diet.
   (4) If there is no bowel movement for 3 to 4 days
      (a) Ask physician for order for stool softener.
      (b) Check for impaction.
      (c) Enema may be given if necessary.
   (5) Check for diarrhea. If present
      (a) Consider request for medication to slow intestinal motility.
      (b) Alter diet (e.g., add cheese).
      (c) Check for impaction. Remove impaction.

v. Be alert for GI or upper respiratory infections.
   (1) Take temperature once per day if fluid intake is markedly restricted.
   (2) Take vital signs once per day unless indicated or ordered more frequently.
   (3) Be sure client has adequate clothing and covering.

w. Hygiene.
   (1) Administer mouth care if fluid intake is restricted. Encourage mouth care by client.
   (2) Encourage a bath every day only if this seems to be pleasing to the client; otherwise, bathing may be every 2 to 3 days if agitation occurs with bath.
   (3) Shave male client or allow client to shave self every day.
   (4) Provide sanitary needs for female client during menses.

x. Observe skin for signs of dryness, edema, reddened bony prominences.
   (1) Observe for pedal edema.
   (2) Encourage increased activity; walk with client.
   (3) Arrange for client to prop up feet while sitting.

(4) Apply lanolin to skin, especially vulnerable areas.

(5) Encourage increase in fluids and decrease in salts in diet and foods naturally having sodium.

3. Therapeutic interventions.
   a. Begin therapeutic sessions with discussion of neutral topics, and progress to feeling topics and then to insight-oriented topics, as client progresses and can cope with this.
   b. Require longer verbalizations as client improves.
   c. Avoid cheerfulness and reassurances that reassure the nurse, not the client.
   d. Avoid agreement with self-deprecating statements of client.
   e. Continue to reinforce worth and rights of client.
   f. Reinforce grooming efforts.
   g. Avoid arguing with client or making light of self statements.
   h. Reinforce increased number of positive statements about self or others.
   i. Encourage the client to engage in activities that may increase feelings of self-esteem (e.g., writing to friends, making objects for family, beginning relationships with others).
   j. Present increasingly more complex decisions for the client to make as the depression lifts.
   k. Ensure that reinforcing statements are honest and not overcomplimentary.
   l. As depression lifts, help client to understand that depression is relatively temporary.
   m. Assist with activities of daily living only as needed.
   n. Provide regular but not rigid schedule of activities.
   o. Encourage activities that can be completed in a relatively short period of time (i.e., one occupational therapy session, to give the patient a sense of accomplishment).
   p. Encourage progress from passive activities to more active ones.
   q. Encourage activities that are noncompetitive (e.g., walks, puzzles, simple projects). These may progress toward more competition and complexity as client improves.
   r. Even more therapeutic is the encouragement of the client to engage in strenuous physical exercise that includes striking motions (e.g., tennis, driving a golf ball, swimming, jogging). Release of body tension, energy, and expression of hostile feelings in socially acceptable and nonverbal manners can be very helpful to the depressed client.
   s. Arrange occupational therapy sessions that emphasize activities that involve gross striking motions (e.g., pounding, hammering, sanding, rubbing, repetitive actions).
4. Teaching interventions. Teaching is focused upon helping the client who has come out of or is in the process of coming out of a depression, to learn from the situation. Teaching also provides the opportunity for the nurse to assess the client's understanding of his or her treatment and enlists the client as a partner in this care. Teaching includes anticipatory guidance to help the client to learn how to prevent or minimize future occurrences of depression.
   a. Suggest that verbalization to identify anger and deal with it appropriately *early* be utilized. Teach modes of coping with internalized anger before it becomes deep depression.
   b. Teach progressive relaxation.
   c. Instruct in behavioral techniques (i.e., thought stopping, leveling of anxiety, and methods that assist in raising self-esteem).
   d. Encourage client to identify individual precipitating factors of depression, and teach how each can be dealt with in a more assertive or more appropriate manner.
   e. Teach tools of self-monitoring and self-control.
      (1) Control of environment.
         (a) Remove stimulus for anger/depression.
         (b) Reinforcements in environment should be enhanced and intensified, if possible.
         (c) Distractions from depressive ideation are helpful.
         (d) Identification of antecedent events may help prevention of depression.

(e) Identification of consequences of depression may help client eliminate these as reinforcers of the depression.

(2) Control of thoughts.

(a) Self-congratulations when client has accomplished a task or reduced negative ideation.

(b) Thought stopping to avoid reinforcing negative thoughts.

(c) Practicing self-talk that is positive.

(d) Disputing negative self-talk (see Intervention 5 under *Anxiety*, above).

(3) Control of feelings.

(a) Relaxation exercises. See Intervention 3 under *Anxiety*.

(b) Breathing exercises. See Intervention 2 under *Anxiety*.

(c) When there are sad feelings or immediately before the onset of crying, ask client to sit up straight quickly and look upward forcefully. This interferes with feelings that are customarily experienced as the client looks downward.

(d) Imagery may be helpful. Ask client to remember a time he or she felt very good, self-assured, loved, happy. Ask client to see clearly that time, hear what was going on, and allow the feelings to come in. When these are intense, take a deep breath and hold it. This pairs the memory of the good feeling with the deep breath, an easily replicable and recurrent behavior.

(4) Control of behavior.

(a) Practice nondepressed behaviors, even though the client does not *want* to do them. After awhile, the enjoyment that previously built the behavior will return, thereby naturally reinforcing engaging in the behavior.

(b) Contract with the self. Rewards, administered by the self, will be contingent upon the client engaging in selected, self-determined, nondepressed behavior.

(c) Select strenuous exercise, preferably to include very brisk walks or jogging.

f. Teach assertive behavior by using role-playing exercises.

g. Teach management of medication and self-observation of effects.

h. Discuss activities and coping skills that client can use to confront anxiety situations effectively.

i. Discuss positive self statements that the client has identified, and encourage client to use these positive statements to reverse negative thoughts.

j. Discuss appropriate expression of tension, frustration, and hostility.

k. Discuss appropriate diet, dress, activities, and so on.

EVALUATION

Outcome Criteria

1. Has client met immediate goals?
2. To what extent have these been met?
3. Has client met long-range goals?
4. To what extent have these been met?
5. Which goals have not been met?
   a. Were these goals realistic?
   b. Why were these goals not met?
   c. What additional interventions might be tried in order to meet these goals?
6. How does the client feel about meeting or not meeting the goals?
7. What additional goals does the client wish to address?
8. What suggestions does the client have that might assist him or her in meeting these goals?

Reevaluation and Follow-up

1. See psychotherapist, physician, and/or counselor regularly.
2. Have first outpatient appointment set up before discharge from hospital.
3. Have medications labeled with name, dosage, time, and precautions.
4. Provide written information as cues to clients (i.e., cards that list what he or she can *do* to control anxiety and depression and to release frustrations).
5. Give client phone number and address of crisis center or emergency referral agency.
6. Expect that the client will take prescribed medications, use what has been learned in

the hospital, and seek natural support systems in own environment.
7. Provide anticipatory guidance; role play potentially stressful situations that are likely to arise after client leaves hospital. Focus on strengths and new coping skills of client.

MILD TO MODERATE DEPRESSION

DESCRIPTION

1. Mild to moderately depressed clients are reacting to frustrations in their life situations (e.g., losses or threatened losses, anger turned inward, physical illness or disability).
2. Clients are sad, indecisive, have little zest for living, look on the dark side of many things, and have lowered self-esteem, but do not require hospitalization.
3. For etiology, incidence, prognosis, and pathophysiology, see *Severe Depression*.

PREVENTION

See *Severe Depression*.

ASSESSMENT

Health History

See Health History under *Anxiety*, above.

Physical and Behavioral Assessment

1. Physical observations or complaints reported by the client may include
   a. Crying.
   b. Slightly less well groomed than usual.
   c. Stooped posture when sitting or standing, much "looking down" behavior.
   d. Sad facies.
   e. Decreased verbalizations.
   f. Eats less or may eat much more.
   g. Recreational activities limited.
   h. Psychomotor retardation.
2. General feelings reported or implied by client may include
   a. Sadness, miserable, decreased enjoyment in living.
   b. Decreased self-esteem and feelings of self-worth.
   c. Negative thoughts about self, world, and future.
   d. Decreased motivation for activities that are customarily reinforcing to client.
   e. Gastrointestinal complaints: nausea, constipation.
   f. Extreme tiredness and fatigue.
   g. Meaninglessness, indecisiveness, withdrawal.
   h. Irritability, loses temper.
   i. Inability to concentrate, does nothing, boredom.
   j. Feelings of helplessness, hopelessness.
   k. Changes in sexual appetite or no interest in sex.

NURSING DIAGNOSES: ACTUAL OR POTENTIAL

1. See Nursing Diagnoses under *Anxiety*.
2. See potential diagnoses under *Severe Depression*.

EXPECTED OUTCOMES

1. Immediate goals. The client will
   a. Decrease number of self-deprecating statements.
   b. Interact with family and/or friends each day.
   c. Begin to engage in previously reinforcing behaviors, whether or not she or he is in the mood to do so.
   d. Begin to release tensions through striking-type sports activities, physical exercise, or work.
   e. Finish tasks that have been started.
   f. Make positive statements about self and others.
   g. Identify situations in life that seem to precipitate depression.
   h. Identify when she or he is feeling sad, angry, frustrated, or anxious.
   i. Identify ways of appropriately relieving tension and anxiety.
   j. Be able to "level" anxiety.
   k. Be able to use progressive relaxation.
   l. Be able to use thought stopping as necessary for negative ideation.
   m. Be able to reduce anxiety through breathing exercises for stress management.
   n. Be able to use esteem-enhancing behavioral techniques as necessary.

o. Express hostility/anger appropriately and interpersonally.
p. Report reduced incidence of suicidal ideation.

2. Long range goals. The client will
a. Associate thoughts with consequent feelings.
b. Measure reality in thought and will not allow one thought to generalize to broad negative feelings.
c. Expand meaningful social contacts.
d. Eliminate all psychoactive drugs.
e. Control anxiety when it begins rather than allowing it to turn into depression.
f. Expand coping behaviors.
g. Eliminate "not helpful thoughts" (e.g., self-deprecating, hopeless, worrying thoughts).
h. Make assertive requests and responses.
i. Express hostility appropriately.
j. Engage in activities previously enjoyed.
k. Identify more behaviors to be used in coping with crisis situations that might lead to depression.
l. Gain insight into own behavior.
m. Identify situations in life that seem to precipitate depression.
n. Identify previous patterns in family or in self in which depression was the lifestyle.
o. Identify alternative behaviors to achieve the secondary gains formerly satisfied by depression.
p. Report a decrease in physical symptoms associated with depression.
q. Become a generally relaxed person.
r. Be a growth-oriented individual.

INTERVENTIONS

1. Refer to Interventions section under *Anxiety.*
2. Refer to therapeutic interventions under *Severe Depression*, above.
3. Refer to teaching interventions under *Severe Depression.*

EVALUATION

See Evaluation section under *Severe Depression* for those appropriate evaluation techniques that are applicable to the moderately depressed individual.

ELATION

DESCRIPTION

Definition

The elated client exhibits euphoric affect, is hyperactive in movement, and may engage in bizarre, grandiose, and extravagant behaviors.

Etiology

1. Dynamically, elation may be seen as a flight from depression.
2. Elated behavior can be learned from family behavior patterns.
3. Elation may be associated with
a. Side effects from drugs.
b. Chemical imbalances.
c. Hormonal imbalances.
d. Any combination of the above.

ASSESSMENT

Health History

See Health History section under *Anxiety.*

NURSING DIAGNOSES: ACTUAL OR POTENTIAL

1. Maladaptive coping patterns.
a. Due to masking of depression, feelings of low self-esteem.
b. Disturbances of mood (e.g., elation, irritability).
c. Acceleration of psychomotor activity.
2. Disruptions in carrying out activities of daily living.
a. Eating.
b. Sleeping.
c. Grooming.
d. Purposeful activity.
3. Disruptions in impulse control.
a. Destructive to property.
b. Potentially destructive to self and others.

EXPECTED OUTCOMES

1. Immediate goals of care. The client will
a. Take in calories in proportion to activity.
b. Extend sleeping time to at least 5 hours per night.
c. Find appropriate outlets for hostility.
d. Verbalize to the nurse for short periods of time.

e. Remain in his or her bedroom for short periods of time.
f. Refrain from destroying property.
g. Occasionally talk with other clients.
h. Engage in tasks assigned (preferably involving much activity, but little concentration).
i. Go to recreational therapy, remaining in the yard without incident.
j. Attend occupational therapy for a short period of time.
k. Wear only necessary items of clothing.
l. Use only one cosmetic at a time.
m. Drink at least 2,500 mL of fluids per day.
n. Be protected from self-inflicted injuries.

2. Long-range goals. The client will
   a. Dress appropriately.
   b. Report decrease in minor physical injuries.
   c. Sleep at least 6 hours per night.
   d. Express hostility and frustration appropriately and interpersonally.
   e. Be assertive (not aggressive) with others.
   f. Gain insight into elation and will understand when it occurs, following which situations, and so on.
   g. Be able to sit and talk about own thoughts and feelings.
   h. Show congruence between words and affect.
   i. Identify life situations that precipitate elation.
   j. Begin and finish tasks or projects assigned or chosen by self.
   k. Remain reality oriented at all times.
   l. Decrease use of psychoactive drugs, as able.
   m. Eat a nutritionally adequate diet.
   n. Remain in psychotherapy and seek therapeutic assistance when stress mounts.
   o. Learn to seek intervention early when depressed behavior begins.
   p. See also Expected Outcomes under *Anxiety*.

INTERVENTIONS

1. General interventions.
   a. Use slow, soft, clear speech, speaking at a slightly slower rate than that used customarily.
   b. Whisper to client occasionally, especially when client is being loud.
   c. Avoid becoming entangled in and affected by the client's hyperactivity.
   d. Provide a calm, pleasant, but firm psychological environment.
   e. Avoid participating in the client's nonreality.
   f. Firmly place limits on client, to avoid destructive behavior.
   g. Divert client's attention from destructive to constructive activities as much, and as quickly, as possible.
   h. Use postponement and substitution to encourage appropriate behavior.
   i. Avoid reasoning or arguing with the elated client.
   j. Attempt to establish a situation in which the client is not the center of attention all the time.
   k. Give short explanations.
   l. Consider all reasonable requests, but try not to be manipulated into treating the elated client differently from other clients on the unit.
   m. Minimize loud noises and loud talking around the elated client, as he or she is overly susceptible to stimuli.
   n. Provide only one cosmetic to use at a time, preferably in subdued shades. More cosmetics and brighter colors may be given when the client demonstrates that she can use them appropriately.
   o. Keep elated clients away from each other, if possible.
2. Environmental interventions.
   a. Assign client a single room, away from the hub of activity.
   b. Furnishings should be pale or monotone in color.
   c. Remove all breakable objects from the room.
   d. Request that the client's valuables be put in a place of safekeeping to avoid their being broken, lost, or given away.
   e. Limit radio, television, magazines, and newspapers, as they provide further stimulation to the elated client.
   f. Keep the client from remaining the center of attention.
   g. Instruct visitors concerning the client, stressing the importance of not breaking rules for the client.
   h. Establish close relationship with visitors,

toward the purpose of their understanding and being helpful, not hurtful to the client.

i. Limit visitors to one or two close family members, who can advise the rest of the family of the client's activities and progress.

j. Read letters written by client before they are mailed, to avoid having the client give away his property or get self into difficulties because of poor judgment.

k. Provide slow, rhythmical music as a soothing factor.

3. Physical interventions.
   a. Provide client with a high-calorie, high-protein diet.
   b. Use plastic dishes, utensils, and cups.
   c. As the elated client may not be able to sit and eat, provide hand foods, such as a banana, apple, protein bar, sandwich.
   d. Provide the client with fluids of choice. Suggest that client take at least one drink of water each time a water fountain is passed. Keep a specially marked cup that is always filled with liquid (e.g., juice) for client to pick up and carry.
   e. Weigh client at least once a week to determine weight loss or gain, more frequently if extremely active.
   f. Inspect client's body frequently for minor cuts, bruises, and joint injuries.
   g. Observe for objective signs of illness, as client may not complain even if in pain.
   h. Insist on at least minimal mouth hygiene. Use oil or lip pomade for cracked lips.
   i. Encourage use of a gargle for hoarseness.
   j. Observe the elderly elated client for signs or symptoms of congestive heart failure, pneumonia, joint injuries, and so on.
   k. Expect the client to eat, drink, and eliminate; convey this expectation to the client.
   l. Provide a warm bath before retiring.
4. Therapeutic interventions.
   a. Attempt to establish a one-to-one relationship with the client, but postpone psychotherapy until the client has progressed through the highly elated stage.
   b. Observe client for swings from elation to depression, at which time suicidal ideation can arise (see Chapter 38).
   c. Encourage client to speak openly to nurse, as one of the best deterrents to suicide is a relationship in which the client can confide these thoughts or apprehensions.
   d. If client is ordered lithium, check blood studies frequently, and provide a high-sodium, high-fluid diet.
   e. Postpone entrance into group psychotherapy until the high state of elation has passed.
   f. Listen to and try to interact with client.
   g. Observe for less-elated behaviors, and, when they occur, reinforce them in a way that is meaningful to the client.
   h. Encourage the client to engage in physical activities (e.g., tearing strips of rags for rag rugs, fingerpainting, painting murals, pounding or sanding objects).
   i. Assign the elated client tasks (e.g., folding linen, raking leaves, digging in the garden, washing walls or floors).
   j. Emphasize the use of continuous action of large muscle groups, avoiding activities that require discrimination or fine muscle activity.
   k. Keep client occupied for extended periods of time writing own life history, a diary of experiences in the hospital or elsewhere, suggestions for improving the activities of the unit, and so on.

EVALUATION

See Evaluation section under *Severe Depression*.

BIBLIOGRAPHY

Baer, E. D., McGowan, M. N., and McGivern, D. O.: "How to Take a Health History," *American Journal of Nursing*, **77**:1190, July 1977. Succinct but comprehensive overview of the health history with emphasis on and examples related to indirect questions and psychologically oriented responses.

Beck, A., Rush, A. J., Shaw, B. F., et al.: *Cognitive Therapy of Depression*, Guilford Press, New York, 1979. Classic and comprehensive work on cognitive approaches in intervention for depression.

Benson, H.: *The Relaxation Response*, Avon Books, New York, 1975. Discusses the physiological responses to stress, interrelationship between emotion and the effect of the relaxation response. Also included are relaxation exercises.

Bernstein, D. A., and Borkovec, T. D.: *Progressive Relaxation Training: A Manual for the Helping Professions,* Research Press, Champaign, Ill., 1973. Comprehensive explanation of progressive relaxation training with accompanying audiorecording.

Burgess, A. W., and Lazare, A.: *Psychiatric Nursing in the Hospital and the Community,* Prentice-Hall, Englewood Cliffs, N.J., 1976. Basic text on psychiatric nursing that can be used as a reference for interventions dealing with depressed, elated, or suicidal clients.

Burns, D. D.: *Feeling Good: The New Mood Therapy,* New American Library, New York, 1980. This comprehensive and excellent best-seller presents theory, research, pharmacological treatment, and psychological interventions. Useful for the interested consumer and the nurse.

Clark, C. C.: *Enhancing Wellness: A Guide for Self-Care,* Springer Publishing, New York, 1981. This excellent resource book focuses on wellness and what the individual can do to achieve it. Numerous applications to affective responses are included.

Clarkin, J., and Glazer, H. (eds.): *Depression: Behavioral and Directive Intervention Strategies,* Garland Publishing Co., New York, 1981. An overview of major treatment strategies for depression, including a self-control therapy program, somatic treatment, and behavioral interventions.

Cline, F. W.: "Dealing with Depression," *Nurse Practitioner,* **2**(3):21, January-February 1977. Emphasis on medications used in depression.

Eggland, E. T.: "How to Take a Meaningful Nursing History," *Nursing '77,* **7**:22, July 1977. Summary of health history with rationale and sample history.

Emory, G.: *A New Beginning: How You Can Change Your Life Through Cognitive Therapy,* Simon & Schuster, New York, 1981. Application of cognitive therapy to anxiety and depression, and a comprehensive overview of the field. Highly readable and practical book.

Horsely, J. A., and Loomis, M. E.: *Interpersonal Change: A Behavioral Approach to Nursing Practice,* McGraw-Hill, New York, 1974. Excellent summary of behavioral management, with many applications to general client care. Useful basic book specifically related to incorporating behavior modification in planning and implementing nursing care.

Knowles, R. D.: "Managing Anxiety," *American Journal of Nursing,* **81**:110, January 1981. Dealing with anxiety by becoming aware of body sensations, leveling the anxiety, and using breathing exercises to lower anxiety. In each of the articles in this series, the problem, intervention, rationale, and evaluation are included.

"Control Your Thoughts," *American Journal of Nursing,* **81**:353, February 1981. The technique of thought stopping is discussed and proposed as a way of overcoming anxiety or depression by controlling selected thoughts.

"Positive Self-Talk," *American Journal of Nursing,* **81**:535, March 1981. How self-talk affects the feeling state and feelings of self-esteem are discussed, with interventions described.

"Disputing Irrational Thoughts," *American Journal of Nursing,* **81**:735, April 1981. Irrational thoughts are dealt with by making "but statement" or disputing irrational statements, utilizing a rational-emotive format.

"Handling Depression by Identifying Anger," *American Journal of Nursing,* **81**:968, May 1981. The interrelationship between anger turned inward and the onset of depression is described, with interventions included.

"Handling Depression Through Activity," *American Journal of Nursing,* **81**:1187, June 1981. Identification of previously reinforcing events, engaging in strenuous activities, such as jogging, are described with rationale.

"Handling Depression with Positive Reinforcement," *American Journal of Nursing,* **81**:1353, July 1981. This article proposes dealing with depression by arranging for reinforcing activities that are antidotes to depression.

"Coping with Lethargy," *American Journal of Nursing,* **81**:1465, August 1981. The cognitive behavioral approach of accomplishing, reinforcing, and sorting for positive occurrences used to counteract depression.

"Overcoming Guilt and Worry," *American Journal of Nursing,* **81**:1663, September 1981. Dealing effectively with anxiety that is produced by guilt and worry through identification of the emotion, determination of its usefulness, and competing interventions.

"Handling Anger: Responding vs. Reacting," *American Journal of Nursing,* **81**:2196, December 1981. Use of appropriate ways to deal with anger, as prevention of its transformation into depression, is presented.

Lewinsohn, P., Muñoz, R. S., Youngren, M. A., et al.: *Control Your Depression,* Prentice-Hall, Englewood Cliffs, N.J., 1978. Utilizing a self approach, this overview of cognitive-behavioral therapy includes self-change methods, relaxation, social skills training, and so on.

Parrino, J. J., and Tanner, B. A.: *Helping Others: Behavioral Procedures for Mental Health Workers,* E-B Press, Eugene, Ore., 1975. Simple overview of behavioral techniques that are applicable to psychiatric and general nursing. Includes relaxation training, thought stopping, and other techniques. Interventions are leveled to the education and experience of the helper.

"Programmed Instruction: Helping Depressed Patients in General Nursing Practice," *American Journal of Nursing,* **77**:1007, June 1977. Programmed instruction with vignettes of depressed clients and varying nursing approaches. Includes test of competency. Excellent review of general approaches to the depressed client.

Rosenbaum, M. S.: "Depression: What to Do, What to Say," *Nursing '80,* **10**:65, August 1980. Application of nursing interventions with the depressed client presented in a concise format.

Sachs, M. L.: "Running Therapy for the Depressed Client," *Topics in Clinical Nursing,* **2**:77, July 1981. Use of strenuous activity, particularly running/jogging, as a treatment for depression is presented with supporting research.

Snyder, J. C., and Wilson, M. F.: "Elements of a Psychological Assessment," *American Journal of Nursing,* **77**:235, February 1977. Organization of the psychological assessment according to various psychological theories. Actual questions to use under categories of the assessment are presented.

37

Interpersonal Problems of Adults

Rhoda L. Moyer and Martha J. Snider

Difficulty in interpersonal relationships is the central factor in persons who have mental health problems. All other problems relate directly to these difficulties. Because of the significance of interpersonal relationships in both the causation and solution of mental health problems, psychiatric–mental health nursing practice includes both the scientific use of theories of human behavior and masterful, artistic use of the self. The therapeutic use of the self is considered such an absolute and essential part of nursing care for *all* clients that it will not be included in any one specific area as an intervention. General aspects of using the self therapeutically include

1. Developing interpersonal trust.
2. Helping to increase the person's self-esteem and autonomous functioning.
3. Promoting the person's ability to maintain him- or herself interdependently with meaningful and satisfying human relationships.
4. Providing a therapeutic milieu that develops the sociopsychological aspects of the person's environment.
5. Accepting and appropriately using the surrogate parental role.
6. Assisting with the here-and-now living problems the person experiences.
7. Teaching emotional health patterns.
8. Behaving as a social agent to improve and promote the person's recreational, occupational, and social competence.
9. Operating within a contractual framework with the person.
10. Adhering to ethical considerations in treatment practices.

ALTERATIONS IN SELF-CARE ACTIVITIES

DESCRIPTION

Alteration in self-care activities is a clinical problem in which a person is unable to be self-directed in the ordinary tasks of eating, drinking, bathing, hygiene and grooming, sleeping, exercising, and eliminating, and in which the assistance of another person to meet these basic needs is required. These alterations may be the result of a variety of factors, either physical and/or social-emotional. Many disorders and normal crises may be accompanied by an alteration in the ability of the person to carry out activities of daily living. It may be among the earliest symptoms to appear in a developing emotional disorder, and it may be part of a syndrome that combines several clinical problems, such as manipulation, dependency, severe anxiety, secondary gains of neurosis, disorientation, and loss of memory. Frequently, alterations in self-care activities are a result of temporary or permanent regression and/or lack of motivation and socialization skills in clients who have been hospitalized or socially isolated for a long period of time. The problem further decreases the client's ability to interact socially with others and move out into the community.

PREVENTION

Crisis Intervention

1. Identify high-stress events.
2. Teach relaxation, self-awareness, and stress reduction skills.
3. Teach concepts of crisis intervention (e.g., realistic perception of event, coping behaviors, and situational supports).
4. Promote understanding of maturational and situational crises.

Population at Risk

1. Persons experiencing maturational and/or situational crisis.
2. Persons experiencing chronic high stress.
3. Persons with low self-esteem.

ASSESSMENT

This general assessment format will be followed in subsequent sections with areas of specific emphasis noted in each section.

Health History

1. Observation and report of client.
2. Family's or significant others' report of behavior.
3. Age.
4. Sex.
5. Socioeconomic data.
   a. Educational level and experience.
   b. Occupational and work history.
   c. Community relationships.
   d. Available and accessible human and material resources.
6. Perception of met and unmet needs.
7. Usual coping behaviors, support system, and strengths.
8. Usual responses to stress, anger, sadness, failure, losses, frustration, success, illness, and threatening situations.
9. Identification of current and potential stressors in personal life.
10. Present level of anxiety: mild, moderate, severe, panic.
11. Social and interpersonal relationships, including patterns, type, quality, and quantity.
12. Alterations and strengths in ego functioning, especially thought, speech, affect, perception, mobility, judgment, and reality-testing abilities.
13. Family history, including health problems, constellation, ways of dealing with stress or threats, interpersonal relationships, early childhood memories, and significant losses.
14. Formulation of growth and developmental level of client.

Physical Assessment

1. Description of performance of activities of daily living.
2. Any physical or intellectual problems or limitations.
3. Neurological exam.

Observations

Observations and emotional responses of nurses or other staff members to the client's behavior, especially related to social functioning and ability to understand instructions and reinforcement.

NURSING DIAGNOSES: ACTUAL OR POTENTIAL

1. Alterations in self-care activities: inability to care for self; refuses to dress self, unable to dress self, or dresses inappropriately; refuses to keep clothes on.
2. Potential nutritional deficit: alterations in food intake.
3. Sleep-rest pattern disturbance: sleeps most of day.
4. Alterations in patterns of elimination: incontinent of urine/feces.
5. Ineffective communication due to inability or unwillingness to interact socially.

EXPECTED OUTCOMES

1. The client will improve personal habits related to activities of daily living.:
   a. Remain continent of feces and urine.
   b. Take interest in grooming, hygiene, and appearance.

   c. Improve eating habits.
   d. Dress self in own clothes appropriately.
   e. Sleep appropriate number of hours.
2. The client will develop social interests outside of self.
3. The client will perform his or her activities of daily living in socially acceptable ways.
4. The client will develop interest in and identification with a group of clients.
5. The client will relate to other people in planned activities.
6. The client will have the minimum necessary social skills and abilities to function in the community.

INTERVENTIONS

1. Take incontinent client to toilet according to a rigid routine (e.g., upon rising, after breakfast, before lunch, after lunch, before dinner, after dinner, and at bedtime).
2. Instruct, remind, or assist client in
   a. Bathing.
   b. Caring for nails.
   c. Use of deodorant.
   d. Brushing teeth regularly.
   e. Combing, washing, and styling hair.
   f. Changing underwear frequently.
   g. Selection of clothes and appropriate attire.
   h. Laundering and ironing clothes.
3. Teach female client appropriate use of cosmetics.
4. Encourage male client to shave regularly.
5. Assist client in setting up routine schedule to meet grooming, dressing, and personal hygiene needs.
6. Teach client to observe proper manners while eating: how to sit, chew with mouth closed, chew a little food at a time, eat with utensils properly.
7. Teach client how to improve orderliness and neatness of room and personal possessions.
8. Reward all appropriate behaviors with verbal recognition.
9. Utilize remotivation techniques to encourage group interactions, including use of food to reinforce pleasure of socializing.
10. Identify group projects and goals with client participation.
11. Encourage individual participation and responsibility in planning and implementing group activities.
12. Assist client in developing and/or expanding interests and skills.
13. Assist clients to hold and participate in ward meetings.
14. Offer work assignments on unit to increase client pride and sense of accomplishment.
15. Provide opportunities for clients to care for other objects or people (e.g., plants, animals, less-socialized patients).
16. Provide opportunities for clients to improve their physical environment through group activities.

EVALUATION

Reassessment

Since alterations in self-care activities are usually a long-term problem, the carefully developed plan will need continuous reassessment and modification to meet the needs and progress of individual clients. Staff will need support and reinforcement from one another and their leaders to assure continued motivation to intervene with clients with chronic regressed patterns of interaction. The goal is to move such clients back into the community as soon as they are able to function self-sufficiently and present minimal levels of social adequacy.

Reevaluation and Follow-up

Clients should be prepared to deal with real-life situations of work, family life, social interactions, and own daily care prior to discharge. If minimally competent, referral to an active day treatment program in a mental health center or halfway house or group home where they can receive support and build their knowledge, skills, and self-confidence is very valuable. A public health nurse could also provide support, ongoing treatment, and be a resource for newly discharged clients.

SELF-IMPOSED SOCIAL ISOLATION

DESCRIPTION

Social isolation is a process in which persons retreat from relationships and contacts with the external world into a world of their own. There is a reduction of external stimuli and an increase in internal stimuli. Usually, this process is a defense against the anxiety related to increased threat or increased stress. Social isolation can range on a behavioral continuum from the unconcern or indifference about others observed at times in "normal" people to the profoundly withdrawn individual who is actively hallucinating.

Dysfunctional social isolation behaviors are a way of coping with threat or stress. Behaviors can include aloofness, detachment, disinterest, active or passive removal of self from others, decreased spontaneity in planning and/or initiating things with others, inability to mingle with others and communicate freely, overt or covert avoidance of others in the environment, use of monosyllables, mutism, working independently rather than cooperatively, and loss of goal-directed behavior. In severe cases, a form of regression in which social relations and external perceptions are eliminated, resulting in hallucinations and delusions, may be observed. Specific behaviors can include refusing to talk with the nurse, being late for or avoiding appointments, answering only when asked direct questions, "forgetting" appointments, remaining in a group to avoid individual contact with the nurse, and verbally or nonverbally engaging in an activity to avoid exploring significant issues with the nurse.

Social isolation may be observed as either a symptom or a syndrome in both acute and chronic forms of dysfunction. In its less severe forms, it may be demonstrated by persons experiencing a crisis, such as loss of a significant person.

PREVENTION

Refer to Prevention section under *Alterations in Self-Care Activities.*

ASSESSMENT

Health History

(Refer to Health History section under *Alterations in Self-Care Activities.*) Note especially interpersonal and social relationships.

1. Number and type of relationships.
2. Length of time knowing friends.
3. Patterns, quantity, and quality of friendships.
4. Sudden changes or recent losses.
5. Recreational interests and pursuits.
6. Relationship patterns during childhood and adolescence.

Staff Reaction to Contact with Client

Note the following:

1. Feeling of talking with a shell or an uninhabited house.
2. Sense of not being heard or of having little or no emotional exchange.
3. Sense of approach-avoidance in the relationship.
4. Experience being "swallowed up" or inappropriate feelings and responses from client.
5. Fear of being close to client (due to client's projections of fear or anger).

NURSING DIAGNOSES: ACTUAL OR POTENTIAL

1. Alterations in pattern of communication: inaudible speech, not responsive to verbal stimuli, uses symbolic language, refuses to talk with others.
2. Alterations in roles and relationships: impulsive (aggressive, hostile) acts against self, others; inappropriate social behavior.
3. Alterations in cognitive/perceptual behavior due to hallucinations, delusions, blocking, loose associations, projection, misinterpretation of environment.

EXPECTED OUTCOMES

1. The client will respond appropriately to here-and-now situations.
2. The client will regain some ability to meet activities of daily living (e.g., sleep, food, hygiene, elimination).
3. The client will establish a positive relationship with one other person.
4. The client will increase contacts and relationships with others.
5. The client will not harm self or others.
6. The client will develop meaningful relationships with others, characterized by trust, acceptance, and closeness.
7. The client will be able to meet own activities of daily living and meet basic needs in an independent manner.
8. The client will understand own social isolation behavior, how and why it was useful, situations that increase anxiety, how to reduce the anxiety, and client will be able to choose selectively to be close to others.

9. The client will maintain self-control over behavior.
10. The client will describe self in a positive way.
11. The client will demonstrate increased ability to communicate with others.

INTERVENTIONS

1. Assist client to identify behaviors used when anxious.
2. Assist client to identify thoughts and feelings in here-and-now situations, and to correlate behaviors used to express these.
3. Point out inappropriate or incongruent behavior.
4. Define and stress reality to client in here-and-now situations.
5. Assist client in naming and exploring feelings and behavior when hallucinating or delusional. (See also Chapter 39.)
6. Observe for and chart behaviors and environmental stimuli that precipitate or relate to client withdrawing into fantasy.
7. Administer medications (e.g., phenothiazines or antidepressants) as prescribed, and observe for side effects and effect of medications on the client.
8. Provide instructions in step-by-step, concrete terms when client is unable to make decisions about personal care.
9. Observe and record fluids and diet consumed daily.
10. Observe and record general physical condition each day.
11. Use silence; share with client that you are willing to be together without talking if that is the client's wish.
12. Acknowledge and respond to client's experiences and feelings when they are expressed.
13. Acknowledge your lack of understanding and wish to understand when client's messages are confused or symbolic.
14. Support client with words and your presence during experiences and activities she or he finds frightening or difficult; role play difficult situations.
15. Teach client communication skills (e.g., how to approach people, how to use topics of interest, and provide opportunity to practice skills).
16. Broaden client's contacts to include other person(s) besides the staff.
17. Assist client to check out perceptions and clarify distortions.
18. Provide opportunities to develop sensual, feeling-type awareness, such as clay modeling, dancing, or music.
19. Set appropriate limits for destructive acts against self and others e.g., tell client that he or she cannot hurt self or others.
20. Ask client to make a contract with you not to hurt self accidentally or on purpose; in case of suicidal feelings, client will ask for protection or will contact a staff member. (See Chapter 38.)
21. Ask client to make a contract with you not to hurt someone else accidentally or on purpose; in case of feelings of anger or violence, client will ask for contact with staff member or for protection (e.g., seclusion).
22. Protect client and others when client is unable to control self by using appropriate means:
    a. Seclusion, to reduce stimuli.
    b. Medication, to reduce anxiety level.
    c. Remove harmful objects from environment. (See Chapter 38.)

EVALUATION

Social isolation requires constant reassessment and evaluation to determine effectiveness of interventions, for example, whether the client is interacting more or is less involved in active living. The nurse must determine whether there are new factors that alter the client's adaptation to and interaction with the environment and/or people. As the client is able to assume increasing levels of responsibility for her or his own personal needs and relationships, the nurse must be willing to relinquish the nurturing role with the client to assure full development. It is also important to assess accurately the client's potential and to accept the client's right to decide on a level of wellness such that unrealistic expectations are decreased.

Reevaluation and Follow-up

1. Refer to community agency and/or outpatient setting, such as a day treatment program, or public health nurse for further support and progression toward goals.
2. Communicate verbally and/or in writing the plan of care and summary of progress:
    a. To agency or person who will follow client.
    b. To significant others in client's life when client requests this.

3. Set up methods to monitor any medication(s) continued on an outpatient basis.
   a. Ask specific questions to assess client's method and regularity of taking medications and attitudes about taking them.
   b. Questions include How many? What time of day? What does client do if a dose is forgotten? Does client ever cut down on the amount? Is client afraid of becoming dependent on drugs? Does taking medications worry client in any way?
4. Upon discharge from hospital or after-care agency, be sure that client
   a. Has a list and schedule of medications, can verbalize importance of taking as scheduled, knows potential side and/or toxic effects, and knows how to obtain refills.
   b. Has an appointment for follow-up with doctor, clinic, or mental health center, and knows how and when to contact them, if needed, before appointment.
   c. Has a plan for maintaining self daily, including adequate diet, personal grooming, and social-interactional needs.
   d. Knows importance of simple communication techniques to facilitate communication and understanding, and to receive support from others.
   e. Has one significant other who is aware of client's communication problems and can work with client during difficult times.

SENSORY-PERCEPTUAL ALTERATION

DESCRIPTION

Sensory-perceptual alteration is a clinical problem that involves an impaired ability to understand temporal, spatial, or personal relationships. Such individuals lose their awareness of the position of themselves in terms of time, space, or other people. They usually appear confused and perplexed and are unable to concentrate on here-and-now situations; they may be unable to identify the date, the place where they are, or who they are.

Sensory-perceptual alteration as a clinical symptom is presented in several psychiatric disorders (e.g., whenever there is severe anxiety or as a result of an emotionally traumatic experience, such as a situational crisis). Sensory-perceptual alteration may also be part of a syndrome involving alterations of memory, judgment, affect, reality testing, and perception, such as occurs in organic brain syndrome. In all cases, there is a related disruption in interpersonal processes.

PREVENTION

Refer to *Alterations in Self-Care Activities.*

ASSESSMENT

Refer to *Alterations in Self-Care Activities.*

Health History

See *Alterations in Self-Care Activities.* Note especially alterations and strengths in client's ego functioning (including any abrupt changes): in thought, recent and remote memory, perception, judgment, reality testing, affect.

Physical Assessment

1. Psychological examination.
2. Laboratory workup related to physical history and findings of examination.
3. Staff observations and responses to client.

NURSING DIAGNOSES: ACTUAL OR POTENTIAL

1. Significant changes in usual patterns of orientation; alteration in recall ability; memory deficit.
2. Orientation to self, time, space, or other people is incongruent with biological age or lifestyle requirements.

EXPECTED OUTCOMES

1. The client will be safe and protected while disoriented.
2. The client will be supported by nursing measures while diagnostic and treatment procedures are followed to identify and correct physical (medical) problems.
3. The client will improve orientation to time, place, and/or person.
4. The client will cope with any permanent disability.

INTERVENTIONS

1. Supervise closely to prevent client from hurting self, wandering off, or exhibiting inappropriate behavior.
2. Decrease agitation and frustration with comforting, relaxing measures, such as warm bath, well-lighted room, soft music.
3. Repeat orienting information frequently in kind, quiet tone of voice.
4. Give simple, short explanations.
5. Use a night-light in client's room during the night.
6. Avoid frequent administration of barbiturates and bromides.
7. Observe client carefully and provide assistance in self-care when it is needed.
8. Do not physically restrain client unless absolutely necessary.
9. Listen carefully to what client says, and correct gently, in a nonpunitive manner, if information is confabulated.
10. Place calendars with large print and clocks with large numbers and hands in client's living area.
11. Label areas, such as bathroom, nurse's station, and client's bedroom, with large-lettered signs.
12. Introduce self to client each time nurse is with client; address client by name frequently.
13. Wear clearly labeled name tags with correct title.
14. Carefully orient client to environment; keep furniture and possessions in same place.
15. Maintain a regular routine and provide a printed schedule of activities for client to follow.
16. Permit client to practice skills in a familiar environment.
17. Tell client when you do not understand her or him.
18. Permit client to bring familiar objects from home to keep with her or him.
19. Place personal items in an area that is easily accessible to client.
20. Teach client to use lists and appointment books to minimize forgetfulness of schedules, people, activities.
21. Tape list of activities of daily care next to client's bathroom mirror.
22. Provide consistent routine and structure for client; introduce change slowly.
23. Encourage client to wear and use watch and to use a pocket calendar.
24. Prevent overstimulation from people or environment.
25. Encourage client to wear own clothes.

EVALUATION

Reassessment and modification of the plan to meet the needs of clients must be continuous and constantly adjusted to their level of functioning. The physical and medical condition of these clients should also be carefully monitored to assure maximum functioning in all spheres of activity.

Reevaluation and Follow-up

1. Prepare clients for any alterations in their environment by giving them simple explanations and by keeping them in contact with familiar people and objects.
2. Have public health nurse visit clients in hospital before their discharge to familiarize them with nurse. Provide nurse with summary of progress and treatment plan at time of client discharge.
3. Teach clients and their family members principles of care before discharge, including the need for medical checkups and the taking of medication, what to expect as a result of the medication, and what to report to the public health nurse and/or physician.
4. Referral to a day treatment program in a mental health center may be helpful for client.
5. Family therapy after client discharge should be recommended.

MANIPULATION

DESCRIPTION

Manipulation is an interpersonal behavioral process designed to meet one's own needs or goals by exploiting and/or controlling the behavior of others without regard for their rights, needs, or goals. It can be either consciously or unconsciously motivated. Usually, an unidentified, misinterpreted, or unmet social need arouses increasing degrees of anxiety that trigger the behavioral patterns known as manipulation.

Manipulation, as a clinical problem, does not include such constructive forms as assertiveness, teaching, selling, guiding, and socializing with other persons. The various forms of destructive manipulation include aggressive, hostile behaviors directed against or toward others and/or oneself; passive, covert behavior to control others or get needs met indirectly; and self-deprecation or deprecation of others.

In interpersonal relationships, manipulation may be observed as a single behavior or group of behaviors. As a symptom, it can be a part of the clinical picture of almost any of the psychiatric diagnoses.

PREVENTION

Crisis Intervention

See *Alterations in Self-Care Activities.*

Population at Risk

1. Persons experiencing maturational and/or situational crisis.
2. Persons experiencing chronic high stress.
3. Persons with low self-, or other, esteem.
4. Persons with chronic feelings of insecurity and powerlessness.
5. Persons with inadequate social learning.
6. Persons with immature personality development.

ASSESSMENT

Refer to *Alterations in Self-Care Activities.* Note especially

1. Communication patterns with and about client.
2. Emotional responses of nurses and other staff members to client's behavior, such as anger, anxiety, defensiveness, embarrassment, frustration, helplessness, withdrawal, indifference, guilt, sympathy, or overprotectiveness.
3. Strengths and weaknesses of nurses and other staff members in own interpersonal relationships, such as attitudes and feelings related to specific types of clients, based on factors including racial, socioeconomic, cultural, religious, national and sexual identity, and type of illness.
4. Behaviors of client demonstrating
   a. Aggressive manifestations, such as
      (1) Organizes other clients to defy or minimize staff authority.
      (2) Makes frequent demands or requests.
      (3) Threatens others, either clients, staff, or family.
      (4) Deliberately breaks rules, routines, procedures, or contracts.
      (5) Requests special attention and/or privileges.
      (6) Attempts to gain power and control in clinical setting.
      (7) Pressures others into meeting requests.
      (8) Reports another client's personal, confidential information.
      (9) Attempts to use others' weaknesses against them.
      (10) Derogates others.
      (11) Acts up when demands are not met or a situation is displeasing.
      (12) Coerces others by secreting articles.
      (13) Forces others to respond by bargaining with them.
   b. Passive manifestations, such as
      (1) Procrastinates or dawdles when required to do something.
      (2) Mumbles and/or avoids direct conversation.
      (3) Changes the subject or activity.
      (4) Breaks a treatment contract jointly established by nurse and client.
      (5) Responds to confrontation with tears and/or helpless behavior.
      (6) Monopolizes the conversation in social and/or therapy situations.
      (7) Is ingratiating or overly solicitous.
      (8) Complies to gain approval or recognition.

NURSING DIAGNOSES: ACTUAL OR POTENTIAL

Disruptions in roles and relationships associated with use of aggressive or passive interpersonal behaviors to meet needs. (See behaviors listed under Assessment, above.)

EXPECTED OUTCOMES

The client will

1. Learn to recognize specific manipulatory patterns.
2. Gain insight into unfulfilled needs that promote manipulatory behavior.
3. Delay immediate need gratification when appropriate.
4. Decrease attempts to manipulate others as measured by a behavior modification tool.

(See tool utilized by Justice and Justice, 1976.)

5. Assume responsibility for expressing needs directly in here-and-now situations.
6. Develop self-control and independence.
7. Develop constructive, appropriate outlets for aggressive needs.
8. Be self-aware and autonomous in relationships.
9. Cooperate, compromise, and collaborate in mutually respectful relationships with others.
10. Recognize how and where manipulatory patterns of behavior were learned (in primary family) and will recognize and develop new options to meet needs as an adult.

INTERVENTIONS

1. Recognize when client is utilizing a manipulative behavior, pattern, or game.
2. Identify own feelings, thoughts, and actions in response to specific behaviors of client.
3. Identify client's tendency to recreate similar manipulations among staff as previously done at home with parents and siblings.
4. Recognize the client's attempt to intimidate staff members.
5. Assess unfulfilled needs that client is trying to meet through manipulation.
6. Assist client in identifying own patterns of manipulative behavior.
7. Assist client in recognizing interpersonal conflicts.
8. Promote idea within client that attainment of self-control is the responsibility of the client.
9. Assist client in identifying consequences of inappropriate behavior.
10. Explore with client possible reasons for inappropriate behavior.
11. Encourage client to explore and express feelings verbally without acting upon them.
12. Encourage client to identify alternative methods of behavior to meet needs appropriately.
13. Teach client how to use direct ways to communicate needs.
14. Teach client the differences between aggressive, assertive, and passive approaches to meet needs.
15. Demonstrate by role playing in specific situations the differences between direct, indirect, adaptive, and manipulative communication.
16. Invite client to help identify real needs if you do not know what is being sought.
17. Teach client to recognize differences between needs that require immediate gratification and those that can be delayed, sublimated, or substituted.
18. Teach and reinforce the idea that experiencing all feelings is okay, but it is not always appropriate to act upon them.
19. Set limits on inappropriate or self-defeating behaviors.
20. Use selective behavior modification program to decrease manipulation. (See tool utilized by Justice and Justice, 1976.)
21. Give direct messages to client.
22. Use verbal and nonverbal reinforcement when client functions within prescribed limits.
23. Point out client's behavior when it is manipulative.
24. Prevent client from manipulating one staff member against another by adhering to agreed-upon limits.
25. Permit freedom within prescribed limits.
26. Avoid demonstrating hostility, negative attitudes, or aggressive or passive behaviors toward client when she or he is being manipulative.
27. Assign consistent staff to client.
28. Develop a plan for dealing with manipulative behavior, and communicate to all staff involved in client's care.
29. Provide opportunities for the client to explore and test alternative behaviors.
30. Explore with client situations in which need is not satisfied.
31. Identify situations in which client lacks control, and point these out.
32. Identify situations in which client demonstrates self-control and independence, and point these out.
33. Teach client to seek out relationships in which he or she is liked and accepted.
34. Utilize peer pressure to modify manipulative behavior.
35. Provide experiences that build self-control and increase independence.
36. Listen to client's requests, and give reasons when requests cannot be met.
37. Allow client an opportunity to verbalize annoyance at restrictions or disappointments.
38. Teach assertive techniques to handle frustrating experiences.
39. Provide opportunity to experience a variety

of methods to express aggression, and evaluate their usefulness with client.

40. Teach client how to verbalize "I" statements.
41. Teach client the difference between "I" and "you" statements in asking for satisfaction of needs or expressing feelings.
42. Be alert to signs of developing anxiety or anger.
43. Give consistent feedback regarding interpersonal behavior patterns; give positive reinforcement for all positive, constructive reactions.

EVALUATION

Manipulative behavior needs constant evaluation to see if the nursing interventions are effective in decreasing such behavior, as it is especially resistant to change. The nurse should evaluate the behavioral changes against a specific set of criteria (expected outcomes). If client behaviors are not changing, it is necessary to reevaluate the entire process of nursing care, paying particular attention to the priorities of care. It is also essential to be sure that the nurse's goals and the client's goals are mutually agreed upon. Renegotiation of the initial agreement may be required if expected behavioral changes are not forthcoming.

Reevaluation and Follow-up

1. Refer to a community agency and/or outpatient setting, such as a day treatment program, for further evaluation of progress toward goals.
2. Communicate verbally and/or in writing the plan of care and summary of progress to agency or person who will follow client.
3. Set up methods to monitor any medication(s) continued on an outpatient basis.

ALTERATIONS IN SELF-CONCEPT

DEPENDENT BEHAVIOR

DESCRIPTION

Dependent behavior is a symptom or syndrome in which a person exhibits difficulty in making independent decisions; a marked tendency to lean on others for support, protection, permission, guidance, and advice; and a compulsive need to unite with a stronger person in order to face life's problems. Increased anxiety is felt when the needed person or object is not available or threatens to be not available. The dependent person may also act or behave in such a manner as not to threaten or disrupt the relationship in order to be taken care of by the significant other.

Initially, a person's survival as an infant depends on the life-sustaining relationship between self and mother in which basic needs for mothering, love, affection, shelter, protection, security, warmth, and food are met without a specific request by the infant. If this normal symbiotic relationship continues, either overtly or covertly, into later years, the person depends on another person as the source of his or her own feeling, thinking, and acting. Therefore, the behavior is such that the person depends upon others or objects for exploitation and the satisfaction of neurotic needs, rather than engaging in cooperative mutual support and affection.

Such dependent persons with dysfunctional symbiosis constantly seek someone or something to meet their needs because they believe that they are unable to meet their own needs and *must* be taken care of by someone or something other than themselves. They deny their own ability to meet their needs directly and demand that someone else meet them. These demands are passive in nature, consisting of several types of behavior:

1. Mobilizing energy to not think or do anything for themselves when a problem arises, solving the problem according to someone else's expectations rather than their own.
2. Performing an activity that is non-goal-directed to relieve tension that avoids solving the problem.
3. Refusing to assume responsibility for themselves and their own decisions, behaviors, feelings, and thoughts.

Dependent behavior includes two main types: (1) dependency on people (referred to as symbiosis), and (2) dependency on drugs. Dependency on drugs is the psychic craving for, habituation to, or addiction to a chemical substance; such dependency creates a lifestyle in which individuals arrange their lives, in whole or in part, to revolve around the need to achieve a specific effect of one or more chemical agents on their mood or state of consciousness. Drug dependency is viewed as the result of altered or ineffective parenting relationships or stagnant family relationships. Drug-dependent individuals experience feelings of being cheated of rightfully deserved parenting within their family of origin. They use their drug dependence as a means of separating from relatedness to family members and as a means of escaping from physical and psychosocial stresses. Both types of dependent behavior—on people and on drugs—are, in part, the result of inadequate symbiotic relationships and cause further relational dysfunction and stagnation. (See also *Compromised Decision Making*.)

PREVENTION

Refer to *Alterations in Self-Care Activities*. In addition, teach assertiveness skills.

Population at Risk

Persons who had a premature separation from parents or neglect, overprotection, or a lack of parental responsiveness.

ASSESSMENT

Refer to *Manipulation*.

Health History

People-dependent symbiosis (refer to *Alterations in Self-Care Activities*). Note especially

1. Family history, including health problems, constellation, ways of dealing with stress, any recent crises, especially losses, early childhood memories, relationship patterns within family, extended family members with drinking problems.
2. Client's description and perception of health status, reasons for hospitalization, expected outcomes of treatment, nutritional patterns.
3. Client's usual responses to stress, anger, sadness, loss, frustration, success, failure, illness.
4. Client's perception of coping patterns and interpersonal relationships (e.g., quality, quantity, type, feelings about these).
5. Client's perceptions of dependence and independence, including people, decision making, daily living experiences.
6. Client's ego function alterations, especially judgment, defense mechanisms (e.g., denial), reality testing, perceptions.
7. Client's report of present and potential stresses in personal life.
8. Use of drugs and/or alcohol in daily life.

Health History

Drug-dependent symbiosis (refer to *Manipulation*). Note especially

1. Family history, including health problems; constellation; ways of dealing with stress; any present or recent crises, especially losses; early childhood memories; relationship patterns within family; extended family members with drinking or drug problems.
2. Client's description/perception of health status, reasons for hospitalization, expected outcomes of treatment, nutritional patterns.
3. Use of drugs and/or alcohol in daily life.
4. For alcohol users, assess the following areas in depth:
   a. *How often* does the client use alcohol: daily, weekly, weekends, holidays, special occasions?
   b. *How* is alcohol used: time of day, to get started or to complete a task, to socialize, mood when drinking, to relax and ease tension, alone or with others, to celebrate an occasion (or is *it* the occasion)?
   c. *How much* does the client drink: type and ounces of liquor, mixed or straight, more or less than friends, daily amount? Has drinking increased or decreased over the past 5 years?
   d. The client's definition of alcoholism ("drinking problem" is often more acceptable to clients).
   e. Relationship problems: who is included as family, description of a typical day?
   f. Work problems: has time been lost and why, how often have there been job changes, does client have salable skills, is client in a vulnerable occupation?
   g. Health problems: any existing physical problems, what relationship exists between drinking and the health problem?
   h. Physical dependence or addiction, measured by tolerance to alcohol and withdrawal symptoms during abstinence: general physical condition, malnutrition

status, presence of seizures, amnesia episodes, blackouts, tremors, anxiety, diaphoresis, anorexia, nausea, vomiting, or hallucinations within 3 days of alcohol abstinence.
   i. Nutritional status; dietary patterns.
5. For drug users, assess the following areas in depth:
   a. How does the client view the world and self in relation to it?
   b. What assets or liabilities does client have in holding a job, handling responsibility, and in maintaining meaningful interpersonal relationships?
   c. Has client ever been, or is client now, involved in criminal and judicial systems?
   d. How does client defend self from making behavioral changes? (Typical patterns include denial, projection, and manipulation.)
   e. What factors in the client's life support the addiction, and what factors bring the client for help?
   f. Is the client currently on drugs, and if so, what kind and how much?

Staff's Responses Related to Dependent Client

1. Feelings, thoughts, behaviors, regarding client: typical negative responses include anger, rejection, punitiveness, frustration, wish to rescue or save the client from problems, taking charge, "doing for" the client, making decisions or setting goals for the client, fear, helplessness, and approach-avoidance behaviors.
2. Attitudes related to alcoholism or drug addicts, use of drugs to cope with life.
3. Personal assessment of strengths and limitations. (This self-evaluation is extremely critical in working with drug abusers.)
   a. Motivation for helping role.
   b. Level of growth and development (resolution of identity and authority issues).
   c. Self-concept.
   d. Personal resources (recreational outlets and sociofamilial relationships).
   e. Past experiences (professional and drug related).
   f. Philosophy about individual choice, accountability, and responsibility for behavioral change.
   g. Level of knowledge about alcoholism, drug addiction, and psychological issues of giving-receiving, victim-victimizer, dependence-independence.

Diagnostic Tests

Drug-dependent symbiosis (refer to *Alterations in Self-Care Activities*). Note especially laboratory workup:

1. Blood alcohol levels.
2. Other blood chemistries.
3. Liver function tests.
4. X-ray films of abdomen.
5. Urine analysis.
6. Note dietary pattern, especially amount of sugar and coffee consumed regularly, and whether food is eaten.

NURSING DIAGNOSES: ACTUAL OR POTENTIAL

1. Alterations in self-concept associated with dependence on people or drugs.
2. Self-care deficit due to significant changes in habits or activities of daily living, self-care activities, and level of independence.

EXPECTED OUTCOMES

The client will

1. Decrease dependent behaviors and increase independent behaviors.
2. Ask for help and assistance when it is needed or desired.
3. Recognize own responsibility and choice for the problem behavior and for making behavioral changes.
4. Develop the ability to think and to feel simultaneously without projecting or manipulating.
5. Develop social skills that increase self-esteem and self-awareness.
6. Give up self-destructive, maladaptive behaviors and maintain a drug-free lifestyle.
7. Develop and maintain a meaningful support system of interpersonal relationships, apart from drug or alcohol users and in addition to family.
8. Develop insight into dependent behaviors and decide to change these behaviors.

INTERVENTIONS

1. Observe for impending delirium tremens in first 24 to 48 hours after hospitalization. Symptoms include extreme agitation, fear,

and auditory hallucinations. (See also Chapter 39.)
2. Treat delirium tremens.
   a. Provide protective setting.
   b. Provide measures to maintain rest and sleep.
   c. Orient to person, place, and time.
   d. Acknowledge fright.
   e. Keep room lighted, and prevent shadows.
   f. Provide sufficient staff to administer prescribed treatments with minimal stress.
   g. Provide simple explanations for tests and procedures.
3. Administer oral fluids for dehydration and electrolyte imbalance.
4. Provide high-protein, high-carbohydrate diet.
5. Observe for symptoms of depression and suicidal ideation or behavior (see Chapters 36 and 38).
6. Begin detoxification program.
7. Observe drug-taking behavior closely.
8. Begin methadone maintenance program, or go "cold turkey," if prescribed.
9. Reassure the client regarding withdrawal symptoms.
10. Treat infections and/or physical complications from drug or alcohol use.
11. Observe and record client's clinical status and signs of drug or alcohol withdrawal.
12. Evaluate ability to perform self-care activities.
13. Educate client regarding physiological and psychological effects of drug abuse.
14. Assist client to recognize that responsibility for behavior and choices lies with him or her alone.
15. Assist client to explore chosen behavior and its consequences.
16. Avoid critical, punitive, or moralistic attitudes.
17. Assist the client in selecting and setting specific goals to work toward attaining.
18. Ask client to contract not to hurt self accidentally or on purpose (i.e., overdose or suicide).
19. Explore with client how her or his basic needs for affection, control, responsibility, and mastery are met.
20. Encourage verbalization of needs, feelings, thoughts, and wants; help to find ways to act on these appropriately.
21. Direct client to cut out or stop self-defeating or socially disruptive actions.
22. Set limits on unrealistic or inappropriate behavior.
23. Communicate expectations and goals to client and staff so all have a clear understanding of what is to be done.
24. Assist client in developing a specific plan to decrease dependency on others and increase ability to meet own needs independently of others (e.g., get own apartment, learn to drive a car, get job).
25. Discuss with client your observations of ways in which he or she manipulates others.
26. Reinforce successful behavior with comment, acknowledgment, and encouragement.
27. Assist client in identifying strengths in area of social functioning (e.g., sense of humor, hobby or special interest, appearance).
28. Explore client's feelings, thoughts, and behaviors related to specific social situations.
29. Role play problematical social situations with client to develop or improve skills.
   a. Encourage client to interact with and relate to other people.
   b. Encourage participation in a group for former drug or alcohol abusers.
   c. Prevent and intervene in the client's discussion of poor self-concept for secondary gains by refocusing conversation.
   d. Provide opportunities for success experiences for client.
   e. Assist client in grieving about giving up drugs, alcohol, or dependent behaviors.
   f. Encourage client to explore life situation and need for drugs and alcohol.
   g. Encourage and support client's ability to think and solve problems.
   h. Invite client to identify and differentiate between feelings, thoughts, and behaviors.
   i. Use a variety of treatment modalities to teach client to think and feel (e.g., group and milieu therapy, poetry, dance, other creative activities, occupational and recreational therapy, bibliotherapy, fantasies, gestalt techniques, individual therapy).
   j. Encourage client to make independent decisions in noncritical areas, such as dress, structuring of time, attendance at meetings and activities.

k. Use the milieu to develop client's responsibility, and provide feedback about client's performance of tasks.

EVALUATION

Dependency is a problem that requires long-term follow-up and continuous evaluation of the effectiveness of the treatment plan. Discharge planning with specific treatment outcomes established should begin at the time of the client's admission to decrease the potential for depending on the staff and hospital setting and deriving secondary gains from hospitalization. The client's ability to meet his or her own basic needs, maintain a relatively stable physical status, and follow through on a community referral are essential factors in preventing the occurrence of the "revolving door" syndrome. Behavioral outcomes of treatment should be evaluated on a regular basis, with goals and plans modified according to the client's status and response to treatment. Relapses of alcohol or drug users should be handled in a matter-of-fact, exploratory manner.

Reevaluation and Follow-up

1. Refer to community agency. It is crucial that alcohol- or drug-dependent clients be referred for long-term follow-up care in the community, such as Alcoholics Anonymous, a day-treatment program, community mental health center, alcoholic rehabilitation unit, or public health nurse. In addition, drug addicts need a new group with which to identify and relate, in order to combat the severe problem of loneliness most drug addicts face. Group therapy can be the supportive link if care is carefully structured. Drug users and nonusers should be in separate groups. The nurse's main role may be as a facilitator or coordinator, rather than as primary therapist.
2. Assist with socioeconomic and family problems. Because the behavior of drug-dependent clients has far-reaching effects and is affected by all those in their system, family therapy is an effective tool for long-term care. This can be initiated before the discharge of clients. Other social and economic factors, such as jobs and new social ties, should also be planned in long-term care if clients are to be rehabilitated. Of course, some clients do not choose to follow through with these long-range plans.
3. Monitor prescribed medications.
   a. Alcoholics may be maintained on Antabuse or a minor tranquilizer after discharge. These clients should be followed and observed regularly for their responses to the medications, and the plan for follow-up should be clearly defined, understood, and agreed upon by the client. Also, in case problems develop before the initial follow-up visit, the client should know whom to see at what location before discharge.
   b. Drug users being maintained on methadone or a narcotic antagonist should know whom to see, when, where, and for what reasons prior to discharge. Unscheduled urinary drug detection tests should be taken periodically when client is using one of these drugs.

MALADAPTIVE COPING PATTERNS

DEMANDING BEHAVIOR

DESCRIPTION

Demanding behavior is manifested in syndromes that involve dysfunctional interpersonal relationships. It usually occurs when individuals believe themselves unable to fulfill their needs and/or have their needs met by making requests in a direct, matter-of-fact manner. Therefore, they tend to coerce others to meet their needs indirectly by making requests with forceful, manipulative behaviors. If others attempt to meet the requested needs without perceiving the real, unspoken needs, or if others attempt to avoid or ignore such clients, the demanding behavior is frequently accelerated as anxiety increases. Demanding behavior may be observed in a variety of behavioral syndromes. (See *Manipulation* and *Dependent Behavior*, above).

PREVENTION

Refer to *Manipulation*.

ASSESSMENT

Refer to *Alterations in Self-Care Activities.*

Health History

See *Alterations in Self-Care Activities.* Note especially client's emotional responses, including withdrawal, anxiety, feelings of being swallowed up, anger, never being able to "do enough," frustration.

Observations

1. Observations of nurses or other staff members of client's emotional responses.
2. Assess behaviors, such as
   a. Makes numerous requests of others.
   b. Asks others to do what could be done by him- or herself.
   c. Detains nurse or staff member in room with additional requests after initial request has been met.
   d. Whines and seems helpless when making a request.
   e. Becomes angry when requests are not met immediately.
   f. Constantly seeks attention from others.
   g. Attempts to coerce others into meeting requests.

NURSING DIAGNOSES: ACTUAL OR POTENTIAL

Alterations in role and relationship patterns associated with demanding behavior.

EXPECTED OUTCOMES

The client will
1. Recognize that many demands are being made.
2. Gain insight into unfulfilled needs and wants that cause demanding behavior.
3. Decrease demands.
4. Ask directly for what is needed or wanted.
5. Develop a variety of options to meet needs.
6. Become more self-aware and autonomous in relationships.

INTERVENTIONS

1. Identify situations in which client is demanding.
2. Reflect client's behavior back to assist her or him in identifying patterns.
3. Share own responses to client's behavior with him or her in a matter-of-fact way.
4. Assess the unfulfilled needs that client is trying to meet via demanding behavior.
5. Identify with client the basic needs he or she believes unmet, and decide together how these will be met (by client or others, at what times, etc.).
6. Point out when client's anxiety is increasing.
7. Identify and point out consequences of inappropriate behavior.
8. Encourage client to explore and express feelings without acting upon them.
9. Assist client in developing new options for meeting needs effectively.
   a. Encourage client to ask directly for what is wanted.
   b. Invite client to use "I" messages for feelings, wants, and needs.
   c. Encourage client to explore feelings if and when demands are not immediately met.
   d. Role play alternative ways to communicate needs other than demanding.
   e. Reinforce appropriate behaviors (e.g., when client asks directly and is independent).
10. Provide safe, consistent limits for behavior.
11. Explain to client clearly defined expectations that are total-staff decisions.
12. Explore client's strengths and liabilities with client.

EVALUATION

It is helpful to use a flow sheet or tool to evaluate the number of times and kinds of situations in which the client is demanding in order to evaluate behavioral changes and the effectiveness of the interventions. Changes should be monitored and evaluated against baseline data developed when the plan is begun. Basic needs, physical, emotional, and social—must be met, while the client is encouraged to achieve both independence and interdependence in meeting the needs. Be sure entire staff is consistent in its expectations and interventions with the client. If behavior does not significantly change within a specified period (no less than 1 week of consistent care), reevaluate all steps in the nursing process.

Reevaluation and Follow-up

To assure positive reinforcement and continuous growth of the client it may be helpful to establish a plan with the client for "spot" checks (e.g., monthly) within the community following discharge. Referral to a community mental health center or public health nurse, with client's consent, is recommended. If referral occurs, the plan of care and earlier progress should be shared with the person or agency for continuity of care. The client should also be taught before discharge to recognize when additional assistance may be needed and how, where, and from whom to obtain it.

COMPULSIVE-RITUALISTIC BEHAVIOR

DESCRIPTION

Compulsive-ritualistic behaviors are involuntary activities performed by a person either to avoid anxiety or to cause an involuntary, irrational, recurring thought to disappear. These behaviors are repetitive, stereotyped, and compelling, even when the individual does not wish to perform these behaviors. Both the obsessive thoughts and the compulsive-ritualistic acts are an attempt to cope with anxiety arising from conflicts that are out of awareness and are often related to hostile, aggressive, or other unacceptable impulses that are in opposition to adult functioning.

Behaviors that are compulsive-ritualistic can range from mild forms, which are viewed as normal and healthy and permit the person to function well in situations requiring orderliness, frugality, and neatness, to those that are severe and cause almost total incapacitation of one's ability to function. Developmentally, these behaviors are normally observed in the stage where autonomy over one's bodily functions and control over one's world are mastered. Compulsive-ritualistic behaviors become a problem in later life when there is restriction of one's creativity, intimacy with others, and ability to experience joy and spontaneous thought, feelings, and actions.

Examples of compulsive-ritualistic behaviors include excessive handwashing or cleaning; returning to one's home to see if the door is locked or lights off; performing tasks in a rigid, never-changing manner; rituals related to activities of daily living; walking, or behaving in certain prescribed ways; and avoiding or relating to persons, situations, or things in a stereotyped, repetitive, and compelling manner. These behaviors may constitute either a symptom or a syndrome in combination with other problem behaviors related to interpersonal dysfunction. These actions may be observed in several diagnostic categories.

PREVENTION

Refer to *Alterations in Self-Care Activities*. Encourage personal autonomy and power over one's own life direction and choices.

ASSESSMENT

Refer to *Alterations in Self-Care Activities.*

Health History

Note especially

1. Description of usual responses to stress, anger, sadness, losses, successes, failures, illnesses, hostility, aggression.
2. Primary concerns and/feelings related to rituals and compulsive behavior, including description of usual patterns.
3. Statement of health goals and concerns related to the problem.

Observations

1. Staff's emotional responses to client's behavior, including pity, disgust, anger, sympathy, empathy, increased anxiety, withdrawal, frustration, and intense discomfort.
2. Recognize behavior patterns, such as
   a. Performs activities of daily living in a rigid, repetitive manner.
   b. Reports having recurring thoughts that cannot be controlled or forgotten.
   c. Becomes severely anxious when repetitive behavior is interrupted or interfered with.
   d. Relates to people or objects in a rigid, stereotyped manner.
   e. Unable to meet basic physical needs due to time invested in complex rituals.
   f. Harms self and/or others by performing compelling acts against own will.
   g. Avoids people or objects consistently due to obsessive thoughts or fears.
   h. Performs activities in a compelling manner, against own wishes.
   i. Has compelling thoughts about killing or harming someone.

NURSING DIAGNOSES: ACTUAL OR POTENTIAL

Ineffective socialization due to increase in time and energy spent in ritualistic patterns of behavior and accompanied by severe anxiety when patterns are interrupted.

EXPECTED OUTCOMES

The client will

1. Maintain good physical health.
2. Control self- or other-destructive patterns.
3. Utilize substitute activities to control anxiety whenever possible.
4. Recognize feelings of anxiety and self-defeating behaviors.
5. Gain some insight into the meaning of own behavior.
6. Resolve the dynamic issues by owning and accepting hostile-aggressive impulses and maintaining control of self and world.
7. Give up obsessive-compulsive-ritualistic behavior.
8. Develop new patterns of behavior that enhance well-being and increase quality of relationships and capacity for intimacy, while maintaining autonomy (i.e., control over self and world).

INTERVENTIONS

1. Provide adequate time and an appropriate place for client to perform compulsive behavior.
2. Assign a patient, tolerant nurse to remain with client.
3. Remain with client during ritualistic activity.
4. Protect client from ridicule of other persons.
5. Provide satisfying channels for substitutions, whenever possible.
6. Protect client from harming self or others with hostile, aggressive behavior.
7. Encourage physical activity that utilizes gross motor movements.
8. Rotate staff to prevent exhaustion from dealing with their own feelings about client's behavior.
9. Provide gloves and/or hand lotion for dermatitis.
10. Ensure adequate rest by permitting adequate time for preretiring rituals and/or administering sedative medications.
11. Observe and record client's activities of daily living to ensure adequacy of meeting physical needs.
12. Provide for nutritional needs of client.
13. Discuss problem behavior with client immediately following completion of ritual, when anxiety level is lowered; encourage discussion of feelings and thoughts.
14. Encourage client to verbalize intense anger instead of acting it out symbolically.
15. Provide protection and limits for safety as client experiences intense rage.
16. Explore the purpose that the behavior fulfills in client's life.
17. Identify situations that increase anxiety and increase use of rituals.
18. Teach client alternative ways of coping with anxiety, such as verbalizing and physical activity.
19. Provide examples of appropriate and effective ways to handle anger.
20. Teach client how to recognize changes in self that indicate impending loss of control.
21. Introduce change slowly.
22. Encourage client to identify strengths, as well as weaknesses.
23. Assist client to increase tolerance of differences, by discussing differences in people as unique strengths.

EVALUATION

Compulsive-ritualistic behaviors are usually severe when they come to the attention of the nurse. Therefore, long-term therapeutic intervention is often required, and it is helpful to measure behavioral changes against a baseline in order to appreciate small changes. A flow chart can be used to indicate the number of times per day or per hour a particular ritualistic behavior occurs. Nurses must frequently evaluate their own responses and feelings to be sure their behavior is not interfering with the treatment or increasing the client's anxiety. Nurses may need supportive relationships with colleagues to deal with their own anger and frustration. Reassessment should go on continually to assure quality care of this challenging client.

Reevaluation and Follow-up

1. Refer the client to a community agency or therapist for continuing support, if client so desires.
2. Provide the agency or therapist with either a written and/or verbal plan of care and summary of progress while hospitalized, so there is continuity of care.
3. Assist the client in developing a plan of action before discharge to meet personal needs and to continue growth.
4. Teach the client to recognize increasing prob-

lematical symptoms early and to know where to go for assistance before incapacitation occurs.
5. Provide for follow-up and supervision if client is on medications at time of discharge.

COMPROMISED DECISION MAKING

DESCRIPTION

Compromised decision making is a clinical problem in which clients demonstrate a lack of ability to make decisions independently, or to choose between two or more alternatives, or who tend to make choices based on the wishes or desires of other individuals regardless of their own wishes or desires. Such clients may agonizingly deliberate over decisions but be unable to use effectively the ego functions of thinking, reality testing, judgment, and affect to sort out the pros and cons of particular choices and decisions. Such behavior results in ineffective relationships and a lack of ability to assume responsibility for oneself in an adult world, as these require constant decision making. Such clients are frequently aware of their difficulty and experience low self-esteem, poor interpersonal relationships, and extreme anxiety as a direct result. Severe anxiety, such as occurs in crisis situations, may also trigger compromised decision making.

The tendency to suffer from compromised decision making begins frequently in early childhood when the developmental task of autonomy versus shame and doubt must be addressed. This clinical problem is present in a variety of psychiatric diagnoses and even in normal life situations in which intense anxiety is present. In addition, it may present as a symptom of acute or chronic organic brain syndrome with physical, emotional, and developmental components.

PREVENTION

Refer to *Alterations in Self-Care Activities*. In addition

1. Encourage independent thinking and decision making appropriate for maturational age.
2. Promote respect for differences in ideas, feelings, values, beliefs.

ASSESSMENT

Health History

Refer to *Alterations in Self-Care Activities*. Note especially estimate of intellectual abilities.

Diagnostic Tests

1. Intellectual testing.
2. Psychological evaluation for organic brain syndrome.

Observations

1. Observations of nurses and other staff members, including such behaviors as confusion, frustration, inability to get an answer to a question, sense of uncertainty.
2. Other behaviors assessed include that client is
   a. Unable to choose between two or more alternatives.
   b. Bases decisions on the opinions and wishes of others rather than on own opinions and wishes.
   c. Lacks ability to make independent decisions.
   d. Depends on other people to make decisions for her or him.
   e. Lacks information necessary to make decisions.
   f. Denies that a problem exists.
   g. Denies the significance of a problem.
   h. Unable to see more than one solution to a problem.
   i. Lacks confidence in own ability to solve problems.
   j. Denies that a problem has a solution.

NURSING DIAGNOSES: ACTUAL OR POTENTIAL

Ineffective coping due to significant changes in ability to make decisions or choices and to think clearly about options.

EXPECTED OUTCOMES

The client will

1. Recognize his or her specific difficulties related to decision making.
2. Alter perceptions of self or the problem to facilitate the decision-making process.
3. Begin to make simple decisions.
4. Improve ability to consider alternatives for specific situations.
5. Improve decision-making skills.

INTERVENTIONS

1. Identify issues or areas of life in which client has difficulty making decisions.
2. Explore with client attitudes about self that help or hinder the ability to make decisions.
3. Assess client's intellectual abilities, level of knowledge, attention span, and physical or organic problems that affect decision making.
4. Explore goals, values, and life purpose with client to provide a framework for decision making in specific situations.
5. Teach client how to test reality and validate perceptions as a part of decision making.
6. Identify and point out previous experiences where client made decisions successfully.
7. Direct client to resources to find necessary information about the problematical situation.
8. Correct misinformation about the problem situation.
9. Teach client how to identify necessary steps to meet activities of daily living and other decisions.
10. Direct client to write down or verbalize to a trusted person the pros and cons related to each decision that must be made.
11. Assist client to identify a variety of alternatives for each decision.
12. Explore with client the consequences of each alternative.
13. Assist client to focus attention on one problem at a time.
14. Teach client assertiveness techniques.
15. Reinforce client in making a decision or voicing independent opinions or ideas.
16. Assure client that it is all right to make mistakes.
17. Teach client that it is okay for one to think and feel for oneself, based on what one wants and needs and not on other's expectations.
18. Permit client to make choices about personal hygiene and dress, attendance at meetings, punctuality, structuring free time.
19. Assist client in transferring learning to new, more complex areas of decision making.

EVALUATION

Evaluation of both the goal being attained and the progress being made in the decision-making process are essentially continuous. It may be necessary to alter the goals or to select new ones as clients gain confidence in their ability to make decisions and develop new skills. Careful evaluation of the process should include both subjective and objective assessments of the client's ability to make increasingly more complex decisions based on life goals, values, and needs.

Reevaluation and Follow-up

1. Refer to community agency or public health nurse, especially if client has a physical or organic limitation for long-term follow-up. Also, refer if client or family requests such support.
2. Provide agency or person referred to with a summary of progress, plan of care, accomplishments, and goals being worked toward.
3. Teach client before discharge about community resources that might be pursued independently for assistance in meeting long-term goals.

REFERENCES

Justice, B., and Justice, R.: *The Abusing Family*, Human Sciences Press, New York, 1976.

BIBLIOGRAPHY

"An Alcohol Manual for Hospital Doctors," *Resident and Staff Physician*, **22:**9, February 1976. Sixteen articles related to diagnosing and treating clients who have alcohol problems. Interdisciplinary, broad community-based treatment focus, including articles on alcoholism in industry and a list of resources with addresses, for additional information and help for clients with a drinking problem.

Arieti, S. (ed.): *American Handbook of Psychiatry*, vol. III: *Adult Clinical Psychiatry*, 2d ed., Basic Books, New York, 1974. A classic text on the diagnosis, symptomatology, and treatment of the syndromes of adult psychopathology from a medical point of view.

Arnold, H. M.: "Working with Schizophrenic Patients," *American Journal of Nursing*, **76:**941, June 1976. An article that focuses on the therapeutic factors in working with withdrawn clients.

Berne, E.: *Games People Play*, Grove Press, New York, 1964. Describes and analyzes from both social and psychological positions 120 games that are frequently played in human transactions. Also presents the "anti-game" for each.

Berne, E.: *What Do You Say After You Say Hello?*, Grove Press, New York, 1972. Based on the principles of transactional analysis, Berne's final book outlines life scripts from a developmental perspective. Provides assessments, interventions, and examples of various scripts, as well as a script check list.

Haber, J., Leach, A. M., Schudy, S. M., and Sideleau, B. F.: *Comprehensive Psychiatric Nursing*, McGraw-Hill, New York, 1982. This is an eclectic nursing text for the advanced learner. Special features include the utilization of psychiatric-mental health nursing principles to formulate an integrated approach to client care across the age span and in a variety of settings, with primary, secondary, and tertiary prevention concepts and a nursing process focus.

James, M., and Jongeward, D.: *Born to Win: Transactional Analysis with Gestalt Experiments*, Addison-Wesley, Reading, Mass., 1971. Presents the theoretical concepts of transactional analysis as a rational method for analyzing and understanding behavior, both in ourselves and in our clients. Excellent tool for developing self-awareness, responsibility, and autonomy.

Justice, B., and Justice, R.: *The Abusing Family*, Human Sciences Press, New York, 1976. Excellent source of knowledge on diagnosing, planning care, intervening, and follow-up care for abusing families, using a psychosocial systems model. Explains the concept of symbiosis and use of the goal attainment guide.

Kneisl, C. R., and Wilson, H. S., (eds.): *Current Perspectives in Psychiatric Nursing*, vol. I: *Issues and Trends*, C. V. Mosby, St. Louis, 1976. A sourcebook providing a collection of articles related to the practice and theoretical framework of the psychiatric-mental health nurse. Includes material on new modes of treatment, including behavior modification, transactional analysis, gestalt therapy, and family mental health.

Meissner, J. E.: "Measuring Patient Stress with the Hospital Rating Scale," *Nursing 80*, **10**(8):70, August 1980. Provides a tool to measure stress in the general hospital client. Could be adapted for psychiatric clients.

Meldman, M. J., McFarland, G., and Johnson, E.: *The Problem-Oriented Psychiatric Index and Treatment Plans*, C. V. Mosby, St. Louis, 1976. Using the nursing history and process as guidelines, this book describes and explains a system for use in health care agencies operating on the problem-oriented record. It is helpful for developing specific written treatment plans for clients experiencing emotional problems.

Morgan, A, J., and Moreno, J. W.: *The Practice of Mental Health Nursing: A Community Approach*, J. B. Lippincott, Philadelphia, 1973. Focusing on clinical practice in the community, the authors have included descriptions and nursing implications for a number of treatment modalities. Written in simple style, it includes an excellent chapter on psychopharmacology, as well as chapters on chronic brain syndrome and drug and alcohol addiction.

Payne, D. B.: *Psychiatric-Mental Health Nursing*, Medical Examination Publishing Company, Garden City, N.Y., 1974. A number of socioenvironmental client problems are described in terms of etiology, dynamics, nursing assessment, and intervention in a simple basic format. Has a section on the nurse's functions and responsibilities to the client.

Reynolds, J. I., and Logsdon, J. B.: "Assessing Your Patient's Mental Status," *Nursing 79*, **9**(8):26, August 1979. Describes a structured format for assessing clients psychosocially and developing a nursing diagnosis. Provides an example of a completed form.

Robinson, L.: *Psychiatric Nursing as a Human Experience*, 2d ed., W. B. Saunders, Philadelphia, 1977. A humanistic approach to clients who have psychosocial problems. Provides an eclectic conceptual basis. Special features include material on transactional analysis applied to nursing situations, care of clients in a large state hospital, alcohol and drug addiction, and organic problems.

Rosenbaum, M. S.: "Depression: What To Do, What To Say," *Nursing 80*, **10**(8):56, August 1980. Describes assessment of and intervention techniques for depressed clients. Applicable to withdrawn clients, too.

Sandroff, R.: "A Skeptic's Guide to Therapeutic Touch," *RN*, 25, January 1980. Provides information about a holistic nursing procedure that may alter anxiety and pain in the client and also protect the care giver's emotional health. Provides insight into mind-body relationships.

Shubin, S.: "Nursing Patients From Different Cultures," *Nursing 80*, **10**(6):78, June 1980. Discusses the value of cultural assessment in providing effective nursing care. Provides examples of specific knowledge areas, including beliefs, values, and lifestyles of various cutures.

Snyder, J. C., and Wilson, M. F.: "Elements of a Psychological Assessment," *American Journal of Nursing*, **77**:235, February 1977. Describes 10 factors that should be included in each psychological assessment, presented as an eclectic approach.

Steiner, C.: *Scripts People Live*, Grove Press, New York, 1974. A potent book describing the role of early decisions, "life scripts," that limit the human potential for intimacy, awareness, and spontaneity. Provides interventions and exercises for changing specific life scripts.

Trail, I. D. (ed.): "Symposium on Alcoholism and Drug Addiction," *The Nursing Clinics of North America* **11**(3), September 1976. A group of eight articles sharing new knowledge and treatments. Applies a problem-solving approach to nursing individuals and families who are coping with the stress of alcoholism and drug addiction.

Wiley, P. L.: "Manipulation," in L. T. Zderad and H. C. Belcher (eds.), *Developing Behavioral Concepts in Nursing*, Southern Regional Education Board, Atlanta, Ga., 1968. Excellent application of the nursing process to the clinical problem of destructivbe manipulation in behavioral terms.

Wyckoff, H.: *Solving Women's Problems Through Awareness, Action, and Contact*, Grove Press, New York, 1977. A book that outlines the theory and practical applications of radical psychiatry to women's problem-solving groups. Useful exercises and applications are included. Special content includes the cooperative contract, sex-role scripting, and mind-body issues.

38

Threats to Survival

Imogene Stewart Rigdon and Karolyn Lusson Godbey

The purpose of this chapter is to describe the nursing process for the client who poses a threat to self-survival and the violent client who poses a threat to the survival of others. Awareness of the impact of the client's threat on the family, significant others, and the nurse is considered to be a part of this process.

A threat is defined as a verbal and/or physical expression of the intention to hurt, destroy, or punish self or others. The client's threat, whether it is self-directed or other-directed, arises out of the client's feelings of hopelessness and helplessness. The client resorts to destructive behaviors in a desperate attempt to obtain relief from these feelings.

When faced with the client's threat, the family and/or significant others are often overwhelmed by their own responses. They are in need of and deserve the attention of a nurse.

Intervening with the threatening client is an anxiety-producing experience for the nurse. The nurse needs to be aware of personal and professional responses, as well as any conflict between the two.

Both suicidal and violent clients may be encountered in every clinical area of nursing. This chapter is designed primarily for the nurse in the hospital but can be adapted for use in other areas. It is our hope that the nursing process presented in this chapter will help the nurse to begin to meet the needs of these clients and their significant others, as well as the nurse.

THE THREAT OF SUICIDE

DESCRIPTION

Suicide is a continuum of self-destructive behaviors that, without intervention, would result in death. This continuum ranges from habitual self-inflicted, life-threatening behaviors to isolated acts that could result in instant death. For the purposes of this section, the suicidal patient is one who (1) is thinking about committing a self-destructive act, (2) is expressing the intent to commit a self-destructive act, or (3) has recently attempted or committed a self-destructive act.

The rate of suicides in the United States in 1979 was 12.0 per 100,000 persons. The ratio between suicide attempts and committed suicides was 8:1. The threat of a suicide is at least as common as the attempts.

There can be three outcomes to the suicidal threat:

1. The threat subsides.
2. The threat remains.
3. The threat becomes a psychiatric emergency (see Chapter 50). Such psychiatric emergencies would include situations in which
   a. The nurse considers the situation beyond control.

b. The client has a lethal weapon, such as a gun or a knife, in hand.
c. The client has made an actual suicide attempt.

PREVENTION

Health Promotion

The client will
1. Develop support systems.
2. Develop self-awareness of strengths and needs.
3. Develop direct communication.
4. Attend life-strategy classes or coping skills training.
5. Seek crisis intervention therapy.

Population at Risk

At some point in nearly everyone's life the thought of suicide is present. People at greatest risk are usually those under stress, without support systems, and without adequate coping mechanisms. The known factors associated with the populations at risk are presented in Table 38-1.

Screening

1. Mental status assessment.
2. Zung Self-rating Depression Scale.
3. Social Readjustment Rating Scale by T. Holmes and R. Rahe.

ASSESSMENT

Health History

1. Assess the client's status in relation to the populations at risk. See Table 38-1.
2. Suicidal plan: ask the client directly about suicidal plan (e.g., "*How* do you plan to kill yourself?"). Assess
   a. Lethality of method. Hanging, jumping from high places, and use of a gun are more lethal and involve higher risk than taking pills or cutting wrist.
   b. Availability of method (e.g., does client have the gun in hand, or must it be purchased?).

TABLE 38-1 POPULATION AT RISK FOR SUICIDE

Sociocultural Variable	Suicide Risk/Rate Increased in Following Populations
Age	Aged—risk increases steadily with age Adolescents—second cause of death among college students
Sex	Male—three times more likely to commit suicide than females; females, however, three times more likely to attempt suicide
Race	White higher than black American Indians three times higher than national rate
Nationality	Americans and Japanese
Occupation	Professionals, especially psychiatrists and lawyers
Religion	Protestants
Family	Divorced, widowed, and single higher than married persons Persons who have nuclear or extended family members who have attempted or committed suicide
Support systems	Persons without support systems
Recent loss	Persons who have lost significant others through divorce, separation, or death Persons commemorating 1 year anniversary of death of significant other Persons who have lost health, job, prestige
Psychiatric problems	Depressed persons Psychotic persons, especially those who hear voices Substance abusers, especially alcoholics Persons who have previously attemtped suicide

   c. Specificity of details. Has preparation been made? Has time been set? Bizarre details are less threatening, unless the client is psychotic.
3. Previous suicide attempts. The person who has made a previous suicide attempt is likely to resort to the same behavior again.
4. Communication that indicates that the client is thinking of suicide.
   a. Verbal.
      (1) Direct statements such as, "I'm going to kill myself!"
      (2) Indirect statements such as, "There isn't any point in going on!" or "Take these golf clubs; I won't be needing them any more."
      (3) Cessation of verbal communication, especially with family and significant others.
   b. Nonverbal.
      (1) Writing letters to ask forgiveness, to forgive others, or to say goodbye.
      (2) Writing a will.
      (3) Unexpectedly buying a life insurance policy.
      (4) Changes in attitudes toward personal possessions (e.g., refusing to spend money for new possessions or giving possessions away).
      (5) Sudden changes in behavior that are uncharacteristic, such as taking walks at midnight or staying in room alone for hours.
5. Evidence of depression (See *Depression* sections in Chapter 36).
   a. Change in sleep patterns, especially awakening in early morning (2 to 5 A.M.).
   b. Loss of appetite.
   c. Weight loss.
   d. Despondency.
   e. Apathy.
   f. Severe feelings of helplessness and hopelessness.
   g. Physical and psychological exhaustion.
   h. Lessening of depression: client has more energy to actually carry out a self-destructive act.
   i. Overtly cheerful behavior for no apparent reason. The decision to kill oneself may be followed by relief and unexplained lessening of depressive symptoms.
6. Strengths: the patient's inner resources can be mobilized to deal with current stress.
   a. Ability to respond by accepting directions.
   b. Ability to reach out to other people for help.
   c. Improvement in mood and thinking during course of conversation.
   d. Past history of success in interpersonal relationships.
7. Support systems. Suicide risk is higher in the absence of support systems. Assess immediately available support systems. Who is with the client now? Who is available to stay with the client?
8. Recent and/or significant losses of persons, status, or health increases suicidal risk.
9. Some conditions can precipitate impulsive acts to obtain relief from anxiety. These conditions warrant special consideration because there may be no other clues to the self-destructive act.
   a. Extreme fear and anxiety.
   b. Hallucinations that are verbally persecutory and self-accusatory or visually tormenting. Client may respond to "voice's" command to kill self. Client may attempt suicide in an effort to silence or get away from threatening, unfriendly voices (see Chapter 39.)
   c. Delusional thinking that is threatening in content (see Chapter 39).
10. Determination. A client who must maintain control over environment, no matter how anguished or incapacitated, could implement suicidal plan even when it seems impossible. A determined client who seems too apathetic to get out of bed, for example, may jump from the window during a change of shifts.

Emergency Assessment

In emergency situations, when a complete assessment of suicidal risk cannot be accomplished, the nurse should assess

1. Suicidal plan. Ask client directly about the suicidal plan (e.g., "How do you plan to kill yourself?"). Assess
   a. Lethality of method. Hanging, jumping from high places, and use of a gun are more lethal and involve higher risk than taking pills or cutting wrist.

b. Availability of method. Does client have gun, pill, and so on, in hand, or must they be obtained?
c. Specificity of details. Has preparation been made? Has time been set? Bizarre details are less threatening, unless client is psychotic.

2. Previous suicide attempts. The client who has made a previous suicide attempt is more likely to resort to the same behavior again.
3. Age: risk increases with age.
4. Sex: men are more likely than women to commit suicide; women are more likely than men to attempt suicide.
5. Precipitating events or stress must be evaluated from the client's point of view. Some stresses to be considered were listed under Health History, above. Ask client questions such as, "What about life seems so intolerable that you want to kill yourself?"
6. Immediately available support systems. Who is with the client now? Who is available to stay with the client? Who is close to the client?

Diagnostic Tests

Only the potential or risk for a suicide attempt can be assessed. There are no specific diagnostic tests.

NURSING DIAGNOSES: ACTUAL OR POTENTIAL

1. Potential for self-injury.
2. Delayed grieving; perceived loss.
3. Impaired verbal communication.
4. Social isolation.
5. Perceptual/cognitive disruptions, e.g., hallucinations, delusions.
6. Diminished support systems.

EXPECTED OUTCOMES

1. The client will be protected from self-destruction until able to assume this responsibility.
2. The client will report suicidal thoughts, delusions, and/or hallucinations each time they occur.
3. The client will engage in at least one easily accomplished task each day.
4. The client will verbalize one positive statement about self and/or one reason for living each day.
5. Within 1 week, the client will begin verbally to identify feelings of anger in response to loss.
6. The client will verbalize alternative behaviors to suicide within 1 week.
7. Within 1 week, the client will begin to reestablish relationships with friends and family or establish new relationships when none are present.
8. Within 1 week, the client will identify stressful life situations that seem to precipitate suicidal thoughts and that can be changed.

INTERVENTIONS

All nursing interventions for the suicidal or self-destructive client are based on the belief that the client is ambivalent, that is, wants to live *and* wants to die.

Interpersonal relationships are the greatest deterrent to suicide. A sense of someone listening and caring is essential to human survival. The nurse is a temporary lifeline. From the first contact with a suicidal person, plan for the establishment or the continuance of the usual social relationships.

1. Have one nurse on each shift establish a one-to-one relationship with the client.
2. Do not leave client alone.
3. As suicide risk decreases, decrease observations to frequent, irregular intervals (every 5 to 10 minutes).
4. Search client's personal belongings.
5. Remove dangerous objects, such as razor blades, drugs, nail files, glass objects, cords, belts, panty hose, and neckties.
6. Explain why personal belongings are removed and that they will be returned.
7. Give the client a semiprivate room near the nurses' station.
8. Notify the family or significant others that the client is suicidal.
9. Do not agree to keep secret the client's reported thoughts or plans of suicide.
10. Give medication in liquid form.
11. Supply nourishment and physical care as needed.
12. Instruct the client warmly and emphatically of the necessity of always delaying any self-destructive impulse and of calling for help.
13. Approach the client with a hopeful attitude. Avoid overly cheerful attitude.
14. Encourage tasks that the client can successfully accomplish in less than 1 hour.

15. Encourage diversional activities that can be an outlet for angry feelings, such as pounding copper in occupational therapy, bowling, working out on a punching bag, and throwing a medicine ball.
16. Avoid contact sports that could provoke the release of stored-up fury and competitive activities that could lead to a sense of failure.
17. Help the client to participate gradually in group activities to prevent isolation and withdrawal.
18. Allow the client to verbalize suicidal thoughts.
    a. Do not ignore or argue about threats.
    b. Take statement seriously; it is communication, not an idle gesture. The idea that people who talk about suicide will not commit suicide is a myth.
    c. Validate the client's feelings.
    d. Do not share your interpretation of the meaning of the suicidal behavior with the client.
19. Remind client that suicide is one alternative and that there are other alternatives available.
20. Help the client's family and significant others identify and share their feelings. Feelings that they may experience are embarrassment, guilt, anger, self-doubt, and confusion.
21. Help client's family and significant others identify support systems that may be useful to them.
22. Observe circumstances under which suicidal behavior occurs.
23. Help client identify the early signs and symptoms of suicidal behavior.
24. Help client identify specific stresses precipitating suicidal behavior.
25. Help client identify solutions, other than suicide, to recognized stresses.
26. Have client list personal strengths to use in coping with stress.
27. Reinforce positive actions and responses to stress.
28. Avoid confronting the client with your observation of improvement. Confronting with improvement, before the client is ready to acknowledge it, may precipitate suicidal response. Allow the client to identify improvement in self.
29. Also see Interventions sections under *Depression* headings in Chapter 36.

Telephone Interventions

The nurse on a psychiatric inpatient unit or in the emergency room may receive a telephone call from a client threatening suicide or self-destructive acts. The following interventions are designed to help the nurse meet this situation.

1. Establish a caring and firm relationship with the suicidal person.
    a. Listen carefully.
    b. Talk and respond. Do not simply reflect feelings.
    c. Make direct and hopeful statements (e.g., "It sounds as if you want to live, and I can and will help you.").
2. Obtain basic information.
    a. Who are you?
    b. Where are you?
3. Complete assessment of suicidal risk can be found under Assessment, above.
4. Assist the person to identify and clarify the perceived focal problem. What is making life intolerable at this moment? Why is client calling at this time?
5. Be directive, and make decisions for the person (e.g., "I am going to send someone to your house now. You keep talking to me.").
6. Involve significant others and all possible support systems. Who is with the client? Do not rely on client to contact this person.
7. Make contact with appropriate resource for follow-up care. Ask client for preference. Options available are crisis center, community mental health center, police, private therapist, private doctor, doctor on call.

Nurse's Feelings and Responses

Other peers and team members are a potential support system that the nurse has for sharing and dealing with feelings about suicidal clients. It is important for the nurse to use this support system. The nurse needs to be aware of personal responses to the suicidal client, especially the client who has already attempted suicide. The nurse may

1. Experience anxiety when faced with a suicidal client, since this brings to consciousness the thoughts or fantasies of suicide that everyone has at one time or another.
2. Feel anger because the nurse was able to control own impulse to escape through suicide and the client was not.
3. Feel burdened by the responsibility for pre-

venting self-destructive behavior, which in turn causes tension and anxiety.
4. Feel frustrated and drained from the dependency of the client on the nurse.
5. Have fantasies of rescuing the client all alone.
6. Feel angry and incompetent if the client attempts suicide in spite of nursing interventions.
7. Judge the client's behavior in the context of the nurse's own life (e.g., a client who attempts suicide to escape marriage may be judged harshly by a nurse whose spouse is dead).

EVALUATION

Outcome Criteria

1. Client is alive.
2. Client has not attempted suicide.
3. Client independently performs activities of daily living.
4. Client verbally and/or physically expresses anger in socially acceptable ways.
5. Client is able to identify and list personal strengths.
6. Client has identified at least one solution, other than suicide, to stressful life situations.
7. Client has identified and made contact with one person who can provide emotional support.

Complications

1. Suicide attempt (see Chapter 50).
2. Death.

Reevaluation and Follow-up

1. Be certain that client has reestablished at least one personal tie.
2. Determine that living arrangements are such that the client will not be alone.
3. Teach significant other the behavioral clues to suicide.
4. Teach significant other, without causing alarm, that the first month after discharge is a critical period for suicide risk.
5. Have client and significant other consider the choice of family therapy, if indicated (see Chapter 43).
6. Reassess with client and significant other their possible support systems in the community: friends, neighbors, relatives, clergy, community mental health center, police, visiting nurses, nurses in college and university health services, emergency referral agencies, social work agencies, legal counsel.
7. Review with client the early signs and symptoms of suicidal behavior.
8. Review with client alternative ways (other than suicide) of dealing with stress.
9. Encourage client to see an outpatient therapist before discharge and to continue with the same therapist.
10. Set up the first appointment for outpatient visit with therapist.
11. Give client the telephone number and address of the suicide prevention center or emergency referral agency.

THE THREAT OF VIOLENCE

DESCRIPTION

Violence is a continuum of physically destructive behaviors that, without intervention, would result in injury, damage, or destruction to other persons or property. This continuum ranges from minor property damage to murder. Violence toward persons demands a life-risking response from the nurse. In violence toward property, the nurse accepts the responsibility of controlling the violence only when there is no life-threatening risk. Violence by the hospitalized client rarely occurs but, understandably, the fear among nurses is that it will occur. Both the client's behavior and the responsibility of the nurse are frightening.

For the purposes of this section, the violent client will be defined as one who is either thinking about committing violence or expressing verbally or physically the intent to commit a violent act. The client who is actually committing a physically destructive act requiring immediate intervention is considered a psychiatric emergency. The nursing process for this client can be found in Chapter 50.

PREVENTION

Health Promotion

The client will

1. Attend anger and/or stress management classes.
2. Attend assertiveness training classes.

Population at Risk

Psychotic disturbances due to either functional or organic states can precipitate impulsive acts of violence.

1. Persons with acute organic brain syndrome, due to
   a. General toxemia.
   b. Intoxication and/or withdrawal from alcohol and/or other drugs.
   c. Trauma.
2. Persons with functional psychotic disturbances (see also Chapter 39), such as
   a. Delusional thinking that is threatening in content.
   b. Hallucinations that are verbally persecutory or visually tormenting.
   c. Bipolar depression, manic phase.

ASSESSMENT

Health History

1. Assess the client's status in relation to the populations at risk.
2. History of previous destructive behaviors or violence. At what point and under what conditions is self-control lost?

Mental Status Assessment

1. Affect.
   a. Intensity is marked.
   b. Angry facial expression is usually present.
   c. Tense facial expression is usually present.
   d. Labile; rapid fluctuation to extremes.
   e. Client may be belligerent.
2. Verbalizations.
   a. Threats, such as "I'm going to hit you."
   b. Apprehension, fear, or concern about losing control, such as "I'm going to blow up," or "I'm afraid I'm going to hit someone."
   c. Indirect threats, such as "I hate you."
3. Motor activity.
   a. Agitation; inability to sit still, pacing.
   b. Sudden cessation of activity; uneasy, tense stillness.
   c. Intensity; pounding, slamming, stomping.
   d. Jumpiness.
   e. Rigid, tense posture.
4. Paranoid delusions may be present.
5. Auditory and visual hallucinations may be present.

Environmental Assessment

The situation in which the threat occurs is usually one in which the client perceives the threat of annihilation either through destruction of physical self, or, perhaps even more frightening, through destruction of self-esteem. The client's threat is a desperate attempt to defend self against this threat of annihilation.

1. Where is client?
2. Who is with client?
3. How lethal is the situation?
4. Is the situation obviously provoking client to threaten violence, and can the situation be changed? Client, for example, is being harassed by roommate, who can be moved to another room until the two of them are able to resolve the problem.
5. How does client perceive the situation?
6. What is clients' relationship to others? To whom does this client relate best?
7. Are alcohol and/or more serious drugs present on the unit?

NURSING DIAGNOSES: ACUTAL OR POTENTIAL

1. Perceived threat to self with violent response.
2. Expression of anger and fear through verbal threats.
3. Potential violent behavior toward others.
4. Delusions (see Chapter 39.)
5. Hallucinations (see Chapter 39.)
6. Potential loss of self-control.
7. Fear.
8. Maladaptive coping patterns.

EXPECTED OUTCOMES

The client will

1. Be prevented from harming others.
2. Discuss threatening situations as they occur and identify the stresses that are perceived as threats to self.
3. Identify ways to avoid recognized stresses.
4. Identify consequences of losing self-control.
5. Identify alternative behaviors to losing self-control.
6. Identify and report feelings of losing control each time these occur.

INTERVENTIONS

Administrative Interventions

Nursing administration has an important responsibility in the control of violent behavior on the nursing unit. This responsibility includes

1. The establishment of a therapeutic milieu staffed by well-trained and caring personnel.
2. The establishment of a standard plan of ac-

tion, with stated expectations for staff responses to violent behavior.

3. Designating one person on each shift as leader/coordinator of the plan of action whose orders must be followed immediately and without question.
4. Educating the staff to the plan of action and to therapeutic interventions in the prevention and control of violence.
5. Providing a "quiet room," a specific room with provisions for privacy, decreased stimulation, and safety.
6. Holding a staff meeting to review staff responses to the threat of violence.

Specific Interventions

1. Take the threat of violence seriously.
2. Remove others who may be in danger as quickly as possible.
3. Look for immediate stresses that could be provoking the threat, such as another person arguing with the client.
4. Allow distance. Touch may be the final threat to loss of control.
5. Speak to the client in a calm, firm, reassuring manner.
6. Call client by name.
7. Explain clearly and directly that client is expected to control own behavior (e.g., "Calm down. You can control yourself.").
8. Verbally acknowledge client's dangerous potential, for example, "Look, you could really have hurt someone with that pool cue." This confirms the client's stance and reduces the need to be defensive.
9. Verbally set limits on behavior (e.g., "I'm not going to let you hit anyone with that pool cue. Put it down and let's talk."). Talking is an effective way of helping client to regain self-control.
10. Verbally acknowledge client's feelings (e.g., "You seem very frightened.").
11. Offer medication. If client refuses, offer again at a later time. If client becomes violent, and medication must be given despite refusal, the nurse needs to be aware of state mental health legislation governing the administration of medications without consent.
12. Do not threaten client with the use of force (e.g., "If you don't do as I say, I'll lock you up."). The threat of force could
    a. Be seen as a challenge and, thus, create a power struggle.
    b. Increase the client's fear and escalate the threat of violence into a violent act.
    c. Decrease the client's confidence in the nurse's ability to control the environment if the nurse is not capable of carrying out the threat.
    d. Result in client's viewing the use of force as a punishment rather than an adjunct to self-control.
13. Give client the opportunity to go to the "quiet room" with one staff member, preferably one to whom client best relates. Other team members should be alerted and prepared to initiate the predetermined plan of action if the need arises.
14. Do not leave client alone.
15. Help client to identify and discuss feelings concerning the incident.
16. Explore with client past feelings and/or events of violence that may have been similar to the present incident.
17. Help client identify early signs of losing control.
18. Help client identify specific stresses that precipitate loss of control.
19. Help client identify the consequences of violent behavior.
20. Help client identify solutions, other than violence, to identified stresses.
21. Provide constructive physical outlets for the expression of feelings (e.g., brisk walks, gardening).
22. Use physical force only if client is actually violent toward another person. The need for the use of physcial force may be greater with the psychotic patient who is less likely to repond to the verbal intervention of the nurse. When the use of force is necessary, it needs to be carried out as swiftly as possible, avoiding physical pain and undue humiliation to client.
23. Apply mechanical restraints only if absolutely necessary. The client fearing loss of control occasionally requests the use of mechanical restraints. This request needs to be respected. The restraints are perceived by client as providing the control he or she is seeking. On the other hand, the nurse needs to be familiar with state mental health legislation before restraining the unwilling client.
24. Use seclusion as an alternative to restraints. The seclusion room is stripped of all furnishings except a mattress. There should be

no exposed light bulbs or glass and no access to the bathroom. Ideally, the room is a neutral or calming color, such as green.

25. Notify client's family or significant others; they may be able to calm client.

Nurse's Feelings and Responses

1. The nurse's fear of personal injury is a natural response to client's threat of violence. The degree of fear will be different for each nurse, depending on how life threatening the client's threat is considered. Feelings of fear can be paralyzing, or they may signal the presence of danger and the need for intervention with client. Fear can also evoke a variety of responses from the nurse. The nurse may
   a. Have the impulse to run away. A wise nurse may leave temporarily to seek the assistance of others. This is not running away.
   b. Feel anger and outrage at client's threat and threaten client in return (e.g., "If you do that, I'll lock you up," or, "I'll take your privileges away"). Such threats of retaliation create a power struggle in which no one wins.
   c. Acquiesce to client's demands even when it is not safe to do so.
   d. Be judgmental and rejecting, since client's behavior is contrary to nurse's values.
   e. Feel anxious that he or she will not be able to control the situation and that actual violence will occur.
   f. Be concerned that peers or supervisor will not approve of the way the nurse intervened.
   g. See in client nurse's own potential for losing control.
2. Being in touch with one's own unique responses to the threat of violence is a prerequisite to effective intervention. Other peers and members of the health team are a potential support system that the nurse has for sharing and dealing with responses.

EVALUATION

Outcome Criteria

1. Client has not harmed others.
2. Number of threatening situations to client and/or others will decrease.
3. Client verbalizes own fear.
4. Client verbalizes consequences of loss of self-control.
5. Client verbally and/or physically expresses anger in socially acceptable ways (e.g., using assertive communications or jogging).

Complications

Acts of violence. (See Chapter 50).

Reevaluation and Follow-up

1. With client. The follow-up care for the client who threatens violence is dependent on the underlying problem (alcoholism, manic depression, elevated blood urea nitrogen (BUN) level, etc.). The nurse will need to identify this problem in order to provide follow-up care for client.
2. With client's family or significant others.
   a. Help them to identify and share their feelings (e.g., guilt, embarrassment, fear of having client return home).
   b. Help them identify support systems that can be useful to them.
3. With other clients. Follow-up with clients against whom the threat was directed or those who witnessed the threat, is a primary action. If the incident creates general agitation among other clients, they would also be included in the follow-up.
   a. Verbally reassure them that the danger is over and that they are safe.
   b. Encourage discussion of their feelings and reactions to the incident.
   c. Validate their feelings concerning the incident.
4. With staff.
   a. Discuss and evaluate what happened and why.
   b. Discuss and share their feelings surrounding the incident.
   c. Discuss questions such as
      (1) Did the staff threaten client with physical force?
      (2) Was the nurse involved in a power struggle?
      (3) Was physical force used as a last resort?
      (4) Was force meant to be punitive or therapeutic?
      (5) Which interventions were most successful?

BIBLIOGRAPHY

Bailey, D. S., and Dreyer, S. O.: *Therapeutic Approaches to the Care of the Mentally Ill*, F. A. Davis, Philadelphia, 1977.

Basic textbook for mental health workers. Concepts of communication are stressed. Interventions with suicidal clients are very specific, and a suicide intervention rating scale is provided. Has helpful chapter on interventions with aggressive clients.

Burgess, A. W.: *Psychiatric Nursing in the Hospital and the Community*, 3d ed., Prentice-Hall, Englewood Cliffs, N.J., 1981. The central focus of this book is humanistic. Attention is paid to stalls in the therapeutic process and the humanness of the nurse. It discusses management of suicidal clients.

DiFabio, S., and Ackerhalt, E. J.: "Teaching the Use of Restraint Through Role Play," *Perspectives in Psychiatric Care*, **16**(5–6):218, September–December 1978. Authors present a seminar program designed to prepare the nurse to intervene therapeutically in an emergency situation with a physically assaultive client.

Farberow, N. L., and Shneidman, E. I. (eds.): *The Cry for Help*, McGraw-Hill, New York, 1961. Focuses on the message of anguish and the plea for help that is expressed by and contained within suicidal behaviors. It presents both community and psychotherapeutic responses to that cry for help.

Grace, H. K., Layton, J., and Camilleri, D.: *Mental Health Nursing*, William C. Brown, Dubuque, Iowa, 1977. Theoretical framework integrates social systems, social-psychological perspectives, growth and development, and crisis concepts. Views suicidal behavior as a severe restriction in the effectiveness of a person's problem-solving activity.

Grosicki, J. P. (ed.), and the Committee on Research in Clinical Nursing of VA Hospital, North Little Rock, Arkansas, Division: *Nursing Action Guides*, U.S. Government Printing Office, Washington, D.C., 1970. This text focuses on nursing interventions and their rationales. Identifies problems that interfere with the accomplishment of goals.

Haber, J., Leach, A., Schudy, S., and Sideleau, B. F.: *Comprehensive Psychiatric Nursing*, McGraw-Hill, New York, 1982. A truly comprehensive book on psychiatric nursing. Develops the nursing process with both suicidal and violent clients.

Hankoff, L. D., and Einsidler, B. (eds.): *Suicide: Theory and Clinical Aspects*, PSG Publishing, Littleton, Mass., 1979. This volume presents the historical background of suicide, contemporary value systems, the biology and psychology of suicidal behavior, specific risk subgroups, and guidelines for the management and prevention of suicide.

Hart, N. A., and Keidel, G. C.: "The Suicidal Adolescent," *American Journal of Nursing*, **79**:80, January 1979. This article focuses on primary and secondary prevention of suicide in the high-risk group of adolescents.

Holmes, T. H., and Rahe, R. H.: "The Social Readjustment Rating Scale," *Journal of Psychosomatic Research*, **11**:213, 1967. Research has established that a cluster of social events requiring a significant change in life adjustment is associated with the onset of illness. This article reports research in which subjects rank a series of life events relative to their degrees of necessary readjustment.

Joel, L. A., and Collins, D. L.: *Psychiatric Nursing: Theory and Application*, McGraw-Hill, New York, 1978. Nursing theory and process are developed for working with clients individually, in groups, and in the family. Crisis intervention and community theory are also included.

Jourard, S. M.: "Suicide, an Invitation to Die," *American Journal of Nursing*, **70**:269, February 1970. Proposes that a person destroys him- or herself in response to an invitation originating from others that he or she stop living and that a person lives in response to the repeated invitation to continue living.

Karshmer, J. F.: "The Application of Social Learning Theory to Aggression," *Perspectives in Psychiatric Care*, **16**(5–6):223, September–December 1978. Compares and contrasts two methods of intervening with the violent client. The methods of intervention are based on drive theory and social learning theory.

Lathrop, V. G.: "Aggression as a Response," *Perspectives in Psychiatric Care*, **16**(5–6):203, September–December 1978. The author defines aggression and gives factors in the staff's approach to a client that may be perceived by the client as threatening.

Lenefsky, B., de Palma, T., and Locicero, D.: "Management of Violent Behaviors," *Perspectives in Psychiatric Care*, **16**(5–6):212, September–December 1978. The authors present an orderly, planned team procedure and rationale for restraining the violent client. Includes photographs showing how to restrain client.

Loughlin, Sister N.: "Suicide: A Case for Investigation," *Journal of Psychiatric Nursing and Mental Health Services*, **18**(2):8, February 1980. Using a case study format, the author presents statistics, causes, clues, and general prevention related to suicide.

Reubin, Richard: "Spotting and Stopping the Suicide Patient," *Nursing '79*, **9**:83, April 1979. This is a concise article on assessment of clues to suicide and nursing interventions.

Ross, E.: "Suicide and the States of Grief," *Death Education*, **2**:407, 1979. A woman's retrospective look at her husband's suicide and her own grieving.

Rumpler, C. H., and Seigerman, C.: "A Behavior Modification Approach to Dealing with Violent Behavior in an Intensive Care Unit," *Perspectives in Psychiatric Care*, **16**(5–6):206, September–December 1978. Presents a case study to describe the use of a token economy system to give the client control of and responsibility for his behavior. Program is described in detail.

Shneidman, E. S.: *Suicidology: Contemporary Developments*, Grune and Stratton, New York, 1976. Currently active suicidologists contributed essays to this book concerning contemporary problems in suicide.

Shneidman, E. S. (ed.): *Death: Current Perspectives*, Mayfield Publishing, Palo Alto, Calif., 1976. A compilation of selected contemporary literature on the subject of death and dying from the cultural, societal, interpersonal, and personal perspectives.

Shneidman, E. S., Farberow, N. L., and Litman, R. E.: *The Psychology of Suicide*, Science House, New York, 1970. This is a collection of writings by the three men who initiated, organized, and administered the first suicide prevention center, the Los Angeles Suicide Prevention Center. It contains a wealth of information derived from the authors' personal experiences and research.

Sletten, I., and Barton, J.: "Suicide Patients in the Emergency Room: A Guide for Evaluation and Disposition," *Hospital and Community Psychiatry,* **30**(6):407, June 1979. The authors summarize three rating scales (J. Tuckman and W. Youngman; A. D. Weisman and J. W. Worden; M. Kovacs, A. Beck, and A. Weissman) for evaluating the suicide potential of clients who have attempted or threatened suicide. The authors cite the original sources for the rating scales.

Stewart, A. T.: "Handling the Aggressive Patient," *Perspectives in Psychiatric Care,* **16**(5–6):228, September–December 1978. Succinctly presents ways to prevent violence as well as ways to defend yourself when the client becomes violent. Includes photographs showing how to restrain client.

Stuart, G. W., and Sundeen, S. J.: *Principles and Practice of Psychiatric Nursing,* C. V. Mosby, St. Louis, 1979. Comprehensively presents the nursing process for problems of self-destructive and violent behaviors.

Whaley, M. S., and Ramirez, L. F.: "The Use of Seclusion Rooms and Physical Restraints in the Treatment of Psychiatric Patients," *Journal of Psychiatric Nursing and Mental Health Services,* **18**(1):13, January 1980. Provides guidelines for the therapeutic use of seclusion and restraints.

Wilson, H. S., and Kneisl, C. R.: *Psychiatric Nursing,* 2d ed., Addison-Wesley, Menlo Park, Calif., 1983. General psychiatric nursing textbook. Deals with suicide as it relates to various groups of people, including adolescents and alcoholics. Gives criteria for assessing lethality of suicide plan.

Zung, W. W. K.: "A Self-Rating Depression Scale," *Archives of General Psychiatry,* **12**:63, 1965. A self-rating scale for the quantitative measurement of depression.

39

Disruptions of Perceptual and Cognitive Functions

Martha J. Snider

The perceptual and cognitive functions of the acutely ill psychiatric client are affected in a plethora of ways. These dysfunctions constitute a wide array of clinical problems and require creative and flexible approaches by nursing staff. The most commonly encountered dysfunctions of perception and cognition are hallucinations and delusions. The two often present simultaneously in clients who are seriously disturbed. The interventions suggested for these clinical problems can be adapted to the individual client and can provide guidelines for dealing with other related problems. It is important to recognize that delusions and hallucinations are highly individualized in content and are directly related to intense psychological needs and to attempts to explain disturbing personal experiences. The hallucinatory and delusional behaviors presented are always purposeful and have meaning to the client.

HALLUCINATIONS

DESCRIPTION

Hallucinations are subjective experiences of sensory perceptions for which there are no corresponding external stimuli. These perceptual experiences may involve any sensorial sphere and usually occur in the presence of a clear consciousness. Perceptual images from the auditory, visual, kinesthetic, olfactory, tactile, and gustatory spheres may be projected onto the environment; that is, the client associates these perceptions as coming from outside the self. The hallucinatory process may characterize clients with sensory deprivation, brain lesions, oxygen deficiency, the chemical effects of psychoactive drugs, insufficient REM sleep, and psychoses.

The auditory sphere is most commonly affected in clients suffering from the group of syndromes known as schizophrenia. Although visual hallucinations are not rare, they usually occur in concert with hallucinations affecting other spheres. *Auditory hallucinations* can take the form of noise, voices that converse with the client, and voices that converse about the client. Voices may be accusatory, critical, comforting, or advising. The client may be able to identify the voices, or the voices may seem to be unfamiliar. Auditory hallucinations may occur occasionally or often at any time during the waking state. The onset of the process may follow a real or fantasized loss of a significant other. Often, the onset may be accompanied by anxiety and be of considerable distress to the client.

The primary stimulus for the hallucinatory experience is the need for psychological self-protection from painful feelings related to guilt, loneliness, anger, fear of abandonment by loved ones, and uncontrollable ego-alien impulses, thoughts, and feelings. In general, anything that seriously threatens self-esteem and the integrity and unity of the familiar self has significance to the process and content of hallucinations. Threats to self-esteem and the integrity of the familiar self result in high levels of anxiety. As anxiety increases, the ability to sort out and organize perceptions and recognize the differences between thoughts and feelings that are generated by the self decreases. Ambiguity of meaning and source increase, and rational processes lose effectiveness. It becomes increasingly difficult to determine which auditory stimuli come from one's own mind and which come from one's environment.

PREVENTION

Health Promotion

1. Encourage conditions that augment integration of ego functions, such as warm and stable home environments.
2. Learn to deal with reality in ways other than fantasy.

Population at Risk

1. All cultures are affected.
2. Some evidence that lower socioeconomic groups are at higher risk.
3. Children of parents who have experienced hallucinations.
4. Persons with difficulty in the ability to initiate and maintain interpersonal relationships that are mutually growth producing.
5. Persons with history of traumatic experiences in childhood, such as rejection, overprotectiveness, or parental aggression.

ASSESSMENT

Health History

Use format suggested in Chapter 36. Note especially the following:

1. Client's memory of onset of sounds not validated by others.
2. Circumstances surrounding onset of hallucinations.
3. Possible relationships between perceptual (hallucinatory) experiences and cognitive (delusional) experiences.
4. Changes in the nature of the auditory experiences (e.g., from critical to comforting, from noise to voice, from unfamiliar to familiar sounds).
5. The duration of the experiences and the diurnal nature of onset.
6. Related changes in the client's life.
7. Drug and other substance use.

Physical Assessment

Neurological examination to rule out definitive organic origin.

Diagnostic Tests

1. Electroencephalogram to rule out frank organic origin.
2. Laboratory studies to rule out metabolic, infectious, or other pathophysiological phenomena that may affect the central nervous system.

NURSING DIAGNOSES: ACUTAL OR POTENTIAL

1. Perceptual alterations associated with loss of contact with reality.
2. Thought impairment coincident with perceptual alteration.

EXPECTED OUTCOMES

1. Decrease in the number of hallucinatory experiences.
2. Decrease in the anxiety level that leads to hallucinations.
3. Identification of needs served by the hallucinatory experience.
4. Increase in the ability to test reality at the onset of a hallucination.
5. Cessation of hallucinatory experiences.
6. Able to intervene in the process without the aid of others.
7. Understand the needs that provoke hallucinatory experiences.
8. Meet interpersonal needs in ways that are more productive.

INTERVENTIONS

1. Assist the client in increasing interpersonal competence through a one-to-one relationship.
2. Arrange a daily schedule with the client so that specific needs are met in a predictable fashion.

3. Teach the client to test reality through seeking consensual validation for perceptual experiences.
4. Indicate doubt as to the reality of a hallucinatory experience.
5. Offer alternative explanations for concrete conclusions that the client develops in support of hallucinations.
6. Indicate in a direct fashion that the hallucination may seem real to the client but is not shared by the nurse.
7. Avoid reflective responses, such as "You hear voices telling you to run away?"
8. Do use declarative responses when discussing feelings evoked by the hallucinatory experience (e.g., "It must be scary to hear voices that no one else can hear").
9. Utilize directive responses when the client hallucinates while talking with you (e.g., "Listen to me, look at me, do not pay attention to the so-called voices right now!").
10. Observe the relationship between evidence of increasing anxiety and the onset of hallucinations. Intervene in the anxiety immediately. (See Chapter 36 for additional ways of dealing with anxiety.)
11. Provide regular physical activity that requires the use of large muscle groups and necessitates concentration.
12. Direct the client to notify staff when he or she fears that an experience of hearing the so-called voices is imminent.
13. Anticipate the situations that seem most likely to evoke hallucinatory behavior.
14. Teach the client to intervene in the hallucinatory experience by active interdiction (e.g., "Go away" or "You are not real").
15. Observe for side effects of psychoactive drugs. Assess the lowest effective dose that will help diminish hallucinations and related symptoms.
16. Help the client assume increasing amounts of responsibility for intervening into the hallucinatory process as he or she becomes less anxious. Focus less and less on the problem as the anxiety level becomes manageable and as interpersonal needs are met in more appropriate ways.
17. Provide the opportunity for group-oriented activities as soon as the anxiety level is consistently below the level evocative of hallucinatory behavior.
18. Reevaluate the entire plan of intervention, particularly in regard to the assessment of self-esteem levels, if elaboration of hallucinatory experiences occurs in terms of the number of affected sensorial spheres and/or if a related delusional system becomes more global and fixed.
19. Provide for continuity of intervention through a mental health clinic.
20. Help develop plans for appropriate social outlets in the community.
21. Provide for consistent monitoring of psychoactive drug regimen.

EVALUATION

Outcome Criteria

1. Hallucinatory experiences decrease in frequency and intensity within 2 weeks.
2. Client is able to employ own devices to defer hallucinatory experiences.
3. Client is able to be free of hallucinatory experiences without the use of psychoactive drugs.
4. Client is able to increase socialization skills to a moderate degree in contrast to baseline data.

Complications

1. Other sensorial spheres become involved in the hallucinatory process.
2. The hallucinatory experience completely replaces contacts with the real world.

Assessment

1. Change route of medication to liquid and observe for 1 week.
2. Reexamine immediate interpersonal environment for reinforcers for the hallucinatory process.

Revised Outcomes

1. Hallucinatory experiences will reconvert to one sensorial sphere.
2. Other goals, as stated above.

Interventions

1. Continue to actively interdict hallucinatory experiences in all spheres.
2. Change route of psychoactive drugs to parenteral only if necessary.

Reevaluation and Follow-up

Psychological deterioration will probably necessitate continued close observation until elaboration of symptoms subside.

DELUSIONS

DESCRIPTION

Delusions are fixed, false beliefs that are maintained regardless of objective evidence and logical argument presented contrary to those beliefs. Further, the beliefs are not shared by others of similar educational and sociocultural background. These beliefs are developed to protect the client from anxiety and insecurity. The trends and themes represented are idiosyncratic in that they are determined by the client's problems and needs. Delusions are considered to be extreme deviations in thought process and content. There is probably some adjustment value in the phenomenon.

The varieties of delusion include those of control or influence, persecution, grandeur, guilt, bodily disorders, or absence of bodily parts. Delusions of persecution are frequently observed among seriously ill psychiatric clients, as are beliefs regarding external control and influence.

It is important to recognize the fixed character of delusions and to understand that the process is representative of attempts to deal with the problems and stresses of the life situation. The stimuli that evoke the delusional system may be concealed by symbolization and obscure language, although occasionally the sources may be surmised through the client's and family's anamnestic report. The situations that combine along some common denominators appear to contain highly affective factors. The cognitive and behavioral responses to these affective factors carry an irrational flavor. It is important to take advantage of any shift in the degree of fixity or elements of doubt that the client presents in regard to delusions. Finally, it is of considerable assistance to the nurse to understand that there is generally a kernel of truth to some delusional systems, obscure though this may be.

PREVENTION

Health Promotion

See under *Hallucinations* and refer also to Chapter 37.

Population at Risk

1. All cultures are affected.
2. Some evidence that lower socioeconomic groups are at higher risk.
3. Children of parents who have utilized projection as a major method of dealing with anxiety and stress.
4. Persons with difficulty assuming responsibility for their own faults whether these are real or imagined faults.
5. Persons with difficulty trusting others, particularly those others who are in perceived or ascribed positions of power.
6. Persons with difficulty initiating and maintaining interpersonal relationships that are mutually growth producing.
7. Persons who depend on others to generate ideas and interpretations of the world.
8. Persons with history of traumatic experiences in childhood, such as maternal or paternal rejection, overprotectiveness, parental aggression, and a seclusive family system.

ASSESSMENT

Health History

Use format presented in Chapter 36. Note especially the following:

1. Client's description of events, circumstances, and situations related to the delusional system. Do this only at the time of the initial assessment so that elaborations can be determined if these occur later.
2. Note the presence or absence of hallucinations. If these are also present, use assessment presented under *Hallucinations*, above.
3. May be useful to have the client read the written history and make any "corrections" desired.

Physical Assessment

1. Neurological examination to rule out definitive organicity and ascertain baseline data for later observation regarding responses to antipsychotic medication.

Diagnostic Tests

1. Electroencephalogram to rule out organic origin.
2. Blood chemistry to rule out organic origin.
3. Include serial 7s and proverbs in mental status workup to assess the extent of thought impairment.

NURSING DIAGNOSES: ACTUAL OR POTENTIAL

1. Conceptual alterations associated with loss of contact with reality.
2. Thought impairment associated with irrationality.
3. Thought impairment associated with fixed, false beliefs about self, others, environment.

EXPECTED OUTCOMES

The client will

1. Interact with the nurse without discussing delusions.
2. Consider an alternative interpretation of a situation without undue anxiety or hostility.
3. Express doubt as to the rationality of her or his delusions.
4. Bring logical thought processes to bear on decisions regarding own behavior.
5. Consider alternative interpretations about phenomena that have personal meaning.
6. Consensually validate interpretations about phenomena that have personal meaning.
7. Recognize the interpersonal needs met by the delusional system and use more appropriate ways to get needs met.
8. Give up the beliefs that cannot be consensually validated.

INTERVENTIONS

1. Avoid the use of logic in an attempt to prove the delusion false.
2. Tell client that you do not share his or her interpretation (delusion).
3. Focus on parts of content that are real.
4. Avoid ignoring client's verbalization of the delusional material.
5. Explain facts and data about phenomena when appropriate, though not in an argumentative manner.
6. Identify the feelings presented when client discusses the delusion.
7. Identify the theme represented by the delusional system.
8. Direct client to describe rather than interpret phenomena related to the delusion.
9. Set limits on the number of times in an interactional session that client may discuss or present the delusional system.
10. Direct client to identify the persons to whom pronouns are attributed.
11. Actively shift conversation from delusional system to another topic when client exceeds limits allowed for discussion of delusions. Tell client why you are shifting topics.
12. Schedule activities that will be likely to provide increased self-esteem through interaction and cooperation with others.
13. Avoid actively soliciting a discussion of delusional content.
14. Avoid argument, and inform client that you will not argue about her or his beliefs.
15. Observe for side effects of psychoactive drugs.
16. Avoid putting medication in food.
17. Provide a brief and honest explanation for changes in milieu or treatment.
18. Support actively any expression of doubt that client presents in regard to the delusional system.

EVALUATION

Outcome Criteria

Acutely ill clients are likely to respond to appropriate psychoactive drugs in approximately 2 weeks following the first dose. Delusions may then lose much of the bizarre, fixed character that was previously observed. Such clients may begin to express doubt and concern regarding the untenable conclusions they reached during the early stages of the disorder. The recognition that one has been "crazy" for a time can have a crisislike effect and may increase anxiety and lower self-esteem. It is crucial that the nurse help clients cope with these feelings so that a return to the delusional system is avoided. Timing is a central factor in assessing whether the status of these clients is supportive of an explanation of their previous need to use delusions for adjustment purposes. A key to the decision to speak directly with them seems to be their own request to do so. In the event that they provide cues that they are ready to attempt to understand their delusional framework, a different set of interventions should be developed. This plan should be geared toward helping them learn to intervene or seek intervention should the problem recur.

Reevaluation and Follow-up

1. Refer to mental health clinic for periodic visits.
2. Refer to an outpatient therapy group.

3. Arrange with after-care personnel for transfer to one person who will consistently handle the medication regimen.
4. Family therapy is an option that should be discussed with client and family. At the least, the family should know the importance of the medication regimen and the group therapy experience.

BIBLIOGRAPHY

Clack, J.: *Nursing Care of the Disoriented Patient*, Monograph 13, American Nurses' Association, New York, 1962, p. 16. An early description of phases of the hallucinatory process in schizophrenic clients. Based on Sullivanian concepts. General approaches to nursing intervention included.

Collins, D. I.: "Some Specific Considerations in the One-to-One Relationship," in L. A. Joel and D. I. Collins (eds.), *Psychiatric Nursing: Theory and Application*, McGraw-Hill, New York, 1978, p. 155. Clinical cases illustrating concepts, including hallucinations and delusions. Provides operational definition of auditory hallucinations. Good presentation of intervention.

Day, M., and Semrad, E. V.: "Schizophrenic Reactions," in A. M. Nicholi, Jr. (ed.), *The Harvard Guide to Modern Psychiatry*, Belknap Press of Harvard University Press, Cambridge, Mass., 1978, p. 199. Lucid overview of contemporary medical opinion regarding etiology, clinical course, and psychiatric treatment of psychoses.

Freedman, A. M., Kaplan, H. I., and Sadok, B. J.: *Modern Synopsis of Comprehensive Textbook of Psychiatry/II*, 3d ed., Williams & Wilkins, Baltimore, 1981. Etiology, clinical features, and symptoms of schizophrenia described. An authoritative work.

Gravenkemper, K. H.: "Hallucinations," in S. F. Burd and M. A. Marshall (eds.), *Some Clinical Approaches to Psychiatric Nursing*, Macmillan, New York, 1963, p. 184. One of the earliest presentations of the application of Sullivanian concepts to the understanding of the hallucinatory process. Brief discussion of case examples presented.

Grosicki, J. P., and Harmonson, M.: "Nursing Action Guide: Hallucinations," *Journal of Psychiatric Nursing and Mental Health Services*, **7**:133, May–June 1969. Development and use of format in planning nursing intervention for hallucinating clients. Some specific approaches suggested.

Haber, J., Leach, A. M., Schudy, S. M., Sideleau, B. F.: *Comprehensive Psychiatric Nursing*, McGraw-Hill, New York, 1982. Outstanding presentation of the nursing process with delusional and hallucinating clients using a systems theory model.

Keup, W.: *Origin and Mechanisms of Hallucinations*, Proceedings of the 14th Annual Meeting of the Eastern Psychiatric Research Association, New York City, November 14–15, 1969, Plenum Publishing, New York, 1970. Research papers related to hallucinations and hallucinosis. A thorough coverage of etiology and process.

Kolb, L. E., and Brodie, H. K. H.: *Modern Clinical Psychiatry*, 10th ed., W. B. Saunders, Philadelphia, 1982, p. 363–369. Excellent discussion of the schizophrenias, including psychodynamics, etiology, symptoms, and treatment.

Salzinger, K.: *Schizophrenia: Behavioral Aspects*, John Wiley, New York, 1973. Presentation of research findings and current theories of schizophrenia. Good illustration of studies pertinent to all aspects of the group of disorders.

Schwartzman, S. T.: "The Hallucinating Patient and Nursing Intervention," in B. A. Backer, P. M., Dubbert, and E. J. P. Eisenman (eds.), *Psychiatric/Mental Health Nursing: Contemporary Readings*, D. Van Nostrand, New York, 1978, p. 140. Presentation of Sullivanian concepts related to hallucinations with use of case examples and discussion of intervention from several other sources.

Spitzer, R. L., et al.: APA; Quick Reference to the Diagnostic Criteria from Diagnostic and Statistical Manual of Mental Disorders, Third Edition, Washington, D.C., APA, 1980. General and concise reference to the more elaborate statistical and diagnostic manual used by clinicians.

Underwood, P. R.: "The Psychotic Disorders" in M. E. Kalkman, and A. J. Davis (eds.), *New Dimensions in Mental Health-Psychiatric Nursing*, 5th ed., McGraw-Hill, New York, 1980, p. 244. Good presentation of clinical problems and nursing care with psychotic clients. Helpful section on hallucinations and delusions.

Wilson, H. S. and Kneisl, C. R.: *Psychiatric Nursing*, 2d ed., Addison-Wesley, Menlo Park, Calif., 1983, p. 341. Excellent clinical presentations presented illustrative of commonly used interventions with psychotic clients.

40

Mental Health Problems of Children

Faye Gary Harris

The purpose of this chapter is to examine the most common difficulties presented by children with emotional problems. Impulsivity and depression categorically include the constellation of behaviors presented by children that usually result in their entry into the mental health care delivery system. Particular emphasis is given to the family system in regard to prevention, assessment, and therapy.

IMPULSIVITY IN CHILDREN

DESCRIPTION

Impulsivity is the manifestation of a drive, an urge, and/or a yearning to express, through verbal or psychomotor modes, actions that are considered nonuseful and harmful to the self and/or others in the environment. This act may have been planned and calculated, or it may have been an "on the spot" response. During the act, the person experiences a relief of tension, which brings on feelings of gratification and pleasure. Following the act, the person may or may not experience remorse, guilt, and/or regret. Impulsivity occurs in all races and ethnic, socioeconomic, and religious groups.

PREVENTION

Health Promotion

1. Environment. Assess for
   a. Disturbances in the family that might be manifested through marital discord, noncommunication between parents and/or parents and child.
   b. Changes in living arrangements within the home.
   c. Frequent moves and migration and immigration patterns.
   d. Lack of verbal skills that have not been mastered that allow for expressions of anger, disappointment, sadness, rejection, and so on.
   e. Adequacy of peer relationships and the opportunities to interact with others.
   f. Family's ability to provide safe and wholesome recreational activities for children.
2. Physical problems. Assess for
   a. Physical discomfort as a result of undiagnosed and untreated problems or syndromes.
   b. Growth and development milestones that should be evident and can be appropriately documented.
   c. Physical limitations that the child might have, thus causing limitations in mobility and physical expression.
   d. Physical limitations that might cause body image problems (e.g., a cast applied to extremities).

e. Medications for physical problems, such as asthma, diabetes, and perhaps renal difficulties.
f. A history of familial physical problems that might exist; frequently children are fearful that they, too, might have the disease.
g. A history of familial emotional problems that might exist. Children usually do not understand outbursts, temperamental dispositions, although they might imitate such aberrant behaviors.
h. Awakening of conflicts revolving around fears of "getting sick" and familial reactions to these fears.
i. Exogenous factors that are available in the household and perhaps used by parents or siblings or the child, such as drugs, alcohol, sedatives, and so forth, that easily induce affective and behavioral changes.
j. A history of organic brain syndromes or disorders in the child, siblings, or parents.

3. Skewed familial values or circumstances. Assess for
   a. Methods of disciplining and limit setting for children, for example, withholding food, affection, or heat (in cold climates).
   b. Sensory overstimulation that might be antecedents to rage, fright, and even delirium.
   c. Sensory deprivation that might also create fears, fright, lack of object-love, and pseudohallucinations.

Population at Risk

These attributes do not necessarily indicate the development of impulsivity in children; however, certain configurations do serve as possible indicators. These include

1. Extended family structures where immediate expression of emotions is acceptable.
2. Families that practice "acting out" rather than "talking out" behaviors.
3. Families that function under intense financial stress.
4. Parents who abuse alcohol and other substances.
5. Families where the ability to relax the superego is not or cannot be practiced.
6. Feelings of isolation and alienation are paramount in the mothering one.
7. Children who have poor socialization and academic skills.
8. Families in which one or both parents and/or their sanguineous kinsmen have histories of assault and impulse control problems, such as gambling.
9. Suspiciousness between parents and among parents and siblings.

Screening

1. Review of school records that might reveal data regarding
   a. Peer relationships.
   b. Management of frustrations.
   c. Response to teachers.
   d. Recreational skills and sports involvement.
   e. Academic performance.
2. Emergency room visits that might indicate impulsive behaviors in family (e.g., broken bones, skin marks, poor nutrition, "nervous and anxious" children and/or adults).
3. A history of threatened abandonment by one or both parents.
4. Crisis center contacts and calls; suicidal threats by one or both parents.
5. Families where there is not a high priority on expressive and verbal language.
6. Children in families where verbal expressions of conflicts, frustrations, fears, and disappointments are not allowed.
7. Saddened and depressed looking children.
8. The child's ability to delay an action, a verbal comment, or an observation.
9. Cutting statements about peers, authority, and self made by the child or parents.

ASSESSMENT

Assessment in children tends automatically to include family members. The purpose of the assessment is to establish the reasons and circumstances that contribute to the child's/family's disorders and behavioral problems; it helps the therapist to establish guidelines and theoretical and practical rationales for intervention and evaluation. This framework incorporates many of the guidelines presented in the Mental Status Examination (Simmons, 1974).

Health History

(When appropriate ask both child and parents or significant others.)

1. Age.
2. Sex.
3. Grade in school.

4. Address.
5. Occupation(s) of parents.
6. Description of any type of physical problem believed to have existed and whether treated or untreated.
7. Physical and neurological examinations.
   a. Specific diagnostic protocols should be used if mental retardation and/or organic involvement are suspected.
   b. A history of any reported syndrome or disability in parents and siblings should be carefully documented.
8. A listing of community agencies that are used by parents and child.
   a. A parental evaluation of the agency and the agent in terms of how their needs were or were not met.
   b. The child's evaluation of the agency and agent in terms of how needs were or were not met.
9. Describe parents' manner of handling themselves under stress.
10. Have parents describe strong and weak points about their personalities.
11. Have parents describe strong and weak points about their child or children.
12. Describe the ways in which parents express aggression.
13. Describe the ways in which the child expresses aggression and sexual impulses.
14. What is the child's level of anxiety at this time?
15. What are the parents' levels of anxiety at this time?
16. Is there a history of stealing or complusive lying associated with the child and/or parents?
17. Do parents trust each other? Do they trust the child?
18. How does the family treat animals (i.e., abusively or kindly).
19. Parents' personal resources to include insurance, transportation, skills, and so on.
20. Identify a support system that the parents might utilize. How does this support system operate?
21. A history of violence in the family.
22. Do parents have a history of psychiatric illness/treatment? Suicidal ideation and/or attempts?
23. A history of homosexuality in the family.
24. Psychosexual perversions, such as paraphilias or gender identity problems?
25. What are the parents ideas and ideals for the child? Can the parents articulate these ideas and ideals?
26. How does the child feel about her or himself?
   a. Is there a perceived problem?
   b. Can the child discuss feelings associated with this problem?

Physical Assessment

Specific concerns regarding the physical assessment for the impulsive child include

1. Bruises on body.
2. Lacerations or lash marks on body.
3. Unkempt, rough-looking skin.
4. Missing teeth.
5. Broken bones.

Diagnostic Tests

1. Complete neurological examination (these examinations might be done by the professionals who will *not* be doing the psychiatric evaluation).
2. If there is a history of specific diseases, such as hyper- or hypothyroidism, hypo- or hyperglycemia, or diabetes, complete laboratory tests are indicated.
3. X-ray films of areas that are determined to be problematical or traumatized.

NURSING DIAGNOSES: ACUTAL OR POTENTIAL

1. Altered activity associated with inappropriate touching, hitting; other destructive acts toward self and others.
2. Lack of compliance with social regulations.
3. Alterations in verbal and expressive abilities.
4. Alterations in control of anger and frustration.
5. Disruptions in family process.
6. Delay in developmental progress associated with eating, elimination, socialization.

EXPECTED OUTCOMES

1. Immediate. The child will
   a. Control enuretic behaviors.
   b. Develop more acceptable sublimatory channels through which impulsivity can be controlled.
   c. Decrease frequency and duration of temper tantrums.

d. Decrease frequency of inappropriate touching and hitting others.
e. Decrease duration and frequency of making "cutting" remarks about staff to other staff members.
f. Decrease frequency and duration of using profane language.
g. Develop better language skills through which frustrations, disappointments, rage, ideals, and ideas might be expressed.
h. Learn more acceptable means of expressing sexual feelings and thoughts.
i. Not destroy property.
j. Learn to participate actively in conversations and group discussions with children and adults without being disruptive or leaving the group.
k. Share time, space, toys, staff with other children.

2. Long range. The child will
   a. Develop a positive relationship with the nurse therapist.
   b. Articulate frustrations and conflicts in an acceptable manner.
   c. Learn to recognize the feeling states accompanying impulsive acts.
   d. Learn to identify thoughts and affective sensations that precede impulsive acts.
   e. Learn to "program in" acceptable control devices that delay, preclude, and prevent the intensity, duration, and frequency of destroying property.
   f. Gain insight into behavior through reviewing videotape and discussing behaviors.
   g. Develop basic socialization skills, such as eating properly, waiting one's turn, and engaging in conversation with peers in an acceptable manner.
   h. Increase the duration and frequency of engaging in tasks that can be completed and/or mastered.
   i. Learn to wait for gratification of needs.
   j. Improve school performance.
   k. Increase effectiveness in communicating with parents.
   l. Develop ideas and ideals for and about him or herself that are realistic and egosyntonic.
   m. Parents and child will learn how to recognize stress and anxiety in the child and parents for the purpose of
      (1) "Nipping problems in the bud."
      (2) Shifting to "talking out" methods before tension becomes expressive.
      (3) Developing feelings of mastery and competency over the situation.
      (4) Planning for continuous learning and familial autonomy.
      (5) Child and/or family will participate in the planned therapies, such as
         (a) Individual play therapy for child.
         (b) Marital therapy for parents.
         (c) Supportive group therapy for parents.
         (d) Possible individual therapy for one or both parents, if indicated.
         (e) Academic programs for child.
         (f) Academic (language skills) program for parents and other significant others.
         (g) Chemotherapy.

INTERVENTIONS

Specific interventions are explicitly or implicitly related to Nursing Diagnoses and Expected Outcomes. A categorization has been implemented to provide for clearer organization and synthesis.

Physical Assertion

1. Identify the specific behavior pattern.
2. Record ecological conditions under which behavior occurs.
3. Observe, recognize, and record duration and frequency of touching behaviors.
4. Identify the nurses' (especially the nurse therapists') feelings about the touching behaviors.
5. Explore with child the meaning the utility of the milieu rules and guidelines.
6. Identify specific situations when child touches staff and other children.
7. Review with child "before" fighting thoughts and feelings.
8. Explore with child thoughts and feelings "during" the fighting period.
9. Explore with child thoughts and feelings "after" the fighting.
10. Discuss the "taking away" of toys, books, and games from other children:
    a. Feelings, thoughts.
    b. Power, control.
    c. Reputation and status in relation to peers and teachers.

d. Anger, guilt, shame.
e. Hopelessness and uselessness.

11. Assist child in recognizing cause-and-effect relationships that arise from each identifiable, physically impulsive act.
12. Explore alternative methods of releasing anger: consider play activities, bag punching, running, and then talking with nurse.
13. Videotape temper tantrum behaviors, hitting behaviors, or any other intimidating behaviors.
14. Review and discuss videotape with child, assisting recall of thoughts and feelings during the identified activity.
15. Solicit from child a reason for the specific behavior(s).
16. Elicit behavioral alternatives.
    a. Direct approach.
        (1) "What could you have done to express yourself without (whatever the identified behavior may be)?"
        (2) "What were you thinking about when you (whatever the identified behavior may be)?"
    b. Indirect approach.
        (1) "I am here to talk with you as soon as you are ready."
        (2) "Throwing chairs is frightening, isn't it?"
17. Ask for clarification when behaviors or verbalizations are not understood.
18. Solicit and encourage positive talk from child about self.
19. Provide situations whereby child can successfully interact with peer group.

Parents and Community

1. Assess and record parents' images of themselves and their perceptions of the identified child (client) as opposed to other sibling(s).
2. Assess and record parents' perceptions of child as opposed to other children in the larger social system.
3. Assess whether parents are likely to facilitate a therapeutic collusion between child and therapist.
4. Explore parents' feelings and thoughts about therapy (e.g., useful, hopeless, mystical).
5. Explore parents' feelings and thoughts about child being mentally sick.
6. Assess whether parents are feeling harassed, embarrassed, humiliated, or rejected by community because of child's difficulties.
7. Explore with parents the formal and informal support systems within their community; encourage and assist parents in mobilizing these resources.
8. Provide parents with appropriate therapeutic modalities.
9. Assess the cultural, religious, socioeconomic, ethnic, sociopolitical, and geographical values and conflicts pertinent to parents, child, family, and community.
10. Assess the degree of comfort or harmony expressed by parents in relation to these values and conflicts.
11. Identify those cultural, religious, socioeconomic, ethnic, sociopolitical, and geographical values and conflicts pertinent to self; then, look for possible opportunities for misinterpretation of conflicts when involved in therapeutic process with child or family.

EVALUATION

Outcome Criteria

When working with children, evaluation of treatment should be done by the team working with the child and family. In addition, a detailed assessment of the daily intervention methods employed should be made. The nurse should consider the following when evaluating intervention:

1. Is the nurse comfortable with the intervention?
2. Does the nurse have the support of the treatment team?
3. Has the nurse communicated appropriately with other members of the care team?
4. Are there patterns in child and family's responses to specific treatment modalities?
5. Does the nurse feel that the child and family are worthy of the time and energy required for treatment?
6. Are the parents and child able to communicate verbally with each other?
7. Do the parents and child actively participate in outlined therapies?
8. Do other siblings and extended family feel comfortable with the child?
9. Do child and parents have improved self-concepts/self-esteem?
10. Can child and parents appropriately and adequately express intimacy?

Reevaluation and Follow-up

1. Make referral to appropriate community agency by providing a summary of therapy, treatment modalities, and progress. Specify any unique and/or unusual attributes of child and family.
2. Terminate treatment with child and parents, providing them with list of agents and agencies where professional help can be obtained.
3. Collaborate with other agencies and institutions that child will, through normal course of development, encounter. The school is probably the most important institution to be considered.
   a. Intervention methods may be shared with teacher and school psychologist.
   b. Rationale for intervention is also helpful and provides a basis for consistency and continuity of those techniques that facilitate the child's and family's positive growth.
   c. Identify self to school personnel as a resource person available for consultation.
4. When necessary, coordinate referrals to other community agencies, such as welfare departments, protective services, and special medical services. Determine the content of clinical summary to be included in each type of referral. The agency receiving the referral and the purpose of the referral will govern the content included.

Complications

1. Staff and parents will feel hopeless, angry, and threatened before improvement is visible.
2. Parents will begin to abuse each other/place blame and possibly separate or divorce.
3. Parents and staff will not communicate productively with each other.
4. Staff will begin to withdraw support from therapist who works with the child.
5. Family members are not comfortable with reuniting with child in the home and community.
6. Child becomes or remains a problem in the school system.
7. Premature discharge from care occurs because parents and extended family members have become threatened.
8. Chemotherapy might produce side effects.
9. Difficulties in the management of accompanying physical problems, such as diabetes or hyperthroidism may occur.

Reevaluation and Follow-up

1. Make referral to appropriate community agency by providing a summary of therapy, treatment modalities, and progress. Specify any unique and/or unusual attributes of child and family.
2. Terminate treatment with child and parents, providing them with list of agents and agencies where professional help can be obtained.

DEPRESSION IN CHILDREN

DESCRIPTION

Depression and sadness are common phenomena in children and their families. Negative self-evaluation and feelings of worthlessness occur. Frequently, the child manifests behaviors such as tantrums, aggression, or sleep disturbances, that lay people usually do not associate with sadness and a depressed mood. Moreover, the child can present with social withdrawal, somatic pain, feelings of rejection, and disturbances in mental and psychomotor functions. These children may or may not have a clear history of "loss" and other precipitating events. See also Chapter 36.

PREVENTION

Health Promotion

1. Environment. Assess for
   a. Value and practice regarding child rearing in the home, day-care centers, and other places where the child spends long hours.
   b. A thorough history from parent(s), both when possible, regarding their perceptions of the child, their aspirations and hopes for the child, and their articulated responsibilities for the child.
   c. Disruption in the parents' lives and how disruptions might have affected the child.
   d. Separation and individuation process practiced by family members and implications for the child.
   e. The nature of peers in the child's immediate and extended environment.

f. The family's value of and time allotment for recreational activities; include a description of these activities, too.
g. The verbalization process. Include
(1) The ability to separate reality from fantasy.
(2) Self-control over one's feelings and emotions.
(3) Articulation of negative and positive feelings and thoughts with corresponding affect.
h. The family's understanding of the need for object constancy, autonomy, and consistency in discipline.
i. The reactions to the child's behaviors, verbalizations, thoughts, and other activities by parents, day-care providers, and peers.
j. Congruence between religious practices, value systems, decision making, and cultural factors among family members.

2. Physical problems. Assess for
a. Physical discomfort as a result of undiagnosed and untreated problems or syndromes.
b. Growth and development milestones that should be evident and can be appropriately documented.
c. Physical limitations that the child might have, thus causing limitations in mobility and physical expressions.
d. Physical limitations that might cause body image problems (e.g., a cast applied to extremities).
e. Medication for physical problems, such as asthma, diabetes, or renal difficulties.
f. A history of familial physical problems that might exist should be recorded; frequently, children are fearful that they, too, might have the disease.
g. A history of familial emotional problems that might exist should be recorded. Children usually do not understand outbursts, tempermental dispositions, though they might imitate such aberrant behaviors.
h. Awakening of conflicts revolving around fears of "getting sick" and familial reactions to these fears—real or imagined.
i. Exogeneous factors that are available in the household and perhaps used by parents/siblings or the child, such as drugs, alcohol, sedatives, that easily induce affective and behavioral changes.
j. A history of organic brain syndrome or disorders in the child, siblings, or parents.
k. Need for specific physical examination and laboratory tests might be indicated, such as endocrine and cardiovascular tests.

3. Skewed familial values and circumstances. Assess for
a. Parents' understanding and perception of withdrawn, shy behaviors; understanding and perception of aggressive types of behaviors and their corresponding reactions to the child.
b. Methods utilized by parents to control the child, such as physical punishment, withholding socialization opportunities, limiting food intake, and requiring that child spend long hours in the dark.
c. The use of religious values and principles in a way that tends to create a punitive superego structure within the child.
d. How information about the child from other sources might be used for or against the child by other family members.

Population at Risk

1. Families that have limited human resources.
2. Families that have few economic resources.
3. Families who are not able to evoke a "caring" response among professionals.
4. Multiple problem families that have the perceived potential for engulfing the nurse.
5. Families that are heavy users of drugs and alcohol.
6. Families that do not encourage children to problem solve.
7. Families that have little tolerance for individual differences and cultural differences within society.
8. Families in which the need for control of self and others is always present.
9. Families in which adult socialization is inadequate and nonuseful.
10. Children who have poor academic skills.
11. Children who become "clowns" or scapegoats in their peer groups.
12. Families that have a history of psychiatric problems (treated or untreated).

Screening

During screening, provide for the potential identification of problems, and include such activities as

1. Contact with school nurses, counselors, and teachers regarding the child's
a. Socialization behaviors.

b. Peer group interaction.
c. Perception of self.
d. Perceptions of how others think and feel about him or her.
e. School performance.
f. Aspirations for the future.
g. Ability to respond to authority.
h. Mastery-competency in specified areas.

2. Children of divorce.
3. Children who live in overcrowded, poorly supervised environments.
4. Children who assume adult roles too early.
5. Children who have little wholesome recreation in their lives.
6. Families who frequently visit emergency rooms because of somatic complaints and perceived disorders, as well as for conditions such as burns, broken bones, anxiety, and drug-related problems.
7. Children of parents who have run away (one or both).
8. Crisis center contacts to include
   a. Frequency.
   b. Precipitating problem.
   c. Name of person making the contact.
   d. Reason for making contact (assess for patterns, cycles, and affect).
9. Families that have different cultural backgrounds and values than the majority population.
10. Visits to day-care centers and schools for assessment of the milieu in which a child must live.
11. Likewise, a home visit for purpose of
    a. Observing communication patterns.
    b. Conflict management.
    c. Tone of environment.
    d. Order/disorder in home.
    e. Father/mother interactions.
    f. Physical space.
    g. Physical resources.
12. The value placed or not placed on verbal expression of happiness, sadness, disappointment, and so forth.
13. The support that parents and other household members (grandparents and other extended family members) provide for each other and the child. Then, what is the nature of the support?
    a. Destructive.
    b. Conflictual.
    c. Facilitative.
    d. Disorganized, with indifference.

ASSESSMENT

A thorough and detailed assessment of a child should include (1) an evaluation of the child, (2) assessment of the home, (3) observations of the school or day-care center, (4) information in detail about nonfamily care providers (extended family, friends), and (5) evaluation of the parents. The purpose of the assessment is to gather data that will aid in the establishment of hypotheses about circumstances that contribute to the child's and family's dysfunctions. These data should be viewed from the perspective of group norms and background of the particular cultural, ethnic, and/or racial group of which the family is a member (e.g., Catholic/Italian, rural). The assessment helps the therapist to establish guidelines, theoretical and practical approaches to treatment, and evaluation.

Health History

See Health History section under *Impulsivity in Children*.

Physical Assessment

Specific concerns regarding physical assessment of the depressed child include

1. Growth and development patterns.
2. Constitutional factors.
3. History of physical problems in parents, sibling groups, and extended family members.
4. Previous disabilities that the child might have had. List them, and include the possible effect on the child/parents/siblings (e.g., a child with a congenital anomaly, such as club foot, that he has outgrown).
5. Body and hygiene care.
6. Bruises and lacerations on body.
7. Weight loss or gain in a rapid fashion.
8. Broken bones.
9. Rashes on skin.
10. History of fevers, nausea, vomiting.
11. History of frequent trips to emergency room, physician's office, other health care facilities.
12. Verbal complaints from the child.
13. Verbal complaints from the parents, sibling group, and extended family members.

Diagnostic Tests

1. Physical examination.
2. Complete neurological examination.
3. Electroencephalogram (EEG).
4. Specific tests are indicated if child has a history of certain physical problems, such as di-

abetes, respiratory problems, cardiac involvement, hypothyroidism, or hypoglycemia. If there are sufficient data in the health history that create suspicion, tests are perhaps indicated to "rule out" these conditions.

5. X-ray films to further study a syndrome, trauma, and/or fractures.

NURSING DIAGNOSES: ACTUAL OR POTENTIAL

1. Disruptions in affective functions associated with sadness, depression, or hopelessness.
2. Disruptions in self-esteem associated with depression.
3. Disruptions in effective coping mechanisms.
4. Disruptions in developmental progress.
5. Disruptions in family process.
6. Potential threat to survival associated with suicide.

EXPECTED OUTCOMES

1. Immediate. The child will
   a. Control suicidal attempts.
   b. Have adequate fluid and food intake.
   c. Become involved in activities; devise a plan for gradual inclusion in activities.
   d. Control encopretic and enuretic behaviors.
   e. Begin to develop a healthier self-appraisal.
   f. Discuss problems, thoughts, and feelings with therapist.
   g. Begin to develop interests in peers, adults, and things in the environment.
   h. Improve sleep patterns.
   i. Not be punished by parents (when this can be controlled).
   j. Begin to learn how to meet some of his own expressed needs.
   k. Learn how to verbalize dissatisfactions and disappointments.
   l. Learn more appropriate ways of expressing sexual needs.
   m. Decrease frequency of runaway behavior.
   n. Begin to learn to experience joy and happiness without fear.
   o. Learn to accept kindness, empathy, and caring.
2. Long-range. The child will
   a. Experience a healthier self-esteem.
   b. Develop a healthier self-appraisal.
   c. Return to highest level of emotional and cognitive functioning.
   d. Begin to problem solve and develop more adequate coping mechanisms.
   e. Not use somatic complaints to verbalize discomforts and disappointments.
   f. Develop adequate and meaningful peer relationships.
   g. Discuss fearful and frightening events with the therapist.
   h. Remain interested in school work and other tasks that are age appropriate.
   i. Discuss the feelings and thoughts associated with fear of punishment.
   j. Develop a futurist reference for self in the world.
   k. Learn to express hostile and angry feelings.
   l. Improve academic performance.
   m. Increase the mastery of skills and tasks.
   n. Increase the mastery of verbalization of needs, thoughts, and feelings in an appropriate manner.
   o. Learn to trust the nurse, other staff, parents, and other authority figures.
   p. Gain insight into manifested behaviors through viewing of
      (1) Videotapes.
      (2) Audiotapes.
      (3) Short story telling.
   q. Learn how to recognize depressive type feelings and thoughts for preventive measures.
      (1) Parents must be taught how to recognize their own depression and then their child's depression.
   r. Become active in therapy.

INTERVENTIONS

1. Observe and identify the behaviors, moods, verbalizations.
2. Observe and record the affect in speech, the frequency of verbalizations, and the expressed thought content.
3. Continually discuss the staff's reactions to
   a. Child.
   b. Child and therapist.
   c. Child's parents.
4. Articulate the case history, upsetting factors, and the here-and-now problems to staff and, selectively, to parents.
5. Assess for hallucinations and delusions.

6. Assist the child in eating appropriately.
7. Explore with child feelings of disappointment, anger, resentment, and rage.
8. Explore with child feelings of isolation and alienation.
9. Discuss feelings and thoughts about suicide.
10. Identify specific situations that make child feel sad, helpless, hopeless.
11. Review with child methods used to handle previous disappointments.
12. Discuss with child and parents the family's method of problem solving. Critique these data in light of racial, ethnic, and religious factors.
13. Observe and record conditions under which child appears to be less sad and depressed. Discuss these conditions with the child and parents.
14. Identify any crises the child may have experienced recently and/or remotely. Detail the situation with the child; later with parents. Observe for misinterpretations, delusions, wrong facts; seek to clarify all misunderstandings and associated feelings.
15. Discuss alternatives to running away.
16. Assist the child to understand cause-effect relationships.
17. Teach mastery over feelings and thoughts.
18. Teach socialization skills to include
    a. Peer relationship skills.
    b. Dating skills.
    c. Conversations with the opposite sex.
    d. Appropriate attire, make-up, and so on.
19. Explore alternatives to internalizing anger.
20. Discuss the future from two points of view:
    a. A depressed one.
    b. A nondepressed one where the child will have mastery skills, decision-making opportunities, and so forth.
21. Assess parents' perceptions of child's treatment.
22. Determine if parents will follow through with recommendations from treatment team.
23. Determine the parents' feelings before and after treatment.
    a. Are they supportive of each other?
    b. Can they trust each other?
    c. Do they like/love the child? Are they willing to invest more time, money, and energy in the child?
24. Discuss the full course of treatment with parents. Highlight their responsibilities, behaviors, feelings, thoughts, and responses that facilitate and inhibit growth of the child.
25. Review cultural, religious, socioeconomic, ethnic, and geographical values and beliefs with parents, highlighting how these impact on the child, the parents, and other siblings.
26. Explore parents' feelings and thoughts about having an emotionally disturbed child.
27. Explore the parents' expectations of the child, the therapist, and the mental health care delivery system.
28. Explore how parents are perceiving themselves in relation to their own reference group. Assess for how they feel the sick child will affect their relationships in regard to
    a. Work.
    b. Recreation.
    c. Religious activities.
    d. Community involvement.
    e. Neighborhood relationships.

EVALUATION

Outcome Critiera

By the end of treatment the child will

1. Be able to control enuresis and encopresis.
2. Manifest no suicidal thoughts, feelings, or ideations.
3. Have developed a trusting relationship with the therapist, one other staff person, and parents.
4. Discuss thoughts and feelings regarding
    a. Previous conflicts.
    b. Crisis situations that evoke anxiety, fear, dread, and depression.
5. Develop alternatives to nonuseful behaviors, such as running away, withdrawing, and isolating one's self.
6. Identify time and events when depression seems to be occurring; identify an appropriate response to the impending depression by knowing how and where to get help.
7. Be able to control all acting-out behaviors.
8. Manifest a level of self-esteem that is congruent with age, sex, and sociocultural factors.

Reevaluation and Follow-up

1. Make referral to appropriate community agency by providing a summary of therapy, treatment modalities, and progress. Specify any unique and/or unusual attributes of child and family.

2. Terminate treatment with child and parents, providing them with list of agents and agencies where professional help can be obtained.
3. Collaborate with other agencies and institutions that child will, through normal course of development, encounter. The school is probably the most important institution to be considered.
   a. Intervention methods may be shared with teacher and school psychologist.
   b. Rationale for intervention is also helpful and provides a basis for consistency and continuity of those techniques that facilitate the child's and family's positive growth.
   c. Identify self to school personnel as a resource person available for consultation.
4. When necessary, coordinate referrals to other community agencies, such as welfare departments, protective services, and special medical services. Determine the content of clinical summary to be included in each type of referral. The agency receiving the referral and the purpose of the referral will govern the content included.

REFERENCES

Simmons, J. E.: *Psychiatric Examination of Children,* Lea & Febiger, Philadelphia, 1974.

BIBLIOGRAPHY

Backer, B., Dubbert, P., and Eiseman, E. (eds.): *Psychiatric/Mental Health Nursing: Contemporary Readings.* Van Nostrand Co., New York, 1978. Excellent resource for diverse clinical issues and problems in the field.

Corfman, E. (ed.): *Families Today: A Research Sampler on Families and Children,* vol. 1, National Institutes of Mental Health, Division of Scientific and Public Information, Superintendent of Documents, U.S. Government Printing Office, Washington, D.C., 1979. This book highlights, through a variety of articles, the force of parents on the total development of children and other family members. It features readings that address specific issues in family and culture through the life span.

The Diagnostic and Statistical Manual of Mental Disorders: Third Edition, The American Psychiatric Association, Washington, D.C., 1980. This manual is an essential resource for all clinicians. Its format, which includes *time axes* in the assessment and diagnostic process, provides a comprehensive base for conceptualizing human behavior; moreover, the descriptions of common emotional problems of children are summarized in a fashion that assists the clinician in the diagnostic process.

Eisenburg, L.: "Hyperkinetic Reactions," in *Basic Handbook of Child Psychiatry,* Basic Books, New York, 1979. The chapter in this book is comprehensive in that the content describes the syndrome, classifies the behaviors, provides information about diagnostic considerations, and concludes with possible therapeutic approaches for treatment.

Enelow, A. L.: *Elements of Psychotherapy.* Oxford University Press, New York, 1977. Provides the clinician with a quick reference to several commonly used treatment modalities. The material is clearly presented and has utility for the novice as well as the expert. Good presentation of the psychotherapist's behavior.

Freedman, A., and Kaplan, H.: *The Child: His Psychological and Cultural Development,* Atheneum, New York, 1976. The book is an excellent reference book that addresses normal growth and development, assessment (mental and neurological), and disturbances of a nonpsychiatric nature (e.g., nail biting). The cultural components of behavior are well integrated in the content.

Group for the Advancement of Psychiatry: *Psychopathological Disorders in Childhood: Theoretical Considerations and a Proposed Classification,* Mental Health Materials Center, Inc., New York, 1968. This document, produced by GAP, details basic knowledge regarding conceptual models and classification systems. The symptom list itemizes terms used in describing deviant and pathological behaviors. Clinicians can easily locate the terminology/symptom list.

Harowitz, M., and Kaltreider, N.: "Brief Therapy of the Stress Response Syndrome," in C. P. Kimball (ed.), *The Psychiatric Clinics of North America,* vol. 2, no. 2, W. B. Saunders, Philadelphia, 1979. This chapter details the theoretical bases of a stress response syndrome. Concepts and examples assist the clinician in understanding behaviors that frequently occur in acute care settings.

Leff, J. P., and Isaacs, A.: *Psychiatric Examination in Clinical Practice,* Blackwell Scientific Publications, Oxford, 1981. An excellent review of the major concepts in psychiatric practice. Of specific utility are the sections that address history taking and the mental status examination of adults and children.

Schubterbrandt, J., and Raskin, A.: *Depression in Childhood: Diagnosis, Treatment, and Conceptual Models,* Raven Press, New York, 1977. A collection of articles written by outstanding clinicians make this an excellent resource for studying theoretical and conceptual materials regarding depression. The clinician's skills are likely to be sharpened as a result of reading this book.

41

Person Abuse

Judy B. Campbell and Noreen King Poole

The perpetration of deliberate and repeated acts resulting in physical and psychological injury to others, and the continual reinforcement of the threat of such acts constitute a social and health problem of immense proportions. The purpose of this chapter is to illustrate the nursing process as it is carried out in cases of spouse abuse, child abuse, sexual abuse, and elder abuse. The nurse who practices in any of the clinical specialty areas may encounter clients and families with severe difficulties in these areas. The interventions suggested as responses to the various forms of person abuse can be implemented in the hospital, community, or in the traditional modes of individual, group, and family therapy.

SPOUSE ABUSE

DESCRIPTION

Spouse abuse is the deliberate and repeated physical injury or threat of bodily harm from a mate, whether legally married or not. It is not to be confused with sadomasochistic behavior between two consenting adults. Persons of all ages, races, ethnic groups, religious affiliations, socioeconomic and educational groups are victims of spouse abuse. The most common form of connubial crime is wife battering, although in some subcultures husband abuse occurs; statistically, husband battering is rare. Conservative estimtes indicate that more than 1 million women are assulted by mates each year; one-fourth to one-half of homicides in the United States occur between spouses.

PREVENTION

Health Promotion

1. Conduct values clarification sessions for engaged couples, emphasizing early warning signs of spouse abuse.
2. Establish and conduct parenting classes in high schools and communities with emphasis on disciplinary techniques other than physical punishment.
3. Educate professionals (teachers, nurses, health care workers, physicians, attorneys, etc.) in assessment, early detection, and intervention skills.
4. Consult law enforcement agencies about recruitment, training, and ongoing in-service programs.
5. Conduct consciousness-raising groups for men and women.
6. Support the establishment of community resources (i.e., local mental health centers, hot lines, emergency shelters, and volunteer training programs).
7. Lobby for legislation making spouse abuse a criminal offense nationwide.
8. Implement programs in public agencies to eliminate gender role stereotyping.
9. Advocate reduction of violence in the media.
10. Help witnessing children to use the family violence as a learning experience.

11. Refer witnessing children to socialization experiences and supportive systems (e.g., YWCA, Alanon, Alateen, school counselors, churches, parents of friends, extended family members).
12. Conduct values clarification classes in grades K through 12 that focus on personal responsibility and problem solving.

Population at Risk

The presence of one or more of the following characteristics does not necessarily indicate that abuse exists; clustering of these characteristics lends a stronger predisposition to conjugal violence.

1. Mates from families of origin in which mother was battered or in which violence or neglect was present.
2. Economically insecure families (real or perceived).
3. Families in which the achievement level of husband (economic, educational, social status) is lower than that of wife.
4. Families isolated from neighbors either geographically or socially.
5. One or both spouses abusing alcohol, mood-altering chemicals, or gambling to excess.
6. Pregnancy unwanted by one or both partners.
7. Partners of different religious faiths.
8. Members of minority religions (i.e., *not* Catholic, Protestant, or Jewish).
9. Families in which abuse or violence was present before conjugal living.
10. Families in which husband has lower occupational status (although not necessarily lower income) than that of neighbors.
11. Families in which husband rigidly adheres to role as "head of family."
12. Jealousy and possessiveness exist in one or both partners.
13. High levels of personality fusion exist among family members (i.e., few differences in feelings, ideas, hopes, fears).
14. Families in which male partner has a criminal record for aggravated assault.
15. Female spouse lacks assertiveness and problem-solving skills.

Screening

1. Records of calls to law enforcement agencies (e.g., "domestic disturbances").
2. Hot line calls.
3. Emergency room visits by battered persons often accompanied by vague explanations of injuries.
4. Petitions to family court (i.e., restraining orders, separation, divorce).
5. Records of family service agencies involving child abuse, neglect, incest.
6. Reports by children to school personnel of "unusual" parental behavior.

ASSESSMENT

The battering victim tends to lack trust in professionals and often is evasive, vague, hesitant, and embarrassed during interview and physical examination. Health professionals who are alert to such client statements as, ". . . Things have been rough lately," or ". . . It's getting worse," might ask, "Have these difficulties ever resulted in physical harm?" The battering victim will feel relief when able to share experiences with a nonjudgmental listener. The client frequently responds physiologically by manifesting symptoms of severe anxiety along with the symptoms of physical battering. When doing the assessment, the nurse will reinforce the client's lowered self-esteem, guilt, and self-blame if he or she expresses surprise that the victim has not sought help sooner. Reinforcement, during this contact, of the positive aspects of the client seeking help is most important.

Health History

See Chapter 36 for format. Note especially the following:

1. Type of relationship: legal marriage or cohabitation.
2. Duration of relationship.
3. Onset of violent behavior.
4. Types of violence: *physical abuse* (slapping, burning, punching, strangulation, kicking, use of weapons, etc.), *verbal abuse* (obscenities, attacks on character), *sexual abuse* (forcible rape, sadistic behavior).
5. Frequency of violence; patterns discerned by client.
6. History of violence in family of origin.
7. History of depression and/or suicidal feelings.
8. Effects of violence on children in family.
9. Help sought from community and results of these contacts (police, family court, friends,

health professionals, religious groups, protective shelters).
10. Have client and partner sought counseling in past?
11. How does client perceive self apart from spouse and marriage?
12. What is client's level of anxiety or fear with respect to current situation and lifestyle?
13. How does client perceive situation (fear, self-blame, guilt, love or sorrow for spouse)?
14. How does client express anger?
15. Client's personal resources (job, skills, finances, transportation).
16. Client's attitudes toward separation and/or divorce.
17. Does client express feelings or desires to exercise control over own life?
18. Under what circumstances will client return home or to spouse?
19. Who knows the client's whereabouts at this time?
20. Patterns of and reactions to separation from partner resulting from abusive episodes.
21. History of tetanus immunization.
22. Brief history of abusive mate, including characteristics, for example.
    a. Stereotyped self-image accompanied by strong feelings of inadequacy, remorsefulness, and needs for nurturing.
    b. Inability to verbalize feelings.
    c. Projection of responsibility for real or perceived failures onto spouse and/or children of family.
    d. Social isolation of family, but not necessarily self.
    e. Control of family and decision making (e.g., money, availability of transportation, movement outside home).
    f. Difficulty forming intimate relationships.
    g. Number of marriages.
    h. History of mental illness, alcohol, drug, or gambling addiction, or personality disorder.
    i. History of temper tantrums in childhood and explosive rage reactions in adolescence and adult life.
    j. Nonacknowledgment of violent behavior as a problem; reluctance to seek help and resistance to intervention.
    k. Demographic factors (e.g., race, education, occupation, and salary).
    l. Criminal record.
    m. Relationship with children.

Physical Assessment

See Chapter 36 for assessment of anxiety and depression. Injuries may be to any part of the body; it is important to examine areas that are normally covered. Note any of the following:

1. Broken bones (rib, jaw, shoulder, etc.).
2. Lacerations: note characteristics of wound; has a weapon (knife, razor, broken bottle, etc.) been used?
3. Soft tissue swellings, bruises, and hematomas: examine back of head, upper thighs, back, abdomen, breasts, and perineum.
4. Burns and scalds.
5. Choke marks.
6. Vomiting with abdominal distension.
7. Broken or missing teeth.
8. Human bite marks.
9. Retinal hemorrhage.
10. Evidence of healed lesions and fractures.
11. General physical condition and grooming, for example, skin color and tonus; nutritional status, and weight.
12. Evidence of pregnancy and/or vaginal bleeding.
13. Evidence of alcohol or drug usage.
14. Pain subjectively related by client (abdominal, back, chest, etc.).
15. Neurotrauma (see Chapter 48).

Diagnostic Tests

1. Provide for immediate physical examination of client.
2. X-ray films of suspected trauma sites.
3. Neurological consult if head injury is suspected.
4. Urinalysis for red blood cell (RBC) count if kidney damage is suspected.
5. Drug screen.
6. Alcohol blood level.
7. Vaginal examination if sexual abuse is suspected.

NURSING DIAGNOSES: ACTUAL OR POTENTIAL

1. Injury due to assault, potential or actual.
2. Anxiety and fear secondary to abuse.
3. Alterations in self-concept associated with verbal and physical abuse.
4. Maladaptive coping patterns associated with multiple dependency needs.
5. Inadequate problem-solving skills due to
    a. Deficiencies in personal resources.

   b. Lack of knowledge of community services.
6. Inadequate family process secondary to impaired verbal communications.
7. Role disturbances secondary to low levels of ego differentiation within the family.
8. Grieving secondary to immediate sense of failure and loss of role as "helpless victim"; potential grief reaction if relationship is terminated.
9. Social isolation due to feelings of shame, jealousy, possessiveness of partner, and learned dependency on partner.
10. Alterations in sexual behaviors and/or methods for sexual gratification.

EXPECTED OUTCOMES

1. Immediate—begin at initial contact with victim. Client will
   a. Seek professional assistance at time assault occurs, resulting in self-protection.
   b. Demonstrate ability to use "survival techniques" to diminish effects of battering in the event client chooses to remain with partner.
   c. Verbalize fears of physical harm to a supportive person (e.g., friend, professional, minister).
   d. Identify personal strengths and support systems following an abusive episode.
   e. Identify his or her role and responsibility in the relationship.
   f. Identify situational characteristics that precipitate battering episodes.
   g. Identify roles accessible to him or her other than role of "helpless victim," for example, student, employee, volunteer, friend.
   h. Attend and participate in group activities designed for battered spouses.
   i. Identify and utilize available community resources until he or she is able to be self-sufficient.
   j. Establish one new same sex relationship in which feelings are shared.
   k. Function as a parent to children of the partnership, using available resources to assist progeny toward optimum growth and development.
2. Intermediate—develop as crisis is stabilized. Client will
   a. Increase independent functioning as evidenced by seeking employment, housing, legal aide, and child care.
   b. Demonstrate assertive behaviors following counseling and assertiveness training, as evidenced by the ability to make decisions, identify options and consequences of actions, and use of "I" messages.
   c. Verbally express feelings of anger to the appropriate person without employing passive-aggressive behaviors (e.g., breaking appointments, rules).
   d. Successfully complete the grieving process as evidenced by realistically identifying the strengths and weaknesses of the lost relationship without necessarily resuming it.
   e. Identify displaced sexual feelings and behaviors (i.e., using child as surrogate spouse for protection, role reversal, and incest) and available options to resolve them.
   f. Decide to remain in or leave the relationship.
   g. Contract for counseling either individually, as a couple, or as a family, and the abusive partner will become involved in problem-oriented counseling.

INTERVENTIONS

1. Immediate—begin these interventions during first 24 to 48 hours.
   a. Assess and treat physical injuries; interview client privately; allow sufficient time for information gathering.
   b. Provide a safe shelter for the client and children; stress confidentiality.
   c. Reinforce client's efforts to end assaults.
   d. Recognize the client's extreme mental and physical fatigue, and provide time for rest, including child care, if needed.
   e. Encourage verbalization of guilt feelings and fears of being seriously hurt or killed.
   f. Communicate an attitude of hopefulness to client.
   g. Provide opportunities for contact with other assault victims to decrease feelings of isolation.
   h. Inform client of legal rights; refer to appropriate agencies.
2. Intermediate—begin these interventions after immediate needs are met.
   a. Assist the client to identify his or her personal strengths, resources, and goals.
   b. Identify expectations and responsibilities

of client while a resident of the protective setting or shelter.

c. Provide concrete information about available financial, occupational, educational, and legal options.
d. Assist client, as needed, in initial encounters with resource agencies, for example, transportation, role playing, job interview.
e. Assist clients with problem solving without making decisions for them.
f. Serve as client's legal advocate if so requested.
g. Provide educational materials and experiences pertinent to spouse abuse (e.g., books, films, and discussion groups).
h. Teach assertive communication skills.
i. Involve the client in a therapeutic one-to-one relationship.
j. Present client with the opportunity to participate in a therapy group.
k. Reinforce behaviors that demonstrate independence (e.g., grooming, job seeking, daily decisions).
l. Encourage client to form a friendship with another person who has had similar experiences.
m. Employ role playing with client for expression of feelings (e.g., anger, frustration, dependency, and sadness); provide feedback.
n. Assist client to identify advantages and disadvantages of resuming relationship with spouse.
o. Teach client how to select a marriage counselor if couple chooses reconciliation.
p. Inform client of available parenting classes, and encourage attendance.
q. Teach client the following survival techniques if relationship with partner is resumed.
    (1) Anticipate another attack, and form a plan of action.
        (a) Prepare one room in the home with secure locks and telephone.
        (b) Identify emergency escape route to a secure place.
        (c) Prepare a secret emergency "get-away kit" that includes extra sets of keys, money, clothing for self and children, important papers (e.g., birth certificates, social security cards) and a list of emergency phone numbers, particularly women's shelters.
        (d) Hide get-away kit with a neighbor or friend.
        (e) Arrange a set of signals with neighbors or friends to notify them of stressful situations.
    (2) Restore, improve, and/or maintain physical health.
    (3) Take classes in self-defense techniques.
    (4) Avoid threatening spouse unless there is intent to take action.
    (5) Learn pattern of factors precipitating abuse, and try to avoid provocative situations.
    (6) Develop a positive self-concept through:
        (a) Counseling.
        (b) Psychotherapy.
        (c) Consciousness-raising groups.
        (d) Assertiveness training.
    (7) Take classes in relaxation techniques.
    (8) Get a job or begin vocational training immediately.
    (9) Leave immediately at first sign of abuse; do not return without police escort.
    (10) Develop at least one close friendship with a sensitive adult who will be available if necessary.
    (11) If personal values prevent consideration of separation, divorce, or legal action, develop a spiritually sustaining philosophy.
r. Involve abusive partner in change-oriented activities if relationship is resumed, such as
    (1) Cognitive-behavioral techniques for developing alternative coping patterns, for example, stress inoculation (Novaco, 1955), sensory relaxation training (Lazarus, 1977). Insight-oriented therapy is resisted by most spouse abusers and statistically has shown minimal behavioral change.
    (2) A.A., N.A., or Gamblers Anonymous if addiction is present; Parents Anonymous if child abuse present.
    (3) Friendships with members of the same sex who do not engage in violent behavior.

(4) Achievement in an area that promotes a feeling of self-satisfaction (e.g., hobbies, sports, clubs).
(5) Participation in consciousness-raising groups.
(6) Recording feelings and thoughts in a journal to be shared with spouse and counselor.
(7) Written assessment of effects of violence on significant others.
(8) Distancing maneuvers for bodily messages of frustration, anger, and rage.
(9) Physical exercise, such as jogging, swimming, and gardening.

EVALUATION

Outcome Criteria

1. The abused client
   a. Makes a decision to remove self and children from family, or the converse.
   b. Verbalizes desire and willingness to change life.
   c. Demonstrates decision-making skills and activities that are enhancing to self-esteem.
   d. Develops a plan of action and utilizes available resources to carry it out.
   e. Participates in group activities designed to develop self-growth and demonstrates changes in activities of daily living that indicate independence.
   f. Establishes one significant relationship with a member of the same sex.
   g. Demonstrates parenting skills that are nonviolent and oriented toward optimal development of children and self.
   h. Secures employment or begins necessary training to develop vocational skills.
   i. Verbalizes feelings and utilizes cognitive skills to develop behavioral options.
   j. Resolves grief process within 1 year, if separation elected.
   k. Develops a sexual relationship with a consenting adult based upon mutual respect and intimacy.
   l. Evaluates own movement toward independence.
   m. Maintains a nonviolent relationship with abusive partner if separation not elected.
2. The abusive spouse changes behaviors and utilizes nonviolent techniques for dealing with frusturation and anger.

Complications

CLIENT RETURNS TO PARTNER BEFORE RESOLUTION OF CRISIS OR DEMONSTRATED CHANGES IN RELATIONSHIP

Assessment
Client leaves shelter to return to home and partner.
Revised Outcome
Client will return to the facility or shelter in the event of further abuse.
Interventions
1. Provide opportunity for client to return to shelter within limits. Many shelters refuse clients if this pattern occurs more than three times.
2. Give client emergency phone numbers to use after the next assault.
3. Inform client of survival techniques.

BATTERING PARTNER THREATENS CLIENT OR UTILIZES LEGAL SYSTEM TO GAIN RETURN OF SPOUSE AND/OR CHILDREN.

Assessment
1. Threatening phone calls, letters, or visits.
2. Breaking into shelter or new residence.
3. Kidnapping.
4. Legal action (e.g., custody conflicts and countersuits).

Revised Outcome
Client will seek protection of legal rights through police, legal counsel, or court system.
Interventions
1. Assist client to obtain legal counsel.
2. Assist client to obtain restraining order, police protection, or whatever is necessary at that time.

PROFESSIONAL HELPER IS PHYSICALLY THREATENED OR INJURED BY ABUSIVE PARTNER

Assessment
1. Refer to 1, 2, and 4 under second Complication, above.
2. Physical assaults on helper.

Revised Outcomes
Professional helper will provide for his or her own safety.
Interventions
1. Maintain confidentiality of shelter.
2. Notify law enforcement agency.
3. Utilize legal system for protection and prosecution.

CLIENT TRANSFERS DEPENDENCY FROM SPOUSE TO HELPING PROFESSIONALS

Assessment
1. Failure to follow through on decisions and/or recommendations.
2. Manipulation of shelter rules, policies, counseling relationships, and so on.

Revised Outcomes
Client will function interdependently with helping professionals.

Interventions
1. Point out dependent behaviors and their consequences.
2. Set limits on manipulative behaviors.
3. Positively reinforce independent functioning.

Reevaluation and Follow-up
1. Provide for continuity of services through shelter and/or mental health clinic.
2. Encourage client to maintain periodic contact as indicated by progress.
3. Communicate with social service agencies utilized by client.
4. Provide client with addresses and phone numbers of shelters elsewhere in the event of a relocation.

CHILD ABUSE

DESCRIPTION

Child abuse is a problem of epidemic proportions characterized by abnormal parenting behaviors. Fewer than 10 percent of abusive parents have serious psychiatric disorders that would preclude their availability for treatment (Steele, 1977). Abusive acts can include neglect, abandonment, and/or physical, mental, verbal, and sexual abuse. "No social class, occupation, education level, race, religion or marital status can claim exemption" (McKeel, 1978). Accurate statistics on child abuse are difficult to obtain due to variations in definitions, interpretations, and the number of unreported cases. It is estimated that the majority of children who die as the result of abuse are known to authorities before their deaths. Child abuse occurs from birth through adolescence; although findings are contradictory, many researchers define the most dangerous period for the child as the years from birth through age 4 years and during adolescence. Abused children frequently become abusive parents* of the next generation. The scope of this problem is such that the Child Abuse Prevention and Treatment Act (PL 93-247) was established in 1974 to provide the 50 states with funds for protective services and federal assistance for identification, diagnosis, and prevention.

PREVENTION

Health Promotion

1. Identify parents in high-risk groups for potential child abuse (see Population at Risk).
2. Establish and conduct parenting classes in high schools and communities; stress normal growth and development, the importance of nurturing, and nonviolent disciplinary measures.
3. Conduct communication skills training and family life education classes beginning at primary school level.
4. Conduct prenatal discussions of parental expectations of unborn child (e.g., sex of child, physical and personality traits, intelligence, and obedience).
5. Educate and actively involve professionals in a multidisciplinary approach (physicians, nurses, health care workers, teachers) in assessment, early detection, intervention, and reporting skills.
6. Encourage formation of child and parent advocacy groups.
7. Establish hot lines to help parents deal with daily crises.
8. Establish Parents Anonymous groups.
9. Establish and publicize crisis centers where children may be brought by overwrought parents before abuse occurs.
10. Educate parents about "time-away" activities available to their children in the community (e.g., library story hours, recreation programs, and museum activities).
11. Organize short-term emergency shelters using families within the community.
12. Develop teams within hospitals that will be prepared to deal with abuse problems (e.g., SCAN) (Helfer, 1977).

* "Parent" will be used to describe any significant caregiver, including babysitters.

13. Establish support groups for mothers of preschool children.
14. Develop child protection agencies within communities to include long-term treatment of abused children and families.
15. Develop prevention programs during the perinatal period in hospitals and birthing centers.
16. Develop policies within newborn nurseries and pediatric facilities that will promote parental involvement in the child's care (i.e., early identification by name, stroking, cuddling, and assisting with care).
17. Teach parents of "special children" attachment behaviors (e.g., eye contact, cuddling on reunion, and games that increase trust levels).
18. Expand services of family courts to allow for earlier intervention and treatment.
19. Help families to develop adaptive life skills (e.g., mate selection, family planning, maximizing individual potentials, social integration, and realistic expectations of family members).
20. Emphasize both the rights and responsibilities of children.
21. Educate police and public that abusive parents are needful people who do love their children and whose abusive behavior can be corrected.

Population at Risk

The National Center for Child Abuse delineates three major components for abuse. First, parents must have potential for abuse. Second, presence of a "special" child. Third, presence of a crisis or series of crises. Not all families will abuse children given these three criteria operating simultaneously; however, it is noteworthy that all identified abusive families have these characteristics (Helfer, 1977).

1. Presence of potential within the family.
   a. Parents have been physically or emotionally abused as children.
   b. Parents who report experiences of having been misunderstood, criticized, worthless, unloved, and overwhelmed by parental demands as children.
   c. Parents with addictive problems, for example, alcohol, drug use, and gambling.
   d. Parents who lack empathy for the problems of their children and their children's rights.
   e. Parents who are physically and socially isolated from support systems.
   f. Parents who lack knowledge of community resources.
   g. Parents who distrust and are antagonistic toward authority, both real and/or perceived.
   h. Parents who have unrealistic expectations of their children (i.e., compliance and age-related behaviors).
   i. Parents with unmet dependency needs seen in role reversal, reluctance to ask for help, and ambivalence.
   j. Parents who are unable to support and/or relieve one another with childrearing tasks.
   k. Parents who project low self-esteem.
   l. Unplanned and/or unwanted pregnancies.
   m. Very young parents with little child rearing knowledge or experience.
   n. Stepparents.
   o. Parents with transitory lifestyles (e.g., military, migrant worker).
2. Presence of a special child.
   a. Results from an unplanned, unwanted, and/or abnormal pregnancy or delivery.
   b. Fails to adequately bond to maternal caregiver at birth due to prematurity, physical impairment, or lack of maternal nurturing.
   c. Viewed as "different" by parents (e.g., sex, intelligence, behavior patterns, appearance).
   d. Fails to meet parents' behavioral expectations and/or learn compliance skills.
   e. Possesses some exceptionality in cognitive, physical, or emotional spheres.
   f. Seemingly normal child with a slight central nervous system dysfunction that impedes empathic concern from others.
   g. Separated from primary caregiver during first 6 months of life.
   h. Illness of either primary caregiver or child during first year of child's life.
   i. Provokes parental aggravation by equating punishment with love.
3. Presence of a crisis or crises. (The situation perceived by the abusive parent is highly subjective).
   a. Physical, for example, unemployment, financial stressors, housing inadequacies, or lack of transportation.
   b. Personal, for example, marital dysfunc-

tions, death, personal loss, legal problems, lack of educational or employment resources, inadequate support systems, or critical remarks from relatives.

Screening

1. Examination of school or medical records with emphasis on locating children with history of developmental lag.
2. Health histories containing discrepancies in degree of illness or injury and parental explanations.
3. Parental attitudes of indifference, belittling, or hostility directed toward injury.
4. Failure to seek medical attention promptly.
5. School absences.
6. Hot line calls.
7. Child abuse registry reports.
8. Repeated emergency room visits.
9. Repeated requests for assistance with normal childhood complaints may be an early sign of potential for parental loss of control.
10. Multidisciplinary conferences involving families who meet criteria for population at risk.
11. Records of family courts, family protective services, child welfare services, mental health clinics, nurse practitioners, pediatricians, and adolescent runaway reports.

ASSESSMENT

Due to the sensitive nature of child abuse, awareness on the part of the practitioner is critical. The possibility that people can and do hurt children must remain ever present in the nurse's mind. It is important to take a complete family history when assessing the child, understanding that the parents may perceive the interview as an interrogation and become angry or hostile.

Health History

See Chapter 36 for complete format of general health history. Note especially the following:

1. Obtain circumstances of and explanations for injury; note response time of parents to injury.
2. Validate history through a second interview; note discrepancies.
3. Parental admission of or history of prior child abuse.
4. Parental expressions of fear of loss of control.
5. Parental concern regarding involvement of legal authorities.
6. Immunization records, allergy history, and medical records of child; note unusual illnesses or injuries and indications of medical or dental neglect.
7. Description of home and social environment (i.e., material values, adequacy of housing, number of family members, social resources, and support systems).
8. Response of parents to child's behavior; note degree of anger generated by behavior.
9. Prior contacts with community agencies.
10. History of family addiction (alcohol, drugs, etc.).
11. Observe for following characteristics of abused child:
    a. Result of unwanted, unplanned, and/or difficult pregnancy.
    b. Prolonged separation from primary caregiver during first year of life.
    c. Perceived as "different" from other children in family.
    d. Neurologically impaired.
    e. Demonstrates developmental lag.
    f. Behavioral responses may include (Kalmar, 1977 and Ortman, 1980)
        (1) Periods of hopeless crying during treatment but generally quiet and withdrawn.
        (2) Resistance to physical contact with parents and others.
        (3) Apprehension when approached by adults.
        (4) Minimal separation anxiety from parents, especially at time of admission.
        (5) Cautious and alert for potential dangers in the environment.
        (6) Seeks structures and routines; asks "what is going to happen next?"
        (7) Seeks attention in form of food, favors, and services.
        (8) Does not express desire to go home.
        (9) Demonstrates flattened affect and withdrawal when discharge is imminent.
        (10) Shows little expectation for adult comforting behaviors, particularly from parents.
        (11) Apprehensive when other children cry; demonstrates curiosity and/or fear at their behaviors.
        (12) Does not reach out to parents for comfort.
        (13) Does not disclose circumstances surrounding injury.

(14) Shows decreased responsiveness during play periods.
(15) Demonstrates minimal locomotion and exploration.
(16) Demonstrates unusual eating habits.
(17) Presents extremes of behavior: excessive aggression or passivity.

g. Presents behavior problems in school or at home.
h. Presents patterns of school absenteeism due to physical signs of abuse.
i. Demonstrates acting out behavior (e.g., drugs, promiscuity, truancy, running away from home).
j. Subjectively reports fatigue—tired and without energy.
k. Somatic symptoms of depression.

12. Observe for following parental behaviors:
    a. Demand behaviors beyond child's ability; may set adult behavioral standards.
    b. Defend violent patterns as "disciplinary measures."
    c. Lack awareness of or disregard for child's needs.
    d. Demonstrate anger, evasiveness, or contradictions in giving accounts of injury.
    e. Fail to seek prompt medical attention for child.
    f. Seek medical attention from many sources for different injuries.
    g. Avoid involvement in child's care and activities.
    h. Give history of having been abused or neglected as children.
    i. Respond inappropriately by lack of concern or overreaction to extent of injury, treatment program, prognosis, and follow-up care.
    j. Express concern regarding what will happen to them.
    k. Leave child quickly at time of admission; may fail to visit child during hospitalization.
    l. May be difficult to locate.
    m. Demonstrate minimal nurturing body contact with child.
    n. Deny involvement in child's injuries; maintain bizarre explanations for serious injuries.
    o. Neglect personal health and grooming.
    p. Express feelings of low self-esteem.
    q. Project own feelings onto child.
    r. Show ambivalence toward child.
    s. Ignore child when attention is sought by child.
    t. Fail to keep appointments.
13. Observe verbal interactions with attention to indifference to child's injuries; for example, parents may
    a. Be critical of child's behaviors.
    b. Fail to positively acknowledge child's achievements.
    c. Present scapegoating, threats of bodily harm and/or abandonment, confusing messages, name-calling, or make derogatory remarks to child.
    d. Demonstrate role reversal between parent and child.

Physical Assessment

Note any of the following:

1. Burns from cigarettes (round, pitted markings) or scalding (redness, blistering).
2. Bruises, welts, fingerprints on arms, legs, or throat.
3. Abrasions, lacerations, scratches, and old scars.
4. Puncture wounds (knives, forks).
5. Sprains and dislocations (especially of shoulders and elbows).
6. Frostbite.
7. Human bite marks (reddened crescent-shaped areas).
8. Internal injuries evidenced by localized tenderness, pain, vomiting, abdominal distension, absent bowel sounds, bleeding from orifices, paradoxical breathing, seizure activity, and changes in level of consciousness.
9. Dismemberment.
10. Emaciated appearance (drawn skin, wasted buttocks, prominent ribs).
11. Recent or healed fractures of long bones, ribs, or skull.
12. Broken or missing teeth; oral lacerations.
13. Poisoning or ingestion of toxic substances.
14. Dehydration.
15. Poor skin hygiene, including feces or dirt in skin folds.
16. Ocular hemorrhage, detached retina, difficulty in focusing eyes.
17. Hearing impairment.
18. Skin pallor.
19. Animal bites.
20. Retarded physical development (low weight and height for age).

21. Localized edema.
22. Genital and anal trauma: vulvitis, vaginitis, venereal disease, ruptured hymen, presence of semen, localized edema and pain, presence of pubic hair in clothing of prepubertal child.
23. Untreated physical problems or abnormalities (e.g., diabetes, strabismus, orthopedic disorders, hernia, cleft lip).
24. Neurotrauma (see Chapter 48).
25. Facial expressions and overall affective responses (sadness, flatness, lethargy).

Diagnostic Tests

A complete physical exam is always indicated and may include some or all of the following:

1. Hematology workup, including platelet count, bleeding time, prothrombin time, blood lead level.
2. X-ray films for trauma: skull, ribs, pelvis, and long bones.
3. Complete blood count.
4. Urinalysis, including culture and drug screen.
5. Stool analysis including pH, occult blood, ova, and parasites.
6. Serum electrolytes.
7. Serum calcium.
8. BUN.
9. Retinal examination.
10. Neurological workup with suspected head injury.
11. Genital and rectal exam with suspected sexual abuse.

NURSING DIAGNOSES: ACTUAL OR POTENTIAL

1. Injury due to assault, actual or potential.
2. Inadequate parent–child bonding.
3. Maladaptive coping patterns associated with multiple dependency needs in child and family.
4. Inadequate family problem-solving skills due to decreased ability to deal with internal and external stress.
5. Anxiety and fear secondary to abuse of child.
6. Inadequate family process secondary to impaired verbal communication.
7. Role disturbances in child and family secondary to diminished awareness of rights and responsibilities of others.
8. Alterations in parenting functions due to inadequate information about child's growth and development.
9. Social isolation secondary to feelings of low self-esteem, distrust, and lack of self-confidence in child and family.
10. Alterations in child's self-concept secondary to physical, cognitive, emotional, or social abuses.
11. Unrealistic perception of problems secondary to family discord.

EXPECTED OUTCOMES

1. Immediate. Begin at initial contact with family and/or when abuse first suspected.
   a. The child's physical condition will be stabilized as evidenced by adequate physiological status, relief of pain and discomfort, and absence of complications.
   b. The child will demonstrate reduction of fear and/or anxiety.
   c. The child will experience protection from further harm, including separation from family, if necessary.
   d. The family will perceive interventions as therapeutic rather than punitive.
   e. Family members will identify and attempt to remedy stressors that precipitate abusive responses.
   f. The abusive parents will identify their legal rights and responsibilities.
2. Intermediate. Begin as crisis stabilizes.
   a. The family will establish and maintain a safe home environment.
   b. The family will recognize the multigenerational cycle of child abuse.
   c. The family will increase social involvement.
   d. The parents will identify and utilize effective parenting techniques.
   e. The parents will delineate realistic expectations for themselves and their children.
   f. The child will be provided with temporary foster care, if necessary.
   g. The family will realistically evaluate assets and liabilities, individually and collectively.
   h. Family members will utilize effective problem-solving skills (i.e., appropriate expression of emotion, nonviolent resolution of family crises, and improved interactions).

i. The family will be involved in ongoing treatment programs.
j. The parents will develop and maintain attachment behaviors with the child (i.e., "bonding").
k. The child will utilize appropriate attention-seeking behaviors.

INTERVENTIONS

1. Immediate. Begin these interventions during the first 24 to 48 hours.
   a. Assess and treat physical injuries.
   b. If abuse is strongly suspected, recommend to treatment team that child remain for observation.
   c. Carefully document and report suspicions of child abuse to appropriate legal agencies.
   d. Protect confidentiality of parents and child from curious staff members and visitors.
   e. Talk openly about the abusive behavior with the parents, focusing on
      (1) The serious nature of the problem.
      (2) Abuse as a means of coping with frustration.
      (3) Availability of treatment programs.
      (4) The varied feelings and concerns of family members.
      (5) Abuse is a modifiable behavior.
   f. Encourage mutual focus on parents and child during all contacts.
   g. Avoid verbal or nonverbal rejection of parents when interacting with child.
   h. Explain all procedures to child and parents; involve parents in child's care.
   i. Encourage description and clarification of factors that trigger abusive behavior (e.g., school problems, mealtime disturbances, crying, bedwetting, separation anxiety).
   j. Inform parents of their legal rights, responsibilities, and reporting procedures.
   k. Make consistent staff assignments to increase security of child and parents.
2. Intermediate. Begin as soon as crisis stabilizes.
   a. Refer family to local child protective services agency for example, SCAN (Helfer, 1977), BCHS (Ortman, 1980).
   b. Inform parents about Parents Anonymous (1-800-421-0353) and other self-help groups; make first contact if necessary.
   c. Assist family in defining and creating a safe home environment.
   d. Assist family members to complete self-assessments, including expectations of self and others.
   e. Provide family with information and phone numbers of available crisis intervention services (hot lines, crisis centers, etc.).
   f. Offer parents information about and opportunities to attend parenting classes and counseling centers.
   g. Inform parents of community resource agencies available to deal with ongoing problems (transportation, housing, employment, health care, addictive disorders, etc.).
   h. Encourage family members to verbalize current problem-solving techniques.
   i. Assist family to accept anger, ambivalence, and jealousy as normal emotions.
   j. Teach family intervention strategies appropriate to emotions of anger and ambivalence.
   k. Conduct or refer family members to family groups and/or individual therapy.
   l. Discuss and model attachment behaviors with child, (e.g., touching, cuddling, eye contact, cooing, talking, and nonverbal communications).
   m. Positively reinforce parental behaviors that demonstrate growth and responsibility (verbalization of negative feelings, effective problem-solving skills, and effective parenting techniques, etc.).
   n. Discuss with family means of decreasing social isolation (e.g., joining social organizations, clubs, trade unions, and cooperatives).
   o. Define, with the family in the presence of the child, the positive behaviors of the child that will be reinforced.
   p. Meet parents' immediate dependency needs (inability to keep appointments, lack of transportation, decreased decision-making skills) while using these encounters to teach adaptive skills via role modeling and information giving.
   q. Encourage abusive parent to maintain and share with nurse and/or therapist a daily journal reflecting stressful periods.
   r. Refer family to health department for continuation of contact following discharge of child from hospital to home.

s. Encourage abusive parent to seek out-of-home interests, especially if parent is a full-time parent.
t. Refer child to evaluation centers if developmental lag or behavior problems are evident.
u. When separation of child from family is indicated, provide adequate adjustment period before transfer; include in discharge planning a visit from potential caretaker while child is hospitalized; involve parents in separation process if possible.

EVALUATION

Outcome Criteria

These may be assessed by nurse, pediatrician, school personnel, or referral agency staff.

1. The abused child
   a. Demonstrates a stabilized health status.
   b. Demonstrates a reduction of fear in his environment as assessed by play, drawings, and behavioral responses.
   c. Is located in a safe environment as determined by the protective service agency.
   d. Utilizes positive behaviors rather than manipulation/provocation to satisfy needs.
   e. Demonstrates mastery of age-appropriate tasks.
   f. Expresses feelings in a constructive manner as observed during play, school, and social interactions.
2. The abusive parent
   a. Demonstrates willingness to cooperate in the treatment program by continued participation in intervention strategies.
   b. Identifies internal and environmental stressors that contribute to abusive behaviors.
   c. Demonstrates parenting skills that promote growth and development of parent and child.
   d. Utilizes treatment facilities for stress reduction (e.g., Parents Anonymous groups, crisis centers, and hot lines).
   e. Maintains a safe home environment.
      (1) Provides adequate food and housing.
      (2) Demonstrates knowledge of child's level of development and potential behaviors.
      (3) Minimizes accident potential within home.
   f. Utilizes appropriate disciplinary skills.
   g. Increases social involvement as evidenced by membership in parent groups, community organizations, clubs, and churches.
   h. Demonstrates ability to solve effectively problems concerned with personal needs, employment, health, transportation, money management.
   i. Demonstrates, in groups or family sessions, impulse control, clear communications, use of "I" messages, and direct rather than indirect expression of frustration.

Complications

NURSE'S RESPONSE TO CHILD ABUSE INTERFERES WITH HIS OR HER ABILITY TO ASSIST EFFECTIVELY IN PROBLEM RESOLUTION

Assessment

1. Inability to accept emotionally the abusive family as worthy of assistance.
2. Anger directed at abusive parent.
3. Lack of objectivity in assessment of family needs.
4. Verbalizes wishes to punish the abusive parent.
5. Overprotects child and has rescue fantasies.

Revised Outcomes

Nurse will develop a nonpunitive, objective attitude toward the abusive family and abused child.

Interventions

1. Provide ongoing opportunities for staff sensitivity groups.
2. Encourage attendance and participation in seminars and continuing education programs.
3. Limit any nurse-therapist to a maximum current caseload of three to four client families.

PARENTAL BEHAVIORS COUNTER-PRODUCTIVE TO THERAPEUTIC INTERVENTIONS

Assessment

1. Superifical compliance with treatment plan.
2. Resentful, negativistic attitudes and behaviors.
3. Inadequate and/or inaccurate information.
4. Transcultural differences predisposing to distrust of those in helping roles.

Revised Outcomes

The abusive parent will develop awareness of their interfering behaviors and will adopt positive behavioral alternatives.

Interventions

1. Consistent limit setting, supervision, and evaluation visits over a prolonged period (up to 5 years).
2. Utilization of at least two team members sharing responsibility for office contacts and home visits.
3. Utilization of medical, legal, and social resources to obtain family data.
4. Assignment of case managers of a similar cultural background when possible.

Reevaluation and Follow-up

1. Systematic review of former clients or suspected cases of abuse.
2. Long- and short-term family contact dependent upon family needs (recommended: 3- to 6-month intervals).
3. Liaison with courts, schools, community service agencies, and child abuse registries to monitor progress of family.

SEXUAL ABUSE

DESCRIPTION

Sexual abuse involves sexual acts without the consent of the victim, who may be too young to give consent or understand the nature of the request. These abusive acts may include rape, incest, oral-genital contact, sodomy, sex-play, and homosexual acts. Sexual assaults may be accompanied by threats of bodily harm or death. The need for sexual gratification is generally not the motivating factor; rather, the behavior occurs to meet nonsexual needs that may be pathological (e.g., rage, feelings of inadequacy, sadism, and antisocial activity). Accurate incidence figures are difficult to obtain due primarily to lack of reporting and/or the clandestine nature of the behaviors. The Federal Bureau of Investigation reports one rape occurring every 9 minutes (Sredl, 1979). Although short-term effects of physical trauma are usually seen, the long-term emotional and sexual effects may lead to serious dysfunction in the victim.

PREVENTION

Health Promotion

1. Disseminate information about sexual abuse, prevention, treatment, and reporting via seminars, media, school health classes, and community groups.
2. Teach protective behaviors and reinforce instructions given by law enforcement agencies (i.e., checking credentials of those attempting entrance into home, avoiding dark streets and parking lots when alone, traveling with companions, limiting information given over phone to strangers, and discernment of manipulative and deceptive behaviors).
3. Teach children to be wary of strangers and/or anyone who makes sexual advances.
4. Teach children their rights with regard to their bodies.
5. Teach potential victims to seek help if approached, threatened, or bribed.
6. Publicize hot line and sexual assault program telephone numbers.
7. Vary daily patterns, (travel, shopping sites, bedtime, etc.).
8. Encourage formation of neighborhood crime watch groups.
9. Educate public that *any* forced sexual activity is sexual abuse.

Population at Risk

1. Adult males and females.
2. Children of both sexes.
3. Physically handicapped, retarded, and intoxicated individuals.
4. Male and female prisoners.

Screening

1. Records of law enforcement agency calls (i.e., prowlers, obscene phone calls, and child molestation reports).
2. Hot line calls.
3. Emergency room visits.
4. Reports by children to school personnel of unusual familial behaviors.
5. Presence of strangers, without visible purpose, in public areas or neighborhoods.

ASSESSMENT

While prompt attention to physical evidence is a priority, it is also important to communicate an attitude that is nonpunitive and concerned.

Health History

See Chapter 36 for format. Note especially the following:

1. Date and time of assault.
2. Time of arrival and examination at health care facility.
3. Hygiene measures taken by client following the assault (e.g., shower, douche, change of clothing, cleansing of wounds, use of mouthwash, and fingernail cleansing).
4. Date of last menstrual period; use of contraceptives, if any; date of last coitus before assault.
5. Identify resources and support systems.

Physical Assessment

Note especially the following:

1. Genital, rectal, or oral evidence of abrasions, tears, ecchymotic areas, and bleeding.
2. Recency of tetanus toxoid immunization.
3. Use of kit to collect specimens: seminal fluid, dried secretions, foreign and victim hairs (pubic and head), blood standards, saliva standards, fingernail scrapings, oral, vaginal, and anal swabs and slides, urethral cultures, and lint. NOTE: Use paper bag for specimens.
4. Photographs of wounds (may be taken next day).
5. Evidence of pregnancy at time of assault.
6. Mental health status: note evidence of denial, blunted affect, slow, slurred, or retarded speech, guilt, shame, fear, paranoia, anger, inability to concentrate, retarded memory for event, distrust (including health team members and law officers), and/or panic states.

Diagnostic Tests

1. Laboratory evaluation of all smears taken, including motile sperm, syphilis, herpes and gonorrhea.
2. Pregnancy test (to be repeated 6 weeks after last menstrual period).
3. Urinalysis, CBC, and VDRL.

NURSING DIAGNOSES: ACTUAL OR POTENTIAL

1. Injury due to assault, potential or actual.
2. Anxiety and fear secondary to abuse.
3. Alterations in self-concept and social isolation secondary to assault and/or rejection by family members.
4. Alterations in sexual patterns due to anxiety, fear, and/or depression.
5. Alterations in interactional patterns secondary to distrust and a sense of vulnerability.

EXPECTED OUTCOMES

1. Client's physical condition will be stabilized as evidenced by
   a. Adequate physiological status.
   b. Relief of pain and discomfort.
   c. Absence of complications.
2. Client will experience reduction of fear and anxiety as evidenced by ability to discuss event and participate in physical examination and interviews.
3. Client will be screened for venereal disease (VD) and treated as necessary.
4. Physical evidence of assault will be documented and secured.
5. Client will participate in plans for follow-up care, including personal counseling and legal proceedings.
6. Client will utilize professional counselors for short- and/or long-term care.
7. Client will share experience with significant others in the support system.
8. Client will demonstrate understanding of legal procedures before formal decision to prosecute offender.
9. Client's spouse, parent, or sexual partner will be involved in counseling.
10. Client will understand options in event of pregnancy.
11. Client will return to normal daily activities when immediate crisis is resolved.
12. Family of client, particularly when children are involved, will resolve anger and grief responses to situation.

INTERVENTIONS

It is of utmost importance that client confidentiality be maintained and the nurse's approach be calm and professional.

1. Assess and treat physical injuries.
2. Assign one staff member per shift to remain with client (adult or child) for duration of stay in emergency treatment facility.
3. Make arrangements for a friend or relative to be with client at time of discharge from treatment facility.
4. If no family member or close friend is avail-

able to client, call the local rape hot line for assistance from an agency representative.
5. Explain each step of all diagnostic and treatment procedures in understandable language; repeat explanations if necessary.
6. Encourage verbalization of event, considering client's readiness.
7. Acknowledge and assist client to verbalize feelings of anger, fear, shame, guilt.
8. Obtain and/or assist with collection of physical evidence for diagnostic and treatment purposes.
9. Administer medications as ordered after obtaining client's allergy history.
10. Document collection of all physical evidence, and arrange for their dispersal to appropriate medical and/or legal authorities; obtain a receipt for evidence following agency policy.
11. Assist with obtaining photographs after securing written permission from client.
12. Make appointments for follow-up care for client at time of discharge.
13. Advise client of resources available for medical-legal assistance and protection, including the process of prosecution.
14. Refer client to sexual assault program for ongoing counseling and/or support group.
15. If the victim of sexual assault is a child, assist family members to
    a. Verbalize feelings of anger, rage, and guilt.
    b. Prepare for possible regressive behaviors on part of the child, including behavioral intervention techniques.
    c. Participate in Parents United.
16. Refer for family therapy.

EVALUATION

Outcome Criteria

1. Client recovers from physical assault and its complications.
2. Client establishs a relationship of trust with the health care provider and legal advocates.
3. Client verbalizes feelings related to assault and becomes involved in ongoing therapy, if indicated.
4. Client resumes activities and relationships.
5. Client learns techniques for future self-protection.
6. Client successfully prosecutes sexual assault offender if identity is established.
7. Client involves self in significant intimate relationships.

Complications

CLIENT DEVELOPS MENTAL HEALTH PROBLEMS, SUCH AS SEXUAL DYSFUNCTIONS, PHOBIC REACTIONS, DEPRESSION, ANXIETY STATES, AND/OR REGRESSIVE BEHAVIORS

Assessment
Objective signs of ego dysfunctioning and/or subjective reports of sexual problems, fears, feelings of worthlessness, and/or inability to resume activities of daily living.

Revised Outcomes
Client will adapt comfortably and satisfactorily to daily living events.

Interventions
1. Assist client to verbalize feelings.
2. Refer for ongoing treatment and/or counseling.

CLIENT IS OVERPROTECTED OR REJECTED BY PARTNER, FAMILY MEMBERS, OR FRIENDS

Assessment
Failure of client to resume normal activities; behaviors of family or friends indicate that client is encouraged to be dependent; verbal and/or nonverbal distancing maneuvers by family or friends.

Revised Outcomes
1. Client will demonstrate appropriate independent behaviors.
2. Client will work through rejection by significant others.

Interventions
1. Assist client to assume increased responsibility in age-appropriate tasks.
2. Encourage partner, family, and/or friends to verbalize concerns and cope with their fears realistically.

NURSE BECOMES INVOLVED IN LEGAL TRANSACTIONS ON BEHALF OF CLIENT

Assessment
Subpoena as a witness and/or expert witness.

Revised Outcomes
The nurse will be a credible witness providing accurate testimony.

Interventions
1. Thoroughly prepare all materials for hearings.
2. Present only facts, not opinions or guesses.

3. Maintain eye contact with legal counselors while being questioned.
4. Maintain professional demeanor in dress, speech, and manner.

Reevaluation and Follow-up
Provide for continuity of service through community resource agencies.

ELDER ABUSE

DESCRIPTION

Elder abuse refers to acts of physical abuse (including neglect), psychological abuse, sexual abuse, material abuse, and violation of the rights of a person 60 years of age or older. It is estimated that more than 2.5 million elderly persons in the United States are abused or neglected. Sometimes the abuse may be no more than a shove, but violent actions can cause great harm or death to an elderly person. As the life span continues to increase, it is predictable that the incidence of elder abuse will rise. Lack of recognition by middle-aged persons of the responsibilities of caring for an elder parent contributes to the rising rate of abused elders. While abusers are generally related to the victims (children, spouses, other relatives), surrogate caretakers and strangers may also victimize the dependent elder. In addition, crime statistics indicate that those persons over age 65 who are disabled, dependent, or lack social supports are frequently victims of neighborhood exploiters. Accurate statistics are difficult to obtain due to the secretive nature of elder abuse.

PREVENTION

Health Promotion

1. Educate to decrease negative stereotypes of ageism and the positive aspects of extended life spans.
2. Encourage intergenerational interactions to decrease misperceptions and distortions of the behaviors characteristic of the aged (e.g., extended family activities and elder volunteers in community agencies and schools).
3. Encourage abolition of mandatory retirement age.
4. Encourage mass media providers to avoid exploitation of ageism and disability.
5. Encourage the elderly to view themselves as independent and able rather than helpless and disabled.
6. Encourage legislation that would provide resources to family caretakers (i.e., home-related services, meal delivery, communal dining programs, adult day-care centers, transportation services, and educational programs for and about the aged).
7. Increase resources available to elders to reduce feelings of uselessness and boredom, for example, retired citizens volunteer organizations and political activist groups.
8. Legislate implementation of state mandatory reporting laws for elder abuse.

Population at Risk

1. Age greater than 60 years.
2. Presence of physical and/or intellectual impairment.
3. Lower and middle income status.
4. Residence with a relative (child, spouse, grandchild, or other family member).
5. Residence in a family in which caretaker is under unusual stress, especially financial.
6. Female, white Protestants.
7. Residents of nursing or boarding homes who are encouraged to be dependent upon caretakers.
8. Elderly persons living alone in low-income areas, especially in large cities.

Screening

1. Reports from professionals and paraprofessionals who have access to the elderly (i.e., doctors, nurses, staff members at senior citizen centers and social service agencies, pharmacists, and other health care workers, attorneys, and financial advisors).
2. Reports from funeral home directors.
3. Reports of law enforcement agency personnel.
4. Reports of suspicions of abuse by neighbors, family members, volunteer workers.
5. Calls to hot lines and person abuse lines.

ASSESSMENT

Health History

See Chapter 36 for format. Note especially the following:

1. Client does not recognize options to remaining in abusive situation.
2. Client denies occurrence of abuse.
3. Needs of the client conflict with expectations of the abuser.
4. Client is overmedicated (with resulting confusion) in attempt to make him or her more manageable.
5. Client reports changing will or signing papers under duress.
6. Client reports theft, misuse of money or property, and/or being forced from home.
7. Client expresses fear, shame, or guilt regarding abusive episode.
8. Presence of physical and/or emotional disability.

Physical Assessment

See Chapter 36. Refer also to preceding sections of this chapter. In addition, note the following:

1. Failure to receive medication as prescribed.
2. Absence of dentures, eyeglasses, hearing aids, or other prosthetic devices if needed.
3. General appearance indicating poor hygiene and nutrition (e.g., urine/feces odors, emaciation).

Diagnostic Tests

Refer to *Spouse Abuse*, above. In addition, note the following:

1. Hearing testing.
2. Ocular examination.
3. Dental examination.

NURSING DIAGNOSES: ACTUAL OR POTENTIAL

1. Injury or impairment due to abuse, actual or potential.
2. Anxiety, fear, and depression secondary to abuse.
3. Alterations in self-concept due to physical and psychological abuse.
4. Maladaptive coping patterns associated with multiple dependency needs.
5. Inadequate problem-solving skills due to deficiencies in personal resources and lack of knowledge of community resources.
6. Social isolation secondary to physical and psychological dependency.
7. Inadequate family process secondary to impaired communications.
8. Role disturbances due to multiple dependency needs.

EXPECTED OUTCOMES

1. Immediate. Begin at initial contact with victim. Client will
   a. Present stabilized physical condition.
   b. Be protected from further physical and/or emotional injury.
   c. Verbalize fears of harm.
   d. Verbalize incidents relating to abusive events and will participate in physical examination.
   e. Identify personal strengths and support systems following an abusive episode.
   f. Identify own role in family dynamics.
   g. Identify and utilize community resources to diminish dependency role within family.
2. Intermediate. Develop as crisis stabilizes.
   a. Client will increase independent functioning within physical and emotional limitations.
   b. Client will participate in individual and/or family counseling.
   c. Client will be offered protective placement outside the home or legal counsel to remove the abuser from the home.
   d. Abuser and client will receive legal counseling.
   e. Abuser will become involved in therapy.

INTERVENTIONS

Elder abuse is a multifaceted problem that shares commonalities with all other forms of person abuse; see Interventions in preceding sections for additional approaches.

1. Immediate.
   a. Assess and treat physical injuries.
   b. Provide protective placement to end threat of abuse.
   c. Document injuries sustained and statements made by client and concerned parties.
   d. Utilize crisis stabilization approaches to assist client to verbalize feelings and fears, discuss abusive episode, and assess client's current assets and liabilities.

e. Inform client of civil and criminal protections available (e.g., restraining orders, formal complaints, rehabilitation programs, and counseling).
f. Discuss social service interventions available to the client and family (e.g., visiting nurse referrals, Meals on Wheels, food stamp program, and visiting homemakers) that may facilitate client remaining in the home.
g. Report cases of elder abuse to local law enforcement agency and/or elder abuse hot line.
h. Inform suspected abuser of his or her legal rights, responsibilities, and reporting procedures.

2. Intermediate.
 a. Refer client and abusive family to the district or regional Department of Health and Human Services for investigation and follow-up after discharge from hospital.
 b. Offer client and suspected abuser counseling options, including individual and family therapy.
 c. Assist in permanent placement of client if return to the home situation is not possible.
 d. Encourage client to explore and act on job and leisure interests, considering available resources.

EVALUATION

Outcome Criteria

1. Abuse ceases.
2. Physical, emotional, and social status of client and abuser are maintained or enhanced.
3. Client seeks protection from further abuse.
4. Client views self as worthy and in control of own life.
5. Client identifies options other than remaining in abusive situation.
6. Abuser continues participation in recommended therapy or counseling.

Complications

Client fears retaliatory response from abuser following disclosure of abuse.

Assessment

Client is reluctant to answer questions.

Revised Outcomes

Client will experience feelings of security following contact with resource agencies.

Interventions

1. Offer protection to client, including temporary placement.
2. Encourage client to verbalize fears and feelings related to living situation.
3. Advise client of social and legal resources e.g., hot lines, family protective services, and legal aid society).
4. Provide privacy and attention to client during interviews and examinations.

Reevaluation and Follow-up

1. Periodic follow-up visits by abuse investigation team.
2. Liaison with courts, community service agencies, and elder abuse registries to monitor client and family progress.

REFERENCES

Helfer, R. E.: *The Diagnostic Process and Treatment Programs,* DHEW Publication No. (OHDS) 77-30069, U.S. Government Printing Office, Washington, D.C., 1977.

Kalmar, R.: *Child Abuse: Perspectives on Diagnosis, Treatment and Prevention,* Kendall/Hunt, Dubuque, Iowa, 1977, p. 101.

Lazarus, A.: *In the Mind's Eye,* Rawson Associates, New York, 1977, p. 193.

McKeel, N. L.: "Child Abuse Can Be Prevented," *American Journal of Nursing,* **78**(9):1478, September 1978.

Novaco, R.: *Anger Control: The Development and Evaluation of an Experimental Treatment,* D. C. Heath, Lexington, Mass., 1955.

Ortman, E.: "Nursing Intervention in Child Abuse," in J. Lancaster (ed.), *Community Mental Health Nursing: An Ecological Perspective,* C. V. Mosby, St. Louis, 1980, p. 121.

———: *Child Abuse/Neglect: A Guide for Detection, Prevention, and Treatment in BCHS Programs and Projects,* DHEW Publication No. (HSA) 77-5220, U.S. Government Printing Office, Washington, D.C., 1977.

Sredl, D. R., Klenkey C., and Rojkind, M.: "Offering the Rape Victim Real Help," *Nursing '79,* Vol. 9, No. 7, July 1979, p. 38.

Steele, B. F.: *Working with Abusive Parents from a Psychiatric Point of View,* DHEW Publication No. (OHD) 77-30070, U.S. Government Printing Office, Washington, D.C., 1977, p. 2.

BIBLIOGRAPHY

Black, M. R., and Sinnott, J. D. (eds.): *The Battered Elder Syndrome: An Exploratory Study*, Center on Aging, University of Maryland, College Park, Md., 1979. This is the first exhaustive study done on the problems of elder abuse in the United States. The authors reviewed the literature on all forms of family violence in preparing the investigation. Societal attitudes toward ageism, self-perceptions of the aged, and the phenomenon of "learned helplessness" are well reviewed. Included are strategies for prevention, assessment, social, and legal interventions. Emphasis is placed on the need for national legislation and central registries for protection of the elderly.

Byme, H. J.: "Crime and Fear: How Inevitable," *Parade Magazine*, February 24, 1980, p. 26. This essay discusses the major problems of elder abuse and lack of social awareness concerning it. The vulnerability of the elderly is discussed, as is the inadequacy of social and/or legal sanctions to prevent and intervene.

Camiglia, P., Lourie, I., James, L., and Dewitt, J.: "Adolescent Abuse and Neglect: The Role of Runaway Youth Programs," *Children Today*, 8(6):27, June 1979. Few articles address the problem of adolescent abuse. Ex-post-facto studies are beginning to reveal relationships between verbal, physical, and sexual abuse and the incidence of adolescent runaways. These authors report that intrafamilial violence is apparent in 30 percent of runaway homes studied. Linkages are made between abuse and the child's view of self as bad and deserving punishment.

Caparo, S., Krell, H., Gundy, J., et al.: "The Stressors of Treating Child Abuse," *Children Today*, 8(1):22, January 1979. Authors delineate eleven problems that professionals deal with when working with abusive families. These include fear of personal harm, lack of professional support, feelings of inadequacy, ambivalence, and need for control. Discussion of the nature of these problems and strategies for resolving them are included.

Carmody, F., Lanier, D., and Bardill, D.: "Prevention of Child Abuse and Negligence in Military Families," *Children Today*, 8(2):16, February 1979. Special social/structural problems of military families (socioeconomic status, isolation, age, mobility, etc.) are discussed in this article, along with known psychodynamics of abusive family members. Protocol established by the military for prevention, detection, and treatment of child abuse is included.

Davidson, T.: *Conjugal Crime*, Hawthorn Press, New York, 1978. A comprehensive book that deals with the problems of spouse abuse pragmatically. Offers shelter directories, hot line numbers, and legal suggestions. Annotated bibliography included.

Dean, D.: "Emotional Abuse of Children," *Children Today*, 8(4):18, April 1979. This article attempts to define emotional (nonphysical) abuse but accedes that this is an intangible problem. Using the model established by the San Diego County government, the author gives examples of differential treatment to children in families where emotional abuse is suspected (e.g., humiliation, scapegoating, rejection, indoctrination).

Ellerstein, N. S.: "Skin Manifestations of Child Abuse," in A. McRedmond (ed.), *Pediatric Nursing Currents*, Ross Laboratories, Columbus, Ohio, **27**(1):1, January–February 1980. Describes lesions recognizable as manifestations of abuse and identifies vehicles inflicting trauma.

Finklegor, D.: "What's Wrong With Sex Between Adults and Children?—Ethics and the Problems of Sexual Abuse," *American Journal of Orthopsychiatry*, **49**(4):692, April 1979. Article discusses need for defining and clarifying ethical issues of immorality of sexual abuse toward children. Denounces intuitive arguments and demands societal delineation of morals and personal rights.

Forward, S., and Buck, C.: *Betrayal of Innocence*, J. P. Tarcher, Los Angeles, 1978. Presents dynamics of incest: family relationships and environmental situations are discussed. Includes several case histories.

Foster, P. H., Lanier, M. W., and Whitworth, J. M.: "Expanding the Role of Nurses in Child Abuse Prevention and Treatment," *Journal of Psychiatric Nursing and Mental Health Services*, **18**(2), February 1980. Discusses the role of the nurse as a member of a multidisciplinary team approach to child abuse. Discusses nursing student involvement on team; offers realistic approaches to problem resolution.

Fuller, S. S.: "Inhibiting Helplessness in Elderly People," *Journal of Gerontological Nursing*, **4**(4):18, April 1978. This article discusses intervention strategies for decreasing dependent behaviors in the elderly client population.

Gelles, R. J.: "Abused Wives: Why Do They Stay?", *Journal of Marriage and the Family*, **38**(4):659, April 1977. Author discusses the factors that contribute to women remaining in situations where they are abused (e.g., infrequent beatings, decreased socioeconomic resources, and a history of having been abused as a child). He suggests that wives seek assistance when they stop believing spouse's promises. Gelles considers larger cultural problems as (1) the view that abuse is the norm, (2) lack of realistic assistance to victims, and (3) the abused spouse's fear of having the family's image tarnished.

Gelles, R. J.: *Family Violence*, Sage Publications, Beverly Hills, 1979. This is the most recent book by this author, who is an authority on intrafamily violence. Essentially a compilation of ten previously published essays, newer material includes a chapter on marital rape, violence during pregnancy, and husband abuse. Methodology for studying family violence is included. Text emphasizes avoidance of using medical/psychological models to study this problem.

Gorline, L. L., and Ray, M. M.: "Examining and Caring for the Child Who Has Been Sexually Assaulted," *Maternal Child Nursing*, **4**:110, March–April 1979. Discusses assessment skills, interviewing techniques, and nursing interventions necessary when working with the sexually assaulted child and family.

Helfer, R. E.: *The Diagnostic Process and Treatment Programs*, DHEW Publication No. (OHDS) 77-30069, U.S. Government Printing Office, Washington, D.C., 1977. This pamphlet discusses the processes involved in developing programs for prevention, early detection, and treatment of child abuse. Serves as a quick reference for information; it is comprehensive in scope but not in depth.

Helfer, R. E., and Kempe, C. H. (eds.): *The Battered Child,* 2d ed., University of Chicago Press, Chicago, 1974. This is an in-depth reference text discussing all aspects of child abuse, including historical perspectives, legal aspects, detection, and treatment.

Hendrix, M. J., LaGodna, G., and Boden, C. A.: "The Battered Wife," *American Journal of Nursing,* **78**(4):650, April 1978. Discusses the phenomenon of battered women and deals with the problems and resistances nurses meet when working with them.

Herjanic, B., and Wilbois, R. P.: "Sexual Abuse of Children: Detection and Management," *JAMA,* **239**(4):331, 1978. This article describes the need for physicians to assess and intervene in cases of childhood sexual abuse. The authors identify a "suspicion index" that might help medical personnel with problem identification. Article also discusses the prevalent physician posture of avoiding legal involvement.

Hilberman, E.: "Overview: The 'Wife-Beater's Wife' Reconsidered," *American Journal of Psychiatry,* **137**(11):1336, November 1980. An extremely well-researched and -documented article that describes the dimensions of spouse abuse; includes guidelines for clinicians in private practice and health clinics that may be used as suspicion indices. The author recommends the use of well-researched concepts for designing health care approaches for victims of spouse abuse.

Illing, M.: "Comment . . . On How We Can Identify Those at Risk," *Nursing Mirror,* **145**(25):34, December 22, 1977. Three areas of elder vulnerability identified by this author are emotional health, physical health, and significant differences over management of finances, for example, the elder may be draining family resources or may be perceived by family members as withholding funds.

Josten, L.: "Out of Hospital Care for a Pervasive Family Problem—Child Abuse, *Maternal Child Nursing,* **3**(2):111, March–April 1978. This article emphasizes the need for a family focus when dealing with problems of abuse. Discusses teaching, counseling, and coordination strategies as these may be utilized by the nurse.

Kalmar, R.: *Child Abuse: Perspectives on Diagnosis, Treatment, and Prevention,* Kendall/Hunt Publishing, Dubuque, Iowa, 1977. Surveys problem of child abuse, using a community approach for detection, prevention, and treatment; presents typology for classification and treatment.

Koch, L., and Koch, J.: "Parent Abuse . . . A New Plague," *Parade Magazine,* January 27, 1980:14. The authors estimate that as many as 1 million elderly are abused yearly. Article draws from research to support four types of prevalent elder abuse: physical, psychological, material, and/or violation of rights. The intergenerational cycle of family violence is also discussed.

Leaman, K.:"Recognizing and Helping the Abused Child," *Nursing 79,* **9**(2):64. The article discusses the role of the nurse in assessment and intervention of child abuse. Emphasis is on careful documentation and reporting.

Loraine, K.: "Battered Women—The Ways You Can Help," *RN,* **44**(1):23, October 1981. Author uses professional experiences to provide guidelines for assisting victims of spouse abuse, particularly in emergency situations.

Martin, D.: *Battered Wives,* Glide Publications, San Francisco, 1976. One of the first major publications reporting the problem of spouse abuse. Comprehensive review of the literature included; text focuses on the historical perspective of male dominance/female subjugation.

McKeel, N. L.: "Child Abuse Can Be Prevented," *American Journal of Nursing,* **78**(9):1478, September 1978. Potential for abuse criteria, case histories, and many nursing interventions discussed in this article; focus on early detection and intervention within hospital environment.

McMillan-Hall, N.: "Group Treatment for Sexually Abused Children," *Nursing Clinics of North America,* **13**(4):701, 1978. The advantages of concurrent group counseling for children who have been abused sexually and their parents are addressed. Children are helped to share feelings, direct punishment for the abuser, and learn assertive skills.

Meiselman, K. C.: *Incest,* Jossey-Bass, San Francisco, 1979. Comparative analysis of incestuous and nonincestuous case histories; comprehensive review of all forms of incestuous relationships; presents guidelines and recommendations for evaluation and treatment.

Neill, K., and Kauffman, C.: "Care of the Hospitalized Abused Child and His Family: Nursing Implications," *Maternal Child Nursing,* **1**(2):117, March–April 1976. This article discusses child abuse as a family problem and utilizes nursing process with a focus on empathic concern for both victim and abuser. Discusses, also, behaviors of the child that may be provocative and negative in gaining need satisfaction.

Ortman, E.: "Nursing Intervention in Child Abuse," in J. Lancaster (ed.), *Community Mental Health Nursing: An Ecological Perspective,* C. V. Mosby, St. Louis, 1980, p. 115. Focus of this article is the failure of adequate parent–child bonding as a contributory factor in child abuse. Report of an experimental study of abused/nonabused children's behaviors and nursing implications are included.

Parker, B.: "Communicating With Battered Women," *Topics in Nursing,* **1**(3):49, October 1979. This article discusses concepts of denial, control, and sexuality as the primary issues underlying the perpetuation of spouse abuse. Very useful techniques for interviewing abused clients are included.

Rist, K.: "Incest: Theoretical and Clinical Views," *American Journal of Orthopsychiatry,* **49**(4):680, April 1979. Theoretical approaches to incest and the dearth of literature on treatment are reported in this article. Author recommends research to increase understanding of incest and to assist in the development of intervention strategies.

Roy, M. (ed.): *Battered Women,* Van Nostrand Reinhold, New

York, 1977. Historical, social, and psychological causes and effects of spouse abuse are examined in this book. Research studies are used to document conclusions. Excellent references offered in appendices.

Rubinelli, J.: "Incest: It's Time We Faced Realty," *Journal of Psychiatric Nursing and Mental Health Services,* **18**(4):17, April 1980. Article focuses on major problems of incestuous relationships, including long-range effects.

Scharer, K.: "Rescue Fantasies: Profession Impediments in Working with Abused Families," *American Journal of Nursing,* **78**(9):1483, September 1978. This article deals with the responses of health professionals to victims of abuse and their families. Focuses on the nurse's need to recognize and handle feelings that may interfere with effective nursing intervention; also alerts the nurse to child behaviors that may need restructuring.

Sredl, D. R., Klenkey, C., and Rojkind, M.: "Offering the Rape Victim Real Help," *Nursing '79,* **9**(7):38, July 1979. The article discusses the immediate and long-term needs of the rape victim; it presents specific clinical, legal, and psychological interventions.

Steele, B. F.: *Working with Abusive Parents from a Psychiatric Point of View,* DHEW Publication No. (OHD) 77-30070, U.S. Government Printing Office, Washington, D.C., 1977. Child abuse is considered a problem of abnormal parenting behaviors in this booklet. Using psychiatric concepts, the author provides a framework for approaches in treating and preventing this phenomenon. Orientation of manual is directed toward altering parenting behavior.

Steinmetz, S. K., and Strauss, M. A.: "The Family As a Cradle of Violence," *Society* **10**(4):50, September–December 1973. Discounts male sex-linked aggression theories of family violence; stresses importance of learned behaviors as responses to stress and habit formation.

Strauss, M. A.: "A Sociological Perspective on the Prevention and Treatment of Wifebeating," *Nursing Dimensions,* **7**(1), Spring 1980. This article discusses prevention and treatment of spouse abuse using as a conceptual framework individual personality characteristics, societal norms and values, and the organization and structure of the family; points out fallacies in using pyschiatric/psychological treatment methods alone.

Walshe-Brennan, K.: "Granny Bashing," *Nursing Mirror,* **145**(25):32, December 22, 1977. This is an often-cited article dealing with the problem of elder abuse identified in Britain. Evidence that elder abuse is accompanied by general family violence, alcohol use, limited cultural/social resources, health, and general socioeconomic status is considered. Article points out reluctance of community to accept elder abuse as a national phenomenon.

Weingourt, R.: "Battered Women: The Grieving Process," *Journal of Psychiatric Nursing and Mental Health Services,* **17**(4):40, April 1979. Comprehensive article discussing the psychological aspects of battering; particular emphasis on the nurse's need to develop intervention skills for assisting the battered spouse to resolve grief.

Woods, F., and Habit, M.: *Strategies for Working with Assaulted Women, Their Families, and the Systems Around Them,* Women Helping Women, Metuchen, N.J., 1976. Pamphlet describing intervention techniques for use with battered spouses, children of battered spouses, and community support agencies.

42

Group Work in Inpatient Settings

Ann Ottney Cain

We are all born into groups and remain a member of a group until our death. Groups influence our interpersonal relationships all through life. In fact, much of our success in life depends on how successful we are in groups.

> Man's first or primary group is the family. . . . It is these early experiences that directly influence and determine a person's behavior in groups, his attitudes toward the leader and group members and the kinds of interpersonal relationships he establishes in general (McManama, 1977).

DESCRIPTION

A group is a congregation of three or more people who can communicate with one another to accomplish common goals. An essential feature is that the members have something in common, and this holds them together. There is interaction between members, and each member is influenced by the behavior and characteristics of the others and by the mood or climate present in the group.

Group dynamics are the forces in the group situation that determine the behavior of the group and its members. One needs to remember that group dynamics are not something that may or may not occur in a group. *Every group* has its own dynamics, its own pattern of forces. Sometimes certain of these forces seem to be at a very minimum in some groups, but their potentiality exists in *any* group situation. "Bad" groups can be examined as productively as "good" groups: one can learn as much about group dynamics from one as from the other. Anytime that three or more people meet, there are interactions, interpersonal relationships, group goals, problems of communication, and many other forces. These forces exist in varying degrees, but they are potentially present in all groups.

ASSESSMENT

1. Distinguishing characteristics of groups. Knowles and Knowles (1972) point out that a group must have a definable membership, a group consciousness, a shared purpose, interaction of some type, and the ability to act in a unitary way. Some other distinguishing characteristics that they suggest are the following and can be used to assess a group:
   a. Group background. In every group situation, there is a history to the group before it even starts. A new group coming together for the first time will have to devote much of its early energy to getting acquainted with one another, with the group's task, and with establishing ways of working together. A group that has met together before will know each other better and will know what to expect from one another, but it may have developed habits

that interfere with its efficiency, such as arguing, dividing into factions, or wasting time. Each member comes to the group with expectations or a "mental set" with reference to the group. They may be looking forward to the meeting or they may be dreading it; they may be deeply concerned about the group's task or indifferent to it. *All* these feelings affect the behavior of the participants and, consequently, influence the group's behavior.

b. Group participation patterns. In every group situation, people are participating in one way or another. There is a distinctive pattern of interaction that is particular to that one group. In some groups certain members overparticipate and dominate the group, and in other groups the leaders do all the talking. Sometimes all group members may talk to the leader directly, or all members may talk to each other, and a real sharing of ideas and opinions may occur. These patterns may tend to be very consistent in any given group, or they may vary over time. Usually, the broader the participation among members of a group, the deeper the interest and involvement will be.

c. Group communication patterns. These demonstrate how well members understand one another and how clearly they communicate their ideas, values, and feelings. Sometimes group members "speak past" each other or attempt to impress one another with elaborate vocabularies. Many feelings are communicated nonverbally; these involve body postures, facial expressions, and gestures.

d. Group cohesion. This is the strength of the bonds that bind the individual members into a unified group. It refers to the morale, the team spirit, and the strength of attraction of the group for its members. High cohesion is present when members of a group can work effectively in a cooperative situation in which all individuals have certain independent responsibilities but are at the same time interdependent. High cohesiveness in a group is evidenced when
   (1) Conflict between members is appropriate and can be tolerated and resolved.
   (2) Support is given to members who are being attacked or criticized.
   (3) Feelings of "we-ness" are evident; when members speak in terms of "we" and not just "I."
   (4) Productivity is high, and agreement concerning new tasks is obvious.

e. Group atmosphere. This is sometimes called the social climate, and it refers to the informality or the freedom of the group situation. Members have certain feelings about the group, and these are reflected in the degree of spontaneity of their interactions. The desirable kind of group atmosphere is one in which members feel free to speak when they have something to say.

f. Group standards or norms. These are the code of ethics by which acceptable behavior is judged within the group. These are ways of behaving that emerge, that can be seen, and that are typical of a certain group. Which subjects may be discussed, which are taboo; how openly members can express their feelings; how long members can talk; whether interruptions are permitted—all these and many other dos and don'ts are part of the group's standards. If standards are clear to group members, group functioning is more effective and members feel freer to participate. Standards are either implicit or explicit, with most groups operating on implicit standards that are rarely shared openly. Group members "just know" what they are.

g. Sociometric pattern. In any group situation, subgroups of one kind or another will develop. These subgroups are sometimes determined on the basis of friendship or common agreement about a particular issue, or they are sometimes determined on the basis of a common dislike of certain persons or situations. These patterns quickly show that certain members begin to identify certain other members they like more than others.

h. Group structure and organization. These can be both visible and invisible. Visibly, there are officers, appointed leaders, or committees. Invisibly, there are behind-the-scenes arrangements of members according to prestige, power, seniority, ability, and so on.

i. Group procedures. These are the ground rules and procedures by which the work of the group is accomplished. Frequently, these are informal, but sometimes very formal procedures, such as *Robert's Rules of Order*, are followed.

j. Group goals. These are sometimes clearly defined and at other times are quite vague and general. Members may be wholly, partially, or not committed at all to these goals.

2. Differences between primary and secondary groups.
   a. Primary groups are characterized by warm, intimate, personal ties with one another. Usually these groups are small and are face-to-face, with interpersonal behavior devoted to mutual ends. Examples of a primary group would be the family or the close friendship group like a high school gang. Earliest experiences in social unity come from the family; therefore, primary groups become the springboards for both individual and social institutions.
   b. Secondary groups are characterized by cool, impersonal, and more formal relationships, where the group is not an end in itself but a means to other ends. These groups are usually large, and members have only intermittent contacts. Examples of a secondary group would be social clubs or professional organizations (Olmstead, 1959).
3. Difference between group content and group process.
   a. Group content refers to the "what." It is what the group is talking about, what they are saying.
   b. Group process includes all the events and interconnecting forces that occur at any given moment in a group. It refers to the "how," It is how the group handles its communication and how members are interacting with each other, that is, who talks how much and to whom? Looking at process means to focus on what is going on in the group and to try to understand what is going on in terms of other things that have occurred previously in the group.
4. Roles of group members. Members play many roles in groups, and these greatly influence group life (Benne and Sheats, 1948).

One thing to remember is that in groups no specific role is assigned to anyone. Individuals move from one role to another in groups, and there may be much shifting around.

a. Functional roles are roles that are helpful in carrying out a group task or that help strengthen and maintain group life and activities. They can be broken down into two kinds: (1) task roles and (2) building and maintenance roles.
   (1) Task roles are those functions required in selecting and carrying out a group task or purpose. Some task roles are
      (a) Initiating activity. Proposing solutions, suggesting new ideas, new definitions of the problem, new attack on the problem, or a new organization of material.
      (b) Seeking information. Asking for clarification or suggestions, requesting additional information or facts; seeking relevant information about the group concern.
      (c) Seeking opinion. Looking for an expression of feeling about something from the members; seeking clarification of values, suggestions, or ideas.
      (d) Giving information. Offering facts or generalizations; relating one's own experiences to the group problem to illustrate a point.
      (e) Giving opinion. Stating an opinion or belief concerning a suggestion or one of several suggestions, particularly concerning its value rather than its factual basis.
      (f) Elaborating. Clarifying; giving examples or developing meanings, trying to envision how a proposal might work out if adopted; clearing up confusion.
      (g) Coordinating. Showing relationships among various ideas or suggestions, trying to pull ideas and suggestions together, trying to draw together activities of various subgroups or members.
      (h) Summarizing. Pulling together related ideas or suggestions; restating suggestions after the group has discussed them; offering a decision or

conclusion for the group to accept or reject.

(i) Testing feasibility. Making application of suggestions to real situations; examining practicality and workability of ideas; preevaluating decisions.

(j) Consensus testing. Sending up trial balloons to see if the group is nearing a conclusion; checking with the group to see how much agreement has been reached.

(2) Building and maintenance roles are those functions required for strengthening and maintaining group life and activities. They deal with the interpersonal and emotional aspects of group life. Some building and maintenance roles are

(a) Encouraging. Being friendly, warm, and responsive to others; praising others and their ideas; agreeing with and accepting contributions of others.

(b) Gate keeping. Attempting to keep communication channels open; facilitating the participation of others (e.g., "We haven't heard from Jim yet?"). Suggesting procedures for sharing opportunities to discuss group problems; bringing a blocked member into the group.

(c) Standard setting. Expressing standards for the group to use in choosing its content or procedures or in evaluating its decisions; reminding the group to avoid decisions that would conflict with group standards.

(d) Following. Going along with decisions of the group; somewhat passively accepting ideas of others; serving as an audience during group discussion and decision making.

(e) Expressing group feeling. Summarizing what group feeling is sensed to be; describing the reactions of the group to ideas or solutions.

(3) Roles seen as both task and group maintenance roles are

(a) Evaluating. Submitting group decisions or accomplishments to comparison with the group standards; measuring accomplishments against goals.

(b) Diagnosing. Determining sources of difficulties and the appropriate steps to take next; determining the main blocks to progress.

(c) Mediating. Harmonizing; attempting to reconcile disagreements and reduce tension; getting people to explore their differences.

(d) Compromising. Offering to compromise one's own position; admitting one's own error in order to maintain the group's cohesion.

(e) Relieving tensions. Draining off negative feeling by jesting or pouring oil on troubled waters; putting a tense situation into broader context.

b. Any group can be viewed from the point of view of what its purpose or function seems to be. When a member says something, certain questions can be asked:

(1) Is he or she primarily trying to get the group's work accomplished (task), or is he or she trying to improve or patch up some relationships among the members (maintenance)? Every group needs both kinds of behavior and needs to work out an adequate balance of task and maintenance activities.

(2) There is another question to ask when a member says something in a group. Is he or she primarily meeting some personal need or goal without regard for the group's problem?

5. Group growth chart (Table 42-1). This is useful to consult when trying to evaluate how any group is functioning. In a new group, interaction is usually relatively superficial, anxiety is fairly high, and the interchange is often stilted and unspontaneous. In a new group, ideas and suggestions are often not followed through. Individuals often seem to see and hear relatively little of what is really going on.

Usually, as groups work together, relationships in the group become more free and open. There is less threat or fear present, and there is a greater probability that the skills and resources of the group members will be utilized effectively. Group members show

TABLE 42-1 GROUP GROWTH CHART

Conditions in Groups Ordinarily Contributing Toward	
Negative Growth	**Positive Growth**
Communication	
1. Superficial, irrelevant.	1. Purposeful, relevant.
2. Differential or specialized language; common meanings not achieved.	2. Understandable language; common meanings achieved.
3. Differences kept hidden or expressed aggressively.	3. Different ideas and points of view expressed freely and positively.
4. Feelings hidden and expressed indirectly through ideas.	4. Feelings expressed directly when essential.
Goals	
1. Individualistic unshared goals.	1. Parellel or commonly shared goals.
2. Use of group for ego satisfaction.	2. Use of group for growth; growth purposes clarified and/or understood.
3. A single group goal is defined and held to at all costs.	3. Both group and individual goals are permitted and encouraged.
Atmosphere	
1. Aggressive, hostile, or overfriendly; demanding.	1. Friendly, accepting but realistic.
2. Prestige seeking.	2. Collaboration seeking.
3. Authorities demanded and accepted.	3. Authorities analyzed and utilized.
4. Hostile to change.	4. Supportive and encouraging of change.
Responsibility and Involvement	
1. Group discourages or denies individual's responsibility for growth; demands dependence.	1. Group allows and encourages individual to take responsibility for own growth.
2. Individual is not personally identified with the group—"It's just another group."	2. Individual is personally identified with the group—its continuance and/or function are important to her or him.
Internal Processes	
1. Group sets up a standard ritual (like "We must always be democratic" or "The leader tells us what to do").	1. Group changes its methods of operation freely and flexibly as needs arise and group development and growth continue.
2. Group sets up demands for a constant and continuting level of productivity.	2. Group varies its tempo of work and allows itself periods of relaxation.
3. Group does not allow any expression of mood other than polite friendliness.	3. Group feels free to express its moods—excitement, enthusiasm, concern, tension, etc.
Standards	
1. Only leader or resource persons help others.	1. Everyone in the group serves as resource to help group and each other.
2. Differences must be kept "out of sight."	2. Differences that are present in the group are useful.
3. Clearly defined and fixed roles are assigned to particular members.	3. Roles defined but may easily move from member to member.
4. Members given no opportunity to test out her or his new insights or skills.	4. Member has chance to try out her or his new insights and skills in the group.

SOURCE: Jenkins, D. H.: "Planning Conditions for Personal Growth," *Adult Leadership*, February 1954, pp. 16–21.

greater openness to information, opinions, and new ideas. Less energy is tied up in protecting and hiding themselves. This energy is freed for constructive group activity, and there is a greater likelihood of finding involvement and satisfaction in the group.

NURSING DIAGNOSES: ACTUAL OR POTENTIAL

1. Ineffectiveness of group growth associated with nonfunctional roles.

   So far, the group processes described deal with the group's attempt to work, but there are many forces active in groups that disturb work. They represent a kind of emotional underworld or undercurrent in the stream of group life. These underlying emotional issues produce a variety of emotional behaviors that interfere with or are destructive to effective group functioning. These are called the *nonfunctional roles*. They cannot be ignored or wished away. They must be recognized, their causes understood, and, as the group develops, conditions must be created that permit these same emotional energies to be channeled in the direction of group effort.

   One thing to guard against is the tendency to blame any person (whether it is self or others) who falls into this nonfunctional category. It is much more useful to regard this kind of behavior as a symptom that all is not well with the group's ability to satisfy individual needs through group-centered activity. As the group grows and as member needs become integrated with the group goals, there will be less of this type of behavior. It is useful to remember that each person interprets things differently. For example, what may appear as "blocking" to one person may seem to be "testing feasibility" to another.
2. Nonfunctional roles associated with negative group growth are
   a. Being aggressive. Working for status by criticizing or blaming others; showing hostility against the group or some individual; deflating the ego or status of others.
   b. Blocking. Interfering with the progress of the group by going off on a tangent, citing personal experiences unrelated to the problem, arguing too much on a point, or rejecting ideas without consideration.
   c. Self-confessing. Using the group as a sounding board, expressing personal, non-group-oriented feelings or points of view.
   d. Competing. Vying with others to produce the best ideas, talk the most, play the most roles, or gain favor with the leader.
   e. Seeking sympathy. Trying to induce other group members to be sympathetic to one's problems or misfortunes; deploring one's own situation or disparaging one's own ideas in order to gain support.
   f. Special pleading. Introducing or supporting suggestions related to one's own pet concerns or philosophies; lobbying.
   g. Horsing around. Clowning, joking, mimicking; disrupting the work of the group.
   h. Seeking recognition. Attempting to call attention to one's self by loud or excessive talking, extreme ideas, or unusual behavior.
   i. Withdrawing. Acting indifferently or passively; resorting to excessive formality, day dreaming, doodling, whispering to others, or wandering from the subject.
3. What are some of the basic issues or causes of this nonfunctional behavior? These are all questions that group members try to answer. Nonfunctional behavior is produced in response to these problems and can be destructive to group functioning. These basic issues are perceived by group members as
   a. The problem of *identity*. Questions asked are: Who am I in this group? Where do I fit in? What kind of behavior is acceptable here?
   b. The problem of *goals and needs*. Questions asked are: What do I want from the group? Can the group goals be made consistent with my goals? What have I to offer to the group?
   c. The problem of *power, control, and influence*. Questions asked are: Who will control what we do? How much power and influence do I have?
   d. The problem of *intimacy*. Questions asked are: How close will we get to each other? How personal? How much can we trust each other and how can we achieve a greater level of trust? ("The Tool Kit," 1953).

EXPECTED OUTCOMES

1. Types of groups and goals. The psychiatric nurse, as well as all other nurses, works with

many kinds of groups. This varied range of groups can include administrative groups, consultative groups, counseling and therapy groups, psychodrama, therapeutic communities, ward meetings, educational or discussion groups, social groups, and many others.

Groups have the potential to promote positive change in people. While no one knows exactly what makes groups work, certain catalysts are almost always present in successful groups. The most significant of these is the willingness of the group members to share themselves with others—their thoughts, ideas, feelings, and perceptions. The attitudes of group members can make or break any group.

Groups can be thought of as falling into three general categories:

a. Task groups. These are work oriented and have specific tasks or goals to accomplish.
b. Psychosocial groups. These focus on the emotional and social needs of people and include social gatherings and therapy groups.
c. Combinations or variations of both.

2. Definition and goals of group therapy. Group therapy is often selected as the method of treatment for many clients. We all live in groups, and these groups influence our interpersonal relationships. If people are having problems with their interpersonal relationships, it stands to reason that part of the healing process could also occur in a group.
   a. There are three things that groups can accomplish that individual therapy cannot:
      (1) The group supplies warmth and cohesion similar to family solidarity with which the individual can identify.
      (2) The group itself exemplifies forms of social adaptation, such as love and friendly competition, that can be directly carried over to larger groups.
      (3) Groups can give the individual the experience of giving as well as receiving help. There is a direct and fundamental fulfillment in being capable of directed love and support controlled by the individual for the benefit of the other group members. This is ego building (Murphy, 1963).
   b. In addition to these the group is
      (1) A laboratory in which to observe the member's behavior (a new milieu).
      (2) A place where members can try out new forms of behavior.
      (3) A place where the facade of defenses can be lifted.
      (4) A place where early unpleasant experiences with groups can be replaced with more pleasant experiences.
      (5) Designed to play up the healthy parts of the personality.
      (6) A place where members can develop a feeling of belonging and increased self-esteem.
      (7) A place where the member gets some validation of feelings, learning that he or she is not alone, and that his or her feelings are not unique.
      (8) Preparing people for handling other situations, such as home situations involving parents, brothers, sisters, spouses, and so on.
      (9) A natural mode of treatment since all humans have a social hunger—they all want to belong.
   c. There are various types of group therapy (Powdermaker and Frank, 1959).
      (1) Didactic groups. These are based on educational material presented by the leader. Any form of structured activity can be used, such as lectures, movies, talks on mental health, anxiety, and so on. The emphasis is placed on developing intellectual insight.
      (2) Repressive-inspirational groups. A wide variety of groups fit in here. These frequently have a planned activity and then a discussion during which members ventilate and realize that other people have similar problems. The emphasis is on morale building and supporting defenses. An example would be Alcoholics Anonymous.
      (3) Therapeutic social clubs. These can be both in and out of the hospital. They can be very structured or very informal and can range from social activities to group discussion of member's problems. They can be organized either by clients or staff. These are social interaction groups that increase the member's skill in social participation.
      (4) Psychodrama. This kind of group uses role playing to act out certain situations. Participants play a part, may

switch roles, and then discuss what happened. Can be used with clients both in and out of the hospital.

(5) Free-interaction groups. These encourage interaction in an atmosphere conducive to free expression of feelings. They are problem centered with no specific activity planned.

(a) Group analysis makes use of the same techniques as in individual analysis but in a group situation (dreams, transference, resistance, free association, etc.). This is conducted primarily with neurotics by analysts in private medical practice.

(b) Group psychotherapy. This is the process which takes place whenever people are gathered together for the consideration of personal emotional problems with the purpose of relieving them, in the presence and with the aid of an individual skilled in both the understanding of the individual personality and the patterns of human interrelationships and group interactions (Neighbor, 1963).

(6) Combination of types. Usually a small group of six to eight members conducted by a psychologist, social worker, psychiatric nurse, and so on. The purpose can be varied: it may be an admission group, a predischarge group, or a client-government group. It may be conducted by cotherapists depending on preference.

d. Groups can also be classified as open and closed groups (Kadis, 1974).

(1) Open groups are groups in which there is a rapid turnover of members, and new members replace the old members when vacancies occur. Certain themes, especially the so-called "birth theme," arise more rapidly in open groups. The kinds of anxieties and hostilities that emerged when a new baby was born or a stepparent entered the family circle, are reexperienced by members in the group. The addition of a new member must be carefully timed to reduce the disruption of the therapeutic process. It will inevitably increase the members' anxiety, and this will be reflected in the group sessions. In most instances the emergence of unconscious material and underlying conflicts is hindered by the presence of a stranger. Open groups have some specific features:

(a) In theory, these groups may perpetuate themselves indefinitely. They are never dissolved. Members who finish their treatment or leave for various reasons are replaced.

(b) Changes can be made to achieve a composition that will facilitate therapeutic movement. Members may be added or transferred at the therapist's discretion.

(c) These groups can be started with only a few members. New members can be added as needed.

(2) Closed groups are defined as having a constant membership, as members are only expected to leave at a definite time. The specific qualities of closed groups almost inevitably lead to specific responses. Separation anxiety and the death theme are very evident. Some of this separation anxiety can be viewed as the primary neurotic problem of separation from the maternal figure. Separation from any important figure, whether it be in the nuclear family, in marriage, or in treatment, may bring back many of these original feelings. The group is compelled to work through the theme that no one is indispensable, and termination is another expression of this inevitability. Carried to its extreme, separation anxiety is a fear of death as the ultimate departure. A member's leaving may be symbolically perceived by the group as a final leavetaking. Closed groups can be broken down into three main types.

(a) Constant membership. Members are not permitted to leave at will but are expected to serve the group's need for a definite period of time. The time is stipulated at the start of treatment.

(b) Family prototype. Members leave one by one when they are ready. They detach themselves as if from their nuclear families. Since no replacements are made, the group goes out of existence when all its members have dropped out.

(c) Occasionally reopened. Members may be added or transferred according to the group's need.

INTERVENTIONS

1. Types of leadership in groups. Group leaders are only as effective as the group members they are leading. The success of any group does not depend on the leader alone; it depends on each individual group member. The following is a description of six different types of leadership (Bonner, 1959). The leader's behavior is described in relation to the group with which he or she is interacting.
   a. Authoritarian leadership. This type of leadership is characterized by power and domination. These leaders value discipline and control of the group. They have no confidence or trust that group members will act independently; consequently, group members act with fear and submission. These leaders discourage interaction and communication between members. They do not assume the responsibility for their own actions and hold the group responsible for any failures. Such groups can only be effective if the members permit their leader to have all the power. When this occurs, the group feels helpless, powerless, and dependent, and there is a low degree of satisfaction among group members. Amazingly, although this type of leadership meets the needs of the individual leader rather than the needs of the group, the task accomplishment of this group is usually highly productive.
   b. Democratic leadership. These leaders encourage members to participate in group activities that enhance group goals. They do not dominate the group but participate as members. They have confidence in, trust, and encourage communication among group members. They share the power of their position and distribute responsibilities to the group. They are friendly, involved, and meet the needs or goals of the group members rather than their individual needs.
   c. Laissez-faire leadership. These leaders facilitate communication among group members and are good listeners who reflect group thoughts back to the group. They are passive, essentially noninvolved, and function somewhat like observers apart from, rather than as a part of, the group. Morale is usually high in such groups; group goals can be achieved in this type of group if the group members are strong enough to collectively achieve them. Essentially, the leadership role is taken over by group members.
   d. Bureaucratic leadership. This type of leadership is characterized by rigidity and inflexibility due to the focus on carrying out the inherent rules of the bureaucracy. These groups are immobilized to define or achieve their own goals, as the group goals must be the rules of the bureaucracy. These leaders are impersonal, aloof, objective, and lack initiative. They do not have to assume the responsibility for their own actions, as they can always blame the rigidity or the rules of the bureaucracy.
   e. Charismatic leadership. These leaders are seen to have supernatural traits, attributed to them by the group members. They must prove themselves to their followers. These groups depend on followers who surrender themselves to the will of their leader.
   f. Shared leadership. These leaders stimulate and facilitate the interaction process among members. All members participate in and share group roles. In this sense, each time a member speaks in a way that facilitates group goals or group process, he or she assumes the leadership role at that point in time. Members are listened to and respected by the group, and there is much interdependence between members. This type of leadership involves all members, facilitates a high degree of group cohesion, and is personally satisfying to group members. This style of leadership does not free leaders from the responsibility of defining and clarifying the group goals initially or whenever needed during the group experience. This group usually has high morale and high productivity.
2. Functions and interventions of group leaders. Gwen Marram (1973) has written about the kinds of things group leaders or therapists do in groups. She has separated functions and

interventions and has emphasized the difference. A *function* is the purpose of the leader in the group. An *intervention* is the specific act or set of activities that leaders employ to accomplish their purpose in the group.

The following functions and interventions apply to leadership in any type of group. Group leaders strive to provide an atmosphere in which group members can express their thoughts and feelings freely, without fear of judgment or retaliation.

a. Leadership functions.
   (1) The group leader facilitates the natural benefits of group membership. Leaders assist members in meeting their needs for security, belonging, and companionship.
   (2) The group leader maintains a viable group atmosphere. Members are free to be present, free to talk about what concerns them, and free to experiment with new behaviors without severe threat.
   (3) The group leader oversees group growth. Most groups have goals. Whatever the goals of the group are, the leader has a direct responsibility to assist the group in meeting those goals. In the role of observer of group growth, the leader keeps members' attention on the goals, clarifies issues in terms of how they relate to goals, and evaluates the group's progress toward the goals periodically and with the assistance of the group members.
   (4) The group leader regulates individual members' growth within the group setting. Individual group members progress at different rates. Sometimes the leader will be concerned with one member's growth so as to further the progress of the total group (e.g., help one member catch up so the entire group can proceed together). Therefore, at times, the leader's interventions may be more individualized and will not be directed solely at the group.
b. Leadership interventions. These actions are carried out both by group leaders and group members.
   (1) Outlines and interprets group objectives. Members need to have an understanding of what is expected of them.
   (2) Manipulates physical and structural arrangements of the group. This includes dealing with numbers of members, room, length of group, duration, and so on.
   (3) Increases interaction between members. Uses basic interviewing and communication skills and assists group members to share and learn from each other.
   (4) Encourages the sharing of common problems. This helps to develop group cohesion.
   (5) Employs strategies with individuals. Plans the use of techniques and experiences to further growth of group members.
   (6) Reduces undue anxiety. The leader is aware of the group's anxiety level and maintains it at a constructive level. Prolonged high anxiety in a group can result in group disintegration and disorganization.
   (7) Summarizes the group's progress toward its goals. This occurs to some extent at the end of each group session and continually throughout the life of the group.

EVALUATION

Reassessment: common problems in groups.

1. Conflict resolution. Conflict is an emotional disturbance resulting from a clash of two opposing forces in operation simultaneously. Conflict is a process, and it is a necessary part of group life; it is unpleasant, full of tension, hostility, and opposing interests.

   Conflict in a group requires at least two members involved in direct interaction with each other. They are involved in a struggle over something that is scarce; there is apparently not enough to go around to satisfy the contending members. This scarcity may apply to material resources, power, status, or values. Those involved usually assume that what their opponents get, they will lose.

   Conflict is normal in groups and is an opportunity for growth rather than something to be avoided at all costs. In the course of dealing with conflict, group members can be helped to see problems and situations in new ways, to call on strengths within themselves that have been dormant, and can develop a set of attitudes and skills that will make a tremendous contribution to their future functioning as mature people. If group leaders grasp these potentialities, they can help their group to realize them and will not be intent upon discouraging all conflicts in the group.

a. There are two kinds of conflict: realistic and nonrealistic.
   (1) Realistic conflicts arise from frustration of specific demands within the relationship and from estimates of gains by each of the members, involving a specific result or issue. Examples would be two members struggling for leadership in the group or members with opposing views as to how to achieve group goals.
   (2) Nonrealistic conflicts do not arise from rival ends or clear issues. They arise from the need for tension release, and they may be directed against members with whom there is no issue. This sort of thing is sometimes at work in scapegoating (e.g., it may be not be safe to vent feelings against the appropriate person and, therefore, they are directed against a weaker, less threatening person.
b. There are particular patterns of conflict resolution (Wilson and Ryland, 1950):
   (1) Elimination. Members may combat each other, each seeking to win, and if necessary to rid the group of the opposing faction.
   (2) Subjugation. The strongest subgroup or individual may force the others to accept its point of view and thus dominate the opposition.
   (3) Compromise. Negotiations take place among competing members or subgroups. Both parties give up something in order to get something else in return. It is essentially a bargaining approach in which costs and rewards are weighed and eventually balanced.
   (4) Alliance. Subgroups or individuals may maintain their independence but combine to achieve a common goal.
   (5) Integration. The group as a whole may arrive at a solution that not only satisfies every member but is better than any of the contending solutions. This is considered the highest achievement in group life.
c. There is another framework that focuses more on how the conflict is handled by group members rather than on its outcome. It can be thought of as a series of levels:
   (1) Physical violence. This is the attempt to beat the opponents into submission.
   (2) Verbal violence. This is the attempt to belittle opponents in order to make them look ridiculous and to turn the feelings of the group and others against them.
   (3) Subtler verbal contention. This is the attempt to belittle and undermine the position of opponents without violently attacking them. It often involves cleverly citing associated or even irrelevant factors.
   (4) Finding allies. This is the attempt to line up others to support one's position. This tends to be a power play. Various motives can be presented to potential allies, but the main point is to gain strength that is greater than that of one's opponents.
   (5) Seeking an authoritative decision. This is the attempt to find someone, probably the leader, who will say definitively who is right and who is wrong.
   (6) Creating diversions and delay. This is the attempt to displace attention on something other than the conflict.
   (7) Respect for differences. There is a desire to understand how the opponent sees the situation, to collect the needed facts, and to attempt to think rationally about the conflict. This level is the highest in the hierarchy. There is a willingness to go beyond the clash of individuals and the desire to win: to be interested in facts, drawing reasonable conclusions from them, and to listen carefully to one's opponents.
d. Group leaders play an important role in dealing with conflict. They try to
   (1) Fully understand the situation and the opposing views.
   (2) Relate to the group as a whole without taking sides. However, they can and should give their opinion without alienating either side.
   (3) Help sort out the issues and clarify areas of agreement and disagreement in the group.

(4) Formulate a strategy for change that includes thinking ahead to anticipate the consequences of each line of possible group action.

2. Decision making. This is a necessary and inherent part of group process, as there must be some mode of operation by which a group can make decisions. It is essential that the group structure be such that the members have the privileges and responsibilities of the management of their own group affairs. A collection of individuals will not develop the characteristics of a productive group unless they have the right and the ability to make decisions that are significant to their own group life.

   Every person in his or her own life is faced with making choices presumed to be based on available alternatives. To make a choice essentially means to select from available alternatives and then to implement that selection. The only "real" alternatives available are those that are within an individual's perceptual field. These are based on personal background, the characteristics of one's own personality, and the social and cultural experiences that have shaped one's personality.

   Decision making ought always to be a rational process, but it is not. Unconscious factors are powerful forces in restricting people from making rational choices. Group leaders need to help members to understand the decision-making process and to assist them in becoming more skillful and rational in arriving at their decisions.

   There are some basic steps in decision making (Lowy, 1965). These steps do not necessarily occur in the order or sequence listed, but they do indicate a process that is inherent in decision making.

   a. Becoming aware of the problem. This includes arriving at a definition of the problem and breaking it down into component parts.
   b. Clarifying and evaluating proposed solutions. This is delineating the alternatives available and evaluating the possible consequences.
   c. Reaching a decision. This is choosing one alternative to the exclusion of all others and evaluating it as to the probable consequences.
   d. Acting upon the decision that has been reached. This is implementing the decision and evaluating the choice.
   e. Examining the results of implementing the decision. This is examining the consequences of a decision and recognizing that the consequences could be quite unanticipated.

3. Adolescent groups. These can present some special problems. One area that can give group leaders difficulty is that of developing realistic expectations of the adolescent. In this age group it is important to keep in mind that the boundaries between normal and abnormal behavior are shifting, often fluid, and frequently a matter of judgment. One may anticipate many swings, such as from rebellion to submission, in a relatively short period of time.

   a. It is essential to have a concept of the developmental tasks of adolescence (Sugar, 1975). These include
      (1) Emancipation from parental attachments.
      (2) Development of satisfying and self-realizing peer attachments, with ability to love and appreciate the worth of others as well as oneself.
      (3) An endurable and sustaining sense of identify in the family, social, sexual, and work-creative areas.
      (4) A flexible set of hopes and life goals for the future.
   b. Some important goals for adolescent groups are listed as follows (Sugar, 1975):
      (1) To support assistance and confrontation from peers.
      (2) To provide a miniature real-life situation for study and change of behavior.
      (3) To stimulate new ways of dealing with situations and to stimulate the development of new skills in human relationships.
      (4) To stimulate new concepts of self and new models of identification.
      (5) To decrease feelings of isolation.
      (6) To provide a feeling of protection from the adult while undergoing changes.
      (7) To allow the swings of rebellion or submission, which will encourage independence and identification with the leader.
      (8) To uncover relationship problems not evident in individual therapy.

c. Everything written previously in this chapter also occurs in adolescent groups, sometimes with a little more intensity. Anyone working with adolescents will have more success if they develop the qualities of empathy, patience, trustfulness, tactfulness, and sensitivity. It is a real challenge to work with this age group and to watch the adolescent moving in the direction of maturity. Adolescence is truly both "the best of times" and "the worst of times."

Reevaluation and Follow-up

Group members are carefully evaluated and referred to community agencies and/or outpatient settings if further treatment or group participation is believed necessary and useful.

Interactions among members of all groups have many similarities—the same basic group dynamics occur in *all* groups. Frequently, their intensity differs in group therapy, but the basic patterns are the same. Conducting group therapy is a specialized skill that requires additional preparation, training, and experience. The therapist needs a theory base in group therapy and a body of knowledge in group dynamics. Clinical practice with groups and supervision of that experience are additional indispensable requirements.

REFERENCES

Benne, K. D.,and Sheats, P.: "Functional Roles of Group Members," *Journal of Social Issues,* **4**:41, Spring 1948.

Bonner, H.: *Group Dynamics: Principles and Application,* Ronald Press, New York, 1959.

Kadis, A. L., Krasner, J. D., Winick, C., and Foulkes, S. H.: *A Practicum of Group Psychotherapy,* Harper & Row, Hagerstown, Md., 1974.

Knowles, M., and Knowles, H.: *Introduction to Group Dynamics,* Association Press, New York, 1972.

Lowy, L.: "Decision-Making and Group Work," in S. Bernstein (ed.), *Explorations in Group Work,* Boston University School of Social Work, Boston, 1965.

Marram, G. D.: *The Group Approach in Nursing Practice,* C. V. Mosby, St. Louis, 1978.

McManama, D.: "Working With Groups," in L. Robinson (ed.), *Psychiatric Nursing as a Human Experience,* W. B. Saunders, Philadelphia, 1977.

Murphy, G.: "Group Psychotherapy in Our Society," in M. Rosenbaum and M. Berger (eds.), *Group Psychotherapy and Group Function,* Basic Books, New York, 1963.

Neighbor, J. E., (et al.): "An Approach to the Selection of Patients for Group Psychiatry," in M. Rosenbaum and M. Berger (eds.), *Group Psychotherapy and Group Function,* Basic Books, New York, 1963.

Olmstead, M.: *The Small Group,* Random House, New York, 1959.

Powdermaker, F., and Frank, J.: "Group Psychotherapy," in S. Arieti (ed.), *American Handbook of Psychiatry,* vol. II, Basic Books, New York, 1959.

Sugar, M. (ed.): *The Adolescent in Group and Family Therapy,* Brunner/Mazel, Publishers, New York, 1975.

"The Tool Kit," *Adult Leadership,* January 1953.

Wilson, G., and Ryland, G.: *Social Group Work Practice,* Houghton Mifflin, New York, 1950.

BIBLIOGRAPHY

Beukenkamp, C.: *Fortunate Strangers,* Grove Press, New York, 1958. An actual report of what happened to eight clients and a doctor during group treatment. Beautifully written, this book conveys the actual human experience of group therapy in a very authentic way.

Johnson, D. W., and Johnson, F. P.: *Joining Together: Group Theory and Group Skills,* Prentice-Hall, Englewood Cliffs, N.J., 1975. An excellent source for the theory of small group dynamics and group leader and participant skills.

Johnson, J.: *Group Therapy: A Practical Approach,* McGraw-Hill, New York, 1963. A significant and practical guide to group therapy and its techniques. Although written some years ago, this book continues to be a clear, concise, down-to-earth description of group therapy. It sets forth a very workable model for anyone using the group method. Dr. Johnson's style of writing is direct, open, and readily understandable.

Kadis A., Krasner, J. D., Winick, C., and Foulkes, S. H. (et al.): *A Practicum of Group Psychotherapy,* Harper & Row, Hagerstown, Md., 1974. Excellent reference. This book covers every aspect of group psychotherapy, from starting a group and its first meeting, through the group's life cycle and its termination. This provides a very useful overview of the group therapy field.

Kaplan, H., and Sadock, B. (eds.): *Comprehensive Group Psychotherapy,* Williams & Wilkins, Baltimore, 1971. This is an excellent book covering a wide range of issues, theories, and techniques related to group therapy.

Knowles, M., and Knowles, H.: *Introduction to Group Dynamics,* Association Press, New York, 1972. A classic writing in group dynamics. This is an excellent primer on group dynamics, what it is, its main ideas, and its practical applications to all groups. It is an easily understood theory-and-practice introduction useful to anyone participating in groups.

Loomis, M.: *Group Process for Nurses,* C. V. Mosby, St. Louis, 1979. This is a concise, very readable book that draws heavily on actual group experiences, as well as group dynamics research and group treatment literature.

Luft, J.: *Group Processes: An Introduction to Group Dynamics,* The National Press, Palo Alto, Calif., 1970. Presents a very useful introduction to group dynamics. Discusses the basic issues in group processes and presents the research in the field. This small text includes an excellent explanation of the Johari window, a graphic model of awareness in interpersonal relations, that is helpful in developing an understanding of groups.

Marram, G.: *The Group Approach in Nursing Practice,* C. V. Mosby, St. Louis, 1978. A well-written book applying the group approach specifically to nursing practice. The author discusses the functions and interventions of group leaders, and these can be applied to any type of group one is leading or participating in.

McManama, D.: "Working with Groups," in L. Robinson (ed.), *Psychiatric Nursing As a Human Experience,* W. B. Saunders, Philadelphia, 1977, p. 275. A well-written and concise presentation of the important aspects of working with groups, including the purposes of specific groups, the group contract, and the phases of group development.

Yalom, I.: *The Theory and Practice of Group Psychotherapy,* Basic Books, New York, 1975. This is a comprehensive, thoroughly up-to-date handbook on group therapy. It contains an excellent bibliography at the end of each chapter and is a very useful guide for the training of group therapists. Also includes a discussion of encounter or sensitivity-training groups and their interface with therapy groups.

43

Family Work in Inpatient Settings

Ann Ottney Cain and Jo Annalee Irving

Families are where we all live. That is where we learn to relate to other people. Early experiences in our family greatly influence our lifestyles and our interpersonal relationships throughout life. Therefore, it is important to assess the family in order to understand both individual and societal functioning.

The purpose of this chapter is to present a framework for conducting family therapy using Bowen's family systems theory as the referent theoretical model. Definitions, propositions, and examples are provided so that a coherent systems approach can be utilized in dealing with families. The interventions suggested can be implemented in both inpatient and outpatient settings.

DESCRIPTION

A family can be defined as a unit of interacting persons related by ties of marriage, birth, or adoption. The central purpose of a family is to cerate and maintain a common culture that promotes the physical, emotional, and social development of each of its members (Duvall, 1971).

A family can be viewed in a number of ways. It is composed of individuals, each with his or her own needs and expectations. It is a primary group, usually small and with considerable emotional involvement and shared goals. A family is a system, and the action of each individual family member has an effect on the family as a whole. It is also a basic unit of society and, therefore, a medium for the transmission of societal values. It is necessary to take all of these views into consideration when thinking about a family (Cain, 1980).

The *nuclear family* is the center of development and consists of two parents and their children. An individual's nuclear family consists of his mother, his father, and his siblings. An individual's nuclear family is sometimes referred to as the *family of origin*, that is, the family one was born into. This is in contrast to the *family of procreation*, which refers to the family that an individual helps to create. If an individual marries and has children, this is the family of procreation.

Extended family refers to the larger family group consisting of parents, children, and all other relatives. This includes grandparents, aunts, uncles, cousins, and all other family members (Cain, 1977).

Every family develops systematic ways of being a family. These include ways of communicating, problem solving, meeting family members' needs for affection and intimacy, resolving conflict, and ways of dealing with loss and change. Observing these processes is essential to the assessment of family functioning.

1. Characteristics of the family as a system. In thinking of families, it is most useful to move away from thinking about individuals and to think, instead, about the entire family system as a whole. Systems theory is useful for viewing the family comprehensively.

a. The family is a system. A system is simply a set of interrelated elements that has a boundary and is comprised of a set of persisting interrelationships between the parts of a whole. There is always interaction or dynamic movement between the parts. Therefore, all parts are interdependent, and if one family member is not functioning, it affects all the other family members.
b. A system is greater than the sum of its parts. The family is a larger whole when viewed together, that is, it is greater than the sum of its individual members.
c. A system strives to maintain a dynamic equilibrium among the various forces operating within it and upon it. A family is constantly striving to maintain this equilibrium and resists change, whenever it is in balance. It constantly exerts energy to maintain the status quo and reacts against any change (Jackson, 1957).
d. In any family system, members compensate for each other, that is, if one family member is underfunctioning in certain areas, another member will compensate by overfunctioning in those areas. Family members constantly deal with each other in specific, reciprocal ways. Eventually mutual patterns of interaction evolve, and these become predictable within the family system.
e. The same elements may be part of more than one system. The family is a member of other, larger systems and also has a variety of subsystems of its own.
f. Each of these larger systems influences the family's functioning, as do its subsystems. Examples of subsystems in the family would be different combinations of members, such as dyads, triangles, and members in stereotyped roles or in intense relationships (e.g., family members who are extremely close to each other or are extremely conflictual). All of these affect the family's functioning.
g. There is no true open or closed system when applied to families.
h. All family systems are open to some degree, but some family systems are more open and some are more closed than others.
i. A family with a greater degree of openness can take in more messages from its environment and can adapt to what it hears, rather than distort the information because it cannot handle change.
j. Some families tend to shut out or distort almost all information coming from the environment in order to avoid upsetting the equilibrium of the system. Systems theory has given us a model of the functioning family—a clear pragmatic concept of what a functional family is and what it is like to be a functioning member of such a family. (Fogarty, 1976)

2. Well-functioning family. A functioning family has the following characteristics:
   a. The family has the kind of balance that can adapt to and even welcome change. This balance is different from homeostasis, which acts to maintain the status quo in the presence of change.
   b. Emotional problems are seen as existing in the unit, with components in each person. There is no such thing as an emotional problem in one person.
   c. Connectedness is maintained across generations with all members of the family.
   d. There is a minimum of fusion, and distance is not used to solve problems.
   e. Each twosome in the family can deal with all problems that occur between them. Triangulating onto a third person who is used to arbitrate or judge or solve the dispute is discouraged.
   f. Differences between people are not only tolerated, but encouraged.
   g. Each person can operate selectively using both thinking and emotional systems with other members of the family.
   h. There is a keen awareness of what each person gets functionally from himself, and what he gets from others. These are the areas of identification and differentiation.
   i. There is an awareness of emptiness in each member of the family, and each person is allowed to have his own emptiness. There is no attempt made to fill it up.
   j. The preservation of a positive emotional climate takes precedence over doing what "should" be done and what is "right."
   k. Function in the family is determined by each member saying that this is a pretty

good family to live in over time. If one or more members say there is a problem, there is a problem.

l. Members of the family can use others in the family as a source of feedback and learning, but not as an enemy (Fogarty, 1976).

3. Basic concepts of family systems theory.
   a. Nuclear family emotional system. This has been previously referred to as the undifferentiated family ego mass. These terms describe the patterns of emotional functioning in a family in a single generation.
      (1) If there is a high fusion between members of a family system, they do not see themselves as separate from one another. What happens to one person is perceived as happening to the whole family.
      (2) Fusion is a blending of self with others—an emotional oneness. Highly fused people do not have a clear definition of their individual boundaries in close emotional relationships; they do not know where they leave off and where others begin. If people get too close to each other, they will seek distance to establish their self-boundaries again. In all families, members are connected to one another and also separate from one another. The degrees of connectedness (fusion) and the degree of separateness (differentiation) are different in every family. Some families are highly fused and others are not. It all depends on the patterns learned in each spouse's family of origin. When fusion is high in families, family members use various methods of gaining distance from each other.
      (3) There are four major ways of handling the anxiety of fusion or undifferentiation in the family:
         (a) Emotional distance. This is the most universal mechanism. People distance from each other by being involved in such things as work, golf, television, extramarital affairs, and so on.
         (b) Marital conflict. Spouses engage in open conflict with each other after a period of intense closeness (fusion). They fight, neither giving in to the other, and neither takes on the adaptive role. This fighting prevents them from a total loss of self by putting distance between them and by easing the anxiety they feel when they think they are going to get lost in fusion.
         (c) Dysfunction in one spouse. One spouse actually dysfunctions in the system. Large amounts of undifferentiation can be absorbed through physical, emotional, or social dysfunction. This is a reciprocal relationship in which one spouse dominates the relationship, while the other is submissive and adaptive. Over time, the adaptive one loses the ability to function and to make decisions for self. This dysfunction may be manifested as drug or alcohol abuse, irresponsible behaviors, poor work history, psychiatric problems, chronic physical illness, or other conditions that seriously affect the individual's functioning.
         (d) Transmission to children. This is the transmission of the anxiety out of the fused marital relationship onto the child and the focus of attention remains there. This is called the family projection process. This is the basic process by which parental problems are projected to one or more of the children and can be observed in such child-related problems as learning difficulties, behavioral problems, psychiatric symptoms, delinquency, and physical illness. The child becomes symptomatic and expresses the conflict for the family. The family projection process is universal and exists in all families to some degree. Impairment in the children is less if the focus is on more than one child (Bowen, 1978).

Depending on the degree of fusion in the marital relationship, spouses may use one or a combination of these four mechanisms to achieve distance in the relationship. Most normal families use all of these mechanisms at various times. Problems usually arise when a family uses one mechanism to the exclusion of the others. The system then becomes rigid and is very difficult to reverse.

b. Differentiation of self or one's level of differentiation is concerned with the individual's ability to distinguish between thinking and feeling. It is also concerned with the degree to which an individual can distinguish his own self, his own desires, wants, needs, and beliefs from those of other people within his relationship system. Differentiation of self refers to getting one's self out of the emotional system of the family, moving away from the deep emotional involvement so that one can improve one's self-functioning. This means being able to pull away emotionally from the family and to become a whole person capable of self direction—with a distinct identity and capable of an increased amount of freedom of choice and action, and at the same time remaining in emotional contact with other family members. This is an ongoing lifetime project, a goal to work for continually.

The differentiation of self scale attempts to classify all levels of human functioning on a single dimension or continuum. (See Table 43-1) One's level of differentiation is the degree to which one self fuses or merges into another self in a close emotional relationship. The scale ranges from 0 to 100. At the lower end of the continuum are those people whose emotions (feelings) and intellect (thinking) are so fused that their lives are dominated by the emotional or feeling system. These individuals are less adaptable and flexible and more emotionally dependent on those around them. They are easily stressed into dysfunction, and they have many human problems. At the higher end of the continuum are those people who are more differentiated, whose intellectual functioning can retain relative control over their emotional system in periods of stress or tension. They are more independent of the emotions around them and are more flexible and adaptable. They are better able to cope with life's stresses and are more free of human problems.

The concepts solid self and pseudoself are also important to the understanding of the concept of differentiation of self. Solid self refers to those principles, beliefs, and convictions that are not negotiable in the relationship system. This is what one really believes in. These life principles have been incorporated from life experiences by a process of intellectual reasoning and careful consideration of alternatives. They are formed and evolved from within the individual without pressure from others. They can only be changed from within self on the basis of new knowledge and experience.

Pseudoself refers to beliefs, principles, and knowledge that are negotiable depending on the emotional climate of the relationship system. They are acquired from others and can be changed by emotional pressure or external influence. Pseudoself is unstable and often contains contradictory elements.

c. Triangles. The basic emotional unit in the family or any other human system is the triangle. The family is a series of interlocking triangles. The triangle is the smallest stable relationship system. A two-person system is smaller, but it is unstable. When it experiences tension, it immediately forms a triangle or a series of interlocking triangles. A triangle is a three-person system that has definite relationship patterns that predictably repeat in periods of calm and stress. In periods of calm. the triangle is composed of a comfortable, close twosome and a less comfortable outsider. The inside position of togetherness is the most desired position, and each person in the triangle moves to attain this inside position when tension is low. In periods of stress, when the tension is high, the outside position is the most comfortable and desirable. Each person in the triangle moves to get the outside position so as to escape the tension of the twosome. Most of the time members of the triangle are able to move and shift within the triangle. If movement is not possible, one of the original twosome will triangle in an-

TABLE 43-1 DIFFERENTIATION OF SELF SCALE

Level	Characteristics	Description
Most mature level		
100	Most differentiation of self Purposeful functioning	Few human problems Temporary illness of short duration Flexibile Principle-oriented More energy for goal-oriented activities Concept of future Have increasingly defined convictions and opinions
75	Characteristics: Increased thinking Decreased feeling	Clear on the difference between thinking and feeling High degree of solid self Low degree of pseudoself
50		Many human problems Chronic illness Rigid Lack of principles Little goal-directed activity
25	Characteristics: Increased feeling Decreased thinking Less differentiation of self Very little purposeful functioning	Make life decisions based on what "feels" right Cannot distinguish between thinking and feeling High degree of pseudoself Low degree of solid self
0		
Least mature level		

SOURCE: Miller, J. R., and Janosik, E. H.: *Family-Focused Care*, McGraw-Hill, New York, 1980. Adapted from Murray Bowen, MD.

other person from the outside, and the emotional forces will duplicate the same patterns in this new triangle.

The emotional forces in a triangle are shifting and moving all the time, even in periods of calm. Each person constantly moves to gain either more comfort, more closeness, or to withdraw from tension; each move requires a compensatory move by another person. A triangle is a system, and a change in one member will result in a change in the system or triangle as a whole.

Over time in families, these emotional forces move from one active triangle to another, finally remaining mostly in just one triangle. The patterns continue to repeat themselves, and the individuals who form the triangle come to have fixed roles in relation to each other (Bowen, 1978).

Family Systems Therapy is based on teaching methods of accurately observing how a triangle operates, determining the part *self* plays in that triangle, and determining how to consciously control this programmed emotional reactiveness.

d. Family projection process. This is a classic example of a triangle and has already been discussed (transmission to children). The basic pattern involves a mother whose emotional energy is directed more toward her children than toward her husband and a father who recognizes his wife's anxiety and supports her emotional involvement with the children. There is usually one child that the mother is overly close to, and this child gets focused on in the family. This triangle consists of the mother and the projected child as the close twosome and the father in the distant position. The child eventually becomes symptomatic, and his emotional functioning is impaired.

e. Multigenerational transmission process. This is the concept of a multiple generational process for the development of schizophrenia which can take several generations. Transmission to children (family projection process) that occurs over a number of generations is the basic component of this concept. One learns the pattern of projection in one's own family or origin and then uses it in one's family of procreation. People marry people at about the same level of differentiation. Consequently, evolution is downward in the less differentiated persons who have been the recipients of the family projection process in their families of origin. Eventually a schizophrenic child can be produced.

f. Sibling position. Essentially, the concept of sibling position depends on the combination of only two characteristics: the sex and age ranks of all the persons in one's immediate family.
   (1) Duplication theorem (i.e., that the kinds of persons one chooses as friends, spouses, and partners of any kind will be determined by the kinds of persons one has lived with the longest and the most intimately).
   (2) The more complete the duplication is, the greater the chance that the relationship will last and be happy.
   (3) Family constellations can be viewed as systems that are influenced by preceding generations and that interact with subsequent generations.
   (4) The early family represents the most important context of life and the family exerts its influence earlier, more regularly, and more extensively than any other cultural system.
   (5) Sibling positions are viewed as roles that a person has learned in his own family and that he tends to assume in future situations outside the family.
   (6) Sibling positions and family configurations imply certain behavior trends, personality traits, and social inclinations.
   (7) There are eight basic sibling positions plus the positions of the only child and twins.
      (a) The oldest brother of brother(s).
      (b) The youngest brother of brother(s).
      (c) The oldest brother of sister(s).
      (d) The youngest brother of sister(s).
      (e) The oldest sister of sister(s).
      (f) The youngest sister of sister(s).
      (g) The oldest sister of brother(s).
      (h) The youngest sister of brother(s) (Toman, 1976).
   (8) There are certain attitudes in each basic sibling position, such as attitudes toward work, property, same-sex and opposite-sex friends, politics, children, religion, philosophy, and losses. All of this information is very useful in gaining a complete picture of the entire family system. Knowledge of a person's sibling position can be very helpful in understanding his functioning.

g. Emotional cutoff refers to a high degree of emotional distance between participants in a relationship. Emotional distance exists when major areas in the thinking and the feeling of participants in a relationship are not communicated, and the relationship remains superficial. This is the opposite of person-to-person relating.
   (1) The term *cutoff* describes the process of separation, isolation, withdrawal, running away, or denying the importance of the parental family.

(2) The life pattern of cutoffs is determined by the way people handle their unresolved emotional attachments to their parents (Bowen, 1978).
(3) The more intense the emotional cutoff with the past, the more likely the person will have an exaggerated version of his own parental family problem in his own marriage, and the more likely his own children will do a more intense cutoff from him in the next generation.
(4) The degree of emotional cutoff is a rough estimate of the differentiation of self (i.e., the higher the degree of emotional cutoff in significant relationships, the lower the differentiation level of the person involved.)
(5) All people have some degree of unresolved emotional attachment to their parents.
(6) The more intense the unresolved emotional attachment, the lower the level of differentiation.
(7) The more an individual or a nuclear family maintains a viable emotional contact with the past generations, the more orderly and less symptomatic the life process will be in both generations.

h. Emotional process in society includes both societal regression and progression and postulates that the emotional problem in society is similar to the emotional problem in the family (Bowen, 1978).
This concept suggests that the principles that operate within family systems also operate within social systems.

PREVENTION

1. Refer engaged couples for counseling about marriage expectations, roles, and goals.
2. Refer conjugal pairs for counseling about roles, expectations, and goals of the couple and the individual.
3. Promote understanding of maturational/situational crises and their effects on the family system.
4. Establish and conduct "rap sessions" for school age children and adolescents about individual and family values.
5. Establish "family life" classes in high school curricula based on well-planned role playing and experiential learning activities.
6. Establish and conduct parenting/family life classes that emphasize the uniqueness of each member, their particular role, and position in the family system.
7. Refer and utilize existing organizations, such as Parents Without Partners, Parents Anonymous, senior citizens, church-related groups, and Parent Effectiveness Training groups.

Population at Risk

1. All family forms.
   a. Conjugal pair.
   b. Nuclear family system.
   c. Extended family system.
   d. Functional family system (communes and groups of unrelated people living together).
   e. Single parent family system.
2. Sibling position.
   a. Oldest sibling.
   b. Youngest sibling.
   c. "Special" child.
3. Family member considered the black sheep (scapegoated member).
4. Family members who are dysfunctional, physically or emotionally.
5. Family system with inadequate communication.
6. Family system experiencing separation or divorce.
7. Family system experiencing death.
8. Family system with stepchildren or adopted children.
9. Family systems with inadequate coping mechanisms and support systems.

ASSESSMENT

Family History

This is an evaluation process to gain factual information about the overall functioning patterns of the family for at least three generations. This is the way to discover how the system has worked over time and how it is working currently. Be sure to include dates for all events of the family history. These data are added to the nursing history data already collected on the individual client.

The family history includes questions about

1. Members of family on maternal and paternal sides.
2. Ages of family members.

3. Sibling positions.
4. Education.
5. Occupation.
6. Divorces and remarriages.
7. Deaths.
8. Adoptions, stepchildren, abortions.
9. Black sheep or outsiders of family system.
10. Family ground rules.
11. Decision makers, leaders of the family system.
12. Family secrets; who "knows"? who doesn't?
13. Past and current living locations.
14. Other individuals living in the family that are not related.
15. Other individuals that are not family members but have significant influence on the family system.
16. Family crisis time(s); when, who was involved, what was the outcome?
17. Last contact, written, phone, and/or visitation with the family (which members were involved and for what purpose?).
18. Client's major concern about self and family.
19. Client's major concern about family.
20. Agencies used by family.

See Figure 43-1 and the Family Diagram section below for how to use this with client and/or family.

Physical Assessment

1. Neurological examination.
2. Note any physical problems, acute or chronic, in any family member. This family history outline is not all-inclusive. Other data deemed important by the interviewer would also be included.

Family Diagram

Figure 43-1 illustrates the extended family system and is an extremely useful tool in teaching families about family systems and how they function. It helps the family to think broadly in terms of the family system.

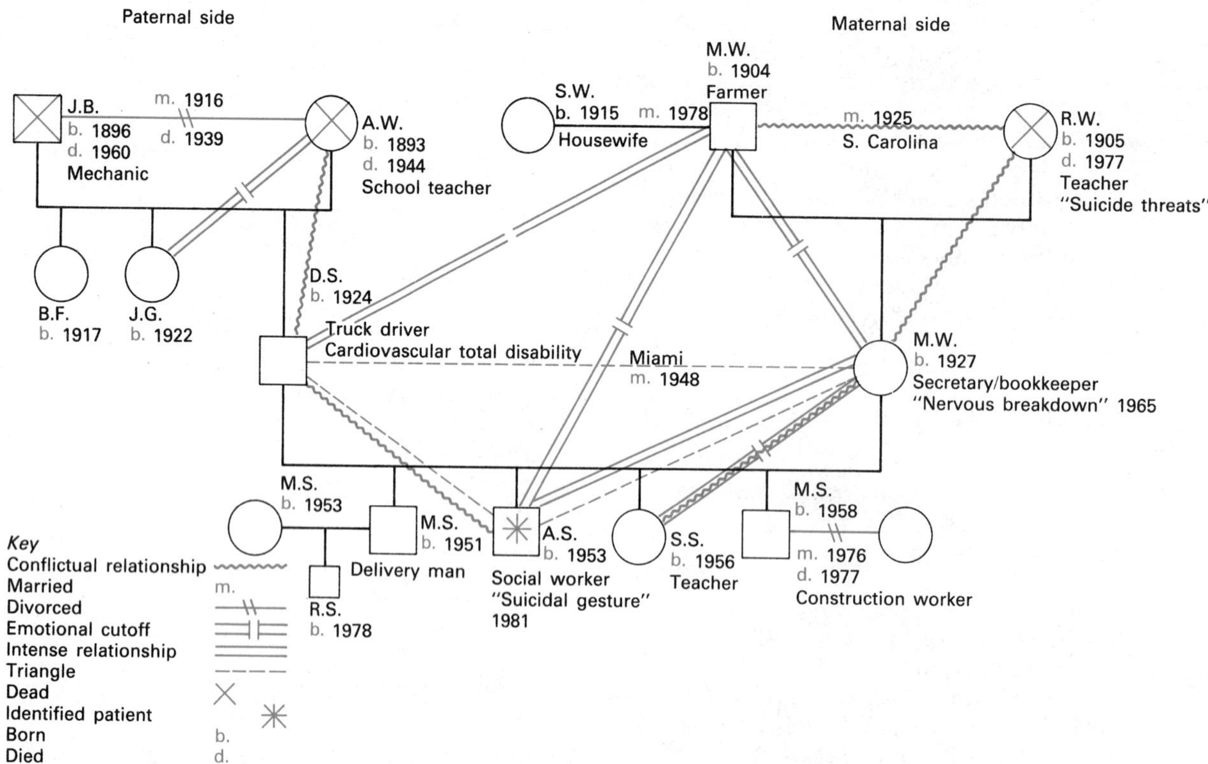

Figure 43-1 Family diagrams. (From Miller, J., and Janosik, E.: *Family Focused Care*, McGraw-Hill, New York, 1979, p. 117. Used with the permission of the publisher.)

NURSING DIAGNOSES: ACTUAL OR POTENTIAL

Dysfunctional family process due to or associated with one or a combination of the following:

1. Emotional distance.
2. Marital conflict.
3. Dysfunction in spouse or child.
4. Use of projective processes.
5. Fusion.
6. Stress.
7. Emotional cutoff.
8. Generally low levels of differentiation.
9. Triangulation.

EXPECTED OUTCOMES

The family will

1. Move toward higher levels of differentiation.
2. Improve communication skills and decision-making processes.
3. Move into roles that are useful and satisfying.
4. Understand, tolerate, and attempt to resolve conflicts.

INTERVENTIONS

1. Stay objective, and do not take sides with any family member.
2. Eliminate the use of "why" questions and use the "how, who, where, and when" style of questioning and thinking to obtain the facts in the situation.
3. Recognize that the family member expressing symptoms is communicating "something" about the family.
4. Pay attention to both the verbal and nonverbal messages coming from all family members.
5. Identify and emphasize areas of family strength, as well as be aware of family weaknesses.
6. Avoid stereotyping of family styles, and have an awareness of a variety of family forms.
7. Relate family developmental tasks to the family circumstances.
8. Teach family members to become astute observers of their own and other family members' interactions.
9. Teach about sibling position profiles and how these may operate in their family.
10. Ask each person to record thoughts and feelings in a log emphasizing the similarities and differences of family members.
11. Facilitate the family process, and increase communication and decision-making skills of family members.
12. Assist the family members to define their own needs and to achieve their family goals.
13. Defuse intense feelings of each family member so that thinking is clearer.
14. Assist family members to define and separate their thinking and feeling reactions and to keep a sense of balance between the two.
15. Point out that feelings are helpful in identifying problems, but they are not enough to solve them. Thinking is the necessary component for this purpose.
16. Assist family members to increase the solid self by having each family member define own principles and values which may be different from other family members.
17. Assist family members in learning to take "I" positions. This is a clear statement, neither offensive nor defensive, of one's thoughts or feelings on a subject. It describes what a person will or will not do and what he believes in and does not believe in.
18. Provide support for the family members' efforts toward change, noting that the process of self-change is a time of high anxiety with feelings of isolation from other family members who are resisting the change.
19. Refuse to keep family secrets, and keep all communication open and available to all family members.
20. Reinforce the sense of humor in family members, and encourage people to not take themselves too seriously.
21. Assist the family members to realize that happiness, as a primary family goal, is not attainable. Happiness usually evolves when each family member is involved in a satisfying pursuit of their individual goals. Many families do not comprehend this and, consequently, search for an abstract state called "happiness," which is often confused with togetherness.
22. Recognize highly charged issues and values in one's own family. Development of this awareness of one's own family system's functioning will assist the helping person to maintain an objective position and in staying de-triangled from the client family system.
23. Accept that a family may not be able to make a commitment to family work. This is the time that the helping person must be willing

to "let the family go" and not attempt to convince them to continue if the family does not see this as a need.

EVALUATION

Outcome Criteria

The family:

1. Shows evidence of increased awareness of how their family functions.
2. Demonstrates ability to be an accurate observer of family interactions.
3. Develops effective communication skills.
4. Demonstrates decision-making skills about self and the family.
5. Demonstrates "I" positions while maintaining continuity with family members.
6. Makes visits to the family based on self-need.
7. Realizes that some conflicts can be resolved whereas others can only be understood and tolerated.
8. Realizes that when stress gets high, family will revert to old patterns of behavior.
9. Realizes that their personal work in their families is a lifetime process.
10. Participates in family therapy, when available.

CASE EXAMPLE

The family unit is the focus of treatment for the helping person in the following case example. The client is viewed as the "symptom bearer" of the family system and is not singled out in family work. Selected data from the family history in this case example will be used to illustrate the family systems theory. The family diagram (Figure 43-1) will be useful to refer to while reading this family history.

The client is a 28-year-old white male admitted to a psychiatric inpatient unit by his parents after a life-threatening gesture of cutting his left wrist. He also attempted an overdose of sleeping medication. He is currently on Antabuse and has a history of alcohol abuse, substance abuse, and depression. (See Chapters 36 through 38 for specifics of these symptoms and interventions.) Family therapy was the recommended treatment for dealing with this crisis.

The client, currently out of a job, lives in the same town as his mother, 54 years old, and father, 57 years old. He has three other siblings. Paternal grandparents are deceased, and the maternal grandmother is deceased with the grandfather remarried.

The father has been on total disability for 8 years and is unemployed and on Social Security benefits. His disability is a result of cardiac problems. He is in an underfunctioning position in the family system. The mother works full time and is in an overfunctioning position in the family system. The aforementioned circumstances support the concept of dysfunction in one spouse. Family history would indicate that the maternal grandparents frequently operated in a similar pattern. The son, who is adaptive, shares an underfunctioning position at times. The mother overfunctions with him and is currently involved in calling up prospective employers for him.

The mother and son have a fused relationship, with the father remaining distant most of the time. The father communicates mostly to his son through the mother. This is a major triangle, mother, father, and son. The son states, "I feel he (father) doesn't respect me. We don't talk much." His anger about this becomes turned inward, resulting in lack of self-respect, increased anxiety, depression, and then fusion over close relationship with his mother. This would demonstrate the *family projection process*. Sometimes this triangle would be son, mother, and substance abuses.

The *multigenerational transmission process* is evidenced by reports from the mother of the maternal grandmother's threats of having a "pill tucked away in a box" that was announced during the grandfather's "bad" drinking periods and during his distancing for periods of days related to work. The mother has a history of depression, suicidal attempts, and a psychiatric hospitalization. These efforts generally resulted from financial problems in the family business and from trying to protect the father from the information. The son has had three suicide attempts. The son was his grandmother's favorite grandchild, looking most like her side of the family. He reports always feeling "different" from his siblings and spent much time in his early years with his mother in the household activities. These experiences increased his lack of *solid self* and reinforced his *fusion* with his mother; this also identifies him as the most projected child.

There are many examples of emotional isolation/cutoff in this family, such as the father and his sisters with their parents and the mother, father, and son with the maternal grandfather. The parents have reconnected with him, but the son still is involved in a major cutoff, and some of the depression revolves around this. He states, "I feel like I lost both grandparents at the same time."

The marriage of the parents may be viewed as not being complimentary because of their rank conflict. At times the son has functioned either in a "third parenting " position or in his position of oldest brother of sisters. This latter position has him functioning as a "caretaker" with his mother and the potential for switching from the underfunctioning position to the overfunctioning position with her. The mother frequently related to her son as her confidant about the family finances and other issues. When she had her "runaway periods" and left suicide notes, they always referred to the son "knowing" how to find her.

According to Bowen's differentiation of self scale, this family would be placed in the "moderate range," which goes from 25 to 50. The father reports he made decisions based on emotions. The mother says, "I know just how my son feels." The son is immobilized about not having a job, has not been able to establish a direction for himself, and responds behaviorally through his symptoms of emotional withdrawal/isolation and depression.

SPECIFIC INTERVENTIONS DIRECTED AT EMOTIONAL ISOLATION OR DEPRESSION

See Chapter 36. The root of depression is emotional isolation, and the depressed person is impinged upon by his emotions. Depression is overpowering, and it represses the thinking structures (i.e., the depressed person is overwhelmed by his or her feelings). A depressed person feels very down, unable to do anything about his or her problems, and is overtaken by a sense of despair. The focus in depression is on one's own self and ends in emotional isolation. The depressed person withdraws from the people around him or her into an inner world. The person's major mechanism for handling tension and stress is distancing. The person is withdrawing from the world to get more comfortable and goes too far and then has difficulty getting back. Decreasing this emotional isolation often decreases the feelings of depression. Therefore, it is very important for the depressed person to stay involved with other people, even though the person will often indicate that he or she prefers to be alone.

Family systems theory views depression as a symptom of family dysfunction, which is determined by one's basic level of self-differentiation and the degree of anxiety in the family system. The symptomology of depression is, in part, a learned response to anxiety and can be understood by exploring the family process and by identifying the behavior patterns present in both the past and the present generations (see Family History, above, and Figure 43-1). The family is the unit of treatment in depression. The family member who is depressed is the "symptom bearer" and is seen as reflecting the disturbances of the family itself. This member learned the pattern of depression in the family.

It is important that each family member gain some awareness of the part he or she plays in the ongoing family process. Teaching motivated family members how family systems operate and assisting them to learn to control their reciprocal roles in the process is essential. Once family members recognize that their patterns have been learned through the generations and that they have the option of doing something different, change can occur. It is then that the family can begin to work together to solve the difficulties they all have.

It is helpful to indicate to the family and to the depressed member that depression is self-limited and that it will decrease in intensity in time. They need support while they ride out the bad times. No matter how bad the depression is, it will someday be history. That knowledge can be comforting during the acute period of depression.

In the case example, the son is in a fused position with his mother in a strong family triangle. When a person maintains this adaptive position for long periods of time, this person gradually loses self, and the ability to function is markedly impaired, as is evidenced in the depressed position of the son. In this instance, the mother is viewed as the "overfunctioner" or dominant one, and the son is viewed as the "underfunctioner" or the adaptive one. Neither position is one that enhances growth within the family system. Unfortunately, once these positions become stable patterns of interaction, the process often becomes chronic and is extremely difficult to reverse.

These individuals have large amounts of pseudoself, and it is the pseudoself that engages in the fusion process and allows for symptom formation. The more pseudoself available, the greater the likelihood of loss of self and depressive dysfunction. Only a moderate amount of stress is necessary to trigger the adaptive individual into dysfunction, due to their relationship orientation and their sensitivity to others.

The more cut off one is from other family members, the more emotionally isolated one can become. The existence of emotional cutoffs increases the amount of emotional investment in the person's present relationships and the chance for fusion in the nuclear family relationships. The depressed person's relationships to extended family members can either perpetuate or decrease the depressive symptoms and, therefore, can have a great impact. If the depressed person's relationships to his or her extended family are open, this absorbs some of the intensity, helps lessen the fusion in the nuclear family, and assists in decreasing the depression. If the extended family relationships are cut off, this increases the emotional investment or fusion in the nuclear family, decreases the personal connectedness of the depressed person, and perpetuates the depression.

The efforts of the helping person when working with families with a depressed member should be directed at decreasing the anxiety in the family, increasing the level of differentiation, and bridging the emotional cutoffs in the family system (Cain, 1977).

In any system people compensate for each other. If one person is underfunctioning in certain areas, someone else in the system will compensate for this by overfunctioning in those areas. In a family with a depressed member, there is usually a seesaw relationship. This means that some member or members of the family are overfunctioning just as much as the depressed family member is underfunctioning. As other family members take on more and more responsibility for family affairs, the depressed member decreases his responsibility and can become almost totally dysfunctional. The aim in working with the family would be to work with members who are overfunctioning and try to get them to do less so that the depressed or underfunctioning member could take back more of the responsibility and gradually increase his functioning. This is very different from focusing on the depressed member to "come up" in functioning—the focus is on the other family members to "let go" or "come down." It is a real error to do too much for someone who is depressed. The more you do, the less the person will do. If no one will do it for the person he or she will eventually begin to do things for him- or herself again.

In working with families, one important role of the helping person is the reeducation of family members (Cain, 1980). One of the common general social values has to do with the concept of togetherness (i.e., the belief that one needs to be merged with other people to be real; one cannot be really alone). This is *not* true, but many families believe that it is, and they strive for a togetherness. As helping persons, it is important to help families to realize that it is okay to think separately and to be different from each other. Differentness is very necessary and useful in the family. It will not destroy closeness but will eventually lead to more satisfying family relationships. It is helpful to assist the family in decreasing the togetherness forces and in increasing the movement toward separateness and individuality. The helping person will want to encourage the depressed person to move out toward other people and to do more things that are personally satisfying to him or her. The more the person is engaged in satisfying activities, the less depressed the person will be.

Another intervention that is helpful is aimed at reversing the depressed person's inner-directed aggression. An individual who is depressed represses much hostility and directs it inward against the self. The depressed person needs to be taught to express anger and aggression constructively—to get it directed outside rather than inside. Physical activities are excellent for this. The helping person should encourage the depressed person to play tennis, Ping-Pong, run, use a punching bag, or any other kind of physical exercise to help work off his or her own feelings. The depression frequently lifts when the person is able to do this. If the person is not the athletic type, suggest that he or she pound on the bed with fists or beat on something indestructible with a hammer. It will definitely help.

REFERENCES

Bowen, M.: *Family Therapy in Clinical Practice*, Jason Aronsoń, New York, 1978.

Cain, A.: "Assessment of Family Structure," in J. Miller, and E. Janosik (eds.), *Family-Focused Care*, McGraw-Hill, New York, 1980.

Cain, A.: "Assisting Depressed Clients and their Families," Proceedings of the Southeastern Regional Conference of Psychiatric-Mental Health Clinical Nurse Specialists. Charleston, S.C., April 1980.

Cain, A.: "Families and Family Therapy," in L. Robinson, *Psychiatric Nursing as a Human Experience*, W. B. Saunders, Philadelphia, 1977.

Duvall, E.: *Family Development*, J. B. Lippincott, Philadelphia, 1971.

Fogarty, T.: "Systems Concepts and Dimensions of Self," in P. Guerin (ed.), *Family Therapy Theory and Practice*, Gardner Press, New York, 1976.

Jackson, D. D.: "The Question of Family Homeostasis," *Psychiatric Quarterly Supplement*, Part I:80, 1957.

Toman, W.: *Family Constellation*, Springer Publishing, New York, 1976.

BIBLIOGRAPHY

Bowen, M.: *Family Therapy in Clinical Practice*, Jason Aronson, New York, 1978. This outstanding volume contains the collected works of Dr. Murray Bowen, a pioneer in the field of family therapy. Dr. Bowen discusses the history and evolution of family therapy and presents clearly the interlocking concepts of his theory. He elaborates on the principles of therapy and provides relevant clinical examples.

Cain, A.: "The Therapist's Role in Family Systems Therapy," *The Family*, **3**:65, 1976. The author discusses the kinds of things that a therapist can do that are helpful for a family experiencing difficulties. Specific interventions are identified with corresponding statements of the theory from which they are derived. This article should be useful to both beginning and experienced family therapists.

Cain, A.: *The Therapist's Role in Family Systems Therapy*, tape recording, Psychotherapy Tape Library, Jason Aronson, New York, 1980. This is a concise, yet complete, discussion of interventions that are useful in family therapy. Each intervention is coupled with corresponding statements of the theory from which it is derived.

Compendium: The Best of the Family, 1973–1978, The Center for Family Learning, New Rochelle, N.Y., 1978. This is an outstanding collection of articles reprinted from *The Family Journal*. They cover a spectrum of topics with examples of clinical application and technique from a family systems theoretical base.

Guerin, P. (ed.): *Family Therapy Theory and Practice*, Gardner Press, New York, 1976. The field of family therapy is covered in depth in this collection. History, theoretical concepts of family systems theory, structural family therapy, communication theory, and clinical change are all presented, along with chapters on social networks, child-focused families, alcoholism, sexual dysfunction, multiple family therapy, and death. Techniques such as family choreography, the use of the arts in family therapy, and the use of video playback in family sessions are also included. An excellent source for anyone working with families.

Haley, J. (ed.): *Changing Families: A Family Therapy Reader*, Grune & Stratton, New York, 1971. An excellent collection of family therapy papers that were published previously in various journals. This presents a wide range of approaches currently being used in family work, conveniently arranged under one cover.

Hall, J., and Weaver, B.: *Nursing of Families in Crisis*, J. B. Lippincott, Philadelphia, 1974. This is a book about families in crisis and nurses who have found ways to help them. Crisis theory is presented well and applied directly to nursing situations. The authors have provided examples of strategies and tactics that should be useful to all nurses in helping families resolve crises, regardless of the area of nursing practice involved.

Lewis, J. M., Beavers, W. R., Gossett, J. T., et al.: *No Single Thread: Psychological Health in Family Systems*, Brunner/Mazel, New York, 1976. This presents the results of a long-term pioneering study of how healthy families function, based on a concept of family systems as an outgrowth of general systems theory. An excellent gathering of significant facts and concepts useful in primary prevention, as well as in treatment intervention with families.

Miller, J., and Janosik, E. (eds.): *Family Focused Care*, McGraw-Hill, New York, 1980. A very useful collection focusing on the family as a system. Contains selected chapters on family structure and interventions. Utilizes the Minuchin and Bowen frameworks in the discussion of families. This should be helpful to all practitioners in the field of nursing.

Miller, J. C.: "Systems Theory and Family Psychotherapy," *Nursing Clinics of North America*, **6**:395, 1971. A useful discussion of the family as a system and the effects of stress upon family systems. The author relates systems theory concepts to family functioning and family psychotherapy and provides clinical examples to illustrate important points.

Minuchin, S.: *Families and Family Therapy*, Harvard University Press, Cambridge, Mass., 1974. This offering includes numerous clinical examples of both effectively functioning families and those seeking therapy. Dr. Minuchin presents structural family therapy and defines its therapeutic goals clearly. Transcripts of family sessions are included and are very instructive.

Satir, V.: *Peoplemaking*, Science & Behavior Books, Palo Alto, Calif., 1972. A very simple and remarkably clear book that deals with family process. Satir emphasizes the important aspects of communication, self-worth, systems, and rules within the family. Her message is that the things in a family that count are changeable and correctable, that is, anything can change.

Sedgwick, R.: "The Family As a System: A Network of Relationships," *Journal of Psychiatric Nursing and Mental Health Services*, **12**:17, 1974. The author discusses the family as a system, emphasizing that the family is a psychosocial unit of relationships. She stresses the importance of having knowledge of organizational and group dynamics and learning theories of behavior in order to deal with the ever-changing family unit.

PART VI

THE NURSING CARE OF THE ELDERLY

PART VI CONTENTS

CHAPTER 44
PHYSICAL CHANGES OF NORMAL AGING 1423

Definition of Aging 1423
Theories of aging 1423
Views of aging 1424

Health Promotion and the Elderly 1425
Preventing injury 1425
Preventing illness 1425
Encouraging good health practices in the elderly 1426
Fulfillment of socialization needs 1426
Obtaining health care 1426
Health teaching 1426

Data Collection and the Elderly Client 1427
Health history 1427
Physical assessment 1428

Physiologic Effects of Aging 1429
Changes in perception and coordination 1429
Cognitive changes 1429
Sensorineural changes 1430
Muscular and skeletal changes 1430
Respiratory changes 1431
Cardiac changes 1431
Changes in blood vessels 1431
Changes in the urinary system 1432
Changes in the reproductive system 1432
Nutritional and metabolic changes 1433
Changes in elimination 1434
Changes in integument 1434
Changes in the immune system 1437

Behavioral Changes and Coping Responses Associated with Aging 1437

Nursing Diagnoses: Actual or Potential 1437
Nutritional deficit: malnutrition 1437
Potential mobility impairment 1438
Constipation 1438
Sleep pattern disturbance 1438
Potential for injury 1439
Altered patterns of sexuality 1439
Other potential nursing diagnoses 1439

Expected Outcomes 1439

Interventions 1440
Nutritional deficit: malnutrition 1440
Potential mobility impairment 1442
Constipation 1442
Sleep pattern disturbance 1443
Potential for injury 1443
Altered patterns of sexuality 1443

Outcome Criteria 1445
Malnutrition 1445
Mobility impairment 1445
Constipation 1445
Sleep pattern disturbance 1445
Potential for injury 1445
Altered patterns of sexuality 1445

Conclusion 1446

CHAPTER 45
COPING WITH LOSS AND AGING 1449

Loss and Grief 1449
Culture 1451

Death 1457
Reactions to death 1457
Religious beliefs and death 1458

CHAPTER 46
COMMON HEALTH PROBLEMS THAT AFFECT THE ELDERLY 1463

Chronic Health Problems 1463

Cardiovascular Disease 1467

Hypertension 1469

Cerebrovascular Disease 1471

Respiratory Disease 1472

Primary Maturity-Onset Diabetes 1473

Osteoarthritis 1475

Osteoporosis 1476

Visual Disturbances 1476

Auditory Disturbances 1478

Medication Effects and the Aged 1478

Organic Mental Disorders 1482

Traumatic Injuries 1486
Accidents 1486

Other Health Problems 1486

44

Physical Changes of Normal Aging

Ann Faas Collard

DEFINITION OF AGING

Individuals "age" at different rates, influenced by inherited genes, lifestyle, emotional well being, physiologic health, nutritional status, psychological health, and many other features. The process of "aging" commences at the moment of conception and continues until death.

Historically, old age was certainly not known, it was simply uncommon. Since the turn of the century, the total U.S. population has nearly tripled while the number of those 65 or older has increased eightfold. By the year 2000, it is projected that nearly one-third of the U.S. population will be over 65 years of age (Dychtwald, 1979).

As we grow older, normal physiologic, psychologic, and social changes accompany the aging process. These changes are not uniform, rather they are unique to each individual and reflect his special style of growing older. The following chapter will examine the components of the "normal" aging process as they occur in the older adult. Coping successfully with these changes can make aging a special time in one's life—a time for self-awareness, wisdom, reflection, fulfillment, and satisfaction.

THEORIES OF AGING

Aging is a process that affects each individual, yet why aging occurs is not clearly understood. Current hypotheses related to aging that are being studied include the following:

1. *Limited cell replication theory* points out that the potential for cellular proliferation is limited by the number of times cells have divided, thus giving an aged organism less potential for new cell growth than a similar organism at a younger age.
2. *Error accumulation theory* states that cellular reproduction is not perfect and that defective cell components may occasionally be generated due to inaccuracies within the synthesis processes. Assuming that these defective parts are stable and passed on to subsequent generations, eventual buildup or impairment of function is thought to result.
3. *Autoimmune theory* postulates that there is growing evidence that autoimmune responses increase with age. These immune bodies attach to cells and lead to the destruction of healthy tissues. Constant demand put on the immune system over the years diminishes its capacity to respond until finally it is unable to deactivate certain chem-

ical processes which can gradually destroy the vital organs and systems.

4. *Irreversible decrement theory* explains that aging is in fact a progressive decline in one's bodily functions that cannot be terminated. It can be viewed as a predictive theory, which attempts to present average functional loss concurrent with aging.
5. *Adaption view* states that even though decline does occur, we should be able to cope with changes and adapt accordingly. Researchers of this theory are also investigating whether aging results from intrinsic or environmental factors.
6. *Genetic theory* suggests that mutations occur within the cell, especially changes related to DNA and RNA. These mutations result in physiologic manifestations of aging.
7. An offshoot of the genetic theory is the *free radical theory*. Free radicals are those parts of molecules from the metabolic process (e.g., pollutants or radiation) not burned in food exchanges with the environment. These radicals interfere with healthy cells. They are specifically injurious to the RNA and DNA cellular components and particularly harmful when the influence of radiation, faulty nutrition, or polluted air is present.
8. *The DNA theory* postulates that DNA can be destroyed by a variety of causative agents and this deterioration of the DNA and RNA is directly responsible for failure of the cell to replicate and repair itself, thus causing aging.
9. *Cross-linking theory* states that a molecule becomes cross linked when an amino acid in it links with an amino acid of another molecule. This creates one large linked molecule that is not as efficient as the former molecules. It can kill healthy cells as well as succumb to attacks by the immune system. These cells arising continually gradually lead to deterioration of normal cells.
10. *Stress theory* is another theory of aging popularized in part by Dr. Hans Selye. His theory holds that replaceable cells constantly stressed and abused by improper nutrition, toxic materials, and overwork simply "wear out" prematurely and are forced to give up their reproductive potential. Those cells which are not replaceable and cannot divide are simply killed off by these stressors.
11. *Neurotransmitter theory* holds that imbalances of the thought-transmitting chemicals in the brain interfere with cell division throughout the body. This is a more recent theory which seems to be gaining momentum.
12. Recent investigations of viruses have led some researchers to postulate a *viral theory* of aging. It is felt that at any time, a slow virus may enter the body and begin to affect any system of the body after a prolonged incubation period of several decades.
13. *Anterior pituitary* release of DECO sometimes called the "death hormone" (decreased oxygen consumption) begins at age 20. It results in decreased thymus function which has been postulated to decrease immunity and decreases the ability of tissue to utilize oxygen.

VIEWS OF AGING

1. Aging by itself does not necessarily connote illness. Many individuals remain healthy well into old age.
2. Aging can increase an individual's risk for illnesses. Often multiple problems, e.g., physical limitations, invalidism, being alone because of widowhood, isolation, poverty and depression are seen.
3. The physical decline that accompanies aging has been well documented, but more than ever, individuals are realizing that their older years need not necessarily be a time of illness and decline but, rather, may represent a time of satisfaction and contentment.
4. The elderly can move toward a state of high-level wellness by emphasizing the physical, psychological and sociological potential the elderly possess, rather than focusing on what has been lost.
5. How older individuals feel about their health is often an accurate predictor of how satisfied they are with their lives (Mezey, 1980).
6. Health is often synonymous with functional ability. If individuals are able to maintain independence and carry out role functions, they will probably view their health as good, even though physiologic limitations are present.
7. Most older people are realistic about their health. The self-evaluation that old people

make of their health is highly correlated with their reports of restrictions in mobility, sensory impairments, and overall incapacity (Shanus, 1980).

HEALTH PROMOTION AND THE ELDERLY

PREVENTING INJURY

1. Accidents are the third leading cause of death and a leading cause of injury to the aged (Abbey, 1973).
2. The most debilitating accidents among the elderly are falls, and most falls and accidents occur in the home.
3. Educating the elderly about home safety includes:
   a. Utilizing good lighting, especially in stairways and landings.
   b. Providing staircases with handrails, preferably one on either side.
   c. Removing loose throw rugs, mats and slippery linoleum. Avoid waxing floors.
   d. Installing special handrails and nonskid mats in the bathtub to prevent injury.
   e. Using non-skid treads on stairs; edges of rugs should be tacked down.
   f. Removing loose extension cords as they can be easily tripped over.
   g. Keeping a flashlight and a telephone at the bedside and lighting to the bathroom easily available.
   h. Assessing the client's visual and auditory changes as they may alter driving habits.
   i. Alerting family members as well as clients to be sensitive to the older individual's diminished reaction time.
   j. Preparing individuals for new situations, e.g., diagnostic procedures, hospitalization, etc., in order to decrease confusion and disruptions in sensory intake.
   k. Compensating for alteration in blood pressure (which may accompany aging), by teaching clients to adjust to changing positions slowly.
   l. Encouraging clients to rest if they feel dizzy or until the uncomfortable feeling passes.
   m. Advising the client to avoid looking up when climbing stairs or making sudden movements of the head to the side. This action may interrupt the blood supply to the brain and cause fainting and a fall could result.
   n. Instructing the client to avoid sedation if at all possible. If it is necessary to take sedation, instruct the client not to attempt to ambulate.
   o. Encourage proper labeling of medications and storing them in a well illuminated place.
   p. Advising the client to wear corrugated soles on shoes and to avoid walking on ice. Rubber-soled firm boots should be worn in the winter and walking in bad weather should be avoided.
   q. Teaching of proper transfer techniques, range of motion exercises, and body positioning necessary to increase overall client mobility and maintain safety.
   r. Utilizing geriatric chairs, well padded with detachable trays and acceptable safety devices. Prosthetic ambulatory devices, such as pick-up or rolling walkers, can also assist the client in independent ambulation.
   s. Encouraging the client to eat slowly and take small bites so the risk of choking will be minimized. This can be a serious problem especially where salivary production is reduced.
   t. Avoiding injury by frequent evaluation of vision, hearing, and foot abnormalities; recommended to help prevent stumbling and falls.
   u. Stressing the importance of never smoking in bed.

PREVENTING ILLNESS

Prevention of illness in the elderly can be achieved by:

1. Providing health teaching regarding risk factor reduction, a crucial factor in illness prevention.

2. Encouraging the elderly to seek more frequent periodic check-ups to detect and treat health problems so they will not become chronic problems.
3. Making multiphasic screening programs available and accessible to the community. Instructing the elderly about the benefits of such programs.
4. Offering prompt treatment for problems before further impairment is sustained.
5. Insuring that the immunizations required for the elderly are up to date.
6. Avoiding exposure to communicable disease whenever possible.
7. Encouraging periodic screening for occult disease that may be asymptomatic.
8. Evaluating deviations from normal found in diagnostic tests, or following a complete evaluation.
9. Participating in periodic screening for vision and hearing losses.
10. Teaching mobility-impaired clients about the importance of position changes in maintaining optimal skin integrity.

ENCOURAGING GOOD HEALTH PRACTICES IN THE ELDERLY

1. Stressing the importance of maintaining an adequate weight.
2. Instructing the client about the necessity for and benefits of eating a well balanced diet. Included in this discussion: the need to avoid the use of concentrated sweets, ingestion of high cholesterol foods, eating unrefined grain products, the value of roughage in diet, and avoidance of salt.
3. Encouraging the client to have good personal hygiene habits, including proper attention to foot care.
4. Stressing the importance of getting adequate rest and sleep.
5. Encouraging active participation in a regular exercise program commensurate with the client's activity tolerance. This will enhance mobility and fluidity of joint movement.
6. Stressing the importance of good dental hygiene and encouraging dental visits at least once yearly.
7. Supporting and assisting the elderly in their efforts to stop smoking.
8. Advising elderly clients to be moderate in their consumption of alcohol.

FULFILLMENT OF SOCIALIZATION NEEDS

1. Encouraging the elderly client to work towards fulfillment in all aspects of life.
2. Assisting clients in preparing for the eventual losses they may experience by addressing these before the loss occurs. (For a more detailed discussion of loss refer to Chapter 45.)
3. Helping to motivate the elderly to invest their time in community activities, hobbies and other areas of interest that may substitute for work in which they may be unable to engage.
4. Encouraging group activities and involvement with others in recreational activities, sharing meals together, and the like.

OBTAINING HEALTH CARE

1. Helping the elderly client to become aware of the resources available within the community that can meet health care needs.
2. Encouraging membership in a health insurance plan if this is financially possible. Instructing clients about Medicare-Medicaid benefits to which they may be entitled.
3. Acquainting the client with the suggested criteria used for selecting a health care provider.

HEALTH TEACHING

1. Contrary to the opinion of many, research has shown that the elderly can learn just as well as young people, given adequate time (Berrin, 1964). It is up to nurses and other health care providers to teach the elderly about maintaining their health, for clearly, the elderly *need* to know more about caring for themselves.
2. Encouraging the elderly to take a more active role in their health care management helps to foster independence.
3. Learning needs should be assessed in terms of content to be learned, learning style, and available teaching strategies.

DATA COLLECTION AND THE ELDERLY CLIENT

Obtaining a health history from an elderly client should yield valuable and relevant information that is essential if the nurse is to assist the client in maximizing health. Special considerations should include an awareness of the following:

1. The nurse must be willing to spend more time in obtaining a complete data base from an older client.
2. The client should be allowed to proceed at his or her own pace. If a detailed history is desired it may be advisable to gather data over several visits.
3. It is helpful to schedule appointments in the morning when fatigue may not be a problem for the older client. Morning appointments should be scheduled as the elderly are often concerned about being out in the late afternoon.
4. Sensory losses which are prevalent in the aging client may impede the history-taking process.
   a. Loss of hearing in clients over 65 years of age may contribute to irritability or suspiciousness during the interview if the client cannot hear what the nurse is saying.
   b. Speaking slowly in a low pitched and well modulated voice is more easily understood by the older client than raising one's voice.
   c. The nurse should face the client so that the client can see the eyes and lips of the examiner. This helps to reduce misinterpretation of data. The room should be as quiet as possible and free of interruptions.
   d. If hearing loss is profound, amplifying equipment may be necessary or the interview may be written.
   e. A well illuminated room without glare may help to compensate for vision loss which is common in the older client.
   f. The aging client may have diminished perception of pain; therefore a more intense stimulus may be required to evoke a pain response.
   g. Questions regarding even minimal pain and discomfort as well as symptomatic complaints should be carefully explored.
5. General intelligence does not decline with age but some specific problem-solving skills may not be as acute as in a younger adult.
6. The learning of new tasks may be difficult for the older client. Direction should be given clearly and simply in language and phrases that are familiar to the client. Questions should be short, concise and to the point.
7. The older client may not be comfortable sharing personal information and answering questions. It is important that the client be as relaxed as possible and the atmosphere be conducive to sharing information. Privacy and confidentiality should be ensured at all times.
8. If a client understands that the information gained during the interview is helpful in planning for health promotion and maintenance activities then the client may be more willing to share this information.
9. Since the elderly often have long and complex medical histories, it is advisable to set a time limit at the beginning of the interview.
10. Utilization of the life review may serve as an excellent way to obtain valuable information about the client.
11. The nurse should choose words that will neither offend nor alienate the client. Attention should be paid to nonverbal behavior as an indicator of the client's comfort level.
12. During the interview the nurse should maintain an open attitude about collecting a sexual history. This shows the client that he or she can freely discuss sexual matters and that the information shared is not only important but is an integral part of the history-taking process.
13. When obtaining a health history, it is important to concentrate on the individual's present and recent past sexual activity, instead of an early sexual history which may be too difficult to recall.

HEALTH HISTORY

In obtaining an accurate history from the elderly client, the nurse should collect data that is concerned with more than the current problem and past medical history. By utilizing a complete functional assessment approach, the nurse will gain far more information about the client that is helpful in planning care. Areas to be considered would include the following:

1. Determine the reliability of the information obtained from the elderly client. If necessary, a family member can be consulted to determine reliability and to supplement the information obtained from the client.
2. Assess client's perception of health status. Determine what "being healthy" means to the client; identify personal health habits.
3. Have the client compare present health with that of one year ago, 2 years, 5 years. Ask the client what he or she does to stay healthy.
4. Question the client about past patterns of health care utilization, e.g., does the individual have a yearly physical or seek health care only when ill? Assess the individual's knowledge of self-breast exam and the seven warning signs of cancer.
5. Encourage the client to describe a particular problem or concern in his or her own words, why he or she believes the problem has occurred, what seems to make the problem better or worse, and how having this problem affects health.
6. Ask clients to describe their past health history, including any significant health problems. Include the significant health problems of family members and assess the impact of these on the client's lifestyle.
7. Question the clients about occupation, retirement plans, current housing, financial concerns, medical insurance, and method of transportation.
8. Obtain a complete diet history; question appetite and eating habits. Assess any recent weight change, determine the individual's ability to eat and chew; question client about meal preparation and shopping.
9. Assess sleep and rest cycle of the client, including the number of hours that the client sleeps, and if the individual feels that this is adequate for him.
10. Assess the client's activity level and exercise limitations. Note the elderly client's satisfaction with this current level of functioning.
11. Determine the client's elimination patterns, both bowel and bladder. Note any use of laxatives and stool softeners, or diuretics.
12. Evaluate any sensory changes, especially hearing, vision and pain response. Inquire about what the client feels is most helpful in assisting him to learn new information. Assess any memory lapses.
13. Assess the client's level of sexual activity and the degree of satisfaction with this activity. Provide opportunity for the widow or widower to discuss the significance of the loss of the sexual partner (Chapter 45).
14. Assess the client's personality traits. Have the individual describe personal strengths and weaknesses. Identify coping patterns previously used to handle stress, evaluate patterns used to deal with loss (refer to Chapter 45).
15. Elicit information about the client's habits and lifestyle, including the use of alcohol, tobacco, salt, foods high in cholesterol, use of hair color, and exposure to sun.
16. Have the elderly client describe a typical week in his or her life. Include information about the use of leisure time, hobbies, etc.
17. Assess the individual's level of satisfaction with his life; assess role performance and level of satisfaction as well as patterns of interaction with life roles and relationships.
18. Identify the number and types of social contact as well as the client's level of satisfaction with these contacts. Identify significant individuals upon whom the client may rely if the need arises.
19. Assess the pattern of interaction with significant others.
20. Identify any religious, ethnic or cultural practices important to the client.
21. Obtain a full history of the medications currently being taken, including any over-the-counter preparations and home remedies. Elicit information about dosage, frequency, compliance and knowledge about the purpose of the medication and potential side effects.
22. Thoroughly explore any symptom, problem or limitation expressed by the elderly client.

PHYSICAL ASSESSMENT

Conducting a physical appraisal of an elderly client is essentially the same as for a client of any age. As in obtaining a health history, several factors must be kept in mind when performing a physical appraisal on an older individual.

APPROACH TO THE CLIENT

1. Comfort and privacy must be ensured at all times.
2. The examining room should be warm enough so that the client isn't chilled.
3. Allow more time to conduct a physical appraisal so that the client will not feel rushed.
4. When positional changes are required, lend assistance to the client when necessary.

GENERAL APPRAISAL OF THE OLDER ADULT

1. Assess the general appearance of the client relative to the chronological age.
2. Observe the overall apparent state of health.
3. Assess the level of awareness and orientation.
4. Evaluate the personal appearance of the client for appropriateness of dress and quality of grooming.
5. Observe the client's posture and gesturing, as these may provide important cues about the client's mood. Nonverbal behaviors are also important as they provide additional valuable information.
6. Describe any tension-releasing behaviors such as tapping or fidgeting.
7. Evaluate the client's affect, level of response and degree of cooperation, noting any unusual behaviors.
8. Measure the client's weight and vital signs, including a blood pressure reading in at least two positions.

PHYSIOLOGIC EFFECTS OF AGING

The aging process is an individual experience. Just as people live differently, so do they age differently and as a result manifest varying signs of aging. The normal changes that commonly accompany aging will be discussed. It should be emphasized that these changes are not necessarily present in all older individuals, nor are they present to the same extent in each individual.

CHANGES IN PERCEPTION AND COORDINATION

1. Alteration in perception and coordination occurs due to increased cell loss from brain tissue, especially the temporal and frontal lobes.
2. Alteration in sleep pattern occurs with less deep sleep required. Older people tend to dream less and have increased periods of wakefulness. Stage four sleep is reduced significantly after age 50, and frequent arousals are common.
3. Reaction time is slowed due to diminished neurotransmitters as well as a decrease in the speed of nerve impulses.
4. There is a delayed overall body response to stressors.
5. Dizziness may occur, as a result of getting up too quickly from a sitting or lying position, resulting from such things as a decrease in cerebral blood flow.
6. There is a decrease in the perception of temperature, vibration, and pain.
7. The threshold for light touch is increased and proprioreception may be impaired.
8. Kinesthetic senses may be less efficient and a parkinsonian gait may be present.

COGNITIVE CHANGES

1. In general, persons of high intellectual capacity experience less decrease in mental efficiency than those of low intellectual capacity (Diekelman, 1977).
2. Many believe that older adults experience less mental decline than was formally thought.
3. More time is required for integration of learning and making responses, reaching a conclusion, or making a decision.
4. Older adults tend to have a poor memory for recent events but a good memory for remote events.
5. It may be more difficult for the elderly to learn

new concepts, therefore longer time may be required for teaching the elderly.

SENSORINEURAL CHANGES

1. All voluntary or automatic reflexes are slowed with a resultant decreased ability to respond to multiple stimuli.
2. Deep tendon reflexes remain intact in the healthy elderly individual.
3. Healthy elderly individual changes in the eye include the following:
   a. Peripheral vision decreases.
   b. Lens accommodation decreases with age and corrective lenses are often required; thickening of the lens may also occur, and focusing for distance and reading may be difficult.
   c. An opaque white ring called an arcus senilis, which is due to fatty deposits, may be visible around the iris.
   d. Opacities of the lens are not uncommon and may be indicative of cataracts.
   e. Visual acuity is often diminished due to macular degeneration. Color differentiation may also be difficult.
   f. Accommodation to light may be diminished; usually changes from light to darkness are more problematic; there may be an inability of the individual to distinguish between various intensities of light. "Night blindness" is not uncommon. There is an increased sensitivity to glare from lights, while at the same time more light may be needed to see.
   g. The conjunctiva thin with age and may appear yellow.
   h. There may be a difference in pupil size (aniseikonia), and volume of tearing may be reduced.
   i. Vascular changes may occur in the retina as part of the aging process.
   j. The muscles of the eye function less efficiently and the pupil aperture narrows.
4. Higher frequency tones are less perceptable to the older individual, resulting in less availability of auditory information and potential language understanding impairment. This may lead to confusion and what may be misperceived by others as a disturbance in thought processing. This hearing loss is more significant in men particularly after age 60 (Carnevali, 1979).
5. About two-thirds of the taste buds die by the time the individual reaches age 70. Decrease in tastes for salt and sugar may be observed.
6. The sense of smell is also considerably diminished due to a decrease of olfactory nerve fibers.
7. Some researchers believe that loss of hearing, taste, and smell is due to a decrease of cellular regeneration of the parietal area (Hughes, 1969).
8. The voice may become higher in pitch, and range, duration, and intensity of the voice may diminish.

MUSCULAR AND SKELETAL CHANGES

1. The most visible physiologic changes in aging relate to decrements in body tissue.
2. There is a widespread decrease in bone mass, frequently resulting in increased stress on weight-bearing areas that become predisposed to fracture (refer to *Osteoporosis* in Chapter 46).
3. Height decreases (1–4 inches) and kyphosis sometimes develops. Scoliosis may intensify the problem. There is thinning or even collapse of intervertebral disks, due to loss of water from the cartilage.
4. Joints lose elasticity and preosteroarthritic degeneration is found in joint cartilage, making the joint less flexible. Ligaments may also become calcified.
5. Muscle size and strength both diminish with age. Muscle tone and strength peaks between ages 20 and 30 with gradual decline thereafter. While regeneration of muscle tissue is still possible in the older person, muscle mass does decrease, gradually but steadily.
6. Decreased muscle strength and increased fatigue exist due to decreased adenosine triphosphate (ATP) and lactic acid production.
7. Alteration in coordination may contribute to disturbance in gait. Fine motor movements may also diminish.
8. Bones become more brittle and tend to break more easily, due to demineralization of bones.
   a. Joint crepitation may be present.

b. Proportion of total fat to body weight increases with age, especially on the trunk, while it diminishes on the legs and arms.

RESPIRATORY CHANGES

1. There is an increase in the anteroposterior diameter of the chest (kyphosis).
2. The number of alveoli is gradually decreased due to a progressive loss of interalveolar septi. This can result in decreased diffusion surface for oxygen and carbon dioxide.
3. The aging lung becomes increasingly rigid and less compliant.
4. Respiratory accessory muscles lose their strength, resulting in increased rigidity of the chest wall.
5. With increasing age there is a measurable reduction in breathing efficiency. Bronchopulmonary movement is decreased due to an increase in fibrous connective tissue and lymphoid elements; both factors lead to a rigid bronchopulmonary tree.
6. The exchange of air between lungs and environment is reduced due to the obstruction of the pulmonary airway and restriction in pulmonary expansion and contraction.
7. Vital capacity decreases, residual air increases, and the respiratory gas exchange functions are diminished. The older individual also takes shorter breaths.
8. Bronchoelimination is decreased due to a diminished cough reflex and lessened effectiveness of the ciliary mechanism.
9. With a decrease in bronchopulmonary function, the oxygen supply needed for cell respiration and assimilation is diminished.
10. Poor posture may decrease the capacity of the thoracic cavity and affect overall oxygenation.
11. Airway resistance increases and there is less ventilation at the base of the lung than at the apex.

CARDIAC CHANGES

1. Cardiac pathology is the number one cause of mortality in the aged (see Chapter 30).
2. The normal physiologic changes in cardiac function result in the heart having to work harder to accomplish less.
3. Peripheral resistance and circulation time increase with age, as well as systolic and sometimes diastolic blood pressure.
4. Physiologic changes related to the heart include the following:
   a. Cardiac output decreases approximately 30 percent by the age of 65.
   b. Prolongation of the period of contraction occurs.
   c. Increased rigidity of valves is observed.
   d. Sudden increased cardiac output caused by nonregular exercise can cause a rise in arterial blood pressure.
   e. Aortic elasticity diminishes considerably with advancing age (Abbey, 1973).
5. Decreased cardiac efficiency and arteriosclerotic and atherosclerotic changes in blood vessels are prime factors in diminished circulation to all parts of the aging body.
6. Increased irritability of the cardiac muscle may result in alteration in rhythm. EKG changes may show such things as smaller and longer QRS complexes and decreased ST waves.
7. Tachycardia may occur in response to stress, but the ability of the heart to increase its rate is generally impaired.
8. Myocardial hypertrophy accompanies the aging process.
9. Kyphoscoliosis may cause a dislocation of the cardiac apex, so that its location loses diagnostic significance.
10. Murmurs are present in more than 60 percent of aged clients and they are most often due to schlerotic changes of the aortic valves (Malasanos, 1977).
11. The older client's response to maximal exercise is not as great as a younger adult's. Cardiac output and heart rate are lower and systolic blood pressure is elevated. See Appendix for listing of ranges for safe maximal pulses.

CHANGES IN BLOOD VESSELS

1. There is a decreased elasticity of blood vessels.
2. Normal calcification of blood vessels (e.g., aortic arch) occurs.
3. Athrogenesis secondary to the aging process is present.

4. Decreased capillary permeability occurs due to sluggish exchange of blood in the capillary bed.
5. Alteration in the vasopressor control mechanism contributes to orthostatic hypertension. These changes may result in dizziness, weakness, and fainting.
6. Pulses are more readily felt due to a loss of adjacent connective tissue. Additionally, the vessels are harder due to atherosclerosis, and they may feel tortuous and rigid.
7. Pedal pulses may be more difficult to obtain due to atherosclerosis. Older clients may complain of cold extremities and these may be present with a cool temperature and somewhat mottled appearance. Neck pulsations may be more observable but caution must be used if they are to be used during palpation.
8. There is a significant increase in the systolic blood pressure due to increased peripheral vascular resistance. The diastolic pressure should increase only slightly, resulting in an increased pulse pressure.
9. Venous circulation remains unchanged in healthy individuals.

CHANGES IN THE URINARY SYSTEM

1. Decreased cardiac output results in diminished renal efficiency, reduced filtration and possible protein loss.
2. Males may have difficulty initiating and ending urinary stream due to prostatic enlargement.
3. A decrease in perineal muscle tone in females results in urgency and stress incontinence.
4. Nocturia increases with age.
5. Bladder capacity is reduced and the volume passed during each voiding episode varies with intake.
6. Incontinence increases with age.
7. Older females are more prone to urinary tract infections associated with sexual activity.

CHANGES IN THE REPRODUCTIVE SYSTEM

1. Changes frequently seen in the aging woman include the following:
   a. Estrogen production declines with menopause.
   b. Glandular breast tissue atrophies and the amount of fat in the breast increases. Breasts become more flaccid due to diminution of connective tissue.
   c. The uterus decreases in size due to a loss of myometerial fibers.
   d. The cervix also decreases in size, mucous secretion is reduced and that which is present is thick and cellular.
   e. The vagina narrows and shortens due to an increase in the amount of submucosal connective tissue; the epithelial lining of the vaginal canal atrophies and the surface appears thin and pale.
   f. A decrease in estrogen production leads to increased alkalinity as glycogen content and acidity decline. This favors the growth of pathogenic organisms.
   g. Dyspareunia may be present due to the loss of vaginal epithelium and associated mucous changes.
2. Changes frequently seen in the aging man include:
   a. Testosterone levels may diminish, but this occurs at a later time in life than that of estrogen decrease in the female. This is somewhat controversial in that a sexually active healthy elderly male may only experience this in a mild way.
   b. There may be a decline in sexual energy associated with an alteration in health.
   c. There is a gradual decline in the strength of the muscles associated with the act of intercourse.
   d. The force of ejaculation is reduced and the refractory phase lengthens.
   e. The testes decrease in size and are less firm on palpation. Thickening in the connective tissue of the tubules also occurs.
   f. Sperm count decreases and the viscosity of seminal fluid diminishes.
   g. Prostatic enlargement is present in some degree in three-fourths of males 65 and over, and secretion may be impaired.
3. Sexuality in the older adult.
   a. Normal physiologic changes accompany the aging process, but do not substantially limit one's sexual capacity.
   b. The phases of intercourse are less intense with a slower excitement phase, longer duration of the plateau and shorter orgasm. Changes noted in the four phases of intercourse in the aging male may be found in Table 44-1.

TABLE 44-1 CHANGES NOTED IN THE FOUR PHASES OF INTERCOURSE IN AGING MALE CLIENT

Phase	Changes
Excitement	Slower increment in excitement; sex flush less in duration and intensity; involuntary spasms diminished; longer time required to achieve erection; less testicular elevation and scrotal sac vasocongestion during erection.
Plateau	Longer duration; increase in penile diameter since less pre-ejaculatory fluid emission.
Orgasmic	Shorter duration. Fewer contractions in expulsion of semen bolus.
Resolution (refractory)	Lasts 12–24 hours as compared to 2 minutes in the youthful client. Loss of erection (return of penis to flaccid state) may take a few seconds as compared to minutes or hours in the youthful client.

SOURCE: Malasanos, L., Barkauskas, V., Moss, M., and Stoltenberg-Allen, K.: *Health Assessment*, 2d ed., C. V. Mosby, St. Louis, 1981, p. 629.

c. At no time in a man's life does he lose the capability of erection, except in rare instances involving injury to or pathology of the central nervous system (Masters and Johnson, 1970).
d. Freeman studied man over 75 years of age and found that over half of those studied reported that coitus was satisfactory for them (Freeman, 1961).
e. Men in every decade of life remain sexually active and the majority suffered no decline in sexual interest (Pfeiffer, 1968).
f. Those studying sexuality in the older adult uniformly agree that proper health and availability of partners are the most important factors for continued sexual activity.
g. The inherent need for closeness and contact with others does not diminish with age. Sexual needs are integral to being human and are a component of one's personality and self concept.
h. Traditionally, the sexual needs of the aged adult have not been viewed as appropriate. Sexual activity viewed as normal in a younger person is sometimes regarded as curious behavior in an older client.
i. Some older individuals do terminate sexual activity but this is most often due to personal preference and is not necessarily physiologic restriction.
j. The older adult may respond to sexual needs by touching, kissing, or embracing. The actual act of coitus is not the only way to fulfill sexual needs.

NUTRITIONAL AND METABOLIC CHANGES

1. Gastric acid secretion declines with advancing age. A reduction in the amount of digestive enzymes may explain why many elderly frequently complain of anorexia and difficulty in digesting meals.
2. Muscle tone in the stomach and intestines is diminished.
3. Hypomotility of the esophagus is a common finding and may contribute to the older client being at risk for aspiration as well as inflammation.
4. Diminishment in the senses of taste and smell may contribute to a decreased appetite, and the older client may not choose a balanced variety of foods to eat.
5. A decrease in appetite and decreased sensitivity to thirst, is at least partially due to reduced hypothalamic efficiency. Medications may also affect appetite.
6. Hiatal hernia is a common finding among the elderly population.
7. Salivation is reduced and swallowing may become more difficult.
8. Achlorhydra prevents vitamin B_{12} absorption, and calcium absorption is also decreased.
9. PH levels, when altered, are slower to return

to normal, and glucose clearance time is increased.

10. Facial changes due to resorption of gum and bony tissue surrounding teeth may also lead to difficulty in mastication.
11. Most clients over 65 years of age are edentulous and loss of teeth and/or poor fitting dentures can lead to malnutrition. Often, insufficient high-bulk foods are ingested because of the difficulty involved in chewing them. Bulky foods help to maintain tonicity of the tract wall, but many people are unaware of this beneficial effect.
12. Malnutrition is of epidemic proportions in the elderly, and may be reflected in generalized weight loss.
13. Obesity may be a problem for women and men over age 50. This may be due to:
    a. Diminishing exercise patterns without altering the caloric intake.
    b. Attempts to compensate for psychologic loss with sweets.
    c. Lifestyle and established food habits.
    d. Reduced or fixed income with frequent use of food high in carbohydrates.
    e. Hormonal changes, especially in women.
    f. Isolation.
14. Men tend to lose weight steadily after age 65, but the majority of women show a tendency toward progressive weight gain.
15. There is a progressive decrease in the basal metabolic rate (BMR), resulting in loss of glycogen deposits and unavailability of glycogen stores. The decreased number of body cells, especially with decreased muscle tissue, also lead to a diminished BMR.
16. The efficiency of the heat production mechanism is reduced and this coupled with the decrease in BMR and loss of fat padding make the elderly susceptible to cold. Decreased hypothalmus function can contribute to this problem.
17. Hormonal changes associated with aging may be found on Table 44-2.

CHANGES IN ELIMINATION

1. There is an overall reduction in the mobility of the gastrointestinal tract, but 90 percent of individuals over 60 have at least one bowel movement daily (Mezey, 1980).
2. Transit time for stool to pass through the gastrointestinal tract is slowed.
3. The urge to defecate may be diminished due to decreased perception of sensory stimuli.
4. Constipation is a frequent complaint and may have multiple etiologies.
5. Rectal sphincter tone may be diminished and involuntary defecation may occur.

CHANGES IN INTEGUMENT

1. Muscle bulk and tone are lost and there is a decrease and redistribution of the total body fat from the periphery to the center of the body.
2. Loss of fat padding over bony prominencies predisposes the elderly with mobility restriction to decubitus ulcers.
3. Thinning of the epithelium occurs and blood vessels are often easily observable.
4. Collagen elastic fibers also shrink in thickness with resultant loss of skin elasticity, and a diminished skin turgor.
5. Sebaceous and sweat glands decrease in number, resulting in thin, dry, and inextensible skin. The amount of perspiration decreases; then drying scaling, called xerosis, is often accompanied by pruritis and flaking. Diminished hormone levels also contribute to these skin changes.
6. Atrophy of apocrine glands makes body temperature regulation more difficult as there is decreased ability of body to rid itself of heat by evaporation. Diminished hypothalmic function also can decrease sweating and vasodilitation.
7. Creases and wrinkle lines appear because of frequent use of muscles and habitual expression.
8. Atrophic changes in subcutaneous tissue also contributes to this wrinkling and laxness of skin is further affected by simple gravitational pull. Exposure to sun is also considered to be a factor that affects skin wrinkling.
9. Pigmentation of skin tends to lighten due to cellular losses of melanocytes. Areas of spotty pigmentation are commonly seen and these "aging spots" are due to a pigment called lipofusion.
10. Evidence of increased bruising and telengiactasias may be apparent due to a decrease

TABLE 44-2 KNOWN HORMONE CHANGES IN THE AGED

Hormones and Controlling Factors	Normal Action	Age Change
	Adrenal Cortex	
Cortisol ACTH	Stimulates protein catabolism, stimulates liver uptake of amino acids and their conversion to glucose, is permissive for stimulation of gluconeogenesis by other tissues, inhibits glucose uptake and oxidation by many body cells	Secretion somewhat decreased in proportion to decreased muscle mass
Aldosterone Angisterin plasma K^+ concentration	Stimulates Na reabsorption, specifically by distal tubules, stimulates transport of Na by other epithelia in the body, e.g., sweat glands, is an "all-purpose" stimulator of Na retention	Young people have been found to have secretion rates for aldosterone that are more than twice as high as those of elderly subjects; metabolic clearance rates and calculated plasma concentrations of aldosterone are also decreased
	Gonads	
Ovaries: Estrogen FSH LH	Maintains the entire female genital tract and the breasts, is responsible for body hair distribution and the general female configuration, is required for follicle and ovum maturation, permits ovulation, and onset of menses	Loss of germinal cells causes decrease in levels of estrogen, which is associated with increase in pituitary activity and a decrease in estrogen levels; source of estrogen in postmenopausal women, adrenal cortex (primarily)
Progesterone FSH LH	Present in significant amounts only during luteal phase of menstrual cycle, has an effect on the endometrium, breasts, oviducts, and uterine smooth muscle	A decrease of 50% of pregnanediol (a byproduct of progesterone breakdown) in urinary excretion of women between 30 and 80
Testes: Testosterone LH	Spermatogenesis, needed for the morphology and function of the entire male duct system, development and maintenance of normal sexual drive and behavior in men, development of secondary sexual characteristics	Is not as abrupt or sudden as in female; loss of geminal cells also occurs when pituitary is functioning at high level

TABLE 44-2 (*continued*)

Hormones and Controlling Factors	Normal Action	Age Change
	Pancreas	
Insulin Plasma Glucose concentrations	Stimulates the facilitated diffusion of glucose into certain cells (muscle and adipose), stimulates protein synthesis, affects liver synthesis	Response of elderly person to insulin is decreased
	Kidneys	
Renin	Catalyzes the reaction in which angiotensiogen becomes angiotensin	Suggested slower response but no evidence
Angiotensin	Profound stimulator of aldosterone, secretion is the primary input into the adrenal gland, which produces aldosterone	Suggested slower response but no evidence
Erythropoietin	Stimulates erythrocyte and hemoglobin synthesis	Suggested slower response but no evidence
	Posterior Pituitary	
ADH: Blood volume Blood pressure Electrolyte levels	Antidiuretic effect on kidney, keeps water permeability of latter nephron segments up, so H_2O reabsorption is able to keep up with Na reabsorption	Kidney (increased) response time
	Thyroid Gland	
Thyroxine TSH	An iodine-containing amino acid, influences metabolic rate, O_2 consumption, and heat production in most body tissues	From 25 years onward there is a slow, gradual decline in thyroid activity (until eighth decade)

SOURCE: Jones, D., Dunbar, C., and Jirovec, M.: *Medical-Surgical Nursing: A Conceptual Approach*, McGraw-Hill, New York, 1982, p. 81.

* Developed by Catherine Kopac, R.N., M.N.

in keratin production, resulting in an increased fragility of vessels.

11. There is a generalized loss of hair from the periphery to the center of the body. Hair on extremities as well as axillary and pubic hair diminishes. Men will also experience a decrease in facial hair.
12. Scalp hair is diminished and it may feel coarse and dry. The scalp itself may also be dry.
13. Graying of the hair occurs due to a loss of pigmentation cells. It may also appear dull, white, or yellow.
14. Women may develop chin whiskers and an increase in facial hair secondary to hormonal changes.

15. The nails, especially on the feet, may become increasingly brittle and thickened, and the growth rate is generally decreased.

CHANGES IN THE IMMUNE SYSTEM

1. Allergic responses appear to increase with aging, particularly in response to drugs.
2. There is marked decrease in the aging liver and kidney functions which delay the elimination and detoxification of chemicals (e.g., medications and allergens).
3. The immune capacity appears to break down with age, as evidenced by the fact that cancer is the number two cause of mortality in people over 65.
4. Studies suggest that infectious processes occur which lymphocytes would have eliminated in persons of younger age.
5. Immunocompetency is one body function in which age-related diminution has occurred, and the immunocompetence of the elderly is very precarious (Carnevali, 1979).
6. Less-than-perfect aging cells are often destroyed by the immune system even though they are still functional.
7. Aging women appear to have increased susceptibility to autoimmune diseases (e.g., arthritis); aging men seem more susceptible to infectious diseases and cancer.

BEHAVIORAL CHANGES AND COPING RESPONSES ASSOCIATED WITH AGING

A complete discussion about the psychological changes, social changes, and the losses experienced by the elderly may be found in Chapter 45.

NURSING DIAGNOSES: ACTUAL OR POTENTIAL

Since the discussion has focused on normal changes and aging, the diagnoses to be discussed are mainly potential nursing problems associated with aging. They include:

1. Malnutrition: nutritional deficit.
2. Potential mobility impairment.
3. Alteration in bowel pattern: constipation.
4. Sleep pattern disturbance.
5. Potential for injury.
6. Altered sexual patterns.

NUTRITIONAL DEFICIT: MALNUTRITION

Population at Risk

1. Low income individuals.
2. Alcohol or drug abusers.
3. Those who have experienced recent losses.
4. Clients who live alone, unable to go to store to purchase food.
5. Individuals who are mentally confused or depressed.
6. Those who are on special diets.
7. Clients with impaired chewing ability or those experiencing difficulty in swallowing.
8. Clients on medications which may cause anorexia.
9. Clients who have a neurological, sensory, or muscular deficit.
10. Decreased ingestion of daily vitamins A, C, and E.

Assessment Data

1. A loss of weight with adequate food intake.
2. 20 percent or more under ideal body weight.
3. Reported inadequate food intake.
4. Weakness of muscles required for swallowing or mastication.
5. Reported or evidence of lack of food.
6. Lack of interest in food.
7. Perceived inability to ingest food.
8. Aversion to eating.
9. Reported altered taste and smell sensations.
10. Satiety immediately after ingesting food.
11. Abdominal pain with or without pathology.
12. Sore, inflamed buccal cavity.
13. Capillary fragility.
14. Abdominal cramping.
15. Diarrhea and/or steatorrhea.
16. Hyperactive bowel sounds.
17. Pale conjunctiva and mucous membranes.
18. Poor muscle tone and poor skin turgor.
19. Loss of hair.
20. Misinformation regarding dietary requirements.

21. Failure to adjust intake during specific life cycle.
22. Adherence to fad diets.
23. Abnormal specific laboratory tests.

POTENTIAL MOBILITY IMPAIRMENT

Population at Risk
1. Persons who are malnourished.
2. Those with arthritic and joint conditions.
3. Persons with foot disorders.
4. Individuals with visual disturbances.
5. Those with decreased perception or neuromuscular deficits.
6. Persons who are depressed.

Assessment Data
1. Inability to move: total body, joint, etc.
2. Reluctance to attempt movement.
3. Perceived inability to move.
4. Goals incongruent with abilities.
5. Altered perception of position of body part(s).
6. Altered perception of presence of body part(s).
7. Alteration in coordination of movement.
8. Limited active range of motion.
9. Decreased muscle strength and/or control.
10. Imposed restrictions of movement.

CONSTIPATION

Population at Risk
1. Persons who eat a low bulk diet.
2. Dehydrated individuals.
3. Individuals with hemorrhoids.
4. Persons with reduced food intake.
5. Confused patients.
6. Individuals who require chronic use of laxatives.
7. Individuals who take medications that are known to cause constipation (opiates, barbiturates, anticholinergics).

Assessment Data
1. Hard-formed stool.
2. Reports of less than three bowel movements weekly.
3. Reported feeling of rectal fullness and pressure.
4. Straining at stool.
5. Palpable mass.
6. Headache.
7. Interference with daily living.
8. Back pain.
9. Reported use of laxatives.
10. Appetite impairment.
11. Reported repetition of the above signs and symptoms.

SLEEP PATTERN DISTURBANCE

Population at Risk
1. Those who are depressed or emotionally troubled.
2. Persons with minimal physical activity.
3. Individuals who are on medication which may alter sleep pattern.
4. Stress responses.

Assessment Data
1. Restless when asleep (females may have increased number of nightmares, sensitive to noise; males have nocturnal micturition).
2. Restless when awake.
3. Decreased daytime activity level.
4. Dozing; increased naps.
5. Insomnia; situational insomnia.
6. Difficult to arouse.
7. Delayed response to stimuli.
8. Increased response to stimuli.
9. Irritability (stage IV sleep decreases: alternate between REM and light sleep).
10. Verbalization of sleep disturbances; decrease in total sleep noted.
11. Verbalization of fatigue.
12. Lethargy.
13. Dream disturbances.
14. Sleep latency.
15. Sleep interruption awakenings increase in frequency and length after 40.
16. Sleep deprivation.
17. Sleep onset disturbance.

Sleep Apnea
A pause in respiration more than 10 seconds and more than 5 awakenings.
1. May awake 20–80 times per night.
2. Increased susceptibility to sudden death.
3. Seen more in males.
4. Increased cooccurrence with hypertension, headaches, smoking, obesity; cardiac pathology.
5. Affects 50–80 percent of the elderly; greater incidence in those who take sleeping medications.

Adaptive Response
When apnea occurs, there is an increase in the production of norepinephrine, blood pressure increases, and there is increased oxygen sent to the tissue.

POTENTIAL FOR INJURY

Population at Risk
1. Persons with a neuromuscular or perceptual deficit.
2. Individuals who live in an unsafe environment.
3. Clients with impaired coordination.
4. Clients who abuse alcohol or drugs.
5. Clients who are on anticoagulant therapy.

Assessment Data
1. Lack of knowledge regarding safety knowledge.
2. An environment (work or home) conducive to injury.
3. Poor vision or hearing.
4. Decreased touch sensation.
5. Balance or coordination deficits.
6. Unavailable or uncomfortable occupational protective gear.
7. Absence of pedestrial crosswalk safeguards.
8. Verbalization of a tendency to bleed easily.

ALTERED PATTERNS OF SEXUALITY

Population at Risk
1. Those clients without adequate role modeling.
2. Individuals who have been physically, psychologically, or socially abused.
3. Clients with a structural or functional alteration or limitation.
4. Those who lack privacy.
5. Individuals without a significant other or available sexual partner.

Assessment Data
1. Verbalization of problem in sexuality.
2. Alterations in achieving perceived sex role.
3. Actual or perceived limitation imposed by disease and/or therapy.
4. Knowledge deficit regarding sexuality.
5. Conflicts involving values.
6. Alteration in achieving sexual satisfaction.
7. Inability to achieve desired sexual satisfaction.
8. Seeking confirmation of desirability.
9. Alteration in sexual relationship with significant other.
10. Change of interest in self and others.

OTHER POTENTIAL NURSING DIAGNOSES

1. *Fluid volume excess: stress incontinence* is a frequently encountered and distressing problem faced by many older clients, particularly female clients. Bladder retraining and the use of Kegal's exercises to strengthen pelvic muscles and sphincter tone are often helpful treatment modalities.
2. *Memory deficit:* older adults tend to have a poorer memory for recent events but a good memory for remote ones. The use of cues is helpful in assisting recall in the older adult. Memory can also be enhanced by coupling a new task such as taking a pill with an already established habit pattern or behavior.
3. *Depression:* depression in the elderly is often overlooked and often undiagnosed. Careful observation by the nurse is required if depression is to be detected. Depression in the elderly may closely resemble an organic brain syndrome and it is imperative that the two be differentiated. For a discussion on organic brain syndrome, refer to Chapter 46. Common signs and symptoms of depression may be regarded as "old age problems" by many health care providers. Careful observation and evaluation of verbal and nonverbal cues, in addition to listening with a sensitive ear while interviewing the older adult, may alert the nurse to the possible existence of depression.

EXPECTED OUTCOMES

1. Clients will maintain their optimal level of wellness through health education, encouragement of healthy behaviors, accident prevention, and prevention and early detection of illnesses.

2. Potential problems that may interrupt the healthy state of the older client and interfere with optimal functioning within the various functional pattern areas will be identified at an early stage.
3. Factors that exist in the environment will be identified to protect the older client from injury, infection, and excessive stress.
4. An individual's coping strategies with the multiplicity of stressful experiences, along with the supports, will be identified to ensure a less stressful lifestyle.
5. Social interaction among the elderly will be promoted to encourage fulfillment of the client's socialization needs.
6. Older individuals will be able to modify their style of living in order to adapt to changes in the physical or psychosocial environment imposed by the aging process.
7. The client's strengths will be stressed and focused upon instead of dwelling on weaknesses or defects.
8. The elderly client will express feelings of self worth, pride, and usefulness, as well as the desire for remaining independent.

INTERVENTIONS

NUTRITIONAL DEFICIT: MALNUTRITION

1. Teach older clients that as they age, their caloric requirements are generally reduced. For the older woman, 1,800 calories per day is average, 2,000 for the older man.
2. Caloric reduction is not synonymous with reduction in essential nutrients. Requirements for protein, vitamins, and minerals are essentially the same as for a younger individual. Vitamin (e.g., E, A, C) requirements may be greater in the elderly population.
3. A proper diet is a necessary factor in preventing disease and in recovery from illness. For a suggested daily diet for the older adult refer to Table 44-3.
4. Small frequent meals often support eating fewer calories as the older patient is less likely to overindulge.
5. Encourage liberal intake of water to facilitate digestion and elimination.
6. Good dental care, gum care, and use of properly fitting dentures are essential to good nutrition.
7. If an older person has a low activity tolerance, a rest before meals will help to conserve the patient's physical energies for eating.
8. Varying the flavor, texture, and appearance of food may help alleviate the gradual diminution of taste and smell.
9. Instruct the client that nutritional supplements are generally not necessary if the diet is adequate and well balanced. However, a regular vitamin supplement may be taken without concern or great expense.
10. The use of wine prior to eating may help to stimulate the appetite.
11. When loneliness is a deterrant to appetite, companionship and socialization at mealtimes helps to make eating a more pleasant experience.
12. Investigate the client's knowledge about nu-

TABLE 44-3 SUGGESTED DAILY DIET FOR THE OLDER ADULT

One or two glasses of milk (preferably skim or low-fat)
At least one large serving of meat, fish, or poultry
At least one serving of green or yellow vegetables
One or two servings of citrus fruit or tomatoes
Possibly a serving of other vegetables such as potatoes
Two or three servings of bread, flour, or cereals
One or two tablespoons of table fat (such as margarine)
Three to five cups of water per day.

SOURCE: Deutsch, D.: "The Family Guide to Better Food and Better Health," in Diekleman, N.: *Primary Health Care of the Well Adult*, McGraw-Hill, New York, 1977, p. 177.

TABLE 44-4 HELPFUL HINTS TO STRETCH FOOD DOLLARS FOR THE ELDERLY

1. Plan your meals and snacks before you shop.
2. If possible, shop for a week at a time for your food needs.
3. Plan to buy staples such as flour, sugar, and corn meal only once or twice a month in larger and less expensive sizes.
4. Eat before you shop! If you are hungry when you go shopping, you will probably "buy on impulse" items you do not need.
5. You can save time by arranging your food list in the same way as the food is found in your store.
6. As you plan your menus, check newspaper ads for weekly specials. However, buy only if you can save money by buying an item you need and if the store is near you. Note: Do not drive three miles to save 3¢.
7. Remember that nonfood items are necessary, perhaps, but they are not a part of your food bill.
8. Use discount coupons if they are for things you really need.
9. Keep a list of commonly purchased food items and compare regular and sales prices. Remember: sometimes so-called specials are not really specials.
10. Learn new ways to use inexpensive high nutritional foods. However, if you will not eat the food and you throw it away, it is not a saving.
11. Beware of some so-called budget recipes in magazines or in the newspaper that start with low-cost main dishes and then "fancy them up" with costly rare spices, nuts, etc.
12. You usually pay more for convenience. Plan to save money whenever possible by doing your own cutting, grating, mixing, seasoning, and cooking.
13. Skillet "helper" dinners are costly. Usually you can put the ingredients together yourself and get twice as much food for the same money.
14. Plan to use moderate-sized portions of high-cost items such as meat.
15. Plan to drink water when you are thirsty. It is the cheapest thirst quencher there is. (Leave the overpriced sugar-loaded or artificially sweetened sodas and fruit drinks on the grocery shelf.)
16. Shop on days when you get the best buys and freshest foods at your store. Often this is toward the end of the week. However, some stores offer savings at the beginning of the week to encourage early shopping.
17. Plan to shop when you are not rushed or distracted.

SOURCE: Carnevali, D., and Patrick, M.: *Nursing Management for the Elderly*, J. B. Lippincott, Philadelphia, 1979, p. 163. Adapted from "Meal Planning for the Golden Years," General Mills, 1966.

trition, access to food and shopping, and ability to prepare meals. In conducting dietary assessment, encourage the use of a diet log for future review.

13. As cost is a significant concern of many elderly, the nurse can suggest alternative less expensive sources of protein.
14. Teach the client to plan ahead, shopping with a list and shopping wisely to help to keep the food cost down. For additional ways of helping the elderly cut food costs, refer to Table 44-4.
15. Refer the client to community resources that are available in the area. Dial a Dietician is a source of nutritional information that the elderly may find very helpful.
16. Feeding programs such as Meals on Wheels provide the elderly with socialization and a well-balanced meal for a nominal fee. Often transportation to the centers is available.

POTENTIAL MOBILITY IMPAIRMENT

1. Assess the client's gait, as this will give the nurse valuable information regarding the client's mobility potential.
2. Put the client's joints through range of motion to determine any impairment.
3. Determine if motion causes the client any discomfort or pain.
4. Teach the client about the positive effects, both physiologic and psychologic, that exercise has on health. Exercise not only improves muscle tone and cardiac status but it enhances sleep, elimination, and digestion, and aids in weight control.
5. Greater flexibility of the musculoskeletal system may permit the older client to engage in more activities and be more self-reliant and satisfied.
6. Encourage older clients to engage in some form of regular exercise of their choice. If clients have not been accustomed to engaging in regular exercise, they should begin slowly and work up to a higher level, allowing for frequent rests.
7. In a recent study of older adults, three health behaviors were examined (inactivity, obesity, and cigarette smoking) and inactivity had the highest correlation with illness indicators (Palmore, 1976).
8. Older adults may enjoy exercising together and many senior citizen centers are offering exercise programs on a regular basis (Figure 44-1).
9. If joint mobility is impaired, clients can be taught new skills that will increase activity. If mobility impairment is severe, prosthetics or supports can be employed to assist the client.
10. Encourage nutritious eating habits that will provide the client with energy levels sufficient to perform activities of his or her choice.

CONSTIPATION

1. An adequate intake of fluids is essential for normal metabolism and elimination. For hospitalized clients, keep a glass of water within the person's reach, offering water with medications and encouraging between-meal fluids.
2. Improved nutrition, balanced diet, and adequate intake help relieve constipation. Stool softeners can be used safely but chronic use of laxatives should be avoided.
3. Encourage a diet that is high in fresh fruits, vegetables and whole grains as these will provide extra bulk and facilitate elimination.

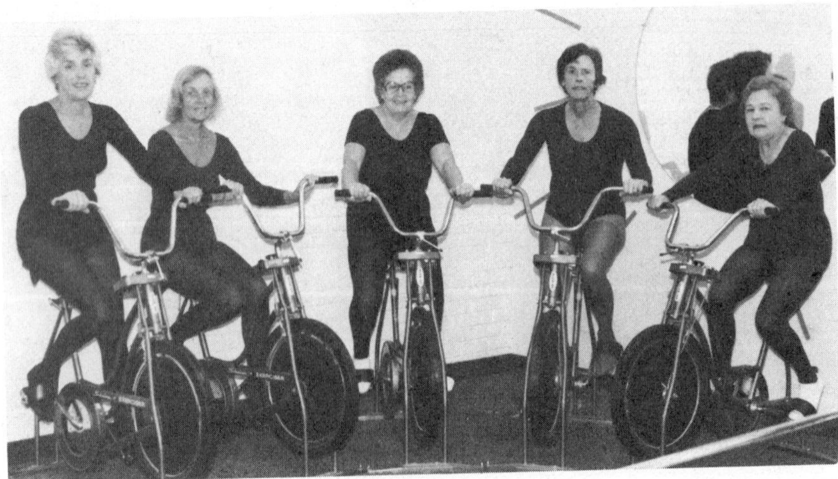

Figure 44-1 Group exercise is often a way for the elderly to engage in activity and to socialize.

4. Clients should be advised to avoid straining at stool but to take adequate time to evacuate the bowel without rushing.
5. At times, a modified squatting position created by placing feet on a stool may help improve defecation.
6. A regular program of moderate exercise is often helpful in preventing constipation.
7. Examine the client's rectum to rule out any obstructive mass.

SLEEP PATTERN DISTURBANCE

1. Teach the client that old age is generally accompanied by a decline in the amount of sleep.
2. More frequent arousals are normal and are not a cause for alarm.
3. Chronic use of sedatives and depressants is strongly not recommended as they quickly lose their therapeutic value and may be addicting.
4. Advise the client to refrain from drinking tea, coffee, or caffeinated products before retiring.
5. Frequent nocturia can be avoided if the client refrains from drinking excessive amounts of fluid in the evening.
6. Advise clients who take diuretics to do so in the late afternoon or early evening in order to avoid frequent nocturia.
7. Eating a large meal before retiring may also interfere with sleep.
8. Many older adults find drinking a warm drink or a weak alcoholic beverage to be relaxing before going to bed.
9. Reading in bed, listening to music, meditation, and taking a few moments to reflect on peaceful thoughts of the day's events are several recommendations that the client may find helpful in promoting sleep.
10. Encourage the client to nap during the day as this may be a beneficial way of compensating for loss of sleep at night.
11. Engaging in regular exercise also promotes rest and sleep in the older adult.
12. A well ventilated room and a quiet environment enhance the client's ability to fall asleep and sleep for longer periods of time.
13. Encourage clients to be aware of their individual needs and to rest when they feel tired, instead of establishing a fixed sleep–rest pattern that may not coincide with ebbing energy levels and fatigue.

POTENTIAL FOR INJURY

Refer to *Preventing Injury* under *Health Promotion and the Elderly*.

ALTERED PATTERNS OF SEXUALITY

1. The nurse must be aware of the sexual needs of the elderly and examine his or her personal feelings regarding this. Staff prejudices may prove to be roadblocks to sexual expression of the older client.
2. Assess the individual's past sexual history, and feelings and attitudes about sexual practices, including sexual preferences.
3. Assess the client's current sexual pattern, number of partners, degree of satisfaction.
4. Explore any concerns or difficulties the client may have related to his or her sexual activity and function.
5. Since the elderly have questions about sexuality, answer them honestly and openly.
6. Encourage the elderly to continue to engage in sexual activity according to the pattern established throughout their life experience.
7. Assist the institutionalized client in his striving for closeness and intimacy. Simple warm human gestures such as the laying on of hands increase the sense of comfort and security.
8. Encouraging the expression of sexual feelings and desire among institutionalized clients may require the nurse to assume a client-advocate posture. Environmental modification may also be required.
9. If a couple have been accustomed to sharing the same bed prior to their institutionalization, wiring their beds together and permitting them to share the room together will help to ensure the continuity of their former lifestyle.
10. If free expression of sexual feelings and desires is to be promoted, traditional rules and regulation, propriety and opinion may need to be reconsidered.

11. Encourage socialization among institutionalized clients by participation in co-ed card parties, bingo, cocktail hours, and dining together. Dancing is also an activity enjoyed by many elders.
12. Encourage clients to discuss the sexual techniques that they find most enjoyable and satisfying. Recommend others that the client may wish to employ.
13. If intercourse is not possible but the sex drive is still present, recommend the use of other sublimating activities such as fantasy, reading sexually explicit literature, and masturbation as an acceptable outlet to decrease sexual tension. "Giving permission" by the nurse may assist the client in his or her acceptance of these activities.
14. Preserve the privacy of the client at all times. Knock before entering a room when the door is closed.
15. Foster Grandparents is a highly successful program that provides the older adult with a sublimated form of intimacy. In addition, it provides society with the valuable contribution made by these senior citizens (Figure 44-2).
16. Teach the client that if sexual function is temporarily diminished due to a particular condition or illness, it is often easily reversed once the cause itself is diagnosed and treated.
17. Clients should be taught that increased heart rate, blood pressure, and breathing at the point of orgasm and ejaculation is quite normal and that these symptoms subside quite rapidly.

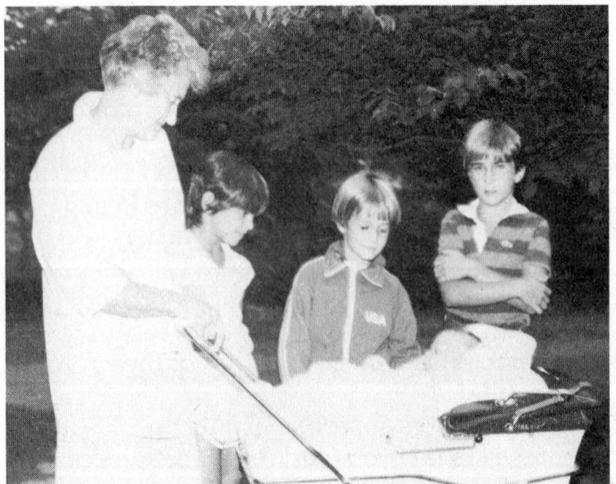

Figure 44-2 The role of a grandparent is one enjoyed by many elderly clients.

18. For those clients with activity tolerance limitations, participation in sexual activity is permissable if they can climb two flights of stairs without experiencing prolonged breathlessness and palpitations (Diekleman, 1977).
19. Individuals with cardiac problems should be instructed to avoid sexual activity if they are fatigued or have eaten or drunk a large amount.
20. Teach clients methods of reducing the demand on their heart:
    a. Take a nap before and after sexual activity.
    b. Engage in sex in the morning when well rested.
    c. Utilize side lying positions having the partner kneel above instead of lying above in the prone position.
    d. Sitting in a chair during sex also tends to decrease the cardiac demand.
    e. Those with angina should take nitroglycerin before initiating sexual activity.
21. Clients with arthritis should plan for sex during the part of the day that is most comfortable for them. Techniques that promote relaxation, like warm tub baths, are helpful, and care should be taken to protect affected joints.
22. For those with chronic pain, taking prescribed analgesics before engaging in sexual activity facilitates comfort.
23. Older women prone to developing urologic problems should be instructed to void before and after sex to flush out any bacteria that enter the urethra during coitus.
24. Since vaginal secretions are diminished in the older female, lubrication should be used so that delicate tissues are not traumatized during sexual activity.
25. Sexual performance is enhanced if older clients eat a well-balanced diet and get adequate sleep and exercise. As with any other age group, encourage those with a sexual dysfunction to seek appropriate counseling.
26. Participation in sexual activity on a regular basis helps to maintain or improve sexual function. Older men have potentially greater ejaculatory control than younger man, and this often enhances the degree of satisfaction experienced by the women.

OUTCOME CRITERIA

MALNUTRITION

The client will:
1. Identify three important reasons why eating a well-balanced diet is so essential.
2. List a sample diet that is both nutritious and mindful of cost.
3. Identify three measures that can enhance appetite.
4. Describe three methods of stretching food dollars.
5. Report eating a well-balanced diet that meets the client's nutritional needs and satisfies the client's individual tastes.

MOBILITY IMPAIRMENT

The client can:
1. List the benefits that can be derived from a regular exercise program.
2. Describe the important role nutrition plays in activity tolerance.
3. Report an interest in participation in a regular exercise program commensurate with the client's age, limitations, and tolerance.

CONSTIPATION

The client can:
1. List three specific measures that help prevent constipation.
2. Report use of specific measures in daily routine and a gradual return of normal bowel patterns.
3. Report cessation or diminishment of constipation.

SLEEP PATTERN DISTURBANCE

The client can:
1. List five specific measures that will promote rest, relaxation, and sleep.
2. Define his or her sleep needs commensurate with his or her level of activity, energy level, nutrition, and biological rhythm.
3. Name foods and beverages to avoid that may interfere with sleep.
4. Report improved to normal sleeping patterns.

POTENTIAL FOR INJURY

The client will:
1. Identify at least five ways that his or her home and work environment can be made safer and will report making the necessary modifications.
2. Report use of safe and appropriate footwear that minimizes the chance of falling.
3. Describe the essential correct body mechanics and transfer technique.
4. Report an accurate understanding of the physiologic basis for changing positions slowly and avoiding sudden movements of the head to the side.
5. Describe a heightened awareness of the tremendous importance of accident and injury prevention in the elderly.

ALTERED PATTERNS OF SEXUALITY

The client will:
1. Feel comfortable discussing sexual matters and demonstrate a willingness to come to the nurse for guidance, facilitation, and support in meeting the client's sexual needs.
2. Verbalize continuation of sexual practice that the client has utilized in the past.
3. Participate in socialization activities and demonstrate participation in acceptable sublimated activities.
4. List the normal cardiac signs that accompany orgastic phenomena.
5. Describe six methods that reduce the cardiac demand during sexual activity.
6. List three ways of conserving energy during sexual activity.
7. Older female clients can describe two methods for reducing discomfort during sexual activity that is associated with the normal aging process.
8. Older male clients can describe some positive aspects of aging that can potentially enhance their sexual function.

CONCLUSION

Working with the elderly can be a challenging and tremendously rewarding experience and so much can be learned from our elders who have the benefit of numerous years of life's experience. Perhaps there is no other group of individuals who need skilled and thoughtful nursing care more than do the elderly. Supporting the elderly as they grow old and assisting them in maintaining an optimal state of wellness is not an easy task. By helping the elderly develop a healthy life perspective and cope with their losses, capitalizing on their strengths and assets, and by encouraging their endeavors to remain self-sufficient and independent, nurses can play a significant role in helping the elderly see that the "older years" can be a wonderfully satisfying time of life.

REFERENCES

Abbey, J. C.: "Physiological Aspect of Aging," unpublished manuscript delivered in lecture at Ethel Peray Andrus Gerontology Center, University of Southern California, Los Angeles, 1973.

Berrin, J. E.: *The Psychology of Aging*, Prentice-Hall, Englewood Cliffs, N.J., 1964.

Burnside, I. M.: "Developmental Reactions in Old Age," in *New Dimensions in Mental Health and Psychiatric Nursing*, McGraw-Hill, New York, 1974.

Butler, R. N., and Lewis, M.: *Aging and Mental Health*, Mosby, St. Louis, 1973, p. 18.

Carnevali, D., and Patrick, M.: *Nursing Management for the Elderly*, Lippincott, Philadelphia, 1979, pp. 75, 227.

"Developmental Patterns of Interaction," in Jones, D. A., et. al. (eds.): *Medical-Surgical Nursing: A Conceptual Approach*, McGraw-Hill, New York, 1982, pp. 78–80.

Diekelman, N.: *Primary Health Care of the Well Adult*, McGraw-Hill, New York, 1977, pp. 156, 194.

Dunn, H. L.: *High Level Wellness*, Beatty Publishing Co., Arlington, Va., 1971, p. 2.

Dychtwald, K.: "The Elder Within: A Lifetime of Aging," *New Age*, February 1979, p. 29.

Freeman, J. T.: "Sexual Capacities in the Aging Male," *Geriatrics*, **16**:37, 1961.

Giorgi, E. A.: "Aging and Mental Health," workshop handout, Los Angeles, February 6, 1971, in Burnside, I.: *Nursing and the Aged*, McGraw-Hill, New York, 1976, pp. 466–470.

Hughes, G.: "Changes in Taste Sensitivity with Advancing Age," *Gerontology Clinics*, **11**:224, 1969.

Malasanos, L., et. al.: *Health Assessment*, Mosby, St. Louis, 1977, pp. 431–439.

Masters, W. H., and Johnson, V.: *Human Sexual Inadequacy*, Little, Brown, Boston, 1970.

Mezey, M.: *Health Assessment of the Older Individual*, Springer, New York, 1980, p. 12.

Palmore, E. (ed.): "Normal Aging II: Reports from the Duke Longitudinal Studies, 1970–1973," in Diekleman, N.: *Primary Health Care of the Well Adult*, McGraw-Hill, New York, 1976, pp. 169–170.

Pfeiffer, E., Veroerdt, A., and Wang, H. S.: "Sexual Behavior in Aged Men and Women, I: Observation of 254 Community Volunteers," *Archives of General Psychiatry*, **19**:753, 1968.

Shanus, E., Townsen, B., Wedderburn, D.: "The Psychology of Health," in Mezey, M.: *Health Assessment of the Older Individual*, Springer, New York, 1980, p. 26.

BIBLIOGRAPHY

Burnside, I. M.: *Nursing and the Aged*, McGraw-Hill, New York, 1980. A good general resource on nursing and the aged. Common problems found in the elderly population are well addressed. Approach to caring for the aged was also helpful as were the sections on the nursing process.

Carnevali, D. L., and Patrick, M.: *Nursing Management for the Elderly*, Lippincott, Philadelphia, 1979. This reference has some good sections where nursing problems are covered in depth. The chapters on oral health maintenance and nutrition are quite complete. Problems encountered in the elderly are well done, and high-risk individuals are identified for each problem. A "quick review" page before each section is also helpful.

Diekleman, N.: *Primary Health Care of the Well Adult*, McGraw-Hill, New York, 1977. This is an excellent resource for care of the adult of any age. The sections on the elderly are particularly excellent, as they focus on common nursing problems encountered in the elderly population. The focus on "normal" and "healthy" is also refreshing.

Jones, D., Dunbar, C. F., Jirovic, M. M. (eds.): *Medical-Surgical Nursing: A Conceptual Approach*, McGraw-Hill, New York, 1982. An excellent chapter, "Developmental Patterns of Interaction," focuses on normal physiologic and psychosocial changes seen in the elderly. Cultural, economic, and family variables, as well as the concept of losses, are also addressed.

Mezey, M.: *Health Assessment of the Older Individual*, Springer, New York, 1980. A reference for assessing the older adult. Besides addressing the physical assessment area, community and home assessment are also stressed. The focus of this text is on the normal aspects of aging. The references are current and the photographic illustrations are helpful.

"Symposium on Gerontological Nursing," *Nursing Clinics of North America*, **11**(1):115, March 1976. This is an excellent symposium that focuses on the multiplicity of needs of the elderly as well as suggesting nursing approaches and interventions for common problems faced by the elderly.

Wardell, S. C.: *Acute Interventions: Nursing Process Throughout the Life Span*, Reston, Va., 1979. Appendix I gives a concise outline on the normal physical assessment findings in the elderly.

45

Coping with Loss and Aging

Cynthia Sarno Yeager

By lengthening the span of life, a greater proportion of the population can count on facing old age. For many, aging can be a time of personal fulfillment and satisfaction. However, regardless of one's ability to cope with the aging process, there are many changes that every individual must face. Many of these changes include physical, emotional, or spiritual losses. Society offers the elderly little in the way of the extended family and emotional social support, while there are many families who offer support to the elderly. Decreased federal support, family mobility, and social trends seemed to limit social support to coping with aging. Cultures that have traditionally esteemed the aged now offer only token respect (Larue, 1976). The aged are often subjected to poverty, stereotyping, and discriminatory treatment. They undergo numerous social, psychological, and physical changes with which they must cope. Embedded in any change is some loss. While dealing with change, there are various developmental tasks that the elderly attempt to accomplish (refer to Table 45-1). Completion of these tasks varies according to individual needs and lifestyles, as well as physical, intellectual, generational, and social factors.

LOSS AND GRIEF

DESCRIPTION

Loss is an individual perception. It will vary from person to person according to how the object lossed is viewed. Loss has been defined as a state of being deprived of or being without something one has had (Peretz, 1970). The aged are subjected to numerous losses (refer to Table 45-2) and present diverse responses in every client. Each loss has consequential losses and often causes many changes in the individual's life.

The loss of replaceable material possessions can evoke feelings of anger, frustration, and the fear that other more serious losses will occur. If the individual fails to find the lost object, activity is then directed toward alternatives that will restore a balance to life. Similar coping patterns used in the past may be used to handle a new loss. These may continue to be effective. However, a loss can be so overwhelming that past coping mechanisms may be inadequate in dealing with the present crisis. New behaviors may

TABLE 45-1 DEVELOPMENTAL TASKS OF THE AGED

A. Concerns centered on:
   1. Health.
   2. Relationships with spouse, friends, and children.
   3. Resignation to the disappointments of life (Gould).

B. Ego integrity versus despair (Erikson).

C. 1. Ego differentiation versus work role preoccupation (retirement).
   2. Body transcendence versus body preoccupation (acceptance of physical changes of aging).
   3. Ego transcendence versus ego preoccupation (facing inevitability of death) (Peck).

D. 1. Regressive tasks: accepting physical, sexual, and social decline and increased dependency.
   2. Compensatory tasks:
      Developing new leisure patterns and new education skills.
      Adjusting to altered environment, altered status, and altered self-concept (Barrett).

E. Receptive tasks: relinquishing power and capacity in physical, social, cultural, and intellectual realms.

F. Expressive tasks: developing a self-transcending philosophy.

G. Dynamic tasks of late life: dying and teaching others how to die.

H. 1. Taking on of new roles (e.g., grandparent) or accepting a greater separation from society.
   2. Adjusting to decreased physical strength and health, retirement, reduced income, death of a spouse.
   3. Establishing an explicit affiliation with one's age group.
   4. Adopting of and adapting to social roles in a flexible way.
   5. Establishing satisfactory living arrangements (Havighurst).

SOURCE: Ebersole, P. P.: "Developmental Tasks in Late Life," in Burnside, I. M., ed., *Nursing and the Aged*, McGraw-Hill, New York, 1976, pp. 69–79.

TABLE 45-2 POTENTIAL LOSSES ASSOCIATED WITH AGING

A. Physical loss may lead to body-image changes:
   1. Loss of youthful appearance.
   2. Sensory losses: can reduce reality testing and can lead to confusion, anxiety, marked suspiciousness, paranoia, depression, and social isolation.
   3. General loss of physical capacity, lessened resilience, and decreased ability to resist stress, trauma, and disease. See the discussion of the physiologic effects of aging in Chapter 40.
   4. Loss of former level of functioning.
   5. Loss of highly valued physical or mental attributes.
   6. Loss of body part.

B. Psychosocial loss may lead to changes in self-esteem:
   1. Role loss.
      Separation from children.
      Death of mate, sibling, child, or friend may involve loss of pattern of daily living, loss of source of human intimacy.
      Retirement may involve loss of income, loss of socially valued position, loss of occupation, loss of sense of significance.
      Divorce.
      Abandonment.
      Loss of well-loved pets.
   2. Institutionalization may involve loss of home and possessions, loss of familiar setting, loss of privacy, loss of significant relationships, loss of independence, loss of self-identity, loss of individuality.
   3. Loss of mobility due to:
      Inadequate or impractical transportation.
      Denial of driver's license.
      Physical inability to travel.
   4. Loss of confidence in cognitive functions.
   5. Loss of sense of security and safety.
      Fear of criminal assaults.
      Fear of falls and fractures.

be incorporated into one's life process and other support systems may be sought.

Separation, or threat of separation, from a loved one through death is a painful loss to the aged person and a reminder of the person's own mortality. It usually evokes grief. *Grief* involves many fluctuating emotions and feelings as well as physiological and behavioral responses to actual or expected significant loss. *Mourning*, or bereavement, involves the intrapsychic processes which are involved in grief and which should lead to integration and healthy resolution of the loss. Otherwise, the grief process is termed unresolved, maladaptive, morbid, or pathological.

Anticipatory grief is the sadness for future losses before they occur. It buffers the shock when a loss is revealed and allows for preparation for coping with loss. Grieving for losses, past and present, is functionally useful, adaptive, and important. When the work of grieving is not completed initially, it tends to reappear. *Unresolved grief* may result in serious physical illness and lasting emotional damage. Research suggests that illness affects individuals more often during the first year after the loss of a loved one, especially a spouse. In addition, there is an increase in mortality among family members during the first year of (mourning) bereavement (Parkes and Brown, 1972). The duration of a grief reaction depends upon the success with which the individual resolves the loss, compensates for it, and readjusts to an environment without the missing object or person. It has been suggested that older persons may experience the death of a spouse in ways different from those who are younger; that men may be at greater risk of physical and emotional deterioration than women (Dimond, 1981). Many factors affect the intensity of the emotional response (refer to Table 45-3).

Each new loss may reactivate the cycle of grieving. The anniversary of the loss may precipitate a grief reaction. This reaction will be brief, however, if grief was previously well resolved. Various rituals, such as furnerals, emphasize reality and finality and thereby allow the grief process to move forward. Most people finally overcome the discomfort of acute grief. They gain renewed control of the present and diminished preoccupation with the past. Energy can then be redirected toward developing new potentials, activities, and relationships.

TABLE 45-3 FACTORS INFLUENCING THE COURSE OF GRIEF

Definition, or significance, of the loss.
Concern about potential losses.
Impact loss has on daily lifestyle.
Responses to past stressors and previous losses.
Relationships to the lost object or person.
Circumstances of the losses: sudden, expected.
Timing of the loss.
Social supports.
Socioeconomic determinants.
Cultural determinants.
Religious determinants.
Quality of physical and emotional health of the bereaved.
Investment in other valued objects, roles, and relationships.

CULTURE

There are many cultural perspectives and variations to the grieving process. Older American blacks tend to rely less on relatives and more on religious persons and symbols for support during experiences with death and dying; they have a very low suicide rate (Kalish and Reynolds, 1980). In the Japanese-American culture, the expression of grief is controlled; the spouse is expected to care for the dying mate at the death bed; and, in this culture, the thought of the death of a man is more tragic than that of a woman (Kalish and Reynolds, 1980). Japanese-Americans are also unlikely to touch the body of a dead spouse at the funeral. Mexican-Americans cry freely over the deaths of loved ones, and they are more likely to touch the body of the deceased. The Chinese express much emotion through wailing and weeping at funerals (Trelease, 1975). In addition, because of a belief in evil spirits, mourners turn their backs when the casket is closed so that the spirits won't follow them home. Jewish tradition views the period of death and dying as a time when loved ones should surround and comfort the dying. A spouse should not leave the bedside of the dying. The laws and traditions of the Jewish culture provide a structure for the mourner to grieve for loss and then become reintegrated into the community. "Judaism organizes the year of mourning into 3 days of deep grief, 7 days of mourning, 30 days of gradual readjustment, and 11 months of remembrance and healing" (Heller, 1975). When the client's response to death is integrated with his or her cultural background, it is considered normal and healthy.

PREVENTION

Health Promotion

1. Early case finding of those individuals who have experienced a loss.
2. Early detection of grief-related signs and symptoms of illness.
3. Preparation and planning for physical and behavioral changes and anticipated losses of aging.
4. Cultivation of varied interests beyond the role of parent and employee at an early age.
5. Lifelong effort to develop constructive methods of coping with losses.
6. Elderly living in close-knit communities that have maintained their values and traditions.
7. Developing preventive or therapeutic interventions to decrease, ameliorate, or prevent the potentially devastating physical and emotional effects of grief.
8. Recognizing and dealing with individuals' reactions to loss, thus preventing more serious problems.
9. Maintaining satisfying interpersonal relationships throughout life.

Population at Risk

1. Persons who have experienced one or more losses of personal significance.
2. Elderly persons who may experience numerous physical and/or psychosocial losses.
3. Persons who have incapacitating physical or emotional illness.
4. Persons who have poor support systems.
5. Persons who have difficulty expressing feelings.
6. Persons who are experiencing role conflicts.
7. Persons who are relocating from a familiar setting to an unfamiliar one (e.g., elderly placement in a nursing home).
8. Persons who are geographically or ethnically isolated, homebound, or psychologically alienated.
9. Persons who have perceptual deficits.
10. Persons who are poverty-stricken, since further socioeconomic loss may be devastating. In addition, loss of a spouse has been found to be most stressful to the poor (Carter, 1976). One out of every four of the elderly lives below the poverty line.
11. Persons who are overinvolved in their jobs, have jobs with mandatory retirement provisions, and/or jobs that demand the total energies of the individual, leaving no time to develop meaningful alternatives and interests.

Screening

Not applicable.

ASSESSMENT

Health History

1. Age (specific).
2. Socioeconomic status: may handle loss differently.
3. Living and transportation arrangements: homebound? Living alone and living in urban area increases risk of loneliness.
4. If institutionalized, attitudes toward facility and toward own family.
5. Sources of support and patterns of interaction with them: family, friends, community.
6. Communication patterns: loss of verbal ability may increase reponse to loss and limit individuals ability to express feelings.
7. Nationality, language spoken, degree of ethnic identity: if client is living in an alien environment, additional social supports and adaptations to health care will be required.
8. Occupation, retirement plans, essential medical insurance.
9. General health of client.
10. Response in coping with stressors and losses, both past and present: overall adaptive ability.
11. Roles and responsibilities of the individual; degree of outside involvement may decrease feelings associated with loss.
12. Recent or reference to past loss: date of the loss (anniversary of the loss may have special significance), definition of the loss, concern about potential losses, impact loss has on daily lifestyle, times of greatest discomfort.
13. Denial of loss: disbelief and refusal to accept the news of the loss may be first response to the crisis.

14. Preoccupation with the loss: thoughts of the lost object or person almost exclusively, visions of the lost object or person, idealization of the lost object or person, fear of approaching insanity.
15. Preoccupation with self: more aware of various bodily sensations.
16. Verbal expression of distress, ability to express saddness or loneliness, helplessness.
17. Expression of guilt (e.g., "If only I had"): self-accusations of negligence, self-recrimination, self-reproach, self-deprecation.
18. Expression of anger: feelings of hostility toward persons or circumstances held to be responsible for the loss, toward friends and relatives, toward lost object or person, and toward self.
19. Expression of dependence: may feel resentful of unchosen dependent role.
20. Traits of lost person appear in behavior of the bereaved: borders on pathological reaction, mood swings described.
21. Complaints or observations reported by the client may include:
    a. Sleep disturbances (e.g., insomnia, nightmares).
    b. Lack of appetite and/or taste, intestinal emptiness, nausea, dysphagia, indigestion, diarrhea, constipation.
    c. Changes in sexual response.
    d. Headaches, dizziness.
    e. Chest pain, palpitations; feeling choked.
    f. Lack of strength and overwhelming exhaustion.
    g. Diminished ability to think, concentrate, and perform even routine activities. Difficulty making decisions.
    h. Increased vulnerability and undue sensitivity to real or imagined slights.
    i. Increased consumption of alcohol, tobacco, or tranquilizers.
    j. Feelings of unreality and numbness, detachment of feelings from persons and things in environment.
    k. Manifestations of intermittent or chronic anxiety may be evident (see discussion of anxiety in Chapter 36). The ability to adapt diminishes as competence diminishes. If a new situation requires an individual to respond beyond capabilities, anxiety results.
    l. Manifestations of depression may be evident (see the discussion of depression in Chapter 36). Depression appears to be a part of even the normal aging process. It is one of the most common reactions to loss. It can be associated with environmental changes, loss of self-esteem, and changes in body image. Apathy is much more characteristic of depression in later life than in early years. Symptoms potentially experienced by the depressed elderly include irritability, constipation, insomnia, and slow movements. It is necessary to distinguish between depression that is realistic, appropriate, and proportionate to the loss that was experienced and extreme depression that persists beyond a reasonable time and interferes with the client's physical and emotional functioning. Remotivation group therapies aid in lessening depression in the aged.

Physical Assessment

1. Client may be crying.
2. Facial expression may show sadness or anger.
3. Skin on forehead may be furrowed.
4. Gestures of helplessness may be observed. "With a fairly brisk motion, the hands are raised before the face, parallel and directly in front, the elbows flexed slightly, the palms facing each other but rotated slightly outward, the fingers spread, and the thumbs extended. This position is held for a second, and then the hands fall limply to the lap with gravity. Abortive and incomplete gestures may also be seen, especially when the person is not in a position in which the full gesture can be executed" (Engel, 1974).
5. Movements may be executed slowly and with apparent difficulty.
6. Movements may be restless. There may be pacing. Speech may be rapid. Actions may appear purposeless.
7. Dyspnea and/or sighing respirations may be present.
8. Auditory and visual acuity may be decreased as a result of normal aging changes.
9. Taste may be diminished as a result of grief response. Cardiac arrhythmias, tachycardia, and/or hypertension may be present.
10. Posture may be stooped with head and shoulder flexion.
11. Muscle strength may be diminished.

Diagnostic Tests

Not applicable.

NURSING DIAGNOSES: ACTUAL OR POTENTIAL

1. Anxiety, mild to moderate, due to potential or actual loss.
2. Alterations in comfort, secondary to grief reaction; pain.
3. Ineffective coping (individual) depression; anger, mood swings.
4. Ineffective family coping: disabling or compromised reaction, secondary to relocation.
5. Grieving: anticipatory unresolved, due to actual or potential loss.
6. Impaired home maintenance management, inability to perform routine activities.
7. Decreased activity tolerance: fatigue due to debilitating physical loss.
8. Nutritional deficit: less than body requirements to nausea, intestinal emptiness.
9. Role disturbance: change in role due to loss of spouse, job, child, friend, sibling.
10. Alterations in self-concept: change in body image due to physical changes.
11. Sensory-perceptual deficit of sensory-perceptual responses to aging (i.e., loss of taste, vision, or hearing or impaired verbalization).
12. Alteration in patterns of sexuality, to loss of mate; grief reaction.
13. Sleep–rest pattern disturbance, insomnia, nightmares, fear of death.
14. Social isolation, decreased social isolation, grief reaction, relocation.
15. Impaired thought processes, altered thinking, decreased concentration, and memory deficit due to grieving.
16. Potential translocation syndrome.
17. Potential independence–dependence conflict unresolved.
18. Knowledge deficit: lack of information concerning the grieving process.

EXPECTED OUTCOMES

1. Personal, physical, role, and/or psychosocial losses that are currently being dealt with are isolated and coping behaviors that will help in dealing with these changes are identified within 3 months following the loss.
2. Feelings about loss (i.e., sadness, guilt, anger, depression) are freely expressed until they are resolved.
3. The client will successfully work through loss and grief process as evidenced by decrease in verbalizations about the loss, verbalizations indicating resolution (e.g., "I feel as though I'm getting over my wife's death") and/or resumption of activities formerly unable to pursue.
4. Gradual decrease in frequency of self-depreciative verbalizations will occur within 6 months following the loss.
5. Conversation will gradually progress from loss to other topics within 6 months following the loss.
6. Excess consumption of alcohol, tobacco, and tranquilizers will lessen ideally to zero, within 6 months following the loss.
7. Sleep pattern will be restored. Client will experience fewer sleep disturbances (insomnia and/or nightmares).
8. Physical complaints, such as headaches and palpitations, will decrease within 3 months following the loss.
9. Nutritional pattern will be restored with fewer digestive disturbances and weight regained or maintained within normal limits within 3 months after the loss.
10. Satisfaction regarding remaining roles and responsibilities will be expressed within 1 year following the loss.
11. Client will compensate for sensory-perceptual and mobility impairments to his/her satisfaction within 1 year following the loss.
12. Client will verbalize perception of increasing independence and decision making within 6 months following the loss.
13. Client will resume contact with family within 1 year following the loss.
14. Social contact outside of home will be initiated. Client will form new relationships within 1 year following the loss.
15. Level of sexual response will resume within 2 years following the loss.

The time period in which goals are to be attained should be individually determined. It is dependent upon initial baseline data as well as the selection of intervention. Frequency of intervention is based upon the severity of the individual's emotional response. There is no generally recognized specific time period for the completion of grief work. The successful work of mourning takes at least 1 year. It has been found that the effects of bereavement in the elderly may be delayed initially and continue into 2 to 4 years after the loss (Gerber and Weiner, 1981).

INTERVENTIONS

1. Health professionals must recognize and work through their own feelings and attitudes about aging and loss.
2. Establish a positive, consistent relationship with the client. Include and support significant others. Present an attitude toward the elderly of understanding and respect; provide privacy.
3. Teach family to recognize the earliest signs of physical or emotional distress in response to loss.
4. Recognize the importance of the need for time to grieve. Indicate to the client that grief is appropriate and necessary for personal growth and health.
5. Be sensitive and respond to the feelings and personal concerns expressed by the client. Let the client know that you recognize his or her feelings. Encourage healthy expression and sorting out of emotions. When a grieving person is allowed to ventilate emotions, there is a release of feeling and the beginning of acceptance of the loss.
6. Respect client's need for denial. Denial is generally considered to be a protective and adaptive defense mechanism in initial period of grieving.
7. Listen and observe carefully and noncritically as clients retell the details of their loss. They need to review their relationship with the lost object or person and share their grief. Often they need reassurance that they did all that was possible to save the lost object or person.
8. Do not provide empty reassurances. Express realistic and hopeful expectations through mutual goal setting.
9. Provide positive reinforcement (praise) for demonstrations of healthy, adaptive coping patterns. Discourage maladaptive behaviors (i.e., consumption of alcohol and tranquilizers), for they tend to suppress and delay grieving.
10. Identify and assess client's strengths and available sources of support. Reassess client's personal goals. Determine realistic alternatives and viable substitutions and compensatory mechanisms for dealing with losses.
11. Give careful consideration to the times of greatest discomfort, particularly anniversaries of losses. Convey this information to staff.
12. Carefully assess client's sensory and perceptual capacity. Assist client in defining realistic individual expectations.
13. Encourage client to postpone major decisions, such as selling a home or drastic alterations in lifestyle, if possible, until judgment and decision-making ability have improved. Afford opportunities for increasing decision-making and independence as abilities are regained.
14. Respect the cultural, religious, and social customs of the client who is grieving. The client identifies with certain values and beliefs and through them finds support and self-worth.
15. For clients who wish to view the body immediately after death, support their choice. Viewing the body as well as revisiting the acute care setting where the death occurred will also facilitate the grief process (McGrory, 1975).
16. Encourage client to decrease isolation and find new patterns of rewarding interaction through participation in activities of interest and in social groups.
17. Provide anticipatory guidance to clients to prepare for life changes and losses before they occur. Emphasize importance of pursuing outside interests and maintaining viable friendships throughout life cycle. Support the expression of anticipated grief reactions for impending losses and suggest appropriate means for its manifestations.
18. Make necessary referrals for financial and legal aid.
19. When appropriate, provide opportunity for mutual help through groups of clients who have sustained similar forms of loss to meet and share together. "Loneliness, anger, and sadness at the loss of a spouse are eased when women are given the opportunity to speak together" (Miles and Hays, 1975).
20. Provide closeness and touch to depressed, aged clients, for they respond well to these

measures, especially following the loss of a significant other (Burnside, 1976).

21. Provide a stimulating and challenging environment to institutionalized clients. If their abilities exceed the demands made by the physical environment, manifestations of understimulation may result (i.e., apathy, sleepiness, aggressive acts).
22. Ensure personal privacy and respect for clients' life patterns in order to help maintain their self-esteem and personal control over the aging process.
23. Arrange support networks for those who are isolated and grieving. Local churches and outreach organizations may offer support by telephone contact or home visits.

EVALUATION

Outcome Criteria

1. Client regains previous affect and resumes normal patterns of daily living.
2. Client reports feeling happier and less sad, guilty, or angry.
3. Mood swings are less pronounced and less frequent.
4. Client is able to think, concentrate, and make decisions more easily.
5. Client reports initiating and completing activities.
6. Nutritional pattern is restored with occasional digestive disturbances and other physical discomforts, and weight is restored within normal limits.
7. Client reports feeling sleep pattern disturbances decrease and less tired and having more energy.
8. Client reports more enjoyable encounters with family or friends and is able to form new relationships that bring personal satisfaction.
9. Client experiences longer periods of calm, satisfaction, and ability to function.

Complications

DELAYED, INHIBITED, ABSENT, OR EXAGGERATED GRIEVING

See Table 45-4.

Assessment

1. Depression may become severe or chronic in nature. Suicide may be attempted. (See the discussion of suicide in Chapter 38.) Conditions that increase the likelihood of suicide are more prevalent in old age. Depression is present in 80 percent of the suicidal attempts in persons over 60 years of age, and 12 percent of these persons may be expected to complete the act within two years. If tried again, the setting is usually identical. Suicide is more prevalent among older individuals than among younger persons (Weiss, 1968). Also, suicidal attempts in the elderly are more vi-

TABLE 45-4 MORBID GRIEF REACTIONS

1. Postponement of reaction: may involve years. Most striking and most frequent reaction.
2. Alteration in client's conduct.
   Overactivity without a sense of loss.
   Manifestations of symptoms of lost person's illness.
3. Psychosomatic illness (i.e., ulcerative colitis, rheumatoid arthritis, and asthma).
4. Conspicuous alteration in relationship to friends and relatives: continued and progressive social isolation.
5. Hostility against specific persons.
6. Lasting loss of patterns of social interaction.
   Lack of decision and initiative.
   Self-punitive acts.
   Agitated depression.
7. Denial of death (i.e., acting and speaking as if the person were still alive).
8. Denial of the loss or of the affect.
9. Use of a vicarious object.
   Feeling sorry for someone else who is mourning instead of oneself.
   Quick replacement of the loss object or person with another.
10. Prolonged unresolved grief, chronic grief: slightest mention of the loss, even many years later, readily evokes crying.

SOURCE: Engel, G., in McGrory, A.: *A Well Model Approach to Care of the Dying Client*, McGraw-Hill, New York, 1978, p. 88. Also Lindemann, E.: "Symptomatology and Management of Acute Grief," *American Journal of Psychiatry*, **101**:141, 1944.

olent and dangerous; the attempt is rarely a gesture.

2. Increased intensity or duration of aforementioned signs and symptoms (e.g., worsening bodily distress, increased dependency on drugs or alcohol).
3. Continued preoccupation with the loss.
4. Fixation in one area of grief reaction (e.g., anger, denial).
5. Exaggeration of the need to fulfill the wishes of the lost person.

Revised Outcomes

1. Client will be protected from self-destruction until able to assume this responsibility.
2. Client will be able to emancipate self from memories of the loss and move toward healthy resolution of the loss.

Interventions

Referral to or more frequent and intensive psychotherapy.

Reevaluation and Follow-up

Establish a specific individualized plan to determine the extent of resolution of the grief reaction.

DEATH

DESCRIPTION

Death is a universal experience. There is, however, no universal definition of death. It can be perceived as the absence of clinically detectable vital signs, the absence of brain wave activity, or an irreversible loss of vital functions. The traditional legal definition of death states that "Death is the final and irreversible cessation of perceptible heartbeat and respiration. Conversely, as long as any heartbeat or respiration can be perceived, either with or without mechanical or electrical aids, and regardless of how the heartbeat and respiration were maintained, death has not occurred" (Halley and Harvey, 1968). At a time when advances in medical technology facilitate the prolongation of life, some individuals are writing "living wills," formally requesting that if recovery is not reasonable, they do not wish to be kept alive by mechanical or heroic means.

TABLE 45-5 FACTORS INFLUENCING ATTRIBUTES TOWARD DEATH

Chronological age.
Mental and physical health.
Distance from death.
Religious beliefs.
Culture.
Involvement in life.
Previous experiences with loss and death.
Behaviors of people caring for client.
Behaviors of significant others.
Self-concept.
Type of treatment required.
Degree of functional loss, disfigurement, and/or discomfort.
How the person is told of impending death.
Time available to prepare for death.
Response to past stressors in earlier life.

Euthanasia is a topic of concern to the elderly. In positive, direct, or active euthanasia there is a deliberate ending of life. Negative, indirect, or passive euthanasia involves the withholding of treatment from a client, who as a result is likely to die somewhat earlier than he or she otherwise would. A distinction is also made between voluntary (e.g., suicide) and involuntary (e.g., "mercy killing") euthanasia.

How persons view death can serve as an important determinant of how they conduct themselves in life. Various influences affect the elderly individual's attitudes toward death. See Table 45-5.

REACTIONS TO DEATH

1. Each person's reaction to death is unique. Our society does not promote open discussion or participation in the dying process.
2. To a great extent, death is feared, denied, dreaded, and evaded.
3. Although there are conflicting views, most elderly fear death less than they fear pain, dependency, rejection, isolation, and loss of social role, dignity, and self-determination.

4. Research by Kalish and Reynolds (1980) produced these conclusions:
   a. The elderly have encountered death more than younger people.
   b. The elderly are more likely to have made out a will and made burial arrangements.
   c. The older person is more likely to indicate acceptance of death, along with more preoccupation with the topic.
   d. The elderly are less concerned about dependents and the termination of life experiences than are the young.
   e. The elderly are not anxious to die and do not feel that death should be precipitated (Weisman, 1974).
5. A proposed program of death education: "to provide a means of helping the elderly grow into old age and the terminal stage of life with the least denial and anxiety. In order to maintain a life style of productivity, autonomy, and participation to the best of their abilities" (Wangsness, 1981).
6. Most people report that they would prefer to die at home; 80 percent of deaths occur in institutions.

RELIGIOUS BELIEFS AND DEATH

1. Religious beliefs influence patterns of living, patterns of dying, and attitudes and values toward death.
2. Older persons often become deeply concerned about religion and the afterlife, although beliefs vary.
3. For Christians, life after death affords heaven and hell as alternatives and also purgatory for Roman Catholics.
4. Some Jews do not believe in a next life and consider death final; Orthodox Jews, however, believe in an afterlife with rewards and punishments. They may pour out deathbed confessions.
5. In some forms of Buddhism, death completes a transition from the world of human beings to the world of spirits in which rewards and punishments are distributed to both living and dead.
6. In Hinduism, judgments are reflected in reincarnation through which a person receives in this life recompense for actions and thoughts in a previous life (Larue, 1976).
7. The Alaskan Indians usually exhibit a willfulness about their death. They not only participate in its planning but also seem to exercise a remarkable power of choice over the timing of its occurrence (Trelease, 1975).
8. There seems to be a growing interest in the client's control over when death will occur. Some aged clients exhibit a fighting will to live; others seem resigned to die.
9. Some may welcome death as an escape from unhappy living conditions (i.e., social deprivation, familial neglect, or pain and physical suffering).
10. Those who are experiencing pain or disablement may interpret their suffering as punishment for past misdeeds, whereas those enjoying health might feel rewarded for adhering to their faith.

PREVENTION

Health Promotion

1. All measures generally considered to prevent illness and promote and restore health.
2. Early case finding of those individuals who are terminally ill.
3. Preparation and planning for dying process.
4. Living each day to the fullest; decrease fear associated with death.

Population at Risk

1. Persons who are terminally ill.
2. Persons who have attempted suicide.
3. Persons who have lost a family member through death.
4. (Refer to mortality statistics.)
5. Accidents.

Screening

Varies according to disease process.

ASSESSMENT

Health History

1. Age.
2. Perception of health and nearness to death. Request for more information regarding prognosis.
3. Objective data regarding health prognosis.
4. Living arrangements: Most people prefer to die at home. "People in homes for the aged look forward to death much more than those living outside of institutions."
5. If institutionalized, attitudes toward facility and family.

6. Nationality, language spoken, degree of ethnic identity.
7. Sources of support and relationships with them: family, friends, community.
8. Response in coping with stressors, both past and present: overall adaptive ability.
9. Covert or overt references to own death.
10. Preparations (social, financial, philosophical, and/or religious) for own death.
11. Perception of life: accomplishments, regrets, unfinished business; religious beliefs.
12. Denial of terminal condition: rejection of any references to death.
13. Expression of anger: toward health care facility and providers, family, friends, God, and/or self; guilt.
14. Expression of dependence: may perceive self as burden to others; preoccupation with self-concerns.
15. Expression of unresolved issues; discomfort (physical, emotional).
16. Manifestations of anxiety may be evident. See Chapter 36.
17. Manifestations of depression may be evident. See Chapter 36 (withdrawal from family, friends).
18. Client may report that family is unable to deal with his or her impending death.

Physical Assessment

See preceding section on loss and grief. Physical findings will vary according to the particular disease process.

1. Client may be crying.
2. Facial expression may show sadness, anger, or pain.
3. Skin or forehead may be furrowed.
4. There may be bodily disfigurement.
5. Muscle strength may be diminished.
6. If withdrawn, head may be turned away; eyes may be closed; client may be verbally noncommunicative.

Diagnostic Tests

These will vary according to the particular disease process.

NURSING DIAGNOSES: ACTUAL OR POTENTIAL

1. Fear of death; anxiety associated with dying.
2. Alterations in comfort, due to illness and emotional distress.
3. Ineffective coping (individual), due to fear of death; loss of control.
4. Ineffective family coping: disabling or compromised.
5. Grieving, anticipatory or dysfunctional.
6. Potential alterations in self-concept, due to physical/emotional change.
7. Potential spiritual distress.
8. Potential independence–dependence conflict, unresolved—unable to care for self.
9. Depression (reactive).
10. Potential self-care deficit, secondary to discomfort, secondary to decreased strength and endurance (Gordon, 1982).

EXPECTED OUTCOMES

1. Grieving for losses that have occurred and for those that will occur is appropriate.
2. Fears, concerns, and feelings about own death are freely expressed.
3. Resolution of unpleasant feelings (i.e., anger, guilt, before death).
4. Client will carry out "life review," with health care provider, and express meaning of his or her life before death.
5. Utilization of remaining strengths before death, maintaining a satisfactory degree of independence for as long as possible.
6. Maximum comfort level maintained until death evidenced by comfortable facial expression and statements indicating absence of pain.
7. Ties with family and/or significant others will be retained until no longer possible.
8. Client will complete own unfinished business and experience death in a manner that he or she requests.

INTERVENTIONS

1. Health professionals must reflect upon and work through their own attitudes, fears, and beliefs about death. Their own fears and concerns may be heightened by contact with the dying. They must avoid confusing their own convictions and desires with the client's needs.
2. Establish a trusting, supportive relationship to promote free expression of feelings and concerns.
3. Respect client's wishes and rights. See Table 45-6.
4. Ensure that the client receives honest, ac-

TABLE 45-6 RIGHTS OF THE TERMINALLY ILL CLIENT

1. Right to know the truth about his or her condition.
2. Right to privacy and confidentiality.
3. Right to consent to treatment.
4. Right to choose place and time of own death.
5. Right to determine the disposition of his or her body after death.

SOURCE: Annas, G.: "Rights of the Terminally Ill Patient," reprinted by permission of the *Journal of Nursing Administration,* **42:**41, March–April 1974.

curate, and complete information about his or her physical condition, diagnosis, prognosis, and life span. Collaboration with physician, family, and client may be helpful. Nurses may need to interpret and explain this information to the client who must make realistic plans and decisions. Whether or not client is aware of the diagnosis is of critical importance to the nurse. The trend seems to be moving toward physicians telling clients the whole truth about their condition. Glaser and Strauss identified types of client and staff awareness (see Table 45-7) and noted the breakdown in communications and detrimental effects on the client of withholding information. These effects include feelings of abandonment, rejection, despair, depression, and distrust.

5. Provide quality physical and personal care—hygiene, positioning, ambulation—not only to prevent further complications but also to convey attitude of caring.
6. Provide analgesia and other comfort measures as ordered and required.
7. Try to facilitate open communication between client and family or significant other. There appears to be a high incidence of guilt and regret among survivors who were unable to talk together and come to an acceptance shared with the dying family member.
8. Support and encourage client, family, and/or significant other to freely express and openly deal with their apprehensions and anxieties about dying as well as their philosophical concerns about death.
9. Be sensitive to and communicate on the client's level of feeling. The dying client grieves for loss of valued persons and objects, including loss of oneself.
10. Reassure client that he or she will not be alone in the process of dying. "Abandonment is feared more than death itself" (Weisman, 1974).
11. Help client to identify and utilize remaining strengths for coping with developmental task of dying.
12. Allow client opportunity to participate in decisions in order to preserve self-esteem, independence, and personal control over the dying process.
13. Help client to identify and complete unfinished business.
14. Seek out spiritual assistance if client desires.
15. Listen attentively to client's life review. Elderly people often enjoy reminiscing about the past. This is a functional task of late life. As the client sorts out accomplishments, failures, appreciations, and regrets, unresolved conflicts may be rekindled or reconciled, comfort and satisfaction may be gained, and there may be a growing awareness of the individual's personal philosophy of life and death.
16. Allow client to spend as much time as desired in familiar and comfortable surroundings. If planning to die at home, provide home visits, education, and ongoing support to client and family. Hospice programs

TABLE 45-7 TYPES OF AWARENESS OF TERMINAL CONDITION

1. Closed awareness context: staff knows client's diagnosis but client does not.
2. Suspicion context: dying person suspects truth, while staff continues to act out pretense that recovery is expected.
3. Pretense context: both client and staff are fully aware of impending death, realize that other is also aware, and yet act as if client will eventually get better.
4. Open awareness: both client and staff are aware of impending death and openly discuss it.

SOURCE: Copyright © 1965 by Barney G. Glaser and Anselm L. Strauss. Reprinted with permission from *Awareness of Dying*, Aldine, New York.

work to preserve the client's control over the process of dying and ties with the familiar. In hospice facilities, unlimited visits from family and pets as well are permitted. Favorite foods and alcoholic beverages are allowed. Palliative care is provided. The prevention of pain is also of prime importance. The hospice movement appears to be taking hold in the United States. Hospice care can be provided through programs based in hospitals, community home care agencies, and hospice facilities themselves.

17. Participate in support systems for health professionals. Death is in conflict with the values of life-saving. Feelings of guilt, depression, helplessness, and failure are common among health care providers. Because of the intense intimacy and emotional impact of the relationship between the nurse and the dying client, nurses must find a means of expressing their own grief for the personal loss of clients who have died (e.g., group discussions, days off).
18. Respect the cultural, religious, and social practices of the client and family.

EVALUATION

Outcome Criteria

1. Client expresses heightened self-awareness and indicates that own affairs are in order.
2. Client is relating to family and/or significant other. Freely expresses concerns and a sense of satisfaction about life.
3. Client appears physically and spiritually comfortable. Expresses sense of peace and strength prior to death.
4. Client expresses readiness to die.
5. Client dies apparently at ease with self and with others.

REFERENCES

Burnside, I. M., ed.: *Nursing and the Aged*, McGraw-Hill, New York, 1976, p. 161.

Carter, F. M.: *Psychosocial Nursing*, Macmillan, New York, 1976, p. 289.

Dimond, M.: "Bereavement and the Elderly: A Critical Review With Implications for Nursing Practice and Research," *Journal of Advanced Nursing*, **6**:461, November 1981.

Engel, G.: "Signs of Giving Up," in Troup, S. B., and Greene, W. A., eds., *The Patient, Death, and the Family*, Scribners, New York, 1974, p. 60.

Gerber, I., and Weiner, A., et al.: in Dimond, M., "Bereavement and the Elderly: A Critical Review With Implications for Nursing Practice and Research," *Journal of Advanced Nursing*, **6**:468, November 1981.

Gordon, M.: *Manual of Nursing Diagnosis*, McGraw-Hill, New York, 1982, pp. 33–226.

Halley, J., and Harvey, A.: "Medical v. Legal Definitions of Death," *Journal of American Medical Association*, **204**:424, 1968.

Heller, Z. I.: "The Jewish View of Death: Guidelines for Dying," in Kubler-Ross, E., ed., *Death: The Final Stage of Growth*, Prentice-Hall, Englewood Cliffs, N.J., 1975, p. 51.

Kalish, R. A., and Reynolds, D. K.: "Death and Ethnicity: A Psychocultural Study," in Esberger, K. K., ed., "Dying and the Aged," *Journal of Gerontological Nursing*, **6**:13, January 1980.

Larue, G. A.: "Religion and the Aged," in Burnside, I. M., ed., *Nursing and the Aged*, McGraw-Hill, New York, 1976, pp. 576–577.

McGrory, A.: *A Well Model Approach to Care of the Dying Client*, McGraw-Hill, New York, 1978, p. 112.

Miles, H. S., and Hays, D. R.: "Widowhood," *American Journal of Nursing*, **75**:280, February 1975.

Parkes, C. M., and Brown, R. J.: "Health After Bereavement: A Controlled Study of Young Boston Widows and Widowers," *Psychosomatic Medicine*, **34**:449, 1972.

Peretz, D.: "Development, Object-Relationships, and Loss," in B. Schoenberg, B., et al., eds., *Loss and Grief: Psychological Management in Medical Practice*, Columbia University Press, New York, 1970, p. 4.

Trelease, M. L.: "Death Through Some Other Windows," in Kubler-Ross, E., ed., *Death: The Final Stage of Growth*, Prentice-Hall, Englewood Cliffs, N.J., 1975, p. 29.

Wangsness, S. I.: "Death Education for the Elderly," *Issues in Mental Health Nursing*, **3**:29, January/June 1981.

Weisman, A. D.: "Care and Comfort for the Dying," in Troup, S. B., and Greene, W. A., eds., *The Patient, Death, and the Family*, Scribners, New York, 1974, p. 100.

Weiss, J. M. A.: "Suicide in the Aged," in Resnik, H. L. P., ed., *Suicide Behaviors: Diagnosis and Management*, Little, Brown, Boston, 1968, pp. 255–267.

BIBLIOGRAPHY

Carnevali, D. L., and Patrick, M., eds.: *Nursing Management for the Elderly*, Lippincott, New York, 1979. This book concerns the normal aging process as well as high-risk health situations. It includes the problems of loneliness, powerlessness, and the losses of aging. Its approach is comprehensive, current, and well organized.

Caughill, R. E., ed.: *The Dying Patient: A Supportive Approach*, Little, Brown, Boston, 1976. This collection of essays provides a practical discussion intended to aid health professionals in their relationships with and care of the terminally ill. Included are issues involved in death (e.g., dying with dignity, society's influence and attitudes toward death, the grieving process, and the experience of death throughout the life span).

Dimond, M.: "Bereavement and the Elderly: A Critical Review With Implications for Nursing Practice and Research," *Journal of Advanced Nursing*, **6**:461, November 1981. This article reviews and summarizes the existing literature on grief and bereavement behavior. Deficiencies and limitations of past studies are identified. New directions and guidelines for nursing practice and research are proposed.

Esberger, K. K.: "Dying and the Aged," *Journal of Gerontological Nursing*, **6**:11, January 1980. This reference reviews three theories regarding death and dying, those of Dr. Elisabeth Kubler-Ross, Dr. Cecily Saunders, and Glaser and Strauss. It further discusses the attitudes of the aged toward death as well as the relationships of religion and culture with these attitudes.

Grollman, E. A.: *Living When a Loved One Has Died*, Beacon Press, Boston, 1977. This book serves as a helpful aide for the grieving. It addresses the physical and emotional reactions of grief in a personalized, supportive, and realistic manner.

McGrory, A.: *A Well Model Approach to Care of the Dying Client*, McGraw-Hill, New York, 1978. The perspective of this book is positive. It focuses on the identification and reinforcement of the client's strengths and potentials in the dying process with a state of maximum well-being as the goal.

McMahon, M., and Miller, P.: "Behavioral Cues in the Dying Process and Nursing Implications," *Journal of Gerontological Nursing*, **6**:16, January 1980. This reference discusses societal and nursing attitudes toward aging and dying. It addresses physical care of the elderly person during the dying process and nursing's role as it pertains to the family.

Murray, R., Huelskoetter, M. M., and O'Driscoll, D.: *The Nursing Process in Later Maturity*, Prentice-Hall, Englewood Cliffs, N.J., 1980. This book utilizes the nursing process in its comprehensive look at the individual in later life. It includes normal aging changes as well as cognitive impairment and emotional illnesses of later life.

46

Common Health Problems That Affect the Elderly

Joanne Kelleher Farley

Aging is an integral part of an individual's growth and development. When disruptions in physical as well as psychosocial components occur, alterations in a person's response to the effects of aging may result. The nurse working in all settings must be able to differentiate those observable changes that are the result of "normal" aging from those that are caused by a major health problem.

This chapter focuses on the impact of selected chronic health problems in the elderly. Since many of these problems are discussed in Part IV, this chapter explores the problem of chronicity and the other unique differences of common health problems in the aged. Implications for modification of the nursing process are also discussed, as relevant.

CHRONIC HEALTH PROBLEMS

DESCRIPTION

Although an elderly person may experience an acute illness, chronic, long-term health problems are common afflictions of the aged. The Commission on Chronic Illness (1949–1956) has identified five criteria, one or more of which must exist in order for a disease to be considered chronic (*Chronic Disease and Rehabilitation*, 1960).

1. The problem must be permanent.
2. The problem must leave a residual disability.
3. The problem must be caused by a nonreversible pathologic condition.
4. The problem must require special rehabilitative training.
5. The problem must require long supervision and care.

Of persons 65 years of age or older, 45.9 percent are limited to some degree in their activity (see Table 46-1). The problems encountered by these individuals may preclude their pursuing a major activity except on a limited basis. (A major activity is defined as those activities related to work or keeping house.) The elderly population has a high degree (U.S. Center for Health Statistics, 1977) of chronic health problems. The major chronic illnesses or problems found in the aged are cardiovascular, respiratory, osteoarthritis and accidents.

There are four distinct phases which the chronically ill go through as they begin to cope with a long-term health problem. They are identified as follows:

1. Denial and disbelief. The client is told of the illness and denies the reality of its happening. Often the impact of the problem and its long-term consequences are so severe that the individual uses this coping mechanism to handle stress at this time.
2. Developing awareness. The client ceases to deny the problem. There is a beginning re-

TABLE 46-1 PERCENT DISTRIBUTION OF PERSONS OVER 65 BY CHRONIC ACTIVITY LIMITATION STATUS

Sex	Total Population	No Limit %	Limited 1%[a]	Limited 2+%[b]	Limited 3++%[c]
Both	23,343	54.0	6.9	22.3	16.9
Male	9,617	50.9	5.2	15.2	28.7
Female	13,726	56.1	8.0	27.2	8.7

SOURCE: National Center for Health Statistics, B. Feller: "Health Characteristics of Persons with Chronic Activity Limitations: United States, 1979," *Vital and Health Statistics* Series 10, No. 137 DHHS Publication No. (HS) 82-1565, PHS, Washington, December 1981.

[a] Limited, but not in major activity

[b] Limited in amount or kind of major activity

[c] Unable to carry on

alization of the consequences of a particular illness, and the client is angry. During this period the person may be argumentative and critical.

3. Reorganization. With the developing awareness of the chronic illness comes a need for reorganization of one's life. Environmental changes are made, and relationships with family members are adjusted. Frequent verbal support for any and all accomplishments is most important during this stage.
4. Resolution or identity change. During this final stage, the client acknowledges the changes that have occurred in the body. The person is usually discharged from a health care facility at this time. After a very careful assessment, the client should be encouraged to become more self-directive until able to tolerate the withdrawal from health care.

Figure 46-1 depicts a model of coping tasks that must be accomplished to various degrees in order to cope with chronic illness. Identifying the clients' coping strategies is essential in determining client needs and plans for future care.

PREVENTION

Health Promotion

1. Maintenance of good health habits, rest, nutrition, etc.
2. Maintenance of current lifestyle within the parameters of the client's health state.

Population at Risk

1. Elderly, particularly females.
2. Older old population.

Screening

1. Chest x-ray.
2. Blood pressure.
3. Annual physical (eye screening).
4. Routine physical.
5. Sputum cultures.
6. Blood sugar analysis.

ASSESSMENT

Health History

1. Usual mode of living: lifestyle which is not conducive to health.
2. Limitations in physical activities and decreased mobility usually are evident; shortness of breath may be evidenced by diminished activity tolerance.
3. Limitations in mental diversions are frequently found; confusion, forgetting may be present.
4. Lack of, or poor, family support.
5. Inappropriate coping mechanisms possible; anxiety and fear associated with living alone; fear of death.
6. Poor nutritional habits frequently present.
7. Possible dehydration; reports of incontinence.
8. Poor health maintenance practices; decreased self-care.
9. Increased fatigue; changes in sleep patterns.

Physical Assessment

Findings would depend upon particular health problem. Refer to appropriate chapters which discuss the particular chronic disease present (e.g., arthritis, cardiovascular disease, respiratory problems, cancer).

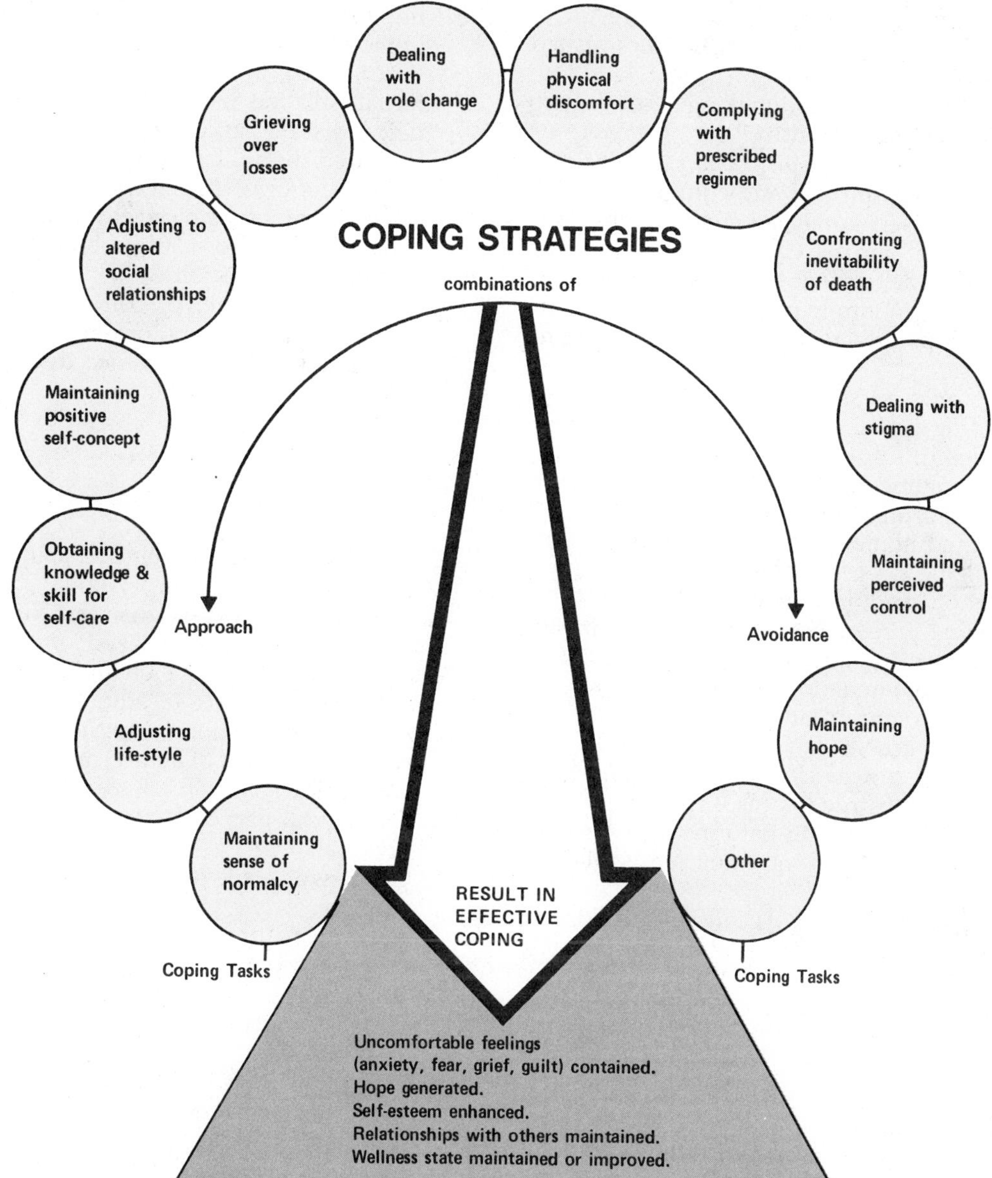

Figure 46-1 Coping with chronic illness. (From Miller, J. F.: *Coping with Chronic Illness: Overcoming Powerlessness*, F. A. Davis, Philadelphia, 1983, p. 32.)

Diagnostic Tests

Tests appropriate to the particular health problem would be performed. Refer to chapter which discusses the particular chronic disease present.

NURSING DIAGNOSES: ACTUAL OR POTENTIAL

1. Activity intolerance due to bed rest and/or generalized weakness.
2. Anxiety (mild to moderate) secondary to bodily changes, fear of death, changes in health status, or changes in environment.
3. Alteration in bowel elimination related to aging and disease processes.
4. Alteration in cardiac output secondary to cardiovascular disease process.
5. Alterations in comfort: pain due to arthritic changes and/or other disease processes.

6. Ineffective individual coping as a result of aging and disease processes and diminished copying strategies.
7. Alterations in decision making secondary to confusion and insecurity.
8. Distress of human spirit as a result of separation from spiritual and cultural ties.
9. Compromised family members coping due to physical and psychological changes and increased dependence of parent.
10. Alteration in family processes, roles and relationships as a result of isolation or aging process.
11. Fear (mild to severe) due to poor understanding of disease process and/or impending death.
12. Fluid volume deficit caused by disease process and/or inadequate fluid intake.
13. Impaired home maintenance resulting from the aging process, disease process, family situation, and/or housing inadequacies.
14. Grieving in response to loss of body image, bodily control, and/or impending death.
15. Health maintenance alteration due to decreased communication ability and perceptual impairment.
16. Ineffective airway clearance secondary to infection or obstruction (COPD).
17. Ineffective breathing patterns as a result of pain, decreased energy, neuromuscular impairment.
18. Potential for injury secondary to loss of strength, loss of visual and auditory acuity, and/or confusion.
19. Knowledge deficit: lack of information about the disease process, medication regime, future changes in physical health status.
20. Impaired mobility due to disease and loss of physical strength.
21. Noncompliance secondary to lack of knowledge, apathy, inability to obtain needed supplies, and/or poor finances.
22. Nutritional alteration: less than body requirements secondary to bodily changes, poor finances and/or disease processes.
23. Powerlessness as a result of the aging process, lifestyle changes, and/or chronic illness.
24. Self-care deficit due to loss of strength, loss of desire, or the disease process.
25. Alteration in self-concept secondary to physical, perceptual and/or social changes.
26. Sensory-perceptual alterations due to cerebrovascular disease and/or sensory impairments.
27. Impairment of skin integrity resulting from immobility, incontinence, and/or dehydration.
28. Social isolation increased because of immobility, disease, and/or poor self-image.
29. Impaired thought processes due to memory deficit and/or confusion.
30. Impairment of urinary elimination due to renal failure, loss of sphinctor control, and/or disorientation.
31. Impairment of verbal communication secondary to sensory motor deficit.
32. Decreased activity tolerance due to lack of regular exercise or fatigue.

EXPECTED OUTCOMES

1. Present activity level is maintained as long as possible.
2. Client will move bowels according to usual pattern of elimination.
3. Level of comfort is maintained; freedom from severe pain verbalized.
4. Client will make decision and problem-solve with the assistance of others.
5. Active participation in spiritual or religious activities (to best of ability) and social events is described.
6. Family will participate in the care of the individual.
7. Client will achieve developmental tasks of age group.
8. Good skin integrity will be maintained as evidenced by:
   a. Healthy skin turgor.
   b. Moist mucous membranes.
   c. Intact skin.
9. Individual will attend to self-care needs, be free from accidents, and verbalize understanding of disease process.
10. Activities of daily living will be performed to the highest level of potential.
11. Compliance with medical/nursing regimens will be evidenced by restoration of physical, emotional and spiritual health.
12. Client will maintain present weight.
13. Client will be free from deformity.
14. Individual will verbalize a sense of being loved and belonging, and decreased fear of death.

INTERVENTIONS

1. Evaluate home for possible modification of environment.

2. Support physical activity as tolerated by the client. Encourage planned activity daily (active and passive exercises). Try to keep client out of bed as much as possible.
3. Encourage family members (especially children and grandchildren or friends) to sit down and visit. Cards, checkers, or other games of interest may be stimulating for the person. The use of environment along with radio and television can also be additional sources of stimulation.
4. Coordinate care at home with the assistance of a homemaker, visiting nurse, or permanent caretaker.
5. Teach client and family all necessary information about a particular health problem and selected intervention.
6. Provide continuous support for family members, and refer them to agencies which will help care for the elderly family member.
7. Monitor fluid intake, output, nutritional intake, and bowel habits on a daily basis. Provide a bowel retraining program if needed. Encourage fluids to prevent dehydration; small but frequent meals may be required to maintain the nutritional status.
8. Maintain range of motion (ROM) and proper body alignment; use of a bed board and footboard may be needed. Maintain client safety and comfort at all times.
9. Position frequently. Observe skin integrity. Prevent skin breakdown by increasing planned activity, keeping client out of bed as much as possible and preventing skin irritation caused by presence of urine or feces. Avoid pressure point(s) by using sheepskin or flotation mattress as needed.
10. Allow the client time to verbalize fears and concerns. Provide support and information in response to questions (see Figure 46-1).
11. Promote regular activity as well as rest periods to stabilize client and improve activity tolerance.
12. Reduce discomfort through use of position change, therapeutic touch and medication, if needed.
13. Provide continued orientation to reality; decrease distractions and promote an environment to decrease confusion.
14. Provide opportunities for client to participate actively in decision to enhance sense of control and self-worth.

EVALUATION

Outcome Criteria

1. Skeletal system is functional and intact; optimal mobility maintained.
2. Bowel pattern restored and maintained.
3. Comfort level achieved; pain absent.
4. Client makes decisions about self and self-care activities.
5. Client has contact with church at least twice a month, or other social activities as tolerated.
6. Family members assist client with care and household chores.
7. Skin integrity maintained, manifested by skin turgor, absence of skin breakdown.
8. Client out of bed 6–8 hours daily, ambulating with assistance.
9. Nutrition level maintained, weight within normal limits; eating at table three times a day.
10. Client dresses self with assistance, showers four times weekly with assistance.
11. Client verbalizes self-worth; decreased fear of loneliness; feels loved and a sense of belonging.
12. Activity tolerance maintained, level of fatigue decreased.

Complications

1. Contractures (refer to Chapter 27).
2. Decubiti, skin breakdown.
3. Dehydration.
4. Accidents (see discussion later in this chapter).
5. Immobility.
6. Decreased self-esteem.
7. Urinary tract infection (refer to chapter 32).
8. Bowel obstruction (refer to Chapter 33).
9. Depression (refer to Chapter 36).
10. Suicide (refer to Chapter 38).

CARDIOVASCULAR DISEASE

DESCRIPTION

The major cause of death in the elderly is cardiovascular disease. Death rates indicate that the primary contributing health problems are alteration in cardiac function, hypertension, cerebrovascular disease and arteriosclerosis (refer to Table 46-2). The following discussion focuses upon alterations in cardiac function.

As individuals age, there are changes in heart size, endocardial tissue, and valve structure. These changes result in specific physiologic effects in the elderly:

1. Decreased cardiac reserve due to increased peripheral resistance and pooling.
2. Decreased cardiac output due to decreased stroke volume and slowed heart rate. Congestive heart failure may result (see Chapter 30).
3. Decreased blood flow through the coronary arteries (35 percent) and decreased utilization of oxygen, resulting in cardiac ischemia and angina.
4. Delayed recovery of myocardial contractility and irritability, resulting in an altered heart rate and rhythm.
5. Elevated peripheral vascular resistance due to atherosclerosis, increased blood viscosity, and/or decreased elasticity of the arteries.
6. Decrease in myocardial sensitivity due to the effects of atropine, and an increased sensitivity to carotid sinus stimulation.

The major cause of cardiac disease in the aged population is coronary atherosclerosis, which frequently results in symptomatic and asymptomatic angina pectoris, coronary thrombosis, and congestive heart failure. There is a lower incidence of angina pectoris in the extremely aged because of reduced activity and greater collateral circulation. However, coronary thrombosis should be suspected if angina persists or progresses. In acute coronary occlusion, the aged person manifests less pain with more dyspnea and congestive heart failure than a younger individual. Although the symptomatology seems to be less severe, the nurse should be aware of the significance of these differences from the younger client (refer to Chapter 30 for a complete discussion of cardiovascular problems).

PREVENTION

Health Promotion

1. Avoid smoking.
2. Avoid situations continuously causing stress.
3. Establish exercise regimen.
4. Eat low cholesterol diet.
5. Maintain desired weight for height.
6. Avoid high consumption of refined sugars, salt.

Population at Risk

1. Smokers.
2. Persons with high blood pressure.
3. Children of parents with cardiovascular disease.
4. Persons employed in stressful occupations.
5. Individuals with elevated cholesterol levels or who eat refined sugars.

Screening

Refer to Chapter 30.

TABLE 46-2 CARDIOVASCULAR DEATH RATES IN THE AGED, UNITED STATES, 1978

<table>
<tr><th>Cause of Death</th><th>Sex</th><th>Age 65–69</th><th>Age 70–74</th><th>Age 75–79</th><th>Age 80–84</th><th>Age 85+</th></tr>
<tr><td>All causes[a]</td><td>Women</td><td>16.9</td><td>27.2</td><td>47.1</td><td>75.1</td><td>135.4</td></tr>
<tr><td></td><td>Men</td><td>34.4</td><td>52.4</td><td>80.7</td><td>116.0</td><td>172.6</td></tr>
<tr><td>Heart disease[b]</td><td>Women</td><td colspan="2">823.1</td><td colspan="2">2,665.6</td><td>6,673.5</td></tr>
<tr><td></td><td>Men</td><td colspan="2">1,761.6</td><td colspan="2">4,064.1</td><td>7,990.6</td></tr>
<tr><td>Cerebrovascular diseases[b]</td><td>Women</td><td colspan="2">207.9</td><td colspan="2">865.5</td><td>2,298.5</td></tr>
<tr><td></td><td>Men</td><td colspan="2">290.0</td><td colspan="2">984.5</td><td>2,244.2</td></tr>
</table>

SOURCE: National Center for Health Statistics, L. Fingerhut: "Changes in Mortality Among the Elderly 1940–1978," in *Vital and Health Statistics*, Series 3, No. 22, DHHS Publication No. (PHS) 82-1406. PHS, Washington, U.S. Government Printing Office, March 1982.

[a] Deaths per 1,000 population

[b] Deaths per 100,000 population

ASSESSMENT

Refer to Chapter 30.

NURSING DIAGNOSES: ACTUAL OR POTENTIAL

1. Anxiety, mild to moderate, due to fear of death.
2. Alteration in cardiac output (decreased) secondary to valvular vessel changes in aging.
3. Alteration in comfort: pain, mild to severe.
4. Alteration in nutritional intake: diminished; decreased sodium and cholesterol intake.
5. Noncompliance with drug therapy due to physiologic effects of aging; forgetting.
6. Decreased activity tolerance: fatigue; diminished muscle strength.

EXPECTED OUTCOME

Refer to *Chronic Health Problems* and Chapter 30.

INTERVENTION

1. Activity programs should be established in view of the client's cardiac status, overall energy reserve, and tolerance.
2. Medications and their use must be carefully discussed and compliance continuously evaluated, especially if the client lives alone. Long-term use of medications may present problems such as misuse of the drugs (e.g., taking several doses of digitalis at one time because the person forgot to take dose for 2 days), or eliminating the drug if client begins to feel better.
3. Emphasize the need for adequate fluids to be sure drugs are adequately excreted, to prevent dehydration (as with diuretics), and to avoid straining at stool. Care should be taken to restrict fluid intake where the risk of congestive heart failure is high.
4. Nutritional counseling to help client restrict sodium and cholesterol intake is important. Because of the alteration in food intake that often accompanies aging, nutritional restrictions may be a problem for the elderly. Careful planning with family and nutritionist is important.
5. Encourage the person to stop smoking. This may be difficult for an elderly person who has established routines. The effects of nonsmoking must be evaluated in light of the stress created during the process of termination.
6. Environmental as well as personal stress should be kept at a minimum to decrease the demand on energy reserves and to prevent vasoconstriction.
7. The perception of chest pain may be affected by aging and decreased activity on the part of the aged individual. The client and family members should be encouraged to contact a physician if antianginal medication is not effective. Oxygen may be used when severe dyspnea is present or to relieve mild pain induced by stress or activity.

EVALUATION

Refer to Chapter 30.

HYPERTENSION

DESCRIPTION

Changes in peripheral resistance are the most significant causes of *hypertension* in the aged. Among persons 65–74, 59% of black females, 50% of black males, 42% of white females, and 35% of white males have hypertension (U.S. Center for Health Statistics, blood pressure levels). Hypertension is not to be considered a normal part of aging; rather, it is a health problem requiring long-term treatment. Isolated systolic hypertension is the most common form of high blood pressure among the elderly. Isolated systolic hypertension is the elevation of only the systolic pressure. It is defined as a systolic pressure of more than 160 and a diastolic pressure of less than 90.

PREVENTION

Refer to Chapter 30.

ASSESSMENT

Refer to Chapter 30.

NURSING DIAGNOSES: ACTUAL OR POTENTIAL

1. Anxiety of the unknown (mild to moderate threat of chronic health problem.)

2. Knowledge deficit: lack of knowledge of health problem; nutritional changes; activity.
3. Noncompliance with medication schedule secondary to lack of knowledge of consequences, apathy, inaccessibility of pharmacy, and/or poor finances.
4. Fear due to possible impending death; threat to survival.
5. Alteration in comfort; headache, nosebleeds.
6. Ineffective coping: increased stress; decreased stress management.

EXPECTED OUTCOME

Refer to *Chronic Health Problems* and Chapter 30.

INTERVENTIONS

1. Explain hypertension slowly and carefully; answer all questions. Provide the client with information to clarify why emotional outbursts or behavioral changes are occurring.
2. Strive to maintain independence and sense of self-worth.
3. Teach client to identify response patterns and encourage avoidance of stressful situations.
4. Provide nutritional counseling, especially in relation to weight reduction and low sodium intake.
5. Avoid dehydration, especially if diuretics are being taken. Be sure client knows signs of electrolyte imbalance, e.g., hyperkalemia or hypokalemia (refer to discussions of fluid loss in Chapters 28 and 32).
6. Monitor blood pressure in both sitting and standing positions.
7. Explain nature of headaches. Teach client to note when they occur and if they are relieved by rest, medication, etc.
8. Prevent nosebleeds. When they do occur, be sure client and family know how to treat them (e.g., Fowler's position, mouth breathing, pinching nostrils to create pressure). Following the episode of a nosebleed, the client should be told to seek medical attention.
9. If excess bleeding is noted, blood loss should be evaluated (e.g., assess hemoglobin and hematocrit levels).
10. The use of drugs to treat hypertension is extensive. Drugs used by the elderly are presented in Table 46-3 and their side effects are discussed. The client should have knowledge of drug action and reactions (particularly behavioral changes) that can accompany drug use. It is important to emphasize the need for continued drug compliance even after symptoms of hypertension are alleviated.
11. Once blood pressure returns to a normal range, a planned exercise and rest program should be developed, based on the client's interests and abilities. Exercises can include walking, swimming, bicycling, golf, etc.
12. Rest periods should be planned periodically throughout the day. Sleep (7 to 8 h per night) is important. Rest after meals may be individualized as necessary.
13. Reducing stress is critical to maintaining

TABLE 46-3 ANTIHYPERTENSIVE DRUG TREATMENT IN THE AGED

Drug	Possible Side Effects in Aged
Antihypertensives:	Muscle weakness
Adrenergics:	Nausea
Methyldopa (Aldomet)	Drowsiness
Clonidine (Catapres)	Mental confusion
Hydralazine (Apresoline)	Orthostatic hypotension
Beta adrenergic blocking agents:	
Propranolol (Inderal)	May precipitate CHF
	May aggravate chronic lung disease
Diuretics:	
Furosemide (Lasix)	Hypokalemia
Ethacrynic Acid (Edecrin)	Decreased ability to exercise
	Forgetfulness
	Incontinence
	Lethargy
	Dehydration
	Muscular weakness

blood pressure levels within normal limits. Teach client how to relax (e.g., procedures such as biofeedback, yoga, etc). The importance of continuing long-term drug compliance to keep blood pressure within normal limits should be emphasized.

EVALUATION

Outcome Criteria

Refer to Chapter 30.

Complications

1. Impairment of circulation in the kidneys. This leads to ischemia of renal tissue, which in turn liberates a pressor mediator that increases arteriolar constriction. (This cycle perpetuates the disorder and can result in irreversible renal damage.)
2. Increased workload on the heart as the left ventricle is forced to work harder to cope with impaired nutrition and oxygenation to the myocardium.
3. Neurologic consequences resulting in cerebral apoplexy due to hemorrhage, thrombosis, or embolism, and eye injury.

CEREBROVASCULAR DISEASE

DESCRIPTION

Cerebrovascular disease is often a major complication of hypertension and is a leading cause of death in the aged (refer to Table 46-2). It is devastating to the aged person because it threatens an individual's independence, dignity, and self-esteem.

Peripheral resistance increases as part of the process of aging. Blood pressure thereby rises, and hypertension can result. Prolonged hypertension can lead to sudden cerebral hemorrhage or infarction (refer to Chapter 30).

PREVENTION

Refer to Chapters 25 and 30 (for discussion of cerebrovascular accident).

ASSESSMENT

Refer to Chapters 25 and 30.

NURSING DIAGNOSES: ACTUAL OR POTENTIAL

1. Impaired mobility secondary to paresis or paralysis, decreased activity tolerance.
2. Self-care deficit due to paresis or paralysis.
3. Grieving (mild to moderate) due to loss and body image changes.
4. Impaired thought processes due to cognitive perceptual deficit.
5. Anxiety due to inability to express self.
6. Impairment of urinary elimination pattern secondary to (paralysis) sensory–motor deficit.
7. Alteration in bowel pattern secondary to sensory–motor deficit.
8. Altered levels of consciousness secondary to decreased cardiovascular perfusion.
9. Nutritional deficit: inability to chew, swallow, etc.
10. Disruption in skin integrity: decreased cardiovascular perfusion.

EXPECTED OUTCOMES

Refer to *Chronic Health Problems* and Chapter 30.

INTERVENTIONS

Refer to Chapters 25 and 30. Additional interventions include:

1. Provide assistance with eating: encourage small, frequent feedings as tolerated. Try to follow individual's eating patterns as closely as possible.
2. Exercise extreme caution in positioning in bed properly to avoid skin breakdown. Prevention of contractures is critical as decreased joint mobility which normally accompanies aging may be intensified with CVA. Early ROM exercise is critical.
3. Meticulous skin care is essential, especially if incontinence is a problem.
4. Use all medications cautiously as the onset of CVA may alter an individual's reaction to a drug (e.g., analgesics).
5. As the client begins to progress, it is important for family members to be patient. The person may be very slow in completing tasks, but when possible, it is important to encourage independent activities.
6. Depression and grieving over the loss of body function is not uncommon (refer to Chapter 45). The nurse must be supportive

of the client and family during this time and encourage all actions that promote independence.
7. Communication difficulties may intensify client's frustration and lead to outbursts of anger. The client needs to be told that speech problems are a result of the CVA and reassured that speech will improve with time. A speech therapist should be enlisted when possible.
8. Stimulation within the environment, including physical therapy and occupational therapy, is important. Rearrangement of the home environment (e.g., use of firm chairs, removal of scatter rugs, bathroom supports, etc.) may be necessary.
9. The client should be told when he or she buys clothes to buy them one size larger, with elastic waists and front fasteners, in order to ease the process of dressing.
10. Teach clients to avoid hot baths; they dilate the cutaneous and muscular vascular bed, allowing blood to pool when patient rises from the tub (Locke). Also, teach clients to avoid straining at stool, as use of the Valsalva maneuver may increase stress and act as a vagal stimulus.
11. Decrease stress within the environment, as the elderly person who has suffered a CVA will have decreased ability to cope with many of the problems of daily living.
12. Bladder retraining and nutritional counseling should be provided, as needed.

EVALUATION

Refer to Chapters 25 and 30 for additional information about CVA.

RESPIRATORY DISEASE

DESCRIPTION

The rigidity of the lungs and reduction of muscle power are prime causes of pulmonary complications in the elderly. The two most prevalent pulmonary diseases found in this population are bronchitis and emphysema. These are collectively known as chronic obstructive lung (or pulmonary) disease (COLD or COPD).

Chronic bronchitis is the leading pulmonary abnormality in the aged. It is clinically evidenced by the presence of persistent cough and sputum production. It relates specifically to clients who cough and raise sputum on most days for a minimum of three consecutive months each year for at least two years.

Many consider emphysema the result of chronic bronchitis, but results of clinical studies indicate that emphysema appears to be a disease distinct from chronic bronchitis. Emphysema increases progressively with age, reaching its highest degree of severity in the seventies. It is defined as the destruction of lung parenchyma distal to the terminal bronchiole (refer to Chapter 31 for a complete discussion of cold, chronic bronchitis and emphysema).

PREVENTION

Refer to Chapter 31.

ASSESSMENT

Health History

1. History of previous respiratory diseases frequent.
2. Employment in area of high dust or fumes.
3. History of frequent cough with sputum.
4. Shortness of breath at rest or with mild exertion.
5. Smokes and has smoked since youth.
6. Decreased energy level.

Physical Assessment

Refer to Chapter 31.

Diagnostic Tests

Refer to Chapter 31.

NURSING DIAGNOSES: ACTUAL OR POTENTIAL

1. Anxiety secondary to dyspnea.
2. Ineffective airway clearance secondary to COPD.
3. Fear secondary to feelings of impending death.
4. Decreased activity tolerance; increased fatigue; decreased energy potential.

EXPECTED OUTCOMES

Refer to *Chronic Health Problems* and Chapter 31 under chronic bronchitis and emphysema.

INTERVENTIONS

1. Clarify problems slowly and clearly, and encourage all improvements.
2. Provide quiet, cheerful, stress-free, supportive environment.
3. Medication should be administered as prescribed. Exercise special precautions with bronchodilators:
   a. Ephedrine compounds may cause urinary retention in elderly men.
   b. Aminophylline preparations are absorbed from gastrointestinal tract erratically in the aged (refer to discussion of medication and the aged).
4. Provide extensive instructions concerning activity, exercise, and breathing exercises (refer to Chapter 31). Plan rest and sleep activities as determined by the client's need and tolerance.
5. Increase energy tolerance (e.g., being of out bed) through intermittent positive pressure breathing (IPPB) treatments.
6. Avoid infections: aged person's perception of heat and cold may be altered, and therefore a fever may go unrecognized. Also, aged persons frequently have an elevation in temperature because they are often dehydrated and unable to perspire. Aged, dyspneic clients may not register a correct oral temperature reading. Person should be instructed to contact a nurse or physician when sputum becomes yellow or green.
7. Instruct client to avoid extremes of heat and cold. Suggest that the person stay indoors when extremes of weather occur. Avoid crowds. Recommend an air-conditioner in extremely hot, humid weather.
8. Encourage fluids, especially in light of dehydration problem.
9. Avoid contact with anyone, including children and family members, who has a cold or respiratory infection.

EVALUATION

Refer to *Chronic Health Problems* and Chapter 31.

PRIMARY MATURITY-ONSET DIABETES

DESCRIPTION

Another chronic problem of the aged is diabetes. Primary maturity-onset diabetes is a "chronic metabolic disease that is evidenced by above-normal blood glucose levels resulting from a deficiency of the pancreatic hormone, insulin. Primary maturity-onset diabetes develops after age 40 and pursues a mild course" (Thomas, 1976).

The incidence of diabetes increases with age and peaks between 65 and 74, occurring in 64.4 percent of 1,000 persons. It is estimated that 20 percent of all diabetics are 60 years or over.

A complete discussion of diabetes is found in Chapter 28. Since several additional problems occur in the aged person with diabetes, the remaining discussion will focus on these important issues.

PREVENTION

Health Promotion

1. Maintain appropriate weight for height.
2. Avoid infection or seek treatment early should infection occur.
3. If genetically predisposed, have periodic blood work (fasting blood sugar).

Population at Risk

1. Persons who are obese.
2. Persons with genetic predisposition.
3. Persons with serious infections.
4. Persons with severe mental anguish.
5. Persons having undergone a surgical procedure.
6. Persons taking diabetogenic drugs (thiazides, cortisone).
7. Persons on prolonged bed rest.

Screening

See Diabetes, Chapter 28.

ASSESSMENT

Refer to Chapter 28. Additional assessment data found in the aged include the following.

Health History

1. Blurred distance vision.
2. Pruritis vulvae.

Physical Assessment

Refer to Chapter 28.

Diagnostic Tests

Blood sugar levels should be drawn 2 h after high carbohydrate meal (100 g).

NURSING DIAGNOSES: ACTUAL OR POTENTIAL

1. Anxiety (mild to severe) secondary to diagnosis of a chronic health problem.
2. Knowledge deficit—lack of knowledge of diabetes secondary to being newly diagnosed.
3. Noncompliance, decreased decision-making abilities, diminished motor abilities and sensory-perceptual abilities.
4. Nutritional alteration: change in dietary and appetite changes.
5. Altered skin integrity due to sensory-perceptual alteration.

ASSESSMENT

Refer to Chapter 24.

EXPECTED OUTCOMES

Refer to Chapter 28. Additional goals in caring for the aged include:

1. Immediate.
   a. Client will perform the necessary perceptual and motor tasks, e.g., administering insulin and urine testing, or have a family member become skilled in performing tasks that the client is unable to manage.
   b. Client will manage to cook food for self, as evidenced by eating meals planned according to dietary regimen, at regular intervals, or have food prepared and delivered according to dietary restrictions.
   c. Client will increase the amount of physical exercise through planning and implementing an activity schedule as tolerated.
2. Long-range.
   Client will cope with the problem of diabetes as it affects lifestyle and incorporate these new behaviors into the way she or he handles the activities of daily living.

INTERVENTIONS

Refer to Chapter 28. Additional interventions in the elderly include the following:

1. Consider all assessed changes when developing the teaching plan for an elderly diabetic.
2. Reinforce all progress made by the client, and make use of repetition. Return demonstration should be supervised by the nurse.
3. Involve family to degree needed, and refer to Visiting Nurse Association or other community health agency to ensure long-term compliance.
4. Begin dietary change by emphasizing the importance of three well-balanced meals taken at regularly spaced times. Limit carbohydrates to 100 g per day.
5. If insulin or oral hypoglycemics are ordered, exchange or food groups will have to be taught. The following components should be considered when planning diet teaching.
   a. Anorexia is common in the elderly.
   b. Food preparation is often difficult for the aged, especially if they live alone or in a setting with limited facilities.
   c. The choice of chewable foods may be limited for the elderly.
   d. Client's usual eating patterns should be preserved and diet planned close to personal eating habits and preferences, including foods especially liked.
6. Exercise should be encouraged as tolerated. Explanation of the relationship between diabetes and exercise should be included in teaching plan. An exercise program should be planned around a patient's regular exercise habits. Encourage walking, as tolerated.
7. Administer and teach the client how to self-administer all medications. Small amounts of insulin are usually preferred with aged [Lente or NPH (isophane insulin suspension) in 100-U doses]. Emphasize the importance of exact compliance; incorporate family into teaching program.
8. Have client utilize a lighted magnifying glass or a preset syringe if visual disturbances interfere with performing the skill of administering insulin.
9. Teach testing of urine by using a second voided specimen before any meal or bedtime. Teach the client to keep a record of sugar and

acetone daily, and increase testing of urine at each meal and bedtime should any illness occur (e.g., fever).

EVALUATION

Outcome Criteria

(Refer to discussions of diabetes in Chapter 28.)

Complications

1. Hypertension (see discussion earlier in this chapter.)
2. Coronary artery disease (see discussion earlier in this chapter.)
3. Cerebrovascular disease (see discussion earlier in this chapter).
4. Peripheral vascular disease (refer to Chapter 30).
5. Retinopathy (refer to Chapter 26).
6. Glaucoma (see discussion on *Visual Disturbances* later in this chapter).
7. Renal disorders (refer to Chapter 32).

OSTEOARTHRITIS

DESCRIPTION

Osteoarthritis is a noninflammatory deterioration of articular cartilages and overgrowth of adjacent bone. There are no systemic manifestations. Advancing age is the major predisposing factor. It is the most common type of arthritis occurring after age 50, and affects approximately 40 million in the United States. (Refer to Chapter 27.)

PREVENTION

Health Promotion

1. Maintain good health habits.
2. Avoid excessive weight gain.
3. Avoid situations of prolonged stress.
4. Decrease trauma to extremeties.

Population at Risk

1. Children of parents who have arthritis.
2. Persons with poor posture.
3. Persons who are obese.
4. Persons who experience occupational stress.

ASSESSMENT

Refer to Chapter 27 for discussion of osteoarthritis.

NURSING DIAGNOSES: ACTUAL OR POTENTIAL

1. Alterations in comfort: pain, backache, due to inflammation.
2. Impaired mobility resulting from stiffness and pain.
3. Decreased self-care activities due to decreased mobility and pain.
4. Alteration in self-concept secondary to disfigurement (e.g., Heberden's nodes): changes in body image.
5. Increased potential for injury: difficulty in mobility and agility.
6. Ineffective coping: depleted strategies to cope with stress.
7. Nutritional excess: obesity.

EXPECTED OUTCOMES

Refer to *Chronic Health Problems* and Chapter 27.

INTERVENTIONS

Refer to Chapter 27. Additional interventions include:

1. Establish exercise–rest program. Consider the following components in plan:
   a. Regularity and consistency of exercise.
   b. Emphasize extension rather than flexion of extremities.
   c. Utilize hydrotherapy before exercises to help decrease inflammation and tenderness and increase movement.
   d. Include active and passive exercises.
   e. Provide daily nap or rest periods as needed.
   f. Use footboard and bed board as needed, depending on the amount of time client is resting.
   g. Provide proper alignment, preventing contractures by placing joints and limbs in the most functional position.
   h. Avoid complete bed rest whenever possible, as this can intensify the problem.

2. Encourage interest in personal appearance, e.g., maintain personal hygiene.
3. Utilize a weight reduction program as needed, explaining the need for weight control in order to reduce stress on joints.
4. Medicate for pain, providing accurate instruction about the use and abuse of medication.

EVALUATION

Refer to Chapter 27.

OSTEOPOROSIS

DESCRIPTION

Osteoporosis is a health problem seen frequently in the elderly, particularly elderly females. It is a progressive problem due to a gradual loss of bone mass. The cause of the disorder is unclear but predisposing factors include genetic factors, postmenopause, white ancestry, low calcium, vitamin C and D intake, lowered levels of sex hormones, and a lack of exercise and activity. Initially, the client is asymptomatic. However, as the disease progresses pain, usually vertebral, may appear as an early symptom. Decrease in height caused by vertebral collapse and diminished spinal mobility may also be present. The diagnosis is confirmed by x-ray and physical examination.

Nursing problems include alteration in comfort, decreased activity tolerance, and nutritional deficits. Interventions focus on replacement of dietary calcium, protein and vitamins C and D on a daily basis. Treatment includes the use of nonspecific estrogens along with a planned physical therapy regime (which includes stress on the bones) and the use of heat. Analgesia is administered in a number of cases to relieve pain. The client should avoid extended periods of rest as this may weaken the muscles and reduce bone stress. The client and the family members must learn to institute maximum safety measures to prevent accidents and falls that can complicate this health problem (see Chapter 27 for additional information).

VISUAL DISTURBANCES

DESCRIPTION

Most aged persons have fair to excellent vision (corrected with glasses). The three major geriatric ocular problems are macular disease, cataracts, and glaucoma.

The macula is the center of retinal vision, and diseases of the macula cause loss of central vision. The cause of the disease is probably any of several vascular changes which occur with age and/or disease.

Cataracts are opaque lenses. If the opacity is near the center of the lens, vision is impaired. Throughout life, the lens grows by laying down new fibers. Compensatory shrinkage or drying of the nucleus occurs simultaneously. In the case of cataracts, the lens capsule thickens and a less permeable lens develops. This progresses with age until the nucleus is too hard and dry to transmit light efficiently. *Central cataracts* are located in the *central area* of the lens; *scattered cataracts* are multiple mini-mirrors in the eye. *Peripheral cataracts* are located in the periphery of the lens.

Glaucoma manifests itself by increased intraocular pressure. The disease worsens with advancing age. The most common form is chronic wide angle glaucoma, due to failure in the facility for outflow of aqueous humor. The symptoms are insidious in onset, and if the disease is undiagnosed and untreated, it will result in vision loss.

PREVENTION

Health Promotion

1. Periodic eye examinations.
2. Frequency of examination increases with age (yearly).

Population at Risk

1. Elderly.
2. Increased incidence in persons with diabetes and hypoparathyroidism.
3. Exposure to radiation, infrared light.

Screening

1. Tonometer examination (glaucoma screening) done on a yearly basis.
2. Annual eye examination.

ASSESSMENT

Refer to *Chronic Health Problems* and Chapter 26. Additional characteristics to be noted include:

1. Macular disease.
   a. Inability to recognize faces.
   b. Inability to read.
   c. Inability to make out detail.
2. Cataracts.
   a. Poor peripheral vision in one or both eyes.
   b. Difficulty walking due to poor eyesight.
   c. Blurred vision in one or both eyes.
   d. Opaque lens in one or both eyes.
3. Glaucoma.
   a. Vague headaches.
   b. Tearing on one or both eyes.
   c. Increased intraocular pressure, determined with a tonometer.

NURSING DIAGNOSES: ACTUAL OR POTENTIAL

1. Anxiety due to threat of impaired vision.
2. Fear (mild or severe) possible impending blindness.
3. Potential for injury due to impaired vision.
4. Impaired mobility due to fear of falling.
5. Alteration in self-concept changes: altered body image.
6. Social isolation: fear and/or inability to leave home.

EXPECTED OUTCOMES

1. Verbalization of the disease process, and prognosis.
2. Maintenance of optimal level of vision by compliance with the therapeutic plan.
3. Ambulate without injury.
4. Maintenance of self-concept by sustained level of independence and social interaction with family and others.

INTERVENTIONS

1. Macular disease. Suggest low-vision aids; magnifying devices, either hand-held (preferred by most aged persons) or in frames.
2. Cataracts.
   a. Reinforce opthalmologist's decision to operate or not to operate.
   b. If surgery is not indicated, instruct client in use and purpose of prescribed miotics. Explain reason for decision to client and family.
   c. Teach client to use increased light to read.
   d. If surgery is performed, give eye care. Refer to Chapter 26, usually postoperative.
   e. Reassure client that an improvement in vision will occur.
   f. Allay fears by describing technical advances (with which client probably is not familiar).
3. Glaucoma.
   a. Administer and teach proper self-administration and action of eye drops. (Pilocarpine or carbachal is usually ordered.)
   b. Encourage client to keep appointments with ophthalmologist.
   c. Teach client and family importance of keeping condition well controlled by following instructions implicitly. A well-controlled glaucoma client usually experiences no symptoms and has a tendency to relax on treatment.
   d. Instruct client about the necessity of telling nurse or physician about any problem with vision, especially prior to surgery.
   e. Teach danger signals of impaired vision:
      (1) Blurring of vision (especially in early morning).
      (2) Halos around artificial lights.
      (3) Pain in or around eyes.

EVALUATION

Outcome Criteria

1. Client verbalizes an understanding of disease process, and prognosis.
2. Client's eyesight remains at same level as previous testing.
3. Maintenance of usual self-care activities unassisted; safety maintained.
4. Eyeglasses worn whenever out of bed.
5. Compliance with the therapeutic plan. Eye medications instilled at appropriate time and in correct dosage as verbalized by patient; appointments kept.

Complications

Increased loss of vision (refer to Chapter 26).

TABLE 46-4 MAJOR AUDITORY DISTURBANCES OF THE AGED

External Ear	Middle Ear	Inner Ear
Partial occlusion with cerumen: This occurs frequently in the aged and interferes with optimum use of a hearing aid. The cerumen can usually be removed by saline irrigation. *Total occlusion with cerumen:* Common in the aged. Impacted cerumen cannot be removed easily by ordinary irrigation. The use of a wax softener or referral to an otologist for curetting may be necessary.	*Atrophic or sclerotic changes of tympanic membrane:* Common to the aged. Severe hearing loss only results when there is marked retraction of the tympanic membrane. *Otosclerosis:* This is the most common middle ear problem. An osseous growth occurs which fixes the footplate of the stapes in the oval window of the cochlea. A conductive hearing loss common to youth, it persists throughout life and eventually produces a sensorineural loss in geriatric patients. *Treatment* includes: Surgical correction (refer to Chapter 26), use of a hearing aid, or both. Surgery in the elderly is frequently discouraged, but each candidate should be individually evaluated.	*Presbycusis* is the most common problem of the inner ear; it is a loss of hearing due to the aging process (refer to Chapter 44).

AUDITORY DISTURBANCES

DESCRIPTION

The majority of older persons develop some form of hearing deficiency (refer to Chapter 44). This results in distorted auditory perception and communication difficulties. The two most common causes of hearing loss are (1) conductive loss, and (2) sensorineural loss. Conductive losses are usually the result of dysfunctions of the external or middle ear and cause a reduction in loudness of speech. Sensorinueral loss is the result of inner ear dysfunction and causes a distortion in sound, making speech unintelligible. Table 46-4 describes the more common auditory problems that affect the elderly.

Nursing care for the client with a hearing loss is discussed in Chapter 26.

MEDICATION EFFECTS AND THE AGED

DESCRIPTION

As the body ages, its ability to metabolize medications is altered. The elderly are particularly vulnerable to drug side effects. As has been seen, elderly persons often experience a chronic disease which requires the use of a large amount of medication. The elderly population uses 25 to 30% of all drugs used in the United States.

The number of drugs administered simultaneously often has a direct bearing on an individual's likelihood of experiencing an adverse drug reaction. The incidence for undesirable drug effects in persons over 60 is $2\frac{1}{2}$ times as high as in those under 60.

It is reported that 60% of the elderly who take medications make some sort of medication error; of this number 90% have some adverse effects and 20% need hospitalization. The physiologic and behavioral changes that occur in elderly persons receiving medications must be carefully evaluated by the nurse.

The plasma level of a drug is directly related to the drug's concentration at its site of action. This, in turn, governs the degree and duration of the body's response to the drug. The factors which influence plasma level and the specific differences in the aged individual are:

1. Absorption. Changes occur in the gastrointestinal tract, e.g., decreased gastric acidity, decreased number of absorbing cells, changes in gastric motility, and decreased blood flow of the gastric intestinal system during the aging process result in an impairment in drug absorption (refer to Chapters 33 and 44).
2. Distribution. Active and functional tissue is replaced by fat as one ages. Drugs which accumulate in the fatty tissues have a more pronounced effect and a longer duration in the elderly.
3. Excretion. Because of a reduced rate of glomerular filtration and renal blood flow in the elderly, there is a delayed elimination of many drugs (refer to Chapters 32 and 44).
4. Metabolism. Animal studies suggest there is a decrease in enzyme activity, especially in the liver, and decreased liver function with aging which is reflected in higher blood levels and longer duration of drug activity.
5. Interaction. There is a decrease in the number of living, active cells in the aged person. Several drug problems result, including decreased activity of stimulants and enhanced activity of depressants.
6. Secondary responses. When a drug is administered for a particular purpose, the body often responds in ways other than intended in order to maintain homeostasis. Often there is a greater secondary effect and a lessened primary response in elderly persons because of the decreased ability to meet certain physiologic demands such as
    a. Poor adjustment to high and low temperatures.
    b. Limited regulation of blood sugar levels.
    c. Decreased restoration of acid-base equilibrium.
    d. Decreased response to orthostatic stress.

The important thing to consider when administering or monitoring medications in elderly persons is a summation of the above: Elderly people have a decreased tolerance to drugs.

PREVENTION

Health Promotion

1. Knowledge of all medications taken (names, purpose, side effects, dosage).
2. Accurate reporting of medications being taken to any new physician.
3. Limited use of over-the-counter (OTC) drugs.
4. Proper disposal of discontinued medications.

Population at Risk

1. Elderly, particularly women.
2. Chronically ill, especially those with two or more chronic conditions.

ASSESSMENT

The phase of the nursing process of utmost importance in terms of the use of medications and the geriatric patient is the assessment. A complete drug assessment is critical in order to prevent complications and to identify the client at risk to develop potentially negative drug reactions.

Health History

1. Identify all drugs being taken and the reason for their use (include over-the-counter drugs).
2. List the amounts (dosages), times, and route of administration used for each drug.
3. Elicit drugs taken in the past; identify reason for termination and any untoward response to any drug.
4. If more than one physician is consulted, ask the client if each doctor has been informed about the other. Aged persons will often see more than one doctor without informing the other, raising the potential for inadvertent drug reactions.
5. Identify drug allergies; also, isolate any allergies to food, animals, etc. If an allergic

reaction has occurred, identify changes noted.
6. Assess client's knowledge of drug action and adverse reactions to current drugs.
7. Assess compliance.
8. Possible financial constraints.
9. Possible physical limitations that may interfere with taking medication. Possible visual impairment that may interfere with reading the label clearly.
10. Possible metabolic, gastrointestinal, or urinary tract problem that may interfere with drug absorption, distribution, or excretion and overall tolerance.
11. Possible behavioral health problem that could be aggravated by a particular medication.

Physical Assessment

Any physical manifestation may be presented, depending on diagnoses, drug interactions, overdoses or noncompliance.

Diagnostic Tests

1. Serum levels (for a particular drug).
2. Digitalis levels (etc.).

NURSING DIAGNOSES: ACTUAL OR POTENTIAL

Any diagnoses related to physical deficits may be identified according to assessment data. In addition, the following diagnoses may be found:

1. Knowledge deficit: lack of knowledge of medications due to apathy, altered memory, confusion and/or lack of information.
2. Noncompliance with medication regimen secondary to poor understanding, financial constraints, apathy, and/or physical limitations.

EXPECTED OUTCOMES

1. Client will verbalize names, dosages, times of administration, purposes, and side effects of all medications being taken.
2. Client will verbalize the importance of compliance with medication regimen.
3. Client will give evidence of compliance with medication regimen by showing written record of having:
   a. taken all prescribed medications
   b. taken correct dosages of all medications
   c. taken prescribed medications at times ordered.
   d. Keep record of "Medicines I Take." NOTE: the following pamphlet is very helpful in assisting the elderly to comply with their medication regimens:
      Using Your Medicines Wisely: A Guide for the Elderly, U.S. Department of Health, Education, and Welfare, PHS, Alcohol, Drug Abuse, and Mental Health Administration, Publication No. (ADM) 80-705, 1979.
4. Client will not dispose of or discontinue medications without physician's order.

INTERVENTIONS

1. Obtain all information about individual's health problem(s) and actions and reactions of all drugs.
2. Review medications at every visit.
3. Listen and observe for any clues to side effects of drugs.
4. Leave specific *written* instructions with client when changes are made.
5. Use innovative techniques to assist individual with proper self-administration of medications:
   a. Egg carton labeled with the 12 hours of the day may be filled every morning to keep the client from forgetting when and if the medication is to be taken (see Expected Outcomes, 3d).
   b. Colored tape on bottle caps can signify a specific time for taking a medication. For example, red is at breakfast, blue is at lunch.
   c. Textures can be pasted to bottle caps for poor-sighted persons (sandpaper, velvet).
   d. Rubber bands around bottles can indicate the time to take the medication (one rubber band means 1:00, two rubber bands mean 2:00, etc.).
6. Observe client when taking medication whenever possible. Safety caps on containers may be difficult to open and may need to be changed.
7. Instruct and monitor client in keeping "Medications I Take" chart.
8. Involve family in teaching plan (or neighbor).
9. Table 46-5 describes drugs commonly used by the aged and potential adverse reactions.

TABLE 46-5 MEDICTIONS COMMONLY TAKEN BY ELDERLY

Medication	Possible Adverse Reactions
Antianxiety agents including sedatives and hypnotics	Oversedation Ataxia Excitement Disorientation Delirium Forgetfulness
Antidepressants	Agitation Confusion Constipation Urinary retention Cardiac arrhythmias Postural hypotension
Cardiovascular agents	
Digitalis	Anorexia Confusion Depression Blurred or hazy vision Arrythmias
Antihypertensives	Refer to Table 42-3
Diuretics	Refer to Table 42-3
OTC Drugs	
Analgesics	Gastrointestinal upset Skin reactions Tinnitus Increased clotting time
Antacids	Increase in serum sodium (Normal = 136–142 mEq/L)
Laxatives	Dehydration Dependency upon drug

EVALUATION

Outcome Criteria

1. Client complies with medication regimen by keeping a written record of medication listing appropriate times in correct amounts.
2. Restoration of normal physical parameters.

Complications

ADVERSE REACTION

Assessment

1. Decreased activity of a particular medication.
2. Enhanced activity of a particular medication.

Revised Outcomes

1. Undesirable effect of combination of medications will be resolved.
2. Other goals remain as stated.

Interventions

1. Report undesired reaction to physician.
2. Instruct client about changes in medication regimen in writing.

Reevaluation and Follow-up

1. Revise plan to ensure that drug interactions cease.
2. Long-term monitoring of client.

NONCOMPLIANCE WITH MEDICATION REGIMEN

Assessment

1. Failure to progress; development of complications.
2. Deterioration of physical condition.
3. Inaccurate record of medication administration.
4. Client verbalizes confusion regarding regimen.
5. Client verbalizes lack of confidence in medications.
6. Client depressed and verbalizes self-destructive clues.
7. Client cannot afford to buy medications.
8. Client's limited mobility inhibits his/her going to pharmacy.
9. Client forgetful; does not keep appointments.

Revised Outcomes

Goals remain as stated.

Interventions

Revise teaching plan to incorporate aspect which was not effective previously.

Reevaluation and Follow-up

Long-term surveillance of client.

ORGANIC MENTAL DISORDERS

DESCRIPTION

Organic brain syndrome is an acute or chronic neuropsychiatric disorder caused by impairment of brain cell function. It is the most common psychiatric disorder in the elderly, occurring more commonly in women than in men. Determination of whether the client's condition is acute or chronic is based on the cause of the problem and the prognosis (Table 46-6). Acute brain syndrome is potentially reversible and may be due to infection, drugs, alcohol, trauma, circulatory disturbances, convulsive disorders, disturbances of metabolism, or neoplasms. Chronic brain syndrome (CBS), also called organic mental syndrome (OMS) is always irreversible and is generally due to congenital anomalies, brain injury, or multiple sclerosis. The most common type of chronic brain disorder is cerebral arteriosclerosis, which results in diffuse brain damage due to a loss in the number of neurons present in the cortex or an increase in the number of nonfunctioning neurons (refer to Chapter 25). This problem should not be confused with a single cerebral episode, such as a stroke, which causes focal damage. It is only when there are repeated cerebrovascular accidents that symptoms of chronic brain syndrome are evidenced. Cerebral thrombosis or carotid artery occlusion are also associated with chronic brain syndrome.

A common manifestation of cerebral arteriosclerosis and other organic brain syndromes is confusion. Organic confusion is caused by physical disturbances: electrolyte imbalance, infection, respiratory disturbances, etc. Functional confusion is brain disorder, resulting in organic changes in brain structures.

TABLE 46-6 CAUSATION OF ORGANIC MENTAL DISORDERS

Categories	Examples
Volatile agents	Gasoline, aerosols, glues, paint removers, solvents, lacquers, varnishes, dry-cleaning agents, home-cleaning products (alone or when mixed)
Heavy metals	Lead (paints, ceramic glazes, moonshine whiskey), mercury, arsenic, manganese
Insecticides	DDT, parathion, malathion, diazine
Circulatory disturbances	Atherosclerosis, infarction, hypoxia, hypoglycemia, hypertensive crisis, postcardiac surgery
Metabolic and endocrine disorders	Hepatic disease, uremic encephalopathy, porphyria, thyroid dysfunction, parathyroid dysfunction, adrenal dysfunction, nutritional disorders, Wernicke-Korsakoff syndrome
Senility	Alzheimer's disease, senile dementia
Progressive degenerative diseases	Parkinsonism, Huntington's chorea, multiple sclerosis
Brain trauma	Concussion, contusion, hemorrhage, thrombosis, penetrating wounds, blast effects, electrical trauma
Drugs	Sedatives, stimulants, psychotropics
Infections	Meningitis, encephalitis, neurosyphilis (tabes dorsalis)
Neoplasms, tumors	Astrocytoma, medulloblastoma, meningioma
Seizures	Petit mal, grand mal, focal seizures, psychic seizures

SOURCE: From Haber, J., Leach, A., Schudy, S., and Sideleau, B.: *Comprehensive Psychiatric Nursing*, 2d ed., McGraw Hill, New York, 1982.

PREVENTION

Health Promotion

1. Avoid adverse drug reactions and interactions by careful supervision of medications.
2. Maintain adequate nutrition, especially foods containing thiamine, riboflavin, ascorbic acid and vitamin A.
3. Provide reality-orientation to institutionalized patients.

Population at Risk

1. Occurs more commonly in women.
2. Aged persons who have metobolic imbalances.
3. Aged persons under acute emotional stress.
4. Aged persons with vitamin deficiencies.
5. Aged persons with cirrhosis of the liver.

Screening

Routine psychological assessments.

ASSESSMENT*

Health History

1. Errors in self-administration of drugs.
2. Nutritional deficiencies.
3. High alcohol intake.
4. Recent trauma to head.
5. Convulsion history.
6. Disturbances of metabolism.
7. History of strokes.
8. Recent emotional stress.
9. Confusion:
   a. Organic confusion.
      (1) Recent memory is more impaired than remote.
      (2) Time disorientation occurs within own lifetime or reasonably near future.
      (3) Disoriented in a familiar, easily accessible place.
      (4) Retains sense of self-identity, but misidentifies others (unknowns) as being familiar.
      (5) Visual and vivid hallucinations, usually of animals and insects, are common.
      (6) The client will describe illusions.
      (7) Expresses delusions about everyday occurrences and people.
      (8) Confusion is erratic. There are moments of clearness mixed with episodes of confusion; more pronounced at night.
   b. Functional confusion.
      (1) No consistent difference between recent and remote memory impairment.
      (2) Time disorientation may not be related to client's lifetime.
      (3) Disoriented in bizarre or unfamiliar places.
      (4) Sense of self-identity is diminished.
      (5) Misidentifies others based on a delusional system. (The nurse is a spy or the family member is an enemy.)
      (6) Bizarre, symbolic auditory hallucinations.
      (7) No illusions described.
      (8) Delusions expressed are bizarre and symbolic.
      (9) Confusion is quite consistent. There is no tendency for it to worsen at night.
10. Poor comprehension.
11. Poor judgment.
12. Shallow affect.

Physical Assessment

1. Circulatory impairments may be evident.
2. Trauma.

Diagnostic Tests

1. Electrolyte profile.
2. Low pH, potassium, magnesium and/or protein may cause irritability and confusion.
3. Increased potassium, and low sodium may lead to hallucinations.
4. Refer to Table 46-7 for additional tests.

NURSING DIAGNOSES: ACTUAL OR POTENTIAL

1. Anxiety, mild to moderate, due to memory lapses.
2. Alteration in nutrition: less than body requirements; disorientation and/or memory lapses.
3. Sensory-perceptual deficit: altered sensory integration, chemical alterations or psychological stress.
4. Impairment of thought processes–memory deficit.
5. Potential for injury due to delusional state, disorientation, and/or tendency to wander.

* The assessment is based on Morris' and Rhodes' differentiation between organic and functional confusion.

TABLE 46-7 DIAGNOSIS OF ORGANIC MENTAL DISORDERS

Type of Test	Description
Face-hand test (FHT)	A series of double simultaneous stimulations of the face and hand. Failure to correctly report the touch on the back of the hand is presumptive of cortical neuronal loss.
Mental status questionnaire (MSQ)	Consists of 10 valid and reliable questions that are indicators of a person's mental status. Questions address: orientation for time, place, and person; memory, recent and remote; and general information or "intellectual capacity."
Electroencephalography (EEG)	Examine brain waves. OMD is usually associated with diffuse slowing of brain activity particularly in the temporal area. Reveals specific brain lesions.
Cerebral angiography	Visualization of cerebral vascular tree. Identification and estimation of cortical atrophy and decreased blood supply.
Dynamic brain scan	Intravenous injection of radioactive substance used to identify gross deficiencies in blood flow of major arteries.
Pneumoencephalography	Injection of air into the subarachnoid space to provide more accurate information regarding extent of cortical atrophy.
Ultrasound	Used to detect flow of underlying arteries and to confirm carotid stenosis.

SOURCE: From Haber, J., Leach, A., Schudy, S., and Sideleau, B.: *Comprehensive Psychiatric Nursing*, 2d ed., McGraw-Hill, New York, 1982.

6. Compromised family coping secondary to state of parent; hallucinations; illusions; delusions.

EXPECTED OUTCOMES

1. Immediate.
   a. Client will be oriented to time, place and person within 2 to 5 days.
   b. Delusions, illusions and hallucinations will be relieved within 48 hours.
   c. Memory deficit will be gradually reduced within 3 days.
2. Long-term
   a. Client will be free from injury.
   b. Present weight will be maintained.
   c. Bowel patterns will be maintained.
   d. Family will identify alternative coping strategies to deal with present altered health state.
   e. Family will participate in patient care.
   f. Client will maintain skin integrity. Refer to *Chronic Illness* earlier in this chapter.

INTERVENTIONS

1. Answer questions in short, simple phrases.
2. Continuously assess mental status in order to identify a possible cause of confusion. If medications are altered or withdrawn, changes in behavior should be noted and evaluated.
3. Evaluate fluid and electrolyte balances, as alterations could potentiate confusion (refer to Chapters 28 and 32).
4. Monitor vital signs. Be aware of signs of infection, as an elevation in temperature may contribute to confusion; withdraw toxic substances if present.
5. Do not support disorientation. Instead, encourage return to reality by providing an environment that is reality orienting. The use

of clocks, calendars, familiar surroundings, and the presence of familiar faces (e.g., family) may help reduce confusion.
6. Reduce the amount of change in an environment by keeping it constant and/or stable. Reducing the number of strangers entering the room, avoiding transfers from one environment to another, and stabilizing personnel may be some measures that can be utilized to orient the client to reality.
7. In order to provide a constant environment for the daily patterns, routines should be established and followed as part of daily activities. In addition, calling individuals by name frequently will also remind them of their identity.
8. Avoid nocturnal sensory deprivation, as this may increase confusion. Provide night light; be sure safety needs are met, e.g., side rails, as needed.
9. Administer and monitor medications as ordered. Carefully monitor the effects of all medications on the client. Careful assessment of the client's reaction to such things as stimulants, sedatives, CNS depressants is essential.
10. Provide mental stimulation (radio, conversation). Do not discuss delusional material as this may support or perpetuate the undesired behavior.
11. Encourage meaningful physical activity (making bed, setting table, etc.). Emphasize individual's capabilities when conversing.
12. Keep client out of bed as much as possible, as physical activity may help stimulate mental activity.
13. Support family. At times this is the most realistic goal to accomplish.
14. Involve family in care of client.
15. Provide a safe environment.
16. For added information about nursing care of the client with delusions, hallucinations, and illusions, refer to Chapter 39.

EVALUATION

Outcome Criteria

1. Immediate
   a. Client verbalizes correct time of day and responds to name when addressed.
   b. Client verbalizes recognition of healthcare provider and family members.
   c. Client verbalizes name of institution and/or home address.
   d. Client verbalizes that he/she is not experiencing any unusual sounds or sights.
   e. Client recalls remote past with 80% accuracy and immediate past with 20% accuracy.
2. Long-term
   a. Client is free from ecchymosis, lacerations, and fractures.
   b. Present weight is maintained.
   c. Bowel patterns return to normal.
   d. Client's family is alternating visits.
   e. One family member visits every other day.
   f. Family members verbalize relief from "guilt."
   g. Family is participating in patient's care, i.e., combing hair, cleaning dentures, feeding, etc.

Complications

INJURY TO SELF

Refer to Chapter 38.

DEPRESSION

Refer to Chapter 36.

SUICIDE

Refer to Chapter 38.

SOCIAL ISOLATION

Assessment
1. Verbalizes loneliness.
2. Family members not visiting.
3. No group involvement.
4. Refusal to leave immediate surroundings.

Revised Outcomes
1. Client will verbalize that he or she is not lonely.
2. Family members will visit twice weekly.
3. Client will join group for meals within 7–10 days.
4. Client will join group in day room between meals within 2–3 weeks.

Interventions
1. Meet with family to assess reason no one is visiting.
2. Explore with family acceptable, manageable visiting schedule.
3. Identify additional visitors who may spell the family.
4. Encourage other clients to visit in room for 5–7 days.
5. Encourage client to dine with the group. Have other clients invite him or her.

Reevaluation and Follow-up
Provide a primary care-giver to ensure consistency of care to client and family.

TRAUMATIC INJURIES

ACCIDENTS

DESCRIPTION

Accidents are a major cause of death in those persons 65 years of age or older. If death does not occur at the time of the accident, severe complications frequently result in the demise of the client. Most injuries to the aged are the result of accidental falls. Fractures occur most frequently in those between 75 and 85 years of age. The most common fracture in the elderly is that of the proximal end of the femur, which occurs three times more often in women than in men.

PREVENTION

Health Promotion

1. Remove potential risk factors present in the home environment.
2. Provide adequate lighting (especially at stairs).
3. Provide hand rails that are securely fastened.
4. Remove all throw rugs unless of nonskid type.
5. Limit the use of floor wax.
6. Remove low-lying objects such as footstools.
7. Wear shoes with corrugated soles. Wear ice grippers in the winter.
8. Avoid walking on snow and ice.
9. Limit snow removal activities.
10. Provide adequate time to complete activities so that there is no need to rush.
11. Avoid driving at night.
12. Avoid application of excessive heat.
13. Avoid overexposure to cold.
14. Maintain weight within normal limits.
15. Subscribe to a daily activity program that will maximize physical fitness.
16. Use hospital or low-lying beds and side rails, if appropriate.

Population at Risk

1. Those with intellectual deterioration.
2. Those with chronic diseases.
3. Those with poor vision.
4. Those with poor hearing.
5. Those who cling to habits and possessions of the past.

ASSESSMENT

Refer to Chapters 47, 48, 49.

NURSING DIAGNOSES: ACTUAL OR POTENTIAL

Refer to Chapters 47, 48, 49.

EXPECTED OUTCOMES

Refer to Chapters 47, 48, 49.

INTERVENTIONS

Refer to Chapters 47, 48, 49.

EVALUATION

Refer to Chapters 47, 48, 49.

OTHER HEALTH PROBLEMS

1. Incontinence: Refer to Chapter 44.
2. Constipation: Refer to Chapter 44.
3. Sleep pattern disturbances: Refer to Chapter 44.
4. Hyperthermia and hypothermia: Refer to Chapters 48 and 49.
5. Diverticulitis: Refer to Chapter 33.
6. Cancer: Discussed in Chapters 25–35.

REFERENCES

Chronic Disease and Rehabilitation, The American Public Health Association, New York, 1960, p. 36.

Health Characteristics of Persons with Chronic Activity Limitation, U.S. Department of Health, Education, and Welfare, Rockville, Md., 1976, p. 11. Raymond Harris, "Cardiopathy of Aging: Are the Changes Related to Congestive Heart Failure?" *Geriatrics,* **32:**42–46, 1977.

Locke, S.: "Cerebrovascular Disorders in Later Life," *Working With Older People: Clinical Aspects of Aging*, U.S. Department of Health, Education, and Welfare, Rockville, Md., 1971, p. 56.

Morris, M., and Rhodes, M.: "Guidelines for the Care of Confused Patients," *American Journal of Nursing*, **72**(9):1630, September 1972.

Thomas, K. P.: "Diabetes Mellitus in Elderly Persons," *Nursing Clinics of North America*, **11**(1):158, March 1976.

U.S. Center for Health Statistics: *Blood Pressure Levels of Persons 60–74 Years, United States, 1971–1974*. Vital and Health Statistics, Ser. 11, No. 203, U.S. Department of Health, Education, and Welfare Publication No. (HRA) 78-1648, Washington, D.C., 1977.

BIBLIOGRAPHY

Burnside, I. M.: *Nursing and the Aged*, McGraw-Hill, New York, 1976. This text is a comprehensive, multidisciplinary approach to the care of the aged. It deals with all aspects of aging and the appropriate nursing responsibilities. Nursing process is outlined.

Clark, C. and Mills, G.: "Communicating with Hearing Impaired Elderly Adults," *Journal of Gerontological Nursing*, **5**:40, May–June 1979. This reference discusses causes, results, and assessment of hearing loss in the elderly.

Daniels, L., and Gifford, R.: "Therapy for Older Adults Who Are Hypertensive," *Geriatric Nursing*, **1**:37, May–June 1980. This is an informative reference which gives current recommendations for helping the elderly lower their blood pressure. It addresses detection, dietary and drug management, and complications.

Gotz, B. E., and Gotz, V.: "Drugs and the Elderly," *American Journal of Nursing*, **78**:1347, August 1978. This gives an overview of physiological changes which are the basis for careful attention to drug administration in the elderly.

Kart, C., Metress, E., and Metress, J.: *Aging and Health: Biologic and Social Perspective*, Addison-Wesley, Reading, Mass., 1978. A good introduction to basic aging, this book addresses common health concerns, health maintenance and illness in the aged. It is multidisciplinary in approach.

Miller, J. F.: *Coping with Chronic Illness*, F. A. Davis, Philadelphia, 1983. Outstanding text focuses upon the general concepts of chronic illness, as related to powerlessness. Strategies to cope with health problems associated with chronic illness well described.

Wolanin, M.: "Physiologic Aspects of Confusion," *Journal of Gerontological Nursing*, **7**(4):236, April 1981. Excellent description of causes, manifestations, prevention and treatment of the confused elderly are provided in this article. "Nursing Home Drug Therapy Improperly Monitored, G.A.O. Asserts," *Geriatric Nursing* 152–156, September/October 1980.

NURSING CARE DURING EMERGENCIES

PART VII

PART VII CONTENTS

CHAPTER 47
GENERAL PRINCIPLES OF EMERGENCY CARE 1493

General Assessment **1493**
Basic guidelines 1493
Focused interview 1494

Triage Nursing **1499**
Airway 1504
Bleeding and shock 1506
Consciousness 1507
Digestive organs 1508
Excretory organs 1509
Fractures 1509

CHAPTER 48
TRAUMATIC INJURIES 1511

Musculoskeletal Injuries **1511**
Fractures 1511
Strains 1516
Sprains 1518
Dislocations 1520
Subluxations 1521
Dental emergencies 1522
Maxillofacial trauma 1524

Environmental Exposure Trauma **1526**
Heat stroke 1526
Heat exhaustion 1527
Heat cramps 1529
Localized hypothermia 1530
Systemic hypothermia 1532
Venomous bites and stings 1534
Drowning and near-drowning 1538
Altitude sickness 1541
Decompression sickness 1543

Wounds **1546**
Abrasions 1546
Avulsions 1547
Contusions 1548
Crush wounds 1550
Lacerations 1552
Punctures 1553

Burns **1555**
Thermal burns 1555
Electrical burns 1560
Chemical burns 1561
Radiation burns 1562

Shock **1565**

Respiratory Trauma **1569**
Upper airway trauma 1569
Lower airway trauma 1573

Cardiac and Great Vessel Trauma **1575**

Abdominal Trauma **1577**

Neurotrauma **1580**

CHAPTER 49
MEDICAL EMERGENCIES 1585

Poisonings **1585**
Overdose 1585
Food poisoning 1593
Carbon monoxide poisoning 1596

Endocrine Emergencies **1597**
Ketoacidosis, nonketotic hyperosmolar coma, and hypoglycemia 1597
Acute adrenal insufficiency 1601
Thyrotoxicosis 1602

Cardiovascular Emergencies **1604**

Abdominal Emergencies **1610**

Fever **1613**

Seizures **1616**
Status epilepticus 1616
Febrile seizures 1619

Emergency Delivery **1621**

CHAPTER 50
PSYCHIATRIC EMERGENCIES 1631

Assaultive Behavior **1631**

Rape **1633**

Suicide **1634**

Acute Alcoholic Intoxication **1636**

Acute Grief Reaction **1637**

47

General Principles of Emergency Care

Mary P. Wieland

Emergency department nursing is rapidly becoming a specialty in itself. The purpose of emergency nursing is to assist the client and family in reaching the client's maximum level of "wellness" or health. Often, these results are not seen within the emergency department or within the medical facility.

Nursing functions and responsibilities within an emergency department are determined by hospital policy and the type of facility. Emergency department nursing is as varied as nursing practice itself. However, certain broad categories of knowledge and skill are common to all emergency department nurses. These include:

1. The ability to perform concise, focused histories. (Focus is on the client's chief complaint.)
2. Ability to set priorities of care (triage).
3. Expertise in delivering basic and advanced life-support measures.
4. Knowledge of all age groups and their various health problems (from delivery to specific problems of the elderly).
5. Rapid, thorough use of observational and assessment skills with appropriate nursing interventions (thinking and acting at the same time).
6. Performance of a wide variety of technical and diagnostic skills in an orderly, rapid fashion.
7. Utilization of crisis intervention techniques.
8. Teaching health care (including discharge instructions and referrals).
9. Advocating for clients and managing care.

The combination of this broad nursing knowledge and skilled technical expertise contributes to the ability of each emergency department nurse to be a specialist in acute nursing care.

This chapter will present some of the basic principles involved in emergency department nursing. Emphasis will be on initial assessments and focused interviewing techniques. Specific nursing interventions are presented in subsequent chapters. In addition, the broad concept of triage will be demonstrated by using a model.

GENERAL ASSESSMENT

BASIC GUIDELINES

1. Obtain a quick overview or primary survey (90 seconds or less) of each client.
   a. Respiratory and circulatory function.
   b. State of consciousness.
   c. Evidence of overt bleeding, obvious deformities.
   d. General appearance of the client.
2. Consider the ABCs of lifesaving first with

each client:
   a. Airway.
   b. Breathing.
   c. Circulation.
3. Recognize that nursing assessment and intervention may occur simultaneously in lifesaving situations.
4. The challenge of emergency room nursing is to maintain a calm, relaxed, and reassuring attitude at all times.

FOCUSED INTERVIEW

1. Data sources:
   a. Client.
   b. Family and/or significant others.
   c. Paramedics/prehospital care providers.
   d. Previous hospital or medical records.
2. General guidelines:
   a. Explain the purpose of this data gathering to obtain the cooperation of the client and family.
   b. Introduce yourself and state your function as a health team member.
   c. Provide privacy.
3. Focused history or principal problem history:
   a. Center or "focus in" on the client's chief complaint: "Why did you come to the emergency department?" "What brings you to the emergency department?"
   b. Take this statement in the person's own words; this would be the *subjective* portion of the assessment record: "My stomach hurts."
   c. Elicit details regarding:
      (1) Onset of the problem: "When did this start?" "Have you experienced this before?"
      (2) The interval history: "Did you do anything to try to relieve this?" "What has been happening since this started?"
      (3) Current status or course of symptom: "How are you feeling now?"
4. If possible, have the client describe the chief complaint as to:
   a. Location and radiation.
   b. Character or quality.
   c. Influence symptom has on activities of daily living.
   d. Aggravating and relieving factors.
   e. Accompanying symptoms: see Table 47–1.
5. In addition to the focused interview, obtain information regarding past history with emphasis on:
   a. Allergies to medications, insect stings, pollen, food.
   b. Medications taken to relieve chief complaint and others taken on a routine basis.
   c. Cardiopulmonary disease.
   d. Diabetes mellitus.
   e. Hypertension.
   f. Stroke.
   g. Renal disease.
   h. Prior surgeries/hospitalizations.
   i. When dealing with trauma, such as lacerations and burns, elicit the date of the last tetanus toxoid booster given.
   j. When dealing with obstetrical and gynecological problems, elicit the date of the last menstrual period (LMP).

Perform a thorough but rapid head-to-toe assessment, depending on the client's chief complaint. This will be a general overview of the nursing assessments involved in evaluating several of the body's systems. Please refer to subsequent chapters dealing with the nursing interventions involved with specific problems.

1. Focused systems: history of (see Table 47–1).
2. Head and spinal assessment. Inspection:
   a. Airway patency.
   b. Level of consciousness.
   c. Orientation to time, place, person.
   d. Pattern of breathing.
   e. Pupillary reaction (PERLA, pupils equally reactive to light and accommodation).
   f. Eye movements, nystagmus.
   g. Visual acuity (if appropriate).
   h. Obvious injury:
      (1) Bleeding, cyanosis of mucous membranes.
      (2) Hematomas.
      (3) Presence of foreign objects, cerebrospinal fluid, or blood from ears, nose.
      (4) Asymmetry, deformity.
   i. Response to verbal, tactile, and painful stimuli.
   j. Breath odor.
   k. Neck:
      (1) Distended neck veins.
      (2) Carotid pulsations.
      (3) Scars, discolorations.
   l. Spinal cord injury level (see Figure 47-1 for summary of brief neurological exam-

TABLE 47-1 SUMMARY CHART FOR THE EMERGENCY REVIEW OF SYSTEMS

GENERAL
Present weight (loss or gain, period of time, contributing factors), weakness, fatigue, malaise, fever, chills, sweats or night sweats

SKIN
Pruritus, pigmentary and other color changes, tendency to bruise, lesions (location), excessive dryness, texture, character of hair and nails, use of hair dyes or other possibly toxic agents

HEAD
Headache, head injury (how, when, where), dizziness

EYES
Pain, vision, glasses, recent change in acuity, diplopia, infection, glaucoma, cataract

EARS
Earaches, hearing, tinnitus, vertigo, discharge, infection, mastoiditis

NOSE AND SINUSES
Sinus pain, epistaxis, nasal obstruction, discharge, postnasal drip, frequent colds, sneezing

ORAL CAVITY
Toothache, recent extractions, state of dental repair; soreness or bleeding of lips, gums, mouth, tongue or throat; disturbance of taste; hoarseness; tonsillectomy

NECK
Pain, limitation of motion, thyroid enlargement

NODES
Tenderness or enlargement of cervical, axillary, epitrochlear, or inguinal nodes

BREAST
Pain, lumps, discharge, operations

RESPIRATORY
Chest pain, pleurisy, cough, sputum (character and amount), hemoptysis, wheezing (location in chest), stridor, asthma, bronchitis, pneumonia, tuberculosis or contact therewith, date of recent x-ray, hypertension, night sweats

CARDIOVASCULAR
Precordial or retrosternal pain or distress, palpitation, dyspnea (relate to effort), orthopnea, paroxysmal nocturnal dyspnea, edema, cyanosis; history of heart murmur, rheumatic fever (enumerate the manifestations), hypertension, coronary artery disease, last ECG, diaphoresis, nausea, vomiting

GASTROINTESTINAL
Appetite, food intolerance, dysphagia (solids, liquids), heartburn, postprandial pain or distress, biliary colic, jaundice, other abdominal pain or distress, belching, nausea, vomiting, hematemesis, flatulence; character and color of stools (bleeding, melena, clay colored, diarrhea, constipation), change in bowel habits; rectal conditions (pruritus, hemorrhoids, fissures, fistula); ulcer, gallbladder disease, hepatitis, appendicitis, colitis, parasites, hernia; date of previous x-rays

TABLE 47-1 *(continued)*

GENITOURINARY
Urinary: Renal colic, frequency of urination, nocturia, polyuria, oliguria, micturition (hesitancy, urgency, dysuria, narrowing of stream, dribbling, incontinence), hematuria, albuminuria, pyuria, kidney disease, facial edema, renal stone, cystoscopy
Male: Testicular pain, change in size of scrotum
Female: Vaginal discharge or itching; intermenstrual or postmenopausal bleeding; dysmenorrhea; dyspareunia; urinary stress, incontinence (involuntary passage of urine on coughing, sneezing, stepping off curbs, etc.); uterine prolapse; date and character of last menstrual period; if menopausal, date of onset
Venereal: Gonorrhea, syphilis, herpes—identify by common name and signs; note date, treatment, complications

EXTREMITIES
Vascular: Intermittent claudication, varicose veins or complications, thrombophlebitis
Joints: Pain, stiffness, swelling (note location, migratory nature, relation to known cardiac involvement); rheumatoid arthritis, osteoarthritis, gout, bursitis
Bones: Flat feet, osteomyelitis, fracture
Muscles: Pain, cramps

BACK
Pain (location and radiation, especially to the extremities), stiffness, limitation of motion, sciatica or disc disease

CENTRAL NERVOUS SYSTEM
General: Syncope, loss of consciousness, convulsions, meningitis, encephalitis, stroke
Mentative: Speech disorders, emotional status, orientation, memory disorders, change in sleep pattern, history of nervous breakdown
Motor: Tremor, weakness, paralysis, clumsiness of movement
Sensory: Radicular or neuralgic pain (head, neck, trunk, extremities), paresthesia

HEMATOPOIETIC
Bleeding tendencies of skin or mucous membrane, anemias and treatment, blood type, transfusion and reaction, blood dyscrasia, exposure to toxic agents or radiation

ENDOCRINE
Nutritional and growth history; thyroid function (tolerance to heat and cold, change in skin, relationship between appetite and weight, nervousness, tremors, results of previous basal metabolism tests, thyroid medication); diabetes or its symptoms (polyuria, polydipsia, polyphagia); hirsuitism, secondary sex characteristics, hormone therapy

SOURCE: "Explanation Outline for Recording a History and Physical," University of Illinois Medical Center, 1972 (unpublished); reproduced from Barry, J.: *Emergency Nursing,* McGraw-Hill, New York, 1978, p. 168.

NOTE: Which systems are evaluated will, of course, depend on the nature of the client's problem. Each emergency department should be equipped with a review-of-systems form, so that the nurse can quickly determine the presence of accompanying symptoms. Medical jargon should be avoided.

ination):
(1) Cervical area:
 (a) C5: Client lifts elbow to shoulder height.
 (b) C6: Bends elbow.
 (c) C7: Straightens elbow from flexed position.
 (d) C8 and T1: Hand grasps.
(2) Lumbar area:
 (a) L3: Lifts leg or flexes hip.
 (b) L4 and L5: Extends knee.
 (c) L5: Wiggles toes backward.
 (d) S1: Pushes toes downward.

m. Palpate:
(1) Scalp, gently running fingers through client's hair, looking for:

(a) Tenderness.
(b) Masses, lesions, or hematomas.
(c) Lacerations.
(d) Decompressions.

(2) Facial bones, looking for bruising, depressions, tenderness.

(3) Neck, looking for:
(a) Tenderness.
(b) Stiffness.
(c) Gland enlargement or pain.
(d) Tracheal deviation.
(e) Subcutaneous emphysema.
(f) Distended neck veins.

(4) Carotid and temporal artery for presence of pulse, equality and quality.

(5) Cervical spine for point tenderness.

3. Cardiopulmonary assessment.
a. Focused history (see Table 47-1).
b. Inspection of:
(1) Client's color: pallor, cyanosis.

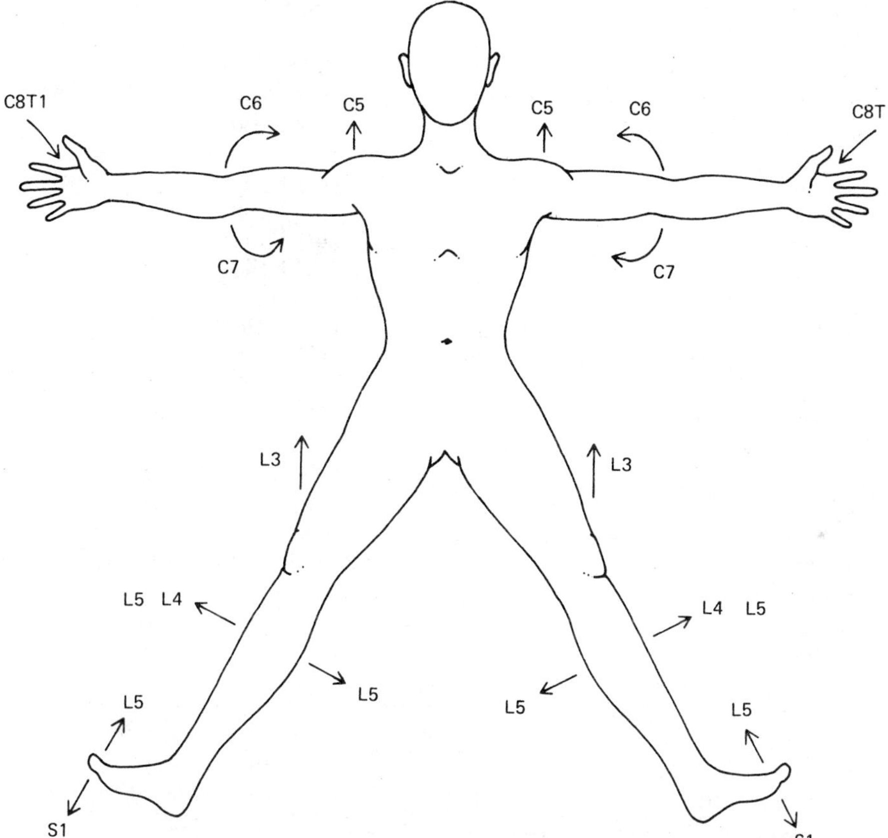

Figure 47-1 Summary chart for brief neurological examination. Starting at the cervical area, ask the client to do the following: (1) *Lift* the elbows up to shoulder height—C5; *bend* the elbow—C6; *straighten* the elbow from a flexed position—C7; *grip*—C8 and T1. (2) *Lift* the leg off the bed or flex the hips—L3; *extend* the knee—L4 and L5; *wiggle* the toes backwards—L5; *push* the toes downward—S1. The client must be checked bilaterally. If the client can do all these, a severe cord injury is not present. If he or she is able to bend the elbows but not extend the elbows, then suspect a lesion between C6 and C7. If the arm function is intact and the chest is moving, but the client is unable to move the legs, then the site of concern is in the upper lumbar area. If the examination shows that one arm moves well but the other arm does not, suspect a nerve root injury on the nonfunctioning side. (From Barry, J.: *Emergency Nursing*, McGraw-Hill, New York, 1978.)

(2) Posture client assumes to facilitate the maximum use of respiratory muscles.
(3) Use of any accessory muscles for breathing.
(4) Rate, character, and depth of respirations.
(5) Bilateral movement of chest wall.
(6) Symmetry of chest wall and contour.
(7) Obvious external injury (abrasions, contusions, scars).

c. Palpate:
(1) Deformities.
(2) Wounds.
(3) Pulses, looking for presence, equality, quality, and PMI (point of maximal intensity).
(4) Contusions.
(5) Abrasions.
(6) Scars.
(7) Evidence of trauma, masses, lesions.
(8) Crepitus.

d. Ascultate:
(1) All lung fields for presence and equality of breath sounds, presence of adventitious sounds.
(2) Heart, noting rate and any abnormalities heard throughout the precordium.

4. Abdominal assessment.
a. Focused history (see Table 47-1).
b. Inspection of:
(1) Texture and color of skin.
(2) Presence of:
(a) Scars.
(b) Wounds.
(c) Rashes.
(d) Striae.
(e) Bruises, discolorations.
(3) Hair distribution.
(4) Abdominal contour (stand at foot of the bed) to check for:
(a) Symmetry.
(b) Bulging, distension.
(c) Hernias.
(5) Abdominal girth.
(6) Noticeable respiratory motion and/or splinting.
(7) Pulsations.
(8) Waves of peristalsis.
(9) Sites of bleeding, including urethral meatus.
c. Auscultate for:
(1) Bowel sounds, noting the quality and rate.
(2) Presence of adventitious sounds, i.e., bruits, friction rubs.
d. Palpate for:
(1) Presence of masses.
(2) Areas of tenderness, rigidity.
(3) Rebound tenderness.
(4) Costovertebral angle (CVA) tenderness.
(5) Deformity.
(6) Quality, equality of femoral pulses.
(7) Pain on symphysis pubis.
(8) Sites of bleeding, including urethral meatus.

5. Skeletal system assessment:
a. Focused history (see Table 47-1).
b. Utilize the five Ps in your evaluation:
(1) Pain.
(2) Pulses.
(3) Paresthesia.
(4) Paralysis.
(5) Pallor.
c. Inspection of:
(1) Color of extremity involved.
(2) Obvious deformities:
(a) Swelling, edema.
(b) Ecchymosis.
(c) Asymmetry.
(3) Voluntary movement.
(4) Open wounds.
(5) Clubbing.
d. Palpate:
(1) Pulses distal to injury for quality and equality.
(2) Areas for:
(a) Pain (with and without manual range of motion).
(b) Tenderness.
(c) Swelling.
(d) Crepitus.
(e) Sensation.
(3) Temperature.

6. Mental (psychological) assessment:
a. Focused history (see Table 47-1).
b. Physical assessment:
(1) Vital signs.
(2) Other specific medical problems.
(3) Nutritional status.
(4) Sleep patterns.
c. Mental assessment:
(1) Behavior:
(a) Social function.
(i) Behavior prior to arrival in the emergency room.
(ii) Change noted.

TABLE 47-2 EXAMPLE OF RAPID ASSESSMENT USING SOAP

S	"I'm having chest pain" (chief complaint). History of sudden onset this morning (onset of the problem) of a sharp, piercing substernal chest pain, nonradiating (location, radiation, character or quality) while climbing a flight of stairs. The pain was not relieved by lying down or by taking aspirin (relieving factors). Denies any dyspnea, diaphoresis, nausea, or vomiting (accompanying symptoms). No prior history of such an incident before, no history of heart disease, respiratory disease, hypertension, or diabetes. Present medications include just ASA prn for an occasional headache.
O	This 40-year-old male appears in good health. VS: BP 138/88, HR 88 regular, RR 16, T 98.6 (oral). Color pale, skin warm and dry. Breath sounds clear in all lung fields. Heart sounds: no observable murmurs. Cardiac monitor—NSR, without ectopic beats. No obvious edema noted.
A	To be evaluated by the ED physician. Follow R/O MI protocol.
P	Carry out R/O MI protocol: lab work, IV, 12-lead ECG, chest x-ray.

(iii) Effect on activities of daily living.

(b) Affect: appropriate or inappropriate expression of emotion.

(c) Speech:

(i) Content, organization.

(ii) Rate, volume.

(2) Internal:

(a) Thought: content and form, e.g., delusions, hallucinations.

(b) Perception.

(c) Cognition.

(d) Orientation.

(e) Memory.

7. Record all data, including:
   a. Focused history.
   b. Vital signs.
   c. Monitoring parameters.
   d. System assessments and interventions: see Table 47-2.

TRIAGE NURSING

The French noun *triage* has been used to define a particular role within the emergency department. Translated, it means "sorting," "choosing," or "setting priorities." The process of setting priorities of care dependent on client assessment is a dynamic one. It occurs throughout the client's stay in the emergency department. Triage may also be done on the telephone.

FUNCTION

1. The function of the triage nurse in the emergency department (see Table 47–3) is to:
   a. Obtain a rapid, concise focused history.
   b. Perform a brief overview of client.
   c. Categorize client as to severity of illness.
   d. Decide proper place of treatment for client.
2. Qualities of the triage nurse:
   a. Accurate clinical judgment.
   b. Tact and efficiency.
   c. Experience in management of emergency clients and their health problems.
   d. Ability to conduct focused interviews with speed and accuracy.
   e. Ability to obtain a quick overview of client's status.
   f. Ability to plan appropriate dispositions of clients by coding the chief complaint as:
      (1) Urgent or nonurgent.
      (2) Critical or routine.
      (3) Emergency or nonemergency.
   g. Knowledge of triage documentation. For example:
      S = "I just cut my finger with a knife about an hour ago."
      O = 1 cm laceration on right middle finger; bleeding controlled with pressure dressing.
      A = Nonurgent; laceration requiring suturing.
      P = To surgical room as soon as suite is available.

TABLE 47-3 RAPID EMERGENCY ASSESSMENT GUIDE

Acute Respiratory Distress

Look for:

Airway obstruction, cyanosis, stridor, chest congestion, decreased heart sounds, rhonchi, rales, diaphoresis, lethargy.

Ask about:

Acute bronchial asthma, chronic obstructive lung disease, trauma, pulmonary edema congestive heart failure.

Emergency actions:

Check for airway obstruction: open airway; remove obstruction, if possible; physician may insert nasotracheal tube or perform emergency cricotracheotomy. Keep client erect if he or she is awake and alert; place client in supine position if he or she is obstructed and not breathing; take vital signs; take ECG; start IV.

Seizure

Look for:

Rhythmic shaking, tonic and clonic motions, eyes rolled back.

Ask about:

Epilepsy, hypoglycemia, head trauma, alcohol ingestion, drug ingestion.

Emergency actions:

Maintain patent airway to prevent lung aspiration. Protect client from injury. Get baseline and follow-up neurological exam. Take vital signs after seizure.

Confirm or rule out:

Epilepsy, electrolyte imbalance, acute alcohol intoxication, drug overdose.

Chest Pain

Look for:

Dyspnea, cyanosis, chest congestion, tachycardia, hypotension or hypertension, vomiting, diaphoresis, tracheal deviation, diminished breath sounds, diminished heart sounds, evidence of chest trauma.

Ask about:

Onset, duration, location of pain; pain quality: stabbing, knife or viselike, burning; activity at onset of trauma; prior history nitroglycerin, rest, nausea.

Emergency actions:

Take vital signs. Start IV fluids. Take ECG. Start oxygen therapy. Give pain medication. Get chest X-ray. Get blood gas workup.

Confirm or rule out:

Myocardial infarction, angina, rib fractures, pulmonary embolus, dissecting aneurysm, pneumothorax.

Suspected Hypovolemic or Cardiogenic Shock

Look for:

Restlessness, cold and clammy skin, pallor, tachycardia, hypotension, mental confusion, disorientation, decreased urine output.

Ask about:

Vomiting, hematemesis; diarrhea, melena, tarry stools; blood loss; history of trauma; history of heart disease; medications; thirst.

Emergency actions:

Start ECG. Start IV fluids (hypovolemic shock). Withhold fluids (cardiogenic shock). Give blood transfusion (hypovolemic shock). Get blood work. Keep warm. Take frequent vital signs. Insert Foley catheter to monitor urine output.

Confirm or rule out:

Severe dehydration, internal hemorrhage, myocardial infarction in progress. Shock: anaphylactic, neurogenic, or septic.

TABLE 47-3 *(continued)*

Suspected Anaphylactic Shock
Look for:
Hives, stridor and chest wheezing, tachycardia, hypotension, dyspnea.
Ask about:
Allergic history, current medications, insect bites.
Emergency actions:
Monitor airway. Start IV. Initiate drug therapy. Take vital signs. Insert Foley catheter. Prepare for intubation.
Confirm or rule out:
Anaphylactic shock, other forms of shock.

Suspected Neurogenic Shock
Look for:
Spinal trauma paralysis.
Ask about:
Length of time since trauma.
Emergency actions:
Keep patient flat. Start IV fluids. Conduct frequent neurological assessment.
Confirm or rule out:
Other forms of shock, severed spinal column.

Suspected Septic Shock
Look for:
High temperature, flushed, dry skin, high or low blood pressure, labored breathing, acidosis, confusion and lethargy.
Ask about:
History of infection.
Emergency actions:
Start IV. Insert Foley catheter. Take blood cultures to find infection source. Administer massive doses broad-spectrum IV antibiotics.
Confirm or rule out:
Source of infection, other forms of shock.

Multiple Trauma
Look for:
Respiratory distress, cardiovascular problems, penetrating wounds, bleeding.
Ask about:
History of events surrounding injury.
Emergency actions:
Assess all systems in this order: resipiratory, vascular, neurologic, gastrointestinal, skeletal. Maintain patent airway. Control hemorrhage. Prevent and treat shock.

Undiagnosed Coma
Look for:
Vomiting, pupillary changes, progressive hemiplegia, decerebrate or decorticate rigidity, convulsions, increased intracranial pressure, bradycardia, widening pulse pressure, respiratory irregularities, dry or clammy skin, fruity breath, alcohol breath, hypothermia, head injury, fever.
Ask about:
How long in coma? History: seizures, diabetes. Drug abuse; type of drug. Trauma or fall, high blood pressure, prescribed medications.
Emergency actions:
Maintain airway. Start IV. Start ECG. Take frequent vital signs. Make frequent neurologic checks. Insert Foley catheter. Prepare for differential diagnosis: dextrose stick, SMA-6,

TABLE 47-3 *(continued)*

drug screen, blood alcohol levels. Administer naloxone (Narcan), if narcotic overdose suspected.

Confirm or rule out:

Diabetic coma, stroke, head trauma, acute alcohol intoxication, drug overdose, electrolyte and acid/base imbalances, hypothermia.

Suspected Acute Alcohol Intoxication

Look for:

Drowsiness, slurred speech, respiratory distress, alcoholic breath, combativeness, hypotension, hypothermia, head injury, pneumonia, contusions, lacerations, hematomas, deformities.

Ask about:

History of alcoholism; how client was found; drug intake.

Emergency actions:

Maintain airway. Start IV fluids. Monitor and observe continuously. Take blood and urine samples. Get x-rays, if indicated.

Confirm or rule out:

Other causes of coma, head trauma, hypertension, seizure disorders.

Suspected Drug Overdose

Look for:

Sedative-hypnotic drugs: respiratory depression, hypotension, hypothermia, dilated pupils, coma, decreased cardiac and renal outputs.

Tranquilizers: respiratory distress, orthostatic hypotension, cardial depression, lethargy, coma, seizure activity (phenothiazines).

Narcotics: respiratory depression, stupor, coma, pinpoint pupils.

Tricyclics: dilated pupils, thirst, decreased bowel sounds, urinary retention, cardiac arrhythmias.

Ask about:

History of drug abuse; what was taken; when it was taken; amount taken.

Emergency actions:

Maintain airway. Administer naloxone (Narcan) to antagonize narcotics. Start IV fluids. Insert Foley catheter. Take vital signs. Start ECG. Make frequent neurological checks. Get blood and urine drug screen. Prepare for peritoneal dialysis.

Confirm or rule out:

Drug or drugs ingested, other forms of coma.

Suspected Diabetic Coma

Look for:

Hypoglycemia: decreased level of consciousness, skin pallor, confusion, weakness, tachycardia, trembling.

Hyperglycemia: malaise, polyuria, fever, hot, dry skin, Kussmaul breathing.

Ask about:

Time of last meal, insulin type and amount, exercise, stress factors.

Emergency actions:

Make dextrose stick glucose level determination.

For hypoglycemia: give immediate bolus of dextrose IV.

For hyperglycemia: give normal saline, not dextrose, IV and insulin (optional). Start constant insulin infusion of correct dosage

Confirm or rule out:

Other forms of coma.

Suspected Electrolyte Imbalance Coma

Look for:

Respiratory distress, hypotension, seizure activity.

TABLE 47-3 *(continued)*

Ask about:
Fluid loss, diuretics, other medications, diabetes, other medical problems.
Emergency actions:
Get SMA-6. Give potassium if indicated.
For acidosis: initiate oxygen therapy as needed. Give bicarbonate if indicated prepare to intubate.
Confirm or rule out:
Other forms of coma.

Severe Abdominal Pain
Look for:
Fever, abdominal distension, hematuria, diaphoresis, diminished or absent bowel sounds, vomiting, abdominal tenderness and rigidity.
Ask about:
Nausea, vomiting, when pain started, exact location, history of radiation therapy, prior history of abdominal pain, whether pain is relieved by eating or drinking milk, whether client has eaten any new or upsetting foods, last bowel movement (fatty, foul, diarrhea, color), pregnancy, vaginal discharge.
Emergency actions:
A differential diagnosis is imperative: management depends on cause; withhold analgesics, which may obscure findings; get pregnancy test.
Confirm or rule out:
Ulcers, gallstones, pancreatitis, appendicitis, abdominal aneurysm, kidney stones, peritonitis, intestinal obstruction, ruptured spleen, ectopic pregnancy.

Lacerations
Look for:
Foreign matter in wound, distal pulses, sensation, ability to move.
Ask about:
Circumstances of injury, whether glass was involved.
For head lacerations: loss of consciousness, period in which unconscious, dizziness, nausea, blurred or double vision, neuro check.
Emergency actions:
Control arterial bleeding; palpate distal pulse.
Confirm or rule out:
Tendon injury, nerve involvement.

Closed and Compound Fractures
Look for:
Edema, ecchymosis, deformity, foreign matter in open wound, diminished distal pulse, loss of sensation (nerve involvement), cyanotic or dusky nail beds.
Ask about:
Circumstances of injury, sensation in affected area, numbness, tingling. Can client move area?
Emergency actions:
Immobilize and keep weight off injury. Elevate limb. Apply ice to closed, swelling fractures. Apply sterile dressing to compound, open wounds. Get x-rays.
Confirm or rule out:
Sprain, strain, tendon involvement, torn ligament, fracture.

Common Nonemergency Complaints
Look for:
Sore throats; upper respiratory tract infections (minor); urinary tract infections; pelvic inflammatory diseases; gastritis; minor injuries to hands, feet, ankles; contusions; sprains; ear infections; mental health disorders (nonviolent).

SOURCE: Ensinger, C.: "Don't Panic!," *RN*, August 1981, 32–36. Copyright © 1981 by Medical Economics Company, Inc., Oradell, N.J. Reprinted by permission.

3. The major components of an effective triage system consist of:
   a. The nature and location of the triage facility in relation to treatment areas.
   b. The personnel performing triage.
   c. The rating system used: see Table 47–4.
4. ABCs of triage with multiple trauma client. Priority order of care (see Table 47–5) modified for any emergency situation: airway, bleeding, consciousness, digestive organs, excretory organs, fractures.
   a. Immediate care = Red alert conditions.
   b. Can wait a short time for care = Yellow alert conditions.
   c. Can be referred to a clinic safely or wait = Green conditions.

AIRWAY

ASSESSMENT

1. Elicit a focused history.
2. Inspection:
   a. Check for patency of airway, tongue occluding pharynx.
   b. Presence of:
      (1) Apnea, dyspnea.

TABLE 47–4 SAMPLE TRIAGE MODEL OR RATING SYSTEM[a]

Category I (Emergency)	Category II (Urgent)	Category III (Nonurgent)
Cardiopulmonary arrests	Unexplained or severe pain	Routine laceration
Unconsciousness	Severe nausea, vomiting; severe diarrhea of infants	Chronic back pain
Obstructed airway	Hemorrhage	Mild headache
Shock	Multiple lacerations	Fatigue
Multiple trauma	Burns: 15% body area in adults; 10% body area in child	Dizziness
Head injuries	Any burns involving face, ears, hands	Nervousness
Spinal injuries	Drug overdose	Minor infection: urinary tract infection (UTI) or upper respiratory infection (URI)
	Poison ingestion	Skin eruptions
	Respiratory distress	Sprains
	Croup in child	Strains
	Asthma	Hernia
	Shortness of breath (SOB)	Gastrointestinal complaints: diarrhea, constipation, hemorrhoids
	Elevated temperature: 103°F in child, 101°F in adult	Dental complaints: abscess, cavities
	Gastrointestinal bleeding	
	Hematuria	
	Oliguria	
	Anuria	
	Suspected fractures of extremities	
	Attempted suicide	
	Pregnancy complications	

[a] Emergency = life-threatening situations; client must be placed in treatment room immediately. Urgent = detrimental to life if not treated within 1–2 h. Nonurgent = stable conditions. This triage model is by no means complete. A triage rating system is based upon the client's chief complaint plus the individual assessment made by the nurse.

TABLE 47-5 MULTIPLE TRAUMA SHEET

Each emergency room should adopt a trauma sheet to standardize assessment and treatment. When completed, the sheet becomes part of the client's medical record. Typically, a trauma sheet contains the following:

Name
Age and sex
Approximate weight and height
Date and time of admission

ASSESSMENT
- History of trauma (time, events, weapons, etc.)
- Pertinent medical history (allergies, medication taken, chronic diseases, disabilities)
- Treatment in progress on admission (check each)
  - ☐ CPR
  - ☐ Airway (oral or nasal)
  - ☐ Intubation
  - ☐ IV therapy
  - ☐ Cardiac monitor
  - ☐ Pressure dressings
  - ☐ Back boards
  - ☐ Splints
  - ☐ Other (explain)

Airway patency
Skin color
Blood pressure (compare to client's normal BP)
Pulse:
- Apical
- Radial

Respiration (regular, tachypneic, apneic)
Breath sounds: left, right (present, diminished, adventitious, absent)
Apparent or possible head injury
Level of consciousness
- ☐ Alert
- ☐ Lethargic
- ☐ Stuporous
- ☐ Unconscious

Pain response
- ☐ Appropriate
- ☐ Decorticate
- ☐ Decerebrate
- ☐ None

Pupillary response to light: left, right
Apparent bleeding sites
Foreign objects (weapons) still in wound
Apparent fractures, dislocations

TREATMENT
- Airway inserted
- Intubation
  - Tube size
  - Oral
  - Nasal
  - Performed by
- Tracheostomy
  - Trach size
  - Performed by
- Diagnostic tests
  - ☐ Complete blood count
  - ☐ Prothrombin time
  - ☐ Partial thromboplastin time
  - ☐ Electrocardiogram
  - ☐ X-ray
  - ☐ Blood type and match
  - ☐ SMA_6
  - ☐ SMA_{12}
  - ☐ Urinalysis
- Fluid therapy
  - Venipuncture or cutdown sites
  - Solutions
  - Amount
- Central venous pressure line inserted
  - Initial reading
- Foley catheter inserted (with Urimeter)
  - Initial amount obtained
  - Color
  - Character
- Peritoneal lavage
  - Intake solution and amount
  - Output (color, character, amount)
- Splints applied
- Medications administered
- Other

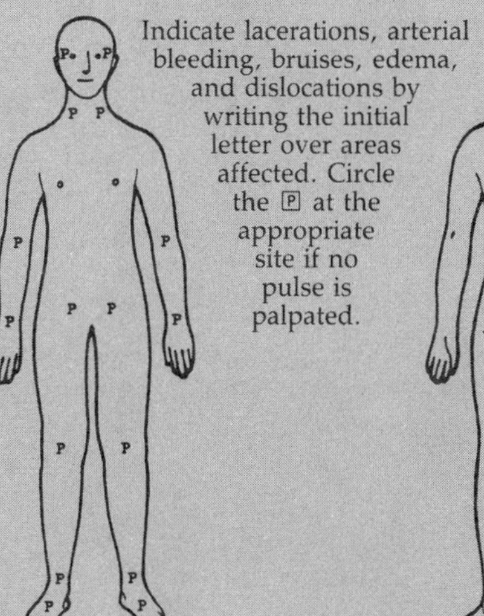

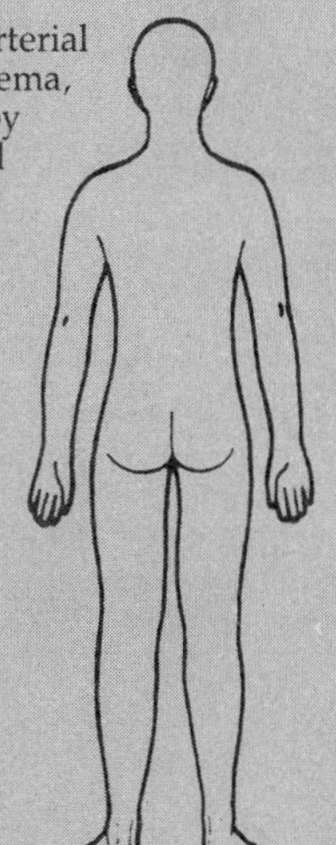

SOURCE: Molyneux-Luick, M.: "The ABC's of Multiple Trauma," *Nursing 77*, **7**(10):30–36, October 1977. Reprinted with permission.

(2) Respiratory rate and rhythm.
(3) Bilateral chest wall movement.
(4) Stridor.
(5) Cyanosis, pallor.
(6) Mucus, blood, misplaced teeth, food particles in oral cavity.
(7) Cough/sputum.

3. Palpation:
   a. For air movement.
   b. For tenderness, crepitus of chest.
4. Auscultation: Listen for breath sounds in all lung fields.
5. Diagnostic tests: Draw and evaluate arterial blood gases.

NURSING DIAGNOSES: ACTUAL OR POTENTIAL

1. Airway clearance, ineffective.
2. Respiratory dysfunction: Breathing pattern, ineffective gas exchange or impaired.

EXPECTED OUTCOMES

1. A patent airway will be provided and maintained.
2. The client will be assisted in optimal ventilation.

INTERVENTIONS

1. Open airway by:
   a. Head tilt/chin lift.
   b. Head tilt/neck lift.
   c. "Modified jaw thrust" for client with head and spinal injuries (see *Neurotrauma* in Chapter 48).
2. With obstructed airway: Perform obstructed airway maneuver (see *Respiratory Trauma* in Chapter 48).
3. Absence of respirations:
   a. Begin rescue breathing:
      (1) Mouth to mouth.
      (2) Mouth to mask.
      (3) Bag mask.
   b. Assist with:
      (1) Endotracheal intubation (or nasotracheal).
      (2) Tracheostomy.
   c. Cricothyroid puncture.
   d. Oxygen therapy.
4. Slow, shallow respirations: Oxygen therapy, evaluate etiology.
5. Faint or absent respirations: Consider hemopneumothorax, assist with chest tube insertion.
6. Noisy, chest wound open: Vaseline dressing to wound.
7. Maintain patent airway with:
   a. Oral airway.
   b. Nasal airway.
   c. Endotracheal tube or tracheotomy.
   d. Frequent suctioning of oral and nasal cavities.
8. Position client for comfort.
9. Provide emotional support to client and family.

EVALUATION

Outcome Criteria

1. Return of spontaneous respirations.
2. Improvement of arterial blood gases.

BLEEDING AND SHOCK

See Chapter 48.

ASSESSMENT

1. Elicit a focused history.
2. Inspection. Look for:
   a. Changes in sensorium, restlessness.
   b. Pallor.
   c. Weakness.
   d. Obvious source (sites) of bleeding.
   e. Decrease in urinary output.
3. Palpation:
   a. Pulses:
      (1) May be irregular, thready, rapid.
      (2) Faint peripheral pulses.
   b. Skin temperature may be cold and clammy.
4. Auscultation:
   a. BP: hypotension dependent on volume.
      (1) Greater than 40 percent of volume lost: moderate to severe hypotension.
      (2) Up to 25 percent of volume lost: moderate hypotension.
      (3) Up to 15 percent of volume lost: slight hypotension.
   b. Listen to breath sounds in all lung fields: Note presence of crackles (rales) or absence of breath sounds.

5. Diagnostic tests.
   a. Type and cross match blood.
   b. CBC; BUN; electrolyte, glucose, hematocrit, and hemoglobin levels.
   c. Appropriate x-rays.

NURSING DIAGNOSES: ACTUAL OR POTENTIAL

1. Cardiac output, alteration in: decreased.
2. Circulation, interruption of.
3. Alteration in fluid volume.
4. Alteration in tissue perfusion.

EXPECTED OUTCOMES

1. Airway management.
2. Bleeding will be controlled or stopped.
3. Tissue and organ perfusion will be improved.
4. Fluid and blood replacement will be provided.
5. Emotional support to client and family will be provided.

INTERVENTIONS

1. See *Airway* for management.
2. Bleeding sites:
   a. Control external hemorrhage with sterile compression dressings.
   b. If wound is on extremity, elevate limb.
   c. Assist with application of hemostats.
   d. Tourniquets are rarely applied.
3. Improve tissue/organ perfusion:
   a. Pulse absent: begin closed chest massage.
   b. Place client on cardiac monitor: assess pulse rate, rhythm.
   c. Deliver supplemental oxygen.
   d. Position client with legs elevated, head flat (if not contraindicated).
   e. Apply MAST trousers (antishock) if ordered (not to be applied if the client is in pulmonary edema).
4. Provide fluid and blood replacement:
   a. Insert at least two large-bore IV catheters.
   b. Administer fluids ordered: Ringer's solution, blood replacement, volume expanders.
   c. Insert Foley catheter.
   d. Monitor fluid status with accurate intake and output recordings.
   e. Assist with insertion of central venous (CVP) lines.

EVALUATION

Outcome Criteria

1. Bleeding stopped or controlled.
2. Hemodynamic status of client returns to pretrauma status.

CONSCIOUSNESS

ASSESSMENT

1. Elicit a focused history.
2. Inspection:
   a. Airway patency.
   b. Respiratory rate and rhythm.
   c. Level of consciousness: describe the behavior of the client.
   d. Pupillary responses: pupils equal and reactive to light and accommodation (PERLA).
   e. Response to verbal, tactile, and painful stimuli.
   f. Movement of extremities.
   g. Temperature rectally or by axilla.
   h. Obvious open wounds, hematomas, drainage of blood or cerebral spinal fluid from ears or nose, presence of foreign bodies.
   i. Any obvious odor of the client's breath (sweet, alcoholic, fetid).
3. Palpation:
   a. Run fingers through hair of scalp looking for lacerations, depressions, foreign bodies, areas of tenderness.
   b. Oral cavity, face, ears, and nose for same.
   c. Pulses noting rate, quality, equality.
   d. Skin temperature.
4. Percussion:
   a. DTRs (deep tendon reflexes) if spinal cord is involved.
   b. Presence of Babinski's reflex.
5. Auscultation. Blood pressure: consider chance of increased intracranial pressure.
6. Diagnostic tests:
   a. X-ray films: skull films, CT scan, cerebral angiography.
   b. Type and cross match blood.

c. CBC, BUN, glucose and electrolyte levels, hemoglobin and hematocrit, and arterial blood gases.

NURSING DIAGNOSES: ACTUAL OR POTENTIAL

Altered level of consciousness.

EXPECTED OUTCOMES

1. Airway management.
2. Frequent assessments will detect increased intracranial pressure and prevent further complications.
3. Emotional support will be provided to the client and family.

INTERVENTIONS

1. Airway maintenance (NOTE: suction with caution).
   a. Assume cervical fracture until x-ray films prove negative. Apply cervical collar, sandbags, backboard; logroll client.
   b. See *Airway* section.
   c. Hyperventilation, to lower the CO_2 and cause cerebral vasoconstriction.
   d. Draw and evaluate arterial blood gases.
   e. Assist with intubation if indicated.
2. Frequent nursing assessments:
   a. Vital signs (BP, pulse, respiration, temperature).
   b. Neurological assessment: consider using Glascow Coma Scale (see Chapter 25).
   c. Response of client to treatments ordered:
      (1) Apply sterile, loose dressing to scalp wounds.
      (2) Assist with debridement of scalp lacerations, Burr holes, and other procedures.
      (3) Monitor response of client to various treatment modalities: steroids, osmotic diuretics, antibiotics.
      (4) Maintain accurate records of intake and output.
      (5) Limit stimulation to the client, provide quiet environment.

EVALUATION

Outcome Criteria

Level of consciousness and integrity of central nervous system are restored.

DIGESTIVE ORGANS

ASSESSMENT

1. Elicit a focused history.
2. Inspection:
   a. Obvious wounds, entrance/exit sites, contusions, abrasions, discolorations.
   b. Protruding organs.
   c. Distension.
   d. Presence of bile, spillage of intestinal contents, abnormal stools.
3. Auscultation:
   a. Bowel sounds: decreasing or absent.
   b. Presence of bruits.
4. Palpation: Areas of pain, tenderness, rigidity.
5. Percussion:
   a. Distention of abdomen.
   b. Rebound tenderness.
6. Diagnostic tests:
   a. CBC, BUN, electolyte, hematocrit, hemoglobin, and amylase levels.
   b. Nasogastric tube insertion.
   c. X-ray: flat plate of the abdomen, perhaps arteriograms.
   d. Peritoneal lavage.

NURSING DIAGNOSES: ACTUAL OR POTENTIAL

1. Alteration in bowel elimination.
2. Impaired digestion.

EXPECTED OUTCOMES

1. Airway management.
2. Fluid and nutritional balance will be maintained.
3. Complications will be prevented.
4. Emotional support to client and family will be provided.

INTERVENTIONS

1. See *Airway*.
2. Restore fluid balance:
   a. Administer IVs ordered.
   b. Deliver blood replacements, if indicated.
   c. Record accurate intake and output.
   d. Provide nutritional support.
      (1) Insert NG tube: note contents and quantity of aspirate.
      (2) Hyperalimentation (not usually instituted in emergency department).
   e. Assist with peritoneal lavage; monitor for vagal response.
3. Prevent complications: Prepare client for sur-

gery, if indicated:
   a. Insert NG tube for gastric decompression.
   b. Assess vital signs frequently.
   c. Administer antibiotics.

EVALUATION

Outcome Criteria

Client is adequately prepared for surgery, if indicated.

EXCRETORY ORGANS

ASSESSMENT

1. Elicit a focused history.
2. Inspection:
   a. Look for contusions, bruises, ecchymosis of flank, areas of bleeding.
   b. Examine color of urine.
   c. Check vital signs.
3. Palpation, looking for:
   a. Areas of tenderness, pain.
   b. Abdominal rigidity.
   c. Presence of flank mass.
   d. CVA tenderness (costovertebral).
4. Diagnostic tests:
   a. CBC, BUN, electrolyte, hemotocrit, and hemoglobin levels.
   b. Urine analysis.
   c. X-ray films: abdominal, IVP.

NURSING DIAGNOSES: ACTUAL OR POTENTIAL

Urinary elimination, alteration in patterns.

EXPECTED OUTCOMES

1. Airway management.
2. Blood volume will be restored.
3. Complications will be prevented.
4. System will be restored to its pretrauma status.
5. Emotional support will be provided to the client and family.

INTERVENTIONS

1. Maintain airway and respiratory status: see *Airway*.
2. Restore blood volume:
   a. Administer IV fluids as ordered.
   b. Insert Foley catheter, if ordered (inform the physician if there is any difficulty passing the catheter).
   c. Maintain adequate intake and output.
   d. Frequent assessments: consider trauma to other systems if client goes into shock.
3. Prevent complications:
   a. Continuous assessment of cardiovascular status, urinary output.
   b. Administer antibiotics as ordered to prevent infection.
4. Assist with radiology studies, preparation for surgery, or admission to the hospital.

EVALUATION

Outcome Criteria

Restoration of pretrauma renal status without complications.

FRACTURES

ASSESSMENT

1. Elicit a focused history.
2. Inspection: Observe all extremities for:
   a. Obvious deformities, asymmetry.
   b. Swelling, color, ecchymosis.
   c. Movement.
3. Palpation:
   a. For pulses.
   b. For pain, tenderness.
   c. For muscle spasm.
   d. For crepitus.
   e. For temperature.
   f. For sensation.
4. Vital signs.
5. Diagnostic tests: Appropriate x-ray films.

NURSING DIAGNOSES: ACTUAL OR POTENTIAL

1. Impaired physical mobility.
2. Potential for further soft-tissue trauma.

EXPECTED OUTCOMES

1. Airway and respiratory status will be maintained.
2. The fracture will be immobilized.
3. Pain will be relieved.
4. Client will return to mobility status he or she had prior to accident.

INTERVENTIONS

1. Maintain airway and respiratory status: see *Airway*.

2. Reduce the fracture:
   a. Immobilize the extremity, splint fractures as they are found:
      (1) Air and traction splints: support above and below the fracture site.
      (2) Apply sterile saline dressings over open fractures.
      (3) Administer tetanus toxoid, antitoxin, or antibiotics if ordered.
   b. Assess vital signs frequently.
   c. Consider potential for blood loss:
      (1) Tibial fracture, can lose as much as 500 to 1,000 mL blood.
      (2) Femur fracture, can lose as much as 1,000 to 2,000 mL blood.
      (3) Pelvic fracture, can lose up to 3,000 mL blood.
   d. Assess frequently the circulatory and sensory status of extremity involved.
3. Relieve pain:
   a. By proper immobilization of fracture.
   b. By changing client's position for comfort.
   c. With analgesics if ordered.
   d. By use of traction devices.
4. Return client to prior status:
   a. Assist with immobilization and reduction.
   b. Prepare client for surgery, if indicated.
5. A multiple trauma sheet (see Table 47-5) may be helpful to provide standardized assessment and intervention.

EVALUATION

Outcome Criteria

Client returns to pretrauma status with few (if any) deficits.

BIBLIOGRAPHY

Barry, J.: *Emergency Nursing*, McGraw-Hill, New York, 1978. This book provides a review of emergency nursing and provides an excellent reference for the physiology, pathophysiology, and assessment information relevant to emergency care.

Budassi, S., and Barber, J.: *Emergency Nursing Principles and Practice*, C. V. Mosby, St. Louis, 1981. An updated presentation on the role of emergency nurses from prehospital to discharge.

Cook County Hospital Nursing Grand Rounds: "Trauma Care: Expect the Unexpected," *Nursing '76*, 6:58–63, June 1976. A thorough presentation of the ABCs of trauma management is provided by this article.

Cosgriff, J. H., and Anderson, D. L.: *The Practice of Emergency Nursing*, Lippincott, Philadelphia, 1975. One of the first and also one of the most comprehensive presentations of emergency nursing, this book covers all the relevant areas of emergency care, including burns.

Estrada, E.: "Triage Systems," *Nursing Clinics of North America*, 16(1):13–24, March 1981. Excellent review of various types of hospital triage systems, roles of triage nurses, and components of triage nursing course.

Mann, J., and Oakes, A.: *Critical Care Nursing of the Multi-Injured Patient*, Saunders, Philadelphia, 1980. Excellent presentation on the use of the nursing process with the multiple trauma client, especially for critical care nurses.

Nelson, D. M.: "Triage in the Emergency Suite," *Hospital Topics*, 32(6):39–41, September 1973. The role of the emergency department nurse as a triage agent is developed in this article.

Slater, R. R.: "Triage Nurse in the Emergency Department," *American Journal of Nursing*, 70(1):127–129, January 1970. This article is considered a classic in emergency nursing literature, as it was probably the first publication to identify the concept of the triage nurse.

Stephenson, H. E.: *Immediate Care of the Acutely Ill and Injured*, Mosby, St. Louis, 1974. Although relatively general in nature, this book presents a comprehensive review of trauma management.

Vayda, E., and Gent, M.: "An Emergency Department Triage Model Based on Presenting Complaints," *Canadian Journal of Public health*, 64(3):246–253, May–June 1973. This article presents a physician's system for classification of emergency problems into categories.

Vickeray, D. M.: *Triage: Problem-Oriented Sorting of Patients*, Robert Brady, Bowie, Md., 1975. This book presents the most comprehensive review of triage according to the problem-oriented medical records approach.

Wells-Mackie, J. J.: "Clinical Assessment and Priority-Setting," *Nursing Clinics of North America*, 16(1):3–12, March 1981. Review of emergency room nursing assessment.

48

Traumatic Injuries

Marilyn de Give and Annalee Oakes

MUSCULOSKELETAL INJURIES

FRACTURES

DESCRIPTION

A fracture is a trauma-induced discontinuity of bone. Fractures are accompanied by soft-tissue damage to adjacent structures, particularly vascular and perivascular tissue. Fracture usually results in immobility; the degree depends on the location, type, and extent of the injury. Figure 48-1 shows varieties of fracture. Other common categories include:

1. *Closed* fracture (also called *simple* fracture): skin remains intact so that bacteria cannot pass through the wound to the bone (opposite of *compound,* or *open* fracture).
2. *Complicated* fracture: the broken bone has damaged an internal organ.
3. *Compound* fracture (also called *open* fracture): the broken bone is exposed to exogenous bacteria, for example, when the bone is driven through the overlying skin or when a foreign body has penetrated to the fracture.
4. *Depressed* fracture: a portion of the bone is displaced inward from its normal position; for example, a depressed skull fracture is one in which a piece of the bony plate is forced inward toward the brain.
5. *Pathologic* fracture (also called *spontaneous* fracture): a fracture that occurs in the presence of some underlying bone disease and results from a mild injury that would not damage normal bone.

Certain injuries produce their own characteristic fractures, so that the history of the incident may help identify what damage the skeletal system has sustained. For example, whiplash sustained during an automobile collision may fracture the second cervical vertebra, while breaks in the patella and the posterior lip of the acetabulum are often caused when the victim strikes the dashboard in a seated position.

PREVENTION

Health Promotion

1. Public education programs: automobile seat belt campaigns, bicycle safety education, driver training courses, and so on.
2. Reduction of exposure to unsafe environments: water spilled on uncarpeted floor should be wiped up, playground hazards should be corrected, icy stairs should be deiced, and so forth.
3. Special safety precautions for high-risk persons: waist belts for people who work on scaffolds, for example.

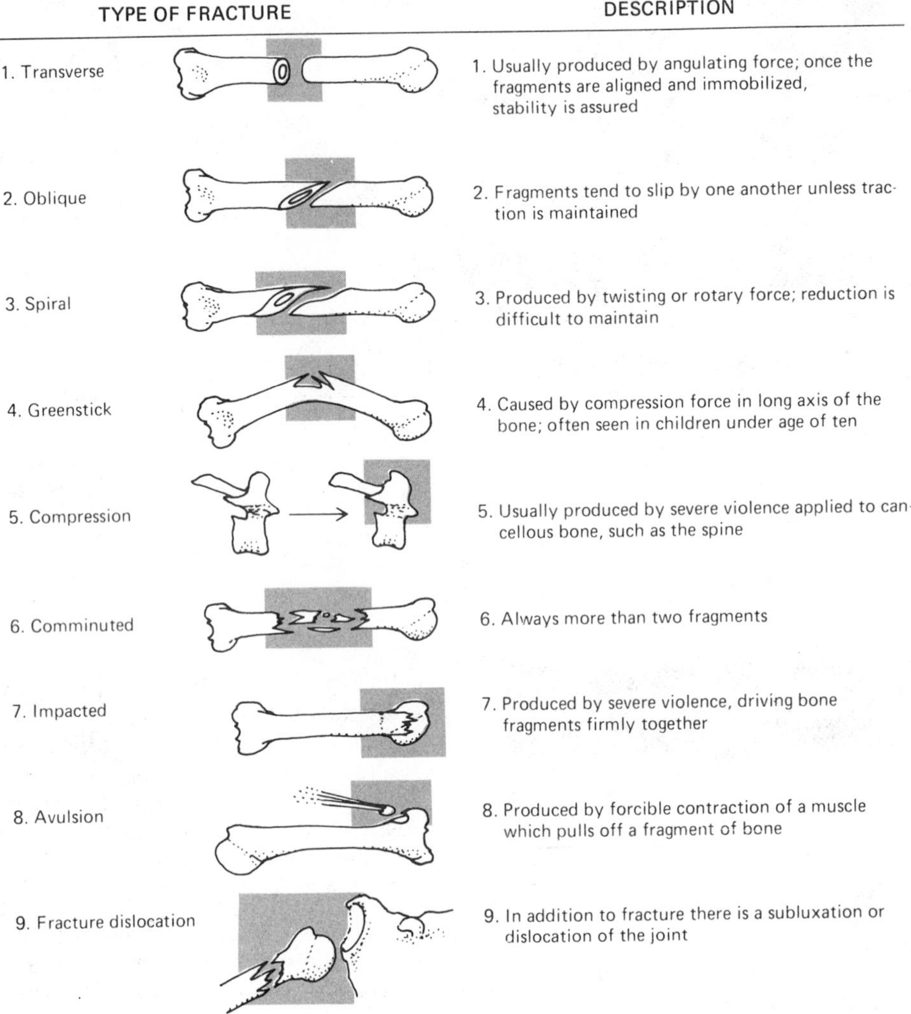

Figure 48-1 Types of fractures. (From Barry, J.: *Emergency Nursing*, McGraw-Hill, New York, 1978.)

Population at Risk

1. Everyone, but particularly those who have impaired coordination, poor judgment, or perceptual limitations such as impaired eyesight.
2. Persons with diminished bone strength, such as elderly women with osteoporosis and persons with bone cancer.
3. Persons who engage in high-risk activities or occupations: mountain climbers, auto racers, athletes, and so forth.
4. Each age group tends to have special risks: school-age children break clavicles and wrists by falling from trees, elderly people break hips and wrists by falling in their homes or yards, and so forth.

Screening

1. History (description of the accident).
2. X-ray films.

ASSESSMENT

Health History

1. History of previous bone or joint disorders and injuries.
2. Extent of disability imposed by this injury.
3. Description of this incident (certain types of trauma produce certain fractures).
4. Pain is usually present.

Physical Assessment

1. Deformity of the injured area (shortening, rotation, abnormal angulation) may be present.
2. Abnormal mobility may occur.
3. Loss of function and intolerance of weight bearing are common.
4. Muscle spasm around fractured bone causes pain, swelling, and shortening of the limb.
5. Fractured bones when palpated may produce a grating sound (bony crepitus) or a rocking motion.
6. Local reactions may include redness and warmth, pallor and coolness, or bruising.
7. Assess integrity of skin and other tissues overlying the fracture: compound fractures are frequently contaminated by dirt, chemicals, or clothing fragments; interstitial air may produce tissue crepitus.
8. Assess sensation: fractures may tear or impinge upon nerves or blood vessels. For example, fracture of the head of the humerus or ulna often causes altered sensation in the fourth and fifth digits or the palmar and dorsal hand surfaces. Vertebral fracture may result in loss of sensation.
9. Assess perfusion: fracture may interfere with blood supply because vessels are torn, pinched, or compressed by swelling (swelling confined within a fascia compartment of a muscle can compress the blood vessels that traverse that compartment, creating ischemia—*compartment syndrome*). Signs of poor perfusion include blanching, slow capillary filling, decreased or absent pulses distal to the injury, and coolness of the extremity as compared to the contralateral extremity.

Diagnostic Tests

1. X-ray films identify the fracture site and type.
2. Complete blood count (CBC) and differential identify extracellular fluid shifts.
3. Urinalysis: myoglobin in the urine indicates extensive skeletal muscle injury.

NURSING DIAGNOSES: ACTUAL OR POTENTIAL

1. Risk of progressive soft-tissue injury secondary to skeletal instability at the fracture site.
2. Alteration of fluid balance secondary to hemorrhage and fluid shift to interstitial tissues.
3. Decreased cardiac output: shock secondary to altered fluid balance.
4. Increased risk of infection secondary to loss of skin integrity.
5. Increased risk of embolus secondary to tissue trauma (e.g., fat embolus or circulating tissue debris).
6. Increased risk of acute cardiorespiratory failure secondary to embolus, shock, or disseminated intravascular coagulation (DIC).
7. Alteration in comfort: pain and discomfort secondary to injury, treatment (immobilization, itching under cast, etc.), or complications.
8. Alteration in mobility and self-care, mild to severe, secondary to injury, treatment (casts, etc.), or complications (nerve damage, etc.).
9. Impaired neurologic function: peripheral nerve damage associated with fracture or due to ill-fitting cast.
10. Altered self-concept secondary to self-care deficit, impaired mobility, or alteration in appearance.
11. Knowledge deficit about self-care and client's role in the treatment regimen.

EXPECTED OUTCOMES

1. Client will be protected against further soft-tissue injury by immobilization of the fracture in proper anatomical position.
2. Shock will be prevented or minimized; client will be adequately hydrated.
3. Infections of the skin, underlying soft tissues, and bone will be prevented or adequately treated.
4. Embolus will not occur or will be promptly recognized and treated.
5. Cardiorespiratory sufficiency will be maintained.
6. Client will be comfortable to the greatest extent compatible with injury.

7. Client will achieve maximum mobility and self-care compatible with the extent of injury and activity tolerance.
8. The prefracture functional capacity of the injured part will be restored.
9. Client will demonstrate acceptance of temporary or permanent body changes.
10. Client will cooperatively and knowledgeably participate in the treatment plan.

INTERVENTIONS

1. Apply protective splints at scene of accident to realign to anatomical position *if possible: great care* must be taken not to disrupt the vasculature. Immobilize with padded splint boards, slings, bandages, air splints, or traction splints, such as Thomas' splint with or without Buck's skin traction (see Figures 48-2 through 48-5). Pad joint protuberances above and below the injury when splinting.
2. Support injured extremity and maintain traction during any repositioning.
   a. Log-roll client with suspected spinal fracture.
   b. Do not flex, extend, or rotate neck if cervical fracture is suspected.
3. Stop open bleeding with pressure dressings or absorbent sterile dressings; estimate blood loss. Place cold packs around affected area and elevate extremity above heart level to minimize swelling.
4. Remove from wound all foreign materials that may be difficult to remove later or that may cause constriction.
5. Monitor vital signs. Monitor capillary filling, pulse, skin temperature and color, and sensation (including pain) of injured extremity; client should be able to move digits of injured extremity.
6. Monitor prescribed intravenous fluids. Withhold oral intake if surgery is anticipated.
7. Monitor wound for indications of infection (induration, drainage, odor); observe client for temperature elevation. Administer antibiotics as prescribed.
8. Monitor client's cardiorespiratory function, especially observing multiple trauma clients for sudden changes associated with pulmonary embolus. If facial fractures are known or suspected, maintain open airway.
9. Assist client to position of comfort permitted by injury. Elevate injured part. Administer analgesia as prescribed. Maintain traction to minimize muscle spasm. Provide general comfort measures, for example, back massage.
10. Maximize client's self-care capacity by rearranging furniture, applying walking heel to leg cast, training client in crutch walking, and so forth. Provide assistance (and help client plan home care) as required.
11. Assess neurologic function (sensation, movement of fingers or toes) and teach client to report immediately any loss of sensation or movement, especially if going home with a new cast.
12. Observe client for self-concept adequacy, watching for and counseling about problematic issues such as guilt, hostility, anxiety, self-absorption, and so forth out of proportion to the real situation.
13. Teach client about the injury and the treatment plan.
    a. Prevention and recognition of common complications.
    b. Care of splinted extremity.
    c. Activity limitations.
    d. Cast care:
       (1) Keep cast dry.
       (2) No autographs for 24 hours; cast takes 24 to 48 hours to dry.
       (3) Symptoms of circulatory or neurological impairment must be reported immediately.
       (4) Cast is not to be painted entirely (paint clogs pores and impedes air circulation to skin).
       (5) Clients casted in outpatient department should return for circulation check the next day.

EVALUATION

Outcome Criteria

1. Fracture is promptly immobilized and avoidable soft-tissue trauma does not occur.
2. Shock is averted and fluid balance is reestablished within 24 hours of the injury.
3. Infection is prevented or successfully treated.
4. Client maintains cardiorespiratory function without evidence of embolus.
5. Muscle spasms are alleviated when traction is applied; other pain and discomfort are decreased.

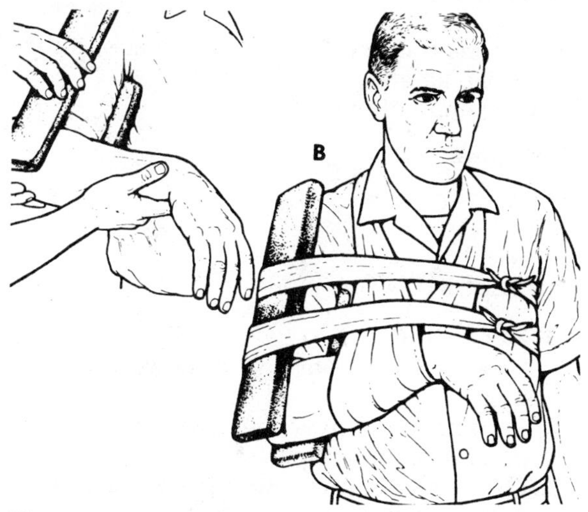

Figure 48-2 Temporary splinting for broken arm, using splints and three cravats. (From Henderson, J.: *Emergency Medical Guide*, 4th ed., McGraw-Hill, New York, 1978. Reproduced with permission.)

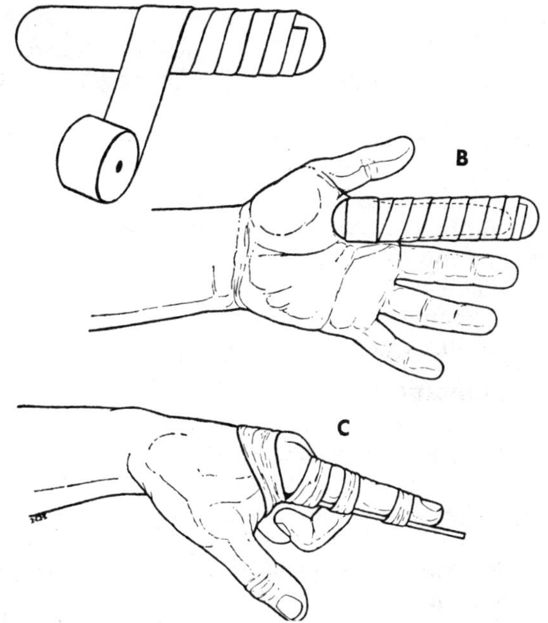

Figure 48-3 Using a tongue depressor to make a finger splint. (From Henderson, J.: *Emergency Medical Guide*, 4th ed., McGraw-Hill, New York, 1978. Reproduced with permission.)

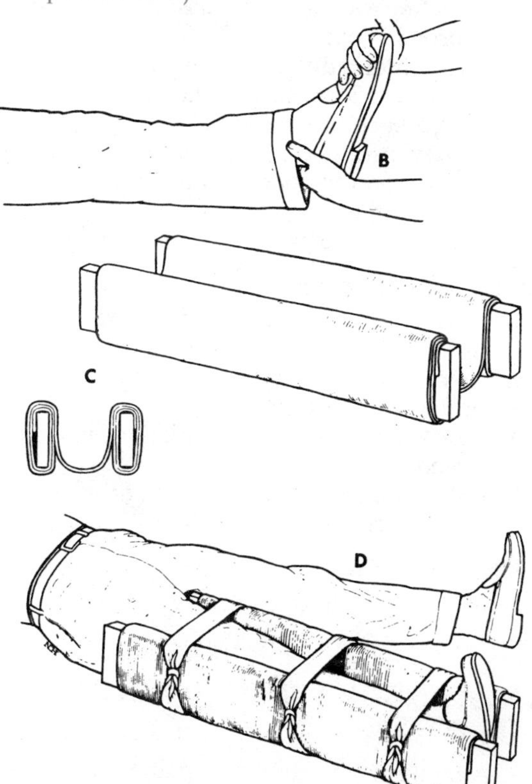

Figure 48-4 Improvised splinting of a fractured leg. Hold the foot and apply gentle traction while splints are being applied. (From Henderson, J.: *Emergency Medical Guide*, 4th ed., McGraw-Hill, New York, 1978. Reproduced with permission.)

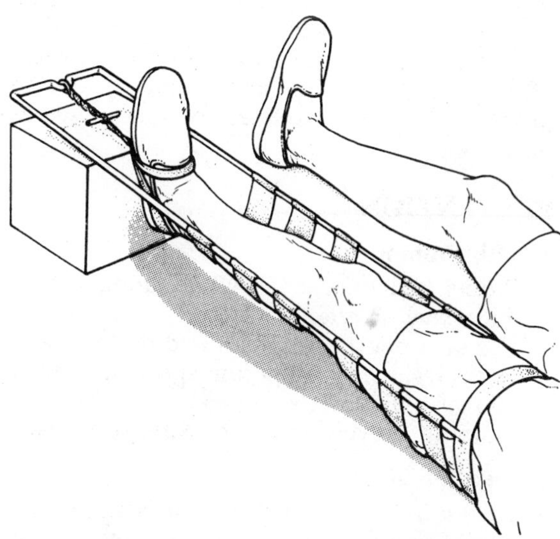

Figure 48-5 Thomas splint applied. (Adapted from Flint, T., and Cain, H.: *Emergency Treatment and Management*, 5th ed., Saunders, Philadelphia, 1980.)

6. Client moves about and provides self-care to the extent safely permitted by physical condition.
7. Fractured part regains normal function after healing is complete.
8. Client demonstrates adequate self-concept and body image by resuming usual activities and interpersonal relations.
9. Client cooperates in plan of care—observes recommended activity restrictions, keeps follow-up appointments, and so on.

Complications

1. Circulatory obstruction.
2. Neurological impairment.
3. Permanent deformity.
4. Permanent impairment of mobility or function.
5. Psychosocial sequelae of the injury or its consequences.
6. Bone or joint infection: osteomyelitis or septic arthritis.

STRAINS

DESCRIPTION

A strain is an overstretching of a single muscle or group of muscles, which results in tearing of the individual fibers or overstretching and rupturing of the related tendon. These injuries are usually due to a violent twisting or pulling movement. The common causes are improper lifting and carrying of heavy loads, sports injuries, and accidents related to work or recreation.

PREVENTION

Health Promotion

1. Proper body mechanics when lifting or moving heavy objects.
2. Use of support equipment and protective devices designed for specific sports and recreational activities.
3. Training for vocational or sports activities.

Population at Risk

1. Heavy industrial workers, for example, loggers, fishermen, and furniture movers.
2. Persons engaged in highly active and competitive sports.
3. Persons training in the physical arts, for example, karate.
4. Weekend gardners.

Screening

None.

ASSESSMENT

Health History

1. Type of work, physical activity, usual lifestyle.
2. Repeated or chronic musculoskeletal injuries (i.e., weakness of part).
3. Use of clothing or shoes particular to occupation or vocation.
4. Age and general physical condition.
5. History of this injury. The client may describe a sprain injury thus:
   a. Characterized by sudden light "pop" or feeling of "tearing" associated with vigorous activity.
   b. In older adults, leg muscle strains may produce forewarning pain a day or two before becoming severe.
   c. May produce no discomfort initially but excruciating pain with first movement after injury.
   d. Pain is described as severe or excruciating.

Physical Assessment

1. Generally, the patient demonstrates limited mobility (or hypermobility); stiffness.
2. There may be swelling, ecchymosis, and tenderness to touch.
3. Muscle spasms and fasciculations may be observed.
4. The client may demonstrate a "drop" or "lag" of the part.

Diagnostic Test

X-ray film to rule out fracture.

NURSING DIAGNOSES: ACTUAL OR POTENTIAL

1. Alteration in comfort: pain secondary to trauma.
2. Reduced mobility secondary to trauma and pain.
3. Altered self-concept secondary to impaired mobility and prosthetic hardware (brace).

EXPECTED OUTCOMES

1. The pain and muscle spasms will be reduced within 2 to 3 hours of initial treatment.
2. Uncomplicated healing will occur as evidenced by gradual and progressive return of function. (Healing time is dependent on extent and severity of injury.)
3. Patient will accept alteration of functional capacity and body image change as demonstrated by consistently complying with the treatment plan.

INTERVENTIONS

1. Rest the strained part in the most comfortable position, preferably anatomical alignment.
2. Immediately treat with cold until hyperemic phase and inflammatory reaction subside (12 to 24 h); follow with heat, preferably dry and constant.
3. Give analgesics such as aspirin, meperidine (Demerol), propoxyphene (Darvon), or phenylbutazone (Butazolidin). Aspirin and Butazolidin reduce inflammation as well as pain.
4. Give muscle relaxants such as diazepam (Valium) or phenylbutazone (Butazolidin) to reduce spasms and fiber shortening.
5. If patient is not allergic to adhesive tape, strap injured part with adhesive tape (elastic bandage is a second choice). Start by fastening the first strip around the affected area but not joining ends; apply subsequent strips parallel and overlapping the preceding strip by 1 to $1\frac{1}{2}$ in. Continue above and below strained area until there is sufficient support (see Figure 48-6). Modify for specific strains. Tell client to keep tape dry and have it removed if blisters develop. Commercially available supports and binders with Velcro fasteners may be used instead of tape or elastic bandage.
6. Elevate extremity for 2 to 3 days to promote lymphatic and circulatory drainage from the traumatized tissue, thus reducing swelling.
7. Teach non-weight-bearing crutch walking if strain is in lower extremity.
8. Using printed instructions and demonstration, teach client how to utilize proper body mechanics when required to lift or move heavy loads. Help client to recognize high risk situations and avoid a repeat strain.
9. Surgery may be required for reattachment or repair of injured tendon.

EVALUATION

Outcome Criteria

1. The strained area becomes relaxed and less hyperemic and swollen under treatment.
2. The client demonstrates a return of full range of motion without discomfort within 3 to 7 days after treatment is started.
3. The patient assumes proper body mechanics

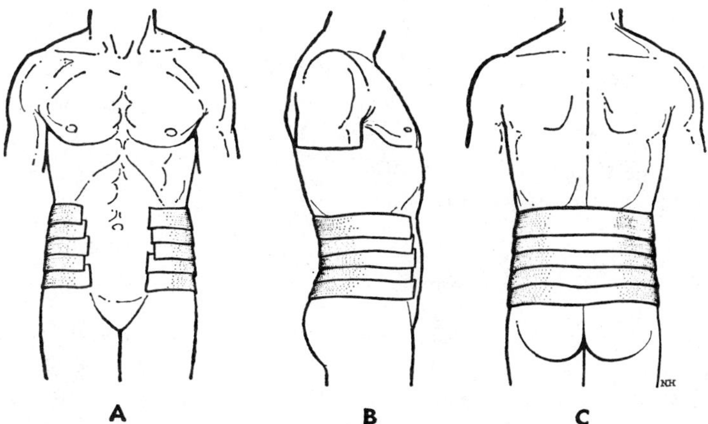

Figure 48-6 Method of providing a firm adhesive tape support for injuries of lower back, particularly useful in treatment of sacroiliac strain. (From Henderson, J.: *Emergency Medical Guide*, 4th ed., McGraw-Hill, New York, 1978. Reproduced with permission.)

throughout all daily activities as indicated by avoidance of repeated injury.
4. The taped region is free of blisters, reddening, or irritation.

Complications

1. Inflammations such as periostitis or myositis ossificans.
2. Circulatory compromise from improper bandaging technique.
3. Blisters and tape burns.
4. Persistent pain and limited movement due to continued irritation of muscle fibers or ruptured tendon.
5. Nonunion of ruptured tendon end and its attachment site on bone.

SPRAINS

DESCRIPTION

Sprains are stretching and/or tearing injuries involving the ligaments of a joint or the joint capsule itself. They may be mild, with only a small amount of ligamentous and soft tissue damage; the client then typically does not seek treatment for 1 or 2 days after the injury. Severe sprains may be difficult to distinguish from fractures, especially avulsion fractures (see Figure 48-1). This differentiation is important, especially in industrial injuries and public liability cases. A sprain may be severe enough to pull off a bone chip, especially in ankle injuries (sprain fracture).

PREVENTION

Health Promotion

1. Comfortable, well-fitting shoes or boots are protective for walking on rough or sloping terrain.
2. Encourage proper and safe training for hazardous sports: track, soccer, basketball, skiing, diving, football, tennis, softball, handball, and so forth.
3. Support the use of seat belts and head rests, which reduce the risk of whiplash injuries accompanying auto accidents, particularly rear-end collisions.
4. Reduce misjudgment of near-vision obstacles (steps, curbs, small animals, rugs, etc.) by recommending periodic eye examinations and corrective lenses as needed.

Population at Risk

Same as for *Fractures* and *Strains*.

Screening

None.

ASSESSMENT

Health History

1. Previous sprains of affected part may indicate a musculoskeletal weakness or propensity for accidental injury.
2. Client actively engages in heavy physical sports.
3. Work patterns suggest high probability for sprains.
4. History of this injury:
   a. Abrupt twisting or stretching injury involving a joint.
   b. Onset and duration of injury are like those for fractures and strains.
5. Severe pain at the site, with or without touch.
6. Pain on movement or weight-bearing at the affected joint.

Physical Assessment

1. Swelling.
2. Discoloration: ecchymosis in 1 or 2 days.
3. Diminished mobility of the joint.
4. Muscle spasms may be present in adjoining musculature.

Diagnostic Test

X-ray examination to rule out fracture.

NURSING DIAGNOSES: ACTUAL OR POTENTIAL

1. Alteration in comfort: pain secondary to trauma.
2. Reduced mobility secondary to trauma and pain.
3. Altered self-concept secondary to impaired mobility and prosthetic hardware (brace).

EXPECTED OUTCOMES

1. The pain and muscle spasms will be reduced within 2 to 3 hours of initial treatment.
2. Uncomplicated healing will take place as evidenced by gradual and progressive return of function.
3. Client will accept alteration of functional capacity and body image as demonstrated by consistently complying with the treatment plan.

INTERVENTIONS

1. Place sprained part at complete rest: immobilize.
2. Elevate extremity.
3. Apply cold packs or ice bags to affected part until swelling stabilizes, approximately $\frac{1}{2}$ to $1\frac{1}{2}$ days. Then follow with heat applications.
4. Apply elastic bandage for support and partial immobility; check circulation frequently (color, warmth, swelling below bandage) (see Figure 48-7).
5. Tape extremity sprains according to accepted protocol and with extremity in proper anatomical alignment.
6. Give prescribed analgesics such as aspirin, Empirin, propoxyphene (Darvon).
7. Restrict activity until firm strapping is applied and swelling reduced.

EVALUATION

Outcome Criteria

1. Pain is promptly decreased with treatment.
2. Swelling gradually decreases. This may take a week or two.
3. Client restricts activity as recommended.
4. Joint function is gradually resumed at preinjury level.

Complications

1. Circulatory compromise caused by incorrect bandaging.
2. Permanent reduction of joint mobility.

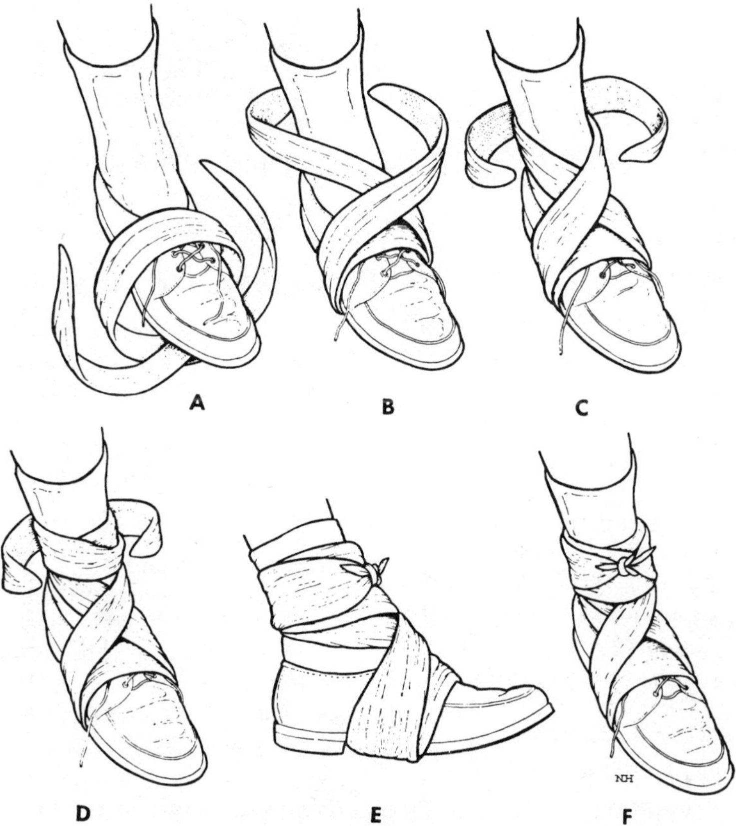

Figure 48-7 Method of applying temporary support to injured ankle by using a figure-eight cravat over a shoe that has been loosened to allow for swelling. (From Henderson, J.: *Emergency Medical Guide*, 4th ed., McGraw-Hill, New York, 1978. Reproduced with permission.)

DISLOCATIONS

DESCRIPTION

Dislocation is displacement of a bone from its joint so that usually articulating surfaces are no longer in proper contact. For example, dislocation at a ball-and-socket joint causes the ball to become dislodged from the cup. Dislocations occur because the joint exceeds the range of motion of which it is capable.

PREVENTION

Health Promotion

1. Prevention of falls.
2. Use of automobile seat belts.
3. Proper training for athletics and use of protective garments (e.g., shoulder pads) while performing.

Population at Risk

1. Athletes.
2. All persons involved in falls, automobile collisions, and other forceful body impact accidents.
3. Abused children and adults.

Screening

X-ray examination to rule out fracture.

ASSESSMENT

Health History

1. History of injury:
   a. Sudden twist forcing joint beyond its usual range of motion.
   b. Sudden impact or blunt injury in which force is transmitted directly to the joint.
2. History of previous dislocations (recurrences are not unusual, especially if therapeutic immobilization is not maintained after the first dislocation).
3. Client may describe joint as "locked."

Physical Assessment

1. Pain is usually severe.
2. Joint deformity: distortion of anatomical positioning and surface landmarks.
3. Inability to move the joint: client usually prefers to hold the dislocated part "hanging" down or free.
4. Swelling of adjacent soft tissues.
5. Muscle spasms.
6. Assess for accompanying fracture of same or adjacent area (see *Fractures*, physical assessment section, earlier in this chapter).

Diagnostic Tests

X-ray films are taken before any attempt to reduce the dislocation.

NURSING DIAGNOSES: ACTUAL OR POTENTIAL

1. Alteration of comfort: pain secondary to trauma.
2. Alteration of mobility: immobility of affected joint due to dislocation.
3. Alteration of self-concept associated with impaired mobility and temporary deformity.

EXPECTED OUTCOMES

1. Joint will be returned to normal anatomical position and preinjury function.
2. Client will be restored to comfort.
3. Client will accept changes in self-concept, including body image, as demonstrated by compliance with treatment (stabilizing bandages, temporary activity restrictions, etc.).
4. Reinjury will not occur.

INTERVENTIONS

1. Refer client immediately to physician so the dislocation can be manually reduced early, while soft-tissue reaction to the injury is minimal.
2. Withhold oral intake if anesthesia is anticipated (for open reduction or difficult closed reduction).
3. Administer analgesia as prescribed (aspirin, muscle relaxants).
4. Immobilize reduced joint by sling, dressing, tape, or chin strap as appropriate; instruct client about recommended activity restrictions.
5. Teach client safety precautions to avoid repeat dislocation.

EVALUATION

Outcome Criteria

1. Dislocation is promptly reduced by physician.
2. Client is pain-free within a few hours of reduction.

3. Client conforms to treatment plan.
4. Full mobility and strength of joint are restored.
5. Dislocation does not recur.

Complications

1. Residual instability of joint.
2. Complications of accompanying fracture.
3. Circulatory or neurological impairment from dislocation.

SUBLUXATIONS

DESCRIPTION

Subluxation is partial dislocation of a joint (dislocation is described immediately above). Some degree of soft-tissue and joint structure damage is usually associated.

PREVENTION

Health Promotion

1. Prevention of falls.
2. Use of automobile seat belts.
3. Training for athletic events and proper use of protective clothing (e.g., football pads).
4. Proper techniques for lifting infants and small children (not by the hands and arms).

Population at Risk

1. Athletes.
2. All persons subject to falls, automobile collisions, and other forceful body impact accidents.
3. Principal victims are young children who have been lifted or jerked by the hands or arms (the radius subluxates at the elbow).
4. Square dancers, especially if elderly (elbow and shoulder subluxations).
5. Young children who swing from gym bars (elbow and shoulder subluxations).
6. Abused children and adults.

Screening

None.

ASSESSMENT

Health History

1. Obtain description of physical force leading to symptoms:
   a. Sudden harsh pull, as when a child is jerked or lifted up a step.
   b. Sustained pull, as from swinging on gym bars or square dancing maneuvers.
   c. Fall or other forceful impact, especially while the affected joint was in extension.
2. Pain may be mild to severe.
3. Impaired mobility: reluctance to use joint.

Physical Assessment

1. Immobility of affected extremity: client may treat extremity as "paralyzed."
2. Distortion of anatomical position and alignment, for example, when radial head is subluxated, the forearm is usually slightly pronated and the elbow slightly flexed.
3. Bulges, creases, dimples, or other surface changes may be present on affected part.
4. Swelling may be present from dependent positioning.
5. Assess for discoloration, paresthesia, or other evidence of circulatory or neurological impairment (see *Fractures* for more detail about neurovascular assessment).

Diagnostic Tests

None (x-ray films are not helpful).

NURSING DIAGNOSES: ACTUAL OR POTENTIAL

1. Alteration in comfort, mild to severe, secondary to displaced joint.
2. Alteration of mobility: diminished mobility of affected joint due to subluxation.
3. Alteration of self-concept associated with impaired mobility and temporary deformity.

EXPECTED OUTCOMES

1. Joint will be returned to anatomic position and preinjury function.
2. Client will be restored to comfort.
3. Client will accept changes in self-concept, including body image, as demonstrated by compliance with treatment (stabilizing bandages, temporary activity restrictions, etc.).
4. Reinjury will not occur.

INTERVENTIONS

1. Promptly refer to physician for manipulations to realign subluxated joint.
2. Provide for joint rest for 12 to 24 hours after malalignment is reduced, by applying sling or appropriate bandage (see Figure 48-8).

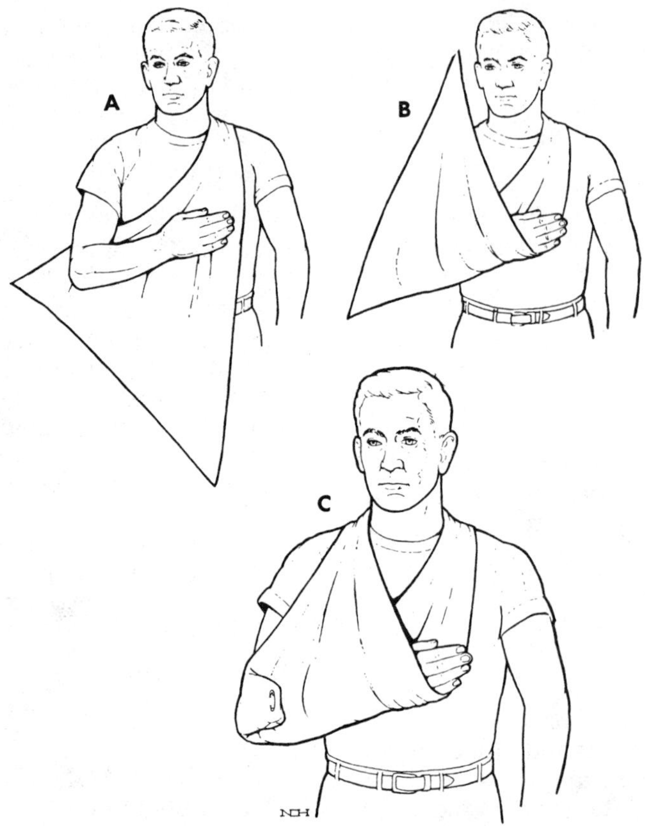

Figure 48-8 Using a triangular bandage as a comfortable arm sling. (From Henderson, J.: *Emergency Medical Guide*, 4th ed., McGraw-Hill, New York, 1978. Reproduced with permission.)

3. Give aspirin or other prescribed analgesic if needed.
4. Encourage use of extremity as soon as pain subsides.
5. Teach client and, if appropriate, family to avoid reinjury. Young children and elderly persons do not have sufficient muscle strength to tolerate forceful swinging or pulling.

EVALUATION

Outcome Criteria

1. Subluxation is promptly reduced by physician.
2. Client is pain-free within a few hours of reduction.
3. Full mobility and strength of joint return.
4. Client complies with treatment plan.
5. Reinjury is avoided.

DENTAL EMERGENCIES

DESCRIPTION

Emergency concerns of the dental skeleton include pain, traumatic fractures and avulsions, and infections. Toothache may be the result of injuries, disease, or extraction.

PREVENTION

Health Promotion

1. Dental self-care: brushing, flossing, mixed diet with minimally refined sugars.
2. Prevention of nursing bottle caries: infants with teeth should not take a bottle to bed with them unless it contains a sugar-free substance (water is all right; milk is cariogenic).
3. Avoidance of dental trauma:
   a. Teach children not to engage in rough play

while they or others are using a drinking fountain, drinking from a beverage bottle, and so forth.
b. Encourage use of automobile seat belts.
c. Encourage use of helmet, mouthguard, and other protective gear as appropriate for hazardous activities such as motorcycling, hockey, and so on.

Population at Risk

1. People with dental caries.
2. People at risk for dental injuries: athletes, active children.

Screening

1. Inspection of mouth.
2. X-ray films.

ASSESSMENT

Health History

1. History of bleeding.
2. Description of onset or event that caused client to seek care at this time (if client has had an accident that broke or avulsed teeth, suspect head injury, cervical fracture, and possible other injuries).
3. Regular dental caretaker, that is, dentist, dental hygienist.
4. Medication allergies.
5. History of anticoagulant therapy.
6. History of medications with anticoagulant effects, such as steroids, phenylbutazone, muscle relaxants, aspirin.

Physical Assessment

1. Swelling, induration.
2. Erythema or other discolorations.
3. Disruption of tooth structure, alveolar ridge, or soft tissue.
4. Hemorrhage.
5. Distortion of facial contour.
6. Difficulty in mastication.
7. Speech impediment.
8. Pain localized or general over face and head; usually sensitive to percussion.
9. Sensitivity to heat and cold.
10. Malodorous mouth.
11. Fever.
12. Dehydration (possible).
13. Assess trauma clients for head injury (neurological checks, etc.).

Diagnostic Tests

X-ray examination.

NURSING DIAGNOSES: ACTUAL OR POTENTIAL

1. Alteration in comfort: pain or discomfort secondary to dental fracture, decay, abscess, or soft-tissue injury.
2. Alteration in fluid balance secondary to blood loss associated with extraction and secondary to diminished oral intake.
3. Alteration in self-concept secondary to changes in appearance.
4. Nutritional deficits due to decreased intake associated with pain and discomfort.

EXPECTED OUTCOMES

1. Client will be relieved of pain and discomfort.
2. Blood loss will be controlled and minimized.
3. Client will take in adequate fluids and nutrients.
4. Client will receive appropriate cosmetic repairs (caps, crowns, etc.) and will adjust to residual body appearance changes.

INTERVENTIONS

1. For toothache:
   a. Provide analgesic as prescribed.
   b. Apply oil of cloves or local anesthesia by ointment or viscous solution.
   c. Pack extraction site with paste of cloves and zinc oxide.
   d. Schedule or instruct client to see dentist regularly. Obtain immediate dental consultation if client is experiencing pulp pain or pressure.
   e. Instruct in routine oral hygiene and preventive self-care of teeth and gums.
2. For trauma:
   a. Inspect mouth carefully, and remove all avulsed teeth.
   b. Immerse avulsed teeth in normal saline for replant: obtain dental consultant immediately.
   c. Reimplant partially avulsed teeth carefully, and immobilize jaw.
   d. Have client consume only soft and liquid foods until teeth are firmly reimplanted.
   e. Provide analgesics as necessary.
   f. Teach client not to suck, use straw, or create negative pressure in mouth.

   g. Instruct client about careful mouth rinses after meals.
   h. Tannic acid (tea bag) applied to bleeding extraction site or tears in gum will promote coagulation.
   i. Use a cavity varnish (Mizzy) for injuries or fractures to tooth enamel only.
   j. For injuries to enamel and dentine (chipped teeth) first use calcium hydroxide compound (Dycal) and then coat with cavity varnish several times to reduce pain and delay for up to 24 hours the need to see a dentist.
3. For abscess:
   a. Reduce acute symptoms through drainage.
   b. Administer prescribed antibiotics (usually penicillin, 250 mg qid for 7 days).
   c. Instruct client in:
      (1) Holding hot saline in the mouth to localize infection.
      (2) Careful mouth rinses after each meal and frequently during day.
4. For surgical or traumatic extraction:
   a. Control bleeding by rolled gauze held firmly by clamped jaw for 30 minutes to 3 hours.
   b. Estimate blood loss.
   c. Monitor vital signs, fluid intake and output, and blood pressure.

EVALUATION

Expected Outcomes

1. Client's pain and discomfort will be promptly reduced and then eliminated.
2. Hydration and nutritional intake will be maintained or quickly restored.
3. Self-concept will be supported by restorative dental work as needed.

Complications

1. Infection.
2. Tooth loss.

Reevaluation and Follow-up

1. Most clients with dental emergencies need to be seen by a dentist or oral surgeon; assist in securing consultation and in explaining to client the necessity for obtaining these specialists' services.
2. Instruct clients in dental self-care (brushing, flossing, diet, and avoidance of trauma).

MAXILLOFACIAL TRAUMA

DESCRIPTION

Blunt trauma to the face, like other head trauma, is potentially very serious because of the possibility of associated intracranial injury (neurological or vascular) or cervical fracture. Brain injury is discussed later in this chapter (see *Neurotrauma*). Airway occlusion is a potential consequence of some facial fractures, either from tissue displacement or from hemorrhage into the airway.

PREVENTION

Health Promotion

1. Use of automobile seat belts.
2. Use of protective helmets for cyclists, auto racers, baseball players, and others.
3. Protective waist belts for linemen, scaffold workers, and so forth.

Population at Risk

1. People in automobile accidents.
2. Cyclists, auto racers, boxers, baseball players, climbers, scaffold workers, and others who are likely to be struck by missiles.

Screening

None.

ASSESSMENT

Health History

1. Heavy impact trauma to face: obtain description of traumatic event in order to assess probable extent of injury, presence or absence of multiple injuries, and likelihood of cervical fracture.
2. Possible loss of consciousness.
3. Bleeding from orifices.

Physical Assessment

1. Ascertain airway adequacy and neurological stability.
2. Check for mandibular fracture:
   a. Palpate the angle of the mandible for a "step-up" (see Figure 48-9).
   b. Sublingual hematoma may be present.
   c. Teeth may be malaligned, broken, or missing; bite may be malocluded.
   d. If mandibular condyle is fractured, the examiner's fingers placed in or immediately anterior to the external ear canals will pal-

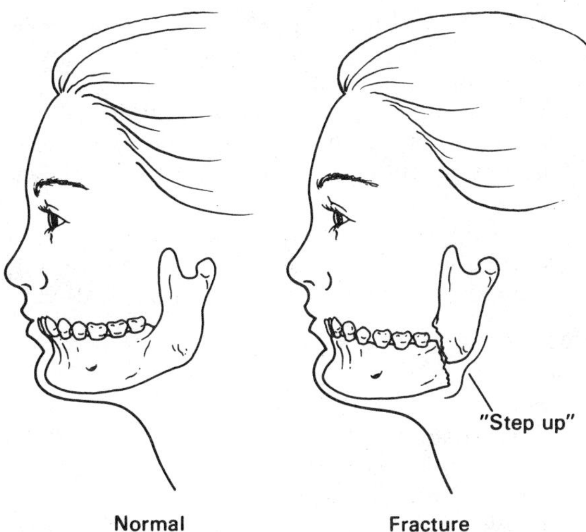

Figure 48-9 Angles of normal and fractured mandibles.

pate only the unfractured condyle moving as client opens and closes the jaw. Lacerations or blood may be noted in the ear canal.

3. Check for maxillary fracture:
   a. Dental arch may move upon palpation, with or without nose.
   b. Bleeding is usually profuse and readily compromises the airway.
   c. Teeth may be broken or malocclusive.
4. Check for zygomatic fracture:
   a. Edema of cheek and lids.
   b. Ecchymosis around eye and in upper buccal pouch.
   c. Subconjunctival hemorrhage.
   d. Dropped or flattened cheek.
   e. Unilateral epistaxis.
   f. Paresthesia of cheek, upper lip, and gingiva.
   g. Step deformity of inferior orbital margin.
   h. Diplopia, slight ptosis, altered position of eyeball (lower than on contralateral side).

NURSING DIAGNOSES: ACTUAL OR POTENTIAL

1. Diminished respiratory exchange due to displaced tissue or hemorrhage impinging on airway.
2. Alteration of comfort: pain secondary to tissue trauma.
3. Alteration in fluid balance and oxygenation secondary to blood loss.
4. Increased risk for progressive soft-tissue damage due to instability of bony structure.
5. Anxiety associated with bleeding, pain, and recent accident.

EXPECTED OUTCOMES

1. Patent airway will be maintained.
2. Blood loss will be controlled.
3. Pain and anxiety will be diminished.
4. Central nervous system trauma will be recognized early.
5. Soft-tissue damage will be controlled by immobilizing fracture.

INTERVENTIONS

1. Insert plastic airway if indicated for nasopharyngeal obstruction; check client at brief intervals for respiratory adequacy.
2. Position client on side for airway drainage if unable to manage own secretions (blood).
3. Apply pressure, padding, and cold for hemostasis; estimate blood loss.
4. Administer analgesia as prescribed (neurological status is a consideration).
5. Reassure client as much as possible, explaining findings and treatment procedures.
6. Monitor for shock: vital signs, color, perfusion, warmth (see *Shock* later in this chapter).
7. Monitor for cervical or brain injury (see *Neurotrauma* later in this chapter).
8. Immobilize fractured mandible (see Figure 48-10).

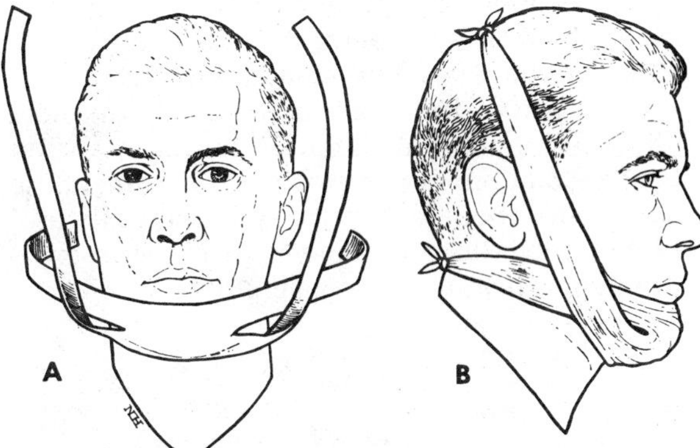

Figure 48-10 Four-tailed bandage for temporarily immobilizing a fractured jaw. (From Henderson, J.: *Emergency Medical Guide*, 4th ed., McGraw-Hill, New York, 1978. Reproduced with permission.)

EVALUATION

Outcome Criteria

1. Airway remains patent; respiratory exchange is adequate.
2. Hemorrhage is controlled.
3. Anxiety is controlled as evidenced by client's ability to cooperate with treatment.
4. Pain is decreased.
5. Neurological injury is recognized and minimized by early treatment.
6. Additional soft-tissue damage is avoided.

Complications

Meningitis due to bacterial infection of central nervous system (see *Meningitis*, in Chapter 25).

ENVIRONMENTAL EXPOSURE TRAUMA

HEAT STROKE

DESCRIPTION

Heat stroke (siriasis, sunstroke, heat hyperpyrexia) is inability to eliminate body heat due to failure of the heat-regulating mechanism as manifested by high fever and cessation of sweating. Heat stroke is a rare disorder but a medical emergency. Without treatment, it is fatal. Even with treatment the prognosis is guarded; The mortality rate is 50 percent, and many of the survivors have residual mental impairment.

Heat stroke has been noted to occur most often during July and August "dog days," when the Dog Star Sirius accompanies the rising of the sun; hence the term *siriasis*. High humidity and physical exertion combine with extreme environmental heat to cause heat stroke.

PREVENTION

Health Promotion

1. Avoid unnecessary exposure to heat.
2. Maintain adequate fluid and salt intake, using 0.1 percent saline for drinking or taking salt tablets and water.
3. Increase level of activity slowly until acclimatized.
4. Wear loose fitting, if possible light-colored or white, clothing, permeable to moisture.
5. Avoid use of alcoholic beverages.
6. Avoid becoming excessively fatigued.
7. Maintain good nutrition, particularly adequate hydration, and salt and caloric intake.
8. Avoid infections.
9. Children and others who may not be able to rescue themselves should *never* be left waiting in a closed car, particularly in hot weather.

Population at Risk

1. Elderly, infants, and children.
2. Men more than women.
3. Alcohol abusers.
4. Para-, hemi- and quadriplegics with impaired perspiration mechanism.
5. People taking medications that inhibit sweating, such as atropine and the phenothiazines.
6. Psychiatric clients whose behavior may camouflage signs and symptoms of impending heat stroke.
7. Athletes, especially football players.
8. Surgical patients draped and under anesthesia.

Screening

None.

ASSESSMENT

Health History

1. Level of consciousness of victim when found.
2. Physical state of victim when discovered, for example, collapse.
3. Working conditions of victim's immediate environment: extremely hot, humid.
4. Temperature of victim's skin on initial contact: abnormally hot.

Physical Assessment

1. Hot, dry, ruddy skin color (early).
2. Pale to gray skin, during circulatory collapse (late).
3. Tachycardia: full, bounding pulse (early).
4. Bradycardia: weak, thready pulse (late).
5. Hyperpyrexia: 104 to 112°F, or above 40°C.
6. Delirium or coma.
7. Deep, slow respirations progressing to Cheyne-Stokes pattern.
8. Dilated pupils (usually).
9. Offensive body odor.

10. Muscle twitching and epileptiform convulsions (early).
11. Rise in blood pressure (early), with drop during circulatory collapse.

Diagnostic Test

Body temperature: fever often rises higher than can be measured by standard thermometers.

NURSING DIAGNOSES: ACTUAL OR POTENTIAL

1. Alteration in body temperature: severe hyperpyrexia secondary to environmental heat and thermoregulatory failure.
2. Alteration in fluid and electrolyte balance: shock, circulatory collapse, and metabolic acidosis secondary to abnormal thermoregulation.
3. Alteration in consciousness: confusion progressing to delirium and coma secondary to abnormal cellular metabolism.
4. Increased risk of injury associated with altered state of consciousness and convulsions.

EXPECTED OUTCOMES

1. Body temperature will be restored to normal range as rapidly as possible.
2. Fluid and electrolyte abnormalities will be corrected.
3. Client will resume consciousness and orientation.
4. Client will not be injured during seizure, coma, or confusion.

INTERVENTIONS

1. Rapidly reduce body temperature by cold baths, ice packs, chilled or iced saline enemas, hypothermia blankets, alcohol sponge baths, and the like. Massage and provide passive range of motion during cooling to enhance circulation and hence speed heat loss from deeper structures. Do not cool below 102°F (39°C), for then shivering is likely to ensue and increase the temperature.
2. Administer intravenous fluids and electrolytes as prescribed. Monitor carefully for pulmonary edema, cerebral edema, and renal failure (see *Congestive Heart Failure, Cerebral Edema,* and *Acute Renal Failure,* in Chapters 30, 25, and 32 respectively).
3. Monitor state of consciousness and protect client as necessary from injury. Pad side rails and remove potentially injurious objects from bed to prevent trauma during seizures. Administer anticonvulsant as prescribed.

EVALUATION

Outcome Criteria

1. Temperature is lowered promptly to 102°F (39°C) and then gradually to normal.
2. Normal hydration and serum electrolyte balance are attained.
3. Normal state of consciousness returns.
4. Client does not become injured from accident or convulsion.
5. Vital signs, intake and output, and blood chemistries are stable within normal limits.

Complications

1. Consequences of hypoperfusion: renal tubular necrosis, disseminated intravascular coagulation (DIC), hepatic failure, cerebrovascular accident, myocardial infarction.
2. Pulmonary edema.
3. Cerebral edema and increased intracranial pressure.
4. Cardiac dysrhythmias.
5. Residual temperature instability.
6. Permanent mental impairment, behavioral or intellectual or both.

Reevaluation and Follow-up

Client will be indefinitely hypersensitive to warm temperatures; teach avoidance of exposure to situations that can cause overheating.

HEAT EXHAUSTION

DESCRIPTION

Heat exhaustion (heat prostration) is due to inadequacy or collapse of the peripheral circulation secondary to dehydration and salt depletion. Heat exhaustion is caused by a sudden shift of blood from circulating volume to skin in an attempt to cool the body when usual mechanisms of sweating are inadequate. Heat exhaustion is less serious than heat stroke (described above). It is rarely fatal if treated.

PREVENTION

Health Promotion

See *Heat Stroke,* immediately above.

Population at Risk

1. People not accustomed to activity in hot weather, such as sporadic gardeners.
2. Young children.
3. People who perspire excessively or are dehydrated for any reason (e.g., diarrhea or use of diuretic drugs for hypertension).
4. Women more than men.
5. Patients with underlying cardiac, cerebral, or systemic disease.

Screening

None.

ASSESSMENT

Health History

1. Determine what client was doing at time of first appearance of symptoms.
2. Elicit whether fainting occurred or not.
3. Note type of working quarters if industrial case.

Physical Assessment

1. Skin cool or cold, and moist.
2. Fatigue, lassitude.
3. Dizziness, stupor, or headache; fainting briefly and recurrently.
4. Body temperature normal, subnormal, or slightly elevated.
5. Hypotension.
6. Tachycardia; weak, thready pulse.
7. Nausea, vomiting.
8. Pupils may be dilated.
9. Slow capillary refill times as noted by depressing the fingernail.

Diagnostic Tests

1. None usually.
2. Hemoglobin and hematocrit to rule out anemia if low red blood cell count is suspected.

NURSING DIAGNOSES: ACTUAL OR POTENTIAL

1. Alteration in body temperature: fever secondary to extreme environmental temperature.
2. Fluid volume deficit due to sweating and vomiting.
3. Altered level of consciousness: syncope secondary to hypotension.
4. Discomfort due to nausea, fever, weakness, and headache.

EXPECTED OUTCOMES

1. If client is febrile, temperature will be returned to normal.
2. Normal fluid volume and distribution, and serum electrolyte balance, will be reestablished as quickly as possible.
3. Client will be returned to normal level of consciousness and state of orientation.
4. Client will be relieved of discomforts.

INTERVENTIONS

1. Remove victim to cool and less humid environment.
2. Place client in supine position with knees bent and feet elevated.
3. Cool body with moist cool compresses to forehead and extremities.
4. If client is able to swallow, give salty solutions such as soups or bouillon or other preferred drinks, including coffee (no alcoholic beverages, which promote vasodilation).
5. If client is unable to take oral fluids, administer IV saline and monitor for fluid acceptance, that is, observe for excessive and rapid blood pressure changes, rales, neck vein distension.
6. Use aromatic spirits of ammonia if victim does not rapidly resume consciousness.
7. As client recovers, do not allow sitting until compensatory mechanisms can stabilize.
8. Monitor urinary output.

EVALUATION

Outcome Criteria

1. Alterations in fluid balance are corrected: vital signs return to normal.
2. Body temperature is reduced if high at outset, and stabilized to normal range.
3. Client regains consciousness and becomes oriented: feelings of faintness are gone.
4. Client is resting comfortably.

Reevaluation and Follow-up

1. Usually client is not hospitalized unless rest and oral fluid therapy are ineffective or additional illness (e.g., chronic heart disease) is present.
2. Teach client how to prevent future occurrences.

HEAT CRAMPS

DESCRIPTION

Heat cramps (muscle spasms, charley horses) are sudden, painful muscle tightenings due to the combination of prolonged exposure to high environmental temperatures, excessive sweating, and large oral intake of water, which lead to vast body salt loss. Prognosis is excellent.

PREVENTION

Health Promotion

1. See *Heat Stroke.*
2. Avoid copious hyptonic (low sodium) fluid intake.

Population at Risk

1. Laborers in heavy industry.
2. People at home who engage in excessive physical work during hot weather.
3. Occasionally athletes.

ASSESSMENT

Health History

1. Excessive oral intake of water or other hypotonic liquids.
2. Strenuous activity (work, sports) preceding attack.
3. Cramping, gripping, prolonged pain; charley horse in legs or abdomen which is not relieved by stopping activity.

Physical Assessment

1. Pale, moist skin.
2. Extreme thirst.
3. Faintness to loss of consciousness.
4. Normal or slightly elevated body temperature.
5. Nausea.
6. Tachycardia: strong, full pulse.
7. Severe muscle cramping with palpable gastrocnemius tightening (lumping).
8. Generalized muscle twitching (possible).
9. Postural blood pressure drop (due to saline deficit).

Diagnostic Tests

1. Serum sodium concentration low (< 140 mg//L).
2. Urine specific gravity low (1.001 to 1.010).
3. Serum chlorides low (< 96 mg/L).

NURSING DIAGNOSES: ACTUAL OR POTENTIAL

1. Alteration in fluid volume and electrolyte balance due to excessive sweating, copious hypotonic fluid intake, and vast body salt loss.
2. Alteration in comfort: pain secondary to uncontrolled muscle cramping.
3. Impairment of mobility due to pain and muscle cramping.
4. Altered levels of consciousness secondary to fainting.

EXPECTED OUTCOMES

1. Fluid and electrolyte balance will be restored.
2. Pain and cramping will be eliminated as quickly as possible.
3. Recurrent attacks will be reduced.

INTERVENTIONS

1. Administer salt solutions such as soup or bouillon, as nausea permits.
2. Reduce water intake by substituting saline solutions.
3. Infuse saline as prescribed.
4. Administer enteric-coated instead of plain salt tablets, to avoid nausea in some people.
5. Provide rest in cool environment.
6. Monitor urinary output.

EVALUATION

Outcome Criteria

1. Fluid and electrolyte balance are returned to normal levels.
2. Pain and cramping are relieved.
3. Client is returned to fully conscious state without recurrent fainting.

Complications

Usually none: client rarely needs hospitalization.

Reevaluation and Follow-up

1. Evaluate client's understanding of condition and long-term preventive measures, that is, decrease exposure to high temperature and take frequent rest periods; avoid excessive fluid intake.
2. Teach client to make oral hypotonic salt solution: 1 tsp table salt and $\frac{1}{2}$ tsp baking soda in 1 qt of water.

LOCALIZED HYPOTHERMIA

DESCRIPTION

Frostbite is injury of the superficial tissues as a result of tissue freezing. This injury occurs most commonly during blizzards, extreme cold, damp, and high wind-chill factor weather, and prolonged subzero temperatures. The temperature of the involved tissue is less than -5.5°C (22°F). Frostbite has been classified into three grades of severity:

1. First degree: freezing without blistering or peeling.
2. Second degree: freezing with blistering or peeling.
3. Third degree: freezing with death of skin and sometimes the deeper tissues (Krupp and Chatton, 1982).

Arteriolar vasoconstriction causes peripheral tissue anoxia, hypothermia, and eventual freezing. Upon thawing, the tissue becomes hyperemic, and this condition (*flare*) is accompanied by intravascular fluid loss (edema) to surrounding interstitial spaces. Wheals (hives) are often part of the flare response, probably because of local release of tissue histamine. In severe frostbite, the thawing appears in phases with the hypermia and interstitial edema followed quickly by a slowing of circulation due to tissue swelling. Dilated vessels become engorged with masses of erythrocytes (RBC). These clumps may be broken up by gentle manipulation early in this phase. Later, arterioles are totally occluded by thrombi.

Chilblains are red, itching skin lesions found most frequently on the extremities. These lesions are due to exposure to cold without actual freezing of the tissues.

Trench foot (immersion syndrome) is caused by prolonged immersion of limb in cool or cold water or mud (freezing of tissue does not occur). The affected parts progress from being cold and anesthetic to hot and burning followed by either paling or cyanosis. Blistering, swelling, redness, heat, hemorrhage, ecchymosis, and gangrene are later developments with lymphangiitis, cellulitis, and thrombophlebitis as secondary complications.

Estimated wind speed mi/h	Actual thermometer reading, °F											
	50	40	30	20	10	0	-10	-20	-30	-40	-50	-60
	Equivalent temperature, °F											
Calm	50	40	30	20	10	0	-10	-20	-30	-40	-50	-60
5	48	37	27	16	6	-5	-15	-26	-36	-47	-57	-68
10	40	28	16	4	-9	-24	-33	-46	-58	-70	-83	-95
15	36	22	9	-5	-18	-32	-45	-58	-72	-85	-99	-112
20	32	18	4	-10	-25	-39	-53	-67	-82	-96	-110	-124
25	30	16	0	-15	-29	-44	-59	-74	-88	-104	-119	-133
30	28	13	-2	-18	-33	-48	-63	-79	-94	-109	-125	-140
35	27	11	-4	-20	-35	-51	-67	-82	-98	-113	-129	-145
40	26	10	-6	-21	-37	-53	-69	-85	-100	-116	-132	-148
(Wind speeds greater than 40 mi/h have little additional effect.)	LITTLE DANGER (for properly clothed person.) Maximum danger of false sense of security.				INCREASING DANGER Danger from freezing of exposed flesh.			GREAT DANGER				

Trenchfoot and immersion foot may occur at any point on this chart.

Figure 48-11 Wind-chill factor chart. (Adapted from Earle, A. S. et al.: *Patient Care*®, copyright © 1972, Patient Care Inc., Darien, Conn. All rights reserved.)

PREVENTION

Health Promotion

1. People should wear warm, dry clothing, preferably several layers, with windproof outer garment.
2. Remove wet clothing, shoes, and stockings as soon as possible and replace with dry ones.
3. Carry extra stockings, mittens, and insoles in a pack when in cold or icy areas.
4. Avoid cramped positions, constricting clothing, and prolonged dependency of the feet.
5. Exercise arms, legs, fingers, and toes to maintain circulation.
6. Maintain good nutrition and skin cleanliness.
7. Avoid wet and muddy ground; keep sheltered from the wind.
8. Avoid use of tobacco and alcohol when danger of frostbite is present.

Population at Risk

1. The old or the very young.
2. People with darkly pigmented skin.
3. People who have experienced previous cold injuries.
4. People in poor physical condition.
5. High altitude climbers who become anoxic.
6. Hunters.
7. Nervous people or those who sweat profusely.
8. Alcoholics.
9. People with prolonged exposure to very cold weather.
10. Occasionally, frostbite occurs in winter sports enthusiasts.
11. People with poor tissue perfusion, as a result of arteriosclerosis, smoking, tight clothing, and so on.

Screening

None.

ASSESSMENT

Health History

1. Description of cold exposure to determine extent of injury, including temperature and wind-chill factor (see Figure 48–11).
2. Description of rewarming measures employed before seeking medical care.
3. History of previous cold injuries and recovery.
4. History of smoking, if any.
5. Past medical history for tissue perfusion abnormalities and general health.
6. Drug history.

Physical Assessment

1. Tingling and numbness of digit and/or extremity (early).
2. Extreme pain with or without external pressure.
3. Violet, deep red hue on digits and extremities. (If untreated, digits progressively deteriorate to white, blanched appearance.)
4. Loss of all sensation in untreated, affected tissue.
5. During thawing, hyperemia and edema appear in affected tissue; skin loses its elasticity and becomes immobile.
6. Visible arteriolar RBC clumping as noted by deep red blotching over skin surface (may occur during thawing).
7. Extreme, sharp pain may occur in affected area during rewarming.
8. Note possible clinical complications:
   a. Thrombi with infarction of affected tissue.
   b. Release of venous thrombi during rewarming.
   c. Development of necrosis and gangrene, with eventual extended loss of function (in some cases).

Diagnostic Tests

Arteriography, though rare, and of questionable value, to ascertain extent of ischemic disease.

NURSING DIAGNOSES: ACTUAL OR POTENTIAL

1. Impairment of circulation to affected body parts due to damage to exposed tissue, and possibly also peripheral infarction.
2. Alteration in comfort: extreme pain in affected limb due to ischemia or tissue expansion by ice crystal formation.
3. Impairment of mobility due to circulatory disruption and pain.
4. Impairment of skin integrity associated with blistering and possible necrosis.
5. Anxiety secondary to potential loss of function and limb itself.

EXPECTED OUTCOMES

1. Tissue perfusion will be reestablished as rapidly as possible.

2. Pain and discomfort will be reduced.
3. Function of affected part will be restored as completely as the extent of the original trauma permits.
4. Residual damage to affected area will be prevented, as much as possible.
5. Fear and anxiety will be reduced.

INTERVENTIONS

1. Place client in recumbent position with head of bed comfortably raised.
2. Rapidly rewarm the injured area with moist heat. Keep solution between 36.7 and 40°C (98 and 104°F). Never use dry heat.
3. Cleanse injured area carefully and separate digits with sterile gauze.
4. Administer analgesics appropriately for pain as prescribed: morphine sulfate in titrated doses IV may be used; codeine sulfate 0.06 g, meperidine hydrochloride (Demerol), 50 to 100 mg orally, or other less potent oral analgesics.
5. Protect affected tissue from further injury by using cradles for bed covers, repositioning frequently, avoiding injections into this area, and so on.
6. Administer tetanus prophylaxis if client's immunization has lapsed.
7. Administer prophylactic antibiotics if prescribed (usually only if frostbite is extensive).
8. Remove smoking materials and discourage smoking during hospitalization and follow-up (vasoconstriction is to be avoided).
9. Keep client warm systemically by encouraging ingestion of hot, stimulating liquids, especially coffee.
10. Do not allow weight bearing or pressure on injured parts.
11. Administer low molecular weight dextran if prescribed, usually in doses of 1 g/kg per day for tissue protection (1,000 mL 6% dextran on day of injury, followed by 500 mL every day for 5 days or 50 mL/h for 3 to 5 days).

EVALUATION

Outcome Criteria

1. Tissue perfusion to affected part is restored.
2. Affected area has minimal residual damage: function is normal, skin is intact, and sensation is normal.
3. Client is no longer experiencing severe pain and discomfort.
4. Client is expressing less fear and anxiety over traumatic injury.

Complications

INFECTION (LOCAL OR SYSTEMIC)

Assessment

1. Elevated body temperature.
2. Purulent drainage from skin blebs after the rewarming process has been completed.
3. Increasing redness, heat, pain in affected area.

Revised Outcomes

Further infection of affected part will be prevented; infection will be treated until cleared.

Interventions

1. Protect skin blebs from physical contact.
2. Treat local infection with mild soaks of soapy water or povidone-iodine (Betadine, etc.).
3. Provide whirlpool therapy at temperatures slightly below body temperature twice daily for 15–20 minutes for a period of 3 or more weeks to help cleanse the skin and debride superficial sloughing tissue.
4. Administer antibiotics as prescribed for deep infections.

SURGICAL AMPUTATION

Usually withheld until line of demarcation is clear between viable and nonviable tissue. It is possible for tissue necrosis (even with black eschar formation) to be quite superficial; underlying skin may heal well spontaneously even after a period of months.

Reevaluation and Follow-up

1. Evaluate level of client understanding regarding care of injuries and prevention of recurrence.
2. Instruct client on etiological factors and preventive measures.
3. Obtain appropriate referrals, such as physical therapy, social work, or psychiatry if indicated for complications necessitating surgical amputation or residual impairment.

SYSTEMIC HYPOTHERMIA

DESCRIPTION

A systemic hypothermic reaction is caused by a chilling of the whole body either from therapeutic procedures such as surgery and some treatments for certain poisonings, or from exposure to cold weather. If left untreated, it progressively slows the physiologic processes, leading to death. Certain factors predict survival from this injury: length of time exposed; the person's innate tolerance of cold; environmental influences of altitude, barometric pressure, and humidity; the person's general physical condition, including nutritional status and previous or chronic disease. The condition is more serious when altered homeostasis is present due to associated debility or disease; in these instances, hypothermia may follow exposure even to ordinary temperatures. Body temperature in accidental hypothermia may range from 25–35°C (77–95°F). (A special rectal thermometer which has readings as low as 25°C [77°F] is required.)

PREVENTION

Health Promotion

1. Avoid exposure to prolonged or extreme cold.
2. Avoid use of alcoholic beverages when exposed to cold (blood vessel dilation increases heat loss).
3. Use extra caution in exposing oneself to extreme cold if on sedative-hypnotic drugs.
4. See also Health Promotion under *Localized Hypothermia*, immediately above.

Population at Risk

1. Mountain climbers, hikers, hunters, and others who become lost or trapped without shelter.
2. Persons experiencing prolonged exposure in water.
3. Industrial workers who work in refrigerator-freezer units.

Screening

None.

ASSESSMENT

Health History

1. Description of exposure, including time interval and type of weather.
2. Past medical history for underlying and/or chronic disease and medication therapy.
3. Type of employment (if applicable).
4. Type of outer wear worn during exposure.

Physical Assessment

1. Progressive chilling.
2. Intense shivering.
3. Apathy.
4. Confusion, delirium, or unconsciousness.
5. Bradycardia.
6. Hypopnea.
7. Progressive freezing of extremities, toward body.
8. Irregular apical and radial pulses.

Diagnost Test

ECG for cardiac arrhythmias: at body temperature approximately 86–88°F, ventricular fibrillation occurs; at 82–86°F, asystole occurs.

NURSING DIAGNOSES: ACTUAL OR POTENTIAL

1. Alteration in body temperature secondary to exposure to prolonged cold.
2. Alteration in cardiac output: arrhythmias associated with metabolic results of hypothermia.
3. Altered levels of consciousness secondary to extreme lowering of core temperature, development of metabolic acidosis with renal impairment, and possible progression to ventricular fibrillation.
4. Alteration in fluid and electrolyte homeostasis secondary to cellular metabolic changes and renal impairment.
5. Impaired thought processes brought on by traumatic exposure to extreme cold and resultant drop in core temperature as well as by impaired renal and cardiac output.
6. Alterations in comfort due to chilling, shivering, and other somatic symptoms.

EXPECTED OUTCOMES

1. Client's body will rewarmed to normal temperature range.
2. Client will return to pretrauma cardiac status with adequate output and no life-threatening arrhythmias.
3. Metabolic functions will be restored to preinjury state.
4. Fluid and electrolyte balance will be restored to normal.
5. Client will regain alert and oriented level of consciousness.
6. Client will become more comfortable and less anxious as symptoms are treated and controlled.

INTERVENTIONS

1. Rapidly rewarm with blankets, others' body heat, and hot oral liquids if victim is in early stages of chilling.
2. If body temperature is near lethal limit, carefully and with frequent monitoring apply electric blankets, warm saline enemas, hot oral liquids (if client can swallow), warm gastric lavage, any heating device to increase room temperature, covered hot water bottles, warmed bricks, and so on.
3. Insert indwelling bladder catheter to monitor kidney function.
4. Record hourly urine output.
5. Monitor urine pH and specific gravity.
6. If ventilation is inadequate, establish airway and ventilation with positive pressure bag, or intubate and place on volumetric respirator.
7. Provide oxygen therapy to maintain arterial blood gases within normal limits (laboratory findings need to be adjusted for hypothermic state).
8. Place client on cardiac monitor and observe for arrhythmias.
   a. If frequent ventricular ectopy occurs, treat with lidocaine, 50 to 100 mg bolus, then IV drip of 1 to 4 mg/min as ordered.
   b. If ventricular fibrillation occurs, treat with direct current countershock (defibrillation) and IV lidocaine at 1 to 4 mg/min as ordered.
   c. If asystole occurs, begin cardiopulmonary resuscitation, and be ready with drugs, usually given in the following order:
      (1) Epinephrine, 0.5 to 1.0 mg of a 1:10,000 solution IV or intracardiac; may be repeated every 5 min.
      (2) Sodium bicarbonate, 0.5 mEq/kg IV, every 10 min or as indicated by blood gases.
      (3) Atropine, 1 to 2 mg IV.
      (4) Calcium chloride, 5 mL of a 10% solution, every 10 min.
9. Do not permit smoking.
10. Watch for mass effects; there are usually unpredictable medication results until client is completely rewarmed.
11. Continue to monitor vital signs, fluid intake and output, level of consciousness, and orientation.
12. Provide emotional reassurance: explain procedures and treatments, and reorient client to place, time, and situation as necessary.

EVALUATION

Outcome Criteria

1. Cardiac status has stabilized; client is no longer experiencing or in danger of developing life-threatening arrhythmias.
2. Client's body temperature has returned to normal range.
3. Metabolic functions are now within normal limits, as evidenced by blood and urine chemistries.
4. Fluid and electrolyte balance is stabilized to near-normal values.
5. Client is conscious, alert, and oriented.
6. Anxiety and fear have been reduced.

Complications

The client may become delirious, then comatose, and may cease breathing and develop metabolic acidosis and ventricular fibrillation; death may ensue. See Chapter 30 for care, including assessment, of clients with life-threatening arrhythmias.

Reevaluation and Follow-up

1. Continue to provide realistic emotional reassurance to client, family, and friends.
2. Teach client and significant others about causes, prevention, and immediate treatment for hypothermia.

VENOMOUS BITES AND STINGS

DESCRIPTION

Insect stings involve piercing of tissue by the insect's stinger and release of venom (toxic, foreign protein antigen). The honeybee's stinger is barbed and readily hooks into the skin. It remains in the skin after the insect flies away or is brushed off. The venom sac, which also may remain, continues contracting for approximately 1 to 3 minutes, thereby injecting additional venom. Other bees, wasps, hornets, yellow jackets, and fire ants retain the stinger after attacking and are able to deliver repeated stings in quick succession. Several chemical compounds in the venoms of these insects are responsible for both direct effects of and allergic reactions to their stings. The insect venoms are similar enough that a person who is allergic to one is likely to be cross-sensitive to the others. It is estimated that 20 percent of the general population are allergic to bee stings. Stinging insects are especially aggressive when their nests or hives are disturbed; a person who unwittingly comes too close may receive dozens or even hundreds of stings in a few seconds.

Spiders of clinical importance are the black widow and the brown recluse. These spiders are found everywhere in the United States except Alaska. Scorpions, botanically related to spiders, are most common in the southwest but live in all states from Florida to California. Most scorpions are nonlethal, but two species found in Arizona and parts of adjoining states are classified as potentially lethal; their stings are seldom fatal but may be so to small children and elderly people.

Poisonous snakes in the United States include pit vipers (rattlesnakes, copperheads, and moccasins) and coral snakes. They inject their venom through hollow fangs, which leave characteristic paired puncture wounds. Venom may not be injected with every bite.

PREVENTION

Health Promotion

1. People at risk to contact poisonous animals should be taught how to recognize them, what their habitats are, and how to avoid provoking an attack.
2. Protective clothing (beekeepers' veils and gloves, snake boots, and the like) should be used by people known to be at risk.

Population at Risk

1. Children who play in areas that are natural habitats for venomous animals (farm fields where bees nest; wooded or rocky areas where snakes, scorpions, or spiders may live).
2. People whose occupations, recreation, or home maintenance activities (lawn mowing, etc.) take place where these animals live (farmers, hunters, hikers, utility company linemen, highway department workers, and so forth).

Screening

None.

ASSESSMENT

Health History

1. Describe the insect, reptile, or arachnid.
2. Note time of incident and ensuing symptoms.
3. Obtain past medical and drug history, especially if client is hypertensive or diabetic or has peripheral vascular disease. There is an enhanced absorption of venom in hypertensives, a development of hypoglycemia in diabetics, and an inhibition of venom absorption in people who have peripheral vascular disease.
4. Obtain a past allergy history and record all previous antigenic agents.
5. Note all care and medications rendered prior to hospital admission.
6. Note if victim is at risk for tetanus.

Physical Assessment

1. Look for signs of anaphylactic reactions (anaphylaxis is discussed later in this chapter; see *Shock*) or angioneurotic edema.
2. Check pulmonary functioning: may have acute cessation of ventilation.
3. Observe for circulatory collapse, neurovasogenic type (see *Shock*).
4. Assess pain and itching.
5. Note local induration, hyperemia, erythema.
6. *Bee, hornet, wasp, and ant stings:* local reactions include pinprick sensation, redness and wheal, pain, itching, and swelling. Toxic reactions include vomiting, diarrhea, faintness, unconsciousness, edema, headache, fever, muscle spasms, and rarely seizures. Delayed reactions, called "serum sickness," are characterized by rash, urticaria, lymphadenopathy, myalgia, arthralgia, and fever. Unusual reactions: nephrotic syndrome; bites around eyes may cause iris atrophy, cataracts, glaucoma, and perforation of globe.
7. *Black widow bite:* on lower extremity, symptoms are extreme pain and rigidity of abdomen; on upper extremity, pain and rigidity in chest, back, and shoulders. Client develops fever, elevated blood pressure, leukocytosis, albuminuria, hematuria, stupor, and convulsions. The venom is neurotoxic, causing ascending motor paralysis and peripheral nerve ending destruction (Rapaport, 1975).

8. *Brown recluse bite:* local symptoms may not develop for 2 to 8 h after bite; area is red, painful, develops blisters and blebs surrounded by ischemia. After several days, center turns dark; after 14 days it becomes depressed, demarcated, and mummified, producing a large open ulcer. Systemic symptoms include fever, chills, malaise, weakness, nausea and vomiting, joint pain, petechial rash, hemolysis, and thrombocytopenia.
9. *Scorpion stings:* stings by nonlethal species produce local swelling, pain, and occasional anaphylaxis. Bites by potentially lethal species have no visible local effects. The client experiences local pain, hyperesthesia followed by hypoesthesia, numbness, and drowsiness; itching of nose, mouth, and throat; slurred speech, muscle spasm, generalized pain, vomiting, incontinence, and seizures. May have respiratory and circulatory collapse. Symptoms last 24 to 48 h.
10. *Bite of pit viper:* local reactions include intense, burning pain, swelling, and copious interstitial bleeding with two puncture wounds; blisters and blebs develop within an hour, becoming extremely large and hemorrhagic. Systemic reactions (due to general circulation absorption and the anticoagulation effects of venom) include muscle fasciculations and twitching, frequently around mouth; gastrointestinal bleeding; nausea; vomiting; diaphoresis; tachycardia; hypotension; syncope and coma; and shallow hypopnea progressing to respiratory arrest.

Diagnostic Tests

None.

NURSING DIAGNOSES: ACTUAL OR POTENTIAL

1. Alteration in comfort: pain or discomfort due to local or systemic toxin, swelling, ischemia, and itching.
2. Alteration in fluid balance associated with edema, hypotension, or anaphylaxis (may include local swelling inside of fascia sheath that causes compression of vessels and nerves passing through that fascia compartment: "compartmental syndrome").
3. Alteration in consciousness, associated with anaphylaxis or toxicity.
4. Alteration in respiratory pattern secondary to shock, hemolysis, or anaphylaxis.
5. Alteration in cardiac output secondary to shock, hemolysis, or anaphylaxis.
6. Loss of skin integrity associated with itching or necrosis.
7. Increased risk of infection at site of injury secondary to toxin, tissue necrosis, and skin breaks.
8. Alteration in self-concept secondary to swelling and other local reactions, which may include necrosis and sloughing (brown recluse, pit vipers).
9. Self-care deficit and alteration in mobility secondary to swelling, pain, and restrictions imposed by therapy.
10. Anxiety associated with exaggerated folklore about death from venomous bites.

EXPECTED OUTCOMES

1. Distribution of the venom in the client's body will be kept to a minimum.
2. Client will maintain adequate cardiorespiratory function, including local tissue perfusion at site of injury.
3. Pain, itching, and swelling will be reduced.
4. Client will not be injured during unconsciousness or seizure.
5. Infection will be prevented or controlled.
6. Client will cope with body image changes.
7. Client's mobility will be restored.
8. Client will be free of unrealistic anxiety (e.g., exaggerated expectations of dire outcome).

INTERVENTIONS

1. Immediately reduce systemic absorption of venom.
   a. Bees, ants, spider, scorpion: apply ice packs or cold compresses (but do not induce frosbite); place victim at rest. If severe allergic reaction is known or suspected (previous history), apply tourniquet above sting site. Carefully scrape stinger away if lodged in skin: *do not pinch* (no tweezers, etc.), for retained venom sac discharges residual venom. Transport to emergency care facility.
   b. Snakebite: ice or cold applications are not recommended because they may worsen

tissue necrosis. If victim is within 4 hours of an emergency care facility, quickly immobilize the bitten extremity and apply tourniquet to reduce lymphatic and venous return (arterial pulses must remain), place client at rest, and transport immediatley. If more than 4 hours from hospital, or if client is unconscious or swelling is rapid, wash skin to remove venom on exterior, apply tourniquet as above to delay venous and lymphatic return, make a 5 mm ($\frac{1}{4}$ inch) linear (not cross-shaped) incision through the skin and into the fat at each fang mark, and apply suction for $\frac{1}{2}$ hour to remove as much venom as possible. NOTE: if available, a snakebite kit, breast pump, or other source of suction is preferable to mouth suction, which may cause wound infection.

2. Maintain ventilation and airway: provide oxygen by mask, and intubate if necessary.
3. Provide analgesia as prescribed, though not morphine unless you are prepared to support ventilation.
4. For anaphylactic reaction:
   a. Administer aqueous epinephrine either SC, IM, or IV as prescribed (fastest route in acute reactions).
   b. Administer prescribed IV or IM antihistamines, such as chlorpheniramine IV or IM.
   c. Administer prescribed IV corticosteroid, such as hydrocortisone sodium succinate.
   d. If antihistamine or epinephrine is not available outside of the hospital, administer cold tablets that have antihistamines and nasal decongestant components. Immediately take victim to hospital or first aid facility for additional therapy. (See discussion of anaphylactic shock under *Shock*, in this chapter.)
5. Antivenin, if available, may be prescribed according to package insert directions. It is mandatory that client be pretested for allergy to the antivenin, since 30 to 50 percent of people are allergic to horse serum (Rapaport, 1975). Follow the manufacturer's instructions for testing for sensitivity, and be prepared to treat anaphylaxis.
6. Administer prescribed buffered isotonic solution (Ringer's lactate) to keep blood pressure at 90 mmHg.
7. If compartmental syndrome develops, assist as required with fasciotomy.
8. Administer prescribed antibiotics (penicillin is usually given for snakebite).
9. Protect client from injury if unconscious or convulsing (apply eye pads, pad bed rails, etc., as appropriate to condition).
10. Monitor vital signs and neurologic status frequently for 24 hours or until stabilized.
11. Administer tetanus prophylaxis if client's immunization is not current.
12. Monitor and record prolonged bleeding times or continued hemorrhage.
13. Assist client in accepting body changes and coping with fear. Provide realistic information about expectations for reversal of edema, formation and healing of ulcerations, general prognosis, and the like.
14. Assist with mobility and self-care as circumstances require: rearrange furniture, teach crutch walking, help with plans for managing at home after discharge, and so forth.

EVALUATION

Outcome Criteria

1. Respiration and tissue perfusion are maintained.
2. Anaphylaxis is prevented or adequately treated.
3. Pain, itching, and swelling are alleviated.
4. Additional injury (e.g., from seizure) does not occur.
5. Infection is prevented or adequately treated.
6. Client verbalizes accurate, realistic prognosis; client accepts body changes as evidenced by verbal expression and cooperative participation in the treatment plan. Signs of excessive anxiety are absent.
7. Self-care and mobility are as good as possible for client's condition.

Complications

1. Circulatory compromise necessitating amputation (snakebite).
2. Cardiac arrhythmias.
3. Shock.
4. Respiratory obstruction from allergic response (bees).
5. Acute renal failure from hemolysis (spiders, snakes).

Reevaluation and Follow-up

1. Desensitization is recommended for persons with allergic responses to bee stings.

2. Instruct persons who are allergic to bee stings:
   a. To avoid bees and wasps by avoiding perfumes and brightcolored clothes when out of doors (scents and colors may simulate flowers and attract bees).
   b. To wear protective clothing: long sleeves and trousers when gardening, shoes whenever out of doors, and so forth.
   c. To carry an emergency sting kit and to use it immediately if stung (without waiting for symptoms). These kits contain a tourniquet, antiseptic, and preloaded one- or two-dose syringe with needle. After self-injection, the client should go to an emergency room for follow-up observation and treatment.

DROWNING AND NEAR-DROWNING

DESCRIPTION

Drowning is death from asphyxiation due to submersion in a fluid; in near-drowning, successful resuscitation is administered or the victim recovers spontaneously. In a typical incident, a swimmer panics, begins to submerge, and spasmodically sucks water into the trachea, which causes gasping and choking. Subsequent events (Figure 48–12) include the aspiration of water ("wet drowning"). Less frequently (10 to 20 percent of incidents) the initial entry of water into the trachea produces reflex laryngotracheal or epiglottic spasms that cause asphyxia; anoxia produces unconsciousness. The victim may die, but does not aspirate water ("dry drowning"). Dry drowning victims have an excellent prognosis for complete recovery if resuscitated before anoxia produces brain injury.

In wet drowning the client's postresuscitation condition is impaired by the presence of fluid and the debris and solvents (mud, sand, salts, chlorine, etc.) it introduces. Osmotic movement of water across the alveolar membrane produces disturbances of body fluid and electrolyte composition. The most severe problem, however, is inadequate pulmonary gas exchange caused by pulmonary edema, which may result from either salt-water or fresh-water near-drowning.

PREVENTION

Health Promotion

1. Water safety in all its forms deserves strong emphasis:
   a. Swim only with a "buddy" and only in places where help is available; do not use a hot tub alone (fainting can result from capillary dilation).
   b. Avoid "horse play" that can cause injury or fatigue.
   c. Teach children to swim (including infants and toddlers, if they live near water).
   d. Supervise infants and children *at all times* when they are in or near a body of water and during bathing.
   e. Avoid alcoholic beverages before and during swimming and hot-tub use.
   f. Boaters need to learn and follow safety regulations for their setting: what to do in the event of a storm, where dangerous subsurface objects are located, how to find their way back to dock or mooring, and so forth.

Population at Risk

1. It is estimated that half the people in the United States are at risk for drowning because of their occupational or recreational use of water. Drowning is, after automobile accident, the leading cause of accidental death; it is the fourth leading cause of accidental death in children.
2. More men than women drown, by a ratio of about 5 to 1.
3. Adolescents 15 to 19 years old show the highest incidence of drowning.
4. People with preexisting health conditions that predispose to medical emergency in the water (e.g., myocardial disease or epilepsy).
5. People who do not know how to swim well (although many drowning victims are excellent swimmers).
6. People with impaired judgment (young children, impetuous or risk-taking adolescents, alcohol abusers, the suicidally depressed, persons with mental retardation).

Screening

None.

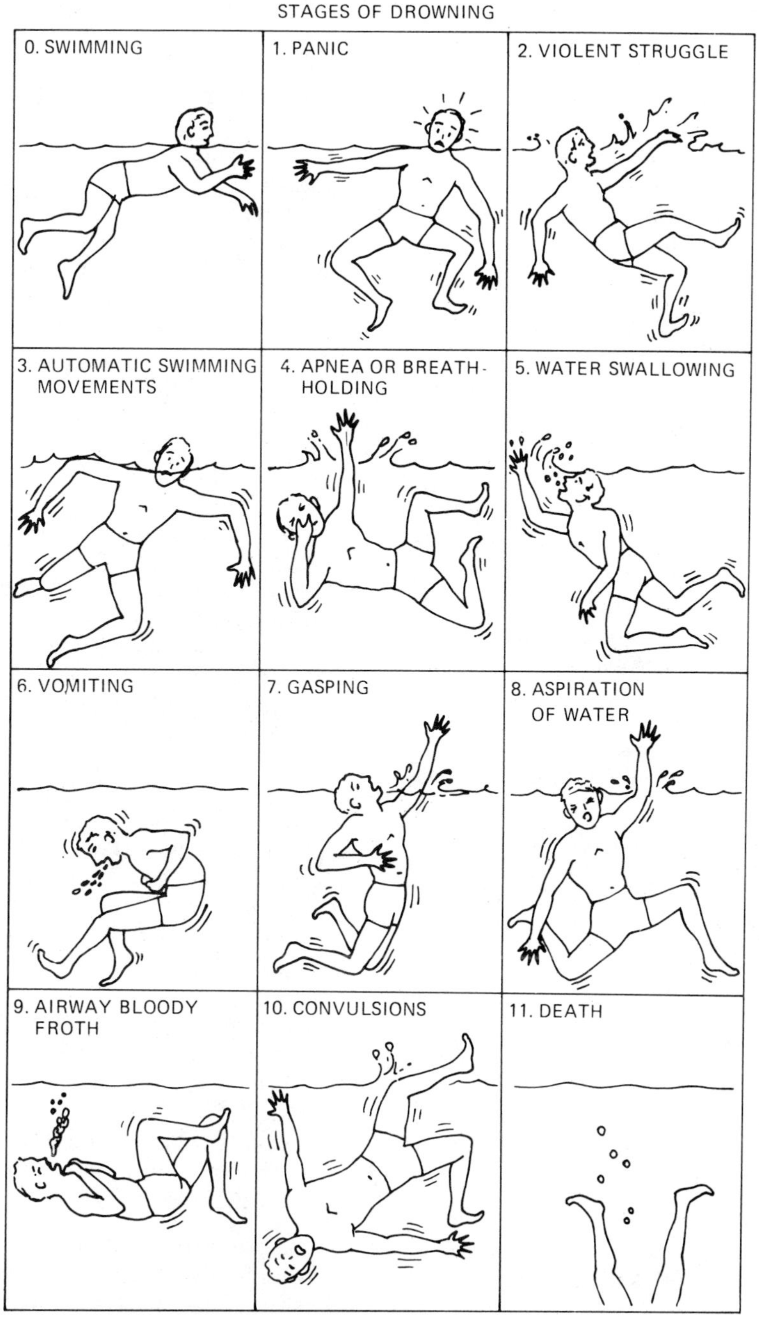

STAGES OF DROWNING

0. SWIMMING
1. PANIC
2. VIOLENT STRUGGLE
3. AUTOMATIC SWIMMING MOVEMENTS
4. APNEA OR BREATH-HOLDING
5. WATER SWALLOWING
6. VOMITING
7. GASPING
8. ASPIRATION OF WATER
9. AIRWAY BLOODY FROTH
10. CONVULSIONS
11. DEATH

Figure 48-12 Stages of drowning and near-drowning. (Adapted from Modell, J. H.: *The Pathophysiology and Treatment of Drowning and Near-Drowning*, courtesy of Charles C Thomas, Publisher, Springfield, Ill., 1971.)

ASSESSMENT

Health History

1. Obtain description of the type of water (salt or fresh) that the victim inhaled.
2. Describe where victim was found: bathtub, quarry, river, mud puddle, and so on.
3. Note time interval of submersion, anoxia, and resuscitation efforts prior to hospitalization.
4. Obtain past medical and drug history; especially note recent respiratory diseases.
5. Note allergy history, especially antibiotics.
6. Question regarding accompanying injuries or causes of drowning event, such as dive into shallow water, sting by aquatic animal.

Physical Assessment

1. Signs of acute pulmonary fluid collection: air hunger, rales, cough, tachypnea.
2. Transient neurologic symptoms of trismus, motor hyperactivity, convulsions, headache, combativeness, speech problems, and fear.
3. Laryngospasm.
4. Pink-red frothy sputum.
5. Inability to take a deep breath.
6. Burning sensation underneath sternum.
7. Pleuritic pain.
8. Some clients are asymptomatic shortly after near-drowning. It is imperative that they be taken promptly to an emergency department for evaluation, since acute pulmonary edema and death can develop in the space of a few minutes during the first 3 or 4 days after the immersion incident. This delayed symptomatology, called *secondary drowning,* is particularly likely following aspiration of fresh water.

Diagnostic Tests

1. Chest x-ray film.
2. CBC and differential, hemoglobin and hematocrit levels (look for leukocytosis).
3. Blood gases and pH.
4. Sputum cultures, if febrile or high index of suspicion regarding contaminants in inhaled fluids.
5. Bacterial cultures on fluid samples immediately, as these cultures give 24 to 72 h advance notice of probable organisms contributing to pneumonia.

NURSING DIAGNOSES: ACTUAL OR POTENTIAL

1. Impaired respiratory exchange, mild to severe, secondary to respiratory arrest or pulmonary edema associated with near-drowning.
2. Impaired circulatory function secondary to fluid and electrolyte imbalances, arrhythmias, congestive failure associated with pulmonary edema, or cardiac arrest.
3. Acid-base imbalance: respiratory acidosis (secondary drowning produces metabolic acidosis) due to fluid shifts at the alveolus and resultant fluid-electrolyte level imbalances.
4. Electrolyte level imbalances, especially hyperkalemia and hypermagnesemia associated with disturbed pulmonary and renal regulation, and ingestion or aspiration of hypertonic sea water.
5. Altered state of consciousness: confusion, delirium, or coma secondary to hypoxia and biochemical imbalances.
6. Increased risk of respiratory infection secondary to lung irritation from foreign substances (including bacteria) in the aspirated fluid.

EXPECTED OUTCOMES

1. Patent airway and adequate gas exchange will be promptly reestablished.
2. Cardiac output and systemic perfusion will be maintained or promptly reestablished.
3. Fluid, electrolyte, and acid-base balance will be reestablished.
4. Client will not sustain injury during confusion, unconsciousness, or seizures.
5. Normal consciousness and intellect will be restored.
6. Sepsis will be treated and controlled.

INTERVENTIONS

1. Begin cardiopulmonary resuscitation immeidately. Mouth-to-mouth resuscitation should begin while victim is still being removed from the water. Do not attempt to remove water from respiratory tract. Such efforts are unproductive and waste critical time. Note: submersion in cold water markedly reduces the metabolic requirements of the brain and other vital organs; successful resuscitation without residual brain damage

has been reported after 20 or 30 minutes of submersion.
2. Suction airway secretions to maintain patency.
3. Oxygenate to maintain arterial Pa_{O_2} within normal range (greater than 80 mmHg) and acid-base in balance (pH 7.35).
4. Collect arterial blood samples frequently to ascertain changes in blood gases.
5. Continuously monitor cardiac status via dynamic ECG.
6. Treat arrhythmias with drugs as prescribed.
7. Position patient for gravity flow of stomach contents to minimize risk of aspirating vomitus.
8. Insert nasogastric tube if stomach contents continue to threaten aspiration.
9. Administer IV fluids as prescribed. Fresh water drowning: use, to keep intravenous line open, 5 percent dextrose in water for medication administration only. Salt water drowning: use 5 percent dextrose in saline, normal saline, or Ringer's solution, if no clinical electrolyte level imbalances exist.
10. Treat accompanying injuries of hemorrhage, seizures, anaphylaxis, allergic reactions, fractures, and so forth with appropriate intervention.
11. Monitor urine for hourly output, specific gravity, pH, and occult blood.
12. Administer broad-spectrum antibiotics until specific culture reports become available.
13. Cleanse and dress all wounds; immunize for tetanus if necessary.
14. Provide rapid, active rewarming for all hypothermia victims.
15. Protect against injury if consciousness is altered: apply protective eye coverings for unconscious client; pad bed rails and remove potentially injurious objects from bed if client is convulsive, and so forth as circumstances dictate.

EVALUATION

Outcome Criteria

1. Cardiopulmonary resuscitation is effected promptly.
2. Blood pressure is maintained above 90/60 to ensure perfusion to vital organs.
3. Pulmonary function is restored to adequate levels, as indicated by blood gases within normal limits.
4. Client does not aspirate stomach contents or become injured by convulsion, confusion, or during unconsciousness.
5. Cerebral function (consciousness and cognition) returns to normal.
6. Infection is controlled and eliminated.

Complications

1. Disseminated intravascular coagulation (DIC).
2. Acute renal failure (acute tubular necrosis) due to hypoxia and inadequate perfusion.
3. Neurological abnormalities secondary to hypoxia.
4. Residual pulmonary disorders: empyema, lung abscess, atelectasis associated with foreign bodies, or the combination of reduced lung compliance and pulmonary edema called adult respiratory distress syndrome.
5. Hemorrhagic diathesis.
6. Secondary drowning.

Reevaluation and Follow-up

1. All victims should be hospitalized and observed for 24 to 48 hours even if they respond immediately to resuscitation. Incidence of fulminating pneumonia and secondary drowning is extremely high, with certain mortality if untreated.
2. All near-drowning victims should be reevaluated in 5 to 14 days for primary amebic meningoencephalitis and leptospirosis meningoencephalitis, if in endemic areas (Sims, 1978).

ALTITUDE SICKNESS (MOUNTAIN SICKNESS)

DESCRIPTION

At altitudes greater than 8,000 feet above sea level, the reduced oxygen saturation of the air produces hypoxemia. Symptoms increase with increasing altitude (and with activity) and range from euphoria to marked loss of cognitive and physical functions and finally to coma. Two severe manifestations of altitude sickness are pulmonary and cerebral edema. The pathophysiology underlying these two problems is obscure. Prognosis is excellent if victim is immediately removed to lower altitude when more than mild clinical symptoms begin.

PREVENTION

Health Promotion

1. Ascents to altitudes over 8,000 ft must be made slowly, climbing no more than 1,000 ft per day, and stopping as necessary for a day or so to become acclimatized before going on.
2. Activities must be adjusted to each person's level of tolerance.

Population at Risk

1. Mountain climbers, hikers, sportspeople, and others who ascend over 8,000 ft above sea level.
2. People under 21 years of age are especially susceptible.
3. People in unpressurized high-altitude vehicles.

Screening

None.

ASSESSMENT

Health History

1. Obtain description of environment where symptoms started.
2. Note precautions employed by victim if seasoned mountain climber.
3. Ascertain past medical history, including medications and allergies.
4. Describe ascent and descent symptomatology.
5. Record all medications administered prior to reaching hospital: doses, frequency, and responses.
6. Note whether oxygen was administered and amount and length of time used.
7. Describe all additional injuries or pathologies.

Physical Assessment

1. Elevated pulse and respiratory rates.
2. Euphoria (initially).
3. Gradually decreasing mental and physical alertness.
4. Oliguria.
5 Nausea, vomiting, poor appetite.
6. Tinnitus and deafness; serous effusions into the middle ear.
7. Lethargy, fatigue.
8. Vertigo.
9. Indications of acute pulmonary edema: severe dyspnea, orthopnea, tachycardia, pallor, red-tinged frothy sputum, wheezing, cyanosis, rales, or bubbling respirations.
10. Indications of cerebral edema: confusion, headache, impaired judgment, staggering, loss of consciousness, or convulsions.

Diagnostic Tests

1. Arterial blood gases.
2. Hemoglobin and hematocrit levels (note increased hematocrit) and CBC (note increase in adhesiveness and aggregability of platelets): these findings indicate risk of thrombus formation.
3. Chest x-ray film.
4. Electrolyte level determinations, if vomiting persists.

NURSING DIAGNOSES: ACTUAL OR POTENTIAL

1. Altered cognitive-perceptual function (thought, vision, hearing) secondary to brain hypoxia.
2. Altered level of consciousness: euphoria, confusion, stupor, or coma due to brain hypoxia.
3. Decreased activity tolerance secondary to hypoxemia.
4. Nutritional and fluid deficits and electrolyte level imbalances secondary to anorexia, nausea, and vomiting.
5. Impaired respiratory function secondary to pulmonary edema.
6. Alterations in comfort: discomfort associated with weakness, nausea, or headache.
7. Increased risk of injury due to impaired judgment, seizures, or unconsciousness.
8. Increased risk of thromboembolic phenomena due to compensatory polycythemia and fluid deficit.

EXPECTED OUTCOMES

1. Client's blood oxygen saturation will be restored, as indicated by relief of symptoms.
   a. Judgment, perception, and thought processes will return to normal.
   b. Level of consciousness will return to normal.
   c. Activity tolerance will be restored.
   d. Vital signs will return to normal.
   e. Comfort will be restored.
   f. Gastrointestinal symptoms will be alleviated.
   g. Hearing impairment and ringing or popping of the ears will be relieved.
2. Fluid balance and electrolyte values will return to normal limits.

3. Respiratory gas exchange will be maintained, and pulmonary function will be restored as indicated by normal blood gases and client's resumption of normal respiratory rate and lung sounds.
4. Client will be protected against injury caused by impaired judgment, convulsion, or coma.
5. Thrombus formation will be prevented or promptly recognized and treated; emboli will not occur.

INTERVENTIONS

1. For mild symptoms, client needs to limit activity to the level of tolerance (bed rest may be required) for a day or so; symptoms should resolve as client makes physiologic adaptations to the altitude.
2. If signs and symptoms are severe, and definitely if they include indications of pulmonary edema or cerebral edema (see Physical Assessment, items 9 and 10 above), the client must be moved immediately to a lower altitude at which he or she has previously been well, and should be placed in a pressurized compartment until transportation becomes available.
3. Provide positive-pressure oxygen by face mask and rebreathing bag at 2 to 4 liters; if respiratory distress is marked, intermittent positive-pressure breathing (IPPB) or continuous end-expiratory pressure (CEEP) may be required. Monitor arterial blood gases.
4. For pulmonary edema, elevate head of bed 45 to 90 degrees; apply rotating tourniquets; and administer IV furosemide (Lasix) as prescribed, often 40 to 80 mg every 5 min for 2 to 3 doses.
5. Protect confused or unconscious person from injury due to poor judgment, convulsion, or coma.
6. Orient client to environment and events as consciousness and lucidity return.
7. Restore nutrient and fluid intake, being judicious about IV fluid administration lest client become underhydrated (which will increase risk of thrombus) or overhydrated (which will worsen pulmonary and cerebral edema). Excessive nausea and vomiting may be treated with dimenhydrinate (Dramamine), 50 to 100 mg orally, or intramuscularly if client is unable to retain oral dosage.
8. Measure intake and output.
9. Discourage thrombosis by positioning for good venous return (e.g., client should not cross legs) and active or passive motion exercises. Monitor for indications of thrombus formation (pain or discomfort in calves or above IV sites, or redness or tenderness along the vein). Monitor hemoglobin and hematocrit for polycythemia, which predisposes to thrombosis.
10. Provide mild analgesia as prescribed for headache (aspirin).
11. Nasal decongestant may be prescribed for middle ear congestion, usually a combination of ephedrine and antihistamine.
12. Continually monitor respiratory effort, arterial oxygen saturation, vital signs, level of consciousness, and orientation in response to treatment.

EVALUATION

Outcome Criteria

1. Neurological, pulmonary, and vital signs indicate return to normal function: judgment, sensorium, cognition, respiratory function, activity tolerance, and vital signs return to pretrauma status within 12 to 36 hours.
2. Client has no continuing discomforts (nausea, headache, hearing problems, sleeplessness, etc.) after 2 to 3 days.
3. Serum electrolyte values, arterial blood gases, and CBC are within normal limits.
4. No injury has occurred during symptomatic phase.
5. Thromboembolic disease has not occurred.

Complications

1. Residual pulmonary deficit (rare).
2. Injury or death from misjudgment (e.g., falling, getting lost), pulmonary or cerebral edema, or associated hypothermia.

DECOMPRESSION SICKNESS (BENDS, CAISSON DISEASE, DIVER'S PARALYSIS)

DESCRIPTION

Decompression sickness is caused by the release of nitrogen bubbles into the bloodstream during too rapid decompression from hyperbaric pressure (i.e., from more than 1 atmosphere of pressure). The quantity of gas that a liquid will absorb increases as pressure increases. Accordingly, when the body is under hyperbaric pressure (during deep sea diving, for example), the body fluids absorb extra nitrogen and oxygen from the inspired air. When the atmospheric pressure is reduced, these excess gases come out of solution. If pressure reduction is gradual, the gases are accommodated by the usual respiratory mechanisms and are simply discharged in exhaled air. But if decompression proceeds too rapidly, the gases form bubbles in the bloodstream that act as air emboli in the capillaries. Nitrogen is the important offender, since oxygen is readily absorbed by the body, including the RBCs. The nitrogen emboli are responsible for the manifestations of the disease. Symptoms appear from minutes up to 10 hours after ascent, usually in 1 to 3 hours. Treatment is to return the victim to hyperbaric pressure so that the nitrogen goes back into solution and decompress gradually, and to provide supportive treatment such as oxygen and analgesia.

PREVENTION

Health Promotion

Adherence to safety specifications for control of compression forces, and of decompression speeds, such as the U.S. Navy standard air decompression tables (obtainable, along with other diving safety literature, from U.S. Navy Experimental Diving Unit, Washington, D.C., 202-433-2790, 24-hour phone).

Population at Risk

1. Persons whose work or recreation involves changes in atmospheric pressure (symptoms may occur even in water as shallow as 10 or 12 feet).
   a. People who work in air locks under increased atmospheric pressure.
   b. Scuba divers and helmet-suit-airhose divers (not shallow-water snorkel divers).
   c. Fliers who ascend rapidly in unpressurized compartments or who lose compression while airborne.

Screening

None.

ASSESSMENT

Health History

1. Note depth of dive (atmospheric pressure doubles with each 33 feet of water depth) and length of time in hyperbaric situation.
2. Describe if victim was scuba diving or in a helmeted deep-diving suit.
3. Describe all therapeutic interventions prior to hospitalization.
4. Note if victim was in salt or fresh water when symptoms began.
5. Obtain past medical history, including medications and allergies.
6. Note if victim is a smoker and approximate number of packs smoked per day.

Physical Assessment

1. Severe throbbing pain which shifts sites frequently from joints, muscles, and bones and may simulate an acute surgical abdomen.
2. Dermatologic symptoms, including intense pruritus, mottling, erythema, and bleb formation.
3. Bladder and bowel incontinence.
4. Bizarre neurologic symptoms of numbness, tingling of extremities, paresthesias, hemi-, para-, and quadriplegia, and paresis.
5. Eye manifestations of strabismus, nystagmus, or diplopia.
6. Vertigo, which may cause staggering gait.
7. Acute dyspnea several hours to days after successful recompression and decompression treatment.
8. Collapse and unconsciousness.
9. Hypothermia.
10. Signs and symptoms of fresh or salt water near-drowning.
11. Rupture of tympanic membranes.
12. Subcutaneous emphysema.
13. Bleeding from the nose or ears.
14. Scuba divers: conjunctival hemorrhages, carbon monoxide poisoning from impure air in the cylinder, and carbon dioxide poisoning.
15. Hemoptysis.
16. Pneumothroax and respiratory arrest.

Diagnostic Tests

1. Arterial blood gases.
2. Oxygen saturation.
3. Chest x-ray film.

NURSING DIAGNOSES: ACTUAL OR POTENTIAL

1. Alteration in comfort: pain due to ischemia from capillary nitrogen gas emboli.
2. Alteration in perception: numbness, tingling, other paresthesias, and visual disturbances

associated with central nervous system ischemia.
3. Alterations in mobility: gait disturbances and even paralysis secondary to central nervous system ischemia.
4. Alterations in skin integrity: erythema, mottling, and intense itching secondary to ischemia.
5. Anxiety secondary to pain, bleeding from nose and ears, and sensorimotor changes.
6. Alterations in consciousness: confusion, disorientation, or unconsciousness secondary to brain ischemia or hypoxia from pulmonary involvement.
7. Respiratory insufficiency ("chokes"): dyspnea, cough, and substernal pain progressing to marked dyspnea and severe hypoxia, secondary to ischemia.
8. Increased risk of thrombosis secondary to obstructed blood flow.

EXPECTED OUTCOMES

1. Client will be recompressed and then gradually decompressed in a hyperbaric pressure chamber.
2. Client will receive respiratory support and oxygen therapy to maintain cardiorespiratory function before and during decompression as necessary.
3. Client's pain will be alleviated.
4. Client will return to normal level of consciousness and sensorimotor function.
5. Client will not sustain injury during period of confusion or unconsciousness.

INTERVENTIONS

1. Provide continuous artificial respiration by mouth-to-mouth, bag-to-mouth, or mechanical support, as feasible.
2. Provide 100% oxygen at 10 liters via face mask.
3. Stop epistaxis and external ear bleeding with firm pressure against ruptured areas and equilibration of sinus pressures with barometric pressure.
4. Stay with victim throughout procedure in decompression chamber to alleviate fears and help orient to reality.
5. Provide analgesia by narcotic as prescribed, such as careful administration of 2 to 10 mg IV of morphine sulfate. Watch respiratory patterns and circulation.
6. Give nasal decongestants and antihistamines as precribed to reduce middle ear fluid accumulation (e.g., Actifed, a combination of triprolidine hydrochloride, 2.5 mg, and pseudoephedrine hydrochloride, 60 mg).
7. Rewarm rapidly to normal body temperature range, and monitor for thermal changes over 24 to 48 h.
8. Monitor vital and neurologic signs frequently until stabilized and victim has completed decompression procedure.
9. Minimize coughing and sneezing until internal head and thoracic pressures are normalized.

EVALUATION

Outcome Criteria

1. Recompression and slow decompression are begun promptly.
2. Cardiopulmonary function is maintained.
3. Pain is reduced by analgesia and thoroughly relieved by recompression.
4. Consciousness, sensation, and motor function are restored to pretrauma level.
5. Client is successfully protected against injury during period of altered consciousness.

Complications

1. Cardiac arrhythmias, shock, and arrest.
2. Residual injury from air embolism (stroke, infarction).
3. Acute pulmonary edema may occur within 24 hours of evidently uneventful recompression and decompression, causing acute dyspnea, and can lead rapidly to death.

Reevaluation and Follow-up

1. Any person with joint pains within 48 hours of diving should be treated (recompressed and decompressed), even though symptoms seem mild, as a precaution against life-threatening late sequelae. The treatment (compression chamber) carries no risk to either the client or the health care staff and should be initiated whenever the possibility of decompression sickness exists.
2. Clients must be observed for 24 hours after compression chamber treatment in order to discern and immediately treat pulmonary complications that may develop even after successful treatment.

WOUNDS

ABRASIONS

DESCRIPTION

An abrasion is a painful, superficial wound, scraping the epidermis and occasionally the upper levels of dermis. Frequently, it is the result of a forceful, skidding motion. A skinned knee is an example of this type of wound. There is an excellent prognosis for complete recovery.

PREVENTION

Health Promotion

1. Prevention of falls and scrapes by general safety measures.
2. Protective clothing when feasible for people at special risk (knee and elbow pads for basketball players and skateboard riders; helmets, boots, and long sleeves and long trousers for motorcyclists, and so forth).

Population at Risk

1. People engaged in vigorous physical activity (e.g., children at play, athletes).
2. People with poor motor coordination (e.g., young children, persons with cerebral palsy).

Screening

None.

ASSESSMENT

Health History

1. Description of incident producing injury.
2. Description of environmental conditions where injury occurred, such as gravel path, sand, cement, and so on.
3. Time interval from injury to request for treatment.
4. History of tetanus immunization.
5. Medication allergies.

Physical Assessment

1. Assess depth of tissue injury (superficial).
2. Look for contaminants and debris ground into wound.

Diagnostic Tests

None.

NURSING DIAGNOSES: ACTUAL OR POTENTIAL

1. Impaired skin integrity secondary to trauma.
2. Alteration of comfort: pain secondary to skin injury.
3. Increased risk of secondary infection due to loss of skin integrity.

EXPECTED OUTCOMES

1. Client's skin will heal with minimal scarring.
2. Client's comfort will be restored.
3. Secondary infection will be avoided.

INTERVENTIONS

1. Before cleansing or debriding, if wound is extensive enough so that substantial pain is anticipated from those procedures, provide anesthesia as prescribed. Lidocaine is preferred; it is available in several forms:
   a. Topical solution (2 or 4 percent): duration of anesthesia approximately 20 min.
   b. Ointment (2.5, 4, and 5 percent); used as vehicle to remove free-floating dirt (not water soluble).
   c. Jelly (2.5, 4, and 5 percent); water soluble.
   d. Injectable, plain ($\frac{1}{2}$ to 2 percent): do not use cardiac lidocaine because deterioration of medication strength is possible (due to lack of preservatives).
2. Scrupulously cleanse wound with saline until dirt and particulate matter are removed.
3. Debride wound with forceps.
4. Apply dressing:
   a. Open: very thin coat of petroleum-base ointment (antibiotics are acceptable, but avoid Neosporin due to high incidence of sensitivity).
   b. Closed: fine-mesh or Owen silk gauze.
5. Teach client to care for wounds by changing dressings daily or as circumstances require and keeping areas free of moisture.
6. Instruct client in periodic use of anesthetic topical applications and oral analgesic (aspirin, etc.) for pain management.
7. Reassure client that though area will be discolored for a period of time, it will not scar if

secondary infection is avoided or promptly treated.

EVALUATION

Outcome Criteria

1. Healing takes place without infection and without permanent scarring or discoloration.
2. Pain is controlled.

Complications

Bacterial infection: purulent drainage, erythema, possible temperature elevation.

AVULSIONS

DESCRIPTION

Avulsion is the tearing away and complete loss of tissue; this injury disallows the approximation of wound edges. It most frequently occurs with nose tip, ear lobe, and fingertip injuries.

PREVENTION

Health Promotion

1. Keep young children and untrained people away from hazardous machinery; teach children safe use of appropriate machines, tools, and so forth.
2. Teach children safety precautions to avoid animal bites (dogs and horses are the domestic animals most often responsible for bite avulsions).

Population at Risk

1. Persons who use tools and machines capable of cutting and tearing away tissue: mechanics, farmers, and many industrial workers.
2. Virtually everyone (fingers can get caught in car doors, feet can be injured by dropped objects, etc.).

Screening

None.

ASSESSMENT

Health History

1. Note time of tissue loss to determine salvageability.
2. Obtain description of forces causing tearing and removal of tissue.
3. Ascertain if injury is job-oriented.
4. Obtain all tissue specimens for preservation and potential reimplanting.

Physical Assessment

1. Extent of tissue loss.
2. Alteration in function of part affected.
3. Hemorrhage.
4. Pain.
5. Disfigurement.
6. Swelling, edema.
7. Local hyperemia.

Diagnostic Tests

1. X-ray film to rule out bone injury (especially in digits).
2. If large avulsion with possible surgical intervention: CBC and differential (including Hb and Hct).

NURSING DIAGNOSES: ACTUAL OR POTENTIAL

1. Impaired skin integrity secondary to trauma.
2. Alteration in comfort: pain secondary to tissue injury.
3. Blood loss secondary to tissue trauma and open wound.
4. Increased risk of infection due to open wound.
5. Self-care deficit due to loss of function in injured body part.
6. Decreased mobility due to loss of function in injured body part.
7. Alterations in self-concept secondary to impaired function and disfigurement.
8. Anxiety associated with impaired function and disfigurement.

EXPECTED OUTCOMES

1. Pain and discomfort will be alleviated.
2. Bleeding will be controlled.
3. Infection will be prevented or adequately treated.
4. Function and appearance of the injured part will be restored to the maximum degree possible.
5. Client will maintain mobility and self-care at the highest level safely permitted by the injury.
6. Client's anxiety will be controlled and alleviated.
7. Self-concept, including body image, will be adequate for good psychosocial function.

Interventions

1. If amputated tissue is being brought from home, roll it so that adipose and subcutaneous tissues are inside to protect from drying, and place in airtight container with ice on outside. *Do not carry tissue in water, antiseptic, or any other solution* except (if available) normal saline.
2. Preserve all avulsed tissue in saline packs or saline solution and keep cool for possible surgical reimplantation.
3. Provide analgesia: topical or nerve block for wound cleaning and repair.
4. Cleanse avulsed area gently with free-flowing saline.
5. Remove all dirt and contaminants with flow of fluids and/or forceps.
6. Do not soak affected tissue in antiseptic solutions.
7. To stop bleeding, apply gentle pressure, gel foam, or topical thrombin.
8. Dress avulsed area with fine-mesh gauze, 2 by 2 inch or 4 by 4 inch fluffs and tube gauze, or with gentle pressure dressing.
9. Provide protective devices (e.g., finger shield or guard).
10. Do not apply tape over injured area.
11. If surgical repair under general anesthesia is anticipated, withhold food and oral fluids.
12. Before discharge, teach client to leave dressing intact for 10 to 14 days and to keep area dry.
13. Teach client to look for regional and systemic indications of infection rather than for local ones.
14. Assist or instruct client in compensatory methods of self-care and mobility, as appropriate to location and type of injury.
15. Instruct client in activity restrictions if any are necessary to avoid infection and to maximize tissue repair.
16. Assist client to reduce anxiety and enhance self-concept by explaining all procedures, realistically informing about treatment plan and prognosis. Teach client about his or her role in treatment and recovery, and listen to client's discussion and questions.

EVALUATION

Outcome Criteria

1. Pain and bleeding are well controlled.
2. Infection does not occur or is effectively and promptly treated.
3. Function and appearance of the injured part are restored.
4. Self-care and mobility are maintained at a safe level with appropriate compensations as required by the injury.
5. Anxiety and self-concept are adequate as evidenced by client's cooperative participation in the treatment plan and maintenance of usual psychosocial function (social interaction patterns, and so forth).

Complications

1. Sepsis.
2. Residual impairment of function or appearance.

Reevaluation and Follow-up

1. Physical therapy, vocational rehabilitation, and home nursing referrals should be arranged if needed.
2. Plastic surgery may be required after healing is complete if tissue regrowth does not fill in avulsed area or if associated scars or contractures need revision.

CONTUSIONS

DESCRIPTION

A contusion is a nonpenetrating injury to soft tissue more commonly called a *bruise*. The injury is produced by a sharp blow to tissue, causing disruption and oozing of tiny blood vessels. Small contusions resulting in mild ecchymosis are nonthreatening and resolve without intervention. Large contusions of extensive tissue mass, such as the thigh or buttocks, have large pools of blood that may become infected and cause abscess formation.

PREVENTION

Health Promotion

1. Avoidance of falls and collisions by general safety measures.
2. Use of automobile seat belts.
3. Special instruction to people at special risk so that they can be aware of their risk and take appropriate precautions.

Population at Risk

1. Everyone at risk for falls or other high-impact injuries (athletes, climbers, children at play,

persons with impaired vision or hearing, cyclists, etc.).
2. Special risk exists for people with bleeding or coagulation disorders: hemophiliacs, persons taking anticoagulants, leukemia patients, and so forth.

Screening

None.

ASSESSMENT

Health History

1. Obtain description of injury force.
2. Note time of injury and interval elapsed before medical care was sought.
3. Question for past medical history and bleeding tendencies.
4. Request medication history.

Physical Assessment

1. Note size and location of contusion.
2. Assess swelling by comparing to uninjured contralateral part.
3. Assess neurovascular function: sensation, movement, and perfusion (pulses, nailbed filling, warmth) distal to the injury.
4. Inspect for areas of trapped interstitial bleeding:
   a. Subungual hematomas.
   b. Compartment syndrome (swelling trapped within a fascia sheath compresses the structures in the sheath so that perfusion and innervation are compromised): pain on passive stretching of the involved area, tenderness on palpation, and diminished peripheral pulses or capillary filling.

Diagnostic Tests

Usually none; bleeding and clotting studies if hemostasis is in question.

NURSING DIAGNOSES: ACTUAL OR POTENTIAL

1. Alteration in comfort: pain and discomfort secondary to bleeding into tissues.
2. Impaired mobility secondary to pain or associated injuries (e.g., sprain).
3. Diminished self-care secondary to decreased mobility.
4. Risk of infection associated with free blood in tissues (excellent culture medium).
5. Risk of circulatory and neurological impairment associated with compartment syndrome or other area of entrapped hemorrhage.

EXPECTED OUTCOMES

1. Interstitial bleeding will be stopped.
2. Pain and discomfort will be reduced and eliminated.
3. Mobility and self-care will be maintained safely.
4. Abscess will be prevented or promptly recognized and treated.
5. Perfusion and neurological function will be maintained.

INTERVENTIONS

1. Apply cold, wet compresses or ice bag, or pack in fresh water ice to prevent further hemorrhage into tissues. Do not use iced saline, because temperature of slush is too low and tends to further damage tissues.
2. Elevate affected area, if possible.
3. Immobilize part, and place affected tissues at rest.
4. Mark ecchymosed area to monitor continued bleeding.
5. Provide mild analgesics orally. Avoid aspirin.
6. Note changes in neurovascular function (diminishing pulses or prolonged capillary refill times); notify physician promptly.
7. Release subungual hematoma by perforating nail with thermolance, heated copper paper clip held on nail just above trapped blood, or short-bevel no. 18 needle; apply bandaid.
8. After 24 h, apply heat to bruise with warm moist packs or heating pad.
9. If abscess develops it will require incision and drainage; assist client through procedure, instruct in aftercare (dressings, soaks, etc.), and administer antibiotics as prescribed.
10. Assist client in achieving required mobility and self-care (planning for home care, arranging alternative transportation, etc.).

EVALUATION

Outcome Criteria

1. Pain and discomfort are alleviated.
2. Bleeding is stopped.
3. Neurovascular function is maintained:

pulses, sensation, and movement are normal in affected area and distal parts.
4. Infection, if it occurs, is recognized and treated.
5. Client maintains mobility and self-care at the highest level compatible with the injury.

CRUSH WOUNDS

DESCRIPTION

Crush wounds give rise to massive edema, extensive interstitial bleeding, and internal and external injuries involving many structures.

PREVENTION

Health Promotion

1. Occupational safety training (and equipment maintenance) for persons who work with hydraulic lifts, block and tackle equipment, railroad car couplings, heavy earth-moving equipment, and so forth.
2. Home safety precautions regarding heavy equipment, including automobiles (e.g., be certain of small children's whereabouts before backing up, and do not work under cars that are insecurely jacked).

Population at Risk

1. Persons who work in construction, in automotive repair, or with presses and wringers of various kinds.
2. Children or others who are in danger of being run over by an automobile.

Screening

None.

ASSESSMENT

Health History

1. Description of forces causing injury.
2. Treatment rendered prior to admission.
3. Estimation of fluid and blood loss prior to admission.
4. Description of additional injuries.

Physical Assessment

1. Arterial insufficiency due to vascular spasm, occlusion, or tears.
2. Nerve deficits of neurotmesis, axonotmesis, neuropraxia.
3. Loss of tendon function due to divisions or ruptures.
4. Massive hematomas within muscles of belly.
5. Shock symptoms.
6. Hyperkalemia with resultant cardiac arrhythmias.
7. Symptoms of sepsis.
8. Accompanying fractures.
9. "Splitting," or "explosion" lacerations.
10. Massive discoloration of area, including ecchymoses.
11. Disfigurement.
12. Pain.

Diagnostic Tests

1. Radiographic evaluation.
2. CBC, differential, hemoglobin, hematocrit, and electrolyte levels.
3. Urinalysis for hemoglobin and RBCs.

NURSING DIAGNOSES: ACTUAL OR POTENTIAL

1. Alteration in fluid balance secondary to possibly massive loss of circulating volume caused by hemorrhage and shift to interstitial fluid compartment.
2. Circulatory impairment associated with interruption of local perfusion or with systemic hypoperfusion (shock).
3. Electrolyte imbalance secondary to fluid shifts, tissue destruction, and possibly renal damage.
4. Alteration in renal function: hematuria, myoglobinuria, or diminished output (acute renal failure) secondary to tubular obstruction from tissue breakdown byproducts (e.g., hemoglobin or myoglobin) or secondary to tubular necrosis from hypoperfusion.
5. Alteration in comfort: pain secondary to trauma.
6. Alteration in perception: sensory disturbances secondary to neurological damage.
7. Sepsis secondary to bacterial invasion of traumatized tissue.
8. Self-care deficit and impaired mobility secondary to trauma.
9. Anxiety and alteration in self-concept, including body image, secondary to disfigurement, impaired mobility, and self-care deficit.

EXPECTED OUTCOMES

1. Cardiorespiratory function will be maintained, as evidenced by vital signs and blood

gases within normal limits (BP 90/60 or above), and perfusion will be adequate in and distal to injured area.
2. Hydration will be maintained.
3. Electrolyte values will remain within normal limits as indicated by blood chemistry reports.
4. Urine output will be adequate for age and hydration (allowing for fluid losses through wounds).
5. Pain will be controlled.
6. Neurological function of affected part, including sensory perception, will be restored.
7. Infection will be prevented or effectively treated.
8. Self-care and mobility will be maintained at the highest safe level compatible with injury.
9. Self-concept will be satisfactory as evidenced by resumption of preinjury social interaction patterns and cooperative participation in the treatment plan.

INTERVENTIONS

1. Lower temperature of affected part (to reduce metabolic requirements) by applying ice packs; no not used iced saline, because its temperature goes so low that it injures tissues.
2. Elevate injured part above heart level to minimize swelling.
3. Immobilize injured area and place client at rest to minimize release of toxic products from traumatized cells.
4. Give analgesic as prescribed.
5. Keep client supine, and monitor vital signs often.
6. Provide salty oral fluids if client is conscious, unless NPO in anticipation of surgery.
7. Monitor IV fluids as prescribed to maintain perfusion pressure at 90 mmHg systolic.
8. Monitor laboratory electrolyte values.
9. Place client on cardiac monitor while hyperkalemic, and observe for myocardial arrhythmias.
10. Monitor pulses and sensation distal to injured area, and observe for swelling and occlusion.
11. Monitor urinary intake and output.
12. Apply light dressings until client is evaluated for definitive treatment.
13. Update tetanus prophylaxis if immunity has expired.
14. Cleanse wounds as directed by physician and administer prescribed antibiotic.
15. Compression dressings may be used for extremity injury: wrap from distal to proximal, and monitor for adequacy of circulation (color, warmth, swelling distal to bandage, pain).
16. Instruct client in prescribed activity restrictions, helping plan adaptations in self-care or mobility patterns so client can be as independent as feasible within the restrictions necessary to prevent further injury to traumatized tissue.
17. Reduce anxiety and support self-concept by explaining all treatments and client's role in the treatment plan and providing realistic information about immediate and long-range prognosis.

EVALUATION

Outcome Criteria

1. Vital signs and hydration remain within normal limits, with blood pressure at least 90/60; pulses, warmth, and capillary filling indicate adequate perfusion.
2. Electrolyte values are within normal limits.
3. Urine output is normal for age and hydration.
4. Pain is controlled.
5. Sensation and movement indicate that neurological function is intact.
6. Infection is avoided or effectively treated.
7. Client is mobile and performs self-help activities to the highest safe level permitted by injury.
8. Client evidences adequate self-concept by complying with recommended therapy and by maintaining usual patterns of social interaction.

Complications

1. Residual deformity or impaired function.
2. Vascular compromise necessitating amputation.
3. Osteomyelitis, septic arthritis, or other prolonged infection.
4. Embolus from tissue debris.

Reevaluation and Follow-up

Referral to physical therapist, visiting nurse, vocational rehabilitation, or psychotherapist may be helpful to client.

LACERATIONS

DESCRIPTION

A laceration is a traumatic opening of skin, mucous membranes, or parenchymal tissue. The lacerated tissue may be contused, avulsed, bevelled, straight or jagged, torn or mangled, and dirty or clean. A laceration occurs when external forces cause incision or other abrupt disruption of tissue, such as splitting. Occasionally, intense internal pressure of tissue will cause eruption-type laceration.

PREVENTION

Health Promotion

1. General accident prevention precautions and preventive teaching, especially where sharp instruments are in use.
2. Use of automobile seat belts reduces the probability of face and head lacerations in auto mishaps.

Population at Risk

1. Industrial workers who deal with glass, sharp instruments, and other materials that produce cuts.
2. People employed in food preparation and food service.
3. People who are involved in most kinds of general accidents, since laceration often accompanies trauma of all sorts: children, alcoholics, athletes, and victims of automobile accidents.

Screening

None.

ASSESSMENT

Health History

1. Ascertain the mechanism of injury, since that will influence the treatment: blow to part, striking head on flat or pointed object, fall into dirt or dung, and so forth.
2. Determine time of injury and interval before seeking medical care (if injury is over 6 to 12 hours old, do not suture, due to probability of infection).
3. Note past medical and drug history, including tetanus prophylaxis.
4. Note medication allergies, especially antibiotics.
5. Determine if injury is work-related.
6. If wounds are extensive, take photographs for later plastic repairs.
7. Note what treatment was initiated prior to admission.
8. Ascertain if client is on anticoagulants or has a bleeding disorder.

Physical Assessment

1. Extent of hemorrhage and body fluid losses.
2. Destruction of tissue and underlying organs relative to mechanism of injury; a blunt blow causing laceration of skin may result in extensive soft tissue injury surrounding site or tear in organ parenchyma.
3. Gross contamination of wound with foreign matter, dirt, hair, pebbles, sand, dung.
4. Irregularity and jaggedness of wound edges, with little blood supply.
5. Assess movement and sensation before anesthetics are given.
6. If laceration has begun to heal, erythema, swelling at wound edge, and purulent drainage may be present.

Diagnostic Tests

1. CBC, including differential.
2. Hemoglobin and hematocrit levels.
3. Partial thromboplastin time (PTT) and prothrombin time (PT) if client is receiving anticoagulation therapy or has history of bleeding.
4. X-ray film of affected part if laceration is deep over bony prominence or if injury is due to fall.
5. Wound culture and sensitivities.

NURSING DIAGNOSES: ACTUAL OR POTENTIAL

1. Impariment of skin integrity due to trauma.
2. Alteration in comfort: pain due to tissue trauma.
3. Increased risk of infection due to loss of skin integrity.
4. Alteration in body fluids secondary to blood loss.
5. Alteration in cardiac output: shock secondary to blood loss.
6. Diminished perfusion at and distal to the site of the injury, due to incised vasculature.
7. Diminished sensation or motor function due to nerve injury.

8. Diminished mobility and self-care deficit secondary to injury.
9. Alteration in self-concept secondary to altered function or appearance.

EXPECTED OUTCOMES

1. Client will heal with minimal scarring or loss of function.
2. Infection will be prevented or adequately treated.
3. Blood loss will be controlled, and blood pressure will not fall below 90/60.
4. Perfusion will be maintained to tissues distal to the laceration, as evidenced by pulses, capillary filling, warmth, and color.
5. Pain will be reduced and eliminated.
6. Client will maintain mobility and self-help activities at the highest safe level compatible with the injury.
7. Adequate self-concept will be maintained as evidenced by compliance with the treatment plan and maintenance of usual social interaction patterns.

INTERVENTIONS

1. Monitor bleeding and blood loss; provide hemostasis by pressure dressings.
2. Use sterile technique in all wound cleansing and repair.
3. Local anesthetic may be needed before cleansing, depending on severity, location, and contamination of the wound.
4. Assist in providing local anesthesia, one of the "caine" anesthetics (e.g., procaine, lidocaine) *without* epinephrine, injected by infiltration or block.
5. Thoroughly cleanse skin around laceration with Betadine scrub solution: do not put into wound.
6. Shave hair around laceration: do not shave eyebrows; they are needed as landmarks for suturing.
7. Profusely irrigate wound with normal saline, not water.
8. Mild soap and scrubbing with sterile brush or plain gauze aid in wound cleansing. Do not use cotton-filled gauze sponges, as cotton debris left in wound causes granulomas. Do not use alcohol or other antiseptic solutions in the wound, because they irritate and kill injured cells, destroy defense cells, and inhibit healing. Do not use peroxide (peroxide uses up oxygen rapidly and is not effective against anaerobes; it causes pain and destroys cells).
9. Irrigation should be done with 50 mL syringe with large needle; Asepto and Toomey syringes and IV tubing should not be used because they provide too weak an ejection force for effective mechanical cleansing action.
10. Assist client and physician during suturing and dressing wound.
11. Monitor perfusion (color, sensation, capillary filling, pulses), sensation, and motor function of affected part.
12. Provide tetanus prophylaxis if client's immunization has expired.
13. Teach client to look for circulatory impairment.
14. Assist client with necessary adaptations in self-care or mobility; instruct about recommended activity restrictions, crutch walking, keeping dressings dry, and so on.
15. Instruct client in use of prescribed antibiotics and analgesia, if any.

EVALUATION

Outcome Criteria

1. Wound heals with full restoration of function and minimal scarring.
2. Infection is prevented or promptly recognized and treated.
3. Systemic and local perfusion are adequate.
4. Pain is relieved.
5. Client maintains self-care and mobility at highest safe level, and continues usual social interaction pattern.
6. Client complies with treatment recommendations.

Complications

1. Sepsis.
2. Neurological or circulatory impairment leading to reduced function.

PUNCTURES

DESCRIPTION

A puncture is a perforation of skin and underlying structures due to a forceful thrust or pressure from a sharp, pointed, narrow object. Common causes of this injury include nails, tacks, staples, ice-pick tools, needles and pins, and intentional or accidental stabbing with knives and daggers. Special types of punctures include animal and human bites, impaled objects, fish hooks, splinters, and needles. Disruption of tissue or organ function depends on depth of wound and degree of contamination.

PREVENTION

Health Promotion

1. Persons at risk (e.g., small children) should be protected from exposure to unsafe objects such as ice picks and fish hooks.
2. Older children need to be instructed in the safe use of tools and equipment.
3. Teach safe behavior around animals to avoid being bitten.
4. Encourage the wearing of shoes.

Population at Risk

Children and adults who do not wear shoes.

Screening

None.

ASSESSMENT

Health History

1. Obtain description of object causing wound and force of entry.
2. Note tetanus immunization history.
3. Note antibiotic allergies.
4. Ascertain if injury is work-related.
5. If animal bite, obtain necessary legal data about species, owner, animal's immunization history, and whether animal is now caged and under observation.
6. If suspicious of details regarding cause of injury, obtain description of surrounding events resulting in puncture wound.

Physical Assessment

1. Foreign body may be retained in puncture tract, "hooked" in skin, or impaled.
2. Bleeding and drainage are minimal.
3. Assess neurovascular and musculoskeletal damage: check motor and sensory function, discoloration, swelling, warmth, and pulses at puncture site and distal to it.
4. Observe for signs of infection: redness, swelling, drainage, and inflammation or tenderness of vessels.

Diagnostic Tests

1. X-ray film or fluoroscopy for identification of needle or other small metal objects.
2. Culture of bite wounds (human and animal).

NURSING DIAGNOSES: ACTUAL OR POTENTIAL

1. Impairment of skin integrity due to puncture wound.
2. Increased risk of infection (including anaerobic infection such as tetanus) due to puncture wound.
3. Alteration in comfort: pain due to tissue trauma.
4. Impairment of circulatory or neurological function due to tissue trauma.
5. Diminished mobility and self-care deficit secondary to injury.

EXPECTED OUTCOMES

Outcome Criteria

1. Infection will be prevented or effectively treated.
2. Pain will be alleviated.
3. Healing will occur with minimal scarring (seldom a problem except in bite wounds with jagged edges that make wound edge approximation difficult).
4. Neurovascular function will be maintained.
5. Client will maintain appropriate mobility and self-care activities.

INTERVENTIONS

1. Thoroughly cleanse and irrigate wound (see *Lacerations*, above).
2. Provide prescribed analgesia as appropriate to wound size, depth, and logistics of cleansing procedure.
3. If wood splinter, do not cleanse wound until foreign body has been removed (wood absorbs water, swells, and falls apart).
4. Administer tetanus prophylaxis.
5. Begin on prophylactic antibiotics depending on wound contamination.
6. Instruct in frequent, warm soaks, at least twice a day.
7. Teach client to apply dry, sterile dressing between soaks.
8. Do not use ointments on puncture wounds.
9. If fish hook is embedded, make small incision over the tip and force tip through. Cut

shaft of hook with wire cutter and pull remainder out (Figure 48–13).

10. Remove splinters with splinter forceps.
11. Leave bite wounds open initially.
12. Give duck embryo vaccine (DEV) if index of suspicion for rabies is high.
13. Apply bulky, fluffy, dry dressings for bites. For face bites, sterile strips may be placed loosely.
14. For industrial accidents, extricate patient from machinery with impaling object intact (protruding ends can be shortened to facilitate movement).
15. When transporting impaled victim, immobilize affected part and stabilize impaling object.
16. Impaling object will be removed surgically, in an aseptic environment, providing for possible massive bleeding or fluid loss.
17. Do not remove impaling object from eye: demands ophthalmologist to protect aqueous and vitreous humors.
18. In emergency, remove impaling object with thorough cleansing and withdrawing along path of entry.
19. Monitor for circulatory or neurological damage to affected part: color, pulses, capillary filling, pain, sensation, and motor function at and distal to wound.
20. Instruct client about activity restrictions, if required, and assist in modifying activity and self-care activities (e.g., teach crutch walking, how to keep dressings dry, and so forth as circumstance require).
21. Teach client about self-administration of prescribed antibiotics and analgesics, if any.

EVALUATION

Outcome Criteria

1. Infections do not occur or are effectively treated.

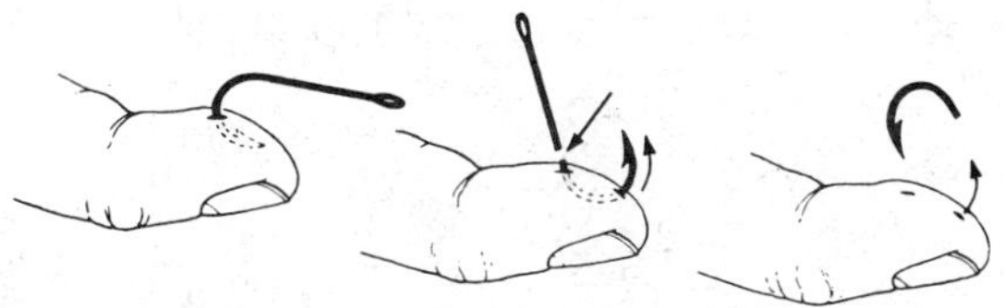

Figure 48-13 Method of removing an embedded fish hook. (From Henderson, J.: *Emergency Medical Guide*, 4th ed., McGraw-Hill, New York, 1978. Reproduced with permission.)

2. Tetanus prophylaxis is brought up to date.
3. Pain is reduced and eliminated.
4. Healing occurs with minimal scarring.
5. Perfusion and neurological function are adequate.
6. Mobility and self-care are carried out at the highest level safely compatible with extent of injury.

Complications

1. Hemorrhage or laceration of internal organs or other deep structures.
2. Sepsis.
3. Tetanus (see Chapter 24).
4. Rabies.

Reevaluation and Follow-up

1. Report to police all stabbings, suspicious penetrating wounds, animal bites, and bites on children if child abuse is suspected.
2. Report to animal control and public health authorities all animal bites. Be aware of the necessity for confining the animal for 15 days for rabies observation. If the animal has been killed, it must not be disposed of until it is examined for rabies.

BURNS

THERMAL BURNS

DESCRIPTION

During a thermal burn, tissue protein is altered, especially after 45°C (113°F). Cells are injured or destroyed by impairment of enzymatic processes, rupture of cell membranes, or frank coagulation of cellular contents.

Burns are categorized according to (1) the depth of the tissue injury and (2) the amount of body surface affected. Depth of the injury is described as first, second, third, or fourth degree, as shown in Figure 48–14. Surface area is estimated according to the well-known "rule of nines" (shown, with a modification for children, in Figure 48–15). Obviously, the deeper the burn and the greater the proportion of body surface affected, the more severe is the injury. The immediate concerns in the emergency care of

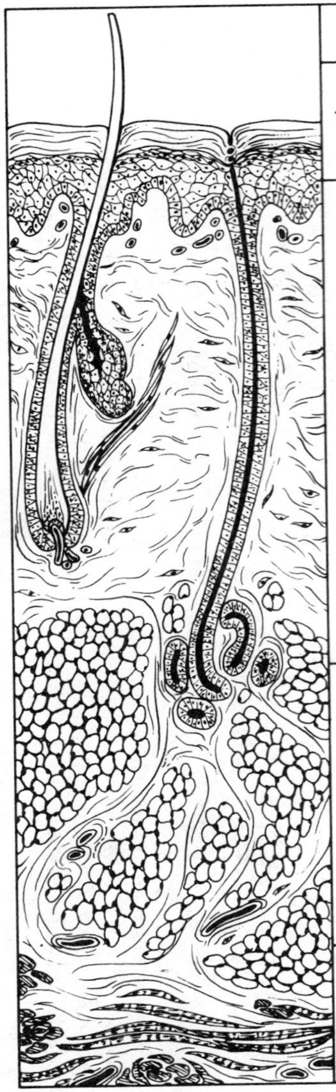

Degree	Depth of burn	Detailed classification	Pain and pinprick sensitivity	Appearance	Healing time	End result of healing	Treatment
1°		Erythema only, no loss of epidermis	Hyperalgesia	Erythema		Normal skin	Allow to heal by natural processes Protect from further injury and infection
2°	Partial skin loss	Superficial, no loss of dermis	Hyperalgesia or normal	Erythema to opaque white blisters are characteristic	6-10 days	Normal skin	Allow to heal by natural processes Protect from further injury and infection
2°	Partial skin loss	Intermediate Healing from hair follicles	Normal to hypo-algesia	Erythema to opaque white blisters are characteristic	7-14 days	Normal to slightly pitted and/or poorly pigmented	Allow to heal by natural processes Protect from further injury and infection
2°	Partial skin loss	Deep Healing from sweat glands	Hypoalgesia to analgesia	Erythema to opaque white blisters are characteristic	14-21 days	Hairless and depigmented Texture normal to pitted or flat and shiny	Elective skin grafting may save time and give better end result
3°	Whole skin loss	Deep dermal Occasionally, healing from scattered epithelium	Analgesia	White opaque to charred coagulated subcutaneous veins may be visible	More than 21 days	Poor texture Hypertrophic scar frequent	Elective skin grafting may save time and give better end result
3°	Whole skin loss	Whole skin loss Healing from edges only	Analgesia	White opaque to charred coagulated subcutaneous veins may be visible	Never, if area is large	Hypertrophic scar and chronic granulations unless grafted	Skin grafting mandatory
4°	Deep tissue loss	Deep structure loss (muscle, tendon, nerve, bone, etc.)	May be some algesia	White opaque to charred coagulated subcutaneous veins may be visible	Never, if area is large	Hypertrophic scar and chronic granulations unless grafted	Skin grafting mandatory

Figure 48-14 Classification of burns according to depth of burn. (From Frank, H. A., and Wachtel, T. L.: "Emergency Management of Burns," in Warner, C. G., ed., *Emergency Care*, 3d ed., Mosby, St. Louis, 1983.)

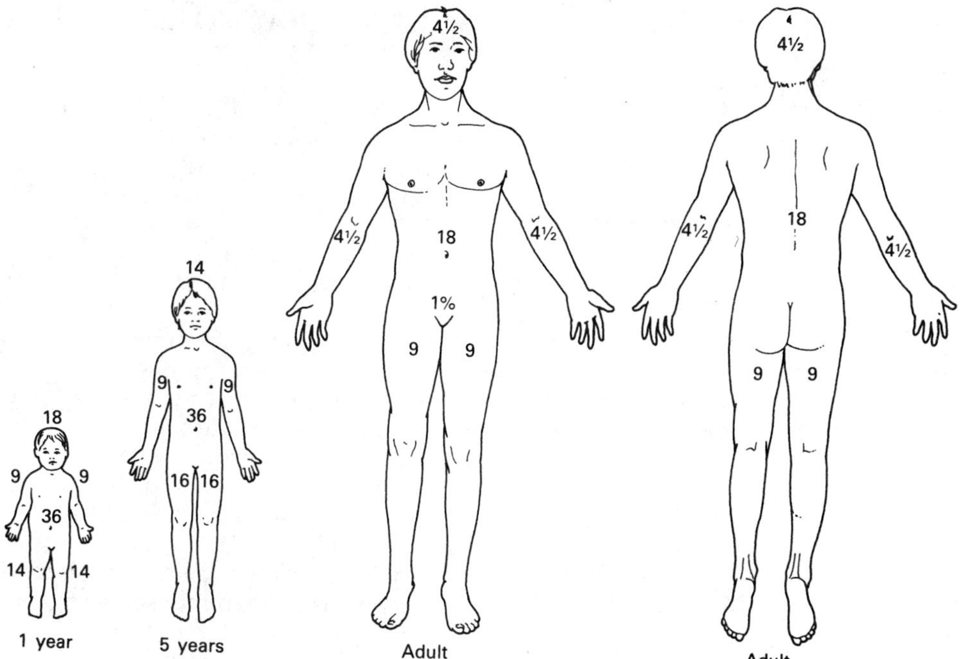

Figure 48-15 Rule of 9s with modification for infants and children. (From Jones, D., et al., *Medical-Surgical Nursing: A Conceptual Approach*, McGraw-Hill, New York, 1978.)

burn victims are:

1. Maintaining respiration (if the client has facial burns or has inhaled hot or irritating gases, edema of the respiratory tract can be life-threatening),
2. Minimizing infection,
3. Combatting shock that readily follows the massive loss of fluid into blisters and through the open burns.

Only the emergency care of persons with burns is outlined here. More complete information is presented in Chapter 35.

PREVENTION

Health Promotion

1. Compliance with occupational safety regulations, building codes, and other public safety specifications that minimize exposure to unsafe equipment and environments.
2. Protection of persons at risk (small children, the mentally retarded, etc.) from open fires, woodstoves, cooking equipment, and so forth.
3. Instruction for children and suitable others (e.g., new employees in certain industries) in the safe use of flame and heat with which they will come into contact.
4. Installation of home smoke detectors and periodic household fire drills.

Population at Risk

1. Persons who work around steam, boiling water, or objects that are fired and retain heat: kitchen workers and other food industry personnel such as bakers, maintenance personnel, metal workers, and so on.
2. Persons who are uninformed or careless about flame: children, careless smokers, confused elderly, and so on.
3. Household cooks.
4. Persons who work with flammable liquids: mechanics, painters, boat operators, and so on.
5. Firefighters.

Screening

Environmental survey for fire hazards (flammable litter, stored flammable or explosive substances, blocked exits, etc.).

ASSESSMENT

Health History

1. Obtain description of thermal source, i.e., dry or wet heat.
2. Note exposure interval and approximate degree of temperature.
3. Obtain description of events associated with injury.
4. Note past medical history and general health.
5. Ascertain medication history and allergies.
6. Determine possible noxious gases produced by fire and client exposure to these.
7. Note if fire occurred in a closed place (increases risk of inhalation injury).
8. Find out whether tetanus immunization is current.

Physical Assessment

1. Classify burn in first-, second-, third-, and fourth-degree categories of tissue destruction (Figure 48–14).
2. Estimate body surface area affected by each type (degree) of burn.
3. Evaluate additional injuries.
4. Assess respiratory effort, cough, and chest sounds. Anticipate airway obstruction if nose, mouth, neck, or face is burned or if smoke or other irritating gases have been inhaled.
5. Note amount of pain (excruciating in first- and second-degree burns).
6. Assess circulatory adequacy, both systemic (vital signs) and local (color, pulse, capillary filling, sensation, and motor function of burned areas and distal areas).
7. Observe dirt or other foreign bodies especially predisposing to sepsis.

Diagnostic Tests

1. CBC, hemoglobin, hematocrit.
2. Urinalysis for myoglobin and casts.
3. Blood chemistries to include: BUN, creatinine, serum electrolyte levels, albumin and globulin levels, blood sugar, bilirubin and alkaline phosphatase levels, calcium and phosphorous levels, carbon monoxide level, and arterial blood gases, if indicated for respiratory tract symptoms.
4. Chest x-ray film in the case of smoke or noxious gas inhalation.
5. May obtain carbon monoxide blood level on admission.
6. Type and cross-match blood.

NURSING DIAGNOSES: ACTUAL OR POTENTIAL

1. Respiratory insufficiency secondary to inhalation of hot or toxic gases.
2. Impaired skin integrity secondary to thermal injury.
3. Infection secondary to loss of skin integrity.
4. Body temperature instability: chilling due to loss of skin (one of whose normal functions is retention of body heat) and due to convection cooling from body fluid seepage from third-degree burns.
5. Alteration in comfort, mild to severe: pain secondary to tissue trauma.
6. Alteration in cardiac output: shock secondary to fluid shift from the intravascular compartment and secondary to pain.
7. Alteration in body fluid composition, especially hypoalbuminemia and hyperkalemia, secondary to wound seepage and cellular damage.
8. Increased fluid and nutrition requirements secondary to fluid shifts and losses and metabolic needs for temperature maintenance, infection resistance, and tissue repair.
9. Impaired mobility and self-care activities secondary to injury.
10. Anxiety secondary to pain, impaired mobility, disfigurement, fear of overwhelming financial burden, fear of death, and so on.

EXPECTED OUTCOMES

1. Airway and respiratory exchange will be maintained.
2. Infection will be prevented (first- and second-degree injury) or effectively treated (third- and fourth-degree burn).
3. Client's body temperature will be maintained within normal limits.
4. Pain will be controlled or eliminated.
5. Perfusion will be maintained as evidenced by blood pressure at least 90/60 and normal peripheral pulses and capillary filling.
6. Electrolyte levels and serum proteins will be maintained within normal limits.
7. Nutritional and fluid requirements will be met.
8. Mobility and self-care will be maintained at the highest level safely compatible with the injury.
9. Anxiety will be controlled and reduced.

INTERVENTIONS

1. Establish airway and maintain respiratory support for all clients with face, head, and neck burns, massive body surface area burns, or known closed-environment entrapment or smoke inhalation. Use oxygen.
2. Combat shock by administering prescribed IV fluids, generally Ringer's lactate or another buffered isotonic solution, based on calculation of body surface area and depth of burn.
3. Insert urinary bladder indwelling catheter and attach to closed drainage system. Monitor hourly urine output.
4. Provide prescribed analgesia, often titrated IV morphine or Demerol. For superficial burns, pain can be reduced by applying cold compress or ice packs for 20 minutes (this treatment can also limit tissue damage if begun immediately after the burn is sustained); but care must be taken if a large body surface is involved, since cooling can lead to dangerous hypothermia.
5. Administer tetanus prophylaxis.
6. Remove jewelry and clothing from affected or potential problem areas.
7. Gently and thoroughly cleanse burned areas with copious amounts of sterile water or saline and a mild soap such as Ivory liquid (fluid may be cooled or slightly warmed for client's comfort). Iodophor soaps can produce iodine toxicity if burns are large.
8. Apply fine-mesh gauze, plain or impregnated, followed with bulky, absorptive fluffs, and even compression dressing of roller gauze or Kling bandage (stockinette may be used over large extremity or torso).
9. Splint burned extremities involving flexor aspects in full extension position, except hand, which should be splinted in functional position.
10. Sodium bicarbonate may be prescribed for addition to IV fluids in order to keep urine pH at 7.0 during the time of great hemoglobin and myoglobin losses, since these substances are more soluble (less damaging to the kidney tubules) in an alkaline urine. The nurse can monitor with urine nitrogen paper; these values should be recorded, along with specific gravity and output. Observe client for urine turbidity or odor, because alkaline urine predisposes to urinary tract infection.
11. Administer prescribed proplylactic antibiotic treatment of penicillin or another broad-spectrum medication.
12. Apply prescribed silver sulfadiazene (Silvadene) or mafenide (Sulfamylon) cream after burned area has been cleansed and debrided. Sulfamylon can cause metabolic acidosis: monitor respirations and blood gases.
13. Keep body temperature in normal range by covering with sterile sheet and sterile light thermal blanket.
14. Administer oral fluids of saline, water, sugar water, or juices if victim is awake, has bowel sounds, and is not vomiting. Add high-calorie, high-carbohydrate, high-protein foods as tolerated.
15. Monitor vital signs frequently, and note orthostatic and nonorthostatic changes.
16. Use sterile mineral oil or bacitracin ointment to "float off" a tar deposit causing burn.
17. Assist client in modifying usual mobility and self-care activities as required by injury, encouraging independence.
18. Reduce anxiety by explaining treatment procedures, treatment plan, and client role in treatment program. Provide supportive, realistic information about prognosis (scarring, limitation of function, and so forth). Listen to client questions and comments. Treat pain.

EVALUATION

Outcome Criteria

1. Respiratory function is adequate as evidenced by clear lung sounds and blood gases within normal limits.
2. Infection is prevented or effectively treated.
3. Body temperature is within normal limits.
4. Client reports pain is effectively reduced by treatment.
5. Blood pressure is within normal limits; pulses and capillary filling are normal at and distal to the injury.
6. Fluid and nutrient intake are adequate for maintenance needs.
7. Client maintains mobility and self-care, as permitted by injury and treatment plan.
8. Client is free of signs of excessive or unrealistic anxiety.

Complications

1. Cardiac arrhythmias associated with shock or potassium imbalance.

2. Acute renal failure due to hypoperfusion.
3. Septic shock.

ELECTRICAL BURNS

DESCRIPTION

An electrical burn can affect any tissue, including bone. An electrical burn creates a local lesion with the following characteristics: a charred black center, a middle area of gray-white coagulation necrosis, and an outer, bright red ring of partial coagulation. The coagulated areas may increase during the first several days after the injury, due to progressive thrombosis. The blood vessels at the burn site are friable, and hemorrhage that is hard to control may occur hours or days after the burn. Electrical injury to bone causes swelling and gradual sequestration with discharge of devitalized areas. Neurological injuries can cover a broad range from paralysis to bizarre pain, aphasia, cerebellar dysfunction, seizures, and psychotic behavior.

The extent of the injury sustained in an electrical burn depends on the duration and voltage, and the parts of the body involved (the pathway taken by the current). Alternating current is more damaging than direct current. Electrical burns are sometimes described as "iceberg" injuries because massive tissue destruction and sloughing can occur even though the skin lesion is small.

PREVENTION

Health Promotion

1. Maintenance and safe use of household appliances (repair of frayed cords, proper grounding, etc.).
2. Protection (wall plug covers) of small children and other persons at risk from sources of current.
3. Instruction of older children and other people about safe use of home and industrial electrical appliances and tools.
4. Instruction on avoiding lightning: during storms, avoid being in or near water, in exposed fields, and under or near solitary trees or water towers or other isolated tall objects that may attract lightning.

Population at Risk

1. Industrial workers who use electrical implements.
2. Many serious electrical burns are caused by lightning; those at risk are golfers, fishermen, swimmers, farmers, and others who may be caught without shelter, particularly in "lightning belts" such as Florida.
3. Homemakers, children, and office and industrial workers.
4. Virtually everyone.

Screening

Periodic inspection and maintenance of electrical implements and appliances.

ASSESSMENT

Health History

1. Establish who can serve as historian regarding the accident.
2. Obtain description of voltage amounts, duration of contact, and type of electrical force.
3. Note past medical and drug history.
4. Ascertain whether injury was related to employment.
5. Establish if client was unconscious and, if so, how long.

Physical Assessment

1. Massive subcutaneous, fascia, and connective tissue destruction in path of current flow.
2. Minimal cutaneous wounds compared to underlying structure destruction.
3. Cardiac standstill, ventricular fibrillation, and respiratory muscle paralysis and/or arrest.
4. Charred markings at current entry site.
5. Hemorrhage and massive fluid losses with muscle tissue injury.
6. Assess consciousness, orientation, and ability to conduct abstract thought.
7. Nausea, vomiting, and paralytic ileus.
8. Violent tetany and uncoordinated muscle contractions.
9. Signs of internal hemorrhage and perforation of abdominal organ (should be suspected in electrical injuries).

Diagnostic Tests

1. Any laboratory tests associated with organs in path of injury.
2. Urinalysis for microscopic blood, myoglobin, and hemoglobin levels.

3. Twelve-lead ECG.
4. Serum potassium level.

NURSING DIAGNOSES: ACTUAL OR POTENTIAL

1. Alteration in cardiac output: cardiac arrhythmia or standstill due to electrical interference with normal cardiac cycle.
2. Respiratory failure: respiratory arrest secondary to electrical shock.
3. Loss of integrity of skin and deeper tissues (muscle, tendon, nerve, vessels, bones, possibly abdominal organs) due to passage of electricity through tissues.
4. Impaired circulation in and distal to the injured tissues, due to vessel coagulation.
5. Impaired systemic perfusion secondary to shock.
6. Alteration in comfort: pain secondary to tissue trauma.
7. Infection due to loss of skin integrity and destruction of deeper tissues.
8. Diminished mobility and self-care due to injury.
9. Alteration in cognition or perception: confusion, personality changes, or coma secondary to electrical shock.

EXPECTED OUTCOMES

1. Cardiopulmonary sufficiency will be restored.
2. Tissue perfusion at and distal to injury will be maintained.
3. Shock will be prevented or treated.
4. Pain will be effectively treated.
5. Infection will be effectively treated.
6. Client will maintain mobility and self-care at maximum safe levels.
7. Client will not be injured during coma, convulsions, or confusion.

INTERVENTIONS

1. Cardiopulmonary resuscitation is frequently necessary.
2. Continuously monitor ECG for dysrhythmia.
3. Intubate, if necessary, or provide oxygen by mask.
4. Monitor IV fluids, usually Ringer's lactate, to maintain blood pressure at least 90/60.
5. Administer prescribed analgesia.
6. Assist client and physician with debridement and cleansing of the wound.
7. Administer prescribed antibiotics and tetanus immunization.
8. Assist client with self-care and mobility as indicated by client's condition.
9. Protect confused, convulsive, or unconscious client from injury.

EVALUATION

Outcome Criteria

1. Vital signs, cardiac rhythm, and blood gas levels are within normal limits.
2. Pulses and capillary filling at and distal to the wound are adequate.
3. Client reports pain treatment is effective.
4. Infection is under treatment with broad-spectrum antibiotic pending report of culture and sensitivity.
5. Client has not been injured by convulsion or during coma or convulsion.
6. Mobility and self-care are being conducted at maximum safe level compatible with injury.

Complications

1. Necrosis and eventual amputation.
2. Peritonitis or other complication of visceral injury.

CHEMICAL BURNS

DESCRIPTION

Chemical burns arise from skin or mucous membrane contact with acid, alkali, or corrosive metal. Alkalis are more dangerous than acids.

PREVENTION

Health Promotion

1. Adherence to occupational safety standards in work settings where caustic chemicals are used.
2. Provision of showers and face bubblers in immediate proximity to science laboratories and other settings in which people handle chemicals.
3. Childproof caps for household caustics and other precautions in storing and handling such chemicals.

Population at Risk

1. Persons who manufacture or apply chemical fertilizers, insecticides, fire retardants, and the like.
2. Students or staff personnel in science laboratories.

Screening

None.

ASSESSMENT

Health History

1. Determine types of chemicals involved in the injury.
2. Ascertain immediate care rendered, including attempts to neutralize chemical agent.
3. Note if accident is work-related.
4. Note past medical history, including drug therapy and allergies.
5. Obtain tetanus immunization status.

Physical Assessment

1. Redness, erythema, severe discoloration of contacted tissue.
2. Swelling and local hyperemia.
3. Pain and paresthesias.
4. Tissue weeping may be present.
5. Affected area feels warm or hot to the touch due to heat of chemical reactions and hyperemia.
6. Excoriated and "raw" appearance.

Diagnostic Tests

Dependent upon extent of injury.

NURSING DIAGNOSES: ACTUAL OR POTENTIAL

1. Impaired skin integrity secondary to chemical injury.
2. Infection secondary to loss of skin integrity.
3. Alteration in comfort: pain secondary to tissue trauma.
4. Alteration in fluid balance: fluid shift or loss associated with edema, blistering, and wound weeping.
5. Impaired mobility and self-care secondary to injury.

EXPECTED OUTCOMES

1. Client's skin will heal with minimal scarring.
2. Infection will be prevented or effectively treated.
3. Pain will be reduced and eliminated.
4. Hydration will be maintained.
5. Client will maintain self-care and mobility at the highest safe level compatible with the injury.

INTERVENTIONS

1. Immediately flush area with copious amounts of water; continue for 20 to 30 minutes. NOTE: Dry chemical should be brushed from skin before water is applied, to minimize the spread of the injury.
2. Apply antibiotic ointment as prescribed.
3. Control restlessness and pain by administering prescribed medications, often diazepam (Valium), meperidine hydrochloride (Demerol), or morphine.
4. Monitor IV fluids, if any; administer oral fluids as desired and tolerated.
5. Assist client in adapting mobility and self-care as required by injury and treatment.

EVALUATION

Outcome Criteria

1. Client's skin heals with minimal scarring and full return of function to the affected part.
2. Infection is prevented or effectively treated.
3. Client's comfort and normal sensation are restored.
4. Fluid balance and hydration are maintained.
5. Mobility and self-care are maintained at the highest safe level compatible with the injury and therapy.

Complications

Contractures or scarring that impair function or appearance.

RADIATION BURNS

DESCRIPTION

Radiation burns are due to radioactive, ionizing effects on all tissue exposed. They may be accompanied by extreme thermal radiation (flash burns) as well as secondary burns from fission products or fall-out in contaminated water or ground, generally caused by bomb blasts or radioactive substance leaks in nuclear plants. Ionizing radiation effects are caused by one or all of the following:

1. Alpha rays, caused or emitted by unfissioned bomb residues of plutonium or uranium. This material may be deposited in bones and cause long-term bombardment of tissue.
2. Beta rays, emitted from fission products, enter body via skin, inhalation, ingestion, or break in skin. Not as penetrating as gamma rays; have similar mechanism of injury as alpha rays, that is, localize in bone tissue and cause severe signs and symptoms. These have delayed but constant bombardment effect.
3. Gamma rays, liberated for very few seconds after high air burst; act like high-energy x-ray machine. Range of effect varies with size of bomb (or spray); can be lethal for several miles from explosion. Rays have extensive and tremendous penetration and are most important cause of radiation injuries.
4. Neutrons, formed by combination of a positively charged proton and an electron; have a short range in comparison to gamma rays. Greatest concern is the fission products, that is, beta and gamma rays, formed when neutrons strike the earth's surface. Victims shielded from initial blast of gamma rays may develop acute symptoms from neutron exposure.
5. Sunburns, a mild type of radiation injury due to overexposure to ultraviolet radiation. Burns can be categorized into first or second degree according to depth of injury. Exposure and extent of injury determine prognosis.

Radiation exposure requires decontamination prior to triage or simultaneously with emergency treatment if rescue personnel are properly protected. Triage teams may face extreme moral and emotional concerns over the necessary decision to withhold treatment from persons with lethal-dose radiation injuries.

PREVENTION

Health Promotion

1. Conformity to medical, biological, industrial, and military regulations for preventing accidental exposure to radiation.
2. Sociopolitical efforts for the avoidance of nuclear war.
3. Sociopolitical efforts to maximize safety of nuclear power installations.

Population at Risk

1. Persons in medical and scientific laboratories where radioactive substances are in use.
2. Hospital personnel, dentists, and others who work with radiography, radiotherapy, and so forth.
3. Employees and neighboring residents of nuclear power installations, nuclear waste transport and storage facilities, and so forth, who may be affected by equipment failures or accidental spills.

Screening

None.

ASSESSMENT

Health History

1. Obtain description of radiation forces, interval of exposure, and events surrounding incident.
2. Obtain information regarding decontamination efforts and relative radioactivity still present.
3. Ascertain from triage officer to which category of care the victim has been assigned.
4. Note past medical and drug history, including allergies.
5. For all hopelessly injured, seek choice of religious caregiver: minister, priest, rabbi.

Physical Assessment

1. Discoloration with initially intact skin and underlying tissue (erythema).
2. Second-degree burn with immediate blister formation accompanying the erythema may be present.
3. Persistent severe vomiting within 2 h after exposure (usually).
4. High fever, diarrhea, tenesmus, and dehydration.
5. Extreme prostration and death due to toxic effects and complete peripheral vascular collapse occurring within a few hours to days.
6. Victim can demonstrate anger, frustration, anxiety, fear, and depression, depending on prognosis and speculated complications.
7. Sunburns:
   a. Dermal hyperemia, with burned surface hot to touch.
   b. Lesser degree of symptoms noted in point 4, above.
   c. Pain unrelated to size of affected area (usually); may be severe.

Diagnostic Tests

1. Initially, radioactive levels as determined by beta-gamma instruments accompanied with audio amplifiers.
2. CBC, hemoglobin and hematocrit levels, platelet count, RBC, differentials.
3. Urinalysis for myoglobinuria and other evidence of tissue destruction.
4. Bone scans for radioactive elements.
5. Electrolyte levels.

NURSING DIAGNOSES: ACTUAL OR POTENTIAL

1. Loss of skin integrity secondary to radiation.
2. Fluid deficit secondary to fluid shift (blisters and edema), or loss (weeping from open wound), and secondary to anorexia, nausea, vomiting, and diarrhea.
3. Decreased cardiac output: shock secondary to fluid deficit.
4. Increased risk of infection secondary to loss of skin integrity, and secondary to leukopenia caused by radiation.
5. Alteration in body temperature: high fever secondary to burn, infection, and toxic byproducts of dying cells.
6. Progressive tissue destruction secondary to radiation.
7. Decreased activity tolerance: extreme fatigue and malaise due to cell death and fluid-electrolyte imbalances.
8. Alteration in comfort: pain secondary to skin damage, and discomfort associated with gastrointestinal symptoms and malaise.
9. Alteration in social interaction patterns: isolation imposed until decontamination is completed.
10. Anxiety secondary to debility and fear or knowledge of impending death.
11. Spiritual distress associated with emotional impact of nuclear disaster and impending death.

EXPECTED OUTCOMES

1. For sunburn:
   a. Pain will be relieved.
   b. Fluid balance will be maintained.
   c. Infection will be prevented or minimized.
2. For other radiation injuries:
   a. Client will be rapidly decontaminated.
   b. Pain will be relieved; discomforts will be reduced as far as possible.
   c. Cardiovascular function and perfusion will be maintained.
   d. Infection will be controlled.
   e. Activity will not exceed tolerance.
   f. Fluid balance will be supported.
   g. Anxiety will be reduced: client will cope effectively with catastrophic changes in his or her life.

INTERVENTIONS

1. For sunburn:
   a. Remove victim from exposure to further sunlight.
   b. Cool affected areas with cool, moist, rotating packs, and by evaporation (moving air).
   c. Treat pain and fever with aspirin.
   d. Provide oral fluids as tolerated: monitor for signs of dehydration (oliguria, loss of turgor in unaffected skin).
2. For other radiation exposure:
   a. Decontaminate immediately, remove all contaminated clothing, and properly isolate victim for protection of others.
   b. Provide analgesia with aspirin or narcotics according to need and extent of injury.
   c. Replace fluids with amount and composition commensurate with losses, as prescribed:
      (1) Saline and other fluids orally as tolerated (1 tsp of table salt and $\frac{1}{2}$ tsp of baking soda dissolved in 1,000 mL water).
      (2) IV normal saline or Ringer's, with caution not to overload the intravascular circulation.
      (3) May administer sodium bicarbonate, 1,000 mL of a 2% solution via rectum every day (Jahre et al., 1975).
   d. Control nausea and vomiting with antiemetics such as chlorpromazine hydrochloride (Thorazine), prochlorperazine (Compazine), or dimenhydrinate (Dramamine).
   e. Support cardiovascular function with ephedrine sulfate, levarterenol (Levophed), or metaraminol (Aramine).
   f. Keep burned areas clean and covered with sterile dressings; may be exposed if in filtered airflow room.
   g. Be observant for any tendency to bleeding and notify chief of care immediately.
   h. Be cautious in use of IM and IV routes due

to increased possiblity of bleeding and lowered resistance to infection.

i. Prepare victim and family for pending terminal state by including family, religious caregiver, and significant others in plan of care.
j. Provide mental health support via nursing staff and consultants.

EVALUATION

Outcome Criteria

1. For sunburned client:
   a. Skin heals without scarring.
   b. Infection does not occur.
   c. Pain is effectively controlled.
   d. Hydration is adequate.
2. For client with other forms of radiation injury:
   a. Pain and other forms of discomfort are effectively treated.
   b. Vital functions are supported.
   c. Client copes adequately.

Complications

1. Bone marrow shutdown.
2. Malignancy.
3. Teratogenesis and mutations.

Reevaluation and Follow-up

1. Survivors of nuclear exposures must be followed throughout their lifetime for residual effects.
2. The social stigma surrounding the nuclear industry and warfare can lead to severe social and psychological repercussions for persons whose radiation injuries are related to sociopolitical issues.

SHOCK (HYPOVOLEMIC, CARDIOGENIC, VASOGENIC, SEPTIC, AND ANAPHYLACTIC)

DESCRIPTION

Shock is a generalized state of severe circulatory inadequacy that causes lowering or cessation of tissue perfusion. Several categories are recognized:

1. Hypovolemic shock. The volume of circulating blood is reduced (e.g., by hemorrhage) to such a degree that blood pressure drops in spite of compensatory vasoconstriction. The goal of treatment is to replace intravascular fluid volume.
2. Cardiogenic shock. The heart does not pump effectively enough to maintain tissue perfusion. The treatment is to restore cardiac function.
3. Vasogenic shock (fainting, also called neurogenic or neurovasogenic shock). The blood vessels dilate so that blood pressure is inadequate to maintain oxygenation to the brain. Fainting episodes are brought on by fright, unexpected bad news, and the like; treatment consists of restoring cerebral blood pressure, which is usually accomplished by having the client lie down. Nervous system regulation of vascular constriction can also be impaired by spinal cord injury, anesthesia, and certain drugs.
4. Septic shock. Hypoperfusion in response to endotoxins related by certain bacteria. Offending organisms are predominantly gram-negative (*Pseudomonas, Escherichia, Klebsiella, Proteus*, etc.) but can include *Staphylococcus* and *Pneumococcus*. Blood pools in the capillaries, fluid seeps from the vessels, and severe biochemical consequences ensue from organ anoxia and acidosis. The treatment is to support vital functions, replace fluid, and treat the underlying infection.
5. Anaphylactic shock (anaphylaxis, allergic shock). An acute allergic phenomenon in which release of histamine and related substances causes vasodilation, airway obstruction, skin manifestations (hives with or without angioedema), and circulatory collapse. Treatment is aimed at relieving dyspnea, combatting hypotension, and reducing allergic manifestations.

Capillary flow is impaired in all types of shock, with both pre- and postcapillary sphincters constricted initially. Eventually, the precapillary sphincters relax, and blood begins to pool in the capillary bed. These events are described as ischemic anoxia progressing to stagnant anoxia. There is a marked drop in pH across the capillary beds, with stasis and backflow causing massive sequestration. Blood viscosity increases in low-flow states due to catecholamine release, lowered pH, and release of lysosomal enzymes. Hypercoagulability follows low-flow states and, with vasoconstriction, helps to reduce further blood loss in hemorrhage.

The progression of cellular events starts with reduction of aerobic metabolism, reduced ATP formation, influx of Na^+ and water causing cellular edema, K^+ leaving the cell, rapid pH change to metabolic acidosis, lysosomal breakdown, destruction of cellular membranes, and bradykinin and histamine release. Activation of certain plasma polypeptides with powerful vasoactive properties, the appearance of proteolytic enzymes, and extracellular acidemia are early signs. Late results include irreversible capillary endothelial damage and intravascular coagulation.

PREVENTION

Health Promotion

Avoidance and prompt, vigorous treatment of the underlying causes of shock:

1. Hypovolemic shock: acute blood loss, major burns, crush injuries, severe gastroenteritis, diabetes insipidus, diabetic acidosis, and so on.
2. Cardiogenic shock: myocardial infarction, congestive heart failure, and outflow obstructions such as dissecting aortic aneurysm or pulmonary embolus.
3. Vasogenic shock: spinal cord injury, heat hyperthermia, insulin overdose, drug overdose (e.g., barbiturates, phenothiazines).
4. Septic shock: septicemia, especially by gram-negative organisms.
5. Anaphylactic shock: bee stings, penicillin, seafood, horse serum preparations, other intensely allergenic substances.

Population at Risk

Everyone susceptible to or afflicted with the causative factors mentioned immediately above.

Screening

1. For anaphylaxis:
   a. Horse serum preparations must never be given without first testing the recipient for allergic response by following the manufacturer's instructions; emergency treatment must be at hand before either testing or administration of these preparations is undertaken.
   b. Skin testing can identify allergies but is rarely necessary for clients who have severe reactions (the offender is usually known).

ASSESSMENT

Health History

1. Obtain description of events leading to shock condition.
2. Note time of onset and duration of symptoms.
3. Obtain past medical history, including medications and allergies.
4. Note all care administered prior to hospital admission and during receiving unit phase.
5. Ascertain last tetanus immunization if shock is due to injury.
6. Note if shock is due to work-related injury.
7. Note if client is wearing emergency-type jewelry or tags that convey relevant information.

Physical Assessment

1. Level of consciousness.
2. Circulatory signs of hypovolemia, hypotension, and decreased tissue perfusion: pallor, BP variable or *below normal for client*, faintness, or slow capillary filling.
3. Anxiety, irritability, personality changes, fear, other emotional changes as shock worsens.
4. Compensatory responses of:
   a. Rapid, shallow respirations.
   b. Tachycardia.
5. Skin is warm and dry with good color in septic shock; and cold, clammy, and cyanotic or pale in cardiogenic and hypovolemic shock. In anaphylaxis, hives (wheals) appear locally at site of sting and/or in a widespread distribution (often in warmer areas such as underarms, groin, neck, and trunk); angioedema (redness and swelling, often of lips and eyelids) may be present; itching is intense.
6. Temperature may be normal or, in septic shock, above or below normal (absence of fever often masks infection).
7. Urine output is reduced or absent.

Diagnostic Tests

1. CBC and differential.
2. Hemoglobin, hematocrit, BUN, blood sugar levels (increased BUN, increased creatinine in septic shock).
3. Electrolyte levels: Na, K, Cl, Ca, Mg.

4. Arterial blood gases for acid-base and oxygenation determination (respiratory alkalosis, early, with metabolic acidosis as shock progresses).
5. Twelve-lead ECG.
6. Blood typing.
7. Platelet count.
8. Coagulation screen.
9. Fibrinogen index, fibrin split products (FSP).
10. Blood cultures and/or other specimen cultures.

NURSING DIAGNOSES: ACTUAL OR POTENTIAL

1. Reduced cardiac output secondary to decreased circulating fluid volume, dilated vascular bed, ineffective cardiac pumping, or biochemical mechanism.
2. Inadequate tissue perfusion secondary to reduced cardiac output.
3. Reduced respiratory exchange secondary to reduced lung perfusion and, in anaphylaxis, upper or lower airway obstruction associated with edema.
4. Fluid and electrolyte level imbalances secondary to fluid loss (hemorrhage, sequestration, or edema) and toxic build-up.
5. Acid-base imbalance: acidosis secondary to circulatory, respiratory, and renal waste product accumulation.
6. Alteration in consciousness: seizures, fainting, or coma secondary to brain hypoxia or toxic build-up.
7. Alterations in body temperature: low or high temperature associated with septicemia and septic shock.
8. Infection: septicemia (in septic shock and clients with trauma).

EXPECTED OUTCOMES

1. Perfusion will be restored, as evidenced by BP, pulse, and respiration within normal limits, return of consciousness, and normal urinary output.
2. Respiratory function will be adequate, as evidenced by normal blood gases and relief of dyspnea (if any).
3. Fluid balance will be restored as evidenced by normal BP, skin turgor, and urine output.
4. Electrolyte values will return to normal limits.
5. Client will return to normal state of consciousness; client will not be injured while confused, convulsive, or unconscious.
6. Body temperature will be returned to normal range.
7. Infection will be prevented or promptly recognized and adequately treated.

INTERVENTIONS

1. For hypovolemic shock:
   a. Place client supine with legs elevated unless head injury or other factor contraindicates.
   b. Ensure patent airway and adequate oxygenation with nasal prongs, mask, or intubation; monitor blood gas determinations.
   c. Stop external bleeding with pressure.
   d. Monitor vital signs continually until stabilized after treatment.
   e. Restore fluid volume with prescribed balanced salt solutions (e.g., Ringer's lactate, Dextran, or normal saline) via two large-bore intravenous lines at rapid rate and in amount necessary to maintain systolic pressure at 90 mmHg.
   f. Type and cross-match for whole blood or packed RBC, if indicated by estimated blood loss and lab reports about hemoglobin and hematocrit.
   g. Insert Foley catheter and monitor hourly output, specific gravity, pH, and presence of hemoglobin or myoglobin.
   h. If prescribed, administer large doses of hydrocortisone preparations once replacement fluids have been given, usually hydrocortisone sodium succinate (Solu-Cortef) or methylprednisolone sodium succinate (Solu-Medrol).
   i. Obtain standard 12-lead ECG and monitor for dysrhythmia.
   j. Administer tetanus prophylaxis if victim is at risk and injuries are massive or contaminated.
   k. Accurately monitor vasopressors and cardiotonics.
   l. Monitor central venous pressure and maintain at 6 to 8 cm H_2O pressure.
   m. Correct acid-base abnormalities with sodium bicarbonate bolus.
   n. Administer prescribed heparin therapy if client develops disseminated intravascular coagulation (DIC).

o. Protect client as required in altered state of consciousness: remove injurious articles from bed of convulsive or comatose client, pad side rails as needed, and so on.

2. For cardiogenic shock:
   a. Administer cardiopulmonary resuscitation if arrest has occurred.
   b. Monitor standard 12-lead ECG for arrhythmias.
   c. Administer 100 percent oxygen continuously.
   d. Correct acid-base abnormalities with sodium bicarbonate bolus.
   e. Administer prescribed analgesic.
   f. Administer prescribed fluid expanders, and vasopressors and cardiotonics.
   g. Correct arrhythmias and prevent ventricular fibrillation by administering prescribed lidocaine.
   h. Insert Foley catheter and monitor hourly output, specific gravity, and pH.
   i. Auscultate lungs frequently to detect and monitor congestion.
   j. Monitor electrolyte levels, BUN, urinalysis, and coagulation screens.
   k. Protect confused, convulsive, or comatose client from injury.
3. For vasogenic shock:
   a. Position client with head at or near heart level so that circulation to brain is increased.
   b. Keep warm but do not apply heat.
   c. Protect against injury while unconscious.
   d. Support cardiorespiratory functions if required, for example, in barbiturate overdose.
4. For septic shock:
   a. Support cardiorespiratory functions: ensure adequate airway and ventilation. Give oxygen, usually under positive pressure.
   b. Monitor 12-lead ECG for arrhythmias.
   c. Correct acidosis by administering prescribed sodium bicarbonate bolus.
   d. Administer prescribed fluids for restoring blood volume, frequently in large amounts (e.g., 10,000 mL in 8 hours) until central venous pressure is normal and BP exceeds 90/60; fluids commonly used are 5 percent dextrose in saline or plasma.
   e. Insert Foley catheter and monitor hourly output, specific gravity, and pH.
   f. Administer prescribed antibiotics.
   g. Accurately administer prescribed vasopressors and cardiotonics, if any.
   h. Auscultate lungs frequently during fluid replacement to detect and monitor congestion.
   i. Administer prescribed large doses of corticosteroids.
   j. If client has fever, support with increased caloric intake (up to 5,000 calories per day, depending on needs).
   k. Protect unconscious or convulsive client from injury.
5. For anaphylactic shock:
   a. Immediately administer prescribed aqueous epinephrine (Adrenalin).
   b. Tourniquet should be applied above injected allergen (bee sting site, penicillin injection site).
   c. Ice applications slow the rate of absorption.
   d. Establish airway and oxygenation (intubation or tracheotomy and positive pressure ventilation may be necessary).
   e. Monitor IV fluids as prescribed.
   f. Administer prescribed corticosteroid, usually hydrocortisone (Solu-Cortef).
   g. Vasopressors may be prescribed: monitor administration and vital signs continually.
   h. Administer prescribed antihistamine, usually diphenhydramine hydrochloride (Benadryl).

EVALUATION

Outcome Criteria

1. Perfusion is restored: vital signs are within normal limits, and client is conscious and oriented.
2. Dyspnea is relieved, and blood gases are within normal limits.
3. Fluid balance is restored: BP, skin turgor, and urine output are normal.
4. Laboratory values for electrolytes are within normal limits.
5. Client has not been injured during confusion, convulsion, or coma.
6. Temperature is normal.
7. Infection has been prevented or adequately treated.

Complications

1. Irreversible shock and death.
2. Disseminated intravascular coagulation (DIC).

3. Acute tubular necrosis (renal failure).
4. Stroke from hypertension induced by therapy.

Reevaluation and Follow-up

Clients with anaphylaxis must be taught about their allergy and ways to avoid potentially fatal reexposure to the allergen. They should wear a medical warning bracelet or neck tag. For client allergic to bees, see *Venomous Bites and Stings,* Reevaluation and Follow-up, earlier in this chapter.

RESPIRATORY TRAUMA

UPPER AIRWAY TRAUMA

DESCRIPTION

The anatomical components of the upper airway include the nose; ethmoid, sphenoid, frontal, and maxillary sinuses; larynx; nasal pharynx and oral pharynx; and trachea. These structures or their functions can be disrupted by obstruction, restriction, avulsion, loss of bony or cartilaginous integrity, tears and penetrations, or paralysis from interruption of nerve supply. Trauma is usually due to foreign bodies; falls; auto accidents; burns or smoke inhalation; industrial accidents; self-inflicted or homicidal gunshot, stabbing, or strangulation; blunt blows; or accidental penetrating wounds. Common foreign bodies are broken dentures, chewing gum, cuds of tobacco, food, vomitus, blood from airway injury, and items of hardware such as nails and pins.

PREVENTION

Health Promotion

1. Proper use of automobile seat belts.
2. Prevention of choking and strangling accidents in infants and small children and others who have difficulty coordinating breathing and swallowing (persons with mental retardation, parkinsonism, etc.).
   a. For pediatric prevention, see Chapter 20, *Foreign Body Aspiration.*
   b. Do not permit force feeding of any client.
   c. Position anesthetized, comatose, severely debilitated, intoxicated, and convulsive persons so that vomitus or other substances will drain away from the airway.
   d. Promote public programs instructing in respiratory first aid (Heimlich maneuver, etc.).
3. Assist potentially suicidal or violent clients to find nonviolent, healthful ways of dealing with their feelings (Chapters 36, 37, 38, and 41).
4. Prevent burns (discussed earlier in this chapter).

Population at Risk

1. Choking on food can happen to anyone, but particularly the very young, the intoxicated, and the debilitated or motorically impaired.
2. Violent or depressed persons.
3. Those at risk for automobile accidents, falls, burns, and other injuries described earlier in this chapter.

Screening

None.

ASSESSMENT

See Table 48–1 for assessment factors that assist in identifying the location of a respiratory obstruction.

Health History

1. Obtain description of mechanism or forces causing injury.
2. Note victim's placement in auto (driver, front passenger, etc.), or position of body during traumatic encounter.
3. Obtain past medical history, particularly respiratory pathology, including medications and allergies.
4. Note if injuries are work-related.
5. Ascertain if victim vomited prior to admission.
6. Note if victim has shown suicidal behavior in recent past.

Physical Assessment

1. Dyspnea, forcible respiratory efforts.
2. Choking, coughing.
3. Shrill, high-pitched noises with inhalation or exhalation suggest foreign body or other obstruction.
4. Sucking or hissing sounds of air movement

TABLE 48-1 GUIDE TO LOCALIZATION OF AIRWAY OBSTRUCTION

Sign or Symptom	Level of Obstruction			
	Pharynx	Larynx	Trachea	Bronchi
Voice changes	Slurred or thick	Hoarse or absent	Decreased volume	Decreased volume
Cough	Persistent, scratchy	Stridulous, "croupy"	Reflex irritative	Reflex irritative
Swallowing	Difficult; drooling present; client juts head forward and down to aid egress	Difficult; may be drooling	Usually normal but occasionally painful	Normal
Dyspnea	Positional	Inspiratory	Inspiratory	Often present with wheezing
Cyanosis	May be present; relieved by position changes	May be present	May be present	Often present
Intercostal reaction	Usually absent	Inspiratory	Inspiratory	If a large bronchus is blocked; may be unilateral
Breath sounds	Normal	Roughened, coarse	Coarse rales and rhonchi	Rhonchi; may be decreased or absent
Restlessness, excitement, apprehension	Intermittent; acute during episodes of dysphagia and dyspnea	Often acute	Variable, depends on % obstruction	Acute if a large bronchus is blocked
X-ray[a]: lateral neck and chest films	"Thumb sign" of swollen epiglottis: retropharyngeal swelling wider than client's little finger	May be normal; esophageal foreign body indentation	May be normal; esophageal foreign body indentation	Acute ball valve obstruction (bilateral expiration decubitas AP film): involved side initially stays expanded, later is collapsed

SOURCE: Cain, H.: *Flint's Emergency Treatment and Management*, 6th ed., Philadelphia, 1980, p. 54.

[a] Obtain portable film or have an experienced person with complete airway equipment accompany patient. Radiopaque or air-displacing foreign bodies may be seen also. All of the films listed may be normal.

through structural disruptions that have more than one passageway.
5. Stertor.
6. Deformities (fractures or dislocations) of nose, face, or neck: asymmetry, depression, crepitus, abnormal mobility, or abnormal angulation.
7. Hemorrhage, external or internal, with resultant hypotension and tachycardia.
8. Subcutaneous emphysema.
9. Visible foreign bodies.
10. Cyanosis or other discolorations of skin and mucous membranes.
11. Fractured, displaced, or avulsed teeth.
12. Edema.
13. Cerebrospinal fluid (CSF) drainage from ears, nose, or oropharynx.
14. Signs of sepsis.
15. Pain.
16. Loss of sensation or of gag and swallow reflexes.
17. Loss of voice.
18. Burns or carbon particles around nostrils or mouth.
19. Emesis.
20. Lacerations or puncture wounds.

NURSING DIAGNOSES: ACTUAL OR POTENTIAL

1. Impaired respiratory exchange secondary to upper respiratory trauma.
2. Acid-base imbalance secondary to impaired respiratory exchange.
3. Impaired integrity of skin or mucous membrane secondary to trauma.
4. Increased risk of infection secondary to loss of integrity of skin or mucous membrane.
5. Hemorrhage associated with trauma.
6. Fluid deficit secondary to blood loss and increased respiratory rate (insensible loss).
7. Alteration in comfort: pain and discomfort associated with trauma.
8. Anxiety secondary to respiratory insufficiency, bleeding, pain, and original trauma.

EXPECTED OUTCOMES

1. Respiratory adequacy will be restored as evidenced by normal blood gases and normal respiratory rate and effort.
2. Infection will be prevented or effectively treated.
3. Blood loss will be minimized.
4. Fluid balance will be restored.
5. Pain and discomfort will be reduced and eliminated.
6. Anxiety will be controlled and reduced.

INTERVENTIONS

1. Establish airway with endotracheal or nasotracheal tube, oral airway, client positioning (chin lift and head tilt unless contraindicated by cervical injury, then jaw thrust), or cricothyrotomy.
2. Remove airway obstruction by encouraging conscious victim to forcefully cough. If unconscious, establish airway and attempt to ventilate. If unable to ventilate, provide victim with four back blows, four manual thrusts, and finger probe through mouth to remove foreign bodies before attempting next ventilation. If still unsuccessful, repeat abdominal or chest thrusts (see Figure 48–16).
3. Aspirate airway, and periodically suction all mucus and drainage to keep airway patent.
4. Provide 5 to 10 L of 100 percent oxygen initially, and follow arterial blood gas results for continued therapy.
5. Place on volumetric respirator if air passages are severely disrupted or significant swelling is expected.
6. Administer muscle relaxant (or respiratory paralyzer) after intubation and under supervision of physician, if unable to remove foreign body due to spasms. Give succinylcholine derivative according to recommended dosages on package insert. Be prepared to support victim's ventilations with positive pressure breathing bag or mechanical ventilation.
7. Stop hemorrhage by nasal or nasopharyngeal packing, cautery, epinephrine spray, ligation of oozing vessel, treatment of underlying cause, or surgical repair, as appropriate.
8. Start large-bore IV line(s) for administration of medications using 1,000 mL of 5 percent dextrose in water.
9. Begin fluid therapy with large-bore IV and 1,000 mL Ringer's solution, and continue with appropriate fluids and/or blood.
10. Cautiously administer analgesia or sedation (morphine sulfate or meperidine hydrochloride [Demerol]) by titrated IV route).
11. Begin broad-spectrum antibiotic therapy if

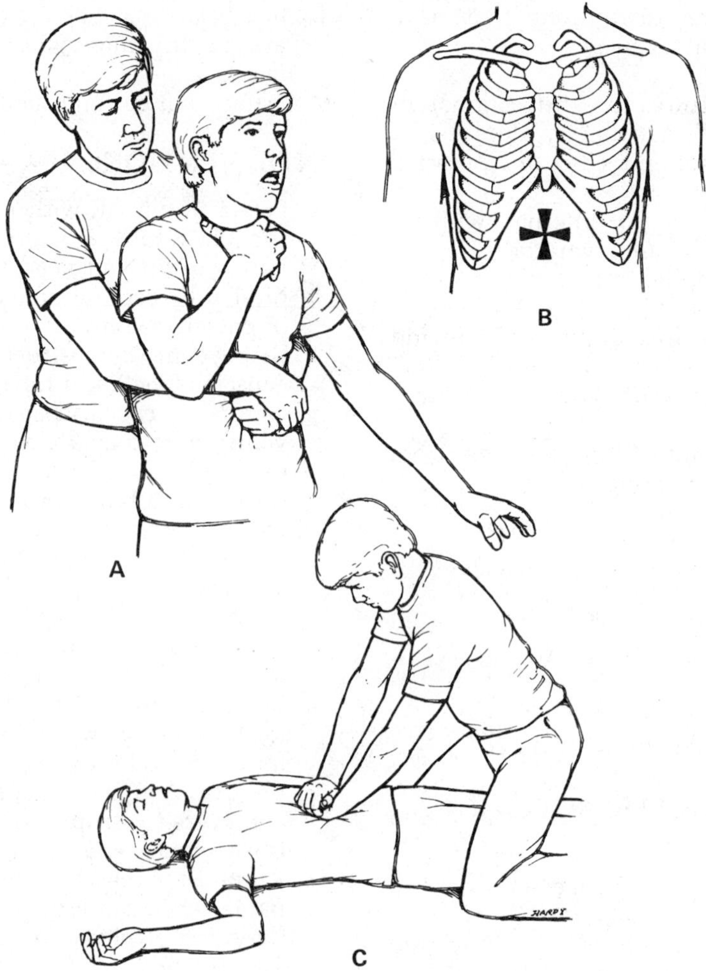

Figure 48-16 The Heimlich maneuver. (*a*) The victim is grasped from behind as quickly as distress is signaled. (*b*) The rescuer's fist should be pressed into the upper abdomen at the spot marked by the cross. (*c*) Correct position of rescuer when client is found lying face up. Note the placement of the hand, which permits a quick upward thrust. (From Henderson, J.: *Emergency Medical Guide*, 4th ed., McGraw-Hill, New York, 1978. Reproduced with permission.)

wounds are contaminated or cerebrospinal fluid drainage is noted.

12. Monitor vital signs frequently, and in particular watch for changes in respiratory patterns and rate.
13. Prepare victims of penetrating neck wounds for immediate surgical debridement, exploration, and repair.
14. Administer tetanus prophylaxis if victim is at risk.
15. Provide emotional support to victim and family.

EVALUATION

Outcome Criteria

1. Blood gases and respiratory rate and effort are within normal limits.
2. Infection is absent or under effective treatment.

3. Fluid balance has been restored.
4. Hemorrhage was quickly controlled.
5. Client reports that analgesia is effective.
6. Anxiety is reduced to manageable and realistic proportions; client cooperates with treatment plan and is free of signs of excessive anxiety.

Complications

1. Shock.
2. Residual respiratory insufficiency.
3. Voice changes.

LOWER AIRWAY TRAUMA

DESCRIPTION

Lower airway trauma includes any disruption of structure or function caused by obstruction, restriction, avulsion, loss of bony integrity, tears and penetrations, or paralysis due to interruption of innervation. The anatomical components of the lower airway include the bronchi, individual lobes of the lung, alveoli, and thorax (ribs and sternum). Trauma is usually due to acceleration-deceleration forces; falls; industrial or auto accidents; blunt blows; and accidental, suicidal, or homicidal penetrating wounds by gunshot, stabbing, or impaling objects. Drivers may have "steering wheel" injuries: sudden sharp pressure changes due to a blow against the steering column can rupture the diaphragm with resultant herniation of the abdominal contents into the pleural cavity. Some foreign bodies in the lower airway may have been dislodged from the upper airway. See *Upper Airway Trauma*, above. Cardiopulmonary resuscitation (CPR) may cause costochondral separations and rib fractures.

PREVENTION

See *Upper Airway Trauma* in this chapter.

ASSESSMENT

Health History

1. Obtain description of mechanism or forces causing injury.
2. Note environmental influences altering mechanism or forces.
3. Note if injuries are work-related.
4. Ascertain past medical history, including medications and allergies.
5. In the case of an auto accident, obtain description of victim's position in car.
6. Ascertain if victim vomited prior to hospital admission.
7. Seek information regarding suicidal or homicidal act causing injuries.

Physical Assessment

1. Signs of inadequate gas exchange and hypoxemia.
2. Hemorrhage, internal or external, with resultant hypotension and tachycardia.
3. Asymmetry of thorax during or between ventilations.
4. Cyanosis, central and peripheral.
5. Sucking or hissing sounds on exhalation.
6. Wheezing, rales, rhonchi, or musical noises on inspiration or expiration.
7. Signs of shock (decreased blood pressure; narrowed pulse pressure; decreased urine output; and increased respiratory rate).
8. Hyperresonance (pneumothorax).
9. Pain.
10. Arrhythmias.
11. Distant, muffled heart sounds.
12. Dull or absent breath sounds on auscultation.
13. Agitation, anxiety, or depressed consciousness.
14. Tracheal deviation to unaffected side.
15. Tachycardia.
16. Fractures, dislocations, or flail chest.
17. Edema, crepitus, or subcutaneous emphysema.
18. Lacerations: abnormal openings to lungs and airways.
19. Scaphoid abdomen: indication of abdominal contents herniation into chest wall.
20. Excessive abdominal movement with respirations: may indicate chest wall damage.
21. Hemoptysis.
22. Mediastinal emphysema, dislocations of mediastinal organs.
23. Bloody froth issuing from wound: tension pneumothorax from penetrating wound.
24. Paradoxical pulse (pulse is weaker during inspiration).

Diagnostic Tests

1. Radiography.
2. Bronchoscopy.

3. CBC, differential, hemoglobin and hematocrit levels.
4. Type and cross-match blood if large blood loss.
5. Arterial blood gas determinations.
6. Continuous 12-lead ECG.
7. Arteriovenous shunt calculations, arteriovenous extraction rates.
8. Diagnostic tap: plunger of moistened glass syringe pushed out by increased intrathoracic pressure.
9. Massive air leak when established on water seal drainage.

NURSING DIAGNOSES: ACTUAL OR POTENTIAL

1. Impaired respiratory exchange secondary to lower respiratory trauma.
2. Acid-base imbalance secondary to impaired respiratory exchange.
3. Impaired integrity of skin or mucous membrane secondary to trauma.
4. Increased risk of infection secondary to loss of integrity of skin or mucous membrane.
5. Hemorrhage associated with trauma.
6. Fluid dificit secondary to blood loss and increased respiratory rate (insensible loss).
7. Alteration in comfort: pain and discomfort associated with trauma.
8. Anxiety secondary to respiratory insufficiency, bleeding, pain, and original trauma.

EXPECTED OUTCOMES

1. Respiratory adequacy will be restored as evidenced by normal blood gases and normal respiratory rate and effort.
2. Infection will be prevented or effectively treated.
3. Blood loss will be minimized.
4. Fluid balance will be restored.
5. Pain and discomfort will be reduced and eliminated.
6. Anxiety will be controlled and reduced.

INTERVENTIONS

1. Cover sucking wound with Vaseline-impregnated gauze during end of exhalation.
2. Immediately establish adequate airway patency with endotracheal or nasotracheal intubation and mechanical ventilation, positive pressure bag-mask and oxygen, or intranasal catheter and pressurized oxygen.
3. Start 100 percent oxygen at 5 to 10 L, and continue therapy based on arterial blood gas reports.
4. Watch for signs of tension pneumothorax, especially if client has been placed on a volumetric respirator: absent breath sounds on affected side and deviated trachea away from tension pneumothorax.
5. Decompress pleural space (for client with tension pneumothorax) with No. 16 or 18 needle and 50-mL moistened syringe and plunger. Cleanse skin over area lateral to the midclavicular line in the second or third interspace on the side of tension pneumothorax. With head of bed at 60 to 90 degrees, insert needle and attached syringe. Allow increased intrapleural pressure to force plunger out of syringe. Withdraw plunger and let air escape. When hissing noise stops, withdraw needle and cover puncture site with dry dressing.
6. Continue to monitor vital signs frequently, particularly rate, depth, and pattern of respirations.
7. Intubate and bag victim with a flail chest who is having respiratory difficulty.
8. Stabilize a flail chest with sandbag, tape, and padding (position victim on affected side); sterile towel forceps may be clamped to flail section and slight traction applied; prepare client for surgical repair.
9. Auscultate chest frequently to ascertain adequacy of ventilations and stasis of secretions.
10. Further support flail by intubation and ventilation with positive end expiratory pressure (PEEP) or continuous positive airway pressure (CPAP). Avoid insertion of chest tube with victim in supine position, as this increases risk of diaphragm injury.
11. For stabbing and gunshot wounds, protect evidence of clothes particles, carbon dust on skin, smoke residue, or other debris as site is cleansed. Lightly scrape specimens into sterile containers before introducing cleansing agents. Avoid irrigating chest wounds caused by gunshot or stabbing.
12. Prior to insertion of water seal or negative pressure chest drainage for atelectatic lung, ask client to deep-breathe in, then forcefully exhale against a closed glottis; quickly cover or stabilize wound with a dry sterile dressing and occlusive dressing. This maneuver may

reinflate atelectatic segment and buy time.
13. Administer prescribed analgesics by IV titration, usually morphine sulfate or meperidine (Demerol). Avoid respiratory depressants if client is not supported with mechanical ventilator. Closely observe responses.
14. Stop external bleeding with pressure dressings and rib belt. Falling blood pressure in the presence of stabilized respiratory function indicates internal bleeding.
15. Start fluid replacement; get blood typed and cross-matched, hemoglobin and hematocrit levels; and prepare client for exploratory surgery.
16. Assess all CPR clients for fractured ribs, costochondral separations, and adequacy of expiratory effort.
17. Massive dose and early administration of methylprednisolone may be given.
18. Protect edematous or ecchymotic skin and soft tissue from further injury (avoid pressure insofar as possible).
19. Administer appropriate broad-spectrum antibiotics if client has aspirated or has high index of suspicion for infection.
20. Administer tetanus prophylaxis if client is at risk.
21. Insert a nasogastric tube to decompress stomach and reduce pressure on diaphragm, hence lungs.
22. Place on cardiac monitor for careful observation of arrhythmias and cardiac arrest.

EVALUATION

Outcome Criteria

1. Blood gases and respiratory rate and effort are within normal limits.
2. Infection is absent or responding to treatment.
3. Fluid balance has been restored.
4. Hemorrhage was quickly controlled.
5. Client reports that analgesia is effective.
6. Anxiety is reduced to manageable and realistic proportions; client cooperates with treatment plan and is free of signs of excessive anxiety.

Complications

1. Shock.
2. Air embolus.
3. Residual respiratory insufficiency.

CARDIAC AND GREAT VESSEL TRAUMA

DESCRIPTION

The structure or function of the heart and great vessels can be disrupted by penetration, avulsion, contusion, rupture, or tearing of cardiac muscle or arteries and veins in the heart, in the superior and inferior vena cava, in the aorta, and in the pulmonary, subclavian, and femoral arteries. The most frequent causes of this trauma include high-speed automobile and motorcycle accidents, heavy industrial equipment accidents, and accidental, suicidal, and homicidal acts. The mechanism involved may be a direct blow, transmitted blow, compression, deceleration, blast overpressure, or a combination of these.

Penetrating wounds of the aorta have a more serious prognosis than cardiac stab wounds due to:

1. High pressure sustained in the aorta.
2. Thinner aortic wall that does not seal as well as the myocardium.
3. The mediastinum is less resistant to the egress of blood than an intact pericardium.
4. Delayed rebleeding of aorta is more common.
5. Survivors of the initial aortic insult are at higher risk for future problems of false aneurysm or arteriovenous fistula.

Prognosis for cardiac contusion is excellent.

PREVENTION

Health Promotion

1. Use of automobile seat belts.
2. Safety instruction of industrial workers.
3. Mental health measures to prevent suicidal and homicidal acts of violence.

Population at Risk

1. Persons in automobile deceleration accidents, especially drivers (because of being thrown against the steering wheel).
2. Suicidally depressed persons.
3. Persons likely to be involved in shootings or other forms of extreme violence: police officers, alcoholics, abused spouses, and so on.

ASSESSMENT

Health History

1. Describe mechanism or forces causing injury.
2. Note if client was driver, wearing shoulder strap or pelvic seat belt, placement in auto, position of body during traumatic encounter.
3. Obtain past medical history, particularly of cardiac pathology, including medications and allergies.
4. Note if injuries are work-related.
5. Note if client has received CPR prior to admission.
6. Ascertain if client is on anticoagulant therapy: look for Medic-Alert or similar medical jewelry.
7. Note if victim has indicated suicidal behavior in recent past.
8. Ascertain tetanus immunization record.

Physical Assessment

1. Hemorrhage: external and internal, with resultant hypotension and tachycardia.
2. Changes in cardiovascular system:
   a. Arrhythmias; ventricular fibrillation; sinus tachycardia; coarse atrial fibrillation, flutter, gallop rhythms; extra sounds of S_3 or S_4; new conduction defects.
   b. Asystole.
   c. Distant, muffled, "mushy" heart sounds.
   d. Mechanical alternans, pulsus paradoxus, pulsus alternans.
   e. Asymmetry of upper and/or lower extremity blood pressures; for example, a rupture of the aorta may produce hypotension in the lower extremities.
   f. Narrowing pulse pressure.
   g. Enlarged and/or displaced point of maximal impulse (PMI).
   h. Distension of jugular veins when the head of the bed is raised more than 45 degrees.
   i. Visible "atrial kick."
   j. May have friction rub from traumatic pericarditis.
   k. Sudden onset of aortic or mitral regurgitation.
   l. Murmurs or bruits (e.g., systolic murmur over precordium or on the back medial to the left scapula with rupture of aorta).
3. Precordial, substernal, diffuse pain; back and subscapular pain (with ruptured aorta).
4. Hoarseness due to hematoma pressure on left recurrent laryngeal nerve.

Diagnostic Tests

1. Serial ECGs.
2. Radiography, looking for:
   a. Widened mediastinum on anteroposterior x-ray film.
   b. Enlarged cardiac silhouette.
3. Arterial pressure monitoring.
4. Hb and Hct, CBC with differential; type and cross-match blood.
5. Arterial blood gases.
6. Arteriography.

NURSING DIAGNOSES: ACTUAL OR POTENTIAL

1. Alteration in cardiac output: decrease due to cardiac arrhythmia or hemorrhage.
2. Shock (cardiogenic or hypovolemic): hypoperfusion due to ineffective cardiac pump or intravascular fluid deficit.
3. Fluid and electrolyte imbalances secondary to blood loss, hypoxia, and cell by-product build-up.
4. Alteration in comfort: pain secondary to tissue trauma.
5. Anxiety secondary to life-threatening injury.
6. Infection secondary to loss of integrity of skin or major vasculature.

EXPECTED OUTCOMES

1. Cardiac function and tissue perfusion will be maintained.
2. Hemorrhage will be controlled.
3. Fluid and electrolyte balance will be restored to normal.
4. Pain will be alleviated.
5. Anxiety will be reduced.
6. Infection will be recognized early and effectively treated.

INTERVENTIONS

1. Immediately establish patent airway with endotracheal tube. Administer 100 percent oxygen until arterial blood gas results become available.
2. Insert two lines with large needles, No. 16 or 18, for IV fluids and medications.
3. Obtain blood type and cross match immediately.
4. Provide fluids with Ringer's lactate, normal

saline, colloid solutions, blood, or blood components commensurate with losses. Be sure massive or exsanguinating bleeds are replaced by fresh whole blood with retained clotting factors or cryoprecipitate.

5. Immediately assist with pericardiocentesis to relieve cardiac tamponade. Be sure fluid replacement has begun.
6. Establish arterial line, and monitor to keep systolic greater than 90 mmHg; however, if victim is known to have been hypertensive prior to accident, keep systolic between 130 and 140 mmHg.
7. Place on continuous cardiac monitoring.
8. Obtain arterial blood gases every 30 to 60 min until oxygen saturation is maintained within normal limits.
9. Obtain electrolyte levels and hemoglobin and hematocrit levels every 4 to 8 h; coagulation screen including PT, PTT, and platelet count when blood replacement passes 10 U of banked blood.
10. Constantly monitor vital signs with comparisons of bilateral blood pressures and pulses.
11. May monitor central venous pressure (CVP) if no arterial lines are available. Maintain pressure between 10 and 12 cmH_20.
12. Insert nasogastric tube to low, intermittent suction to decompress stomach. Calculate fluid and electrolyte losses; monitor pH of gastric contents every 4 to 8 h.
13. Insert Foley bladder catheter, and monitor output, specific gravity, and pH every hour.
14. Obtain chest x-ray film only if condition is stable; repeat x-rays will be done to assess changes.
15. Prepare for immediate surgical intervention in the operating room in cases of penetrating cardiac trauma or rupture of aorta.
16. If victim has blunt cardiac trauma, treat much like acute myocardial infarction with arrhythmia monitoring, bed rest, serial enzymes, and appropriate drugs.
17. Administer prescribed analgesics, and monitor vital sign responses as well as effectiveness of pain relief.
18. Reduce anxiety by reassuring client about what is being done: explain that there will be time to ask questions after the immediate measures are taken.
19. Administer prescribed antibiotic.

EVALUATION

Outcome Criteria

1. Blood pressure, pulse, and respiration are stabilized within normal limits.
2. Electrolyte values and fluid intake and output are within normal limits.
3. Client reports that analgesia is effective.
4. Client's anxiety is controlled: client is able to cooperate with treatment.
5. Infection is absent or responding to treatment.

Complications

1. Irreversible shock.
2. Acute renal failure, brain damage, or other organ damage due to hypoperfusion.
3. Transfusion reaction or other complication of transfusion.
4. Late hemorrhage.

ABDOMINAL TRAUMA

DESCRIPTION

Abdominal trauma includes any disruption of structure or function of the abdominal viscera or abdominal wall caused by penetration, rupture, tear, contusion, avulsion, or ingestion of corrosive agents or foreign bodies.

The anatomical components that may be injured include small bowel; stomach; colon; mesentery and omentum; spleen; diaphragm; pancreas; duodenum; biliary system, including liver and gallbladder; pancreas; kidneys; uterus; sciatic plexus; urinary bladder; ovary; adrenals; vagina; and muscles. The trauma may be due to high-velocity auto and motorcycle accidents, causing injuries by sharp and blunt objects; seat belt syndrome; penetrating wounds of stabbing and gunshot; crush injury; blast injury from air or immersion (which usually affects air-filled organs more severely); corrosive gastritis from hydrochloric, nitric, trichloroacetic, sulfuric, and carbolic acids or alkalis affecting the esophagus; and ingested foreign bodies. Iatrogenic causes of abdominal injury include endoscopy with biopsy; CPR; paracentesis or thoracentesis; peritoneal dialysis; barium enema; sigmoidoscopy; peritoneoscopy; liver biopsy; and radiation therapy producing corrosion of bowel or other organ. Mortality of abdominal trauma is generally correlated with the number of abdominal organs injured and the severity of insult to each.

PREVENTION

Health Promotion

1. Correct use of automobile seat belts: belt is to be strapped across the flexed hip joint, never up over the abdomen. Shoulder belt is to be in front of the shoulder, never under the arm.
2. Prevention of accidental ingestion of nonfoods (see Chapter 22, *Ingestion of Corrosive Substance*, Prevention).
3. Prevention of ingestion of foreign bodies: teach children and others not to place inedible items in the mouth.
4. Assist depressed or potentially violent persons to find nonviolent ways to deal with their feelings (see Chapters 36, 37, 38, and 41).
5. Ensure that all clients void before abdominal paracentesis (to reduce risk of bladder perforation).

Population at Risk

1. Persons in automobile or motorcycle accidents.
2. Persons who fall onto traumatizing objects.
3. The suicidally depressed.
4. Potentially violent persons and their victims.
5. Victims of accidental or intentional ingestion of corrosives or foreign bodies.
6. Persons who have had CPR with associated rib fractures.
7. Persons who have had intrusive diagnostic or therapeutic procedures such as paracentesis, peritoneal dialysis, and so on.
8. Persons receiving abdominal radiotherapy.

Screening

Physicial assessment (see below).

ASSESSMENT

Health History

1. Obtain description of mechanisms or forces causing injury.
2. If auto accident, inquire whether client was wearing seat belt and what type.
3. Describe speed or abruptness of onset of symptoms.
4. Note previous medical history, including medications, allergies, and abdominal surgical history.
5. Describe drinking history, cultural mores.
6. Note if injuries are work-related.
7. Note if victim received CPR prior to admission.
8. Ascertain additional and/or associated injuries.

Physical Assessment

1. Hemorrhage.
2. Symptoms of hypovolemic shock with resultant compensatory tachycardia, hypotension, oliguria, peripheral vasoconstriction, increased circulating catecholamines, increased blood glucose, normal range hemoglobin and hematocrit progressing to hemodilution, and tissue ischemia leading to total organism death.
3. Signs of sepsis.
4. Pain: diffuse, burning, peristaltic, rebound tenderness, referred.
5. Findings on abdominal examination:
   a. Absence of bowel sounds, abnormal location of sounds, bruits with major vessel disruption.
   b. Rigid and guarded abdomen.
   c. Spillage and loss of intraluminal contents, such as bile, gastric juices, proteolytic enzymes.
   d. Abdominal mass.
   e. Tympany of abdomen.
   f. Girth size increases rapidly.
6. Degrees of unresponsiveness.
7. Percussion reveals loss of dullness over major organs.
8. Less common signs: priapism, testicular pain.
9. Kehr's sign (left shoulder pain associated with rupture of the spleen).
10. Associated rib fractures: posterior left, 9 to 12, suggests spleen injury.

Diagnostic Tests

1. Culdocentesis.
2. Vaginal and bimanual examinations.
3. Rectal examination.
4. Hemoglobin, hematocrit levels, CBC, including WBC and differential, serial hematocrit.

5. Radiography.
6. Peritoneal lavage with laboratory analysis for RBC, WBC, bile, amylase, and bacteria; paracentesis.
7. Radionuclide photo images (spleen injuries).
8. Serum albumin, prothrombin, serum transaminases, lactic dehydrogenase (LDH), serum bilirubin, serum amylase, BUN, blood glucose.
9. Electrolyte levels.
10. Urinalysis.
11. Radiography: flat plate of abdomen and kidneys, ureter, and bladder, then for free air, dilatation, and extravasation of contrast media.
12. Liver and spleen scans.

NURSING DIAGNOSES: ACTUAL OR POTENTIAL

1. Fluid volume deficit secondary to hemorrhage or due to cellular or intravascular fluid shift into interstitial space.
2. Decreased cardiac output and hypoperfusion associated with fluid volume deficit.
3. Electrolyte and acid-base imbalances secondary to fluid deficit and hypoperfusion (toxic cellular byproduct build-up).
4. Infection secondary to gastrointestinal spillage, mucous membrane break-down, puncture wound, and so on.
5. Alteration in comfort: pain secondary to trauma.

EXPECTED OUTCOMES

1. Shock will be avoided or corrected.
2. Electrolyte values and acid-base balance will be restored to normal.
3. Infection will be prevented or promptly treated.
4. Client will be relieved of pain.

INTERVENTIONS

1. Establish patent airway with intubation, and provide adequate ventilation to maintain arterial oxygenation at Po_2 = 80 mmHg.
2. Insert two large-bore needles, no. 16 or 18, to administer IV fluids and medications.
3. Provide fluid replacement with Ringer's lactate, normal saline, colloid solutions, blood, or blood components commensurate with losses. Be sure massive or exsanguinating bleeds are replaced by fresh whole blood with retained clotting factors or cryoprecipitate.
4. Obtain blood type and cross match immediately.
5. Insert Foley catheter to straight drainage, and monitor output hourly until stable.
6. Insert nasogastric tube and connect to intermittent suction.
7. Continue to obtain serial electrolyte levels, BUN, hemoglobin and hematocrit levels, and arterial blood gas levels.
8. Help physician establish a CVP line and/or pulmonary wedge pressure monitoring.
9. Establish careful intake and output records.
10. Mark abdomen at point of greatest girth, and measure and record girth for baseline data.
11. Stabilize associated injuries, such as pneumothorax, hemothorax, life-threatening disruption of cardiac function.
12. Obtain baseline weight.
13. Administer electrolyte therapy to begin one-half correction of losses plus regular basic allowances. This should be 24-h plan.
14. Assist with peritoneal lavage by obtaining trochar and/or knife handle and blades of varying sizes and shapes, peritoneal dialysis catheter, and 1 L of normal saline or balanced salt solution for flush, tape, and dry dressings.
15. Give prescribed analgesia by IV titration and provide careful observation of victim if in danger of shock or in distress.
16. Administer tetanus prophylaxis if client is at risk.
17. Administer prescribed antibiotics.
18. Monitor for vagal response.

EVALUATION

Outcome Criteria

1. Vital functions are maintained.
2. Shock is averted or reversed: blood pressure is stabilized at or above 90/60, and urine output is adequate for size and state of hydration.
3. Electrolyte levels and acid-base laboratory values are within normal range.
4. Infection is averted or is responding to treatment.
5. Client reports relief of pain.

Complications

1. Irreversible shock (hypovolemic or septic).
2. Acute renal failure secondary to hypoperfusion.
3. Organ necrosis necessitating surgical removal.
4. Blood transfusion reaction or other complication of transfusion.

NEUROTRAUMA

DESCRIPTION

The structure or function of the nervous system can be disrupted by penetration, avulsion, contusion, concussion, rupture, shearing, or laceration. The damage may occur in the dura, brain parenchyma, vessels, spinal cord, or peripheral nerves entering or leaving the spinal cord. Anatomical components from topmost to caudal include:

1. Cerebral hemispheres, including sensory and motor strips, basal nuclei, and lateral ventricles.
2. Diencephalon, with thalamus, hypothalamus, pineal body, and foramen of Monro connecting to third ventricle.
3. Mesencephalon (midbrain), which includes cerebral aqueduct of Sylvius, cerebral peduncles, oculomotor (III) cranial nerves, trochlear (IV) cranial nerves, and corpora quadrigemina (which are reflex centers for visual, auditory, and tactile impulses).
4. Pons, a bridge between cell bodies, the pontine nuclei, and each half of the cerebellum. Included are nerve roots of the trigeminal (V) cranial nerve; at the pons base, abducens (VI), facial (VII), and acoustic or auditory (VIII) cranial nerves arise.
5. Medulla includes the reticular formation, the glossopharyngeal (IX), vagus (X), accessory (XI), and hypoglossal (XII) cranial nerves.
6. Spinal cord. Other structures essential to normal function are the meninges and blood vessels, and the protective bony encasement of the skull and vertebral column.

Neurotrauma usually results from high-speed automobile and motorcycle accidents; falls; heavy industrial equipment accidents; and suicidal or homicidal acts. The mechanisms of injury include acceleration-deceleration; blows from blunt objects; crushing; penetration by bullets or impaling objects; twisting with subsequent shearing, tearing, or rupture; "whiplash" of cervical spine (acceleration); cord compression with associated mechanical distortion of neural tissue and local cord ischemia and contusion; vascular insufficiency that develops as a complication of contusion and some fractures; and combinations of these.

PREVENTION

Health Promotion

1. Avoidance of falls from heights by use of safety belts for linemen, and instruction of children about how to climb safely (recognition and avoidance of dead tree limbs, use of non-skid shoes, and so forth), and similar precautions.
2. Proper use of automobile seat belts and car seat restraints for infants and children.
3. Use of protective helmets for cyclists and contact-sport athletes, hard hats for construction workers, and so on.
4. Counseling or teaching to help depressed or potentially violent persons to find nonviolent ways of dealing with their feelings.

Population at Risk

1. Persons whose work or recreation involves climbing or the risk of being struck by falling objects.
2. Persons in automobile accidents.
3. Athletes, cyclists.
4. The suicidally depressed.
5. Persons who abuse alcohol or other psychotropic drugs.
6. Potentially violent people and their victims.

Screening

None.

ASSESSMENT

Health History

1. Obtain description of mechanism or forces causing injury, such as speed, impact.
2. Note victim's initial complaints and level of consciousness, particularly before hospitalization if there is a reliable historian.
3. Note if motorcyclist wore helmet.
4. Ascertain if victim was thrown from car,

how many feet, and the position in which victim was found.

5. Ascertain if victim was wearing seat belt or shoulder belt.
6. Obtain past medical history, including medications and allergies. Note particularly if victim abuses alcohol or other drugs.
7. Ascertain if victim has recently had:
   a. Ingestion, inhalation, or injection of alcohol or other abused drug.
   b. Hypoglycemic state or other physiological disruption (arrhythmia, myocardial infarction, seizure, etc.).
   c. Cessation of respiration for any reason.
   d. Fainting.
   e. Abrupt onset of neurologic or special sensory deficit.
8. Obtain description of victim's cultural, educational, and social background (for aid in assessing speech, cognition, and other aspects of behavior).
9. Note if victim wears glasses or contact lenses.
10. Ascertain tetanus immunization record.
11. Look for medical identification tag or bracelet.
12. Note if injuries are work-related.
13. Note if victim has shown suicidal behavior in recent past.

Physical Assessment

1. Respiratory pattern may be abnormal in rate, depth, and rhythm.
2. Level of consciousness and orientation to time and date, surroundings, recognition of family, and self.
3. Other signs of neurological deficit:
   a. Speech: aphasia or dysphasia.
   b. Eyes: pupillary reflexes, nystagmus, corneal reflex, photophobia, diplopia, coordination of extraocular movements.
   c. Motor reflexes:
      (1) Pyramidal or motor tract responses, upper motor neuron: Babinski reflex, clonus.
      (2) Deep tendon reflexes.
   d. "Frontal lobe" release signs (elicit by tapping upper lip): rooting, snorting, sucking, teeth grinding, or cortical thumb.
   e. Ciliospinal reflex (pinch sternocleidomastoid muscle and victim's eyes jerk toward the side of stimulus).
   f. Deep pain, Melnick triad: comatose person may respond to (1) pressure of examiner's knuckles on sternum, (2) pressure against optic nerve as it courses through a foramen in the medial supraorbital ridge; and (3) to pinching of testicle or nipple. Client with diffuse irritation of meninges will have violent headache (if awake to tell examiner) and nuchal rigidity.
   g. Decorticate posturing (rigidity): flexion of upper extremities and extension of lower extremities with "toeing in."
   h. Decerebrate posturing (rigidity): extension and internal rotation of upper extremities and extension of lower extremities and "toeing in."
   i. Areflexic: no response to any stimuli (flaccidity).
   j. Weakness of muscle strength or asymmetry of movement of facial muscles or extremities.
   k. Drifts of extremities when placed in extension.
   l. Battle's sign: bleeding into mastoid sinus with obvious ecchymosis due to fracture of temporal bone.
   m. Dermatographia: a fingernail scratch on abdominal skin produces a raised, welted line indicating that the victim has lost sympathetic nervous system innervation.
   n. Altered pain, pressure, touch, and thermal sensations.
   o. Altered body temperature control.
4. Rising systolic blood pressure and falling diastolic blood pressure.
5. Hemorrhage: through open wounds, as space-occupying lesion, into orbital space, ear canal, nose, and so on.
6. Cerebrospinal fluid rhinorrhea or otorrhea as noted by spot test (bloody center with peripheral clear ring) or positive glucose strip test.
7. Cushing triad:
   a. Projectile vomiting.
   b. Papilledema.
   c. Vital sign changes.
8. Victim may have "traumatic" diabetes insipidus with copious urine output of very low specific gravity (below 1.001).
9. Lateralizing signs.
10. Crepitance, false motion, and tenderness over cervical spine fracture.
11. Pain or selected loss of sensation; loss of voluntary movement with spinal injury.

12. Loss of bladder or bowel control; priapism.
13. Extreme agitation, restlessness, or depression may accompany head trauma.
14. Pain: headache.
15. Movable fractures, dislocations, and changes in the bony structure of skull or face.
16. Edema of injured cervical or thoracolumbar muscles.
17. Rigidity and splinting of neck and back muscles with spinal fractures.
18. Initial loss of consciousness, followed by lucid interval with rapid deterioration as arterial bleed progresses (indicates epidural bleed).

Diagnostic Tests

1. Radiography: most common types are anteroposterior and lateral skull, Towne (half-axial view), and cervical views including the odontoid for C1 to C2 fractures. Pineal gland shifts of greater than 2 mm from midline are significant.
2. Cerebral angiography to identify intracranial space-occupying lesions.
3. Trephine (burr holes) to locate subdural hematomas (craniectomy).
4. Computerized tomography (CT scan).
5. Radioactive scan (may diagnose intracerebral hematoma and subdural or extradural hematoma).
6. Echoencephalography (ultrasound technique) to detect midline shift.
7. Questionable use or relevance of EEG (electroencephalogram).
8. Questionable use or relevance of ventriculography or pneumoencephalography.
9. Lumbar puncture: rarely or never used with head injury due to risk of herniation.
10. Urinalysis.
11. CBC, differential, hemoglobin, hematocrit, and electrolyte levels.
12. Blood cultures.
13. Secretion cultures for pyogens gaining entrance into dura or cranial vault.

NURSING DIAGNOSES: ACTUAL OR POTENTIAL

1. Impaired perfusion of brain tissue secondary to disruption (e.g., tearing or laceration) of blood supply, swelling that compresses vessels, or systemic shock.
2. Compromise of vital functions (especially respiration), secondary to increased intracranial pressure associated with trauma.
3. Fluid imbalances secondary to blood loss, fluid shift to interstitial space (edema, shock), vomiting, or diabetes insipidus.
4. Electrolyte level and pH imbalances secondary to fluid imbalance, hypoperfusion, and respiratory disturbances (e.g., Cheyne-Stokes syndrome or Biot's respirations).
5. Alteration in consciousness: lethargy, stupor, or coma secondary to brain hypoxia associated with trauma.
6. Alteration in sensation and perception: paresthesia, visual disturbances, and other sensory or perceptual distortions secondary to nervous system trauma.
7. Alteration in cognitive function: agitation, confusion, or impaired thought secondary to brain hypoxia (from laceration, swelling, etc.) associated with trauma.
8. Alteration in motor function: paralysis, paresis, clonus, spasticity, and so forth associated with nervous system trauma.
9. Impaired mobility and self-care deficits secondary to motor, perceptual, and cognitive alterations.
10. Increased risk of infection secondary to open or communicating traumatic wounds.
11. Increased risk of injury due to disturbances of consciousness, thought, motor control, and perception.
12. Alteration of comfort: pain associated with laceration, fracture, contusion, and so forth, and with meningeal irritation.
13. Alteration in body temperature: hyperthermia secondary to thermostatic impairment.

EXPECTED OUTCOMES

1. Vital functions will be stabilized within normal limits as evidenced by vital signs.
2. Fluid and electrolyte levels will be restored and maintained in normal balance.
3. Client's preinjury alertness, orientation, sensory functions, perception, and motor skills will be restored.
4. Mobility and self-care activities will be restored.
5. Infection will be prevented or promptly recognized and effectively treated.
6. Client will not be injured during periods of altered consciousness or by convulsions or sensory-motor impairments.

7. Pain will be alleviated.
8. Body temperature will be restored to normal.

INTERVENTIONS

1. Immediately establish patent airway, intubating if necessary, and ventilate as needed to maintain acceptable serial arterial blood gases.
2. Immediately triage for cervical spine injury, immobilize with back board, collar, sand bags, or any material that keeps neck and head from moving.
3. Prevent aspiration or obstruction by careful suctioning and positioning to encourage gravity drainage.
4. Stop or reduce hemorrhage of all external wounds by packing and pressure dressings. Note increasing ecchymosis of mastoid area, orbital space, and so on, and report it.
5. Continually monitor neurologic status (especially level of consciousness); vital signs; cardiac rhythm; and increasing CSF drainage or ecchymoses, and record every 15 min until stable. Watch for signs of increasing intracranial pressure.
6. Carefully administer isotonic IV fluids to maintain blood pressure and urine output. Limit intake to keep patient "on the dry side."
7. Maintain careful recording of intake and output. Prevent fluid overload to minimize cerebral edema.
8. Obtain serum electrolyte and hematocrit levels as needed, at least every 24 h.
9. Maintain quiet, reality-oriented environment. Avoid or limit stimulation and hyperactivity. Do not allow client to initiate Valsalva's maneuver (coughing, straining at stool, etc.), as it can dangerously increase intracranial pressure.
10. Elevate head of bed 30 degrees to aid in venous return, or maintain preset height if ventriculostomy tube is in place.
11. Observe for bladder and gastric distention, especially if catheter and nasogastric tubes have not been inserted.
12. Monitor hourly urines for amount, specific gravity, and pH in any serious head injury. Note change indicating traumatic diabetes insipidus (increased output with low specific gravity).
13. Watch for any occlusion of jugular venous return (e.g., from tight dressings or tape); reduced cerebral venous return worsens brain edema.
14. Carefully observe acid-base balance to avoid hypercarbia (ventilate by bagging a tidal volume that does not reduce venous return from the head).
15. Protect client against neurologic deficit pressure areas, and position and reposition to avoid skin breakdown. If client is placed on "egg carton" mattress or low-pressure mattress, touch his or her body to stimulate different sensation (keeps client from feeling weightless and sensory-deprived: "floating out of reality").
16. Maintain positions of function for feet, wrists, and hands by placing bolsters, foot board, hand rolls and other supports. Provide passive range-of-motion four times a day. Keep body properly aligned.
17. Provide mental health consultation and psychosocial, emotional, and spiritual support to client and family.
18. If client is on circle bed, Bradford frame, or other special bed, constantly orient and protect.
19. Meticulously monitor all rhinorrhea or otorrhea, and maintain reverse isolation to avoid sepsis.
20. Diuretics (osmotic type such as mannitol or urea) may be administered; they are of limited use except to "buy time" when cerebral edema is present.
21. Corticosteroids may be administered for cerebral edema.
22. May assist with internal decompression (partial temporal lobe resection) for cerebral edema refractory to conservative treatment.
23. In cerebral edema, hyperventilate client to keep Pa_{CO_2} approximately 30 to 32 to promote cerebral vasoconstriction.
24. Administer prophylactic diphenylhydantoin (Dilantin) to avoid seizure activity (necessary for victims with trauma, including disrupted dura). Implement seizure precautions to protect against injury.
25. For high fever, place client on hypothermia mattress and gradually decrease temperature to approximately 100°F (38°C).
26. For febrile states, may administer acetominophen (Tylenol) or acetylsalicylic acid (aspirin) orally or by suppository.
27. Medicate with antibiotics prescribed accord-

ing to culture and sensitivity reports. Initially, may begin broad-spectrum antibiotic before organism is identified, but only *after* first cultures are obtained.

28. Keep hyperchlorhydria to minimum by administering prescribed antacids via nasogastric tube, with clometidine to maintain gastric pH greater than 6. Check gastric contents for positive guaiac.
29. Observe victim carefully for signs of neurogenic pulmonary edema and inappropriate ADH release (antidiuretic hormone) causing expanded extracellular and intracellular volume leading to decreased aldosterone output. This causes urinary salt loss, known as "cerebral salt wasting."
30. If oral intake is possible, give prescribed Tegretol to client with diabetes insipidus; if not, administer injectable Pitressin.
31. Carefully maintain ventriculostomy tube and any intracranial pressure monitor probes at exactly the angle specified by the physician.
32. Constantly orient client to surroundings, procedures, time, date, and personnel. Be sensitive to unspoken and uncommunicated needs. Consult with social worker and mental health personnel for special needs.
33. Administer tetanus prophylaxis if at risk.
34. Assist client to maximum allowable mobility and self-care: rearrange furniture to accommodate one-sided weakness, provide helping devices, and so forth.

EVALUATION

Outcome Criteria

1. Vital signs, blood gases, and electrolyte levels are within normal limits.
2. Consciousness, orientation, sensory functions, perception, and motor activities are restored to preinjury level.
3. Mobility and self-care are carried out by client at maximum level compatible with safety and with treatment plan restrictions.
4. Infection is absent or responding to treatment.
5. Injury due to unconsciousness, seizure, motor or sensory deficit, or cognitive impairment has not occurred.
6. Client reports relief of pain.
7. Body temperature is normal.

Complications

1. Meningitis.
2. Pulmonary edema.
3. Irreversible shock.
4. Brain stem herniation.
5. Residual neurological impairment (motor deficits, sensory limitation, loss of intellect, etc.).

Reevaluation and Follow-up

A range of rehabilitative services may be required by clients who have less than complete recovery.

REFERENCES

Jahre, J., et al.: "Medical Approach to the Hypertensive Patient and the Patient in Shock," *Heart and Lung*, **4**:577–587, July–August 1975.

Krupp, M. A., and Chatton, M. J. (eds.): *Current Medical Diagnosis and Treatment*, 3d ed., Lange, Los Altos, California, 1982.

Rapaport, H.: "Disarming Insect Stings," *Drug Therapy*, **5**:272–277, May 1975.

Sims, J. K.: "Drowning and Near-drowning," in Barry, J. (ed.), *Emergency Nursing*, McGraw-Hill, New York, 1978.

BIBLIOGRAPHY

Budassi, S. A., and Barber, J. M. (eds.): *Emergency Nursing: Principles and Practice*, Mosby, St. Louis, 1981. A comprehensive and clear anthology dealing with nursing in emergency settings. Includes not only treatments and procedures and the rationales for them, but also excellent material about more general topics, such as communication in crisis, client assessment, emergency department management, legal factors, and working with child clients.

Cain, H.: *Flint's Emergency Treatment and Management*, 6th ed., Saunders, Philadelphia, 1980. A treatment manual for common emergency care situations. Very concise, accurate account of problems and the immediate *medical* intervention required.

Hazlett, C. B.: *Primary Care Nursing: A Manual of Clinical Skills*, F. A. Davis, Philadelphia, 1977. This is an outstanding compilation of solid intervention techniques, developed from a curriculum devised for nurses who practice in the remote areas of Canada. Much of the information can be readily adapted for nursing use in emergency stiuations inside or outside a major institution.

49

Medical Emergencies

Marilyn de Give

POISONINGS

Cases of poisoning can be divided into three specific categories: (1) Exposure to a *known* poison; (2) exposure to an unknown substance which *may* be a poison; and (3) disease of unknown etiology, in which poisoning *should be considered* as part of the differential diagnosis.

OVERDOSE

DESCRIPTION

An overdose is any intoxication created by a greater than therapeutic level of medication ingested, inhaled, injected, or otherwise consumed without prescription or without the supervision of medical personnel. Taking or administering a medication with the ultimate result of toxic and/or greater than normal range levels and for other than therapeutic reasons may be accidental or intentional. Therefore, a misdemeanor may have been committed, and the nurse is legally required to report all incidences of drug overdoses where certain drugs are identified. The most common overdosed medications include salicylates, narcotics, sedatives, tranquilizers, mood elevators, and antipsychotics. To give an example: a hypertensive client presents in shock and is thought to have sustained a myocardial infarction. Instead, this client has, in fact, taken too much hypotensive medication.

Recognition is given to Annalee Oakes, who was coauthor of this chapter in the previous edition of this book.

PREVENTION

Health Promotion

1. Education of high risk groups within the general population: to prevent drug abuse in school children; to prevent children at home from ingesting medication left accessible to them, and so on.
2. Community involvement in ongoing local projects: to support suicide victims and their families; to offer work or school alternatives to students or others involved with drugs; to establish legal guidelines to deal with local drug selling and distribution.
3. Awareness on part of public regarding manifestations of drug overdosage and appropriate assessments and interventions required to initiate first aid.

Population at Risk

The entire population is at risk. Some specific examples are:

1. Children, of all ages, left unsupervised or experiencing extreme stress.
2. School age children and young adults, college and university students in particular, who are likely to experiment with amphetamines, sedatives, hypnotics, tranquilizers, and hallucinogens.
3. Persons with chronic illness and pain requiring continual medication for relief of symptoms.

4. Persons with previous history of drug ingestion.
5. Persons who have threatened or previously attempted suicide.
6. Persons with history of psychiatric illness leading to decreased self-esteem, depression, and possible self-destructive tendencies.
7. Confused, disoriented persons with limited understanding of health regimen and dosages of prescribed medicines.
8. Health workers who have easy access to drugs and who work under high stress conditions.
9. Persons with history of alcoholism.

Screening

1. Elicit thoughts about depression and suicide from general client interview and health history.
2. Complete neurological examination as part of regular physical exam, with attention to levels of consciousness, pupillary responses, eye movements.
3. Discuss with parents the precautions in the home to avoid poison ingestion, especially if the victim shows unusual stress or change in lifestyle.
4. Draw blood samples for toxicology studies or for blood levels of medication in question, particularly in persons who repeatedly request medication refills or those in chronic pain or in disoriented states.
5. Attention to case findings in families of chronic drug abusers or alcoholics to note formation of similar patterns in behavior before drug abuse becomes established. Research indicates increased risk of alcoholism among children of alcoholic parents over the general population.

ASSESSMENT

Health History

1. Ascertain victim's previous drug abuse and the type of drug. What drugs are available to this person?
2. Ascertain multiple doses and kinds of drugs for combination effects. For example, a person who has ingested large amounts of Dilantin, atropine, aspirin, Nembutal, thyroid extract, and Percodan will be apneic, comatose, hyperthermic, and hypertensive.
3. Ascertain initial symptoms that may provide clues as to type of drug and/or suggest additional pathologic processes (diseases). For example, a young woman was thought to have an aspirin overdose until friends reported that she had had a sudden onset of excruciating headache and immediately ingested a large amount of aspirin; the subsequent diagnosis was subarachnoid hemorrhage.
4. Ascertain from a review of systems particular symptoms that might relate directly to the ingested drug. For example,
   a. Delirium, hallucinations: alcohol, atropine, cocaine, amphetamines.
   b. Eyes:
      (1) Blurred vision: atropine, cocaine.
      (2) Double vision: alcohol, barbiturates.
   c. Ears:
      (1) Tinnitus: quinine, salicylates, quinidine.
      (2) Deafness/disturbances in equilibrium: gentamycin, quinine, streptomycin. (See listing in this chapter of commonly abused drugs for other symptomatic manifestations of overdosage.)

Physical Assessment

1. Initially, note respirations and blood pressure, and treat if these vital signs are falling.
2. Do a careful general and neurologic examination. Pay particular attention to the following:
   a. Levels of consciousness.
   b. Pupil responses.
   c. Eye movements and extraocular movements.
   d. Corneal reflexes.
   e. Optic fundi.
   f. Gag reflex.
   g. Response to pain.
   h. Deep tendon reflexes (DTR).
   i. Evidence of focal weakness.
   NOTE: Pressure neuropathies and myopathies are common in patients who have not moved for several hours.
3. Assess following systems:
   a. Skin: cyanosis, dryness, perspiration, jaundice, redness, rash, loss of hair, skin lesions, signs of trauma, ecchymoses (document for medico-legal implications in the future).
   b. HEENT:
      (1) Eyes: dilated or contracted pupils, pigmented scleras, pallor of optic disc (quinine, nicotine).

(2) Nose: perforated nasal septum.
(3) Mouth: gingival inflammation, salivation, breath odor.

c. Chest and lungs: respirations, wheezing, signs of pulmonary edema.
d. Musculoskeletal system: muscle twitching, weakness, or paralysis.

4. Be aware of diseases that masquerade as overdoses, such as subdural hematoma, meningitis, subarachnoid hemorrhage, and brain tumor; particularly look for head trauma.
5. Watch for associated additional pathology accompanying the client with drug intoxication:
   a. Aspiration pneumonia.
   b. Pulmonary edema.
   c. Cardiac arrhythmias.
   d. Hepatitis.
   e. Stabbing or gunshot wounds.
   f. Subacute bacterial endocarditis.
6. If client is a woman, is she pregnant?

Diagnostic Tests

Routine studies include:

1. Hematocrit.
2. White blood count.
3. Urinalysis.
4. Electrolyte levels.
5. Liver function tests.
6. Blood sugar.
7. Arterial blood gases.
8. Electrocardiogram.
9. Chest x-ray film.
10. Appropriate blood toxicology studies. Since the common screen includes only aspirin and barbiturates, others must be requested when overdose of a particular drug is suspected. Provide information to laboratory regarding drug categories or amounts, and so on.
11. Send specimen samples of urine and gastric contents for toxicology screen.
12. If special chemical examinations for depressants, tranquilizers, alkaloids and so on are required, the following laboratories are recommended. Usually prior arrangements with these facilities are needed in order to have them accept samples for analysis (Krupp and Chatton, 1978).
    a. County coroner's laboratory: blood alcohol, barbiturates.
    b. City, county, state police laboratories: barbiturates, blood alcohol.
    c. Federal Bureau of Investigation Laboratory, Washington, D.C. (only through local police).
    d. County hospital laboratory: barbiturates, blood alcohol.

NURSING DIAGNOSES: ACTUAL OR POTENTIAL

1. Respiratory dysfunction secondary to aspiration or depressed respirations.
2. Altered levels of consciousness secondary to depression of the vasomotor centers.
3. Alteration in cardiac output secondary to myocardial damage, arrhythmias.
4. Impairment of urinary elimination due to shock, dehydration, electrolyte imbalance.
5. Alteration in fluid volume secondary to fluid and blood loss.
6. Impairment of mobility secondary to muscular paralysis.
7. Alteration in emotional and social stability due to possible drug abuse and familial stress.

EXPECTED OUTCOMES

1. Adequate ventilation will be reestablished and patent airway will be maintained.
2. Client will be returned to consciousness; neurologic status will be closely monitored for change.
3. Cardiac output will be reestablished with appropriate management of cardiac arrhythmias and supportive measures to lessen impact of any myocardial damage.
4. Renal function will return gradually to preoverdose levels via dialysis or forced diuresis.
5. Fluid volume will be restored to pretrauma levels and electrolyte balances will be restored.
6. Emotional and social supports will be provided to both client and family within three days of the resolution of an acute episode, via direct intervention and appropriate referral.

INTERVENTIONS

1. Do not discharge patient if in doubt about consciousness or orientation status.
2. Intubate if shallow respirations, cyanosis, or absent gag reflex is noted, or if prognosis indicates respirations may deteriorate.
3. Obtain skull films for all patients presenting with one or more of the following signs (look for pineal shifts):
   a. Coma.

b. Lethargy.
c. Confusion.
d. Signs of head trauma.
e. Papilledema.
f. Focal neurologic findings.

4. Use syrup of ipecac or gastric lavage as follows:
   a. Ipecac is useful in purging drugs from stomach only if administered before they are absorbed. Use judiciously with adequate oral fluids to allow for "flushing" of stomach. Guard against aspiration of contents during vomiting. Never administer ipecac to victim who is known to have ingested a fast-acting depressant (e.g., Valium), as victim will become obtunded as he or she begins to vomit. *Do not* administer ipecac to a client who:
      (1) Is lethargic.
      (2) Has absent reflex.
      (3) Has ingested hydrocarbon-type compounds, corrosive poisons, or convulsants.
   b. Lavage should be performed on all obtunded and comatose drug-intoxication victims, even several hours after ingestion. Procedure of choice:
      (1) Insert into stomach large-bore, red rubber tube with multiple holes at gastric end.
      (2) Place head lower than waist.
      (3) Initially *intubate* if client is comatose or if gag reflex is absent.
      (4) Use copious amounts of normal saline, 100 to 200 mL at a time (intermittent flow and drainage).
      (5) Do not cool normal saline, in order to avoid lowering body temperature.
      (6) Continue lavage until return is clear, which may require 10 L or more (usually 2 to 5 L is sufficient).
      (7) Look at gastric contents for drug particles.
      (8) Send sample (20 to 50 mL) of gastric contents to toxicology laboratory for analysis.
5. General management for any drug intoxication should include:
   a. Frequent observation at 15- to 30-min intervals, to note changes in:
      (1) Levels of consciousness.
      (2) Vital signs.
      (3) Pupils.
      (4) Signs of focal neurologic deficit.
   b. Postural drainage of secretions, frequent tracheal suctioning (provision for meticulous airway care and patency).
   c. Intravenous (IV) line with 5 percent dextrose in water for medications and fluid resuscitation.
   d. Turning and repositioning of victim at frequent intervals (at least every 2 h) to reduce pressure areas and neuropathies.
   e. Protective eye care if unconscious (i.e., methylcellulose eye drops).
6. The question of *hypoxic brain damage* should not be a determining factor in emergency room treatment. Certain drugs may produce fixed pupils and cause neurologic depression bordering on death, and the victim may fully recover. If after several days have passed and drug levels have dropped to zero the neurologic deficits persist, then hypoxic brain damage may be a factor (Flint and Cain, 1975).
7. Assist with dialysis or forced diuresis.
   a. *Dialysis* is life-saving in ethylene glycol poisoning and when deep coma is prolonged (e.g., phenobarbital or Placidyl); it is also indicated for victims with severe renal, pulmonary, cardiac, or hepatic disease or if the victim is pregnant.
   b. *Diuresis* (forced) and alkalization of the urine is of little value generally and may be dangerous, especially in victim with renal or heart failure. *May be helpful in aspirin intoxications.*
8. *Withdrawal syndrome* may follow acute intoxication. This can be manifested by only slight agitation and brisk tendon reflexes, progressing to gross delirium and convulsions resembling alcohol withdrawal. Look for other causes of delirium, such as electrolyte imbalance and infection (elevated temperature). Withdrawal may be treated with intravenous fluids, restraints, and sedation.
9. If victim's vital signs worsen after initial 24 h, look for another cause of coma.
10. Obtain *psychiatric consultation* for all drug intoxication victims. Clients should be restrained until it is determined they are not an immediate danger to self or others (Flint and Cain, 1975).

11. Obtain neurology consultation on all people in stupor or coma.

EVALUATION

Outcome Criteria

1. Client's respiratory function is no longer compromised; a patent airway is being maintained.
2. Client has regained consciousness.
3. Cardiac output and adequate circulation are restored to pretrauma levels.
4. Client's renal function is reestablished and adequate urinary output is being attained.
5. Fluid and electrolyte balance is reestablished.
6. Client and family are following through on referrals and ongoing social support measures suggested by the professional.

Complications

1. See individual drug listing for complications related to specific product.
2. Withdrawal.

Assessment

There are generally separate phases for minor withdrawal and major withdrawal

1. Minor withdrawal usually begins at zero h after intoxication and lasts approximately 40 to 45 h. May peak in 20 to 25 h with the following symptoms:
   a. Tremor.
   b. Hallucinations.
   c. Seizures.
   d. Minimal disorientation.
   e. Rising blood pressure.
   f. Increased heart rate, increased respiration.
   g. Nystagmus, a fine movement in lateral gaze, elicited during examination of visual fields.
   h. Increased temperature.
2. Major withdrawal (delerium tremens) has onset approximately 30 h after being intoxicated, peaks between 70 and 90 h after "drinking binge," and may last to 130 h or 4½ days after intoxication with the following symptoms:
   a. Psychomotor activity.
   b. Tremors.
   c. Autonomic activity with profuse sweating.
   d. Hallucinations (e.g., victim cannot tell he or she is whole, suffers loss of reality, becomes psychotic).
   e. Grand mal seizures.
   f. Profound disorientation (see Chapter 39).

Revised Outcomes

1. Seizures will be treated appropriately and will cease.
2. Other goals as originally stated.

Intervention

1. May include careful and judicious use of Valium, Librium, and so on.
2. Watch respirations and support airway ventilation.

Reevaluation and Follow-up

Establish a plan of care that provides for ongoing treatment (through clinic; hospital; drug rehabilitation facility; halfway house; self-help group such as Alcoholics Anonymous, Narcotics Anonymous, or Al-Anon; and/or private psychotherapist) so that complications do not recur and appropriate support will be provided to client and family.

COMMONLY ABUSED DRUGS

The following is a list, by category, of drugs that are commonly abused. Key concepts of the most notorious drugs, selected laboratory data, and accepted management are provided as general guidelines for the nurse who delivers early and emergency care to the drug-intoxicated client.

Sedatives, Hypnotics, and Tranquilizers

LONG ACTING: PHENOBARBITAL; INTERMEDIATE ACTING: SECOBARBITAL, PENTOBARBITAL, TUINAL (SECOBARBITAL AND AMOBARBITAL)

Key Concept

Produce profound CNS depression of several days' duration. Onset is relative to drug; the intermediate acting have a more rapid onset and shorter duration of action. The longer acting may have a gradual progression of lethargy to coma.

Assessment

1. Deep tendon reflexes are usually depressed or absent but may be hyperactive.
2. Respiratory arrest.
3. Hypotension.
4. Hypothermia.
5. May lose brainstem reflexes (doll's eyes, corneals, cold calorics).
6. Victims may have an early period of "paradoxical agitation."

Interventions
1. Intubate.
2. Mechanical ventilation.
3. Intravenous saline for hypotensives if heart and kidneys can tolerate load.
4. Give vasopressors in severely depressed cases; dopamine or Levophed to help support blood pressure to 90 mmHg systolic.
5. Assist with dialysis if in prolonged coma and if barbiturate level is high.

PLACIDYL (ETHCHLORVYNOL), CHLORAL HYDRATE

Key Concept
Obtundation and sweet breath (like Juicy Fruit chewing gum).
Assessment
1. Chloral hydrate and alcohol ("Mickey Finn") may cause:
   a. Sudden loss of consciousness.
   b. Irritation of gastric mucosa.
   c. Liver damage.
   d. Renal cell damage.
2. Placidyl or overdose exhibits in addition:
   a. Associated respiratory depression.
   b. Hypotension.
   c. Hypothermia.
   d. Bradycardia and seizures (exacerbated by alcohol).

Interventions
1. Basically supportive.
2. Client may need dialysis.

QUAALUDE (METHAQUALONE)

Key Concept
A popular drug with college, university, and some high-school populations (so-called "heroin for lovers").
Assessment
1. Stupor, coma, and/or death in similar manner to barbiturates.
2. Pulmonary edema.
3. Cutaneous edema.
4. Hypotension.
5. Liver and renal damage.
6. Bleeding disorders.

Interventions
Basically supportive.

VALIUM (DIAZEPAM), LIBRIUM (CHLORDIAZEPOXIDE)

Key Concept
Valium may produce loss of consciousness in 10 to 30 min; Librium has a slower reaction and obtundation lasting several days.
Assessment
Initial symptoms:
1. Drowsiness.
2. Ataxia.
3. Slurred speech.
4. Nystagmus.
5. Respiratory depression. These drugs, combined with alcohol, can cause synergistic effect.

Interventions
1. Support respirations.
2. Assist with gastric lavage, if early (relative to each drug).
3. NOTE: *do not use ipecac with Valium.*

Opiates

HEROIN, METHADONE, CODEINE, MORPHINE

Assessment
1. Severe respiratory depression, cyanosis.
2. Pinpoint, nonreactive pupils.
3. Injection scars ("tracks"), thrombophlebitis, superficial abscesses.
4. Pulmonary edema (may be due to contaminants).
5. Atrial fibrillation.
6. Other associated complications (endocarditis, hepatitis, jaundice, hepatomegaly).
7. Look for other drug-mixing symptoms: strychnine, which may have been used to dilute the powder, can produce hyperthermia and convulsions.

Interventions
1. Intubate, and support respirations as necessary; use oxygen.
2. Administer appropriate dose of Nalline (nalorphine), that is, 5 mg IV to produce pupillary dilation and improved respirations.
3. May have to repeat Nalline in 20 to 30 min. Do not use unless you are quite sure this is an opiate overdose, as Nalline causes respiratory depression. Note: If patient does not respond to a total dose of 15 mg of Nalline, narcotic overdose is probably not the cause of the coma.
4. Narcan (naloxone) is a morphine antagonist at 0.4 mg IV but can also produce primary respiratory depression.
5. Pulmonary edema and atrial fibrillation usually resolve spontaneously (Flint and Cain, 1978).

DARVON (PROPOXYPHENE)

Member of opiate family; treat accordingly.

Assessment
1. Stupor progressing to coma plus respiratory depression.
2. Pupils pinpoint, unreactive.
3. Seizures.
4. Metabolic acidosis.

Interventions
1. Narcan (see above).
2. Nalline (see above).
3. Oxygen.
4. Intubate if necessary.
5. Sodium bicarbonate if necessary.

Stimulants

AMPHETAMINES: RITALIN (METHYLPHENIDATE)

Assessment
1. Produces agitated hyperactivity progressing to syndrome resembling heat stroke.
2. Tremulousness.
3. Flushing.
4. Tachycardia.
5. Mydriasis.
6. Hypertension
7. Hyperactive tendon reflexes.
8. Vivid, threatening, visual hallucinations.
9. Muscular twitching.
10. Dry mouth, nausea, vomiting, abdominal cramps.
11. Convulsions, hyperthermia, coma.
12. Coagulopathies. NOTE: Look for other drugs that may be complicating situation, for example, barbiturates and strychnine (amphetamine abusers use barbiturates to "level out the highs"). Watch known amphetamine abusers who present in depressed state, as they may have inadvertently overdosed on barbiturates. Monoamine oxidase (MAO) inhibitors may increase severity of amphetamine-induced hyperthermia and hypertension.

Interventions
1. Provide supportive care.
2. Provide cooling blanket for hyperthermia.
3. Sedatives may be used, cautiously; monitor level of consciousness.
4. When signs of severe central nervous system stimulation are present, chlorpromazine 0.5 mg/kg IM may be given. Dose may be repeated at 30 min intervals if indicated by continuation of excitatory symptoms (Johns, et. al., 1972).
5. Initiate ice baths and packs if fever is over 106°F.
6. Administer antihypertensives in hypertensive crises, if necessary.

Hallucinogens

LSD

Assessment
1. May present anticholinergic state:
   a. Agitation.
   b. Hot, flushed.
   c. Delirium.
   d. Hallucinations (lasting 12 to 18 h).
2. Cardiovascular shock and death when combination of LSD, phenothiazines, and some other hallucinogen has been taken.

Interventions
1. Support and observation.
2. *Very cautiously* provide sedation with diazepam or chlordiazepoxide (Valium or Librium) *only when absolutely* necessary.

PHENCYCLIDINE (ANGEL DUST)

Key Concept
A veterinary anesthetic; on the street, it can be ingested or injected.

Assessment
1. Victim is agitated or depressed.
2. Respiratory failure.
3. Pinpoint pupils that do not respond to Nalline or Narcan.
4. Effects last 2 to 4 days, with paradoxical excitement in various stages of withdrawal.
5. Overdose facilitated by alcohol.
6. If taken IV, may cause sudden death.

Interventions
Support and observation.

Anticholonergics (Atropinics)

COGENTIN, KEMADRIN, ARTANE, OVER-THE-COUNTER SLEEPING PILLS (E.G., SLEEP-EZE, COMPOZ, COPE)

Assessment
1. Delirious.
2. Flushed.
3. Hyperthermic.
4. Dilated pupils and poor accommodation.
5. Absent perspiration.
6. Seizures.
7. Urinary retention.
8. Paralytic ileus.
9. Tachycardia. Note: Psychotic patients on phenothiazines are often taking anticholinergics for their antiparkinsonian effects.

Interventions

1. Use cooling blanket, ice baths, ice packs, for hyperthermia (fever higher than 106°F).
2. Avoid sedatives unless absolutely necessary.
3. Insert Foley catheter.
4. Support with intravenous fluids as necessary.

Psychotherapeutic Drugs

THORAZINE (CHLORPROMAZINE), STELAZINE (TRIFLUOPERAZINE), MELLARIL (THIORIDAZINE), COMPAZINE (PROCHLORPERAZINE), HALDOL (HALOPERIDOL, A-BUTYROPHENONE), TRILAFON (PERPHENAZINE)

Assessment

1. Lethargy.
2. Hypotension (crthostatic).
3. Stupor and frank hypotension.
4. Pulmonary edema.
5. Cardiac arrhythmias (Mellaril).
6. Lowered seizure threshold (all phenothiazines).
7. Urinary retention.
8. Hyperthermia.
9. May produce idiosyncratic extrapyramidal symptoms of rigidity, dystonic movements, opisthotonus, oculogyric crises. NOTE: Clients taking these drugs usually have a baseline psychotic personality.

Interventions

1. Observation, supportive care.
2. Administer intravenous fluids for hypotension (usually normal saline, if heart and kidneys can tolerate it).
3. Victim must remain flat in bed until hypotension is resolved.
4. Assist with administration of intravenous lidocaine or Dilantin (diphenylhydantoin) for victims with Mellaril-induced cardiac arrhythmias.
5. Provide Benadryl, 50 mg IV, for extrapyramidal symptoms.

TRICYCLIC ANTIDEPRESSANTS ("MOOD ELEVATORS")

1. Elavil (amitriptyline).
2. Tofranil (imipramine).
3. Norpramin (desipramine).
4. Vivactyl (protriptyline).
5. Aventyl (nortriptyline).

Assessment

1. Cardiac arrhythmia and sudden death.
2. Victim arrives excited with progression to lethargy, obtundation with tachycardia, and hypotension.
3. ECG changes show marked conduction defects with alterations of terminal phase of the QRS-T complex.
4. Atrial and ventricular arrhythmias.
5. Variable degrees of atrioventricular block.
6. Seizures.
7. Hyperthermia.
8. Hypotension or hypertension.
9. Victim may have anticholinergic or extrapyramidal effects.

Interventions

1. Provide constant ECG monitoring.
2. ECG changes require Dilantin coverage: 250 mg diphenylhydantoin given *slowly* intravenously every 15 to 30 min to total of 1 g, then 300 mg orally per day for 1 week (Flint and Cain, 1975); intravenous Dilantin can cause hypotension.
3. Monitor blood pressure carefully.
4. *Do not use phenobarbital to counteract seizures,* as it exacerbates the effect of tricyclics.

TRIAVIL (PERPHENAZINE AND AMITRIPTYLENE)

Key Concept

A combination of a phenothiazine and a tricyclic (Elavil).

Assessment

1. Obtundation.
2. Hypotension.
3. Cardiac arrhythmias.
4. Seizures.
5. Hyperthermia.
6. Anticholinergic and extrapyramidal symptoms.

Intervention

1. Same as for the group of psychotherapeutic drugs discussed immediately above.
2. Dilantin therapy for arrhythmias may aggravate hypotension.

Aspirin

Key concept

1. Produces metabolic acidosis and respiratory alkalosis.
2. Blood levels of greater than 40 to 50 mg per 100 mL are considered serious. Blood level may not peak for several hours after ingestion.

Assessment

1. Tinnitus.
2. Headache.
3. Nausea.
4. Hyperventilation.

5. Increased perspiration.
6. Thirst.
7. Lethargy.
8. Agitation.
9. Delirium.
10. Convulsions.
11. Coma.
12. Hyperthermia.
13. Petechiae (usually not serious hemorrhage).
14. Vertigo.

Interventions

1. Intubate as necessary.
2. Assist with gastric lavage with normal saline.
3. Administer syrup of ipecac, if early.
4. Assist with forced diuresis, including acetazolimide, bicarbonate, sodium chloride, and potassium. Do not overcorrect the metabolic acidosis.
5. Frequently monitor arterial blood gases and aspirin levels.
6. Place patient on cooling blanket.

Alcohol

Ethanol or methanol (methyl alcohol is metabolized to formaldehyde and formic acid); ethylene glycol (antifreeze, metabolized from ethylene glycol to oxalic acid, which then combines with calcium to form an insoluble calcium oxalate which precipitates in kidneys).

Assessment

1. Ataxia.
2. Slurred speech.
3. Nystagmus.
4. Agitated state.
5. Stupor, respiratory depression (which is associated with cold clammy skin and hypothermia).
6. While awake, victim may have increased pain threshold.
7. Watch for associated head trauma, pneumonia, meningitis, liver failure.
8. Onset of blurred vision, headache, delirium, nausea, vomiting, and abdominal pain (methyl alcohol).
9. Optic disks hyperemic (methyl alcohol leads to irreversible retinal and optic nerve damage).
10. Elevated serum amylase with associated pancreatitis.
11. Coma with hyperventilation and profound metabolic acidosis.
12. Pulmonary edema, followed by renal failure (ethylene glycol).
13. Seizures and hypocalcemia (ethylene glycol).
14. Oxalate crystals on microscopic urinalysis (ethylene glycol).

Interventions

1. Supportive, with respiratory assistance as necessary.
2. Rapid intervention to correct acidosis with intravenous bicarbonate and intravenous ethyl alcohol to block metabolism of methanol by alcohol dehydrogenase (methanol abuse), that is, titrate a 10 percent solution of ethanol to maintain blood level at approximately 100 to 150 mg per 100 mL.
3. Treat ethylene glycol poisoning as methanol poisoning with the following addition: provide supplemental calcium as necessary.

FOOD POISONING

DESCRIPTION

Food poisoning is a general term denoting the syndrome of acute nausea, vomiting, diarrhea, and anorexia related to food intake. It is usually unaccompanied by fever, and, in most instances, affects groups of people.

Botulism occurs 18 to 36 hours after eating improperly processed canned foods. Time lapse can be longer in some instances. Prognosis is dependent upon the amount of toxin ingested in relation to body weight. Bacterial food poisoning occurs 2 to 6 h after ingestion of staphylococcic enterotoxins that form in food 2 to 12 h after streptococcic contamination. In poisoning from organisms, for example, *Salmonella*, symptoms come on 8 h or more after ingestion.

Chemical food poisoning results from ingestion of acid foods that were placed in containers lined with antimony, cadmium, lead, or zinc and from eating unwashed fruits or vegetables sprayed with preparations containing the metal salts listed above; also from food preservatives, sugar substitutes, and salt substitutes.

PREVENTION

Health Promotion

1. Support community education on appropriate safe home canning and preservation methods, careful food preparation and refrigeration techniques, prevention of food spoil-

age in large group picnics or gatherings, especially during warm weather.
2. Provide information to groups, businesses, professionals on sanitation and possible prevention of transmission of bacterial contaminants in food prepared for mass consumption.
3. Educate community groups in first-aid procedures for large outbreaks of nausea, vomiting, diarrhea to prevent possible complications of dehydration and shock, especially in infants and elderly persons.
4. Reinforce methods of formula preparation, proper food selection and preservation in the feeding of newborns and young infants.

Population at Risk

1. Large groups of people participating in church picnics, outings, potluck suppers, especially in warm weather, where questionable refrigeration and preservations methods are utilized.
2. Families relying heavily on preserved fruits, vegetables, meats, and fish without utilizing safe methods of food canning and smoking.
3. Young infants and newborns with formula as primary source of nourishment.
4. Any persons consuming foods that permit organisms to multiply and form toxin, such as potato salad, cream fillings in pastries.
5. Food preparers.
6. Travelers.

Screening

1. Cultures of suspected food.
2. Stool cultures.
3. Blood test for toxin in botulism, demonstrated by mouse inoculation.

ASSESSMENT

Health History

1. Note food intake over last 1–36 hours. Ask specifically about intake of:
   a. Canned, smoked or vacuum packed anaerobic foods, such as home-canned vegetables, smoked meats, vacuum packed fish (botulism).
   b. Meat cooked previously and allowed to cool slowly or tinned meats.
   c. Custards, cream fillings, foods such as potato salad that have mayonaise as a main ingredient (staphylococcal food poisoning).
2. Check for general health history, including allergies, current medications, chronic diseases.
3. Question on the duration and severity of GI and associated symptoms:
   a. Weakness, malaise, dizziness.
   b. Cramps.
   c. Muscle pain.
   d. Nausea, vomiting.
   e. Diarrhea.

Physical Assessment

1. Botulism:
   a. Gastrointestinal upset.
   b. Dimness of vision, double vision.
   c. Drooping eyelids.
   d. Decreased blood pressure.
   e. Afebrile.
   f. Difficulty in talking, swallowing.
   g. Shortness of breath.
   h. Paralysis of throat muscles (late).
   i. Coma and death from respiratory paralysis.
2. Bacterial food poisoning:
   a. Vertigo.
   b. Weakness.
   c. General malaise.
   d. Salivation.
   e. Nausea, vomiting.
   f. Gastric pain.
   g. Tenesmus.
   h. Diarrhea.
   i. Muscular cramps.
   j. Shock.
3. Chemical food poisoning:
   a. Nausea, vomiting.
   b. Diarrhea.

Diagnostic Tests

1. Culture of suspected food.
2. Stool cultures.
3. Tests on patient serum and in suspected food demonstrated by mouse inoculation for botulism.
4. Urinalysis.
5. CBC with differential.

NURSING DIAGNOSES: ACTUAL OR POTENTIAL

1. Respiratory dysfunction secondary to inadequate ventilation if lethargy or coma is present.
2. Alteration in fluid and electrolyte balance due

to nausea, anorexia, vomiting, diarrhea, possible dehydration, and shock.
3. Alterations in consciousness secondary to coma, convulsions, possible shock.
4. Alterations in comfort due to pain, discomfort, fear, and anxiety.
5. Knowledge deficit regarding food preparation and handling, as well as food preservation techniques.

EXPECTED OUTCOMES

1. Respiratory function will be maintained and adequate ventilation will result as emergency treatment and fluid replacement are provided for acute symptoms.
2. Fluid and electrolyte balance will be restored via appropriate fluid replacement for body losses resulting from severe vomiting and diarrhea.
3. Patient will be returned to consciousness once underlying cause of loss of consciousness is treated; for example, anti-convulsant therapy.
4. Patient will become more comfortable as acute GI symptoms lessen and fluid replacement is provided. Once episode has subsided, client and family are instructed in proper food preservation and preparation.

INTERVENTIONS

1. Assist with ventilating efforts as appropriate, such as nasal cannula with oxygen, cardiopulmonary resuscitation (CPR), mechanical ventilation.
2. See discussion of coma (Chapter 25) and shock (Chapter 48) for appropriate interventions.
3. Treatment of individual types of food poisoning as follows:
   a. Botulism:
      (1) Hospitalize at once for treatment with trivalent botulinum antitoxin.
      (2) Provide relief of symptoms and supportive care as indicated.
      (3) Note: emetics and lavage are of no value because 12 h (or even several days) elapse before symptoms arise.
      (4) Stimulants and oxygen therapy are usually indicated.
   b. Bacterial food poisoning:
      (1) Empty stomach at once by use of emetics and gastric lavage followed by activated charcoal.
      (2) Administer caster oil, 30 mL, or 0.2 g calomel (mercurous chloride) by mouth.
      (3) Control pain with morphine sulfate. Administer subcutaneously; intramuscular and intravenous administration is also effective.
      (4) Relieve tenesmus, diarrhea with 1 g bismuth subcarbonate or 7.5 g PO of kaolin. Paregoric (tincture of opium), 4 to 8 mL, may be given orally after each loose bowel movement.
      (5) Hospitalize if severe shock or dehydration is present.
   c. Chemical food poisoning:
      (1) Provide emetics, followed by gastric lavage (if profuse vomiting has not taken place).
      (2) Consider activated charcoal in water by mouth.
      (3) Provide as indicated:
         (a) Saline cathartics.
         (b) Atropine sulfate, 0.5 mg SC.
         (c) Bismuth subcarbonate PO.
      (4) Specific treatment as outlined under specific metals.
4. Teach victim and family appropriate food storing, preparation, foods likely to be contaminated (e.g., poultry, frankfurters, by *Salmonella*, etc.).

EVALUATION

Outcome criteria

1. Respiratory function is restored and ventilation is adequate.
2. Fluid and electrolyte balance is being maintained.
3. Client is conscious and increasingly responsive.
4. Client is experiencing less pain and discomfort.
5. Education is being provided to client and family about proper food preservation and preparation techniques.

Complications

1. Shock (see Chapter 48 for treatment).
2. Coma (see Chapter 25 for treatment).

Reevaluation and Follow-up

1. Public health nurse follow-up is indicated at client's home for reinforcement of teaching and assessment of patient recovery.

2. All cases of food poisoning should be reported to the local department of health.

CARBON MONOXIDE POISONING

DESCRIPTION

Carbon monoxide poisoning is caused by inhalation of the colorless, odorless gas, carbon monoxide, which results from incomplete combustion. Such inhalation may take place in the presence of improperly functioning or inadequately vented equipment, especially burning, heating, or illuminating gas appliances. A common source is automobile exhaust fumes; another is open circuit diving apparatus (Flint and Cain, 1975).

PREVENTION

Health Promotion

1. Avoid exposure to inadequately vented combustion devices.
2. Seek appropriate professional guidance and support for depression, low self-esteem, and anxiety—all possible precursors to a suicidal attempt utilizing CO poisoning from auto exhaust fumes.
3. Educate public about dangers of use of automobile power to run heaters, radios, and so on, in an unventilated area.

Population at Risk

1. Persons involved in occupations or who frequent areas that allow for persistent exposure to carbon monoxide fumes. For example, subclinical toxicity has been reported in dense traffic situations.
2. Persons with possible suicidal thoughts or those who have attempted suicide previously and are depressed and anxious.
3. Teenagers or others with old or malfunctioning cars that might leak carbon monoxide into the passenger section if windows are shut.

ASSESSMENT

Health History

1. Note history of exposure.
2. Note length of time exposed, immediate treatment given.
3. Obtain history of depression, suicide attempts.
4. Note previous medical history, allergies, use of medication.
5. Note complaints of headache, faintness, giddiness, tinnitis, loss of memory.

Physical Assessment

Common findings include:

1. Cherry red color to lips (may be absent or transient).
2. Peaceful expression.
3. Facial twitchings.
4. Elevated temperature.
5. Pale skin with blisters and bullous lesions.
6. Brownish-red stippling on arms or trunk.
7. Vertigo.
8. Paralysis.
9. Unconsciousness.

Diagnostic Tests

1. Arterial blood gas levels.
2. Carboxyhemoglobin.
3. CBC with differential.
4. Serum electrolyte levels.
5. ECG.

NURSING DIAGNOSES: ACTUAL OR POTENTIAL

1. Respiratory dysfunction associated with tissue anoxia and high level of circulating carboxyhemoglobin.
2. Alterations in level of consciousness secondary to coma and convulsions caused by inadequate ventilation and tissue anoxia.
3. Decreased cardiac output due to myocardial irritability.
4. Fluid volume deficit due to possible loss of blood or other fluids through injury, skin lesions, and vomiting.
5. Ineffective coping patterns secondary to emotional instability, possible past psychiatric history, previous suicide attempts.

EXPECTED OUTCOMES

1. Adequate ventilatory function will be restored as soon as possible after client comes under treatment.
2. Client will be returned to normal neurological status and full consciousness.
3. Cardiac output will be restored to pretrauma levels.

4. Fluid and electrolyte imbalance will be corrected gradually as client's ventilatory function improves and he or she regains consciousness.
5. Emotional support and appropriate referral to needed psychiatric services will be instituted once client's physical condition has stabilized.

INTERVENTIONS

1. Institute immediate mouth to mouth resuscitation after removing victim from exposure and determining that the airway is clear (Flint and Cain, 1975). Provide 95 to 100 percent oxygen under positive pressure using endotracheal catheter or face mask for at least one hour.
2. Insert IV line; use dextrose solution (50 percent), 100 mL, slowly, and prednisone IV for cerebral edema as needed.
3. Prevent chilling, excitement.
4. Hospitalize for observation, supportive treatment (including transfusions).
5. Consider induction of hypothermia in severe cases.
6. Do not administer cardiac stimulants unless there is no alternative.
7. Do not give morphine, atropine sulfate, or synthetic narcotics.
8. Do not let the client go home after recovery from the immediate postexposure phase. Certain myocardial and neurologic effects are delayed and may be life-threatening (Flint and Cain, 1975).

EVALUATION

Outcome Criteria

1. Client's respiratory function becomes more stable; patent airway is maintained.
2. Client regains consciousness.
3. Cardiac irritability has decreased and cardiac output has returned to pretrauma levels.
4. Client's fluid and electrolyte balance has been restored.
5. Client is following through on obtaining psychological support and guidance.

Complications

1. Residual neurological damage (see Intervention 4).
2. Possible repeat of suicide attempt (see Chapter 50).

Reevaluation and Follow-up

Assist with formulation of plan for patient and family to overcome long-term physical and emotional problems.

ENDOCRINE EMERGENCIES

KETOACIDOSIS, NONKETOTIC HYPEROSMOLAR COMA, AND HYPOGLYCEMIA

Chapters 17 and 28 contain complete discussions of diabetes mellitus as it affects children and adults, respectively. Emergency care for hyperglycemia and hypoglycemia are presented below.

DESCRIPTION

Hyperglycemic emergencies are of two types: diabetic ketoacidosis and hyperglycemic hyperosmolar nonketotic coma (HHNC). Ketoacidosis is almost exclusively a disorder of insulin-dependent diabetes, while HHNC primarily affects non-insulin-dependent diabetics.

Ketoacidosis arises when, in the absence of sufficient insulin for glucose metabolism, proteins and fats are broken down as alternative sources of energy. Ketones, by-products of fat metabolism, accumulate in the bloodstream and begin to be excreted by the lungs (detectable as a characteristic fruity odor of the breath) and kidneys (as ketonuria). In the urinary excretion of glucose and ketones, water and electrolytes are lost in large quantities. The resulting dehydration and acidosis account for the signs and symptoms (see Assessment, below) and, unless reversed by effective treatment, lead to coma and death. Ketoacidosis is usually caused by failure to take prescribed insulin, but physical or psychological upsets (e.g., influenza, surgery, emotional trauma) can produce ketoacidosis even when insulin intake is maintained. Signs and symptoms develop over a period of 24 to 48 h. Treatment consists of restoring acid-base balance and hydration, providing life support measures as necessary if the client is comatose, and correcting underlying problems that precipitated the episode.

HHNC is also a life-threatening hyperglycemic emergency. By mechanisms not well understood, hypoglycemia and glycosuria in elderly diabetics can produce diuresis, dehydration, stupor, and coma *without* ketones or significant acidosis. HHNC is triggered by various situations that induce hyperglycemia and uncompensated diuresis; commonly a systemic infection is the cause, but diuretics, corticosteroids, tube feedings, major illness such as stroke or myocardial infarction, and peritoneal dialysis can also produce this syndrome. Treatment consists of correcting the profound dehydration, correcting hyperglycemia, providing life support as required by coma, and treating the precipitating cause.

Hypoglycemia (hyperinsulinism, insulin shock) occurs when insulin is present in larger amounts than can be balanced by blood glucose. The insulin excess may result from dosage errors, excessive exercise, or failure to eat scheduled meals. Because the brain is highly sensitive to hypoglycemia, disturbances of thought, behavior, and consciousness develop within minutes or a few hours following insulin injection (speed of onset depends on type of insulin). Hypoglycemia is dangerous because it can produce lasting brain damage (as well as personal injury resulting from the client's confusion and misjudgment or coma). Treatment consists of correcting hypoglycemia by administration of glucose or glucagon.

The *Somogyi phenomenon* is serial fluctuation between hypoglycemia and hyperglycemia. An episode of hypoglycemia occurs first (often during the night, when intermediate or long-acting insulin peaks) and induces a counterresponse from the body (release of catecholamines, glucagon, and corticosteroids) that overcompensates and produces hyperglycemia. The hypoglycemic period may go unnoticed because the client is asleep. The hyperglycemic phase that follows is detected in the morning urine sample and may easily lead to the erroneous assumption that the insulin dose needs to be increased. Treatment consists of reregulating the insulin at a lower dosage.

PREVENTION

Health Promotion

1. Help diabetics learn how to maximize control of their diabetes and how to recognize and respond *early* to hyperglycemic and hypoglycemic episodes and the conditions that precipitate them. See *Diabetes Mellitus* in Chapters 17 and 28 for information about diet, insulin use, activity regulation, foot care, and other aspects of self-care for diabetic control. See Chapter 3 for guidelines about client teaching.
2. Encourage close health supervision for all clients with diabetes, especially pregnant women and insulin-dependent diabetics, to avoid hyperglycemia and hypoglycemia or recognize them before they become dangerous.
3. Prevent infections insofar as possible (by avoiding exposure to infected persons, avoiding catheterization, etc.); vigorously treat infections that do occur, taking special precautions to monitor glycosuria and prevent dehydration.
4. Drugs that alter fluid balance and electrolyte levels (e.g., corticosteroids, diuretics) must be taken only with close professional supervision and careful attention to urinary glucose and acetone.

Population at Risk

1. Persons with undiagnosed diabetes mellitus or those who have been diagnosed but are in poor control of their disease.
2. Diabetics who suffer trauma, acute illness, infection, or unusual stress of any kind.
3. Insulin-dependent diabetics whose insulin requirements are changing, e.g., young adolescents who are growing rapidly, pregnant women, and people whose activity is undergoing marked increase or decrease.

Screening

1. Urine for glucose and acetone. Note: Certain agents interfere with both Clinitest tablets and Clinistix test papers. Ascorbic acid, salicylates, methyldopa (Aldomet), and levodopa, if taken in large doses, cause positive Clinitest results. With the Clinistix methods (those using glucose oxidase and a chromogen system), negative results occur with these same medications (Krupp and Chatton, 1978).

ASSESSMENT

Health History

1. Obtain description of onset of symptomatology, that is, slow and gradual or abrupt and acute.

2. Obtain past medical history, including medications, allergies.
3. Obtain information regarding recent surgery, other stress events.
4. Note family history regarding endocrine disturbances.
5. Where did incident (symptoms) occur, and what were immediate treatments?
6. Note recent ingestion of food, drugs, alcohol, other substances.
7. Note if client is insulin-dependent or not and, if not, what oral hypoglycemic is used.
8. Note occurrence of specific symptoms, duration, time when first noted, and extent.
   a. Polyuria, polydipsia, polyphagia, recurrent blurred vision, fatigue, nocturnal enuresis in children (suggestive of hyperglycemia).
   b. Night sweats, nightmares, sleep walking, tremor, hunger, yawning, nausea, confusion (suggestive of hypoglycemia).

Physical Assessment

See Table 49-1.

1. Ketoacidosis.
   a. Dehydration: dry skin with "tenting" (poor turgor, inelasticity), dry mucous membranes, hypotension relative to the client's usual blood pressure, flat jugular veins when supine.
   b. Depressed level of consciousness: drowsiness, stupor progressing to coma.
   c. Deep and rapid respirations (Kussmaul's respirations), a physiological mechanism to "blow off" excess carbonate (acid).
   d. Fruity breath odor.
2. Hyperglycemic hyperosmolar nonketotic coma: same as *a* and *b* under ketoacidosis, above. Kussmaul's respirations and acetone breath are not present, since the client is not ketotic.
3. Hypoglycemia.
   a. Sweating.
   b. Pallor.
   c. Anxiety.
   d. Weakness.
   e. Tachycardia.
   f. Irritability, headache, mental confusion, feelings of vagueness.
   g. Possible respiratory arrest.
4. Somogyi effect.
   a. Signs and symptoms of hypoglycemia (see above), although these may not be detected because they may occur during sleep.
   b. Night sweats, nightmares, sleepwalking.

TABLE 49-1 DIABETES EMERGENCIES

	Insulin Insufficiency–Glucagon Excess		
	Ketoacidosis	Hyperosmolarity	Insulin Excess
Duration of diabetes	Variable	Recent onset	Uncontrolled, variable
Precipitating events	Infection, stress	Burns, steroids, stress, diuretics, particularly chlorothiazide	Recent insulin injection
Age	All ages	Fifth to seventh decades	All ages, particularly insulin-dependent clients
Dehydration	Variable	Severe	Not primary problem
pH	Low	Normal	Low: lactic acidosis and anaerobic metabolism
Acetone	Present	Absent	Absent at onset
Breathing	Kussmaul	Normal	Shallow, absent
Blood sugar	400–800 mg per 100 mL	900+ mg per 100 mL	20–50 mg per 100 mL
Mortality	<5–10%	>50%	——

c. Early morning headache (before breakfast).

Diagnostic Tests

1. Blood sugar: postprandial, serial, fasting, taken at various times and in response to various stimulations.
2. Urinalysis for sugar and acetone (negative glucose with positive ketones suggests Somogyi phenomenon).
3. Electrolyte levels (blood and urine).
4. Blood urea nitrogen (BUN).
5. Hematocrit.
6. ECG.
7. Serum osmolarity, osmolality.
8. Serum acetone.
9. Arterial blood gases.
10. Serum cholesterol and triglycerides.

NURSING DIAGNOSES: ACTUAL OR POTENTIAL

1. Altered levels of consciousness secondary to hyperglycemia and ketoacidemia, both due to insulin lack associated with hyperglucagonemia.
2. Respiratory dysfunction (inadequacy of ventilation) due to ketoacidemia and lactic acidosis evidenced by rapid, deep breathing.
3. Imbalance in electrolyte levels and fluid volume secondary to dehydration due to diuresis, nausea, anorexia, diarrhea, and vomiting.

EXPECTED OUTCOMES

1. Client will be returned to consciousness within 12–24 hours after initial treatment has begun. If client is experiencing stupor, lethargy, confusion, these symptoms will dissipate within 24 hours.
2. Respiratory function will be reinstated and adequate ventilation will be reestablished from time of initiation of treatment.
3. Fluid and electrolyte balance will be reestablished within 24 hours of admission for acute episode.

INTERVENTIONS

1. Ensure airway patency and adequate ventilation with oral airway and oxgenation or, in more severe respiratory depression, intubation and mechanical ventilation.
2. Fluid resuscitate immediately (use no. 16 to 18 intravenous needles) with normal saline for extracellular fluid deficit and 5 percent dextrose in water for cellular water deficit.
3. Cautiously administer potassium replacement in IV fliud when kidney function is established. Monitor for cardiac and vessel reactions.
4. Administer small intravenous doses of regular insulin (10-U increments), and monitor blood sugar level every hour until within 250 to 350 mg per 100 mL (for client with insulin insufficiency; watch for insulin sticking to IV tubing and glass bottle).
5. Administer intravenous glucose, 50 mL of 50 percent glucose, to maintain blood glucose over 100 mg per 100 mL or 300 g carbohydrate daily (for client with insulin excess).
6. Monitor acid-base imbalance by arterial blood gases every 30 min during rapid fluid resuscitation, and every 4 h until stable.
7. Monitor serum electrolyte levels every 4 h until fluid and electrolyte balances remain relatively stable (usually within 24 hr).
8. One sodium bicarbonate ampule in 1 L of water over 3 to 4 h may be administered and discontinued when serum bicarbonate level is 15 mEq/L.
9. Obtain urine specific gravity, sugar, and acetone testing every hour until client has stable acid-base status, then every 4 h until blood sugar is within 250 to 350 mg per 100 mL.
10. Monitor vital signs and neuromuscular checks every hour.
11. Auscultate breath sounds, and observe ventilatory patterns every hour until acid-base balance returns to compensated, normal range.
12. Immediately and frequently assess level of consciousness and mentation status.
13. Insert Foley bladder catheter and attach to straight drainage.
14. Monitor intake and output, with urine measured every hour.
15. Institute meticulous skin protection and care.
16. Reestablish insulin coverage according to individual needs.
17. If client is unconscious, insert nasogastric tube and attach to low intermittent suction.

EVALUATION

Outcome Criteria

1. Client is conscious with decreased lethargy, confusion, and fatigue.
2. Respirations are normal and ventilation is adequate.

3. Client is mobile and ambulatory within limitations imposed by trauma or vascular complications.
4. Client is experiencing little if any discomfort.
5. Fluid and electrolyte levels are restored to normal.
6. There are no further acute episodes of ketoacidosis or hypoglycemia that require hospitalization within 6 months of time of discharge.

Complications

1. Convulsions.
2. Injury sustained during coma or convulsion.
3. Permanent brain damage from hypoglycemia.

Reevaluation and Follow-up

After the crisis, assess client for understanding of diabetic control. With community health nurses, social workers, other professionals, establish a plan for client education regarding precipitating factors in crisis episodes, such as alcohol intake, other drugs, medications, insulin dosage and activity levels, and so on.

ACUTE ADRENAL INSUFFICIENCY (ADRENAL CRISIS)

DESCRIPTION

Acute adrenal insufficiency is caused by either an insufficient endogenous supply of adrenocortical hormones or a sudden marked deprivation of exogenous supplements of these same hormones. It generally occurs in the following patients:

1. Those who have been on large doses of glucocorticoids that have been discontinued.
2. Those experiencing stress, such as surgery, trauma, infection.
3. Those with injury to the adrenals from infection, anticoagulant therapy, hemorrhage, and trauma.
4. Those who have had a bilateral adrenalectomy or who have had a unilateral tumorous adrenal gland removed that was suppressing the other adrenal.

PREVENTION

Health Promotion

1. Educate patients taking glucocorticoids and anticoagulant therapy about prodromal symptoms of adrenal crisis, so early treatment can be instituted.
2. Establish plans of care that minimize physical and emotional stress for surgical and trauma patients, to avoid the possibility of adrenal crisis.

Population at Risk

See description above.

Screening

1. Serum electrolyte levels (decreased Na, increased K, hypochloremic acidosis).
2. Blood pressure (decreased BP).
3. BUN (increased).
4. Blood glucose levels (decreased).
5. CBC (eosinophilia and relative neutropenia).

ASSESSMENT

Health History

1. Note past medical history including medications and allergies.
2. Note recent high-stress events.
3. Note nonspecific symptoms such as:
   a. Headache.
   b. Lassitude.
   c. Personality changes.
4. Note GI symptoms such as:
   a. Abdominal pain.
   b. Nausea and vomiting.
   c. Diarrhea.
5. Note miscellaneous symptoms such as:
   a. Weight loss.
   b. Salt craving.
   c. Menstrual abnormalities.

Physical Assessment

1. Increased skin pigmentation with sparse axillary hair.
2. Hypotension.
3. Abdominal pain.
4. Apathy and confusion.
5. Extreme weakness.
6. Tachycardia.
7. Fever.

Diagnostic Tests

1. See screening tests above.
2. Serum cortisol and aldosterone levels (may be low or within normal range).
3. Serum ACTH (increase in primary adrenal insufficiency).
4. Urinary electrolyte levels (increased Na and decreased K).

5. Urinary 17–hydroxycorticosteroids.
6. Abnormal metyrapone test.

NURSING DIAGNOSES: ACTUAL OR POTENTIAL

1. Ineffective coping in stress situations, secondary to loss of adrenal reserve.
2. Circulatory insufficiency secondary to volume depletion.
3. Disturbances in electrolyte levels due to aldosterone insufficiency, dehydration caused by nausea, vomiting, weight loss, fever.
4. Altered levels of consciousness (lethargy, confusion, and possible coma) secondary to shock and electrolyte imbalance.
5. Alteration in comfort: discomfort due to abdominal pain, nausea and vomiting, CNS disturbances, fever.
6. Disturbances in cardiovascular function secondary to hypotension and tachycardia.

EXPECTED OUTCOMES

1. Response to stress situations will return to preillness levels as soon as treatment of acute crisis is completed.
2. Fluid volume will be restored to normal.
3. Electrolyte balance will be restored as treatment for adrenal crisis is carried out. This will be accomplished within the first 24 hours of therapy.
4. Patient will be returned to consciousness with lessened signs of lassitude and confusion within 24 hours.
5. Patient will be at precrisis level of comfort once emergency therapy is completed.

INTERVENTIONS

1. Immediately institute antishock measures (see Chapter 48). *Do not give narcotics or sedatives.*
2. Administer normal saline with 5 percent dextrose to maintain vascular volume.
3. Administer hydrocortisone as prescribed.
4. Identify and treat underlying cause(s).
5. Keep client supine until orthostatic blood pressure is stable at 90 to 110 mmHg systolic.

EVALUATION

Outcome Criteria

1. Adrenal gland functions are reestablished.
2. Normal fluid and electrolyte balance is maintained.
3. Patient is alert and responsive.
4. Patient is comfortable.

Complications

1. Hyperpyrexia (see *Fever* later in this chapter).
2. Loss of consciousness.
3. Generalized edema with hypertension (due to excessive use of IV fluids and corticosteroids).
4. Flaccid paralysis due to low K^+.
5. Psychotic reactions may occur with cortisone therapy.

Reevaluation and Follow-up

1. Be aware that certain clients may need periodic replacements of corticosteroids if adrenals are permanently damaged.
2. Establish guidelines for teaching clients about stress precipitators, such as infections, trauma, surgery. Initiate educational program as soon as client is alert and cooperative.
3. Refer to community health nurse for follow-up and reinforcement of preventive counseling.

THYROTOXICOSIS ("THYROID STORM")

DESCRIPTION

Thyrotoxicosis is an excessive outpouring of thyroid hormone and catecholamine release. It is usually precipitated in persons who have high levels of thyroxine and are subject to stress (Barry, 1978). Thyroid storms are indicated by:

1. Pulse greater than 120 per minute.
2. Temperature greater than 100°F.
3. Confused mental state.

PREVENTION

Health Promotion

1. Prepare client properly before thyroidectomy, so that stored hormone will not be released into the circulation by the manual manipulation of the gland. (This is now a rare occurrence because of careful preoperative preparation).
2. Be aware of possible occurrence in a client who has received therapeutic radio-iodine administration.

Population at Risk

1. Persons undergoing a subtotal thyroidectomy.
2. Persons receiving ^{131}I therapy.

3. Persons with thyrotoxicosis who are untreated and who are exposed to the stress of trauma, infection, or an independent illness.

Screening

1. T_3, T_4.
2. CBC (lymphocytosis).

ASSESSMENT

Health History

1. Obtain previous medical history, with medications and allergies included.
2. Note precipitating factors to present condition, such as stress induced by infection, trauma, illness.
3. Ask about ingestion of other over-the-counter medications, street drugs, alcohol.

Physical Assessment

1. Profuse sweating; sticky, hot, moist skin over inner aspect of arms; face flushed.
2. Hyperpyrexia (over 100°F or 38°C).
3. Tachycardia (> 120/minute).
4. Widening pulse pressure.
5. Enlarged thyroid gland.
6. Exophthalmos.
7. Restlessness and agitation.
8. Muscle jerking and uncontrolled "jitters."
9. Delirium, frank psychosis, coma.
10. Symptoms of dysfunctions of GI system: pernicious diarrhea, abdominal cramps.

Diagnostic Tests

1. Thyroid scan.
2. Serum electrolyte levels.
3. Thyroid levels (blood chemistries): T_3 or T_4.

NURSING DIAGNOSES: ACTUAL OR POTENTIAL

1. Impairment of cardiovascular system secondary to excessive release of thyroid hormone causing cardiac stress and potential vascular collapse.
2. Alteration in levels of consciousness secondary to agitation, delirium, frank psychosis, and coma.
3. Alterations in comfort secondary to agitation, restlessness, cardiac dysfunction evidenced by increased heart rate, possible arrthymias, and fever.
4. Endocrine system dysfunction due to excessive outpouring of thyroid hormone.
5. Impairment of mobility due to alterations in level of consciousness and musculoskeletal symptoms, such as tremors, jerking.
6. Nutritional deficit due to symptoms relating to GI tract disturbances, such as abdominal cramps, pernicious diarrhea.
7. Disruption in skin integrity secondary to profuse sweating.
8. Alteration in body temperature due to excessive metabolic activity produced by hormonal excess.
9. Changes in emotional stability secondary to fear of impending death, frank psychosis, confusion.

EXPECTED OUTCOMES

1. Cardiovascular impairment will be corrected immediately upon client's admission to emergency room.
2. Client will be returned to precrisis level of consciousness and mental status.
3. Client will become more comfortable as symptoms from acute episode gradually recede.
4. The endocrine system with adequate treatment and long-term follow-up will become stabilized.
5. The client will have full mobility restored.
6. Symptomatic problems with digestion, skin, and fever will recede as condition is successfully managed.
7. Client's emotional stability will improve with correction of overproduction of thyroid hormone and with ongoing professional support.

INTERVENTIONS

1. Correct underlying cause, such as sepsis, with appropriate antibiotics, and so on.
2. Administer O_2 via mask or nasal cannula.
3. Suppress hormone production with propylthiouracil, 80 to 120 mg daily in three divided doses or methimazole (Tapazole), 80 to 120 mg daily in three divided doses. Medications may be given orally or via nasogastric tube.
4. Block hormone release: 30 min after antithyroid drugs have been started, begin sodium iodide, 1 g in 1,000 mL 5 percent dextrose in water or normal saline over 8 to 12 h. May give Lugol's solution (30 drops in 1 L of 5 percent glucose in water) as an alternative if client is sensitive to other drugs or shows no improvement with other measures.
5. Block adrenergic response by administration of following: guanethidine, 100 to 150 mg IV or PO in a single dose to block catecholamine discharge (may cause orthostatic hypoten-

sion); or, propranolol (Inderal), 1 to 5 mg IV or 20 to 80 mg PO every 4 h (use cautiously, especially in patients with congestive heart failure, diabetes mellitus, or asthma).
6. Meet metabolic needs; provide carbohydrates, calories, and vitamin supplementation.
7. May use peritoneal dialysis for refractory cases.
8. Provide alcohol sponge baths to lower body temperature.
9. Digitalis preparations may be prescribed for intractable sinus tachycardia or congestive heart failure.

EVALUATION

Outcome Criteria

1. Cardiovascular function is stabilized.
2. Client is alert and oriented.
3. Client is experiencing no discomfort and is less affected by skin, GI, CNS symptoms.
4. The level of circulating thyroid hormone has decreased and is returning to normal.
5. The client is ambulatory.
6. Emotional stability has been restored to precrisis state.

Complications

See *Hyperthyroidism* in Chapter 28.

1. Exophthalmos.
2. Cardiac complications (tachycardia, CHF, atrial fibrillation). See discussion of treatment of these clinical entities in Chapter 30.
3. Posttreatment hypothyroidism (see Chapter 28).

Reevaluation and Follow-up

1. Client education about disease entity, effects of stress, avoidance or better management of stressful situations. Long-term management involves surgery or radioactive iodine.

CARDIOVASCULAR EMERGENCIES

DESCRIPTION

Cardiovascular emergencies include angina pectoris, myocardial infarction, congestive heart failure, and cardiogenic shock. Angina pectoris is characterized by impaired blood flow through coronary arteries due to atherosclerosis and/or arteriosclerosis. It may also occur as a result of severe aortic insufficiency or stenosis, with severe anemia, after thyroid therapy, and with hyperthyroidism.

It is precipitated by exertion, causing disparity between oxygen consumption and availability. Angina is most common in people with predisposing risk factors of familial history, high cholesterolemia and lipidemia, smoking history, hypertension, and associated diseases, such as diabetes mellitus.

Myocardial infarction is the interruption of the body supply to a localized portion of the heart muscle with necrosis resulting. The pain of infarction is similar to angina in radiation and location, but differs in the following ways.

1. It may begin during rest as well as during activity.
2. It is more severe.
3. It does not subside with rest.
4. Nitroglycerin has little effect.

Congestive heart failure is characterized by insufficiency of contractile power coupled with inadequate blood flow. Increasing left ventricular and diastolic pressure with resultant back pressures cause the systemic venous pressure to increase. Ultimately, there is venous pooling and occlusion with resultant systemic engorgement, edema, and hypertension.

Cardiogenic shock is ultimate contractile deficit with little or no perfusion of cardiac or systemic tissue.

PREVENTION

Health Promotion

1. Establish regular exercise program.
2. Maintain weight within normal limits for age, height, and sex.
3. Follow diet low in saturated fats and cholesterol.
4. Stop smoking.
5. Learn to deal constructively with stress-inducing events in daily life.
6. Continue regular health care for treatment and prevention of associated illness, such as diabetes mellitus, hypertension.

Population at Risk

1. Smokers.
2. Persons in high stress occupational and personal situations.

3. Obese people.
4. Persons with family history of heart disease, hypercholesterolemia.
5. Persons with high cholesterol and triglyceride levels on laboratory examination.
6. Persons performing limited or little daily exercise; those with sedentary work habits.
7. Persons with other chronic diseases, such as arterial hypertension, diabetes mellitus.
8. Entire population, but especially men age 50–60 and women age 60–70.

Screening

1. Cholesterol and triglyceride levels.
2. ECG exercise test to determine ischemic changes.

ASSESSMENT

Health History

1. Obtain description of precipitating events.
2. Note past medical history, medications, and allergies.
3. Obtain description of lifestyle, especially for myocardial infarction client.
4. Note any treatment instituted before client was brought to hospital.
5. Question about pain characteristics.
   a. Location?
   b. Radiation?
   c. Duration?
   d. Similar pain experienced before?
   e. Nature of pain?
   f. What preceeded pain?
   g. What helps pain: nitroglycerine, rest, breathing slowly, change of position?
6. Note associated symptoms (see Chapter 30). for full listing of presenting symptoms of myocardial infarction (MI), congestive heart failure (CHF), angina pectoris.
   a. Sweating.
   b. Shortness of breath, coughing, orthopnea, paroxysmal nocturnal dyspnea.
   c. Fatigue, weakness.
   d. Nocturia.
   e. Anorexia, right upper quadrant pain, nausea.
   f. Dependent edema.

Physical Assessment

1. Vital signs. Look for:
   a. Hypertension or hypotension.
   b. Arrhythmias.
   c. Narrowing pulse pressure.
   d. Tachycardia or bradycardia.
   e. Weak pulse.
   f. Dyspnea, increased respiratory rate.
2. Pallor.
3. Pain: precordial, chest, jaw, left arm, neck (left side).
4. Venous engorgement: distended neck veins.
5. Fatigue, lassitude, weakness.
6. Diaphoresis.
7. Chest and lungs: basilar rales.
8. Heart: gallop rhythm, S_3 or S_4, arrhythmias, increased or decreased rate, lower sternal heave independent of apical impulse (right-sided failure), faint S_1 and S_2 (acute MI).
9. Abdomen: enlarged, tender liver.

Diagnostic Tests

1. Twelve-lead ECG and dynamic monitoring.
2. Serum electrolyte levels.
3. Arterial blood gas levels.
4. Chest x-ray film.
5. Cardiac enzymes (CPK-MB, SGOT, LDH).
6. CBC with hemoglobin, hematocrit, differential.
7. Digitalis level.
8. Blood glucose, cholesterol, triglyceride levels.
9. Sedimentation rate.
10. Urinalysis.
11. BUN.

NURSING DIAGNOSES: ACTUAL OR POTENTIAL

1. Alteration in comfort secondary to pain, anxiety, respiratory difficulties, immobilization.
2. Compromised cardiovascular function with inadequate tissue perfusion due to cardiac damage, ischemia, failure evidenced by shortness of breath, rales, arrhythmias, sinus tachycardia/bradycardia, and so on.
3. Alterations in fluid and electrolyte balance secondary to anorexia, nausea, vomiting, lack of fluid intake, or retention of fluids due to cardiac failure or inadequate renal function.
4. Impairment of respiratory function secondary to left-sided failure, leading to increased pulmonary vasculature congestion and accompanying symptom of shortness of breath.
5. Alterations in mobility due to weakness, fatigue, pain, anxiety.
6. Impairment in coping ability secondary to ex-

treme fear, anxiety, possible depression, anger, and denial.

EXPECTED OUTCOMES

1. Client will become more comfortable within first hours of treatment as pain is relieved and respiratory and cardiovascular symptoms are treated.
2. Cardiovascular function will become stabilized within first 24 h after treatment is initiated, so that tissue perfusion will be improved.
3. Fluid and electrolyte levels will be compensated during ongoing treatment, so that adequate balance will be maintained.
4. Adequate ventilation will be reestablished immediately on admission and symptoms of respiratory dysfunction will diminish gradually.
5. Client will regain mobility once the acute cardiovascular crisis has been resolved and he or she has remained stable without complications. Such increases in mobility will depend on the individual client, the extent of myocardial damage, and continuous observation for possible complications.
6. Client will show increased emotional stability and concomitant ability to cope as his or her physical condition improves. Signs of overt hostility, denial, and anxiety will decrease.

INTERVENTIONS

ANGINA PECTORIS

1. Administer glyceryltrinitrate (nitroglycerin, NTG), 0.3 to 0.6 mg, repeated every 5 min (sublingual lozenges). If three doses do not cause marked relief of symptoms, suspect myocardial infarction.
2. Place client at rest, seated or supine as tolerated.
3. Start intravenous (no. 16 to 18 needle) infusion of 5 percent dextrose in water for medications (keep-open rate).
4. Obtain 12-lead ECG and look for ischemic changes.
5. Monitor vital signs every 15 min until stable.

MYOCARDIAL INFARCTION AND CARDIAC ARREST

1. Establish adequate airway and ventilation.
2. Administer external cardiac compression if victim is pulseless (see Tables 49-2 and 49-3 and Figures 49-1 and 49-2). Myocardial infarction and sudden cardiac arrest victims have lowest morbidity and mortality when CPR begins within 4 min after incident. Brain damage is relative to length of anoxic-anaerobic period.
3. Provide oxygen by intubation and positive pressure bag, or mechanical ventilation.
4. Place electrodes for monitoring and assess cardiac rhythms.
5. Defibrillate if ventricular fibrillation or ventricular tachycardia is present and client is unconscious.
6. Start intravenous (no. 16 to 18 needle) infusion of 5 percent dextrose in water for medications.
7. Provide lidocaine, 50–100 mg IV followed by IV infusion at a rate of 1 to 2 mg/min for ventricular ectopy. Assist with administration of Bretylium for life-threatening ventricular arrhythmias unresponsive to adequate dosages of a first line anti-arrhythmic agent, such as lidocaine.
8. Provide bed rest, keep client supine.
9. Administer morphine sulfate, 5 to 15 mg IV in 2- to 5-mg aliquots; meperidine hydrochloride (Demerol), 50 to 100 mg in 25-mg aliquots; hydromorphone (Dilaudid), 10 mg in 2 to 4 doses. Watch for respirations $<12/$minute, hypotension. $P_{CO_2} > 45$ mmHg.
10. Monitor vital signs and mentation every 30 to 60 min until stable.
11. Carefully record intake and output.
12. Obtain serial ECG and enzymes every 3 days.
13. Place on continuous cardiac monitoring.
14. Attempt to allay apprehension and anxiety.

CONGESTIVE HEART FAILURE

1. Provide furosemide (Lasix) 40–50 mg IV and watch for diuresis responses.
2. Keep head of bed at 90 degrees or in position of comfort with client's legs dangling.
3. Apply tourniquets serially to proximal portions of three of the four extremities with periods of release of one tourniquet at a time for 15 min. Obstruct venous return and not arterial flow. Generally inflate to 60 to 80 mmHg, and use blood pressure cuffs for equal pressure distribution. May phlebotomize 200 to 500 mL, especially if patient has polycythemia vera.
4. Administer digitalis (if client has not been on digitalis) with 1.5 mg Digoxin and start with intravenous dose, 0.25 to 0.5 mg, 4 to 8 h intervals.
5. Use Swan-Ganz pressure monitoring.

TABLE 49-2 BASIC LIFE SUPPORT PROCEDURES INCLUDING UNWITNESSED CARDIAC ARREST (ONE OR TWO RESCUERS)

Preparation Time	What to Do First	General Procedure	Remarks
4–10 s	Make sure victim is unconscious and not breathing	Turn victim face up; shout at victim to see if he or she responds	Make sure victim is not suffering from some disease that does not require resuscitation (simple fainting, diabetic coma, etc.)
7–15 s	Establish patent airway	Place one hand under neck, other hand on forehead to tilt head back and extend neck	In this way, neck can be extended, nostrils closed, and jaw jutted forward for mouth-to-mouth inflation
10–20 s	Give four quick inflations	Make sure nostrils are pinched off, neck is extended, mouth seal is tight	Volume of each inflation should be about 800 mL, enough to give quick supply of oxygen; check chest for expansion
15–20 s	Check for presence or absence of carotid pulse on each side	This is most easily found in the groove just to one side of the larynx	Time is of the essence, and sometimes pulse may be weak and difficult to find
75–90 s	Start cardiac pulmonary resuscitation in the ratio of 15 compressions to two inflations	Make sure you and the victim are properly positioned and in trying to do two things at once there is no air leakage	During compression it is particularly important that both hands and arms be correctly positioned. When there is a single rescuer, give 80 compressions per minute with two very fast lung inflations after each 15 chest compressions. When there are two rescuers, give 60 chest compressions per minute; after rescuer no. 1 delivers five compressions, rescuer no. 2 performs one respiration.[a]
80–100 s	Determine if breathing and pulse have returned	Continue efforts until a satisfactory CPR function is established	The pupil size (beginning contraction) will give a good hint of returning function

SOURCE: This material is reproduced in condensed form from *Instructors' Manual of Basic Cardiac Life Support*, by permission of the American Heart Association.

[a] Functions may be switched as fatigue requires; it is important not to get in each other's way or interfere with either rhythm. When a second rescuer arrives on the scene, the change in rhythm to 60 compressions per minute is accomplished as follows: Rescuer No. 1 says: "one-one thousand, two-one thousand, three-one thousand, four-one thousand, five-one thousand," and so on until the second person is ready. Then Rescuer No. 1 says "We switch on next breath." The inflator takes over at the count of three-one thousand and the new compressor begins and picks up the count without pause. Rescuer No. 1 then quickly checks for pulse and pupils.

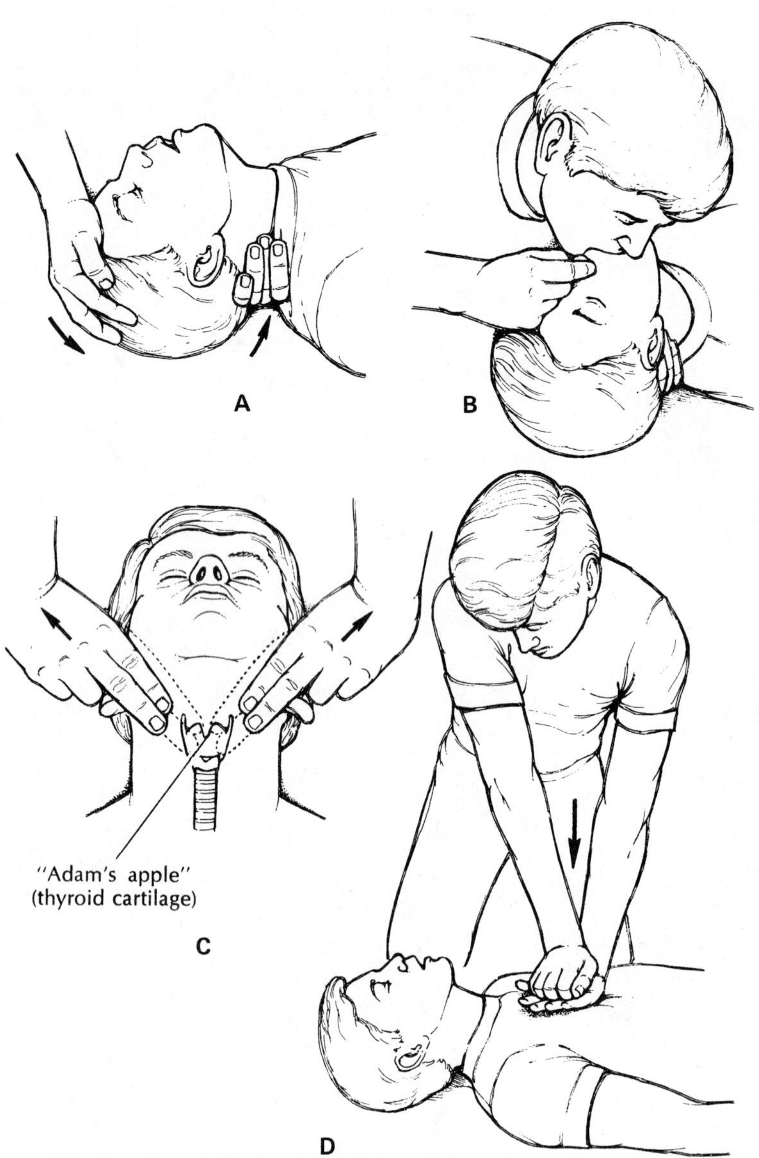

Figure 49-1 Major steps in cardiopulmonary resuscitation. (*a*) Make certain the victim has an open airway. (*b*) Start respiratory resuscitation immediately. (*c*) Feel for the carotid pulse in the groove alongside the Adam's apple or thyroid cartilage. (*d*) If pulse is absent, begin cardiac massage. Two rescuers use 60 compressions a minute with one lung inflation after each group of five chest compressions; a single rescuer uses 80 compressions a minute with two inflations after every five compressions. Note: Do not palpate both carotid pulses simultaneously, as this maneuver can decrease cerebral blood flow. (From Henderson, J.: *Emergency Medical Guide*, 4th ed., McGraw-Hill, New York, 1978.)

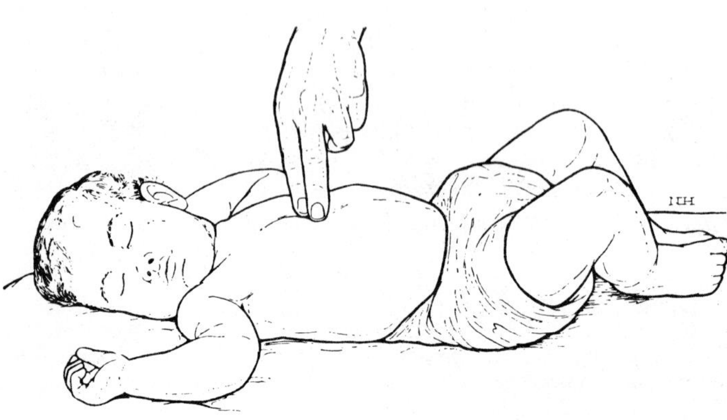

Figure 49-2 For external cardiac massage in children, gentle pressure is exerted midsternum (between the nipples) with tips of fingers rather than with the heel of hand. (From Henderson, J.: *Emergency Medical Guide*, 4th ed., McGraw-Hill, New York, 1978.)

TABLE 49-3 INFANT RESUSCITATION

Preparation Time	What to Do First	General Procedure	Remarks
3–5 s	Make sure infant is unconscious	Place infant in horizontal position	Make sure that cardiac arrest has taken place
6–10 s	Establish patent airway	Do not overextend the neck	Simply tilt head gently backward
9–15 s	Give four gentle puffs into mouth	In infants do not breathe as forcefully as in adults	Horizontal position facilitates cardiac massage, if necessary
14–25 s	Determine lack of pulse	Use carotid or precordial pulse	Overextension of head may block airway (collapsed trachea) rather than help it
44–55 s	If cardiac arrest is present, begin cycles of five compressions to one inflation	Use two fingers for compression gently, as sternum is very flexible; pressure is exerted about midsternum, as in infants the heart lies higher than in adults; danger to liver is also greater for the same reason	In infants, rate should be 80–100 compressions per minute with rapid inflation after five compressions (this equals about five compressions every 3 s with one inflation every 3 s, i.e., 5:1 ratio.)

SOURCE: This material is reproduced in condensed form from the *Instructors' Manual of Basic Cardiac Life Support*, by permission of the American Heart Association.

6. Listen to heart sounds for appearance of gallop rhythm, friction rub murmurs.

CARDIOGENIC SHOCK

1. Use vasodilator drugs such as sodium nitroprusside or phentolamine given by IV drip. (Note: these drugs tend to lower blood pressure, so systolic blood pressure should be more than 100 mmHg when drug is initiated). These drugs assist with decreasing the impedance to left ventricular ejection, decreasing the myocardial O_2 consumption, and improving tissue perfusion.
2. Use vasopressor agents to maintain blood pressure; dopamine (drug of choice) according to prescribe doses and based on blood pressure, urine output responses. Use intravenous pumps or drip-monitoring regulators.
3. Administer inotropic agents such as digitalis (according to medication levels described immediately above in section on *Congestive Heart Failure*).
4. Maintain meticulous intake and output records.
5. Watch peripheral circulation and tissue oxygenation: arterial blood gases.
6. Protect skin and pressure areas with sheep skin and frequent turning.
7. Assist with treatment with aortic balloon counter-pulsation if indicated to raise arterial pressure.

8. Monitor arterial pressures and pulmonary artery and capillary wedge pressures.
9. Auscultate heart sounds for gallops and murmurs.

EVALUATION

Outcome Criteria

1. Client is more comfortable, less anxious, experiencing less pain.
2. Cardiovascular function is stabilized as client is transferred to the coronary care unit for close observation and follow-up.
3. Fluid and electrolyte balance continues to improve.
4. Adequate ventilation is established.
5. Client is gradually becoming more mobile and is following a progressive ambulation regimen.
6. Client is able to cope better with realization of illness, is able to communicate anxiety and is receiving ongoing support.

Complications

See Chapter 30.

ANGINA PECTORIS

1. Myocardial infarction.
2. Congestive heart failure.
3. Arrhythmias and conduction defects.

ACUTE MYOCARDIAL INFARCTION

1. Cardiac failure and cardiogenic shock (see Tables 49-2, 49-3 and Figures 49-1, 49-2 for procedures for cardiopulmonary resuscitation).
2. Arrhythmias.
3. Thromboembolic complications.
4. Stokes-Adams attack with heart block.

CONGESTIVE HEART FAILURE

1. Pulmonary edema.
2. Pulmonary embolism secondary to venous thrombosis in lower extremities.

Reevaluation and Follow-up

1. Prepare client for transfer to cardiac unit.
2. Be aware that clients with 40 percent or more myocardial damage are certain candidates for cardiogenic shock and have an exceedingly poor prognosis.
3. Refer appropriately to chaplain, social service department, coronary care nurse-clinician for emotional support and rehabilitative interventions for client and family.

ABDOMINAL EMERGENCIES

DESCRIPTION

Abdominal emergency is a general term indicating diverse conditions that necessitate immediate care. Such conditions may be traumatic (see Chapter 48). Examples of acute abdominal conditions include infection, torsion, or obstruction of gut; hemorrhage; peritonitis; space-occupying masses; and vascular problems. Life-threatening situations arising from other body systems can first present as pain in the abdomen, for example, myocardial infarction, dissecting aortic aneurysm, and ruptured ectopic pregnancy.

1. Inflammation: appendicitis, cholecystitis, diverticulitis, pancreatitis, ulcerative colitis, viral gastroenteritis.
2. Perforation: duodenal and gastric ulcers, cancer of the colon, ovarian cyst, ectopic tubal pregnancies, appendicitis.
3. Trauma (see Chapter 48).
4. Vascular problems: abdominal aortic aneurysms, mesenteric vascular occlusions, volvulus of the intestine (loss of circulation to part of the bowel, with necrosis).
5. Obstruction: causative agents such as tumor, a torsion (volvulus), adhesions, hernias, foreign bodies.
6. Bleeding: ulcers of upper gastrointestinal tract, tumors of stomach, colon; inflammatory disease, such as ulcerative colitis.

PREVENTION

Health Promotion

1. Obtain regular physical care for complaints involving GI tract to avoid emergency complications. For instance, vigorous, early treatment of ulcers may make perforation unlikely.
2. Encourage diets high in fiber, low in refined sugar (to reduce the incidence of diverticulitis, cancer of the colon). Encourage weight control.
3. Offer alternative methods of dealing with high-stress situations (to reduce the incidence of psychologic gastrointestinal disorders.

4. Avoid exposure to people with symptoms of acute viral gastroenteritis.
5. Encourage treatment for clients with history of alcoholism to prevent complications such as esophageal varices and other causes of massive upper GI hemorrhage, acute or chronic pancreatitis, cirrhosis.
6. Reinforce early case-finding for colonic cancer, by annual rectal exams, stool for guaiac test.

Population at Risk

1. Persons indulging in dietary or alcoholic excesses.
2. Persons not eating high residue diet.
3. Persons involved in high-stress situations with inadequate or poorly developed coping abilities.
4. Persons with history of gastrointestinal disease, cardiovascular disease, or gynecologic problems, such as repeated ectopic pregnancies.
5. Persons with history of emotional or psychiatric problems.
6. Persons with genetic background indicative of sickle cell disease.

Screening

1. CBC with hemoglobin, hematocrit levels, differential (check for anemia, leukocytosis, neutrophils, eosinophils).
2. Stool guaiac tests (three tests one week apart).
3. Sickle cell preparation.

ASSESSMENT

Health History

1. Age of client.
2. Ascertain sexual and menstrual history.
3. Question about pain.
   a. Location and radiation.
   b. Character: constant, localized, dull ache, colicky with or without pain-free episodes, cramping, migrating.
   c. Onset and course.
   d. Related to:
      (1) Meals.
      (2) Defecation.
      (3) Stress.
      (4) Time of day or season.
      (5) Activity and position.
   e. Severity.
4. Note any associated symptoms:
   a. Bleeding.
   b. Change in bowel or digestive habits.
   c. Anorexia, nausea, vomiting, diarrhea.
   d. Weight loss.
   e. Jaundice.
   f. Flatulence, eructation, bloating, heartburn.
   g. Fever, chills.
   h. Cardiovascular, gynecological, genitourinary, or respiratory symptoms.
5. Ask about:
   a. Past operations, illnesses, medications (especially aspirin, alcohol, or steroids).
   b. History of allergies.
   c. Bleeding tendencies.
   d. Recent exposure to hepatitis or different geographic areas.
   e. Recent trauma.
   f. Family history (important with gallbladder disease, ulcer, pancreatic problems, cancer).

Physical Assessment

1. Check vital signs: note fever, signs of shock.
2. Evaluate general appearance, color of skin, posture.
3. Note anxiety, nervousness, depression.
4. Examine the abdomen. Note the following:
   a. Pain, tenderness. "The general rule can be laid down that the majority of severe abdominal pains which ensue in clients who have been previously fairly well, and which last as long as six hours, are caused by conditions of surgical import" (Cope, 1968).
      (1) Location and character of pain.
      (2) Referred pain, such as fractured lumbar vertebra causing abdominal pain.
      (3) Tenderness on coughing.
      (4) Rebound tenderness (a test for peritoneal irritation) (Barry, 1978).
      (5) Rectal, pelvic examination (usually done last).
      (6) Check for pain over flank and costovertebral angles over kidney.
   b. Distension and peristalsis.
      (1) Increased bowel sounds (gastroenteritis).
      (2) High-pitched bowel sounds with quiet intervals (intestinal obstruction).

(3) Decreased bowel sounds (generally peritonitis).

c. Rigidity, spasm of abdominal wall, such as an voluntary spasm in early appendicitis, involuntary spasm of advanced disease of the abdomen.

d. Vomiting.

(1) Type: is it projectile?

(2) What is vomited?

(3) Amount and frequency.

5. Be aware of need to examine genitourinary system, cardiovascular system, chest and lungs for possible etiological findings:
   a. Pain radiating to pelvis caused by infection of seminal vesicle.
   b. Hepatomegaly from right-sided failure causing abdominal pain due to stretching of liver capsule.

Diagnostic Tests

1. CBC with differential, hemoglobin and hematocrit levels.
2. Urinalysis.
3. X-ray film of patient in erect and supine positions.
4. BUN.
5. Possible paracentesis.
6. Possible gastrointestinal series, if indicated; gallbladder series.
7. Serum amylase.
8. Typing and cross match.
9. Sickle cell prep if indicated by family history.
10. Vaginal or urethral discharge: Gram stain, wet prep, culture.
11. Liver function tests (bilirubin, SGOT, SGPT, alkaline, phosphatase).
12. Erythrocyte sedimentation rate.
13. ECG. May demonstrate cardiovascular site of pain.

NURSING DIAGNOSES: ACTUAL OR POTENTIAL

1. Pain, fear, and anxiety secondary to gastrointestinal complaints, fever.
2. Alteration in cardiac output and tissue perfusion due to loss of blood and other body fluids.
3. Alterations in fluid and electrolyte balance associated with vomiting, anorexia, diarrhea, blood loss.
4. Impairment of mobility due to discomfort and anxiety.
5. Fear and anxiety secondary to pain, blood loss, sudden onset of discomfort, lack of knowledge.

EXPECTED OUTCOMES

1. Client will be made as comfortable as possible pending results of diagnostic tests in preparation for admission and possible surgical intervention.
2. Cardiac output and tissue perfusion will be maintained at adequate levels and restored to normal functioning as the acute abdominal crisis is resolved.
3. Fluid and electrolyte balance will be gradually reinstated following appropriate therapy or surgical intervention.
4. Once acute situation subsides or surgery is over, client mobility will improve and return to pretrauma level of functioning.
5. Client's and family's fear and anxiety will be diminished through ongoing professional support during hospitalization.

INTERVENTIONS

1. For shock, see Chapter 48.
2. Insert large-gauge intravenous needle. For dehydrated patients with history of vomiting, fluid resuscitate with a balanced salt solution.
3. Assess extent (if any) of hemorrhage, have blood typed and crossmatched in preparation for transfusion (a client with hypotension, rapid pulse, and history of GI bleeding should have a minimum of 3 U of blood cross matched (Eckert, 1976).
4. Insert nasogastric tube.
5. Insert indwelling Foley catheter to straight drainage. Maintain accurate input and output record. Observe urine for blood, cloudiness, and so on.
6. Prepare client for surgical intervention, if indicated.
7. Provide ongoing support to client and family.

EVALUATION

Outcome Criteria

1. Client is becoming more comfortable and experiencing less pain as he or she is prepared for admission or for surgical intervention.
2. Cardiovascular function is compensated and adequate to allow for full tissue perfusion.

3. Fluid and electrolyte balance is returning to within normal limits.
4. Client is gradually becoming more mobile.
5. Client's fear and anxiety are lessened and he or she is becoming more communicative.

Complications

Complications might result from the use of surgical intervention, such as wound infection, sepsis, paralytic ileus, etc.

Reevaluation and Follow-up

Place certain clients under observation for at least 24 hours if diagnosis remains unclear. During this time, patient should be hydrated with intravenous fluids, given nothing by mouth and observed frequently (Eckert, 1976).

FEVER

DESCRIPTION

Fever is an elevation of body temperature from the usual so-called normal of 98.6°F. However, normal body temperatures range, rectally, from 97.2 to 100.4°F and orally from 96.5 to 99.2°F (see Table 49–4). Activity, emotion, ambient temperature, dress, can all cause variations within these normal ranges. The causes of fever are many, but the usual cause is infection. Fevers may be classified according to patterns (see Figure 49–3).

The hypothalamus is the thermoregulatory center for the body. In disease, fever-producing (pyrogenic) substances of either exogenous (e.g., microbes) or endogenous origin act upon this center. In addition, the hypothalamus is triggered by blood warmed by the fever to stimulate peripheral dilatation and sweating in order to dissipate heat (Krupp and Chatton, 1978).

TABLE 49-4 NORMAL RANGE OF BODY TEMPERATURE

	Oral	Rectal	Axillary
Farenheit °F	96.5–99.2	97.2–100.4	96.5–98.5
Celsius °C	35.8–37.3	36.2–38	35.8–37

PREVENTION

Health Promotion

1. Avoid exposure to people with infections of viral, rickettsial, bacterial, and fungal origins.
2. Be aware of familial tendency to acquire certain fever-producing diseases, such as rheumatoid arthritis, systemic lupus erythematosus (SLE).
3. Avoid exposure to environmental heat loads that exceed normal heat loss mechanisms, for example, overuse of sauna.
4. In all acutely ill clients, maintain adequate fluid balance and close monitoring of intake and output to prevent fever-inducing conditions of dehydration, acidosis.

Population at Risk

1. People exposed to infections in daily activities: children in day-care settings or school, teachers, professional health workers.
2. Persons working or living in densely populated settings with little or no ventilation, where associates experience repeated viral or bacterial infections.
3. Persons with family history of certain fever producing clinical entities, such as SLE, rheumatoid arthritis.
4. Persons traveling in unfamiliar areas where they may be exposed to different local, systemic infections, unusual foods, or inadequate hygiene.
5. Allergic persons with history of drug reactions or anaphylaxis.

Screening

1. Rectal or oral temperature over 24-h period (see Table 49–4).
2. CBC with differential.
3. Urinalysis.

ASSESSMENT

Health History

1. Obtain history of exposure to infection (travel, drugs).
2. Note past medical history.
3. Ask about allergies and any medications.
4. Ascertain:
   a. Age of client.
   b. History of seizures.

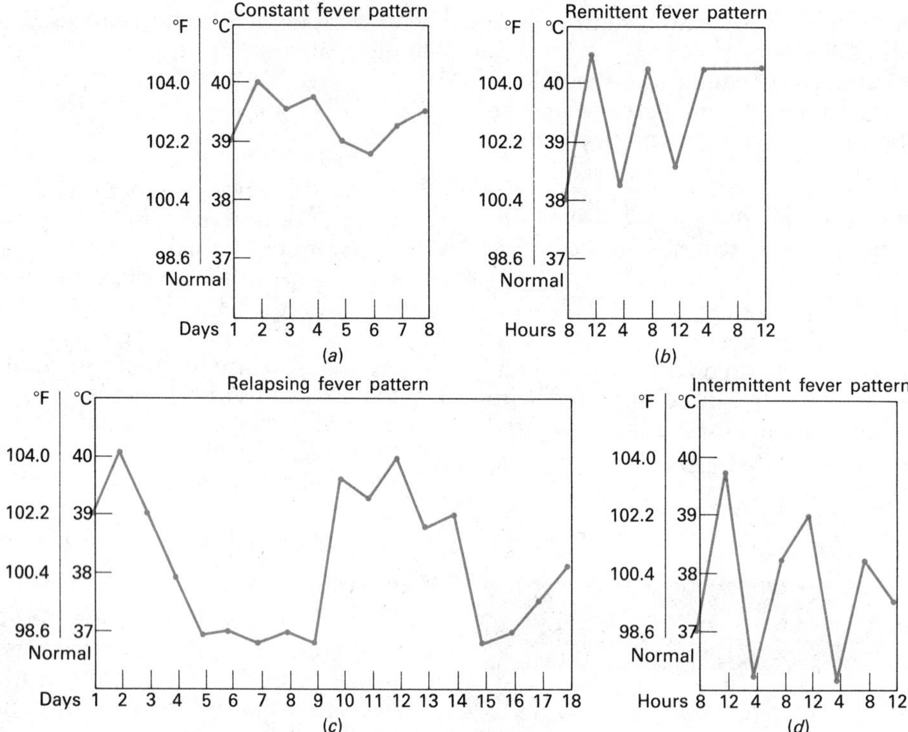

Figure 49-3 Patterns of fever. (*a*) Constant: temperature elevation of nearly constant level, e.g., typhoid fever. (*b*) Remittent: daily fluctuations of more than 2°F, e.g., septicemia, lymphomas. (*c*) Relapsing or recurrent: initial febrile period followed by normalization for several days, only to rise again to its previous height, e.g., Pel-Ebstein fever of Hodgkin's disease. (*d*) Intermittent: drops to below normal and then rises to previous height, e.g., malaria, juvenile rheumatoid arthritis.

c. Duration, pattern, extent of fever.
d. Presence of sweating.
e. Presence of chills.
f. Anorexia, vomiting, diarrhea, weight loss.
g. Headaches.
h. Myalgias.
i. Associated symptoms related to cardiovascular, gastrointestinal, genitourinary, gynecologic, musculoskeletal systems.

Physical Assessment

1. Temperature: remember that the degree of the fever does not necessarily correspond directly to the severity of the cause. Sepsis in newborns, for example, presents with subnormal temperatures.
2. Pulse rate.
3. Respiratory rate.
4. General physical examination for infectious etiology, including rectal and pelvic examination on adults where indicated. For infants under 6 months of age or newborns, the presence of fever requires a systematic and thorough evaluation. Look for the following:
   a. Anorexia.
   b. Lethargy, especially in young children and infants.
   c. Irritability, especially in young children and infants.
   d. Rashes.
   e. Petechiae.
   f. Adenopathy.
   g. Inflamed joints.
   h. Abdominal findings.
   i. Upper and lower respiratory tract findings.

Diagnostic Tests

1. CBC with differential.
2. Urinalysis and culture if indicated.

3. Erythrocyte sedimentation rate.
4. Chest x-ray film. Tachypnea out of proportion to the fever in an infant, for example, may be a clue to the presence of infiltrate on a chest film. In addition, extensive laboratory tests may be required to rule out clinical entities. Examples are:
   a. Infections:
      (1) Throat culture with pharyngitis.
      (2) Blood cultures.
      (3) Electrolyte levels with septicemia.
   b. Cardiovascular disease or acute MI:
      (1) ECG.
      (2) Arterial blood gases.
      (3) Serum enzymes.
   c. Collagen disease, rheumatoid arthritis:
      (1) Joint x-ray films, latex fixation test.
      (2) Erythrocyte sedimentation rate, serum protein tests.
   d. Malignant neoplastic disease:
      (1) Appropriate x-ray films.
      (2) Studies to determine tumor site.
      (3) Proctoscopy, stool for guaiac.

NURSING DIAGNOSES: ACTUAL OR POTENTIAL

1. Fluid volume deficit secondary to sweating, chills, anorexia, vomiting and diarrhea, dehydration, possible weight loss.
2. Inadequate tissue perfusion and impaired cardiovascular functioning due to dehydration, electrolyte and fluid imbalances, etiologic basis for fever elevation (acute MI, septicemia).
3. Alterations in comfort associated with fever, chills, pain, nausea, and vomiting.
4. Fear secondary to anxiety, loss of control, need for emergency treatment.
5. Impairment of mobility due to the debilitating effects of fever and associated symptoms.
6. Alteration in body temperature secondary to various etiologic agents, such as infection; physical or chemical agents; or central nervous system, cardiovascular, gastrointestional, hematologic, endocrine, neoplastic, and pulmonary disease.

EXPECTED OUTCOMES

1. Fluid and electrolyte balance will be restored and maintained during treatment of acute fever and attempt to diagnose its cause.
2. Cardiovascular function and adequate tissue perfusion will be restored, as adequate intervention to control fever is instituted.
3. Client will become more comfortable as fever is brought within normal limits and as relief for pain and other symptoms is provided.
4. Client will be less fearful with ongoing support and careful explanation of treatment and diagnostic procedures within first few hours of admission.
5. Client's mobility will increase, as fever and causative agent(s) are controlled.
6. Body temperature will return to normal range after appropriate treatment is provided for causative agent(s).

INTERVENTIONS

1. Remove unneeded clothing to allow radiation of heat. However, children can become overcooled and develop chills if undressed and may therefore need to remain lightly clothed.
2. Measures for reducing heat:
   a. Sponge patient with tepid water. Do not use cold water or cold, wet towels, for they produce peripheral vasoconstriction with conservation of body heat. They may also cause shivering, which causes increased heat production.
   b. The skin may be rubbed briskly to increase both heat loss and skin capillary circulation. Do not sponge infants or small children for longer than a half hour q2h.
   c. Ice packs, fanning, and cooling blankets may also be used.
   d. Avoid use of alcohol with infants.
3. Antipyretic drugs:
   a. Acetylsalicylic acid (aspirin). Give aspirin (60 mg for every year of age up to 5 years, q4h). For 5 to 10 year old child, 300 mg suffices; 600 mg suffices for older children. If vomiting occurs, give dose rectally. The rectal preparation can irritate the rectal mucosa. For adults, 0.3–0.6 g q4h as needed.
   b. Acetaminophen. Advantage is less gastric irritation than aspirin. In children, the dose is 5–10 mg/kg q 4–6 h. For adults, use 300–600 mg every 4 h.
   c. Aspirin and acetaminophen may be alternated in children to reduce the risk of Reye's syndrome.
   d. Chlorpromazine. In small doses (0.1 mg/z kg/24 h) for children, this does reduce fever via surface vasodilatation and inhi-

bition of shivering. Its use is reserved for patients in hospital with core temperatures > 104°F.

4. Fluid replacement. Administer oral or parenteral fluids in amounts adequate to make up for extra fluid losses from perspiration and other causes. Accurately measure fluid intake and output, as well as fluid loss through wound drainage, stool volume, blood loss, nasogastric suction. Weigh patient daily.
5. Other interventions as appropriate for etiologic agent of fever.

EVALUATION

Outcome Criteria

1. Fluid and electrolyte balance is maintained as treatment progresses, and cause for the elevated body temperature is found.
2. Cardiovascular function is adequate and full tissue perfusion is restored.
3. Client is resting comfortably.
4. Client is less anxious and fearful.
5. Patient is able to move around more freely and is working toward a progressively increasing level of activity.
6. Body temperature is returning to within normal limits.

Complications

For treatment of dehydration and shock, see Chapter 48.

Reevaluation and Follow-up

1. Provide for continuity of care with adequate follow-up for reevaluation of fever if client is sent home.
2. If the client is a child or infant, teach parents how to read a thermometer and what to do if fever recurs.

SEIZURES

STATUS EPILEPTICUS

DESCRIPTION

Status epilepticus is the state of prolonged seizures, when two or more major seizures occur without intervening return of consciousness. Over 50 percent of these cases are associated with tumor, vascular disease, infection, or trauma. The largest single cause is idiopathic. One must search for metabolic causes: hypoglycemia, hyponatremia, hypocalcemia, hypomagnesemia, hepatic dysfunction, uremia, and endocrine disorder.

Status epilepticus may also be precipitated by a number of other conditions, particularly abrupt withdrawal of anticonvulsant medications, such as barbiturates, and also by withdrawal of alcohol by chronic alcoholics. Death or brain damage is possible from the continuous seizures and accompanying anoxia.

PREVENTION

Health Promotion

1. Avoid sudden cessation or withdrawal from long-term anticonvulsant therapy. Anticonvulsants should always be tapered off over a period of 2–3 weeks under close supervision.
2. Promote ongoing supportive programs for chronic drug abusers to allow for gradual withdrawal from drugs and alcohol under close supervision.
3. Encourage education of clients with seizures and their families, especially where young children are involved. Emphasize chronic nature of epilepsy and the need for the client to remain on anticonvulsant medication indefinitely.
4. Give appropriate counsel to persons with a family history of seizures (although the role of heredity in seizures is poorly understood).
5. Reduce extreme physical or emotional stress in persons with history of recurrent seizures.
6. Be aware that fluid retention, common in many women before menstruation and also in both men and women when they consume too much fluid, can mean that an increase in anticonvulsant medications is required (Swift, 1978).
7. Persons with a history of seizures need to avoid those environmental influences, such as direct sunlight or flashing lights, that tend to precipitate their episodes.
8. Provide ongoing support and counseling to clients and families to combat the social stigma associated with seizures. Often, denial and poor control of seizures arise from the stigma.

Population at Risk

1. Persons with family history of seizures.
2. Persons presently under therapy for seizures who might need adjustments in anticonvulsant therapy or who have stopped such therapy.
3. Chronic alcohol abusers who suddenly stop consumption of alcohol.
4. Chronic drug abusers who are withdrawing from drug use, especially barbiturates.
5. Persons with history of seizures exposed to extreme physical or emotional stress or to sudden infection or trauma.
6. Children and adolescents with history of seizures whose medication and treatment are not being carefully supervised.
7. Children who have experienced severe birth trauma or postnatal trauma.
8. Persons exposed to high level of toxins, such as lead, alcohol.
9. Persons with neoplastic, vascular, metabolic, or infectious diseases.

Screening

None.

ASSESSMENT

Health History

1. History of seizure disorder.
2. Medications, if any. Ask about street drugs. With anticonvulsant therapy, ask for time of last dose. Was the client taking the medication on schedule?
3. Associated illnesses, such as hypertension.
4. Acute illness prior to seizure.
5. Description of seizure:
   a. Localized, generalized.
   b. Cyanosis.
   c. Duration.
   d. Incontinence.
   e. Activity before and after attack.
   f. Onset (sudden or gradual).
   g. How did eyes, body position, face look during seizure (e.g., skin flushed or clammy, eyes open, pupil size)?
   h. What was breathing like (gasping and noisy)?

Physical Assessment

1. Determine adequacy of airway.
2. Obtain vital signs.
3. Perform brief physical exam with special attention to neurologic system. Look for a Medic-alert tag or identification card in the client's wallet.
4. Observe seizures. Pay attention to:
   a. Onset (usually abrupt with tonic muscular contraction).
   b. Sequence of spread.
   c. Lateralizing signs.

Diagnostic Tests

1. Electrolyte levels.
2. BUN.
3. Blood sugar level.
4. Calcium, phosphorus levels.
5. Blood gases.
6. Toxicology screen.
7. Blood lead level.
8. Lumbar puncture.
9. Urinalysis.
10. Serologic test for syphilis.
11. Chest x-ray film.
12. Skull films.
13. EEG.
14. CT scan to rule out neoplasm as causative agent.

NURSING DIAGNOSES: ACTUAL OR POTENTIAL

1. Respiratory dysfunction due to seizures, possible aspiration, leading to possible respiratory arrest. Respiratory arrest secondary to airway obstruction by vomitus, saliva, or tongue.
2. Fluid volume deficit associated with decreased fluid intake, dehydration, vomiting, fever.
3. Impairment in cardiovascular functioning secondary to cardiac arrthymias, respiratory depression, inadequate ventilation, and fluid loss, leading to inadequate tissue perfusion and shock.
4. Alterations in levels of consciousness associated with lethargy, disorientation, or coma and secondary to seizures and respiratory depression.
5. Alterations in level of comfort due to pain, fear, and possible physical damage during seizures.
6. Fear associated with anxiety and social embarrassment about disorder.
7. Possible lack of drug compliance due to lack of knowledge about need for continuous an-

ticonvulsant therapy and to social embarrassment.

EXPECTED OUTCOMES

1. A patent airway will be maintained and adequate ventilation will be sustained during acute period while seizures are being brought under control.
2. Fluid and electrolyte balance will be reinstated during ongoing therapy for seizure control.
3. Cardiovascular functioning will be maintained within normal limits and adequate tissue perfusion will result.
4. Client will return to consciousness with minimal residual neurological deficit, as acute seizure episode is brought under control.
5. Client will become more comfortable as therapeutic intervention continues and seizures are controlled.
6. Ongoing counseling and support will allow client's fears and anxiety to decline by the time he or she is discharged from the hospital.
7. Client will demonstrate increased compliance with drug regimen on reevaluation at 2 weeks, 3 months, 6 months, and one year.

INTERVENTIONS

1. Assure adequate ventilation:
   a. Resuscitate, if indicated.
   b. Suction at regular intervals.
   c. Administer oxygen whether or not cyanosis is present.
   d. Possibly begin early intubation because of respiratory depression due to use of anticonvulsant drugs.
2. Start a slow intravenous infusion of 5 percent dextrose.
3. Insert indwelling Foley catheter and monitor carefully intake and output at 15-min intervals.
4. Administer appropriate drugs as ordered: Note: the major cause of death with status epilepticus is respiratory or cardiac failure after IV use of a hypnotic agent. It is necessary to continuously monitor vital signs every 5–10 min and note all medications administered.
   a. Diazepam (Valium), 5 to 10 mg IV at a rate of no more than 5 mg/min. If seizure has not stopped within 10 min, another 5 to 10 mg may be given 10 to 20 min after the second dose. If not controlled after 25 to 30 mg, other therapy must be considered. Monitor blood pressure and respirations closely, since hypotension and respiratory depression may accompany high cumulative doses of diazepam. For children: IV diazepam in doses of 2 mg every 3–5 min up to 10 mg. This is supplied as 5 mg/mL and given undiluted close to the infusion site (Graef and Cone, 1980).
   b. Phenobarbital: initial dose, 150 mg (never more than 200 mg) IV, at a rate of 25 to 50 mg/min; additional doses may be given after 15 to 20 min. In clients responding to diazepam, a single dose of 150 to 200 mg phenobarbital IV at 25 mg/min will give longer acting epileptic coverage. Also produces hypotension and respiratory depression.
   c. Phenytoin: usual loading dose 750–1500 mg (15–18 mg/kg body weight); give in divided doses every few hours. Must be given directly into vein since it does not mix with usual IV solutions. Do not administer at rate exceeding 50 mg/min. Monitor vital signs; watch for hypotension, cardiac arrthymias, apnea. *Do not give IM* (Freitag and Miller, 1980).
   d. For children, 8–10 mg/kg diphenylhydantoin (Dilantin) is given slowly in saline (not to exceed 25 mg/min). In addition, 3 mg/kg is given IM. Dilatin given IV may have toxic cardiac effects, slowing conduction velocity and heart rate.
   e. Paraldehyde: give intravenously, intramuscularly, or rectally if above drugs fail. Respiratory depression may occur.
5. Monitor neurologic status and vital signs carefully.
6. Make sure client's bed is well padded, with side rails up, to prevent injury during seizure. If possible at outset of seizure, a padded tongue blade should be placed between the teeth at the back of the mouth to prevent damage to cheeks, tongue, or teeth. Do not attempt to force tongue blade between clenched jaws.
7. Provide ongoing emotional support to family and client. Call appropriate clergy if indicated.
8. Assist in establishing an ongoing teaching

plan once client's condition has stabilized. Include information on:

a. Rest, avoidance of extreme stress.
b. Anticonvulsant therapy, doses, side effects.
c. Emergency care during seizures.

EVALUATION

Outcome Criteria

1. Adequate ventilation is established and respiratory function is corrected.
2. Fluid and electrolyte balance is reestablished, as client is well-hydrated, fluid loss is decreased, fever is controlled.
3. Cardiovascular functioning is maintained and adequate tissue perfusion is evident.
4. Client is conscious, oriented, and communicating appropriately.
5. Client is experiencing less discomfort and pain.
6. Teaching and support are continuing to decrease client's and family's fears and increase compliance with health regimen.

Complications

1. Respiratory arrest (see Chapter 48).
2. Shock (see Chapter 48).
3. Aspiration.
4. Cardiac arrhythmias (see Chapter 30 for assessment and intervention).
5. Hyperthermia (See discussion under *Fever*, above, for assessment and interventions).

Reevaluation and Follow-up

Reevaluate ongoing teaching and compliance with drug regimen at regular intervals. It is important to continue to explore with client and family their ideas about seizures and the chronic nature of the disorder. Reassurance about prognosis and social as well as genetic implications should be provided.

FEBRILE SEIZURES

DESCRIPTION

A febrile seizure is an occurrence of convulsions in infancy or childhood (usually between the ages of 3 months and 5 years) and is associated with fever. The victim demonstrates no evidence of intracranial infection of defined cause (Consensus Development Panel, 1981). Three to 5 percent of children have febrile convulsions. These seizures merely represent an initial symptom of an acute benign febrile illness and are self-limiting in nature. There is, at present, no evidence of mental or neurologic impairment due to a febrile seizure. However, any child presenting with a seizure should be evaluated for the possibility of some other etiology, such as, tetany, lead encephalopathy, hemorrhage, tumor, hypoglycemia, asphyxia, epilepsy, acute nephritis, and so on.

PREVENTION

Health Promotion

1. Educate parents in temperature taking and reading the thermometer, and in giving tepid baths, aspirin and acetaminophen, and other basic methods of fever reduction.
2. Provide basic information in health care settings and in the community regarding emergency treatment of a seizure and how to obtain assistance.
3. Emphasize need to continue on therapeutic regiment and to obtain close health supervision for children with history of febrile seizures or with a family history of nonfebrile seizures.

Population at Risk

1. Children who have had one febrile seizure and who do not receive prophylactic therapy.
2. Infants who have experienced a febrile seizure during the first year of life.
3. Children with a family history of nonfebrile seizures.
4. Children with history of abnormal neurologic or development status.

Screening

None.

ASSESSMENT

Health History

1. History of previous seizures.
2. Family history of febrile seizures.
3. Medications child is taking.
4. Illnesses that may be associated with seizures, such as hypertension.
5. Acute illness prior to the seizure.

6. Description of the seizure:
   a. Localized or generalized.
   b. Symptoms immediately preceeding, such as hyperirritability, headache, vomiting, dizziness, fever.
   c. Duration.
   d. Incontinence.
   e. Cyanosis.

Physical Assessment

Perform complete pediatric and neurologic examination. Note especially:

1. Signs of the febrile illness, such as hyperirritability and lethargy with meningitis.
2. Degree of temperature elevation.
3. Signs of fear, anxiety.

Diagnostic Tests

1. Lumbar puncture (if CNS infection suspected).
2. CBC with differential.
3. Serum electrolyte levels.
4. Calcium and glucose levels.
5. Skull x-ray film.
6. Computed tomography (CT) scan of brain.
7. Throat culture; urinalysis; and chest x-ray film, where indicated, to find site of infection.
8. EEG.

NURSING DIAGNOSES: ACTUAL OR POTENTIAL

1. Possible respiratory dysfunction secondary to possible obstruction of the airway with vomitus, saliva, or tongue.
2. Imbalance in fluid and electrolyte levels secondary to dehydration, anorexia, fever resulting from infectious process.
3. Alteration in levels of consciousness associated with seizure and its resulting disorientation, fatigue, and lethargy.
4. Central nervous system dysfunction secondary to febrile seizures and underlying infectious process.
5. Alteration in levels of comfort due to seizures, associated symptoms of infection, fever, and anxiety.
6. Fear associated with parent's and child's anxiety and social embarassment.
7. Poor compliance with health regimen due to lack of knowledge of appropriate treatment for the disorder.

EXPECTED OUTCOMES

1. Patent airway and adequate ventilation will be restored and maintained as soon as the child comes under emergency care.
2. Fluid and electrolyte balance will be maintained during acute phase of treatment until stabilized.
3. Client will return to consciousness with decreased lethargy and disorientation.
4. Child will become more comfortable as seizure is treated, fever is controlled, and infection is diagnosed and appropriate therapy instituted.
5. Child and parents will demonstrate decreased fear and anxiety once ongoing supportive counseling is provided. Such improvement will be evident within three months from date of initial febrile seizure.
6. Compliance with recommended health regimen will be evident at regular follow-up intervals after the acute incident: 4 weeks, 2 months, 6 months.

INTERVENTIONS

1. Monitor vital signs carefully.
2. Determine adequacy of airway; provide suctioning, oxygen if indicated.
3. Make sure child is protected from falls and bruising during seizure.
4. Continue to provide emotional support to parents and child.
5. Begin fever control with tepid water sponging and rectal aspirin 60 mg per year of age, up to 600 mg.
6. Give as ordered:
   a. Phenobarbital: usually 2–3 mg/kg IV. If not effective in 10 min, give additional 2 to 3 mg/kg IM. Maximum dose of 120 mg advised.
   b. Use of diazepam with children is under investigation. It must not be used with phenobarbital.
   c. Paraldehyde: either initially or in conjunction with phenobarbital. Administer via high rectal tube, 0.3 mL/kg, up to 6.0 mL; mix with equal volume of mineral oil, inject in tube, and follow with 10 mL of normal saline (used to flush mixture through tube) (Graef and Cone, 1980).
7. After acute episode, anticonvulsant prophylaxis should be considered in the following

conditions and is continued for at least two years:

a. When febrile seizure lasts longer than 15 min or if it is focal or followed by persistent neurologic abnormalities.
b. If abnormal neurologic development is present; for example, microcephaly, cerebral palsy.
c. If there is a family history of nonfebrile seizures.
d. If multiple febrile seizures occur.
e. If seizures occur in an infant under the age of 12 months.

Otherwise, the consensus is that due to the benign nature and outcome of most febrile seizures, *no* medication is needed on a continuing basis (Consensus Development Panel, 1981).

EVALUATION

Outcome Criteria

1. Adequate ventilation is maintained.
2. Fluid and electrolyte balance has been reestablished via appropriate fluid replacement and rehydration.
3. Client is awake and less lethargic.
4. Child is more comfortable and less fearful.
5. Compliance with recommended therapeutic regimen is evidenced by family's continued communication with professional and support groups and no recurrence of febrile seizures.

Complications

In rare cases, febrile seizures precede epilepsy.

Reevaluation and Follow-up

1. Refer to appropriate social service or community health agencies for home follow-up, further emotional support, and parent teaching on:
   a. Medication, if prescribed, compliance, and side effects.
   b. Recognition and appropriate home treatment of future high fevers.
   c. Use of antipyretic medications.
   d. First aid for a seizure.
   e. How to obtain emergency assistance if needed.
2. As already noted, long-term treatment of children who have experienced febrile seizures with daily phenobarbital, 30–60 mg at bedtime, is not recommended except in certain situations. Parents may expect this preventive treatment and may need to be reassured if it is not prescribed.

EMERGENCY DELIVERY

DESCRIPTION

Any delivery occurring outside of a planned, prepared environment is considered an emergency. Women who deliver this way generally fall into three groups: those with unexpected preterm labor, those with unusually rapid progress through the first and second stages, or those who are uninformed or uncomprehending (for example, women with a language barrier or mental retardation, or terrified teenagers). Thus, obstetric and psychosocial problems almost always complicate the nursing care. Delivery enroute to the hospital in a car or taxi may be due to uncontrollable external events, such as traffic patterns, car breakdowns, and the like. Finally, emergency delivery during a disaster may be due to the pregnant woman's being sequestered in shelters or marooned in isolated places. Health personnel should be informed about steps of support and care during emergency delivery, just as they are for cardiopulmonary resuscitation. There are four basic principles:

1. Labor *always* progresses through a step-by-step pattern to delivery. In many emergency cases, the progress is merely more rapid through one or more phases than in normal labor.
2. Panic in the mother and the assistants must be avoided. The most knowledgeable person should take charge. Send volunteers for equipment and for help. It is most important to maintain a calm atmosphere. Get the mother to focus on helping herself by correct breathing and position.
3. Cooperate with the natural forces of labor, since skill in manipulation or instruments are absent. Do not do vaginal assessments of dilatation. External signs are clearly recogniz-

able. Position the mother to facilitate delivery: a semisitting or squatting position to push, and a Sims' position or semisitting for delivery.
4. The infant must be protected against respiratory dysfunction and cold stress; mother and infant must have their fluid and nutritional needs anticipated and fulfilled.

PREVENTION

Health Promotion

1. Encourage early health supervision for all women of child-bearing age, so that complications during pregnancy and the puerperium will be avoided.
2. Provide services within the community that offer fewer barriers to poor, very young, and less-educated women, so that continuous monitoring of a pregnancy is available to them.
3. Increase educational groups open to prospective parents in both early and late pregnancy. Discussions should cover signs of labor, stages of labor, preparation for childbirth, danger signs and symptoms, how to obtain emergency care if needed, and parenting after birth.
4. Be aware of multiparous women with history of brief labors and counsel these women to seek professional assistance at the first signs of impending labor.

Population at Risk

1. Multiparous women with or without history of precipitous labor.
2. Adolescents, single women, women wanting no "medical interference," and so on, who have not sought previous health care during pregnancy from embarrassment, lack of funds, inaccessibility of services, or those who are not well informed on the normal progression of labor.
3. Women whose labor is precipitous either from an abnormally low resistance of the soft parts, from unusually strong uterine or abdominal contractions, or in rare instances from the absence of painful sensations during labor (Hellman and Pritzhard, 1971).
4. Women in sparsely populated areas in which health care facilities are a long distance away.
5. Women living in areas of severe weather conditions.
6. Women who prefer for personal, financial, religious, or other reasons to give birth at home, but have no professional resources available to aid them if complications or difficulties arise during labor and delivery.

Screening

1. Perform Nitrazine test for rupture of membranes.
2. Check for evidence of bloody show.

ASSESSMENT

Health History

If possible, obtain from woman or family the following:

1. Pregnancy status (gravida, para, full term, premature, abortions, number of living children).
2. Expected date of delivery.
3. Marital status: if single, is she keeping baby?
4. Does the mother plan bottle or breast feeding? (Since some mothers wish to breastfeed right after delivery, this is important to note.)
5. Allergies to drugs or foods.
6. History of kidney or bladder infection.
7. Varicose veins or hemorrhoids.
8. When the woman last slept.
9. Contractions:
   a. When started?
   b. Where does she feel the discomfort?
   c. Start written record.
10. Membrane:
    a. Intact or broken?
    b. When ruptured?
    c. Odor, color.
11. Bloody show if any; frank clots or blood.
12. Any preparation for childbirth.
13. When woman last voided.

Physical Assessment

1. Obtain vital signs.
2. Check for fetal heart sounds every 5–10 min. Note:
   a. Character.
   b. If membranes ruptured, check fetal heart rate during and then immediately after contraction to detect compression or prolapse of cord.
   c. Rate (120–160, average 140; at height of contraction, may fall to 100 transiently, but returns rapidly to normal value as contraction diminishes).

3. Assess type, duration, strength and frequency of uterine contractions and keep a record.
4. Palpate abdomen for position, presentation by means of Leopold's maneuvers.
5. Watch for signs that the second stage of labor is imminent:
   a. Woman begins to bear down by herself as fetal head starts to press on perineal floor.
   b. A sudden increase in bloody show might become apparent.
   c. Woman complains she needs to defecate, due to pressure of fetal head on perineal floor.
   d. Perineum starts to bulge, anal orifice begins to dilate.

Diagnostic Tests

Diagnostic tests are not available under usual emergency delivery circumstances.

NURSING DIAGNOSES: ACTUAL OR POTENTIAL

1. Alterations in comfort due to pain of contractions, fear, and anxiety.
2. Impairment in coping ability secondary to extreme pain, loss of control, fear about health of baby.
3. Decreased resistance to infection associated with precipitate delivery, inadequate time for preparation of woman for labor, possible tears and lacerations of birth canal, premature rupture of membranes.
4. Fear due to lack of knowledge about labor and delivery, inability to get to health facility in time, loss of control, pain, lack of training in prepared childbirth.
5. Impairment in cardiovascular functioning associated with hemorrhage, loss of fluid volume, and resulting inadequate tissue perfusion.
6. Increased risk to health of newborn due to lack of preparation for delivery, inadequate facilities for controlled birth.
7. Increased risk to health of mother secondary to possible complications of hypotonic uterus, incomplete delivery of placenta, lacerations of birth canal.

EXPECTED OUTCOMES

1. Client will gain confidence during labor and delivery and will be more comfortable immediately after delivery of infant and placenta.
2. Client's ability to cope will improve gradually during the immediate recovery and postpartum period.
3. Increased resistance to infection will be reestablished as client recovers from delivery and is appropriately treated if any symptoms of infection occur.
4. Cardiovascular functioning will return to normal after appropriate treatment is given if complications do occur.
5. Newborn will be appropriately treated for any health problems at birth.

INTERVENTIONS

1. Continue to obtain vital signs of laboring woman at regular intervals.
2. Continue to check for fetal heart rate every 5–10 min.
3. Monitor type, duration, strength, and frequency of contractions.
4. Continue to provide instruction on coping with contractions and pushing effectively.
5. Assist woman with comfort measures, such as keeping perineum clean and dry, moistening her lips, offering verbal reassurance, encouragement.
6. Position mother in physiologic position: space between perineum and surface must be obtained to allow manipulation of the infant's shoulders and head:
   a. Position away from drafts, crowds. Maintain shielding for privacy.
   b. Place rolled up newspapers under buttocks, pad area to receive amniotic fluid and blood at delivery.
   c. Allow mother to assume any position during first and second stages: Sims', semisitting, squatting.
7. Direct volunteers to seek aid if available and to gather equipment from environment (see Table 49–5). Obtain plastic bag for placenta.
8. Provide for asepsis as possible: Cleanse hands, using any available liquid; wipe down perineum, with the mother's underclothes if nothing else is available. Use clean newspaper as a barrier between perineum and surface of car seat, bench, floor.
9. Once crowning occurs—distension of perineum by fetal head to diameter of 6–8 cm (see Figures 49–4,5)—place towel over hand

TABLE 49-5 ENVIRONMENTAL EQUIPMENT FOR EMERGENCY DELIVERY: DISASTER PLANNING

For cleansing the mother	Alcohol, dish washing liquid, or wipe down with underclothes
For padding or protection during delivery	Newspapers (unused), brown paper, large plastic bags, old sheets, towels, shower curtain
To clear infant's airway	Ear bulb syringe, meat basting syringe, paper or plastic straw, manual milking of nose and throat
For the cord	Strong cotton thread, yarn, new razor blade, scissors or knife (flame sterilized)
To warm the baby	Mother's clothes, skin-to-skin contact, blanket, towel, sheet, clean newspapers, padded box
To feed the baby	Milk powder, bottle, nipple

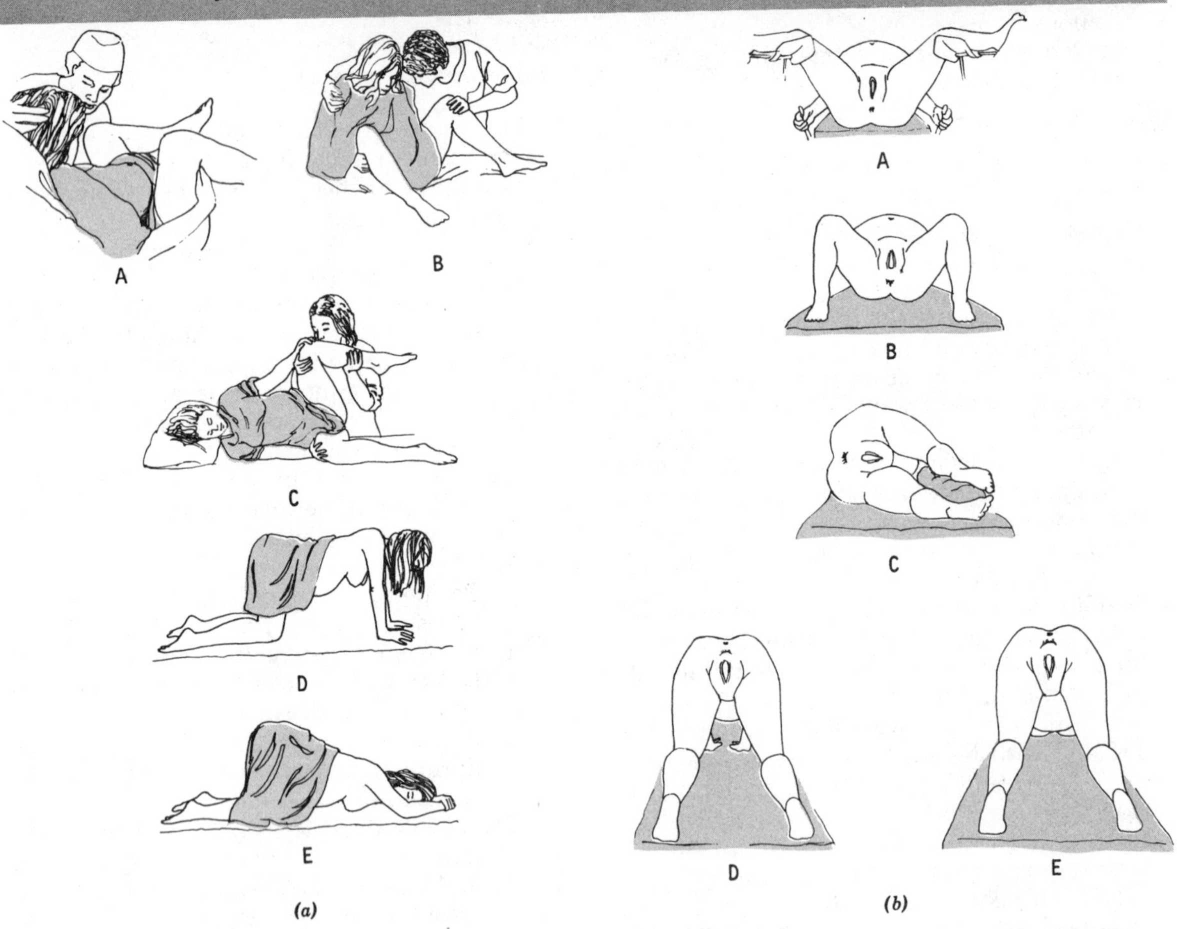

Figure 49-4 (*a*) Position for pushing during the second stage. (A) Lithotomy but with head elevated. (B) Dorsal position. (C) Side-lying position. (D) All fours, up on hands and knees. (E) Knee-chest position. (*b*) Vaginal opening as seen in the various positions for delivery. (A) Lithotomy, the usual position for delivery room. (B) Dorsal elevated, usually the most comfortable position (with head and shoulders elevated). (C) Side-lying position. An attendant should support the upper leg. (D) All-fours, upon hands and knees. An attendant at her head should help with support if fatigue becomes evident. (E) Knee-chest is very uncomfortable if delivery is prolonged. A pillow or padding is necessary for her chest. (From Buckley, K., and Kulb, N. W.: *Handbook of Maternal-Newborn Nursing*, John Wiley & Sons, New York, 1983.)

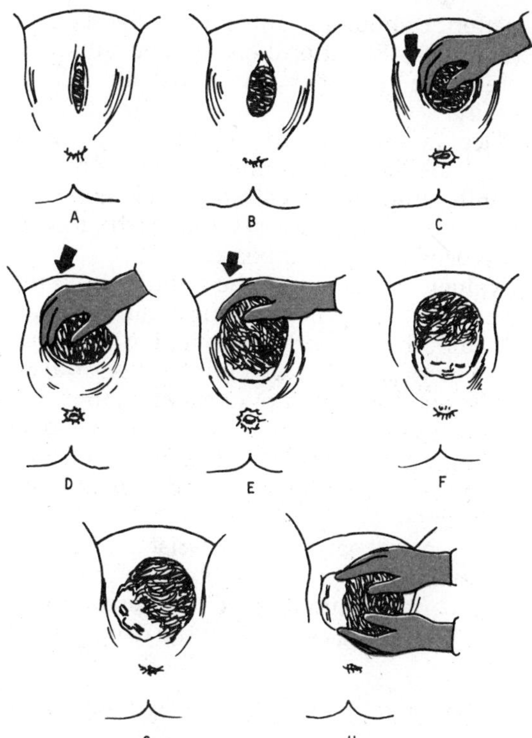

Figure 49-5 Normal sequence of birth when minimal assistance is needed. (*a*) Vaginal opening reveals baby's hair and scalp. (*b*) Vulva distends and bulges. (*c*) Head appears, encircled by vulva. At this point, apply cupped fingers to head and exert light downward pressure. (Ask woman not to push; if the pressure is too strong now, lacerations may occur.) (*d*) Slow the rate of delivery by gentle downward pressure as head emerges. (*e*) Extension of the head. (*f*) Face emerges, "sweeping the perineum." (*g*) External rotation of the head as it returns to the position assumed after internal rotation. (*h*) Begin to exert downward pressure on the whole head in order to deliver the shoulders (see next Figure). (From Buckley, K., and Kulb, N. W.: *Handbook of Maternal-Newborn Nursing*, John Wiley & Sons, New York, 1983.)

to protect it from anus and exert forward pressure on chin of baby's head. At the same time, with the other hand, exert pressure on the occiput (Ritgen maneuver, see Figure 49–6). Deliver head between contractions as slowly as possible (see Figure 49–7).

10. When head is delivered, milk nose and throat, free the cord.

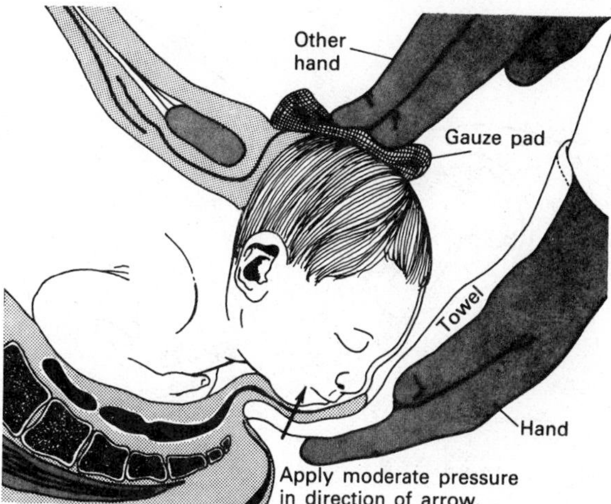

Figure 49-6 Assistance may be needed if head does not extend smoothly (Ritgen's maneuver). Exert hand pressure downward on the occiput, with forward pressure applied to the obstetric perineum, just between the vaginal and anal openings. Feel for the baby's chin and exert forward pressure on the chin through the distended tissue of the perineum. Use an article of the mother's clothing, the cleanest material available in an emergency, as skin will be slippery.

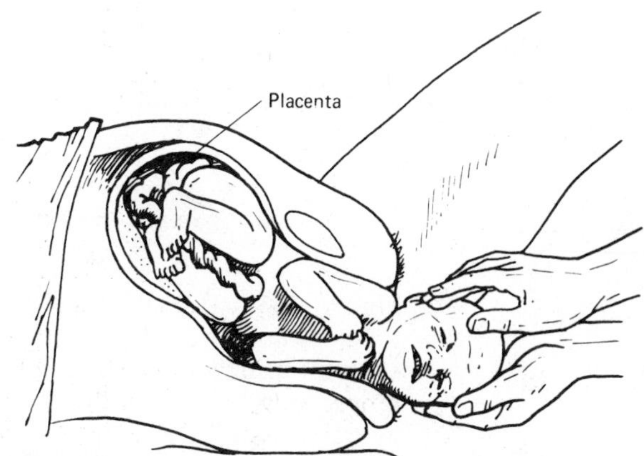

Figure 49-7 The baby's head is gently directed downward to help partial delivery of the anterior (upper) shoulder past the symphysis pubis, before proceeding with the delivery of the lower shoulder. (From Henderson, J.: *Emergency Medical Guide*, 4th ed., McGraw-Hill, New York, 1978.)

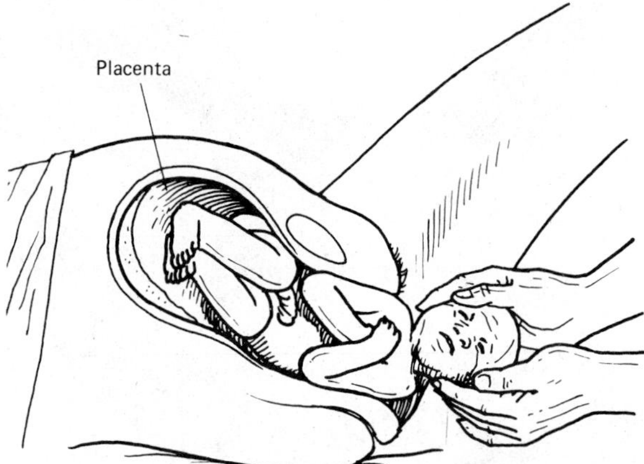

Figure 49-8 The lower (posterior) shoulder is delivered by very gently directing the axis of the baby's head and neck upward. Never pull hard in an attempt to drag the baby out; this would cause permanent damage to the baby or lacerate the mother's perineum. (From Henderson, J.: *Emergency Medical Guide,* 4th ed. McGraw-Hill, New York, 1978).

11. Anterior shoulder is usually delivered first (Figure 49–8). After the shoulders are delivered, the rest of the body usually follows easily.
12. Place infant in head dependent position, skin to skin on mother's abdomen, and gently stimulate breathing. Milk nose and throat again if necessary. Show the mother the baby as soon as possible.
13. Evaluate condition at one minute. If no respirations, wrap infant warmly and prepare for mouth-to-mouth resuscitation. First suction with a straw, or bulb syringe if available, and then attempt to expand lungs with a positive puff of pressure. It is the deep gasping breath that is critical in establishing neonatal circulatory and respiratory changes.
14. If no heartbeat, get an assistant to apply pressure in correct rhythm for CPR while you continue mouth-to-mouth breathing.
15. Cord clamping can wait. If the deep gasping

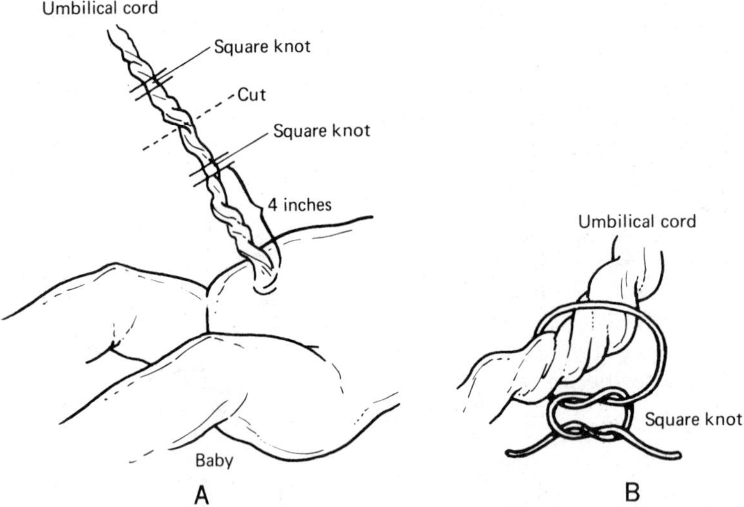

Figure 49-9 The cord is firmly tied off. (*a*) Use two strips of tape, clean torn cloth, or heavy yarn. Cut between the tapes with a sterilized knife or scissors, usually unavailable during an emergency, or a razor blade that has never been out of its package; or leave cord attached until a clean instrument can be found. Neonatal tetanus or other infection may result from use of contaminated instruments or ties. Do *not* use shoelaces. (*b*) The cord is tied with a square knot, which will not slip. However, if the infant has established adequate respirations, tying the cord is of secondary importance; circulation has ceased because of the cardiodynamics of fetal-to-newborn circulation. (From Henderson, J.: *Emergency Medical Guide,* 4th ed., McGraw-Hill, New York, 1978.)

breath has occurred, the cord has probably collapsed to a thin, limp, nonengorged connection. Such a state indicates that fetal circulation has changed and the fetal structures are closing in the normal patterns.

a. If nothing clean is available to tie cord, do not tie it; place placenta in a plastic bag, or wrap in newspaper and lay alongside baby for trip to hospital or clinic.
b. If there is no possibility of medical help, use cleanest available material to tie cord in two places (see Figure 49–9) and sever with a flame-sterilized knife or scissors, or a new, out-of-the-package razor blade.

16. Placental delivery should follow birth within 15 to 30 min. Encourage this by placing infant to nipple to lick and attempt to feed. Nipple stimulus causes the reflex "let down" with pitocin secreted from posterior pituitary. If baby cannot suck, ask the mother to roll the nipples, making them erect, to achieve same effect.
17. Examine all surfaces of placenta to determine if it and membranes are intact. Massage fundus to aid in firm contraction *after* breast feeding (see Figure 49–10). Assess amount of bleeding.
18. Assess state of perineum; if lacerated, apply external pressure to obtain hemostasis. Obtain ice, if available, to reduce swelling of hematoma.
19. Give the mother sweet and salty liquids to drink in adequate amounts. Infant can wait for feeding for 2–4 h.
20. Watch uterus constantly for the hour following delivery and massage fundus at the slightest sign of relaxation (Figure 49–10).
21. At regular intervals, note amount and kind of vaginal bleeding.
22. Obtain medical help as quickly as possible.
23. Monitor newborn carefully for signs of respiratory distress, fall in body temperature, cyanosis. Perform Apgar evaluation at 1 min and at 5 min after birth (Table 49–6).

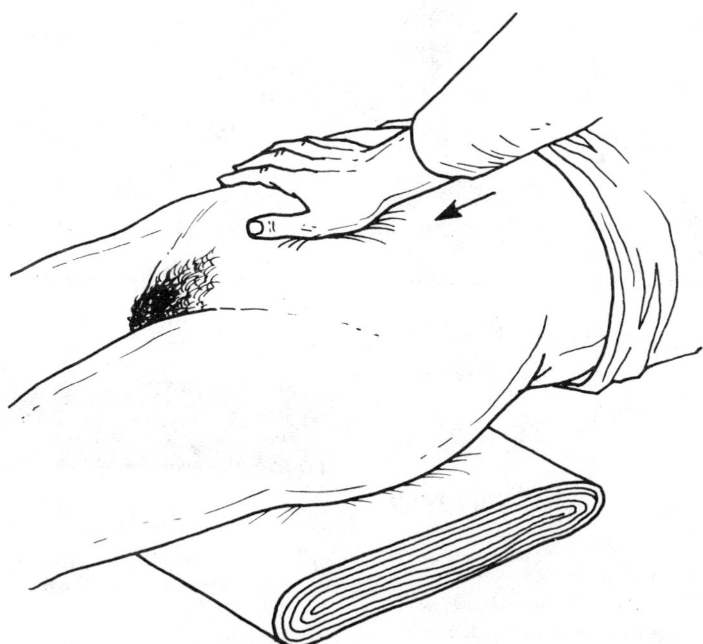

Figure 49-10 Position of hand for compressing the uterus (which is easily felt as something like a football) to stimulate contraction and thus help to control postpartum bleeding. In the absence of drugs to keep the uterus contracted, gentle manual kneading must be maintained for at least an hour or until medical help becomes available. (From Henderson, J.: *Emergency Medical Guide,* 4th ed., McGraw-Hill, New York, 1978.)

TABLE 49-6 APGAR SCORING SYSTEM

Sign	0	1	2
Heart rate	Absent	Slow	Over 100
Respiratory effort	Absent	Slow, irregular	Good, crying
Muscle tone	Flaccid	Some flexion of extremities	Active motion
Reflex irritability	No response	Cry	Vigorous cry
Color	Blue, pale	Body pink, extremities blue	Completely pink

SOURCE: Hellman, L., and Pritzhard, J.: *Williams' Obstetrics,* 14th ed., Appleton-Century-Crofts, New York, 1971, p. 479.

EVALUATION

Outcome Criteria

1. Woman is resting comfortably; infant is stabilized.
2. Woman is visibly able to cope with situation.
3. Woman is receiving treatment appropriate for any infection resulting from delivery.
4. Client is no longer fearful.
5. Cardiovascular functioning is within normal limits.
6. Newborn is responding appropriately to any therapy required.

Complications

LACERATIONS OF BIRTH CANAL

Assessment

1. First degree lacerations involve fourchette, perineal skin, vaginal mucous membrane.
2. Second degree lacerations involve above plus muscles of perineal body but exclude rectal spincter.
3. Third degree lacerations involve above and rectal spincter.

Interventions (in Medical Facility)

1. Suturing and specialized techniques for repair.
2. Assist with repair, provide heat lamp, analgesia as needed.

Reevaluation and Follow-up

Check repair site often if pain is severe or persistent to detect possible hematoma or abscess.

POSTPARTUM HEMORRAGE

Description

Loss of more than 500 ml of blood during the first 24 h after birth. There are three major causes of postpartum hemorrhage:

1. Vaginal and cervical lacerations.
2. Uterine atony.
3. Retention of placenta fragments.

NOTE: In postpartum hemorrhage, pulse and BP do not undergo major alterations until large amounts of blood have been lost.

Interventions (in Medical Facility)

1. Treat immediately for shock (See Chapter 48).
2. Begin transfusion of blood.
3. Assist as necessary with application of bimanual compression, exploration of uterine cavity for retained placental fragments, and visual inspection of cervix for missed lacerations.
4. Assist with administration of 0.2 mg ergonovine IV or IM or 10 or 20 units of oxytocin IV or IM.
5. Continue to massage fundus.

Reevaluation and Follow-up

1. Continue to monitor vital signs, assess consistency of fundus, and note amounts of blood lost.
2. Provide ongoing reassurance to client.

REFERENCES

Barry, J.: *Emergency Nursing,* McGraw-Hill, New York, 1978.

Consensus Development Panel: "Febrile Seizures: Long Term Management of Children with Fever-associated Seizures," *Pediatrics in Review,* American Academy of Pediatrics, Vol. 2, No. 7, January 1981.

Cope, Z.: *The Early Diagnosis of the Acute Abdomen,* Oxford University Press, New York, 1968.

Eckert, C.: *Emergency Room Care,* 3d ed., Little, Brown, Boston, 1976.

Flint, T., and Cain, H. D.: *Emergency Treatment and Management,* 5th ed., Saunders, Philadelphia, 1975.

Freitag, J., and Maller L. (eds.): *Manual of Medical Therapeutics,* Little Brown, Boston, 1980.

Graef, J., and Cone, T.: *Manual of Pediatric Therapeutics*, Little, Brown, Boston, 1980.

Hellman, L., and Pritzhard, J.: *Williams Obstetrics*, 14th ed., Appleton-Century-Crofts, New York, 1971.

Johns, H., Owens, and Ross: *The Principles and Practice of Medicine*, 18th ed., Appleton-Century-Crofts, New York, 1972.

Krupp, M., and Chatton, M.: *Current Medical Diagnosis and Treatment*, Lange Medical Publications, Los Altos, 1978.

Swift, N.: "Helping Patients Live with Seizures," *Nursing 78*, Vol. 8, No. 6, June 1978.

BIBLIOGRAPHY

Cope, Z.: *The Early Diagnosis of the Acute Abdomen*, Oxford University Press, London, 1968. This is the classic textbook on the acute abdomen. The first four chapters alone give the practitioner the necessary skills and knowledge to assess an abdominal emergency. Varied, individual entities are also described in detail in subsequent chapters, ending with diseases that may simulate the acute abdomen.

Freitag, J., and Miller, L. (eds.): *Manual of Medical Therapeutics*, Little, Brown, Boston, 1980. This text is the looseleaf "Washington Manual," a compendium of medical situations, including both medical and neurologic emergencies, their diagnoses, appropriate laboratory tests, signs and symptoms, and immediate treatment. A very clear set of guidelines for the practitioner in surgical and emergency nursing.

Graef, J., and Cone, T.: *Manual of Pediatric Therapeutics*, Little, Brown, Boston, 1980. A looseleaf reference book dealing with the management and assessment of pediatric diseases and emergencies. Etiology, evaluation, treatment, follow-up, and prevention of each entity is handled concisely. An excellent resource for immediate information needed to assess pediatric situations.

50

Psychiatric Emergencies

Sherry W. Honea and Beverly H. Durrett

ASSAULTIVE BEHAVIOR

DESCRIPTION

Although rare in occurrence, assaultive episodes are perhaps the most disturbing and disruptive situations encountered by emergency room personnel. Often the person who is or has been harmful to others is brought into the emergency room by the police, and therefore has already been subdued, at least to some extent. More difficult to deal with is the person who goes out of control after arriving at the emergency room; this person may be coming in for treatment or may have accompanied someone else for treatment. (Factors—including Health Promotion, Population at Risk, and Screening—contributing to violent behavior are enumerated in Chapter 38, Threats to Survival.)

ASSESSMENT

Due to the difficulties in this situation, assessment may have to be done very quickly, followed by a more detailed assessment after the immediate situation is brought under control. Factors to be considered immediately include:

1. Is the person armed?
2. Are sufficient personnel available to subdue the person?
3. Are others in the environment in danger?

NURSING DIAGNOSES: ACTUAL OR POTENTIAL

1. Physical trauma, threat of.
2. Anxiety, moderate to panic, both in assaultive person and in staff, other clients, family members.
3. Fear secondary to threat of physical injury.

EXPECTED OUTCOMES

1. The client will cause no injury to self or others.
2. The client will regain control of behavior.
3. The client will identify and discuss factors that precipitated out-of-control behaviors.
4. Staff and significant others involved in the situation will discuss their fear and other responses to the assaultive episode.

INTERVENTIONS

1. Telephone, signal by emergency button, or shout for additional staff assistance. Sources for assistance may include emergency room staff, security guards, staff from other areas of the hospital and, as a last resort, visitors to the emergency room.
2. Talk with the violent person and keep talking throughout management of the situation. Often, conveying the expectation that the situation is under control and that the client will behave well is enough to end the crisis.

3. Relatives and friends of the client may serve to either calm or inflame the situation. If their presence is calming, make use of this influence; if inflaming, remove them from the area as quickly as possible.
4. If there is immediate danger to the violent person or others, staff must intervene regardless of personal risk; if violence is destructive only to property, staff should intervene when this can be done at no personal risk.
5. As quickly as possible remove any others who may be in danger.
6. If initial attempts at verbal intervention are not sufficient, move quickly to bring physical measures to bear. Gather as much physical force as will be necessary to subdue the client (at least four people for an adult male). This "show of force" is frequently all that is necessary.
7. When it is obvious that physical control is necessary, limit the client's range of movement and work him or her into a corner if possible.
8. Throwing a blanket over the head or pinning the client to the wall with a lightweight mattress are very effective ways to immobilize a violent person, especially if he or she is armed.
9. After immobilizing the client, bring him or her to the floor in a face down position.
10. Medication (most often phenothiazines) may be administered to effect control. Physical restraint should be maintained until medication takes effect. Close monitoring of vital signs must be maintained, as hypotension is a frequent side effect of phenothiazines.
11. Mechanical restraints should be used only if medication does not sufficiently control the client's behavior. If restraints are necessary, the following precautions should be observed:
    a. Protect skin from abrasion by using padded restraints.
    b. Constant attendance of the client is preferred. If this is not possible, he or she should be checked at least every 15 minutes.
    c. Check circulation of extremities frequently; loosen or reposition restraints as necessary.
    d. If the client is maintained in restraints for more than 2 h, provisions should be made for exercising the extremities. Remove restraint from one extremity at a time, provide range of motion exercises, replace restraint, and repeat procedure for other extremities. If the client is still fighting restraints, at least two staff members should be present when even one extremity is removed from restraint. Repeat every 2 h.
    e. Provide skin care and change position if necessary when the range of motion exercises are performed.
    f. Offer fluids frequently but in small amounts. To prevent aspiration, assist client to a sitting position, if possible, before offering nourishment.
    g. Offer urinal and/or bedpan at frequent intervals.
    h. The decision to remove restraints should be based on careful assessment of the client's physical and mental status. Calming of physical activity and verbalization of intent to cooperate may indicate that the client may be released from restraints. Sufficient personnel should be available to control unpredictable behavior before restraints are removed. Assist the client to walk slowly; postural hypotension may cause initial dizziness and unsteadiness.
12. Seclusion may be necessary to remove the person from stimuli with which he or she cannot cope. If so, the following precautions should be observed.
    a. The room should be "safe," that is, few or no furnishings, protected electrical outlets, recessed light fixtures and a smooth non-toxic finish on walls and floors. If this environment is not available, the client must be constantly attended.
    b. Frequent or constant observation of the client is essential, minimally every 15 minutes.
    c. Staff members should never enter the seclusion room alone, even after the aggressive behavior has subsided.
    d. Food and fluids should be served in nonbreakable, preferably paper, dishes.
    e. The decision to allow the client to come out of the seclusion room to use the toilet will depend on its location. Initially, it

may be advisable to use a portable commode chair or urinal. If the client is allowed to go to the toilet, he or she must be constantly attended. *Providing privacy is not appropriate at this point.*

f. After giving care, always check the room before leaving to be sure you are taking all equipment with you.

g. When the decision is made to allow the client out of seclusion, he or she should be constantly attended until assessment is made of his or her ability to handle additional stimulation.

EVALUATION

Expected Outcome

The person's behavior is brought under control.

Reevaluation and Follow-up

1. Interview of client, if appropriate, to identify precipitating events. If a family member or friend is available, he or she may be able to provide this information.
2. Review of health history for:
   a. Previous record of assaultive behavior.
   b. History of alcohol or drug abuse.
   c. History of psychiatric illness such as schizophrenia, antisocial personality, or paranoid state.
   d. Symptoms suggestive of temporal lobe epilepsy and/or cerebral lesion, such as changes in mental functioning, general change in behavior, and/or adult onset of convulsions without a history of trauma.
   e. Difficulties in interpersonal relationships such as explosive personality, domestic quarreling, general social maladjustment.
3. Assessment of the potential for future incidents of violence. Is this person going back into the same situation that precipitated the current episode? Is he or she experiencing command hallucinations of a homicidal nature?
4. Further treatment will depend on the findings from the assessment. Alternatives may include:
   a. Admission to an inpatient facility for psychiatric and/or medical evaluation.
   b. Referral for treatment of alcohol or drug abuse.
   c. Referral for psychotherapy on an outpatient basis.
5. For all involved in the life-threatening situation, it is essential to provide time for discussion of reactions to the incident. Staff members, as well as other clients, need an opportunity to ventilate their feelings of fear, anger, and frustration generated by the event.
   a. For families or significant others of the client, staff members can offer their time and a private place to discuss the feelings aroused and to make realistic plans for dealing with a similar situation should it arise.
   b. For staff members, it is important to set aside time after particularly stressful episodes to discuss feelings about the client, about their own performance in the situation, and about colleagues' responses to the events. It is particularly helpful if a mental health professional is available to act as a facilitator in such discussions. Regular meetings of emergency room staff with such a facilitator are desirable.

RAPE

See also *Sexual Abuse,* Chapter 41.

DESCRIPTION

Rape is most often defined as sexual intercourse with a woman without her consent. Intercourse may be effected by force or intimidation or the woman may be too young or without sufficient intelligence to give consent. While most rape victims are young women, the elderly and the pregnant woman are also frequent victims, as well as children of both sexes and, occasionally, men. For all victims, rape is an encounter with life-threatening violence. It is not necessarily perceived as primarily a sex crime. Although physical trauma is frequently seen, psychological trauma is usually far more devastating to the victim. Emotional responses include shock, anger, guilt, shame, and fear of rejection by friends and family. Lasting impairment of sexual functioning may be a frequent result of unresolved psychological trauma. (See *Sexual Abuse,* Prevention, Chapter 41.)

ASSESSMENT

Physical Assessment

1. Particularly note bruises, lacerations, general condition of victim's clothing and body.
2. Vaginal examination should be performed with water-moistened speculum. Note any evidence of trauma to external or internal genitalia. Check for anal trauma in male victims.

Psychological Assessment

1. Note mental status.
2. Identify victim's major concerns.
3. Identify social supports available to victim (spouse, family, friends).

Diagnostic Tests

1. Provide for immediate examination of smears from vulva and fornix for presence of motile sperm in women and in anus for both men and women.
2. Culture for *Neisseria* and *Treponema.*
3. Take fingernail scrapings.
4. Comb pubic hair for free hairs.

NURSING DIAGNOSES: ACTUAL OR POTENTIAL

1. Physical trauma.
2. Anxiety, moderate to panic.
3. Alteration in self-concept: potential.
4. Alterations in patterns of sexuality: potential.
5. Exposure to venereal disease.
6. Exposure to unwanted pregnancy.

EXPECTED OUTCOMES

1. The client will recover from physical injuries without sequelae.
2. The client will discuss with staff the fears generated by the assault.
3. The client will identify ongoing support available to her (or him) for counseling.
4. The client will receive prophylactic treatment for venereal disease.
5. The client will be given a choice of prophylaxis against pregnancy.

INTERVENTIONS

1. Make certain that victim is not left alone. If she (or he) comes to the agency alone, stay with her (or him) until arrangements are made for a friend, relative, or rape crisis counselor to be with victim. (Know how to contact the rape crisis center in your community.)
2. Encourage the victim to talk. Assist in identifying feelings, fears, available social supports.
3. Explain physical examination; stay with victim, repeating explanations as necessary.
4. Emphasize the need for preservation of physical evidence in case of prosecution. Do not allow bath or shower before examination.
5. Assist victim in explanation to family or friends if they are available.
6. Provide full information on prophylaxis available for prevention of pregnancy and venereal disease.
7. Arrange escort home. If available, rape crisis counselors may provide this service.
8. Make certain that all findings are accurately recorded in the medical record, including results of the physical examination, description of the victim's appearance and responses, and a description of the assault in her (or his) own words.

EVALUATION

1. Before discharge from the facility, make arrangements for follow-up. A phone call or home visit within a few days to evaluate victim's coping and need for further assistance is appropriate.
2. Counseling may be indicated for the victim and family as they attempt to integrate the experience into their lives. Problems with resuming sexual functioning are common.
3. Long-term therapy may be indicated for the victim who develops phobic reactions, persistent sexual dysfunctions, chronic anxiety, and depression.
4. Staff members may also need assistance in discussing feelings stimulated by working with the rape victim. Staff meetings or one-to-one peer discussions may serve this purpose.

SUICIDE

DESCRIPTION

The term *suicide* is applied to all cases of death resulting directly or indirectly from a positive or negative act of the victim that he or she knew would produce death. *Attempted suicide* is an act so defined, but falling short of actual death. The person who either presents a suicidal risk or who has actually made a suicide attempt is the most common emergency in psychiatric practice. See Chapter 38.

The client may present him or herself to a health agency requesting help in dealing with suicidal impulses or stating she or he has ingested a potentially lethal substance such as pills, household chemicals, pesticides, poison. She or he may be brought into an emergency facility in coma or with self-inflicted physical trauma from any number of causes. A number of factors are positively correlated with high suicide risk. Depression is the most common of these factors. Also included are a history of previous suicide attempts or violent episodes, recent real or perceived loss of personal significance, chronic medical illness, alcohol or drug abuse, and chronic lack of resources such as significant people, money, or purpose.

ASSESSMENT

Physical Examination

1. Trauma.
2. Level of consciousness.
3. Vital signs.

Psychological Assessment

If client's condition permits:

1. Expressed intent. Did this person want to die? Was he or she using the gesture as a cry for help?
2. What are this person's feelings about the outcome of the attempt? Is he or she glad to have been found? Does he or she express wish to have died?
3. What are the client's plans for the future? Does he or she talk about "doing a better job" next time? Can he or she express any hope?

Medical and Psychiatric History

May have to be obtained from family or friends.

1. Previous suicide attempts.
2. Previous episodes of violence.
3. Chronic medical or psychiatric illness.
4. Alcohol or drug use.
5. Prescribed medications. (Some that may cause depression as a side effect include steroids, hormones, antihypertensives.)

Social Assessment

1. Marital status.
2. Living arrangements.
3. Job situation.
4. Financial status.
5. Tangible losses.
6. Blows to self-concept.
7. Friends.

NURSING DIAGNOSES: ACTUAL OR POTENTIAL

1. Physical trauma; self-inflicted.
2. Maladaptive coping patterns: self-destructive behavior.
3. Social isolation.

EXPECTED OUTCOMES

1. The client's physiologic status will stabilize.
2. The client will be protected from further self-harm.
3. The client will discuss with staff member the feelings that led to the suicide attempt.
4. The client will identify alternatives to harming self in coping with current life situation.
5. The client will establish an on-going supportive relationship with professional person or organization.

INTERVENTIONS

1. *Do not leave the victim alone.*
2. Treat physical trauma as indicated (suturing, lavage, setting fractures, oxygen, prepare for surgery, etc.).
3. Encourage expression of feelings.
4. Provide care in a manner to enhance self-esteem. Provide privacy; listen to and acknowledge the feelings of hopelessness and despair.
5. Assist in identifying strengths and resources.
6. Assist in identifying situations that precipitate thoughts of suicide; discuss consequences of self-destructive behavior and more positive alternative coping behaviors based on identified strengths and resources.
7. Avoid guilt-inducing statements such as, "But you have so much to live for," or "Don't you care anything about how your family (friends) feel?"
8. Prepare for dealing with the responses of significant others, which are likely to be anger, guilt, feelings of responsibility for causing the act.
9. In the case of the completed suicide, the family or friends of the victim will need supportive care.

a. Do not leave them alone after they are given the news of the death.
b. Encourage them to talk about their feelings.
c. Acknowledge the difficulty in dealing with grief, anger, and sense of responsibility for the death.
d. Provide assistance in making arrangements for the body.

EVALUATION

Outcome Criterion

Client recovers from suicidal act. See also *The Threat of Suicide*, Expected Outcomes, Chapter 38.

Reevaluation and Follow-up

1. Hospitalization is indicated for management of the continuing high-risk client. Commitment may be necessary and can be effected on the basis of "imminent danger to self" in all jurisdictions.
2. If discharge is planned when client is physiologically stable, provision must be made to ensure that he or she is not alone; family, friends, YWCA, YMCA, Salvation Army are all possible resources.
3. Before releasing client, confirm plans for follow-up, such as referral to personal physician or mental health center.
4. Educate client on availability of emergency services in the community, such as hot line or suicide prevention service.
5. Explore with the client the possibility of family therapy.
6. Assist client in identifying social outlets in the community such as clubs, church groups, volunteer work.

ACUTE ALCOHOLIC INTOXICATION

DESCRIPTION

Alcoholic intoxication may be defined as a state in which the ingestion of alcohol has resulted in noticeable impairment of speech and coordination or in alteration in behavior. The acutely intoxicated client often presents to the emergency room because the impariment in his or her behavior has resulted in accidental injury or has brought him or her to the attention of the police.

ASSESSMENT

It is important to rule-out other medical conditions that may result in behavior that looks like acute intoxication. Assuming that persons who are disoriented or uncoordinated and smell of alcohol are drunk may result in tragedy for those suffering from such conditions as subdural hematoma, other cerebral trauma, hypoglycemia, hepatic failure, diabetic coma, barbiturate overdose, toxic psychosis secondary to mixing alcohol and other drugs. See Assessment, *Alterations in Self-Concept*, Chapter 37.

Physical Examination

1. Vital signs: close monitoring of respiratory rate and depth is essential.
2. Reaction of pupils.
3. Reflexes.
4. Evidence of physical trauma, such as bruises, abrasions, and lacerations.

Health History

May have to be obtained from family or friends.

1. Chronic medical or psychiatric illness.
2. Other drugs ingested or available.
3. History of falls and head trauma.

Drinking History

May have to be obtained from family or friends.

1. Description of this episode. When did drinking start? How much alcohol was consumed? Was there any concomitant food intake?
2. What is the client's usual behavior when drinking?
3. Are any situational factors associated with client's excessive drinking?

Diagnostic Tests

1. Blood alcohol level.
2. Blood sugar level.
3. Blood urea nitrogen.
4. Urine screen for drugs.

NURSING DIAGNOSES: ACTUAL OR POTENTIAL

1. Altered level of consciousness secondary to alcohol ingestion.
2. Respiratory dysfunction: potential.

3. Physical trauma: actual or potential.
4. Maladaptive coping patterns.

EXPECTED OUTCOMES

1. The client will be maintained in physiologically stable condition.
2. The client will recover from physical trauma without sequelae.
3. The client will be protected from any further physical trauma.
4. Before leaving the facility, the client will verbalize understanding of the physiological effects of ingestion of alcohol.
5. Before leaving the facility, the client will identify community resources available to assist with long-term resolution of maladaptive coping patterns.

INTERVENTIONS

1. Treat trauma and acute medical problems, as indicated.
2. Control disruptive behavior.
   a. Nonstimulating environment.
   b. Soft restraints.
   c. Tranquilizing drugs are indicated only in otherwise unmanageable situations. Diazepam (Valium) or chlordiazepoxide (Librium) would be the drug of choice.
   d. Potentially synergistic depression of vital functions requires close monitoring of vital signs.
3. Anti-emetics may be ordered parenterally for nausea.
4. Nonjudgemental attitude is essential on part of care providers. Avoid labeling client as "just another drunk," as the needs for care are legitimate.
5. Attempts at reasoning with the client are likely to be ineffective during intoxicated state. Act to bring situation under control as quickly as possible and then talk with client.
6. When client is sober, attempt to provide information on effects of alcohol, other medical problems, and alternatives for dealing with anxiety and tension, such as meaningful leisure time activities, psychotherapy.

Reevaluation and Follow-Up

1. Hospitalization is indicated if there are serious medical problems.
2. Release to family or friends is first choice if not hospitalized; refer to community facility such as YWCA, YMCA, or Salvation Army if no personal resources exist.
3. Jail may be appropriate if a crime was committed while the client was under the influence of alcohol or if he or she poses a continuing threat to society.
4. Arrange follow-up appointment with health professional or mental health agency to assess extent of alcohol problem and need for long-term therapy.

ACUTE GRIEF REACTION

DESCRIPTION

For purposes of this discussion, an acute grief reaction is one following a sudden unexpected loss of a significant person or persons in one's life. This is likely to be encountered in the emergency room when a friend or relative of a victim of death by trauma, as in an automobile accident, or sudden death from natural causes, such as myocardial infarction or cerebral hemorrhage, is present. The grief reaction may appear in one of several guises, ranging from no apparent emotional reaction to severe emotional outburst. Feelings of anger and guilt are often expressed in self-blaming, such as, "If only I hadn't . . . ;" or blaming health care personnel, such as "Why wasn't there a doctor here sooner? Wasn't there anything else you could do? Don't you care at all?"

ASSESSMENT

1. Is the bereaved person alone?
2. Is this person openly expressing grief?
3. What was the person's relationship with the deceased? How close was the emotional attachment?
4. Is any information available on the physical condition of the bereaved person?
5. What social supports are immediately available?

NURSING DIAGNOSES: ACTUAL OR POTENTIAL

1. Grieving.
2. Maladaptive coping patterns: potential.

EXPECTED OUTCOMES

1. The bereaved person will be assisted to express feelings openly and without guilt.
2. The bereaved person will be assisted in identifying sources of support immediately available to him or her.

INTERVENTIONS

1. Do not leave the bereaved person alone. Staff members should leave only if family members are present and request to be left alone.
2. Provide privacy: take the person away from the mainstream of hospital activity. If a hospital chapel is available, it is ideal. If not, any quiet area can be used.
3. Acknowledge the feelings of sadness, loss, guilt, and anger. Do not encourage the person to blame him- or herself, if this is occurring. Remain as objective as possible.
4. Encourage expression of feelings through verbalization and/or crying.
5. Allow and encourage the bereaved person to see the body of the deceased. This may later be a significant aspect of accepting the reality of the loss of the significant other.
6. If requested, call a minister and/or relative. If not requested, ask the bereaved person if there is anyone he or she wishes to have called.
7. Assist with arrangements for the body: explain basis for autopsy if one is required or requested. Call the undertaker chosen by the bereaved person.
8. Often medications such as sedatives and hypnotics can be given to assist the bereaved to temporarily control intense feelings. Watch for immediate side effects of sedation, such as oversedation and hypotension; monitor vital signs.

EVALUATION

Outcome Criterion

Individual will be supported in the immediate shock phase of grief reaction.

Reevaluation and Follow-Up

1. Do not allow the person to leave the emergency room alone, if this can be avoided. If family, friends, or minister are not available, or if the person is a stranger to the area, contact local social service agencies to provide immediate arrangements for companionship, lodging, and food.
2. Reassess physical condition, particularly if any medical or psychiatric problems are known to exist. Treat any exacerbation of symptoms.
3. Assess suicide risk. This is particularly important if the bereaved person is alone and/or is showing little apparent reaction to the loss. If there is significant suicide risk, and there is no one to stay with the person, hospitalization is indicated.
4. Provide appropriate information to the person about the use and side effects of drugs prescribed to be taken at home. If drugs are given, make sure the person is not driving.
5. Plan time for staff members to deal with their own feelings in response to the death of clients. Group discussions, facilitated by a mental health professional, should be scheduled on a regular basis. Staff members are then better prepared to offer support to one another in times of crisis.

BIBLIOGRAPHY

Ciuca, R. G., Downie, C. S., and Morris, M.: "When a Disaster Happens," *American Journal of Nursing*, **77**:3, March 1977. This is an excellent, objective treatment of an emotion-laden occurrence. It emphasizes the need for every hospital to have a workable disaster plan that includes a mental health team, since emotional support for survivors is as important as medical care for victims. The role of the mental health team is described as one of crisis intervention in the initial phase of shock and grief reactions, with the primary goal being to facilitate the emotional expression of grief.

Gutheil, T. G.: "Observations on the Theoretical Bases for Seclusion of the Psychiatric Inpatient," *American Journal of Psychiatry*, **135**:3, 325–328, March 1978. A convincing argument for the use of seclusion for certain psychiatric inpatients. Dr. Gutheil offers a brief review of the theoretical and clinical rationale for this kind of treatment. He concedes that it is indeed possible to misuse or abuse seclusion, but points out that it can also be very therapeutic when used conservatively and appropriately. He elaborates some alternatives and points out some of its effects.

Lindemann, E.: "Symptomatology and Management of Acute Grief," *American Journal of Psychiatry*, **101**:141–148,

September 1944. This article, a classic of its kind, is as relevant today as when it was written. Dr. Lindemann is a pioneer in the study of bereavement. His theoretical formulations on grief and crisis intervention have been of invaluable assistance to counselors in understanding and treating grief responses, both normal and abnormal. A basic premise is that abnormal grief may be transformed to normal grief through the use of appropriate techniques or preventive intervention. His inquiry has encouraged other investigators to test and observe and has stimulated other studies on crisis.

Loy, W. (ed.): "Confronting Alcoholism: How One Medical/ Surgical Unit Faced the Problem," *Nursing '77*, 54–61, May 1977. A panel of health professionals from Kissimmee, Florida reviews the hospitalization of a woman alcoholic patient. Because the primary problem is an orthopedic one, medical aspects of care are accented; however, there is also a realistic appraisal of the client's emotional needs.

Maynard, C. K., and Chitty, K. K.: "Dealing with Anger: Guidelines for Nursing Intervention," *JPN and Mental Health Services*, **17**:36–42, June 1979. Unexpressed anger often becomes internalized and leads to feelings of powerlessness and frustration. These feelings can in turn precipitate a psychiatric emergency. These authors offer a step-by-step intervention procedure, based on the nursing process, which is designed to help clients deal more effectively with their anger.

Nadelson, C. C., and Notman, M. T.: "Emotional Repercussions of Rape," *Medical Aspects of Human Sexuality*, **11**:16–31, March 1977. The authors discuss many traumatic reactions to rape and elaborate the stages of the rape trauma. Some physiological reactions and emotional responses are predictable and universal; others will vary according to many factors. Regardless of the circumstances, crisis counseling and follow-up are essential for recovery.

Reubin, R.: "Spotting and Stopping the Suicide Patient," *Nursing, '79*, **9**:83–85, April 1979. An interesting article in which the author offers the nurse 10 signs to assess a client's suicide potential, and 10 guidelines to help manage suicidal crisis.

APPENDIXES

APPENDIX CONTENTS

APPENDIX A
DIAGNOSTIC TABLES 1645

Categories of Nursing Diagnoses 1645

DSM-III Classification: Axes I and II Categories and Codes 1679

APPENDIX B
CONVERSION TABLES 1684

Fahrenheit and Celsius Equivalents: Body Temperature Range 1684

Celsius and Fahrenheit Equivalents: Body Temperature Range 1685

Length Conversions 1685

Weight Conversions (Metric and Avoirdupois) 1686

Weight Conversions (Metric and Apothecary) 1686

Volume Conversions (Metric and Apothecary) 1686

Commonly Used Metric and Apothecary Equivalents 1687

Approximate Household Measurement Equivalents (Volume) 1687

Pound-to-Kilogram Conversion 1688

Gram Equivalents for Pounds and Ounces: Conversion for Weight of Newborns 1689

APPENDIX C
CLINICAL LABORATORY VALUES 1690

Critical Laboratory Values 1690

Blood Parameters of Acid–Base Balance during Uncompensated and Compensated States 1692

APPENDIX D
NOMOGRAMS AND GROWTH CHARTS 1693

Body Surface Area of Children: Nomogram for Determination of Body Surface Area from Height and Weight 1693

Body Surface Area of Adults: Nomogram for Determination of Body Surface Area from Height and Weight 1694

Girls: Birth to 36 Months, Physical Growth NCHS Percentiles 1695

Girls: Birth to 36 Months, Physical Growth NCHS Percentiles 1696

Boys: Birth to 36 Months, Physical Growth NCHS Percentiles 1697

Boys: Birth to 36 Months, Physical Growth NCHS Percentiles 1698

Girls: 2 to 18 Years, Physical Growth NCHS Percentiles 1699

Girls: Prepubescent, Physical Growth NCHS Percentiles 1700

Boys: 2 to 18 Years, Physical Growth NCHS Percentiles 1701

Boys: Prepubescent, Physical Growth NCHS Percentiles 1702

APPENDIX E
COMMUNICABLE DISEASE TABLE 1703

Communicable and Infectious Diseases 1703

APPENDIX F
DIETARY TABLES 1713

Mean Heights and Weights and Recommended Energy Intake 1713

Recommended Daily Dietary Allowances 1714

APPENDIX CONTENTS *(continued)*

Estimated Safe and Adequate Daily Dietary Intakes of Additional Selected Vitamins and Minerals 1716

Canadian Dietary Standards 1717

Guide to Good Nutrition: Basic Four Food Groups 1719

Formula for Full-Term Infants 1720

Formula for Low-Birth-Weight Infants 1721

Food Exchange Lists 1722

Cultural Food Habits 1725

APPENDIX G
VITAL STATISTICS 1733

Birth and Death Rates, 1960 to 1980 1733

Deaths and Death Rates for the 10 Leading Causes of Death in Specified Age Groups: United States, 1979 1734

Appendix A

Diagnostic Tables

CATEGORIES OF NURSING DIAGNOSES

The categories of nursing diagnoses listed in the tables below are those currently accepted by the Third, Fourth, and Fifth National Conferences on Nursing Diagnoses (reproduced from Kim, M. J., McFarland, G. K., and McLane, A. M.: *Classification of Nursing Diagnoses: Proceedings of the Fifth National Conference*, Mosby, St. Louis, 1984). It is important to note that these are working documents with research and revision in progress. National Conferences gather nurses together every two years, but research in new categories and for accepted categories is an ongoing priority.

ACTIVITY INTOLERANCE

Etiology	Defining Characteristics
Bedrest/immobility	Verbal report of fatigue or weakness[a]
Generalized weakness	Abnormal heart rate or blood pressure response to activity
Sedentary lifestyle	Exertional discomfort or dyspnea
Imbalance between oxygen supply/demand	Electrocardiographic changes reflecting arrhythmias or ischemia

[a] Critical defining characteristics.

AIRWAY CLEARANCE, INEFFECTIVE

Etiology	Defining Characteristics
Decreased energy/fatigue	Abnormal breath sounds [rales (crackles), rhonchi (wheezes)]
Tracheobronchial	Changes in rate or depth of respiration
Infection	Tachypnea
Obstruction	Cough, effective/ineffective; with or without sputum
Secretion	Cyanosis
Perceptual/cognitive impairment	Dyspnea
Trauma	

ANXIETY

Definition: A vague, uneasy feeling the source of which is often nonspecific or unknown to the individual.

Etiology	Defining Characteristics: Subjective	Defining Characteristics: Objective
Unconscious conflict about essential values/goals of life Threat to self-concept Threat of death Threat to or change in health status Threat to or change in socioeconomic status Threat to or change in role functioning Threat to or change in environment Threat to or change in interaction patterns Situational/maturational crises Interpersonal transmission/ contagion of unmet needs	Increased tension Apprehension Painful and persistent increased helplessness Uncertainty Fearful Scared Regretful Overexcited Rattled Distressed Jittery Feelings of inadequacy Shakiness Fear of unspecified consequences Expressed concerns about change in life events Worried Anxious	Sympathetic stimulation: cardiovascular excitation, superficial vasoconstriction, pupil dilation[a] Restlessness Insomnia Glancing about Poor eye contact Trembling/hand tremors Extraneous movement (foot shuffling, hand/arm movements) Facial tension Voice quivering Focus on "self" Increased wariness Increased perspiration

[a] Critical defining characteristic.

BOWEL ELIMINATION, ALTERATION IN: CONSTIPATION

Etiology	Defining Characteristics	Other Possible Defining Characteristics
To be developed	Decreased activity level Frequency less than usual pattern Hard formed stool Palpable mass Reported feeling of pressure in rectum Reported feeling of rectal fullness Straining at stool	Abdominal pain Appetite impairment Back pain Headache Interference with daily living Use of laxatives

BOWEL ELIMINATION, ALTERATION IN: DIARRHEA

Etiology	Defining Characteristics	Other Possible Defining Characteristics
To be developed	Abdominal pain Cramping Increased frequency Increased frequency of bowel sounds Loose, liquid stools Urgency	Changes in color

BOWEL ELIMINATION, ALTERATION IN: INCONTINENCE

Etiology	Defining Characteristics
To be developed	Involuntary passage of stool

BREATHING PATTERN, INEFFECTIVE

Etiology	Defining Characteristics
Neuromuscular impairment Pain Musculoskeletal impairment Perception/cognitive impairment Anxiety Decreased energy/fatigue	Dyspnea Shortness of breath Tachypnea Fremitus Abnormal arterial blood gas Cyanosis Cough Nasal flaring Respiratory depth changes Assumption of 3-point position Pursed-lip breathing/prolonged expiratory phase Increased anteroposterior diameter Use of accessory muscles Altered chest excursion

CARDIAC OUTPUT, ALTERATION IN: DECREASED

Etiology	Defining Characteristics	Other Possible Defining Characteristics
To be developed	Variations in blood pressure readings Arrhythmias Fatigue Jugular vein distension Color changes, skin and mucous membranes Oliguria Decreased peripheral pulses Cold, clammy skin Rales Dyspnea Orthopnea Restlessness	Change in mental status Shortness of breath Syncope Vertigo Edema Cough Frothy sputum Gallop rhythm Weakness

COMFORT, ALTERATION IN: PAIN

	Defining Characteristics	
Etiology	Subjective	Objective
Injuring agents: Biological Chemical Physical Psychological	Communication (verbal or coded) of pain descriptors	Guarding behavior, protective Self-focusing Narrowed focus (altered time perception, withdrawal from social contact, impaired thought process) Distraction behavior (moaning, crying, pacing, seeking out other people and/or activities, restlessness) Facial mask of pain (eyes lack luster, "beaten look," fixed or scattered movement, grimace) Alteration in muscle tone (may span from listless to rigid) Autonomic responses not seen in chronic stable pain (diaphoresis, blood pressure and pulse rate change, pupillary dilatation, increased or decreased respiratory rate)

COMMUNICATION, IMPAIRED VERBAL

Etiology	Defining Characteristics
Decrease in circulation to the brain	Unable to speak dominant language[a]
Physical barrier, brain tumor, tracheostomy, intubation	Speaks or verbalizes with difficulty[a]
Anatomical deficit, cleft palate	Does not or cannot speak[a]
Psychological barriers, psychosis, lack of stimuli	Stuttering
Cultural difference	Slurring
Developmental or age-related	Difficulty forming words or sentences
	Difficulty expressing thought verbally
	Inappropriate verbalization
	Dyspnea
	Disorientation

[a] Critical defining characteristic.

COPING, INEFFECTIVE INDIVIDUAL

Definition: Ineffective coping is the impairment of adaptive behaviors and problem-solving abilities of a person in meeting life's demands and roles.

Etiology	Defining Characteristics
Situational crises	Verbalization of inability to cope or inability to ask for help[a]
Maturational crises	Inability to meet role expectations
Personal vulnerability	Inability to meet basic needs
	Inability to problem-solve[a]
	Alteration in societal participation
	Destructive behavior toward self or others
	Inappropriate use of defense mechanisms
	Change in usual communication patterns
	Verbal manipulation
	High illness rate
	High rate of accidents

[a] Critical defining characteristic.

COPING, INEFFECTIVE FAMILY: COMPROMISED

Definition: A usually supportive primary person (family member or close friend) is providing insufficient, ineffective, or compromised support, comfort, assistance, or encouragement which may be needed by the client to manage or master adaptive tasks related to his or her health challenge.

	Defining Characteristics	
Etiology	**Subjective**	**Objective**
Inadequate or incorrect information or understanding by a primary person Temporary preoccupation by a significant person who is trying to manage emotional conflicts and personal suffering and is unable to perceive or act effectively in regard to client's needs Temporary family disorganization and role changes Other situational or developmental crises or situations the significant person may be facing The client providing little support in turn for primary person Prolonged disease or disability progression that exhausts the supportive capacity of significant people	Client expresses or confirms a concern or complaint about significant other's response to his or her health problem Significant person describes preoccupation with personal reactions, e.g., fear, anticipatory grief, guilt, anxiety, to client's illness, disability, or to other situational or developmental crises Significant person describes or confirms an inadequate understanding or knowledge base which interferes with effective assistance or supportive behaviors	Significant person attempts assistive or supportive behaviors with less than satisfactory results Significant person withdraws or enters into limited or temporary personal communication with the client at time of need Significant person displays protective behavior disproportionate (too little or too much) to the client's abilities or need for autonomy

COPING, INEFFECTIVE FAMILY: DISABLING

Definition: The behavior of a significant person (family member or other primary person) disables his or her own capacities and the client's capacities to effectively address tasks essential to either person's adaptation to the health challenge.

Etiology	Defining Characteristics
Significant person with chronically unexpressed feelings of guilt, anxiety, hostility, despair, etc. Dissonant discrepancy of coping styles being used to deal with the adaptive tasks by the significant person and client or among significant people Highly ambivalent family relationships Arbitrary handling of a family's resistance to treatment which tends to solidify defensiveness as it fails to deal adequately with underlying anxiety	Neglectful care of the client in regard to basic human needs and/or illness treatment Distortion of reality regarding the client's health problem, including extreme denial about its existence or severity Intolerance Rejection Abandonment Desertion Carrying on usual routines, disregarding client's needs Psychosomaticism Taking on illness signs of client Decisions and actions by family which are detrimental to economic or social well-being Agitation, depression, aggression, hostility Impaired restructuring of a meaningful life for self, impaired individualization, prolonged overconcern for client Neglectful relationships with other family members Client's development of helpless, inactive dependence

COPING, FAMILY: POTENTIAL FOR GROWTH

Definition: The family member has effectively managed adaptive tasks involved with the client's health challenge and is exhibiting desire and readiness for enhanced health and growth in regard to self and in relation to client.

Etiology	Defining Characteristics
The person's basic needs are sufficiently gratified and adaptive tasks effectively addressed to enable goals of self-actualization to surface	The family member attempts to describe growth impact of crisis on his or her own values, priorities, goals, or relationships Family member is moving in direction of health-promoting and enriching lifestyle which supports and monitors maturational processes, audits and negotiates treatment programs, and generally chooses experiences which optimize wellness Individual expresses interest in making contact on a one-to-one basis or on a mutual-aid group basis with another person who has experienced a similar situation

DIVERSIONAL ACTIVITY, DEFICIT

Etiology	Defining Characteristics
Environmental lack of diversional activity Long-term hospitalization Frequent, lengthy treatments	Patient's statements regarding: Boredom Wish there were something to do, to read, etc. Usual hobbies cannot be undertaken in hospital

FAMILY PROCESSES, ALTERATION IN

Etiology	Defining Characteristics
Situation transition and/or crisis Development transition and/or crisis	Family system unable to meet physical needs of its members Family system unable to meet emotional needs of its members Family system unable to meet spiritual needs of its members Parents do not demonstrate respect for each other's views on child-rearing practices Inability to express/accept wide range of feelings Inability to express/accept feelings of members Family unable to meet security needs of its members Inability to accept/receive help appropriately Family does not demonstrate respect for individuality and autonomy of its members Inability of the family members to relate to each other for mutual growth and maturation Family uninvolved in community activities Rigidity in function and roles Family inability to adapt to change/deal with traumatic experience constructively Family fails to accomplish current/past developmental task Unhealthy family decision-making process Failure to send and receive clear messages Inappropriate boundary maintenance Inappropriate/poorly communicated family rules, rituals, symbols Unexamined family myths Inappropriate level and direction of energy

FEAR

Definition: Fear is a feeling of dread related to an identifiable source which the person validates.

Etiology	Defining Characteristics
To be developed	Ability to identify object of fear

FLUID VOLUME DEFICIT, ACTUAL

Etiology	Defining Characteristics	Other Possible Defining Characteristics
Failure of regulatory mechanisms Active loss	Dilute urine Increased urine output Sudden weight loss Decreased urine output Concentrated urine Output greater than intake Decreased venous filling Hemoconcentration Increased serum sodium	Possible weight gain Hypotension Decreased venous filling Increased pulse rate Decreased skin turgor Decreased pulse volume/ pressure Increased body temperature Dry skin Dry mucous membranes Hemoconcentration Weakness Edema Thirst Change in mental state

FLUID VOLUME DEFICIT, POTENTIAL

Etiology	Defining Characteristics
Extremes of age Extremes of weight Excessive losses through normal routes, e.g., diarrhea Loss of fluid through abnormal routes, e.g., indwelling tubes Deviations affecting access to, intake of, or absorption of fluids, e.g., physical immobility Factors influencing fluid needs, e.g., hypermetabolic states Knowledge deficiency related to fluid volume Medications, e.g., diuretics	Increased output Urinary frequency Thirst Altered intake

FLUID VOLUME, ALTERATION IN: EXCESS

Etiology	Defining Characteristics
Comprised regulatory mechanism Excess fluid intake Excess sodium intake	Edema Effusion Anasarca Weight gain Shortness of breath (SOB), orthopnea Intake greater than output S_3 heart sound Pulmonary congestion: chest x-ray Abnormal breath sounds: crackles (rales) Change in respiratory pattern Change in mental status Decreased hemoglobin and hematocrit Blood pressure changes Central venous pressure changes Pulmonary artery pressure changes Jugular vein distention Positive hepatojugular reflex Oliguria Specific gravity changes Azotemia Altered electrolytes Restlessness and anxiety

GAS EXCHANGE, IMPAIRED

Etiology	Defining Characteristics
Ventilation, perfusion imbalance	Confusion Somnolence Restlessness Irritability Inability to move secretions Hypercapnea Hypoxia

GRIEVING, ANTICIPATORY

Etiology	Defining Characteristics	
To be developed	Potential loss of significant object Expression of distress at potential loss Denial of potential loss Guilt Anger Sorrow	Choked feelings Changes in eating habits Alterations in sleep patterns Alterations in activity level Altered libido Altered communication patterns

GRIEVING, DYSFUNCTIONAL

Etiology	Defining Characteristics	
Actual or perceived object loss (object loss is used in the broadest sense). Objects include people, possessions, a job, status, home, ideals, parts and processes of the body, etc.	Verbal expression of distress at loss Denial of loss Expression of guilt Expression of unresolved issues Anger Sadness Crying Difficulty in expressing loss Alterations in: Eating habits Sleep patterns Dream patterns Activity level Libido	Idealization of lost object Reliving of past experiences Interference with life functioning Developmental regression Labile affect Alterations in concentration and/or pursuits of tasks

HEALTH MAINTENANCE, ALTERATIONS IN

Definition: Inability to identify, manage, and seek out help to maintain health.

Etiology	Defining Characteristics
Lack of, or significant alteration in, communication skills (written, verbal, and gestural)	Demonstrated lack of knowledge regarding basic health practices
Lack of ability to make deliberate and thoughtful judgments	Demonstrated lack of adaptive behaviors to internal/external environmental changes
Perceptual/cognitive impairment, complete/partial lack of gross and fine motor skills	Reported or observed inability to take responsibility for meeting basic health practices in any or all functional pattern areas
Ineffective individual coping, dysfunctional grieving	History of lack of health seeking behavior
Unachieved developmental tasks	Expressed client interest in improving health behaviors
Ineffective family coping: spiritually disabling	Reported or observed lack of equipment, financial, and other resources
Lack of material resources	Reported or observed impairment of personal support system

HOME MAINTENANCE MANAGEMENT, IMPAIRED

Definition: The client is unable to independently maintain a safe, growth-promoting immediate environment.

	Defining Characteristics	
Etiology	Subjective	Objective
Individual/family member disease or injury	Household members express difficulty in maintaining their home in a comfortable fashion[a]	Disorderly surroundings
Insufficient family organization or planning	Household requests assistance with home maintenance[a]	Unwashed or unavailable cooking equipment, clothes, or linen[a]
Insufficient finances	Household members describe outstanding debts or financial crises[a]	Accumulation of dirt, food wastes, or hygienic wastes[a]
Unfamiliarity with neighborhood resources		Offensive odors
Impaired cognitive or emotional functioning		Inappropriate household temperature
Lack of knowledge		Overtaxed family members, e.g., exhausted, anxious family members[a]
Lack of role modeling		Lack of necessary equipment or aids
Inadequate support systems		Presence of vermin or rodents
		Repeated hygienic disorders, infestations, or infections[a]

[a] Critical defining characteristic.

INJURY: POTENTIAL FOR

Etiology

Interactive conditions between individual and environment which impose a risk to the defensive and adaptive resources of the individual

Internal Factors, Host	External Environment
Biological	Biological
Chemical	Chemical
Physiological	Physiological
Psychological perception	Psychological
Developmental	People/provider

Defining Characteristics

Internal	External
Biochemical:	Biological:
Regulatory function:	Immunization level of community
Sensory dysfunction	Microorganism
Integrative dysfunction	Chemical:
Effector dysfunction	Pollutants
Tissue hypoxia	Poisons
Malnutrition	Drugs:
Immune-autoimmune	Pharmaceutical agents
Abnormal blood profile:	Alcohol
Leukocytosis/leukopenia	Caffeine
Altered clotting factors	Nicotine
Thrombocytopenia	Preservatives
Sickle cell	Cosmetics and dyes
Thalassemia	Nutrients (vitamins, food types)
Decreased hemoglobin	Physical:
Physical:	Design, structure and arrangement of community, building and/or equipment
Broken skin	Mode of transport/transportation
Altered mobility	Nosocomial agents
Developmental:	People-provider:
Age:	Nosocomial agent
Physiological	Staffing patterns
Psychosocial	Cognitive, affective, and psychomotor factors
Psychological:	
Affective	
Orientation	

A. Poisoning, Potential for

Definition: The client has accentuated risk of accidental exposure to or ingestion of drugs or dangerous products in doses sufficient to cause poisoning.

Defining Characteristics

Internal (Individual) Factors	External (Environmental) Factors
Reduced vision Verbalization of occupational setting without adequate safeguards Lack of safety or drug education Lack of proper precaution Cognitive or emotional difficulties Insufficient finances	Large supplies of drugs in house Medicines stored in unlocked cabinets accessible to children or confused persons Dangerous products placed or stored within the reach of children or confused persons Availability of illicit drugs potentially contaminated by poisonous additives Flaking, peeling paint or plaster in presence of young children Chemical contamination of food and water Unprotected contact with heavy metals or chemicals Paint, lacquer, etc., in poorly ventilated areas or without effective protection Presence of poisonous vegetation Presence of atmospheric pollutants

B. Suffocation, Potential for

Definition: The client has accentuated risk of accidental suffocation (inadequate air is available for inhalation).

Defining Characteristics

Internal (Individual) Factors	External (Environmental) Factors
Reduced olfactory sensation Reduced motor abilities Lack of safety education Lack of safety precautions Cognitive or emotional difficulties Disease or injury process	Pillow placed in an infant's crib Propped bottle placed in an infant's crib Vehicle warming in closed garage Children playing with plastic bags or inserting small objects into their mouths or noses Discarded or unused refrigerators or freezers without removed doors Children left unattended in bathtubs or pools Household gas leaks Smoking in bed Use of fuel-burning heaters not vented to outside Low-strung clothesline Pacifier hung around infant's head Person who eats large mouthfuls of food

C. Trauma, Potential for

Definition: The client has accentuated risk of accidental tissue injury, e.g., wound, burn, fracture.

Defining Characteristics		
Internal (Individual) Factors	**External (Environmental) Factors**	
Weakness Poor vision Balancing difficulties Reduced temperature and/or tactile sensation Reduced large- or small-muscle coordination Reduced hand-eye coordination Lack of safety education Lack of safety precautions Insufficient finances to purchase safety equipment or effect repairs Cognitive or emotional difficulties History of previous trauma	Slippery floors, e.g., wet or highly waxed Snow or ice collected on stairs, walkways Unanchored rugs Bathtub without hand grip or antislip equipment Use of unsteady ladders or chairs Entering unlighted rooms Unsturdy or absent stair rails Unanchored electric wires Litter or liquid spills on floors or stairways High beds Children playing without gates at the top of stairs Obstructed passageways Unsafe window protection in homes with young children Inappropriate call-for-aid mechanisms for bed-resting client Pot handles facing toward front of stove Bathing in very hot water, e.g., unsupervised bathing of young children Potential igniting gas leaks Delayed lighting of gas burner or oven Experimenting with chemicals or gasoline Unscreened fires or heaters Wearing plastic aprons or flowing clothing around open flame Children playing with matches, candles, cigarettes Inadequately stored combustibles or corrosives, e.g., matches, oily rags, lye	Highly flammable children's toys or clothing Overloaded fuse boxes Contact with rapidly moving machinery, industrial belts, or pulleys Sliding on coarse bed linen or struggling within bed restraints Faulty electrical plugs, frayed wires, or defective appliances Contact with acids or alkalis Playing with fireworks or gunpowder Contact with intense cold Overexposure to sun, sun lamps, radiotherapy Use of cracked dishware or glasses Knives stored uncovered Guns or ammunition stored unlocked Large icicles hanging from roof Exposure to dangerous machinery Children playing with sharp-edged toys High-crime neighborhood and vulnerable client Driving a mechanically unsafe vehicle Driving after partaking of alcoholic beverages or drugs Driving at excessive speeds Driving without necessary visual aids Children riding in the front seat in car Unrestrained babies riding in car Nonuse or misuse of seat restraints

Defining Characteristics		
Internal (Individual) Factors	**External (Environmental) Factors**	
	Smoking in bed or near oxygen Overloaded electrical outlets Grease waste collected on stoves Use of thin or worn pot holders or mitts	Nonuse or misuse of necessary headgear for motorized cyclists or young children carried on adult bicycles Unsafe road or road-crossing conditions Play or work near vehicle pathways, e.g., driveways, laneways, railroad tracks

KNOWLEDGE DEFICIT

Etiology	Defining Characteristics
Lack of exposure Lack or recall Information misinterpretation Cognitive limitation Lack of interest in learning Unfamiliarity with information resources	Verbalization of the problem Inaccurate follow-through of instruction Inadequate performance of test Inappropriate or exaggerated behaviors, e.g., hysterical, hostile, agitated, apathetic

MOBILITY, IMPAIRED PHYSICAL

Etiology	Defining Characteristics
Intolerance to activity/decreased strength and endurance Pain/discomfort Perceptual/cognitive impairment Neuromuscular impairment Musculoskeletal impairment Depression/severe anxiety	Inability to purposefully move within the physical environment, including bed mobility, transfer, and ambulation Reluctance to attempt movement Limited range of motion Decreased muscle strength, control, and/or mass Imposed restrictions of movement, including mechanical, medical protocol Impaired coordination

Suggested Code for Functional Level Classification

0	Completely independent
1	Requires use of equipment or device
2	Requires help from another person, for assistance, supervision or teaching
3	Requires help from another person *and* equipment or device
4	Is dependent, does not participate in activity

SOURCE: Adapted from Jones, E., et al. *Patient Classification for Long-Term Care: User's Manual,* HEW, Publication No. HRA-74-3107, November 1974.

Comment: Use of a scale applicable when patients are rated from dependence to independence is suggested.

NONCOMPLIANCE (SPECIFY)

Definition: Noncompliance is a person's informed decision not to adhere to a therapeutic recommendation.

Etiology	Defining Characteristics
Patient value system: Health beliefs Cultural influences Spiritual values Client-provider relationships	Behavior indicative of failure to adhere by direct observation, statements by patient or significant others[a] Objective tests (physiological measures, detection of markers) Evidence of development of complications Evidence of exacerbation of symptoms Failure to keep appointments Failure to progress

[a] Critical defining characteristic.

NUTRITION, ALTERATIONS IN: LESS THAN BODY REQUIREMENTS

Etiology	Defining Characteristics	
Inability to ingest or digest food or absorb nutrients due to biological, psychological, or economic factors	Loss of weight with adequate food intake 20% or more under ideal body weight Reported inadequate food intake less than RDA[a] Weakness of muscles required for swallowing or mastication Reported or evidence of lack of food Lack of interest in food Perceived inability to ingest food Aversion to eating Reported altered taste sensation	Satiety immediately after ingesting food Abdominal pain with or without pathology Sore, inflamed buccal cavity Capillary fragility Abdominal cramping Diarrhea and/or steatorrhea Hyperactive bowel sounds Pale conjunctiva and mucous membranes Poor muscle tone Excessive loss of hair Lack of information, misinformation Misconceptions

[a] RDA, Recommended Daily Allowance.

NUTRITION, ALTERATIONS IN: MORE THAN BODY REQUIREMENTS

Etiology	Defining Characteristics
Excessive intake in relationship to metabolic need	Weight 10% over ideal for height and frame Weight 20% over ideal for height and frame[a] Triceps skin fold greater than 15 mm in men and 25 mm in women[a] Sedentary activity level Reported or observed dysfunctional eating patterns: Pairing food with other activities Concentrating food intake at end of day Eating in response to external cues such as time of day, social situation Eating in response to internal cues other than hunger, e.g., anxiety

[a] Critical defining characteristic.

NUTRITION, ALTERATIONS IN: POTENTIAL FOR MORE THAN BODY REQUIREMENTS

Etiology	Defining Characteristics
Hereditary predisposition Excessive energy intake during late gestational life, early infancy and adolescence Frequent, closely spaced pregnancies Dysfunctional psychological conditioning in relationship to food Membership in lower socioeconomic group	Reported or observed obesity in one or both parents[a] Rapid transition across growth percentiles in infants or children[a] Reported use of solid food as major food source before 5 months of age Observed use of food as reward or comfort measure Reported or observed higher baseline weight at beginning of each pregnancy Dysfunctional eating patterns: Pairing food with other activities Concentrating food intake at end of day Eating in response to external cues such as time of day, social situation Eating in response to internal cues other than hunger such as anxiety

[a] Critical defining characteristic.

ORAL MUCOUS MEMBRANE, ALTERATIONS IN

Etiology	Defining Characteristics
Pathological condition: oral cavity radiation to head and/or neck, dehydration Trauma: Chemical, e.g., acidic foods, drugs, noxious agents, alcohol Mechanical, e.g., ill-fitting dentures, braces, endotracheal/nasogastric tubes, oral cavity surgery Nothing by mouth for more than 24 hours Ineffective oral hygiene Mouth breathing Malnutrition Infections Lack of or decreased salivation Medication	Oral pain/discomfort Coated tongue Xerostomia (dry mouth) Stomatitis Oral lesions or ulcers Lack of or decreased salivation Leukoplakia Edema Hyperemia Oral plaque Desquamation Vesicles Hemorrhagic gingivitis Carious teeth Halitosis

PARENTING, ALTERATIONS IN: ACTUAL OR POTENTIAL

Definition: Parenting is the ability of a nurturing figure(s) to create an environment which promotes the optimum growth and development of another human being. It is important to state as a preface to this diagnosis that adjustment to parenting in general is a normal maturational process that elicits nursing behaviors of prevention of potential problems and health promotion.

Etiology	Defining Characteristics
Lack of available role model	*For actual and potential*
Ineffective role model	Lack of parental attachment behaviors[a]
Physical and psychosocial abuse of nurturing figure	Inappropriate visual, tactile, auditory stimulation
Lack of support between/from significant other(s)	Negative identification of infant/child's characteristics
Unmet social/emotional maturation needs of parenting figures	Negative attachment of meanings to infant/child's characteristics
Interruption in bonding process, i.e., maternal, paternal, other	Constant verbalization of disappointment in gender or physical characteristics of the infant/child
Unrealistic expectation for self, infant, partner	Verbalization of resentment towards the infant/child
Perceived threat to own survival, physical and emotional	Verbalization of role inadequacy
Mental and/or physical illness	Inattention to infant/child needs[b]
Presence of stress: financial, legal, recent crisis, cultural move	Verbal disgust at body functions of infant/child
Lack of knowledge	Noncompliance with health appointments for self and/or infant/child
Limited cognitive functioning	Inappropriate caretaking behaviors (toilet training, sleep/rest, feeding)[b]
Lack of role identity	Inappropriate or inconsistent discipline practices
Lack of or inappropriate response of child to relationship	Frequent accidents
Multiple pregnancies	Frequent illness
	Growth and development lag in the child
	History of child abuse or abandonment by primary caretaker[b]
	Verbalizes desire to have child call him/herself by first name versus traditional cultural tendencies
	Child received care from multiple caretakers without consideration for the needs of the infant/child
	Compulsively seeking role approval from others
	For actual
	Abandonment[a]
	Runaway
	Verbalization cannot control child[a]
	Evidence of physical and psychological trauma

[a] Highly critical factor.
[b] Critical defining characteristic.

POWERLESSNESS

Definition: The perception that one's own action will not significantly affect an outcome. Powerlessness is a perceived lack of control over a current situation or immediate happening.

	Defining Characteristics		
Etiology	**Severe**	**Moderate**	**Low-Passivity**
Health care environment Interpersonal interaction Illness related regimen Lifestyle of helplessness	Verbal expressions of having no control or influence over situation Verbal expressions of having no control or influence over outcome Verbal expressions of having no control over self-care Depression over physical deterioration which occurs despite patient compliance with regimens Apathy	Nonparticipation in care or decision making when opportunities are provided Expressions of dissatisfaction and frustration over inability to perform previous tasks and/or activities Does not monitor progress Expression of doubt regarding role performance Reluctance to express true feelings fearing alienation from care givers Passivity Inability to seek information regarding care Dependence on others that may result in irritability, resentment, anger, and guilt Does not defend self-care practices when challenged	Expressions of uncertainty about fluctuating energy levels

RAPE-TRAUMA SYNDROME

Definition: Rape is forced, violent sexual penetration against the victim's will and without the victim's will and consent. The trauma syndrome which develops from this attack or attempted attack includes an acute phase or disorganization of the victim's lifestyle and a long-term process of reorganization of lifestyle.

A. Rape Trauma

Defining Characteristics

Acute Phase	Long-term Phase
Emotional reactions Anger Embarassment Fear of physical violence and death Humiliation Revenge Self-blame Multiple physical symptoms Gastrointestinal irritability Genitourinary discomfort Muscle tension Sleep pattern disturbance	Changes in lifestyle (changes in residence; dealing with repetitive nightmares and phobias; seeking family support; seeking social network support)

B. Compound Reaction

Defining Characteristics

All defining characteristics listed under rape trauma
Reactivated symptoms of previous conditions, i.e., physical illness, psychiatric illness
Reliance on alcohol and/or drugs

C. Silent Reaction

Defining Characteristics

Abrupt changes in relationships with men
Increase in nightmares
Increasing anxiety during interview, i.e., blocking of associations, long periods of silence, minor stuttering, physical distress
Marked changes in sexual behavior
No verbalization of the occurrence of rape
Sudden onset of phobic reactions

SELF-CARE DEFICIT: FEEDING, BATHING/HYGIENE, DRESSING/GROOMING, TOILETING

Etiology

Intolerance to activity, decreased strength and endurance
Pain, discomfort
Perceptual or cognitive impairment
Neuromuscular impairment
Musculoskeletal impairment
Depression, severe anxiety

A. Self-Feeding Deficit (Level 0 to 4)

Defining Characteristics

Inability to bring food from a receptacle to the mouth

B. Self-Bathing/Hygiene Deficit (Level 0 to 4)

Defining Characteristics

Inability to wash body or body parts[a]
Inability to obtain or get to water source
Inability to regulate temperature or flow

C. Self-Dressing/Grooming Deficits (Level 0 to 4)

Defining Characteristics

Impaired ability to put on or take off necessary items of clothing[a]
Impaired ability to obtain or replace articles of clothing
Impaired ability to fasten clothing
Inability to maintain appearance at a satisfactory level

D. Self-Toileting Deficit (Level 0 to 4)

Etiology (Broad Categories)	Defining Characteristics
Impaired transfer ability Impaired mobility status Intolerance to activity, decreasing strength and endurance Pain, discomfort Perceptual or cognitive impairment Neuromuscular impairment Musculoskeletal impairment Depression, severe anxiety	Unable to get to toilet or commode[a] Unable to sit or rise from toilet or commode[a] Unable to manipulate clothing for toileting[a] Unable to carry out proper toilet hygiene[a] Unable to flush toilet or empty commode

Suggested Code for Functional Level Classification

0	Completely independent
1	Requires use of equipment or device
2	Requires help from another person, for assistance, supervision or teaching
3	Requires help from another person *and* equipment or device
4	Is dependent, does not participate in activity

SOURCE: Adapted from Jones, E., et al.: *Patient Classification for Long-Term Care: Users' Manual*, HEW, Publication No. HRA-74-3107, November 1974.

[a] Critical defining characteristic.

Comment: Use of a scale applicable when patients are rated from dependence to independence is suggested.

SELF-CONCEPTS, DISTURBANCE IN: BODY IMAGE, SELF-ESTEEM, ROLE PERFORMANCE, PERSONAL IDENTITY

Definition: A disturbance in self-concept is a disruption in the way one perceives one's body image, self-esteem, role performance, and/or personal identity. These four subcomponents, in turn, have their own etiologies and defining characteristics.

A. Body Image, Disturbance in

Etiology	Defining Characteristics	
Biophysical Cognitive perceptual Psychosocial Cultural or spiritual	Either A or B must be present to justify the diagnosis of body image, alteration in: A. Verbal response to actual or perceived change in structure and/or function[a] B. Nonverbal response to actual or perceived change in structure and/or function[a] The following clinical manifestations may be used to validate the presence of A or B	
	Objective	**Subjective**
	Missing body part Actual change in structure and/or function Not looking at body part Not touching body part Hiding or overexposing body part (intentional or unintentional) Trauma to nonfunctioning part Change in social involvement Change in ability to estimate spatial relationship of body to environment	Verbalization of: Change in lifestyle Fear of rejection or of reaction by others Focus on past strength, function, or appearance Negative feelings about body Feelings of helplessness, hopelessness, or powerlessness Preoccupation with change or loss Emphasis on remaining strengths, heightened achievement Extension of body boundary to incorporate environmental objects Personalization of part or loss by name Depersonalization of part or loss by use of impersonal pronouns Refusal to verify actual change

SELF-CONCEPTS, DISTURBANCE IN: BODY IMAGE, SELF-ESTEEM, ROLE PERFORMANCE, PERSONAL IDENTITY *(continued)*

B. Self-Esteem, Disturbance in

Etiology	Defining Characteristics
To be developed	Inability to accept positive reinforcement Lack of follow-through Nonparticipation in therapy Not taking responsibility for self-care (self-neglect) Self-destructive behavior Lack of eye contact

C. Role Performance, Disturbance in

Etiology	Defining Characteristics
To be developed	Change in self-perception of role Denial of role Change in others' perception of role Conflict in roles Change in physical capacity to resume role Lack of knowledge of role Change in usual patterns or responsibility

D. Personal Identity, Disturbance in

Definition: Inability to distinguish between self and nonself.

Etiology	Defining Characteristics
To be developed	To be developed

[a] Critical defining characteristic.

SENSORY-PERCEPTUAL ALTERATIONS: VISUAL, AUDITORY, KINESTHETIC, GUSTATORY, TACTILE, OLFACTORY PERCEPTION

Etiology	Defining Characteristics	Other Possible Defining Characteristics
Altered environmental stimuli, excessive or insufficient	Disoriented in time, in place, or with persons	Complaints of fatigue
Altered sensory reception, transmission and/or integration	Altered abstraction	Alteration in posture
Chemical alterations, endogenous (electrolyte), exogenous (drugs, etc.)	Altered conceptualization	Change in muscular tension
Psychological stress	Change in problem-solving abilities	Inappropriate responses
	Reported or measured change in sensory acuity	Hallucinations
	Change in behavior pattern	
	Anxiety	
	Apathy	
	Change in usual responses to stimuli	
	Indication of body-image alteration	
	Restlessness	
	Irritability	
	Altered communication patterns	

SEXUAL DYSFUNCTION

Etiology	Defining Characteristics
Biopsychosocial alteration of sexuality:	Verbalization of problem
Ineffectual or absent role models	Alterations in achieving perceived sex role
Physical abuse	Actual or perceived limitation imposed by disease and/or therapy
Psychosocial abuse, e.g., harmful relationships	Conflicts involving values
Vulnerability	Alteration in achieving sexual satisfaction
Misinformation or lack of knowledge	Inability to achieve desired satisfaction
Values conflict	Seeking confirmation of desirability
Lack of privacy	Alteration in relationship with significant other
Lack of significant other	Change of interest in self and others
Altered body structure or function: pregnancy, recent childbirth, drugs, surgery, anomalies, disease process, trauma, radiation	

SKIN INTEGRITY, IMPAIRMENT OF: ACTUAL

Etiology		
External (Environmental)	**Internal (Somatic)**	**Defining Characteristics**
Hyper- or hypothermia	Medication	Disruption of skin surface
Chemical substance	Altered nutritional state: obesity, emaciation	Destruction of skin layers
Mechanical factors:	Altered metabolic state	Invasion of body structures
Shearing forces	Altered circulation	
Pressure	Altered sensation	
Restraint	Altered pigmentation	
Radiation	Skeletal prominence	
Physical immobilization	Developmental factors	
Humidity	Immunological factors	
	Alterations in turgor (change in elasticity)	

SKIN INTEGRITY, IMPAIRMENT OF: POTENTIAL

	Defining Characteristics[a]	
Etiology	**External (Environmental)**	**Internal (Somatic)**
Not applicable	Hypo-/hyperthermia	Medication
	Chemical substance	Alterations in nutritional state (obesity, emaciation)
	Mechanical factors:	Altered metabolic state
	Shearing forces	Altered circulation
	Pressure	Altered sensation
	Restraint	Altered pigmentation
	Radiation	Skeletal prominence
	Physical immobilization	Developmental factors
	Excretions/secretions	Alterations in skin turgor (change in elasticity)
	Humidity	Psychogenic
		Immunologic

[a] Presence of one or more risk factors (something which increases the possibility of a condition's occurring).

SLEEP PATTERN DISTURBANCE

Definition: Disruption of sleep time which causes a client discomfort or interferes with the desired lifestyle.

Etiology	Defining Characteristics
Sensory alterations: Internal factors: Illness Psychological stress External factors: Environmental changes Social cues	Verbal complaints of difficulty falling asleep[a] Awakening earlier or later than desired[a] Interrupted sleep[a] Verbal complaints of not feeling well rested[a] Changes in behavior and performance: Increasing irritability Restlessness Disorganization Lethargy Listlessness Physical signs: Mild, fleeting nystagmus Slight hand tremor Ptosis of eyelid Expressionless face Thick speech with mispronunciation and incorrect words Dark circles under eyes Frequent yawning Changes in posture

[a] Critical defining characteristic.

SOCIAL ISOLATION

Definition: Condition of aloneness perceived as imposed by others and as a negative or threatening state.

	Defining Characteristics	
Etiology	**Objective**	**Subjective**
Factors contributing to the absence of satisfying personal relationships: Delay in accomplishing developmental tasks Immature interests Alteration in physical appearance Alterations in mental status Unaccepted social behavior Unaccepted social values Altered state of wellness Inadequate personal resources Inability to engage in satisfying personal relationships	Absence of supportive significant others: family, friends, group Sad, dull affect Inappropriate or immature interests/activities for developmental age/stage Uncommunicative, withdrawn, no eye contact Preoccupation with own thoughts, repetitive, meaningless actions Projects hostility in voice, behavior Seeks to be alone, or exists in a subculture Evidence of physical/mental handicap or altered state of wellness Shows behavior unaccepted by dominant cultural group	Expresses feelings of aloneness imposed by others[a] Expresses feelings of rejection[a] Experiences feelings of difference from others Inadequacy in or absence of significant purpose in life Inability to meet expectations of others Insecurity in public Expresses values acceptable to the subculture but unacceptable to the dominant cultural group Expresses interests inappropriate to the developmental age/stage

[a] Critical defining characteristic.

SPIRITUAL DISTRESS (DISTRESS OF THE HUMAN SPIRIT)

Definition: Distress of the human spirit is a disruption in the life principle which pervades a person's entire being and which integrates and transcends one's biological and psychosocial nature.

Etiology	Defining Characteristics
Separation from religious/cultural ties Challenged belief and value system, e.g., due to moral/ethical implications of therapy, due to intense suffering	Expresses concern with meaning of life/ death and/or belief systems[a] Anger toward God Questions meaning of suffering Verbalizes inner conflict about beliefs Verbalizes concern about relationship with deity Questions meaning for own existence Unable to participate in usual religious practices Seeks spiritual assistance Questions moral/ethical implications of therapeutic regimen Gallows humor Displacement of anger toward religious representatives Description of nightmares/sleep disturbances Alteration in behavior/mood evidenced by anger, crying, withdrawal, preoccupation, anxiety, hostility, apathy, etc.

[a] Critical defining characteristic.

THOUGHT PROCESSES, ALTERATION IN

Etiology	Defining Characteristics	Other Possible Defining Characteristics
To be determined	Inaccurate interpretation of environment Cognitive dissonance Distractibility Memory deficit/problems Egocentricity Hyper/hypovigilance	Inappropriate/nonreality-based thinking

TISSUE PERFUSION, ALTERATION IN: CEREBRAL, CARDIOPULMONARY, RENAL, GASTROINTESTINAL, PERIPHERAL

	Defining Characteristics with Estimated Sensitivities and Specificities		
Etiology	Characteristic	Chance Defining Characteristic Will Be Present Given Diagnosis	Chance Defining Characteristic Not Explained by Any Other Diagnosis
Interruption of flow, arterial	Skin temperature: cold extremities	High	Low
Interruption of flow, venous	Skin color:	Moderate	Low
	Dependent, blue or purple		
Exchange problems	Pale on elevation, and color does not return on lowering leg[a]	High	High
Hypervolemia	Diminished arterial pulsations[a]	High	High
Hypovolemia	Skin quality: shining	High	Low
	Lack of lanugo	High	Moderate
	Round scars covered with atrophied skin		
	Gangrene	Low	High
	Slow growing, dry, thick brittle nails	High	Moderate
	Claudication	Moderate	High
	Blood pressure changes in extremities		
	Bruits	Moderate	Moderate
	Slow healing of lesions	High	Low

[a] Critical defining characteristic.

URINARY ELIMINATION, ALTERATION IN PATTERNS

Etiology	Defining Characteristics
Multiple causality, including: Anatomical obstruction Sensory motor impairment Urinary tract infection	Dysuria Frequency Hesitancy Incontinence Nocturia Retention Urgency

VIOLENCE, POTENTIAL FOR (SELF-DIRECTED OR DIRECTED AT OTHERS)

Etiology	Defining Characteristics	Other Defining Characteristics
Antisocial character Battered women Catatonic excitement Child abuse Manic excitement Organic brain syndrome Panic states Rage reactions Suicidal behavior Temporal lobe epilepsy Toxic reactions to medication	Body language; clenched fists, facial expressions, rigid posture, tautness indicating intense effort to control Hostile threatening verbalizations; boasting of prior abuse to others Increased motor activity, pacing, excitement, irritability, agitation Overt and aggressive acts; goal-directed destruction of objects in environment Possession of destructive means; gun, knife, weapon Rage Self-destructive behavior/active, aggressive suicidal acts Substance abuse/withdrawal Suspicion of others, paranoid ideation, delusions, hallucinations	Increasing anxiety levels Fear of self or others Inability to verbalize feelings Repetition of verbalizations: continued complaints, requests, and demands Anger Provocative behavior: argumentative, dissatisfied, overreactive, hypersensitive Vulnerable self-esteem Depression (specifically, active, aggressive, suicidal acts)

DSM-III CLASSIFICATION: AXES I AND II CATEGORIES AND CODES

All official DSM-III codes and terms are included in ICD-9-CM. However, in order to differentiate those DSM-III categories that use the same ICD-9-CM codes, unofficial non-ICD-9-CM codes are provided in parentheses for use when greater specificity is necessary.

The long dashes indicate the need for a fifth-digit subtype or other qualifying term.

DISORDERS USUALLY FIRST EVIDENT IN INFANCY, CHILDHOOD, OR ADOLESCENCE

Mental retardation

(Code in fifth digit: 1 = with other behavioral symptoms [requiring attention or treatment and that are not part of another disorder], 0 = without behavioral symptoms.)

317.0(x) Mild mental retardation, ______
318.0(x) Moderate mental retardation, ______
318.1(x) Severe mental retardation, ______
318.2(x) Profound mental retardation, ______
319.0(x) Unspecified mental retardation, ______

Attention deficit disorder

314.01 With hyperactivity
314.00 Without hyperactivity
314.80 Residual type

Conduct disorder

312.00 Undersocialized, aggressive
312.10 Undersocialized, nonaggressive
312.23 Socialized, aggressive
312.21 Socialized, nonaggressive
312.90 Atypical

Anxiety disorders of childhood or adolescence

309.21 Separation anxiety disorder
313.21 Avoidant disorder of childhood or adolescence
313.00 Overanxious disorder

Other disorders of infancy, childhood, or adolescence

313.89 Reactive attachment disorder of infancy
313.22 Schizoid disorder of childhood or adolescence
313.23 Elective mutism
313.81 Oppositional disorder
313.82 Identity disorder

Eating disorders

307.10 Anorexia nervosa
307.51 Bulimia
307.52 Pica
307.53 Rumination disorder of infancy
307.50 Atypical eating disorder

Stereotyped movement disorders

307.21 Transient tic disorder
307.22 Chronic motor tic disorder
307.23 Tourette's disorder
307.20 Atypical tic disorder
307.30 Atypical stereotyped movement disorder

Other disorders with physical manifestations

307.00 Stuttering
307.60 Functional enuresis
307.70 Function encopresis
307.46 Sleepwalking disorder
307.46 Sleep terror disorder (307.49)

Pervasive developmental disorders

Code in fifth digit: 0 = full syndrome present, 1 = residual state.

299.0x Infantile autism, ______
299.9x Childhood onset pervasive developmental disorder, ______
299.8x Atypical, ______

Specific developmental disorders
Note: These are coded on Axis II.

315.00 Developmental reading disorder
315.10 Developmental arithmetic disorder
315.31 Developmental language disorder
315.39 Developmental articulation disorder
315.50 Mixed specific developmental disorder
315.90 Atypical specific developmental disorder

ORGANIC MENTAL DISORDERS

Section 1. Organic mental disorders whose etiology or pathophysiological process is listed below (taken from the mental disorders section of ICD-9-CM).

Dementias arising in the senium and presenium

Primary degenerative dementia, senile onset
290.30 With delirium
290.20 With delusions
290.21 With depression
290.00 Uncomplicated
Code in fifth digit: 1 = with delirium, 2 = with delusions, 3 = with depression, 0 = uncomplicated.
290.1x Primary degenerative dementia, presenile onset ______
290.4x Multi-infarct dementia, ______

Substance-induced

Alcohol
303.00 Intoxication
291.40 Idiosyncratic intoxication
291.80 Withdrawal
291.00 Withdrawal delirium
291.30 Hallucinosis
291.10 Amnestic disorder
Code severity of dementia in fifth digit: 1 = mild, 2 = moderate, 3 = severe, 0 = unspecified.
291.2x Dementia associated with alcoholism, ______
Barbiturate or similarly acting sedative or hypnotic
305.40 Intoxication (327.00)
292.00 Withdrawal (327.01)
292.00 Withdrawal delirium (327.02)
292.83 Amnestic disorder (327.04)
Opioid
305.50 Intoxication (327.10)
292.00 Withdrawal (327.11)
Cocaine
305.60 Intoxication (327.20)
Amphetamine or similarly acting sympathomimetic
305.70 Intoxication (327.30)
292.81 Delirium (327.32)
292.11 Delusional disorder (327.35)
292.00 Withdrawal (327.31)
Phencyclidine (PCP) or similarly acting arylcyclohexylamine
305.90 Intoxication (327.40)
292.81 Delirium (327.42)
292.90 Mixed organic mental disorder (327.49)
Hallucinogen
305.30 Hallucinosis (327.56)
292.11 Delusional disorder (327.55)
292.84 Affective disorder (327.57)
Cannabis
305.20 Intoxication (327.60)
292.11 Delusional disorder (327.65)
Tobacco
292.00 Withdrawal (327.71)
Caffeine
305.90 Intoxication (327.80)
Other or unspecified substance
305.90 Intoxication (327.90)
292.00 Withdrawal (327.91)
292.81 Delirium (327.92)
292.82 Dementia (327.93)
292.83 Amnestic disorder (327.94)
292.11 Delusional disorder (327.95)
292.12 Hallucinosis (327.96)
292.84 Affective disorder (327.97)
292.89 Personality disorder (327.98)
292.90 Atypical or mixed organic mental disorder (327.99)

Section 2. Organic brain syndromes whose etiology or pathophysiological process is either noted as an additional diagnosis from outside the mental disorders section of ICD-9-CM or is unknown.

293.00 Delirium
294.10 Dementia
294.00 Amnestic syndrome
293.81 Organic delusional syndrome
293.82 Organic hallucinosis
293.83 Organic affective syndrome
310.10 Organic personality syndrome
294.80 Atypical or mixed organic brain syndrome

SUBSTANCE USE DISORDERS

Code in fifth digit: 1 = continous, 2 = episodic, 3 = in remission, 0 = unspecified
305.0x Alcohol abuse, ______
303.9x Alcohol dependence (Alcoholism), ______
305.4x Barbiturate or similarly acting sedative or hypnotic abuse, ______
304.1x Barbiturate or similarly acting sedative or hypnotic dependence, ______
305.5x Opioid abuse, ______

304.0x Opioid dependence, ______
305.6x Cocaine abuse, ______
305.7x Amphetamine or similarly acting sympathomimetic abuse, ______
304.4x Amphetamine or similarly acting sympathomimetic dependence, ______
305.9x Phencyclidine (PCP) or similarly acting arylcyclohexylamine abuse, ______ (328.4x)
305.3x Hallucinogen abuse, ______
305.2x Cannabis abuse, ______
304.3x Cannabis dependence, ______
305.1x Tobacco dependence, ______
305.9x Other, mixed or unspecified substance abuse, ______
304.6x Other specified substance dependence, ______
304.9x Unspecified substance dependence, ______
304.7x Dependence on combination of opioid and other nonalcoholic substance, ______
304.8x Dependence on combination of substances, excluding opioids and alcohol, ______

SCHIZOPHRENIC DISORDERS

Code in fifth digit: 1 = subchronic, 2 = chronic, 3 = subchronic with acute exacerbation, 4 = chronic with acute exacerbation, 5 = in remission, 0 = unspecified

Schizophrenia
295.1x Disorganized, ______
295.2x Catatonic, ______
295.3x Paranoid, ______
295.9x Undifferentiated, ______
295.6x Residual, ______

PARANOID DISORDERS

297.10 Paranoia
297.30 Shared paranoid disorder
298.30 Acute paranoid disorder
297.90 Atypical paranoid disorder

PSYCHOTIC DISORDERS NOT ELSEWHERE CLASSIFIED

295.40 Schizophreniform disorder
298.80 Brief reactive psychosis
295.70 Schizoaffective disorder
298.90 Atypical psychosis

NEUROTIC DISORDERS: These are included in Affective, Anxiety, Somatoform, Dissociative, and Psychosexual Disorders. In order to facilitate the identification of the categories that in DSM-II were grouped together in the class of Neuroses, the DSM-II terms are included separately in parentheses after the corresponding categories. These DSM-II terms are included in ICD-9-CM and therefore are acceptable as alternatives to the recommended DSM-III terms that precede them.

AFFECTIVE DISORDERS

Major affective disorders

Code major depressive episode in fifth digit: 6 = in remission, 4 = with psychotic features (the unofficial non-ICD-9-CM fifth digit 7 may be used instead to indicate that the psychotic features are mood-incongruent), 3 = with melancholia, 2 = without melancholia, 0 = unspecified.

Code manic or mixed episode in fifth digit: 6 = in remission, 4 = with psychotic features (the unofficial non-ICD-9-CM fifth digit 7 may be used instead to indicate that the psychotic features are mood-incongruent), 2 = without psychotic features, 0 = unspecified.

Bipolar disorder,
296.6x Mixed, ______
296.4x Manic, ______
296.5x Depressed, ______

Major depression,
296.2x Single episode, ______
296.3x Recurrent, ______

Other specific affective disorders

301.13 Cyclothymic disorder
300.40 Dysthymic disorder (or Depressive neurosis)

Atypical affective disorders

296.70 Atypical bipolar disorder
296.82 Atypical depression

ANXIETY DISORDERS

Phobic disorders (or Phobic neuroses)
300.21 Agoraphobia with panic attacks
300.22 Agoraphobia without panic attacks
300.23 Social phobia

300.29 Simple phobia
Anxiety states (or Anxiety neuroses)
300.01 Panic disorder
300.02 Generalized anxiety disorder
300.30 Obsessive compulsive disorder (or Obsessive compulsive neurosis)
Post-traumatic stress disorder
308.30 Acute
309.81 Chronic or delayed
300.00 Atypical anxiety disorder

SOMATOFORM DISORDERS

300.81 Somatization disorder
300.11 Conversion disorder (or Hysterical neurosis, conversion type)
307.80 Psychogenic pain disorder
300.70 Hypochondriasis (or Hypochondriacal neurosis)
300.70 Atypical somatoform disorder (300.71)

DISSOCIATIVE DISORDERS (OR HYSTERICAL NEUROSES, DISSOCIATIVE TYPE)

300.12 Psychogenic amnesia
300.13 Psychogenic fugue
300.14 Multiple personality
300.60 Depersonalization disorder (or Depersonalization neurosis)
300.15 Atypical dissociative disorder

PSYCHOSEXUAL DISORDERS

Gender identity disorders

Indicate sexual history in the fifth digit of Transsexualism code: 1 = asexual, 2 = homosexual, 3 = heterosexual, 0 = unspecified.

302.5x Transsexualism, ______
302.60 Gender identity disorder of childhood
302.85 Atypical gender identity disorder

Paraphilias

302.81 Fetishism
302.30 Transvestism
302.10 Zoophilia
302.20 Pedophilia
302.40 Exhibitionism
302.82 Voyeurism
302.83 Sexual masochism
302.84 Sexual sadism
302.90 Atypical paraphilia

Psychosexual dysfunctions

302.71 Inhibited sexual desire
302.72 Inhibited sexual excitement
302.73 Inhibited female orgasm
302.74 Inhibited male orgasm
302.75 Premature ejaculation
302.76 Functional dyspareunia
306.51 Functional vaginismus
302.70 Atypical psychosexual dysfunction

Other psychosexual disorders

302.00 Ego-dystonic homosexuality
302.89 Psychosexual disorder not elsewhere classified

FACTITIOUS DISORDERS

300.16 Factitious disorder with psychological symptoms
301.51 Chronic factitious disorder with physical symptoms
300.19 Atypical factitious disorder with physical symptoms

DISORDERS OF IMPULSE CONTROL NOT ELSEWHERE CLASSIFIED

312.31 Pathological gambling
312.32 Kleptomania
312.33 Pyromania
312.34 Intermittent explosive disorder
312.35 Isolated explosive disorder
312.39 Atypical impulse control disorder

ADJUSTMENT DISORDER

309.00 With depressed mood
309.24 With anxious mood
309.28 With mixed emotional features
309.30 With disturbance of conduct
309.40 With mixed disturbance of emotions and conduct
309.23 With work (or academic) inhibition
309.83 With withdrawal
309.90 With atypical features

PSYCHOLOGICAL FACTORS AFFECTING PHYSICAL CONDITION

Specify physical condition on Axis III.

316.00 Psychological factors affecting physical condition

PERSONALITY DISORDERS

Note: These are coded on Axis II.

301.00 Paranoid
301.20 Schizoid
301.22 Schizotypal
301.50 Histrionic
301.81 Narcissistic
301.70 Antisocial
301.83 Borderline
301.82 Avoidant
301.60 Dependent
301.40 Compulsive
301.84 Passive-Aggressive
301.89 Atypical, mixed or other personality disorder

V CODES FOR CONDITIONS NOT ATTRIBUTABLE TO A MENTAL DISORDER THAT ARE A FOCUS OF ATTENTION OR TREATMENT

V65.20 Malingering
V62.89 Borderline intellectual functioning (V62.88)
V71.01 Adult antisocial behavior
V71.02 Childhood or adolescent antisocial behavior
V62.30 Academic problem
V62.20 Occupational problem
V62.82 Uncomplicated bereavement
V15.81 Noncompliance with medical treatment
V62.89 Phase of life problem or other life circumstance problem
V61.10 Marital problem
V61.20 Parent-child problem
V61.80 Other specified family circumstances
V62.81 Other interpersonal problem

ADDITIONAL CODES

300.90 Unspecified mental disorder (nonpsychotic)
V71.09 No diagnosis or condition on Axis I
799.90 Diagnosis or condition deferred on Axis I

V71.09 No diagnosis on Axis II
799.90 Diagnosis deferred on Axis II

SOURCE: *Diagnostic and Statistical Manual of Mental Disorders*, 3rd ed., American Psychiatric Association, Washington, D.C., 1980.

Appendix B

CONVERSION TABLES

FAHRENHEIT AND CELSIUS EQUIVALENTS: BODY TEMPERATURE RANGE

F°	C°	F°	C°	F°	C°	F°	C°	F°	C°
94.0	34.44	97.0	36.11	100.0	37.78	103.0	39.44	106.0	41.11
94.2	34.56	97.2	36.22	100.2	37.89	103.2	39.56	106.2	41.22
94.4	34.67	97.4	36.33	100.4	38.00	103.4	39.67	106.4	41.33
94.6	34.78	97.6	36.44	100.6	38.11	103.6	39.78	106.6	41.44
94.8	34.89	97.8	36.56	100.8	38.22	103.8	39.89	106.8	41.56
95.0	35.00	98.0	36.67	101.0	38.33	104.0	40.00	107.0	41.67
95.2	35.11	98.2	36.78	101.2	38.44	104.2	40.11	107.2	41.78
95.4	35.22	98.4	36.89	101.4	38.56	104.4	40.22	107.4	41.89
95.6	35.33	98.6	37.00	101.6	38.67	104.6	40.33	107.6	42.00
95.8	35.44	98.8	37.11	101.8	38.78	104.8	40.44	107.8	42.11
96.0	35.56	99.0	37.22	102.0	38.89	105.0	40.56	108.0	42.22
96.2	35.67	99.2	37.33	102.2	39.00	105.2	40.67		
96.4	35.78	99.4	37.44	102.4	39.11	105.4	40.78		
96.6	35.89	99.6	37.56	102.6	39.22	105.6	40.89		
96.8	36.00	99.8	37.67	102.8	39.33	105.8	41.00		

CELSIUS AND FAHRENHEIT EQUIVALENTS: BODY TEMPERATURE RANGE

C°	F°	C°	F°	C°	F°	C°	F°	C°	F°
34.0	93.20	35.5	95.90	37.0	98.60	38.5	101.30	40.0	104.00
34.1	93.38	35.6	96.08	37.1	98.78	38.6	101.48	40.1	104.18
34.2	93.56	35.7	96.26	37.2	98.96	38.7	101.66	40.2	104.36
34.3	93.74	35.8	96.44	37.3	99.14	38.8	101.84	40.3	104.54
34.4	93.92	35.9	96.62	37.4	99.32	38.9	102.02	40.4	104.72
34.5	94.10	36.0	96.80	37.5	99.50	39.0	102.20	40.5	104.90
34.6	94.28	36.1	96.98	37.6	99.68	39.1	102.38	40.6	105.08
34.7	94.46	36.2	97.16	37.7	99.86	39.2	102.56	40.7	105.26
34.8	94.64	36.3	97.34	37.8	100.04	39.3	102.74	40.8	105.44
34.9	94.82	36.4	97.52	37.9	100.22	39.4	102.92	40.9	105.62
35.0	95.0	36.5	97.70	38.0	100.40	39.5	103.10	41.0	105.80
35.1	95.18	36.6	97.88	38.1	100.58	39.6	103.28		
35.2	95.36	36.7	98.06	38.2	100.76	39.7	103.46		
35.3	95.54	36.8	98.24	38.3	100.94	39.8	103.64		
35.4	95.72	36.9	98.42	38.4	101.12	39.9	103.82		

LENGTH CONVERSIONS

Meters	Centi-meters	Yards	Feet	Inches
1	100	1.094	3.281	39.37
.01	1	.01094	.0328	.3937
.9144	91.44	1	3	36
.0348	30.48	1/3	1	12
.0254	2.54	1/36	1/12	1

WEIGHT CONVERSIONS (METRIC AND AVOIRDUPOIS)

Grams	Kilograms	Ounces	Pounds
1	.001	.0353	.0022
1,000	1	35.3	2.2
28.35	.02835	1	1/16
454.5	.4545	16	1

WEIGHT CONVERSIONS (METRIC AND APOTHECARY)

Grams	Milligrams	Grains	Drams	Ounces	Pounds
1	1,000	15.4	.2577	.0322	.00268
.001	1	.0154	.00026	.0000322	.00000268
.0648	64.8	1	1/60	1/480	1/5,760
3.888	3,888	60	1	1/8	1/96
31.1	31,104	480	8	1	1/12
373.25	373,248	5,760	96	12	1

VOLUME CONVERSIONS (METRIC AND APOTHECARY)

Milliliters	Minims	Fluid Drams	Fluid Ounces	Pints
1	16.2	.27	.0333	.0021
.0616	1	1/60	1/480	1/7,680
3.697	60	1	1/8	1/128
29.58	480	8	1	1/16
473.2	7,680	128	16	1
Liters	**Gallons**	**Quarts**	**Fluid Ounces**	**Pints**
1	.2642	1.057	33.824	2.114
3.785	1	4	128	8
.946	1/4	1	32	2
.473	1/8	1/2	16	1
.0296	1/128	1/32	1	1/16

COMMONLY USED METRIC AND APOTHECARY EQUIVALENTS

Grains	Grams	Milligrams
1/300	.0002	0.2
1/200	.0003	0.3
1/150	.0004	0.4
1/120	.0005	0.5
1/100	.0006	0.6
1/60	.001	1
1/30	.002	2
1/12	.005	5
1/6	.010	10
1/4	.015	15
3/8	.025	25
1/2	.030	30
3/4	.050	50
1	.060	60
1½	.100	100
2	.120	120
3	.200	200
5	.300	300
7½	.500	500
10	.600	600
15	1	1,000
30	2	2,000
60	4	4,000

APPROXIMATE HOUSEHOLD MEASUREMENT EQUIVALENTS (VOLUME)

						1 tsp =	5 mL
					1 tbsp =	3 tsp =	15 mL
				1 fl oz =	2 tbsp =	6 tsp =	30 mL
			1 cup =	8 fl oz		=	240 mL
		1 pt =	2 cups =	16 fl oz		=	480 mL
	1 qt =	2 pt =	4 cups =	32 fl oz		=	960 mL
1 gal =	4 qt =	8 pt =	16 cups =	128 fl oz		=	3,840 mL

POUND-TO-KILOGRAM CONVERSION[a]

Pounds	0	1	2	3	4	5	6	7	8	9
0	0.00	0.45	0.90	1.36	1.81	2.26	2.72	3.17	3.62	4.08
10	4.53	4.98	5.44	5.89	6.35	6.80	7.25	7.71	8.16	8.61
20	9.07	9.52	9.97	10.43	10.88	11.34	11.79	12.24	12.70	13.15
30	13.60	14.06	14.51	14.96	15.42	15.87	16.32	16.78	17.23	17.69
40	18.14	18.59	19.05	19.50	19.95	20.41	20.86	21.31	21.77	22.22
50	22.68	23.13	23.58	24.04	24.49	24.94	25.40	25.85	26.30	26.76
60	27.21	27.66	28.12	28.57	29.03	29.48	29.93	30.39	30.84	31.29
70	31.75	32.20	32.65	33.11	33.56	34.02	34.47	34.92	35.38	35.83
80	36.28	36.74	37.19	37.64	38.10	38.55	39.00	39.46	39.91	40.37
90	40.82	41.27	41.73	42.18	42.63	43.09	43.54	43.99	44.45	44.90
100	45.36	45.81	46.26	46.72	47.17	47.62	48.08	48.53	48.98	49.44
110	49.89	50.34	50.80	51.25	51.71	52.16	52.61	53.07	53.52	53.97
120	54.43	54.88	55.33	55.79	56.24	56.70	57.15	57.60	58.06	58.51
130	58.96	59.42	59.87	60.32	60.78	61.23	61.68	62.14	62.59	63.05
140	63.50	63.95	64.41	64.86	65.31	65.77	66.22	66.67	67.13	67.58
150	68.04	68.49	68.94	69.40	69.85	70.30	70.76	71.21	71.66	72.12
160	72.57	73.02	73.48	73.93	74.39	74.84	75.29	75.75	76.20	76.65
170	77.11	77.56	78.01	78.47	78.92	79.38	79.83	80.28	80.74	81.19
180	81.64	82.10	82.55	83.00	83.46	83.91	84.36	84.82	85.27	85.73
190	86.18	86.68	87.09	87.54	87.99	88.45	88.90	89.35	89.81	90.26
200	90.72	91.17	91.62	92.08	92.53	92.98	93.44	93.89	94.34	94.80

[a] Numbers in the farthest left column are 10-pound increments; numbers across the top row are 1-pound increments. The kilogram equivalent of weight in pounds is found at the intersection of the appropriate row and column. For example, to convert 54 pounds, read down the left column to 50 and then across that row to 4: 54 pounds = 24.49 kilograms.

GRAM EQUIVALENTS FOR POUNDS AND OUNCES: CONVERSION FOR WEIGHT OF NEWBORNS[a]

Pounds	Ounces 0	1	2	3	4	5	6	7	8	9	10	11	12	13	14	15	Pounds
0	—	28	57	85	113	142	170	198	227	255	283	312	340	369	397	425	0
1	454	482	510	539	567	595	624	652	680	709	737	765	794	822	850	879	1
2	907	936	964	992	1021	1049	1077	1106	1134	1162	1191	1219	1247	1276	1304	1332	2
3	1361	1389	1417	1446	1474	1503	1531	1559	1588	1616	1644	1673	1701	1729	1758	1786	3
4	1814	1843	1871	1899	1928	1956	1984	2013	2041	2070	2098	2126	2155	2183	2211	2240	4
5	2268	2296	2325	2353	2381	2410	2438	2466	2495	2523	2551	2580	2608	2637	2665	2693	5
6	2722	2750	2778	2807	2835	2863	2892	2920	2948	2977	3005	3033	3062	3090	3118	3147	6
7	3175	3203	3232	3260	3289	3317	3345	3374	3402	3430	3459	3487	3515	3544	3572	3600	7
8	3629	3657	3685	3714	3742	3770	3799	3827	3856	3884	3912	3941	3969	3997	4026	4054	8
9	4082	4111	4139	4167	4196	4224	4252	4281	4309	4337	4366	4394	4423	4451	4479	4508	9
10	4536	4564	4593	4621	4649	4678	4706	4734	4763	4791	4819	4848	4876	4904	4933	4961	10
11	4990	5018	5046	5075	5103	5131	5160	5188	5216	5245	5273	5301	5330	5358	5386	5415	11
12	5443	5471	5500	5528	5557	5585	5613	5642	5670	5698	5727	5755	5783	5812	5840	5868	12
13	5897	5925	5953	5982	6010	6038	6067	6095	6123	6152	6180	6209	6237	6265	6294	6322	13
14	6350	6379	6407	6435	6464	6492	6520	6549	6577	6605	6634	6662	6690	6719	6747	6776	14

[a] 1 pound = 453.59 grams. 1 ounce = 28.35 grams. Grams can be converted to pounds and tenths of a pound by multiplying the number of grams by .0022.

Appendix C

Clinical Laboratory Values

CRITICAL LABORATORY VALUES

Test	Low	Possible Effect	High	Possible Effect
Packed cell volume	<15 vol %	Heart failure and anoxemia	None	
Blood hemoglobin	<5 g %	Heart failure and anoxemia	None	
Blood platelets	<30,000 cu mm	Hemorrhage	None	
Blood platelets (newborn and pediatrics)	<20,000 cu mm	Hemorrhage	None	
Prothrombin time	None		>40 s	Hemorrhage
Serum bilirubin, total (newborn)	None		>18 mg/dL	Brain damage
Serum calcium	<6 mg/dL	Tetany and convulsions	>13 mg/dL	Coma
Serum calcium (newborn)	<6 mg/dL	Tetany and convulsions	>13 mg/dL	Coma
Serum glucose	<40 mg/dL	Brain damage	>700 mg/dL	Diabetic coma
Serum glucose (newborn)	<30 mg/dL	Brain damage	>300 mg/dL	Diabetic coma
Serum phosphate	<1 mg/dL	Seizures and coma	None	
Serum potassium	<2.5 mEq/L	Muscle weakness, paralysis, cardiac arrhythmias	>6.5 mEq/L	Cardiotoxicity with arrhythmias
Serum potassium (hemolyzed)	<2.5 mEq/L	Muscle weakness, paralysis, cardiac arrhythmias	>8.0 mEq/L	Cardiotoxicity with arrhythmias

Serum potassium (newborn)	<2.5 mEq/L	Muscle weakness, paralysis, cardiac arrhythmias	>8.0 mEq/L	Cardiotoxicity with arrhythmias
Serum salicylate	None		>700 µg/mL	Continuing untreated toxicity
Serum sodium	<120 mEq/L	Extremes of dehydration, vascular collapse, or edema; hypervolemia, heart failure	>160 mEq/L	Extremes of dehydration, vascular collapse, or edema; hypervolemia, heart failure
Serum bicarbonate	<10 mEq/L	Complex interwoven patterns of acidosis, alkalosis, and anoxemia	>40 mEq/L	Complex interwoven patterns of acidosis, alkalosis, and anoxemia
Arterial or capillary blood P_{CO_2}	<20 mm Hg	Complex interwoven patterns of acidosis, alkalosis, and anoxemia	>70 mmHg	Complex interwoven patterns of acidosis, alkalosis, and anoxemia
Arterial or capillary blood pH	<7.2 U	Complex interwoven patterns of acidosis, alkalosis, and anoxemia	>7.6 U	Complex interwoven patterns of acidosis, alkalosis, and anoxemia
Arterial or capillary blood P_{O_2}	<40 mm Hg	Complex interwoven patterns of acidosis, alkalosis, and anoxemia	None	
Positive blood culture		Worsening sepsis		
Positive CSF gram stain		Untreated bacterial meningitis		
Positive CSF culture		Untreated bacterial meningitis		

SOURCE: Reprinted by permission from Lundberg, G. D.: *Clinical Laboratory Reference*, copyright © 1982 and published by Medical Economics Co., Inc.

A critical laboratory value is a value at such variance with normal as to represent a pathophysiological state that is life threatening unless some action is taken in a very short time and for which an appropriate action is possible. It is a laboratory responsibility to communicate these values immediately and flawlessly to the responsible clinicians.

BLOOD PARAMETERS OF ACID–BASE BALANCE DURING UNCOMPENSATED AND COMPENSATED STATES

	Uncompensated	Compensated
Respiratory acidosis		
pH	↓	Low normal
Pa_{CO_2}	↑	↑
HCO_3	Normal	↑
Respiratory alkalosis		
pH	↑	High normal
Pa_{CO_2}	↓	↓
HCO_3	Normal	↓
Metabolic acidosis		
pH	↓	Low normal
Pa_{CO_2}	Normal	↓
HCO_3	↓	↓
Metabolic alkalosis		
pH	↑	High normal
Pa_{CO_2}	Normal	↑
HCO_3	↑	↑

SOURCE: McFarland, M. B., and Grant, M. M.: *Nursing Implications of Laboratory Tests,* John Wiley, New York, 1982.

Appendix D

Nomograms and Growth Charts

BODY SURFACE AREA OF CHILDREN: NOMOGRAM FOR DETERMINATION OF BODY SURFACE AREA FROM HEIGHT AND WEIGHT[a]

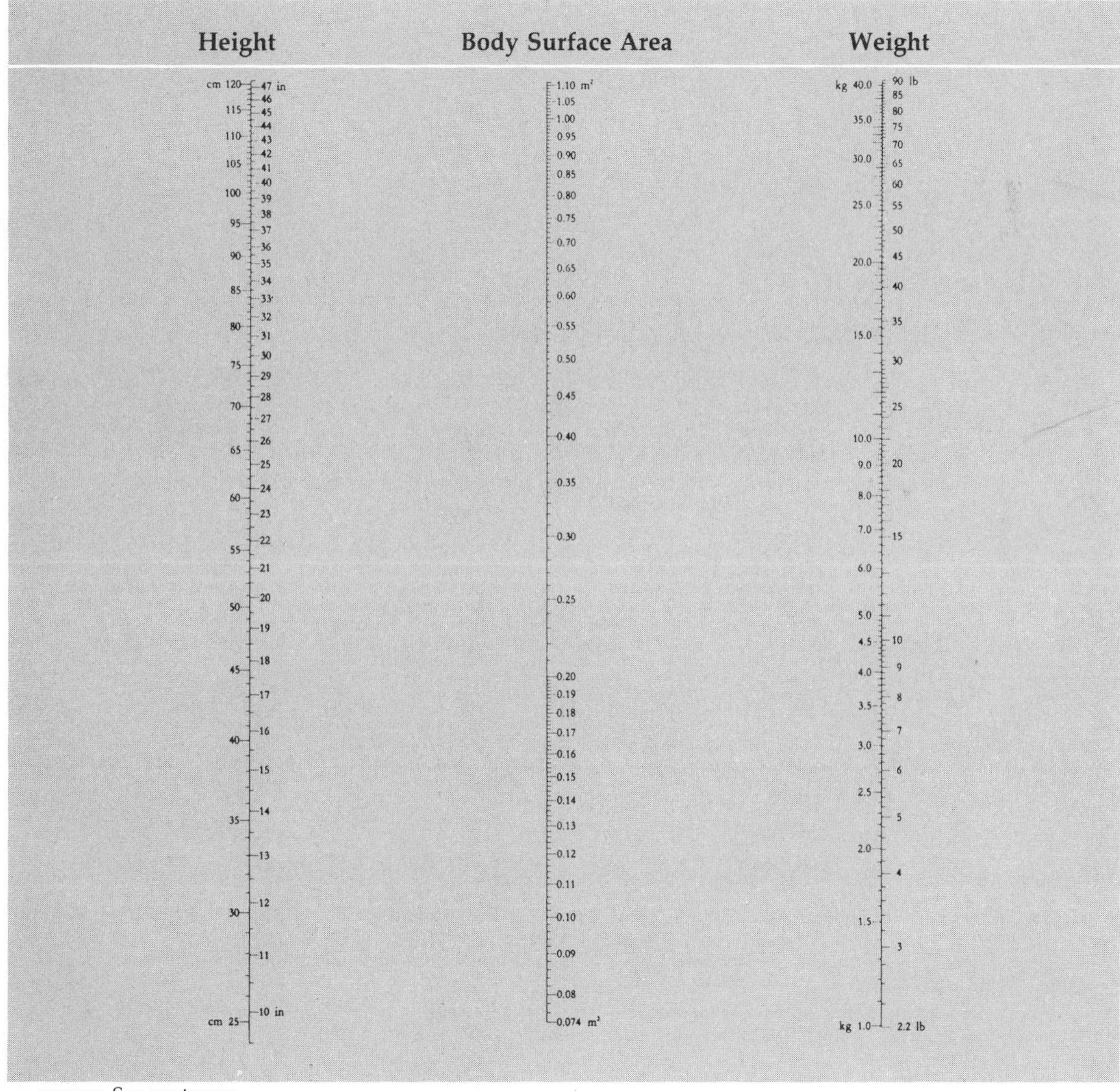

SOURCE: See next page.

[a] See next page.

BODY SURFACE AREA OF ADULTS: NOMOGRAM FOR DETERMINATION OF BODY SURFACE AREA FROM HEIGHT AND WEIGHT[a]

Height **Body Surface Area** **Weight**

Height: cm 200, 195, 190, 185, 180, 175, 170, 165, 160, 155, 150, 145, 140, 135, 130, 125, 120, 115, 110, 105, cm 100; 79 in, 78, 77, 76, 75, 74, 73, 72, 71, 70, 69, 68, 67, 66, 65, 64, 63, 62, 61, 60, 59, 58, 57, 56, 55, 54, 53, 52, 51, 50, 49, 48, 47, 46, 45, 44, 43, 42, 41, 40, 39 in

Body Surface Area: 2.80 m², 2.70, 2.60, 2.50, 2.40, 2.30, 2.20, 2.10, 2.00, 1.95, 1.90, 1.85, 1.80, 1.75, 1.70, 1.65, 1.60, 1.55, 1.50, 1.45, 1.40, 1.35, 1.30, 1.25, 1.20, 1.15, 1.10, 1.05, 1.00, 0.95, 0.90, 0.86 m²

Weight: kg 150, 145, 140, 135, 130, 125, 120, 115, 110, 105, 100, 95, 90, 85, 80, 75, 70, 65, 60, 55, 50, 45, 40, 35, kg 30; 330 lb, 320, 310, 300, 290, 280, 270, 260, 250, 240, 230, 220, 210, 200, 190, 180, 170, 160, 150, 140, 130, 120, 110, 105, 100, 95, 90, 85, 80, 75, 70, 66 lb

SOURCE: Nomograms for children and adults from the formula of Du Bois and Du Bois: *Arch Inter Med* **17:**863, 1916: $S = W^{0.425} \times H^{0.725} \times 71.84$, or $\log S = \log W \times 0.425 + \log H \times 0.725 + 1.8564$ (S = body surface in cm², W = weight in kg, H = height in cm). Reproduced from Documenta Geigy Scientific Tables, 8th edition, Volume I (1981). Courtesy CIBA-GEIGY Limited, Basle, Switzerland.

[a] For both nomograms, a straight edge is placed from the patient's height in the left column to his weight in the right column; this intersect on the body surface area column indicates body surface area.

GIRLS: BIRTH TO 36 MONTHS, PHYSICAL GROWTH NCHS PERCENTILES

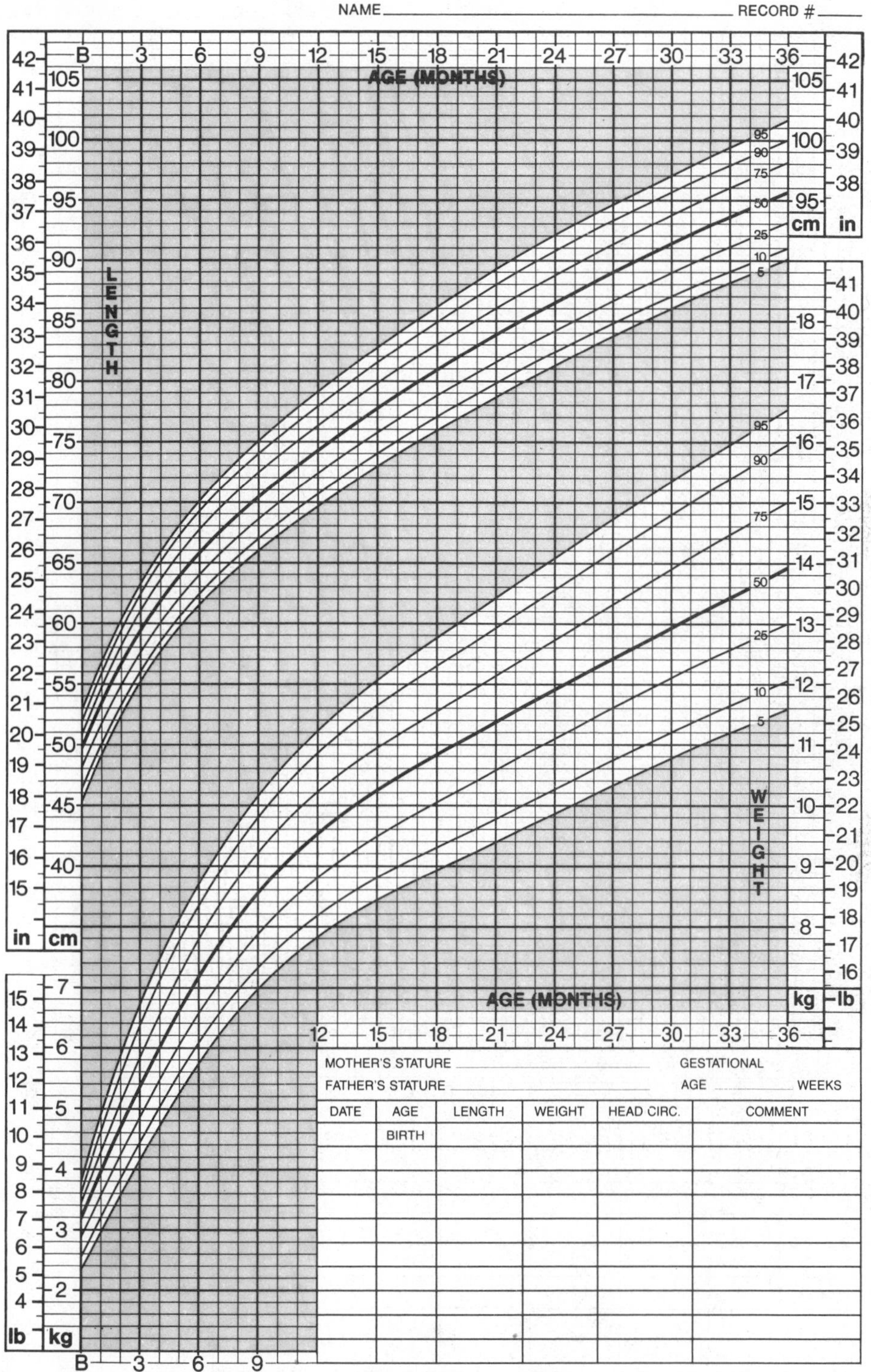

SOURCE: Adapted from: Hamill PVV, Drizd TA, Johnson CL, Reed RB, Roche AF, Moore WM: Physical growth: National Center for Health Statistics percentiles. *Am J Clin Nutr* **32**:607–629, 1979. Data from the Fels Research Institute, Wright State University School of Medicine, Yellow Springs, Ohio. © 1982 Ross Laboratories. Courtesy of Ross Laboratories, Columbus, Ohio.

GIRLS: BIRTH TO 36 MONTHS, PHYSICAL GROWTH NCHS PERCENTILES

NAME ____________________ RECORD # ______

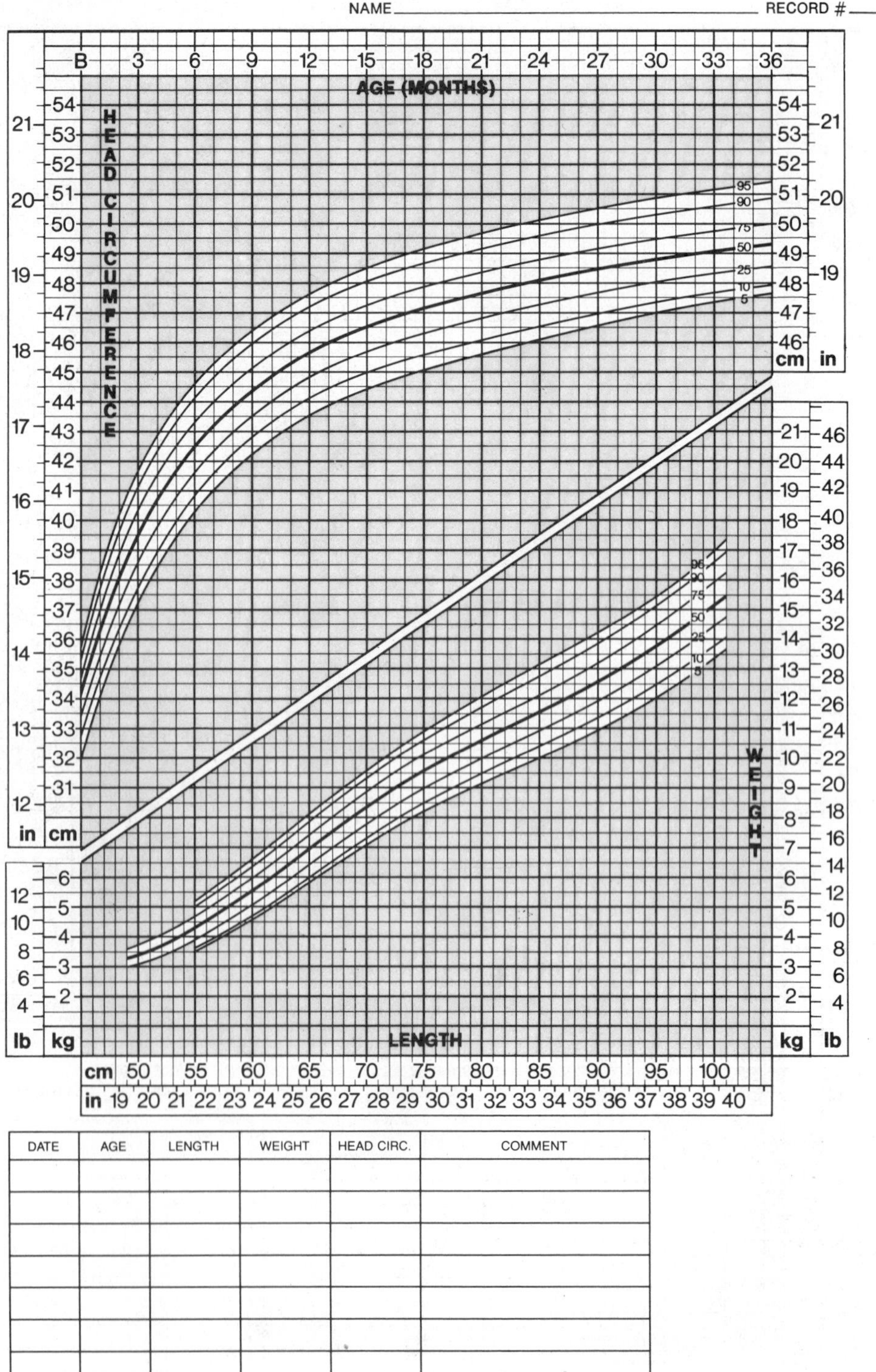

DATE	AGE	LENGTH	WEIGHT	HEAD CIRC.	COMMENT

SOURCE: Adapted from: Hamill PVV, Drizd TA, Johnson CL, Reed RB, Roche AF, Moore WM: Physical growth: National Center for Health Statistics percentiles. *Am J Clin Nutr* **32:**607–629, 1979. Data from the Fels Research Institute, Wright State University School of Medicine, Yellow Springs, Ohio. © 1982 Ross Laboratories. Courtesy of Ross Laboratories, Columbus, Ohio.

BOYS: BIRTH TO 36 MONTHS: PHYSICAL GROWTH NCHS PERCENTILES

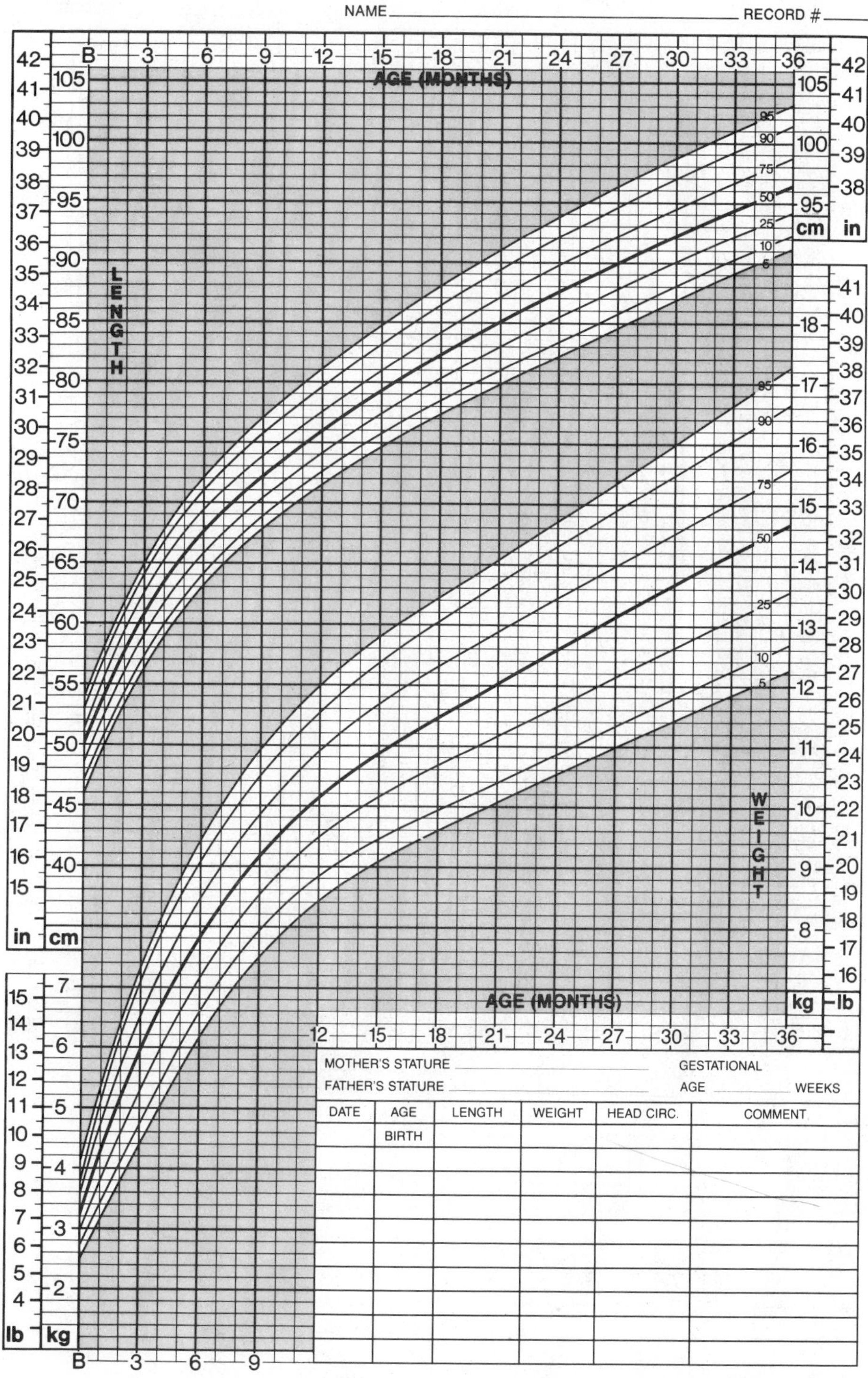

SOURCE: Adapted from: Hamill PVV, Drizd TA, Johnson CL, Reed RB, Roche AF, Moore WM: Physical growth: National Center for Health Statistics percentiles. *Am J Clin Nutr* **32**:607–629, 1979. Data from the Fels Research Institute, Wright State University School of Medicine, Yellow Springs, Ohio.

BOYS: BIRTH TO 36 MONTHS, PHYSICAL GROWTH NCHS PERCENTILES

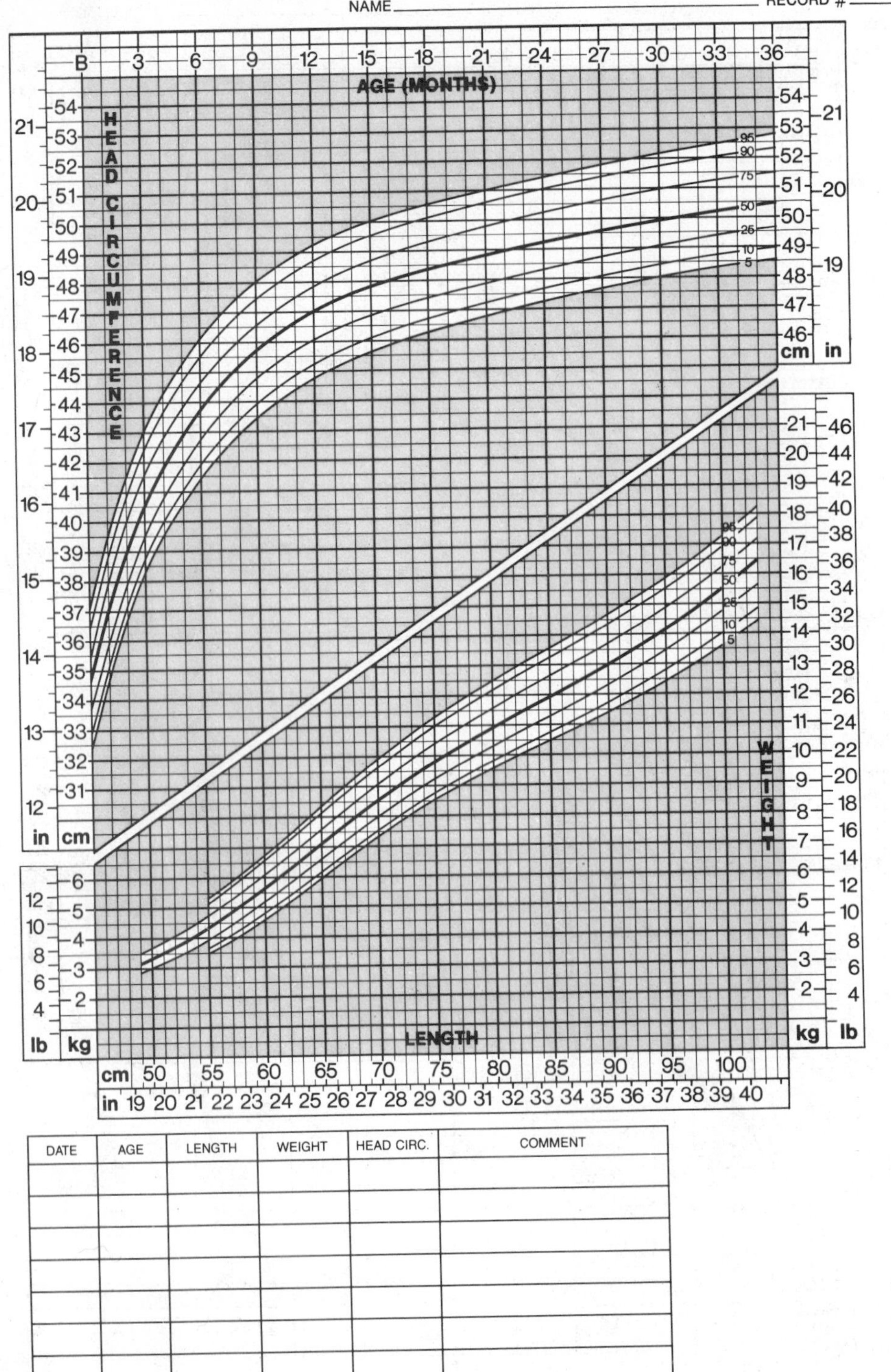

DATE	AGE	LENGTH	WEIGHT	HEAD CIRC.	COMMENT

SOURCE: Adapted from: Hamill PVV, Drizd TA, Johnson CL, Reed RB, Roche AF, Moore WM: Physical growth: National Center for Health Statistics percentiles. *Am J Clin Nutr* **32**:607–629, 1979. Data from the Fels Research Institute, Wright State University School of Medicine, Yellow Springs, Ohio. © 1982 Ross Laboratories. Courtesy of Ross Laboratories, Columbus, Ohio.

GIRLS: 2 TO 18 YEARS, PHYSICAL GROWTH NCHS PERCENTILES

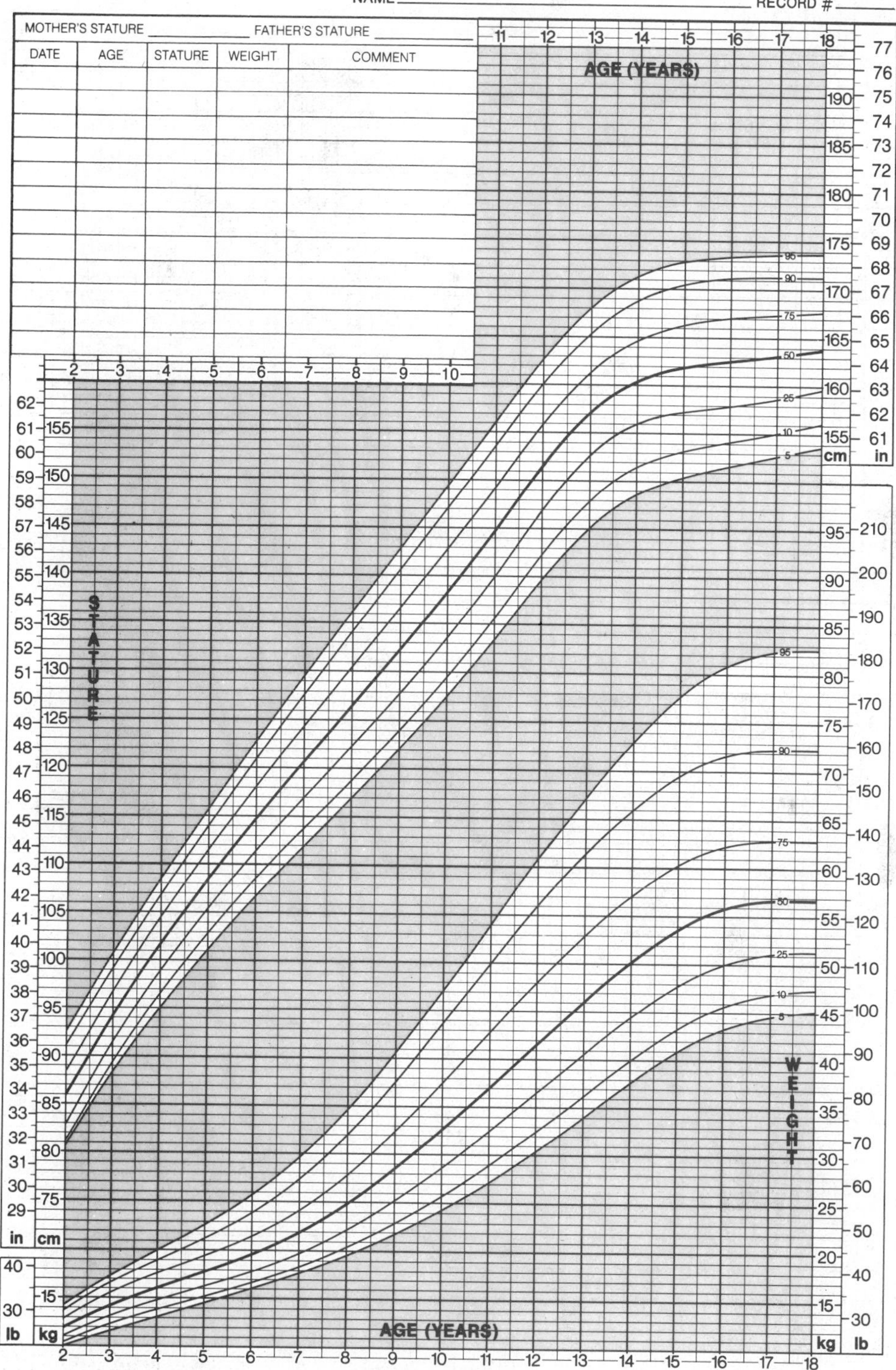

SOURCE: Adapted from: Hamill PVV, Drizd TA, Johnson CL, Reed RB, Roche AF, Moore WM: Physical growth: National Center for Health Statistics percentiles. *Am J Clin Nutr* **32:**607–629, 1979. Data from the Fels Research Institute, Wright State University School of Medicine, Yellow Springs, Ohio. © 1982 Ross Laboratories. Courtesy of Ross Laboratories, Columbus, Ohio.

GIRLS: PREPUBESCENT, PHYSICAL GROWTH NCHS PERCENTILES

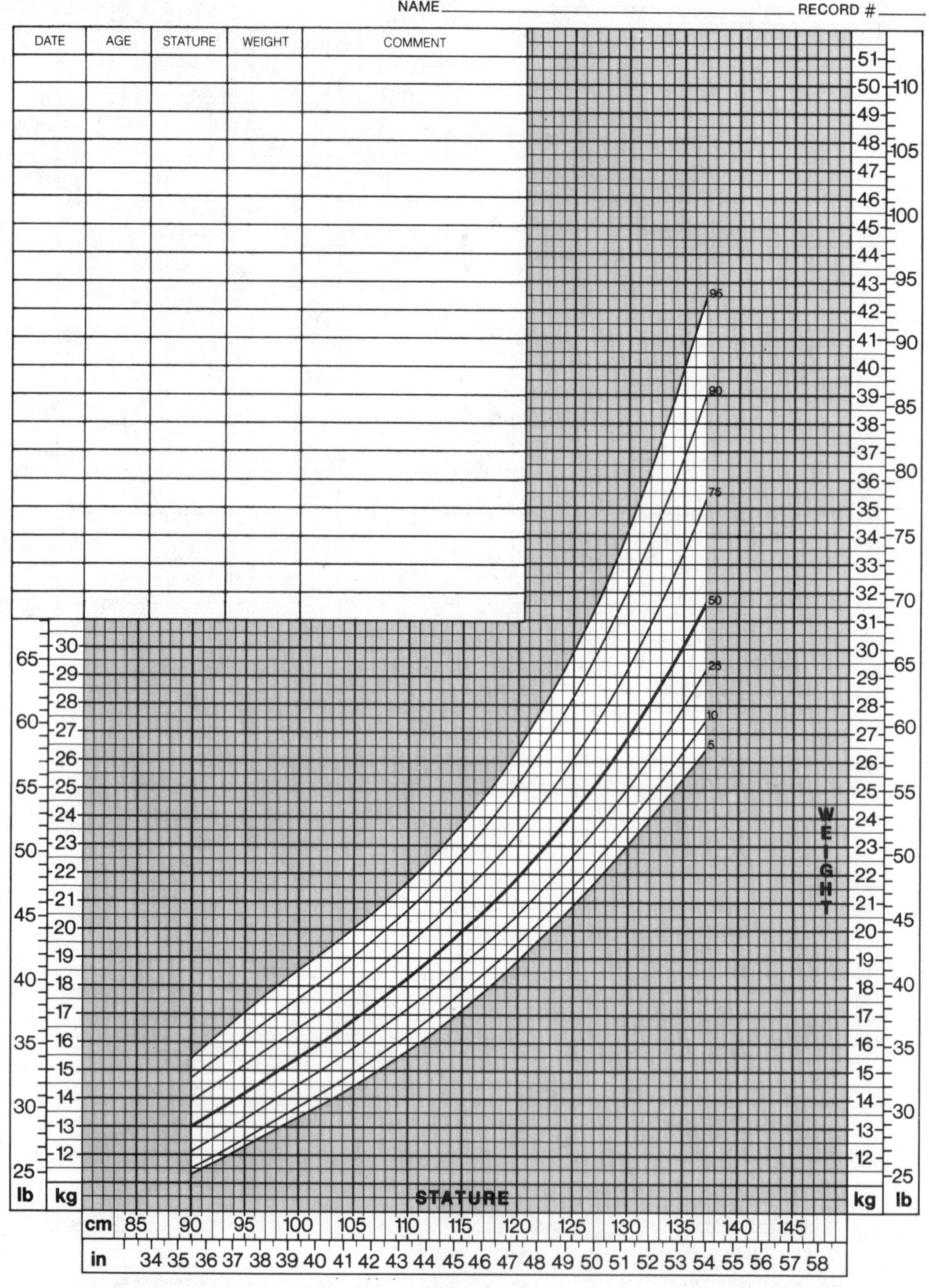

SOURCE: Adapted from: Hamill PVV, Drizd TA, Johnson CL, Reed RB, Roche AF, Moore WM: Physical growth: Nationa. Center for Health Statistics percentiles. *Am J Clin Nutr* **32**:607–629, 1979. Data from the Fels Research Institute, Wright State University School of Medicine, Yellow Springs, Ohio. © 1982 Ross Laboratories. Courtesy of Ross Laboratories, Columbus, Ohio.

BOYS: 2 TO 18 YEARS: PHYSICAL GROWTH NCHS PERCENTILES

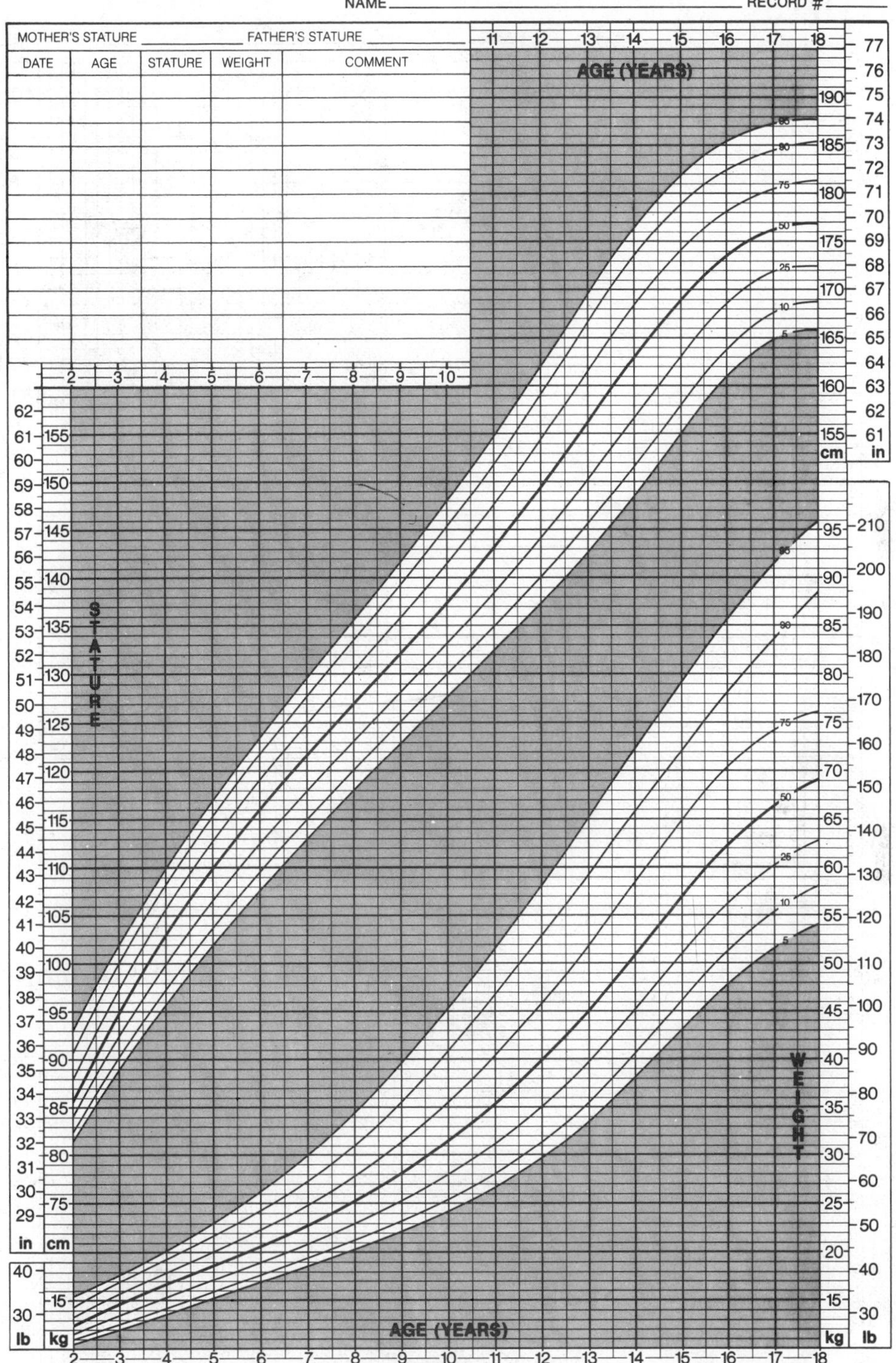

SOURCE: Adapted from: Hamill PVV, Drizd TA, Johnson CL, Reed RB, Roche AF, Moore WM: Physical growth: National Center for Health Statistics percentiles. *Am J Clin Nutr* **32:**607–629, 1979. Data from the Fels Research Institute, Wright State University School of Medicine, Yellow Springs, Ohio. © 1982 Ross Laboratories. Courtesy of Ross Laboratories, Columbus, Ohio.

BOYS: PREPUBESCENT, PHYSICAL GROWTH NCHS PERCENTILES

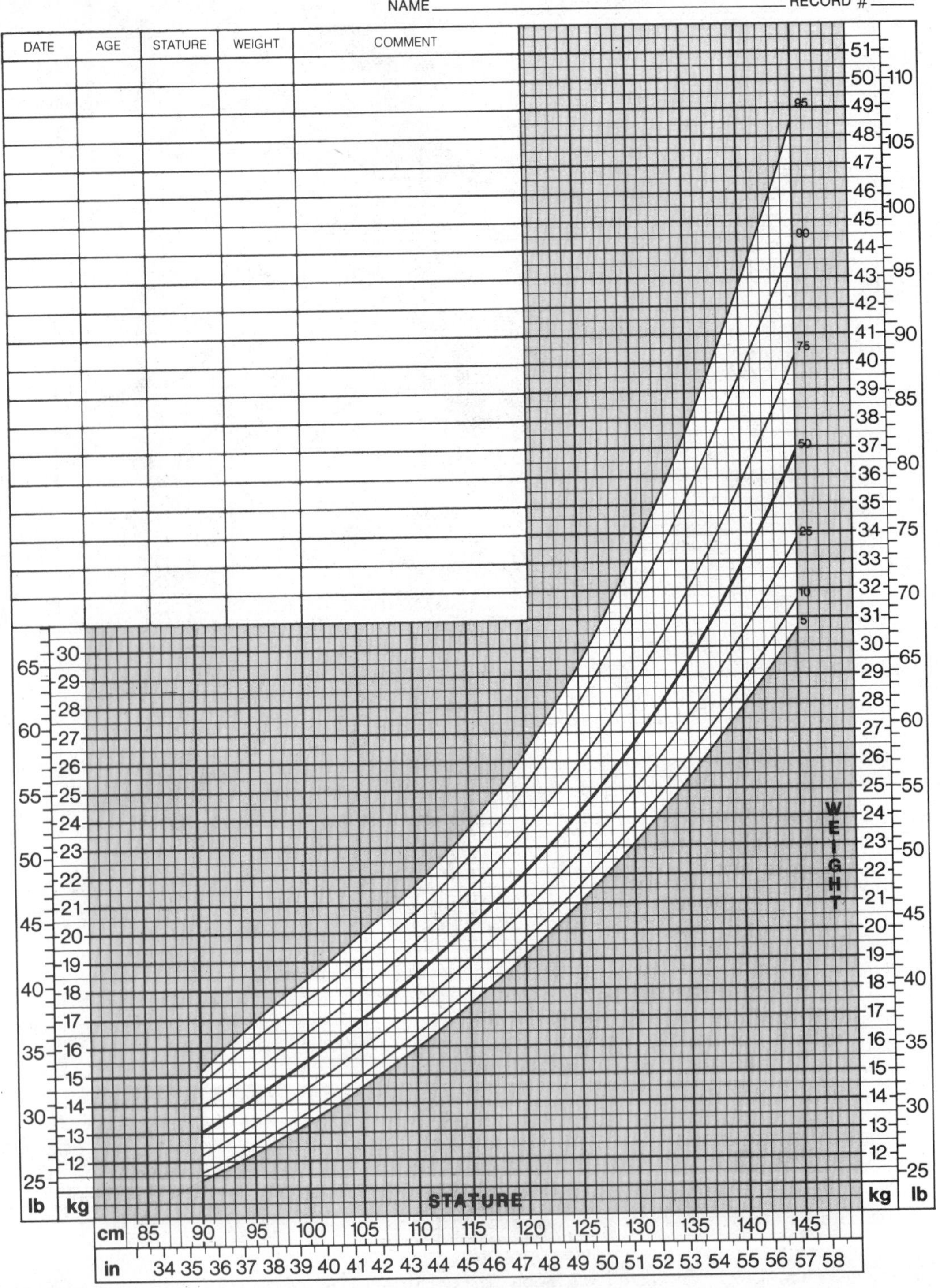

SOURCE: Adapted from: Hamill PVV, Drizd TA, Johnson CL, Reed RB, Roche AF, Moore WM: Physical growth: National Center for Health Statistics percentiles. *Am J Clin Nutr* **32**:607–629, 1979. Data from the Fels Research Institute, Wright State University School of Medicine, Yellow Springs, Ohio. © 1982 Ross Laboratories. Courtesy of Ross Laboratories, Columbus, Ohio.

Appendix E

Communicable Disease Table

COMMUNICABLE AND INFECTIOUS DISEASES

Name	Incubation Period	Period of Communicability	Mode of Transfer
Amebic dysentery (amebiasis)	2–4 weeks	During period of passing of feces contaminated with protozoan cysts; may continue for years	Food or water contaminated with the feces of infected persons
Anthrax	2–5 days, at least within 7 days	No evidence of transmission from person to person; articles and soil contaminated with spores may remain infective for years	Skin contact with tissue, wool, hides, and hair of infected animals and with soil contaminated by infected animals; inhalation of spores; ingestion of contaminated undercooked meat
Bacillary dysentery (shigellosis)	Usually less than 4 days, range 1–7 days	During acute infection and until infectious agent no longer present in feces (usually within 4 weeks of illness)	Fecal-oral transmission from infected individual or carrier, either by direct contact or contamination of food, water, or fomites; spread of contaminated feces by flies
Brucellosis	5–21 days, occasionally several months	No evidence of communicability from person to person	Contact with body fluids, tissues, aborted fetuses, and placentas of infected animals; ingestion of milk and dairy products from infected animals; inhalation of infectious agent
Candidiasis (moniliasis, thrush)	Variable, 2–5 days for thrush	While lesions persist	Contact with excretions from mouth, skin, vagina, and with feces of patients or carriers; during birth via contact with vaginal secretions; contact with contaminated bladder catheters and IV tubing
Chancroid	3–5 days, up to 14 days; can be as short as 24 h if mucous membranes not intact	While infectious agent present in original lesion or in discharging regional lymph nodes; can last for weeks	Sexual contact with discharges from open lesions or buboes; may be asymptomatic infection in women

COMMUNICABLE AND INFECTIOUS DISEASES *(continued)*

Name	Incubation Period	Period of Communicability	Mode of Transfer
Chickenpox (varicella) shingles (herpes zoster)	13–17 days; may extend to 21 days	As long as 5 days before eruption of chickenpox and not more than 6 days after last crop of vesicles	Spread of respiratory secretions of infected persons by direct, droplet, or airborne route; indirect spread by fomites freshly soiled with discharges from vesicles and mucous membranes of infected persons; scabs are not infective; susceptible persons may contract chickenpox from individuals with herpes zoster
Cholera	2–3 days; range from a few hours to 5 days	Not definitely known, presumed to last for duration of stool-positive carrier state which lasts for a few days after recovery	Ingestion of food or water contaminated with feces or vomitus of infected persons or with feces of carriers
Coccidioidomycosis	1–4 weeks	Not directly transmitted from persons or animals to man	Inhalation of spores from soil or culture media
Common cold	24 h; range 12–72 h	24 hours before onset to 5 days after onset	Direct oral contact or spread by droplet Fomites freshly soiled by nasal and oral discharges of infected persons
Dengue fever	5–6 days; range 3–15 days	Not directly transmitted from person to person	Bite of infective mosquito
Diphtheria	2–5 days	Usually 2 weeks or less, but seldom more than 4 weeks Until virulent bacilli are no longer present in discharges and lesions Carrier may disseminate organisms for 6 months or longer	Contact with droplets from mouth, nose, or throat of infected person or carrier Rarely by articles soiled with discharges from lesions of infected person
Encephalitis			
Mosquito-borne	5–15 days	Not directly transmitted from person to person	Bite of infective mosquito
Tick-borne	7–14 days	Same as above	Bite of infective ticks, milk from certain infected animals
Flukes			
Blood (schistosomiasis)	4–6 weeks after infection systemic manifestations usually begin	Usually 1–2 years or as long as eggs are discharged in urine or feces of infected person; may be 25 years or longer	Penetration of skin by free-swimming larvae

COMMUNICABLE AND INFECTIOUS DISEASES *(continued)*

Name	Incubation Period	Period of Communicability	Mode of Transfer
Intestinal (fasciolopsiasis)	Approx. 7 weeks from ingestion of infective larvae; eggs found in stool 1 month after infection	As long as viable eggs are discharged by patient: not directly transmitted from person to person	Ingestion of uncooked freshwater plants and snails containing the encysted larvae
Liver (clonorchiasis)	Undetermined; flukes reach maturity within 16–25 days after person ingests encysted larvae	Viable eggs may be passed by infected individual for up to 30 years, not directly transmitted from person to person	Ingestion of freshwater fish containing encysted larvae
Food Poisoning			
Botulism	Usually 12–36 h, sometimes several days	Not directly transmitted from person to person	Ingestion of improperly processed and inadequately cooked foods (usually from cans or jars) containing the toxin
Clostridium perfringens	10–12 h; range 8–22 h	Same as above	Inadequately heated meats containing feces or soil in which organism has multiplied
Salmonellosis	12–36 h; range 6–72 h	Several days to several weeks; occasionally a temporary carrier state continues for months, but rarely for over 1 year	Ingestion of food contaminated by feces of infected man or animals; inadequately cooked meat, poultry, and egg products; pharmaceuticals made from animal products
Staphylococcal	2–4 h; range 1–6 h	Not directly transmitted from person to person	Ingestion of contaminated food in which toxin-producing staphylococci from humans or cows have multiplied; food left standing before serving
German measles (rubella)	18 days; range 14–21 days	1 week before and at least 4 days after onset of rash	Droplet spread or direct contact with nasopharyngeal secretions of infected persons or with articles freshly soiled with discharges from nose and throat; may also be spread by urine, blood, and feces of infected persons
Giardiasis	Variable, usually 6–22 days	Entire period of infection	Water contaminated by feces; hand-to-mouth transfer of cysts from feces of infected persons

COMMUNICABLE AND INFECTIOUS DISEASES *(continued)*

Name	Incubation Period	Period of Communicability	Mode of Transfer
Gonorrhea	Usually 2–5 days, may be as long as 9 days	Months or years if untreated, especially in females who are often asymptomatic	Sexual contact with exudate from mucous membranes of infected persons
Granuloma Inguinale	Unknown, presumably 8–80 days	Unknown; presumably during period of open lesions on skin and mucous membranes	Sexual contact with lesions
Hepatitis			
Infectious (type A)	28–30 days; range 15–50 days	From latter half of incubation period to a few days after onset of jaundice	Person to person transmission via fecal-oral route; ingestion of contaminated food and water containing infective human feces, blood, or urine; parental administration of infected blood or blood products
Serum (type B) (homologous serum jaundice)	60–90 days; range 45–160 days	From several weeks before onset of symptoms through clinical course of disease; carrier state may last for years	Parenteral administration of infected blood and blood products; contaminated needles, syringes, and IV equipment
Herpes simplex	Up to 2 weeks	Up to 7 weeks after recovery from stomatitis for HSV type 1	HSV Type 1: Direct contact with virus in saliva of carriers HSV Type 2: Sexual contact
Histoplasmosis	10 days; range 5–18 days	Not usually transmitted from person to person	Inhalation of spores on dust particles
Infectious mononucleosis	2–6 weeks	Unknown	Spread from person to person via oral-pharyngeal route
Influenza	1–3 days	3 days from onset	Direct contact, droplet infection, or contact with articles freshly contaminated with discharges from nose and throat of infected persons
Keratoconjunctivitis, epidemic	5–12 days	From late in incubation period until 14 days after onset	Direct contact with eye secretions of infected persons or with instruments or solutions contaminated with these secretions
Leishmaniasis, visceral (kala azar)	2–4 months; range 10 days–2 years	While parasite remains in circulating blood or skin of mammalian reservoir host	Bite of infective sandflies; direct transmission from person to person and via blood transfusion has been reported
Lockjaw	See Tetanus		
Leptospirosis	10 days; range 4–19 days	Direct transmission from person to person is rare	Contact with water, moist soil, or vegetation contaminated with urine of infected animals; direct contact with infected animals

COMMUNICABLE AND INFECTIOUS DISEASES *(continued)*

Name	Incubation Period	Period of Communicability	Mode of Transfer
Lymphogranuloma venereum	5–30 days	Variable; while active lesions persist; may be weeks or years	Sexual contact with open lesions; indirect contact with articles contaminated by discharges
Malaria			
Benign Tertian (vivax malaria)	14 days	1–3 years	*For all:* Bite of infective female anopheline mosquito; injection or transfusion of blood of infected person; use of contaminated syringes
Quartan	30 days	Indefinitely	
Malignant tertian (falciparum malaria)	12 days	Not more than one year *For all:* patient infective for mosquitoes for as long as plasmodia gametocytes are present in blood	
Measles (rubeola)	10 days; range 8–13 days from exposure to onset of fever; 14 days until rash appears	From beginning of prodromal period until 14 days after rash appears	Droplet spread or direct contact with nose and throat discharges or urine of infected persons; less commonly transmitted by fomites freshly soiled with nose and throat secretions or by airborne spread
Meningococcal meningitis	3–4 days; range 2–10 days	Until organisms no longer present in secretions from nose and mouth; communicability ceases within 24 h after start of appropriate chemotherapy	Droplet spread and direct contact with discharges from nose and throat of clinically infected persons and carriers
Moniliasis	See Candidiasis		
Mumps	18 days; range 12–26 days	Height of communicability occurs approximately 48 h before swelling begins; virus has been found in saliva from 6 days before salivary gland involvement to 9 days after	Droplet spread and direct contact with saliva of an infected person
Paratyphoid fever	1–10 days for gastroenteritis, 1–3 weeks for enteric fever	1–2 weeks or as long as organism exists in excreta	Direct or indirect contact with urine or feces of patient or carrier; commonly spread by milk products or shellfish contaminated by hands of a carrier

COMMUNICABLE AND INFECTIOUS DISEASES *(continued)*

Name	Incubation Period	Period of Communicability	Mode of Transfer
Pediculosis	Eggs of lice hatch in 1 week under optimal conditions; sexual maturity is reached in 2 weeks	While lice remain alive on infested person or in clothing and until eggs in hair and clothing have been destroyed	Direct contact with an infested person, indirect contact with clothing, linen, and headgear on which lice or eggs exist
Pertussis	See Whooping cough		
Plague	2–6 weeks	Bubonic plague not directly transmitted from person to person; pneumonic plague highly communicable in conditions of overcrowding	Bubonic plague transmitted by bite of oriental rat flea (*Xenopsylla cheopsis*) and by contact with tissues of infected animals; pneumonic plague spread by airborne droplets from respiratory tract of an infected person
Pneumonia			
Pneumococcal and other bacterial	1–3 days	While infectious agent present in oral and nasal discharges	Spread by droplet or direct oral contact; indirect transmission through articles freshly soiled with respiratory discharges of infected persons
Primary atypical (mycoplasmal)	14–21 days	Usually less than 10 days; occasionally may last longer with persisting fever	Same as above
Poliomyelitis	7–12 days; range 3–21 days	7–10 days before and after onset of symptoms	Direct contact with feces or secretions from pharynx of infected persons
Q Fever	14–21 days	Direct transmission from person to person is rare	Inhalation of the rickettsiae in dust particles contaminated with excreta of infected animals; direct contact with infected animals and associated materials such as straw, fertilizer
Rabies	2–8 weeks	In biting animals for 3–5 days before onset of symptoms and throughout course of the disease	Virus transmitted in the saliva from the bite of an infected animal
Ringworm			
Body (tinea corporis)	4–10 days	While lesions present on body and viable spores exist on fomites	Contact with skin lesions of infected persons and animals and with contaminated furniture, bathroom fixtures, floors, and shower stalls

COMMUNICABLE AND INFECTIOUS DISEASES *(continued)*

Name	Incubation Period	Period of Communicability	Mode of Transfer
Foot (tinea pedis, athlete's foot)	Unknown	Same as above	Contact with skin lesions of infected persons or with contaminated floors, shower stalls, and other articles used by infected persons
Scalp (tinea capitis)	10–14 days	Same as above	Contact with infective lesions and with articles such as seats, toilet articles, or clothing contaminated with hair from infected persons or animals
Rocky mountain spotted fever	3–10 days	Not directly transmitted from person to person; tick remains infective for life, often as long as 18 months	Bite of an infected tick which has been attached to the skin for at least 4–6 h; contamination of the skin with crushed tissue or excreta of the tick
Roundworms			
Giant intestinal roundworm (ascariasis)	Worms reach maturity about 2 months after embryonated eggs are ingested by humans	As long as fertilized female worms live in intestine; adult worm usually lives less than 10 months; embryonated eggs may live in soil for months	Ingestion of soil containing infective eggs in human feces; not directly transmitted from person to person
Hookworm (ancylostomiasis)	A few weeks to several months	Potentially for several years if infected person not treated	Penetration of skin (usually of foot) by larvae in moist soil contaminated with feces
Pinworm (enterobiasis)	Life cycle of worm is 3–6 weeks	As long as gravid females remain in intestine; frequently reinfection by self or family members occurs	Direct transfer of eggs from anus to mouth by unwashed hands; indirect transfer of eggs via food, clothing, bedding, toilet seats Inhalation of eggs on dust particles
Threadworm (strongyloidiasis)	Indefinite and variable	As long as living worms remain in intestine	Penetration of skin (usually of foot) by larvae in moist soil contaminated with feces
Trichinosis	9 days after ingestion of infective meat; range 2–28 days	Not directly transmitted from person to person	Ingestion of insufficiently cooked pork containing encysted viable larvae
Whipworm (trichuriasis)	Indefinite	Same as above	Ingestion of soil contaminated with eggs from human feces
Rubella	See German Measles		
Rubeola	See Measles		
Salmonellosis	See Food Poisoning		

COMMUNICABLE AND INFECTIOUS DISEASES *(continued)*

Name	Incubation Period	Period of Communicability	Mode of Transfer
Scabies	Several days to weeks before itching occurs	Until mites and eggs are destroyed by specific treatment	Direct contact with skin of an infected person; to a small extent by bedding and clothing used by an infected person
Scarlet fever	1–3 days	10–21 days in untreated cases	Droplet spread by patient or carrier
Shigellosis	See Bacillary Dysentery		
Shingles (herpes zoster)	See Chickenpox		
Smallpox (variola)	10–12 days to onset of illness; range 7–17 days; 2–4 more days to onset of rash	Approx. 3 weeks; from development of first lesions to disappearance of all scabs; most communicable during first week	Direct contact with respiratory discharges, mucous membranes, and skin lesions of infected persons; indirect contact with articles contaminated by infected person; airborne spread
Streptococcal sore throat	1–3 days	10–21 days in untreated cases; transmission generally eliminated in 24 h with adequate penicillin therapy	Direct contact with respiratory discharges of an infected person; ingestion of contaminated milk or other food
Syphilis	21 days; range 10 days—10 weeks	Variable; intermittently communicable for 2–4 years during primary and secondary stages and during mucocutaneous recurrence; infectiveness ends within 24 h with adequate treatment with penicillin	Direct contact during sexual activity with saliva, semen, vaginal discharges, blood, and exudates from moist skin lesions and mucous membranes; placental transfer after 4th month of pregnancy; occasionally transferred by blood transfusion
Tapeworms			
Beef	8–14 weeks	Not directly transmitted from person to person	Ingestion of inadequately cooked beef containing the infective larvae
Fish	3–6 weeks	Same as above	Ingestion of inadequately cooked fish
Pork	8–14 weeks	Eggs remain viable for months and are discharged in feces for as long as worms live in intestines	Ingestion of inadequately cooked pork containing infective larvae; direct transfer of eggs in feces to mouth; ingestion of food or water containing eggs
Tetanus (lockjaw)	10 days; range 4–21 days	Not directly transmitted from person to person	Tetanus spores enter body via puncture wounds contaminated with soil which contains the feces of infected persons or animals

COMMUNICABLE AND INFECTIOUS DISEASES *(continued)*

Name	Incubation Period	Period of Communicability	Mode of Transfer
Tinea	See Ringworm		
Trachoma	5–12 days	While active lesions are present in conjunctivae and surrounding mucous membranes	Direct contact with discharges from the eye and possibly discharges from nasal mucous membranes of infected persons; contact with articles contaminated with these discharges
Trichomoniasis	7 days; range 4–20 days	While infection persists	Sexual contact with vaginal and urethral secretions of infected persons; during birth via contact with vaginal secretions
Tuberculosis	4–12 weeks from infection to primary lesion	As long as infectious tubercle bacilli are discharged in sputum	Airborne and droplet spread from sputum of infected persons
Tularemia	3 days; range 1–10 days	Not directly transmitted from person to person	Handling diseased animals or their hides; ingestion of undercooked infected wild rodents; bite of insects which have fed on infected animals
Typhoid fever	7–21 days	Until typhoid bacilli no longer appear in excreta; approx. 10% of patients discharge bacilli for 3 months after onset of symptoms; 2–5% become carriers	Ingestion of food or water contaminated by feces or urine of a patient or carrier
Typhus fever			
Epidemic louse-borne	12 days; range 7–14 days	Not directly transmitted from person to person	Rubbing crushed lice or their feces into bitten area on skin
Flea-borne (murine)	Same as above	Same as above	Bite of infective rat fleas
Mite-borne (scrub typhus, tsutsugamushi disease)	10–12 days; range 6–21 days	Same as above	Bite of infective mites during the larval stage
Varicella	See Chickenpox		
Variola	See Smallpox		
Whooping cough (pertussis)	7 days, not longer than 21 days	7 days after exposure to 3 weeks after onset of paroxysmal cough	Direct contact with respiratory secretions of infected persons; droplet spread; indirect contact with fomites freshly soiled with respiratory discharges of infected persons

COMMUNICABLE AND INFECTIOUS DISEASES *(continued)*

Name	Incubation Period	Period of Communicability	Mode of Transfer
Yellow fever	3–6 days	Not directly transmitted from person to person; highly communicable where many susceptible persons and mosquito vectors concurrently exist	Bite of infective mosquitoes
Yaws	2 weeks–3 months	Variable; while moist lesions are present	Direct contact with exudates from early skin lesions of infected persons

Appendix F

Dietary Tables

MEAN HEIGHTS AND WEIGHTS AND RECOMMENDED ENERGY INTAKE

Category	Age (years)	Weight (kg)	Weight (lb)	Height (cm)	Height (in)	Energy Needs (with range) (kcal/day)	Energy Needs (with range) (MJ)
Infants	0.0–0.5	6	13	60	24	kg × 115 (95–145)	kg × .48
	0.5–1.0	9	20	71	28	kg × 105 (80–135)	kg × .44
Children	1–3	13	29	90	35	1300 (900–1800)	5.5
	4–6	20	44	112	44	1700 (1300–2300)	7.1
	7–10	28	62	132	52	2400 (1650–3300)	10.1
Males	11–14	45	99	157	62	2700 (2000–3700)	11.3
	15–18	66	145	176	69	2800 (2100–3900)	11.8
	19–22	70	154	177	70	2900 (2500–3300)	12.2
	23–50	70	154	178	70	2700 (2300–3100)	11.3
	51–75	70	154	178	70	2400 (2000–2800)	10.1
	76+	70	154	178	70	2050 (1650–2450)	8.6
Females	11–14	46	101	157	62	2200 (1500–3000)	9.2
	15–18	55	120	163	64	2100 (1200–3000)	8.8
	19–22	55	120	163	64	2100 (1700–2500)	8.8
	23–50	55	120	163	64	2000 (1600–2400)	8.4
	51–75	55	120	163	64	1800 (1400–2200)	7.6
	76+	55	120	163	64	1600 (1200–2000)	6.7
Pregnancy						+300	
Lactation						+500	

SOURCE: Reproduced from *Recommended Dietary Allowances*, 9th Edition (1980), with the permission of the National Academy of Sciences, Washington, D.C.

The energy allowances for the young adults are for men and women doing light work. The allowances for the two older age groups represent mean energy needs over these age spans, allowing for a 2% decrease in basal (resting) metabolic rate per decade and a reduction in activity of 200 kcal/day for men and women between 51 and 75 years, 500 kcal for men over 75 years and 400 kcal for women over 75. The customary range of daily energy output is shown for adults in parentheses, and is based on a variation in energy needs of ±400 kcal at any one age, emphasizing the wide range of energy intakes appropriate for any group of people.

Energy allowances for children through age 18 are based on median energy intakes of children of these ages followed in longitudinal growth studies. The values in parentheses are 10th and 90th percentiles of energy intake, to indicate the range of energy consumption among children of these ages.

RECOMMENDED DAILY DIETARY ALLOWANCES[a]

							Fat-Soluble Vitamins			Water-Soluble			
	Age (years)	Weight (kg)	Weight (lbs)	Height (cm)	Height (in)	Protein (g)	Vitamin A (μ R.E.)[b]	Vitamin D (μg)[c]	Vitamin E (mg α T.E.)[d]	Vitamin C (mg)	Thiamin (mg)	Ribof-lavin (mg)	Niacin (mg N.E.)[e]
Infants	0.0–0.5	6	13	60	24	kg × 2.2	420	10	3	35	0.3	0.4	6
	0.5–1.0	9	20	71	28	kg × 2.0	400	10	4	35	0.5	0.6	8
Children	1–3	13	29	90	35	23	400	10	5	45	0.7	0.8	9
	4–6	20	44	112	44	30	500	10	6	45	0.9	1.0	11
	7–10	28	62	132	52	34	700	10	7	45	1.2	1.4	16
Males	11–14	45	99	157	62	45	1000	10	8	50	1.4	1.6	18
	15–18	66	145	176	69	56	1000	10	10	60	1.4	1.7	18
	19–22	70	154	177	70	56	1000	7.5	10	60	1.5	1.7	19
	23–50	70	154	178	70	56	1000	5	10	60	1.4	1.6	18
	51 +	70	154	178	70	56	1000	5	10	60	1.2	1.4	16
Females	11–14	46	101	157	62	46	800	10	8	50	1.1	1.3	15
	15–18	55	120	163	64	46	800	10	8	60	1.1	1.3	14
	19–22	55	120	163	64	44	800	7.5	8	60	1.1	1.3	14
	23–50	55	120	163	64	44	800	5	8	60	1.0	1.2	13
	51 +	55	120	163	64	44	800	5	8	60	1.0	1.2	13
Pregnant						+30	+200	+5	+2	+20	+0.4	+0.3	+2
Lactating						+20	+400	+5	+3	+40	+0.5	+0.5	+5

SOURCE: Reproduced from *Recommended Dietary Allowances*, 9th Edition (1980), with the permission of the National Academy of Sciences, Washington, D.C.

[a] The allowances are intended to provide for individual variations among most normal persons as they live in the United States under usual environmental stresses. Diets should be based on a variety of common foods in order to provide other nutrients for which human requirements have been less well defined.

[b] Retinol equivalents. 1 retinol equivalent = 1 μg retinol or 6 μg β-carotene.

[c] As cholecalciferol. 10 μg cholecalciferol = 400 I.U. vitamin D.

[d] α tocopherol equivalents. 1 mg d-α-tocopherol = 1 α T.E.

Vitamins			Minerals					
Vitamin B6 (mg)	Folacin[f] (μg)	Vitamin B12 (μg)	Calcium (mg)	Phosphorus (mg)	Magnesium (mg)	Iron (mg)	Zinc (mg)	Iodine (μg)
0.3	30	0.5[g]	360	240	50	10	3	40
0.6	45	1.5	540	360	90	15	5	50
0.9	100	2.0	800	800	150	15	10	70
1.3	200	2.5	800	800	200	10	10	90
1.6	300	3.0	800	800	250	10	10	120
1.8	400	3.0	1200	1200	350	18	15	150
2.0	400	3.0	1200	1200	400	18	15	150
2.2	400	3.0	800	800	350	10	15	150
2.2	400	3.0	800	800	350	10	15	150
2.2	400	3.0	800	800	350	10	15	150
1.8	400	3.0	1200	1200	300	18	15	150
2.0	400	3.0	1200	1200	300	18	15	150
2.0	400	3.0	800	800	300	18	15	150
2.0	400	3.0	800	800	300	18	15	150
2.0	400	3.0	800	800	300	10	15	150
+0.6	+400	+1.0	+400	+400	+150	*h*	+5	+25
+0.5	+100	+1.0	+400	+400	+150	*h*	+10	+50

[e] 1 N.E. (niacin equivalents) is equal to 1 mg of niacin or 60 mg of dietary tryptophan.

[f] The folacin allowances refer to dietary sources as determined by *Lactobacillus casei* assay after treatment with enzymes ("conjugases") to make polyglutamyl forms of the vitamin available to the test organism.

[g] The RDA for vitamin B12 in infants is based on average concentration of the vitamin in human milk. The allowances after weaning are based on energy intake (as recommended by the American Academy of Pediatrics) and consideration of other factors such as intestinal absorption.

[h] The increased requirement during pregnancy cannot be met by the iron content of habitual American diets nor by the existing iron stores of many women; therefore the use of 30–60 mg of supplemental iron is recommended. Iron needs during lactation are not substantially different from those of nonpregnant women, but continued supplementation of the mother for 2–3 months after parturition is advisable in order to replenish stores depleted by pregnancy.

ESTIMATED SAFE AND ADEQUATE DAILY DIETARY INTAKES OF ADDITIONAL SELECTED VITAMINS AND MINERALS[a]

		Vitamins			Trace Elements[b]						Electrolytes		
	Age (years)	Vitamin K (μg)	Biotin (μg)	Panto-thenic Acid (mg)	Copper (mg)	Man-ganese (mg)	Fluoride (mg)	Chromium (mg)	Selenium (mg)	Molyb-denum (mg)	Sodium (mg)	Potassium (mg)	Chloride (mg)
Infants	0–0.5	12	35	2	0.5–0.7	0.5–0.7	0.1–0.5	0.01–0.04	0.01–0.04	0.03–0.06	115–350	350–925	275–700
	0.5–1	10–20	50	3	0.7–1.0	0.7–1.0	0.2–1.0	0.02–0.06	0.02–0.06	0.04–0.08	250–750	425–1275	400–1200
Children	1–3	15–30	65	3	1.0–1.5	1.0–1.5	0.5–1.5	0.02–0.08	0.02–0.08	0.05–0.1	325–975	550–1650	500–1500
and	4–6	20–40	85	3–4	1.5–2.0	1.5–2.0	1.0–2.5	0.03–0.12	0.03–0.12	0.06–0.15	450–1350	775–2325	700–2100
Adoles-	7–10	30–60	120	4–5	2.0–2.5	2.0–3.0	1.5–2.5	0.05–0.2	0.05–0.2	0.1–0.3	600–1800	1000–3000	925–2775
cents	11+	50–100	100–200	4–7	2.0–3.0	2.5–5.0	1.5–2.5	0.05–0.2	0.05–0.2	0.15–0.5	900–2700	1525–4575	1400–4200
Adults		70–140	100–200	4–7	2.0–3.0	2.5–5.0	1.5–4.0	0.05–0.2	0.05–0.2	0.15–0.5	1100–3300	1875–5625	1700–5100

SOURCE: Reproduced from *Recommended Dietary Allowances*, 9th Edition (1980), with the permission of the National Academy of Sciences, Washington, D.C.

[a] Because there is less information on which to base allowances, these figures are not given in the main table of the RDA and are provided here in the form of ranges of recommended intakes.

[b] Since the toxic levels for many trace elements may be only several times usual intakes, the upper levels for the trace elements given in this table should not be habitually exceeded.

CANADIAN DIETARY STANDARDS

Age	Sex	Weight (kg)	Protein (g/day)[c]	Fat-Soluble Vitamins: Vitamin A (RE/day)[d]	Vitamin D (μg/day)[e]	Vitamin E (mg/day)[f]	Water-Soluble Vitamins: Vitamin C (mg/day)	Folacin (μg/day)[g]	Vitamin B_{12} (μg/day)	Minerals: Calcium (mg/day)	Magnesium (mg/day)	Iron (mg/day)	Iodine (μg/day)	Zinc (mg/day)
Months														
0–2	Both	4.5	11[h]	400	10	3	20	50	0.3	350	30	0.4[i]	25	2[j]
3–5	Both	7.0	14[h]	400	10	3	20	50	0.3	350	40	5	35	3
6–8	Both	8.5	16[h]	400	10	3	20	50	0.3	400	45	7	40	3
9–11	Both	9.5	18	400	10	3	20	55	0.3	400	50	7	45	3
Years														
1	Both	11	18	400	10	3	20	65	0.3	500	55	6	55	4
2–3	Both	14	20	400	5	4	20	80	0.4	500	65	6	65	4
4–6	Both	18	25	500	5	5	25	90	0.5	600	90	6	85	5
7–9	M	25	31	700	2.5	7	35	125	0.8	700	110	7	110	6
	F	25	29	700	2.5	6	30	125	0.8	700	110	7	95	6
10–12	M	34	38	800	2.5	8	40	170	1.0	900	150	10	125	7
	F	36	39	800	2.5	7	40	170	1.0	1000	160	10	110	7
13–15	M	50	49	900	2.5	9	50	160	1.5	1100	220	12	160	9
	F	48	43	800	2.5	7	45	160	1.5	800	190	13	160	8
16–18	M	62	54	1000	2.5	10	55	190	1.9	900	240	10	160	9
	F	53	47	800	2.5	7	45	160	1.9	700	220	14	160	8
19–24	M	71	57	1000	2.5	10	60	210	2.0	800	240	8	160	9
	F	58	41	800	2.5	7	45	165	2.0	700	190	14	160	8
25–49	M	74	57	1000	2.5	9	60	210	2.0	800	240	8	160	9
	F	59	41	800	2.5	6	45	165	2.0	700	190	14[k]	160	8
50–74	M	73	57	1000	2.5	7	60	210	2.0	800	240	8	160	9
	F	63	41	800	2.5	6	45	165	2.0	800	190	7	160	8
75 +	M	69	57	1000	2.5	6	60	210	2.0	800	240	8	160	9
	F	64	41	800	2.5	5	45	165	2.0	800	190	7	160	8

continued on next page

CANADIAN DIETARY STANDARDS *(continued)*

				Fat-Soluble Vitamins			Water-Soluble Vitamins			Minerals				
Age	Sex	Weight (kg)	Protein (g/day)[c]	Vitamin A (RE/day)[d]	Vitamin D (µg/day)[e]	Vitamin E (mg/day)[f]	Vitamin C (mg/day)	Folacin (µg/day)[g]	Vitamin B_{12} (µg/day)	Calcium (mg/day)	Magnesium (mg/day)	Iron (mg/day)	Iodine (µg/day)	Zinc (mg/day)
Pregnancy (additional)														
1st Trimester			15	100	2.5	2	0	305	1.0	500	15	6	25	0
2nd Trimester			20	100	2.5	2	20	305	1.0	500	20	6	25	1
3rd Trimester			25	100	2.5	2	20	305	1.0	500	25	6	25	2
Lactation (additional)			20	400	2.5	3	30	120	0.5	500	80	0	50	6

SOURCE: From *Recommended Nutrient Intakes for Canadians,* copyright © 1983 by Minister of Supply and Services, Canada. Reproduced by permission.

[a] Recommended intakes of energy and of certain nutrients are not listed in this table because of the nature of the variables upon which they are based. The figures for energy are estimates of average requirements for expected patterns of activity. For nutrients not shown, the following amounts are recommended: thiamin, 0.4 mg/1000 kcal (0.48 mg/5000 kJ); riboflavin, 0.5 mg/1000 kcal (0.6 mg/5000 kJ); niacin, 7.2 NE/1000 kcal (8.6 NE/5000 kJ); vitamin B_6, 15 µg, as pyridoxine, per gram of protein; phosphorus, same as calcium.

[b] Recommended intakes during periods of growth are taken as appropriate for individuals representative of the mid-point in each age group. All recommended intakes are designed to cover individual variations in essentially all of a healthy population subsisting upon a variety of common foods available in Canada.

[c] The primary units are grams per kilogram of body weight. The figures shown here are only examples.

[d] One retinol equivalent (RE) corresponds to the biological activity of 1 µg of retinol, 6 µg of β-carotene or 12 µg of other carotenes.

[e] Expressed as cholecalciferol or ergocalciferol.

[f] Expressed as *d*-α-tocopherol equivalents, relative to which β- and γ-tocopherol and α-tocotrienol have activities of 0.5, 0.1 and 0.3 respectively.

[g] Expressed as total folate.

[h] Assumption that the protein is from breast milk or is of the same biological value as that of breast milk and that between 3 and 9 months adjustment for the quality of the protein is made.

[i] It is assumed that breast milk is the source of iron up to 2 months of age.

[j] Based on the assumption that breast milk is the source of zinc for the first 2 months.

[k] After the menopause the recommended intake is 7 mg/day.

GUIDE TO GOOD NUTRITION: BASIC FOUR FOOD GROUPS

	Recommended Number of Servings				
Food Group	Child	Teenager	Adult	Pregnant Woman	Lactating Woman
Milk 1 cup milk, yogurt, or **Calcium Equivalent:** 1½ slices (1½ oz) cheddar cheese[a] 1 cup pudding 1¾ cups ice cream 2 cups cottage cheese[a]	3	4	2	4	4
Meat 2 ounces cooked, lean meat, fish, poultry, or **Protein Equivalent:** 2 eggs 2 slices (2 oz) cheddar cheese[a] ½ cup cottage cheese[a] 1 cup dried beans, peas 4 tbsp peanut butter	2	2	2	3	2
Fruit-Vegetable ½ cup cooked or juice 1 cup raw Portion commonly served such as medium-size apple or banana	4	4	4	4	4
Grain Whole grain, fortified, enriched 1 slice bread 1 cup ready-to-eat cereal ½ cup cooked cereal, pasta, grits	4	4	4	4	4

SOURCE: *Guide to Good Eating . . . A Recommended Daily Pattern,* Courtesy of National Dairy Council.

[a] Count cheese as serving of milk or meat, not both simultaneously.

"Others" complement but do not replace foods from the Four Food Groups. Amounts should be determined by individual caloric needs.

FORMULA FOR FULL-TERM INFANTS

	SMA with Iron	Enfamil with Iron	Similac with Iron
Protein	Nonfat milk and demineralized whey	Nonfat milk and demineralized whey	Nonfat milk
Fat (oils)	Oleo: 33% Oleic: 25% Coconut: 27% Soy: 15%	Coconut: 55% Soy: 45%	Coconut: 40% Soy: 60%
Carbohydrate	Lactose	Lactose	Lactose
Constituents (per liter)			
Protein (g)	15	15	15.0
Fat (g)	36	38	36.3
Carbohydrate (g)	72	69	72.3
Ash (g)	2.50	3.00	3.3
Vitamin A (IU)	2640	2100	2000
Vitamin D (IU)	423	420	400
Vitamin E (IU)	9.5	21	20
Vitamin C (mg)	58.2	55	55
Thiamine (mg)	0.71	0.53	0.65
Riboflavin (mg)	1.05	1.06	1.0
Niacin (mg equiv)	10.1	8.5	7.0
Pyridoxine (mg)	0.42	0.42	0.40
Pantothenic acid (mg)	2.1	3.2	3.0
Folacin (μg)	52.8	106	100
Vitamin B_{12} (μg)	1.05	1.6	1.5
Vitamin K_1 (μg)	58.1	58	55
Calcium (mg)	443	460	510
Phosphorus (mg)	330	320	390
Sodium (mg)	150	210	230
Potassium (mg)	560	690	800
Chloride (mg)	375	420	500
Magnesium (mg)	53	53	41
Manganese (mg)	0.16	0.11	0.03
Copper (mg)	0.50	0.63	0.60
Zinc (mg)	3.7	5.3	5.0
Iodine (μg)	69	106	100
Iron (mg)	12.7	12.7	12
Choline (mg)	106	106	—
Inositol (mg)	—	32	—
Biotin (μg)	15	16	10
Estimated renal solute load, mOsm/L	91.2	99.0	105
Osmolality, mOsm/kg H_2O	300	300	290

SOURCE: Courtesy of Wyeth Laboratories.

FORMULA FOR LOW-BIRTH-WEIGHT INFANTS

	SMA "Preemie"	Enfamil Premature	Similac Special Care
Components			
Protein	Nonfat milk and demineralized whey	Nonfat milk and demineralized whey	Nonfat milk and demineralized whey
Fat (oils)	MCT: 10% Oleo: 20% Oleic: 25% Coconut: 27% Soy: 18%	MCT: 40% Corn: 40% Coconut: 20%	MCT: 50% Corn: 30% Coconut: 20%
Carbohydrate	Lactose: 50% Glucose polymers: 50%	Lactose: 40% Glucose polymers: 60%	Lactose: 50% Glucose polymers: 50%
Constituents (per liter)			
Protein (g)	20	24	22
Fat (g)	44	41	44
Carbohydrate (g)	86	89	86
Ash (g)	4.00	5.00	6.50
Vitamin A (IU)	3200	2500	5500
Vitamin D (IU)	510	510	1200
Vitamin E (IU)	15	16	30
Vitamin C (mg)	70	69	300
Thiamine (mg)	0.80	0.62	2.00
Riboflavin (mg)	1.30	0.73	5.00
Niacin (mg equiv)	12.2	10.1	40
Pyridoxine (mg)	0.50	0.50	2.00
Pantothenic acid (mg)	3.60	3.80	15.00
Folacin (μg)	100	240	300
Vitamin B_{12} (μg)	2.0	2.5	4.5
Vitamin K_1 (μg)	70	76	100
Calcium (mg)	750	950	1440
Phosphorus (mg)	400	480	720
Sodium (mg)	320	320	380
Potassium (mg)	750	900	1120
Chloride (mg)	530	690	710
Magnesium (mg)	70	85	100
Manganese (mg)	0.20	0.21	0.10
Copper (mg)	0.70	0.73	2.0
Zinc (mg)	5	8	12
Iodine (μg)	83	64	150
Iron (mg)	3	1.3	3
Choline (mg)	127	57	80
Inositol (mg)	30	38	45
Biotin (μg)	18	190	300
Estimated renal solute load, mOsm/L	128	152.4	154.0
Osmolality, mOsm/kg H_2O	268	300	300

SOURCE: Courtesy of Wyeth Laboratories.

FOOD EXCHANGE LISTS

Food Product	Amount in 1 Exchange
Milk Exchanges	
Whole milk products (also count as 2 fat exchanges)	
Whole milk	1 cup
Canned, evaporated whole milk	½ cup
Buttermilk	1 cup
Yogurt (unflavored)	1 cup
Low-fat milk products	
1% fat-fortified milk (also counts as ½ fat exchange)	1 cup
2% fat-fortified milk (also counts as 1 fat exchange)	1 cup
Yogurt made from 2% fat-fortified milk, unflavored (also counts as 1 fat exchange)	1 cup
Nonfat milk products	
Skim milk	1 cup
Powdered milk in dry form	⅓ cup
Canned, evaporated skim milk	1 cup
Yogurt made from skim milk (unflavored)	1 cup
One milk exchange contains 12 g carbohydrate, 8 g protein, a trace of fat, and 80 calories	
Vegetable Exchanges	
Asparagus	½ cup
Bean sprouts	½ cup
Beets	½ cup
Broccoli	½ cup
Brussels sprouts	½ cup
Cabbage	½ cup
Carrots	½ cup
Cauliflower	½ cup
Celery	½ cup
Cucumber	½ cup
Eggplant	½ cup
Greens (beet, chard, collards, kale, mustard, spinach, turnip)	½ cup
Mushrooms	½ cup
Okra	½ cup
Onion	½ cup
Rhubarb	½ cup
Rutabaga	½ cup
Sauerkraut	½ cup
String beans	½ cup
Summer squash	½ cup
Tomato or tomato juice	½ cup
Turnip	½ cup
Vegetable juice cocktail	½ cup
Zucchini	½ cup
The following may be used raw in any amount desired	
Chicory	
Chinese cabbage	
Endive	
Escarole	
Lettuce	
Parsley	
Radish	
Watercress	
One vegetable exchange contains approximately 5 gm carbohydrate, 2 g protein, and 25 calories (See Bread Exchange List for the starchy vegetables)	
Fruit Exchanges (without sugar added)	
Apple	1 small
Apple juice	⅓ cup
Applesauce, unsweetened	½ cup
Apricot, fresh	2 medium
Apricot, dried	4 halves
Banana	½ small
Berries	
Blackberries	½ cup
Blueberries	½ cup
Raspberries	½ cup

FOOD EXCHANGE LISTS *(continued)*

Food Product	Amount in 1 Exchange
Strawberries	$\frac{3}{4}$ cup
Cherries	10 large
Cider	$\frac{1}{3}$ cup
Dates	2
Figs, fresh	1
Figs, dried	1
Grapefruit	$\frac{1}{2}$
Grapefruit juice	$\frac{1}{2}$ cup
Grapes	12
Grape juice	$\frac{1}{4}$ cup
Mango	$\frac{1}{2}$ small
Melon	
Cantaloupe	$\frac{1}{4}$ small
Honeydew	$\frac{1}{8}$ medium
Watermelon	1 cup
Nectarine	1 small
Orange	1 small
Orange juice	$\frac{1}{2}$ cup
Papaya	$\frac{3}{4}$ cup
Peach	1 medium
Pear	1 small
Persimmon	1 medium
Pineapple	$\frac{1}{2}$ cup
Pineapple juice	$\frac{1}{3}$ cup
Plums	2 medium
Prunes	2 medium
Prune juice	$\frac{1}{4}$ cup
Raisins	2 tbsp
Tangerine	1 medium
One fruit exchange contains 10 g carbohydrate and 40 calories	
Bread Exchanges	
Breads	
White, including French or Italian)	1 slice
Whole wheat	1 slice
Rye or pumpernickel	1 slice
Raisin	1 slice
Bagel, small	$\frac{1}{2}$
Plain roll, bread	1
Frankfurter roll	$\frac{1}{2}$
Hamburger bun	$\frac{1}{2}$
Dry bread crumbs	3 tbsp
Tortilla, 6 in.	1
Cereals	
Bran flakes	$\frac{1}{2}$ cup
Other ready-to-eat, unsweetened cereal	$\frac{3}{4}$ cup
Puffed cereal, unsweetened	1 cup
Cooked cereal	$\frac{1}{2}$ cup
Grits, cooked	$\frac{1}{2}$ cup
Rice or barley, cooked	$\frac{1}{2}$ cup
Macaroni, noodles, or spaghetti, cooked	$\frac{1}{2}$ cup
Popcorn, popped, no fat added	3 cups
Cornmeal, dry	2 tbsp
Flour	$2\frac{1}{2}$ tbsp
Wheat germ	$\frac{1}{4}$ cup
Crackers	
Arrowroot	3
Graham, $2\frac{1}{2}$ in. square	2
Matzoth, 4 in. × 6 in.	$\frac{1}{2}$
Oyster	20
Pretzels, $3\frac{1}{8}$ in. long × $\frac{1}{8}$ in. diameter	25
Rye wafers, 2 in. × $3\frac{1}{2}$ in.	3
Saltines	6
Soda, $2\frac{1}{2}$ in. square	4
Beans, peas, lentils (dried and cooked)	$\frac{1}{2}$ cup
Baked beans without pork, canned	$\frac{1}{4}$ cup
Starchy vegetables	
Corn	$\frac{1}{3}$ cup
Corn on the cob	1 small
Lima beans	$\frac{1}{2}$ cup
Parsnips	$\frac{2}{3}$ cup
Green peas, canned or frozen	$\frac{1}{2}$ cup
Potato, white	1 small
Potato, white, mashed	$\frac{1}{2}$ cup
Pumpkin	$\frac{3}{4}$ cup
Winter squash, acorn or butternut	$\frac{1}{2}$ cup
Yam or sweet potato	$\frac{1}{4}$ cup

FOOD EXCHANGE LISTS *(continued)*

Food Product	Amount in 1 Exchange
Prepared foods (also count as 1 fat exchange)	
Biscuit, 2 in. diameter	1
Cornbread, 2 in. × 2 in. × 1 in.	1
Corn muffin, 2 in. diameter	1
Crackers, round, butter type	5
Muffin, plain, small	1
Potatoes, French fried, 2 in. to 3½ in. long	8
Potato chips or corn chips (also counts as 2 fat exchanges)	15
Pancake, 5 in. × ½ in.	1
Waffle, 5 in. × ½ in.	1
One bread exchange contains 15 g carbohydrate, 2 g protein, and 70 calories	
Meat Exchanges	
Lean meats	
Beef: baby beef, chipped beef, chuck, flank steak, tenderloin, top round, bottom round, rump, spare ribs, tripe	1 oz
Lamb: leg, rib, sirloin, loin roast, loin chops, shank, shoulder	1 oz
Pork: leg (whole rump, center shank), ham, smoked center slices	1 oz
Veal: leg, loin, rib, shank, shoulder, cutlets	1 oz
Poultry: (meat without skin): chicken, turkey, Cornish hen, guinea hen, pheasant	1 oz
Fish: any canned or frozen	1 oz
canned salmon, tuna, mackerel, crab, and lobster	¼ cup
clams, oysters, shrimp, scallops	5 or 1 oz
sardines, drained	3
Cheeses containing less than 5% butterfat	1 oz
Cottage cheese, dry or 2% butterfat	¼ cup
Dried beans and peas (also counts as 1 bread exchange)	½ cup
One lean meat exchange contains 7 g of protein, 3 g of fat, and 55 calories	
Medium-fat meats (also count as ½ fat exchanges)	
Beef: ground (15%) fat, canned corned beef, rib eye, round	1 oz
Pork: tenderloin (all cuts), picnic shoulder, shoulder blade, Boston butt, Canadian bacon, boiled ham	1 oz
Liver, heart, kidney, and sweetbreads	1 oz
Cottage cheese, creamed	¼ cup
Cheese: mozzarella, ricotta, farmer's cheese, neufchatel	1 oz
Parmesan cheese	3 tbsp
Egg	1
Peanut butter (also counts as 2½ fat exchanges)	2 tbsp
High-fat meats (also count as 1 fat exchange)	
Beef: brisket, corned beef brisket, ground beef (more than 20% fat), hamburger (commercial), chuck (ground commercial), rib roasts, club and rib steaks	1 oz
Lamb: breast	1 oz
Pork: spare ribs, loin (back ribs), ground pork, country ham, deviled ham	1 oz
Veal: breast	1 oz
Poultry: capon, domestic duck, goose	1 oz

FOOD EXCHANGE LISTS *(continued)*

Food Product	Amount in 1 Exchange
Cheese: cheddar types	1 oz
Cold cuts $4\frac{1}{2}$ in. × $\frac{1}{8}$ in. slice	$\frac{1}{2}$ in. × $\frac{1}{8}$ in. slice
Frankfurter	1 small
Fat Exchanges	
Unsaturated fats	
Margarine, soft	1 tsp
Avocado, 4 in. diameter	$\frac{1}{8}$
Oil: corn, cottonseed, olive, peanut, safflower, soy, sunflower	1 tsp
Olives	5 small
Almonds	10 whole
Pecans	2 large whole
Peanuts, Spanish	20 whole
Peanuts, Virginia	10 whole
Other nuts	6 small
Saturated fats	
Margarine, regular stick	1 tsp
Butter	1 tsp
Bacon fat	1 tsp
Bacon, crisp	1 strip
Cream, light or sour	2 tbsp
Cream, heavy	1 tbsp
Cream cheese	1 tbsp
Salad dressings, French or Italian style	1 tbsp
Lard	1 tsp
Mayonnaise	1 tsp
Salad dressing, mayonnaise-type	2 tsp
Salt pork	$\frac{3}{4}$ in. cube
One fat exchange contains 5 g fat and 45 calories	

SOURCE: Adapted from *Exchange Lists for Meal Planning,* prepared by Committees of the American Diabetes Association, Inc., and The American Dietetic Association, in cooperation with the National Institute of Arthritis, Metabolism and Digestive Diseases and the National Heart and Lung Institute, National Institutes of Health, Public Health Service, U.S. Department of Health, Education and Welfare.

CULTURAL FOOD HABITS

Chinese Food Habits

Milk: Considered luxury item, even disliked. Cheese rarely used, except in Northern China a cheese-type product from goat's or cow's milk.

Suggestions: Encourage use of milk in cereals or steamed eggs (pudding). Encourage milk cheese, ice cream, and bean curd.

Meat: Limited, mostly pork, fish and eggs, some chicken, shellfish; sometimes excluded from diet of children.

Suggestions: Encourage increased use of meat, fish, poultry, and eggs. Introduce "baby food meat" for children.

Vegetables and fruits: Spinach, broccoli, leeks, greens, bok toy (cabbage), carrots, pumpkin, sweet potatoes, mushrooms, soybeans, brussel sprouts, turnips, radishes, kohlrabi, white eggplant, yautia, eggplant, bambo shoots, and snowpeas.

Fruits considered a delicacy–snack food, some reserved for men. Fruits common: persimmon, peaches, plums, pears, large dates, apples, figs, winter melon, bananas, mango, red tangerines, papaya, pineapple, orange, litchee nuts, small dates.

Suggestions: Increased use of fruits or vegetables high in vitamin C as snack or "dessert."

Breads and cereals: Millet and rice predominant; wheat products include noodles and steamed bread.

Suggestions: Encourage use of brown rice.

Miscellaneous: Soybean oil, peanut oil, and lard are used.

Suggestions: Affirm practice of limited use of fats but encourage liquid types.

Italian Food Habits

Milk: Adults use little except in coffee. Seldom thought of as food. Children may or may not get recommended amounts.

Cheese used frequently, and in preparation of cooked foods.

Suggestions: Encourage use of milk for all the family. Greater use of dry skim milk and evaporated can be encouraged. Encourage wider use of cheeses at end of meal with fruit and in cooking.

Meat: Veal, beef, pork, and chicken are most popular. All parts are eaten including organ meats. Highly seasoned meats are common. All kinds of fish, both fresh and canned, some fried in oil, used in stews or chowders.

Eggs are liked, the most expensive grades preferred.

Dried beans and peas are used in soups with pasta and served in salads.

Suggestions: Encourage cooking methods other than frying. Discourage the use of highly seasoned fatty and fried meats for small children.

Fish, eggs, dried peas and beans, and ricotta cheese make good meat substitutes.

Vegetables and fruits: Large quantities of escarole, swiss chard, mustard greens, dandelion greens, and broccoli are popular. Salads are part of most meals. Peppers and tomatoes are used in preparation of foods. Eggplant, zucchini, artichokes, mushrooms, and fava beans are favorites.

Fruits liked: Grapes, oranges, tangerines, figs, persimmons, and pomegranates.

Suggestions: Less cooking time and less use of oil. Encourage use of canned tomatoes when fresh are out of season.

Selection of fresh fruit in season and canned fruit juices when less expensive than fresh.

Bread and cereal: Pasta and rice are staples eaten each meal. Use of oatmeal and farina has increased.

Suggestions: Encourage use of whole grain bread.

Miscellaneous: Olive oil preferred for cooking. Lard and salt pork are flavoring for soups and tomato sauce. Butter preferred for baking.

Suggestions: Urge families to use soybean, cottonseed, and corn oils.

Japanese Food Habits

Milk: Milk fresh and canned is used in small amounts, in coffee and milk desserts, such as ice cream.

Cheese is used in only small amounts.

Suggestions: Encourage increased consumption of all forms of milk, including use of cheese.

Meat: Variety of salt and fresh water fish eaten, baked, boiled, and in soups. Raw fish consumed on occasion. Smoked, dried, and canned fish consumed. Beef, pork, and poultry preferred to lamb and veal, mixed with vegetables and seasoned with soy sauce. Eggs eaten raw, fried, boiled, scrambled, and in soups.

Suggestions: Encourage use of highly nutritious variety meats, hard and soft cheeses and cottage cheese for protein. Discourage eating raw eggs. Use of pea and bean dishes as well as peanut butter can be encouraged.

Vegetables and fruits: Commonly used vegetables are spinach, broccoli, carrots, green beans, peas, cauliflower, tomatoes, cucumbers, eggplant, peppers, and squash. May be prepared with meat, fish, and chicken. Fruits eaten are oranges, tangerines, grapefruit, apples, pears, and melons.

Suggestions: Encourage cooking procedures to preserve nutrients. Discourage par-cooking and draining of water. Emphasize use of fruits high in vitamin C.

Breads and cereals: Polished white rice is the staple. Consumption of wheat products is a post–World War II practice.

Suggestions: Encourage use of restored rice and discourage washing prior to cooking. Suggest more frequent inclusion of potatoes cooked in skin in place of rice. Urge use of whole grain breads and cereals.

Miscellaneous: Butter used in small amount. Fat used in food only for deep fat frying. Simple cakes and cookies of sugar and rice flour contain little or no fat.

Seasonings are soy sauce or Miso sauce. Pickles with high salt content eaten in variety.

Suggestions: Seasonings and pickles should be used in moderation.

Jewish Food Habits

Milk: Dietary Laws prohibit using meat and milk at the same meal. (Six hours must elapse after a meat meal before dairy foods may be eaten; half an hour must elapse after a dairy food before meat may be eaten).

Cheeses—American, Muenster, and Swiss—well liked. Cottage cheese and pot cheese eaten plain or in blintzes and noodle puddings.

Suggestions: Encourage use of milk at breakfast and lunch times to insure adequate milk intake. Explain that cream cheese is a fat, not a milk substitute and encourage cheeses high in protein and calcium.

Meat: Separate dishes and utensils must be used for preparing and serving meat and dairy products.

Orthodox Jews use only the forequarters (rib section forward) of quadrupeds with a cloven hoof who chew their cud, i.e., cattle, sheep, goat, and deer. Animals and poultry must be slaughtered by a ritual slaughterer (shochet) according to specified regulations. Before cooking, meat is koshered by one of two methods: (1) soaking it in cold water for half an hour; salting it with coarse salt (koshering salt); and draining it to let blood run off. It is then thoroughly washed under cold running water and drained again before cooking. (2) Quick searing. Liver, for example, cannot be koshered by soaking and salting because of its high blood content. It is, therefore, rinsed, drained well, and broiled on a grill. It may then be fried, chopped, or combined with other foods. The second method is preferred for patients on salt restricted diets.

Meat is usually broiled, boiled, roasted, or stewed with vegetables added. Fish that have fins and scales may be used, such as whitefish (fresh and as gefilte fish); smoked sable; karp, lox (salmon); and caviar.

Shellfish (such as oysters, crab, and lobster) and scavenger fish such as sturgeon and catfish are not allowed.

Fish and eggs are considered "pareve" or neutral and may be eaten as dairy or meat.

Eggs are eaten in abundance. An egg with a clot of blood must be discarded.

Dried beans, peas, lentils are eaten liberally, especially as soup.

Suggestions: Discourage excessive use of delicatessen-type meats, such as corned beef, pastrami, and salami.

Urge use of fish, cheese, and other sources of protein.

Vegetables and fruits: Greens, spinach, sorrel leaves are used for Schav, a soup. Use is made of broccoli, carrots, chicory, sweet potatoes, and yams. Green peppers often stuffed with meat or dairy mixture. Green cabbage is cooked slightly and stuffed with beef and raisin mixture with tomato sauce. Root vegetables and potatoes are liberally used. Noodles as a potato substitute are preferred to rice. Beets are used in soup (borscht).

Oranges or grapefruit used for breakfast. Cooked dried fruits (prunes, raisins, apples, peaches, pears, apricots) are commonly served with meat meal.

Suggestions: Stress more variety in use of dark green leafy and deep yellow vegetables, their correct method of cooking with small amount of water, covered pot and short cooking time.

Point out high caloric value of dried fruits.

Breads and cereals: Water rolls (bagel), rye bread, and pumpernickel are often used, as these do not have milk or milk solids and, therefore, can be eaten with meat or dairy meals. They are considered "pareve" or neutral. Matzoth, also "pareve," is the only bread product allowed during Passover, but is commonly used throughout the year. Whole grains such as oatmeal, barley, brown rice, buckwheat groats (kasha) are used.

Suggestions: Encourage use of whole wheat bread at dairy meals. Matzoth, crackers, and saltines are not enriched and make little contribution to diet, other than Calories.

Miscellaneous: Sweet (unsalted) butter, usually whipped, is preferred to salted butter. Vegetable oils and shortenings are considered "pareve" or neutral. Chicken fat is often the choice for browning meats and frying potato pancakes.

Danish pastries, coffee cakes, homemade cakes and cookies may be eaten in large quantities. Honey cakes are served for various holidays.

There may be an overuse of relishes.

Soup may be used at every meal.

Soft drinks are served with meat meals when milk is forbidden.

Suggestions: The code "U" on a package indicates it is permissible. If in doubt check with local rabbinical authorities. Encourage greater use of vegetable oils.

Encourage desserts such as milk puddings, ice milk, ice cream, for dairy meals and fruit with meat meals.

Encourage soups high in daily nutrient needs. Discourage overuse of soft drinks.

Polish Food Habits

Milk: Children drink fresh milk, while adults may prefer buttermilk. Sour cream is also popular, used in soup, salad dressings, with berries, and raw vegetables.

Cheese is well liked. Cottage cheese is well liked and may be served with sour cream.

Suggestions: Encourage recommended intake of milk or milk products for whole family.

Meat: Meat commonly consumed—beef, pork, pigs' knuckles, sausages, smoked and cured pork, chicken, goose, duck and variety meats (liver, tripe, tongue, brains). Small amounts used in soups and stews. Fish, fresh, smoked, dried, or pickled, is used. Eggs well liked and also used in pancakes, noodles, dumplings and soups, along with legumes.

Suggestions: For economy greater use of meat substitutes and less expensive cuts of meat in the preparation of stews and soups. Greater amounts of meat may be desirable in mixed dishes.

Vegetables and fruits: Potatoes are a very important part of diet. Other popular vegetables include carrots, beets, turnips, cauliflower, kohlrabi, broccoli, sorrel, green pepper, peas, spinach, and green beans.

Vitamin C–rich fruits are not traditionally popular but citrus fruits may be used more today than in previous years. Dried fruits are liked.

Suggestions: Encourage retention of vitamin A in use of broccoli, kale, sorrel, green peppers, raw cabbage, fresh tomato in season, and canned and frozen citrus juices in off-season may be stressed for vitamin C.

Encourage proper cooking methods for retention of vitamin C in vegetables.

Stress use of root vegetables and fruits and vegetables in season.

Breads and cereals: Bread eaten with each meal. Pumpernickel, sour rye bread, and white bread are well liked. Sweet buns are common. Oatmeal, rice, noodles, dumplings, cornmeal, porridge and kasha are prominent.

Suggestions: Encourage whole grains.

Miscellaneous: Wide variety of fats and oils are used. Fond of candy, sweet cakes, and other sweets such as honey.

Coffee with cream and sugar is a favorite beverage. Tea is infrequent.

Polish foods are highly salted and seasoned.

Suggestions: Suggest more frequent use of fruits as desserts.

Puerto Rican Food Habits

Milk: Milk may be used in insufficient quantities due to economic conditions rather than because it is not liked. Although milk may not be consumed as such, a cup of cafe con leche may contain two to five ounces of milk.

The domestic American cheese is used in limited quantities. Native white cheese (resembling farmer cheese, but firmer and saltier) is used, but is expensive.

Suggestions: Use of milk as a beverage and in cooking may need to be encouraged, including evaporated milk, nonfat dry milk and in puddings and cereals.

Greater emphasis can be placed on use of cheese.

Meat: Chicken in combination with other foods is frequently eaten. Expensive cuts of pork and beef are usually fried. Ham butts and sausage used to flavor different dishes. The intestine of the pig is eaten either fried (cuchifritos) or stewed with native vegetables (salcocho) and chick-peas.

Fish is used in limited amounts, salt codfish is common. Eggs used in cooking and fried and scrambled eggs are popular.

Beans are eaten either cooked or served with rice daily. A sauce called "refrito" (green pepper, tomato, garlic, and lard) is served with beans and rice. Pigeon and chick-peas are popular.

Suggestions: Variety meats may be used in increased amounts. Emphasize lean, tender, and lower cost cuts with slow cooking methods.

Suggest that use of cuchifritos be limited to holidays. Encourage larger quantities of vegetables and meat as well as peas in salcocho.

More consumption of fresh, frozen, or canned fish.

Greater use of eggs as a main dish and meat substitute. Suggest larger amounts of beans than rice. Milk, meat, chicken, cheese, or fish should be eaten with the bean meal for protein. Pigeon peas are more expensive than chick-peas, and chick-peas protein is almost as good as that of the soybean.

Vegetables and fruits: Expensive imported vegetables, such as yautia, apio, malanga, name, plantain are frequently used. These viandas are high in starch and have fair amounts of B vitamins, iron, and vitamin C. Pumpkins, carrots, green pepper, tomatoes, and sweet potatoes are well liked. Pumpkin is used to thicken and flavor foods. Potatoes are eaten in small amounts in stews, soups, or are fried. Head lettuce, cabbage, fresh tomatoes, and onions are often salad ingredients. Long cooking of vegetables in stews is common.

Imported fruits are used often. Fruit cocktail, canned pears, and peaches are liked. Peach, apricot, and pear nectar are commonly used.

Suggestions: Encourage use of less expensive vegetables such as carrots, beets, yellow squash, turnips. Root vegetables may be prepared and served same way as tubers (plantain, yautia, yucca, name).

Urge use of more cooked and raw green leafy vegetables. Stress greater intake of other salad greens and cabbage. Emphasize correct cooking methods of vegetables, small amount of water, covered pot and short time.

Greater use of potatoes cooked in skin can be suggested.

Greater amount of citrus juices, fresh, frozen, or canned can be used. Encourage use of bananas and pineapple in season, also apples and pears. Recommend use of fruits canned in light rather than heavy syrup.

Breads and cereals: Bread used in only small amounts. Plantain is often eaten in place of bread. French bread, rolls, and crackers are most frequent choices.

Breakfast cereals—oatmeal, farina, cornmeal, and cornflakes—are increasing. Cereals are often cooked in milk instead of water.

Suggestions: Encourage use of whole grain breads, enriched or brown rice. Encourage cooking cereal in milk. Use of sugar-coated cereals should be discouraged.

Miscellaneous: Butter is used in small amounts on bread. Lard and salt pork are used for flavoring in large amounts. Olive oil is favorite for salads.

Sugar is liberally used in beverages and desserts. Cakes, pies, guava, orange and mango pastes, and boiled papaya preserves are favored often between meals.

Black malt beer is a favorite beverage, and is combined with beaten egg for convalescents and pregnant women. It contains a fair amount of iron and some B vitamins and is high in Calories.

Canned soups are often served as main dish.

Suggestions: Suggest margarine in place of butter. Corn, cottonseed, or soybean oils in seasoning vegetables and other dishes rather than lard and salt pork.

Encourage less frequent use of sugar. Recommend use of other nourishing beverages such as milk and fruit juices.

Stress meal planning around a main dish made of a protein food rather than soups of low protein value.

Southern United States Food Habits

Milk: Limited amounts of milk are consumed. Buttermilk often preferred.

Cheese is well liked in sandwiches and baked macaroni.

Suggestions: Encourage use of evaporated and nonfat dry milk for both cooking and drinking, and greater use of cheese.

Meat: Chicken as "company" dish is enjoyed. Pork and variety meats are popular. Pigs' feet, hog jowls, ham hocks, cured ham, and heart are often eaten, stewed, boiled with vegetables, or fried. Spareribs are baked or barbecued. Lungs, kidneys, and brains are floured and fried. Chitterlings (intestines) are cut, dredged with cornmeal or flour, and fried crisp.

Beef is used in hash or stewed with vegetables. Cured tongue is also eaten.

Fish and shellfish, fresh, and canned, Swannee River catfish dipped in cornmeal and fried, boiled shrimp, fried scallops, and fried, stewed or raw oysters are popular.

Game—rabbit, squirrel, opossum—are usually used in a stew.

Eggs are usually fried.

Legumes and nuts—dried black-eyed peas and beans cooked with salt pork—are prominent part of meal. Peanuts and peanut butter are consumed.

Suggestions: Emphasize the lean, economical cuts of meat and stress that salt pork and bacon are fats not meats. Encourage stewing, baking, roasting, and boiling as methods of cookery.

Stress that white or brown eggs are equally nutritious, Grade B for cooking.

Urge that milk or cheese be served with the "bean meal."

Vegetables and fruits: Vegetables are liked but few eaten raw. Leafy greens, turnip greens, mustard greens, collards, cabbage, and green beans are cooked in water with bacon, ham hocks or salt pork. The cooking liquid may be eaten with cornbread. Tomatoes, fresh and canned, white potatoes, sweet potatoes, fried, baked, or candied with syrup are popular.

Fruits, although little citrus fruit, may be eaten. Fruits in season are eaten between meals and watermelon and lemonade are favorites in the summer.

Suggestions: Discuss quick-cooking of vegetables in little water to save vitamins. Note that addition of baking soda to water in which vegetables are cooked destroys the vitamins.

Stress that cooked or raw vegetables should be served in addition to potatoes or legumes.

Point out value of fruits. For limited budgets encourage serving citrus fruit or juice as well as cheaper grades of canned tomatoes, raw cabbage, "greens," and potatoes for vitamin C.

Breads and cereals: Few whole grain cereals are used. Hominy grits with gravy, hot biscuits with molasses, and cornbread are eaten.

White or polished rice cooked and combined with ham fat, tomatoes, onion, and okra is popular. Dumplings, pancakes, and hoecakes (originally baked on a hoe) are favorites.

Suggestions: Teach use of whole grain breads and cereals. Stress use of cooked cereals such as oatmeal.

Emphasize inclusion of protein food such as meat or milk when casserole is served.

Miscellaneous: Bacon and salt pork are liberally used. Lard used for baking and frying. Butter for preparing desserts. Gravies are used generously.

Sweets in cakes, cookies, pies, other pastries, and sweet breads are popular. Molasses and cane syrup are employed as sweeteners. Ice cream, jams, and jellies are eaten. Soft drinks consumed by children.

Suggestions: Discourage use of large amounts of bacon and salt pork where overweight and salt restrictions are factors. Suggest methods of cooking other than frying. Encourage use of margarine and oil.

Since rich desserts may tend to displace protective foods, especially in the low-income food budget, they should be used only in moderation. Excessive intake of sweets should be avoided, especially by small children.

Spanish American—Mexican Food Habits

Milk: Milk may be limited due to availability and economy.

Limited amounts of cheese are used.

Suggestions: Utilize various forms of milk in cookery, as a beverage—dried, evaporated or fresh milk.

Increase use of cheeses to improve quality of protein in diet.

Meat: Chicken, pork chops, weiners and cold cuts and hamburgers usually used only once or twice a week.

Eggs used frequently fried. In rural areas, many have their own chickens.

Beans are usually eaten with every meal, cooked, mashed, or refried with lard.

Suggestions: Emphasis on variety of lower cost meats and cooking methods may provide more frequent use of meats.

Eggs are good meat substitute and daily consumption is encouraged.

Beans and lentils provide good source of protein and calcium. Their protein is enhanced when eaten with animal proteins such as milk, meat, eggs, or cheese.

Vegetables and fruits: Fried potatoes are basic, maybe three times a day.

Chilies from green and red peppers are popular each meal. These items are good sources of vitamin A even when dried. Green peppers are usually called "mangoes."

Fresh tomatoes are purchased the year round and most popular vegetable. Occasionally canned tomatoes are used.

Pumpkin, corn, field greens, onions, and carrots are used frequently.

Bananas, melons, peaches, and canned fruit cocktail are popular. Oranges and apples are used as snacks.

Suggestions: Encourage wide variety of vegetables. Different cooking methods could be used. Encourage use of peppers but stress caution in home canning methods.

Recommend a variety of fruit canned in light syrup as economical. Use of citrus fruits could be encouraged. Fruit drinks should not be substituted for fruit juices.

Melons (cantaloupe in particular) are encouraged due to high vitamin C content.

Breads and cereals: Bread is a popular item. Tortillas from enriched wheat flour are made daily. Sweet rolls are purchased. Purchased bread for sandwiches in sack lunches is a status symbol.

Breakfast cereals are usually prepared type with emphasis on sugar coated. Occasionally oatmeal is used.

Fried macaroni is prepared and served with beans and potatoes.

Suggestions: Continue use of enriched flour. In some sections where corn tortillas are used, encourage use of dried skim milk.

Encourage whole grain cereals. Cooked cereals more economical.

Encourage use of vegetables rather than excessive starch foods.

Miscellaneous: Lard, salt pork, and bacon fat are used liberally. Most foods are fried.

Soft drinks, popsicles, and sweets of all kinds are used liberally.

Suggestions: Encourage a variety of cookery procedures.

Purchased cookies, soft drinks, and sweets are expensive and do not contribute to nutritional needs. Utilizing more milk, ice cream, and juices would be helpful.

SOURCE: Adapted from *Cultural Food Patterns in the U.S.A.*, published by the American Dietetic Association, 1976.

Appendix G

Vital Statistics

BIRTH AND DEATH RATES, 1960 TO 1980

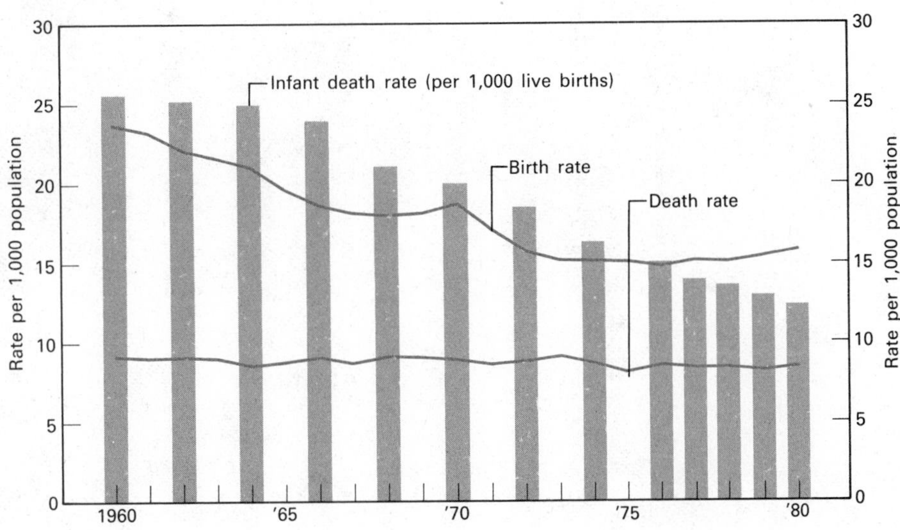

SOURCE: *Statistical Abstract of the United States,* 1981. U.S. Department of Commerce, Bureau of the Census, Washington, D.C.

DEATHS AND DEATH RATES FOR THE 10 LEADING CAUSES OF DEATH IN SPECIFIED AGE GROUPS: UNITED STATES, 1979

Rank Order	Cause of Death and Age (Ninth Revision International Classification of Diseases, 1975)	Number	Rate
	1–4 years		
...	All causes	8,108	65.6
1	Accidents and adverse effects . . . E800–E949	3,349	27.1
...	Motor vehicle accidents E810–E825	1,239	10.0
...	All other accidents and adverse effects . . . E800–E807, E826–E949	2,110	17.1
2	Congenital anomalies 740–759	1,021	8.3
3	Malignant neoplasms, including neoplasms of lymphatic and hematopoietic tissues . . . 140–208	578	4.7
4	Homicide and legal intervention . . . E960–E978	314	2.5
5	Diseases of heart. . . 390–398, 402, 404–429	265	2.1
6	Pneumonia and influenza 480–487	258	2.1
7	Meningitis . . . 320–322	183	1.5
8	Meningococcal infection 036	107	0.9
9	Certain conditions originating in the perinatal period . . . 760–779	75	0.6
10	Anemias . . . 280–285	73	0.6
...	All other causes . . . Residual	1,885	15.2
	5–14 years		
...	All causes	11,146	32.2
1	Accidents and adverse effects . . . E800–E949	5,689	16.5
...	Motor vehicle accidents E810–E825	2,952	8.5
...	All other accidents and adverse effects . . . E800–E807, E826–E949	2,737	7.9
2	Malignant neoplasms, including neoplasms of lymphatic and hematopoietic tissues . . . 140–208	1,552	4.5
	25–44 years		
...	All causes	105,664	176.3
1	Accidents and adverse effects . . . E800–E949	26,097	43.5
...	Motor vehicle accidents E810–E825	15,658	26.1
...	All other accidents and adverse effects . . . E800–E807, E826–E949	10,439	17.4
2	Malignant neoplasms, including neoplasms of lymphatic and hematopoietic tissues . . . 140–208	16,918	28.2
3	Disease of heart . . . 390–398, 402, 404–429	14,420	24.1
4	Homicide and legal intervention . . . E960–E978	10,130	16.9
5	Suicide . . . E950–E959	9,733	16.2
6	Chronic liver disease and cirrhosis . . . 571	4,714	7.9
7	Cerebrovascular diseases 430–438	3,224	5.4
8	Diabetes mellitus 250	1,417	2.4
9	Pneumonia and influenza 480–487	1,337	2.2
10	Congenital anomalies 740–759	774	1.3
...	All other causes . . . Residual	16,900	28.2
	45–64 years		
...	All causes	422,231	961.7
1	Diseases of heart . . . 390–398, 402, 404–429	149,384	340.3
2	Malignant neoplasms, including neoplasms of lymphatic and hematopoietic tissues . . . 140–208	133,689	304.5
3	Cerebrovascular diseases 430–438	20,671	47.1
4	Accidents and adverse effects . . . E800–E949	18,346	41.8
...	Motor vehicle accidents E810–E825	8,162	18.6

Rank	Cause	ICD code	Number	Rate
3	Congenital anomalies	740–759	578	1.7
4	Homicide and legal intervention	E960–E978	394	1.1
5	Diseases of heart	390–398, 402, 404–429	289	0.8
6	Pneumonia and influenza	480–487	212	0.6
7	Suicide	E950–E959	152	0.4
8	Cerebrovascular diseases	430–438	104	0.3
9	Benign neoplasms, carcinoma in situ, and neoplasms of uncertain behavior and of unspecified nature	210–239	91	0.3
10	Anemias	280–285	83	0.2
...	All other causes	Residual	2,002	5.8
	15–24 years			
...	All causes		48,719	117.7
1	Accidents and adverse effects	E800–E949	26,574	64.2
...	Motor vehicle accidents	E810–E825	19,369	46.8
...	All other accidents and adverse effects	E800–E807, E826–E949	7,205	17.4
2	Homicide and legal intervention	E960–E978	6,156	14.9
3	Suicide	E950–E959	5,246	12.7
4	Malignant neoplasms, including neoplasms of lymphatic and hematopoietic tissues	140–208	2,581	6.2
5	Diseases of heart	390–398, 402, 404–429	1,117	2.7
6	Congenital anomalies	740–759	576	1.4
7	Cerebrovascular diseases	430–438	379	0.9
8	Pneumonia and influenza	480–487	341	0.8
9	Diabetes mellitus	250	170	0.4
10	Anemias	280–285	145	0.4
...	All other causes	Residual	5,434	13.1
...	All other accidents and adverse effects	E800–E807, E826–E949	10,184	23.2
5	Chronic liver disease and cirrhosis	571	15,887	36.2
6	Chronic obstructive pulmonary diseases and allied conditions	490–496	10,762	24.5
7	Diabetes mellitus	250	7,594	17.3
8	Suicide	E950–E959	7,357	16.8
9	Pneumonia and influenza	480–487	5,145	11.7
10	Homicide and legal intervention	E960–E978	4,000	9.1
...	All other causes	Residual	49,396	112.5
	65 years and over			
...	All causes		1,271,656	5,157.2
1	Diseases of heart	390–398, 402, 404–429	566,924	2,299.1
2	Malignant neoplasms, including neoplasms of lymphatic and hematopoietic tissues	140–208	247,922	1,005.4
3	Cerebrovascular diseases	430–438	144,891	587.6
4	Chronic obstructive pulmonary diseases and allied conditions	490–496	38,249	155.1
5	Pneumonia and influenza	480–487	36,598	148.4
6	Atherosclerosis	440	27,521	111.6
7	Accidents and adverse effects	E800–E949	24,032	97.5
...	Motor vehicle accidents	E810–E825	5,887	23.9
...	All other accidents and adverse effects	E800–E807, E826–E949	18,145	73.6
8	Diabetes mellitus	250	23,948	97.1
9	Nephritis, nephrotic syndrome, and nephrosis	580–589	11,966	48.5
10	Chronic liver disease and cirrhosis	571	8,956	36.3
...	All other causes	Residual	140,649	570.4

SOURCE: National Center for Health Statistics **31:6** (supplement), September 30, 1982.

Rates per 100,000 population in specified group.

INDEX

Abdomen:
emergency conditions of, 1503, 1610–1613
postpartum exercises for, 187–189
trauma, 1577–1580
Abortion:
among adolescents, 270
classification of types, 129–130
complications, 278–279
criminal, 270
elective, 269–280
emotional response to, 278–279
legislation about, 269–270
methods, 274–277
self-induced, 270
spontaneous, 129–130
Abrasions, 1546–1547
Abruptio placentae, 144
Abstinence syndromes (*see* Withdrawal, from alcohol or other drugs)
Abuse:
alcohol, 1328–1332
effects on neonate, 218–221
intoxication, 713–714
emergency care, 1502, 1593, 1636–1637
visual changes, 811
withdrawl syndromes, 684–691, 1330–1331, 1588, 1599
child, 1375–1382
(*See also* Abuse, sexual)
drug, 1328–1332
effects on neonate, 218–221
overdose, 1585–1593
substances commonly involved in, 1589–1593
withdrawal syndromes, 684–691, 1588, 1589
elder, 1385–1387
person, 1369–1390
sexual, 1382–1385, 1633–1634
spouse, 1369–1375
A-butyrophenone, overdose, 1592
Accident prevention (*see* Safety)
Achalasia, 1189–1190
Acne, 607–609, 1269–1272
Acoustic neuroma, 680
Acquired hemolytic anemia, 412–413, 960–964
Acquired immune deficiency syndrome (AIDS), 942–943
Acromegaly, 374–375, 868–873
Activities of daily living, mental health problems with, 1319–1321
Activity:
restriction of: in anemia, 408
for child with heart disease, 465
in thrombocytopenia, 407
Activity-exercise pattern, 20, 30
Addisonian crisis, 388, 389, 908–910, 1601–1602
Addison's disease, 379–380, 388, 907–910, 1601–1602
Adenocarcinoma (*see* Cancer)
Adolescent(s):
abortions, 270
development, 60–63
sexual: delayed, 378
precocious, 375–377, 389
developmental tasks, 68, 1402
group work with, 1402–1403
health teaching strategies for, 37–38
hospitalized, 63–65, 68–71
pregnancy, 131–132
Adoption, 213, 214
Adrenal crisis, 388, 389, 908–910, 1601–1602
Adrenal glands:
functions, 387
tumors, 876–879
Adrenocortical hyperplasia, 388–391
Adrenogenital syndrome, 388–391
Adult (*see* Middle adult; Older adult; Young adult)
Adult respiratory distress syndrome, 1092–1093
Affect, disorders of, 1297–1318, 1681
Agammaglobulinemia, 434–435
Aged (*see* Older adult)
Ageusia, 813–814
Aging:
cognition and, 1429–1430
coping with, 1449–1462
definition, 1423
health problems common to, 1463–1487
physical changes of, 1423–1447
theories of, 1423–1424
(*See also* Older adult)
Agranulocytosis, 941–942
AIDS (acquired immune deficiency syndrome), 942–943
Air embolism, 410
and intravenous fluids, 491
Airway (*see* Respiratory system)
Alcohol:
dependency, 1328–1332
effect on neonate, 218–221
intoxication, 713–714
emergency care, 1502, 1593, 1636–1637
visual changes, 811
withdrawal syndrome, 684–691, 1330–1331, 1588, 1589
Altitude sickness, 1541–1543
Alzheimer's disease, 742–747
Ambiguous genitalia, 254–255, 389
Amenorrhea, 285
American Nurses' Association:
definition of nursing, 15–18, 33
social policy statement, 15–18
standards of practice, 18–30
nursing process and, 19–28
Amitriptyline, overdose, 1592
Amniocentesis, 133, 142, 265–266
Amphetamines, overdose, 1591
Amputation, 854–857
Amyotrophic lateral sclerosis, 747–751
Analgesics, overdose, 714
(*See also* Aspirin, overdose)
Anaphylactoid purpura, 455–456, 955
Anaphylaxis, 1565–1569
following venomous bite or sting, 1537
Anemia:
activity guidelines for, 408
aplastic, 405–408, 411, 936–941
Cooley's (*see* Thalassemia major)
Diamond-Blackfan, 414–415
Fanconi's, 411–412
folic acid deficiency, 415–417, 945, 946, 948–950, 952
in pregnancy, 146
glucose-6-phosphate dehydrogenase (G-6-PD) deficiency, 146, 256, 419–420, 960–964
heart disease secondary to, 1001–1002
hemolytic, 412–413, 960–964
types of, 962
iron deficiency, 417–419, 950–953
Mediterranean (*see* Thalassemia major)
megaloblastic nutritional, 415–417, 944–950, 952
pernicious, 416, 713, 944–948
in pregnancy, 140–141, 146
sickle cell, 435–439, 960–964
guidelines for client management, 438
inheritance patterns, 256, 437
in pregnancy, 146
vitamin B_{12} deficiency, 415–417, 944–948
Aneurysm:
aortic, 1040–1042, 1610
cerebral, 767, 768
Angel dust, overdose, 1591
Anger, depression and, 1416
Angina pectoris, 976, 1025–1029, 1468, 1604–1610
Ankylosing spondylitis, 837–838
Anomalies, congenital (*see* Birth defects)
Anorexia nervosa, 1194–1195
Anosmia, 814–815
Ant bites, venomous, 1534–1538
Anticholinergic drugs, overdose, 1591–1592
Antidiuretic hormone (ADH):
inappropriate secretion, 882–884
(*See also* Diabetes insipidus)
Antipsychotic drugs, overdose, 716–717
Anus:
imperforate, 589–591
stenotic, 590
Anxiety, 1297–1306, 1681–1682
behavior checklist to assess, 1300
during drug withdrawal, 684–691
hallucinations due to, 1351–1352
of hospitalized child or adolescent, 65–71

during labor, 156–157
leveling of, 1302
of parents of hospitalized child, 69–71
pathophysiology related to, 1298
separation, 56, 58, 65–67
teaching for control of, 1302–1306
Aorta:
aneurysm, 1040–1042, 1610
coarctation, 475–479, 971–973
stenosis, 479–481, 976–982
trauma, 1024–1025, 1575–1577
Aorticopulmonary window, 475
Aortic valve:
insufficiency, 503, 976–982
stenosis, 479–481, 976–982
Apgar newborn scoring system, 199, 1628
Aplastic anemia, 405–408, 411, 936–941
causes, 936–937
Apnea:
infant, 238, 239
neonate, 238–239
Appendicitis, 577, 1610
Arnold-Chiari malformation, 318–319
Arrhythmias, 981, 1002–1014
drugs for, 1010, 1013
interpretation of, 1005–1009
Arsenic, intoxication from, 718–719, 1482
Artane, overdose, 1591–1592
Arteriosclerosis, peripheral arterial disease in, 1029–1031
Arteriovenous malformation (AVM), 319–320, 767, 768
Arteritis, temporal, 733–734
Arthritis:
degenerative, 858–862
gouty, 828–830
rheumatoid, 838, 858
eye changes due to, 812
juvenile, 357–359
septic, 355–357
Arthroplasty, hip, 861–862
Artificial insemination, 300–301
Ascariasis, 656–658
Aspiration of foreign body, 511–513, 1569–1575
Aspirin, overdose, 1592–1593
Assault:
threat of, as psychiatric emergency, 1344–1347, 1631–1633
(*See also* Person abuse)
Assertiveness, for anxiety reduction, 1305–1306
Assessment:
as step in nursing process, 19–20
(*See also* Health history; Physical assessment)
Asthma, 519–524, 1102–1105
breathing exercises for, 521
drugs used for, 522–523, 1105
Astrocytoma, cerebellar, 320–324
Atelectasis, following pneumonia, 1063
Atherosclerosis:
of coronary arteries, 1025
peripheral artery disease in, 1029–1031
Athetosis, 761
Athlete's foot, 615–617, 1272–1273
Atopic dermatitis, 604–606, 1273–1275
Atrial septal defect, 482–486
Atrioventricular canal, 486
Atropinic drugs, overdose, 1591–1592
Attachment, parent-child, 179–180, 185, 209–210, 231–232
disturbances of, 213–216
Autonomic dysreflexia, 786–787
Autonomic hyperreflexia, 786–787
Aventyl, overdose, 1592
Avulsion injuries, 1547–1548
Azotemia, 561, 1140
encephalopathy from, 561, 699
(*See also* Renal failure)

Back:
emergency assessment, 1494, 1496, 1497
pain, 852–854
(*See also* Spinal cord injury)
Bacterial endocarditis, 1018–1020
Barbiturates, overdose, 714–715, 1589–1590
Barium enema, 1197
Basic four food groups, 185, 1719
Battering (person abuse), 1369–1390
Beckwith's syndrome, 373
Bee stings, 1534–1538
Behavioral states of infant, 54, 55, 197, 198
Beliefs, and health, 20, 26, 39–44, 46
Bellevue bridge for scrotal support, 554
Bell's palsy, 733
Bends, 1543–1545
Benign essential tremor, 691
Benign prostatic hypertrophy, 1160–1163, 1254
Beriberi, 710–712
Billroth gastrectomy, 1188
Birth (*see* Delivery; Labor)
Birth control (*see* Contraception)
Birth defects:
chromosomal and genetic factors, 253–257
environmental factors, 257–263
family of infant with, 253–268
Birth injuries, 260–263
Birthmarks, 597–600, 1259
Bites, venomous, 1534–1538
Black lung disease (*see* Pneumoconiosis)
Black widow spider bites, 1534–1538
Bladder:
indwelling catheter, 542, 1122–1123
inflammation, 1152–1154
neurogenic, 554–556
self-catheterization of, 555
stones, 1163, 1166, 1167
trauma, 1174–1175
tuberculosis, 1159–1160
tumors, 1128–1133
Blalock-Hanlon atrial septectomy, 496
Blalock-Taussig anastomosis, 490, 500
Blepharitis, 802
Blindness, 341–342
color, 256
(*See also* Cranial nerves, trauma; Eyes, disorders)
Blood:
composition, 921, 923
disorders, 405–458, 921–965
signs and symptoms of, 925
(*See also particular diseases and disorders*)
laboratory tests and interpretations, 1690–1692, 938–939, 957, Appendix C
Blood incompatibility:
mother-infant, 145, 216–217, 245–247
in transfusion reaction, 408–409
Blood pressure:
norms of, for children, 462
newborn, 205, 462
(*See also* Hypertension; Shock)
Blood transfusion:
exchange, 246, 247
reactions, 408–410
Bonding (*see* Attachment)
Bone(s)
aging and, 1430
tumors, 352–355, 823–828
(*See also* Musculoskeletal system *and particular diseases and disorders*)
Bone marrow:
aspiration, 926
biopsy, 926
Bottle feeding, 211
formulas for, 1720–1721
Botulism, 717, 718, 1593–1596
Bowel:
obstruction, 567–575, 587–591, 1218–1222, 1508–1509, 1610–1613
tumors, 1182–1183, 1610
Bradycardia, 1006, 1010–1013
Brain:
abscess, 722–725
edema, 700–701
hemisphere functions and deficits, 737–738
herniation, 672–674, 707–708
trauma, 328–331, 770–778, 1580–1584
hypoxic, 697–698
tumors, 320–324, 669–676
(*See also* Encephalitis; Encephalocele; Encephalomyelitis; Encephalopathy; Increased intracranial pressure)
Brainstem glioma, 320–324

Breast(s):
cancer, 1237–1241
after delivery, 178, 183–184
emergency assessment, 1495
infection, 194
Breastfeeding, 184, 210–211
during breast infection, 194
Breathing:
for anxiety reduction, 1302–1303
exercises for, in asthma, 521
Breath sounds, 507
Brittle bone disease, 350–352
Brock procedure for pulmonary valvulotomy, 493
Bromides, overdose, 715–716
Bronchiectasis, 1097–1100
Bronchiolitis, 514–516
Bronchitis, chronic, 1105–1108, 1472–1473
Bronchopneumonia, 529–530
Bronchopulmonary dysplasia (BPD), 527–529
Bronchoscopy, fiberoptic, 1047, 1048
Brown lung disease (*see* Pneumoconiosis)
Brown recluse spider bites, 1534–1538
Bryant's traction, 349
Buchwald-Vasco operation for intestinal bypass, 1193
Buck's extension traction, 845–846
Buerger's disease, 1034–1036
Bulimia, 1196
Burns, 1280–1286, 1555–1565
chemical, 1561–1562
of esophagus, 578–579, 1216–1217
classification, by depth, 1283, 1555–1556
electrical, 1560–1561
estimation of body surface area of, 1557
fluids for treatment of, 1282–1284
radiation, 1562–1565
from sun, 1562–1565
Bursitis, 838–840
Butyrophenone, overdose, 716–717, 1592
Bypass operations:
arterial: for peripheral artery disease, 1033–1034
coronary, 1027–1028
extracranial, 734, 741, 1033
intracranial, 734, 741
intestinal, for obesity, 1193–1194

Caisson disease, 1543–1545
Calories:
of children, 229, 463, 1713
in first year of life, 210
requirements for, 1713
Cancer:
bladder, 1128–1133
bone, 352–355, 823–828
bowel, 1182–1183, 1610
breast, 1237–1341
cervix, 1231–1237
drugs for, 354, 934
antileukemic, 445–447, 930, 931
esophagus, 1181–1182
fallopian tube, 1244–1245
kidney, 548–550, 1117–1128
larynx, 1049–1054
lip, 1177–1180
liver, 1183
lung, 1045–1049
mouth, 1177–1180
ovary, 1245
pancreas, 1183–1184
penis, 1255
prostate, 1133–1135, 1254–1255
radiation therapy for, in leukemia, 445, 930, 931
salivary gland, 1181
skin, 1259–1261
stomach, 1182
testicle, 1255
tongue, 1177–1180
uterus, 1242, 1244–1245
vagina, 1242
vulva, 1241–1242
Candidiasis, 128, 609–610, 1246–1250
Canker sores, 1213
Carbamazepine, overdose, 715–716
Carbon monoxide poisoning, 1596–1597
Carcinoma (*see* Cancer)
Carcinoma in situ:
cervix, 1231
larynx, 1049
vulva, 1241
Cardiac arrest, treatment of, 1013, 1014, 1606–1609
Cardiac catheterization:
care following, 474–475
complications, 975, 1025
Cardiac monitoring, 1003–1009
Cardiac pacemaker, 1010–1013
Cardiac tamponade, 470, 1024–1025
Cardiopulmonary resuscitation, 1606–1609
Cardiospasm, 1189–1190
Cardiovascular accident (*see* Stroke)
Cardiovascular system, 459–504, 967–1043
abnormal cellular growth, 466–502, 971–984
aging and, 1431–1432, 1467–1472
anxiety and, 1298
degenerative disorders, 1037–1042
emergencies, 1604–1610
emergency assessment, 1495, 1497–1498
hyperactivity and hypoactivity, 459–466, 984–997
inflammations, 502–503, 1018–1024
metabolic disorders, 997–1018
obstructions, 1025–1037
trauma, 1024–1025, 1575–1577
(*See also particular organs, structures, diseases, and disorders*)
Cardioversion, 1013, 1014
Caries, dental, 593–595
Carotid endarterectomy, 734, 741
Case study:
college student with hepatitis, 28
family of malformed neonate, 264
family of psychiatric client, 1414–1415
Cast care, 350, 843–844, 1514
Cataracts, 806–807, 1476–1477
Catheter:
intra-arterial, 994–997
balloon, 994–997
Swan-Ganz, 994, 995
nephrostomy, 1167–1169
suprapubic, collection harness for, 545
ureteral, 542, 1169
urethral, 542, 1122–1123
Catheterization:
bladder, by client, 555
cardiac: care following, 474–475
complications, 975, 1025
Cat-scratch disease, 648–649
Causalgia, 819
Cecostomy, 1200
Celiac disease, 591–593, 1195
Cellophane tape test for pinworms, 655
Cerebral edema, 700–701
Cerebral palsy, 338–339
Cerebrovascular accident (*see* Stroke)
Cervical spondylosis, 765–767
Cervix:
cancer, 1231–1237
inflammation, 1253
polyps, 1245
Cesarean section, 190–195
Chalazion, 803
Charley horses, 1529
Chart, client, 30
in emergency care, 1499, 1505
problem oriented, 30, 1499
Chédiak-Higashi syndrome, 424–425
Chemical burns:
of esophagus, 578–579, 1216–1217
of skin, 1561–1562
Chemotherapy (*see* Drugs)
Chest:
exercises for, in asthma, 521
flail, 1087, 1088, 1573–1575
pain, emergency assessment, 1500
sucking wound, 1573–1575
trauma, 1087–1093, 1569–1575
Chest physical therapy, 236, 237, 1099
Chest tube, 466–467, 1076, 1574–1575
Chickenpox, 636–638
Chilblains, 1530–1532
Child abuse, 1375–1382
(*See also* Sexual abuse)

Children:
caloric requirements for, 229, 463, 1713
in first year of life, 210
and death of family, 89
depression in, 1362–1367
fluid requirements for, 464
full-term infant, 210
high-risk infant, 229, 232
as focus of family anxiety, 1407
growth norms for, 1695–1702
newborn, 205, 1695–1698
health teaching of, 36–37, 70–71
heart rate norms for, 461
newborn, 461, 205
impulsivity in, 1357–1362
mental disorders of, 1357–1367, 1679
respiratory rate norms for, 461
newborn, 205, 461
responses to hospitalization, 63–71
(*See also* Adolescent; Infant; Neonate; Preschooler; School-age child; Toddler)
Chlamydia, 1253
Chloral hydrate, overdose, 715–716, 1590
Chlordiazepoxide, overdose, 715–716, 1590
Chlorpromazine, overdose, 716–717, 1592
Chlorprothixene, overdose, 716–717
Choking, 511–513, 1569–1573
Cholecystectomy, 1202–1203
Cholecystitis, 1200–1203, 1610
Cholecystotomy, 1202–1203
Cholelithiasis, 1200–1203
Cholestasis, 1195
Chorea, 761
Huntington's, 743, 759–760
Chorioretinitis, 805–806
Christmas disease, 429–433, 958
Chromosome(s):
abnormalities, 255
and birth defects, 253–256
hormonal disorders related to, 399–403
Philadelphia, 923–924, 926
(*See also* Genetics)
Chronic discoid lupus erythematosus, 1269
Chronic familial jaundice, 442–444
Chronic granulomatous disease, 424–425
Chronic obstructive pulmonary disease (*see* Bronchitis, chronic; Emphysema)
Chylothorax, 499–500
Circumcision, 212
Cirrhosis of liver, 1223–1229
Cleft lip, 580–581
Cleft palate, 580–581
Client:
health care record, 30
in emergency care, 1499, 1505
problem oriented, 30, 1499
health teaching of, 33–52
role in health care, 13, 21, 26
Climacteric, 1253–1254
Closed-heart surgery, 466–470, 978
Clubfoot, 346–348
Coarctation of the aorta, 475–479, 971–973
Codeine, overdose, 1590
Cogentin, overdose, 1591–1592
Cognition:
disturbances of, 1351–1356
(*See also* Dementia; Development, cognitive; Mental retardation; Organic brain syndrome)
Cognitive-perceptual pattern, 20, 24
Cold, common, 1077–1079
Coldsores, 612, 1087, 1213
Colitis, ulcerative, 1196–1200, 1610
Colonoscopy, 1197
Color blindness, 256
Colostomy, 1200, 1221–1222
Coma, 692–696
in diabetic ketoacidosis, 392, 398–399, 1597–1601
emergency assessment, 1501–1503, 1507–1508
hepatic, 698–699, 1227–1228
hyperglycemic hyperosmolar nonketotic, 1597–1601
myxedema, 896, 898
undiagnosed, 1501–1503
Compazine, overdose, 1592
Compoz, overdose, 1591–1592
Compromised decision making, 1336–1337
Compulsive-ritualistic behavior, 1334–1336
Concussion, 328–331, 771
of spinal cord, 779
Condyloma acuminatum, 1253, 1262, 1263
Conflict, in groups, 1400–1402
Confusion:
in dementia, 742–747
in organic brain syndrome, 1482–1485
in sensory-perceptual alteration, 1324–1325
Congenital anomalies (*see* Birth defects)
Congenital hemolytic jaundice, 960–964
Congestive heart failure, 459–466, 984–991, 1604–1610
Conjunctivitis, 803–804
Constipation, 1198, 1438, 1442–1443, 1445
Contact dermatitis, 602, 1275
Continuous ambulatory peritoneal dialysis (CAPD), 562, 1142–1145, 1149
Continuous cycle peritoneal dialysis (CCPD), 562
Contraception, 97–113
choice of method, 97–99, 109
permanent methods, 99, 106
temporary methods, 99–105
Contract, nurse-client, 20, 21
Contractions, uterine, in labor, 151, 167, 170, 172
Contrecoup injury of brain, 771, 776
Contusion, 1548–1550
brain, 328–331, 771
heart, 1025
spinal cord, 779
Convulsions (*see* Seizures)
Cooley's anemia (*see* Thalassemia major)
Coordination:
aging and, 1429
disturbance of, 672
Cope, overdose, 1591–1592
Coping:
with aging, 1449–1462
with chronic illness, 1463–1464, 1467
compulsive-ritualistic behavior as maladaptive pattern of, 1334–1336
demanding behavior as maladaptive pattern of, 1332–1334
Coping-stress-tolerance pattern, 20, 25
Copperhead snake bite, 1534–1538
Coral snake bite, 1534–1538
Corneal ulcer, 804–805
Coronary artery bypass surgery, 1027–1028
Coronary heart disease, 1025–1029, 1468
(*See also* Angina pectoris)
Cor pulmonale, 991–993
Corrosives, ingestion of, 578–579, 1216–1217
Cortical syndrome, 818–819
Cor vaginale vaginitis, in pregnancy, 128
Coughing, client instruction about, 1073
Coup injury of brain, 771
Crab lice, 617–618
Cradle cap, 606–607
Cranial nerves:
assessment, in children, 322
degeneration, 764–765
trauma, 776–778, 1580–1584
Craniopharyngioma, 320–324
Craniosynostosis, 319
Credé's method, in neurogenic bladder, 555
Cretinism, 384–386
Creutzfeldt-Jacob disease, 742–747
Cri-du-chat syndrome, 255
Crohn's disease, 1215
Croup, 516–518
Crush wounds, 1550–1551
Crutch walking, 845
Crying of neonate, 54, 197, 198
Cryptorchidism, 547–548
Cultural differences:
and diet, 1725–1732
in grief, 1451–1452

health teaching and, 39–44
Curling's ulcer, 1184–1189
Cushing's disease, 387–388, 899–904
Cushing's syndrome, 388, 899–904
Cushing's ulcer, 1184–1189
Cutoff, emotional, in family systems theory, 1410–1411
Cyanosis, polycythemia accompanying, 413–414
systemic consequences of, 490–491
Cystic fibrosis, 256, 524–527
Cystitis, 1152–1154
Cystoscopy, 1120
Cytomegalic inclusion disease, 257–260, 652–654

Dacryocystitis, 803
Dalmane, overdose, 715–716
Darvon, overdose, 1590–1591
Data base, development of, 19–20
(*See also* Health history; Physical assessment)
Deafness, 340–341, 779
(*See also* Cranial nerves, trauma)
Death:
attitudes of older adult toward, 1457–1458
client rights concerning, 1460
definition, 1457
family coping with, 89–91
of fetus, 130
Decision making:
in groups, 1402
impaired capacity for, 1336–1337
Decompression sickness, 1543–1545
Defibrillation, 1013, 1014
Degenerative joint disease, 858–862, 1475–1476
Delirium tremens, 684–691, 1330–1331, 1589
Delivery:
cesarean, 190–195
estimated date of, 127
vaginal, 175–189
(*See also* Labor)
Delusions, 1351, 1354, 1356
in organic brain syndrome, 1483–1485
Demanding, as behavior pattern, 1332–1334
Dementia, 742–747
causes, 743
reversible, 743–744
(*See also* Organic brain syndrome)
Dental caries, 593–595
Dependency:
as behavior problem, 1328–1332
on drugs, 1328–1332
Depression, 1306–1314, 1415–1416
aging and, 1439
anger and, 1416
in children, 1362–1367
and suicide potential, 1365–1366
in family systems theory, 1415–1416
pathophysiology related to, 1307
postpartum, 179, 195
De Quervain's thyroiditis, 917–918
Dermatitis:
contact, 602, 1275
diaper, 600–601, 609–610
Dermatologic conditions, 597–620, 1259–1290
support measures for children with, 603
(*See also particular diseases and disorders*)
Dermatophytosis, 614–617, 1272–1273
Dermatosis, 1273–1275
Desipramine, overdose, 1592
Detached retina, 809–810
Development:
cognitive: adolescent, 61
infant, 55–57
middle adult, 73
neonate, 54
older adult, 75, 1429–1430
preschooler, 58–59
school-age child, 60
toddler, 57–58
young adult, 71
family life cycle, 80–83
fetus and embryo, 116–118, 125–126
infant, 55–57
hospitalization and, 66
middle adult, 72–74
neonate, 53–55
gestational age and, 199, 200, 202–203
older adult, 74–77, 1450
physical: adolescent, 60–61
infant, 55–57
middle adult, 72–73
neonate, 53
older adult, 74–75, 1423–1447
preschooler, 58
school-age child, 59–60
toddler, 57
young adult, 71
preschooler, 58–59
hospitalization and, 67
psychosocial: adolescent, 61–62
infant, 55–57
middle adult, 73
older adult, 75
preschooler, 59
school-age child, 60
toddler, 58
young adult, 71–72
school-age child, 59–60
hospitalization and, 68
sexual: of adolescent, 61
delayed, 378
middle adult, 73, 74
older adult, 76, 1432, 1434, 1438, 1442–1443, 1445
precocious, 375–377, 389
toddler, 57–58
young adult, 71–72
Developmental tasks:
adolescent, 68
family, 80–82
hospitalization and, 66–68
infant, 66
older adult, 1450
in pregnancy, 118–124
preschooler, 67
school-age child, 68
toddler, 67
Deviated septum, 1100–1102
Diabetes insipidus, 382–383, 884–886
Diabetes mellitus, 392–399, 887–892, 1473–1475
eye changes due to, 813
food exchange lists for, 1722–1725
hyperglycemic hyperosmolar nonketotic coma (HHNC) in, 1597–1601
hypoglycemia in, 397–398, 1598–1601
insulin shock in, 397–398, 1598–1601
ketoacidosis in, 392, 398–399, 1597–1601
during labor, 166–167
in pregnancy, 138–140
Dialysis, 562–563, 1142–1147, 1149
hemo-, 562–563, 1145–1147, 1149
peritoneal, 562, 1142–1145, 1149
continuous ambulatory, 562, 1142–1145, 1149
continuous cycle, 562
Diamond-Blackfan syndrome, 414–415
Diaper dermatitis, 600–601, 609–610
Diaper rash, 600–601, 609–610
Diapers, weighing to measure urinary output, 538
Diaphragmatic hernia, 505–510
Diarrhea, in gastroenteritis, 577–578, 1215, 1610
Diazepam, overdose, 715–716, 1590
Diet:
basic four food groups and, 185, 1719
caloric requirements for, 1713
for children, 229, 463, 1713
cultural variations in, 1725–1732
diabetic: food exchange lists for, 1722–1725
for older adult, 1433–1434, 1437–1438, 1440–1441, 1445
in pregnancy, 134
for weight control, 140
recommended daily allowances for, 1714–1715
(*See also* Eating; Nutritional-metabolic pattern)
Digitalis, administration and dosage, 462–463, 987–988
Di Guglielmo syndrome, 444
Diphtheria, 621–625, 717, 718
Disease prevention, 13–15
(*See also* Health, promotion and maintenance)
Dislocations, 1520–1521
hip, congenital, 348–350
vertebrae, 778

Disorientation:
  organic brain syndrome, 1483–1485
  sensory-perceptual alteration, 1324–1325
Disseminated intravascular coagulation, 957–958
Diuretics, dosage for children, 464
Diver's paralysis, 1543–1545
Diverticulitis, 1215–1216, 1610
Doriden, overdose, 715–716
Down's syndrome, 253–254
  heart disease in, 486–489
Drowning, 1538, 1541
Drugs:
  abuse, 1328–1332
    substances commonly involved, 1589–1593
    withdrawal syndromes, 684–691
  for arrhythmias, 1010, 1013
    (*See also* Digitalis)
  for asthma, 522–523, 1105
  and birth defects, 258, 260–263
  for cancer, 323, 354, 934
    (*See also* Drugs, for leukemia)
  contraceptive, 99–102, 107–110, 112
  diuretic, for children, 464
  eye disorders caused by, 811–812
  for fever, 1615–1616
  for hypertension, 999–1000, 1470
  for infertility, 290–292
  for juvenile rheumatoid arthritis, 359
  during labor and delivery, 158–162, 260–263
  for leukemia, 445–447, 930, 991
  overdose, 713–717, 1585–1593
    emergency assessment, 1502
  for psoriasis, 1265
  for seizures, 326, 1618, 1620
  for tuberculosis, 1069, 1070
  use by older adult, 1478–1481
Dubowitz examination for neonatal gestational age, 225–226
Duchenne's muscular dystrophy, 256, 364–366
Dumping syndrome, 1188–1189
Duodenal ulcers, 1184–1189, 1610
Dwarfism, 377–379
Dysentery, 577–578, 1215, 1610
Dystocia, 157, 163–164
Dystonia, 761

Eardrum, perforation of, 792–793
Ears:
  anatomy, 790
  emergency assessment, 1495–1497
  foreign body, 513–514, 791–792
  furunculosis, 792
  obstruction, 791–792
  removal of wax, 791–792
  (*See also* Hearing impairment)
Eating, mental health problems with, 1194–1196, 1319–1321
Eclampsia, 137
Eczema, 604–606, 1273–1275
Edema:
  cerebral, 700–701
  posttraumatic, 820
  pulmonary, 989–991
Education (*see* Teaching)
Edward's syndrome, 254
Eisenmenger's syndrome, 488
Elation, 1314–1316
Elavil, overdose, 1592
Elder abuse, 1385–1387
Elderly (*see* Older adult)
Electrocardiography, 1002–1009
Elimination pattern, 20, 23
Elliptocytosis, heredity, 444
Embolism:
  air, 410
    and intravenous fluids, 491
  arterial, 1031–1034
  in bacterial endocarditis, 1020
  fat, 848–849
  in heart trauma, 1025
  following heart valve surgery, 981–982
  pulmonary, 1093–1097
  surgical treatment, 1033
Embryo:
  in vitro transfer of, 301
  (*See also* Fetus)
Emergency nursing:
  general assessment in, 1493–1504
  general principles of, 1493–1510
  for medical disorders, 1585–1629
  for psychiatric disorders, 1631–1639
  record keeping (charting) in, 1499, 1505
  for traumatic injuries, 1511–1585
E.M.G. (exomphalos, macroglossia, and giantism) syndrome, 373
Emotional cutoff, in family systems theory, 1410–1411
Emotional isolation from social interaction, 1321–1324, 1415–1416
Emphysema, 1108–1111, 1472–1473
Empyema, 1063–1064
Encephalitis, 333, 725–726
Encephalocele, 319
Encephalomyelitis, 733
Encephalopathy:
  from heavy metals, 718–720
  hepatic, 698–699
  hypercapnic, 698
  hypoxic, 697–698
  portosystemic, 698–699
  uremic, 561, 699
  Wernicke's, 708–710
Endarterectomy, 734, 741, 1033
Endocardial cushion defect, 486–489
Endocarditis, bacterial, 1018–1020
Endocrine system, 371–403, 865–919
  abnormal cellular growth, 866–881
  assessment of disorders, 865–866
  classification of disorders, 372
  emergencies, 1597–1604
  emergency assessment, 1496
  hyperactivity and hypoactivity, 371–403, 882–912
  inflammations, 917–918
  metabolic disorders, 912–917
  (*See also* Hormones *and particular diseases and disorders*)
Endometriosis, 1242–1244
Endometritis following abortion, 278
End-stage renal disease, 560–564, 1140–1149
Enterobiasis, 654–655
Enterocolitis, necrotizing, 240–241, 575–577
Eosinophilic granuloma, 454–455
Ependymoma, 320–324
Epididymitis, 1256
Epidural hematoma, 328–331
Epiglottitis, 518
Epilepsy, 325–328, 680–684
  classification, 681
  drugs used for, 326
  (*See also* Seizures)
Epinephrine, effects of, 877
Epiphysis:
  fracture, 366–368
  slipped, 368–369
Epispadias, 546–547
Epistaxis, 1093
  in hypertension, 998, 999, 1470
Equanil, overdose, 715–716
Equinovarus, 346–348
Erb's spastic paraplegia, 731–732
Erythema infectiosum, 613
Erythema multiforme, 1278–1279
Erythroleukemia, 444
Esophagus:
  atresia, 581–585
  cancer, 1181–1182
  chemical burns, 578–579, 1216–1217
  fistula, 581–585
  inflammation, 1214
  spasm, 1189–1190
  stenosis, 582
  tumors, 1181–1182
  varices, 1228
Estimated date of delivery (EDD), 127
Estriols, in pregnancy, 142
Ethchlorvynol, overdose, 1590
Euphoria, 1314–1316
Eustachian tube, blockage, 794
Euthanasia, 1457
Evaluation:
  as step of nursing process, 19, 21, 26, 29
  of teaching-learning plan, 51
Ewing's sarcoma, 352–355
Exchange transfusion, 246, 247
Exercise:
  breathing, for asthma, 521
  postpartum, 187–189
Exercise-activity pattern, 20, 23
Expected outcomes, as step of nursing process, 19, 20

Extracranial bypass grafting, 734, 741, 1033
Extremities, emergency assessment, 1496
Eyes:
aging and, 1430
anatomy, 800
assessment, 800–802
in coma, 693
in emergency, 1495–1497
disorders, 256, 341–342, 645, 800–813, 1476–1477
(*See also* Cranial nerves, injury)

Face, trauma, 1524–1526
Factor VIII deficiency, 429–433, 958, 959
Factor IX deficiency, 429–433, 958, 959
Fainting, 1565–1569
Fallopian tube:
cancer, 1244–1245
occlusion, 295–296
Family:
abusive, 1369–1390
assessment, 79–92, 1411–1412
of child or adult with mental health problems, 1357–1367, 1391–1418
chronic illness or rehabilitation and, 87–89
cohesion and adaptability, 87–89
common problems, 80–82
death in, 89–91
definition, 79–80, 1405
developmental stages, 80–83
developmental tasks, 80–82
functions 79, 1405–1407
health teaching for, 43, 70–71, 1405
of hospitalized person, 63–71, 84–87, 1405–1418
of infant with birth defects, 253–268
influence on health, 79–80
self-differentiation in, 1408, 1409
types of, 80, 82
Family planning (*see* Contraception)
Family systems theory, 1407–1411
Family therapy, 1405–1418
Fanconi's anemia, 411–412
Febrile seizures, 325–328, 1619–1621
Fecal diversion (*see* Colostomy; Ileostomy)
Ferning of cervical mucus, 288, 293
Fertilization:
double, 254–255
in vitro, 301
Fetal alcohol syndrome, 218–221
Fetus:
death of, 130
gestational age and, 223, 224
growth and development of, 116–118, 125–126
heart rate of, 133
decelerations in, 155–156
monitoring of, 142
decelerations detected by, 155–156
positions in labor and delivery, 163–164, 168, 169
presentation at delivery, 150–151, 163, 164
station of, 151, 169
Fever, 1613–1616
drugs for, 1615–1616
in labor, 165
patterns of, 1614
postpartum, 193–194
seizures from, 325–328, 1619–1621
following transfusion, 409–410
Fever blisters, 612, 1087, 1213
Fibrillation, 1007, 1008
Fibroid tumors, 1245–1246
Fifth disease, 613
FIMI (Funke-Irbe Mother Infant Interactional Assessment), 214–215
Fish hook, removal, 1555
Flail chest, 1087, 1088, 1573–1575
Fluid requirements:
children, 464
full-term infant, 210
high-risk neonate, 229, 232
Flurazepam, overdose, 715–716
Folic acid deficiency anemia, 415–417, 945, 946, 948–950, 952
in pregnancy, 146
Fontan procedure for tricuspid atresia, 495
Food poisoning, 717, 718, 1593–1596
Foreign body:
aspiration of, 511–512, 1569–1575
in ear, 513–514, 791–792
Foster care, 213, 214
Fracture-dislocation, 1512
of vertebrae, 778
Fractures, 841–853, 1509–1516
casts for, 843
care of, 843–844, 1514
emergency assessment of, 1503
epiphyseal plate, 366–368
healing of, 844
hip, 850–852
jaw and face, 1524–1526
nose, 1093
skull, 328–331, 771
(*See also* Fracture, jaw and face)
splints for, 1515
types, 842, 1511–1512
vertebrae, 778
(*See also* Spinal cord injury)
Frostbite, 1530–1532
Frozen shoulder, 838–840
Functional health patterns, 20
assessment, 22–26
Funke-Irbe Mother Infant Interactional Assessment (FIMI), 214–215
Furunculosis of ear, 792
Fusion, in family systems theory, 1407
Gallbladder:
inflammation, 1200–1203, 1610
removal, 1202–1203
(*See also* Bowel, obstruction)
Gallstones, 1200–1203
Ganglioneuromas, 876–879
Gardnerella vaginalis vaginitis, 1246–1250
Gastric ulcer, 1184–1189, 1610
Gastritis:
acute, 1214
chronic, 1214–1215
Gastroenteritis, 577–578, 1215, 1610
Gastrointestinal system, 564–595, 1177–1230
abnormal cellular growth, 580–591, 1177–1184
aging and, 1433–1434, 1437–1438, 1440–1441, 1445
anxiety and, 1298
degenerative disorders, 1223–1229
emergency assessment, 1495
hyperactivity and hypoactivity, 1184–1190
inflammations, 575–578, 1196–1216
metabolic disorders, 591–593, 1191–1196
obstructions, 567–575, 1218–1222, 1508–1509, 1610–1613
trauma, 578–579, 1216–1217, 1508–1505
(*See also particular organs, structures, diseases, and disorders*)
Gastroschisis, 585–587
Gaucher's disease, 456–458
Genetics:
autosomal dominant disorders, 255
autosomal recessive disorders, 255–256
and birth defects, 253–257
polygenic disorders, 257
sex-linked disorders, 256
of sickling diseases, 256, 437
(*See also* Chromosomes)
Genital herpes, 257–260, 1250–1252
in pregnancy, 128, 257–260
Genitalia, amgibuous, 254–255, 389
German measles, 257–260, 632–634
Gestational age:
classifications, by size of infant, 199–200, 202–203, 224
estimation, 199–200, 202–203, 225, 226
and mortality, 223, 224
Giantism, 374–375, 868–873
Gigantism, 373
Gingivitis, 1213
Glaucoma, 807, 1476–1477
Glenn procedure for tricuspid atresia, 495
Glioma, brainstem, 320–324
Glomerulonephritis:
acute poststreptococcal, 551–553, 1156–1159
chronic, 1170

Glucocorticoids, functions of, 899
Glucose-6-phosphate dehydrogenase (G-6-PD) deficiency, 256, 419–420, 960–964
  in pregnancy, 146
Glue ear, 795–796
Gluten-induced enteropathy, 591–593, 1195
Glutethimide, overdose, 715–716
Goals of care (*see* Expected outcomes)
Goiter, 386–387
  in Graves' disease, 893, 894
  toxic multinodular, 893
Gonadotropins:
  deficiency of, 380–381, 886–887, 910–912
    (*See also* Klinefelter's syndrome; Turner's syndrome)
Gonorrhea, 644–646
  cervicitis from, 1253
  ophthalmia neonatorum from, 645
  in pregnancy, 128
  (*See also* Urethritis)
Gout, 828–830
Granulomatous disease, chronic (disorder of phagocytosis), 424–425
Granulomatous thyroiditis, 917–918
Graves' disease, 384, 893
Gravida:
  definition, 125
  elderly, 132
Great vessels:
  congenital malposition, 495–502
  trauma, 1024–1025, 1575–1577
Grief:
  abnormal, 1456
  after abortion, 278–279
  aging and, 1449–1462
  cultural variations, 1451–1452
  of dying child or adult, 452–453, 930
  in family: of dying child or adult, 89–91, 452–453
    of ill child, 64–65
    of malformed infant, 64–65, 253–268
  as psychiatric emergency, 1637–1638
  stages, 90–91, 452–453
Grooming, mental health problems and, 1319–1321
Groups:
  adolescent, 1402–1403
  conflict in, 1400–1402
  decision making in, 1402
  dynamics of, 1391–1396, 1400–1403
  growth chart for, 1394–1396
  leadership in, 1399–1400
Group therapy, 1397–1399
Growth:
  of children, norms of, 1695–1702
  delayed, 377–379
  of diabetic child, 395
  prenatal, 116–118, 125–126
Growth and development (*see* Development)
G-6-PD (glucose-6-phosphate dehydrogenase) deficiency, 256, 419–420, 960–964
  in pregnancy, 146
Guillain-Barré syndrome, 728–731
Gynecologic examination, support during, 110–111

Habit spasm, 761
Haldol, overdose, 716–717, 1592
Hallucinations, 1351–1353
  in organic brain syndrome, 1483–1485
  in withdrawal from alcohol or other drugs, 684–691
Hallucinogens, overdose, 1591
Haloperidol, overdose, 716–717, 1592
Hand-Schüller-Christian syndrome, 454–455
Hashimoto's thyroiditis, 386–387, 917–918
Headache:
  after brain trauma, 775
  migraine, 699–700
Head injury, 328–331, 770–778, 1580–1584
  closed, 770–771
  emergency assessment, 1495–1497
  open, 771–776
Health:
  client role, 13, 21, 26
  definition, 13, 46
  family influence, 79–80
  functional patterns, 20
    assessment, 22–26
  holistic, 13
  national goals, 8, 13–14
  nursing and, 15–30
  promotion and maintenance, 9, 14
    middle adult, 73–74
    older adult, 75–76, 1425–1426
    young adult, 72
    (*See also* Safety)
Health education (*see* Teaching)
Health history, 19, 22–26
  of child or adolescent, 64–65
  in emergency, 1494–1499
  format, 22–26
  of older adult, 1427–1428
Health perception–health management pattern, 20, 22
Health teaching (*see* Teaching)
Hearing impairment, 340–341, 799
  aging and, 1430, 1478
  (*See also* Cranial nerves, trauma to)
Heart:
  aging and, 1431, 1467–1469
  arrhythmias, 1002–1014
  assessment, 967–971
  monitoring, 1003–1009
  physiology, 984–985, 1002–1009
  trauma, 1024–1025, 1575–1577
  (*See also* Cardiovascular system)
Heart block, 1008–1009
Heart disease:
  from anemia, 1001–1002
  functional classification of client with, 968
  in labor, 166
  in pregnancy, 147
  pulmonary, 991–993
  (*See also particular diseases and disorders*)
Heart rate:
  children, 461
    newborn, 461, 205
  fetus, 133
    decelerations in, 155–156
Heart sounds, 969–971
Heart surgery:
  closed, 466–470, 978
  hypothermia for, 470
  open, 470–472, 978
Heat cramps, 1529
Heat exhaustion, 1527–1528
Heat hyperpyrexia, 1526–1527
Heat prostration, 1527–1528
Heat rash, 607
Heat stroke, 1526–1527
Heavy metals, intoxication from, 334–336, 718–720, 1482, 1593–1596
Heberden's nodes, 858
Heights and weights:
  adults, 1192
  children, 1695–1702
    newborn, 205, 1695–1698
Heimlich maneuver, 1571–1572
Hematocrit, normal values for children, 469
Hematologic system, 405–458, 921–965
  abnormal cellular growth, 435–455, 921–936
  degenerative disorders, 958–964
  diseases:
    signs and symptoms, 925
    (*See also particular diseases and disorders*)
  emergency assessment, 1496
  hyperactivity and hypoactivity, 405–435, 936–943
  inflammations, 455–456, 954–955
  laboratory tests and interpretations, 938–939, 957, 1690–1692
  metabolic disorders, 456–458, 944–954
  obstructions, 955–958
  trauma, 1506–1507
Hematoma:
  of birth canal, 173
  epidural, 328–331
  subdural, 328–331, 771
Hemodialysis, 562–563, 1145–1147, 1149
Hemoglobin AS disease, 146, 437, 439
Hemoglobin CA trait, 146
Hemoglobin CC disease, 146, 439–440
Hemoglobin SC disease, 146, 439–440
Hemoglobin SF disease, 439–440

Hemoglobin SS disease, 146, 245, 435–439, 960–964
Hemolytic diseases, 412–413, 960–964
  classification, 962
Hemophilia, 256, 429–433, 958–960
Hemorrhage:
  puerperal, 192–193
  subarachnoid, 767–770
  (*See also* Shock, hypovolemic)
Hemorrhoids, 1223
Hemosiderosis, 414, 440–441
Hemothorax, 1087
Henoch-Schönlein purpura, 455–456
Hepatic cirrhosis, 1223–1229
Hepatitis, 1207–1212
  case study about, 28
Hereditary elliptocytosis, 444
Hereditary ovalocytosis, 444
Hereditary spherocytosis, 442–444, 960–964
Hermaphroditism, 254–255
  (*See also* Ambiguous genitalia)
Hernia, 1222–1223
  diaphragmatic, 505–510
  inguinal, 573–574
  umbilical, 575
Heroin, overdose, 1590
Herpes simplex:
  genital, 257–260, 1250–1252
    in pregnancy, 128, 257–260
  oral, 612, 1087, 1213
Herpes zoster, 613, 726–728
Hip:
  congenital dislocation, 348–350
  fracture, 850–852
  replacement, 861–862
  subluxation, 348
  unstable, 348
Hirschsprung's disease, 587–589
Histiocytosis, 454–455
Hives, 601–602
Hookworms, 655–656
Hordeolum, 802–803
Hormones:
  chromosomal disorders affecting, 399–403
  at menopause, 1253
  of older adult, 1435–1436
  in pregnancy, 142
  (*See also* Endocrine system *and particular glands*)
Hornet stings, 1534–1538
Hospice, 1460–1461
Hospitalization:
  effects: on children and adolescents, 63–71
    on family members, 63–71, 83–87
Hot flash, 1253
Housemaid's knee, 838
Human chorionic gonadotropin (HCG), normal values of, 130
Hunner's ulcer, 1152
Huntington's chorea, 743, 759–760
Husband, abuse of, 1369–1375
Hyaline membrane disease, 233–237, 527
Hydatidiform mole, 130–131
Hydramnios, 145
Hydrocele, 1255
Hydrocephalus, 316–318, 742
Hydronephrosis, 1168–1170
Hygiene:
  mental health problems interfering with, 1319–1321
  oral, 594
Hyperactivity:
  in elation, 1314–1316
  in minimal brain dysfunction, 339–340
  (*See also* Impulsivity in children)
Hyperaldosteronism, 904–907
Hyperbilirubinemia of neonate, 216–217, 244–247
Hypercapnia, encephalopathy from, 698
Hypercortisolism, 387–388, 889–904
Hyperemesis gravidarum, 131
Hyperglycemia, diabetic, 392, 398–399, 1597–1601
Hyperglycemic hyperosmolar nonketotic coma (HHNC), 1597–1601
Hypernephroma, 1117
Hyperoxia of high-risk neonate, 234
Hyperparathyroidism, 912–915
Hypersomnias, 821–822
Hypertension, 997–1001, 1469–1471
  drugs for, 999–1000, 1470
  intracranial, 704
    (*See also* Increased intracranial pressure)
  during labor, 165
  in pregnancy, 137–138
  retinopathy due to, 812, 813
Hyperthyroidism, 384, 873–875, 892–896, 1602–1604
Hypertrophic obstructive cardiomyopathy, 982–984
Hypnotic drugs, overdose, 715–716, 1589–1590
Hypocalcemia of neonate, 242–243
Hypogammaglobulinemia, 434–435
Hypogeusia, 813–814, 1430
Hypoglycemia, 392
  in diabetes mellitus, 397–398, 1598–1601
  of neonate, 210, 241–242
Hypogonadism, 380–381, 886–887, 910–912
  (*See also* Klinefelter's syndrome; Turner's syndrome)
Hypoparathyroidism, 915–917
Hypoplastic left-heart syndrome, 502
Hypoprothrombinemia, 954
Hyposmia, 814–815, 1430
Hypospadias, 546–547
Hypotension:
  during labor, 169
  (*See also* Shock)
Hypothalamus:
  functions, 371, 865, 882
  hormones of, 867
Hypothermia:
  for heart surgery, 470
  localized, 1530–1532
  of neonate, 243–244
  systemic, 1532–1534
Hypothyroidism:
  acquired, 386–387, 896–898
  congenital, 384–386
Hypoxia, encephalopathy from, 697–698

Idiopathic hypertrophic subaortic stenosis (IHSS), 982–984
Idiopathic thrombocytopenic purpura, 425–426, 955–957
Ileal conduit, 555–556, 1131
Ileostomy, 1199–1200
Ileus:
  meconium, 524
  paralytic, 1218
  spastic, 1218
Illness:
  adaptation to, 40, 46–51
  chronic: coping with, 40, 46–51, 1463–1464, 1467
    definition, 1463
Imagery, for anxiety reduction, 1306
Imipramine, overdose, 1592
Immersion syndrome, 1530–1532
Immunity:
  of older adult, 1437
  principles of, 626
Immunization:
  schedules, 622, 623
  sites, 624
Immunoglobulin deficiency, 434–435
Immunoglobulins, classification of, 1104
Imperforate anus, 589–591
Impetigo, 610–612
Impulsivity:
  in children, 1357–1362
  (*See also* Hyperactivity)
Inappropriate antidiuretic hormone (ADH) secretion syndrome, 882–884
Incest (*see* Sexual abuse)
Increased intracranial pressure, 701–708
  (*See also* Brain, tumors; Hydrocephalus)
Infant:
  apnea, 238, 239
  attachment behavior, 179–180, 185, 209–210, 231–232
    disturbances, 213–216
  behavioral states, 54, 55, 197, 198
  birth defects, 253–268
    (*See also particular defects and disorders*)

birth injuries, 260–263
development, 55–57
gestational age, 199, 200, 202–203
hospitalization, 66
developmental tasks, 66
feeding, 55
by bottle, 211
formulas for, 1720–1721
by breast, 184, 210–211
during breast infection, 194
fluid and calorie requirements, 210
full-term, 197–221
gestational age: assessment, 199–200, 202–203, 225, 226
classification, by size, 199–200, 202–203, 224
and mortality, 223, 224
high-risk, 223–252
feeding, 229, 230, 232
transport, 249–251
(*See also particular diseases and disorders*)
jaundice, 216–217, 244–247
hospitalized, 66
large for gestational age, 223, 224
low-birth-weight, 223–251
formulas for, 1721
maternal diabetes mellitus, 139
maternal drug abuse, 218–221
maternal smoking, 218–221
postmature, 247–249
premature, 223–247
reflexes, 206
safety, 55–57
separation anxiety, 56
septicemia, 239–240
small for gestational age, 223, 224
Infantile paralysis, 638–641, 732–733
Infantile spasms, 325–328
Infectious mononucleosis, 651–652, 954–955
Infertility, 281–303
causes, 282
drugs for, 290–292
female factors in, 285–296
guidelines for overcoming, 301–302
male factors in, 297–300
Ingestion of corrosive substance, 578–579, 1216–1217
(*See also* Overdose; Poisoning)
Inguinal hernia, 573–574, 1222–1223
Inheritance (*see* Genetics)
Insect stings, 1534–1538
Insemination, artificial, 300–301
Insomnia, 820–821
in mental disturbance, 1319–1321
Insulin:
peaks and durations of, 397
in pregnancy, 139
Insulinoma, 392, 879–881
Insulin shock, 397–398, 1598–1601
Integumentary system, 597–620, 1259–1290
abnormal cellular growth, 597–600, 1259–1263
aging, 1434, 1436–1437
anxiety, 1298
degenerative disorders, 1286–1290
emergency assessment, 1495
hyperactivity and hypoactivity, 1263–1269
inflammations, 600–619, 1269–1279
trauma, 1279–1286, 1546–1565
(*See also particular diseases and disorders*)
Interpersonal relationships, problems in, 1319–1338
Interventions as step in nursing process, 19, 21
Intestinal bypass for obesity, 1193–1194
Intestine (*see* Bowel *and particular diseases and disorders*)
Intoxications (*see* Overdose; Withdrawal; *and particular substances*)
Intra-aortic balloon, 996
Intracranial bypass grafting, 734, 741
Intracranial pressure, increased, 701–708
(*See also* Brain, tumors; Hydrocephalus)
Intravenous fluids, air embolism from, 491
Intravenous pyelogram, 1120–1121
Intussusception, 570–572
(*See also* Bowel, obstruction)
Involuntary movement disorders, 761
Ipecac, administration of, 1588
Iridocyclitis, 805–806
Iron:
administration of, 953
dietary requirements for, 951, 1715, 1717–1718
tissue deposits of, 414, 440–441
Iron deficiency anemia, 417–419, 950–953
Isolation, social or emotional, 1321–1324, 1415–1416
"Itch," 618–619, 1276–1277
Itching:
arm and hand restraints for, 606
support measures for child with, 603
Itch-scratch cycle, 604, 1274

Jatene procedure for great vessel transposition, 497
Jaundice:
chronic familial, 442–444
congenital hemolytic, 960–964
of neonate, 216–217, 244–247
Jaw, fracture, 1524–1526
Jock itch, 1272–1273
Johnson, Dorothy, 15, 17
Joint replacement, 861–862

Kegel exercise, 182, 183
Kemadrin, overdose, 1591–1592
Keratitis, 804
Kernicterus, 216–217, 245
Ketoacidosis, diabetic, 392, 398–399, 1597–1601
Kidney:
benign tumors, 550, 1117
cancer, 548–550, 1117–1128
stones, 1163–1168
tests of function, 1121
transplantation, 1147–1148
trauma, 558, 1172–1174, 1577–1580
tuberculosis, 1159–1160
Kidney disease:
encephalopathy from, 699
end-stage, 560–564, 1140–1149
in pregnancy, 145
retinopathy due to, 812
Kidney failure:
acute, 558–560, 1170
chronic, 560–564, 1140–1149, 1170
Klinefelter's syndrome, 254, 401–403, 910–912
Korsakoff's psychosis, 708–710

Labor, 149–196
anoxia during, 263
anxiety during, 156–157
and cesarean delivery, 190–195
contractions during, 151, 167, 170, 172
diabetes mellitus and, 166–167
drugs used in, 158–162, 260–263
in emergency, 1621–1628
equipment for, 1624
estimated date of confinement, 127
fever during, 165
first stage of, 149–167
complications, 156–167
definition, 149
fourth stage, 172–173
complications, 173
definition, 149, 172
heart disease and, 166
hypertension during, 165
hypotension during, 169
ineffective, 157, 164, 169, 170–171
laceration from, 171–172, 1628
premature, 166
second stage, 167–169
definition, 149
third stage, 170–173
definition, 149
and vaginal delivery, 175–189
Laceration, 1552–1553
of birth canal, 171–172
in emergency delivery, 1628
of brain, 328–331, 771
emergency assessment, 1503
of spinal cord, 779
Lactation, 178, 211
(*See also* Breastfeeding)
Lactose intolerance, 256

Landry-Guillain-Barré syndrome, 728–731
Laparoscopy, for infertility, 295–296
Large for gestational age neonate, 223
Laryngitis, 1086–1087
Laryngotracheal malacia, 510–511
Laryngotracheobronchitis (LTB), 516–518
Larynx, cancer, 1049–1054
Lavage, procedure, 1588
Leadership in group work, 1399–1400
Lead poisoning, 334–336, 718, 1482
Learning:
  affective, 46–47, 51
  by client, 33–52
  cognitive, 46–47, 51
  cultural differences, 39–44
  developmental differences, 36–39, 59, 1426
  domains, 46–47, 51
  locus of control and, 43–44
  psychomotor, 46–47, 51
  sex differences, 34–36
  socioeconomic differences, 40, 45
  (*See also* Teaching)
Learning disability, 339–340
Legg-Perthes disease, 359–361
Leiomyoma, 1245–1246
Leptomeningitis, 720–722
Letterer-Siwe disease, 454–455
Leukemia, 444–454, 921–931
  acute granulocytic, 922–924, 926–931
  acute lymphocytic, 444–454, 922, 927–931
  acute monocytic, 922, 927–931
  acute myelocytic, 444–454, 922–924, 926–931
  chronic granulocytic, 922–924, 926–931
  chronic lymphocytic, 921, 922, 924, 926–931
  chronic monocytic, 921, 922, 927–931
  chronic myelocytic, 921, 922, 927–931
  classification, 922
  drugs used for, 445–447, 930, 931
  radiation therapy in, 445, 930, 931
    side effects of, 354–355
  remission, 444–445, 448
Leukoplakia, 1180–1181
Librium, overdose, 715–716, 1590
Lice, 617–618
Life review, 1459, 1460
Lip:
  cancer, 1177–1180
  cleft, 580–581
  fever blisters, 612, 1087, 1213
Liver:
  biopsy, 1225
  cirrhosis, 1223–1229
  tests of function, 1209–1211
  tumors, 1183
Liver disease, stupor or coma due to, 698–699, 1227–1228
Living will, 1457
Lochia, 178
"Lockjaw," 625–628, 717
Locus of control, and health teaching, 43–44
Loss, coping with in aging, 1449–1462
  (*See also* Grief)
Low-birth-weight neonate, 223–251
  formulas for, 1721
Lower airway trauma, 1573–1575
Lower back pain, 852–854
LSD, overdose, 1591
Lung(s):
  abscess, 1071–1074
  aging and, 1431
  cancer, 1045–1049
  lobes (location), 506
  tests of function, 1103
  (*See also* Respiratory system *and particular diseases and disorders*)
Lupus erythematosus:
  chronic discoid, 1269
  eye changes due to, 813
  systemic, 145, 1016–1018, 1267–1269
Luteal phase defects, 294
Lye, ingestion of, 578–579, 1216–1217
Lymph nodes, emergency assessment, 1495

Malabsorption syndromes, 1195–1196
Malignant melanoma, 810–811, 1260–1261
Malrotation of the bowel, 569–570
Mandible, fracture of, 1524–1526
Manganese poisoning, 719, 1482
Mania (*see* Elation)
Manipulation in interpersonal behavior, 1325–1328
Maple syrup disease, 336
Marie-Strümpell disease, 837–838
Mason operation for intestinal bypass, 1193
Mastitis, 194
Mastoiditis, 795–796
Maturity (*see* Older adult)
Maxilla, fracture of, 1524–1526
McCune-Albright syndrome, 376
Measles, 630–632
  German, 257–260, 632–634
Meconium aspiration syndrome, 248–249
Meconium ileus, 524
Medication:
  overdose, 1585–1593
  use by elderly, 1478–1481
  (*See also* Drugs)
Mediterranean anemia (*see* Thalassemia major)
Medulloblastoma, 320–324
Megacolon, 587–589
Megaloblastic nutritional anemia, 415–417, 944–950, 952
Melanoma, 810–811, 1260–1261
Mellaril, overdose, 716–717, 1592
Membranes, rupture of fetal, 150
Memory:
  aging and, 1439
  in dementia, 742–747, 1324–1325, 1483–1485
Meniere's syndrome, 797–798
Meningitis, 331–333, 720–722
Meningocele, 311–316
Menopause, 1253–1254
Menstrual cycle, 98
Menstruation, precocious, 375–377
Mental retardation, 336–338
Mental status, emergency assessment, 1498–1499
Meprobamate, overdose, 715–716
Mercury, poisoning, 719, 1482
Metals, toxicity, 334–336, 718–720, 1482, 1593–1596
Methadone, overdose, 1590
Methaqualone, overdose, 715–716, 1590
Methylphenidate, overdose, 1591
Microcephaly, 319
Middle adult:
  development of, 72–74
  health teaching for, 38
Migraine, 699–700
Miliaria rubra, 607
Miltown, overdose, 715–716
Minimal brain dysfunction, 339–340
Mites, 618–619, 1226–1227
Mitral valve insufficiency, 503, 976–982
Mitral valve stenosis, 503, 976–982
Moccasin (snake) bite, 1534–1538
Mole:
  hydatidiform, 130–131
  pigmented, 1259
Mongolian spots, 599–600
Moniliasis, 128, 609–610, 1246–1250
Mononeuropathy, 764
Mononucleosis, 651–652, 954–955
Monosomy, 253
Mood elevators, overdose, 1592
Morphine, overdose, 1590
Mosaicism, 254
Motion sickness, 798–799
Mountain sickness, 1541–1543
Mourning (*see* Grief)
Mouth:
  cancer, 1177–1180
  emergency assessment, 1495
  inflammations, 612, 1087, 1213–1214
Multiple myeloma, 825–828, 931–935
Multiple sclerosis, 760–764
Multiple trauma, client record sheet for, 1505
Mumps, 634–636, 1213
Muscular dystrophy, Duchenne's, 256, 364–366
Muscular subaortic stenosis, 982–984
Musculoskeletal system,
  abnormal cellular growth, 345–355, 823–828
  aging and, 1430–1431
  anxiety and, 1298

degenerative diseases, 364–366, 858–862
diagnostic procedures, 826
emergency assessment, 1496, 1498
hyperactivity and hypoactivity, 359–364
inflammations, 355–359, 834–841
metabolic disorders, 828–834
obstructions, 854–858
trauma, 366–369, 841–854, 1496, 1498, 1509–1526
(*See also particular structures, diseases, and disorders*)
Mustard procedure for great vessel transposition, 496–497
Myasthenia gravis, 755–759
Myeloma, multiple, 825–828, 931–935
Myelomeningocele, 311–316
Myocardial infarction, 1025–1029, 1604–1610
Myocarditis, 1020–1022
Myoclonus movement disorder, 761
Myringoplasty, 792
Myringotomy, 534
Myxedema coma, 896, 898

Narcan, 714
Narcolepsy, 821–822
Near-drowning, 1538–1541
Neck:
emergency assessment, 1494–1495
whiplash injury, 1580–1584
(*See also* Spinal cord injury)
Necrotizing enterocolitis (NEC), 240–241, 575–577
Neonate:
apnea, 238–239
attachment behavior, 179–180, 185, 209–210, 231–232
disturbances of, 213–216
behavioral states, 54, 55, 197, 198
with birth defects, 253–268
(*See also particular defects and disorders*)
body measurements, 205
care of, 185–187
crying, 54, 197, 198
development, 53–55
gestational age and, 199, 200, 202–203
diagnostic tests for, 207–208
effects of labor drugs on, 158–160, 260–263
feeding: by bottle, 211
formulas for, 1720–1721
by breast, 184, 210–211
during breast infection, 194
fluid and calorie requirements, 210
for high-risk neonate, 229, 232
gestational age: assessment, 199–200, 202–203, 225, 226
classification by size, 199–200, 202–203, 224
and mortality, 223, 224
high-risk, 223–252
feeding, 229, 230, 232
transport, 249–251
(*See also particular diseases and disorders*)
hypocalcemia, 242–243
hypoglycemia, 210, 241–242
hypothermia, 243–244
jaundice, 216–217, 244–247
large for gestational age, 223
low-birth-weight, 223–251
formulas for, 1721
maternal diabetes and, 139
maternal drug abuse and, 218–221
maternal infection and, 128
maternal smoking and, 218–221
ophthalmia neonatorum, 645
physical assessment, 199–205
polycythemia, 413
postmature, 165–166, 247–249
premature, 223–247
reflexes, 206
safety for, 212
septicemia, 239–240
small for gestational age, 223, 224
vital signs, 205
Nephrectomy, 1124
Nephritic syndrome, 551–553, 1156–1159
Nephritis, acute poststreptococcal, 551–553, 1156–1159
Nephroblastoma, 548–5550
Nephrolithiasis, 1163–1168
Nephrosis, 553–554, 1170–1171
Nephrostomy tube, care of, 1167–1169
Nephrotic syndrome, 553–554, 1170–1171
Nerve impairment after fracture, 849
Nerve tumors, 680
Nervous system, 311–343, 669–788
abnormal cellular growth, 311–325, 669–680
aging and, 1430
degenerative diseases, 742–770
developmental disorders, 336–342
emergency assessment, 1494–1497
hyperactivity and hypoactivity, 325–328, 680–696, 1500, 1616–1621
inflammations, 331–334, 720–734
metabolic disorders, 334–336, 696–720
obstructions, 734–742
signs and symptoms of disorders, 332
trauma, 328–331, 770–787, 1507–1508, 1580–1584
(*See also particular organs, structures, diseases, and disorders*)
Nesidioblastosis, 392
Neurinoma, 680
Neuroblastoma, 324–325, 876–879
Neurogenic bladder, 554–556
Neuropathic bladder, 554–556
Neurosyphilis, 731–732, 816–817, 1288
Neurotrauma, 1580–1584
(*See also* Brain, trauma; Cranial nerves, trauma; Spinal cord injury)
Neutropenia, 420–424
cyclic, 421
Nevi, 597–600, 1259
in cirrhosis, 1224
New York Heart Association functional classification of cardiac client, 968
Niemann-Pick disease, 456–458
Nonketotic hyperosmolar coma, 1597–1601
Norepinephrine, effects, 877
Norpramin, overdose, 1592
North American Nursing Diagnosis Association, 20
Nortriptyline, overdose, 1592
Nose:
deviated septum, 1100–1102
emergency assessment, 1495–1497
fracture, 1093
inflammation, 1077–1079
polyps, 1057–1059
submucous resection, 1101–1102
Nosebleed, 1093
in hypertension, 998, 999, 1470
Nuclear accident (*see* Radiation burns)
Nursing:
conceptual frameworks for, 15–18
definition, 15–18
and health, 15–30
Nursing audit, 28–30
Nursing diagnoses, 19–21
defining characteristics, 27, 1645–1678
definition, 9, 20–21
formulation of, 27
list of accepted, 27–28, 1645–1678
Nursing goal (*see* Expected outcomes)
Nursing models, 15–18, 31
Nursing practice, 13–32
defining characteristics, 31
standards, 18–30
Nursing process, 13–32
and standards of practice, 19–28
steps of, 19–28
Nursing science, 15
Nursing theory, 15–18, 31
Nutrition (*see* Diet)
Nutritional-metabolic pattern, 20, 22–23

Obesity, 1191–1194
aging and, 1434
intestinal bypass for, 1193–1194
Obsessive thought, and compulsive-ritualistic behavior, 1334–1336

Older adult,
abuse of, 1385–1387
attitudes toward death, 1457–1458
development, 74–77
developmental tasks, 1450
diet, 1433–1434, 1437–1438, 1440–1441, 1445
drug effects on, 1478–1481
health problems, 1463–1487
health promotion for, 1425–1426, 1478–1481, 1486
health teaching strategies for, 38–39, 1426
hormonal changes, 1435–1436
losses and grieving, 1449–1462
memory, 1439
physical assessment, 1428–1429
physical changes, 1423–1447
safety for, 76, 1425, 1439, 1445, 1486
and medication usage, 1478–1481
Omphalocele, 585–587
Open-heart surgery, 470–472, 978
Ophthalmia neonatorum, gonococcal, 645
Opiates, overdose, 714, 1590
Optic neuritis, 810
Orchitis, 1256
Orem, Dorothea, 15, 17
Organic brain syndrome:
causes, 1482
classification, 1680
confusion in, 1482–1485
delusions in, 1483–1485
diagnostic tests, 1484
sensory-perceptual alteration in, 1324–1325
(*See also* Dementia)
Organogenesis, 115–118
Ortolani test for congenital hip dislocation, 348
Osteitis deformans, 832–833
Osteoarthritis, 858–862, 1475–1476
Osteoclastoma, 823
Osteogenesis imperfecta, 350–352
Osteogenic sarcoma, 352–355, 823–828
Osteomalacia, 833–834
Osteomyelitis, 355–357, 834–836
Osteoporosis, 830–832, 1476
Ostium primum defect, 482
Ostium secundum defect, 482
Otitis externa, 789–791
Otitis media, 533–534, 794–796
Otosclerosis, 796–797
Outcome criteria, 21
(*See also* Evaluation, as step of nursing process)
Ovalocytosis, hereditary, 444
Ovary:
cancer, 1245
cysts, 293, 1246, 1610
hyperstimulation, 294
Overdose, 713–717, 1585–1593
emergency assessment, 1502
(*See also* Withdrawal *and particular substances*)
Oviducts, occlusion, 295–296
Ovulation, multiple, 134–137, 293
Oxyuriasis, 654–655

Pacemaker, cardiac, 1010–1013
Paget's disease, 832–833, 1241
Pain, 819–820
abdominal, emergency assessment, 1503
chest, emergency assessment, 1500
lower back, 852–854
phantom limb, 856–857
Palate, cleft, 580–581
Pancreas:
cystic fibrosis, 256, 524–527
hormonal functions, 391–392
tumors, 1183–1184
Pancreatic insufficiency, 1195
Pancreatitis:
acute, 1203–1206, 1610
chronic, 1206–1207
Para, definition, 125
Paracentesis, 1226
Paraldehyde, overdose, 715–716
Paralysis:
familial periodic, 691–692
hypokalemic periodic, 691–692
Paralysis agitans, 751–755
Paraplegia, 779
Erb's spastic, 731–732
(*See also* Spina bifida; Spinal cord injury; Stroke)
Parathyroid gland, disorders, 912–917
Parathyroid hormones, functions, 913
Parent-infant interaction (*see* Attachment)
Parents:
of hospitalized child or adolescent, 63–71
teaching for, 70–71
Parietal syndrome, 818–819
Parity, classification, 150
Parkinson's disease, 751–755
Parkland formula for fluids for burned client, 1284
Parosmia, 814–815
Parotitis, 634–636, 1213–1214
Patau's syndrome, 254
Patent ductus arteriosus, 472–475
Patterns of health-related behavior, 20, 22–26
Payne-DeWind operation for intestinal bypass, 1193
Pediculosis, 617–618
Peer review, 28–30
Pellagra, 713
Pelvic examination, support during, 110–111
Penis:
cancer, 1255
circumcision, 212
Peptic ulcer, 1184–1189, 1610
Perception:
aging and, 1429, 1430
disturbances of, 1324–1325, 1351–1356
Pericarditis, 1022–1023
Periodic breathing, 238, 239
Periodontitis, 1213
Peripheral arterial diseases, 1029–1037
Peripheral nerve degeneration, 764–765
Peripheral vascular disease, 854–857
Peritoneal dialysis, 562, 1142–1145, 1149
continuous ambulatory, 562, 1142–1145, 1149
continuous cycle, 562
Peritonitis, 1610–1613
Pernicious anemia, 416, 713, 944–948
Perphenazine, overdose, 1592
Person abuse, 1369–1390
Pertussis, 628–630
Phagocytosis, disorders of, 424–425
Phantom pain sensations, 856–857
Pharyngitis, 531–533, 1085–1086
Phencyclidine, overdose, 1591
Phenothiazine, overdose, 716–717
Phenylketonuria (PKU), 256, 336
Pheochromocytoma, 876–879
Philadelphia chromosome, 923–924, 926
Phlebothrombosis, 1023
Phosphate intoxication, 719
Photo therapy, 246, 247
Physical assessment, 19–20
child and adolescent, 63, 65
neonate, 199–205
older adult, 1428–1429
Physical therapy, chest, 236, 237, 1099
Pica, 334–418
Pick's disease, 742–747
Pinworms, 654–655
Pituitary gland:
anterior: functions and hormones of, 371, 373, 866–867
hyperactivity and hypoactivity, 371–381
posterior: functions and hormones of, 381, 866–867, 887
hyperactivity and hypoactivity, 381–383
tumors, 866–873
Pit viper, 1534–1538
Pityriasis rosea, 613–614
Placenta:
abruption of, 144
delivery of, 170
hormones of, 142
Placenta previa, 143–144
Placidyl, overdose, 1590
Plantar warts, 1262–1263
Platelets, deficiency of (*see* Thrombocytopenia)
Pleurisy, 1074–1077
Plumbism, 334–336, 718, 1482
Plummer's disease, 893
Pneumoconiosis, 1111–1113

Pneumonia, 529–530, 1059–1064
 aspiration, 530–531
 causes, 1059–1060
 chemical, 530–531
 hydrocarbon, 530–531
Pneumothorax, 1087–1093, 1574
Poisoning, 1585–1597
 (*See also* Overdose; Withdrawal; *and particular substances*)
Poison ivy, 602, 1275
Poison oak, 602–603, 1275
Poliomyelitis, 638–641, 732–733
Polycystic disease of the kidney, 537–541, 1171–1172
Polycystic ovarian disease, 293
Polycythemia:
 of cyanotic heart disease, 413–414
 of newborn, 413
 systemic consequences, 490–491
Polycythemia vera, 935–936
Polyhydramnios, 145
Polyneuritis, acute idiopathic, 728–731
Polyneuropathy, 765, 815–816
 nutritional, 710–712
 types, 815
Polyploidy, 254
Polyps:
 cervical, 1245
 nasal, 1057–1059
Posterior urethral valves, 544–546
Postmature neonate, 165–166, 247–249
Postpartum period (*see* Puerperium)
Posttraumatic edema, 820
Posttraumatic pain syndrome, 819–820
Posttraumatic syndrome, following head injury, 775
Postural drainage, 1099
 for neonate, 236, 237
Preeclampsia, 137–138
Pregnancy, 115–148
 adolescent, 131–132
 anemia in, 140–141, 146
 blood incompatibility in, 145, 216–217
 concerns of woman during, 118–124, 135
 developmental tasks, 118–124
 diabetes mellitus in, 138–140
 diagnosis of, 127
 diet, 134, 140
 ectopic, 131, 1610
 effects of previous abortion, 278
 first trimester, 115–132
 after 40 years of age, 132
 fourth trimester, 175–196
 gonorrhea in, 128
 health care during, by trimester, 116–118
 heart disease in, 147
 hemoglobinopathies in, 146
 herpes simplex type 2 in, 128, 257–260
 hormones in, 142
 hyperemesis gravidarum in, 131
 hypertension in, 137–138
 multiple, 134–137, 293
 polyhydramnios in, 145
 recovery, 175–196
 renal disease in, 145
 second trimester, 116–117, 121–123, 132–141
 syphilis in, 128
 systemic lupus erythematosus in, 145
 third trimester, 117–118, 123–124, 141–147
 thrombophlebitis in, 141
 unplanned, 112–113
 urinary tract infection in, 141
 vaginal bleeding in, 143–144, 147
 vaginal infection in, 128–131
 varicose veins in, 141
 weight gain in, 126
  abnormal, 140
  with preeclampsia, 137
 (*See also* Fetus; Delivery)
Prematurity (*see* Neonate)
Preschooler:
 development, 58–59
 developmental tasks, 67
 hospitalized, 67
 safety for, 59
Prevention of disease, 13–15
 (*See also* Health, promotion and maintenance)
Prickly heat, 607
Problem-oriented record, 30
 in emergency, 1499
Prochlorperazine, overdose, 1592
Profession, functions and responsibilities, 18
Professional organization, functions, 18
 (*See also* American Nurses' Association)
Professional standard review organization, (PSRO), 28
Promazine, overdose, 716–717
Propoxyphene, overdose, 1590–1591
Prostaglandin E_1, for patent ductus arteriosus, 473, 496
Prostate:
 benign hypertrophy, 1160–1163, 1254
 cancer, 1133–1135, 1254–1255
Protriptyline, overdose, 1592
Pseudogout, 828
Pseudoself, 1408, 1416
Pseudotruncus, 500–501
Psoriasis, 1263–1267
Psychosis, Korsakoff's, 708–710
Puberty:
 delayed, 378
 precocious, 375–377, 389
Puerperium, 175–196
 complications, 192–195
 depression in, 179, 195
 emotional adjustments of, 179
 exercises for, 187–189
 fever during, 193–194
Pulmonary artery banding, 484–485
Pulmonary edema, 989–991
Pulmonary embolism, 1093–1097
Pulmonary emphysema, 1108–1111, 1472–1473
Pulmonary function tests, 1103
Pulmonary heart disease, 991–993
Pulmonary valvular atresia, 493–494
Pulmonary valvular stenosis, 493–494
Puncture wounds, 1553–1555
Pupils, assessment in coma, 693
Purpura:
 activity guidelines for thrombocytopenia in, 407
 anaphylactoid, 455–456, 955
 classification, 955
 Henoch-Schönlein, 455–456
 idiopathic thrombocytopenic, 425–426, 955–957
Pyelonephritis, 1154–1156
Pyloric stenosis, 567–569
Pyruvate kinase, in pregnancy, 146

Quaalude, overdose, 715–716, 1590
Quadriplegia, 779
 (*See also* Spinal cord injury)
Quality assurance, 28–30

Rabies, 732
Radiation burns, 1562–1565
Radiation therapy, in leukemia, 445, 930, 931
 side effects, 354–355
Ramstedt pyloromyotomy, 567
Rape, 1382–1385, 1633–1634
Rashkind balloon septostomy, 494, 496
Rattlesnake bites, 1534–1538
Rauwolfia alkaloids, overdose, 716–717
Raynaud's disease, 1036–1037
Recommended daily dietary allowances, 1713–1718
Record, client, 30
  in emergency care, 1499, 1505
  problem oriented, 30, 1499
Reevaluation as step of nursing process, 27
Reflexes of neonate and infant, 206
Reflex sympathetic dystrophies, 819–820
Refraction, errors of visual, 801
Regional enteritis, 1215
Rehabilitation, family counseling about, 87–89
Relaxation, techniques, 1303–1304
Renal artery thrombosis, 588
Renal disease:
 encephalopathy from, 699

end-stage, 560–564, 1140–1149
in pregnancy, 145
retinopathy from, 812
(*See also* Kidney *and particular disorders*)
Renal failure:
acute, 1135–1140, 1170
chronic, 560–564, 1140–1149, 1170
Renal transplantation, 1147–1148
Renal tubular acidosis, 564–565
Renal vein thrombosis, 556–558
Reproductive system, 1231–1258
aging and, 1432–1433
female: abnormal cellular growth, 1231–1246, 1610
degenerative changes, 1253–1254
hyperactivity and hypoactivity, 253–254, 375–378, 380–381, 388–391, 399–401, 886–887, 910–912
inflammatory disorders, 1246–1253
male, 1254–1256
abnormal cellular growth, 546–547, 1133–1135, 1160–1163, 1254–1256
hyperactivity and hypoactivity, 375–378, 380–381, 388–391, 401–403, 886–887, 910–912
inflammation, 1256
(*See also* Sexuality)
Reserpine, overdose, 716–717
Respirations, assessment, 507–509
Respiratory distress syndrome (RDS), 233–237, 527
adult, 1092–1093
Respiratory insufficiency, 1107–1108
following crushed chest injuries, 1090
Respiratory rate, for children, 461
newborn, 205, 461
Respiratory system, 505–535, 1045–1115
abnormal cellular growth, 505–511, 1045–1059
aging and, 1431, 1472–1473
anxiety and, 1298
emergency assessment, 1495, 1497–1498, 1500
inflammations, 527–534, 1059–1087
obstructions, 511–527, 1093–1113, 1569–1575
trauma, 1087–1093, 1504, 1506, 1538–1541, 1569–1575
(*See also particular organs, structures, diseases, and disorders*)
Restraints:
elbow, for child, 606
for violent client, 1346
Retina, detachment of, 809–810
Reye's syndrome, 334
Rheumatic fever, 502–503, 973
Rheumatic heart disease, 502–503, 973–975
Rheumatoid arthritis, 838, 858
eye changes due to, 812
juvenile, 357–359
Rhinitis, 1077–1079
Rhinoplasty, 1101–1102
Rh_0D immune globulin, 217
for abortion client, 273
Rickets, adult, 833–834
Riedel's thyroiditis, 917
Riehl, Joan, 15
Rights of client with terminal illness, 1460
Ringworm, 614–617, 1272–1273
Ritalin, overdose, 1591
Ritualistic behavior, 1334–1336
Rocky Mountain spotted fever, 649–650
Rogers, Martha, 15, 16
Role and relationship pattern, 20, 24
Roles, in groups, 1393–1394
nonfunctional, 1396
Rotating tourniquets, 990
Roy, Calista, 15, 16
Rubella, 257–260, 632–634
Rubeola, 630–632
Rule of nines for estimating burn area, 1557
Rum fits, 684–691
Russell's traction, 845, 846

Safety:
for infant, 55–57
for neonate, 212
for older adult, 76, 1425, 1439, 1445, 1486
in medication usage, 1478–1481
for preschooler, 59
for toddler, 58
Salivary glands:
inflammation, 1213–1214
tumors, 1181
Salmonella, 1593–1596
Salt-losing syndrome in adrenal disease, 388–391
Sarcoidosis, 732, 1054–1057
Sarcoma:
Ewing's, 352–355
osteogenic, 352–355
Scabies, 618–619, 1276–1277
Schick test for susceptibility to diphtheria, 621
Schmidt's disease, 388
School-age child:
development, 59–60
hospitalization and, 68
developmental tasks, 68
health teaching for, 60
hospitalized, 68
Schwannoma, 680
Scleroderma, 1014–1016
Scoliosis, 361–364
Scorpion stings, 1534–1538
Scott operation for intestinal bypass, 1193
Seborrhea, 606–607, 1275–1276
Sedatives, overdose, 715–716, 1589–1590
Seizures, 325–328, 680–684, 1616–1621
causes, 682
emergency assessment, 1500
febrile, 325–328, 1619–1621
after head trauma, 775–776
in pregnancy, 137
Self:
differentiation of, in family, 1408, 1409
pseudo-, 1408, 1416
solid, 1408
therapeutic use of, 1319
Self-care, mental problems with, 1319–1321
Self-catheterization, 555
Self-concept, dependency as alteration of, 1328–1332
Self-esteem, improvement of, in anxiety, 1305
Self-perception–self-concept pattern, 20, 25
Self-statements, for anxiety reduction, 1305
Semen, laboratory analysis of, 297, 298
Senning procedure for great vessel transposition, 496–497
Sensation, disorders, 815–820
Sensory-perceptual alteration, 1324–1325
Sensory systems, 789–822
(*See also* Ears; Eyes; Hearing impairment; Taste; *and particular diseases and disorders*)
Separation anxiety:
of infant, 56
stages of, 66
support during, 65–67
of toddler, 58
Septicemia:
neonatal, 239–240
(*See also* Shock, septic)
Septostomy, Rashkind, 494, 496
Severe combined immunodeficiency (SCID), 434–435
Sexual abuse, 1382–1385, 1633–1634
Sexuality:
in adolescence, 61
delayed development, 378
and pregnancy, 131–132
of middle adult, 73, 74
of older adult, 76, 1432, 1434, 1438, 1442–1443, 1445
Sexuality-reproductive pattern, 20, 25
Sheehan's syndrome, 379–380
Shingles, 613, 726–728
Shock, 1506–1507, 1565–1569
allergic, 1537, 1565–1569
anaphylactic, 1537, 1565–1569
cardiogenic, 993–997, 1565–1569, 1604–1610
electrical (*see* Burns, electrical)
emergency assessment, 1500–1501, 1506–1507

hypovolemic, 1565–1569
neurogenic, 1565–1569
septic, 1565–1569
vasogenic, 1565–1569
Shoulder, frozen, 838–840
Shoulder-hand syndrome, 819–820
Shunt:
for hydrocephalus, 317, 318
peritoneal-jugular for ascites, 1226
portosystemic for cirrhosis, 1229
Sibling position, in family systems theory, 1410
Sickle cell anemia, 435–439, 960–964
guidelines for client management, 438
inheritance patterns, 256, 437
in pregnancy, 146
Sickle cell trait, 439
inheritance patterns, 437
in pregnancy, 146
Sigmoidoscopy, 1197
Simmonds' disease, 379–380
Sinus, paranasal, emergency assessment, 1495–1497
infection, 1079–1083
Sinusitis, 1079–1083
Sinus venosus defect, 482
Siriasis, 1526–1527
Skin (*see* Integumentary system, *and particular diseases and disorders*)
Skull fractures, 328–331, 771
(*See also* Face, trauma)
Slapped cheek syndrome, 613
Sleep:
disorders, 820–822
mental health, 1319–1321
of middle adult, 73, 74
of neonate, 54, 197, 198
of older adult, 76, 1438–1439, 1443, 1445
of toddler, 57
(*See also* Sleep-rest pattern)
Sleep-Eze, overdose, 1591–1592
Sleep-rest pattern, 20, 23
Sling, for arm, 1522
Small for gestational age neonate, 223, 224
Smell, disorders of sense of, 814–815
Smoke inhalation (*see* Burns, thermal; Upper airway trauma)
Smoking:
effect on neonate, 218–221
visual changes due to, 811
Snake bite, 1534–1538
Snellen eye chart, 800
SOAP format for charting, 30
in emergency setting, 1499
Social isolation, 1321–1324, 1415–1416
Somogyi phenomenon, 1598–1600
Sparine, overdose, 716–717
Spermatocele, 1255
Spherocytosis, hereditary, 442–444, 960–964
Spica cast, incontinent child in, 350
Spider bites, 1534–1538
Spina bifida, 311–316
Spinal cord injury, 331, 778–787, 1580–1584
emergency assessment, 1494, 1496, 1497
spinal shock in, 779, 781–782
Spinal cord tumors, 324–325, 677–680
Spinnbarkeit, 286, 293
Spirometry, 1103
Spleen, trauma, 1577–1580
Splenectomy:
for aplastic anemia, 941
in hemolytic anemia, 964
Splint(s)
for first aid, 1515
Thomas, with Pearson attachment, 847
Spondylitis, ankylosing, 837–838
Spondylosis, cervical, 765–767
Spouse abuse, 1369–1375
Sprains, 1518–1519
Sprue, 591–593, 1195
Standards of nursing practice, 18–30
and nursing process, 19–28
Status asthmaticus, 1102, 1104–1105
Status epilepticus, 684, 1616–1619
Stelazine, overdose, 716–717, 1592
Sterility, 281
(*See also* Infertility)
Steroid synthesis, 388–389
Stillbirth, 130
Stimulants, overdose, 1591
Stings, venomous, 1534–1538
Stomach:
cancer, 1182
inflammation, 1214–1215
ulcer, 1184–1189, 1610
Stomatitis, 1213
(*See also* Fever blisters)
Stones:
of gallbladder, 1200–1203
of urinary tract, 1163–1168
Storage diseases, 456–458
Strains, 1516–1518
Stroke, 734–742, 1030, 1471–1472
Stroke-in-evolution, 734, 740
Sty, 802–803
Subarachnoid hemorrhage, 767–770
Subdural hematoma, 328–331, 771
Subluxations, 348, 1521–1522
Submucous resection of the nose, 1101–1102
Substance abuse (*see* Abuse, alcohol; Abuse, drug)
Sudden infant death syndrome (SIDS), 238, 239
Suicide, 1339–1344, 1634–1636
emergency care of client's family or friends after, 1635–1636
factors indicating probability, 1307
potential for in depressed children, 1365–1366
telephone intervention for threat, 1343
Sunburn, 1563–1565
Sunstroke, 1526–1527
Survival techniques for abused spouse, 1373
Swan-Ganz catheter, 994, 995
Swimmer's ear, 789–791
Symbiosis, dysfunctional, 1328–1332
Sympathalgia, 819–820
Syndrome of inappropriate antidiuretic hormone (ADH) secretion, 882–884
Synovitis, 828
Syphilis, 646–648, 1286–1290
congenital, 646–648
neurological sequelae, 731–732, 816–817, 1288
in pregnancy, 128
Syringomyelia, 765
Syrup of ipecac, administration of, 1588
Systemic lupus erythematosus (SLE), 1016–1018, 1267–1269
in pregnancy, 145
Systems theory, family and, 1405–1406

Tabes dorsalis, 731, 732
sensory disorders of, 816–817
(*See also* Neurosyphilis)
Tachycardia, 1006, 1007, 1013
Talipes, 346–348
Tamponade, cardiac, 470, 1024–1025
Taractan, overdose, 716–717
Taste, sense of:
aging and, 1430
disorders of, 813–815
Tay-Sachs disease, 256, 336
Teaching, 33–52
for anxiety reduction, 1302–1306
of child, 36–37, 70–71
of depressed client, 1311–1312
evaluation of, 51
for infertile couple, 301–302
and locus of control, 43–44
for parents of hospitalized child or adolescent, 70–71
strategies for: age differences and, 36–39, 59, 1426
cultural differences and, 39–44
sex differences and, 34–36
socioeconomic differences and, 40, 45
(*See also* Learning; Teaching-learning plan; Teaching-learning transaction)
Teaching-learning plan, 46, 48–51
Teaching-learning transaction (TLT), 46, 48–51
Teeth:
caries of, 593–595
emergencies involving, 1522–1524
of infant, 56, 57
of preschooler, 58, 59
of school-age child, 59
of toddler, 57, 58

Tegretol, overdose, 715–716
Temperature, body:
of neonate, 205
and fertility, 286, 288, 289, 293
Temporal arteritis, 733–734
Tennis elbow, 838
Teratogenesis, 253–260
Testicle(s):
cancer, 1255
inflammation, 1256
undescended, 547–548
Tetanus, 625–628, 717
Tetralogy of Fallot, 489–493
"Tet" spells in tetralogy of Fallot, 490–492
Thalamic syndrome, 818
Thalassemia major, 440–442, 960–964
in pregnancy, 146
Thalassemia minor, 440, 960–964
in pregnancy, 146
Thallium intoxication, 719–720
Therapy:
family, 1405–1418
group, 1397–1399
radiation: in leukemia, 445, 930, 931
side effects of, 354–355
(*See also* Drugs)
Thiamine deficiency, 710–712
Thioridazine, overdose, 716–717, 1592
Thioxanthine, overdose, 716–717
Thomas splint, 847
Thorazine, overdose, 716–717, 1592
Thought-stopping techniques for anxiety control, 1304–1305
Thromboangiitis obliterans, 1034–1036
Thrombocytopenia:
acquired, 425–426, 955
activity guidelines for, 407
idiopathic, 425–426, 955–957
immune, 426, 955
Thrombophlebitis, 1023–1024
postpartum, 194–195
in pregnancy, 141
Thrombosis:
following heart valve surgery, 981–982
renal artery, 558
renal vein, 556–558
Thrush, 609, 610
Thyroid gland, functions, 383–384
Thyroiditis, 917–918
Hashimoto's, 386–387, 917–918
subacute, 386–387, 917–918
Thyroid storm, 1602–1604
Thyroid tumors, 873–876
(*See also* Goiter)
Thyrotoxicosis, 892–896, 1602–1604
Tic (habit spasm), 761
Tic douloureux, 817–818
Ticks, and Rocky Mountain spotted fever, 649–650
Tinea capitis, 614–616, 1272–1273
Tinea circinata, 615, 616, 1272–1273
Tinea corporis, 615, 616, 1272–1273
Tinea cruris, 1272–1273
Tinea pedis, 615–617, 1272–1273
Toddler:
development, 57–58
developmental tasks, 67
hospitalized, 67
safety for, 58
separation anxiety, 58
Tofranil, overdose, 1592
Tongue, cancer, 1177–1180
Tonsillitis, 531–533, 1083
TORCH syndrome, 245, 257–260
Torticollis, 345–346
Total anomalous pulmonary venous return, 501–502
Total hip replacement, 861–862
Total parenteral nutrition (TPN), 229
Tourniquets, rotating, 990
Toxoplasmosis, 257–260
Tracheobronchitis, 1083–1085
Tracheoesophageal fistula, 581–585
Tracheostomy, care of, 1091
Traction:
balanced suspended, 844–845, 847
Bryant's, 349
Buck's extension, 845–846
care of client with, 844–847
for cervical injury, 784–785
Russell's, 845, 846
Thomas splint and Pearson attachment with, 847
Tranquilizers, overdose, 1589–1590
Transfusion:
exchange, 246, 247
reactions to, 408–410
Transient ischemic attack (TIA), 734
Transmission, in family systems theory, 1407, 1410
Transport of high-risk neonate, 249–251
Transposition of great vessels, 495–500
Trauma:
during birth, 260–263
in child abuse, 1378–1379
client record in emergency care, 1499, 1505
multiple, emergency assessment for, 1501
in spouse abuse, 1371
(*See also* Emergency nursing *and particular organs and structures*)
Travis, John, 13
Tremor(s):
benign essential, 691
familial, 691
senile, 691
table of, 686–687
in withdrawal from alcohol and other drugs, 684–691
Trench foot, 1530–1532
Trench mouth, 1213
Triage, 1499–1504
Triangles, in family systems theory, 1408–1410
Triavil, overdose, 1592
Trichomonas vaginal infection, 1246–1250
in pregnancy, 128
Trichuriasis, 658–659
Tricuspid atresia, 494–495
Tricuspid insufficiency, 977–982
Tricuspid stenosis, 977–982
Tricuspid antidepressants, overdose, 1592
Trifluoperazine, overdose, 716–717, 1592
Trigeminal neuralgia, 817–818
Trilafon, overdose, 1592
Trisomy, 253–254
Truncus arteriosus, 500–501
Tuberculosis, 641–644, 1064–1071
of bones, 840–842
classification, 1065
drugs for, 1069, 1070
of genitals, 1160
skin testing for, 1066
interpretation of, 1067
schedule for, 622, 623, 642
of urinary tract, 1159–1160
Tuboplasty, for infertility, 295
Tubular necrosis (renal), acute, 558–560
Tumors (*see particular organs, body systems, diseases, and disorders*)
Turner's syndrome, 253–254, 399–401, 910–912
Twins, 134–137, 293
Type A behavior, 1298

Ulcer:
corneal, 804–805
Curling's, 1184–1189
Cushing's, 1184–1189
duodenal, 1184–1189, 1610
gastric, 1184–1189, 1610
Hunner's, 1152
peptic, 1184–1189, 1610
varicose, 1039–1040
Ulcerative colitis, 1196–1200, 1610
Ultrasonography, in pregnancy, 133
Undescended testicles, 547–548
Upper airway trauma, 1569–1573
Uremia, 561, 1140
encephalopathy from, 561, 699
(*See also* Renal failure)
Ureteral reflux, 541–543
Urethra:
inflammation, 1149–1152
stones in, 1163, 1166
stricture, 1152
(*See also* Benign prostatic hypertrophy)
Urethritis, 1149–1152
Urinary diversion, 555–556, 1131–1133
Urinary system, 537–566, 1117–1176
abnormal cellular growth, 537–550, 1117–1135

aging and, 1432
assessment findings in disorders of, 1118–1119
degenerative diseases, 1170–1172
emergency assessment, 1496
hyperactivity and hypoactivity, 558–564, 1135–1149
inflammations, 550–554, 1149–1160
metabolic disorders, 564–565
obstructions, 554–558, 1160–1170
trauma, 558, 1172–1175, 1509
(*See also particular organs, structures, diseases, and disorders*)
Urinary tract infection, 550–551
in pregnancy, 141
postpartum, 194
Urine:
laboratory tests, 539
methods of obtaining specimens, 540, 541
Urticaria, 601–602
Uterus:
atony, 170–171, 192
cancer, 1242, 1244–1245
(*See also* Cervix, cancer)
fibroid tumors, 1245–1246
inertia, 164
Uveitis, 805–806

Vagina:
cancer, 1242
hematoma, 173
infections, 1246–1250
during pregnancy, 128, 131
laceration from labor, 171–172, 1628
Vaginal bleeding, in pregnancy, 143–144, 147
Vaginal delivery, 175–189
Vaginitis, 1246–1250
in pregnancy, 128, 131
Valium, overdose, 715–716, 1590
Value-belief pattern, 20, 26, 39–44, 46
Varicella, 636–638
Varices, 1037–1040
esophageal, 1228
Varicocele, 1255–1256
Varicose ulcers, 1039–1040
Varicose veins, 1037–1040
esophageal, 1228
in pregnancy, 141
Vascular rings, 481–482
Veins, varicose, 1037–1040
of esophagus, 1228
in pregnancy, 141
Vena cava syndrome, 169
Venereal warts, 1253, 1262, 1263
Ventricular septal defect, 484–486
Verrucae, 1261–1263
Vertebrae:
dislocation, 778
fracture, 778
(*See also* Spinal cord injury)
Vesicoureteral reflux, 541–543
Vincent's angina, 1213
Violence:
threats of, 1344–1347, 1631–1633
(*See also* Abuse of persons)
Viruses, and birth defects, 257–260
Vision (*see* Eyes)
Vital signs:
of children and adolescents, 65
of newborns, 205
Vitamin B_1 deficiency, 710–712
Vitamin B_{12} deficiency anemia, 415–417, 713, 944–948
Vitamin K deficiency, 954
Vivactyl, overdose, 1592
Voices, hallucinations of, 1351–1353
Volvulus, 569–570, 1610
(*See also* Bowel, obstruction)
Von Willebrand's disease, 433–434
Vulva:
cancer, 1241–1242
inflammation, 1252–1253
Vulvectomy, 1241–1242
Vulvitis, 1252–1253

Warts, 1261–1263
venereal, 1253, 1262, 1263
Wasp stings, 1534–1538
Water intoxication, 883–884
Waterston shunt for tetralogy of Fallot, 490
Weight:
control in pregnancy, 140
gain in pregnancy, 126
abnormal, 140
with preeclampsia, 137
loss following delivery, 175, 177
Weights and heights:
for adults, 1192
for children, 1695–1702
newborn, 205, 1695–1698
Wernicke's encephalopathy, 708–710
Wet lung syndrome, 1092
Wheals, 601–602
Whiplash injury, 1580–1584
Whipple's disease, 1195
Whipworms, 658–659
White blood cells, deficiency of, 420–424
Whooping cough, 628–630
Wife battering, 1369–1375
Will, living, 1457
Wilms' tumor, 548–550
Wind-chill factor chart, 1530
Wiscott-Aldrich syndrome, 428–429
Withdrawal:
from alcohol or other drugs, 684–691, 1330–1331, 1588, 1589
violence associated with, 1344–1347
social or emotional, 1321–1324, 1415–1416
Worms, infestation with, 654–659
Wounds, 1546–1555
abrasion, 1546–1547
avulsion, 1547–1548
contusion, 1548–1550
crush, 1550–1551
laceration, 1552–1553
puncture, 1553–1555
Wry neck, 345–346

X-ray procedures for orthopedic diagnosis, 826

Yellow jacket stings, 1524–1538
Young adult:
development, 71–72
health teaching of, 38